CURRENT
Diagnosis & Treatment
Surgery

FIFTEENTH EDITION

Edited by

Gerard M. Doherty, MD

Moseley Professor of Surgery, Harvard Medical School
Surgeon-in-Chief, Brigham Health & Dana-Farber Cancer Institute
Crowley Family Distinguished Chair, Department of Surgery
Brigham and Women's Hospital
Boston, Massachusetts

Mc
Graw
Hill

New York   Chicago   San Francisco   Athens   London   Madrid   Mexico City
Milan   New Delhi   Singapore   Sydney   Toronto

Current Diagnosis & Treatment: Surgery, Fifteenth Edition

Previous editions copyright © 2015, 2010, 2006, 2003 by the McGraw-Hill Companies, Inc.; © 1994, 1991 by Appleton & Lange; ©1973–1985 by Lange Medical Publications.

2 3 4 5 6 7 8 9   LCR   25 24 23 22

ISBN 978-1-260-12221-3
MHID 1-260-12221-2
ISSN 0894-227

Notice

Medicine is an ever-changing science. As new research and clinical experience broaden our knowledge, changes in treatment and drug therapy are required. The authors and the publisher of this work have checked with sources believed to be reliable in their efforts to provide information that is complete and generally in accord with the standards accepted at the time of publication. However, in view of the possibility of human error or changes in medical sciences, neither the authors nor the publisher nor any other party who has been involved in the preparation or publication of this work warrants that the information contained herein is in every respect accurate or complete, and they disclaim all responsibility for any errors or omissions or for the results obtained from use of the information contained in this work. Readers are encouraged to confirm the information contained herein with other sources. For example and in particular, readers are advised to check the product information sheet included in the package of each drug they plan to administer to be certain that the information contained in this work is accurate and that changes have not been made in the recommended dose or in the contraindications for administration. This recommendation is of particular importance in connection with new or infrequently used drugs.

This book was set in Minion Pro by Cenveo® Publisher Services.
The editors were Andrew Moyer and Christie Naglieri.
The production supervisor was Catherine H. Saggese.
Project management was provided by Garima Poddar, Cenveo Publisher Services.

This book is printed on acid-free paper.

Contents

Authors

Marco Ettore Allaix, MD, PhD
Department of Surgery
University of Turin
Turin, Italy

Sherif Aly, MD
Resident
Department of Surgery
Boston Medical Center
Boston, Massachusetts

Reza Askari, MD
Assistant Professor
Department of Surgery
Harvard Medical School
Brigham and Women's Hospital
Boston, Massachusetts

Edward L. Bove, MD
Professor
Department of Cardiac Surgery
University of Michigan
Ann Arbor, Michigan

Melissa Brackmann, MD
Assistant Professor
Department of Obstetrics and Gynecology
University of Michigan
Ann Arbor, Michigan

Peter A. Burke, MD
Professor
Department of Surgery
Boston University School of Medicine
Boston, Massachusetts

Michael R. Cassidy, MD
Assistant Professor
Department of Surgery
Boston University School of Medicine
Boston, Massachusetts

Andrew C. Chang, MD
Professor
John Alexander Distinguished Professor of Thoracic Surgery
University of Michigan
Ann Arbor, Michigan

Antonia Chen, MD, MBA
Assistant Professor
Department of Orthopedic Surgery
Harvard Medical School
Brigham and Women's Hospital
Boston, Massachusetts

Nancy L. Cho, MD
Assistant Professor
Department of Surgery
Harvard Medical School
Brigham and Women's Hospital
Boston, Massachusetts

Daniel I. Chu, MD, FACS, FASCRS
Assistant Professor of Surgery
Department of Surgery
University of Alabama-Birmingham
Birmingham, Alabama

Yoon S. Chun, MD
Associate Professor
Department of Surgery
Harvard Medical School
Brigham and Women's Hospital
Boston, Massachusetts

Thomas E. Clancy, MD
Assistant Professor
Department of Surgery
Harvard Medical School
Brigham and Women's Hospital
Boston, Massachusetts

Jessica N. Cohan, MD
Assistant Professor
Department of Surgery
University of Utah
Salt Lake City, Utah

Juliane Y. Cruz, MD
Surgeon
Pasadena, California

Ana C. De Roo, MD
Resident
Department of Surgery
University of Michigan
Ann Arbor, Michigan

Kristopher B. Deatrick, MD
Assistant Professor
Department of Surgery
University of Maryland
Baltimore, Maryland

Tracey Dechert, MD, FACS
Associate Professor
Department of Surgery
Boston University School of Medicine
Boston, Massachusetts

Karen E. Deveney, MD
Professor
Department of Surgery
Oregon Health & Science University
Portland, Oregon

Gerard M. Doherty, MD
Moseley Professor of Surgery
Harvard Medical School
Crowley Family Surgeon-in-Chief
Brigham and Women's Hospital and Dana-Farber Cancer
    Institute
Boston, Massachusetts

Quan-Yang Duh, MD
Professor
Department of Surgery
University of California
San Francisco, California

J. Englebert Dunphy, MD
Formerly Professor of Surgery Emeritus (deceased)
University of California
San Francisco, California

Alessandro Fichera, MD
Professor
Department of Surgery
Baylor Scot & White Health
Dallas, Texas

Michael G. Franz, MD, FACS
General Surgeon
Bay Pines Veterans Healthcare System
Bay Pines, Florida

Armando E. Giuliano, MD
Executive Vice Chair
Department of Surgery
Samuel Oschin Comprehensive Cancer Institute
Cedars-Sinai Medical Center
Los Angeles, California

Jonathan W. Haft, MD
Associate Professor
Department of Cardiac Surgery
University of Michigan
Ann Arbor, Michigan

Scott L. Hansen, MD
Professor
Department of Surgery
University of California
San Francisco, California

David A. Harris, MD
Resident
Department of Surgery
Brigham and Women's Hospital
Boston, Massachusetts

Michael S. Harris, MD
Assistant Professor
Department of Otolaryngology
Medical College of Wisconsin
Milwaukee, Wisconsin

Joaquim M. Havens, MD
Assistant Professor
Harvard Medical School
Brigham and Women's Hospital
Boston, Massachusetts

Mark R. Hemmila, MD
Professor
Department of Surgery
University of Michigan
Ann Arbor, Michigan

Jonathan L. Hills-Dunlap, MD, MPH
Resident
Department of Surgery
Brigham and Women's Hospital
Boston, Massachusetts

Sameer Hirji, MD
Resident
Department of Surgery
Brigham and Women's Hospital
Boston, Massachusetts

Jennifer C. Hirsch-Romano, MD, MS
Associate Professor
Department of Cardiac Surgery
University of Michigan
Ann Arbor, Michigan

Kevin T. Huang, MD
Resident
Department of Neurosurgery
Brigham and Women's Hospital
Boston, Massachusetts

Sara A. Hurvitz, MD
Associate Professor
Department of Medicine, Division of Hematology Oncology
University of California
Los Angeles, California

Kamal M. F. Itani, MD
Professor
Departments of Surgery
Boston University School of Medicine
Harvard Medical School
VA Boston Healthcare System
Boston, Massachusetts

William R. Jarnagin, MD
Professor
Department of Surgery
Memorial Sloan-Kettering Cancer Center
Weill Medical College of Cornell University
New York, New York

Joshua S. Jolissaint, MD
Resident
Department of Surgery
Brigham and Women's Hospital
Boston, Massachusetts

Haytham M. A. Kaafarani, MD, MPH
Associate Professor
Harvard Medical School
Department of Surgery
Massachusetts General Hospital
Boston, Massachusetts

Mark H. Katz, MD
Assistant Professor
Department of Urology
Boston University School of Medicine
Boston, Massachusetts

Lindsay E. Kuo, MD, MBA
Assistant Professor
Department of Surgery
Temple University
Philadelphia, Pennsylvania

Pui Man Rosalind Lai, MD
Resident
Department of Neurosurgery
Brigham and Women's Hospital
Boston, Massachusetts

Chienying Liu, MD
Professor
Department of Medicine
University of California
San Francisco, California

James N. Luo, MD
Resident
Department of Surgery
Brigham and Women's Hospital
Boston, Massachusetts

Heather G. Lyu, MD
Resident
Department of Surgery
Brigham and Women's Hospital
Boston, Massachusetts

David McAneny, MD, FACS
Professor
Department of Surgery
Boston University School of Medicine
Boston, Massachusetts

Kris M. Mogensen, MS, RD-AP, LDN, CNSC
Specialist Dietitian
Brigham and Women's Hospital
Boston, Massachusetts

Matthew A. Nehs, MD
Assistant Professor
Department of Surgery
Harvard Medical School
Brigham and Women's Hospital
Boston, Massachusetts

Stephanie Nitzschke, MD
Instructor
Department of Surgery
Harvard Medical School
Brigham and Women's Hospital
Boston, Massachusetts

Andrea T. Obi, MD
Assistant Professor
Department of Surgery
University of Michigan
Ann Arbor, Michigan

Richard G. Ohye, MD
Professor
Department of Cardiac Surgery
University of Michigan
Ann Arbor, Michigan

Sean B. Orenstein, MD
Assistant Professor
Department of Surgery
Oregon Health Sciences University
Portland, Oregon

Marco G. Patti, MD
Professor
Department of Surgery
University of North Carolina
Chapel Hill, North Carolina

Ian Pitha, MD, PhD
Assistant Professor
Wilmer Eye Institute
Johns Hopkins University
Baltimore, Maryland

Michael Poulson, MD
Resident
Department of Surgery
Boston Medical Center
Boston, Massachusetts

Erika Rangel, MD, MS, FACS
Assistant Professor
Department of Surgery
Harvard Medical School
Brigham and Women's Hospital
Boston, Massachusetts

Shawn J. Rangel, MD, MSCE
Associate Professor
Department of Surgery
Harvard Medical School
Boston Children's Hospital
Boston, Massachusetts

R. Kevin Reynolds, MD
George W. Morley Professor
Department of Obstetrics and Gynecology
The University of Michigan
Ann Arbor, Michigan

Malcolm K. Robinson, MD
Associate Professor
Department of Surgery
Harvard Medical School
Brigham and Women's Hospital
Boston, Massachusetts

Jennifer E. Rosen, MD
Chief of Endocrine Surgery and Vice Chair for Research
Medstar Washington Hospital Center
Washington, DC

Michael S. Sabel, MD
Professor
Department of Surgery
University of Michigan
Ann Arbor, Michigan

Sabrina E. Sanchez, MD, MPH
Assistant Professor
Department of Surgery
Boston University School of Medicine
Boston, Massachusetts

Theodore J. Sanford Jr, MD
Professor of Clinical Anesthesiology
University of Michigan
Ann Arbor, Michigan

Francisco Schlottmann, MD, MPH
Fellow
Department of Surgery
University of North Carolina
Chapel Hill, North Carolina

Carolyn Dacey Seib, MD, MAS
Assistant Professor
Department of Surgery
Stanford University
Palo Alto, California

Stephen M. Sentovich, MD, MBA
Professor
Department of Surgery
City of Hope Cancer Center
Duarte, California

Anupamaa Seshadri, MD
Fellow
Department of Surgery
University of Pittsburgh
Pittsburgh, Pennsylvania

Samir K. Shah, MD
Assistant Professor
Department of Surgery
University of Florida
Gainesville, Florida

Gaurav Sharma, MD
Fellow
Department of Surgery
Brigham and Women's Hospital
Boston, Massachusetts

Eric G. Sheu, MD
Assistant Professor
Department of Surgery
Harvard Medical School
Brigham and Women's Hospital
Boston, Massachusetts

Douglas Smink, MD, MPH
Associate Professor
Department of Surgery
Harvard Medical School
Brigham and Women's Hospital
Boston, Massachusetts

Timothy R. Smith, MD, PhD
Assistant Professor
Department of Neurosurgery
Harvard Medical School
Brigham and Women's Hospital
Boston, Massachusetts

Kevin C. Soares, MD
Surgeon
Memorial-Sloan Kettering Cancer Center
Weill Medical College of Cornell University
New York, New York

Ian Tafel, MD
Resident
Department of Neurosurgery
Brigham and Women's Hospital
Boston, Massachusetts

Ali Tavakkoli, MD
Chief, Division of General and GI Surgery
Brigham and Women's Hospital
Associate Professor of Surgery
Harvard Medical School
Boston, Massachusetts

Erin M. Taylor, MD
Fellow
Department of Surgery
Brigham and Women's Hospital
Boston, Massachusetts

Linda M. Tsai, MD
Professor
Department of Ophthalmology and Visual Sciences
Washington University
St. Louis, Missouri

Stefan G. Tullius, MD, PhD
Professor
Department of Surgery
Harvard Medical School
Brigham and Women's Hospital
Boston, Massachusetts

Pablo A. Valdes, MD, PhD
Resident
Department of Neurosurgery
Brigham and Women's Hospital
Boston, Massachusetts

Madhulika G. Varma, MD
Professor
Department of Surgery
University of California
San Francisco, California

Thomas W. Wakefield, MD
Stanley Professor of Surgery
Department of Surgery
University of Michigan
Ann Arbor, Michigan

Lawrence W. Way, MD
Professor
Department of Surgery
University of California
San Francisco, California

William Weir, MD
Resident
Department of Cardiac Surgery
University of Michigan
Ann Arbor, Michigan

Kyle Wu, MD
Resident
Department of Neurosurgery
Brigham and Women's Hospital
Boston, Massachusetts

David M. Young, MD
Professor
Department of Surgery
University of California
San Francisco, California

Joseph Zenga, MD
Assistant Professor
Department of Otolaryngology
Medical College of Wisconsin
Milwaukee, Wisconsin

Rui Zheng-Pywell, MD
Resident
Department of Surgery
University of Alabama-Birmingham
Birmingham, Alabama

Preface

Current Diagnosis & Treatment: Surgery is a ready source of information about diseases managed by surgeons. Like other books in this Lange series, it emphasizes quick recall of major diagnostic features and brief descriptions of disease processes, followed by approaches for definitive diagnosis and treatment. Epidemiology, pathophysiology, and pathology are discussed to the extent that they contribute to the ultimate purpose of the book, which is guidance for patient care. About one-third of the book is focused on general medical and surgical topics important in the management of all patients.

The book also includes limited current references to literature for the reader who wishes to pursue specific additional detail. Because of the concise nature of this text, more focused exploration may be useful to gain detail in specific areas.

OUTSTANDING FEATURES

- To maintain currency of the information, this text is revised and updated frequently. The most recent edition was published in 2015. With each revision, particular subjects are completely, substantially, partially, or minimally rewritten as indicated by the progress in each field. New authors and chapters are introduced for the text as needed.
- This edition includes major revisions of many chapters, and entirely new chapters on:
  - Neurosurgery
  - Weight Management

INTENDED AUDIENCE

- Students: This is an authoritative introduction to surgery as the discipline is taught and practiced at major teaching institutions.
- Residents: This is a ready reference for concise discussions of the diseases faced each day, as well as the less common ones calling for quick study.
- Medical practitioners: Those who have occasion to counsel patients needing surgical referrals appreciate the concise readability of this book.
- Practicing surgeons: A most useful guide to current management strategies.

ORGANIZATION

This book is arranged chiefly by organ system. Early chapters provide general information about the relationship between surgeons and their patients (Chapter 1), training and professionalism (Chapter 2), preoperative care (Chapter 3), postoperative care (Chapter 4), and surgical complications (Chapter 5). Subsequent chapters deal with wound healing, inflammation, infection, antibiotics, fluid and electrolyte management, and surgical metabolism and nutrition. The main series of body systems topics begins with the chapter on head and neck tumors and ends with the chapter on hand surgery. Further chapters on pediatric surgery, oncology, weight management, and organ transplantation complete the coverage.

MULTIPLE CHOICE QUESTIONS

Along with the customary revision of all sections as called for by changing concepts in each field covered, in this edition, multiple choice questions and answers have been added to supplement each chapter.

ACKNOWLEDGMENTS

The editor and contributors continue to acknowledge their gratitude to J. Englebert Dunphy, MD, for the inspiration to begin the first edition of this text, and his lifetime of service to the practice and teaching of surgery, and to Lawrence W. Way, the long-time editor of editions 2 through 12, and the conscience of the UCSF surgical training program. I have witnessed that same dedication to surgical students and trainees from faculty members at Washington University in St. Louis, the University of Michigan, Boston Medical Center, and Brigham and Women's Hospital as well as at dozens of other universities and hospitals that I have visited. At each institution, I have appreciated the diligence and curiosity of our trainees, and the energy that they bring to our daily work.

I am particularly grateful for the important contributions that the staff at McGraw-Hill has made to ensuring an accurate, high-quality text. I am also grateful to colleagues and readers who have offered comments and criticisms to guide preparation for future editions. I hope that anyone with an idea, suggestion, or criticism regarding this book will contact me.

Finally, I thank my wife, Faith Cuenin, our children Kevin and Megan, and our grandson Christopher for their constant love and support.

Gerard M. Doherty, MD
Boston, Massachusetts
January 2020

Approach to the Surgical Patient

J. Englebert Dunphy, MD
Lawrence W. Way, MD

The management of surgical disorders requires not only the application of technical skills and training in the basic sciences to the problems of diagnosis and treatment, but also a genuine sympathy, and indeed love, for the patient. The surgeon must be a doctor in the old-fashioned sense: an applied scientist, an engineer, an artist, and a minister to his or her fellow human beings. Because life or death often depends upon the validity of surgical decisions, the surgeon's judgment must be matched by courage in action and by a high degree of technical proficiency.

▼ THE HISTORY

At their first contact, the surgeon must gain the patient's confidence and convey the assurance that help is available and will be provided. The surgeon must demonstrate concern for the patient as a person who needs help and not just as a "case" to be processed. This is not always easy to do, and there are no rules of conduct except to be gentle and considerate. Most patients are eager to like and trust their doctors, and respond gratefully to a sympathetic and understanding person. Some surgeons are able to establish a confident relationship with the first few words of greeting; others can only do so by means of a stylized and carefully acquired bedside manner. It does not matter how it is done, so long as an atmosphere of sympathy, personal interest, and understanding is created. Even under emergency circumstances, this subtle message of sympathetic concern must be conveyed.

Eventually, all histories must be formally structured, but much can be learned by letting the patient ramble a little. Discrepancies and omissions in the history are often due as much to overstructuring and leading questions as to the unreliability of the patient. The enthusiastic novice asks leading questions, the cooperative patient gives the answer that seems to be wanted, and the interview concludes on a note of mutual satisfaction with the wrong answer thus developed.

BUILDING THE HISTORY

History taking is detective work. Preconceived ideas, snap judgments, and hasty conclusions have no place in this process. The diagnosis must be established by inductive reasoning. The interviewer must first determine the facts and then search for essential clues, realizing that the patient may conceal the most important symptom—for example, the passage of blood by rectum—in the hope (born of fear) that if it is not specifically inquired about or if nothing is found to account for it in the physical examination, it cannot be very serious.

Common symptoms of surgical conditions that require special emphasis in the history taking are discussed in the following paragraphs.

▷ Pain

A careful analysis of the nature of pain is one of the most important features of a surgical history. The examiner must first ascertain how the pain began. Was it explosive in onset, rapid, or gradual? What is the precise character of the pain? Is it so severe that it cannot be relieved by medication? Is it constant or intermittent? Are there classic associations, such as the rhythmic pattern of small bowel obstruction or the onset of pain preceding the limp of intermittent claudication?

One of the most important aspects of pain is the patient's reaction to it. The overreactor's description of pain is often obviously inappropriate, and so is a description of "excruciating" pain offered in a casual or jovial manner. A patient who shrieks and thrashes about is either grossly overreacting or suffering from renal or biliary colic. Very severe pain—due to infection, inflammation, or vascular disease—usually forces the patient to restrict all movement as much as possible.

Moderate pain is made agonizing by fear and anxiety. Reassurance of a sort calculated to restore the patient's confidence in the care being given is often a more effective analgesic than an injection of morphine.

Vomiting

What did the patient vomit? How much? How often? What did the vomitus look like? Was vomiting projectile? It is especially helpful for the examiner to see the vomitus.

Change in Bowel Habits

A change in bowel habits is a common complaint that is often of no significance. However, when a person who has always had regular evacuations notices a distinct change, particularly toward intermittent alternations of constipation and diarrhea, colon cancer must be suspected. Too much emphasis is placed upon the size and shape of the stool—for example, many patients who normally have well-formed stools may complain of irregular small stools when their routine is disturbed by travel or a change in diet.

Hematemesis or Hematochezia

Bleeding from any orifice demands the most critical analysis and can never be dismissed as due to some immediately obvious cause. The most common error is to assume that bleeding from the rectum is attributable to hemorrhoids. The character of the blood can be of great significance. Does it clot? Is it bright or dark red? Is it changed in any way, as in the coffee-grounds vomitus of slow gastric bleeding or the dark, tarry stool of upper gastrointestinal bleeding? The full details and variations cannot be included here but will be emphasized under separate headings elsewhere.

Trauma

Trauma occurs so commonly that it is often difficult to establish a relationship between the chief complaint and an episode of trauma. Children in particular are subject to all kinds of minor trauma, and the family may attribute the onset of an illness to a specific recent injury. On the other hand, children may be subjected to severe trauma though their parents are unaware of it. And the possibility of trauma having been inflicted by a parent must not be overlooked.

When there is a history of trauma, the details must be established as precisely as possible. What was the patient's position when the accident occurred? Was consciousness lost? Retrograde amnesia (inability to remember events just preceding the accident) always indicates some degree of cerebral damage. If a patient can remember every detail of an accident, has not lost consciousness, and has no evidence of external injury to the head, brain damage can be excluded.

In the case of gunshot wounds and stab wounds, knowing the nature of the weapon, its size and shape, the probable trajectory, and the position of the patient when hit may be very helpful in evaluating the nature of the resultant injury.

The possibility that an accident might have been caused by preexisting disease such as epilepsy, diabetes, coronary artery disease, or hypoglycemia must be explored.

When all of the facts and essential clues have been gathered, the examiner is in a position to complete the study of the present illness. By this time, it may be possible to rule out (by inductive reasoning) all but a few diagnoses. A novice diagnostician asked to evaluate the causes of shoulder pain in a given patient might include ruptured ectopic pregnancy in the list of possibilities. The experienced physician will automatically exclude that possibility on the basis of gender or age.

Family History

The family history is of great significance in a number of surgical conditions. Polyposis of the colon is a classic example, but diabetes, Peutz-Jeghers syndrome, chronic pancreatitis, multiglandular syndromes, other endocrine abnormalities, and cancer are often better understood and better evaluated in the light of a careful family history.

Past History

The details of the past history may illuminate obscure areas of the present illness. It has been said that people who are well are almost never sick, and people who are sick are almost never well. It is true that a patient with a long and complicated history of diseases and injuries is likely to be a much poorer risk than even a very old patient experiencing a major surgical illness for the first time.

In order to make certain that important details of the past history will not be overlooked, the system review must be formalized and thorough. By always reviewing the past history in the same way, the experienced examiner never omits significant details. Many skilled examiners find it easy to review the past history by inquiring about each system as they perform the physical examination on that part of the body.

In reviewing the past history, it is important to consider the nutritional background of the patient. There is a clear awareness throughout the world that the underprivileged malnourished patient responds poorly to disease, injury, and operation. Malnourishment may not be obvious on physical examination and must be elicited by questioning.

Acute nutritional deficiencies, particularly fluid and electrolyte losses, can be understood only in the light of the total (including nutritional) history. For example, low serum sodium may be due to the use of diuretics or a sodium-restricted diet rather than to acute loss. In this connection, the use of any medications must be carefully recorded and interpreted.

A detailed history of acute losses by vomiting and diarrhea—and the nature of the losses—is helpful in estimating the probable trends in serum electrolytes. Thus the patient who has been vomiting persistently with no evidence of bile in the vomitus is likely to have acute pyloric stenosis associated with benign ulcer, and hypochloremic alkalosis must be anticipated. Chronic vomiting without bile—and particularly with evidence of changed and previously digested food—is suggestive of chronic obstruction, and the possibility of carcinoma should be considered.

It is essential for the surgeon to think in terms of nutritional balance. It is often possible to begin therapy before the results of laboratory tests have been obtained, because the specific nature and probable extent of fluid and electrolyte losses can often be estimated on the basis of the history and the physician's clinical experience. Laboratory data should be obtained as soon as possible, but knowledge of the probable level of the obstruction and concentration of the electrolytes in the gastrointestinal fluids will provide sufficient grounds for the institution of appropriate immediate therapy.

▶ The Patient's Emotional Background

Psychiatric consultation is seldom required in the management of surgical patients, but there are times when it is of great help. Emotionally and mentally disturbed patients require surgical operations as often as others, and full cooperation between psychiatrist and surgeon is essential. Furthermore, either before or after an operation, a patient may develop a major psychotic disturbance that is beyond the ability of the surgeon to appraise or manage. Prognosis, drug therapy, and overall management require the participation of a psychiatrist.

On the other hand, there are many situations in which the surgeon can and should deal with the emotional aspects of the patient's illness rather than resorting to psychiatric assistance. Most psychiatrists prefer not to be brought in to deal with minor anxiety states. As long as the surgeon accepts the responsibility for the care of the whole patient, such services are superfluous.

This is particularly true in the care of patients with malignant disease or those who must undergo mutilating operations such as amputation of an extremity, ileostomy, or colostomy. In these situations, the patient can be supported far more effectively by the surgeon and the surgical team than by a consulting psychiatrist.

Surgeons are increasingly aware of the importance of psychosocial factors in surgical convalescence. Recovery from a major operation is greatly enhanced if the patient is not worn down with worry about emotional, social, and financial problems that have nothing to do with the illness itself. Incorporation of these factors into the record contributes to better total care of the surgical patient.

▼ THE PHYSICAL EXAMINATION

The complete examination of the surgical patient includes the physical examination, certain special procedures such as gastroscopy and esophagoscopy, laboratory tests, x-ray examination, and follow-up examination. In some cases, all of these may be necessary; in others, special examinations

and laboratory tests can be kept to a minimum. It is just as poor practice to insist on unnecessary thoroughness as it is to overlook procedures that may contribute to the diagnosis. Painful, inconvenient, and costly procedures should not be ordered unless there is a reasonable chance that the information gained will be useful in making clinical decisions.

THE ELECTIVE PHYSICAL EXAMINATION

The elective physical examination should be done in an orderly and detailed fashion. One should acquire the habit of performing a complete examination in exactly the same sequence, so that no step is omitted. When the routine must be modified, as in an emergency, the examiner recalls without conscious effort what must be done to complete the examination later. The regular performance of complete examinations has the added advantage of familiarizing the beginner with what is normal so that what is abnormal can be more readily recognized.

All patients are sensitive and somewhat embarrassed at being examined. It is both courteous and clinically useful to put the patient at ease. The examining room and table should be comfortable, and drapes should be used if the patient is required to strip for the examination. Most patients will relax if they are allowed to talk a bit during the examination, which is another reason for taking the past history while the examination is being done.

A useful rule is to first observe the patient's general physique and habitus and then to carefully inspect the hands. Many systemic diseases show themselves in the hands (cirrhosis of the liver, hyperthyroidism, Raynaud's disease, pulmonary insufficiency, heart disease, and nutritional disorders).

Details of the examination cannot be included here. The beginner is urged to consult special texts.

Inspection, palpation, and auscultation are the time-honored essential steps in appraising both the normal and the abnormal. Comparison of the two sides of the body often suggests a specific abnormality. The slight droop of one eyelid characteristic of Horner syndrome can only be recognized by comparison with the opposite side. Inspection of the female breasts, particularly as the patient raises and lowers her arms, will often reveal slight dimpling indicative of an infiltrating carcinoma barely detectable on palpation.

Successful palpation requires skill and gentleness. Spasm, tension, and anxiety caused by painful examination procedures may make an adequate examination almost impossible, particularly in children.

Another important feature of palpation is the laying on of hands that has been called part of the ministry of medicine. A disappointed and critical patient often will say of a doctor, "He hardly touched me." Careful, precise, and gentle palpation not only gives the physician the information being sought but also inspires confidence and trust.

When examining for areas of tenderness, it may be necessary to use only one finger in order to precisely localize the extent of the tenderness. This is of particular importance in examination of the acute abdomen.

Auscultation, once thought to be the exclusive province of the physician, is now more important in surgery than it is in medicine. Radiologic examinations, including cardiac catheterization, have relegated auscultation of the heart and lungs to the status of preliminary scanning procedures in medicine. In surgery, however, auscultation of the abdomen and peripheral vessels has become absolutely essential. The nature of ileus and the presence of a variety of vascular lesions are revealed by auscultation. Bizarre abdominal pain can easily be ascribed to anxiety on the basis of a negative physical examination and x-rays of the gastrointestinal tract. Auscultation of the epigastrium, however, may reveal a murmur due to obstruction of the celiac artery.

▶ Examination of the Body Orifices

Complete examination of the ears, mouth, rectum, and pelvis is accepted as a part of complete examination. Palpation of the mouth and tongue is as essential as inspection. Every surgeon should acquire familiarity with the use of the ophthalmoscope and sigmoidoscope and should use them regularly in doing complete physical examinations.

THE EMERGENCY PHYSICAL EXAMINATION

In an emergency, the routine of the physical examination must be altered to fit the circumstances. The history may be limited to a single sentence, or there may be no history if the patient is unconscious and there are no other informants. Although the details of an accident or injury may be very useful in the total appraisal of the patient, they must be left for later consideration. The primary considerations are the following: Is the patient breathing? Is the airway open? Is there a palpable pulse? Is the heart beating? Is massive bleeding occurring?

If the patient is not breathing, airway obstruction must be ruled out by thrusting the fingers into the mouth and pulling the tongue forward. If the patient is unconscious, the respiratory tract should be intubated and mouth-to-mouth respiration started. If there is no pulse or heartbeat, start cardiac resuscitation.

Serious external loss of blood from an extremity can be controlled by elevation and pressure. Tourniquets are rarely required.

Every victim of major blunt trauma should be suspected of having a vertebral injury capable of causing damage to the spinal cord unless rough handling is avoided.

Some injuries are so life threatening that action must be taken before even a limited physical examination is done.

Penetrating wounds of the heart, large open sucking wounds of the chest, massive crush injuries with flail chest, and massive external bleeding all require emergency treatment before any further examination can be done.

In most emergencies, however, after it has been established that the airway is open, the heart is beating, and there is no massive external hemorrhage—and after antishock measures have been instituted, if necessary—a rapid survey examination must be done. Failure to perform such an examination can lead to serious mistakes in the care of the patient. It takes no more than 2 or 3 minutes to carefully examine the head, thorax, abdomen, extremities, genitalia (particularly in females), and back. If cervical cord damage has been ruled out, it is essential to turn the injured patient and carefully inspect the back, buttocks, and perineum.

Tension pneumothorax and cardiac tamponade may easily be overlooked if there are multiple injuries.

Upon completion of the survey examination, control of pain, splinting of fractured limbs, suturing of lacerations, and other types of emergency treatment can be started.

▼ LABORATORY & OTHER EXAMINATIONS

▶ Laboratory Examination

Laboratory examinations in surgical patients have the following objectives:

1. Screening for asymptomatic disease that may affect the surgical result (eg, unsuspected anemia or diabetes)

2. Appraisal of diseases that may contraindicate elective surgery or require treatment before surgery (eg, diabetes or heart failure)

3. Diagnosis of disorders that require surgery (eg, hyperparathyroidism or pheochromocytoma)

4. Evaluation of the nature and extent of metabolic or septic complications

Patients undergoing major surgery, even though they seem to be in excellent health except for their surgical disease, should have age-appropriate laboratory examination. A history of renal, hepatic, or heart disease requires detailed studies. Medical consultation may be helpful in the total preoperative appraisal of the surgical patient. It is essential, however, that the surgeon not become totally dependent upon a medical consultant for the preoperative evaluation and management of the patient. The total management must be the surgeon's responsibility and is not to be delegated. Moreover, the surgeon is the only one with the experience and background to interpret the meaning of laboratory tests in the light of other features of the case—particularly the history and physical findings.

▶ Imaging Studies

Modern patient care calls for a variety of critical radiologic examinations. The closest cooperation between the radiologist and the surgeon is essential if serious mistakes are to be avoided. This means that the surgeon must not refer the patient to the radiologist, requesting a particular examination, without providing an adequate account of the history and physical findings. Particularly in emergency situations, review of the films and consultation are needed.

When the radiologic diagnosis is not definitive, the examinations must be repeated in the light of the history and physical examination. Despite the great accuracy of x-ray diagnosis, a negative gastrointestinal study still does not exclude either ulcer or a neoplasm; particularly in the right colon, small lesions are easily overlooked. At times, the history and physical findings are so clearly diagnostic that operation is justifiable despite negative imaging studies.

▶ Special Examinations

Special examinations such as cystoscopy, gastroscopy, esophagoscopy, colonoscopy, angiography, and bronchoscopy are often required in the diagnostic appraisal of surgical disorders. The surgeon must be familiar with the indications and limitations of these procedures and be prepared to consult with colleagues in medicine and the surgical specialties as required.

Training, Communication, Professionalism, & Systems-Based Practice

Gerard M. Doherty, MD

TRAINING

The process of medical education and surgical training in the United States is overseen by an interconnected group of organizations. Each of these organizations has its specific focus; however, the common theme is continuous process improvement encouraged by intermittent external review (Table 2–1). The ultimate goal is the provision of a consistent, qualified, and professional work force for medical care in the United States.

Medical Student Education

The Liaison Committee on Medical Education (LCME) is the group that provides accreditation for medical schools in the United States and Canada. *Accreditation* is the process of quality assurance in postsecondary education that assesses whether an institution meets established standards. Accreditation by the LCME is effectively necessary for schools to function in the United States. Without accreditation, the schools cannot receive federal grants for medical education or participate in federal loan programs. Graduation from an LCME-accredited school enables students to sit for medical licensing examinations (the USMLE) and to achieve licensure in most states around the country. Graduation from a LCME-accredited medical school is also necessary for acceptance into an ACGME-accredited residency program (see below) for graduates of U.S. medical schools. The authority for the LCME to provide this accreditation is delegated by the United States Department of Education and the Committee on Accreditation of Canadian Medical Schools (CACMS).

Each accredited medical school is reviewed annually for appropriateness of their function, structure, and performance. Formal site visits are conducted periodically with more in-depth review and reaccreditation at that time. The usual period of full accreditation is 8 years. At the time of this in-depth accreditation visit, and in the intervals between, the LCME works to disseminate best practices and approve the overall quality of education leading to the MD degree.

Graduate Medical Education

The Accreditation Council for Graduate Medical Education (ACGME) is responsible for the accreditation of post-MD medical training programs within the United States. Accreditation is accomplished through a peer review process based on established standards and guidelines. The member organizations of the ACGME as an accrediting group are the American Board of Medical Specialties (ABMS), the American Hospital Association (AHA), the American Medical Association (AMA), the Association of American Medical Colleges (AAMC), and the Council of Medical Specialty Societies. The ACGME creates and ensures a basic set of standards for training in residencies and fellowships. The ACGME sets and reviews the institutional clinical learning environment requirements for development of the skills, knowledge, and attitudes necessary to take personal responsibility for the individual care of patients. These requirements are designed to facilitate an environment where residents and fellows can interact with patients under the guidance and supervision of qualified faculty members who give value, context, and meaning to those interactions. ACGME-accredited residency programs must adhere to the ACGME common program requirements that apply to all residencies, as well as specific program requirements that apply to each training program. The institutional requirements that must be met for overall accreditation of the institution to house training programs are reviewed periodically as a part of Clinical Learning Environment Reviews (CLER site visits).

The ACGME has identified six general competency areas that must be addressed during every graduate residency training program (Table 2–2). The specific application of these competency areas varies widely among training programs. However, each rotation of each residency must

Table 2–1. U.S. organizations with medical education oversight.

Organization	Acronym and Website	Purpose
Liaison Committee on Medical Education	LCME www.LCME.org	Accreditation of medical schools in United States and Canada
Accreditation Council for Graduate Medical Education	ACGME www.ACGME.org	Accreditation of post-MD training programs in some specialties
American Board of Surgery	ABS www.absurgery.org	Certifies and recertifies individual surgeons who have met standards of education, training, and knowledge
American College of Surgeons	ACS www.facs.org	Scientific and educational association of surgeons to improve the quality of care for the surgical patient

include attention to, and assessment of, progress in fulfilling the general competency requirements. The ACGME has established *milestones* for programs to use in the clinical competency assessments of trainees.

The review and accreditation of specialty residency programs is undertaken by a committee specific for that field. In surgery, the group is the Residency Review Committee for Surgery (RRC-S). The RRC-S assesses program compliance with accreditation standards both at the common program requirement level and at the program-specific level. The Residency Review Committees also control the number of positions that each program is accredited to have. This effectively sets the maximum number of graduates who can finish from a given training program in any given year.

American Board of Surgery

The American Board of Surgery (ABS) is an independent, nonprofit organization with the purpose of certifying individual surgeons who have met defined standards of education, training, and knowledge. The distinction between the ACGME and the ABS is that the ACGME accredits training institutions and programs, while the ABS certifies individuals. This distinction is similar for specialty boards in other disciplines as well. The ABS also recertifies practicing surgeons, and has made a recent fundamental philosophical

Table 2–2. ACGME general competencies for graduate medical education.

General Competency
- Patient care
- Medical knowledge
- Interpersonal and communication skills
- Professionalism
- Practice-based learning
- Systems-based practice

change from periodic retesting for recertification to a more continuous maintenance of certification (MOC) plan.

The ACGME and the specialty boards interact. The success of individuals in achieving board certification is considered an important measure of graduate medical education program success, and the measures that can be required of an individual for board certification must somehow also reflect the education that is offered to them through their graduate medical education. Thus though these entities have different purposes, they must, optimally, mesh their efforts constructively.

Board certification within a defined period after completing residency is necessary for privileging to perform surgery in many hospitals in the United States. Thus the most straightforward route into surgical practice in the United States includes graduation from an LCME-accredited medical school, completion of an ACGME-accredited residency training program, and satisfactory completion of the Qualifying Examination (written boards) and Certifying Examination (oral boards) of the American Board of Surgery.

There are other entry points into surgical practice in the United States, most prominently by physicians who have graduated from medical schools in countries outside the United States and Canada. These graduates can be certified by the Educational Commission for Foreign Medical Graduates (ECFMG). Once an individual graduate has been certified by the ECFMG, then he or she is eligible to train in an ACGME-approved residency training program, and can thus be eligible for board certification.

American College of Surgeons

The American College of Surgeons (ACS) is a scientific and educational association of surgeons whose mission is to improve the quality of care for the surgical patient by setting high standards for surgical education and practice. The American College of Surgeons has members, known as fellows, who are entitled to use the letters "FACS" after their name. Membership as a fellow implies that the surgeon has met standards of education, training, professional qualifications, surgical competence, and ethical conduct. However, despite these requirements, the ACS is a voluntary professional membership group, and does not certify individuals for practice. The ACS does sponsor a wide variety of educational and professional support programs both for practicing surgeons and trainees. In addition, they have membership categories for surgeons in training (Resident Membership) and students (Medical Student Membership), and for those surgeons who have completed training but have not yet met all the requirements for fellowship (Associate Fellow). The ACS also engages in important advocacy roles on behalf of patients and the surgeon members.

COMMUNICATION

Efficient and effective communication skills are a critical resource for all clinicians including surgeons. A surgeon must be capable of establishing rapport with the patient and family quickly and reliably. This mutual respect is critical to a therapeutic relationship. The patient and family must be confident of the competence of the surgeon in order to participate in the recommended management and recovery. Judgments about surgeon competence frequently come within the first few moments of interaction based on the surgeon's ability to communicate. In addition to communicating with patients, clinicians must communicate with referring and collaborating physicians, and also within their own healthcare teams.

▶ Communicating With Patients

Communication with patients requires attention to several aspects. First, the clinician must demonstrate respect for the patient as a person. Second, the clinician must display effective listening to the patient's message, followed by demonstrated empathy to their situation or concerns. Finally, the clinician must have clarity in the response. If any of these items are omitted, then the interaction will be less effective than it could be. Many surgeons try to jump straight to a very clear, concise statement of the plan; however, unless the first three steps have occurred, the patient may not listen to the plan at all.

Respect

It is critically important to show respect for the patient and family as people. The healthcare environment is often inconvenient and encountered during a time of stress. The patients are out of their normal venue and comfort zone. They are often frightened by the prospect of what they may learn. Showing respect for their identity will place the patient at more ease and encourage their trusting communication with the clinician. Failing to show respect will have the contrary effect. Thus meeting an adult for the first time and addressing them by their first name can immediately put many patients

on guard with respect to their personal independence and control. Similarly, referring to the mother of a pediatric patient as "Mom" rather than using her name implies lack of attention to her as an individual worthy of learning her identity. On initial meetings, the clinician should use the patient's last name preceded by an honorific title (eg, Mr. Smith, or Ms. Jones). If you are not certain if a woman prefers Mrs. or Ms., then ask her. In contemporary U.S. society, a woman over 18 years of age is never referred to as Miss.

In addition, engaging in brief small talk regarding some aspect of a patient's life other than the medical matter at hand can further put them at ease ("It must be interesting to be a dog trainer. What is your favorite breed?"). These efforts will be rewarded by a more trusting patient and a more efficient interview, with a better therapeutic relationship over the long term.

Listening

Listening to the patient is critical to establishing a correct diagnosis and appropriate therapeutic plan for the individual. Every patient who comes to the medical system with a problem has a story that they have thought through and decided to tell. It is important to let them do so. Not only is the patient likely to reveal critical issues regarding the clinical matter, but they are also often determined to tell the story eventually, whether they are allowed to do so at the outset or not. Allowing, and in fact encouraging them, to tell the story at the beginning of the interview relieves them of this burden of information, and allows the clinician to move on to interpretation.

Listening should be an active, engaged activity. The clinician should appear comfortable, settled, and upon as much of an even eye level with the patient as possible. It is important not to appear rushed, inattentive, or bored by their account. Interjecting questions for clarity or intermittent, brief verbal encouragements will let the patient know that the clinician is engaged with the problem.

It may be helpful at the outset of the listening phase to let the patient know what materials have been reviewed. For example, telling the patient that the clinician has reviewed the referral letter from the primary physician, the results of the last two operations, and their recent laboratory work, may help the patient to be more concise in their discussion.

Empathy

Once the patient has recounted their history and the other aspects of examination and data review have been completed, it is important to review this material with the patient in a way that demonstrates empathy with their situation. A surgeon's understanding of the problem is important for the patient, but the problem is not confined to the medical issue; the problem must be understood in the context of the patient. For this reason, demonstration of empathy is important to the patient's trust of the physician. Establishing this connection with the patient is crucial to their engagement in the process of care.

Clarity

Having established respect for the patient, heard and understood their story, and empathized with their situation, the physician must speak clearly, using vocabulary understood by the individual, about the recommendations for further evaluation or care. This portion of the conversation should include a clear distinction between what is known about the patient's diagnosis or condition and what is not known but might be anticipated. When appropriate, likelihoods of various outcomes should be estimated in a way that the patient can grasp. The recommended approach to next steps should be listed clearly, along with alternative approaches. Patients always have at least one alternative to the recommended choice, even if this is only to decide not to have further medical care. This portion of the conversation can be augmented with illustrations or models that may improve the patient's understanding. Often reviewing radiologic studies directly with the patient or family at this time can help their understanding.

The risk taken by failing to establish this relationship with the patient is great. This can lead to errors in judgment about diagnosis or management. It also precludes the opportunity to engage the patient as an ally in his or her care. If things go badly, it also can make subsequent communication about problems or complications difficult or impossible. Finally, the surgeon who communicates poorly excludes him or herself from enjoying a personally and professionally satisfying physician–patient relationship.

▶ Communication With Collaborating Physicians

Surgeons often work with other physicians in collaboration of care for patients. Communication in these settings is important to the overall patient outcome, particularly when the surgeon will be involved in the patient's care for some defined interval that has been preceded and will be followed by the ongoing care provided by the primary care physician. The communication in these settings can be separated into two basic types: routine and urgent. Routine communication can take place in a variety of ways depending on the healthcare setting. This communication is typically asynchronous and written. It may take the form of a note in the patient's electronic medical record, or a letter sent to the physician's office. This is an appropriate way to communicate reasonably expected information that does not need to be acted on urgently. For example, a patient who is referred to a surgeon for cholecystectomy and who has a plan made for cholecystectomy can have routine communication back to the referring physician.

Urgent communication should occur to the collaborating physicians when there are unexpected or adverse outcomes. Again, there are a variety of communication modes that may be utilized for this, but the communication is more often synchronous via a direct conversation either in person or by telephone. The communication is more than courtesy to the collaborating physician, as knowledge of these events allows them to participate constructively on behalf of the patient. Examples of situations that warrant more urgent communication include new diagnosis of significant cancers, life-altering complications from interventions, and certainly death of the patient.

Clarity in transfer of care responsibility is critical to the continuous optimal care of the patient. For that reason, any communication with the collaborating physicians should indicate either the ongoing role of the surgeon in the patient's care, or the deliberate transfer of responsibility for ongoing care issues back to other collaborating physicians.

▶ Communications Within Teams

Surgical care is often provided in a team setting, and communication within these teams has become a recent focus of several groups. Systems have been built to both teach and assess these skills, the most predominant being the Nontechnical Skills for Surgeons (NOTSS) work done in Scotland and the United States. Current surgical teams typically include physicians, non-physician mid-level providers (often physician assistants or nurse practitioners), and a variety of students. The student trainees may include students in medical school, physician assistant programs, and nursing school. These teams have become increasingly complex, and the information that they manipulate as a team to provide patient care is voluminous. In addition, the transfer of information from one provider to another as shifts or rotations change is recognized as a weak point in the patient care continuum.

With these complex teams and extensive information, the keys to efficient and effective team processes appear to be clarity of roles and designing processes that involve writing things down only once. The advent of electronic medical records has allowed the generation of electronic tools to transfer information from team member to team member. This may be useful to facilitate this process. Careful attention to transfers of care from one provider to another, and explicit recognition that this is a potential time for errors, is important.

PROFESSIONALISM

Professionalism denotes a series of behaviors that demonstrate that a person has achieved status as a professional. A *professional* in this context is implied to possess the specialized knowledge and have gone through long and intensive academic preparation for their vocation. These behaviors affect the interactions that professionals have both with

Table 2–3. AMA principles of medical ethics.

1. A physician shall be dedicated to providing competent medical care, with compassion and respect for human dignity and rights.
2. A physician shall uphold the standards of professionalism, be honest in all professional interactions, and strive to report physicians deficient in character or competence, or engaging in fraud or deception, to appropriate entities.
3. A physician shall respect the law and also recognize a responsibility to seek changes in those requirements which are contrary to the best interests of the patient.
4. A physician shall respect the rights of patients, colleagues, and other health professionals, and shall safeguard patient confidence and privacy within the constraints of the law.
5. A physician shall continue to study, apply, and advance scientific knowledge, maintain a commitment to medical education, make relevant information available to patients, colleagues, and the public, obtain consultation, and use the talents of other health professionals when indicated.
6. A physician shall, in the provision of appropriate patient care, except in emergencies, be free to choose whom to serve, with whom to associate, and the environment in which to provide medical care.
7. A physician shall recognize a responsibility to participate in activities contributing to the improvement of the community and the betterment of public health.
8. A physician shall, while caring for a patient, regard responsibility to the patient as paramount.
9. A physician shall support access to medical care for all people.

Table 2–4. Principles of medical ethics.

Principle	Definition
Autonomy	Deliberated self-rule; the patient has the right to choose or refuse their treatments; requires physicians to consult and obtain patient agreement before doing things to them.
Beneficence	A practitioner should act in the best interest of the patient, without regard to physician self-interest.
Nonmaleficence	Do no harm; the practitioner should avoid treatments that harm the patient.
Justice	Rendering what is due to others; affects the distribution of medical care among patients and populations.

patients and other healthcare professionals. For optimal effectiveness, the surgeon should behave in a professional way both with patients and within their healthcare institutions. The American Medical Association has promulgated a set of medical ethical principles that apply equally well to surgical practice, and that can help to guide professional behavior (Table 2–3).

The ethics of surgical practice are complex, and can be approached from a variety of theoretical frameworks. The most commonly applied framework for the evaluation of ethical dilemmas for individual patient decisions in medicine, known as "The Principles Approach," involves four principles: Autonomy, Beneficence, Nonmaleficence, and Justice, as promulgated by Beauchamp and Childress (Table 2–4). A detailed analysis of these principles is beyond the scope here; however, the need for a code of medical ethics that is distinct from general societal ethics is the basis for medical professionalism. There are five features of medical relationships that provide the moral imperatives underlying the profession and the requirement for a separate ethical code from other forms of business.

1. The inequality in medical knowledge, and attendant vulnerability, of the patient.
2. The requirement for the patient to trust the physician, known as the fiduciary nature of the relationship.
3. The moral nature of medical decisions that encompass both the technical aspects of health management and the ultimate effect on the patient's life.
4. The nature of medical knowledge as a public property that physicians receive in order to apply to the practical improvement of patients' lives.
5. The moral complicity of the physician in the outcome of the prescribed care, in that no formal medical care can take place without the physician's collusion.

Because of these characteristics of the relationship between physicians and their patients, physicians must adhere to a set of ethical constraints specific to their profession.

Although these imperatives are not generally understood explicitly by patients, patients can clearly grasp when these principles are in danger. They may even be suspicious that their physician or surgeon has motives that compete with the patient's best interest. One of the goals of the physician–patient interaction is to allay these fears, and construct a trusting relationship based on the patient's needs, within the principles noted above.

▶ Interaction With Patients

The interactions with patients should be characterized by polite and possibly somewhat formal manners. These manners will aid the professional in their communication efforts, as noted above. In order to meet the patient's expectations of what the physician or surgeon should be, proper socially acceptable manners should be observed. The purpose of these manners is to put the patient at ease that the physician is an empathetic person with the self-awareness to recognize the way that he or she appears to other people. The manners that the physician projects affect the credibility of the subsequent interactions. These conventions extend to the type of dress that is worn in a professional setting. The details of whether a physician wears a white coat or formal business clothing (suits, ties, pantsuits, blouses, skirts, and so on) are best left to local custom and practice. However, the mode of dress in general should be neat, clean, and formal rather than casual, and not distracting to the interaction.

Another aspect of professionalism is the capability of the physician to do the right thing for the patient and the family even when that course is difficult or unpleasant. This includes such situations as frankly and openly disclosing errors made during care, or delivering bad news about new or unexpected diagnoses. Although human nature can make these interactions difficult, the professional must rise to the task and perform it well. Avoiding the opportunity to do so not only obviates the professional's role as advisor on the issue at hand, but affects the physician's credibility in the remainder of that therapeutic relationship.

▶ Interactions With Healthcare Personnel

Surgeons frequently work in complex, multilayered organizations. The behavior of the surgeon within this group should always remain productive and patient centered. In any complex organization with multiple people and personalities, conflicts arise. In that context, it is not appropriate for the surgeon to necessarily shrink from the conflict, but rather the surgeon should take up the role of constructive evaluator and team builder to resolve the issue. At all times, the surgeon must avoid personal attacks on people based upon their personal characteristics, but may legitimately criticize behavior. Professional comportment in these matters will be rewarded with progress in resolving the issue.

Reputation is a fragile and valuable commodity. All healthcare professionals have a reputation, and it works either for or against them in achieving their patient care and professional goals. Careful adherence to professional behavior in dress, speech, manners, and conflict resolution will create the professional reputation that is most advantageous for the surgeon. With a positive reputation, the surgeon's behavior in ambiguous situations will be interpreted in a benevolent way. The reputation of any clinician is as valuable as their education or certification.

SYSTEMS-BASED PRACTICE

Systems-based practice is one of the core competencies defined by the ACGME as a necessary skill to be developed by graduate medical trainees. These residents must demonstrate an awareness of, and responsiveness to, the larger context and system of healthcare and the ability to effectively call on system resources to provide care that is of optimal value. The process of teaching and learning systems-based practice has been in place for many years. This is what might be considered the practical part of graduate medical training. However, it is only more recently that it has become a focus and metric for performance by training programs.

As a part of training, then, residents must learn how different types of medical practice and healthcare delivery systems differ from one another, including methods that they use to control healthcare costs and allocate resources. They must use this knowledge to practice cost-effective healthcare and resource allocation that limits the compromise of quality of care. They must advocate for quality patient care, and assist patients in dealing with complexities of the healthcare delivery system. They must also understand how to work with healthcare managers and other collaborating healthcare providers to assess, coordinate, and improve healthcare for patients.

In practice, this is easier to understand. The role of the resident in identifying both the healthcare needs of the patient and the capability of the system to meet those needs is well established. Surgery residents in their senior years are often important resources for hospital systems by understanding how to manipulate the system to meet the needs of the patient. Medical students and surgical trainees must also recognize their role as a part of these complex systems.

▶ Reference

Nontechnical skills for surgeons (NOTSS). https://www.notss.org. Accessed January 2, 2019.

MULTIPLE-CHOICE QUESTIONS

1. All of the following are true of the Principles of Medical Ethics, *except:*

    A. Beneficence and nonmaleficence are synonyms.

    B. Justice addresses the distribution of medical care among patients and populations.

    C. Autonomy includes the concept that the patient has the right to choose or refuse their treatments.

    D. Beneficence asserts that a practitioner should act in the best interest of the patient, without regard to physician self-interest.

    E. Autonomy requires physicians to consult and obtain patient agreement before doing things to them.

2. The LCME and the ACGME:

   A. Both accredit institutions to provide education or training.
   B. Provide diplomas and credentialing to individual practitioners.
   C. Conduct periodic reviews to ensure that institutions maintain their programs.
   D. Are units of the U.S. Department of Commerce.
   E. Both A and C are true.

3. ACGME general competencies include all of the following, *except:*

   A. Interpersonal and communication skills.
   B. Professionalism.
   C. Technical skills.
   D. Practice-based learning.
   E. Systems-based practice.

4. The American Board of Surgery and the American College of Surgeons:

   A. Are both a part of the American Medical Association.
   B. Both report directly to the Surgery RRC of the ACGME.

C. Work together to accredit individuals to practice general surgery.
D. Are separate organizations that credential surgeons, and educate surgeons, respectively, as primary parts of their missions.
E. A and C.

5. Effective communication with patients requires:

   A. Demonstrated respect for the patient as a person.
   B. Effective listening to the patient's message.
   C. Clarity in the physician's response to the patient.
   D. Family members who can reinforce the messages.
   E. A, B, and C.

Preoperative Preparation

Michael R. Cassidy, MD
David McAneny, MD, FACS

INTRODUCTION

The preoperative management of any patient is part of a continuum of care that extends from the surgeon's initial consultation through the patient's full recovery. Although this care generally involves multidisciplinary collaboration, surgeons lead the team to ensure that the best care is provided to all patients. This involves the establishment of a culture of quality care and patient safety with high, uniform standards. In addition, the surgeon is responsible for balancing the hazards of the natural history of the condition if left untreated versus the risks of an operation. A successful operation depends upon the surgeon's comprehension of the biology of the patient's disease and keen patient selection.

This chapter will consider preoperative preparation from the perspectives of the patient, operating room facility and equipment, operating room staff, and surgeon. The surgeon is the only professional present for each perioperative phase of care, including the preoperative evaluation, the immediate preoperative setting, the intraoperative phase, the early postoperative recovery, and the postdischarge convalescence. Therefore the surgeon bears the ultimate responsibility for meticulous planning and coordination throughout the phases to ensure the best outcome for the patient.

PREPARATION OF THE PATIENT

▶ History & Physical Examination

The surgeon and team should obtain a proper history from each patient. The history of present illness includes details about the presenting condition, including establishing the acuity, urgency, or chronic nature of the problem. Inquiries will certainly focus on the specific disease and related organ system. Questions regarding pain can be guided by the acronym "OPQRST," relating to Onset (sudden or gradual), Precipitant (eg, fatty foods, movement), Quality (eg, sharp, dull, or cramps), Radiation (eg, to the back or shoulder), Stop (what offers relief?), and Temporal (eg, duration, frequency, crescendo-decrescendo). The presence of fevers, sweats, or chills suggests the possibility of an acute infection, whereas significant weight loss may imply a chronic condition such as a tumor. The history of present illness is not necessarily confined to the patient interview. Family members or guardians provide useful information, and outside records can be indispensable. Documents might include recent laboratory or imaging results that preclude the need for repetitive, costly testing. The surgeon should request CD-ROM disks of outside imaging, if appropriate. In the case of reoperative surgery, prior operative reports and pathology reports are essential (eg, when searching for a missing adenoma in recurrent primary hyperparathyroidism).

The past medical history should include prior operations, especially when germane to the current situation, medical conditions, prior venous thromboembolism (VTE) events such as deep vein thromboses (DVT) or pulmonary emboli (PE), bleeding diatheses, prolonged bleeding with prior operations or modest injuries (eg, epistaxis, gingival bleeding, or ecchymoses), and untoward events during surgery or anesthesia, including airway problems. One must secure a list of active medications, with dosages and schedule. Moreover, it is beneficial to inquire about corticosteroid usage within the past 6 months, even if not current, to avoid perioperative adrenal insufficiency. Medication allergies and adverse reactions should be elicited, although knowledge about environmental and food allergies is also valuable and should be recorded so that these exposures are avoided during the hospital stay. Some anesthesiologists are reluctant to use propofol in patients with egg allergies, and reactions to shellfish suggest the possibility of intolerance of iodinated contrast agents.

The social history classically involves inquiries into tobacco, alcohol, and illicit drug usage, but this moment also offers the opportunity to establish a personal relationship with patients (and their loved ones). It is fun and often stimulating to learn about patients' occupations, avocations, exercise, interests and accomplishments, fears and expectations, and family lives. Patients' regular activities offer insight into physiologic reserve; an elite athlete should tolerate nearly any major operation, whereas a frail, sedentary patient can be a poor candidate for even relatively minor operations.

A family history includes queries pertinent to the patient's presenting condition. For example, if a patient with a colorectal cancer has relatives with similar or other malignancies, genetic conditions such as familial adenomatous polyposis or hereditary nonpolyposis colorectal cancer could be implicated. This scenario would have screening implications for both the patient and family members. In addition, one should also elicit a family history of VTE complications, bleeding disorders, and anesthesia complications. For example, a sudden and unexpected death of a relatively young family member during an operation could suggest the possibility of a pheochromocytoma, particularly in the setting of a medullary cancer or related endocrine disorder. A strong family history of allergic reactions might imply hypersensitivity to medications.

A review of systems assesses the patient's cardiovascular, pulmonary, and neurologic status, including questions about exertional chest pain or dyspnea, palpitations, syncope, productive cough, or central nervous symptoms. It is also important to have a basic understanding of the patient's symptoms relative to other major organ systems. For example, while one might not necessarily expect an orthopedic surgeon to have an interest in a patient's gastrointestinal or genitourinary habits or problems, these issues may bear grave consequences if a patient experiences postoperative incontinence following joint replacement. Regardless of degree of specialization, surgeons and their designated teams are capable of identifying and investigating potentially confounding conditions.

A thorough physical examination is also an essential part of the patient assessment. Even if the surgeon already knows from imaging that there will be no pertinent physical findings, human touch and contact are fundamental to the development of a trusting physician–patient relationship. In addition to the traditional vital signs of pulse, blood pressure, respiratory rate, and temperature, for many operations it is also important to record the patient's baseline oxygen saturation on room air, weight, height, and body mass index (BMI). The physical examination includes an assessment of general fitness, exercise tolerance, cachexia or obesity, as well as focusing on the patient's condition. Additional observations may detect findings such as cardiopulmonary abnormalities, bruits, absent peripheral pulses, adenopathy, skin integrity, incidental masses, hand-dominance, neurologic deficits, or deformities. A thorough abdominal exam may include digital anorectal and pelvic examinations. The surgeon should also appreciate potential airway problems, particularly if general anesthesia is anticipated.

▶ Preoperative Testing

Laboratory and imaging investigations are tailored to the individual patient's presenting condition, as discussed in later chapters. However, there should be no "routine" battery of preoperative laboratory studies for all patients. In fact, published data do not support an association between routine studies and outcome. In addition, laboratory tests are costly and may result in harm due to false-positive and fortuitous findings. Instead, tests should be selected based upon the patient's age, comorbidities, cardiac risk factors, medications, and general health, as well as the complexity of the underlying condition and proposed operation. For example, children uncommonly require preoperative lab tests for most operations. On the other hand, a complete blood count, chemistries, and electrocardiogram are proper for high-risk patients before complex operations. Algorithms and grid matrices are available to individualize the selection of preoperative tests (Table 3–1). Importantly, each system should establish a practice for managing abnormal test results, whether germane to the patient's active condition or a serendipitous finding.

A complete blood cell count and basic chemistries are reasonable for some operations, but their likelihood of predicting abnormal or meaningful results should be considered. Coagulation factors such as prothrombin time (PT), international normalized ratio (INR), and partial thromboplastin time (PTT) are not routinely indicated but should be pursued when patients report prolonged bleeding or the usage of anticoagulants. Moreover, INR and PTT may be warranted for operations that have little threshold for intraoperative or postoperative bleeding, such as those on the brain, spine, or neck. Bile duct obstruction, malnutrition, or an absent terminal ileum can affect vitamin K absorption, and a preoperative assessment of INR is important in those instances as well. A pregnancy test (eg, urine beta-human chorionic gonadotropin [beta-HCG]) should be performed shortly before operations upon women with childbearing potential. Other laboratory testing will be dictated by specific conditions, including liver chemistries, tumor markers, and hormone levels. A blood bank specimen should be selectively submitted in advance of operations that are associated with significant hemorrhage or in the setting of anemia with prospects for further blood loss. The preparation of blood for transfusion is costly, so blood-typing alone may suffice without actual cross-matching.

Routine preoperative testing of blood glucose is an intriguing concept, given the relationship between elevated blood sugars and surgical site infections (SSIs), although hemoglobin A1C levels have not been correlated with postoperative infections. Some reckon that nondiabetic patients

Table 3–1. Sample preoperative testing grid.

	CBC	Basic Chemistries	INR or PT	PTT	Liver Chemistries	Urinalysis	ECG	CXR	Urine Pregnancy Test
Cardiac disease (MI, CHF, pacemaker/AICD, coronary stents)	X						X		
Pulmonary disease (COPD, active asthma)	X						X	X	
End-stage renal disease on dialysis	X	X					X		
Renal insufficiency	X	X							
Liver disease	X	X	X		X				
Hypertension							X		
Diabetes		X					X		
Vascular disease	X						X		
Symptoms of urinary tract infection						X			
Chemotherapy	X	X							
Diuretics		X							
Anticoagulants			X	X					
Major operation (eg, cardiac, thoracic, vascular, or abdominal)	X	X					X	X	
Menstruating women									X

AICD, automated implantable cardioverter-defibrillator; CBC, complete blood count; CHF, congestive heart failure; COPD, chronic obstructive pulmonary disease; CXR, chest radiograph; ECG, electrocardiogram; INR, international normalized ratio; MI, myocardial infarction; PT, prothrombin time; PTT, partial thromboplastin time.
Used with permission of Boston Medical Center.

comprise 30%-50% of cases with perioperative hyperglycemia, perhaps constituting an argument for measuring preoperative glucose levels in all candidates for major operations. Although it is accepted that diabetic patients require close monitoring of perioperative glucose levels, including immediately before the operation, the value of doing this for all patients is evolving and warrants thoughtful consideration.

Some investigators have advocated routine nasal swab screening to identify carriers of *Staphylococcus aureus*. The results can guide decontamination measures such as intranasal application of antibiotic ointment (eg, mupirocin) and local hygiene with 2% chlorhexidine showers for 5 days before surgery. Patients with methicillin-resistant *S aureus* (MRSA) receive appropriate antibiotic prophylaxis and contact precautions. Although the issue of routine MRSA screening is not fully resolved, this practice may be conducted at least for immunocompromised patients and for those undergoing open cardiac operations and implantations of foreign bodies, particularly in orthopedics and neurosurgery. Prospective

wound or abscess culture results should also influence decisions about perioperative antibiotics.

Electrocardiograms are not routinely performed but are justified for patients older than 50 years, those having vascular operations, and patients with a history of hypertension, cardiac disease, significant respiratory disease, renal dysfunction, and diabetes mellitus. Chest radiographs are no longer performed on a regular basis but are primarily reserved for patients with malignancies or perhaps with significant pulmonary disease. Further special tests are selectively obtained when clinically indicated and often with guidance from consultants; these tests may include echocardiography, cardiac stress testing, baseline arterial blood gases, and pulmonary function tests. Carotid ultrasonography may be valuable in patients with carotid bruits or histories of cerebrovascular accidents or transient ischemia attacks. Noninvasive venous studies may be considered in patients who have had prolonged immobility and/or hospital stays before surgery.

Preoperative Process

At its simplest, the process of preparing a patient for an operation can involve a rapid assessment in the clinic or emergency room followed by an expeditious trip to the operating room. However, like most care in the contemporary healthcare system, the process is more commonly complex and involves a formal series of integrated steps to ensure best outcomes. It is incumbent upon the surgery team to create an efficient and cost-effective preoperative system and scheduling protocol that result in optimally prepared patients, rare cancellations of operations, and few disruptions of the operating room schedule. A systemic approach to patient preparation focuses upon risk assessment and reduction, as well as education of the patient and family. This effort begins during the first encounter with the surgeon and continues through the moments before the operation. Ideal preoperative systems assign risk based upon evaluations that are derived from sound published evidence and best practices and driven by standardized algorithms to identify, and then modify, hazards before operations.

▶ Risk Assessment & Reduction

A. Overview

The essence of preparing a patient for an operation regards considering whether the benefits of the operation justify the risks of doing harm, along with deciding how to minimize or eliminate those hazards. The American Society of Anesthesiologists (ASA) classification system (Table 3–2) stratifies the degree of perioperative risk for patients. Although somewhat rudimentary, this system has faithfully served anesthesiologists and surgeons in predicting how well patients might tolerate operations, and the scores have been validated by several recent publications. The Acute Physiology and Chronic Health Evaluation (APACHE II and III) is an example of a severity of illness scoring system that may be applied to critically ill patients to predict mortality. The value of such assessments lies in numerically designating the severities of patients' conditions, permitting comparisons of outcomes.

Some analyses, such as that provided by Vizient (formerly University Health-Systems Consortium), derive from inpatient administrative and financial data-sets to predict risk-adjusted outcomes for mortality, length of stay, and cost of care. The vagaries of medical coding can result in discrepancies, and this system does not monitor patients after hospital discharge. Nevertheless, these data can identify deficiencies in practice. Although clinical databases are more costly and challenging to implement than commercially available products, they provide more robust risk-adjusted outcomes data. Examples of clinical databases include those from the Society of Thoracic Surgeons and the National Surgical Quality Improvement Program (NSQIP). In NSQIP, dedicated nurses prospectively collect and validate an established panel of defined patient variables, comorbidities, and outcomes, and they pursue surveillance for 30 days after hospital discharge. The NSQIP analysis considers patient factors, effectiveness of care, and random variation; and logistic regression models calculate risk-adjusted 30-day morbidity and mortality. These data are reported as odds ratios for comparison with expected

Table 3–2. American Society of Anesthesiologists (ASA) classification system.

ASA Classification	Preoperative Health Status	Example
ASA 1	Normal healthy patient	No organic, physiologic, or psychiatric disturbance; excludes the very young and very old; healthy with good exercise tolerance.
ASA 2	Patients with mild systemic disease	No functional limitations; has a well-controlled disease of one body system; controlled hypertension or diabetes without systemic effects, cigarette smoking without chronic obstructive pulmonary disease (COPD); mild obesity, pregnancy.
ASA 3	Patients with severe systemic disease	Some functional limitation; has a controlled disease of more than one body system or one major system; no immediate danger of death; controlled congestive heart failure (CHF), stable angina, former heart attack, poorly controlled hypertension, morbid obesity, chronic renal failure; bronchospastic disease with intermittent symptoms.
ASA 4	Patients with severe systemic disease that is a constant threat to life	Has at least one severe disease that is poorly controlled or at end stage; possible risk of death; unstable angina, symptomatic COPD, symptomatic CHF, hepatorenal failure.
ASA 5	Moribund patients who are not expected to survive without the operation	Not expected to survive > 24 hours without surgery; imminent risk of death; multiorgan failure, sepsis syndrome with hemodynamic instability, hypothermia, poorly controlled coagulopathy.
ASA 6	A declared brain-dead patient whose organs are being removed for donor purposes	

outcomes, allowing for the severity of the patients' illnesses. Immediate benefits of NSQIP present the ability to identify true risk-adjusted data and local opportunities for improvement. For example, Veterans Administration (VA) surgeons reduced postoperative mortality from 3.2% in 2003 to 1.7% in 2005, while the complication rate declined from 17% to 10% ($p < 0.0001$). Similarly, the odds ratio of postoperative morbidity in General Surgery at our medical center declined from 1.22 to 0.88 over an 8-year interval as a result of programs that are specifically designed to decrease the likelihood of VTE and pulmonary complications, where opportunities were identified by NSQIP reports. Databases such as NSQIP have focused upon systems of care, providing reliable information to assess and reduce risks associated with operations. When compared to administrative data programs, NSQIP is much more likely to identify complications because its surveillance of patients extends 30 days beyond hospital stays.

The NSQIP program has also generated a tremendous repository of data to develop "risk calculators" for a variety of operations and conditions, allowing preoperative risk assessments and hopefully facilitating significant reductions of preoperative hazards. Finally, NSQIP participants have fostered a culture of sharing best practices and processes, both within the published literature and through formal and personal collaborations.

Beyond the obvious physical and emotional implications of adverse outcomes for patients and their families, the financial costs of postoperative complications to the healthcare system are staggering. It has been postulated that a major postoperative complication adds over $11,000 to the cost of the hospital care of an affected individual and significantly extends the duration of the inpatient confinement. In fact, the total cost of care increases by more than half when a complication develops. Notably, respiratory complications may increase the cost of care by more than $52,000 per patient. Strikingly, data from NSQIP have demonstrated that the occurrence of a serious complication (excluding superficial wound infections) after major operations is an independent risk factor for decreased long-term survival. Therefore, it is crucial that efforts focus upon reducing and eliminating postoperative complications.

Well-designed, systematic preoperative assessment programs can prospectively identify predictors of various complications and drive the ability to attenuate risks and improve outcomes. The perspective of teams of surgeons, physicians, nurses, and others with expertise in managing standardized, algorithm-driven preoperative evaluations, often with checklists, is a departure from traditional care that primarily involved solitary surgeons with disparate practices. The new paradigm recognizes that variability in practice is the enemy of efficiency.

The financial dividends appreciated from enhanced results and diminished death and complication rates more than compensate for the expenditures associated with quality improvement efforts and participation in auditing programs such as NSQIP. It is essential that surgeons monitor their patients' outcomes, preferably in a risk-adjusted fashion, to understand their practices and to demonstrate opportunities for improvement.

Operative risk factors may be conceptually categorized as modifiable, inherent, or prohibitive. Modifiable risks may be attenuated by careful planning and patient optimization. Formal programs identify risk factors and intervene with efforts such as supervised weight loss and smoking cessation. However, certain hazards may be inherent to the patient or to the operation, and thus are not amenable to correction. In those instances, careful patient and family counseling is needed to ensure comprehension of the potential risks and the possibility of unavoidable adverse outcomes. Finally, prohibitive risk factors are those that pose an unacceptable likelihood of adverse outcomes. In these cases, the surgeon has no obligation to proceed with an operation that is more likely to do harm than good.

B. Cardiovascular

In 1977, Goldman published a multifactorial index for assessing cardiac hazards among patients undergoing noncardiac operations. The same group issued a Revised Cardiac Risk Index (RCRI) in 1999, reporting six independent predictors of cardiac complications. These include a history of ischemic heart disease, congestive heart failure (CHF), cerebrovascular disease, a high-risk operation, preoperative treatment with insulin, and a preoperative serum creatinine greater than 2.0 mg/dL. The likelihood of major cardiac complications increases incrementally with the number of factors present. Contemporary NSQIP data have led to the development of a risk calculator to predict postoperative cardiac complications. A multivariate logistic regression analysis determined five prognostic factors for perioperative myocardial infarction (MI) or cardiac arrest: the type of operation, dependent functional status, abnormal creatinine, ASA class, and increasing age. The analysis has been validated and has led to the composition of an interactive risk calculator.

Another multivariate model demonstrated criteria that predict adverse cardiac events among patients who have had elective vascular operations, and it also suggested improved predictive accuracy among these patients compared to the RCRI. Independent hazards include increasing age, smoking, insulin-dependent diabetes, coronary artery disease, congestive heart failure (CHF), abnormal cardiac stress test, long-term beta-blocker therapy, chronic obstructive pulmonary disease, and creatinine ≥ 1.8 mg/dL. Conversely, the analysis demonstrated a beneficial effect of prior cardiac revascularization. There is obviously overlap among the factors identified in these models.

The determination of an increased chance of a patient developing postoperative cardiac complications will certainly influence the tenor of preoperative discussions with patients and their family members, especially if the surgeon can present validated data regarding the actual likelihood of a cardiac complication or death. In addition, correctable hazards may be addressed, including smoking cessation, optimal control of diabetes, blood pressure control, fluid status, and assurance of compliance with medical measures. Finally, formal risk assessments guide cardiologists with respect to cardiac stress testing, echocardiography, and coronary catheterization among higher-risk patients. Selected patients may be candidates for preoperative revascularization, either with coronary artery stent placement or surgical bypass.

The American College of Cardiology (ACC) Foundation and the American Heart Association (AHA) periodically issue joint recommendations about the cardiac evaluation and preparation of patients in advance of noncardiac operations. These guidelines are evidence based, include an explanation of the quality of the data, and provide comprehensive algorithms for the propriety of testing, medications, and revascularization to ensure cardiac fitness for operations. As important as preoperative cardiac risk stratification is, a cardiology consultation also lays the groundwork for postoperative risk assessment and later modifications of coronary risk factors.

Noninvasive and invasive preoperative testing should be performed only when the results will influence patient care. Noninvasive stress testing before noncardiac operations is indicated in patients with active cardiac conditions (eg, unstable angina, recent MI, significant arrhythmias, or severe valve disease) or in patients who require vascular operations and have clinical risk factors and poor functional capacity. Good data support coronary revascularization before noncardiac operations in patients who have significant left main coronary artery stenosis, stable angina with three-vessel coronary disease, stable angina with two-vessel disease and significant proximal left anterior descending coronary artery stenosis with either an ejection fraction < 50% or ischemia on noninvasive testing, high-risk unstable angina; non–ST-segment elevation MI, or acute ST-elevation MI. However, current data do not support routine preoperative percutaneous revascularization among patients with asymptomatic coronary ischemia or stable angina.

The role of beta-blockers for cardiac protection is evolving, and these agents are no longer empirically advised for all high-risk patients due to potential adverse consequences. Beta-blockers should be continued perioperatively among those patients who are already taking them and among those having vascular operations and at high cardiac risk, including known coronary heart disease or the presence of ischemia on preoperative testing. The role of beta-blockers is uncertain for patients with just a single clinical risk factor for coronary artery disease. Cardiac complication risk calculators may become beneficial in the stratification of patients who should receive beta-blockers to reduce perioperative cardiac complications.

Preoperative aspirin usage should continue among patients at moderate to high risk for coronary artery disease, unless the risk of resultant hemorrhage definitely outweighs the likelihood of an atherothrombotic event. Thienopyridines, such as ticlopidine or clopidogrel, are administered in concert with aspirin as dual antiplatelet therapy following placement of coronary artery stents. They are intended to inhibit platelet aggregation and resultant stent thrombosis, although they certainly increase the risk of hemorrhage. Therefore, if an operation can be anticipated, the surgeon and cardiologist must coordinate efforts regarding the sequence of the proposed operation and coronary stenting, weighing the hazards of operative bleeding while on antiplatelet therapy for a stent versus potential postoperative coronary ischemia. Elective operations with a significant risk of bleeding should be delayed 12 months before the discontinuation of the thienopyridine in the presence of a drug-eluting stent, at least 4-6 weeks for bare-metal stents, and 4 weeks after balloon angioplasty. Therefore, if a patient requires percutaneous coronary artery intervention prior to noncardiac surgery, bare-metal stents or balloon angioplasty should be employed rather than drug-eluting stents. Even when thienopyridines are withheld, aspirin should be continued, and the thienopyridine is to be resumed as soon as possible after the operation. In circumstances such as cardiovascular surgery, the dual antiplatelet agents are continued throughout the perioperative course to minimize the likelihood of vascular thrombosis.

C. Pulmonary

Postoperative pulmonary complications (PPC), such as the development of pneumonia and ventilator dependency, are debilitating and costly. They are associated with prolonged lengths of hospital stay, an increased likelihood of readmission, and increased 30-day mortality. Therefore, it is critical to identify patients at greatest risk for PPC. Established risk factors for PPC include advanced age, elevated ASA class, congestive heart failure, functional dependence, known chronic obstructive pulmonary disease, and perhaps malnutrition, alcohol abuse, and altered mental status. In addition, hazards are greater for certain operations (eg, aortic aneurysm repair, thoracic or abdominal, neurosurgery, head and neck, and vascular), prolonged or emergency operations, and those done under general anesthesia. A risk calculator was devised to predict the likelihood of PPC occurrence, indicating seven independent risk factors: low preoperative arterial oxygen saturation, recent acute respiratory infection, age, preoperative anemia, upper abdominal or thoracic operations, duration of operation over 2 hours, and emergency surgery.

A multivariable logistic regression has affirmed that active smoking is significantly associated with postoperative pneumonia, SSI, and death, when compared to nonsmokers or those who have quit smoking. Moreover, this is a dose-dependent phenomenon, predicated upon the volume and duration of tobacco consumption. The benefits of preoperative smoking cessation seem to be conferred after an interval of at least 4 weeks. Conversely, the risk of developing PPC is the same for current smokers as for those who quit smoking for less than 4 weeks before an operation. Smoking cessation also confers favorable effects on wound healing. Therefore, patients should be encouraged to stop smoking at least 1 month before operations, ideally with programmatic support through formal counseling programs and possibly smoking cessation aids such as varenicline or transdermal nicotine.

A recent analysis of patients having general surgery and orthopedic operations demonstrated that sleep apnea is an independent risk factor for the development of PPC. A simple "STOP BANG" questionnaire can screen patients for sleep apnea. The acronym queries Snoring, Tired during day, Obstructed breathing pattern during sleep, high blood Pressure, BMI, Age over 50 years, Neck circumference, and male Gender. Patients with sleep apnea may be managed with continuous positive pressure (CPAP) or bilevel positive airway pressure (BiPAP) devices, both before and after operations. The presence of sleep apnea may also influence anesthesia techniques.

Patients identified as being at highest risk for the development of PPC may benefit from preoperative consultations with Respiratory Therapy and Pulmonary Medicine experts. Pulmonary function tests and baseline arterial blood gas tests guide the care of select patients, especially those anticipating lung resections. In addition to smoking cessation, asthma should be medically controlled. Our group has implemented the "I COUGH" protocol that focuses upon Incentive spirometry (to promote inspiratory muscle usage), Coughing and deep breathing, Oral hygiene (tooth-brushing and mouthwashes), Understanding (patient and family education), Getting out-of-bed (mobilization), and Head of bed elevation. This decade-long program is specified in the perioperative order sets and has markedly reduced the odds ratio of patients developing any pulmonary complication. Respiratory therapists can provide expertise with CPAP and BiPAP systems for patients with sleep apnea. Surgeons and anesthesiologists should collaborate regarding plans for neuromuscular blocking agents and strategies to reduce pain, including the administration of epidural analgesics and the consideration of minimally invasive techniques to avoid large abdominal or thoracic incisions. Finally, formal intensive care unit protocols can liberate patients from ventilator support.

D. Venous Thromboembolism

Venous thromboembolism (VTE) events such as DVT or PE are major complications that can lead to death or serious long-term morbidity, including chronic pulmonary hypertension and postthrombotic limb sequelae. Scoring systems stratify patients by their probability of developing a postoperative VTE to guide preventative measures. In the 2012 American College of Chest Physicians (ACCP) recommendations, the patient's score selects the alternatives of early ambulation alone (very low risk), mechanical prophylaxis with intermittent pneumatic compression (IPC) devices (low risk), options of low-molecular-weight heparin (LMWH) or low-dose unfractionated heparin or IPC (moderate risk), and IPC in addition to either LMWH or low-dose heparin (high risk). Furthermore, an extended course (4 weeks) of LMWH may be indicated among patients undergoing resections of abdominal or pelvic malignancies. Of course, the surgeon must entertain the hazards of pharmacologic prophylaxis when bleeding poses the likelihood of even greater harm than VTE, in which case IPC alone may suffice. Heparin prophylaxis is associated with a 4%-5% chance of wound hematomas, 2%-3% incidence of mucosal bleeding and the need to stop the anticoagulation, and a 1%-2% risk of reoperation. The ACCP 2012 guidelines do not advocate routine vein surveillance with ultrasonography or the insertion of inferior vena cava filters for primary VTE prevention. Notably, antiembolism graduated compression stockings do not promote venous blood flow from the leg and can violate skin integrity and result in the accumulation of edema. The efficacy of stockings for VTE prevention is unproven.

Caprini has developed a more elaborate risk calculation that has been validated in a variety of clinical settings and specialties and is adaptable to standardized order sets (Figure 3-1). This scoring system acknowledges the gravity of individual hazards, including personal and family histories of VTE, the diagnosis of a malignancy, a history of obstetrical complications or known procoagulants, and prolonged operations, among several other factors. It also identifies patients who may either entirely avoid anticoagulation or benefit from an extended duration of LMWH. There is no doubt that the cumulative incidence of VTE extends many weeks after operations, particularly for malignancies and in an era when the duration of hospital stays (and inpatient prophylaxis) has declined. In fact, about one-third to one-half of patients who manifest a VTE after cancer operations do so following hospital discharge. A randomized trial showed that an extended duration of outpatient prophylaxis with enoxaparin after operations for cancer resulted in a statistically significant reduction in VTE events, compared with inpatient administration only, with no increase in bleeding complications. Therefore, regimens of pharmacologic prophylaxis should be maintained after the discharge of patients who have elevated risk scores. Our center has embedded a mandatory Caprini protocol in the perioperative order sets, including "extended prophylaxis" for high-risk patients, for nearly 10 years and has experienced a dramatic and sustained reduction in the odds ratio of postoperative VTE. We are also developing a protocol for "enhanced prophylaxis"

Venous Thromboembolism (VTE) Risk Factor Assessment

Assessments in Last 30 Days	Assessment #1: 10/3/2012 LOC: E8EOF-1 Score: 3 Moderate Risk	
Previously Selected Safety Considerations	Patient taking oral anticoagulants, platelet inhibitors (eg, NSAIDS, Clopidogrel, Salicylates)	Use This Previous Assessment
Previously Selected Risk Factors	Age 40-59 years, Major surgery (>45 minutes)*	Clear Assessment

Today's Assessment   MRN:

Date: 10/3/2012   Location: E8EOF-1   Score: 3   Level: Moderate Risk

Anticoagulants: Factors Associated with Increased Bleeding
- ☐ Patient is experiencing active bleeding
- ☐ Patient has (or has had history of) heparin-induced thrombocytopenia
- ☐ Patient's platelet count <100,000/mm3
- ☑ Patient taking oral anticoagulants, platelet inhibitors (eg, NSAIDS, Clopidogrel, Salicylates)
- ☐ Patient's creatinine clearance is abnormal. Value:

Potential contraindications to Intermittent Pneumatic Compression (IPC)
- ☐ Patient has severe peripheral Arterial disease
- ☐ Patient has congestive heart failure
- ☐ Patient has an acute superficial/deep vein thrombosis

A1: Each Risk Factor Represents 1 Point
- ☑ Age 40-59 years
- ☐ Minor surgery planned*
- ☐ History of prior major surgery (<1 month)
- ☐ Varicose veins
- ☐ History of inflammatory bowel disease
- ☐ Swollen legs (current)
- ☐ Obesity (BMI > 30)
- ☐ Acute myocardial infarction (<1 month)
- ☐ Congestive heart failure (<1 month)
- ☐ Sepsis (<1 month)
- ☐ Serious acute lung disease incl. pneumonia (<1 month)
- ☐ Abnormal pulmonary function (chronic obstructive pulmonary disease)
- ☐ Medical patient currently at bed rest

B: Each Risk Factor Represents 2 Points
- ☐ Age 60-74 years
- ☑ Major surgery (>45 minutes)*
- ☐ Arthroscopic surgery*
- ☐ Laparoscopic surgery (>45 minutes)*
- ☐ Leg plaster cast or brace
- ☐ Central Venous access
- ☐ Prior cancer (except non-melanoma skin)
- ☐ Present Cancer (except breast or thyroid)
- ☐ Patient confined to bed (>72 hrs)

C: Each Risk Factor Represents 3 Points
- ☐ Age 75 years or more
- ☐ History of DVT/PE
- ☐ Family History of DVT/PE
- ☐ Present chemotherapy
- ☐ Positive Factor V Leiden
- ☐ Positive Prothrombin 20210A
- ☐ Elevated serum homocysteine
- ☐ Positive Lupus anticoagulant
- ☐ Elevated anticardiolipin antibodies
- ☐ Heparin-induced thrombocytopenia (HIT)
- ☐ Other thrombophilia-Type

D: Each Risk Factor Represents 5 Points
- ☐ Major Surgery lasting over 6 hours*
- ☐ Elective major lower extremity arthroplasty
- ☐ Hip, pelvis or leg fracture (<1 month)
- ☐ Stroke (<1 month)
- ☐ Multiple trauma (<1 month)
- ☐ Acute spinal cord injury (paralysis) (<1 month)

A2: For Women Only (Each Represents 1 Point)
- ☐ Oral contraceptives or hormone replacement therapy
- ☐ Pregnancy or postpartum (< 1 month)
- ☐ History of unexplained stillborn infant, recurrent spontaneous abortion (≥ 3), premature birth with toxemia of pregnancy or growth restricted infant

Save and Close   Cancel

▲ **Figure 3–1.** Sample order set page with "Caprini" calculation of venous thromboembolism risk. The total value of checked-off factors indicates the proper preoperative and postoperative prophylaxis regimens, including upon discharge from hospital. (Used with permission of Boston Medical Center.)

among patients who are at an increased risk of VTE despite standard prophylaxis; candidates have perioperative sepsis, multiple operations, or emergency operations. The ACCP and Caprini systems are two among several VTE risk assessments tools, each of which has advantages and disadvantages. The system adopted in any hospital or surgery center will be a function of local resources and culture, but it is ideal that surgeons develop and maintain a local standard to minimize the threat of postoperative VTE. Prospective identification of patients who may be at increased risk for VTE will allow for individualized counseling of patients and setting expectations about efforts to reduce their risks.

E. Diabetes Mellitus

Patients with diabetes mellitus are more likely to undergo operations than those without diabetes, and their care is associated with longer lengths of hospital stay, increased rates of postoperative death and complications, and relatively greater utilization of healthcare resources. It has been established that elevated postoperative blood glucose levels in diabetic patients translate to progressively greater chances of SSIs following cardiac operations, as well as a greater likelihood of postoperative infections and prolonged hospital stays in patients with noncardiac operations. In fact, increased perioperative glucose levels have been correlated with a higher risk of SSIs in general surgery, cardiac surgery, colorectal surgery, vascular surgery, breast surgery, hepatobiliary and pancreatic surgery, orthopedic surgery, and trauma surgery. The relative risk of an SSI seems to incrementally increase in a linear pattern with the degree of hyperglycemia, with glucose levels greater than 140 mg/dL being the sole predictor of SSI upon multivariate analysis. In one study, the likelihood of an adverse postoperative outcome increased by 30% for every 20 mg/dL increase in the mean intraoperative glucose level. Interestingly, about one-third of patients with perioperative hyperglycemia are not diabetics. Furthermore, the risk of death relative to perioperative hyperglycemia among patients undergoing noncardiac operations has been shown to be greater for those *without* a history of diabetes than for those with known diabetes. Nevertheless, these data pertain to intraoperative and postoperative blood sugars, not preoperative values.

Current recommendations for desirable glucose ranges in critically ill patients are commonly about 120-180 mg/dL, but the best range for perioperative glucose levels is not yet established, and low levels may result in harm when clinicians try to achieve "tight" control of blood sugars. In fact, trials and meta-analyses have failed to prove a clinical benefit of maintaining glucose levels in the normal laboratory reference range (80-110 mg/dL). Although *preoperative* blood sugar and hemoglobin A1C levels are inconsistently associated with adverse outcomes, good control of glucose before operations likely facilitates blood sugar management during and after operations. An abundance of data support *postoperative* glucose control as a major determinant of postoperative complications, with emerging data also indicating an adverse effect of intraoperative hyperglycemia. Curiously, surgeons may actually be more influential than are patients' primary care physicians in terms of encouraging preoperative compliance with diabetes medications, at least in the short term. Patients are commonly motivated to attend to medical conditions such as diabetes to enhance chances of postoperative success.

Patients having operations that require fasting status are advised about oral antihyperglycemic medications on the day of surgery in accordance with Table 3–3. Injectable medications, such as exenatide and pramlintide, are not administered on the day of surgery, and insulin therapy is determined by the duration of action of the particular preparation, as outlined in Table 3–4. Patients with type 1 diabetes require basal insulin at all times. Patients with insulin pumps may temporarily reduce their basal rates starting at midnight prior to the operation and continuing until they are able to eat again.

Multidisciplinary teams—including endocrinologists, surgeons, anesthesiologists, nurses, pharmacists, information technology experts, and others—have developed formal protocols and algorithms for perioperative glycemic control, and an example of a preoperative order set is given in

Table 3–3. Instructions for preoperative management of oral antihyperglycemic medications.

Medication	Prior to Procedure	After Procedure
Short-acting sulfonylureas • Glipizide (Glucotrol) • Glyburide (DiaBeta, Glynase, Micronase)	Do not take the morning of procedure.	Resume when eating.
Long-acting sulfonylureas • Glimepiride (Amaryl) • Glipizide XL (Glucotrol XL)	Do not take the evening prior to or the morning of procedure.	Resume when eating.
Biguanides • Metformin (Glucophage) • Metformin ER (Glucophage XL)	Do not take the morning of procedure. Do not take the day prior to procedure if receiving contrast (or if unsure about contrast).	Resume when eating. After contrast injection, wait 48 hours and repeat creatinine prior to resuming.
Thiazolidinediones • Pioglitazone (Actos) • Rosiglitazone (Avandia)	Do not take the morning of procedure.	Resume when eating.
Alpha-glucosidase inhibitors • Acarbose (Precose) • Miglitol (Glyset)	Do not take the morning of procedure.	Resume when eating.
DPP-4 inhibitors Alogliptin (Nesina), Linagliptin (Tradjenta), Saxagliptin (Onglyza), Sitagliptan (Januvia)	Do not take the morning of procedure.	Resume when eating.
Meglitinides • Nateglinide (Starlix) • Repaglinide (Prandin)	Do not take the morning of procedure.	Resume when eating.
SGLT-2 inhibitors • Canagliflozin (Invokana), Dapagliflozin (Farxiga), Empagliflozin (Jardiance), Ertugliflozin (Steglatro)	Do not take the morning of procedure AND do not take the day prior to procedure.	Resume when eating.

Used with permission of Boston Medical Center.

Table 3–4. Instructions for preoperative management of injectable antihyperglycemic medications and insulin.

Medication	Prior to Procedure	After Procedure
Injectable Non-insulin Medications		
GLP-1 analogs Dulaglutide (Trulicity), Exenatide (Byetta or Bydureon), Liraglutide (Victoza), Semaglutide (Ozempic) insulin glargine/lixisenatide (Soliqua)	Do not take the morning of procedure.	Resume when eating.
Amylin analogs Symlin (Pramlintide)	Do not take the morning of procedure.	Resume when eating.
Insulins		
Ultra long-acting Degludec (Tresiba) U100 and U200, Glargine (Lantus) U 300	Reduce dose by 20%. Dose reductions should be started 2 nights prior to procedure.	Resume usual schedule after procedure.
Long-acting Basaglar, Detemir (Levemir), Glargine (Lantus) U100	Reduce dose by 20% the night prior and/or morning of the procedure.	Resume usual schedule after procedure.
Intermediate-acting NPH (Humulin N, Novolin N)	Take half of usual dose the morning of procedure.	Half of usual dose while NPO; resume usual schedule when eating.
Mixed insulins Humalog mix 75/25, Novolog 70/30, Humulin 70/30, 50/50, Novolin 70/30	Do not take the morning of procedure.	Resume usual schedule when eating.
Short-acting Regular insulin (Humulin R, Novolin R)	Do not take the morning of procedure.	Resume when eating.
Rapid/ultra-rapid acting Aspart (Novolog), Fiasp, Glulisine (Apidra), Lispro (Humalog) U100 and U200	Do not take the morning of procedure.	Resume when eating.
Subcutaneous insulin infusion pumps	In general, it is appropriate to temporarily reduce basal rate by 20% starting at midnight prior to the procedure until the time when the patient is able to eat a meal. If questions arise, the patient may also contact his or her usual outpatient diabetes provider.	
Concentrated insulins U500 Regular insulin (Humulin R U500)	Reduce dose by 30% the night prior to procedure. Reduce dose by 50% morning of the procedure.	Resume usual schedule after procedure.

Used with permission of Boston Medical Center.

Table 3–5. A typical protocol is nurse-driven and involves checking glucose levels on all diabetic patients in the holding area shortly before operations. As an example of one protocol, glucose values ≤ 180 mg/dL are satisfactory and require no treatment. Glucose levels of 181-300 mg/dL prompt the nurse to begin an infusion of IV insulin before the operation, along with a 5% dextrose solution to minimize the chances of hypoglycemia. Endocrinologists are automatically consulted to assist with postoperative insulin management in these patients and in those with insulin pumps. In general, insulin pump therapy may be continued with the infusion of a dextrose solution for procedures and operations of short duration. Patients with pumps may also require the addition of IV insulin, as per the protocol.

Patients with glucose levels > 300 mg/dL are assessed for ketones or for acidosis prior to starting an insulin infusion.

Markedly elevated preoperative blood sugars warrant special deliberation by all involved. Matters to be considered include the urgency of the operation, whether the underlying condition itself may be contributing to hyperglycemia, metabolic consequences such as the presence of ketoacidosis, the risks of proceeding with an operation at that moment, the likelihood of establishing better control at a later date, and the dangers imposed by postponing the operation. Dramatic elevations of glucose levels (eg, > 300 mg/dL) are typically indicative of chronic poor glucose control, but the clinician often does not have the luxury of perfectly managing diabetes before operations.

Intravenous insulin is best for perioperative glucose control due to its rapid onset of action, short half-life, and immediate availability (as opposed to subcutaneous absorption). Insulin may be administered with an IV bolus

Table 3-5. Example of adult perioperative glycemic control protocol.

Adult 120–180 mg/dL
Perioperative Insulin Infusion Guideline
*** Not to be used in patients in acute diabetic ketoacidosis or hyperglycemic hyperosmolar syndrome ***
Goal: To maintain whole blood glucose levels and/or fingersticks between 120 and 180 mg/dL.

Glucose level	Below Desired Range			Desired Range		Above Desired Range			
	< 80 mg/dL	80-99 mg/dL	100-119[b] mg/dL	120-180 mg/dL[b]	181-220[b] mg/dL	221-250 mg/dL	251-300 mg/dL	301-350 mg/dL	> 350 mg/dL
Infusion rate of 1 U/h	Stop insulin infusion. Give 25 mL of D50 IVP, maintain continuous dextrose source.	Stop insulin infusion. Maintain continuous dextrose source.	Decrease infusion rate by 50%.	Once in range, if glucose ↑ over 2 consecutive checks, ↑ infusion by 0.5 U/h.[a]	↑ infusion by 1 U/h.	Give 2 units insulin IVP and ↑ infusion by 1 U/h.	Give 3 units insulin IVP and ↑ infusion by 1 U/h.	Give 4 units insulin IVP and ↑ infusion by 1 U/h.	Give 5 units insulin IVP and ↑ infusion by 1 U/h.
Infusion rate of 2-5 U/h	Call MD.			Once in range, if glucose ↑ over 2 consecutive checks, ↑ infusion by 0.5 U/h.[a]	↑ infusion by 1 U/h.	Give 2 units insulin IVP and ↑ infusion by 1 U/h.	Give 3 units insulin IVP and ↑ infusion by 1 U/h.	Give 6 units insulin IVP and ↑ infusion by 1 U/h.	Give 8 units insulin IVP and ↑ infusion by 1 U/h.
Infusion rate of 6-10 U/h	Check glucose level in 15 min. If >120 mg/dL, restart insulin at ½ previous rate.	Check glucose level in 15 min. If >120 mg/dL, restart insulin at ½ previous rate.		Once in range, if glucose ↑ over 2 consecutive checks, ↑ infusion by 1 U/h.[a]	↑ infusion by 1.5 U/h.	Give 2 units insulin IVP and ↑ infusion by 2 U/h.	Give 3 units insulin IVP an ↑ infusion by 2 U/h.	Give 6 units insulin IVP and ↑ infusion by 2 U/h.	Give 8 units insulin IVP and ↑ infusion by 2 U/h.
Infusion rate of 11-16 U/h	Resume fingersticks every hour until stable.	Resume fingersticks every hour until stable.		Once in range, if glucose ↑ over 2 consecutive checks, ↑ infusion by 2 U/h.[a]	↑ infusion by 2 U/h.	Give 2 units insulin IVP and ↑ infusion by 3 U/h.	Give 3 units insulin IVP and ↑ infusion by 3 U/h.	Give 6 units insulin IVP and ↑ infusion by 3 U/h.	Give 8 units insulin IVP and ↑ infusion by 3 U/h.
Infusion rate of > 16 U/h	Restart infusion as above any time glucose is > 120	Restart infusion as above any time glucose is > 120			Call MD.				

Monitoring: Check glucose every hour.
[a]"Once in range" example:

Glucose	190	140 (in range now)	130 (drop #1)	120 (drop #2)	130
U/h	4	4	4	↑3.5	3.5

[b] If the glucose drops by > 100 mg/dL/h, consider decreasing infusion rate or discontinuing infusion if BG declining rapidly and < 150 mg/dL.
IVP = IV push.
Used with permission of Boston Medical Center.

technique or via continuous IV infusion, but regular glucose monitoring (eg, hourly for continuous insulin infusions) is necessary in either system to ensure adequate control and to avoid hypoglycemia. The insulin administration method before, during, and after an operation (infusion versus bolus) is a function of local resources (eg, glucose meters, blood sample processing, and staffing), as well as the patient's individual circumstances. After the operation, a patient should be assessed for an insulin infusion regimen if being transferred to a critical care setting, a basal-bolus insulin program, or the resumption of the patient's usual diabetes medications.

F. Surgical Site Infection

Surgical site infections (SSIs) are major contributors to postoperative morbidity, and their incidence can be reduced by multiple complex interventions that are institution-specific. Excellent surgical technique is obviously a major factor in eliminating SSIs, and this involves limiting wound contamination, blood loss, the duration of the operation, and local tissue trauma and ischemia (eg, using sharp dissection rather than excessive electrocoagulation). However, a variety of adjuvant preoperative measures, beyond glycemic control described above, also contribute to the prevention of SSIs. Antibiotics should be administered during the 1-hour period before incision for certain clean operations and for all clean-contaminated, contaminated, and dirty operations (unless the patient is already receiving scheduled antibiotics). In addition, further dosages of the antibiotics should be infused about every two half-lives during the operation (eg, every 4 hours for cefazolin). Correct antibiotic choices are determined by several factors such as the bacterial flora that are most likely to cause an infection, local bacterial sensitivities, medication allergies, the presence of MRSA, and the patient's overall health and ability to tolerate an infection and to metabolize antibiotics. In clean operations with low rates of infections, the surgeon should contrast the cost and hazards of antibiotics with the likelihood, cost, and morbidity of a postoperative infection. Antibiotic choices for prophylaxis against SSIs are cited in Table 3–6 for a variety of operations. Operations that involve bacteroides should prompt the addition of metronidazole to the regimen, and operations with a dirty wound classification may be guided by culture results and hospital-specific bacterial sensitivities. When antibiotics are administered for SSI prophylaxis rather than for treatment of an established or suspected infection, they are typically not continued after surgery, except in special circumstances such as vascular grafts, cardiac surgery, or joint replacements. Even then, prophylaxis should expire within 1-2 days. Order sets, automated reminders, and team vigilance are essential to ensure the consistent usage of the correct antibiotics at the right time and for the proper duration.

Wound perfusion and oxygenation are also important to minimize the likelihood of SSIs. A sufficient intravascular blood volume provides end-organ perfusion and oxygen (and antibiotic) delivery to the surgical site. The maintenance of perioperative normothermia also has salutary effects on wound oxygen tension levels and can consequently reduce the incidence of SSIs. Therefore, the application of warming blankets immediately prior to the operation may support the patient's temperature in the operating room, especially for high-risk operations such as bowel resections that often involved a prolonged interval of positioning and preparation when a broad surface area of the patient is exposed to room air. Similarly, some data support hyperoxygenation with $FiO_2 \geq 80\%$ during the first 2 hours after a major colorectal operation.

Several other adjuvant measures are employed at the surgical site to reduce the incidence of SSIs. Protocols with mupirocin nasal ointment application and chlorhexidine soap showers have reduced the incidence of SSIs among patients colonized with methicillin-sensitive *S aureus*. During an operation, wound protectors may be deployed to minimize the chances of a superficial or deep SSI developing. Some surgeons (and their teams) change gloves and gowns and may use a separate set of instruments (that have not come into contact with potential contaminants) for wound closure.

▶ Fluid Management & Blood Volume

Likely out of concerns about incurring renal insult, surgeons and anesthesiologists have traditionally advocated liberal perioperative fluid resuscitation during recent decades, often overestimating insensible and "third-space" fluid losses. As a result, patients can develop significant volume and salt overload that are associated with serious complications. Recent data instead support goal-directed (or protocol-based) fluid management as likely resulting in a decreased incidence of cardiac and renal events, pneumonia, pulmonary edema, ileus, wound infections, and anastomosis and wound healing problems, as well as shorter durations of hospital stay. Unfortunately, traditional vital signs, even including central venous pressure, do not reliably correlate with intravascular volume or cardiac output. Moreover, pulmonary artery catheterization has actually been associated with increased mortality, and its implementation for the optimization of hemodynamic status is rarely required. Pulmonary artery catheterization is valuable for a few, highly selected patients who exhibit clinical cardiac instability along with multiple comorbid conditions. Newer, minimally invasive modalities for monitoring cardiac output offer promise to determine optimal preload volume and tissue oxygen delivery before and during operations, including esophageal Doppler and analyses of stroke volume variation and pulse pressure variation. The precise standards of goal-directed volume

Table 3–6. Examples of prophylactic antibiotic selections for various operations.[a]

Operation	Standard Selection	Penicillin Allergy	MRSA Colonization
Clean			
Adrenalectomy	Cefazolin	Clindamycin +/− gentamicin	Vancomycin +/− gentamicin
Breast	Cefazolin	Clindamycin +/− gentamicin	Clindamycin +/− gentamicin
Cardiac surgery	Cefazolin	Clindamycin + gentamicin	Cefazolin + vancomycin
Distal pancreatectomy	Cefazolin	Clindamycin + gentamicin	Cefazolin
Hernia	Cefazolin	Clindamycin	Vancomycin
Neurosurgery	Cefazolin	Clindamycin	Vancomycin
Orthopedic arthroscopy ORIF	Cefazolin	Clindamycin + gentamicin	Cefazolin + vancomycin
Plastic surgery	Cefazolin	Clindamycin + gentamicin	Vancomycin +/− gentamicin
Renal transplantation	Cefazolin	Clindamycin + gentamicin	Cefazolin +/− vancomycin
Splenectomy	Cefazolin	Clindamycin + gentamicin	Vancomycin +/− gentamicin
Thoracotomy or laparotomy	Cefazolin	Clindamycin	Vancomycin
Thyroid/parathyroid	None	None	None
Vascular (no foreign body)	Cefazolin	Clindamycin	Vancomycin
Vascular (with foreign body)	Cefazolin	Clindamycin + gentamicin	Cefazolin + vancomycin
Clean-Contaminated			
Bariatric surgery	Cefazolin	Clindamycin + gentamicin	Cefazolin
Biliary	Cefazolin	Clindamycin + gentamicin	Cefazolin
Colorectal surgery (elective)	Cefazolin + metronidazole	Clindamycin + gentamicin	Cefazolin + metronidazole
Gastroduodenal resection	Cefazolin	Clindamycin + gentamicin	Cefazolin
Gynecology	Cefazolin +/− metronidazole	Clindamycin + gentamicin	Add vancomycin
Head and neck (incision through the oral or pharyngeal mucosa)	Cefazolin + metronidazole	Clindamycin	Cefazolin + metronidazole
Lung resection	Cefazolin	Clindamycin	Vancomycin
Urology (no entry into urinary tract or intestine)	Cefazolin	Clindamycin	Cefazolin
Urology (entry into urinary tract or intestine)	Cefoxitin +/− metronidazole	Clindamycin + gentamicin	Cefoxitin +/− metronidazole
Whipple resection	Cefazolin + metronidazole	Clindamycin + gentamicin	Cefazolin + metronidazole
Contaminated or Dirty			
Gastrointestinal (emergency)	Ceftriaxone + metronidazole	Clindamycin + gentamicin	

[a]These recommendations differ depending upon local antibiotic resistance patterns.

resuscitation remain elusive, but surgeons and anesthesiologists should prospectively collaborate regarding plans for both volume resuscitation and the type of anesthesia. This is especially so during the management of challenging problems such as pheochromocytomas, when patients require preoperative vasodilatation and then intravascular volume expansion for a couple of weeks. Another clinical dilemma involves patients with end-stage renal failure. Dialysis should be performed within about 24-36 hours before an operation to avoid electrolyte disturbances, but the surgeon should confer with the nephrologist to minimize intravascular blood volume depletion.

Blood transfusions may be necessary before operations, especially in the setting of active hemorrhage or profound anemia. However, transfusions have been associated with increased operative mortality and morbidity, decreased long-term survival, greater lengths of hospital stay, and higher chances of tumor recurrence due to immunosuppressive effects imparted by transfused blood. The benefits of transfusions must be balanced against their hazards. Of course, bleeding diatheses require preoperative correction, including transfusions of blood products such as fresh frozen plasma, specific clotting factors, or platelets. Hematology consultations are invaluable when blood incompatibilities or unusual factor deficiencies are present or under special circumstances such as exchange transfusions for sickle-cell anemia.

Nutrition

Preoperative nutritional status bears a major impact on outcome, especially with respect to wound healing and immune status. A multivariate analysis recognizes hypoalbuminemia (albumin < 3.0 mg/dL) as an independent risk factor for the development of SSIs, with a fivefold increased incidence versus patients with normal albumin levels, corroborating the results of previous studies. Among moderately to severely malnourished patients, efforts may be focused upon preoperative feedings, ideally via the gut, although at least 1 week of the regimen is necessary to confer benefit. Total parenteral nutrition is an option for select patients in whom the gut cannot be used, but it conveys potential hazards. Immune modulating nutrition (IMN), with agents such as L-arginine, L-glutamine, ω-3 fatty acids, and nucleotides, can enhance immune and inflammatory responses. A meta-analysis of randomized controlled trials suggests that perioperative IMN with open, elective gastrointestinal operations is associated with fewer postoperative complications and shorter lengths of hospital stay compared to results for patients with standard enteral nutrition. However, the value of preoperative IMN is not firmly established.

At the other end of the spectrum, investigators have demonstrated that severe obesity is associated with increased rates of postoperative mortality, wound complications, renal failure, and pulmonary insufficiency, as well as greater durations of operative time and hospital stays. The AHA has issued guidelines for the assessment and management of morbidly obese patients, including an obesity surgery mortality score for gastric bypass. Unfavorable prognostic elements include BMI ≥ 50 kg/m², male sex, hypertension, PE risks (eg, presence of a VTE event, prior inferior vena cava filter placement, history of right heart failure or pulmonary hypertension, findings of venous stasis disease), and age ≥ 45 years. Bariatric surgeons typically enforce a preoperative regimen of weight reduction before proceeding with surgery to enhance outcomes and to ensure the patient's commitment to the process.

Endocrine

Endocrine deficiencies pose special problems. Patients may have either primary adrenal insufficiency or chronic adrenal suppression from corticosteroid usage. Inadequate amounts of perioperative steroids can result in an Addisonian crisis, with hemodynamic instability and even death. The need for perioperative "stress" steroid administration is a function of the duration of steroid therapy and the degree of the physiologic stress imposed by the operation. Supplemental corticosteroids should definitely be administered for primary or secondary adrenal insufficiency, for a current regimen of more than the daily equivalent of 20 mg of prednisone, or for those with a history of chronic steroid usage and a Cushingoid appearance. Perioperative steroids should be considered if the current regimen is 5-20 mg of prednisone for 3 weeks or longer, for a history of more than a 3-week course of at least 20 mg of prednisone daily during the past year, for chronic usage of oral and rectal (eg, for inflammatory bowel disease) steroid therapy, or for a significant history of chronic topical steroid usage (> 2 g daily) on large areas of affected skin. Increased amounts of corticosteroids are not necessary for patients who have received less than a 3-week course of steroids. Patients having operations of moderate (eg, lower extremity revascularization or total joint replacement) and major (eg, cardiothoracic, abdominal, central nervous system) stress should receive additional corticosteroids as outlined in Table 3–7. Minor or ambulatory operations, especially those under local anesthesia, do not require supplemental steroids. Excessive amounts of steroids can have adverse consequences, including increased rates of SSIs, so hydrocortisone should not be indiscriminately prescribed. Of course, glucose levels should be closely monitored while patients receive steroids. Conversely, patients with advanced Cushing syndrome require expeditious medical and perhaps surgical treatment due to the potential for rapid deterioration, including fungal sepsis. Cushing syndrome is addressed in another chapter.

Thyrotoxicosis must be corrected to avoid perioperative thyroid storm. Management includes antithyroid medications (eg, methimazole or propylthiouracil), beta-blockers,

Table 3–7. Guidelines for perioperative corticosteroid management.

Type of Operation	Corticosteroid Administration
Minor/ambulatory operation[a] Example: inguinal hernia repair or operation under local anesthesia	Take usual morning steroid dose; no supplementary steroids are needed.
Moderate surgical stress[a] Example: lower extremity revascularization, total joint replacement	Day of surgery: Take usual morning steroid dose. Just before induction of anesthesia: Hydrocortisone 50 mg IV, then hydrocortisone 25 mg IV every 8 hours × 6 doses. When able to take oral steroids, change to daily oral prednisone, at a dosage equivalent to the recommended hydrocortisone, or to the preoperative steroid dosage if that was higher.[b] On the second postoperative day: Resume prior outpatient dose, assuming the patient is in stable condition.[a]
Major surgical stress[a] Example: major cardiac, brain, abdominal, or thoracic surgery Inflammatory bowel disease[c]	Day of surgery: Take usual morning steroid dose. Just before induction of anesthesia: Hydrocortisone 100 mg IV, then hydrocortisone 50 mg q8h × 6 doses (or until able to take oral steroids). On the second postoperative day: Reduce to hydrocortisone 25 mg q8h if still fasting, or oral prednisone 15 mg daily (or the preoperative steroid dosage if that was higher). Postoperative day 3 or 4: Resume preoperative steroid dose if the patient is in stable condition.[a]

[a]For patients who have a complicated postoperative course or a prolonged illness, consider an Endocrinology consultation for dosing recommendations. If the steroid-requiring disease may directly impact the postoperative course (eg, autoimmune thrombocytopenia [ITP] or hemolytic anemia), specific dosing programs and tapers should be determined prior to surgery and in consultation with the appropriate service (eg, Hematology for ITP patients) during the hospital stay.
[b]100 mg hydrocortisone = 25 mg prednisone = 4 mg dexamethasone.
[c]For patients with inflammatory bowel disease in whom all affected bowel was resected, taper to prednisone 10 mg daily (or IV equivalent) by discharge (or no later than postoperative day 7), followed by an outpatient taper over the next 1-3 months, depending upon the duration of prior steroid usage and assuming that there are no concurrent indications for steroids (eg, COPD).
Used with permission of Boston Medical Center.

and possibly corticosteroids; saturated solution of potassium iodide controls hyperthyroidism and reduces the vascularity of the gland in patients with Graves disease. On the other hand, significant hypothyroidism can progress to perioperative hypothermia and hemodynamic collapse and thus requires preoperative hormone replacement. This is normally accomplished with daily oral levothyroxine, but greater doses of IV thyroid hormone may be necessary to acutely reverse a significant deficit. Large goiters can affect the airway and require collaboration between surgeon and anesthesiologist, including a review of imaging to demonstrate the extent and location (eg, substernal) of the goiter. When possible, computed tomography contrast should be avoided in patients with significant goiters as the iodine load may provoke thyrotoxicosis.

Geriatric Patients

As the elderly demographic expands, surgeons are confronted with increasingly frail patients who have multiple comorbidities. Simple, noninvasive, yet focused elements from the patient's history and physical examination serve as prognostic factors based upon the patient's well-being or frailty. Makary has reported graded scores (allowing for BMI, height, and gender) that are predicated upon degree of weight loss, diminished dominant grip strength, self-reported description of exhaustion levels, and weekly energy expenditure in the course of routine activities, along with walking speed. Fried and associates recognized frailty as a clinical syndrome in which three or more of the above criteria are present. Another method of assessing frailty is timed stair climbing. Reddy and coworkers observed that longer climbing times among patients preparing for abdominal operations were significantly associated with increased postoperative morbidity, adjusting for other factors such as age, COPD, serum albumin, and hypertension.

Preoperative frailty is predictive of an increased chance of falls, worsened mobility, postoperative complications, prolonged lengths of hospital stay, and discharge to a skilled or assisted-living facility after having previously lived at home. A multivariate analysis demonstrated that among more than 58,000 patients undergoing colon resection, independent predictors of major complications were an elevated frailty index, an open (versus laparoscopic) operation, and ASA Class 4 or 5, but interestingly not wound classification or emergency status.

The care of the elderly requires thoughtful considerations of their diminished physiologic reserve and tolerance of the insult of an operation. Interventions may include preoperative and early postoperative physical therapy, prospective discharge planning, and the introduction of elder-specific order sets. Simple scoring systems can provide valuable information for the surgeon to present to the patient and family so that they can anticipate the nature of the postoperative care and recovery, including potential transfer to a rehabilitation facility and long-term debility.

Programs to improve the perioperative management of older adults have successfully reduced perioperative morbidity. An integrated care coordination clinic convened specialists in geriatric medicine, geriatric nursing, social work, and anesthesia to complete perioperative risk assessments and modifications for older adults who were about to undergo elective abdominal operations. A geriatrics consult team also visited these patients during their hospital stays. Perioperative decision-making, discharge planning, and postoperative care were orchestrated by a multidisciplinary team that included surgeons and geriatricians and engaged the patients and their families. McDonald and colleagues demonstrated that the program resulted in fewer postoperative complications, shorter hospital stays, more frequent discharges to home (rather than to a rehabilitation facility), and fewer readmissions, when compared to a control group of older adults who received standard care.

▶ Illicit Drug & Alcohol Usage

The value of routine testing for the presence of illicit drugs, at least among patients with suggestive histories, is uncertain. The presence of drugs in blood or urine might result in a cancellation of an operation, particularly if it is not immediately required. Conversely, some clinicians are not concerned about proving recent drug usage as long as the patient does not exhibit current evidence of toxicity or a hypermetabolic state. The confirmation of illicit drug usage obviously heightens awareness of the possibility of postoperative withdrawal. In general, patients should be advised to refrain from taking illicit drugs for at least a couple of weeks before an operation. Similarly, a history of heavy alcohol consumption raises the possibility of a postoperative withdrawal syndrome, which can be associated with significant morbidity and even death. It is best if patients can cease drinking alcohol for at least 1 week before an operation. Regardless of whether the patient can suspend alcohol consumption, the surgeon must closely monitor for symptoms of withdrawal among these patients and consider the regular administration of a benzodiazepine during recovery to prevent or treat acute withdrawal.

▶ Cancer Therapy

Many patients undergo neoadjuvant therapy for malignancies involving the breast, esophagus, stomach, pancreas, rectum, soft tissues, and other sites. The surgeon is responsible for restaging the tumor before proceeding with a resection. In general, the interval between the completion of external-beam radiation and an operation is commensurate with the duration of the radiation therapy. Similarly, a reasonable amount of time should elapse after systemic therapy to permit restoration of bone marrow capacity and nutrition, to the extent possible. Angiogenesis inhibitors such as bevacizumab disrupt normal wound perfusion and healing. The duration of time between biologic therapy and an operation is not firmly established. However, it is probably best to allow 4-6 weeks to elapse after treating with bevacizumab before proceeding with an operation, and the therapy should not be resumed until the wound is fully healed, perhaps 1 month later.

▶ Emergency Operations

Emergency operations generally permit little time for risk reduction, although fluid and blood resuscitation can be instituted and antibiotics administered. Emergency operations on patients who have undergone chemotherapy within the past month are associated with increased rates of major complications and death. In patients with profound neutropenia, operations should be deferred to the extent possible due to severely impaired wound healing and the likelihood of irreversible postoperative sepsis. We have determined that emergency operations pose a significantly increased risk for VTE complications, which may factor into decisions about enhanced VTE prophylaxis protocols during the perioperative period.

INFORMED CONSENT

The informed consent process is far more that a signed document or "permission slip." Consent involves a conversation between the surgeon and patient (and perhaps family members or a legal guardian) that extends from the initial consultation through subsequent clinic visits or correspondence and into the preoperative holding area. The discussion addresses indications for the operation and its expected outcome, alternative treatments, the natural history of the underlying condition without intervention, timing of the operation, the basic mechanics and details of the operation, potential risks, the impact of the operation on the patient's health and quality of life, the extent of hospitalization and recuperation (including possible rehabilitation care), the timing of resumption of normal activities, and residual effects. The informed consent process may also indicate that a resident will participate in the patient's care, under the supervision of the teaching surgeon and with an appropriate level of competence. Spouses and other family members should be included in the consent process for major operations that present chances of death or major debility.

In some circumstances, the patient may not be able to provide consent and no family members or guardians may be available. The surgeon should consider the acuity of the patient's condition and whether it requires an immediate operation. If emergency surgery is indicated, the surgeon should document the situation and advise a hospital administrator or lawyer, if possible. Some unusual, nonacute scenarios may require seeking legal consent for an operation through the judicial process.

PATIENT ENGAGEMENT

Patient engagement in care considers the patient's priorities, goals, values, and understanding to reach a shared decision. Shared decision-making goes beyond informed consent and considers the patient's knowledge about and comprehension of the proposed operation and its risks, benefits, and alternatives. In elective circumstances, patients should be allowed time to reflect upon their choices before rendering a decision. Shared decision-making considers social, cultural, and financial issues that may affect the outcomes of operations. Even when clinically indicated, operations may not confer benefits to some patients if these issues are not thoughtfully entertained during the preoperative phase of care. Therefore, patients should be empowered to express their personal values and preferences while decisions about their care are being made.

Expectations for the postoperative period should be stated during preoperative counseling, and patients should understand their engagement in the recovery process. Counseling may include setting goals for postoperative mobilization and how pain will be managed. This approach should enhance efforts to limit narcotics.

In frail or older adults, standards to achieve optimal goals and decision-making should be followed. The patient and family should have the opportunity to discuss several essential concepts, and that conversation should be documented in the medical record. This includes a review of the patient's health goals, which may be to live as long as possible, to live independently, to be comfortable and symptom-free, to cure a condition, to survive until a special event, or to accomplish other outcomes. The primary purpose of the operation should be articulated and aligned with the patient's goals. The surgeon's purpose for an operation may include cure, prolongation of life, preservation of function, relief of symptoms, diagnosis alone, or other goals. If the surgeon's purpose and anticipated outcome of the operation are not concordant with the patient's goals, then matters need to be reconciled, and nonoperative approaches could be more appropriate.

The patient's decision-making capacity is determined during preoperative counseling. If the patient cannot make decisions, a healthcare proxy should be established, if possible. Preferences for specific intensive treatments—such as mechanical ventilation, cardiopulmonary resuscitation, dialysis, blood transfusion, and parenteral nutrition—should be expressed and documented. Involving the patient's primary care physician in preoperative deliberations may be beneficial and can provide meaningful insight to the surgeon.

PREOPERATIVE INSTRUCTIONS

In some settings, all preoperative preparation is conducted by surgeons and their office staffs. Conversely, more robust systems may employ an elaborate process to prepare patients for operations. Regardless of the preoperative process, education constitutes a major component. In addition to learning about the actual operation, patients (and family members or caretakers) need to understand both preparation for and recovery from the operation.

Consistent information should be provided about how long a patient should fast and what medications are to be taken on the morning of the operation. The American Society of Anesthesiologists has issued guidelines about preoperative fasting. To minimize retained gastric volume and maximize gastric pH, anesthesiologists advise adults and children to refrain from drinking clear liquids for at least 2 hours before general anesthesia, regional anesthesia, or sedation/analgesia (versus 4 hours for infants taking breast milk, or 6 hours for infant formula). Patients should avoid eating light meals for at least 6 hours and fatty meals for 8 hours before receiving anesthetics or sedatives.

In general, it is ideal for patients to take their usual critical medications with sips of water on the morning of an operation, including beta-blockers, calcium channel blockers, nitrates, certain other hypertension-control agents, alpha agonists or alpha antagonists, statins, hormones such as levothyroxine, psychotropic agents, oral contraceptives, and medications for cardiac rhythm problems, chronic obstructive pulmonary disease, gastroesophageal reflux, peptic diatheses, and neurologic disorders. Some surgeons and anesthesiologists advise patients to not take angiotensin-converting enzyme (ACE) inhibitors or angiotensin II receptor blockers (ARBs) on the day of surgery due to the possibility of patients developing refractory hypotension during general anesthesia, although these medications should generally be resumed shortly after the operation. Similarly, diuretics are commonly withheld on the morning of operations that involve potentially significant amounts of fluid losses and resuscitation. Of course, these recommendations are tempered by individual circumstances and clinical judgment. For example, patients probably should take their ACE inhibitors and diuretics before operations that do not require general anesthesia or much IV fluid, and when inadequately controlled hypertension could postpone the operation. Glucose and corticosteroid management have already been addressed.

Chronic narcotics (eg, methadone) are continued on the day of surgery to avoid possible withdrawal. Monoamine oxidase (MAO) inhibitors are associated with drug interactions with indirect sympathomimetics such as ephedrine (resulting in severe hypertension) or with tramadol, methadone, dextromethorphan, propoxyphene, and phenylpiperidine opioids such as meperidine or fentanyl (causing a serotonin syndrome with potential coma, seizures, or even death). Acute withdrawal of MAO inhibitors can provoke major depression, so they can be maintained preoperatively but without the concomitant usage of confounding medications.

The management of aspirin and thienopyridines for active coronary (or cerebrovascular) disease was reviewed earlier. Aspirin taken for other reasons, nonsteroidal antiinflammatory agents, herbal preparations, and vitamin E can disrupt normal coagulation and should be stopped 1 week before an operation. Epoprostenol is a prostaglandin that is used to treat pulmonary hypertension; it also inhibits platelet aggregation and behaves like "IV aspirin." The discontinuation of epoprostenol will provoke pulmonary hypertension, so it is best to continue the infusion, accepting possible surgical site oozing that can be controlled with standard measures. Estrogen receptor antagonists (eg, tamoxifen) can be associated with an increased risk of VTE. Therefore, the surgeon should consider stopping these medications 2-4 weeks before an operation and resuming them after a similar postoperative interval, especially in patients at a heightened risk of developing VTE.

Patients receiving anticoagulants require consideration of the indication for this therapy, the potential hazards of thrombosis developing while the anticoagulation is suspended, and the dangers of perioperative hemorrhage while anticoagulated. Stopping warfarin 5 days in advance will ordinarily allow normalization of the INR for an operation, and the surgeon and consultants will determine if a "bridge" of a quickly reversible unfractionated heparin infusion or of low-molecular-weight heparin injections is necessary to minimize the duration of time during which anticoagulation is withheld.

Patients should bring bronchodilator inhalers to the hospital for usage shortly before being anesthetized. Similarly, eye drops, particularly those with beta-blockade properties, should be taken in accordance with their usual schedule.

Additional preoperative instructions include skin hygiene (eg, preoperative chlorhexidine showers, although their benefit is not absolutely proven) and local care of preexisting wounds or ulcers, as well as discussions about tobacco, drug, or alcohol cessation, glucose management, and nutrition. Nurses may mark potential sites for bowel stomae. Some patients will require vaccinations when a splenectomy is possible.

Education also addresses what patients can expect during convalescence. This includes the importance of early postoperative mobilization and ambulation, pulmonary toilet, pain management, oral care, wound care, diet, physical therapy, rehabilitation, later adjuvant care, and even complementary or alternative options. Patients may be shown videos or provided brochures, which can be produced in multiple languages. The team should definitely provide details about the logistics of the operation, including when and where the patient will report for preoperative visits and tests and for the operation itself. Finally, patients should know whom to contact with questions.

PREOPERATIVE HOLDING AREA

The time in the preoperative holding unit offers a final opportunity to educate the patient and family and to coordinate care before proceeding into the operating room. Patients (and their loved ones) are commonly anxious before operations and will be reassured by an organized, professional, and collegial environment. Members of the surgery team should introduce themselves and discuss the proposed operation and the anticipated postoperative care and recovery, including the possibilities of transfer to an intensive care unit or later to a rehabilitation facility. Vital signs are recorded, including baseline oxygen saturation. Special instructions address postoperative mobilization and pulmonary care for those patients undergoing general anesthesia or at high risk for PPC, and might involve breathing exercises with incentive spirometry. This setting definitely provides a good moment to formally mark the correct site and laterality of the operation, when pertinent, and to confirm fasting status, medications taken during the past 24 hours (especially beta-blockers), allergies, recent corticosteroid usage, and pregnancy status. Checklists (Figure 3–2) have become an important mechanism to ensure the application of standard practices, and a section can be devoted to the preoperative unit. In addition, order sets greatly contribute to the delivery of consistent and correct care, including the administration of prophylactic antibiotics, adequate VTE prophylaxis (including the application of compression boots), and hydrocortisone for those patients with a recent history of significant corticosteroid usage. The infusion of antibiotics is not necessarily begun in the holding area, as it may still be more than 1 hour before the actual incision, but antibiotics can be secured for delivery to the operating room with the patient. Glycemic control protocols are begun in the holding area, as outlined earlier. For patients having bowel resections, the effectiveness of any mechanical prep may be investigated, and warming blankets can be applied to promote perioperative euthermia. Finally, surgeons and anesthesiologists have the chance to discuss blood volume status and strategies for fluid administration, which may begin in the holding area.

The surgeon should use the immediate preoperative period for a final review of critical information in the medical record, including an update of the history and physical examination and an examination of laboratory and imaging results. The surgeon should also verify the availability of family or representatives to be contacted after the operation, if the patient wishes, or even during the operation if unexpected findings require a change in plans.

Before Entering OR	Before Inducing Anesthesia	Final Pause Before Incision	Before Leaving OR	Post Operative Destination
PATIENT CHECK-IN ☐ PATIENT STATES NAME AND D.O.B. ☐ PATIENT CONFIRMS ID BAND/CONSENT ☐ PATIENT STATES PROCEDURE, SITE, SIDE ☐ PATIENT NAMES HIS/HER SURGEON ☐ PATIENT ASKED WHEN THEY LAST ATE ☐ DETERMINE NEED FOR INTERPRETER ☐ ALLERGIES REVIEWED/RECORDED ☐ VERIFY WITH OR BOARD ☐ SITE MARKED IF APPLICABLE AND CONFIRMED* ☐ H & P UPDATED AND IN CHART ☐ CONSENTS UP-TO-DATE/SIGNED ☐ ANESTHESIA PREOP/CONSENT DONE ☐ ASA STATUS VERIFIED/DOCUMENTED ☐ ANTIBIOTIC ORDERED IF APPLICABLE ☐ VTE PROPHYLAXIS IF APPLICABLE ☐ PRECAUTIONS IDENTIFIED ☐ PREOP RN/CIRCULATOR BRIEFING ☐ IMPLANTS, SPECIAL EQUIPMENT, BLOOD AND TISSUE AVAILABLE IF APPLICABLE ☐ DETERMINE POTENTIAL NEED FOR UNIT BED ☐ CONFIRM B BLOCKER USAGE AND DOCUMENT IF APPLICABLE ☐ STEROID PROTOCOL IF APPLICABLE **HAND OFF** PREOP RN:_____ CIRCULATOR:_____ DATE:_____ TIME:_____ (mm/dd/yyyy) *ATTENDING SURGEON'S INITIALS	**UPON OR ENTRY** ☐ STRETCHER/TABLE LOCKED FOR TRANSFER ☐ SAFETY BELT IN PLACE ☐ TEAM MEMBERS INTRODUCED ☐ PATIENT IDENTITY CONFIRMED ☐ CONFIRM RECORD LABELING ☐ ALLERGIES VERBALIZED ☐ CONFIRM PROCEDURE(S) BEING PERFORMED ☐ PATIENT POSITIONING CONFIRMED ☐ EMERGENCY EQUIPMENT AVAILABLE ☐ SPECIAL EQUIPMENT AVAILABLE ☐ IMAGING DISPLAYED AND REVIEWED **REVIEW PRIOR TO INDUCTION** ☐ FIRE RISK ASSESSMENT ☐ PULSE OXIMETER ON/FUNCTIONING ☐ RISK OF DIFFICULT AIRWAY/ASPIRATION ☐ SURGEON REVIEWS DURATION, IRRIGATION FLUIDS AND RISK OF RETAINED FOREIGN BODY ☐ BLOOD AVAILABLE IF APPLICABLE ☐ **ALL** DRUGS/SOLUTIONS LABELED ☐ COMPRESSION BOOTS IF APPLICABLE ☐ ANTIBIOTICS DOSE/REDOSING ☐ B-BLOCKER/GLUCOSE CONTROL ☐ TEMPERATURE CONTROL MEASURES ☐ FLUID MANAGEMENT STRATEGY **PERFORM OR TIMEOUT** Patient, procedure, site, side, level, implants, structures, position and consents reviewed and verified STOP ALL ACTIVITY ATTENDING SURGEON:_____ ATTENDING ANESTHESIOLOGIST:_____ CIRCULATOR:_____ TIME:_____	**ALL STAFF REVIEW CRITICAL EVENTS BEFORE INCISION** ☐ ATTENDING SURGEON REVIEWS CRITICAL/ADDITIONAL STEPS AND ANTICIPATED BLOOD LOSS ☐ ANESTHESIA PROVIDER REVIEWS PATIENT SPECIFIC CONCERNS/ISSUES ☐ CIRCULATOR REVIEWS STERILITY AND EQUIPMENT ISSUES ☐ TISSUE AND IMPLANTS CHECKED AND VERIFIED ☐ NEUTRAL ZONE ESTABLISHED **FINAL PAUSE** ☐ STOP ALL ACTIVITY ☐ ATTENDING SURGEON PRESENT ☐ PREP DRIED ☐ SURGEON SITE MARKING VISIBLE AND CONFIRMED AFTER PREP AND DRAPE AND PRIOR TO INCISION WHEN APPLICABLE ☐ REMARK SITE AND REDO TIMEOUT IF INITIALS NOT VISIBLE ☐ INCISION TIME CONFIRMED AND RECORDED **FOR ADDITIONAL SURGEONS OR TIMEOUT** Patient, procedure, site, side, level, implants, structures, position and consents reviewed and verified ATTENDING SURGEON:_____ ATTENDING ANESTHESIOLOGIST:_____ CIRCULATOR:_____ TIME:_____ ☐ N/A	**NURSE VERBALLY REVIEWS WITH THE TEAM** **FINAL COUNT PAUSE** ☐ INSTRUMEN, SPONGE, NEEDLE COUNTS PERFORMED PER POLICY ☐ SPECIMENS RECONCILED BY RN ☐ FINAL DIAGNOSIS CONFIRMED AND RECORDED ☐ NAME OF PROCEDURE(S) ☐ WOUND CLASSIFICATION VERIFIED WITH SURGEON ATTENDING SURGEON:_____ DATE:_____ TIME:_____ (mm/dd/yyyy) RN:_____ DATE:_____ TIME:_____ (mm/dd/yyyy) **REVIEW CRITICAL EVENTS** ☐ ANESTHESIA PROVIDER, NURSE AND SURGEON REVIEW THE KEY CONCERNS FOR RECOVERY AND MANAGEMENT OF THE PATIENT ☐ DISCUSSION OF POST OPERATIVE ANALGESIA/BLOCK ☐ PROCEDURE NOTE BY SURGEON ☐ DETERMINE IF THERE WERE ANY EQUIPMENT ISSUES ☐ STEPS TO EXIT INITIATED ☐ CALL POSTOP DESTINATION WITH ANY PRECAUTIONS AND EQUIPMENT	**UPON ARRIVAL** ☐ O₂ SATURATION ☐ TEAM MEMBERS INTRODUCED ☐ VITAL SIGNS AND TEMPERATURE ☐ OR NURSE/SURGEON REVIEW CONCERNS FOR RECOVERY ☐ ORDERS BY SURGEON **ANESTHESIA REPORT** ☐ ALLERGIES VERBALIZED ☐ PATIENT HISTORY ☐ LAST OR VITAL SIGNS ☐ DRUGS ADMINISTERED ☐ URINE OUTPUT/BLOOD LOSS ☐ FLUIDS/BLOOD PRODUCTS **PRIOR TO FINAL SIGN OUT** ☐ PROCEDURE NOTE IN CHART ☐ ANESTHESIA DRUG/DISCHARGE ORDERS ☐ NEED FOR CONSULTS/X-RAYS/LABS ☐ POST ANESTHESIA PROGRESS NOTE ☐ TIMING OF ANTIBIOTICS IF APPLICABLE ☐ FINAL DISPOSITION RN:_____ DATE:_____ TIME:_____ (mm/dd/yyyy)

▲ **Figure 3–2. Sample of Universal Checklist for perioperative care.** (Used with permission of Boston Medical Center.)

OPERATING ROOM

Preparation of the patient continues in the operating room, up to the moment of the incision. When local hair removal is necessary for exposure, this should be done immediately before the operation with electric clippers. Razors traumatize skin and have been associated with a greater chance of infection. Most surgical site skin preparations contain iodine-based compounds or chlorhexidine, but the addition of isopropyl alcohol to either of these agents seems to confer the best outcomes. Regardless of the agent selected, it is important that the skin prep be applied in a standard fashion—ideally by an assigned, trained individual to ensure consistency—and that it dries prior to the application of the sterile drapes. Iodine-impregnated adherent drapes can also be used to cover the skin surrounding the surgical site. The role of mechanical bowel preparations and antibiotic prophylaxis (oral and/or parenteral) in colorectal operations is addressed in another chapter. The placement of urinary catheters in the operating room merits special comment. Urinary tract infections (UTIs) are costly and can be reduced in frequency by restricting catheter placement to relatively few patients. When catheters are necessary, they should be sterilely placed and then removed as soon as possible. The routine practice of two people (one for exposure and one for insertion) catheterizing obese women can also decrease the incidence of UTI.

Proper positioning of the patient for an operation is critical to enhance exposure, to protect potential pressure points or muscle compartments, and to avoid traction injuries to nerves. Surgeons, nurses, and anesthesia staff share responsibility for patient safety during operations and should concur about how the patient is situated on the operating room table. The same principle applies to the end of the operation, when team members remain vigilant at bedside until the patient has been safely transported to the recovery unit.

PREPARATION OF THE OPERATING ROOM FACILITY

Beyond the hazards for SSIs discussed earlier, wound sepsis is also related to the bacteriologic status of both the hospital setting in general and the operating room in particular. The entire hospital environment must be protected from undue contamination to avoid colonization and cross-infection of patients with virulent strains of microorganisms that could invade surgical sites despite practices of asepsis, antisepsis, and sterile surgical technique. *All* staff should diligently wash their hands before and after contact with patients, regardless of location (ie, in the operating room or elsewhere in the facility). Patients with especially dangerous or resistant organisms (eg, *Clostridium difficile*, MRSA, and vancomycin-resistant *Enterococcus*) may warrant special precautions such as isolation and staff wearing gowns and gloves during direct contact with the patient and secretions. Notably, alcohol-based hand sanitizers are not effective against *C difficile*.

In the United States, it is standard for members of the operating room team to wear issued "scrub" clothes, caps, shoe covers, and masks, although this practice is less dogmatic in other countries. Surgeons and staff who perform the operation and handle sterile instruments wear sterile gowns, gloves, and protective eye gear. "Universal precautions" are practiced for the safety of the team, under the presumption that any patient's blood or fluids can convey communicable diseases such as human immunodeficiency virus or hepatitis. Formal procedures and policies should be developed locally for injured staff or those exposed to blood or other potential hazards during operations.

▶ Sterilization

Items used during an operation are sterilized to destroy microorganisms on the surface of the instrument or in a fluid. Current sterilization methods include steam autoclave, hydrogen peroxide gas plasma, gamma irradiation, ethylene oxide gas, and dry heat. An autoclave system uses saturated steam under pressure. This is the most widely used method due to its ability to rapidly sterilize devices while being relatively inexpensive and nontoxic. The two most common types of steam autoclaves are gravity displacement, which must reach temperatures of 121°C, and prevacuum sterilizers, which must reach temperatures of 132°C. Minimum exposure periods for wrapped devices are 30 minutes for the former technique and 4 minutes for the latter system. Of course, the implementation of steam is limited by its corrosive effect on heat-sensitive items.

Liquid hydrogen peroxide is a nontoxic sterilizing agent that initiates the inactivation of microorganisms on a heat-sensitive device within 75 minutes. Liquid hydrogen peroxide is vaporized and diffused through the sterilization chamber to contact the surfaces of the device. An electrical field is created within the chamber, changing the vapor to gas plasma. Microbicidal free radicals are generated in the plasma, rendering the device sterile.

Gamma sterilization utilizes Cobalt-60 radiation to inactivate microorganisms on single-use medical supplies, pharmaceuticals, and biological-based products, although the United States Food and Drug Administration does not approve gamma irradiation in healthcare facilities. Liquid and gaseous ethylene oxide is a toxic, flammable sterilizing agent that initiates the inactivation of microorganisms on a heat-sensitive device within 1-6 hours, with 8-12 hours required for aeration. Ethylene oxide gas is diffused through the sterilization chamber at temperatures between 37°C and 63°C and a relative humidity of 40%-80%. The gas bonds with water molecules to reach the device surfaces and render the device sterile. Due to the extended aeration time requirement and high level of toxicity, ethylene oxide gas sterilization is being replaced with nontoxic systems that have shorter process times.

Dry heat sterilization utilizes heating coils to raise the temperature of the air inside the sterilization chamber to sterilize surfaces of devices. It is appropriate only for items that have a low moist heat tolerance but high temperature tolerance. The most common time–temperature relationships for dry heat sterilization are 170°C for 1 hour, 160°C for 2 hours, and 150°C for 2.5 hours.

Operating Room Plans

Surgeons should prospectively communicate with the operating room staff about the operation to be performed, including its anticipated duration and all necessary items, to enhance efficiency and avoid delays. "Case cards" contain information about standard equipment, devices, and sutures. Surgeons must also anticipate special needs such as unusual instruments or hardware, prosthetic materials for implantation, coagulation devices (eg, electrocautery, ultrasound or radiofrequency energy devices, lasers), intraoperative laboratory testing (eg, glucose, hematocrit, parathyroid hormone), imaging (eg, fluoroscopy, ultrasonography), nerve monitoring, and other details specific to the operation. The primary surgeon is responsible for coordinating teams when multiple consultants and allied professionals collaborate in a patient's care, including fellow surgeons, anesthesiologists, nurses, technicians, and others. A checklist hopefully promotes communication about these matters to ensure that it is safe to proceed with the operation. In fact, our group has added "fire risk assessment" to the Universal Protocol (Figure 3–2). Beyond establishing actions to douse a fire (eg, basin with water or saline on the sterile field or awareness of the nearest fire extinguisher), a safety risk score for fire can be calculated based upon proximity of the operation to the airway, presence of an open oxygen source, usage of an ignition source (eg, cautery, fiber-optic light source, laser, drills, or saws), and the application of a skin prep solution that contains alcohol or other volatile chemicals. Special considerations are given to patients with high fire risk scores.

Preparations also include the development of contingency plans for a variety of dangerous scenarios in the operating room. These include potentially catastrophic environmental problems (eg, fire, loss of humidity control, ventilation, or air conditioning systems, disruption or contamination of water supply, flooding, destruction of structural integrity, computer failure, even threat of physical violence to patient or staff) or potentially fatal clinical conditions (eg, massive hemorrhage, cardiac arrest, air embolus, failed airway, malignant hyperthermia). Plans can be composed as algorithms and documented on paper or online and even projected on monitors for the entire team to review.

PREPARATION OF THE SURGERY TEAM

Attention is being increasingly focused upon the development of teams in the operating room. Much of this work has been modeled upon the concepts of Crew Resource Management (CRM), as promulgated by the aviation profession. Psychologists analyzed behaviors of flight crews in the 1970s and proposed measures to improve safety, including reducing the hierarchy of that time, empowering junior team members to express concerns about potential problems, and training senior crew members to listen to the perspectives of other team members while accepting questions as honest communication rather than insubordination. This approach encourages the crew to participate in the enterprise and offer their expertise and talents, while the captain remains the ultimate authority.

As in the airline industry, the implementation of CRM in the operating room is supported by a series of activities before the main event. The ideal preoperative briefing establishes the team leader, facilitates communication, outlines the team's work, and specifies protocols, responsibilities, expectations, and contingency plans. This collaboration can result in improved outcomes, greater patient satisfaction, and better morale among team members. Checklists should not merely be perfunctory recitations of goals; they should promote a culture of teamwork. These checklists can be modified to suit local circumstances, resources, and cultures, and they codify critical steps, such as having necessary materials and medications on hand as well as indicating the appropriate location and site of the operation in instances when wrong-site mistakes could be made. Simulation training is also becoming more readily available, particularly regarding rare, complex, or high-risks scenarios as well as the introduction of new members to teams.

PREPARATION OF THE SURGEON

The professional development of a surgeon is a privilege and an enduring pursuit involving emotional and intellectual growth, discipline, creativity, dedication, equanimity, technical talent, and formal education. College, postgraduate, and medical school curricula are certainly preludes to accredited surgery residencies and fellowships. That certain personalities are drawn to different surgical specialties is part of the joy and wonder of the profession.

Board certification confirms that a surgeon has completed the requisite years of residency and passed a rigorous examination to indicate competence. Learning continues well beyond formal training, as exemplified by specialty board certification and the recent Continuous Certification program that the American Board of Surgery instituted to ensure lifelong professional development. The surgeon must be familiar with contemporary literature and willing to adapt to emerging technologies and operative techniques, building upon established knowledge and skills. Moreover, the surgeon critically assesses data to decide the wisdom and value of new developments—for the individual patient, the surgeon, and the prevailing healthcare system. Fellowship in the American College of Surgeons (or comparable organizations outside the United States and Canada) endorses that the surgeon has successfully completed a thorough evaluation of professional competence and ethical fitness. The qualifications include board certification, commitment to the welfare of patients above all else, and pledges regarding appropriate compensation and the avoidance of unjustified operations.

The surgeon must also be versed in—and a leader of—quality improvement within the process of caring for patients. Naturally, the proficiency provided by performing large numbers of certain high-risk operations results in improved outcomes. This is a matter of designing excellent systems that support surgical care, rather than the exclusive talents of a solitary surgeon. Ideal care involves a coordinated series of steps and collaborations—bundles of care—among teams of professionals so that the system and culture are sustained despite the loss of any individual, and the surgeon is the leader of that team. Crew Resource Management, as described earlier, has defined seven characteristics of leaders of high-performance teams:

1. **Command:** One person retains the ultimate authority and responsibility for the team and outcomes.

2. **Leadership:** The leader establishes a culture of open communication, accountability, and teamwork, serves as a mentor, manages conflict, and establishes high standards of excellence and professionalism. An effective leader inspires the team with strength and humanity.

3. **Communication:** A work environment thrives upon an effective and timely exchange of ideas among professionals to create the essential bond within the team. Members of the team should be empowered to raise concerns and to ask questions, particularly when doing so might prevent harm to a patient.

4. **Situational awareness:** This involves a comprehension of the present circumstances through active communication with team members and knowledge of preceding events.

5. **Workload management:** Tasks are delegated among team members commensurate with their skills and training so that everybody is doing the right job in synergy with others.

6. **Resource management:** This trait prospectively identifies the local resources to result in optimal outcomes.

7. **Decision-making:** This process includes collecting data from the environment and soliciting opinions from team members to permit informed judgments.

Leadership traits are not necessarily intuitive, and they require introspection, training, and practice. The surgeon remains the proverbial captain of the ship regarding the care of patients having operations, but as a consultative leader among trusted colleagues.

CONCLUSIONS

Perioperative management and thoughtful decision-making are necessary to optimize patient outcomes and experiences through the phases of care by aligning four elements:

1. **The right patient:** Thorough risk assessment, shared decisions, and meticulous preoperative preparation.

2. **The right operation:** The best treatment for the disease, based upon the best available evidence.

3. **The right provider:** A surgeon who has the training, skills, and judgment to safely and expertly care for the patient's condition.

4. **The right place:** A healthcare facility with the necessary resources.

▶ References

American Society of Anesthesiologists Committee. Practice guidelines for preoperative fasting and the use of pharmacologic agents to reduce the risk of pulmonary aspiration: Application to healthy patients undergoing elective procedures. An updated report by the American Society of Anesthesiologists Committee on Standards and Practice Parameters. *Anesthesiology.* 2011;114:495-511.

Ata A, Lee J, Bestle SL, et al. Postoperative hyperglycemia and surgical site infection in general surgery patients. *Arch Surg.* 2010;145:858-864.

Bahl V, Hu HM, Henke PK, et al. A validation study of a retrospective venous thromboembolism risk scoring method. *Ann Surg.* 2010;251:344-350.

Bergqvist D, Agnelli G, Cohen AT, et al. Duration of prophylaxis against venous thromboembolism with enoxaparin after surgery for cancer. *N Engl J Med.* 2002;346(13):975-980.

Berian JR, Rosenthal RA, Baker TL. Hospital standards to promote optimal surgical care of the older adult: A report from the Coalition for Quality in Geriatric Surgery. *Ann Surg.* 2018;267: 280-290.

Bertges DJ, Goodney PP, Zhao Y, et al. The Vascular Study Group of New England Cardiac Risk Index (VSG-CRI) predicts cardiac complications more accurately than the Revised Cardiac Risk Index in vascular surgery patients. *J Vasc Surg.* 2010; 52:674-683.

Bode LG, Kluytmans JA, Wertheim HF, et al. Preventing surgical-site infections in nasal carriers of *Staphylococcus aureus. N Engl J Med.* 2010;362:9-17.

Canet J, Gallart L, Gomar C, et al. Prediction of postoperative pulmonary complications in a population-based surgical cohort. *Anesthesiology.* 2010;113:1338-1350.

Cassidy MR, Macht R, Rosenkranz P, Caprini JA, McAneny D. Patterns of failure of a standardized perioperative venous thromboembolism prophylaxis protocol. *J Am Coll Surg.* 2016;222: 1074-1080.

Cassidy MR, Rosenkranz P, McAneny D. Reducing postoperative venous thromboembolism complications with a standardized risk-stratified protocol and mobilization program. *J Am Coll Surg.* 2014;218:1095-1104.

Cassidy MR, Rosenkranz P, McCabe K, Rosen JE, McAneny D. ICOUGH: Reducing postoperative pulmonary complications with a multidisciplinary patient care program. *JAMA Surg.* 2013;148:740-745.

Cooper Z, Sayal P, Abbett SK, et al. A conceptual framework for appropriateness in surgical care: Reviewing past approaches and looking ahead to patient-centered shared decision making. *Anesthesiology.* 2015;123:1450-1454.

Corcoran T, Rhodes JEJ, Clarke S, et al. Perioperative fluid management strategies in major surgery: A stratified meta-analysis. *Anesth Analg.* 2012;114:640-651.

Darouiche RO, Wall MJ, Itani KMF, et al. Chlorhexidine-alcohol versus povidone-iodine for surgical-site antisepsis. *N Engl J Med.* 2010;362:18-26.

Fried LP, Tangen CM, Walston J, et al. Frailty in older adults: Evidence for a phenotype. *J Gerontol A Biol Sci Med Sci.* 2001; 56(3):M146-M156.

Frisch A, Chandra P, Smiley D, et al. Prevalence and clinical outcome of hyperglycemia in the perioperative period in noncardiac surgery. *Diabetes Care.* 2010;33:1783-1788.

Gould MK, Garcia DA, Wren SM, et al. Prevention of VTE in nonorthopedic surgical patients: Antithrombotic therapy and prevention of thrombosis, 9th ed. American College of Chest Physicians evidence-based clinical practice guidelines. *Chest.* 2012;141(2 suppl):e227S-e277S.

Gupta PK, Gupta H, Sundaram A, et al. Development and validation of a risk calculator for prediction of cardiac risk after surgery. *Circulation.* 2011;124:381-387.

Hawn MT, Houston TK, Campagna EJ, et al. The attributable risk of smoking on surgical complications. *Ann Surg.* 2011; 254:914-920.

Hennessey DB, Burke JP, Ni-Dhonochu T, et al. Preoperative hypoalbuminemia is an independent risk factor for the development of surgical site infection following gastrointestinal surgery: A multi-institutional study. *Ann Surg.* 2010;252:325-320.

Makary MA, Segev DL, Pronovost PJ, et al. Frailty as a predictor of surgical outcomes in older patients. *J Am Coll Surg.* 2010; 210:901-908.

Marimuthu K, Varadhan KK, Ljungqvist O, et al. A meta-analysis of the effect of combinations of immune modulating nutrients on outcome in patients undergoing major open gastrointestinal surgery. *Ann Surg.* 2012;255:1060-1068.

McDonald SR, Heflin MT, Whitson HE, et al. Association of integrated care coordination with postsurgical outcomes in high-risk older adults: The Perioperative Optimization of Senior Health (POSH) Initiative. *JAMA Surg.* 2018;153(5):454-462.

Memtsoudis S, Liu SS, Ma Y, et al. Perioperative pulmonary outcomes in patients with sleep apnea after noncardiac surgery. *Anesth Analg.* 2011;112:113-121.

Merkow RP, Bilimoria KY, McCarter MD, et al. Post-discharge venous thromboembolism after cancer surgery. *Ann Surg.* 2011; 254:131-137.

Obeid NM, Azuh O, Reddy S, et al. Predictors of critical care-related complications in colectomy patients using the National Surgical Quality Improvement Program: Exploring frailty and aggressive laparoscopic approaches. *J Trauma Acute Care Surg.* 2012;72:878-883.

Pannucci CJ, Bailey SH, Dreszer G, et al. Validation of the Caprini risk assessment model in plastic and reconstructive surgery patients. *J Am Coll Surg.* 2011;212:105-112.

Poirier P, Alpert MA, Fleisher LA, et al. Cardiovascular evaluation and management of severely obese patients undergoing surgery: A science advisory from the American Heart Association. *Circulation.* 2009;120:86-95.

Reddy S, Contreras CM, Singletary B. Timed stair climbing is the single strongest predictor of perioperative complications in patients undergoing abdominal surgery. *J Am Coll Surg.* 2016; 222:559-566.

Rutala WA, Weber DJ; the Healthcare Infection Control Practices Advisory Committee. Guideline for disinfection and sterilization in healthcare facilities, 2008. http://www.cdc.gov/hicpac/pdf/guidelines/disinfection_nov_2008.pdf.

Shuman AG, Hu HM, Pannucci CJ, et al. Stratifying the risk of venous thromboembolism in otolaryngology. *Otolaryngol Head Neck Surg.* 2012;146:719-724.

Swenson BR, Hedrick TL, Metzger R, et al. Effects of preoperative skin preparation on postoperative wound infection rates: A prospective study of 3 skin preparation protocols. *Infect Control Hosp Epidemiol.* 2009;30:964-971.

Wong J, Lam DP, Abrishami A. Short-term preoperative smoking cessation and postoperative complications: A systematic review and meta-analysis. *Can J Anaesth.* 2012;59:268-279.

MULTIPLE-CHOICE QUESTIONS

1. The American Society of Anesthesiologists patient classification system:

   A. Is an approach to preoperatively categorizing patients to assess their risk for an operation.

   B. Requires specific measures of certain laboratory values in order to complete the scoring system.

   C. Can be used to decide upon whom not to operate. For example, no ASA 5 patients should undergo operations.

   D. Includes categories ASA1 through ASA5.

   E. Both A and C are true.

2. After the decision to operate has been made, the evaluation regarding safety to proceed:

   A. Is the sole province of the anesthesiologist.

   B. Should not take into account the planned operation.

   C. Is best performed by specialists not directly invested in the planned operation.

   D. Should include a pain assessment to aid in the management of postoperative pain.

   E. Both A and C are true.

3. Venous thromboembolism risk:

   A. Has no relationship to the family history.

   B. Is assessed using the RCRI score.

   C. Can be modified by risk-based interventions.

   D. Has few long-term consequences as long as a pulmonary embolus is not fatal.

   E. Frequently should be modified by placement of an inferior vena cava filter preoperatively.

4. Diabetes mellitus patients require more operations than patients without diabetes, and if not carefully controlled have increased risks of:

   A. Surgical site infection.
   B. Perioperative adrenal insufficiency.
   C. Perioperative hypoglycemia.
   D. A, B, and C are all true.
   E. Both A and C are true.

5. Geriatric patients:

   A. Are a limited portion of a general surgery practice now and in the near future.
   B. Can have perioperative risks closely estimated by chronological age.
   C. Can have frailty measured by a variety of means that predict the risk of complications.
   D. Require limited special assessment other than modification of drug dosages.
   E. Both A and C are true.

Postoperative Care

Jennifer E. Rosen, MD

The modern surgeon is involved with the management of a patient from preoperative evaluation, through the conduct of the operation into the postoperative care period, and often into generating a long-term plan. As the operating surgeon, he or she is best situated to apply evidence-based scientific knowledge and a deep understanding of potential complications to that patient's care. The recovery from major surgery can be divided into three phases: (1) an immediate, or post anesthetic, phase; (2) an intermediate phase, encompassing the hospitalization period; and (3) a convalescent phase. During the first two phases, care is principally directed at maintenance of homeostasis, treatment of pain, and prevention and early detection of complications. The convalescent phase is a transition period from the time of hospital discharge to full recovery. The trend toward earlier postoperative discharge after major surgery has shifted the venue of this period. We often say "postop starts preop," which essentially means that the postoperative plan should be considered and discussed before surgery to set expectations for the patient and their family.

THE IMMEDIATE POSTOPERATIVE PERIOD

The primary causes of early complications and death following major surgery are acute pulmonary, cardiovascular, and fluid derangements. The post anesthesia care unit (PACU) is staffed by specially trained personnel and provided with equipment for early detection and treatment of these problems. All patients should be monitored in this specialized unit initially following major procedures unless they are transported directly to an intensive care unit. While enroute from the operating room (OR) to the PACU, the patient should be accompanied by a physician and other qualified attendants. In the PACU, the anesthesiology service generally exercises primary responsibility for cardiopulmonary function. The surgeon is responsible for the operative site and all other aspects of the care not directly related to the effects of anesthesia. The patient can be discharged from the recovery room

when cardiovascular, pulmonary, and neurologic functions have returned to baseline, which usually occurs 1-3 hours following operation. Patients who require continuing ventilatory or circulatory support, or who have other conditions that require frequent monitoring, are transferred to an intensive care unit. In this setting, nursing personnel specially trained in the management of respiratory and cardiovascular emergencies are available, and the staff-to-patient ratio is higher than it is on the wards. Monitoring equipment is available to enable early detection of cardiorespiratory derangements. Some hospitals may also have intermediate sites of care, either with telemetry or so-called "stepdown" units where the staff-to-patient ratio may be higher than on a regular floor with increased capabilities for monitoring of cardiorespiratory function, administration of specialty medications, and so on.

Postoperative Orders

Detailed treatment orders are necessary to direct postoperative care. The transfer of the patient from OR to PACU requires reiteration of any patient care orders. Unusual or particularly important orders should also be communicated to the nursing team orally. The nursing team must also be advised of the nature of the operation and the patient's condition. Errors in postoperative orders, including medication errors and omission of important orders, are diminished by electronic order entry systems that contain postoperative order sets. Careful review of order sets is still warranted, as individual patients require specialized attention. Postoperative orders should cover the following.

A. Monitoring

1. Vital signs—Blood pressure, pulse, and respiration should be recorded frequently until stable and then regularly until the patient is discharged from the recovery room. The frequency of vital sign measurements thereafter depends upon the nature of the operation and the course in the PACU.

When an arterial catheter is in place, blood pressure and pulse should be monitored continuously. Continuous electrocardiographic monitoring is indicated for most patients in the PACU. Any major changes in vital signs should be communicated to the anesthesiologist and attending surgeon immediately. Call parameters for major changes should be explicit, as should parameters for cardiac or glucose management medications to be given or withheld.

2. Central venous pressure—Central venous pressure should be recorded periodically in the early postoperative period if the operation has entailed large blood losses or fluid shifts, and invasive monitoring is available. Invasive Swan–Ganz catheters or alternative noninvasive measurements of pulmonary artery wedge pressure may be indicated under these conditions if the patient has compromised cardiac or respiratory function.

3. Fluid balance—The anesthetic record includes the type and volume of fluid administered as well as blood loss and urine output during the operation. This record should be continued in the postoperative period and should also include fluid losses from drains and stomas. This aids in assessing hydration and helps to guide intravenous fluid replacement. A bladder catheter can be placed for frequent measurement of urine output. In the absence of a bladder catheter, the surgeon should be notified if the patient is unable to void within 6-8 hours after operation to determine whether intermittent catheterization may be warranted. Noninvasive bladder scanning may assist in avoiding chronic indwelling catheter placement.

4. Other types of monitoring—Depending on the nature of the operation and the patient's preexisting conditions, other types of monitoring may be necessary. Examples include measurement of intracranial pressure and level of consciousness following cranial surgery, monitoring of distal pulses following vascular surgery or in patients with casts, and evaluating for expanding hematoma in patients after thyroid surgery.

5. The "postoperative check"—Most patients who remain in the hospital beyond the immediate postoperative period require an evaluation by a physician or adjunct during the 4-6 hours following surgery. This evaluation should include a review of the patient's overall subjective status, any objective alterations during that time period, an assessment of whether the postoperative orders are appropriate and adequate, and an evaluation of whether the patient has developed any signs or symptoms indicative of a complication related to their particular procedure or the anesthesia and medications administered since that time. A thorough understanding of the patient's history and surgical course will help in anticipating, preventing, and identifying any complications. Any worrisome findings should be directly and quickly communicated to the attending surgeon, who is in the best position to determine if an intervention is warranted. Proper documentation

of the postoperative check is important as patients change hands during team turnover and legal issues can arise if the plan of care is not explicitly laid out or executed as intended.

B. Respiratory Care

In the early postoperative period, the patient may remain mechanically ventilated or be treated with supplemental oxygen by mask or nasal prongs, preferably with humidification. These orders should be specified. For intubated patients, tracheal suctioning or other forms of respiratory therapy must be specified as required. Patients who are not intubated should be instructed on how to cough and do deep breathing exercises frequently to prevent atelectasis. Proper dual use of an incentive spirometer includes setting a goal for volume and maintaining that volume intake to allow the bead to "hover."

C. Position in Bed and Mobilization

The postoperative orders should describe any required special positioning of the patient. Unless doing so is contraindicated, the patient should be turned from side to side every 30 minutes until conscious and then hourly for the first 8-12 hours to minimize atelectasis. Early ambulation is encouraged to reduce venous stasis; the upright position helps to increase diaphragmatic excursion. Venous stasis may also be minimized by intermittent compression of the calf by pneumatic stockings. Safety considerations are paramount, including special alerts to fall risk (such as using red socks and bed rails), one-on-one monitoring, and assistance with all transfers. Support under the knees and heels can help reduce back pain and tension from immobility during surgery. Certain procedures may require the head of bed to be upright at 30 or 45 degrees, for patients to be upright during eating or drinking, or for avoiding any inadvertent loss of crucial drains or catheters.

D. Diet

Patients at risk for emesis and pulmonary aspiration should have nothing by mouth until some gastrointestinal (GI) function has returned (usually within 4 days). Most patients can tolerate liquids by mouth shortly after return to full consciousness. Patients with neurologic deficits may need evaluation by a "speech and swallow" team to determine their ability to tolerate liquids and solids of varying thicknesses. The plan for progression to a regular diet should be laid out in advance, and it is not uncommon to see that patients have remained on a liquid diet when solids could be tolerated or were given a solid food tray in error.

E. Administration of Fluid and Electrolytes

Orders for postoperative intravenous fluids should be based on maintenance needs, operative losses, and the replacement of gastrointestinal losses from drains, fistulas, or stomas. These orders should be reviewed frequently to avoid over hydration, inappropriate hydration, or under hydration of the patient.

F. Drainage Tubes

Drain care instructions should be included in the postoperative orders. Details such as type and pressure of suction, irrigation fluid and frequency, skin exit site care, and support during ambulation or showering should be specified. The surgeon should examine drains frequently, since the character or quantity of drain output may herald the development of postoperative complications such as bleeding or fistulas. Careful positioning and reinforcement of anchors can prevent the dreaded early loss of key placement of nasogastric tubes, chest tubes, and drains. If patients have multiple drains or catheters, each one should be clearly labeled to avoid confusion. No drain should be pulled without the clear and express permission of the attending surgeon.

G. Medications

Orders should be written where appropriate for antibiotics, analgesics, gastric acid suppression, deep vein thrombosis prophylaxis, and sedatives. If appropriate, preoperative medications should be reinstituted. Medication reconciliation is important, as interactions are possible and potentially harmful. For example, antithyroid medication such as methimazole should not be routinely restarted after surgery for Graves' disease, and thyroid hormone supplementation may sometimes not be started until 4-5 days afterwards. Route of administration of medications and medication substitution should be discussed with the pharmacy when necessary. Careful attention should be paid to replacement of corticosteroids in patients at risk, since postoperative adrenal insufficiency may be life threatening, but over-supplementation can affect wound healing. Other medications such as antipyretics, laxatives, and stool softeners should be used selectively as indicated. Prophylaxis for postoperative nausea and vomiting can be useful; the type and route of medication remains controversial and should be tailored to the patient.

H. Laboratory Examinations and Imaging

Postoperative laboratory and radiographic examinations should be used to detect specific abnormalities in high-risk groups. The routine use of daily chest radiographs, blood counts, electrolytes, and renal or liver function panels is not useful. Patients who have had central venous line placement may require chest x-rays for confirmation of placement and to identify a pneumothorax if this was not already done in the operating room. Identification and treatment of hyperglycemia should be instituted in patients who require management.

I. Enhanced Recovery After Surgery

Enhanced Recovery After Surgery (ERAS) programs have become increasingly common. These protocols are intended to be evidence-based and designed to standardize and streamline medical care. In their best use, they can expedite recovery, reduce confusion, improve postoperative pain, and reduce complications. Many of these protocols include optimal use of parenteral analgesia, operative approach, early mobilization and progression of diet, removal of lines and catheters as soon as appropriate, and planning for discharge. Early adopters were colorectal surgeons, but nearly every surgical specialty has some form of ERAS program either published or underway. Key to successful ERAS implementation in an institution is leadership support, multidisciplinary team involvement, and a commitment to audits, assessment and, reiteration of ERAS protocols as new data develop.

THE INTERMEDIATE POSTOPERATIVE PERIOD

The intermediate phase begins with complete recovery from anesthesia and lasts for the rest of the hospital stay. During this time, the patient recovers most basic functions and becomes self-sufficient and ready to continue convalescence at home. Transfer from the PACU/SICU to a less monitored setting usually occurs at the start of this period. Communication within the care team is important during this transition; this team can include surgeons; nurses; nutritionists; social workers and case managers; respiratory, physical, and occupational therapists; residents; and consulting physicians. Isolation and specialized management of patients colonized or infected with drug-resistant organisms or highly contagious infectious agents continues from the OR through the stay in the PACU and then, with appropriate barrier devices and room determination, throughout the hospital stay. Nursing staff and patient care managers should be included early on to be certain that patients know when they may be ready for discharge and their disposition is planned (discharge to home, plan for travel home, discharge to a subacute nursing facility, etc). The earlier the plan is in place, the earlier the care team can get the plan on track.

▶ Care of the Wound

Within hours after a wound is closed, the wound space fills with an inflammatory exudate. Epidermal cells at the edges of the wound begin to divide and migrate across the wound surface. By 48 hours after closure, deeper structures are completely sealed off from the external environment. Sterile dressings applied in the operating room provide protection during this period.

Removal of the dressing and handling of the wound during the first 24 hours should be done with aseptic technique. Medical personnel should wash their hands before and after caring for any surgical wound. Gloves should always be used when there is contact with open wounds or fresh wounds.

Dressings over closed wounds should be removed by the third or fourth postoperative day. If the wound is dry, dressings need not be reapplied; this simplifies periodic inspection. Dressings should be removed earlier if they are wet or placed in a contaminated setting, because soaked dressings increase bacterial contamination of the wound. Dressings should also be removed if the patient has new manifestations of infection (such as fever or increasing wound pain). The wound should then be inspected and the adjacent area gently compressed. Any drainage from the wound should be examined by culture and Gram-stained smear.

Vacuum dressings should usually be replaced within 24-72 hours. Pain management around the time of dressing change is important to consider, as proper prophylaxis can make the procedure less difficult for both the patient and the surgical team.

Generally, skin sutures or skin staples may be removed by the fifth postoperative day and replaced by tapes. Sutures should be left in longer (eg, for 2 weeks) for incisions that cross creases (as in the groin or popliteal area), for incisions closed under tension, for some incisions in the extremities (eg, the hand), and for incisions of any kind in debilitated patients. Sutures should be removed if suture tracts show signs of infection. If the incision is healing normally, the patient may be allowed to shower or bathe by the seventh postoperative day (and often sooner, depending on the incision).

Glue or other dermal bonding may be used in lieu of traditional gauze dressings, and should usually be left in place without removal after surgery until the appropriate postoperative visit. Most of these bonding products still allow for showering and light use of soap around the area. Patients should be cautioned to avoid use of lotions, creams, antiseptic or antibiotic ointment, or any other mechanical scrubbing to avoid removing or dissolving the dressing.

Patients with ostomies should have careful wound care and be instructed in the care of their ostomy. Ideally, an ostomy nurse can assist both in the hospital and after discharge. The skin surrounding an ostomy should be pristinely prepared for appliance placement, and proper appliance placement can avoid skin erosion or injury to the new or revised stoma. Here is another area where preoperative preparation can mean the difference between an ostomy that was marked for ideal placement where the patient can view and care for it, and an ostomy that sits deep within a fold and cannot be pouched or cared for without difficulty. The patient also may need psychologic preparation for their ostomy, whether it will be temporary or permanent, and to have supplies in place at home for care.

▶ Management of Drains

Drains are used either to prevent or to treat an unwanted accumulation of fluid such as pus, blood, or serum. Drains are also used to evacuate air from the pleural cavity so that the lungs can reexpand. When used prophylactically, drains are usually placed in a sterile location. Strict precautions must be taken to prevent bacteria from entering the body through the drainage tract in these situations. The external portion of the drain must be handled with aseptic technique, and the drain must be removed as soon as it is no longer useful. When drains have been placed in an infected area, there is a smaller risk of retrograde infection of the peritoneal cavity, since the infected area is usually walled off. Drains should usually be brought out through a separate incision, because drains through the operative wound increase the risk of wound infection. Closed drains connected to suction devices (Jackson–Pratt or Blake drains are two examples) are preferable to open drains (such as Penrose) that predispose to wound contamination. The quantity and quality of drainage should be recorded and contamination minimized. When drains are no longer needed, they may be withdrawn entirely at one time if there has been little or no drainage, or may be progressively withdrawn over a period of a few days.

Sump drains (such as Davol drains) have an airflow system that keeps the lumen of the drain open when fluid is not passing through it, and they must be attached to a continuous suction device. Sump drains are especially useful when the amount of drainage is large or when drainage is likely to plug other kinds of drains. Some sump drains have an extra lumen through which saline solution can be infused to aid in keeping the tube clear. After infection has been controlled and the discharge is no longer purulent, the large-bore catheter may be progressively replaced with smaller catheters as the cavity closes.

Drains that have clot or thick material within them or that have lost their drainage capacity can be stripped or flushed to restore function; this should be performed only under the supervision and approval of the attending surgeon, as doing so could disrupt the operative bed in some circumstances.

▶ Postoperative Pulmonary Care

The changes in pulmonary function observed following anesthesia and surgery are principally the result of decreased vital capacity, functional residual capacity (FRC), and pulmonary edema. Vital capacity decreases to about 40% of the preoperative level within 1-4 hours after major intra-abdominal surgery. It remains at this level for 12-14 hours, slowly increases to 60%-70% of the preoperative value by 7 days, and returns to the baseline level during the ensuing week. FRC is affected to a lesser extent. Immediately after surgery, FRC is near the preoperative level, but by 24 hours postoperatively it has decreased to about 70% of the preoperative level. It remains depressed for several days and then gradually returns to its preoperative value by the tenth day. These changes are accentuated in patients who are obese, smoke heavily, or have preexisting lung disease. Elderly patients are particularly vulnerable because they have decreased compliance, increased closing volume, increased residual volume, and increased dead space, all of which enhance the risk of postoperative atelectasis. In addition, reduced forced expiratory volume in 1 second (FEV1) impairs the aged patient's ability to clear secretions and increases the chance of infection postoperatively.

The postoperative decrease in FRC is caused by a breathing pattern consisting of shallow tidal breaths without periodic maximal inflation. Normal human respiration includes inspiration to total lung capacity several times each hour. If these maximal inflations are eliminated, alveolar collapse begins to occur within a few hours, and atelectasis with transpulmonary shunting is evident shortly thereafter. Pain is thought to be one of the main causes of shallow breathing postoperatively. Complete abolition of pain, however, does not completely restore pulmonary function. Neural reflexes, abdominal distention, obesity, and other factors that limit diaphragmatic excursion appear to be as important.

The principal means of minimizing atelectasis is deep inspiration and cough. Periodic hyperinflation can be facilitated by using an incentive spirometer. This is particularly useful in patients with a higher risk of pulmonary complications (eg, elderly, debilitated, or markedly obese patients). Early mobilization, encouragement to take deep breaths (especially when standing), and good coaching by the nursing staff suffice for most patients.

Postoperative pulmonary edema is caused by high hydrostatic pressures (due to left-ventricular failure, fluid overload, decreased oncotic pressure, etc), increased capillary permeability, or both. Edema of the lung parenchyma narrows small bronchi and increases resistance in the pulmonary vasculature. In addition, pulmonary edema may increase the risk of pulmonary infection. Adequate management of fluids postoperatively and early treatment of cardiac failure are important preventive measures.

Systemic sepsis increases capillary permeability and can lead to pulmonary edema. In the absence of deranged cardiac function or fluid overload, the development of pulmonary edema postoperatively should be regarded as evidence of sepsis. Signs and symptoms of pulmonary complications include fever, tachypnea, tachycardia, and an alteration in mental status. Development of atrial fibrillation or an abnormal cardiac rhythm can often precede identification of pulmonary complications.

Patients who smoked tobacco up until the time of surgery should be considered at higher risk for postoperative pulmonary complications. Symptoms of withdrawal from nicotine can be managed with a nicotine patch or gum.

Many patients undergoing surgery are offered vaccination against pneumococcal or influenza infection during their hospital stay; these should be considered where there are no contraindications.

RESPIRATORY FAILURE

Most patients tolerate the postoperative changes in pulmonary function described above and recover from them without difficulty. Patients who have marginal preoperative pulmonary function may be unable to maintain adequate ventilation in the immediate postoperative period and may develop respiratory failure. In these patients, the operative trauma and the effects of anesthesia reduce respiratory reserve below levels that can provide adequate gas exchange. In contrast to acute respiratory distress syndrome (see Chapter 12), early postoperative respiratory failure (which develops within 48 hours after the operation) is usually only a mechanical problem; that is, there are minimal alterations of the lung parenchyma. However, this problem is life threatening and requires immediate attention.

Early respiratory failure develops most commonly in association with major operations (especially on the chest or upper abdomen), severe trauma, and preexisting lung disease. In most of these patients, respiratory failure develops over a short period (minutes to 1-2 hours) without evidence of a precipitating cause. By contrast, late postoperative respiratory failure (which develops beyond 48 hours after the operation) is usually triggered by an intercurrent event such as pulmonary embolism, abdominal distention, or opioid overdose.

Respiratory failure is manifested by tachypnea of 25-30 breaths per minute with a low tidal volume of less than 4 mL/kg. Laboratory indications are acute elevation of P_{CO_2} above 45 mm Hg, depression of P_{O_2} below 60 mm Hg, or evidence of low cardiac output. Treatment consists of immediate endotracheal intubation and ventilatory support to ensure adequate alveolar ventilation. As soon as the patient is intubated, it is important to determine whether there are any associated pulmonary problems such as atelectasis, pneumonia, or pneumothorax that require immediate treatment.

Prevention of respiratory failure requires careful postoperative pulmonary care. Atelectasis must be minimized using the techniques described above. Patients with preexisting pulmonary disease must be hydrated carefully to avoid hypovolemia or hypervolemia. These patients must hyperventilate in order to compensate for the inefficiency of the lungs. This extra work causes greater evaporation of water and dehydration. Hypovolemia leads to dry secretions and thick sputum, which are difficult to clear from the airway. High fraction of inspired oxygen (F_{IO_2}) in these patients removes the stabilizing gas nitrogen from the alveoli, predisposing to alveolar collapse. In addition, it may impair the function of the respiratory center, which is driven by the relative hypoxemia, and thus further decrease ventilation. The use of epidural blocks or other methods of local analgesia in patients with chronic obstructive pulmonary disease (COPD) may prevent respiratory failure by relieving pain and permitting effective respiratory muscle function.

Postoperative Fluid & Electrolyte Management

Postoperative fluid replacement should be based on the following considerations: (1) maintenance requirements, (2) extra needs resulting from systemic factors (eg, fever, burns, loss during surgery), (3) losses from drains, and (4) requirements resulting from tissue edema and ileus (third-space losses). Daily maintenance requirements for sensible and insensible loss in the adult are about 1500-2500 mL depending on the patient's age, gender, weight, and body surface area. A rough estimate can be obtained by multiplying the patient's weight in kilograms times 30 (eg, 1800 mL/24 h in a 60-kg patient). Maintenance requirements are increased by fever, hyperventilation, and conditions that increase the catabolic rate.

For patients requiring intravenous fluid replacement for a short period (most postoperative patients), it is not necessary to measure serum electrolytes at any time during the postoperative period, but measurement is indicated in patients with extra fluid losses, sepsis, preexisting electrolyte abnormalities, renal insufficiency, or other factors. Assessment of the status of fluid balance requires accurate records of fluid intake and output and is aided by obtaining the patient's body weight prior to surgery and weighing the patient daily.

As a rule, 2000-2500 mL of 5% dextrose in normal saline or in lactated Ringer solution is delivered daily (Table 4–1). Potassium should usually not be added during the first 24 hours after surgery, because increased amounts of potassium enter the circulation during this time as a result of operative trauma and increased aldosterone activity.

In most patients, fluid loss through a nasogastric tube is less than 500 mL/d, and can be replaced by increasing the infusion used for maintenance by a similar amount. About 20 mEq of potassium should be added to every liter of fluid used to replace these losses. However, with the exception of urine, body fluids are isosmolar, and if large volumes of gastric or intestinal juice are replaced with normal saline

solution, electrolyte imbalance will eventually result. Whenever external losses from any site amount to 1500 mL/d or more, electrolyte concentrations in the fluid should be measured periodically, and the amount of replacement fluids should be adjusted to equal the amount lost. Table 4–1 lists the compositions of the most frequently used solutions.

Losses that result from fluid sequestration at the operative site are usually adequately replaced during the operation, but in a patient with a large retroperitoneal dissection, severe pancreatitis, etc, third-space losses may be substantial and should be considered when postoperative fluid needs are assessed.

Fluid requirements must be evaluated frequently. Intravenous orders should be evaluated every 24 hours or more often if indicated by special circumstances. Following an extensive operation, fluid needs on the first day should be reevaluated every 4-6 hours. Potassium administration can be added to the intravenous infusion only if the patient has good urine flow, has a demonstrated deficiency after significant pathologic fluid losses, and is not anticipated to start enteral feedings shortly. Postoperative ionized serum calcium in patients who have undergone thyroid or parathyroid surgery should be monitored and replaced as per the operating surgeon.

Postoperative Care of the Gastrointestinal Tract

Following laparotomy, gastrointestinal peristalsis temporarily decreases. Peristalsis returns in the small intestine within 24 hours, but gastric peristalsis may return more slowly. Function returns in the right colon by 48 hours and in the left colon by 72 hours. After operations on the stomach and upper intestine, propulsive activity of the upper gut can remain disorganized for 3-4 days. In the immediate postoperative period, the stomach may be decompressed with a nasogastric tube. Nasogastric intubation was once used in almost all patients undergoing laparotomy to avoid gastric

Table 4–1. Composition of frequently used intravenous solutions.

Solution	Glucose (g/dL)	Na$^+$ (mEq/L)	Cl (mEq/L)	HCO$_3$ (mEq/L)	K$^+$ (mEq/L)
Dextrose 5% in water	50	...	...	...	...
Dextrose 5% and sodium chloride 0.45%	50	77	77	...	...
Sodium chloride 0.9%	...	154	154	...	...
Sodium chloride 0.45%	...	77	77	...	...
Lactated Ringer solution	...	130	109	28	4
Sodium chloride 3%	...	513	513	...	...

distention and vomiting, but it is now recognized that routine nasogastric intubation is unnecessary and may contribute to the occurrence of postoperative atelectasis and pneumonia. For example, following cholecystectomy, pelvic operations, and colonic resections, nasogastric intubation is not needed in the average patient, and it is probably of marginal benefit following operations on the small bowel. On the other hand, nasogastric intubation is probably useful after esophageal and gastric resections and should always be used in patients with marked ileus or a very low level of consciousness (to avoid aspiration) and in patients who manifest acute gastric distention or vomiting postoperatively.

The nasogastric tube should be connected to low intermittent suction and assessed frequently to ensure patency. The tube should be left in place for 2-3 days or until there is evidence that normal peristalsis has returned (eg, return of appetite, audible peristalsis, or passage of flatus). Suture placement is usually unnecessary, but careful placement of the tube and tape fixation in a natural curve can enable the patient to move their head without risk of inadvertent removal. The nasogastric tube enhances gastroesophageal reflux, and if it is clamped for a period to assess residual volume, there is a slight risk of aspiration. Most tubes are used as a "sump" where one port is for suction and the other left open to air to allow for continuous flow. This sump port should not be clamped, tied, or flushed with saline unless clogged with material.

Once the nasogastric tube has been withdrawn, fasting is usually continued for another 24 hours, and the patient is then started on a liquid diet. Opioids may interfere with gastric motility and should be limited if possible for patients who have slow gastric emptying beyond the first postoperative week. Routine use of promotility agents or chewing gum has not demonstrated benefit in terms of quicker return to GI function.

Gastrostomy and jejunostomy tubes should be connected to low intermittent suction or dependent drainage for the first 24 hours after surgery. Absorption of nutrients and fluids by the small intestine is not affected by laparotomy, and enteral nutrition through a jejunostomy feeding tube may be started on the second postoperative day even if motility is not entirely normal. Gastrostomy or jejunostomy tubes should not be removed before the third postoperative week once firm adhesions have developed between the viscera and the parietal peritoneum. The length of tube from its point of entry into the abdominal cavity should be measured and similar between the time of insertion and the time of use; dislodgement of the tubes can be catastrophic if unrecognized before use. Any pills or medication used through the tube should be crushed (and crushable) and flushed carefully to ensure that the tube is not clogged and rendered unusable.

After most operations in areas other than the peritoneal cavity, the patient may be allowed to resume a regular diet as soon as the effects of anesthesia have completely resolved. Short-term use of parenteral nutrition in patients with good preoperative nitrogen balance and caloric intake is ill-advised; patients with preoperative catabolic states may benefit from longer-term nutritional support.

Identification & Management of Perioperative Hyperglycemia

Patients should be assessed at admission for history of diabetes and should undergo blood glucose testing on admission. Point-of-care assessment should be made in cases of elevated blood glucose for patients with known diabetes regarding monitoring, testing schedules, and glycemic targets to allow for careful coordination of blood glucose control and return to reinstitution of preadmission regimens. For patients not previously known to have diabetes or those who may have new glucocorticoid- or surgery-induced diabetes, discharge planning may need to include management of this new diagnosis. There is a well-established link between perioperative hyperglycemia and adverse outcomes, which can be improved by treatment.

TRANSFUSION THERAPY

Determination of the need for transfusion and what type of transfusion is necessary can do much to improve patient outcome, or can obfuscate a complication when performed without consideration of the underlying etiology of the patient's need. Knowledge of the patient's preoperative status, the course of the operation and any complications, and proper preparation for potential complications should help the physician who is considering transfusion. Restrictive transfusion thresholds may minimize patient exposure to adverse outcomes. Ultimately, the attending surgeon should determine the need for transfusion, as patients can have deficits even when laboratory values appear transiently normal.

Whole Blood

Whole blood is composed of 450-500 mL of donor blood, containing Red blood cells (RBCs) (hematocrit, 35%-45%), plasma, clotting factors (reduced levels of labile factors V and VIII), and anticoagulant. Platelets and granulocytes are not functional. It is indicated for red cell replacement in massive blood loss with pronounced hypovolemia. However, whole blood for transfusion is not routinely available.

Red Blood Cells

RBCs are obtained by apheresis collection or prepared from whole blood by centrifugation and removal of plasma, followed by supplementation with 100 mL of adenine-containing red cell nutrient solution. The hematocrit is 55%-60%, and the volume is 300-350 mL. RBCs collected in CPDA-1 anticoagulant have a hematocrit of 65%-80% and a storage volume of 250-300 mL. RBC transfusions are indicated to increase oxygen-carrying capacity in anemic patients. Hemoglobin levels of 7-9 g/dL are well tolerated by most asymptomatic patients. A transfusion trigger of 7 g/dL is commonly used in most stable patients. Symptomatic patients with cardiac, pulmonary, or cerebrovascular disease may require RBC transfusions to achieve higher hemoglobin levels. In a nonbleeding 70-kg recipient, transfusion of 1 unit of RBCs should increase hemoglobin level by 1 g/dL and the hematocrit by 3%. Patients can donate autologous blood in the month before surgery when appropriate; directed donors do not necessarily reduce the risk of transfusion or transfusion reaction.

Washed Red Blood Cells

RBCs are washed with saline to remove more than 98% of plasma proteins and resuspended in approximately 180 mL of saline, at an approximate hematocrit of 75%. Anemic patients with recurrent or severe allergic reactions benefit from washed RBCs. Patients with severe IgA deficiency who test positive for anti-IgA antibodies should receive RBCs washed with 2-3 L of saline or receive blood collected from IgA-deficient donors.

Leukocyte-Reduced Red Blood Cells

Third-generation leukocyte reduction filters remove more than 99.9% of the contaminating leukocytes, leaving less than 5×10^6 white blood cells per unit. Filtration done soon after collection (prestorage leukoreduction) is more effective than bedside filtration. Patients experiencing recurrent febrile nonhemolytic transfusion reactions (FNHTRs) to RBCs or platelets should receive leukocyte-reduced products. The prophylactic use of leukoreduced RBCs and platelets in patients with long-term transfusion needs decreases the likelihood of human leukocyte antigens (HLA) alloimmunization and protects from immune platelet refractoriness and recurrent FNHTRs. Leukoreduction also decreases the risk of transmission of cytomegalovirus (CMV) infection in immunosuppressed CMV-seronegative patients.

Irradiated Red Blood Cells

RBCs are irradiated with 25 Gy of gamma irradiation. All cellular products should be irradiated for patients who are at risk for transfusion-associated graft versus host disease (TA-GVHD). Adult patients at risk for TA-GVHD include, but are not limited to, those with congenital severe immunodeficiency, hematologic malignancy receiving intensive chemoradiotherapy, Hodgkin and non-Hodgkin lymphoma, certain solid tumors (neuroblastoma and sarcoma), peripheral blood stem-cell and marrow transplants, recipients of fludarabine-based chemotherapy, and those receiving directed donations from blood relatives or HLA-matched platelets. Acellular products such as fresh frozen plasma (FFP) and cryoprecipitate are not irradiated. Leukoreduction is not an acceptable substitute for irradiation.

Frozen-Deglycerolized Red Blood Cells

RBCs frozen in glycerol are washed extensively in normal saline to remove the cryoprotectant and then resuspended in saline at a hematocrit of approximately 75%. More than 99.9% of the plasma is removed, and few leukocytes remain in the product. Patients who are alloimmunized to multiple antigens or those with antibodies against high-frequency antigens are supported with blood collected from donors with rare phenotypes. Most patients with severe IgA deficiency can safely receive RBCs washed with 2 L or more of saline. Frozen-deglycerolized RBCs are an equally safe and effective, albeit more cumbersome, alternative for these patients. Rarely, patients may require RBCs collected from IgA-deficient donors. A national rare donor program facilitates the collection and storage of rare blood types.

Platelets

Apheresis platelets are collected from single donors by apheresis and contain at least 3×10^{11} platelets in 250-300 mL plasma. Random-donor platelets (RDP) are platelet concentrates prepared from whole blood and contain 5.5×10^{10} platelets suspended in approximately 50 mL of plasma. Five to six units of RDP are pooled into a single pack to provide an adult dose. Platelet transfusions are indicated for the management of active bleeding in thrombocytopenic patients. Nonthrombocytopenic patients with congenital or acquired disorders of platelet function may also require platelets to stop bleeding. Platelet transfusions are also indicated prophylactically in patients requiring line placement or minor surgery when the platelet counts are less than 50,000/μL and in patients undergoing major surgical procedures when the count falls below 50-75,000/μL. Patients scheduled for ophthalmic, upper airway, or neurosurgical procedures should have platelet counts above 100,000/μL. Platelets are not usually recommended for the correction of thrombocytopenia in patients with heparin-induced thrombocytopenia (HIT), type IIB von Willebrand disease (vWD), idiopathic thrombocytopenic purpura (ITP), or thrombotic thrombocytopenic purpura (TTP). The clinical indications for the use of washed, irradiated, and leukoreduced platelets are analogous to those described in the section on RBCs. Patients with platelet refractoriness secondary to HLA alloimmunization should be supported with HLA-matched platelets.

Fresh Frozen Plasma

Fresh frozen plasma (FFP) is obtained by apheresis or prepared by centrifugation of whole blood and frozen within 8 hours of collection. It contains normal levels of all clotting factors, albumin, and fibrinogen. FFP is indicated for the replacement of coagulation factors in patients with deficiencies of multiple clotting factors as occurs in the coagulopathy of liver disease, disseminated intravascular coagulation (DIC), warfarin overdose, and massive transfusions. One milliliter of FFP contains one unit of coagulation factor activity; soon after the infusion of a 10-15 mL/kg dose, the activity of all coagulation factors is increased by 20%-30%. Coagulation tests should be monitored to determine efficacy and appropriate dosing intervals. FFP should be used only if the international normalized ratio (INR) is greater than 1.5 or the prothrombin time/activated partial thromboplastin time (PT/aPTT) are elevated more than 1.5 times the normal. Patients with liver disease who have minimally altered PT/aPTT and nominal bleeding should initially be managed with vitamin K replacement. Similarly, most patients with warfarin overdose can be managed by stopping warfarin for 48 hours and monitoring coagulation tests until they return to baseline levels. FFP is indicated only for active bleeding or if there is a risk for bleeding from an emergent procedure. FFP is the only replacement product currently available for patients with rare disorders such as isolated factor deficiencies (V, X, XI) or C-1 esterase inhibitor deficiency. Patients with severe IgA deficiency should be supported with IgA-deficient plasma. FFP is the first choice for fluid replacement in patients with TTP undergoing therapeutic plasma exchange. FFP is not indicated for volume replacement, nutritional support, or replacement of immunoglobulins.

Cryoprecipitate

Cryoprecipitate is the cold-insoluble precipitate formed when FFP is thawed at 1-6°C. This is then resuspended in 10-15 mL plasma. It contains 150 mg or more of fibrinogen, 80 IU or more of factor VIII, 40%-70% of vWF and 20%-30% of factor XIII present in the initial unit of FFP, and 30-60 mg of fibronectin. Each unit (bag) of cryoprecipitate increases fibrinogen level by 5-10 mg/dL. Eight to 10 bags are pooled and infused as a single dose in a 70-kg adult. Cryoprecipitate is indicated for the correction of hypofibrinogenemia in dilutional coagulopathy and the hypofibrinogenemia/dysfibrinogenemias of liver disease and DIC. Cryoprecipitate improves platelet aggregation and adhesion and decreases bleeding in uremic patients. It has been used for the correction of factor XIII deficiency, and it is the source of fibrinogen in the two-component fibrin sealant (Tisseel). Cryoprecipitate is no longer used to treat patients with hemophilia A or vWD.

Granulocyte Transfusions

Granulocytes are collected by leukapheresis from donors stimulated with granulocyte colony-stimulating factor (G-CSF) and steroids to mobilize neutrophils from the marrow storage pool into peripheral blood. On average they contain 1×10^{10} or more granulocytes suspended in 200-300 mL plasma. About 1-3×10^{11} platelets and 10-30 mL RBCs are also present in the product. Granulocyte transfusions are indicated in severely neutropenic (absolute neutrophil count $< 0.5 \times 10^3/\mu L$) patients with bacterial sepsis who have not responded to optimum antibiotic therapy after 48-72 hours, provided there is a reasonable expectation of recovery of bone marrow function. Transfusions are given daily until clinical improvement or neutrophil recovery occurs.

Erythropoietin-Stimulating Agents & Other Blood Substitutes

Routine use of erythropoietin stimulating agents for patients undergoing surgery is not recommended. Selective use in patients with anemia undergoing major elective surgery is under investigation. Likewise, the effectiveness of recombinant human factor VIIa and other coagulation factor replacement for routine prophylactic use in general surgery in patients without hemophilia remains unproven.

Postoperative Pain

Severe pain is a common sequela of intrathoracic, intra-abdominal, and major bone or joint procedures. About 60% of such patients perceive their pain to be severe, 25% moderate, and 15% mild. In contrast, following superficial operations on the head and neck, limbs, or abdominal wall, less than 15% of patients characterize their pain as severe. The factors responsible for these differences include duration of operation, degree of operative trauma, type of incision, and magnitude of intraoperative retraction. Gentle handling of tissues, expedient operations, and good muscle relaxation help lessen the severity of postoperative pain. Objective measures of pain remain elusive.

Although factors related to the nature of the operation influence postoperative pain, it is also true that the same operation produces different amounts of pain in different patients. This varies according to individual physical, emotional, and cultural characteristics. Much of the emotional aspect of pain can be traced to anxiety. Feelings such as helplessness, fear, and uncertainty contribute to anxiety and may heighten the patient's perception of pain.

It was once thought that anesthesia and analgesia in neonates and infants were too risky, and that these young patients did not perceive pain. It is now known that reduction of pain with appropriate techniques actually decreases morbidity from major surgery in this age group.

The physiology of postoperative pain involves transmission of pain impulses via splanchnic (not vagal) afferent fibers to the central nervous system, where they initiate spinal, brainstem, and cortical reflexes. Spinal responses result from stimulation of neurons in the anterior horn, resulting in skeletal muscle spasm, vasospasm, and gastrointestinal ileus. Brainstem responses to pain include alterations in ventilation, blood pressure, and endocrine function. Cortical responses include voluntary movements and psychologic changes, such as fear and apprehension. These emotional responses facilitate nociceptive spinal transmission, lower the threshold for pain perception, and perpetuate the pain experience.

Postoperative pain serves no useful purpose and may cause alterations in pulmonary, circulatory, gastrointestinal, and skeletal muscle function that contribute to postoperative complications. Pain following thoracic and upper abdominal operations, for example, causes voluntary and involuntary splinting of thoracic and abdominal muscles and the diaphragm. The patient may be reluctant to breathe deeply, promoting atelectasis. The limitation in motion due to pain predisposes to venous stasis, thrombosis, and embolism. Release of catecholamines and other stress hormones by postoperative pain causes vasospasm and hypertension, which may in turn lead to complications such as stroke, myocardial infarction, and bleeding. Prevention of postoperative pain is thus important for reasons other than the pain itself. Effective pain control may improve the outcome of major operations.

A. Communication

Close attention to the patient's needs, frequent reassurance, and genuine concern help to minimize postoperative pain. Spending a few minutes with the patient every day in frank discussions of progress and any complications does more to relieve pain than many physicians realize. Patients with preoperative drug and substance abuse still have postoperative pain needs and may require more medication than others. Communication among the patient care team can help in the understanding of specific pain-control needs.

B. Parenteral Opioids

Opioids are the mainstay of therapy for postoperative pain. Their analgesic effect is via two mechanisms: (1) a direct effect on opioid receptors and (2) stimulation of a descending brainstem system that contributes to pain inhibition. Although substantial relief of pain may be achieved with opioids, they do not modify reflex phenomena associated with pain, such as muscle spasm. Opioids administered intramuscularly, while convenient, result in wide variations in plasma concentrations. This, as well as the wide variations in dosage required for analgesia among patients, reduces analgesic efficacy. Physician and nurse attitudes reflect a persistent misunderstanding of the pharmacology and psychology of pain control. Frequently, the dose of opioid prescribed or administered is too small and too infrequent. When opioid usage is limited to temporary treatment of postoperative pain, drug addiction is extremely rare.

Morphine is the most widely used opioid for treatment of postoperative pain. Morphine may be administered intravenously, either intermittently or continuously. Except as discussed below in the section on patient-controlled analgesia (PCA), continuous intravenous administration requires close supervision and is impractical except in the PACU or intensive care unit. Side effects of morphine include respiratory depression, nausea and vomiting, and clouded sensorium. In the setting of severe postoperative pain, however, respiratory depression is rare, because pain itself is a powerful respiratory stimulant.

Meperidine is an opioid with about one-eighth the potency of morphine. It provides a similar quality of pain control with similar side effects. The duration of pain relief is somewhat shorter than with morphine. Like morphine, meperidine may be given intravenously, but the same requirements for monitoring apply.

Other opioids useful for postoperative analgesia include hydromorphone and methadone. Hydromorphone is usually administered in a dose of 1-2 mg intramuscularly every 2-3 hours. Methadone is given intramuscularly or orally in an average dose of 10 mg every 4-6 hours. The main advantage of methadone is its long half-life (6-10 hours) and its ability to prevent withdrawal symptoms in patients with morphine dependence. Patients who use methadone preoperatively should be continued postoperatively on their usual dose to avoid withdrawal; most clinics maintain records on their patients and should be consulted to confirm the appropriate replacement.

C. Nonopioid Parenteral Analgesics

Ketorolac tromethamine is a nonsteroidal antiinflammatory drug (NSAID) with potent analgesic and moderate antiinflammatory activities. It is available in injectable form suitable for postoperative use. In controlled trials, ketorolac (30 mg) demonstrated analgesic efficacy roughly equivalent to that of morphine (10 mg). A potential advantage over morphine is its lack of respiratory depression. Gastrointestinal ulceration, impaired coagulation, and reduced renal function—all potential complications of NSAID use—have not yet been reported with short-term perioperative use of ketorolac.

D. Oral Analgesics

Within several days following most abdominal surgical procedures, the severity of pain decreases and oral analgesics suffice for control. Aspirin is often avoided as an analgesic postoperatively, since it interferes with platelet function, prolongs bleeding time, and interferes with the effects of anticoagulants; however, in some settings aspirin is used to diminish the risk of cardiovascular complications by these mechanisms. For most patients, a combination of acetaminophen with codeine (eg, Tylenol No. 3) or propoxyphene (Darvocet-N 50 or -N 100) suffices. Hydrocodone with acetaminophen (Vicodin) is a synthetic opioid with properties similar to those of codeine. For more severe pain, oxycodone is available in combination with aspirin (Percodan) or acetaminophen (Percocet, Tylox). Oxycodone is an opioid with slightly less potency than morphine. As with all opioids, tolerance develops with long-term use.

E. Patient-Controlled Analgesia

Patient-controlled analgesia (PCA) puts the frequency of analgesic administration under the patient's control but within safe limits. A device containing a timing unit, a pump, and the analgesic medication is connected to an intravenous line. By pressing a button, the patient delivers a predetermined dose of analgesic (usually morphine, 1-3 mg). The timing unit prevents over dosage by interposing an inactivation period (usually 6-8 minutes) between patient-initiated doses. The possibility of over dosage is also limited by the fact that the patient must be awake in order to search for and push the button that delivers the morphine. The dose and timing can be changed by medical personnel to accommodate the needs of the patient. This method appears to improve pain control and even reduces the total dose of opioid given in a 24-hour period. The addition of a background continuous infusion to the patient-directed administration of analgesic appears to offer no advantage over PCA alone.

F. Continuous Epidural Analgesia

Opioids are also effective when administered directly into the epidural space. Topical morphine does not depress proprioceptive pathways in the dorsal horn, but it does affect nociceptive pathways by interacting with opioid receptors. Therefore, epidural opioids produce intense, prolonged, segmental analgesia with relatively less respiratory depression or sympathetic, motor, or other sensory disturbances. In comparison with parenteral administration, epidural administration requires similar dosage for control of pain, has a slightly delayed onset of action, provides substantially longer pain relief, and is associated with better preservation of pulmonary function. Epidural morphine is usually administered as a continuous infusion at a rate of 0.2-0.8 mg/h with or without the addition of 0.25% bupivacaine. Analgesia produced by this technique is superior to that of intravenous or intramuscular opioids. Patients managed in this way are more alert and have better gastrointestinal function. Side effects of continuous epidural administration of morphine include pruritus, nausea, and urinary retention. Respiratory depression may occur.

G. Intercostal Block

Intercostal block may be used to decrease pain following thoracic and abdominal operations. Since the block does not include the visceral afferent nerve fibers, it does not relieve pain completely, but it does eliminate muscle spasm induced by cutaneous pain and helps to restore respiratory function. It does not carry the risk of hypotension—as does continuous epidural analgesia—and it produces analgesia for periods of 3-12 hours. The main disadvantage of intercostal blocks is the risk of pneumothorax and the need for repeated injections. These problems can be minimized by placing a catheter in the intercostal space or in the pleura through which a continuous infusion of bupivacaine 0.5% is delivered at a rate of 3-8 mL/h.

H. Direct Infiltration

Direct administration of a combination of short- and long-acting local anesthetics can help significantly in management of postoperative pain in a variety of settings. Optimally, wound infiltration or local nerve block should occur following the induction of intravenous anesthesia and prior to skin incision but may still be beneficial after incision.

▶ Special Considerations

Patients at the extreme of ages, who underwent acute/emergency surgery or had a poor preoperative functional and nutritional status, require special postoperative consideration.

Infants and children can be both more easily taken out of equilibrium and yet can return to health more quickly. Reassessment should occur more frequently with calculation of fluid needs tailored to their body surface area and losses. The nursing ratio is expected to be higher for more critically ill children. Elderly patients tend to have more complex preoperative medical issues, require a careful preoperative functional assessment of their nutritional reserve, and may have a more sensitive response to sedatives and other medications with a prolonged return to full mental function. Careful attention to even small changes in status should trigger thoughtful appraisal of the patient. Cognitive modalities and transcutaneous electrical nerve stimulation (TENS) units may offer additional benefits in patients with chronic pain or those who are expected to have long-lasting pain symptomatology.

THE CONVALESCENT PHASE

Determination and planning for discharge should start even before the operation and should be modified accordingly. It is not uncommon for patients to be discharged to a setting other than home; emergency or acute care surgery is more likely to lend itself to a change in disposition of the patient. Plans should be made early for home assistance in the activities of daily living and in assisting recovery from surgery including education on the care of ostomies, new tubes/drains, and intravenous or intramuscular medications.

Daily rounds should include a plan for discontinuation of drains, supplemental oxygen, nasogastric tubes, indwelling urinary catheters, medications including antibiotics, and the need for ongoing antithrombotic therapy. Transition of medication to the oral route where possible should occur early; otherwise, preparation for home administration of IV or SQ/IM medication should be made.

BIBLIOGRAPHY

▷ Postoperative Outcomes

Cronin J, Livhits M, Mercado C, et al. Quality improvement pilot program for vulnerable elderly surgical patients. *Am Surg.* 2011;77(10):1305-1308.
Guillamondegui OD, Gunter OL, Hines L, et al. Using the National Surgical Quality Improvement Program and the Tennessee Surgical Quality Collaborative to improve surgical outcomes. *J Am Coll Surg.* 2012;214(4):709-714; discussion 714-716.
Ingraham AM, Richards KE, Hall BL, Ko CY. Quality Improvement in Surgery: The American College of Surgeons National Surgical Quality Improvement Program Approach. *Adv Surg.* 2010;44:251-267.
Ljungqvist OL, Scott M, Fearon KC. Enhanced recovery after surgery: A review. *JAMA Surg.* 2016;152(3):292-298.
Vonlanthen R, Slankamenac K, Breitenstein S, et al. The impact of complications on costs of major surgical procedures. *Ann Surg.* 2011;254:907-913.

▷ Fluid Therapy

Myles PS, Andrews S, Nicholson J, Lobo DN, Mythen M. Contemporary approaches to perioperative IV therapy. *World J Surg.* 2017;41(10):2457-2463.

▷ Transfusion Therapy

American Association of Blood Banks. *Technical Manual*, 18th ed. Bethesda: AABB; 2014.
American Society of Anesthesiologists Task Force on Perioperative Blood Transfusion and Adjuvant Therapies. Practice Guidelines for Perioperative Blood Management. *Anesthesiology.* 2015; 122(2):241-275.
Carson JL, Grossman BJ, Kleinman S, et al; Clinical Transfusion Medicine Committee of the AABB. Red blood cell transfusion: A clinical practice guideline from the AABB. *Ann Intern Med.* 2012;157(1):49-58.
Society of Thoracic Surgeons Blood Conservation Guideline Task Force; Ferraris VA, Brown JR, Despotis GJ, et al; Society of Cardiovascular Anesthesiologists Special Task Force on Blood Transfusion; Shore-Lesserson LJ, Goodnough LT, Mazer CD, Shander A, Stafford-Smith M, Waters J; International Consortium for Evidence Based Per Baker RA, Dickinson TA, FitzGerald DJ, Likosky DS, Shann KG. 2011 update to the Society of Thoracic Surgeons and the Society of Cardiovascular Anesthesiologists blood conservaclinical practice guidelines. *Ann Thorac Surg.* 2011;91(3):944-982.

Gunter OL, Au BK, Isbell JM, Mowery NT, Young PP, Cotton BA. Optimizing outcomes in damage control resuscitation: Identifying blood product ratios associated with improved survival. *J Trauma.* 2008;65(3):527-534.
Napolitano LM, Kurek S, Luchette FA, et al. EAST Practice Management Workgroup; American College of Critical Care Medicine (ACCM) Taskforce of the Society of Critical Care Medicine (SCCM). Clinical practice guideline: Red blood cell transfusion in adult trauma and critical care. *Crit Care Med.* 2009; 37(12):3124-3157.
Qaseem A, Humphrey LL, Fitterman N, Starkey M, Shekelle P; Clinical Guidelines Committee of the American College of Physicians. Treatment of anemia in patients with heart disease: A clinical practice guideline from the American College of Physicians. *Ann Intern Med.* 2013;159(11):770-779.

▷ Postoperative Analgesia

Gordon DB, de Leon-Casasola OA, Rosenberg JM, et al. Management of Postoperative Pain: A Clinical Practice Guideline from the American Pain Society, the American Society of Regional Anesthesia and Pain Medicine, and the American Society of Anesthesiologists Committee on Regional Anesthesia, Executive Committee, and Administrative Council. *J Pain.* 2016;17(2):131-157.
Practice guidelines for acute pain management in the perioperative setting: An updated report by the American Society of Anesthesiologists Task Force on Acute Pain Management. *Anesthesiology.* 2012;116(2):248-273.

▷ Hyperglycemia

Duggan EW, Carlson K, Umpierrez GE. Perioperative hyperglycemia management: An update. *Anesthesiology.* 2017;126(3):547-560.
Umpierrez GE, Hellman R, Korytkowski MT, et al. Management of hyperglycemia in hospitalized patients in non-critical care setting: An Endocrine Society clinical practice guideline. *J Clin Endocrinol Metab.* 2012;97(1):16-38.

MULTIPLE-CHOICE QUESTIONS

1. A 65-year-old woman undergoes a thyroid lobectomy for a follicular neoplasm. She has a history of coronary artery disease, hypertension, insulin-dependent diabetes, and stroke. The procedure lasted 2 hours, during which the patient required occasional neosynephrine for brief intraoperative hypotension. Two hours after the procedure, the nurse called from the post anesthesia care unit to report that the patient is agitated and hypertensive. Which of the following is *not likely* to be the cause for her agitation?

   A. Hypoxia.
   B. Stroke.
   C. "Unmasking" of cognitive dysfunction.
   D. Hyperglycemia.
   E. Hypocalcemia.

2. A 43-year-old man with a distant history of intravenous drug use is now status post right inguinal hernia repair and is complaining of severe groin pain on the side of the operation. All of the following are appropriate actions *except:*

   A. Evaluate the patient for necrotizing fasciitis.
   B. Reassure the patient that his use of preoperative Suboxone that morning may have blocked his postoperative response to narcotics.
   C. Allow the nurse to administer a postoperative parenteral nonopioid analgesic.
   D. Discharge the patient with a prescription for pain medication and a plan for follow-up in 2 weeks.
   E. Perform a nerve block with local anesthetics.

3. A 56-year-old woman is being prepared for an elective ventral hernia repair in the preoperative care unit. She is overweight, with a history of non–insulin-dependent diabetes, hypertension, and smoking. Her fingerstick glucose is 326, and you note that her most recent HgA1c was 8.4%. She wants to proceed with the operation, and has traveled a long distance to see you and has taken the day off from work. The most appropriate choice of management is to:

   A. Proceed with the operation and plan for an intraoperative insulin drip.
   B. Repeat the fingerstick after insulin administration and proceed with the operation if the glucose is improved, with the plan for consultation of the diabetes team postoperatively for management.
   C. Cancel the operation with the plan for improved preoperative preparation.
   D. Admit the patient for preoperative glucose management and reschedule the operation for several days from now.

4. Which of the following are routine components of an ERAS protocol in patients who have undergone colon resection?

   A. Vital signs including heart rate, blood pressure, oxygen saturation.
   B. Wound evaluation including assessment of drain output and content.
   C. Assessment of the adequacy of pain management.
   D. Plan for removal of the nasogastric tube, Foley catheter, and advancement of diet.
   E. All of the above.

5. A 72-year-old man underwent resection of hepatic segments 5/6 for a hepatoma in the setting of hepatocellular carcinoma 2 days ago and was recently discharged to the floor. Perioperatively, he required a large volume of fluid resuscitation. He now has bloody output from his two Jackson–Pratt drains that are seated in the liver bed, his hematocrit has fallen 7 points to 23, his INR is 2.7, he is febrile to 102.8°F, and he is confused. Which of the following is the most appropriate order and choice of management?

   A. Evaluation of the patient, transfer to higher level of care, transfusion with 2 units of unmatched packed red blood cells, return to the operating room for surgical control of bleeding.
   B. Evaluation of the patient, transfusion with two packs of fresh frozen plasma and 2 units of matched packed red blood cells, computed tomography with angiography for possible embolization.
   C. Evaluation of the patient, intubation for protection of airway, transfer to higher level of care, transfusion with cryoprecipitate, antibiotic administration, return to the operating room for surgical control of bleeding.
   D. Evaluation of the patient, intubation for protection of airway, transfer to a higher level of care, transfusion with 2 units of fresh frozen plasma and 2 units of matched packed red blood cells, antibiotic administration, and computed tomography of the abdomen.

5

Postoperative Complications

Rui Zheng-Pywell, MD
Daniel I. Chu, MD, FACS, FASCRS

INTRODUCTION

All operations come with inherent risks for postoperative complications. These range from relatively common complications, such as superficial wound infections, to other systemic complications, such as cerebrovascular accidents. All complications, however small or big, matter and increase the risk of patient mortality, longer length of stay, and readmissions. Agencies such as the Centers for Medicare & Medicaid Services (CMS) recognize the significance of these events and now tie financial reimbursements to surgical quality through several complication metrics (Table 5–1). Postoperative complications therefore impact not only patients, but also providers and healthcare systems. To reduce these complications, surgeons must be cognizant of patient risk factors, facile in diagnosing the complication, and well-versed in managing them.

This chapter will systematically discuss both minor and major complications that may occur postoperatively. The aim will be to equip readers with the knowledge to identify, understand, and reduce postoperative complications with nonoperative and operative strategies. Such knowledge is necessary to achieve the best possible outcome for all surgical patients.

WOUND COMPLICATIONS

Wound complications are common causes of early and late postoperative complications. Disruptions in the steps of the healing process may lead to the formation of seromas and hematomas, surgical site infections (SSIs), anastomotic leaks, and even wound dehiscence.

▶ Seroma

A seroma is a localized fluid collection not containing pus or blood. Seromas are composed of serous fluid that fills an empty space following elevation of skin flaps and transection of lymphatic channels (eg, mastectomy, hernia repairs). These fluid collections delay healing and increase the risk of wound infection. Seromas may self-resolve, but if problematic, they can be electively evacuated by needle aspiration. Repeat needle aspirations may be necessary for recurrent seromas. Compression dressings can be applied to occlude lymphatic leaks and limit reaccumulation. Seromas of the groin, which are common after vascular operations, are best left to resorb without aspiration, since the risks of introducing a needle are greater than the risk associated with the seroma itself. However, should seromas persist with incisional drainage, wound reexploration is recommended with ligation of the primary source.

▶ Hematoma

A hematoma is a collection of blood and clot, typically adjacent to the surgical incision. It is a common wound complication following inadequate hemostasis. It typically presents as an elevated discoloration around the wound edges associated with swelling and discomfort. Sometimes there is bloody drainage along the incision. The incidence is higher in patients with intrinsic coagulopathy (eg, cirrhosis) or anticoagulation (eg, on antiplatelet therapy). Even patients receiving aspirin or low-dose heparin have an increased risk of developing this complication.

Small hematomas often self-resolve. Like seromas, however, incisional hematomas increase the incidence of wound infection. Of note, neck hematomas following thyroid, parathyroid, or carotid artery surgery can be particularly dangerous due to the risk of airway compromise from external compression secondary to rapid enlargement of the hematoma in a finite space. Treatment in most cases consists of evacuation of the clot under sterile conditions, ligation of bleeding vessels, and reclosure of the wound.

Table 5–1. Complications tracked by the Centers for Medicare & Medicaid Services.

Surgical Complications
Iatrogenic pneumothorax
Respiratory failure
Pulmonary embolism
Unrecognized abdominopelvic accidental puncture/laceration
Acute kidney injury
Sepsis
Deep vein thrombosis
Perioperative hematoma/hemorrhage
Wound dehiscence
In-hospital fall
Pressure ulcers

▶ Surgical Site Infection

A surgical site infection (SSI) is an infection that occurs in areas where surgery was performed. SSIs develop in 3%-20% after an operation. Classically, SSIs are categorized as (1) superficial incisional—limited to skin/subcutaneous tissues; (2) deep incisional—involve muscle/fascia; and (3) organ space.

Risk factors for SSIs include patient factors (eg, age, nutritional status, diabetes, smoking, obesity, coexistent infection at another site, microorganism colonization, altered immune response, and duration of postoperative stay) and operative factors (eg, preoperative antiseptic preparation, antimicrobial prophylaxis, duration of operation, operation room venting, use of foreign materials, surgical site, and surgical technique).

Prevention of SSIs includes use of antiseptic technique (eg, preoperative skin preparation, appropriate duration of surgical scrub, preoperative shaving), meticulous surgical techniques (adequate hemostasis, closing of dead space, and minimizing tissue trauma), and administration of appropriate preoperative antibiotics as determined by the type of operation being performed. Clean cases would only necessitate antibiotic coverage of skin flora (eg, cefazolin for inguinal hernia repair) while clean-contaminated cases involving the gastrointestinal tract would require additional Gram-negative and anaerobic coverage (eg, cefazolin and metronidazole for colectomy).

SSIs are diagnosed clinically and supplemented by culture data. Typical symptoms include localized pain, warmth, and erythema in line with cellulitis. Often they are accompanied by purulent drainage from the incision. Deep and organ space SSIs may require radiologic examination or wound exploration. Sometimes SSIs can lead to wound dehiscence or anastomotic breakdown (to be discussed below).

Treatment is source control. For superficial infections, the treatment may be performed at bedside and typically involves opening the incision, exploring the space, irrigating, and debriding the wound with subsequent regular wound care. Deep incisional and organ-space infections may necessitate a return to the operation room for exploration, washout, drainage, and debridement. Should implanted material be involved (eg, infected mesh after an umbilical hernia repair), then it must be removed. Alternatively, if the patient has medical comorbidities that make reoperation risky, the infection is localized and accessible, or the patient is in the postoperative window with extensive adhesive disease, percutaneous drainage may be pursued under image guidance. Antibiotics alone do not usually address the underlying nidus of infection.

▶ Wound Dehiscence

Wound dehiscence is a partial or complete disruption of any or all layers of the operative wound. Evisceration is defined as rupture of all layers of the abdominal wall and extrusion of abdominal viscera. Wound dehiscence occurs in 1%-3% of abdominal surgical procedures. Eviscerations, however, are rare and considered surgical emergencies. Systemic and local factors contribute to the development of this complication.

Certain comorbid conditions lead to slow wound healing or poor tissue integrity, that increases overall risk of dehiscence (eg, diabetes mellitus, uremia, impaired immune function, steroid use, jaundice, sepsis, poor nutritional status, cancer, obesity, and smoking). Three important local factors (usually in combination) predispose to wound dehiscence: (1) inadequate closure, (2) increased intra-abdominal pressure, and (3) deficient wound healing. The type of incision (transverse, midline, etc) does not influence the incidence of dehiscence.

Proper wound closure is one of the most important and modifiable factors. The fascia is the strength layer, and failure to accurately approximate this layer leads to increased wound disruption. Steps taken to avoid inadequate wound closure include a clean initial incision, appropriate tissue handling (avoid devitalization of fascial edges), appropriate suture material, and adequate spacing of the sutures. Placement of retention stitches should be considered in high-tension wounds or patients with increased risk factors. Although they do not prevent dehiscence, they may prevent evisceration and the morbidity and mortality associated with it. Increased abdominal pressure increases wound intension, leading to risk of dehiscence. Valsalva maneuvers are common culprits: coughing and straining. These may be regularly encountered in the postoperative period when dealing with atelectasis and constipation; thus preventative measures should to be taken (eg, holding a pillow while coughing, using abdominal binders, and regular administration of stool softeners). Finally, any factor that disrupts wound healing increases risk of wound dehiscence, such as the presence of foreign materials (eg, drains) or peri-incisional fluid collections (eg, seromas/hematomas and patients with ascites).

Although wounds can dehisce at any time, it most commonly occurs between postoperative days 5 and 8 (when the strength of the healing tissue is at a minimum). Early findings include drainage from the incision. Rarely, there is sudden evisceration, associated with a popping sensation following severe coughing or retching. Fascial dehiscence without evisceration is managed electively with prompt reclosure. If a partial disruption is stable and the patient is at poor operative risk, treatment may be delayed (though there will be an incisional hernia). Should the wound be infected, elective closure should be delayed until the infection is controlled, the wound has healed, and 6-7 months have elapsed. Then antibiotics specific for the organisms isolated from the previous wound infection must be given at the time of incisional hernia repair. Patients who eviscerate need to be taken emergently back to the operating room.

Anastomotic Leak

Anastomotic leaks are a form of wound dehiscence that occurs as a result of disrupted wound healing between visceral anastomoses. They occur in 1%-24% of anastomoses, and higher frequencies occur in low pelvic anastomoses compared to more proximal ones in the abdomen. The morbidity and mortality are increased threefold for a patient with an anastomotic leak, making these complications one of the most feared in gastrointestinal surgery.

The risk factors for developing an anastomotic leak are the same as those for wound dehiscence. Systemic risk factors include age, malnutrition, vitamin deficiencies, steroid use, obesity, and comorbid conditions such as diabetes, smoking, inflammatory bowel disease (Crohn disease and ulcerative colitis), previous radiation/chemotherapy, and anemia. Local risk factors include tension, poor blood flow, hypotension, radiation, and contamination.

There are several technical variations to consider when making an anastomosis: hand-sewn versus stapled anastomoses, continuous versus interrupted sutures, and single- versus double-layer hand-sewn anastomoses. The rate of anastomotic leak is not associated with the technique chosen. Aside from the risk factors of the patient, care should be made to avoid tension at the suture line and ensure adequate blood flow to the two ends of the anastomosis. Of note, stapled end-to-end anastomoses may lead to higher rates of anastomotic strictures in long-term follow-up.

The diagnosis of an anastomotic leak can be made clinically, radiographically, and intraoperatively. Clinically, the patient may present with pain, fever, peritonitis and drainage of purulent material, bilious succus, or fecal material. Radiographically, fluid and gas-containing collections may be seen tracking to an anastomosis. Should the patient be given oral contrast or a contrasted enema, leakage may be seen out of the bowel. Intraoperatively, there may be gross contamination from gastrointestinal contents and evidence of anastomotic disruption.

Management of anastomotic leaks depends on the patient's clinical status, the time from initial operation, and the location and severity of the leak. The management strategies can range from nonoperative (observation, bowel rest, antibiotics, and percutaneous drainage of abscesses) to, more commonly, operative intervention (wide drainage, proximal diversion, and/or revision of anastomosis).

NEUROLOGIC COMPLICATIONS

Perioperative Cerebrovascular Accidents

Perioperative strokes occur infrequently, but are associated with significant perioperative morbidity and mortality. The most common mechanism is thromboembolic and occurs within the initial 72-hour postoperative period. Patients are typically asymptomatic leading up to the event. Less common causes of perioperative strokes include air embolism, fat embolism, paradoxical embolism, cervical arterial dissections, hemorrhagic stroke, lacunar ischemic stroke, and spinal cord infarctions.

Risk factors include the type of surgery performed, history of previous stroke, atrial fibrillation, valvular heart disease, hypertension, coronary artery disease, peripheral vascular disease, chronic obstructive pulmonary disease (COPD), renal disease, advanced age, neoplastic disease, and smoking. Intraoperative hypotension also increases the rate of stroke due to the ischemia and dysregulation of cerebral blood flow. Cessation of anticoagulation including antiplatelet therapy increases the risk of stroke, but these risks need to be balanced with the underlying risks for bleeding. High-risk conditions for stroke with cessation of anticoagulation include mechanical heart valves (mitral and atrial), atrial fibrillation with a previous history of stroke, hypercoagulable state, and deep venous thrombosis diagnosed within 30 days.

The risk of stroke is higher in some surgeries than others. There is a 10% risk with multivalve replacement surgeries, < 1% risk with hemicolectomy, and up to 6% risk with carotid endarterectomies or stents. In cardiac surgery, the use of an extracorporeal circulatory pump increases the risk of microemboli that bypass the lungs. In carotid surgery, stroke risk varies by patient symptomatology (highest risk with symptomatic stroke followed by transient ischemic attacks, and lowest risk with asymptomatic patient), plaque anatomy, and degree of stenosis. Causative factors for strokes include atherosclerotic plaque embolization, ischemic duration from clamping, postoperative thrombosis at an arteriotomy site, or intimal flap development.

Cerebrovascular events usually present with an acute neurologic change (eg, weakness, facial droop, slurred speech). Workup involves getting a noncontrasted computed tomography (CT) of the head to identify whether the stroke is ischemic or hemorrhagic. There should be simultaneous workup to rule out other possible causes of acute change in mental status (eg, low blood sugar, hypoxia, or acute electrolyte derangements). For ischemic stroke, patients should be started on aspirin and a statin. If the stroke was identified < 4.5 hours from the known time of onset, and the patient is not at significant risk for bleeding, recombinant tissue plasminogen activator (tPA) may be given. In the acute phase of the stroke, patients may have permissive hypertension with a target systolic blood pressure < 185 mm Hg and diastolic blood pressure < 110 mm Hg. Additional studies must be obtained to identify possible causes of stroke (eg, ECG to rule out an acute cardiac event or arrhythmia, cardiac echocardiogram to evaluate for cardiac of vascular thrombus/embolus or patent foramen ovale, or carotid ultrasound for atherosclerotic buildup). For hemorrhagic stroke, attempts should be made to discontinue anticoagulation/antiplatelets, give reversal agents (vitamin K, fresh frozen plasma [FFP], etc), and start aggressive blood pressure management with target systolic blood pressures < 50 mm Hg. For those exhibiting depressed mental status with findings of intracranial mass effect on imaging, neurosurgery should be involved for hematoma decompression. Close attention should be paid to intracranial pressure monitoring (ICP).

▶ Paraplegia

Spinal cord ischemia is a rare but possible complication that has devastating consequences. Patients most at risk of this complication are those with manipulation of the descending thoracic aorta through both open and endovascular procedures due to the involvement of the artery of Adamkiewicz. Rare cases of injury from epidural placement have been seen in patients with predisposition due to vascular disease, spinal stenosis, and intraoperative hypotension. Patients with a history of aortic aneurysms have also been found to be at increased risk with perioperative hypotension. The extent of spinal cord injury is determined by several factors: ischemic duration, severity of ischemia, success of reestablishing blood supply, and reperfusion injury. The risk of spinal cord injury can be minimized by using cerebrospinal fluid drainage, hypothermia, partial bypass of the blood flow, and maintaining normotension.

▶ Sexual Dysfunction

Sexual problems commonly occur after certain types of operations for patients of both genders. Typically, they involve surgeries in the deep pelvis (eg, prostatectomy, hysterectomy, and rectal cancer resections) or relate to surgeries affecting perfusion (eg, cardiac surgery and aortic reconstruction). The pathogenesis can be due to injury to nerves necessary for sexual function, though in other cases the etiology is

unclear. After abdominoperineal resection, transection of the peripheral branches of the sacral plexus, a part of the pelvic autonomic nerves, may cause impotence. It is important to discuss this possibility with the patient before any operation. When sexual dysfunction is psychogenic, reassurance is usually all that is needed. If impotence persists beyond 4-6 weeks, appropriate consultation is indicated.

PSYCHIATRIC COMPLICATIONS

▶ Postoperative Delirium

Delirium is a condition associated with a waxing and waning consciousness ranging from hypoactive to hyperactive states complicated by symptoms of psychosis. Postoperative delirium (POD) is a form of delirium that occurs after a surgical procedure and anesthesia. It affects between 37% and 46% of postsurgical patients, with rates as high as 87% in patients requiring care in an intensive care unit (ICU). It is not to be confused with emergence delirium, which occurs in 8%-20% of patients after awakening from anesthesia.

Risk factors can be broken down to two categories: predisposing and precipitating. Predisposing factors include reduced cognitive reserve from preexisting comorbidities (eg, dementia, depression, and advanced age), reduced physical reserve, sensory impairment, malnutrition, dehydration, and substance abuse. Precipitating factors include use or withdrawal of certain types of medications (general anesthetics, anticholinergics, benzodiazepines, muscle relaxants, antihistamines, etc), pain, hypoxemia, electrolyte abnormalities, sleep–wake cycle disturbances, and environmental change (eg, prolonged hospitalization or ICU stay). Overall, the cause of postoperative delirium is likely multifactorial, and there are several hypotheses regarding the cause: acute central cholinergic deficiency, decreased GABA-ergic activity, abnormalities in serotonin and melatonin pathways, noradrenergic hyperactivity, inflammatory state leading to neuronal damage, or cerebral hypoperfusion. It has been shown that patients who suffer from delirium are at double the risk of requiring institutionalization postdischarge and a tenfold increase in the risk of dementia. Higher rates are associated with vascular and cardiac surgeries.

Delirium presents on a spectrum ranging from hypoactive to hyperactive. Symptoms can change as the patient oscillates between states. Hyperactive delirium is characterized by restlessness, agitation, hallucinations, and delusions. Hypoactive delirium has reduced movement, minimal communication, and overall unresponsiveness that may be confused for depression, anxiety, or even calmness. As a result, hypoactive delirium can often go unrecognized.

Preventative measures can be taken, including frequent and deliberate orientation of patient to place, time, and reason of hospitalization, early postoperative mobilization, and consistent use of home devices while hospitalized (eg, hearing aids and glasses). For patients in the ICU, sedative medication should be carefully titrated between patient comfort and oversedation. Studies have looked at sedating agents with findings that suggest dexmedetomidine is less likely to cause delirium. Treatment involves the use of typical and atypical antipsychotics.

Early psychiatric consultation should be obtained when delirium is suspected. The earlier the condition is recognized, the easier it is to correct. Metabolic derangements or early sepsis (especially in burn patients) must be evaluated and treated if present. Severe postoperative emotional disturbances may be avoided by appropriate preoperative counseling of the patient by the surgeon. This includes a thorough discussion of the operation and the expected outcome, and acquainting the patient with the intensive care unit. Postoperatively, the surgeon must attend to the patient's emotional needs, offering frequent reassurance, explaining the postoperative course, and discussing the prognosis and the outcome of the operation.

Alcohol Withdrawal

Alcohol is a commonly abused substance. Patients who have a physical dependence, tolerance, and compulsive use of alcohol are chronic alcoholics. They are at high risk of developing alcohol withdrawal syndrome (AWS) in the perioperative periods. Patients typically become symptomatic 6-24 hours after the last drink and peak within 24-48 hours. The most common features include tremulousness, sweating, nausea, vomiting, anxiety, and agitation. Patients may even experience epileptiform seizures within 12-48 hours after their last drink. Some patients do progress to delirium tremens, which is a life-threatening consequence of alcohol withdrawal.

Delirium tremens, which is the worst form of alcohol withdrawal, occurs after the initial prodrome of alcoholic withdrawal. Readaptation to ethanol-free metabolism requires about 2 weeks, and it is during this period that alcoholics are at greatest risk of developing delirium tremens. Symptoms include development of auditory and visual hallucinations, confusion, altered mental status, and autonomic hyperactivity (hypertension, tachycardia, tachypnea, and diaphoresis). Diaphoresis and dehydration are common. If left untreated, delirium tremens can lead to death from cardiovascular collapse or respiratory collapse. Cardiac index, oxygen delivery, and oxygen consumption double during delirium tremens and return to normal 24-48 hours after resolution.

Patients at risk of developing AWS can be prophylactically treated. First-line agents are benzodiazepines. Alternatives include chlormethiazole or giving alcohol directly. Symptomatic treatment is determined by the CIWA-AR score, which looks at ten different categories: nausea/vomiting, tremor, paroxysmal sweats, anxiety, agitation, tactile disturbances, auditory disturbances, visual disturbances, headaches, and change in patient orientation/altered mental status. Vitamin B_1 (thiamine) and magnesium sulfate should also be given. The aims of treatment are to reduce agitation and anxiety as soon as possible, and to prevent the development of other complications (eg, seizures and aspiration pneumonia). General measures should include frequent assessment of vital signs, restoration of nutrition, administration of vitamin B, correction of electrolyte imbalance or other metabolic derangements, and adequate hydration. Physical restraint, though necessary for seriously violent behavior, should be as limited as possible. With proper care, most patients improve within 72 hours.

Pain

Pain occurs after surgery. In the setting of the opioid epidemic, studies looking at persistent opioid use after both major and minor surgical procedures found that approximately 6% of opioid-naïve patients have persistent use (> 90 days) postoperatively. Surgery itself is an inherent risk factor for chronic opioid use. Other risks include male gender, age > 50 years, preoperative history of substance abuse, and depression. Excessive analgesic leads to oversedation, respiratory suppression, delirium, and ileus. Prolonged used also leads to opioid tolerance, dependence, immunosuppression, opioid-induced endocrinopathy (eg, sexual dysfunction, depression, and decreased energy), and increased inpatient mortality. Steps can be taken to assist with opioid cessation after surgery using multimodal analgesia. This includes using neuraxial, regional, and/or local anesthesia, perioperative ketamine, and nonopioid analgesics (acetaminophen, gabapentin, selective COX-2 inhibitors, and nonsteroidal antiinflammatory drugs).

The adoption of multimodal analgesia has been more recently incorporated into Enhanced Recovery Programs (ERPs) and Enhanced Recovery After Surgery (ERAS) for elective surgeries. These recovery pathways hasten postoperative recovery by minimizing the surgical stress response and organ dysfunction that occurs after major surgery. Although ERP/ERAS focus on all three perioperative phases of surgery, these pathways limit the use of narcotics in the postoperative phase. Instead, the pathways emphasize use of scheduled acetaminophen and antiinflammatory drugs such as ibuprofen for baseline pain control. Narcotics are only available should pain remain uncontrolled, with escalation as needed to patient-controlled analgesia. These principles of ERP/ERAS have led to decreased postoperative use of opioids.

CARDIAC COMPLICATIONS

Cardiac complications following surgery may be life threatening. Patients with risk factors of cardiac disease need to be identified preoperatively and undergo the appropriate cardiovascular testing and intervention prior to surgical intervention. Patients are typically evaluated preoperatively via the Revised Cardiac Risk Index (RCRI), which looks at six independent risk factors for patients over 50 years of age that put them at increased risk for cardiac complications with elective surgery: high-risk surgery, history of ischemic cardiac disease, history of congestive heart failure, history of cerebrovascular disease, insulin dependence, and elevated Cr > 2.0. An additional tool for evaluating risk is the American College of Surgeons National Surgical Quality Improvement Project (ACS-NSQIP) calculator. Exercise tolerance is an important factor affecting operative risk since it is a predictor of underlying ischemic heart disease. It can be determined through history taking by asking the patient their ability to walk a mile without excessive fatigue and dyspnea, or asking the number of flights they are able to climb or blocks they can walk without symptoms. The Duke Activity Status Index looks at metabolic equivalents (METs) attributed to set activities and it is a good method of predicting activity tolerance.

In general, oral anticoagulant drugs should be stopped 3-5 days before surgery, and the prothrombin time should be allowed to return to normal. Patients at high risk of thromboembolic disease should receive heparin until approximately 6 hours before the operation, when heparin should be stopped. If needed, heparin can be restarted 36-48 hours after surgery along with oral anticoagulation. Beta-blockers should only be used if they are a home medication the patient consistently used preoperatively.

Noncardiac complications may affect the development of cardiac complications by increasing cardiac demands in patients with a limited reserve. Common examples include postoperative sepsis and hypoxemia. Excessive use of postoperative fluids can lead to volume overload and acute left-ventricular failure. Patients with coronary artery disease, dysrhythmias, or low cardiac output should be monitored postoperatively in an intensive care unit.

Perioperative Myocardial Infarction

Approximately 0.4% of all patients undergoing an operation in the United States experience a postoperative myocardial infarction. The incidence increases to 5%-12% in patients undergoing operations for forms of atherosclerotic disease (eg, carotid endarterectomy, grafts for peripheral vascular disease). Other important risk factors include preoperative congestive heart failure, preoperative ischemia confirmed during a cardiac stress test, and advanced age (> 70 years). In select patients with angina, consideration should be given to coronary revascularization before proceeding with a major elective operation on another organ.

Postoperative myocardial infarction may be precipitated by factors such as hypotension or hypoxemia. Clinical manifestations include chest pain, hypotension, and cardiac dysrhythmias. Patients may also be asymptomatic, and may

be due to the residual effects of anesthesia and to analgesics administered postoperatively.

Diagnosis is made with electrocardiographic changes and elevated cardiac enzymes (specifically troponin-I). The mortality rate of postoperative myocardial infarction is as high as 67% in high-risk groups. The prognosis is better if it is the first infarction. Outcomes are worse if the patient has a history of previous infarctions. Prevention of this complication includes postponing elective surgery up to 6 months after a myocardial infarction, treating congestive heart failure preoperatively, and controlling hypertension perioperatively.

Patients with postoperative myocardial infarction should be monitored in the intensive care unit and provided with adequate oxygenation and precise fluid and electrolyte replacement. Anticoagulation, though not always feasible after major surgery, limits the risk of mural thrombosis development and arterial embolism after myocardial infarction. Definitive treatment requires restoration of myocardial blood flow. Should a patient be diagnosed within 120 minutes of presentation, the optimal intervention is via percutaneous coronary intervention (PCI) for cardiac stent placement. However, should the patient be outside that window but within 12 hours of the event, they can receive fibrinolysis. Only when the patient fails PCI or fibrinolysis, or when there are mechanical considerations against intravascular treatment (eg, ruptured of ventricular free wall or acute valvular dysfunction), should coronary artery bypass graft (CABG) surgery be considered due to high perioperative mortality within the initial postoperative week. Patients who receive cardiac stents will need to be on dual antiplatelet therapy and lifelong statin therapy.

Postoperative Cardiac Failure

Left-ventricular failure and pulmonary edema appear in 4% of patients over age 40 undergoing general surgical procedures with general anesthesia. Fluid overload in patients with limited myocardial reserve is the most common cause. Postoperative myocardial infarction and dysrhythmias producing a high ventricular rate are other causes. Clinical findings include progressive dyspnea, hypoxemia, and diffuse pulmonary edema on chest x-ray. Confounding factors for diagnosis include factors that also predispose the patient to be risk for pulmonary edema (ie, massive trauma, multiple transfusions, and sepsis). The diagnosis may be suspected from a decreased PaO_2, abnormal chest x-ray, or elevated pulmonary artery wedge pressure.

The treatment of left-ventricular failure depends on the hemodynamic state of the patient. Those who are in shock require transfer to the intensive care unit, placement of a pulmonary artery line, monitoring of filling pressures, and immediate preload and afterload reduction. Preload reduction is achieved by diuretics (and nitroglycerin if needed); afterload reduction, by administration of sodium nitroprusside.

Angiotensin-converting enzyme (ACE) inhibitors and beta-blockers have been demonstrated to reduce mortality. Patients should undergo fluid restriction and diuresis, if appropriate. Respiratory insufficiency calls for ventilator support with escalation to either noninvasive positive pressure ventilation or endotracheal intubation and a mechanical respirator. Although pulmonary function may improve with the use of positive end-expiratory pressure (PEEP), hemodynamic derangements and decreased myocardial reserve preclude it in most cases.

Dysrhythmias

General anesthesia depresses the myocardium, and some anesthetic agents predispose to dysrhythmias by sensitizing the myocardium to catecholamines. Monitoring of cardiac activity and blood pressure during the operation detects dysrhythmias and hypotension early. In patients with a high cardiac risk, regional anesthesia may be safer than general anesthesia for procedures below the umbilicus. Most dysrhythmias appear during the operation or within the first 3 postoperative days. They are especially likely to occur after thoracic procedures.

The overall incidence of intraoperative cardiac dysrhythmias is 20%, though most are self-limited. They occur in patients with preexisting dysrhythmias and known heart disease (35%) and tend to accompany use of anesthetic agents (eg, halothane, cyclopropane), sympathomimetic drugs, or induction-associated hypercapnia. Postoperative dysrhythmias are generally related to reversible factors (eg, electrolyte abnormalities, hypoxemia, and stress during emergence from anesthesia). Occasionally, postoperative dysrhythmias may serve as a sign of myocardial infarction. Most patients remain asymptomatic, but occasionally the patient complains of chest pain, palpitations, or dyspnea.

Supraventricular dysrhythmias decrease cardiac output and coronary blood flow, occasionally leading to hypotension and cardiac hypoperfusion. Two of the most common forms include atrial fibrillation and atrial flutter with rapid ventricular response (RVR). Those who are hemodynamically unstable require immediate cardioversion. If they are hemodynamically stable, pharmacologic agents (eg, betablockers, calcium channel blockers, or digoxin) should be tried. Premature ventricular beats (PVCs) are often precipitated by hypercapnia, hypoxemia, pain, or fluid overload. They should be treated with oxygen, sedation, analgesia, and correction of fluid losses or electrolyte abnormalities. When they are sustained, they lead to ventricular dysrhythmias. Ventricular dysrhythmias (ventricular tachycardia or ventricular fibrillation) carry a high risk of sudden cardiac death. With ventricular tachycardia, as with supraventricular dysrhythmias, those who are hemodynamically unstable require synchronized cardioversion. Those who are stable may receive adenosine in an attempt to break the rhythm. Should adenosine fail, then second-line agents include lidocaine, procainamide, amiodarone, or sotalol for chemical conversion. Ventricular fibrillation is a nonperfusing rhythm and should be treated the same as pulseless ventricular tachycardia. Per Advanced Cardiac Life Support (ACLS), the mainstay therapy are defibrillation and chest compressions. For both supraventricular and ventricular dysrhythmias, all underlying electrolyte abnormalities need to be treated.

Heart Block

There are various types of heart block. When the patient suffers a complete (third-degree) heart block, it is indicative of serious underlying disease, and a pacemaker is necessary. Patients with heart block are at risk of symptomatic bradycardia with potential for serious consequences due to hypoperfusion from poor cardiac output as a result of bradycardia. First-degree or second-degree heart block is usually well tolerated.

PULMONARY COMPLICATIONS

Respiratory complications are the most common single cause of morbidity after major surgical procedures and the second most common cause of postoperative deaths in patients older than 60 years. Patients undergoing chest and upper abdominal operations are particularly prone to pulmonary complications. They are more common after emergency operations. Common postoperative pulmonary complications include atelectasis, pneumonia, prolonged intubation, and need for reintubation. Factors that contribute to increased risk include older age, poor functional status, prolonged operative duration, preexisting lung disease (eg, COPD, interstitial lung disease [ILD]), and medical comorbidities (eg, ascites, preoperative shock, and smoking). Elderly patients are at much higher risk because they have decreased compliance, increased closing and residual volumes, and increased dead space, all of which predispose to atelectasis.

Postoperative Respiratory Failure

Postoperative respiratory failure is usually defined as postoperative ventilation for > 48 hours or patient reintubation. Severity can range from acute lung injury (ALI), where the PaO_2/FiO_2 (P/F ratio) is greater than 200 but less than 300, to acute respiratory distress syndrome (ARDS), where the P/F ratio is less than 200. Causes can be multifactorial, and this may occur even in a healthy preoperative patient. Risks include preoperative lung function, age, concomitant comorbidities (eg, obstructive sleep apnea, pulmonary hypertension, cardiovascular disease), and smoking. Furthermore, risk is increased with intraoperative lung injury or postoperative aspiration. Several steps can be taken to avoid postoperative pulmonary failure. Preoperative respiratory training, medication optimization, smoking cessation, and close screening of functional status may help identify and mitigate postoperative complications. Intraoperative factors include duration of surgery, volume management, gas anesthesia, pain therapy, and avoidance of blood transfusions. Postoperatively, preventative measures include fast-track extubation, effective pain therapy, breathing training, physiotherapy, noninvasive ventilation, use of bronchodilators, appropriate volume resuscitation, thrombosis prophylaxis, and antibiotics as needed.

Treatments include early tracheostomy (decreases dead space), protective ventilation (tidal volume 6 mL/kg body weight), lowered peak pressures (< 30 mm Hg), increased positive end-expiratory pressure (PEEP goal 10-20 mm H_2O), early patient mobilization, and bronchoscopy as needed. Critical cases may lead to use of extracorporeal membrane oxygenation (ECMO). Both ALI and ARDS are inflammatory pulmonary processes; however, no benefits have been found with antiinflammatory, steroid, or antibiotic drug use. Care should be made to avoid excessive fluids.

▶ Pulmonary Embolisms

Perioperative pulmonary embolism (PE) is a condition where pulmonary arterial flow is obstructed and may lead to a possibly life-threatening condition. Incidence varies from 0.3% to 30% after surgery, with a mortality rate of 16%-31%. Causes include thrombus (most common), tumor, air, fat, and amniotic fluid.

Pulmonary embolisms can cause pulmonary infarction, abnormal gas exchange, and cardiovascular compromise. The most common symptom is sinus tachycardia. Pulmonary infarction may occur with occlusion of the pulmonary artery or its segmental branches. Patients may complain about pleuritic chest pain or hemoptysis. With complete mechanical obstruction of the vasculature, patients can have functional change with decreased ventilation-to-perfusion ratio (leads to hypoxia), increased local inflammation, surfactant dysfunction, and atelectasis. Patients tend to become tachypneic, leading to respiratory alkalosis. In the worst-case scenario, patients develop cardiopulmonary compromise from increased pulmonary vascular resistance leading to decreased right-ventricular output (increased ventricular pressure and flattening of the septum). Decreased right-sided output leads to reduced left-ventricular preload. Thus there is a decrease in stroke volume and cardiac output.

Patients who develop PEs can be managed according to their hemodynamic stability. Those who are hemodynamically stable require supportive measures (eg, oxygen supplementation) with anticoagulation. Should patients not be a candidate for anticoagulation, an inferior venous cava (IVC) filter can be placed to prevent future PEs. Those who are hemodynamically unstable (systolic blood pressure < 90 mm Hg for > 15 minutes or requirement for vasopressors) typically go into shock from obstructed pulmonary flow from location

or size of the PE. If patients are stable enough, computed tomographic pulmonary angiography (CTPA) is first choice to look for a filling defect suggestive of a PE. However, if the patient cannot undergo a CTPA due to contrast allergy or limited kidney function, then a ventilation-perfusion (V/Q) scan can be performed. At some centers, V/Q scans can be portable and may be preferable for patients who cannot be safely taken for CTPA. However, should neither be an option, the next step is an echocardiogram to look at right-ventricular function. If workup if inconclusive, anticoagulation can be started empirically for concern of underlying PE. If hemodynamically unstable, other treatments include systemic thrombolysis or suction embolectomy.

There are several different origins of pulmonary emboli. The most common are thromboembolisms formed in the distal proximal veins (iliac, femoral, and popliteal). The more proximal the deep venous embolism, the greater the risk for embolization. Thrombi form due to Virchow's triad: venous stasis, endothelial injury, and a hypercoagulable state. Risk factors are inherent (genetic) and acquired (eg, immobilization from surgery/trauma, cancer, hormone therapy, obesity, and smoking).

Another source of pulmonary emboli is fat. Though fat particles are relatively common, they rarely cause symptoms. Fat particles can be found in the pulmonary vascular bed in 90% of patients who have had fractures of long bones or joint replacements. Fat embolism can also be caused by exogenous sources of fat, such as blood transfusions, intravenous fat emulsion, or bone marrow transplantation. Fat embolism syndrome can also lead to neurologic dysfunction, respiratory insufficiency, and petechiae of the axillae, chest, and proximal arms. Symptoms typically begin 12-72 hours after injury, but may be delayed for several days, and diagnosis is made off clinical findings. Patients may have decreased hematocrit, thrombocytopenia, and other changes in coagulation parameters. Once symptoms develop, supportive treatment should be provided until the symptoms subside.

▶ Atelectasis

Atelectasis is the most common pulmonary complication and affects 25% of patients who have abdominal surgery. It is more common in smokers, the elderly, the obese, and those with underlying respiratory disease. It appears most frequently in the first 48 hours after operation, and is responsible for over 90% of febrile episodes during that period. In most cases, the course is self-limited and recovery uneventful.

Atelectasis develops due to obstructive and nonobstructive factors. Obstruction may be caused by secretions (mucous and occasional blood clots), sedation, and malposition of the endotracheal tube. Most causes of atelectasis are nonobstructive from closure of the bronchioles. Small bronchioles (≤ 1 mm) are prone to close when lung volume reaches a critical point (closing volume). Portions of the lung that are dependent or compressed are the first to experience bronchiole closure, since their regional volume is less than that of nondependent portions. Poor respiratory effort can lead to shallow breathing, with failure to periodically hyperinflate the lung. This leads to smaller alveolar size and decreased volume. The closing volume is higher in older patients and smokers due to the loss of elastic recoil of the lung. Other nonobstructive factors include loss of pulmonary surfactant, which can occur with alveolar damage from pneumonia.

The immediate effect of atelectasis is decreased oxygenation of blood. Even though there is air in the atelectatic portion of the lung, there is minimal perfusion leading to a ventilation–perfusion mismatch. There is greater risk for infection in parts of the lung that remain atelectatic for more than 72 hours.

Symptoms of atelectasis may include fever, tachypnea, and tachycardia. Physical examination may show elevation of the diaphragm, scattered rales, and decreased breath sounds. Postoperative atelectasis can be largely prevented by early mobilization, frequent changes in position, encouragement to cough, and use of an incentive spirometer. Preoperative teaching of respiratory exercises and postoperative execution of these exercises prevents atelectasis in patients without preexisting lung disease. Intermittent positive pressure breathing is expensive and less effective than these simpler exercises.

Treatment consists of clearing the airway by chest percussion, coughing, or deep suctioning. Bronchodilators and mucolytic agents given by nebulizer may help in patients with severe chronic obstructive pulmonary disease. Obstructive atelectasis may require intrabronchial suction through an endoscope, a procedure that can usually be performed at the bedside with mild sedation.

▶ Pulmonary Aspiration

Aspiration of oropharyngeal and gastric contents is normally prevented by several important structures of the aerodigestive apparatus: pharynx, upper esophageal sphincter, esophageal body, glottis and vocal cords, and the airway. Three key reflexes are also important: the laryngeal adductor reflex (vocal cord closure), esophagoglottal closure reflex, and pharyngoglottal closure reflex. These normal protections are compromised by depression of mental status and the presence of a foreign body (eg, nasogastric or endotracheal tubes). Two-thirds of aspiration cases follow thoracic or abdominal surgery. Half the patients proceed to have pneumonia. The death rate for grossly evident aspiration and subsequent pneumonia is about 50%.

The magnitude of pulmonary injury from aspiration is determined by the volume aspirated, pH content, and frequency of event. If the aspirate has a pH of 2.5 or less, it causes immediate chemical pneumonitis, which results in local edema, inflammation, and an increased risk of secondary infection. Aspiration of solid matter can produce airway obstruction, which may lead to pulmonary abscess formation. The basal segments are affected most often (right side more often than left side). Tachypnea, rales, and hypoxia are usually present within hours. Less frequently, cyanosis, wheezing, and apnea may appear. In patients with massive aspiration, hypovolemia caused by excessive fluid and colloid loss into the injured lung may lead to hypotension and shock.

Aspiration can be limited by preoperative fasting, proper positioning of the patient, and careful intubation. A single dose of H_2-blocker or proton pump inhibitor before induction of anesthesia may have value when the risk of aspiration is high. Treatment of tracheobronchial aspiration involves reestablishing patency of the airway and preventing further damage to the lung. Immediate treatment includes endotracheal suctioning, which is both diagnostic and therapeutic. Endotracheal bronchoscopy may be required to remove solid matter. Fluid resuscitation and antibiotics should be started concomitantly.

▶ Postoperative Pleural Effusion & Pneumothorax

Formation of a very small pleural effusion is common immediately after upper-abdominal operations and is of no clinical significance. Patients with free peritoneal fluid at the time of surgery with postoperative atelectasis are at higher risk of developing pleural effusions. Patients without underlying cardiac failure or pulmonary disease that develop late postoperative effusions suggest subdiaphragmatic inflammation (subphrenic abscess, acute pancreatitis, etc). Effusions that do not compromise respiratory function do not require intervention. If there is a suspicion of infection, a sample can be collected via needle aspiration. Symptomatic effusions require thoracostomy tube placements that can be discontinued once rate of accumulation decreases.

Postoperative pneumothorax may occur following central venous line (CVL) placement or may spontaneously occur in a patient with underlying lung disease under positive-pressure ventilation. Sometimes, patients develop a pneumothorax after the pleura has been injured (eg, during a paraesophageal hernia repair, nephrectomy, or adrenalectomy). Pneumothorax should be treated with a small-caliber thoracostomy tube because there is no need for draining viscous fluid.

GASTROINTESTINAL COMPLICATIONS

Gastrointestinal complications are very common after major abdominal operations and range from nausea/vomiting to complete bowel obstructions. The severity of complications is often determined by the type of operation performed, such as minimally invasive versus open.

Table 5–2. Common causes and terms for bowel obstructions.

	Small Bowel	Large Bowel
Functional obstruction	Ileus	Pseudo-obstruction
		Ogilvie syndrome
Mechanical obstruction	Adhesions	Cancer
	Hernias	Diverticular disease
	Cancer	Volvulus

Functional Bowel Obstruction (Ileus & Pseudo-obstruction)

The presence, strength, and direction of normal peristalsis are governed by the enteric nervous system. Anesthesia and surgical manipulation result in a decrease of the normal propulsive activity of the gut, or postoperative ileus (for small bowel) and pseudo-obstruction (for large bowel) (Table 5–2). Several factors can slow the return of bowel function including medications (ie, opioids), electrolyte abnormalities, inflammatory conditions (ie, pancreatitis or peritonitis), pain, and degree of operative manipulation. Patients typically present with symptoms of nausea, bloating, burping, and hiccups in the absence of flatus or bowel movements. Abdominal distension and accompanied tympani are usually observed on physical exam. Abdominal X-rays usually show dilated loops of bowel.

Gastrointestinal peristalsis typically returns within 24 hours after nonabdominal operations. Minimally invasive surgery causes less ileus than open procedures. After laparotomy, gastric peristalsis usually returns in about 48 hours. Colonic activity returns after 48 hours, starting at the cecum with progression caudally. Small-bowel function then returns. For those with symptomatic nausea and vomiting, a therapeutic nasogastric tube may be placed to decompress the bowel while awaiting return of bowel function. Return of peristalsis is often noted by the patient as mild cramps, passage of flatus, and return of appetite. Although previous dogma held that feedings should be withheld until return of normal gastrointestinal motility, current recovery pathways (eg, ERAS) encourage early feeding as soon as postoperative day 0. There is no definitive therapy for postoperative ileus and pseudo-obstruction and treatment is supportive.

Mechanical Bowel Obstruction

Most postoperative patients have return of bowel function. Failure to do so is usually due to functional (eg, ileus and pseudo-obstruction) or mechanical obstruction. For small bowel, mechanical obstruction is most often caused by postoperative adhesions or an internal (mesenteric) hernia (Table 5–2). Most of these patients experience a short period of apparently normal intestinal function before manifestations of obstruction supervene. About half of cases of early postoperative small-bowel obstruction follow abdominal surgery.

Diagnosis may be difficult because the symptoms are difficult to differentiate from those of paralytic ileus. Abdominal plain film may show air-fluid levels in loops of small bowel for mechanical obstruction. A small-bowel series with barium sulfate may aid diagnosis. Strangulation is uncommon from inflammatory bands, but extent of distension can lead to bowel necrosis. With bowel dilation from obstruction, there is increased mural tension, which decreases mucosal perfusion. This accompanies bacterial proliferation and increases bowel perforation risks. Mortality from small-bowel dilation is approximately 10% and increases to 30% with necrosis and perforation. Treatment can initially be conservative with nasogastric suction. However, if the obstruction does not resolve spontaneously, then the patient may require surgical laparotomy.

Bowel Intussusception

Small-bowel intussusception is an uncommon cause of early postoperative obstruction in adults but accounts for 10% of cases in the pediatric age group. Approximately 90% of postoperative intussusceptions occur within the first 2 postoperative weeks, and more than 50% occur in the first week. They tend to occur after retroperitoneal and pelvic surgeries. Unlike idiopathic ileocolic intussusception, most postoperative intussusceptions are ileoileal or jejunojejunal. Symptoms include vomiting, distention, and abdominal pain after laparotomy in children. Early reoperation prevents perforation and peritonitis. Operative intervention is the only treatment, and if the bowel is viable, reduction of the intussusception is all that is needed.

Postoperative Constipation & Fecal Impaction

Postoperative constipation is common after surgery due to opioid use for pain control. If left unaddressed, it may lead to fecal impaction as a result of colonic ileus and impaired perception of rectal fullness. Risk factors include predisposing conditions (eg, megacolon or paraplegia), age, and anticholinergic and narcotic medications. Early symptoms are anorexia, obstipation, or diarrhea. In advanced cases, marked distention may cause colonic perforation. Diagnosis is made by rectal examination. The impaction should be manually removed, and enemas are given with repeat digital examination.

Barium remaining in the colon from an examination done before surgery may harden and produce barium impaction.

This typically involves the right colon, where water absorption occurs, and it is a more difficult management problem than fecal impaction. Barium impaction has the same symptoms of bowel obstruction. Treatment includes enemas and polyethylene glycol-electrolyte solutions (Colyte, GoLYTELY). Diatrizoate sodium (Hypaque), a hyperosmolar solution that stimulates peristalsis and increases intraluminal fluid, may be effective by enema if other solutions fail. Operation is rarely necessary.

Abdominal Compartment Syndrome

Abdominal compartment syndrome is a rare but life-threatening complication that may result from aggressive resuscitation of patients leading to increased abdominal pressure (eg, burn or trauma patients). Similar to compartment syndrome of the extremities, the fascia resists stretch exerted by the muscle and other tissue with resuscitation leading to the elevated pressures. Unlike the extremities, patients with abdominal compartment syndrome do not exhibit the 5 Ps (pain, paresthesia, pallor, paralysis, and pulselessness). However, a high index of suspicion, rapid diagnosis, and expeditious treatment result in restoration of flow and prevention of morbidity in both scenarios. Intra-abdominal hypertension, as measured by bladder pressure, is generally self-limiting but it can become dangerous when pressures exceed 30 mm Hg. Increased abdominal pressure limits cardiac venous return via the inferior vena cava (IVC).

Additionally, venous outflow from the bowel and kidney may become compromised. Respiratory complications may occur from the pressure exerted on the diaphragm. It leads to decreased tidal volume, elevated peak inspiratory pressures, and respiratory acidosis. With elevated abdominal pressure, the compartment must be rapidly decompressed to reestablish flow from the viscera, usually via abdominal laparotomy. With decompression, symptoms tend to resolve.

Postoperative Pancreatitis

Postoperative pancreatitis accounts for 10% of all cases of acute pancreatitis. It occurs in 1-3% of patients who have operations in the vicinity of the pancreas and with higher frequency after operations on the biliary tract—1% of patients undergoing cholecystectomy and 8% of patients undergoing common bile duct exploration unrelated to intraoperative interventions. Pathogenesis is typically from mechanical trauma, pancreatic manipulation (ie, biopsy or resection), or compromised blood supply. Postoperative pancreatitis after biliary surgery is worse in patients who have had preoperative biliary pancreatitis. It is frequently necrotizing and may lead to insufficiency. Complications from pancreatic necrosis occur three to four times more often in postoperative pancreatitis compared to biliary and alcoholic pancreatitis. Postoperative pancreatitis is associated with a mortality rate of 30%-40%.

Postoperative Hepatic Dysfunction

Hepatic dysfunction, ranging from mild jaundice to life-threatening hepatic failure, follows 1% of surgical procedures performed under general anesthesia. The incidence is greater following pancreatectomy, biliary bypass operations, and portacaval shunt. Postoperative hyperbilirubinemia may be categorized as prehepatic jaundice, hepatocellular insufficiency, and posthepatic obstruction.

Prehepatic jaundice can be caused by bilirubin overload, most often from hemolysis or reabsorption of hematomas. Factors that impair biliary function in the postoperative period include fasting, malnutrition, hepatotoxic drugs, and anesthesia. Increased hemolysis can result from incompatible blood transfusion, hemolysis, ECMO, congenital hemolytic disease (eg, sickle-cell disease), and drugs.

Hepatocellular insufficiency is the most common cause of postoperative jaundice and occurs as a consequence of hepatic cell necrosis, inflammation, or massive hepatic resection. Drugs, hypotension, hypoxia, and sepsis are among the injurious factors. Benign postoperative intrahepatic cholestasis is a vague term used to denote jaundice following operations that often involve hypotension and multiple transfusions. They may also develop in patients receiving total parenteral nutrition (TPN). Serum bilirubin ranges from 2 to 20 mg/dL and serum alkaline phosphatase is usually high, but the patient is typically afebrile with a smooth postoperative course. It is usually a diagnosis of exclusion. Jaundice typically resolved by the third postoperative week.

Posthepatic obstruction can be caused by direct surgical injury to the bile ducts, retained common duct stones, tumor obstruction of the bile duct, or pancreatitis. Acute postoperative cholecystitis is associated with jaundice in up to one-third of cases even when mechanical obstruction of the common duct is not usually apparent. It is important to determine if a patient with postoperative jaundice has a correctable cause that requires treatment. Sepsis may lead to decreased liver function. Otherwise, levels may be elevated from obstructed bile duct or postoperative cholecystitis. Liver function tests are not helpful in determining the cause and do not usually reflect the severity of disease. Liver biopsy, ultrasound and CT scans, and transhepatic or endoscopic retrograde cholangiograms are the tests most likely to sort out the diagnostic possibilities. Renal function must be monitored closely, because renal failure may develop in these patients. Treatment is otherwise expectant.

Postoperative Cholecystitis

Acute postoperative cholecystitis may follow any kind of operation, but it is more common after gastrointestinal procedures. In 3%-5% of patients, acute cholecystitis develops after endoscopic sphincterotomy. Chemical cholecystitis occurs in patients undergoing hepatic arterial chemotherapy with mitomycin and floxuridine with such frequency that cholecystectomy should always be performed before infusion of these agents is begun. Fulminant cholecystitis with gallbladder infarction may follow percutaneous embolization of the hepatic artery for malignant tumors of the liver or for arteriovenous malformation involving this artery.

Postoperative cholecystitis differs in several respects from the common form of acute cholecystitis. It is frequently acalculous (70%-80%), more common in males (75%), progresses rapidly to gallbladder necrosis, and is not likely to respond to conservative therapy. The cause is clear in cases of chemical or ischemic cholecystitis but not in other forms. Factors thought to play a role include biliary stasis (with formation of sludge), biliary infection, and ischemia.

GENITOURINARY COMPLICATIONS

▶ Perioperative Kidney Injury

Acute kidney injury (AKI) describes a decrease in renal function over a course of hours to days. As defined by ACS-NSQIP, it is a change in serum creatinine greater than 2 mg/dL. Acute renal injury is a common complication in the postoperative setting and is associated with increased mortality and risk of developing chronic renal failure. Major causes include ischemia (shock), sepsis, hypovolemia, bleeding, toxins, and cardiovascular failure. Preventative measures include avoidance of nephrotoxic drugs, hemodynamic stabilization, and early identification. Kidney injury can be broken down into three types: prerenal, intrinsic, and postrenal.

A common form of postoperative kidney dysfunction is acute tubular necrosis (ATN). Its pathophysiology progresses across multiple phases, starting with a prerenal insult leading to an intrinsic injury. Prerenal causes of renal injury are a result of poor perfusion. The most common cause is hypovolemia causing hypoperfusion; treatment is therefore focused on fluids. However, other causes include obstruction of renal flow (eg, from renal artery dissection or thrombus, external compression) or poor cardiac function. ATN occurs as a result of prolonged or severe ischemia, leading to renal tubular epithelial necrosis, sloughing, and cast formation and excretion. Typically, it takes time to recover, and treatment consistent of avoiding further nephrotoxic agents. While in the prerenal phase, patient should be appropriately rehydrated to decrease duration and severity of ischemia. Postsurgical patients are also at risk of postrenal AKI, typically in the form of urinary retention (discussed in the next section). Treatment requires relieving the obstruction.

▶ Postoperative Urinary Retention

Inability to void postoperatively is common, especially after pelvic and perineal operations or patients with spinal anesthesia. Factors responsible for postoperative urinary retention are interference with the neural mechanisms responsible for normal emptying of the bladder and over-distention of the urinary bladder. Although its normal capacity is about 500 mL, when the volume is exceeded, bladder contraction is inhibited. An indwelling Foley catheter should to be placed whenever an operation is likely to last 3 hours or longer or where large volumes of intravenous fluids are anticipated. The catheter can be removed at the end of the operation if the patient is expected to be able to ambulate within a few hours. When bladder catheterization is not performed, the patient should be encouraged to void immediately before coming to the operating room and as soon as possible after the operation, with close monitoring for complete emptying. During abdominoperineal resection, operative trauma to the sacral plexus alters bladder function enough so that an indwelling catheter should be left in place for 4-5 days. Patients with inguinal hernia who strain to void as a manifestation of prostatic hypertrophy should have the prostate treated before the hernia.

The treatment of acute urinary retention is catheterization of the bladder. In the absence of factors that suggest the need for prolonged decompression, such as the presence of 1000 mL or more of urine, the catheter may be removed.

OTHER INFECTIOUS COMPLICATIONS

Besides wound complications, as previously discussed, additional postoperative infectious complications are common. A wide range of organisms are involved in these infections, but what is very concerning is the increasing prevalence of antibiotic-resistant bacteria, such as methicillin-resistant *Staphylococcus aureus* (MRSA) and vancomycin-resistant *Enterococcus* (VRE).

▶ Postoperative Pneumonia

Pneumonia is the most common pulmonary complication among patients who die after surgery. Overall mortality rates for postoperative pneumonia vary from 20% to 40%. Atelectasis, aspiration, and copious secretions are important predisposing factors.

After surgery, cough is usually weak and may not effectively clear the bronchial tree. The mucociliary transport mechanism is damaged by endotracheal intubation, and the functional ability of the alveolar macrophage is compromised by a number of factors that may be present during and after surgery (oxygenation, pulmonary edema, tracheobronchial aspiration, corticosteroid therapy, etc). In addition, squamous metaplasia and loss of ciliary coordination further hamper antibacterial defenses. More than half of the pulmonary infections that follow surgery are caused by gram-negative bacilli. Pneumonias are frequently polymicrobial and usually acquired through aspiration of oropharyngeal secretions. Aggravating factors are azotemia, prolonged endotracheal intubation, and severe associated infection.

Patients may also be exposed to nosocomial infections acquired from inhalation (eg, mechanical respirators). *Pseudomonas aeruginosa* and *Klebsiella* are common causes of pneumonia in ICUs. These pathogens can survive in the moist reservoirs of ventilators. Rarely, the lung may become contaminated directly from hematogenous spread from distant septic foci.

Clinical findings suggestive of postoperative pneumonia include fever, tachypnea, increased secretions, and physical exam suggestive of pulmonary consolidation. Chest x-rays may use patchy opacification or localized consolidation.

Secretion management is important in the prevention of postoperative pneumonia. Respiratory exercises, deep breathing, and coughing help prevent atelectasis, which is a precursor of pneumonia. Postoperative pain is thought to contribute to shallow breathing; thus postoperative pain control is tantamount. The prophylactic use of antibiotics does not decrease the incidence of gram-negative colonization of the oropharynx or that of pneumonia. Sputum obtained directly from the trachea, usually by endotracheal suctioning, is required for specific identification of the infecting organism.

Urinary Tract Infection

Urinary tract infections (UTIs) are the most frequently acquired nosocomial infection. Preexisting contamination of the urinary tract, urinary retention, and instrumentation are the principal contributing factors. Although clinical symptoms of UTIs only occur in 1% of patients, bacteriuria is suspected to be present in about 5% of patients who undergo short-term (< 48 hours) bladder catheterization. Symptoms of cystitis include dysuria and mild fever. Pyelonephritis is characterized by high fever, flank tenderness, and occasionally ileus. Diagnosis is made by examination of the urine with confirmation by cultures. Prevention involves treating urinary tract contamination before surgery, prevention or prompt treatment of urinary retention, and careful instrumentation when needed. Treatment includes adequate hydration, proper drainage of the bladder, and specific antibiotics.

Clostridium difficile Colitis

Postoperative diarrhea due to *Clostridium difficile* is a common nosocomial infection in surgical patients. It ranges from asymptomatic colonization to severe, toxic colitis. Transmission from hospital personnel probably occurs. The major risk factor is perioperative antibiotic use. Diagnosis is established by identification of a specific cytopathic toxin in the stool or culture of the organism from a stool sample. In severely affected patients, colonoscopy reveals pseudomembranes. Prevention is accomplished by strict handwashing, enteric precautions, and minimizing antibiotic use. Treatment of established infection is first line with vancomycin by mouth due to increasing resistance of the organism.

Drug-Resistant Organisms

An increase in the prevalence of multi-drug-resistant organisms has been noted over the past two decades, particularly methicillin-resistant *Staphylococcus aureus* (MRSA) and vancomycin-resistant *Enterococcus* (VRE). Although routine screening of patients has found the prevalence as high as 30% in the community, these organisms are much more frequently found in the hospital or other institutions (nursing homes, prisons, gymnasiums, etc). Increased antibiotic usage in the inpatient and outpatient settings has been speculated to be the cause of the drug resistance; however, the spread within institutions has been demonstrated to be due to direct patient contact. Continuous surface decontamination, utilization of barrier techniques when examining patients, and assiduous hand hygiene have been shown to decrease transmission. Furthermore, discontinuation of inappropriate antibiotics has been shown to limit the colonization of patients with most drug-resistant organisms, including *Clostridium difficile*.

Postoperative Fever

Fever occurs in about 40% of patients after major surgery. In most patients, the fever self-resolves. However, a postoperative fever may indicate serious infection, and it is therefore important to evaluate the patient clinically. Features often associated with an infectious origin of the fever include preoperative trauma, ASA class above 2, fever onset after the second postoperative day, an initial temperature elevation above 38.6°C, a postoperative white blood cell count greater than 10,000/μL, and a postoperative serum urea nitrogen of 15 mg/dL or greater. If three or more of the above are present, the likelihood of associated bacterial infection is nearly 100%.

Fever within 48 hours after surgery is usually caused by atelectasis (as discussed in detail under the pulmonary section). Reexpansion of the lung causes body temperature to return to normal. When fever appears after the second postoperative day, atelectasis is a less likely explanation. The differential diagnosis of fever at this time includes catheter-related phlebitis, pneumonia, and urinary tract infection. A directed history and physical examination complemented by focused laboratory and radiologic studies usually determine the cause. Patients without infection are rarely febrile after the fifth postoperative day. Fever this late suggests wound infection, anastomotic breakdown, intra-abdominal leak, or intra-abdominal abscesses. A diagnostic work-up directed to the detection of intra-abdominal sepsis is indicated in patients who have high temperatures (> 39°C) and wounds without evidence of infection 5 or more days

Table 5–3. Timing and causes of postoperative fever.

Postoperative Day	Fever Sources
1-2	Atelectasis
3-5	Urinary tract infection, pneumonia, phlebitis
5-7	Wound infection, anastomotic breakdown, intra-abdominal infection, deep vein thrombosis
Anytime	Drug reaction, transfusion reaction, bacteremia

postoperatively. CT scan of the abdomen and pelvis is the test of choice and should be performed early, before overt organ failure occurs.

Fever is rare after the first week in patients who had a normal convalescence. Allergy to drugs, transfusion-related fever, septic pelvic vein thrombosis, and intra-abdominal abscesses should be considered (Table 5–3).

HEMATOLOGIC COMPLICATIONS

Besides the risk of bleeding, major surgery such as abdominal and trauma operations alter the fine balance of the hematologic system, especially with regards to the coagulation pathway.

Venous Thromboembolism

Virchow's triad defines the underlying risk factors for venous thromboembolism (VTE): hypercoagulable state, stasis, and vessel damage. Patients are at higher risk of developing a VTE with prolonged immobilization from trauma, cancer operations, or dissections of the pelvis. Postoperative patients should be monitored for lower extremity swelling, hypoxia, or new-onset pleuritic chest pain, suggestive of embolization to the pulmonary artery.

Diagnosis can be made by duplex ultrasound. Alternative, more costly or invasive, alternatives include computed tomography, magnetic resonance imaging, or venography. Prevention of VTE is much more effective than treatment of this complication. The CHEST guidelines are a useful adjunct to stratifying risk and assigning appropriate preventive therapy. This usually requires heparin therapy with regular or low-molecular-weight heparin, sequential compression stockings, and early ambulation. Inferior vena cava (IVC) filters may be considered as a preventive method in patients who have contraindications to anticoagulation or have progression of disease despite adequate anticoagulation.

Heparin-Induced Thrombocytopenia

Thrombocytopenia commonly occurs in the postoperative period and has several causes. Postoperative thrombocytopenia is defined to be a 50% reduction in total platelet volume. Heparin-induced thrombocytopenia (HIT) is generally seen within 1 week after initiation of heparin therapy, and it is more commonly associated with unfractionated heparin than low-molecular-weight heparin. Although generally associated with thrombocytopenia, the initial phase is procoagulative and thrombotic with many patients experiencing VTE, myocardial infarction, or stroke. Thrombocytopenia is a later finding. Once suspicious of HIT, all heparin, including flushes and coated catheters, should be discontinued and an antibody assay should be performed. If the diagnosis of HIT is confirmed, then further use of heparin and heparin-coated products should be avoided. If anticoagulation is necessary, lepirudin or argatroban should be considered. The choice of agent is generally made by patient factors: lepirudin should be avoided in patients with renal failure and argatroban should be avoided in patients with hepatic failure. Long-term anticoagulation may be transitioned to warfarin; however, it must not be administered during the acute phase of HIT as it may lead to an increased risk of procoagulation.

Disseminated Intravascular Coagulation

A condition with abnormal, diffuse activation of the coagulation system with excessive thrombin production, disseminated intravascular coagulation (DIC) leads to fibrin and platelet activation, fibrinolysis, and depletion of the coagulation factors. Typical causes include sepsis, shock, trauma, burns, fat/cholesterol/amniotic embolism, and large-volume bleed. Clinical findings include petechiae, ecchymoses, bleeding around lines and injection sites, and even frank hemorrhage from orifices and surgical sites. Treatment includes replacement of appropriate blood products (FFP, platelets, and cryoprecipitate) that can be directed by looking at thromboelastograph (TEG) results to see what components are low. In states with inappropriate thrombosis, heparin may be used to decrease fibrin formation. Use of fibrinolysis inhibitors are not recommended due to risk of diffuse intravascular thrombosis.

Hemoperitoneum

Bleeding is the most common cause of shock in the first 24 hours after abdominal surgery. Postoperative hemoperitoneum is defined as a rapidly evolving, life-threatening complication that is the result of a technical problem with hemostasis. However, coagulation disorders need to be considered. Causes of possible coagulopathy include intravenous dilution with fluid resuscitation after massive blood loss, mismatched transfusion, or administration of anticoagulation.

Hemoperitoneum usually becomes apparent within 24 hours after operative intervention. Symptoms are related to intravascular depletion leading to tachycardia, hypotension, decreased urine output, and peripheral vasoconstriction. An increase in abdominal girth may be noted along with intra-abdominal hypertension or abdominal compartment syndrome. Changes in the hematocrit may not be reflected in blood work for the first 4-6 hours due to loss of whole blood.

With the presentation of postoperative circulatory collapse, the initial differential includes PE, cardiac dysrhythmias, pneumothorax, myocardial infarction, and severe allergic reactions. Infusions to expand the intravascular volume should be started as soon as other diseases have been ruled out. Should symptoms of hypovolemic shock persist, the patient will need to be taken back to the operating room for source control. Intraoperatively, the source ought to be localized, clots evacuated, and the peritoneal cavity washed with saline solution.

COMPLICATIONS OF LINES, DRAINS, & RETAINED FOREIGN BODIES

▶ Lines

Complications due to central line placement and maintenance are preventable with adequate preparation, technique, and experience. Choice of site, utilization of ultrasound, and adherence to sterile technique decreases infection, decreases mechanical complications, and increases successful placement.

Peripheral venous complications include phlebitis, which is inflammation at the site of a peripheral intravenous catheter. It is one of the most common causes of fever after the third postoperative day. The triad of findings includes induration, edema, and local tenderness. Venous catheters should be removed at the first sign of redness, induration, or edema. Removal of the catheter is adequate treatment. Phlebitis occurs more frequently with lower-extremity veins; thus upper-extremity veins are preferable. Suppurative phlebitis occurs from an infected thrombus at the site of the venous catheter. The most common causative agent is *Staphylococcus*. Unlike phlebitis, pus may be expressed from the venipuncture site. High fever and positive blood cultures are common. Treatment consists of excising the affected vein, extending the incision proximally to the first open collateral, and wound care with healing by secondary intention.

Complications from central venous lines (CVLs) include pneumothorax with placement, line infection from indwelling line, and air embolus with removal. Pneumothorax occurs with CVL placement into the subclavian or internal jugular veins in approximately 1% of the lines. Use of ultrasound decreases the complication rate with CVL placement. It decreases the rate of arterial injury, which can prevent pseudoaneurysm, bleeding, or stroke. There is a very low risk of right-atrial perforation with cardiac tamponade. Complications associated with the use of the flow-directed balloon-tipped (Swan-Ganz) catheter include cardiac perforation (usually of the right atrium), intracardiac knotting of the catheter, and cardiac dysrhythmias. Pulmonary hemorrhage may result from disruption of a branch of the pulmonary artery during balloon inflation and may be fatal in patients with pulmonary hypertension. Steps in prevention include careful placement, advancement under continuous pressure monitoring, and checking the position of the tip before inflating the balloon. With placement or removal, there is a risk of introducing an air embolism. Intravenous air lodges in the right atrium, preventing adequate filling, leading to hypotension, jugular venous distention, and tachycardia. This complication can be avoided by placing the patient in the Trendelenburg position with insertion and removal of a CVL. Emergency treatment consists of aspiration of the air with a syringe. If this is unsuccessful, the patient should be positioned right side up and head down, which will help dislodge the air from the right atrium and return circulatory dynamics to normal.

There are also complications with arterial line placements. An arterial line allows continuous perioperative monitoring of blood pressure. There is an associated risk of thrombosis, bleeding, or aneurysmal formation from the artery accessed. If the artery thrombosis, then there is the risk for acute limb ischemia, which will require immediate revascularization. With the wrist, this serious complication may be limited by evaluating the patency of the ulnar artery (Allen test) before establishing the radial line.

▶ Drains

Intraoperative drainage of the peritoneal cavity is indicated to prevent accumulation of fluid (eg, bile or pancreatic fluid from cholecystectomy, splenectomy, or colectomy). Postoperatively, a drain may also be placed to drain new collections or abscesses. Strict documentation of drain outputs help dictate when they can be removed. Latex Penrose drains, which were used frequently in the past, should generally be avoided because of the risk of introducing infection. Large, rigid drains may erode into adjacent viscera or vessels and cause fistula formation or bleeding. This risk is lessened with the use of softer Silastic drains, and removing them as early as possible. Drains should not be left in contact with intestinal anastomoses, as they may promote anastomotic leakage and fistula formation.

▶ Retained Foreign Bodies

Studies based on hospital claims data estimate that cases of retained objects, which include sponges and instruments, occur at least once a year in those hospitals where 8000-18,000 major procedures are performed annually. Although mortality is low, the morbidity is high due to the almost universal need for reoperation. The most common body cavity involved is the abdomen, followed by the thoracic cavity. Improving communication within the operating room, formal sponge and instrument counts, and appropriate use of radiography all contribute to a decrease in this complication.

CONCLUSIONS

Complications are an inherent risk to performing surgery. They lead to increased morbidity, mortality, duration of hospitalization, and rates of readmission. It is critical to be aware of the patient's risk factors and be vigilant for complications that occur in the postoperative period. Surgeons need to recognize them early, respond in an expedient manner, and administer the appropriate treatment to rescue the patient and achieve the best possible outcome.

▶ References

Brummett CM, Waljee JF, Goesling J, et al. New persistent opioid use after minor and major surgical procedures in US adults. *JAMA Surg.* 2017;152(6):e170504.

Khuri SF, Henderson WG, DePalma RG, Mosca C, Healey NA, Kumbhani DJ. Determinants of long-term survival after major surgery and the adverse effect of postoperative complications. *Ann Surg.* 2005;242(3):326-341; discussion 341-343.

Lawson EH, Hall BL, Louie R, et al. Association between occurrence of a postoperative complication and readmission: Implications for quality improvement and cost savings. *Ann Surg.* 2013; 258(1):10-18.

Schilling PL, Dimick JB, Birkmeyer JD. Prioritizing quality improvement in general surgery. *J Am Coll Surg.* 2008;207(5):698-704.

Wick EC, Grant MC, Wu CL. Postoperative multimodal analgesia pain management with nonopioid analgesics and techniques: A review. *JAMA Surg.* 2017;152(7):691-697.

MULTIPLE-CHOICE QUESTIONS

1. All the following are true of surgical site infections *except:*

   A. Antiseptic technique helps prevent surgical site infections.
   B. Development of an intra-abdominal phlegmon is indicative of poor wound healing.
   C. Surgical technique does not play a role in leading to infection.
   D. Wound dehiscence is a consequence of surgical site infection.

2. A 45-year-old woman developed fever, chills, and worsening abdominal pain 7 days after a small-bowel resection for Crohn disease. She complained of persistent nausea and vomiting. Her abdomen was distended and diffusely firm with peritonitis on examination. Her vital signs are a temperature of 102.3°F, heart rate of 117 beats/min, blood pressure of 98/56 mm Hg, and respiratory rate of 23 breaths/min on 2L nasal cannula. CT of the abdomen/

pelvis showed anastomotic stranding with trace free fluid. What is the next best step?

   A. Take her back to the operating room.
   B. Consult interventional radiology for drain placement.
   C. Initial management requires a nasogastric tube placement, IV fluids, and supportive management.
   D. Start empiric antibiotics.
   E. Both A and D.
   F. Both B and C.
   G. None of the above.

3. A 74-year-old 100-kg man with rectal cancer underwent a laparoscopic low anterior resection with diverting loop ileostomy. Preoperatively, he received a regional block per ERAS protocol. Intraoperatively, he received 2-L of IV crystalloid for a 5-hour case and received multimodal pain control with Toradol and Tylenol. On postoperative day 1, 200 mL of urine was collected from his Foley catheter over 12 hours, accompanied by an elevation from his baseline creatinine. He was given 40 mL/h of crystalloid over the same time period. What is the most likely cause of his oliguria?

   A. Inadequate fluid resuscitation.
   B. High ileostomy output.
   C. Urinary tract obstruction.
   D. Low cardiac output.
   E. Bladder dysfunction.

4. A 25-year-old man is 6 hours postoperative from emergent laparotomy after blunt abdominal trauma from a motor vehicle accident. His spleen was removed, and the hepatic laceration was repaired primarily with sutures and packed with topical procoagulants. There was tearing in his mesentery leading to a small partial bowel resection and a notable retroperitoneal hematoma. The duration of the operation was 5 hours, and he received 3 L of crystalloid, 15 U of blood, 15 U of fresh frozen plasma, and 10 U of platelets. His abdominal wall was lax enough to be closed primarily. He remained intubated and was transferred to the ICU postoperatively for further resuscitation. His urine output dropped from 50 mL/h to 15 mL/h over the past 3 hours. His abdomen appears distended and his breaths appear more labored on the ventilator with increased peak pressures and decreased tidal volumes. Further steps in his management should include:

   A. Paralyzing the patient for better ventilation.
   B. Trial of diuresis to improve renal function.
   C. Additional fluid resuscitation, given the large-volume blood loss.
   D. Bladder pressure measurement to assess for increased abdominal pressures.
   E. Obtain CT of the chest/abdomen/pelvis to evaluate for further bleeding.

5. An 82-year-old woman with dementia who is otherwise healthy presented to the emergency department with a strangulated umbilical hernia. Her initial vital signs were a temperature of 102.1°F, heart rate of 112 beats/min, blood pressure of 102/46 mm Hg, and respiratory rate of 22 breaths/min on 2 L nasal cannula. On exam, she had a large, nonreducible bulge that was erythematous and tender to palpation. Lab work showed leukocytosis to 23 with a lactic acid of 3.1. She was emergently taken for exploratory laparotomy and hernia repair, with subsequent normalization of her labs and vital signs. On postoperative day 3, she became confused and combative, requiring restraints. She reported new low abdominal pain and was found to have a low-grade fever. What is the most likely cause?

A. Atelectasis.
B. Postoperative delirium.
C. Urinary tract infection.
D. Abdominal abscess.
E. Nosocomial pneumonia.

Wound Healing

Michael G. Franz, MD, FACS

ACUTE WOUNDS

Acute wounds result from the sudden loss of anatomic structure in tissue following some form of injury with the transfer of kinetic, thermal, or chemical energy. Physiologically, an acute wound progresses predictably through the phases of wound healing and results in complete and sustained repair (Figure 6–1). Acute wounds typically occur in recently uninjured and otherwise normal tissue. Acute wound healing continuously advances completing the entire process within 6-12 weeks. Most surgical wounds are acute wounds.

CHRONIC WOUNDS

The continuum of wound healing fails in a chronic wound. The process of tissue repair is prolonged and pathologic. The usual mechanism is dysregulation of one of the classic phases of normal acute wound healing. Most often, healing is delayed due to a prolonged inflammatory phase. A protracted inflammatory phase may be due to wound infection or another form of chronic irritation. Tissue and wound hypoxia is the other important mechanism for the development of a chronic wound. Failed epithelialization due to repeat trauma or desiccation may also result in a chronic partial thickness wound. Chronic wounds may be surgically converted to acute wounds by sharp excision of the abnormal wound tissue.

GENERAL CONSIDERATIONS

▷ Clinical Wound Healing

Surgeons often describe wound healing as primary or secondary. *Primary healing* occurs when tissue is cleanly incised and anatomically reapproximated. It is also referred to as healing by primary intention, and tissue repair usually proceeds without complication. *Secondary healing* occurs in wounds left open through the formation of granulation tissue and eventual coverage of the defect by migration of epithelial cells. Granulation tissue is composed of new capillaries, fibroblasts, and a provisional extracellular matrix that forms at the base of the early wound. This process is also referred to as healing by secondary intention. Most infected wounds or contaminated wounds heal in this manner. Primary healing is most efficient physiologically, requiring less time and tissue synthesis than secondary healing. A wound healing primarily repairs a smaller volume than an open wound healing secondarily. The principles of primary and secondary healing are combined in *delayed primary closure*, when a wound is left open to heal under a carefully maintained, moist wound healing environment for approximately 5 days and is then closed as if primarily. Wounds treated with delayed primary closure are less likely to become infected than if closed immediately because bacterial balance is achieved and oxygen requirements are optimized through capillary formation in the granulation tissue.

▷ The Mechanism of Wound Healing

The complex but well-coordinated processes of wound healing normally progresses from coagulation and inflammation through fibroplasia, matrix deposition, angiogenesis, epithelialization, collagen maturation, and finally wound contraction (Figure 6–1). Wound healing signals include peptide growth factors, complement, cytokine inflammatory mediators, and metabolic signals such as hypoxia and accumulated lactate. Many of these cellular signaling pathways are redundant and pleiotropic.

New tissue formation occurs within the wound about 2-10 days after injury. A fibrous coagulum (eschar or scab) is present on the surface of the wound. The platelet and neutrophil numbers fall within the wound while macrophages now infiltrate along with new blood vessels. Epithelial cells also begin to migrate from the wound edge across its surface beneath the eschar. Remodeling of the mature wound matrix

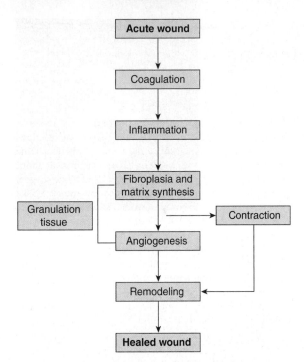

▲ Figure 6–1. Acute wound healing normally proceeds from coagulation and inflammation, through angiogenesis, fibroplasia, matrix deposition (granulation tissue formation), collagen maturation, epithelialization, and finally wound contraction. A chronic wound fails to heal anywhere along this wound healing pathway.

or scar occurs for a year or longer. Disorganized collagen has been deposited by infiltrating fibroblasts and wound contraction occurs at the surface. The newly healing wound does not contain normal skin appendages due to limitations in human tissue regeneration.

A. Hemostasis and Inflammation

Hemostasis and inflammation initiate the classic stages of wound repair. Following injury, a wound must stop bleeding in order to heal and for the injured host to survive. It is therefore not surprising that cellular and molecular elements involved in hemostasis also signal an inflammatory response and fibroplastic tissue repair. This stage lasts until about 48 hours after injury. The wound environment is hypoxic (ischemic) and occupied by a fibrin clot, bacteria, platelets, and neutrophils. Immediately after injury, the coagulation products fibrin, fibrinopeptides, thrombin split products, and complement components attract inflammatory cells into the wound. Platelets activated by thrombin release insulin-like growth factor 1 (IGF-1), transforming growth factor α (TGF-α), transforming growth factor β (TGF-β), and platelet-derived growth factor (PDGF), which attract leukocytes,

particularly macrophages, and fibroblasts into the wound. Damaged endothelial cells respond to a signal cascade involving the complement products C5a, tumor necrosis factor α (TNF-α), interleukin-1 (IL-1), and interleukin-8 (IL-8), and express receptors for integrin molecules on the cell membranes of leukocytes. Circulating leukocytes then adhere to the endothelium and migrate into the wounded tissue. Interleukins and other inflammatory components, such as histamine, serotonin, and bradykinin, cause vessels first to constrict for hemostasis and later to dilate, becoming porous so that blood plasma and leukocytes can migrate into the injured tissue.

The very early wound inflammatory cells increase metabolic demand. Because the local microvasculature is also damaged, a local energy sink results, and tissue O_2 concentrations fall while CO_2 accumulates. Tissue lactate also accumulates and serves a critical role in signaling acute wound healing, because its source is mainly anaerobic and its level is tightly regulated by dropping tissue oxygen levels. Relative and moderate tissue hypoxia is another important signal for angiogenesis and tissue repair. These early wound conditions trigger reparative processes and stimulate their propagation.

Macrophages assume a dominant role in the synthesis of wound healing molecules as coagulation-mediated tissue repair signal levels fall. Again, macrophages, stimulated by fibrin, continue to release large quantities of lactate. This process continues even as oxygen levels begin to rise, thereby maintaining the "environment of injury." Lactate alone stimulates angiogenesis and collagen deposition through the sustained production of growth factors. Unless the wound becomes infected, the granulocyte population that dominated the first days diminishes. Macrophages now cover the injured surface. Fibroblasts begin to organize, mixed with buds of new blood vessels. It has been shown that circulating stem cells, such as bone marrow–derived mesenchymal stem cells, contribute fibroblasts to the healing wound, but the extent of this process is as yet unknown.

B. Fibroplasia and Matrix Synthesis

1. Fibroplasia—Throughout wound healing, fibroplasia (the replication of fibroblasts) is stimulated by multiple mechanisms, starting with PDGF, IGF-1, and TGF-β released by platelets and later by the continual release of numerous peptide growth factors from macrophages and even other fibroblasts within the wound. Growth factors and cytokines shown to stimulate fibroplasia and wound healing include fibroblast growth factor (FGF), IGF-1, vascular endothelial growth factor (VEGF), IL-1, IL-2, IL-8, PDGF, TGF-α, TGF-β, and TNF-α. Dividing fibroblasts localize near the wound edge, an active tissue repair environment with tissue oxygen tensions of approximately 40 mm Hg in normally healing wounds. In cell culture and clinically, this is the optimum concentration of oxygen fibroblast replication and wound healing. Smooth muscle cells are also likely progenitors

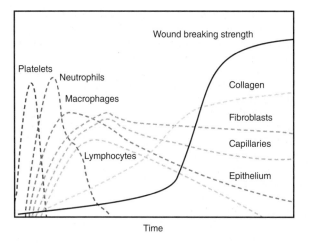

▲ Figure 6–2. The fundamental cellular and molecular elements activated during normal wound healing.

because fibroblasts seem to migrate from the adventitia and media of wound vessels.

2. Matrix synthesis—Fibroblasts secrete the collagen and proteoglycans of the forming connective tissue matrix that holds wound edges together and embeds cells of the healing wound matrix. These extracellular molecules polymerize, form a scaffold, and become the physical basis of wound strength (Figure 6–2). Collagen synthesis is not a constitutive property of fibroblasts but must be signaled. The mechanisms that regulate the stimulation and synthesis of collagen are multifactorial and include both growth factors and metabolic inputs such as lactate. The collagen gene promoter has regulatory binding sites for stress corticoids, the TGF-β signaling pathway, and retinoids, which control collagen gene expression. Other growth factors regulate glycosaminoglycans, tissue inhibitors of metalloproteinase (TIMP), and fibronectin synthesis. The accumulation of lactate in the extracellular environment is shown to directly stimulate transcription of collagen genes as well as posttranslational processing of collagen peptides. The redox state and energy stores of repair cells occupying the wound are a fundamental mechanism regulating collagen synthesis.

The increase in collagen messenger RNA (mRNA) leads to an increased procollagen peptide. This, however, is not sufficient to increase collagen deposition because procollagen peptide cannot be transported from the cell to the extracellular space until, in a posttranslational step, a proportion of its proline amino acids is hydroxylated. In this reaction, catalyzed by prolyl hydroxylase, an oxygen atom derived from dissolved O_2 is inserted (as a hydroxyl group) into selected collagen prolines in the presence of the cofactors ascorbic acid, iron, and α-ketoglutarate. Thus, accumulation of lactate, or any other process that decreases the nicotinamide adenine dinucleotide (NAD^+) pool, leads to

production of collagen mRNAs, increased collagen peptide synthesis, and (provided enough ascorbate and oxygen are present) increased posttranslational modification and secretion of collagen monomers into the extracellular space.

Another enzyme, lysyl hydroxylase, hydroxylates many of the procollagen lysines. A lysyl-to-lysyl covalent link then occurs between collagen molecules, maximizing mature collagen fiber strength. This process, too, requires adequate amounts of ascorbate and oxygen. These oxygenase reactions (and therefore collagen depositions) are rate limited by tissue oxygen levels, (Pao_2). The rates are half-maximal at about 20 mm Hg and maximal at about 200 mm Hg of tissue oxygen. Hydroxylation can be "forced" to supernormal rates by tissue hyperoxia. Collagen deposition, wound strength, and angiogenesis rates may be increased and accelerated as tissue Pao_2 is elevated, the likely significant mechanism for benefits in wound healing seen clinically with hyperbaric oxygen.

C. Angiogenesis

Angiogenesis is required for wound healing. It is clinically evident about 4 days following injury, but begins earlier when new capillaries sprout from preexisting venules and grow toward the injury in response to chemoattractants released by platelets and macrophages. In primarily closed wounds, budding vessels soon meet and fuse with counterparts migrating from the other side of the wound, establishing blood flow across the wound. In wounds left open, newly forming capillaries connect with adjacent capillaries migrating in the same direction, and granulation tissue forms. Numerous growth factors and cytokines are observed to stimulate angiogenesis, but animal experiments indicate that the dominant angiogenic stimulants in wounds are derived first from platelets in response to coagulation and then from macrophages in response to hypoxia or high lactate, fibrin, and its products.

D. Epithelialization

Epithelial cells respond to several of the same stimuli as fibroblasts and endothelial cells within the mesenchymal area of a wound. A variety of growth factors also regulate epithelial cell replication. TGF-α and keratinocyte growth factor (KGF), for instance, are potent epithelial cell mitogens. TGF-β tends to inhibit epithelial cells from differentiating and thus may support cell division and fibroplasia, though it is itself not a mitogen for these cells. During wound healing, maximal cell proliferation occurs in the epithelium a few cells away from the wound edge. The new cells migrate over cells at the wound edge and into the unhealed area and then anchor to the first unepithelialized matrix position encountered. The Pao_2 on the underside of the cell at the anchor point is usually low. Low Pao_2 stimulates squamous epithelial cells to produce TGF-β, likely suppressing terminal differentiation and again supporting further mitosis. This process of epidermal-mesenchymal communication repeats itself until the wound is closed.

Squamous epithelialization and differentiation proceed maximally when surface wounds are kept moist. Even short periods of drying impair this process, and therefore wounds should not be allowed to desiccate. The exudates from acute, uninfected superficial wounds also contain growth factors and lactate and therefore may serve as markers for the growth environment found at the base of the wound.

E. Collagen Fiber Remodeling and Wound Contraction

Remodeling of the wound extracellular matrix is also a well-regulated process. First, fibroblasts replace the provisional fibrin matrix with collagen monomers. Extracellular enzymes, some of which are oxygen dependent, quickly polymerize these monomers, initially in a pattern that is more random than in uninjured tissue, predisposing the early wound to mechanical failure. Progressively, the very early provisional matrix is replaced with a more mature one by forming larger, better organized, stronger, and more durable collagen fibers. If mechanically strained, the very early wound provisional matrix usually fails within the matrix itself (days 0-5). Subsequent mechanical failure occurs at the matrix-tissue interface or fusion point (Figure 6–3). The mechanism for ultimately connecting the wound matrix to the uninjured tissue border is poorly understood.

Reorganization of the new matrix is an important feature of healing, and fibroblasts and leukocytes secrete collagenases that catalyze the lytic component. Turnover occurs rapidly at first and then more slowly. Even in simple wounds healing normally, wound matrix turnover can be detected chemically for as long as 18 months. Healing is successful when a net excess of matrix is deposited despite concomitant lysis. Lysis, in contrast to anabolic synthesis, is less dependent upon energy and nutrition. If synthesis is impaired, however, lysis weakens wounds.

During rapid turnover, wounds normally gain strength and durability but are vulnerable to contraction or stretching.

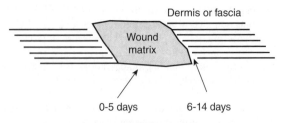

▲ **Figure 6–3.** The very early wound matrix is weak and susceptible to mechanical failure, especially in load-bearing tissues like the abdominal wall. After 5 days, mechanical failure occurs at the interface of the wound matrix and the uninjured surrounding tissue.

Fibroblasts exert the force for contraction. Fibroblasts attach to collagen and each other and pull the collagen network together when the cell membranes shorten as the fibroblasts migrate. The wound myofibroblast, a specialized phenotype, expresses intracellular actin filaments that also contribute force to fibroblast-mediated wound contraction. The collagen fibers are then fixed in the packed positions by a variety of cross-linking mechanisms. Both open and closed wounds tend to contract if not subjected to a superior counterforce. The phenomenon is best seen in surface excisional wounds, which may close 90% or more by contraction alone in loose skin. For example, the residual of a large open wound on the back of the neck may be only a small area of epithelialization. On the back, the buttock, or the neck, this is often a beneficial process, whereas in the face and around joints, the results may be disabling or disfiguring. Pathologic wound contraction is usually termed a contracture or a stricture. Skin grafts, especially thick ones, may minimize or prevent disabling wound contractures. Dynamic splints, passive or active stretching, or insertion of flaps containing dermis and subdermis also counteract scar contraction. Prevention of a stricture often depends on ensuring that opposing tissue edges are well perfused so that healing can proceed quickly to completion and contraction stops. Healing wounds may also stretch during active turnover when tension overcomes contraction. This may account for the laxity of scars in ligaments of injured but unsplinted joints, and the tendency for incisional hernia formation in abdominal wounds of obese patients.

F. Healing of Specialized Tissues

Tissue other than skin heals generally by the same fundamental pathways. Although tissue structure may be specialized, the initial repair processes are shared. It does appear that the rate and efficiency of wound healing in different tissue types depends in large part on total collagen content, collagen organization, and blood supply.

1. Gastrointestinal tract—The rate of repair varies from one part of the intestine to the other in proportion to blood supply. Anastomoses of the colon and esophagus heal least reliably and are most likely to leak, whereas failure of stomach or small intestine anastomoses is rare. Intestinal anastomoses regain strength rapidly when compared to skin wounds. After 1 week, bursting strength may exceed the uninjured surrounding intestine. However, the surrounding intestine also participates in the reaction to injury, initially losing collagen by lysis, and as a result losing mechanical strength. For this reason, leakage can occur a few millimeters from the anastomosis. A tight suture line causing ischemia will exacerbate this surgical problem.

The mesothelial cell lining of the peritoneum also is important for healing in the abdomen and gastrointestinal tract (GI) tract. The esophagus and retroperitoneal colon lack a serosal mesothelial lining, which may contribute to failed wound healing. There is evidence that mesothelial cells signal healing of peritoneal linings and are a source of repair cells.

Comorbidities that delay collagen synthesis or stimulate collagen lysis are likely to increase the risk of perforation and leakage. The danger of leakage is greatest from the fourth to seventh days, when tensile strength normally would rise rapidly but may be impeded by impaired collagen deposition or increased lysis. Local infection, which most often occurs near esophageal and colonic anastomoses, promotes lysis and delays synthesis, thus increasing the likelihood of perforation.

2. Bone—Bone healing is controlled by many of the same mechanisms that control soft-tissue healing. It too occurs in predictable, morphologic stages: inflammation, fibroplasia, and remodeling. The duration of each stage varies depending on the location and extent of the fracture.

Injury (fracture) causes hematoma formation from the damaged blood vessels of the periosteum, endosteum, and surrounding tissues. Within hours, an inflammatory infiltrate of neutrophils and macrophages is recruited into the hematoma as in soft-tissue injuries. Monocytes and granulocytes debride and digest necrotic tissue and debris, including bone, on the fracture surface. This process continues for days to weeks depending on the amount of necrotic tissue. As inflammation progresses to fibroplasia, the hematoma is progressively replaced by granulation tissue that can form bone. This bone wound tissue, known as callus, develops from both sides of the fracture and is composed of fibroblasts, endothelial cells, and bone-forming cells (chondroblasts, osteoblasts). As macrophages (osteoclasts) phagocytose the hematoma and injured tissue, fibroblasts (osteocytes) deposit a collagenous matrix, and chondroblasts deposit proteoglycans in a process called enchondral bone formation. This step, prominent in some bones, is then converted to bone as osteoblasts condense hydroxyapatite crystals at specific points on the collagen fibers. Endothelial cells form a vasculature structure characteristic of uninjured bone. Eventually the fibrovascular callus is completely replaced by new bone. Unlike healing of soft tissue, bone healing has features of regeneration, and bone often heals without leaving a scar.

Bone healing also depends on blood supply. Following injury, the ends of fractured bone are avascular. Osteocyte and blood vessel lacunae become vacant for several millimeters from the fracture. New blood vessels must sprout from preexisting ones and migrate into the area of injury. As new blood vessels cross the bone ends, they are preceded by osteoclasts just as macrophages precede them in soft-tissue repair. In bone, this unit is called the cutting cone because it bores its way through bone in the process of connecting with other vessels. Excessive movement of the bone ends during this revascularization stage will break the delicate new vessels and delay healing. Osteomyelitis originates most often in ischemic bone fragments. Hyperoxygenation optimizes fracture healing and aids in the cure (and potentially the prevention) of osteomyelitis. Acute or chronic hypoxia slows bone repair.

Bone repair may occur through primary or secondary intention. Primary repair can occur only when the fracture is stable and aligned and its surfaces closely apposed. This is the goal of rigid plate fixation or rod fixation of fractures. When these conditions are met, capillaries can grow across the fracture and rapidly reestablish a vascular supply. Little or no callus forms. Secondary repair with callus formation is more common. Once the fracture has been bridged, the new bone remodels in response to the mechanical stresses upon it, with restoration to normal or near-normal strength. During this process, as in soft tissue, preexisting bone and its vascular network are simultaneously removed and replaced. Increased bone turnover may be detected as long as 10 years after injury. Although remodeling is efficient, it cannot correct deformities of angulation or rotation in misaligned fractures. Careful fracture reduction is still important.

Bone repair can be manipulated. Electrical stimulation, growth factors, and distraction osteogenesis are three tools for this purpose. Electrical currents applied directly (through implanted electrodes) or induced by external alternating electromagnetic fields accelerate repair by inducing new bone formation in much the same way as small piezoelectric currents produced by mechanical deformation of intact bone controls remodeling along lines of stress. Electrical stimulation has been used successfully to treat nonunion of bone (where new bone formation between bone ends fails, often requiring long periods of bed rest). Bone morphogenetic protein (BMP)-impregnated implants have accelerated bone healing in animals and have been used with encouraging results to treat large bony defects and nonunions, including during spinal fusion.

The **Ilizarov technique,** linear distraction osteogenesis, can lengthen bones, stimulate bone growth across a defect, or correct defects of angulation. The Ilizarov device is an external fixator attached to the bones through metal pins or wires. A surgical break is created and then slowly pulled apart (1 mm/d) or slowly reangulated. The vascular supply and subsequent new bone formation migrate along with the moving segment of bone.

Gurtner GC, Warner S, Barrandon Y, Longaker MT. Wound repair and regeneration. *Nature.* 2008;453;15:314-321.
Young A, McNaught CE. The physiology of wound healing. *Surgery.* 2011;29(10):475-479.

PATHOGENESIS

▶ Effect of Tissue Hypoxia

Impaired perfusion and inadequate oxygenation are the most frequent causes of healing failure. Oxygen is required for successful inflammation, bactericidal activity, angiogenesis, epithelialization, and matrix (collagen) deposition. The critical collagen oxygenases involved have Km values (half of maximum catalytic velocity) for oxygen ranging from

20 mm Hg and maximum of about 200 mm Hg, meaning that reaction rates are regulated by Pao_2 and blood perfusion throughout the entire physiologic range. The Pao_2 of wound fluid in human incisions is about 30-40 mm Hg, suggesting that these enzymes normally function just beyond half capacity. Wound Pao_2 is reduced by hypovolemia, catecholamine infusion, stress, and hypothermia. Under ideal conditions, wound fluid Pao_2 can be raised above 100 mm Hg by improved perfusion and inhaled oxygen therapy. Human healing is profoundly influenced by local blood supply, vasoconstriction, and all other factors that govern perfusion and blood oxygenation. Wounds in well-vascularized tissues (eg, scalp, mouth, anal canal) heal rapidly and are remarkably resistant to infection (Figure 6–4).

▲ **Figure 6–4.** Tissue oxygen concentration ($TcPO_2$) is a critical determinant of wound healing. Human healing is profoundly influenced by local blood supply, vasoconstriction, and all other factors that govern perfusion and blood oxygenation. Despite raising FiO_2 to 50% or 100%, the $TcPO_2$ remains in the ischemic range when flow is reduced to less than 25% of baseline. Supplementing the FiO_2 of oxygen will not benefit healing of ischemic ulcers. Flow must be increased to improve the $TcPO_2$.

Dysregulated Inflammation During Impaired Wound Healing

Molecular growth signals and lytic enzymes released by inflammatory cells are necessary for repair. Inhibited or excessive inflammatory responses lead to wound complications. Failure to heal is common in patients taking antiinflammatory corticosteroids, immune suppressants, or cancer chemotherapeutic agents that inhibit inflammatory cells. Open wounds are more effected than primarily repaired wounds. Antiinflammatory drugs impair the wound less after the third day of healing, as the normal level of inflammation in wound healing is reduced. Inflammation may also be pathologically excessive. Increased wound inflammation (eg, in response to infection and endotoxin or foreign bodies like suture material or mesh implants during hernia repair) can stimulate inflammatory cells to produce cytolytic cytokines and excessive proteases with the consequence of pathologic lysis of newly formed tissue. A pathologic cycle of prolonged wound healing may ensue and result in an impaired quantity and quality of wound scar.

Impaired Healing Due to Malnutrition

Malnutrition impairs healing by limiting nucleic acid and protein synthesis that is required for cell replication and extracellular matrix production. Weight loss and protein depletion have been shown experimentally and clinically to be risk factors for poor healing. Deficient healing is seen mainly in patients with acute malnutrition (ie, in the weeks just before or after an injury or operation). Even a few days of starvation measurably impairs healing, and an equally brief period of repletion can reverse the deficit. Wound complications increase in severe malnutrition. A period of preoperative corrective nutrition is generally helpful for patients who have recently lost 10% or more of their body weight.

Scar Formation Versus Regeneration

In excessive healing or proliferative scarring, it is as if the equilibrium point between collagen deposition and collagen lysis is never reached. It is unclear why some wounds seem to continue in the dysregulated repair process. Upregulation of fibroplastic growth factors like TGF-β is implicated during hypertrophic or keloid scar formation. Because the mechanism of excessive scar formation is unknown, there is no universally accepted treatment regimen. In a meta-analysis of pathologic scar treatments, the mean amount of improvement to be expected was only 60%. Hypertrophic scars are generally self-limited, are related to residual inflammation, and may regress after a year or so. Keloids by definition extend beyond the borders of the wound and are most common in pigmented skin. The last areas of a burn to heal are most often hypertrophic, possibly due to traction, reinjury, and tension. Immune mechanisms may also contribute to pathologic scar. Prolonged inflammatory reactions potentiate scar. Therapy includes intralesional injection of anti-inflammatory steroids and dressing with Silastic sheets, which are shown to increase protease-based lytic activity in the scar. Excessive or hypertrophic scarring is rare in burn injuries that heal within 21 days. Pressure garments or compression dressings are effective in decreasing scarring in burn injuries that require more than 21 days to heal. The exact mechanism by which pressure is effective is unknown.

Rafehi H, El-Osta A, Karagiannis TC. Genetic and epigenetic events in diabetic wound healing. *Int Wound J*. 2011;8(1):12-21.

Wild T, Rahbarnia A, Kellner M, Sobotka L, Eberlein T. Basics in nutrition and wound healing. *Nutrition*. 2010;26(9):862-866.

CLINICAL FINDINGS

Impediments to wound healing may be broadly categorized as those local to the wound and those that are systemic comorbidities and diseases. Often, a clinical intervention is possible to minimize or eliminate these obstacles to tissue repair (see Table 6–1).

▶ Acute Wounds

Acute wounds express normal wound healing pathways and are expected to heal. Over days and weeks, the undisturbed acute wound can be observed to progress reliably through the phases of hemostasis, normal inflammation, normal fibroplasia, and ultimately scar maturation with epithelialization. The most common acute wound complications are pain, infection, mechanical dehiscence, and hypertrophic scar.

▶ Chronic Wounds

Chronically unhealed wounds, especially on the lower extremity, are common in the setting of vascular, immunologic, and neurologic disease. Venous ulcers, largely of

Table 6–1. Local and systemic impediments to wound healing.

Systemic	Local
Obesity	Wound infection
Malnutrition	Wound necrosis
Diabetes mellitus	Foreign bodies
Drugs (steroids, cytotoxins)	Wound hypoperfusion and hypoxia
Shock	Repeat trauma
Immunodeficiency	Irradiated tissue
Renal failure	Neoplasm

the lower leg, reflect poor perfusion as a result of draining venous hypertension and perivascular leakage of plasma into surrounding tissues. The extravasation of plasma proteins into the soft tissue stimulates chronic inflammation. The venous hypertension occurs because of incompetent venous valves. Most venous ulcers will heal if the venous congestion and edema are relieved by leg elevation, compression stockings, or surgical procedures that eliminate or repair incompetent veins or their valves.

Arterial or ischemic ulcers, which tend to occur on the lateral ankle or foot, are best treated by revascularization. Hyperbaric oxygen, which provides a temporary source of enhanced oxygenation to the wound tissue that stimulates angiogenesis, is an effective although expensive alternative when revascularization is not possible. Useful information can be obtained by transcutaneous oximetry. Tissues with low Pao_2 will not heal spontaneously. However, if oxygen tension can be raised into a relatively normal range by oxygen administration even intermittently, the wound may respond to oxygen therapy.

Sensory loss, especially of the feet, can lead to ulceration. Bony deformities due to chronic fractures, like the Charcot deformity, cause pathologic pressure on wounded tissue. Ulcers in patients with diabetes mellitus may have two causes. Patients with neuropathic ulcers usually have good circulation, and their lesions will heal if protected from trauma by off-loading, special shoes, or splints. Recurrences are common, however. Diabetics with ischemic disease, whether they have neuropathy or not, are at risk for gangrene, and they frequently require amputation when revascularization is not possible.

In pyoderma gangrenosum, granulomatous inflammation, with or without arteritis, causes skin necrosis, possibly by a mechanism involving excess cytokine release. These ulcers are associated with inflammatory bowel disease and certain types of arthritis and chondritis. Corticosteroids or other antiinflammatory drugs are helpful. However, antiinflammatory corticosteroids can also contribute to poor healing by inhibiting cytokine release and collagen synthesis.

▶ Decubiti

Decubitus ulcers can be major complications of immobilization. The morbidity of decubitus ulcers lengthens hospital stays and increases healthcare costs. They result from prolonged pressure that reduces tissue blood supply, irritative or contaminated injections, and prolonged contact with moisture, urine, or feces. Most patients who develop decubitus ulcers are also poorly nourished. Pressure ulcers are common in paraplegics, immobile elderly patients following fractures, and intensive care unit patients. The ulcers vary in depth and often extend from skin to a bony pressure point such as the greater trochanter, the sacrum, the heels, or the head. Most decubitus ulcers are preventable. Hospital-acquired ulcers are nearly always the result of immobilization, unprotected positioning on operating tables, and ill-fitting casts or other orthopedic appliances.

COMPLICATIONS

▶ Wound Infection

A wound infection results when bacterial proliferation and tissue invasion overcomes wound immune defense mechanisms. This is more than just the presence of bacteria in a wound. When an imbalance in this quantitative equilibrium results in infection, a delay in wound healing occurs. Therefore, prevention and treatment of wound infection involves maintenance or reestablishment of the balanced equilibrium.

Wounds containing more than 10^5 bacteria/gram of tissue or any tissue level of β-hemolytic streptococci are at high risk for wound infection if closed by direct wound edge approximation, skin graft, pedicled, or free flap. Clean-contaminated and contaminated wounds result in high rates of postoperative infection (6%-15%), while clean cases have lower infection rates (1%-3%). When wounds are considered at risk for having a significant bacterial bioburden (clean-contaminated or contaminated cases), prophylactic operative antibiotics reduce wound infection rates. Wounds following clean cases with negligible bacterial bioburden do not clearly benefit from prophylactic antibiotics except when implanted prosthetic materials are used.

▶ Mechanical Wound Failure

Mechanical factors play an important role in acute wound healing. Primary closure of an incision stabilizes distractive forces to allow wound healing and an optimized anatomic result (HW, Figure 6–5). Cellular response and synthesis of a wound matrix is impaired and delayed within the mechanically failing wound (FW). Cellular studies confirm that mechanical load forces are an important signal for acute wound repair. When anatomic stability of a wound is achieved, a particular suture material or suturing technique is of secondary importance. The increased use of foreign material implants, like meshes for hernia repair, is suggested to manipulate the mechanical environment of the acute wound, even to the point of promoting "tension-free" wound healing. Negative pressure wound therapy is increasingly applied to stabilize acute wounds and to support acute wound healing. Mechanical microdeformation of repair cells in the wound bed is thought to stimulate acute wound healing.

Mechanical signaling pathways are important for the regulation of tissue repair, especially in load-bearing structures like the abdominal wall and Achilles tendon. From this perspective, the midline fascia behaves more like a ligament or tendon than skin, for example. It is observed that scars placed under mechanical loads ultimately will assume the morphology and function of tendons and, conversely, that incisions placed under abnormally "low" loads organize scars with reduced tensile strengths. The empiric observation that a suture length (SL)–wound length (WL) ratio of 4:1 results in the most reliable midline abdominal wall closure may reflect the technique resulting in establishing the optimal acute wound healing–load set point for the abdominal wall. When a laparotomy wound mechanically fails, a fundamental repair signal may be lost, contributing to the biology of hernia formation. Clinically, laparotomy dehiscence of only 12 mm on postoperative day 30 predicts a 94% incisional hernia rate after 3 years.

A.

B.

▲ **Figure 6–5.** **A.** In a healing laparotomy wound (HW), fibroplasia, matrix synthesis, and angiogenesis stabilize the rectus muscles at the wound edges until repair is complete. **B.** When laparotomy wounds fail to heal (FW), there is an absence of fibroplasia and herniated preperitoneal fat occupies the wound space.

Franz MG. The biology of hernia formation. *Surg Clin North Am.* 2008;88:1.

Franz MG, Steed DL, Robson MC. Optimizing healing of the acute wound by minimizing complications. *Curr Prob Surg.* 2007;44:1.

Sanchez-Manuel FJ, Lozano-García J, Seco-Gil JL. Antibiotic prophylaxis for hernia repair. *Cochrane Database Syst Rev.* 2007;3:CD003769.

Sørensen LT. Wound healing and infection in surgery: The pathophysiological impact of smoking, smoking cessation, and nicotine replacement therapy. A systematic review. *Ann Surg.* 2012;255(6):1069-1079.

TREATMENT

▶ Acute Wounds

A. Sutures

The ideal suture material is flexible, strong, easily tied, and securely knotted. It stimulates little tissue reaction and does not serve as a nidus for infection.

Silk is an animal protein but is relatively inert in human tissue. It is commonly used because of its historical reliability and favorable handling characteristics. It loses strength over long periods of time and is unsuitable for suturing arteries to plastic grafts or for insertion of prosthetic cardiac valves. Silk sutures are multifilament, providing mechanical immune barriers for bacteria. Occasionally, silk sutures form a focus for small abscesses that migrate and "spit" through the skin, forming small sinuses that will not heal until the suture is removed.

Synthetic nonabsorbable sutures are generally inert polymers that retain strength. However, their handling characteristics are not as good as those of silk, and they must usually be knotted at least four times, resulting in increased amounts of retained foreign material. Multifilament plastic polymer sutures may also become infected and migrate to the surface like silk sutures. Monofilament polymers will not harbor bacteria. Nylon monofilament is extremely nonreactive, but it is difficult to tie. Monofilament polypropylene is intermediate in these properties. Vascular anastomoses to prosthetic vascular grafts rely indefinitely on the strength of sutures; therefore, use of absorbable sutures may lead to aneurysm formation.

Synthetic absorbable sutures are strong, have predictable rates of loss of tensile strength, incite a minimal inflammatory reaction, and have special usefulness in gastrointestinal, urologic, and gynecologic operations that are contaminated. Polyglycolic acid and polyglactin retain tensile strength longer in gastrointestinal anastomoses. Polydioxanone sulfate and polyglycolate are monofilament and lose about half their strength in 50 days, thus solving the problem of premature breakage in fascial closures. Poliglecaprone monofilament synthetic sutures have faster reabsorption, retaining 50% tensile strength at 7 days and 0% at 21 days. This suture is suitable for low-load soft-tissue approximation such as in plastic surgery or ophthalmology procedures, but is not intended for fascial closure. There is no reliable evidence that absorbable sutures lead to more incisional hernias or gastrointestinal anastamotic leaks.

Stainless steel wire is inert and maintains strength for a long time. It is difficult to tie and may have to be removed late postoperatively because of pain. It does not harbor bacteria, and it can be left in granulating wounds, when necessary, and will be covered by granulation tissue without causing abscesses. However, sinuses due to motion and wire fracture are fairly common.

Catgut (now made from the submucosa of bovine intestine) will eventually resorb, but the resorption time is highly variable. It stimulates a considerable inflammatory reaction due to its biologic origin and tends to potentiate infections. Catgut also loses strength rapidly and unpredictably in the intestine and in infected wounds as a consequence of acid and enzyme hydrolysis.

Staples, whether for internal use or skin closure, are mainly steel–tantalum alloys that incite a minimal tissue reaction. The technique of staple placement is different from that of sutures, but the same basic rules pertain. There are no real differences in the healing that follows sutured or stapled closures. Stapling devices tend to minimize errors in technique, but at the same time, they do not offer a feel for tissue and have limited ability to accommodate to exceptional circumstances, such as anatomic constraints to stapler placement. Staples are often used for skin closure following contaminated cases, since this allows opening only part of the wound should infection occur. Newer barbed suture materials now also make it possible to partially open and drain a postoperative wound infection without complete wound dehiscence.

Surgical glues or tissue adhesives are now established as safe and effective for the repair of skin incisions. The most common forms are cyanoacrylate-based glues. Tissue adhesives are often less painful than sutures or staples, and the seal can serve as the wound dressing as well.

▶ Surgical Technique

Primarily closed wounds are of a smaller volume and heal mainly by the synthesis of a new matrix. Wound contraction and epithelialization, as in an open wound healing by secondary intent, contribute only a small part to primary wound healing. An open wound, healing by secondary intent, must synthesize granulation tissue to fill in the wound bed, contract at the wound periphery, and cover the surface area with epithelial cells. Wounds heal faster following delayed primary closure than by secondary intent, as well. The mechanical load forces transmitted through a primarily reconstructed wound will stimulate repair. Successful delayed primary closure requires that the acute wound be in bacterial balance. Primary repair should approximate, but not strangulate, the incision. The type of suture material used does not matter, as long as the primary repair is anatomic and perfused.

The most important means of achieving optimal healing after operation is good surgical technique. Many cases of surgical wound failure are due to technical errors. Tissue should be protected from drying and contamination. The surgeon should use fine instruments; should perform clean, sharp dissection; and should make minimal, skillful use of electrocautery, ligatures, and sutures. All these precautions contribute to the most important goal of surgical technique, gentle handling of tissue. Anatomic tissue approximation should be achieved when possible but optimum tissue perfusion preserved.

A. Wound Closure

As with many surgical techniques, the exact method of wound closure may be less important than how well it is performed. The tearing strength of sutures in fascia is no greater than 4 kg. There is little reason to use sutures of greater strength than this. Excessively tight closure strangulates tissue, often leading to hernia formation or infection.

The most reliable laparotomy closure uses a continuous technique at SL-WL ratio of 4:1, which allows for the normal 10% strain that occurs along the length of the incision, while maintaining mechanical integrity. A 4:1 SL-WL ratio is achieved with suture placed 1 cm deep on normal fascia (the bite) followed by 1 cm of progress. The depth of the suture-line bite must extend beyond the wound lytic zone. Normal collagen lysis occurs for approximately 5 mm perpendicular to the incision, weakening the adjacent fascia. The most common technical causes of dehiscence are an SL-WL ratio less than 4:1, infection, and excessively tight sutures. Tight suture lines impair wound perfusion and oxygen delivery that is required for wound healing. If wound healing is impaired, wider, interrupted internal retention sutures may be added, although improved outcomes are not proven (Figure 6–6).

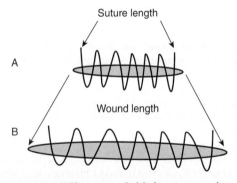

Suture length

A

Wound length

B

▲ **Figure 6–6. A.** The most reliable laparotomy closure uses a continuous technique at a suture length–wound length ratio of 4:1. **B.** This allows for the normal 10% strain that occurs along the length of the incision, while maintaining mechanical integrity.

Delayed primary closure is a technique by which the subcutaneous portion of the wound is left open for 3-5 days prior to primary repair. During the delay period, angiogenesis and fibroplasia start, and bacteria are cleared from the wound. The success of this method depends on the ability of the surgeon to detect the signs of wound infection. Merely leaving the wound open for 4 days does not guarantee that it will not become infected. Some wounds (eg, fibrin-covered or inflamed wounds) should not be closed but should be left open for secondary closure. Quantitative bacterial counts less than 10^5 non-β-hemolytic streptococcus organisms per gram of wound tissue predict successful healing after delayed primary closure. Any level of β-hemolytic streptococcal wound infection predicts delayed wound healing.

▶ Implantable Materials

Soft-tissue prostheses reduce the incidence of wound failure and recurrence following hernia repair. The recurrence rate following inguinal hernia repairs using autologous tissues ranges from 5% to 25% in most series. The recurrence rate following primary incisional hernia repair using autologous tissues is even worse, ranging from 20% to 60%. The introduction of synthetic soft-tissue prostheses to inguinal and incisional hernia repair has significantly reduced recurrence rates across general surgery. The prevailing view is that the mechanism for the reduced hernia recurrence rates is the reduction of tension along suture lines when using mesh and the replacement abnormal tissue.

No implantable prosthesis is ideal in regard to tissue compatibility, permanent fixation, and resistance to infection. Two principles are paramount: biocompatibility and a material that is incorporated into tissue. Both specific and nonspecific immune mechanisms are involved in the inflammatory reaction to foreign materials. Highly incompatible materials, such as wood splinters, elicit an acute inflammatory process that includes massive local release of proteolytic enzymes (inflammation). Consequently, the foreign body is never incorporated and instead is isolated loosely in a fibrous pocket. In less severe incompatibility, rejection is not so vigorous and proteolysis not so prominent. Mononuclear cells and lymphocytes, the major components of wound inflammatory tissue, direct a response that creates a fibrous capsule that may be acceptable in a joint replacement but may distort a breast reconstruction (encapsulation). Newer biologic prostheses are composed of acellularized tissue to abrogate the immune response. The expectation is that these materials recellularize with host cells and blood vessels during incorporation and assume a more physiological function (regeneration).

Most implants must become anchored to adjacent normal tissues through fibrous tissue ingrowth. This process requires biocompatibility and interstices large enough to permit repair fibroblast migration, just as in a wound, and to allow pedicles of vascularized tissue to enter and join similar units. In bone, this tissue incorporation imparts stability. In vascular grafts, the invading tissue supports neointima formation, which retards mural thrombosis and distal embolization. Soft tissue will grow into pores larger than about 50 μm in diameter. Of the vascular prostheses, woven Dacron is best for tissue incorporation. In bone, sintered, porous metallic surfaces are best. Large-screen polypropylene mesh can be used to support the abdominal wall or chest and is usually well incorporated into the granulation tissue that penetrates the mesh. Mesh porosity is increasingly recognized as an important design element for reliable implantation and wound healing. Microporous polytetrafluoroethylene (PTFE) sheets are often not well incorporated and are not suitable for use in infected tissues.

The implantation space remains vulnerable to infection for years and is a particular problem in implants that cross the body surface. Mesh cuffs around vascular access devices that incite incorporation have successfully forestalled infection for months, but infections that arise from bacteria entering the body along "permanently" implanted foreign bodies traversing the skin surface, such as ventricular assist devices, remain an unsolved problem.

Because incisional hernia is now the most common complication of abdominal operations, there is growing interest in using meshes prophylactically to stabilize the laparotomy closure and prevent incisional hernias from forming. A recent randomized, controlled trial (the PRIMA Study) showed that the use of a prophylactic mesh to reinforce an abdominal wall primary closure is both safe and effective in reducing the high incidence if incisional hernias in high-risk patients who are obese or have arterial aneurysmal disease. Obesity contributes to laparotomy wound failure through increased mechanical loads and aneurysmal disease due to a defect in the extracellular matrix formed within the healing wound scar.

Negative Pressure Wound Therapy

Negative pressure wound therapy (NPWT) mechanically stabilizes the distractive forces of an open acute wound and supports healing. Distractive tissue forces keep a wound open with force vectors that oppose wound contraction, thereby delaying healing. NPWT also reduces periwound edema and improves wound perfusion. NPWT may directly stimulate repair fibroblast activity through mechanical microdeformation of the cell surface.

NPWT can also stabilize a therapeutically open abdomen (laparostomy), minimizing wound size and supporting closure of the abdominal wall. Distractive force from the rectus muscle components and lateral oblique muscles act to keep the laparostomy open, leading to incisional hernia formation and potentially loss of abdominal, peritoneal volume (domain) (Figure 6–7).

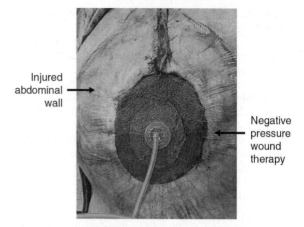

Injured abdominal wall

Negative pressure wound therapy

▲ **Figure 6–7.** Negative pressure dressings oppose distractive soft-tissue vectors and mechanically stabilize a wound. NPWT also improves wound healing through the reduction of periwound edema and stimulation of repair fibroblast activity.

The successes of NPWT in improving open wound healing lead to its application for closed wound healing. Clinical trials have shown shorter times to complete wound healing and lower wound infection rates for NPWT applied to closed incisions. This was first shown in studies of clean wounds after median sternotomy closure and primary repairs following total knee arthroplasty and abdominoplasty. A recent randomized controlled trial also showed significantly shorter times until complete wound healing and lower wound infection rates when applying NPWT to primarily closed wounds in contaminated fields. This important observation challenges the traditional surgical approach of leaving such wounds open for frequent dressing changes and allow secondary wound healing to occur with or without open NPWT in these Class III wounds. Caution remains in the application of primary wound closure and NPWT for dirty surgical wounds (Class IV) with most surgeons recommending serial wound debridements, including the use of open abdominal management, converting a dirty surgical wound to a contaminated surgical wound before performing a delayed primary closure with closed NPWT. Here again randomized studies observed shorter times until complete wound healing and lower surgical wound site infection rates.

Chronic Wounds

The first principle in managing chronic wounds is to diagnose and treat tissue hypoxia, such as underlying circulatory disease. The second principle is never to allow open wounds to dry—ie, use moist dressings, which may also relieve pain. A third principle is to control any infection with topical or systemic antibiotics. A fourth principle is to recognize that chronically scarred or necrotic tissue is usually poorly perfused. Debridement of unhealthy tissue, often followed by skin grafting, may be required for healing. A fifth principle is to reduce autonomic vasoconstriction by means of warmth, moisture, and pain relief.

A number of growth factors have been shown to accelerate healing of acute wounds in laboratory studies. They include FGFs, TGF-β, IGF-1, PDGF, and epidermal growth factor (EGF). However, in the setting of chronic human wounds, with the perfusion problems noted above and the hostile wound environment with elevated tissue protease levels, proof of efficacy has been difficult, and no clear-cut advantage to any formulation has yet been convincingly demonstrated. The one exception is the randomized, prospective, double-blind, placebo-controlled multicenter trial by the Diabetic Ulcer Study Group, which demonstrated that daily topical application of recombinant human PDGF-BB homodimer moderately accelerated healing and resulted in more wounds that healed completely.

▶ Ducubiti

The first principle is to incise and drain any infected spaces or debride necrotic tissue. Dead tissue is debrided until the exposed surfaces are viable. Sources of pressure must again be unloaded. Many will then heal spontaneously. However, deep ulcers may require surgical closure, sometimes with removal of underlying bone, again to reduce tissue pressure. The defect may require closure by judicious movement of thick, well-vascularized tissue into the affected area. Musculocutaneous flaps are the treatment of choice when chronic infection and significant tissue loss are combined. However, recurrence is common because the flaps are usually insensate.

POSTOPERATIVE CARE

Optimum postoperative care of the wound requires cleanliness, maintenance of a moist wound environment, protection from repeated trauma, and support of the patient. Even closed wounds can be infected by surface contamination, particularly within the first 2-3 days. Bacteria gain entrance most easily through suture tracts. If a wound is likely to be traumatized or contaminated, it should be protected during this time. Such protection may require special dressings such as occlusive dressings or sprays, tissue adhesives, or repeated cleansing.

Moderate, physiologic mechanical stress enhances healing. Even bone fracture callus formation is greater if slight motion is allowed. Early ambulation and return to normal activity are, in general, good for repair. Patients should be instructed to avoid excess loads, such as heavy lifting and coughing, or to stabilize their wounds when unavoidable.

The appearance of delayed wound infections, weeks to years after operation, reinforces that all wounds are contaminated and may harbor bacteria. Most frequently, poor tissue perfusion and oxygenation of the wound during the postoperative period weakens host resistance. Regulation of perfusion is largely due to sympathetic nervous activity. The major stimuli of vasoconstriction are cold, pain, hypovolemia, cigarette smoking, and hypoxemia. Recent studies show that efforts to limit these impediments to wound healing reduce the wound infection rate by more than half. Maintenance of intraoperative normothermia and blood volume is particularly important. Appropriate assurance that peripheral perfusion is adequate is best obtained from peripheral tissues rather than urine output, central venous pressure, or wedge pressure, none of which correlate with peripheral wound tissue oxygenation. What does correlate with tissue oxygenation is the capillary refill time on the forehead or patella, which should be less than 2 s and 5 s, respectively. Collagen deposition is increased also by the addition of oxygen breathing (nasal prongs or light mask) but only in well-perfused patients.

The ideal care of the wound begins in the preoperative period and ends only months later. The patient must be prepared so that optimal conditions exist when the wound is made. Surgical technique should minimize tissue trauma and repairs should approximate normal anatomic structure whenever possible. Nutrition should be optimized preoperatively. Cessation of cigarette smoking will improve wound outcomes. Postoperatively, wound care includes maintenance of nutrition, blood volume, oxygenation, and careful restriction of immunosuppressant drugs when possible. Although wound healing is in many ways a local phenomenon, ideal care of the wound is essentially ideal care of the patient.

▶ References

Deerenberg EB, Harlaar J, Steyerberg EW. Small bites versus large bites for closure of abdominal midline incisions (STITCH): A double-blind, multicenter, randomized controlled trial. *Lancet.* 2015;386:1254-1260.

Frazee R, Manning A, Abernathy S, et al. Open vs closed negative pressure wound therapy for contaminated and dirty surgical wounds: A prospective randomized comparison. *J Am Coll Surg.* 2018;226:507-512.

Jairam AP, Timmermans L, Eker HH, et al. Prevention of incisional hernias with prophylactic onlay and sublay mesh reinforcement versus primary suture only in midline laparotomies (PRIMA): Two-year follow-up of a multicenter, double-blind, randomized controlled trial. *Lancet.* 2017;390:567-576.

Park H, Copeland C, Henry S, Barbul A. Complex wounds and their management. *Surg Clin North Am.* 2010;90:1181-1194.

Perez D, Wildi S, Demartines N, et al. Prospective evaluation of vacuum-assisted closure in abdominal compartment syndrome and severe abdominal sepsis. *J Am Coll Surg.* 2007;205:586.

World Health Organization 2016. Global Guidelines for the Prevention of Surgical Site Infection. Available at: http://apps .who.int/bitstream/handle/10665/250680/9789241549882-eng .pdf?sequence=1. Accessed March 25, 2018.

Wu SC, Marston W, Armstrong DG. Wound care: The role of advanced wound healing technologies. *J Vasc Surg.* 2010; 52(3 suppl):59S-66S.

MULTIPLE-CHOICE QUESTIONS

1. Which phase of acute wound healing is prolonged during progression to a chronic wound?

   A. Coagulation.
   B. Inflammation.
   C. Fibroplasia.
   D. Angiogenesis.
   E. Remodeling.

2. Which cell is most important for signaling wound healing?

   A. Platelet.
   B. PMN.
   C. Macrophage.
   D. Fibroblast.
   E. Endothelial cell.

3. Which is the most predictive direct measure of impaired or delayed wound healing?

   A. Vitamin C deficiency.
   B. Low serum albumin.
   C. Irradiated tissue.
   D. Smoking.
   E. $Tco_2 < 30$ mm Hg.

4. Which of the following is not a clinical impediment to wound healing?

   A. Repeated trauma.
   B. Wound infection.
   C. A moist wound environment.
   D. Foreign bodies.
   E. Obesity.

5. The fundamental mechanism for incisional hernia formation is:

   A. Long-term fascial scar failure.
   B. Suture failure.
   C. Suture pulling through the fascia.
   D. Early fascial dehiscence and wound failure.
   E. Poor technique.

Power Sources in Surgery

Kristopher B. Deatrick, MD

INTRODUCTION

Modern surgery has been enhanced by powered instruments that have revolutionized the delicacy, precision, and accuracy of operations. Yet many people who use these implements every day have very little understanding of the technology behind them. Although a complete treatise on the electromagnetic generation of heat and the physics of current generation are beyond the scope of this chapter (and are available elsewhere), understanding some fundamental rules governing the behavior of electrical currents and some relatively straightforward principles helps guide the use of these technologies.

ELECTROSURGERY

▶ Principles of Electricity

An electrical **circuit** is any pathway that allows the uninterrupted flow of electrons. Electrical **current** is the flow of electricity (the number of electrons) in a given circuit over a constant period of time and is measured in **amperes** (A). Current can be supplied either as **direct current** (DC), with constant positive and negative terminals, or as **alternating current** (AC), with constantly reversing poles. The electromotive force, or **voltage,** is a measurement of the force that propels the current of electrons and is related to the difference in potential energy between two terminals. The **resistance** is the tendency of any component of a circuit to oppose the flow of electrons, and applies to DC circuits. The equivalent of this tendency in an AC circuit is known as **impedance**. Any electromagnetic wave, from household electricity to radio broadcasts to visible light, can be described by three components: speed, frequency, and wavelength. These three characteristics are defined by the equation:

$$c = f\lambda$$

where c is the speed of light, 2.998×10^8 m/s.

Because the speed of light is constant, frequency (f) and wavelength (λ) are inversely related; that is, as frequency increases, wavelength decreases, and vice versa. Frequency is measured in cycles/second, reported as Hertz (Hz), and wavelength in meters. Although there are many electrical currents, including nerve impulses, in the human body, high-frequency current can pass through it easily. The ability of high-frequency current to pass through the human body without causing excess damage makes electrosurgery possible.

▶ Electrocautery

Electrosurgery is sometimes incorrectly called electrocautery, a separate technique. **Electrocautery** is a closed-circuit DC device in which current is passed through an exposed wire offering resistance to the current (Figure 7–1). The resistance causes some of the electrical energy to be dissipated as heat, increasing the temperature of the wire, which then heats tissue. In true electrocautery, *no current passes through the patient.* Electrocautery is primarily used in microsurgery, such as ophthalmologic procedures, where a very small amount of heat will produce the desired effect or where more heat or current may be dangerous. These devices also have use in customization of woven or knitted vascular grafts.

▶ Principles of Electrosurgery

Electrosurgery, colloquially referred to as the "Bovie" (following its inventor, William T. Bovie, engineer and collaborator of Harvey Cushing), is perhaps the most ubiquitous power source in surgery. Although the principle of using heat to cauterize bleeding wounds dates back to the third millennium BC, the directed use of electrical current to produce these effects is a far more recent development. Bovie refined the electrical generator and made it practical and applicable to everyday surgery. Electrosurgery uses high-frequency (radiofrequency) electromagnetic waves to produce a localized heating of tissues, leading to localized tissue destruction.

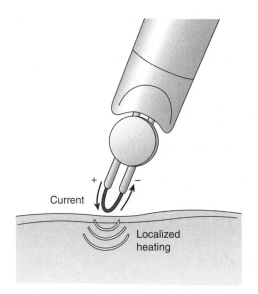

+ Current −

Localized
heating

▲ **Figure 7–1.** In electrocautery, current passes through a wire loop and heats it. This heat cauterizes tissue. No current passes through the patient.

The effect produced (cutting vs. coagulation) depends on how this energy is supplied.

A useful way to understand the way electrosurgery works is to follow the flow of current from the power outlet as it travels through the patient and returns to the wall outlet. By convention, charge is depicted as moving from positive (cathode) to negative (anode). These descriptions are based on that convention, following the flow of positive charge.

Monopolar Circuits

The electrosurgical circuit consists of four primary parts: the electrosurgical generator, the active electrode, the patient, and the return electrode. Current from the power outlet flows to the electrosurgical generator, where it is modulated to a high frequency and short wavelength. From the machine, it travels through the handpiece, out the tip of the device, to the patient. In the patient, current flows through the body to the return electrode, and back to the generator, completing the circuit. Although there are two poles (the active and return electrodes) in this circuit, it is called monopolar electrosurgery, as only one pole is directly utilized by the surgeon at the surgical site. It is distinguished from bipolar electrosurgery in which both electrodes are under the surgeon's direct control (Figure 7–2A).

Bipolar Circuits

The essential components of the bipolar electrosurgical circuit are the same as those in the monopolar circuit; however, in this system, the active and return electrodes are in the same surgical instrument. In this technique, high-frequency

current is passed through the active electrode and through the patient to heat and disrupt tissue. In this arrangement, however, the return electrode is in the handpiece, as the opposite pole of the active electrode. This method enables the surgeon pass current through a smaller, discrete amount of tissue (Figure 7–2B).

The Electromagnetic Spectrum & Tissue Effects

The current that powers the electrosurgical generator is supplied at a frequency of 60 Hz. This type of electromagnetic energy can cause very strong (potentially lethal) neuromuscular stimulation, making it unsuitable for use in its pure form. Muscle and nerve stimulation ceases at around 100 kHz, and current with a frequency above this threshold can be delivered safely, without the risk of electrocution. The outputs of modern electrosurgical generators deliver current with a frequency greater than 200 kHz. Current at this frequency is known as **radiofrequency** (RF); it is in the same portion of the spectrum as some radio transmitters.

Applying electrosurgical current to a patient produces localized tissue destruction via intense heat production, yet no other lesions are produced during application of this technique. The effect is exerted only at the site where the surgeon is operating and not at the site of the return electrode, because the surface area by which the charge is delivered is much smaller than that to which it returns. Thus, there is a far greater **density of charge** at the site of the handpiece ("active" electrode) contact than there is at the site of return. If there is another connection between the patient and ground that offers less resistance to the flow of current, in a relatively small surface area, the patient could be in danger of suffering an electrosurgical burn. Similarly, if the return electrode were to be damaged, or if contact was not maintained, a burn could occur in this area. The possibility of a burn at the site of the return electrode is eliminated in most modern machines by the presence of a monitoring system that assesses the completeness of contact (by maintaining a smaller, secondary circuit) and automatically disables power if full contact of the pad is lost (as could be caused by tripping over a wire and tearing the return pad).

Types of Electrosurgery

All types of electrosurgery exert their effects via the localized production of heat and the subsequent changes in the heated tissue. Therefore, the different effects produced by electrosurgical instruments are created by altering the manner in which this heat is produced and delivered. Adjustment is made possible by altering the wave pattern of the current.

A. Cutting

Cutting is produced by delivery of a continuous sine wave of current (Figure 7–3A). Compared with coagulation current (discussed later), cutting current has a relatively low

A

Generator

Current flow

Bovie electrode

Current passes through body

Return electrode

Ground

B

▲ **Figure 7–2. A.** In monopolar electrosurgery, current from an electrosurgical generator passes from an active electrode (the "Bovie" tip) through the patient to a return electrode of greater area. **B.** In bipolar electrosurgery, the active and return electrodes are in the handpiece, and current only flows through the surgical site.

voltage and a relatively high crest factor, the ratio of the peak voltage to the mean (root mean square) voltage of the current. Additionally, it has a relatively high "duty cycle"—that is, once the current is applied, the current is actively flowing during the entire application. In this technique, the tip of the electrode is held just slightly off the surface of the tissue. The flow of the high-frequency current through the resistance of the patient's tissue at a very small site produces intense heat, vaporizing water and exploding the cells in the immediate vicinity of the current. Thus, cutting occurs with minimal coagulum production and consequently minimal hemostasis. A combination of coagulation and cutting can be produced by setting the electrosurgical generator to

blend, which damps down a portion of the waveform, allowing greater formation of a coagulum and consequently more control of local bleeding.

B. Coagulation: Desiccation and Fulguration

In contrast with cutting currents, **coagulation** currents do not produce a constant waveform. Rather, they rely on spikes of electric wave activity (Figure 7–3B). Although these currents produce less heat overall than the direct sine wave, enough heat is produced to disrupt the normal cellular architecture. Because the cells are not instantly vaporized, however, the cellular debris remains associated with the edge of the wound, and the heat produced is enough to denature the cellular

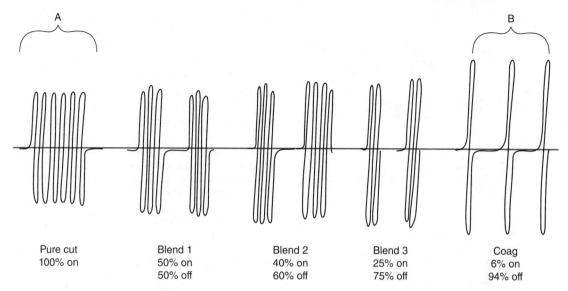

▲ **Figure 7–3.** Electrosurgical waveforms. **A.** Cutting current. **B.** Coagulation current.

protein. This accounts for the formation of a coagulum, a protein-rich mixture that allows sealing of smaller blood vessels and control of local bleeding. Compared to cutting, coagulation currents have a higher crest factor and a shorter duty cycle (94% off, 6% on). In part, the increased voltage is necessary to overcome the impedance of air during the process of arcing current to the tissues. Coagulation can be accomplished in one of two ways. With **desiccation,** the conductive tip is placed in direct contact with the tissue. Direct contact of the electrode with tissue reduces the concentration of the current; less heat is generated, and no cutting action occurs. A relatively low power setting is used, resulting in a limited area of tissue ablation with coagulation. The cells dry out and form a coagulum rather than vaporize and explode.

In **fulguration,** the tip of the active electrode is not actually brought into contact with the tissues but rather is held just off the surface, and following activation, the current arcs through the air to the target. Again, this process disrupts normal cellular protein to form a coagulum; the tissue is charred, and a black eschar forms at the site of operation. It is possible to cut with the coagulation current and, conversely, to coagulate with the cutting current by holding the electrode in direct contact with tissue. It may be necessary to adjust power settings and electrode size to achieve the desired surgical effect. The benefit of using the cutting current is that far less voltage is needed, an important consideration during minimally invasive procedures.

C. Variables

Just as the power setting and the waveform affect the results of the current application, any change in the circuit that influences the impedance of the system will influence the tissue effect. These include the size of the electrode, the position of the electrode, the type of tissue, and the formation of eschar.

1. Size of the electrode—The smaller the electrode, the higher the current concentration. Consequently, the same tissue effect can be achieved with a smaller electrode, even though the power setting is reduced. At any given setting, the longer the generator is activated, the more heat is produced. The greater the heat, the farther it will travel to adjacent tissue (thermal spread). (See the various electrodes shown in Figure 7–4.)

2. Placement of the electrode—Placement can determine whether vaporization or coagulation occurs. Which one occurs is a function of current density and the heat produced while sparking to tissue versus holding the electrode in direct contact.

3. Type of tissue—Tissues vary widely in resistance.

4. Eschar—Eschar is relatively high in resistance to current. Electrodes should be kept clean and free of eschar, maintaining lower resistance within the surgical circuit.

D. Disadvantages and Potential Hazards

1. Alternate site burns—Early electrosurgical generators used a **ground-referenced** circuit design. In this type of construction, grounded current from the wall outlet was directly modulated, and it was assumed that it would return to the generator via the return electrode. With this type of system, however, any path of low resistance to ground, including metal instruments, ECG leads, and other wire and

▲ **Figure 7–4. A.** Knife electrode. **B.** Ball electrode.
C. Needle electrode. **D.** Loop electrode. **E.** Wire electrode.

conductive surfaces, can complete the circuit. The ground-referenced circuit design presented a relatively high hazard for alternate site burns when current was not distributed over a great enough area to dissipate the current.

Modern electrosurgical units use isolated generator technology. The isolated generator separates the therapeutic current from ground by referencing it within the generator circuitry. In an isolated electrosurgical system, the circuit is completed by the generator, and electrosurgical current from isolated generators will not recognize grounded objects as pathways to complete the circuit. Isolated electrosurgical energy recognizes the patient return electrode as the preferred pathway back to the generator. Since the ground is not the reference for completion of the circuit, the potential for alternate site burns is greatly reduced. However, if the return electrode were to become partially disconnected, a burn could occur at the site of the return electrode if the area was too small to distribute the current widely enough to prevent heating of the tissue or if the impedance was too high. It is important to place the return electrode over a well-vascularized tissue mass, not over areas of vascular insufficiency or over bony prominences where contact might be compromised. Therefore, some electrosurgical generators use a monitoring system that assesses the quality of the contact between the return electrode and the patient by monitoring impedance, which is related to surface area. Any loss of contact between the electrode and the generator results in interruption of the circuit and deactivation of the system.

2. Surgical fires—In any setting with high heat sources and an ample supply of oxygen, vigilance against combustion is essential. Drapes, gowns, gas (particularly in bowel surgery

and cases involving the upper airway), and hair, for example, are flammable and must be kept away from heat sources. Careful application of electrosurgery and use of a protective holster to store the electrode while not in use are important to minimize the risk of fire.

3. Minimally invasive surgery—Several safety concerns are unique to minimally invasive surgery, given the limited and relatively tight environment in which operations occur. One potential danger is that of direct coupling between the electrode and other conductive instruments, leading to inadvertent tissue damage. Another is the risk, with the use of high-voltage currents (especially those used for coagulation), of breakdown in the insulation, resulting in arcing from an exposed conductor to adjacent tissue, again, causing unwanted tissue damage. The risk can be reduced by using cutting current instead of coagulation current to lower the voltage used.

Yet another unique hazard is the potential for creating a capacitor with the cannula. A capacitor is any conductor separated from another conductor by a dielectric. The conductive electrode separated from either a metal cannula or the abdominal wall (both good conductors) can induce capacitance in either of these structures. For maximum safety, an all-metal cannula (by which current can escape to the rest of the body) rather than a combination of metal and plastic should be used, and vigilance must be maintained at all times.

E. Principal Applications for Electrosurgery

Electrosurgery is ubiquitous in its presence within the modern operating room. In its earliest use by Dr. Cushing, it allowed surgery on previously inoperable vascular tumors in neurosurgery. Today, electrosurgery is an essential component of all types of surgery. Applications include dissection in general and vascular surgery, allowing tissue to be resected with minimal blood loss. Additionally, use in urology facilitates transurethral prostatectomy (TURP) and other procedures. In gynecologic practice, electrosurgical instruments are essential in cervical resections and biopsies.

▶ Related Electrosurgical Devices

A. Aquamantys

The Aquamantys device is an electrosurgical device that features a proprietary bipolar radiofrequency energy with saline to produce an effect called transcollation, a form of saline-enhanced thermal sealing. The use of the saline irrigation at the tip of a bipolar electrosurgical handpiece reduces the temperature generated at the tissue level to 100°C. Per the manufacturer, this results in heat-induced collagen contraction and vascular occlusion. This can be used for partial hemostasis prior to further tissue division. A particular advantage of this approach is that this device can treat vessels that have retracted into tissue.

B. Applications

This can be especially beneficial for areas of diffuse bleeding, such as the chest wall following division of dense pleural adhesions, lung parenchyma, or liver parenchyma in hepatic resections.

C. Vessel Sealing Devices (Ligasure, EnSeal)

A number of devices primarily marketed as vessel or tissue sealing instruments are electrosurgical instruments. In principle, these devices combine both tissue apposition and energy, delivered as bipolar current via the opposite jaws of the instrument. The jaws of the instrument provide pressure, and bipolar current generates heat, leading to fusion of native collagen and elastin fibers in the tissue to be divided, whether fat, parenchyma, or vessel walls. A feedback circuit determines the time of energy delivery necessary to provide sealing of the tissue being manipulated. The Ligasure device (Medtronic) has been evaluated to provide sealing and division of vessels up to 7 mm in diameter, with a burst pressure of over 360 mm Hg. The EnSeal (Ethicon) device also relies on the pressure of tissue apposition and delivery of bipolar energy to allow tissue division, and has been evaluated to provide sealing of vessels up to 7 mm in diameter. These devices differ in proprietary circuit design, and have different characteristics as described by sealing time (Ligasure is generally faster) and lateral thermal spread (EnSeal generally has less). A wide variety of generators and handpieces are available, for both open and endoscopic applications, each with particular advantages and disadvantages for different approaches and operations.

▶ Argon Beam Coagulation

A. Principles

Argon beam coagulation is closely related to basic electrosurgery. Argon beam coagulation uses a coaxial flow of argon gas to conduct monopolar RF current to the target tissue. Argon is an inert gas that is easily ionized by the application of an electrical current. When ionized, argon gas becomes far more conductive (has less impedance) than normal air and provides a more efficient pathway for transmitting current from the electrode to tissues (Figure 7–5). The current arcs along the pathway of the ionized gas, which is heavier than both oxygen and nitrogen, and thereby displaces air. Whereas current can sometimes follow unpredictable pathways while arcing through the air, the argon gas allows more accurate placement of current flow. Once the current arrives at the tissue, it produces its coagulating effect in the same manner as conventional electrosurgery. Argon beam coagulation devices can operate only in two modes: pinpoint coagulation and spray coagulation. The method does not cut even the most delicate tissue.

▲ **Figure 7–5.** Ionized argon gas facilitates the flow of current from the handpiece to the tissue.

B. Advantages

There are multiple advantages to this type of electrosurgical current delivery. First, it allows use of the coagulation mode without contact of the electrode. This prevents buildup of eschar, which diminishes electrode efficiency, on the electrode tip. Second, there is generally less smoke and less odor from coagulating with this type of current. Third, tissue loss and tissue damage are reduced when the current is more accurately targeted. Fourth, because the argon gas is delivered at room temperature, there is less danger of the instrument igniting gowns or drapes. Finally, the beam of coagulation generally improves coagulation and reduces blood loss and the risk of rebleeding.

C. Disadvantages

Argon beam coagulation cannot be used to produce a cutting effect in the same manner as other types of electrosurgical equipment. Also, the nozzle for gas delivery can become clogged, reducing its efficiency, and just as with other electrosurgical instruments, if it is used for a prolonged period of time, it may overheat and cause inadvertent damage when set aside.

D. Applications

Argon beam coagulation is especially useful for procedures in which the surgeon must rapidly and efficiently coagulate a wide area of tissue. It is especially suited to dissecting very vascular tissues and organs, such as the liver. Its efficient delivery of a consistent current load and its inability to become occluded with eschar are advantageous for operation with a significant risk of hemorrhage.

MECHANICAL (ULTRASONIC) TISSUE DISRUPTION

Apart from passing current through the patient to produce localized heating and tissue destruction (either cutting or coagulation), there are other means of transforming electrical potential energy into energy for surgery. Two of the most prominent technologies depend on the production of ultrasonic vibrations, although each produces its effect in a different manner.

▶ Ultrasonic Scalpels and Clamps

A. Principles

Several types of ultrasonic "scalpels," such as the Harmonic Scalpel, and clamps allow cutting and coagulation of tissue in a technique completely different from that employed in electrosurgery. In this type of an instrument, electrical energy from a power source is transformed into ultrasonic vibrations by a transducer, a unit that expands and contracts in response to electrical current at a frequency of up to 55.5 kHz/s. The vibration is amplified in the shaft of the instrument to magnify the vibrating distance of the blade, which moves longitudinally. The blade tip vibrates through an amplitude of around 200 μm. As the blade tip vibrates, it produces cellular friction and denatures proteins. The denatured proteins form a coagulum, which allows sealing of coapted blood vessels. With longer instrument applications, significant secondary heat is produced, and larger blood vessels may be sealed by coagulation of tissue at a small distance from the instrument. By producing cellular disruption in this fashion, the temperatures achieved are between 50°C and 100°C. In contrast, in conventional electrosurgery, tissues are subjected to temperatures between 150°C and 400°C. Thus with an ultrasonic device, tissues can be dissected without burning or oxidizing tissues and without producing an eschar; there is also less potential to disrupt the coagulum when removing the instrument. When cutting using the clamp portion of the instrument, energy is transferred to the tissue through the active blade under applied force, minimizing lateral spread. Additionally, the motion of the blade induces cavitation along the cell surfaces, whereby low pressure causes cell fluid to vaporize and rupture (Figure 7–6).

▲ **Figure 7–6.** Ultrasonic scalpel.

Clamp   Transducer

Blade vibration

Piezoelectric ceramic or magnetostrictive device

B. Advantages

The advantages of an ultrasonic scalpel system are clearest when operating in tight spaces with the attendant risks of damage to adjacent structures. Ultrasonic instruments are especially suited for laparoscopic and other types of minimally invasive procedures. Although the potential still exists for damaging adjacent tissue by inadvertently touching it with an active tip, there is no risk of current inadvertently arcing to adjacent structures, because the current is converted into mechanical energy in the handpiece. Further, there is no neuromuscular stimulation produced, since no current passes through the patient. Because the tissue effects are exerted through mechanical disruption of the cells, and coagulation occurs at much lower temperatures than used in conventional electrosurgery, lateral thermal tissue damage is minimized. And because tissue is not heated to the point of combustion or carbonization of proteins, there is no eschar formation on the blade, and less smoke is produced.

C. Disadvantages

Primary disadvantage of ultrasonic scalpels and clamps is that the components are more expensive than those used for conventional electrosurgery; and with more mechanical parts, there are more potential points of equipment failure. Further, whereas electrosurgery can be applied throughout an operation, ultrasonic scalpels are typically used for more controlled dissection around the site of interest.

D. Applications

The primary applications of ultrasonic instruments are found when traditional electrosurgery is unsuitable or undesirable. As mentioned, they are particularly useful during minimally invasive procedures because they mitigate the risk of running an active electrode through a cannula and into a body cavity. Additionally, the reduced smoke production by instruments of this type is advantageous in this setting. When electrophysiology is involved (such as in patients with implantable cardiac defibrillators or pacemakers), ultrasonic instruments eliminate a source of concern by avoiding the hazard of passing current through the patient's body.

▶ Cavitational Ultrasonic Surgical Aspiration

A. Principles

Cavitational ultrasonic surgical aspirators work on many of the same principles as ultrasonic scalpels. In the handpiece, current passes through a coil and induces a magnetic field. The magnetic field excites a transducer of a nickel alloy (either a piezoelectric or magnetostrictive device), expanding and contracting to produce an oscillating motion (vibration) in the longitudinal axis with a frequency of 23 or 36 kHz.

These ultrasonic mechanical vibrations are magnified over the length of the handpiece. The amount of oscillation varies: with low frequency, there is greater amplitude; with high frequency, there is lower amplitude. The oscillating tip, when brought into contact with tissue, causes fragmentation of tissue by producing cavitation at the cell surface, with low pressure outside the cell leading to cellular disruption. This high-frequency vibration produces heat, which is reduced via a closed, recirculating cooling-water system. This system maintains the temperature of the tip at approximately 40°C. As tissue is fragmented, the debris must be carried away, which is another function of the cavitational ultrasonic surgical aspirator, as its name implies. For irrigation, intravenous (IV) fluid (water or saline) is fed through tubing to the handpiece, where it irrigates the surgical site and suspends the fragmented tissue debris. Removal of this debris is possible because the instrument contains a vacuum pump that provides suction. Suction pulls irrigation fluid, fragmented tissue, and other material through the distal tip of the handpiece. The material is contained in a separate canister.

Some ultrasonic surgical aspirator instruments enable the surgeon to influence the selectivity of the disruption induced by the instrument itself. Some surgeons attempt to gain extra control by lowering the amplitude of the tip oscillations. Lowering amplitude to gain greater selectivity when fragmenting tissue near critical structures, however, only results in reduced speed of tissue removal. By using a mode in which on/off power intervals are supplied, the reserve power (which governs the tip response when encountering tissue) is reduced. The total amount of power in the oscillating hollow tip is determined by the amount of reserve power available. Reserve power maintains tip oscillation when a resistive load is placed on the tip, as occurs when it contacts tissue. As the resistance increases, more power is supplied to the tip (Figure 7–7).

B. Applications

Ultrasonic surgical aspirator systems are primarily applicable in situations where fragmentation, emulsification, and aspiration of a significant amount of tissue are desirable. Because minimal additional hemostasis is provided, this instrument is not as versatile in its application to general surgery as electrosurgery or the more high-powered ultrasonic scalpel. In general surgery, its primary application is in liver resection, where it can disrupt parenchyma while leaving major vasculature and the biliary ducts intact.

▶ Radiofrequency Ablation

In addition to facilitating open tissue dissection, electromagnetic radiation in the form of RF current can be used for a number of ablative approaches, both surgically and percutaneously. In radiofrequency ablation (RFA) of a tumor, RF (350-500 kHz) is delivered via a bipolar probe inserted via imaging (ultrasound or CT) guidance into the lesion of interest. As current flows through the RF probe, localized heating of cells occurs, and as the temperature approaches 60°C, tissue destruction occurs, leading to coagulative necrosis. Because of the localized effects of RF, it causes less collateral damage and lateral thermal spread than other forms of ablative therapies. In general, tumors smaller than 2.5 cm can be treated with one application of RFA, whereas larger tumors can be addressed with multiple applications of RF energy.

A. Applications

In surgical oncology, RFA has been applied with varying degrees of success in pulmonary, esophageal, hepatic, pancreatic, biliary, and renal tumors, among others, and the results of these approaches are addressed in their respective chapters. Endoscopically, it has also demonstrated efficacy in the treatment, via localized tissue ablation, of premalignant lesions such as Barrett esophagus. In cardiac and vascular surgery, RFA is used for elimination of accessory pathways contributing to arrhythmias, and can be used for surgical correction of atrial fibrillation as part of the Cox-Maze procedure. RFA has also been used for ablation of varicose veins.

▶ References

Feldman LS, et al, eds. *The SAGES Manual on the Fundamental Use of Surgical Energy (FUSE)*. Springer, 2012.

Jones DB, et al. Safe energy use in the operating room. *Curr Probl Surgery*. 2015;52(11):447-468.

Medtronic, Covidien. Electrosurgery self-study guide. Principles of electrosurgery online. 2019. Available at: https://www.medtronic.com/covidien/en-us/clinical-education/catalog/electrosurgery-self-study-guide.html

Taheri A, et al. Electrosurgery: Part I. Basics and principles. *J Am Acad Dermatol*. 2014;70(4):591.e1-591.e14.

▲ **Figure 7–7.** Cavitational ultrasonic surgical aspirator.

MULTIPLE-CHOICE QUESTIONS

1. All of the following are true about electrosurgery *except*:

   A. In monopolar electrosurgery, the current flows through the patient from the active electrode to the return electrode.
   B. In bipolar electrosurgery, the current flows from the handpiece to the return electrode.
   C. The cutting mode of monopolar electrosurgery utilizes a continuous sine wave of current.
   D. The coagulation mode of monopolar electrosurgery relies on spikes of electric wave activity.

2. A bipolar surgical instrument differs from a monopolar instrument in:

   A. The source of energy.
   B. The number of applications permitted in an operation.
   C. The length of the path between the two poles in the circuit.
   D. The number of poles in the circuit.

3. Which is true regarding electrosurgery and fire in the operating room?

   A. Fire is preventable by keeping the oxygen levels used for ventilation low.
   B. Fire depends upon the presence of an oxygen source, an ignition source, and fuel.
   C. Alcohol from skin prep solutions is not flammable.
   D. Fire cannot be caused by electrosurgical instruments.

4. Which is *not* an important safety factor in electrosurgery?

   A. Return electrodes have a wide surface, dispersing the density of charge.
   B. Low voltage prevents serious electrical injury.
   C. Muscle and nerve stimulation ceases at 100 kHz.
   D. Return electrodes include a separate "safety circuit," assuring complete contact over a wide area.

5. Radiofrequency ablation:

   A. Causes tissue destruction by heating tissues to 500°C.
   B. Cannot be used for tumors over 2.5 cm.
   C. Destroys tumor tissue by generating heat with the application of electromagnetic waves.
   D. Can only be applied via an open surgical incision.

Inflammation, Infection, & Antimicrobial Therapy in Surgery

Haytham M.A. Kaafarani, MD, MPH

Kamal M.F. Itani, MD

▼ INTRODUCTION

TERMINOLOGY

Surgery and infection are unfortunately intimately intertwined. For the purpose of this chapter, we will differentiate between infections resulting from surgery (*surgical site infections*) and those resulting from other disease processes but *requiring surgical management*. Surgical incisions involve a breach of the skin and immune barriers, and can thus be complicated by infection. The term "wound infection" has been replaced by the more accurate term "surgical site infection" (SSI), to emphasize that the infection can occur anywhere within any of the areas accessed surgically (not exclusively at the skin level) and to differentiate it from "traumatic wound infection."

As opposed to SSI, the term "surgical infection" is used to indicate infections that are unlikely to respond to medical and antimicrobial treatments and require surgical intervention or management. Common examples include abscesses, empyema, intra-abdominal infections, and necrotizing skin and soft-tissue infections (NSSTIs). Surgical decision making involves, at its core, the knowledge and experience to determine the timing of surgery and a right balance between surgery and other adjunct therapy such as antibiotic therapy, resuscitative efforts, and nutritional optimization, in order to provide the patient with the best chances to cure the infection with the best overall outcomes.

▶ Pathogenesis

The development of a surgical infection involves a close interplay between three elements: (1) a susceptible host, (2) an infectious agent, and (3) a suitable medium or environment (Figure 8–1). The degree of contribution of each of the three factors to the eventual occurrence of the infection depends on the individual patient and the specific nature and site of the infection. Whether a given inoculum of bacteria results in

an established infection or not depends on the virulence of the bacteria, the strength of the immune and inflammatory host response (eg, chemotaxis, phagocytosis, B- and T-lymphocyte activation), and the amount of blood perfusion and oxygen tension in the medium where the inoculum resides.

A. The Susceptible Host

Many surgical infections occur in patients with no evidence of decreased immune defenses. However, with the major advances in medicine and healthcare services in recent decades, more immunocompromised patients (eg, transplant, HIV, and diabetic patients) are presenting with infections requiring surgical management or with SSIs following surgical interventions. Table 8–1 delineates a list of patient-related conditions associated with decreased immunity and potential predisposition to surgical infections. The mechanisms by which the listed conditions affect a host's immunity are diverse in nature. For example, diabetic patients have suboptimal neutrophil adherence, migration, and antibacterial functions, making them less able to fight an occult infection. Such effect of diabetes on immunity is much more pronounced in patients whose glucose levels are poorly controlled than in those with appropriate and consistent management of their diabetes. The current Centers for Disease Control (CDC) 2017 guidelines strongly recommend maintaining perioperative glucose control levels below 200 mg/dL in diabetic and nondiabetic patients to decrease the risk of SSIs.

B. The Infectious Agent

Identification of the organism causing the infection is crucial. This is often achieved through the use of Gram stains and cultures of the tissue or purulent material at the site of infection. A recent report published in the *New England Journal of Medicine* suggests that the six most common pathogens responsible for hospital-acquired infections in surgical and nonsurgical patients are *Clostridium difficile*

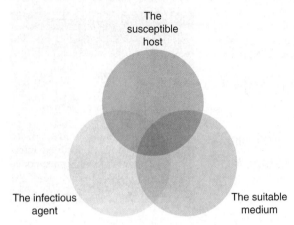

▲ Figure 8–1. The interaction between host, infectious agent, and suitable medium to result in infection.

(12%), *Staphylococcus aureus* (11%), *Klebsiella pneumoniae* or *oxytoca* (10%), *Escherichia coli* (9%), *Enterococcus species* (9%), and *Pseudomonas aeruginosa* (7%). *Staphylococcus aureus* is the most common pathogen in SSIs, and its ability to develop resistance to antimicrobial therapy continues to be one of the biggest challenges currently faced by the medical community. *Staphylococcus epidermidis* is one of the other 33 known species of the genus *Staphylococcus* and is usually a skin and mucous membrane nonpathogenic colonizer. Nonetheless, in immunosuppressed individuals and those with indwelling surgical catheters or implants,

Table 8–1. Patient-related conditions associated with decreased immunity and a higher risk for surgical infections.

Advanced age
Diabetes mellitus
Malnutrition (eg, albumin less than 3.5 mg/dL)
Smoking
Obesity
Alcoholism
Immunosuppressive therapy (eg, posttransplant)
Systemic corticosteroid use
Peripheral vascular disease
Malignancy and antineoplastic treatment (eg, chemotherapy, radiotherapy)
Concomitant remote site infection
Human immunodeficiency virus/acquired immunodeficiency syndrome (HIV/AIDS)
Liver failure
Renal failure

Staphylococcus epidermidis can cause serious infections requiring treatment. In necrotizing skin and soft-tissue infections, the etiology is often polymicrobial, with gram-positive, gram-negative, and anaerobic bacteria involved. Monobacterial necrotizing infections can result from either clostridial species (especially *Clostridium perfringes*) or *Streptococcus pyogenes*. Streptococci are well known for their ability to invade even minor breaks in the skin, and to cause superficial skin and skin structure infections by spreading through connective tissue planes and lymphatic channels. When surgical procedures involve the small or large intestines, gram-negative and anaerobic bacteria are implicated in a significant proportion of the SSIs in addition to the regular gram-positive colonizers. Among these, *E. coli, K. pneumoniae, Enterobacter,* and *Bacteroides* species are the most commonly isolated pathogens. In immunocompromised or critically ill patients, fungi (eg, *Candida, Aspergilla, Histoplasma*) may result in localized or systemic life-threatening infections. *Candida* species account for up to 6% of hospital-acquired infections. Parasites such as amebas and *Echinococcus* may also cause abscesses in internal organs, especially the liver.

C. The Suitable Medium

A suitable medium for bacteria consists of a closed space with poor vascular perfusion, low oxygen tension, and a low pH. Ischemic and necrotic tissues are perfect examples of such a medium where microorganisms can thrive. For example, a sacral pressure ulcer that harbors necrotic tissue that does not get promptly debrided presents an acidic medium with minimal vascular perfusion, and low oxygen tension that will almost always evolve to become a wound infection and even sacral osteomyelitis. The appendix, with its narrow orifice, presents another classic example. When an appendicolith blocks the orifice of the appendix, the intraluminal pressure increases and eventually blocks lymphatic and venous outflow. As the vascular perfusion of the appendix diminishes, the tissue oxygen tension decreases, the milieu becomes acidotic, and the appendix becomes ischemic and necrotic. Unless removed, the inflamed appendix and its blocked lumen contain colonic bacteria that will result in an appendiceal infection followed by perforation and a periappendiceal abscess and/or peritonitis.

A foreign body such as a joint prosthesis can become seeded in the event of a systemic infection. As with necrotic tissue, the lack of vascularity decreases the formation of free oxygen radicals within a prosthesis and prevents the immune system from readily fighting microorganisms in that area.

SURGICAL SITE INFECTION

▶ Definition

The Centers for Disease Control and Prevention (CDC) define SSI as an infection that occurs at or near the surgical incision. The CDC further classifies SSI as being (1) superficial incisional, (2) deep incisional, or (3) organ/space SSI

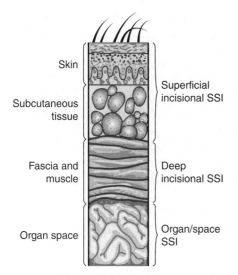

Skin

Subcutaneous tissue

Superficial incisional SSI

Fascia and muscle

Deep incisional SSI

Organ space

Organ/space SSI

▲ **Figure 8–2.** The three types of surgical site infections.

(Figure 8–2). The time-frame given for those infections is within 30 days for all infections and up to 90 days for deep and organ space infections occurring after certain surgeries. Table 8–2 illustrates the criteria that define each of these

three classes of SSIs. It is noteworthy that a skin infection at or around the site of a traumatic wound is classified as a skin and skin structure infection, not a surgical site infection.

▶ Epidemiology

At least 234 million surgical procedures are performed globally each year, including more than 16 million in the United States alone; SSIs develop in 2%-5% of these patients. SSIs account for 22%-31% of all hospital-acquired infections, and as such are considered, along with pneumonia, the most common nosocomial infections. The rate of SSI depends on the nature of the surgical procedure performed and the extent of concomitant intraoperative contamination. In an attempt to quantify the inoculum of bacteria typical of certain surgical procedures, a wound classification was developed in 1964 by the National Academy of Sciences (Table 8–3). This classification divides wounds into clean (eg, inguinal hernia repair), clean-contaminated (eg, right hemicolectomy), contaminated (eg, laparotomy for penetrating injury to small intestines), and dirty (eg, laparotomy for peritonitis and intra-abdominal abscesses) wounds. Several studies have emerged since the conception of the classification confirming that, with reasonable risk adjustment, the classes of contamination correlate well with the incidence

Table 8–2. Criteria and definitions of surgical site infection.

Superficial Incision

Must meet the following criteria:

Date of event for infection occurs within 30 days after any NHSN operative procedure (where day 1= the procedure date)

and

Involves only skin and subcutaneous tissue of the incision

and

Patient has at least *one* of the following:

  a. Purulent drainage from the superficial incision.

  b. Organisms identified from an aseptically obtained specimen from the superficial incision or subcutaneous tissue by a culture or nonculture-based microbiologic testing method, which is performed for purposes of clinical diagnosis or treatment (for example, not Active Surveillance Culture/Testing (ASC/AST).

  c. Superficial incision that is deliberately opened by a surgeon, attending physician,[a] or other designee.

    and

    Culture or nonculture-based testing is not performed.

    and

    Patient has *at least one* of the following signs or symptoms:

      Pain or tenderness

      Localized swelling

      Erythema

      Heat

  d. Diagnosis of a superficial incisional SSI by the surgeon or attending physician[a] or other designee.

Comments:

There are two specific types of superficial incisional SSIs:

1. Superficial Incisional Primary (SIP): A superficial incisional SSI that is identified in the primary incision in a patient who has had an operation with one or more incisions (for example, C-section incision or chest incision for CBGB).

2. Superficial Incisional Secondary (SIS): A superficial incisional SSI that is identified in the secondary incision in a patient who has had an operation with more than one incision (for example, donor site incision for CBGB).

(Continued)

Table 8–2. Criteria and definitions of surgical site infection. (*Continued*)

Reporting Instructions for Superficial SSI:

The following do not qualify as criteria for meeting the NHSN definition of superficial SSI:

- Diagnosis/treatment of cellulitis (redness/warmth/swelling), by itself, does not meet criterion "d" for superficial incisional SSI. Conversely, an incision that is draining or that has organisms identified by culture or nonculture-based testing is not considered a cellulitis.
- A stitch abscess alone (minimal inflammation and discharge confined to the points of suture penetration).
- A localized stab wound or pin site infection. Such an infection might be considered either a skin (SKIN) or soft tissue (ST) infection, depending on its depth, but not an SSI.
  Note: A laparoscopic trocar site for an NHSN operative procedure is not considered a stab wound.
- Circumcision is not an NHSN operative procedure. An infected circumcision site in newborns is classified as CIRC and is not an SSI.
- An infected burn wound is classified as BURN and is not an SSI.

Deep Incisional SSI

Must meet the following criteria:

Date of event for infection occurs within 30 or 90 days after the NHSN operative procedure (where day 1 = the procedure date)

and

Involves deep soft tissues of the incision (eg, fascial and muscle layers)

and

Patient has at least *one* of the following:

  a. Purulent drainage from the deep incision.
  b. A deep incision that spontaneously dehisces, or is deliberately opened or aspirated by a surgeon, attending physician,[a] or other designee
    and
    Organism is identified by a culture or nonculture-based microbiologic testing method that is performed for purposes of clinical diagnosis or treatment (eg, not Active Surveillance Culture/Testing (ASC/AST) or culture or nonculture-based microbiologic testing method is not performed
    and
    Patient has *at least one* of the following signs or symptoms:
      Fever (> 38°C)
      Localized pain or tenderness
Note: A culture or nonculture-based test that has a negative finding does not meet this criterion.
  c. An abscess or other evidence of infection involving the deep incision that is detected on gross anatomic or histopathologic exam, or imaging test.

Comments:

There are two specific types of deep incisional SSIs:

1. Deep Incisional Primary (DIP): A deep incisional SSI that is identified in a primary incision in a patient who has had an operation with one or more incisions (eg, section incision or chest incision for CBGB).
2. Deep Incisional Secondary (DIS): A deep incisional SSI that is identified in the secondary incision in a patient who has had an operation with more than one incision (eg, donor site incision for CBGB).

Organ/Space SSI

Must meet the following criteria:

Date of event for infection occurs within 30 or 90 days after the NHSN operative procedure (where day 1 = the procedure date)

and

Infection involves any part of the body deeper than the fascial/muscle layers that is opened or manipulated during the operative procedure

and

Patient has at least *one* of the following:

1. Purulent drainage from a drain that is placed into the organ/space (eg, closed suction drainage system, open drain, T-tube drain, CT-guided drainage).
2. Organisms are identified from fluid or tissue in the organ/space by a culture or nonculture-based microbiologic testing method which is performed for purposes of clinical diagnosis or treatment—for example, not Active Surveillance Culture/Testing (ASC/AST).
3. An abscess or other evidence of infection involving the organ/space that is detected on gross anatomic or histopathologic exam, or imaging test evidence suggestive of infection.

and

Meets at least *one* criterion for a specific organ/space infection site.

[a]The term "attending physician," for the purposes of application of the NHSN SSI criteria, may be interpreted to mean the surgeon(s), infectious disease specialist, other physician on the case, emergency physician, or physician's designee (nurse practitioner or physician's assistant). Modified with permission from Surgical Site Infection (SSI) Event. Centers for Disease Control (CDC), January 2019 https://www.cdc.gov/nhsn/pdfs/pscmanual/9pscssicurrent.pdf. Accessed August, 2019.

Table 8–3. Wound classification.

Clean	These are uninfected operative wounds in which no inflammation is encountered and the respiratory, alimentary, genital, or uninfected urinary tracts are not entered.
Clean/contaminated	These are operative wounds in which the respiratory, alimentary, genital, or urinary tract is entered under controlled conditions and without unusual contamination.
Contaminated	These include open, fresh, accidental wounds, operations with major breaks in sterile technique or gross spillage from the gastrointestinal tract, and incisions in which acute, nonpurulent inflammation is encountered.
Dirty	These include old traumatic wounds with retained devitalized tissue and those that involve existing clinical infection or perforated viscera.

Data from User Guide for the 2008 Participant Use Data File. American College of Surgeons National Surgical Quality Improvement Program, July 2009.

of postoperative SSI. A 2012 American College of Surgeons-National Surgical Quality Improvement (ACS-NSQIP) study of more than 600,000 patients, suggested that the rates of SSI increase as the degree of contamination increases: 2.58% for clean wounds, 6.67% for clean-contaminated wounds, 8.61% for contaminated wounds, and 11.80% for dirty wounds.

Attributable Cost & Impact

In addition to the morbidity incurred by patients, the healthcare and economic burden of SSIs is significant. Multiple studies have consistently documented that SSIs lead to a considerable increase in length of hospital stay (LOS), hospital charges, and societal health services cost. It is estimated that 11 days of hospitalization are added for each SSI that occurs, and that SSIs account for $3.2 billion in attributable cost per year in acute care hospitals. The excess cost results from the additional procedures (eg, incision and drainage, wound washout, skin grafts), antibiotics, and increased hospital LOS. In addition, even when SSI patients are successfully discharged, their rate of hospital readmission is at least doubled. Another study using patient-centered surveys and large administrative databases suggested almost a threefold increase in the total cost for patients *diagnosed with SSI following discharge* from the hospital compared to those who do not develop SSI. The increased costs were accounted for by a significant increase in the use of visiting nurses for wound care, diagnostic imaging, and an increase in readmissions to emergency departments and to the hospital.

Pathophysiology

The etiology of SSI is multifactorial; the patient's comorbidities, the nature of the surgical procedure and technique, and the perioperative environment including infrastructure and processes of care all interact to result in, or prevent, an SSI. It is thought that most SSIs are directly caused by the patient's endogenous flora at the time of surgery. This is further supported by the fact that, in clean wounds, SSIs are most commonly caused by *Staphylococcus aureus* or coagulase-negative *Staphylococcus*, both abundantly present on patients' skin. On the other hand, SSIs following bowel surgery are usually caused by endogenous intestinal flora. When a surgical device or implant is left in place, bacteria can secrete special glycolyx-based biofilms that can potentially shield the offending bacteria from the body's immune defenses. One of the immediate sequelae of such a phenomenon is the fact that the inoculum needed to cause an SSI in the presence of a foreign body such as a surgical implant or device is typically smaller than the inoculum needed to cause the same infection in the absence of a foreign body.

Despite the belief that most SSIs originate from endogenous microbes, there is convincing literature suggesting that nonendogenous sources are implicated in the occurrence of SSIs as well. Breach of the strict sterile surgical field, undetected surgical glove perforations, increased personnel traffic through the operating room (OR), suboptimal air flow and ventilation in the operating room, and poor surgical technique with excessive tissue injury or tension are some of the many factors implicated in SSI that will be discussed further in the next few sections.

Risk Factors

Many risk factors have been implicated as predictors of SSI. Some are directly related to the patient's health status, immune system, and comorbidities, while others are inherent to the nature of the procedure being performed and therefore are not easily modifiable. A few risk factors reflect suboptimal healthcare system design and less than reliable processes of care delivery; and their importance lies in the possibility of subjecting them to improvement and optimization strategies.

A. Patient-Related Risk Factors

Several studies have shown that advanced age, diabetes mellitus, obesity, smoking, alcoholism, malnutrition, and immunosuppression (eg, chronic steroid use, HIV/AIDS, posttransplant) are all risk factors for the development of SSI (Table 8–1). Most of these factors are not amenable to immediate preoperative modification or prevention, although long-term and perioperative control of glucose levels, smoking cessation, and attempts to improve nutrition may help in the overall performance of the patient perioperatively and may also decrease complications, including SSI.

B. Procedure-Related Risk Factors

The nature of the procedure, especially the wound classification (Table 8–3) and the expected inoculum of bacteria into the surgical site, are key factors that influence the risk of developing an SSI. For example, the rate of SSI complicating eye surgery, where the inoculum of bacterial contamination is minimal, is almost nonexistent. In comparison, the rate of SSI complicating colorectal surgery remains closer to 20% despite strategies and efforts aimed at prevention. In early 1990s, the National Healthcare Safety Network (NHSN) risk index, previously called the National Nosocomial Infections Surveillance System (NNIS), was developed in an attempt to better define a priori a patient's risk of developing SSI. This index considered the following three factors: (1) An American Society of Anesthesiologists (ASA) score ≥ 3, (2) a surgical wound classification as either contaminated or dirty, and (3) a prolonged duration of procedure over a certain number of hours (T), where T depends on the nature of the procedure being performed. The analysis of the CDC data by Culver and colleagues revealed that the rates of SSIs are 1.5%, 2.9%, 6.8%, and 13% in the presence of none, 1, 2, or 3 of the above risk index factors, respectively. The NHSN has introduced improved SSI risk adjustment models for specific operations based on easily traceable patient risk factors.

C. Process- and System-Related Risk Factors

Several process- and system-related risk factors have been identified over the years as potential factors contributing to a higher rate of SSI.

1. Suboptimal choice and timing of perioperative antibiotics—In a systematic review of more than 30,000 Medicare patients, Bratzler and colleagues found that fewer than 56% of patients undergoing surgery received their perioperative antibiotics within the recommended 60-minute window before incision. In the same study, up to 10% of patients did not receive the appropriate antibiotic regimen that would cover the type of pathogens specific to the procedures the patients were undergoing. Based on this study, the Surgical Care Improvement Project (SCIP) was initiated in 2004 and addressed SSI prevention by addressing, among other factors, components of prophylactic perioperative antibiotics, namely choice and timing (Table 8–6). SCIP was successful in achieving its goal of increasing compliance with evidence-based strategies and was discontinued in 2016.

2. Unrecognized breach of asepsis—Operating room staff, including nursing, anesthesia, and surgical personnel, are strongly encouraged to immediately report to the surgeon when suspecting a potential breach of the sterile field (eg, inadequate skin preparation, soiled clothes or equipment, glove perforation). In a study of gynecologic laparotomies, glove perforations were found to occur in 27 out of 29 laparotomies. The relationship between the rates of SSIs and glove perforation is less evident when the data are analyzed. In a study of more than 4000 procedures, the rates of SSIs increased with glove perforation only in the absence of appropriate antibiotic prophylaxis.

3. Preoperative hair removal—Preoperative hair removal has been correlated in several studies with a higher rate of SSI, even when the procedure involves the scalp or the patient has abundant hair at the surgical site. A 2006 Cochrane database systematic review and meta-analysis concluded that preoperative shaving increases the rate of SSI at least twofold; it is noteworthy that there was no difference in the rates of SSI when hair clipping was compared to no hair removal. Therefore, if hair removal is deemed necessary, preoperative hair clipping is preferred to shaving.

4. Surgical technique—The use of "rough" surgical techniques with unnecessary or excessive tissue disruption and trauma, whether resulting from electrocautery, traction, or blunt dissection, is believed to lead to higher rates of SSI. Even though most surgeons and common sense suggest this correlation, strong evidence supporting a cause–effect relationship has not been demonstrated.

5. Operating room design and traffic—It is well established that the burden of airborne bacteria in a closed space is directly related to the number of people in the space, as well as to the number of people entering and exiting a closed space such as the operating room (OR). The link between poor air flow due to OR design or increased traffic through the OR doors and SSIs has been studied mostly in the orthopedic literature, but has not been clearly established.

▶ Prevention Strategies

Prevention of SSI relies primarily on optimizing the patient's comorbidities and creating a systematic method to ensure that all modifiable risk factors are addressed. All processes of care proven or arguably thought to prevent SSIs should be executed in all patients at all times. Table 8–4 lists potential measures to minimize the risk of SSI. In addition, the World Health Organization, the American College of Surgeons, the Surgical Infection Society, and the CDC all published guidelines between 2016 and 2017 highlighting specific recommendations for prevention of SSI and the strength of the evidence behind such recommendations (Table 8–5). Although level-one evidence is lacking for many of those measures, inclusion of some or all in a bundle might prove to be a beneficial strategy. The surgical improvement project (SIP), established in 2004 and folded within the surgical care improvement program (SCIP) in 2006, created performance measures out of several of these preventative measures based on best evidence in the literature (Table 8–6). Whether the SCIP measures resulted in a national decrease in SSI incidence or not remains controversial, and a detailed discussion

Table 8–4. Potential[a] measures to prevent surgical site infections.

Optimizing the patient's nutritional status
Appropriate perioperative antibiotic prophylaxis (choice, dosing, and timing)
Adequate glucose level control in diabetic patients
Maintenance of perioperative normoglycemia in all patients
Maintenance of strict asepsis
Preoperative skin preparation with alcohol-based solutions
Gentle skin handling and minimization of cautery-related tissue damage
Improving ventilation and laminar air flow in the OR
Maintenance of perioperative normothermia
Avoiding hair removal; clipping instead of shaving, if necessary
Perioperative oxygen supplementation
Preoperative antibacterial soap showers
Antibacterial coated sutures
Antibacterial irrigation solutions
Operative wound barriers
Antibacterial dressings

[a]Many of these measures have shown controversial and nondefinitive results in the prevention of SSI.

of SCIP is beyond the scope of this text. Perioperative antibiotics and the choice of the skin preparation solution are discussed below.

A. Perioperative Antibiotics

The timing of prophylactic antibiotic administration and the choice of the appropriate perioperative antibiotic are key components in the strategy to prevent SSI. The choice of the prophylactic antibiotic should be dictated by the procedure and pathogens most likely to cause SSI. It is also crucial to achieve bactericidal concentration at time of incision. To do that, the infusion should be complete within 1 hour prior to incision (2 hours for vancomycin or fluoroquinolone). No additional prophylaxis is needed after skin closure, even in the presence of drains. This will also prevent side effects of the antibiotic and the emergence of drug resistance. Proper antibiotic dosing based on the patient's weight and manufacturer's recommendation for the antibiotic is a key consideration in prophylaxis. In addition, redosing of the antibiotic during surgery based on the antibiotic half-life and the amount of fluid administration and blood loss should be strongly considered if the procedure is lengthy. Table 8–7 is a practical guide into dosing and time for redosing for commonly used prophylactic antibiotics.

Table 8–5. Summary of the 2017 CDC Guidelines for Prevention of Surgical Site Infection.

Recommendation	Strength of Evidence
Parenteral Antimicrobial Prophylaxis	
Administer antimicrobials only when indicated based on published guidelines. Time administration such that bactericidal concentration is established in serum and tissues at initial incision.	Category IB
For caesarean sections, administer the appropriate agent prior to skin incision (versus at cord clamping).	Category IA
Nonparenteral Antimicrobial Prophylaxis	
Consider use of triclosan-coated sutures.	Category II
Glycemic Control	
Implement perioperative glycemic control using blood glucose target levels ≤ 200 mg/dL in both diabetic and nondiabetic patients.	Category IA
Normothermia	
Maintain perioperative normothermia.	Category IA
Oxygenation	
Administer increased fraction of inspired oxygen intraoperatively and in the immediate postoperative period following extubation for all patients with normal pulmonary function undergoing general anesthesia with endotracheal intubation.	Category IA
Antiseptic Prophylaxis	
Instruct patients to perform full body shower or bath the night before surgery (with either soap or an antiseptic agent).	Category IB
Intraoperative skin preparation should be performed with an antiseptic agent containing alcohol unless contraindicated.	Category IA
Consider intraoperative irrigation of deep or subcutaneous tissues with aqueous iodophor solution.	Category II

B. Antiseptic Skin Preparation

Based on a prospective randomized trial and an observational study, the National Quality Forum has recommended the use of alcohol containing solutions for the preparation of patient's skin prior to surgery.

C. Adhesive Drapes

The CDC guidelines currently state that the use of adhesive drapes, with or without antibiotics, is not necessary (weak recommendation).

Table 8–6. Surgical care improvement project (SCIP) measures aimed at prevention of surgical site infections[a].

SCIP Infection Measure 1	Prophylactic antibiotic received within 1 h prior to surgical incision
SCIP Infection Measure 2	Appropriate prophylactic antibiotic selection for the surgical patient
SCIP Infection Measure 3	Prophylactic antibiotic discontinued within 24 h after surgery end-time (within 48 h after cardiac surgery end-time)
SCIP Infection Measure 4	Blood glucose level at 6 AM < 200 mg/dL on postoperative days 1 and 2 in cardiac surgery
SCIP Infection Measure 6	No or appropriate hair removal (clippers, not shaving)
SCIP Infection Measure 7	Immediate postoperative normothermia (temperature > 96.8°F within 15 min postoperatively) in colorectal surgery

[a]Although the SCIP measures were retired in 2016, they remain essential components of the prevention of SSI and are part of the CDC Prevention Guidelines.

D. Maintaining Normoglycemia

Maintenance of perioperative normoglycemia, specifically keeping glucose levels below 200 mg/dL, is strongly recommended in the perioperative phase, for both diabetic and nondiabetic patients. From a long-term glucose-control perspective, an optimal HBA1C level that can be achieved preoperatively has not been identified yet.

E. Perioperative Oxygen Supplementation

Based on level-one evidence, it is now strongly recommended to use 80% oxygen intraoperatively and for 2-6 hours postoperatively to decrease the risk of SSI. Achieving a specific oxygenation level target and the best mode of delivery of oxygen, especially after removal of the endotracheal tube, remain unknown.

F. Maintaining Normothermia

Maintenance of normothermia perioperatively with the use of warming devices is strongly recommended based on moderate to high evidence, although the duration needed for such intervention postoperatively remains unclear.

G. Other Prevention Strategies

Preoperative antibacterial soap showers, antibacterial coated sutures, antimicrobial irrigants, and antibacterial dressings are additional measures that remain controversial in the prevention of SSI. Mechanical bowel preparation and oral antibiotics in patients undergoing colorectal surgery are the subjects of renewed controversy and discussion but remain an important strategy in the prevention of SSI in this field. At present, the combination of mechanical and antibiotic (PO) preparation is recommended for all elective colorectal surgeries.

▶ Treatment

The treatment of an established SSI consists of opening the incision, draining the purulent material, and debridement of any necrotic tissue. Adjunctive antimicrobial treatment is given when the patient has systemic symptoms, associated cellulitis, or a deep SSI with risk for fascial and subcutaneous spread. Cultures are important to track emergence of resistant organisms, to deescalate from broad-spectrum empiric antibiotics, and for epidemiologic surveillance. In the case of an organ/space SSI, percutaneous drainage using radiologic guidance, along with adequate antibiotic coverage, is the preferred approach.

INFECTIONS NEEDING SURGICAL MANAGEMENT

When infections fail to respond or are deemed unlikely to respond to medical and antimicrobial treatments alone, surgical intervention might be needed. The list of surgical infections necessitating surgical management is long, but the most common ones include abscesses, empyema, necrotizing skin and soft-tissue infections (NSSTIs), intra-abdominal infections, and *Clostridium difficile* (*C. difficile*) colitis. Many of these surgical infections can become life threatening by causing sepsis, septic shock, and multiple organ dysfunction syndrome (MODS) if not controlled and treated promptly. Spreading can occur through tissue planes (necrotizing infections), abscess/fistulae formation, or the lymphatic system and the bloodstream. Spread of an infection through the bloodstream (bacteremia) can lead to distant seeding of bacteria and subsequent abscess formation (eg, brain, liver, adrenal glands, heart valves).

▶ Inflammation, Sepsis, & Septic Shock

Microbial infection results in tissue damage that leads to an inflammatory response at the local tissue level in an effort by the patient's immune system to overcome the infection. At the site of injury, endothelial cells and leukocytes coordinate the local release of mediators of the inflammatory response, including cytokines (tumor necrosis factor-α), interleukins, interferons, leukotrienes, prostaglandins, nitric oxide, reactive oxygen species, and products of the classic inflammatory pathway (complement, histamine, and bradykinin) (Table 8–8). Once these mediators reach the infected site, they are extremely effective at recruiting and priming cells of both the innate and adaptive

Table 8–7. Suggested initial dose and time to redosing for antimicrobial drugs commonly utilized for surgical prophylaxis.

| Antimicrobial | Renal Half-Life (h) | | Recommended Infusion Duration | Standard Dose | Weight-Based Dose Recommendation[a] | Recommended Redosing Interval (h)[b] |
	Patients with Normal Renal Function	Patients with End-Stage Renal Disease				
Aztreonam	1.5-2	6	3-5 min,[c] 20-60 min[d]	1-2 g IV	2 g maximum (adults)	3-5
Ciprofloxacin	3.5-5	5-9	60 min	400 mg IV	400 mg	4-10
Cefazolin	1.2-2.5	40-70	3-5 min,[c] 15-60 min[d]	1-2 g IV	20-30 mg/kg (if < 80 kg, use 1 g; if > 80 kg, use 2 g)	2-5
Cefuroxime	1-2	15-22	3-5 min,[c] 15-60 min[d]	1.5 g IV	50 mg/kg	3-4
Cefamandole	0.5-2.1	12.3-18[e]	3-5 min,[c] 15-60 min[d]	1 g IV		3-4
Cefoxitin	0.5-1.1	6.5-23	3-5 min,[c] 15-60 min[d]	1-2 g IV	20-40 mg/kg	2-3
Cefotetan	2.8-4.6	13-25	3-5 min,[c] 20-60 min[d]	1-2 g iv	20-40 mg/kg	3-6
Clindamycin	2-5.1	3.5-5[f]	10-60 min (do not exceed 30 mg/min)	600-900 mg IV	If < 10 kg, use at least 37.5 mg; if > 10 kg, use 3-6 mg/kg	3-6
Erythromycin base	0.8-3	5-6	NA	1 g po 19, 18, and 9 h before surgery	9-13 mg/kg	NA
Gentamicin	2-3	50-70	30-60 min	1.5 mg/kg IV[g]	...[g]	3-6
Neomycin	2-3 (3% absorbed orally)	12-24 or longer	NA	1 g po 19, 18, and 9 h before surgery	20 mg/kg	NA
Metronidazole	6-14	7-21; no change	30-60 min	0.5-1 g IV	15 mg/kg initial dose (adult); 7.5 mg/kg on subsequent doses	6-8
Vancomycin	4-6	44.1-406.4 (CCl < 10 mL/min)	1 g over 60 min (use longer infusion time if dose > 1 g)	1 g IV	10-15 mg/kg (adult)	6-12

Note. CCl, creatinine clearance.

[a]Data are primarily from published pediatric recommendations.

[b]For procedures of long duration, antimicrobials should be readministered at intervals of 1-2 times the half-life of the drug. The intervals in the table were calculated for patients with normal renal function.

[c]Dose injected directly into vein or via running IV fluids.

[d]Intermittent IV infusion.

[e]In patients with a serum creatinine level of 5-9 mg/dL.

[f]The half-life of clindamycin is the same or slightly increased in patients with end-stage renal disease, compared with patients with normal renal function.

[g]If the patient's body weight is > 30% higher than their ideal body weight (IBW), the dosing weight (DW) can be determined as follows: DW = IBW + (0.4 × (total body weight − IBW)).

Data from McEvoy GK, ed. AHFS drug information. 43rd ed. Bethesda, MD: American Society of Health-System Pharmacists, 2003; Nissen D, ed. Mosby's drug consultant. 2nd ed. St. Louis: Elsevier Science, 2003; Anderson PO, Knoeben JE, Troutman WG, eds. *Handbook of clinical drug data.* 10th ed. New York: McGraw-Hill, 2002.

Table 8–8. Cytokines and growth factors.

Peptide	Site of Synthesis	Regulation	Target Cells	Effects
G-CSF	Fibroblasts, monocytes	Induced by IL-1, lipopoly-saccharide (LPS), IFN-α	Committed neutrophil progenitors (CFU-G, Gran)	Supports the proliferation of neutrophil-forming colonies. Stimulates respiratory burst.
GM-CSF (IL-3 has almost identical effects)	Endothelial cells, fibroblasts, macrophages, T-lymphocytes, bone marrow	Induced by IL-1, TNF	Granulocyte-erythrocyte-monocyte-megakaryocyte progenitor cells (CFU-GEMM, CFU-MEG, CFU-Eo, CFU-GM)	Supports the proliferation of macrophage-, eosinophil-, neutrophil-, and monocyte-containing colonies.
IFN-α, IFN-β, IFN-γ	Epithelial cells, fibroblasts, lymphocytes, macrophages, neutrophils	Induced by viruses (foreign nucleic acids), microbes, microbial foreign antigens, cancer cells	Lymphocytes, macrophages, infected cells, cancer cells	Inhibits viral multiplication. Activates defective phagocytes, direct inhibition of cancer cell multiplication, activation of killer leukocytes, inhibition of collagen synthesis.
IL-1	Endothelial cells, keratinocytes, lymphocytes, macrophages	Induced by TNF-α, IL-1, IL-2, C5a; suppressed by IL-4, TGF-β	Monocytes, macrophages, T-cells, B cells, NK cells, LAK cells	Stimulates T-cells, B-cells, NK cells, LAK cells. Induces tumoricidal activity and production to other cytokines, endogenous pyrogen (via PGE$_2$ release). Induces steroidogenesis, acute-phase proteins, hypotension, chemotactic neutrophils. Stimulates respiratory burst.
IL-1ra	Monocytes	Induced by GM-CSF, LPS, IgG	Blocks type 1 IL-1 receptors on T-cells, fibroblasts, chondrocytes, endothelial cells	Blocks type 1 IL-1 receptors on T-cells, chondrocytes, endothelial cells. Ameliorates animal models of arthritis, septic shock, and inflammatory bowel disease.
IL-2	Lymphocytes	Induced by IL-1, IL-6	T-cells, NK cells, B-cells, activated monocytes	Stimulates growth of T-cells, NK cells, and B-cells.
IL-4	T-cells, NK cells, mast cells	Induced by cell activation, IL-1	All hematopoietic cells and many others express receptors	Stimulates B-cell and T-cell growth. Induces HLA class II molecules.
IL-6	Endothelial cells, fibroblasts, lymphocytes, some tumors	Induced by IL-1, TNF-α	T-cells, B-cells, plasma cells, keratinocytes, hepatocytes, stem cells	B-cell differentiation. Induction of acute-phase proteins, growth of keratinocytes. Stimulates growth of T-cells and hematopoietic stem cells.
IL-8	Endothelial cells, fibroblasts, lymphocytes, monocytes	Induced by TNF, IL-1, LPS, cell adherence (monocytes)	Basophils, neutrophils, T-cells	Induces expression of endothelial cell LECAM-1 receptors, β$_2$ integrins, and neutrophil transmigration. Stimulates respiratory burst.
M-CSF	Endothelial cells, fibroblasts, monocytes	Induced by IL-1, LPS, IFN-α	Committed monocyte progenitors (CFU-M, mono)	Supports the proliferation of monocyte-forming colonies. Activates macrophages.
MCP-1, MCAF	Monocytes; some tumors secrete a similar peptide	Induced by IL-1, LPS, PHA	Unstimulated monocytes	Chemoattractant specific for monocytes.
TNF-α (LT has almost identical effects)	Macrophages, NK cells, T-cells, transformed cell lines, B-cells (LT)	Suppressed by PGE$_2$, TGF-β, IL-4; induced by LPS	Endothelial cells, monocytes, neutrophils	Stimulates T-cell growth. Direct cytotoxin to some tumor cells. Profound proinflammatory effect via induction of IL-1 and PGE$_2$. Systemic administration produces many symptoms of sepsis. Stimulates respiratory burst and phagocytosis.

immune systems to identify and attack invading pathogens. In addition, these inflammatory mediators initiate the damaged tissue healing processes. However, if the degree of the infectious or traumatic insult overwhelms the ability of the body to control it, the inflammatory mediators might trigger a systemic inflammatory reaction of serious damaging consequences. Such a quasi-maladaptive systemic response can disrupt normal cellular metabolism and jeopardize tissue perfusion at the cellular level. From a terminology perspective (Table 8–9), when the systemic response occurs in the absence of a documented infection (eg, burns, trauma, pancreatitis), it is called systemic inflammatory response syndrome (SIRS). The term "sepsis" is used when the systemic response results from a documented infection rather than systemic inflammation alone. Septic shock occurs when severe sepsis is associated with hypotension or hemodynamic instability. Septic shock can lead to progressive dysfunction of multiple organs such as the brain (delirium), lungs (hypoxia and respiratory failure), heart (hypotension, pulmonary edema), and kidneys (oliguria and renal failure). Bacteremia is the presence of viable bacteria in blood, often documented through blood cultures. Transient bacteremia (eg, following dental work) is common, benign, and self-limited. It usually has no clinical implications except in patients with damaged heart valves; cardiac, vascular, or orthopedic implants; or impaired immunity. Bacteremia happening in a patient with an uncontrolled source of infection can be devastating and may result in sepsis, septic shock, and organ dysfucntion.

A. Diagnosis

Localizing the source of the suspected infection or sepsis is crucial, and a good and thorough physical examination is indispensable. Laboratory evaluation often shows leukocytosis, but leukopenia is not infrequent in cases of severe infection or sepsis. Acidosis is occasionally present and might be helpful in making the diagnosis. Radiologic examinations—including plain films for suspected pneumonia, computed tomography or ultrasound for suspected intra-abdominal or intra-thoracic abscesses, and bone scans or magnetic resonance imaging (MRI) for suspected osteomyelitis—are often essential for making the diagnosis and establishing the source of infection.

Identifying the causative organism by culturing the infected site, followed by testing the implicated pathogen's sensitivity to diverse antimicrobial agents, are the two next key steps. If infection is suspected but the source remains unclear, cultures of blood, sputum, and urine should be performed. Culturing other body fluids (eg, cerebrospinal fluid, pleural and joint effusions, ascites) can be performed if warranted based on the patient's history, physical examination, and the degree of clinical suspicion.

B. Treatment

Infectious source control and antibiotics constitute the mainstay of surgical infection treatment. When patients are septic with or without shock, "goal-directed" management of the sepsis with prompt patient resuscitation and immediate initiation of the appropriate empiric antibiotics are of ultimate importance, and have been shown by high-level evidence to improve patient survival. The *Surviving Sepsis Guidelines* emphasize the systematic and evidence-based approach to treating sepsis and septic shock patients. These guidelines can be found at www.survivingsepsis.org.

▶ Surgical Skin & Skin Structure Infections

Surgical cutaneous infections span the spectrum of the superficial skin abscesses such as furuncles and carbuncles to the devastating and often fatal necrotizing deeper soft-tissue infections.

A. Furuncle

1. Pathophysiology—A furuncle (boil) is a superficial skin abscess usually caused by *Staphylococcus aureus* infection

Table 8–9. Definitions of sepsis, severe sepsis, septic shock, and systemic inflammatory response syndrome (SIRS).

Systemic Inflammatory Response Syndrome (SIRS)
Two or more of the following Temperature > 38.3°C or < 36°C Heart rate > 90 beats/min Respiratory rate > 20 breaths/min or paCO$_2$ < 32 mm Hg WBC > 12,000 cells/mm^3, < 4000 cells/mm^3, or > 10% immature (band) forms
Sepsis
Sepsis is defined as life-threatening organ dysfunction caused by a dysregulated host response to infection. Sepsis clinical criteria: Organ dysfunction is defined as an increase of 2 points or more in the Sequential Organ Failure Assessment (SOFA) score for patients with infections. An increase of 2 SOFA points gives an overall mortality rate of 10%. Patients with suspected infection who are likely to have a prolonged ICU stay or to die in the hospital can be promptly identified at the bedside with SOFA ("HAT"); ie, 2 or more of: - Hypotension: SBP ≤ 100 mm Hg - Altered mental status (any GCS < 15) - Tachypnea: respiratory rate ≥ 22
Septic Shock
Septic shock is a subset of sepsis in which underlying circulatory and cellular/metabolic abnormalities are profound enough to substantially increase mortality. Patients with septic shock can be identified with a clinical construct of sepsis with persisting hypotension requiring vasopressors to maintain mean arterial pressure (MAP) ≥ 65 mm Hg and having a serum lactate level > 2 mmol/L (18 mg/dL) despite adequate volume resuscitation. With these criteria, hospital mortality is in excess of 40%.

at the level of the hair follicle. Bacteria asymptomatically inhabit most hair follicles, but it is thought that obstruction of the pilosebaceous apparatus is the triggering event for the formation of furuncles.

2. Risk factors—Some of the identified risk factors include puberty, male gender, obesity, diabetes, poor hygiene, as well as living in a climate characterized by a high level of humidity.

3. Causative organisms—Even though staphylococci are the most common causative organisms, streptococci, gram-negative organisms, and anaerobic diphteroids can also cause furuncles.

4. Clinical presentation—Furuncles present as itchy, indurated small abscesses, surrounded by skin erythema. A small white area of skin necrosis is often notable at the top of the abscess.

5. Treatment—Most furuncles resolve spontaneously, although larger lesions require incision and drainage. The use of antibiotics following incision and drainage is not routinely necessary and remains controversial, even though a recent randomized controlled trial suggested a 7-day course could improve cure rates. We recommend antibiotics only in the presence of concomitant extensive surrounding cellulitis. Antibacterial soap showers might be helpful in both treatment and prevention of recurrence.

B. Carbuncle

1. Pathophysiology—Carbuncles are rare and result when several furuncles coalesce, extend into the subcutaneous tissue, and/or form a "network" of multilocular interconnected abscesses and tracts.

2. Risk factors—Carbuncles on the back of the neck are seen almost exclusively in diabetic or relatively immunocompromised patients. In addition to obesity and diabetes, chronic steroid intake and malnutrition are potential risk factors for carbuncles.

3. Causative organism—Similar to furuncles, *Staphylococcus aureus* remains the most common organism involved in carbuncles.

4. Clinical presentation—Carbuncles often have the appearance of multiple large furuncles with several openings draining pus. As carbuncles enlarge, the blood supply to the skin is destroyed and the tissue over the top of the abscess becomes white in color and necrotic in appearance. Patients might show some systemic signs such as fever and malaise.

5. Treatment—Carbuncles often require incision and drainage; occasionally, a more extensive excision is required. When appropriate, the excision is continued until many associated deep sinus tracts are removed. Antibiotics are usually needed in view of the associated extensive skin

cellulitis and induration. In patients with recurrent and multiple skin abscesses due to *Staphylococcus aureus,* consideration should be given to a decolonization regimen with chlorhexidine showers and nasal mupirocin with or without oral antibiotics.

C. Hidradinitis Suppurativa

1. Pathophysiology—Hidradinitis suppurativa is a serious skin condition characterized by blockage and infection of the apocrine sweat glands. Hidradinitis most commonly involves the axilla or the groin. Since apocrine glands develop postpuberty, prepubertal disease is very rare. Even though hidradinitis often becomes chronic with serious patient morbidity and disability, systemic complications and constitutional signs and symptoms are uncommon.

2. Risk factors—Obesity, puberty, female gender, and smoking are some of the identified risk factors associated with hidradinitis.

3. Causative agents—Hidradinitis is a polymicrobial infection involving gram-positive, gram-negative, and anaerobic organisms. Superinfection with fungal organisms is not uncommon, especially in patients with chronic or recurrent hidradinitis.

4. Clinical presentation—Hidradinitis can affect any area where apocrine glands exist, most commonly the axilla and groin, but also the perineum, inframammary folds, gluteal folds, areola, and scrotum. On exam, erythematous tender skin nodules characterize early stages. This can quickly progress to deeper indurated abscesses with interconnected sinuses, purulent drainage, and associated regional lymphadenopathy.

5. Treatment—Drainage of the individual abscesses and their associated sinuses is needed. If healing is delayed, fungal superinfections should be suspected and, if confirmed, should be treated as well. With chronic and recurrent infections, the involved skin and apocrine glands can be excised, and the underlying soft tissue left to heal by secondary intention. Skin flaps and grafts might be needed in later stages, as the resultant scarring can be severe. Topical clindamycin, systemic tetracycline, and isotretinoin are potential adjunctive therapies. Weight loss and hygiene-focused interventions should be encouraged to decrease the risk of recurrence.

D. Necrotizing Skin and Soft-Tissue Infections (NSTIs)

1. Introduction—Accurate data on the incidence of necrotizing skin and soft-tissue infections (NSTIs) are lacking, and most existing data are based on single-institution experiences, suggesting a large variability in clinical presentation, severity, and outcome. NSTIs are skin and soft-tissue infections characterized by widespread and severe tissue necrosis resulting from aggressive and life-threatening bacteria that are often able to secrete toxins. NSTIs are also known as gas gangrene, necrotizing fasciitis (when involving fascial layers), Fournier gangrene (when involving the perineum and genitalia), and Ludwig angina (when involving the floor of the mouth).

2. Pathophysiology—NSTIs can be caused by single agents such as clostridia or streptococci species, but most are polymicrobial in etiology. An inciting site (eg, puncture wound, insect bite) can occasionally be discovered by history or physical exam. In the perineum, a perirectal/perianal abscess or manipulation of the urogenital tract and diabetes are known to be associated with NSTIs. The infection is classically one of sudden onset and rapid progression through ischemic tissue planes, occasionally with air formation at deeper layers. Small-vessel thrombosis occurs along the infection progression pathway, and thus the underlying deeper tissue damage is almost always much more pronounced than what the overlying skin appearance suggests.

3. Causative agents—By definition, type I NSTIs are monomicrobial (eg, streptococci, clostridia), while type II NSTIs are polymicrobial. Type III NSTIs are rare, caused by *Vibrio vulnificus,* often found in saltwater. *Clostridium perfringens* secretes exotoxins (eg, lecithinases, collagenases, proteases, hemolysins) that lead to small-vessel thrombosis and allow for rapid progression and aggressive invasion of fascial and muscle planes. These toxins contribute to the serious deep-tissue destruction and the overlying skin grayish discoloration. The alpha toxin (a lecithinase) is believed to be an essential contributor to clostridial virulence. In addition to their local effect, these toxins may lead to severe sepsis, pronounced SIRS, and not uncommonly MODS. Streptococci can also secrete several exotoxins with similar virulence leading to fascial and deeper plane disruptions. *Streptococcus pyogenes* (group A strep), although rare, is classically described to secrete a superantigen toxin that can result in toxic shock syndrome with resultant organ failure. NSTIs are often caused by mixed nonclostridial, nonstreptococcal bacteria including staphylococci, gram-negatives, and anaerobes.

4. Risk factors—Immunocompromised (eg, HIV, diabetes), intravenous drug abuse and cancer patients are at a particularly higher risk of developing NSTIs, as well as malnourished, diabetic, and obese patients.

5. Clinical presentation—Prompt suspicion and early diagnosis of NSTIs are essential. In early stages, patients often have fever and pain out of proportion to physical examination findings. Erythema, induration, hemorrhagic skin bulla, blisters, and vesicles are occasionally present. Grayish discoloration of the underlying skin and pain beyond the affected skin area are especially suggestive of deeper underlying tissue involvement. "Dishwasher-like" gray discharge might be seen and should raise suspicion for NSTIs. Patients

Table 8–10. The laboratory risk indicator for necrotizing fasciitis (LRINEC) score.

Variable	Points
C-Reactive protein (mg/L) > 150	4
WBC count ($\times 10^6$ per mm^3)	
< 15	0
15-25	1
> 25	2
Hemoglobin (g/dL)	
> 13.5	0
11-13.5	1
< 11	2
Sodium (mmol/L) < 135	2
Creatinine (μmol/L) > 141	2
Glucose (mmol/L) > 10	1

can quickly develop systemic signs of toxicity with hypotension, tachycardia, electrolyte imbalances, lethargy, and even organ failure. Laboratory workup typically shows leukocytosis (with or without bandemia) or leucopenia, hyponatremia, and acidosis. Several models have been developed over the years in an attempt to predict the probability of a skin infection being a NSTI versus a more benign superficial skin infection. The Laboratory Risk Indicator for Necrotizing Fasciitis (LRINEC) score assigns different point scores to each of six laboratory values (Table 8–10). A LRINEC score of six or more was found in a study of 89 NSTIs to have a positive predictive value of 92% and a negative predictive value of 96% for NSTI, but later studies have failed to find such high accuracy. Radiologically, plain films showing deep soft tissue air are very rare but pathognomonic. CT scan is the standard of care when difficulty arises in differentiating between "benign" skin or soft-tissue infection, and NSTIs and are almost 100% sensitive when interpreted carefully and expertly. CT images often show inflammation and edema at the deeper fascial or muscular layers, and occasionally will show gas between these tissue layers. Although crepitus as felt on physical examination and/or deep tissue air as diagnosed by plain radiography or CT imaging have been classically described with several (but not all) clostridial species, they may occur with non-clostridial infections as well. When the clinical picture and the radiologic imaging fail to differentiate between benign soft-tissue infection and NSTIs, diagnostic surgical exploration of the area in question is required. Operative findings suggestive of NSTIs include pale and/or necrotic deep tissue, "dishwasher" nonpurulent gray discharge, nonbleeding soft tissue, and thrombosed microvessels. Easy separation with unopposed finger "sliding" between the tissue planes (the "finger test") is highly suggestive of

NSTIs. Pathologic examination will reveal severe inflammation and tissue necrosis.

6. Treatment—A NSTI is a surgical emergency and requires immediate wide surgical debridement, broad-spectrum antibiotics, and hemodynamic and fluid resuscitation.

1. *Wide surgical debridement.* All tissue that appears pale, ischemic or necrotic, "lifts off" easily, or does not bleed appropriately needs to be removed. This should include the overlying skin, even when it appears viable, as studies have documented severe vasculitis and microvessel thrombosis that eventually lead to loss of skin, if not adequately debrided. Extensive debridement is usually needed, with one or more repeat trips to the operating room, until viable tissue is ensured. When an extremity is involved, amputation might be required, although attempts at debridement and limb salvage, with a planned "second look" are reasonable and might be preferred. Perirectal NSSSI and Fournier gangrene occasionally necessitate creation of an ostomy and/or urinary diversion. Depending on the extent and location of debridement, many patients, if they survive and recover, will need reconstructive surgery ranging from simple split-thickness skin grafts to major flap reconstructions.

2. *Antibiotics.* As soon as an NSSSI is suspected, broad-spectrum antibiotics should be initiated. Gram-positive, gram-negative, and anaerobic organisms need to be covered. A combination of a penicillin-based agent or cephalosporin with an aminoglycoside or fluoroquinolone and an antianaerobic agent (eg, metronidazole or clindamycin) is a reasonable starting empiric regimen. Clindamycin has been shown by in-vitro studies to have antiinflammatory and toxin-neutralizing effects, in addition to its antibacterial effects. If methicillin-resistant *Staphylococcus aureus* (MRSA) is suspected, vancomycin, linezolid, or daptomycin can be added. Aminoglycosides can be replaced by third- or fourth-generation cephalosporins (eg, cefepime, cefotaxime) or by carbapenems (eg, imipenem, meropenem, ertapenem), if indicated (eg, in patients with acute renal failure). Antimicrobials should be deescalated as soon as culture results and sensitivities are available. Antibiotics should be continued until the patient's clinical condition has stabilized, fever has subsided, and white blood cell count is normal.

3. *Hyperbaric oxygen.* The usefulness of hyperbaric oxygen in the treatment of NSSTI is controversial. A large Nationwide Inpatient Sample study has suggested decreased mortality with hyperbaric therapy, but the absence of supportive level-one evidence, combined with the logistical difficulties in critically ill patients, remain the main obstacles to recommend its routine utilization.

4. *Intravenous immunoglobulins.* A very small randomized controlled trial that was terminated early mainly due to slow patient recruitment suggested that intravenous immunoglobulins might decrease mortality in patients with group A streptococcus NSTIs. AB-103 is a peptide mimetic of CD-28, and its use in NSTIs is currently undergoing further investigation.

7. Prognosis—NSSSI has a poor prognosis, with reported mortality as high as 20%-35%, and an even higher morbidity rate. Diabetic patients and/or those presenting with septic shock and/or multisystem organ failure are at a particularly higher risk of mortality. Shorter time from onset of infection to operative debridement has been shown consistently to correlate with better survival.

▶ Organ/Space Infections

Organ/space infections are often deep infections resulting from uncontrolled infection or perforation of an internal organ. Internal postoperative abscesses are termed organ/space SSIs, and have been discussed previously. In addition to antibiotic treatment, many of these organ/space infections will need drainage.

A. Intra-abdominal Abscesses and Infections

In the era of high-resolution CT imaging, diseases such as acute diverticulitis and acute perforated appendicitis are more likely to be successfully managed nonoperatively in the acute clinical setting. When patients have no signs of diffuse peritonitis, periappendiceal, pericolonic abscesses, and other contained intraperitoneal abscesses may be drained percutaneously under radiologic guidance when accessible. With the combination of percutaneous drainage and adequate antibiotic coverage, patients' intra-abdominal infections can be treated adequately, allowing for the inflammation to resolve with potentially one-stage and less complicated surgical intervention at a later time to address the diseased organ. When percutaneous drainage is not possible, usually because of the abscess location and its inaccessibility to radiologic interventions, surgical drainage with removal of the infected organ (eg, appendectomy, colectomy) is warranted. If the abscess is less than 3-4 cm in diameter, an attempt at treatment with antibiotics alone without percutaneous or surgical drainage is a reasonable option in the stable patient without peritoneal signs. The management of complicated intra-abdominal infections, whether community-acquired or health-care associated, whether originating from the hepatobiliary system or the gastrointestinal system, is beyond the scope and goal of this chapter, but the emphasis should always be on (1) source control (surgical or percutaneous drainage), (2) early and appropriate antibiotics coverage, (3) fluid resuscitation, and (4) microbiologic evaluation, when feasible. The current recommended course of antibiotics following surgical or percutaneous source control is 4 days only, based on the recently published *New England*

Journal of Medicine STOP-IT trial results. An online application addressing the management and preferred antibiotics for various intra-abdominal infections can be downloaded from the Surgical Infection Society website at www.sisna.org.

B. Empyema

Empyema is a collection of pus in the pleural cavity, most commonly related to bacterial pneumonia and resulting parapneumonic effusions. Occasionally, empyemas occur postprocedurally, such as following thoracentesis, chest-tube placement, or lung resection. When empyema occurs, drainage is needed. In addition to antibiotics, tube thoracostomy is the recommended initial management. Unfortunately, chest-tube lumens often get clogged with thick pus, leading to placement of additional tubes, and not infrequently, failure to completely drain the pleural cavity and reexpand the lung. When that occurs, surgical drainage with decortication using a video-assisted thoracoscopic approach or an open thoracotomy is indicated. In cases of recurrent or persistent empyema despite surgical management, creation of an Eloesser flap or window with an open track between the pleural cavity and the outside skin might be needed to allow adequate and definitive drainage of the empyema.

C. *Clostridium difficile* Colitis

Clostridium difficile as an organism can be recovered in the feces of 5% of healthy individuals. The use of antibiotics can alter the colonic flora allowing for *C. difficile* overgrowth and colonization of the colon. The result is *C. difficile* colitis with severity ranging from simple watery diarrhea to life-threatening sepsis. *C. difficile* is currently considered one of the most common and most serious healthcare-associated infections.

1. Risk factors—Antibiotic intake is the single most important risk factor for *C. difficile* colitis, and has been described even following a single antibiotic dose administration as with SSI prophylaxis. Although all antibiotics can be implicated, fluoroquinolones, clindamycin, penicillins, and cephalosporins are the most frequently encountered culprits, partly because of their widespread utilization. A Canadian study conducted during a relatively recent *C. difficile* outbreak in Quebec strongly suggested that fluroquinolones are currently the antibiotics most commonly associated with *C. difficile* infections rather than clindamycin as classically and historically described.

Table 8–11 lists the different antibiotics classified into those with high, moderate, and small risk of *C. difficile* infection.

Transmission of *C. difficile* by healthcare providers caring for patients with *C. difficile* colitis has resulted in outbreaks of *C. difficile* among patients within hospitals and the emergence of multidrug-resistant organisms. These epidemics are addressed and prevented by proper hand hygiene among health care providers and the isolation of patients with *C. difficile* colitis.

2. Clinical presentation—The presentation of *C. difficile* colitis can range from the asymptomatic carrier state that requires no treatment, and the mild diarrhea state that can easily be treated with oral antibiotics as an outpatient, to the severely toxic, septic, and MODS patient presentation. Across all the severity range, watery diarrhea and abdominal distention remain the essential characteristics of *C. difficile* colitis. Lower abdominal pain may be also present, and is usually of a crampy nonspecific nature. Constitutional symptoms such as fever and malaise are also frequently reported. The presence of peritoneal signs such as rebound tenderness or guarding may be indicative of colonic perforation (rare) or severe and/or fulminant *C. difficile* colitis. Leukocytosis is often present and not infrequently elevated above 20K. In fact, it is not unreasonable to test the hospitalized patient with unclear etiology of leukocytosis for occult *C. difficile* infection, even in the absence of diarrhea. In a small study of inpatients with white blood cell counts above 15K, and without a clear etiology of the leukocytosis, Wanahita and coworkers found that 58% of the patients tested positive for *C. difficile*. Fecal leukocytes are also often present, but nonspecific. On colonoscopy, when performed, patients with *C. difficile* colitis frequently show mucosal ulcerations with pathognomonic pseudomembranes, often described as raised yellow plaques composed of fibrinous exudates.

Table 8–11. Antibiotics associated with *Clostridium difficile* colitis.

Association with *C. difficile*	Very Strong	Strong	Moderate	Weak/Rare
Antibiotic class	Fluoroquinolones Lincosamides	Cephalosporins Penicillins Carbapenems	Sulfonamides Macrolides	Aminoglycosides Nitroimidazoles Glycopeptides
Common examples	Ciprofloxacin Levofloxacin Clindamycin	Ceftriaxone Cefoxitin Imipenem Amoxicillin	Trimethoprim-sulfamethoxazole Erythromycin Azithromycin	Gentamicin Amikacin Vancomycin (IV) Metronidazole

Abdominal x-rays may show "thumbprinting" suggestive of colonic inflammation, but are often nonspecific. CT examination of the abdomen shows thickening of the colonic wall. In fulminant *C. difficile* colitis, the abdominal x-rays and CT may show toxic megacolon with a diffusely dilated colon.

3. Diagnosis—In addition to the clinical patient presentation described above, diagnostic tests for *C. difficile* currently consist of either *C. difficile* organism detection (eg, anaerobic stool culture, antigen testing) or toxin A or B detection tools (eg, cytotoxin assays, enzyme immunoassays, or polymerase chain reaction (PCR) testing). The best approach to diagnose *C. difficile* remains controversial and institution-dependent. The stool culture is a sensitive test but has a long turnover time (2-3 days) that is suboptimal in the critically ill patient who needs a fast and accurate diagnosis. Antigen detection is a reasonable screening test, but needs further confirmation when positive. The diagnosis of *C. difficile* has become a complicated area with lots of alternative tests, and there has been considerable uncertainty about which are the best tests to use. The most sensitive test (considered standard by many) is the cytotoxin assay. Its sensitivity is above 95%, and its specificity approaches 100%, but it is an expensive test with a 24- to 48-hour turnover time. PCR testing for toxins A and B gives the most rapid results.

4. Treatment—Treatment of asymptomatic patients is not indicated. On the other hand, the clinical, laboratory, and radiologic presentation of the patient might carry a sufficient suspicion for *C. difficile* infection that empiric antibiotics are justified pending *C. difficile* organism or toxin detection tests. For patients with mild disease, level-one evidence suggests the safety and equivalency of single-agent oral antibiotic treatment with PO fidoxamicin or PO vancomycin. A 10- to 14-day course of either antibiotic is recommended. Metronidazole may be used as an alternative if neither medication is available. Patients might still test positive for *C. difficile* for many weeks despite treatment, and therefore retesting these patients for *C. difficile* when the antibiotic course is done and the patient signs and symptoms resolved, is not recommended. Adjunct therapies for *C. difficile* such as probiotics, toxin-binding resins, and immunoglobulins, have been used, but the evidence for their utility is still controversial. In a randomized clinical trial, stool transplantation was shown to be very efficacious in recurrent *C. difficile* infections and is currently being investigated as a treatment for severe infections as well. Vancomycin enemas are particularly useful in patients with ileus (questionable adequate intracolonic concentration from PO vancomycin alone), those with PO intolerance, and possibly those with severe distal colonic inflammation (rectosigmoid colon). Fidoxamicin (200 mg every 12 hours) is a relatively new bactericidal antibiotic with promising results as an alternative therapy. In a randomized clinical trial comparing fidoxamicin and vancomycin, the cure rates were equivalent. Patients with refractory severe *C. difficile* colitis,

those who progress to toxic megacolon, or those with hemodynamic instability or showing signs of early MODS, should be considered for prompt surgical intervention. The timing and decision to operate are controversial, but there is certainly value in earlier intervention in critically ill patients, as the mortality of fulminant *C. difficile* infection remains as high as 30%-50%. Independent predictors of mortality include age more than 70 years, leukocytosis more than 35K, leucopenia less than 4K, hemodynamic instability, and respiratory failure. When surgery is indicated, the procedure of choice is a subtotal colectomy with end-ileostomy. A single-center study has recently demonstrated improved outcomes in severe *C. difficile* colitis using an alternative approach where a loop ileostomy was created and subsequent intraoperative colonic washout was performed with polyethelene glycol solution. In this small study of fewer than 50 patients, the new approach was associated with decreased mortality and more than 90% colon preservation, when compared to the traditional subtotal colectomy approach, but that treatment remains controversial and its practice is very limited in the United States.

ANTIMICROBIAL MANAGEMENT

▶ General Principles

Antibiotic optimal management includes the following guiding principles:

1. Establishing a clinical diagnosis of infection and/or sepsis.
2. Establishing an "evidence-based-guess" of the likely nature of the involved pathogen(s).
3. Attempting to obtain microbiologic data (Gram stain and culture), when possible.
4. Prompt initiation of broad-spectrum empiric antibiotics likely to cover the culprit pathogen(s).
5. Selectively narrowing the antibiotic regimen to cover the pathogen recovered in microbiologic testing.

The decisions to initiate, continue, or tailor the antibiotic choices for each patient should be carefully balanced against the increasingly serious challenge facing healthcare, namely the epidemic emergence of multidrug-resistant organisms such as methicillin-resistant *Staphylococcus aureus* (MRSA), vancomycin-resistant enterococcus (VRE), and multidrug-resistant gram-negative organisms. The above principles are the pillars of every antibiotic stewardship program currently mandated within each healthcare setting.

▶ Empiric & Pathogen-Directed Antibiotic Selection

Selecting the appropriate empiric antibiotics entails an understanding of the nature of the infectious process affecting the patient, the most likely organisms causing the infection, as well as awareness of the antibiotic resistance map at the local healthcare institution level. For example, simple skin infections are most likely caused by skin flora such as staphylococci and streptococci, and therefore an appropriate empiric treatment should at least cover gram-positive organisms. Acute diverticulitis with a pericolonic abscess is more likely to be caused by colonic flora, such as gram-negative and anaerobic bacteria, and therefore empiric treatment should focus on covering these pathogens. Once a specific organism has been recovered from the tested microbiologic specimen, it is often possible to narrow the antibiotic regimen, even before the specific data on antibacterial susceptibilities are available using the microbiologic properties of antibiotics and the currently available clinical experience. The use of local antibiograms is crucial and highly encouraged, as the patterns of bacterial susceptibilities and resistance vary not only from one region to the other, but also from one institution to the other. Susceptibility testing methods include disk-diffusion and dilution (broth microdilution, plates, and E-tests) procedures. Disk-diffusion tests indicate whether a microbial culture is susceptible or resistant to serum-achievable, in-vivo drug concentrations with conventional dosage regimens. In contrast, dilution procedures allow report of the minimal inhibitory concentration (MIC) and minimal bactericidal concentration (MBC). The MIC is the lowest concentration of a specific antimicrobial agent that inhibits the test organism, while the MBC is the lowest concentration of a specific antimicrobial agent that kills the test organism. Tailoring therapy based on reported susceptibility via disk diffusion or MIC is recommended.

Antibiotic Duration of Therapy

If all cultures are found to be negative, and the suspicion for continuing infection is low, empiric antibiotics should be discontinued, as unnecessary antibiotic therapy clearly increases the risk of multidrug-resistant bacteria, *C. difficile* colitis, and other side effects. The duration of antibiotic treatment depends on the nature of the infection and the severity of the clinical presentation. Evidence-based guidelines for type of antibiotics and duration in the treatment of various infections have been developed and should be followed when possible. Most antibiotic regimens are now limited, although more difficult infections such as liver abscesses, brain abscesses, endocarditis, septic arthritis, or osteomyelitis require prolonged antibiotic therapy.

Failure of Clinical Response

Upon failure of clinical response to initial surgical intervention and antibiotic therapy, the clinician is encouraged to think of all the following possibilities for failure of therapy:

1. The existence of another organism.
2. The presence of an uncontrolled source of infection needing additional interventions.

3. The presence of a concomitant superinfection (with fungal organisms, for example).
4. The development of a new drug resistance by the same isolated organism.
5. Failure of the chosen antibiotic medication (despite favorable susceptibility data) to penetrate the site of infection.

The latter may be due to the properties of the antibiotic itself, the chosen route of administration, or the specific physiology and morbidity of the patients themselves.

Antibiotic Side Effects

Adverse antibiotic reactions may occasionally mimic infection by causing fever, skin rashes, and mental status changes. Clinicians should consider this possibility in patients with persistent fevers despite appropriate antibiotic coverage and seeming resolution of the infectious process. In addition, antibiotics can result in microbial superinfections (eg, fungi, *C. difficile*), emergence of new bacterial drug resistance, or organ toxicity.

Antibiotics in Renal or Hepatic Failure

Several antibiotics may induce or exacerbate existing organ dysfunction, most commonly renal or hepatic, and thus require intermittent assessment of kidney and liver function. Aminoglycosides and renal failure is a classical example.

In addition, decreased creatinine clearance at baseline or due to critical illness has an important influence on antimicrobial drug dosage, since most of these drugs are excreted, at least partially, by the kidneys. Therefore, many of these medications, such as vancomycin, penicillins, and aminoglycosides, require adjustments in dosage or frequency of administration in the presence of renal insufficiency to prevent toxicity.

CONCLUSION

In conclusion, surgery can result in infection (ie, SSI), but may also be the primary treatment to achieve source control in many infectious processes (ie, surgical infections). In the former, prevention by implementing processes of care (eg, timely provision of perioperative antibiotics, maintenance of strict sterile techniques) and patient risk-factor optimization prior to surgery should be the goal of every surgeon, as SSI remains one of the biggest healthcare-associated postoperative challenges. For the latter (surgical infections), source control is the cornerstone in the prevention of systemic progression of the infection into sepsis, septic shock, and/or MODS. Alongside surgical treatment of infections, antibiotic stewardship with appropriate timing, duration, and choice of antibiotics is needed now more than ever to prevent the emergence of resistant organisms as well as *C. difficile* infection.

References

Boltz MM, Hollenbeak CS, Julian KG, Ortenzi G, Dillon PW. Hospital costs associated with surgical site infections in general and vascular surgery patients. *Surgery*. 2011;150(5):934-942.

Bratzler DW, Houck PM, Richards C, et al. Use of antimicrobial prophylaxis for major surgery: Baseline results from the National Surgical Infection Prevention Project. *Arch Surg*. 2005;140(2):174-182.

Cohen SH, Gerding DN, Johnson S, et al. Society for Healthcare Epidemiology of America; Infectious Diseases Society of America. Clinical practice guidelines for *Clostridium difficile* infection in adults: 2010 update by the Society for Healthcare Epidemiology of America (SHEA) and the Infectious Diseases Society of America (IDSA). *Infect Control Hosp Epidemiol*. 2010;31(5):431-455.

Darenberg J, Ihendyane N, Sjölin J, et al. Intravenous immunoglobulin G therapy in streptococcal toxic shock syndrome: A European randomized, double-blind, placebo-controlled trial. *Clin Infect Dis*. 2003;37(3):333-340.

Darouiche RO, Wall MJ Jr, Itani KM, et al. Chlorhexidine-alcohol versus povidone-iodine for surgical-site antisepsis. *N Engl J Med*. 2010;362(1):18-26.

Daum RS, Miller LG, Immergluck L, et al. A placebo-controlled trial of antibiotics for smaller skin abscesses. *N Engl J Med*. 2017;376(26):2545-2555.

Edwards JR, Peterson KD, Mu Y, et al. National Healthcare Safety Network (NHSN) report: Data summary for 2006 through 2008, issued December 2009. *Am J Infect Control*. 2009; 37(10):783-805.

Fry DE. Colon preparation and surgical site infection. *Am J Surg*. 2011;202(2):225-232.

Fukuda H, Morikane K, et al. Impact of surgical site infections after open and laparoscopic colon and rectal surgeries on postoperative resource consumption. *Infection*. 2012. Epub ahead of print.

Hospital acquired infections. The Centers for Disease Control (CDC). Available at: http://www.cdc.gov/HAI/pdfs/toolkits/SSI_toolkit021710SIBT_revised.pdf. Last accessed November 3, 2012. 11/3/2012.

Kaafarani HM, King DR. Necrotizing skin and soft tissue infections. *Surg Clin North Am*. 2014;94(1):155-163.

Keely Boyle K, Rachala S, Nodzo SR. Centers for Disease Control and Prevention 2017 Guidelines for Prevention of Surgical Site Infections: Review and Relevant Recommendations. *Curr Rev Musculoskelet Med*. 2018;11(3):357-369.

Louie TJ, Miller MA, Mullane KM, et al. OPT-80-003 Clinical Study Group. Fidaxomicin versus vancomycin for *Clostridium difficile* infection. *N Engl J Med*. 2011;364(5):422-431.

Magill SS, Edwards JR, Bamberg W, et al. Multistate point-prevalence survey of health care-associated infections. *N Engl J Med*. 2014;370(13):1198-1208.

Manjunath AP, Shepherd JH, Barton DP, Bridges JE, Ind TE. Glove perforations during open surgery for gynaecological malignancies. *BJOG*. 2008;115(8):1015-1019.

Martinez M, Peponis T, Hage A, et al. The role of computed tomography in the diagnosis of necrotizing soft tissue infections. *World J Surg*. 2018;42(1):82-87.

Misteli H, Weber WP, Reck S, et al. Surgical glove perforation and the risk of surgical site infection. *Arch Surg*. 2009;144(6):553-558; discussion 558.

Mu Y, Edwards JR, Horan TC, Berrios-Torres SI, Fridkin SK. Improving risk-adjusted measures of surgical site infection for the national healthcare safety network. *Infect Control Hosp Epidemiol*. 2011;32(10):970-986.

Neal MD, Alverdy JC, Hall DE, Simmons RL, Zuckerbraun BS. Diverting loop ileostomy and colonic lavage: An alternative to total abdominal colectomy for the treatment of severe, complicated *Clostridium difficile* associated disease. *Ann Surg*. 2011;254(3):423-427; discussion 427-429.

Ortega G, Rhee DS, Papandria DJ, et al. An evaluation of surgical site infections by wound classification system using the ACS-NSQIP. *J Surg Res*. 2012;174(1):33-38.

Panahi P, Stroh M, Casper DS, Parvizi J, Austin MS. Operating room traffic is a major concern during total joint arthroplasty. *Clin Orthop Relat Res*. 2012 Feb 3. Epub ahead of print.

Sailhamer EA, Carson K, Chang Y, et al. Fulminant *Clostridium difficile* colitis: Patterns of care and predictors of mortality. *Arch Surg*. 2009;144(5):433-439; discussion 439-440.

Sawyer RG1, Claridge JA, Nathens AB, et al. Trial of short-course antimicrobial therapy for intraabdominal infection. *N Engl J Med*. 2015;372(21):1996-2005.

Soh CR, Pietrobon R, Freiberger JJ, et al. Hyperbaric oxygen therapy in necrotising soft tissue infections: A study of patients in the United States Nationwide Inpatient Sample. *Intens Care Med*. 2012;38(7):1143-1151.

Solomkin JS, Mazuski JE, Bradley JS, et al. Diagnosis and management of complicated intra-abdominal infection in adults and children: Guidelines by the Surgical Infection Society and the Infectious Diseases Society of America. *Surg Infect (Larchmt)*. 2010;11(1):79-109.

The Surviving Sepsis Guidelines. Available at: www.survivingsepsis.org. Last accessed November 3, 2012.

Swenson BR, Hedrick TL, Metzger R, et al. Effects of preoperative skin preparation on postoperative wound infection rates: A prospective study of three skin preparation protocols. *Infect Control Hosp Epidemiol*. 2009;30(10):964-971.

van Nood E, Vrieze A, Nieuwdorp M, et al. Duodenal infusion of donor feces for recurrent *Clostridium difficile*. *N Engl J Med*. 2013;368(5):407-415.

Weiser TG, Regenbogen SE, Thompson KD, et al. An estimation of the global volume of surgery: A modelling strategy based on available data. *Lancet*. 2008;372(9633):139-144.

Zimlichman E, Henderson D, Tamir O, et.al. Health care-associated infections: A meta-analysis of costs and financial impact on the U.S. health care system. *JAMA Intern Med*. 2013;173(22):2039-2046.

MULTIPLE-CHOICE QUESTIONS

1. Deescalation of antibiotics consists of:

   A. Stopping antibiotics.

   B. Narrowing the spectrum of antibiotic coverage based on cultures.

   C. Adjusting antimicrobial dose based on renal function.

   D. Changing antimicrobial therapy based on location of therapy in the hospital.

   E. Adjusting antimicrobials based on hospital antibiogram.

2. Established processes to prevent surgical site infection:

    A. Do not include antibiotic timing and dosing as long as delivery occurs prior to skin closure.
    B. Do not address the choice of antibiotic prophylaxis.
    C. Requires the use of alcohol-containing skin preparation solutions.
    D. Are similar in hospitals around the world.
    E. Are currently well known, and best practices are no longer controversial.

3. The treatment of surgical site infection includes:

    A. Opening the incision for superficial SSI.
    B. Antibiotics in every case.
    C. Debridement of necrotic tissues, if present.
    D. Avoidance of wound cultures.
    E. A and C.

4. All of the following are true about necrotizing skin and skin structure infections (NSSSIs), except:

    A. NSSSI are generally self-limited and nonthreatening.
    B. They can be caused by single or polymicrobial infections.
    C. Small-vessel thrombosis occurs along the infection progression pathway.
    D. Immunocompromised (eg, HIV, diabetes), IV drug abuse, and cancer patients are at a particularly higher risk of developing NSSSIs.
    E. Grayish discoloration of the underlying skin and pain beyond the affected skin area are especially suggestive of deeper underlying tissue involvement.

Fluid, Electrolyte, & Acid–Base Disorders

Michael Poulson, MD

Sherif Aly, MD

Tracey Dechert, MD, FACS

Fluid status, electrolyte homeostasis, and acid–base balance are clinical parameters of critical significance in surgical patients. As a surgeon, it is crucial to understand normal physiology and pathophysiology related to these parameters.

FLUIDS & ELECTROLYTES

Surgical patients are at a high risk for derangements of body water distribution and electrolyte homeostasis. These disturbances may be secondary to trauma, surgical or medical conditions that may alter normal physiology, or the nature of the surgery itself.

▶ Body Water Distribution & Composition

Total body mass is 45%-60% water. The percentage in any individual is influenced by age and lean body mass; therefore the percentage is higher in men compared to women, in children compared to adults, and in people of normal body habitus compared to the obese (Table 9–1). Two-thirds of total body water (TBW), 30%-40% of body mass, is intracellular; one-third, 15%-20% of total body mass, is extracellular. The extracellular fluid (ECF) is divided into two compartments, with 80% (12%-16% of total body mass) in the interstitial compartment and 20% (3%-4%) in the intravascular compartment. One-fifth of intravascular fluid is proximal to the arterioles; the remaining four-fifths is distal to the arterioles.

The intracellular, interstitial, and intravascular compartments each hold fluid characterized by markedly different electrolyte profiles (Figure 9–1). The main intracellular cation is the potassium ion (K^+), while the main extracellular cation is the sodium ion (Na^+). Not only the electrolyte profile, but also the protein composition of the fluids, differs; intracellular cations are electrically balanced mainly by the polyatomic ion phosphate (PO_4^{3-}) and negatively charged proteins, while extracellular cations are balanced mainly by the chloride ion (Cl^-). The intravascular fluid has a relatively higher concentration of protein and lower concentration of organic acids than the interstitial fluid. This higher concentration of protein, chiefly albumin, is the main cause of the high colloid osmotic pressure of serum, which in turn is the chief regulator of the fluid distribution between the two extracellular compartments. The relationship between colloid osmotic pressure and hydrostatic pressure governs the movement of water across the capillary membrane, and is modeled by the Starling equation.

The body's volume status and electrolyte composition are regulated largely by the kidneys. The kidneys maintain a constant volume and osmolality by modulating how much Na^+ and free water are reabsorbed from the renal filtrate. Na^+, along with the accompanying anions Cl^- and HCO_3^-, account for most of the extracellular osmolality. Since almost 90% of available Na^+ is in the extracellular fluid, the amount of total body Na^+ is an important determinant of total body water. Na^+ is freely filtered in the renal glomerulus. Most filtered Na^+ (60%-70%) is reabsorbed in the proximal tubule. A further 20%-30% of filtered Na^+ is reabsorbed in the thick ascending limb of the loop of Henle. The remaining distal tubule and collecting ducts reabsorb 5%-10% of filtered Na^+. The exact percentage of Na^+ reabsorbed and subsequently excreted by the kidneys is tightly regulated and is influenced by the Na^+ load initially filtered and a variety of hormonal factors, particularly aldosterone and natriuretic peptides. Under normal circumstances the kidneys will adjust excreted water and Na^+ to match a wide spectrum of dietary intake.

Antidiuretic hormone (ADH), also known as arginine vasopressin, is the chief regulator of osmolality and free-water reabsorption. The peptide hormone is released from the posterior pituitary in response to increased serum osmolality. ADH induces translocation of aquaporin channels to the collecting duct epithelium, increasing permeability to water and causing reabsorption of free water from the renal filtrate. Thus water is retained, and the urine concentrated.

Table 9–1. Approximate percentage water of total body mass.

Patient	%
Children	60
Non-elderly males	60
Non-elderly females	50
Elderly males	50
Elderly females	45

In the absence of ADH, the collecting duct is impermeable to water, leading to water loss and production of dilute urine. At high physiologic levels ADH has a direct vasoconstrictive effect on arterioles.

Although the movement of ions and proteins between the different fluid compartments is normally restricted, water itself is freely diffusible between them. Consequently, the osmolality of the different fluid compartments is identical, normally approximately 290 mOsm/kg. Control of osmolality occurs through regulation of water intake through diet and excretion through urine and insensible loses.

Volume Disorders

Hypo- and hypervolemia commonly occur in surgical patients, both following elective surgery and in the setting of trauma and emergency surgery. Volume disturbances run the gamut from being clinically insignificant to being immediately life-threatening. The underlying cause of any volume disorder must be sought and addressed while the volume disorder itself is managed.

A. Hypovolemia

1. Etiology—Hypovolemia is common in surgical patients. It is typically caused by loss of isotonic fluids in the setting of hemorrhage, gastrointestinal losses (eg, gastric suctioning, emesis, and diarrhea), sequestration of fluids in the gut lumen (eg, bowel obstruction, ileus, and enteric fistulas), burns, or excessive diuretic therapy. In resource-poor settings, sweat is often an additional important source of fluid loss, as in a non–air-conditioned operating room. In all of these cases, loss of isotonic fluid results in loss of Na^+ and water without significantly affecting the osmolality of the extracellular fluid compartment; thus there is very little shift of water into or out of the intracellular compartment. Hypovolemia results in decreased kidney perfusion, which in turn activates the renin–angiotensin–aldosterone system. This stimulates aldosterone secretion from the zona glomerulosa of the

▲ **Figure 9–1.** Electrolyte composition of human body fluids. Note that the values are in mEq/L of water, not of body fluid. (Reproduced with permission from Newburgh LH, Leaf A: *Significance of the Body Fluids in Clinical Medicine.* Springfield, IL: Charles C Thomas; 1950.)

adrenal cortex, leading to increased reabsorption of Na^+ and water from the renal filtrate and excretion of low volumes (oliguria) of hypertonic urine with a low Na^+ concentration. Decreased renal perfusion will also result in decreased glomerular filtration rate (GFR) and a subsequent elevation in blood urea nitrogen (BUN) and serum creatinine (Cr).

Fractional excretion of Na^+ (FENa) is a useful tool for differentiating causes of oliguria:

$$FENa = 100 \times \frac{(Na_U \times Cr_P)}{(Cr_U \times Na_P)}$$

where U = urine, P = plasma, Na = sodium, and Cr = creatinine.

FENa $\leq$ 1% usually indicates prerenal azotemia. However, FENa $\leq$ 1% may be found in patients with oliguria secondary to hepatorenal syndrome, as the liver does not effectively metabolize aldosterone. In patients already receiving diuretic therapy, fractional excretion of urea nitrogen (FEUN) is more helpful than FENa. FEUN is calculated analogously; FEUN $\leq$ 35% indicates prerenal azotemia.

2. Presentation—Hypovolemia is suggested by a patient's history, physical exam, and laboratory data. Diagnosis by physical exam alone in the immediate postoperative setting is difficult, especially when volume loss is mild to moderate, and especially in very old and very young patients. One review found that longitudinal furrows on a patient's tongue and dry oral and nasal mucous membranes are 85% sensitive for hypovolemia; increased capillary refill time, unclear speech, upper or lower extremity weakness, a dry axilla, and postural hypotension were all relatively specific indicators of hypovolemia. The same review found that a postural (supine to standing) increase in heart rate of at least 30 beats per minute or severe postural dizziness that prevented the patient from standing had 6%-48% sensitivity for mild to moderate hypovolemia but 91%-100% sensitivity for severe hypovolemia. Laboratory evidence of hypovolemia includes elevated BUN:Cr ratio, as hypovolemia decreases renal perfusion, causing prerenal azotemia characterized by a disproportionate rise in BUN compared to Cr. However, an elevated BUN:Cr ratio may also be associated with renal failure and gastrointestinal bleeding, independent of volume status. No single highly sensitive test to diagnose hypovolemia exists; thus the diagnosis must be made by examining all available data with a high index of suspicion.

3. Treatment—Hypovolemia is corrected with IV administration of an isotonic fluid. Recent studies have suggested the superiority of balanced crystalloids (ie, lactated Ringer's) in resuscitation over normal saline solution. Normal saline has a higher concentration of Na^+ and Cl^-, which in high-volume resuscitations, can result in hyperchloremic metabolic acidosis and kidney failure. This is less likely to occur with balanced crystalloids, as their electrolyte composition closely mimics that of plasma. Coexistent electrolyte abnormalities should also be addressed during resuscitation. Care must be taken in patients in renal or heart failure not to exacerbate these conditions. If hypovolemia is allowed to worsen unimpeded it will eventually lead to circulatory collapse and shock, which is covered elsewhere.

B. Hypervolemia

1. Etiology—Hypervolemia is also common in surgical patients. It often occurs after treatment of shock with colloid and crystalloid fluids, with or without attendant renal failure as well as in the postoperative period, as ADH is secreted in response to nonphysiologic stimuli, disrupting its role in regulation of osmolality. High physiologic levels of ADH have a vasoconstrictive effect, leading to a decreased filtered Na^+ load and thus greater Na^+ and water retention. This secretion of ADH typically ceases 2-3 days after the surgical insult, after which ADH levels return to an appropriate level and patients experience a so-called "autodiuresis." Heart failure, liver disease, renal disease, and malnutrition all exacerbate hypervolemia in the surgical patient. Preexisting heart failure decreases the range across which a patient will adequately compensate for increased intravascular volume. Liver disease decreases metabolism of circulating ADH and aldosterone, increasing the homeostatic set point for intravascular volume and thus decreasing the physiologic reserve remaining to respond to surgical insults. Renal disease disrupts all aspects of volume regulation. Syndrome of inappropriate ADH hypersecretion (SIADH) causes hypervolemia secondary to a sustained ADH release independent of the normal physiologic triggers. SIADH typically occurs in the setting of traumatic brain injury, brain tumors and abscesses, pneumonia, lung abscesses, as a paraneoplastic syndrome associated with small-cell lung cancer and other neoplasia, and with a variety of drugs including morphine and the chemotherapeutic agents, cyclophosphamide and vincristine.

2. Presentation—Like hypovolemia, hypervolemia is often suggested by the patient's history and physical exam. Signs include hypertension, decreased arterial oxygen saturation and basilar crackles, jugular venous distention, dependent soft-tissue edema, gallop rhythms on cardiac auscultation, and rapid weight gain. Examination of recorded fluid administration may assist in the diagnosis. Eventually a hypervolemic patient may show signs of pulmonary edema, easily diagnosed on chest x-ray, or even congestive heart failure (CHF).

3. Treatment—If the hypervolemic patient develops CHF or pulmonary edema, treatment with diuretics, or in extreme cases hemodialysis, may be required. Mechanical ventilation may be lifesaving if pulmonary edema and/or CHF have progressed to the point of respiratory failure.

ELECTROLYTE DISORDERS

Electrolyte derangements may occur independently of each other, but are often closely linked. Like volume disorders, disturbances of electrolyte homeostasis run the gamut from mild and inconsequential to severe and immediately life-threatening.

The underlying cause of any electrolyte disorder must be sought while the electrolyte disorder itself is managed. Special care must always be taken when repleting electrolytes in patients with renal insufficiency. These patients require slower repletion and more frequent monitoring of electrolyte levels.

▶ Sodium

Hypo- and hypernatremia reflect excessive gain or loss of TBW, respectively. Significant derangements of Na^+ homeostasis result in significant changes to plasma tonicity and eventually whole-body osmolality, with potentially devastating consequences for the central nervous system (CNS).

A. Hyponatremia

1. Etiology—Hyponatremia is a sign of relative water gain; total body Na^+ may be decreased, normal, or even increased. Hyponatremia is common in surgical patients postoperatively, as ADH is secreted in response to pain, nausea, and vomiting, opiate administration, and positive-pressure ventilation. Typically, this hyponatremia is mild and inconsequential; however, it may be exacerbated by rapid parenteral administration of hypotonic fluids. Hyponatremia may result from severe hyperglycemia, or any other condition in which an osmotically active solute draws water from the intracellular space to the extracellular space. In the setting of hyperglycemia, a corrected Na^+ is calculated as:

$$Na^+_{corrected} = Na^+_{measured} + 0.016 \text{ (plasma glucose in mg/dL} - 100)$$

The correction factor 0.016 accounts for the unit conversion from mg/dL to mmol/L. Some investigators believe a correction factor of 0.024 is more appropriate.

Other causes of hyponatremia include cerebral salt-wasting syndrome, liver disease, congestive heart failure, and SIADH.

2. Presentation—The signs of hyponatremia are varied and related to the rate of change in sodium levels. With acute changes, one can develop CNS dysfunction, as brain cells swell in a fixed-volume space (the Monro–Kellie hypothesis). Mental status changes, obtundation, coma, and seizures typically are not seen until serum Na^+ is less than 120 mmol/L. Such hyponatremia is a medical emergency requiring immediate intervention. Chronic changes are often asymptomatic, but may be necessary to correct as in those patients with increased intracranial pressure.

3. Treatment—Generally with chronic hyponatremia, free water restriction and salt tabs are sufficient to raise sodium levels, particularly in those with SIADH. Sodium should be corrected slowly to reduce the risk of osmotic demyelination, with a correction rate of no more than 4-6 mEq/L/d.

In those with acute hyponatremia and CNS signs and symptoms attributable to hyponatremia, sodium needs to be corrected more quickly. Hypertonic saline is used sparingly until correction of CNS symptoms, at which point more conservative measures are used. No consensus exists on the appropriate rate of correction. One review recommended correction by no more than 8 mmol/L/d, starting with correction of 1-2 mmol/L/h in patients with severe manifestations. Sodium levels should not be corrected beyond what is needed to alleviate CNS disturbances. Correction of Na^+ does not replace pharmacologic intervention in a seizing patient.

One formula used to calculate the expected change in Na^+ from IV administration of 1 L of any fluid is:

$$\text{Change in serum } Na^+ = \frac{(\text{fluid } Na^+ + \text{fluid } K^+ \text{ in mmol/L}) - \text{serum } Na^+}{\text{TBW in L} + 1}$$

TBW is estimated as a fraction of body mass (Table 9–1). Hyponatremia causing CNS disturbances should prompt admission to an intensive care unit given the close monitoring needed in such patients, the need for rapid intervention, and the potentially devastating consequences of delays in management.

B. Hypernatremia

1. Etiology—Loss of free water alone occurs when patients do not have access to water (eg, preverbal, bedbound, or otherwise incapacitated patients), in diabetes insipidus, in the setting of high fevers, and in patients in whom enteral feeds do not contain adequate water. Hypernatremia typically occurs simultaneously with volume derangements, and total body Na^+ may be increased, normal, or even decreased. Induced hypernatremia is a useful treatment modality in patients with traumatic brain injury to reduce cerebral edema, decrease intracranial pressure, and increase cerebral perfusion pressure.

2. Presentation—As with hyponatremia, the signs and symptoms of hypernatremia are caused by CNS dysfunction: lethargy, fatigue, hyperactive deep tendon reflexes, seizure, and coma may occur. Signs and symptoms are rare with Na^+ less than 158 mmol/L.

3. Treatment—Development of CNS symptoms requires parenteral administration of free water, typically as 5% dextrose in water or free water if enteral access is available. As with hyponatremia, correction of hypernatremia should be done slowly. Rapid lowering of plasma Na^+ concentration can result in cerebral edema, resulting in worsened encephalopathy. If the patient's hypernatremia developed over a period of hours it may safely be corrected at a rate of 1-2 mmol/L/h with a goal of normonatremia within 24 hours. In patients whose hypernatremia developed more slowly, a rate of 0.5 mmol/L/h is safe. As derangements in Na^+ are caused by derangements in TBW, the concept of a "water deficit" is a useful one in guiding correction of hypernatremia. The free water deficit is calculated as:

$$\text{Water deficit} = TBW \times (1 - [140/Na^+ \text{ in mmol/L}])$$

This formula is accurate when calculating the water deficit in patients with pure water loss, but is inaccurate in patients with hypernatremia caused by loss of hypotonic fluid. Using the formula in the section above on hyponatremia, one may calculate the estimated correction 1 L of any fluid will have on Na^+. As with hyponatremia, hypernatremia with clinical manifestations warrants admission to an intensive care unit so that correction may be achieved safely and effectively.

▶ Potassium

Potassium is the major intracellular cation. Plasma potassium ion (K^+) concentration is determined primarily by two factors. The first is acid–base homeostasis. Hydrogen ion (H^+) and K^+ are exchanged between the intracellular and extracellular spaces; thus disturbances of acid–base balance (see below) tend to cause disturbances in serum K^+. The second factor is the size of the total body K^+ pool. Intracellular stores of K^+ are large, but may be exhausted, especially in the setting of prolonged ketoacidosis.

A. Hypokalemia

1. Etiology—In the surgical setting, total body K^+ is typically decreased by gastrointestinal losses, excessive diuretic administration, and prolonged malnutrition, particularly in alcoholic patients. Prolonged alkalosis (see below) that also results in hypokalemia (eg, due to gastric losses of hydrochloric acid and K^+) results in a so-called "paradoxical aciduria" as the nephron conserves K^+ at the expense of H^+, which maintains the alkalosis instead of correcting it in an attempt to prevent life-threatening hypokalemia (see below for details).

2. Presentation—The hallmark signs of hypokalemia are decreased muscle contractility eventually leading to diaphragmatic paralysis, ECG changes including a flattened or inverted T-wave and a prominent U-wave, and cardiac arrhythmias, which may present an immediate threat to life.

3 Treatment—When hypokalemia develops acutely it should be corrected with parenteral supplementation. Parenteral administration of K^+ must be done carefully so as not to cause iatrogenic hyperkalemia. Hypomagnesemia may cause

hypokalemia refractory to parenteral administration. In such cases hypomagnesemia should be corrected along with hypokalemia (see below). In cases of chronic hypokalemia in which neuromuscular and cardiac manifestations are absent, oral supplementation (either through dietary changes or oral potassium chloride administration) should suffice.

B. Hyperkalemia

1. Etiology—In the surgical setting, hyperkalemia is often caused by crush injuries, burns, other catabolism-inducing events, renal insufficiency, adrenal insufficiency, and excessive K^+ administration. Acidosis may cause hyperkalemia, as the intracellular space buffers acidemia by exchanging H^+ from the extracellular space for K^+ from within cells (see below). Hemolysis during venipuncture and the resultant release of intracellular K^+ can lead to a falsely elevated K^+ on laboratory testing. One must take care in these cases as the patient may still be hyperkalemic, so repeat testing is often necessary.

2. Presentation—Hyperkalemia has few outward signs and symptoms until potentially lethal cardiac arrhythmias manifest. Initial ECG changes include flattened P-waves and peaked T-waves. Widening of the QRS complex is a later finding and demands immediate intervention, as it portends the imminent onset of ventricular fibrillation.

3. Treatment—A serum K^+ of 6.5 mmol/L or greater is a medical emergency and must prompt immediate intervention. The patient must be placed on continuous ECG monitoring. Initial treatment should consist of IV administration of 50% dextrose in water, 10 units of regular insulin, and calcium gluconate, as well as inhaled β-adrenergic agonists like albuterol. Insulin, glucose, and β-agonists drive K^+ from the extracellular space into the intracellular space, while calcium gluconate increases the excitability threshold of the myocardium, protecting against arrhythmias. Sodium bicarbonate, on the other hand, was not shown to be beneficial. These measures are rapidly acting, temporizing treatments that provide time for the initiation of more definitive therapies to remove excess K^+ from the body. In patients with intact kidney function, loop or thiazide diuretics can be used to promote urinary excretion of K^+. On the other hand, if renal function is severely impaired, then hemodialysis may be the only way to adequately remove excess K^+. Slowly developing hyperkalemia not severe enough to warrant IV interventions may be treated with oral sodium polystyrene sulfonate, which causes a slow enteral K^+ wasting or potassium-wasting diuretics. It is also important to treat the underlying cause of hyperkalemia to prevent further episodes of electrolyte abnormalities.

▶ Magnesium

The magnesium ion (Mg^{2+}) is an essential cofactor in many of the most important biochemical reactions in the body. Adenosine triphosphate (ATP) must be bound to Mg^{2+} to be biologically active. Mg^{2+} is required for every step of DNA transcription and translation, nerve conduction, ion transport, and Ca^{2+} channel activity. Approximately 50%-60% of total body magnesium is found in the bones. The large majority of the rest is intracellular, and approximately 1% is extracellular. A constant proportion of dietary Mg^{2+} is absorbed by the gut. If gut absorption exceeds Mg^{2+} needs, the excess is excreted by the kidneys. If dietary intake is insufficient, the kidney retains Mg^{2+}, with urinary levels dropping to nearly zero.

A. Hypomagnesemia

1. Etiology—Hypomagnesemia occurs in the setting of malnutrition (especially malnutrition associated with alcoholism), gastrointestinal losses (especially prolonged diarrheal loses), diuretic or aminoglycoside use, hyper- or hypocalcemia, and hypophosphatemia.

2. Presentation—In the surgical setting, hypomagnesemia most commonly presents as hypokalemia refractory to parenteral K^+ administration. Hypomagnesemia may cause sedation, muscle paralysis, tetany, seizures, and coma.

3. Treatment—Parenteral administration of Mg^{2+} is generally preferred to oral supplementation, as orally administered magnesium is a cathartic agent.

B. Hypermagnesemia

1. Etiology—Hypermagnesemia is rare in the surgical setting, but may develop in acute renal failure.

2. Presentation—At high concentrations, Mg^{2+} acts as a Ca^{2+} antagonist. Thus although hypermagnesemia may cause lethargy, weakness, and diminished deep tendon reflexes, it most often presents as cardiac arrhythmias. Peaked T-waves and widening of the QRS complex occur, which may progress to complete heart block, arrhythmias, and eventually asystole.

3. Treatment—If hypermagnesemia is mild and caused by supplementation, withdrawal of supplementation and close monitoring should be sufficient treatment. If hypermagnesemia is significant and causing ECG changes, calcium gluconate should be administered IV so as to overwhelm the Ca^{2+}-antagonizing effect of Mg^{2+} in neuromuscular function. Diuretic therapy with loop or thiazide diuretics may be required. In severe cases and in patients with significant renal failure, hemodialysis may be required.

▷ Calcium

Calcium (Ca^{2+}) is involved in a wide variety of physiologic processes, from maintenance of bone strength to neuromuscular function. Half of serum Ca^{2+} is protein-bound, chiefly to albumin. The unbound fraction is physiologically active, while the bound fraction is not; this unbound (or "ionized")

fraction is normally held constant across a wide range of plasma Ca^{2+}. Ca^{2+} homeostasis is influenced by vitamin D, parathyroid hormone, calcitonin, acid–base balance, and PO_4^{3-} homeostasis.

Standard laboratory tests measure total serum Ca^{2+}, including the fraction bound to albumin. Thus, a low Ca^{2+} value on a serum chemistry may reflect hypoalbuminemia rather than true hypocalcemia. Many formulas exist to correct Ca^{2+} in the setting of hypoalbuminemia. The most commonly used is:

$$Ca^{2+}_{corrected} = 0.8(4 - \text{serum albumin in g/dL}) + Ca^{2+}_{measured}$$

This and other such formulas are inaccurate in the setting of hemodialysis. In dialyzed patients, the uncorrected Ca^{2+} should be used to determine if the patient is hypo- or hypercalcemic. If doubt exists, an ionized Ca^{2+} measurement should be obtained.

A. Hypocalcemia

1. Etiology—Hypocalcemia in the surgical setting is often caused by hypothyroidism and hypoparathyroidism (either organic or iatrogenic after thyroid or parathyroid surgery), pancreatitis, renal insufficiency, crush injuries, severe soft-tissue infections, and necrotizing infections like necrotizing fasciitis.

2. Presentation—Hypocalcemia manifests as neuromuscular dysfunction, causing hyperactive deep tendon reflexes, Chvostek sign, muscle cramps, abdominal pain, and in severe cases tetany and cardiac arrhythmias.

3. Treatment—In persistent hypocalcemia, whole-blood pH must be determined, and any alkalosis corrected. In symptomatic patients, those with prolonged QT, or with rapid drops in calcium level, parenteral calcium is necessary. In milder cases, enteral calcium is sufficient. Chronic hypoparathyroidism and hypothyroidism require chronic vitamin D and Ca^{2+} supplementation, and may require aluminum hydroxide to decrease PO_4^{3-} absorption from the gut.

B. Hypercalcemia

1. Etiology—Hypercalcemia in the surgical setting is often caused by primary or tertiary hyperparathyroidism, hyperthyroidism, bony cancer metastases, paraneoplastic syndromes in which parathyroid hormone-related peptide is elaborated, and as a complication of thiazide diuretic use.

2. Presentation—Signs and symptoms of acute hypercalcemia include anorexia, nausea and vomiting, polydipsia, polyuria, depression, confusion, memory loss, stupor, coma, psychosis, and cardiac arrhythmias. Dyspepsia, constipation, acute pancreatitis, nephrolithiasis, osteoporosis, osteomalacia, and osteitis fibrosa cystica are indicative of chronic hypercalcemia. Untreated longstanding hypercalcemia, especially in conjunction with untreated hyperphosphatemia and especially in patients with chronic renal failure, may lead to calciphylaxis and high morbidity and mortality. Calciphylaxis, or more specifically calcific uremic arteriolopathy, is a serious, often fatal condition involving the calcification of arterioles in the skin and subcutaneous tissue. This results in plaques of skin ischemia, necrosis, and ulceration, which frequently become superinfected, leading to significant morbidity and mortality.

3. Treatment—In a patient with healthy kidneys, administration of large volumes of normal saline over 1-3 days will often correct even a profound hypercalcemia. In severe cases, IV fluids are supplemented with calcitonin and bisphosphonates, while targeting a urine output of 2-3 mL/kg/h and monitoring serum Ca^{2+} levels closely. Loop diuretics (eg, furosemide) inhibit Ca^{2+} reabsorption in the nephron, and will aid in calciuresis, but should not be used until the patient is clinically euvolemic. Calcitonin increases osteoblastic activity and inhibits osteoclastic activity, locking Ca^{2+} into the skeleton. In severe hypercalcemia or hypercalcemia secondary to renal failure, hemodialysis may be required. In patients whose hypercalcemia is caused by malignancy, bisphosphonates may provide a means of controlling Ca^{2+} levels in the medium and long term. In hypercalcemia caused by hyperparathyroidism, parathyroidectomy is potentially curative, but is reserved for the elective setting unless the patient is in hypercalcemic crisis which is refractory to optimal medical management.

▶ Phosphate

Like Ca^{2+} and Mg^{2+}, the majority of PO_4^{3-} is found in the skeleton. The large majority of the remainder is found intracellularly, where it functions as a constituent of ATP. Like Mg^{2+}, it is essential to energy metabolism.

A. Hypophosphatemia

1. Etiology—As with hypomagnesemia, chronic hypophosphatemia is typically found in malnourished patients, especially alcoholic patients. It may also occur in patients who consume large amounts of antacids, and following liver resection. An important and often overlooked cause of hypophosphatemia is refeeding syndrome. This syndrome occurs after a patient who has been without significant caloric intake for at least 5 days begins to eat again. Severe hypophosphatemia may occur as phosphofructokinase binds PO_4^{3-} to glucose to begin glycolysis, and as PO_4^{3-} is consumed in production of large amounts of ATP. The syndrome usually manifests within 4 days of starting refeeding.

2. Presentation—Hypophosphatemia results in muscular and neurologic dysfunction. Muscle weakness, diplopia,

depressed cardiac output, respiratory depression due to diaphragmatic weakness, confusion, delirium, coma, and death may all develop. An uncommon presentation is with rhabdomyolysis. Hypophosphatemia may leave patients ventilator-dependent, as they are unable to replenish ATP stores for proper functioning of the muscles of respiration.

3. Treatment—Severe hypophosphatemia is a medical emergency, requiring parenteral administration of Na_3PO_4 or K_3PO_4, depending on the patient's electrolyte profile. Mild hypophosphatemia may be treated with oral supplementation, either with sodium phosphate/potassium phosphate or with high-phosphate foods like milk.

B. Hyperphosphatemia

1. Etiology—Hyperphosphatemia is unusual in the surgical setting, typically developing in the setting of severe renal disease or after severe trauma.

2. Presentation—Hyperphosphatemia is usually asymptomatic, but it may cause hypocalcemia as calcium phosphate precipitates and is deposited in tissues.

3. Treatment—Hyperphosphatemia is treated by diuresis, administration of phosphate-binders like aluminum hydroxide, or hemodialysis in the setting of renal failure.

ACID–BASE BALANCE

The body's handling of hydrogen ion (H^+) is a particularly complex example of electrolyte management. It involves not only dietary intake and renal excretion, but also encompasses extracellular and intracellular buffer systems, as well as respiratory regulation.

▶ Normal Physiology

An acid is a chemical that donates a H^+ in solution, eg, HCl or H_2CO_3. A base is a chemical that accepts H^+ in solution, eg, Cl^- or HCO_3^-. The concentration of H^+ in a solution determines the acidity of the solution. Acidity of a solution is measured by pH, which is the negative logarithm of H^+ concentration expressed in mol/L. The strength of an acid is determined by its degree of dissociation into H^+ and the corresponding base, as expressed in the Henderson–Hasselbach (H-H) equation:

$$pH = pK \times \log [A\text{-}]/[HA]$$

where K = dissociation constant, [A-] = concentration of acid, and [HA] = concentration of base. Stronger acids have a higher K than weaker acids.

The main buffer system in human blood is a carbonic acid/bicarbonate (H_2CO_3/HCO_3^-) system. Using the H-H equation, the pH of this buffer system is calculated as:

$$pH = pK \times \log [HCO_3^-]/[H_2CO_3]$$

Table 9–2. Estimated arterial to venous blood gas conversions.

$pH_a = pH_v \times 1.005$
$PaCO_2 = pvCO_2 \times 0.8$
$HCO_3^-_a = HCO_3^-_v \times 0.90$

a = arterial, v = venous, p = partial pressure.

H_2CO_3 in the blood exists mostly as CO_2 (the so-called "volatile acid"); conversion of one to the other is catalyzed by the enzyme carbonic anhydrase. The dissociation constant of CO_2 is 0.03. Making these substitutions into the equation above, we have:

$$pH = pK \times \log [HCO_3^-]/[pCO_2 \times 0.03]$$

where pCO_2 is the partial pressure of CO_2.

The pK for this buffer system is 6.1. In arterial blood, HCO_3^- normally ranges from 21 to 37 mmol/L, while pCO_2 ranges from 36 to 44 mm Hg. Thus, arterial pH normally ranges from 7.36 to 7.44. Venous blood is easier to sample than arterial blood (Table 9–2). Venous blood gas sampling varies significantly between institutions, and between central, mixed, and different peripheral sites of sampling, and thus must be interpreted with caution.

Acid–base homeostasis is maintained by pulmonary excretion of CO_2 and renal excretion of non-volatile acids, which is discussed in further sections.

▶ Acid–Base Disorders

The fundamental acid–base disorders are:

- Acidemia: pH below the normal range.
- Alkalemia: pH above the normal range.
- Acidosis: A process that lowers the pH of the extracellular fluid.
- Alkalosis: A process that raises the pH of the extracellular fluid.

There are four primary or simple (as opposed to mixed) acid–base disorders:

- Metabolic acidosis: A disorder in which decreased HCO_3^- causes decreased pH.
- Metabolic alkalosis: A disorder in which increased HCO_3^- causes increased pH.
- Respiratory acidosis: A disorder in which increased pCO_2 causes decreased pH.
- Respiratory alkalosis: A disorder in which decreased pCO_2 causes increased pH.

Table 9–3. Changes in HCO_3^- and pCO_2 in primary acid–base disorders.

Disorder	pH	HCO_3^-	pCO_2
Metabolic acidosis	⇓	⇓	⇓ (compensatory)
Metabolic alkalosis	⇑	⇑	⇑ (compensatory)
Respiratory acidosis	⇓	⇑ (compensatory)	⇑
Respiratory alkalosis	⇑	⇓ (compensatory)	⇓

Acid–base disorders are classified as simple or mixed. In a simple acid–base disorder, only one primary acid–base disorder is present, and the compensatory response is appropriate. In a mixed acid–base disorder, more than one primary acid–base disorder is present. Mixed acid–base disorders are suspected from a patient's history, from a lesser or greater than expected compensatory response, and from analysis of the serum electrolytes and anion gap (AG; see below).

The use of a systematic approach to identifying and diagnosing acid–base disorders is essential. One must first determine alkalemia or academia based on pH. One must then determine whether a metabolic derangement with respiratory compensation or a respiratory derangement with metabolic compensation exists, based on the HCO_3^- and pCO_2 values (Table 9–3).

Whether the disturbance is primarily respiratory or metabolic, some degree of compensatory change occurs in an attempt to maintain normal pH. Changes in pCO_2 (respiratory disorders) are compensated for by changes in HCO_3^- (metabolic/renal compensation), and vice versa.

Acute respiratory disorders may develop in a matter of moments. Such circumstances may not allow sufficient time for renal compensation, resulting in severe pH changes without significant compensatory changes. By contrast, chronic respiratory disturbances allow the full range of renal compensatory mechanisms to function. In these circumstances, pH may remain normal or nearly normal despite wide variations in pCO_2. By contrast, respiratory compensation for metabolic disorders occurs quickly. Thus there is little difference in respiratory compensation for acute and chronic metabolic disorders.

A. Metabolic Acidosis

Metabolic acidosis is caused by increased production of H^+ or by excessive loss of HCO_3^-. In the surgical setting, metabolic acidosis is commonly encountered in trauma, critically ill and postoperative patients, and especially in patients in shock.

1. The anion gap—The serum anion gap (AG) is vital to determining the cause of any metabolic acidosis. AG may help differentiate between metabolic acidosis caused by accumulation of acid and that caused by loss of HCO_3^-.

AG represents the difference between the primary measured serum cation, Na^+, and the primary measured serum anions, Cl^- and HCO_3^-:

$$AG = Na^+ - (Cl^- + HCO_3^-)$$

The AG is normally less than 12; however, the highest normal value varies by institution.

Increased acid production causes an increased AG, as unmeasured anions electrically neutralize Na^+. Thus metabolic acidosis caused by increased H^+ production is associated with a high AG. The most common causes of an anion gap metabolic acidosis include methanol ingestion, uremia/renal failure, diabetic ketoacidosis, polypropylene glycol ingestion, isoniazid ingestion, lactic acidosis, ethylene glycol ingestion, and salicylate poisoning. In the surgical setting, lactic acidosis is by far the most common cause, seen in hypoperfused states like shock and sepsis.

A non-anion gap metabolic acidosis is caused by excessive HCO_3^- loss. The nephron maintains electrical neutrality by reabsorbing Cl^- as HCO_3^- is lost, hence the normal AG. Non-anion gap metabolic acidosis in the surgical setting typically results from diarrhea or high small-bowel output, eg, from an ileostomy. Non-anion gap acidosis also occurs in renal tubular acidosis, as the nephron fails to reabsorb HCO_3^-. Iatrogenic hyperchloremia, especially from administration of large amounts of normal saline to trauma and postoperative patients, may induce a non-anion gap metabolic acidosis.

The anion gap may be influenced by phenomena unrelated to acid–base balance, which must be kept in mind. Hypoalbuminemia may lower AG, as Cl^- and HCO_3^- increase to electrically balance Na^+ that was previously balanced by albumin. Similarly, hyper- or hypo- states of positively charged ions like calcium, magnesium, and potassium may affect the anion gap.

Treatment of metabolic acidosis involves identifying the underlying cause of the acidosis and correcting it. Often, this is sufficient. It is often unnecessary to correct acidosis with $NaHCO_3^-$ unless a patient has renal insufficiency, either chronic or acute. The degree of restoration is estimated by subtracting the plasma HCO_3^- from the normal value (24 mmol/L at our institution) and multiplying the resulting number by half TBW. This is a useful empiric formula, as in practice it is unwise (and unnecessary) to administer enough $NaHCO_3^-$ to completely correct pH. Doing so will likely cause fluid overload from the large Na^+ load delivered, and will likely overcorrect the acidosis. In patients with a chronic metabolic acidosis, often seen in chronic renal failure, alkali may be administered chronically as oral $NaHCO_3^-$. Efforts to minimize the magnitude of HCO_3^- loss in these patients must be undertaken as well.

2. Compensation—The body's response to metabolic acidosis is respiratory hyperventilation, "blowing off" H_2CO_3 as CO_2 and correcting the acidosis. This response is rapid, beginning within 30 minutes of the onset of acidosis and reaching full compensation within 24 hours. The adequacy of the respiratory response to metabolic acidosis is evaluated using Winter's formula:

$$pCO_2 = (1.5 \times HCO_3^- \text{ in mmol/L}) + (8 \pm 2)$$

If compensation is inadequate or excessive—ie, if pCO_2 is not within the range predicted by Winter's formula—one must evaluate for a mixed acid–base disorder (see below).

B. Metabolic Alkalosis

Metabolic alkalosis is often encountered in surgical patients. The pathogenesis is complex, but often involves (1) loss of H^+, usually via gastric losses of HCl; (2) hypovolemia, and (3) total body K^+ depletion. All three are commonly encountered with vomiting or gastric suctioning, diuretic use, and renal failure.

HCl is secreted by chief cells in the gastric mucosa; simultaneously, HCO_3^- is absorbed into the blood. $NaHCO_3$ is then secreted by the pancreas into the lumen of the duodenum, neutralizing the gastric acid, after which the neutralized acid and base are reabsorbed by the small intestine. Thus, under normal circumstances there is no net alteration of acid–base balance in the function of the gastrointestinal tract. However, when H^+ is lost from the gastric lumen—eg, through emesis, gastric suctioning, or gastric drainage—the result is loss of H^+ from the gastric lumen and a corresponding gain of HCO_3^- in the blood, leading to metabolic alkalosis.

Normally, the kidneys excrete excess HCO_3^-. However, if volume depletion accompanies HCO_3^- excess, the kidneys attempt to maintain normovolemia by increasing tubular reabsorption of Na^+, which is reabsorbed in an electrically neutral fashion by increasing reabsorption of Cl^- and HCO_3^-. This impairs HCO_3^- excretion, perpetuating the metabolic alkalosis.

Severe K^+ depletion further exacerbates metabolic alkalosis. To preserve K^+, Na^+ is exchanged for H^+ in the kidney, through the Na^+-K^+ and Na^+-H^+ ATPases in the distal renal tubule. This explains why severe metabolic alkalosis with hypokalemia results in paradoxical aciduria. In such cases, urine Na^+, K^+, and Cl^- concentrations are low, and the urine is acidic. In simple volume depletion, urine Cl^- alone is low and the urine is alkaline. Severe metabolic alkalosis may lead to tetany and seizures, as seen in hypokalemia and hypocalcemia.

Treatment of metabolic alkalosis includes fluid administration, usually normal saline. With adequate fluid repletion, tubular reabsorption of Na^+ is diminished, and the kidneys will excrete excess HCO_3^-. K^+ must be repleted, both to allow for correction of the alkalosis and to prevent life-threatening hypokalemia. Repletion of volume with normal saline and of potassium with KCl also provides the nephron with needed

Cl^-, allowing for reabsorption of K^+ and Na^+ with Cl^- instead of HCO_3^-. Acetazolamide, a carbonic anhydrase inhibitor diuretic, may also be used to treat metabolic alkalosis as long as the patient is euvolemic. Administration of exogenous acid in the form of HCl may be employed in the case of profound alkalosis.

1. Compensation—Adequate respiratory compensation for metabolic alkalosis should raise pCO_2 by 0.7 mm Hg for every 1 mmol/L elevation in HCO_3^-. Generally, respiratory compensation will not raise pCO_2 beyond 55 mm Hg. Thus a pCO_2 greater than 60 mm Hg in the setting of metabolic alkalosis suggests a mixed metabolic alkalosis and respiratory acidosis.

C. Respiratory Acidosis

Acute respiratory acidosis occurs when ventilation suddenly becomes inadequate. CO_2 accumulates in the blood, and as carbonic anhydrase coverts it to H_2CO_3, acidosis develops.

Acute respiratory acidosis is most common in conditions where gas exchange is physically impaired, resulting in decreased ventilation. These conditions typically involve decreased oxygenation as well. They include respiratory arrest, acute airway obstruction, pulmonary edema, pneumonia, saddle pulmonary embolus, aspiration of intraoral contents, and acute respiratory distress syndrome. Hypoventilation may occur in patients postoperatively who are oversedated (eg, from narcotics or benzodiazepines, or as they recover from general anesthesia). Pain, especially pain from large abdominal incisions or from rib fractures, leads to respiratory splinting and hypoventilation. Excess ethanol ingestion decreases respiratory drive, thereby impairing ventilation. Head trauma, either by direct damage to central nervous system respiratory centers or by global brain damage and brainstem herniation, may impair ventilation.

Patients with obesity hypoventilation syndrome and obstructive sleep apnea may develop a periodically recurring acute respiratory acidosis, leading eventually to some renal compensation. True chronic respiratory acidosis arises from chronic respiratory failure in which impaired ventilation leads to persistently elevated pCO_2, eg, as seen in chronic obstructive pulmonary disease. Chronic respiratory acidosis is usually well tolerated with adequate renal compensation; thus pH may be normal or near normal.

Treatment of respiratory acidosis involves restoration of adequate ventilation by treating the underlying cause. Aggressive chest physical therapy and pulmonary toilet should be instituted on all postsurgical patients. Patients with pulmonary edema should receive appropriate diuretic therapy, and patients with pneumonia should receive appropriate antibiosis. Naloxone or flumazenil should be used as needed in the setting of narcotic or benzodiazepine overdose, respectively. If necessary, endotracheal intubation and mechanical ventilation should be employed in order to correct pCO_2.

Acute respiratory acidosis should be corrected rapidly. However, too-rapid correction of chronic respiratory acidosis risks causing posthypercapneic metabolic alkalosis syndrome, characterized by muscle spasms and by potentially lethal cardiac arrhythmias.

1. Compensation—Over 80% of increased acid produced in respiratory acidosis is buffered by the body's tissues and intracellular hemoglobin. The remaining minority is buffered by HCO_3^- in the blood, which the kidney reclaims and reabsorbs. Thus metabolic (renal) compensation for respiratory disorders is a much slower process than respiratory compensation for metabolic disorders. Furthermore, in acute respiratory acidosis, renal mechanisms may not have had time to function at all, and HCO_3^- may be within normal limits. Adequate renal compensation for respiratory acidosis involves an increase in HCO_3^- of 1 mmol/L for every 10 mm Hg increase in pCO_2.

D. Respiratory Alkalosis

Hyperventilation decreases pCO_2 (hypocapnia), leading to respiratory alkalosis. In the surgical setting, anxiety, agitation, and pain are common causes of respiratory alkalosis. Hyperventilation and respiratory alkalosis may be early signs of sepsis and of moderate pulmonary embolism. Chronic respiratory alkalosis occurs in chronic pulmonary and liver disease.

Acute respiratory alkalosis is treated by addressing the underlying cause. Patients may require pain control, sedation/anxiolytics, and even paralysis with mechanical ventilation if necessary. Well-compensated chronic respiratory alkalosis does not require treatment. In these cases, rapid correction of pCO_2 leads to so-called post-hypocapneic hyperchloremic metabolic acidosis, which is often severe.

1. Compensation—The renal response to respiratory alkalosis is decreased resorption of filtered HCO_3^- and increased urinary HCO_3^- excretion. HCO_3^- decreases as Cl^- increases, since Na^+ is reabsorbed with Cl^- instead of with HCO_3^-. This same pattern is seen in hyperchloremic metabolic acidosis; the two are distinguished only by pH measurements.

Adequate renal compensation for respiratory alkalosis involves a decrease in HCO_3^- of 2 mmol/L for every 10 mm Hg decrease in pCO_2.

E. Mixed Acid–Base Disorders

Many common pathophysiologic processes cause mixed acid–base disorders. In these situations, pH may be normal or near normal, but compensatory changes are either inadequate or exaggerated. One way of determining the presence of a simple versus mixed disorder is to plot the patient's acid–base disorder on a nomogram (Figure 9–2). If the data fall outside one of the confidence bands, then by definition the patient has a mixed disorder. If the acid–base data fall

Hydrogen ion concentration (meq/L)

▲ Figure 9–2. Acid–base nomogram for use in evaluation of clinical acid–base disorders. Hydrogen ion concentration (top) or blood pH (bottom) is plotted against plasma HCO_3^- concentration; curved lines are isopleths of CO_2 tension ($PaCO_2$, mm Hg). Knowing any two of these variables permits estimation of the third. The circle in the center represents the range of normal values; the shaded bands represent the 95% confidence limits of four common acid–base disturbances: I, acute respiratory acidosis; II, acute respiratory alkalosis; III, chronic respiratory acidosis; and IV, sustained metabolic acidosis. Points lying outside these shaded areas are mixed disturbances and indicate two primary acid–base disorders.

within one of the confidence bands, the patient more likely has a simple acid–base disorder.

As with simple acid–base disorders, a systematic approach to mixed acid–base disorders is essential. First, determine the primary acid–base disorder. Next, determine whether or not adequate compensation has occurred, using the equations and rules given above (Table 9–4). If compensation is

Table 9–4. Expected compensation in primary acid–base disorders.

Metabolic acidosis	Winter's formula: $pCO_2 = 1.5 \times HCO_3^- + (8 \pm 2)$
Metabolic alkalosis	⇑ pCO_2 0.7 mm Hg for every 1 mmol/L increase in HCO_3^-
Respiratory acidosis	⇑ HCO_3^- 1 mmol/L for every 10 mm Hg increase in pCO_2
Respiratory alkalosis	⇓ HCO_3^- 2 mmol/L for every 10 mm Hg decrease in pCO_2

Table 9–5. Common laboratory values distinguishing between oliguric prerenal and intrinsic renal failure.

Test	Prerenal Value	Intrinsic Venal Value	Postrenal Value
FENa	< 1%	≥ 1%	
FEUN	< 35%	≥ 35%	
BUN:Cr ratio	> 20	< 10	10-20

"inadequate," meaning too little or too much, the patient has a mixed acid–base disorder.

An additional step is needed in the case of metabolic acidosis. After AG has been calculated, the "delta-delta" or "delta ratio" or "gap-gap" (three names for the same parameter) should be calculated:

$$\Delta\Delta = \Delta AG / \Delta HCO_3^-$$

where $\Delta\Delta$ = delta-delta; ΔAG = AG – maximum normal AG; and ΔHCO_3^- = normal HCO_3^- – HCO_3^-. At our institution, maximum normal AG is 12 mmol/L and normal HCO_3^- concentration is 24 mmol/L; thus $\Delta\Delta = (AG - 12)/(24 - HCO_3^-)$.

$\Delta\Delta < 1$ indicates the coexistence of an AG and a non-AG metabolic acidosis, ie, a metabolic acidosis caused by increased production of acid *and* by renal loss of HCO_3^-. This may occur in the setting of diabetic ketoacidosis.

$\Delta\Delta > 1$ indicates the coexistence of an AG metabolic acidosis and a metabolic alkalosis. This can occur in the intensive care unit in patients who have an underlying AG metabolic acidosis and are also undergoing diuresis or gastric suctioning, leading to the concurrent metabolic alkalosis.

The most common mixed acid–base disorder in surgical patients is a metabolic acidosis superimposed on a respiratory alkalosis. This occurs in patients with septic shock and hepatorenal syndrome, and also in the case of salicylate poisoning. Since the two acid–base disorders disrupt H^+ homeostasis in opposite directions, the patient's pH may be normal or near normal. Mixed respiratory acidosis and metabolic alkalosis is less common, occurring in the setting of cardiorespiratory arrest, which is a medical emergency.

▶ **References**

Adrogué HJ, Madias NE. Secondary responses to altered acid-base status: The rules of engagement. *J Am Soc Nephrol.* 2010;ASN-2009121211.

Ayers P, Warrington L. Diagnosis and treatment of simple acid-base disorders. *Nutr Clin Pract.* 2008;23(2):122-127.

Calvi LM, Bushinsky DA. When is it appropriate to order an ionized calcium? *J Am Soc Nephrol.* 2008;19(7):1257-1260.

Cengiz M, Ulker P, Meiselman HJ, Baskurt OK. Influence of tourniquet application on venous blood sampling for serum chemistry, hematological parameters, leukocyte activation and erythrocyte mechanical properties. *Clin Chem Lab Med.* 2009;47(6):769-776.

Gennari FJ. Pathophysiology of metabolic alkalosis: A new classification based on the centrality of stimulated collecting duct ion transport. *Am J Kid Dis.* 2011;58(4):626-636.

Jaber S, Paugam C, Futier E, et al. Sodium bicarbonate therapy for patients with severe metabolic acidaemia in the intensive care unit (BICAR-ICU): A multicentre, open-label, randomised controlled, phase 3 trial. *Lancet.* 2018;392(10141):31-40.

Jung B, Rimmele T, Le Goff C, et al. Severe metabolic or mixed acidemia on intensive care unit admission: Incidence, prognosis and administration of buffer therapy. A prospective, multiple-center study. *Crit Care.* 2011;15(5):R238.

Kraut JA, Madias NE. Differential diagnosis of nongap metabolic acidosis: Value of a systematic approach. *Clin J Am Soc Nephrol.* 2012;7(4):671-679.

Moritz ML, Ayus JC. Water water everywhere: Standardizing postoperative fluid therapy with 0.9% normal saline. *Anesth Analg.* 2010;110(2):293-295.

Semler MW, Self WH, Wanderer JP, et al. Balanced crystalloids versus saline in critically ill adults. *N Engl J Med.* 2018; 378(9):829-839.

Song ZF, Gu WH, Li HJ, Ge XL. The incidence and types of acid-base imbalance for critically ill patients in emergency. *Hong Kong J Emerg Med.* 2012;19(1):13-17.

Spasovski G, Vanholder R, Allolio B, et al. Clinical practice guideline on diagnosis and treatment of hyponatraemia. *Nephrol Dial Transplant.* 2014;29(suppl 2):i1-i39.

MULTIPLE-CHOICE QUESTIONS

1. A 28-year-old man with a history of depression is found down and brought to the emergency department. He responds to voice, moves his extremities spontaneously, and opens his eyes to pain only. Initial vital signs: temperature 98.0°F, pulse 72 beats/min, blood pressure 118/65 mm Hg, respiratory rate 28 breaths/min, and O_2 saturation 99% on a non-rebreather mask. Primary survey is within normal limits. Secondary survey reveals only superficial abrasions. Initial laboratory data include ABG: pH 7.36, pCO_2 38 mm Hg, paO_2 173 mm Hg, and HCO_3^- 20 mmol/L.

$$\begin{array}{c} 14.1 \\ 13.2 \diagdown \diagup 285 \\ 41.1 \end{array} \qquad \begin{array}{c|c|c} 145 & 102 & 18 \\ \hline 4.2 & 21 & 0.82 \end{array} \diagup 97$$

CPK 125
Serum salicylate 824 mg/L (normal 30-300 mg/L)

Based on this patient's history, exam findings, and laboratory data, what is this patient's acid–base derangement?

A. No disorder.
B. Respiratory acidosis with appropriate renal compensation.
C. Anion gap metabolic acidosis with appropriate respiratory compensation.

D. Non-anion gap metabolic acidosis with appropriate respiratory compensation.
E. Mixed metabolic acidosis and metabolic alkalosis.

2. A 54-year-old alcoholic man is discovered to have a new gastric cancer. He reports 15-lb weight loss over the past month. Laboratory data include an albumin of 2.4 g/dL, indicating significant longstanding malnutrition. Postoperatively, which of the following electrolyte derangements would be of initial concern, especially when he starts to eat or receive some other form of nutrition?

A. Hypophosphatemia.
B. Hyperphosphatemia.
C. Hypermagnesemia.
D. Hyponatremia.
E. Hyperkalemia.

3. A 70-year-old man undergoes a laparoscopic cholecystectomy for acute cholecystitis. On postoperative day 1 he complains of lightheadedness while attempting to transfer from his bed to a chair. His vital signs are temperature 99.1°F, pulse 82 beats/min, blood pressure 109/63 mm Hg, respiration rate 14 breaths/min, and O_2 saturation 99% on room air. The nurse informs you that he has had poor enteral intake since the operation, and his urine output has diminished to 10 mL/h. The nurse also informs you that his IV access was lost soon after his surgery and was never reestablished. His BUN and Cr preoperatively were 16 mg/dL and 0.8 mg/dL, respectively. Laboratory data include:

$$\begin{array}{c|c|c} 139 & 99 & 32 \\ \hline 3.6 & 24 & 1.47 \end{array} \diagup 88$$

Urine Na 153 mmol/L, Urine Cr 284 mg/dL

You suspect the cause of his orthostasis and oliguria is hypovolemia. Which of the following findings would most strongly confirm your hypothesis?

A. BUN:Cr ratio < 20.
B. Fractional excretion of sodium (FENa) > 1%.
C. FENa < 1%.
D. Renal ultrasonography demonstrating normal kidney parenchyma and vasculature.
E. Fractional excretion of urea nitrogen (FEUN) > 35%.

4. A 19-year-old woman arrives in the trauma bay after a helmeted motorcycle crash. She is hemodynamically unstable, and immediately taken to the operating room. Exploratory laparotomy reveals 3 L of hemoperitoneum, a grade 5 splenic laceration, and a grade 3 liver laceration. A splenectomy is performed and the liver laceration is packed. Inspection of the rest of her abdomen reveals no additional injuries. During the case, her

temperature is 93°F and her pH is 7.2; thus you decide to suspend the operation, leave her abdomen open, and admit her to the surgical intensive care unit (SICU) for resuscitation before returning to the operating room. Despite aggressive resuscitation with packed red blood cells (pRBCs) and other blood products, she remains hemodynamically unstable. Pelvic angiography reveals a bleeding right inferior gluteal artery, which is embolized. She is returned to the SICU for further resuscitation. You take over her care at this point, and notice that she has received 21 units of pRBCs, 19 units of fresh frozen plasma, and 20 units of platelets, but has not had her serum electrolytes checked in 5 hours. Which of the following electrolyte disorders is she most at risk for?

A. Hypocalcemia.
B. Hypomagnesemia.
C. Hyperkalemia.
D. All of the above.
E. None of the above.

5. A 61-year-old woman undergoes a sigmoid colectomy for perforated sigmoid diverticulitis. Postoperatively she is transferred to the surgical intensive care unit, still intubated and mechanically ventilated. On postoperative day 3 she develops an ileus, and her orogastric tube is put to low wall suction. On postoperative day 8 she develops hypotension and tachycardia to 140 beats/min, and requires a norepinephrine infusion to maintain adequate mean arterial blood pressure. Laboratory data includes ABG 7.32/40/154/20.

$$\begin{array}{c} 8.1 \\ 13.4 \diagdown\!\!\!\!\diagup 147 \\ 25.2 \end{array} \quad \begin{array}{c|c|c} 139 & 101 & 34 \\ \hline 3.4 & 22 & 1.2 \end{array} \diagdown 88$$

What is the most likely explanation for her acid–base disorder?

A. Anion-gap metabolic acidosis with adequate respiratory compensation.
B. Mixed metabolic alkalosis and anion-gap metabolic acidosis.
C. Metabolic alkalosis with respiratory compensation.
D. Mixed metabolic alkalosis and respiratory acidosis.
E. Mixed anion-gap metabolic acidosis and respiratory alkalosis.

Surgical Metabolism & Nutrition

Kris M. Mogensen, MS, RD-AP, LDN, CNSC

Malcolm K. Robinson, MD

The human body responds to surgical trauma, infection, and critical illness in a complex manner. The response is designed to provide energy and essential substrates for reparative processes while protecting the host from microbial infection and optimizing vital organ function. Compounds are released from peripheral tissues and taken up by visceral organs for use in these functions, which expedites recovery once the primary pathologic process has been controlled. The flow of substrates is initiated and maintained by the neuroendocrine milieu as well as a multitude of inflammatory mediators. The catabolic response appears well orchestrated but favors—sometimes too exuberantly—abundant delivery. Hence, the response may be deleterious when prolonged or severe. There may be significant degradation of lean body mass, which can result in debility and death if nutritional and cardiopulmonary reserves are exhausted. The magnitude and extent of the catabolic state is proportional to the incipient injury. One goal of surgeons and others who care for seriously ill patients is to support the salutary components of the response to injury while mitigating the detrimental elements. This can be accomplished in part through appropriate nutritional management of the critically ill patient.

This chapter will focus on the metabolic responses to starvation, traumatic injury, and sepsis, with emphasis on the nutritional management of the surgical patient.

METABOLIC RESPONSE TO STARVATION

▶ Basal Metabolic Rate & Resting Energy Expenditure

Daily energy expenditure is comprised of basal metabolic rate (BMR), the thermic effect of exercise, and thermogenesis of food intake. BMR, the major component of daily energy expenditure, is the amount of energy expended under complete rest, shortly after awakening, in a fasting state for 12-18 hours. BMR depends on age, gender, and body size.

It is proportional to lean body mass—not fat—and correlates roughly with body surface area. The thermic effect of exercise is the energy used in physical activity. BMR increases by approximately 20%-30% in those who are ambulating but may increase significantly more in those who are vigorously exercising. In contrast, ventilated patients who are paralyzed have very low activity levels because the ventilator performs the work of breathing and there is little muscle activity. The thermogenic effect of feeding relates to the increase in BMR that follows food intake. The digestion and metabolism of nutrients by mouth increase the metabolic rate and accounts for 5%-10% of the daily energy expenditure, depending on the amount and composition of the diet.

Resting energy expenditure (REE), which often, but incorrectly, is used synonymously with BMR, represents the amount of energy expended 2 hours after a meal under conditions of rest and thermal neutrality. REE is generally 10% higher than the BMR. Those suffering from starvation, but otherwise healthy, usually have an REE less than 90% of predicted values and are therefore hypometabolic. This affords an advantage for the starved individual, because it decreases the need for exogenous calories and therefore the need to break down endogenous substrates such as protein for fuel. Note that those who are both starved and ill are usually hypermetabolic due to the metabolic response to injury, as will be discussed later.

▶ Protein Metabolism During Starvation

There is a lack of exogenous nutrients during starvation, which leads to a fall in plasma glucose and insulin levels. This results in decreased protein synthesis, while protein catabolism remains unchanged (Figure 10–1). The net effect is the difference between synthesis and catabolism, which results in breakdown of body protein and release of amino acids into the plasma. It is important to note that there are no protein "stores" in the human body. All body protein has a functional

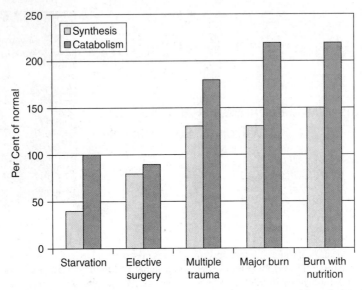

▲ **Figure 10–1.** Protein synthetic and catabolic rates in starvation and varying severities of critical illness and the impact of exogenous nutritional support.

or structural purpose. Thus, any loss of body protein results in degradation of body function or structure, which increases morbidity and risk of death when severe or prolonged.

Skeletal muscle is the major source of protein loss during starvation, and two amino acids, glutamine (GLN) and alanine (ALA), are key in protein metabolism during catabolic states. These amino acids account for 70% of the free amino acid pool in skeletal muscle and greater than 50% of the amino acids released during catabolic states, even though they only account for 13% of amino acids in intact muscle protein. GLN and ALA are synthesized de novo in skeletal muscle from alpha-ketoglutarate, pyruvate, and other amino acids obtained from muscle proteolysis as well as branched-chain amino acids (BCAAs) derived from the liver. Peripherally released GLN is primarily used as a fuel source by the gastrointestinal (GI) tract and rapidly dividing cells such as stimulated leukocytes. GLN is also used to a lesser degree in the liver for gluconeogenesis. ALA is the major amino acid used for hepatic gluconeogenesis. The GI tract and kidney also release ALA for hepatic glucose production. Most of these biological processes, which are largely initiated by decease in insulin during starvation, obligate nitrogen loss from the body and thus total body protein degradation (Figure 10–2).

Protein is degraded at a rate of approximately 75 grams/day primarily to derive amino acids for hepatic gluconeogenesis in the early stages of starvation. Otherwise healthy individuals would die in a few weeks at this rate of protein loss. However, healthy individuals who have adequate water can survive for months without exogenous food intake due to several adaptive responses that are initiated as starvation becomes prolonged. First, the metabolic rate decreases,

which decreases the need for the body to degrade protein. Secondly, most tissues in the body preferentially use fatty acids or ketone bodies for fuel rather than glucose. The process of switching from glucose utilization to ketones for fuel is known as ketoadaptation. Once the body ketoadapts, the quantity of amino acids consumed in gluconeogenic pathways is markedly reduced. Notably, the central nervous system (CNS) decreases its glucose requirement by 50%-70% of normal during prolonged starvation, as it increases its use of ketones for fuel. The CNS ability to ketoadapt has a profound protein-sparing effect. Finally, those tissues that require glucose obtain it by incompletely oxidizing glucose to lactate rather than complete oxidation to water and carbon dioxide. The resulting lactate is transferred to the liver and kidney, where it is converted back into glucose for use by glycolytic tissues. The cycling of lactate and glucose in this fashion is known as the Cori cycle, and the energy required for glucose resynthesis is derived from fat oxidation. This effectively means that lipid-derived calories are shuttled to glycolytic tissues in the form of glucose, thus minimizing irreversible glucose consumption (Figure 10–2).

Overall, the adaptive responses of prolonged starvation decrease protein needs by as much as 75% compared to normally fed individuals. This allows people to maintain vitality for months if adequate hydration is provided.

▶ Carbohydrate Metabolism During Starvation

Glucose is stored as glycogen in the liver and skeletal muscle, but only in limited amounts. This is because glucose intake in excess of that needed to fulfill energy requirements

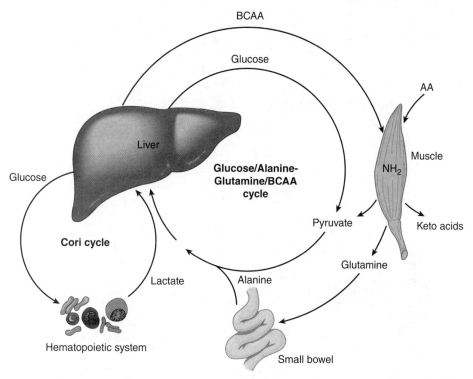

▲ **Figure 10–2.** The cycles that preserve metabolic intermediates during fasting. Lactate is recycled to glucose via the Cori cycle, while pyruvate is transaminated to alanine in skeletal muscle and converted to glucose via hepatic gluconeogenesis.

is primarily converted to fat. Glycogen stores are rapidly depleted within the first 24 hours of starvation, and the subsequent glucose needs of the body must be supplied via gluconeogenic pathways. The decreased insulin levels found in starvation favor glycogenolysis and hepatic gluconeogenesis. In addition, glucagon levels increase during starvation as glucose levels fall. Glucagon promotes hepatic glycogenolysis. Finally, cortisol is released in higher concentrations during starvation. Cortisol promotes hepatic gluconeogenesis while preventing peripheral uptake of amino acids, which consequently preserves circulating amino acids for the liver to use for glucose production. The presence of thyroid hormone has a permissive effect on hepatic gluconeogenesis and free fatty acid mobilization. Thus, there is a coordinated response of decreased insulin secretion and increased glucagon and cortisol secretion during starvation, which favors hepatic release of glucose. Eighty percent of the glucose is utilized by the nervous system in short-term starvation until the body ketoadapts as starvation becomes prolonged (Figure 10–3).

▶ Fat Metabolism During Starvation

The major source of fuel during prolonged starvation is derived from fat stored in adipose tissue. Insulin inhibits

lipase and therefore lipolysis. Insulin levels are depressed in starved individuals, which results in increased lipase activity and therefore increased lipolysis. Glucagon, which is increased during starvation, increases lipase activity, accelerates release of lipid from fat stores, and inhibits triglyceride storage in the liver. The glycerol moiety of triacylglycerol (ie, fat) can be converted to glucose. However, mammals do not possess the enzymatic machinery necessary to convert fatty-acid side chains to glucose. Instead, fatty acids generated from lipolysis serve as precursors to acetoacetate, beta-hydroxybutyrate, and acetone known as ketone bodies. Ketone bodies are water-soluble byproducts of triglycerides that can be easily circulated throughout the body for use by various tissues. Fatty acids are converted into ketone bodies in the liver, and these fat metabolites serve as another important signal to the body to decrease glucose utilization. The sum of the changes found during prolonged starvation is that fat becomes the primary energy source while carbohydrate and protein utilization is minimized.

In summary, prolonged starvation is characterized by accelerated skeletal muscle protein breakdown with movement of amino acids—primarily GLN and ALA—from the periphery to the viscera. The viscera uses peripherally derived amino acids for gluconeogenesis to supply glucose

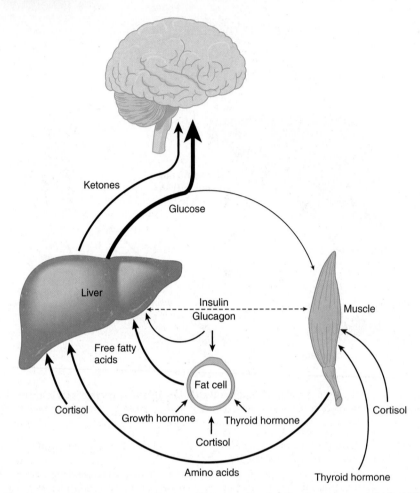

▲ **Figure 10–3.** The plasma substrate concentrations and hormone levels following an overnight fast. The brain is dependent on glucose, which is supplied predominantly by hepatic glycogenolysis until glycogen supplies are exhausted.

for those tissues that require it for fuel. The body adapts as starvation continues to minimize glucose needs and therefore protein breakdown. These adaptive processes include the slowing of the metabolic rate, preferential use of ketone bodies instead of glucose for energy, and increasing release of fat from adipose tissue to serve as the primary fuel source. These metabolic changes are primarily under hormonal control (Figure 10–4).

METABOLIC RESPONSE TO TRAUMATIC INJURY & CRITICAL ILLNESS

▶ Acute Injury Response

The response to traumatic injury over time is not static but changes to meet ongoing requirements of the body. Sir David Cuthbertson first described the response in the 1930s, and

divided it into two phases: the ebb and flow phases. The injury response is characterized by release of the counterregulatory hormones cortisol, glucagon, and catecholamines, which orchestrate many of the physiologic changes observed in both phases. Insulin levels are depressed in the ebb phase, and while glucose production remains the same, there is hyperglycemia related to catecholamine-induced hepatic glycogenolysis. Catecholamines also induce lipolysis, leading to increased plasma free fatty acids. The ebb phase is further characterized by depressed cardiac output, lactic acidosis, hypothermia, and depressed oxygen consumption. Once the traumatized individual is resuscitated and as time from the initial injury progresses, the host enters the flow phase.

The flow phase represents the hyperdynamic phase of the response to injury and begins 24-48 hours after injury. Cardiac output and oxygen consumption are increased. Lactate levels normalize in the fully resuscitated individual.

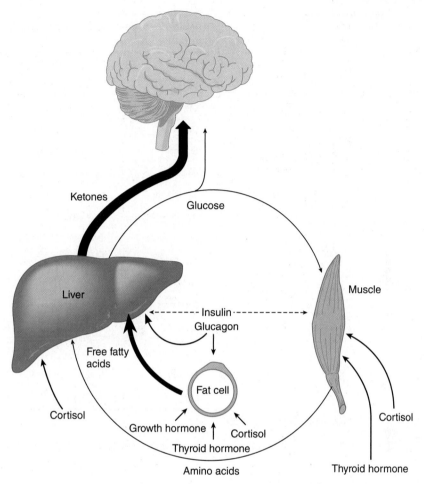

▲ Figure 10–4. The metabolic adaptation to chronic starvation whereby the brain shifts its substrate preference to ketones produced by the liver. Hepatic gluconeogenesis falls and protein breakdown is diminished, thus preserving lean tissue.

Insulin levels become normal or can be increased in those who exhibit insulin resistance. The injured have an increase in resting energy expenditure (REE). The increase in REE can vary from 10% to 15% above normal in those undergoing elective surgeries to over 100% above normal in those recovering from major burns (Figure 10–5). Body core temperature rises as well. There are changes in protein, carbohydrate, and fat metabolism that are similar to that observed during simple starvation without injury. This is because the hormonal changes that occur following injury are similar to that observed during starvation.

Following injury, neural impulses stimulate the hypothalamus. Norepinephrine is released from sympathetic nerve endings, epinephrine from the adrenal medulla, aldosterone from the adrenal cortex, antidiuretic hormone (ADH) from the posterior pituitary, insulin and glucagon from the

pancreas, and corticotropin, thyrotropin, and growth hormone from the anterior pituitary. This results in elevation of serum cortisol, thyroid hormone, and somatomedins. The characteristics of the ebb and flow phases are summarized in Table 10–1.

One of the major differences between simple starvation and traumatic injury is the presence of an inflammatory focus. This focus consists of devitalized tissue, microbial infection, or endogenous autodigestion of surrounding tissue, as observed in patients with severe pancreatitis. The focus leads to priming and activation of inflammatory and other cells that release a host of compounds that have potent metabolic effects. The compounds are collectively referred to as inflammatory mediators, and include cytokines, prostaglandins, leukotrienes, complement, and platelet-activating factor. In uncomplicated or "simple" starvation, where the host is uninjured

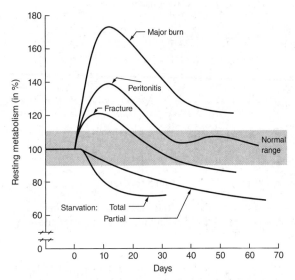

▲ **Figure 10–5.** Protein (ie, nitrogen) excretion and resting metabolic rate in starvation and individuals with varying degrees of disease severity.

Table 10–1. Features of the ebb and flow phases of the response to injury.

	Ebb Phase	Flow Phase
Hormones		
Catecholamines	Increased	Normal–increased
Cortisol	Increased	Increased
Glucagon	Increased	Increased
Insulin	Decreased	Normal–increased
Metabolism		
Oxygen consumption	Decreased	Increased
Cardiac output	Decreased	Increased
Body temperature	Decreased	Increased
Glucose production	Normal	Increased
Substrates		
Glucose	Increased	Normal–increased
Protein balance	Negative	Very negative
Fatty acids	Increased	Normal–increased
Lactic acid	Increased	Normal

▶ Protein Metabolism During Critical Illness

As in starvation, there is a net loss of protein from the body during critical illness. In those with mild to moderate injury, total body protein synthesis decreases while protein catabolism remains unchanged or slightly depressed, leading to net loss of protein (Figure 10–1). In those with severe injury or infection, both protein synthesis and catabolism are accelerated but protein catabolism exceeds synthesis, which again results in net loss of protein from the body. Hence, patients recovering from illness lose large quantities of protein from the body. The magnitude of protein loss correlates with the severity of illness (Figure 10–5). Protein loss invariably represents degradation of body structure and function, as there are no protein stores in the body. Degradation of the protein-rich lean body mass is associated with debility and mortality. The loss of protein from the body can be mitigated by appropriate nutrition management, which is why nutritional care of the critically ill patient is so important.

Under the control of the counter-regulatory hormones and inflammatory mediators, there is a shift of amino acids from skeletal muscle to visceral tissues, and glutamine (GLN) and alanine (ALA) play key roles in this process.

and otherwise well, the metabolic changes are primarily under hormonal control. In contrast, the cellular changes that produce the metabolic response to traumatic injury and critical illness are under the control of both the classic hormones and inflammatory mediators. The inflammatory mediators add a dimension to the metabolic response to illness that make it distinct from the metabolic response to simple starvation.

The degradation of muscle protein serves to supply amino acids (primarily ALA) for gluconeogenesis as well as for the synthesis of proteins needed for reparative processes and host defense against microbial invasion. GLN is the preferred fuel of enterocytes and other rapidly dividing cells.

Many tissues are obligate users of glucose for fuel. When glucose stores run out, amino acids from the periphery and glycerol from lipid are used in gluconeogenic processes to produce glucose for the body's ongoing fuel needs. In starvation, the body ketoadapts, preferentially using ketone bodies derived from lipid for fuel rather than glucose. Ketoadaptation markedly reduces glucose consumption and has a profound protein-sparing effect in those with uncomplicated starvation.

However, critically ill patients have a markedly reduced capacity to ketoadapt. This represents one of the most important differences between the metabolic response to starvation and the metabolic response to critical illness. As a consequence, the length of survival in critically ill individuals without nutrition is markedly reduced compared to those with simple starvation. Why the ketoadaptation response in the critically injured is attenuated compared to the catabolic state of starvation is unknown.

Carbohydrate Metabolism During Critical Illness

Glucose stored as glycogen is depleted within 24 hours in critically injured individuals. Thus the body uses muscle amino acids, lipid-derived glycerol, lactate, and pyruvate to generate glucose via hepatic gluconeogenesis for use by glycolytic tissues. The increased glucose production is primarily under hormonal control. Although insulin levels are elevated under such conditions, there is profound tissue insulin resistance mediated in part by epinephrine and glucocorticoids. The glucose produced is used by the central nervous system, kidneys, and for reparative processes.

Fat Metabolism During Critical Illness

There is a significant increase in fuel consumption in the critically ill individual secondary to hypermetabolism, accelerated gluconeogenesis, mobilization of peripheral substrates, and elevated core body temperature. To meet the body's increased energy needs, glycerol and free fatty acids are released from adipose tissue. Free fatty acids cannot be used by all tissues for energy, as some tissues are obligate glucose users. The glycerol generated from fat can be used for glucose production. However, free fatty acids cannot, as the human body cannot synthesize glucose from fatty acids. This means that the body cannot solely rely on its largest depot of energy (ie, fat) to meet the high energy demands of critical illness. Accordingly, protein, glucose, and fat supplies are all rapidly depleted during

traumatic injury and critical illness unless adequate nutrition support is supplied (Figure 10-6 and Table 10-2).

NUTRITION ASSESSMENT

▶ Nutrition Screening

The metabolic response to critical illness leads to degradation of lean body mass and increased risk of nutritionally related complications. Malnourished patients, or those who become malnourished during hospitalization, are particularly vulnerable. Hence, it is imperative to identify nutritionally compromised patients to develop a comprehensive plan for nutrition intervention.

Nutrition screening is the process of identifying patients who are either malnourished or at risk for developing malnutrition. Nutrition screening should ideally be done by healthcare professionals who are experts in clinical nutrition. However, most hospitals do not have the resources to provide such personnel to screen 100% of patients admitted to inpatient services. Hence, screening is often done based on admission labs, which can be very unreliable, or by the admitting nurse using a nutrition screening tool.

Several tools have been developed for nutrition screening. For example, the malnutrition universal screening tool (MUST) detects protein–energy malnutrition and identifies individuals at risk of developing malnutrition using three independent criteria: current weight status, unintentional weight loss, and acute disease effect. The patient's current body weight is determined by calculating the body mass index (BMI) (kg/m^2). Weight loss over the past 3-6 months is determined by looking at the individual's medical record. An acute disease factor is then included if the patient is currently affected by a pathophysiologic condition and there has been no nutritional intake for more than 5 days. A total score is calculated placing the patients in a low, medium, or high category for risk of malnutrition.

An alternative is the malnutrition screening tool (MST). The MST assesses patient answers to questions about eating and weight loss. A MST score of 0-1 is considered not at risk for malnutrition, while a score of 2 or greater indicates risk (Tables 10-3 and 10-4).

Patients who are found to be malnourished or at risk for malnourishment based on a nutrition screening tool are referred for a more detailed evaluation. Nutrition screening tools have the advantage of simplicity, making them usable by non-nutrition experts. However, screening tools have two caveats. First, the screening is only as good as compliance with utilization of the tool. For institutions that faithfully use the tool on admission and throughout the inpatient stay as necessary, the likelihood of identifying most of the at-risk population can be quite good. For hospitals that do not make faithful use of the tools, many malnourished patients may be

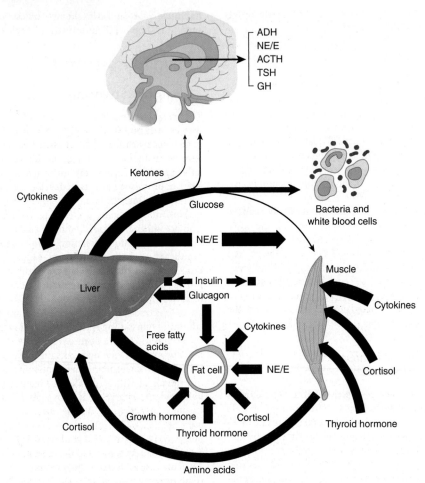

▲ **Figure 10–6.** During sepsis, cytokines (IL-1, IL-2, TNF) released by lymphocytes and macrophages contribute to catabolism of muscle and adipose tissue and amplify the neurohormonal response to antecedent trauma.

Table 10–2. Metabolic responses to starvation and injury.

	Starvation	Critical Illness
Resting energy expenditure	Decreased	Increased
Glucose utilization	Minimized	Accelerated
Fatty acid utilization	Increased	Increased
Protein degradation	Minimized	Accelerated
Ketone utilization	Increased	Decreased
Gluconeogenesis	Initially increased, then decreased	Increased
Hormonal control	Yes	Yes
Inflammatory mediators	No	Yes

unknown and therefore untreated. Second, nutrition screening must trigger a referral for formal nutrition assessment and result in development of a comprehensive nutrition plan. Screening does no good if it is not acted upon.

Table 10–3. Malnutrition universal screening tool (MUST).

BMI score: Weight loss score (unplanned weight loss):
   BMI > 20 (> 30 obese) = 0; weight loss < 5% = 0
   BMI 18.5-20 = 1; weight loss 5.10% = 1
   BMI < 18.5 = 2; weight loss > 10% = 2
Acute disease effect: Add 2 if there has been or is likely to be no nutritional intake for > 5 days.
Risk of malnutrition: 0 = low risk; 1 = medium risk; ≥ 2 = high risk

Table 10–4. Malnutrition screening tool (MST).

Question 1: Have you recently lost weight without trying?
  No, 0 points; Unsure, 2 points
  If Yes, how much weight have you lost:
    2-13 lb: 1 point
    14-23 lb: 2 points
    24-33 lb: 3 points
    34 lb or more: 4 points
Question 2: Have you been eating poorly because of a poor appetite?
  No, 0 points; Yes, 1 point
Add up scores from questions 1 and 2
MST score of 0-1 point: No risk
MST score of 2 or more: At risk for malnutrition and should undergo nutrition
  assessment

Nutrition Evaluation

The formal process for minimizing nutrition-related issues begins with nutrition evaluation. The components of nutritional evaluation include assessment of past energy intake and weight loss as part of a comprehensive medical history. The medical history should explore conditions that may impair normal oral intake, swallowing, or intestinal absorption. A complete history of current medications is essential to alert caregivers to potential underlying deficiencies and drug–nutrient interactions. There should be a nutrition-focused physical assessment to evaluate for decrease in muscle mass, loss of subcutaneous fat, and presence of edema. Particular attention should be paid to skin changes that may indicate a nutritional deficiency or a medical condition with skin conditions that may be improved with targeted nutrition therapy (Figure 10–7). The physical exam should also focus on abdominal pathology which may or

may not inform the clinician about the likelihood of tolerating enteral nourishment. This may include, for example, enterocutaneous fistulae. The functional status is also assessed.

Anthropometric Measurements

Anthropometry is the science of assessing body size, weight, and proportions. Anthropometric measurements gauge body weight and composition with the intent of providing specific information about lean body mass and fat stores. Body composition studies may be used to determine total body water, fat, nitrogen, and potassium levels. Anthropometric measurements that can be easily performed in the clinic or at the bedside include determination of height and weight, with calculation of body mass index (BMI). Additional measurements such as arm span, body part summation, or knee-height measurement can also be used in nutrition assessment. More advanced techniques allow the clinician to assess the patient's visceral and somatic protein mass and fat reserve. Accurate weight is important, as is current weight expressed as a percentage of ideal body weight. Ideal body weight values are taken from the 1983 Metropolitan Height-Weight Tables. Other methods to determine ideal body weight are also used. Another frequenty used method is the Hamwi Formula, which is a calculated ideal body weight (for women, 100 lb for the first 5 feet and 5 lb for every inch after; for men, 106 lb for the first five feet and 6 points for every inch after).

The body mass index (BMI) is used in a weight classification scheme based on weight relative to height, and is independent of gender. A BMI between 18.5 and 24.9 is considered normal in most Western countries. Less than 18.5

| Panel A | Panel B | Panel C |

▲ **Figure 10–7.** Rashes with nutrition implications. Panel A demonstrates a patient with essential fatty acid deficient who had the classic scaly skin rash. Panel B demonstrates a patient with necrolytic migratory erythema of the back, the characteristic rash associated with glucagonoma syndrome. Panel C demonstrates the patient in Panel B after treatment with amino acid and fatty acid infusions.

is considered underweight. Overweight is defined as a BMI from 25 to 29.9, and a BMI greater than 30 defines obesity.

- BMI is calculated as follows:

$$BMI = \frac{Weight\,(kg)}{Height\,(m)^2} = 703 \times \frac{Weight\,(lb)}{Height\,(in)^2}$$

Dual-energy x-ray absorptiometry (DEXA) is increasingly available in hospitals and can be used to assess various body compartments (mineral, fat, and lean muscle mass). Most protein resides in skeletal muscle. Somatic (skeletal) protein reserve is estimated by measuring the mid-humeral circumference. This measurement is corrected to account for subcutaneous tissue, yielding the mid-humeral muscle circumference (MHMC). The result is compared with normal values for the patient's age and gender to determine the extent of protein depletion. Fat reserve is commonly estimated from the thickness of the triceps skin fold (TSF). Reliability of anthropometric measurements is dependent on the skill of the person performing the measurement, and is subject to error if performed by different caregivers on the same patient.

▶ Nutrition Classification

In 2012, the Academy of Nutrition and Dietetics and the American Society for Parenteral and Enteral Nutrition (ASPEN) published new guidelines to define malnutrition in adults. The guidelines recognize the impact of chronic disease and acute inflammation on nutritional status, and new categories of malnutrition were recommended that include the degree of inflammation. The specific characteristics of malnutrition are based on clinical scenarios: acute illness or injury-related illness; chronic disease-related illness; or social or environment-related malnutrition. The criteria are summarized in Tables 10–5 to 10–7.

Serum biomarkers such as albumin, prealbumin (transthyretin), and transferrin are not used in the new malnutrition characteristics, as these measures are often unreliable, especially in acute and critically ill patients. Such biomarkers are altered by the degree of inflammation, infection, and hydration independent of the host's nutritional status.

▶ Nutritional Status & Risk of Complications

Several indices have attempted to assess the risk of complications based on patient nutritional status. This in theory provides a guide for identifying patients who require nutrition intervention. There are several risk equations to assist with this. For example, the prognostic nutrition index (PNI) has been validated in patients undergoing either major cancer or gastrointestinal surgery, and found to accurately identify a subset of patients at increased risk for complications.

Table 10–5. Classification of acute illness- or injury-related malnutrition.

Clinical Characteristic	Nonsevere (Moderate) Malnutrition	Severe Malnutrition
Energy intake	< 75% estimated energy requirements for > 7 days	≤ 50% of estimated energy requirements for ≥ 5 days
Interpretation of weight loss	1%-2% loss in 1 week, 5% loss in 1 month, 7.5% loss in 3 months	> 2% loss in 1 week, > 5% loss in 1 month, > 7.5% loss in 3 months
Loss of subcutaneous fat	Mild	Moderate
Loss of muscle mass	Mild	Moderate
Presence of edema	Mild	Moderate to severe
Reduced hand grip strength	Not applicable	Measurably reduced

Furthermore, preoperative nutritional repletion has been shown to reduce postoperative morbidity in this patient group. The PNI has also been widely adapted to identify patients at risk in nonsurgical populations, who may benefit from nutritional support (Table 10–8).

The nutritional risk index (NRI) was used by the VA TPN Cooperative Study Group for determining preoperative

Table 10–6. Chronic disease-related malnutrition.

Clinical Characteristic	Nonsevere (Moderate) Malnutrition	Severe Malnutrition
Energy intake	< 75% estimated energy requirements for ≥ 1 month	≤ 75% of estimated energy requirements for ≥ 1 month
Interpretation of weight loss	5% loss in 1 month, 7.5% loss in 3 months, 10% loss in 6 months, 20% loss in 1 year	> 5% loss in 1 month, > 7.5% loss in 3 months, > 10% loss in 6 months, > 20% loss in 1 year
Loss of subcutaneous fat	Mild	Severe
Loss of muscle mass	Mild	Severe
Presence of edema	Mild	Severe
Reduced hand grip strength	Not applicable	Measurably reduced

Table 10–7. Social- or environment-related malnutrition.

Clinical Characteristic	Nonsevere (Moderate) Malnutrition	Severe Malnutrition
Energy intake	< 75% estimated energy requirements for ≥ 3 months	≤ 50% of estimated energy requirements for ≥ 1 month
Interpretation of weight loss	5% loss in 1 month, 7.5% loss in 3 months, 10% loss in 6 months, 20% loss in 1 year	> 5% loss in 1 month, > 7.5% loss in 3 months, > 10% loss in 6 months, > 20% loss in 1 year
Loss of subcutaneous fat	Mild	Severe
Loss of muscle mass	Mild	Severe
Presence of edema	Mild	Severe
Reduced hand grip strength	Not applicable	Measurably reduced

malnutrition, and it has since been prospectively cross-validated against other nutritional indices with good results (Table 10–9). The index successfully stratifies perioperative morbidity and mortality using serum albumin and weight loss as predictors of malnutrition. Those with severe malnutrition based on the NRI may benefit from preoperative feeding to reduce postoperative complications. Preoperative feeding with enteral nutrition (EN) or parenteral nutrition (PN) should be considered for such individuals if they are clinically stable and can wait for 7-10 days of preoperative feeding required for it to have an impact. Of note, the NRI is not a tool for monitoring the adequacy of nutritional support, since supplemental nutrition often fails to improve serum albumin levels.

The NUTRIC (NUTrition Risk In Critically ill) score is a relatively new tool designed by Heyland and colleagues in 2011 (Table 10–10). The score helps to quantify the risk of critically ill patients developing adverse events that may

Table 10–8. Prognostic nutrition index (PNI).

$$PNI = 158 - [16.6 \times Alb^1] - [0.78 \times TSF^2] - [0.2 \times TFN^3] - [5.8 \times DH^4]$$
Note: for DH, > 5 mm induration = 2;
1-5 mm induration = 1;
anergy = 0

[1]Alb, albumin (g/dL).
[2]TSF, triceps skin fold (mm).
[3]TFN, transferrin (mg/dL).
[4]DH, delayed cutaneous hypersensitivity.

Table 10–9. Nutritional risk index (NRI).

NRI = [15.19 × Alb] + 41.7 × [actual weight (kg)/ideal weight (kg)]	
Well-nourished	> 100
Mild malnutrition	97.5-100
Moderate malnutrition	83.5-97.5
Severe malnutrition	< 83.5

be modified by aggressive nutrition therapy, in the general population of an ICU. The NUTRIC score accounts for the fact that not all ICU patients will respond the same to nutritional intervention. The score accurately identifies those patients who have higher mortality rates or survivors with longer lengths of stay. In addition, patients with NUTRIC scores of 6 or higher benefit the most from increasing nutritional intake. The original NUTRIC score included measurement of serum IL-6 levels, which is not easily done

Table 10–10. NUTRIC scoring system.

Variables in NUTRIC Score	NUTRIC Scoring System	
	Range	Points
Age	< 50	0
	50-< 75	1
	≥ 75	2
APACHE II	< 15	0
	15-< 20	1
	20-28	2
	≥ 28	3
SOFA	< 6	0
	6-< 10	1
	≥10	2
# Co-morbidities	0-1	0
	2+	1
Days from hospital to ICU admit	0-< 1	0
	1+	1
IL6*	0-< 400	0
	400+	1

APACHE II, Acute Physiology and Chronic Health II score, which is a severity-of-disease classification scoring system calculated within 24 hours of ICU admission. SOFA, Sequential Organ Failure Assessment score, which is used to track patient status during an ICU stay. IL-6 measurement and scoring is optional by most hospital clinical laboratories. Hence, a modified NUTRIC score without use of the IL-6 variable has been validated for use.

Determining Nutrient Needs

A cornerstone of nutrition intervention is estimating energy needs to reduce the risk of overfeeding or inappropriate underfeeding, both of which have known risks that may affect outcome. Hence the last step in the nutrition assessment process is determination of nutrient needs. The easiest way to estimate calorie needs is based on body weight and the severity of clinical illness, as indicated in Table 10–11.

Caloric needs can also be estimated using a variety of predicative equations. There are several predictive equations that one may use based on a variety of clinical scenarios. However, possibly the most famous equation for estimating caloric needs is the Harris–Benedict equation (Table 10–12).

This Harris–Benedict equation has four variables: height (cm), weight (kg), gender, and age (y). This allows one to determine basal energy expenditure (BEE). Daily caloric needs are then determined by multiplying BEE by a stress factor, which varies per disease severity; and then a physical activity factor, which varies from 1.0 to 1.3. Ventilated and paralyzed patients have an activity factor of 1.0, while those who are ambulating in the hospital may have an activity factor of 1.3. Thus estimated daily caloric intake is determined by the following formula:

Daily Calorie Needs = BEE × Stress Factor × Activity Factor

Some believe that predictive equations such as the Harris–Benedict equation overestimate BEE. Hence they do not use the activity factor when determining daily caloric needs.

Predictive equations for estimating caloric needs can be highly inaccurate—at times by more than 50%. The gold standard for determining needs is indirect calorimetry. Using a metabolic cart, a trained technician determines oxygen consumption ($\dot{V}O_2$) and carbon dioxide production ($\dot{V}CO_2$) from the patient's pulmonary gas flow. Based

Table 10–11. Energy requirements.

Clinical Condition	Energy Requirements (kcal/kg)
Maintenance/minimal metabolic stress	20
Mild metabolic stress	25
Initial phase of critical illness	25
Moderate metabolic stress	25-30
Moderate to severe stress	30-35
Large wounds	35-40

Table 10–12. Harris–Benedict equation.

Basal energy expenditure (BEE) in kcal/day	
Male: 66.4 + [13.7 × weight (kg)] + [5.0 × height (cm)] − [6.8 × age (yrs)]	
Female: 655 + [9.6 × weight (kg)] + [1.7 × height (cm)] − [4.7 × age (yrs)]	

Stress factors	
Starvation	0.80-1.00
Elective surgery	1.00-1.10
Peritonitis	1.05-1.25
Adult respiratory distress syndrome (ARDS) or sepsis	1.30-1.35
Bone marrow transplant	1.20-1.30
Cardiopulmonary disease (uncomplicated)	0.80-1.00
Cardiopulmonary disease with dialysis or sepsis	1.20-1.30
Cardiopulmonary disease with major surgery	1.30-1.55
Acute renal failure	1.30
Liver failure	1.30-1.55
Liver transplantation	1.20-1.50
Pancreatitis or major burns	1.30-1.80

on these measurements and the amount of nitrogen excreted in the urine, the resting energy expenditure (REE) can be derived using the Weir formula, as follows:

$$REE\ (kcal/day) = [3.94\ (\dot{V}O_2) + 1.1(\dot{V}CO_2)] \times 1.44 - 2.17(UN)$$

where $\dot{V}O_2$ and $\dot{V}CO_2$ are expressed in mL/min and urine nitrogen is in g/min.

The utility of this technique is limited by the expense and cumbersomeness of the metabolic cart, as well as lack of trained personnel to operate it. Hence, many institutions cannot reliably perform metabolic cart studies. In addition, it is not clinically practical to measure urine nitrogen in most patients, and hence an abbreviated Weir equation that does not factor in urine nitrogen excretion may be used. Note that the metabolic cart studies already account for the disease severity of the patient, as the measurements are performed on individual patients who are ill. Thus determining daily caloric needs does not require multiplication by a stress factor and can be determined by the following formula:

Daily Calorie Needs = REE × Activity Factor

Additionally, the metabolic cart provides information for calculation of the respiratory quotient (RQ). The RQ is the ratio of carbon dioxide production to oxygen consumption in the metabolism of fuels by the body. When the RQ is 1, pure carbohydrate is being oxidized. Patients metabolizing lipids only will have an RQ of 0.67. Lipogenesis occurs in patients with excess caloric intake (overfeeding). When excessive calories are ingested or administered, the RQ is greater than 1 and can theoretically approach 9. The excess production of CO_2 may impair ventilator weaning in patients, particularly

Table 10–13. Protein requirements.

Condition	Protein Requirements (g/kg)
Well nourished	0.8
Well nourished, elderly	1.2
Wound healing	1.3-1.5
Burn < 20% total body surface area	1.5
Burn > 20% total body surface area	2.0
High-dose steroids	1.5
Hemodialysis	1.1-1.4
Peritoneal dialysis	1.2-1.6
Continuous renal replacement therapy	1.8-2.5

those with intrinsic lung disease (eg, chronic obstructive pulmonary disease, COPD). Those who have an RQ greater than 1 may be receiving excessive energy delivery and should have calories reduced.

Because metabolic cart studies depend on the accurate measurement of oxygen consumption and carbon dioxide production, there are clinical circumstances in which such studies should not be used as they are highly inaccurate. This includes patients with chest tubes who may have an air leak and are losing an unmeasured amount of oxygen. It also includes patients who are dialyzed, as they may lose an unmeasured amount of CO_2. Finally, metabolic cart studies are not accurate in patients who are receiving high concentrations of oxygen (eg, FiO_2 > 60%).

In contrast to caloric determination, there are no predictive equations or direct measurement modalities for determining protein needs during critical illness. Instead, protein needs are largely determined by the clinical situation and body weight, as described in Table 10–13. It should be noted that the weight used for determination of needs should be a dry or estimated dry weight, so that excessive protein is not given to grossly edematous individuals.

NUTRITION INTERVENTION

The appropriate nutrition intervention depends on many factors, including preexisting nutrition status, metabolic demands of the current illness and postoperative status, ability to take oral nutrition, and functional status of the GI tract. The simplest and most desired nutrition intervention will involve the oral diet when possible. Oral intake, unless contraindicated, is the most natural and is associated with the fewest complications compared to other forms of nutrition intake.

Patients with adequate functional swallowing ability should be able to take an oral diet, and if intake is inadequate, oral nutritional supplements may be helpful to meet energy and protein requirements. Clinicians should consider ordering the least restrictive oral diet as possible, which in some cases will allow for improved intake. The least restrictive oral diet is a "regular" or "house" diet, which carries no restrictions. Depending on the patient's comorbidities, a more restricted diet may be appropriate. For example, a patient with diabetes may require a consistent carbohydrate diet to assist with glucose control, or a patient with heart failure may require a sodium restriction. Clinical judgment is required to determine if the oral diet restriction is necessary or can be lifted in the initial postoperative period to assure adequate energy and protein intake to support wound healing and recovery.

▶ Indications for Nutrition Support Therapy

Enteral nutrition (EN) or parenteral nutrition (PN) may be required for patients who are unable to take adequate oral nutrition. EN and PN are the two forms of nutrition support. The American Society for Parenteral and Enteral Nutrition (ASPEN) has published several clinical guidelines to assist with the decision process for initiating enteral or parenteral nutrition. In general, patients who cannot take an oral diet either because of a swallowing problem or GI dysfunction, cannot take enough oral nutrients, or cannot digest and absorb oral/enteral nutrients properly, would be candidates for nutrition support therapy. One algorithm for determining when nutrition support is necessary, and the route of nutrition support, is given in Figure 10–8.

▶ Enteral Versus Parenteral Nutrition

Enteral nutrition (EN) is the provision of nutrients through a tube into the GI tract, and parenteral nutrition (PN) is the provision of nutrients intravenously. The decision to select one therapy over the other lies in (1) the ability to safely access the GI tract with a feeding tube and (2) if the GI tract is functioning normally (or normally enough) to allow safe administration and absorption of tube feeds. The adage "If the gut works and can be used safely, use it" is a key consideration when deciding to initiate nutrition support. Clinicians should make every effort to select EN over PN for nutrition support therapy, as EN generally carries a lower risk of complications than PN and EN is associated with lower costs. Table 10–14 provides a more detailed analysis of typical indications for EN and PN and should be considered in concert with Figure 10–8.

Use of EN also offers physiologic and immunologic benefits. Infusing complex nutrients (intact protein, carbohydrate, fiber, and fat) into the GI tract provides a stimulus for hepatic synthetic function of proteins. In contrast, PN bypasses the portal circulation and decrease this stimulus. EN

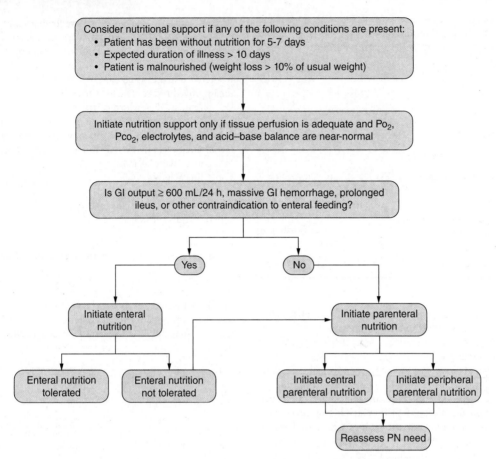

Consider nutritional support if any of the following conditions are present:
- Patient has been without nutrition for 5-7 days
- Expected duration of illness > 10 days
- Patient is malnourished (weight loss > 10% of usual weight)

Initiate nutrition support only if tissue perfusion is adequate and Po_2, Pco_2, electrolytes, and acid–base balance are near-normal

Is GI output $\geq$ 600 mL/24 h, massive GI hemorrhage, prolonged ileus, or other contraindication to enteral feeding?

Yes | No

Initiate enteral nutrition | Initiate parenteral nutrition

Enteral nutrition tolerated | Enteral nutrition not tolerated | Initiate central parenteral nutrition | Initiate peripheral parenteral nutrition

Reassess PN need

▲ **Figure 10–8.** Indications for nutrition support intervention and the route of feeding.

also has beneficial local effects on gastrointestinal mucosa, including trophic stimulation and maintenance of absorptive structures by nourishing the enterocytes directly, thus supporting epithelial cell repair and replication. The presence of nutrients in the gut, particularly protein and fat,

Table 10–14. Indications for enteral and parenteral nutrition.

Indications for Enteral Nutrition	Indications for Parenteral Nutrition
Swallowing difficulty/dysphagia	Impaired absorption or loss of nutrients
Inability to take oral nutrition for other causes (eg, head/neck cancer, facial trauma)	Mechanical bowel obstruction
Hypermetabolism with inability to take adequate oral nutrition	Need for bowel rest
Mechanical ventilation with functional GI tract	GI motility disorders
Severe malnutrition	Inability to place enteral access or maintain enteral access in place

triggers feeding-dependent neuroendocrine activity. This activity stimulates the transport of immunoglobulins into the gut, particularly secretory immunoglobulin A, which is important for preventing bacterial adherence to gut mucosa and bacterial translocation. Enteral nutrition also prevents villus atrophy, minimizing subsequent loss of epithelial border function and helping to maintain normal gut pH and flora, diminishing opportunistic bacterial overgrowth in the small bowel. In recent animal studies, EN has been shown to reverse the aberrant cytokine profile associated with parenteral nutrition that is believed to lead to enterocyte apoptosis.

When EN is not feasible or contraindicated, then PN should be considered. Parenteral nutrition was developed in the late 1960s by Wilmore and colleagues and remains an important therapy today for patients with significant GI dysfunction and inability to digest and absorb enteral nutrients. Consensus recommendations were recently published by ASPEN addressing appropriate use of PN. Indications for PN include impaired absorption or loss of nutrients, mechanical bowel obstruction, need for bowel rest, motility disorders, or inability to achieve or maintain enteral access. Parenteral nutrition does carry a higher risk of complications compared to EN. These risks include complications associated with the central venous access device and metabolic complications.

In the early days of PN, there was a much higher risk of infectious complications with this therapy. Although there is still some risk of infectious complications, the use of central line care and insertion bundles, avoiding overfeeding, and controlling blood glucoses have had a major impact on reducing the risk of infection with PN. In fact, three large randomized trials comparing EN to PN showed no significant differences in infectious complications. The safety of both therapies has improved significantly, and ASPEN has published safety recommendations for both EN and PN.

▶ Enteral Nutrition

A. Enteral Access

The selection of enteral access devices depends on the anticipated duration of EN therapy. The oral or nasal routes are used for short-term therapies, generally up to 6-8 weeks. Beyond that period, long-term access devices, inserted directly into the stomach or jejunum, should be considered.

Orogastric tubes (OGTs) are typically used in the intensive care unit setting and are most appropriate for patients who are sedated and have a secure airway. In an awake patient, an OGT is uncomfortable and may stimulate the patient's gag reflex. For patients who are awake and alert, nasally inserted tubes are more appropriate. These tubes can be placed into the stomach (ie, nasogastric tubes, NGTs) or beyond the pylorus, either as a nasoduodenal tube (NDT) or a nasojejunal tube (NJT). Long-term enteral access devices should be considered early in a patient's course if it is anticipated that the patient will require long-term EN. The clinician may want to consider insertion of a long-term enteral access device at the time of surgery for presenting pathologic process. For example, one may consider insertion of a feeding jejunostomy tube at the time of esophagectomy for esophageal cancer, or insertion of a gastrostomy tube at the time of surgery for head/neck cancer. Types of feeding tubes are listed in Table 10–15.

Table 10–15. Enteral access devices.

Short-term enteral access devices	Long-term enteral access devices
Orogastric tube	Gastrostomy
Nasogastric tube	Gastro-jejunostomy
Nasoenteric tube	Jejunostomy

B. Types of Enteral Nutrition

Enteral nutrition formulas are generally divided into four broad categories: polymeric, chemically defined (or "elemental"), disease specific (may include polymeric and elemental formulas), and modular formulas. The patient's clinical status, type of feeding tube, cost, and institutional availability are all factors in deciding the most appropriate formula for the patient.

Polymeric EN formulas are generally composed of intact protein (often whey protein, casein, and/or soy protein), complex carbohydrates (some including dietary fiber), and an appropriate fat source to meet essential fatty acid requirements, such as canola oil. Almost all polymeric enteral formulas are lactose free. These formulas are appropriate for patients with normal digestive and absorptive capacity.

Chemically defined, or elemental, formulas are provided in a predigested and readily absorbed form. The protein source is typically small peptides or amino acids; the carbohydrates are often smaller glucose polymers; and a large proportion of the fat is from medium-chain triglyceride (MCT) oil. These formulas are often used for patients with malabsorption or maldigestion (eg, pancreatitis). Chemically defined EN formulas are more expensive than standard polymeric enteral formulas, and are often hyperosmolar, and thus may cause abdominal cramping and diarrhea. Therefore use of these formulas should be limited in patients in whom diarrhea has been a clinical issue. Of note, providing such formulas to those with intestinal failure or short bowel syndrome may exacerbate stool output and inhibit adaptive processes.

Disease-specific EN formulas are designed for a specific disease state, such as those with renal, pulmonary, hepatic, or cardiac dysfunction. Generally speaking, disease-specific formulas have not been shown to improve outcome. Hence, ASPEN does not recommend these formulas because they tend to be more expensive.

Modular formulations may contain one or two macronutrients, as with a product that is only a protein supplement or a combination of carbohydrate and fat to increase energy density of a formula. These products are used to customize an EN regimen to meet the individual needs of a patient.

C. Initiating and Advancing EN

In the past, elaborate protocols for initiating tube feedings were used, including diluting the EN formula and taking many days to get to a goal rate. Now it is recommended that feedings be started with full-strength formula at a slow rate and steadily advanced. It is not recommended to dilute EN formulas because it increases the risk of microbial contamination. A more rapid advancement schedule allows for achievement of full nutrient intake earlier. A typical EN initiation and advancement regimen is to start full-strength formula at 10-40 mL/h, and then advanced by increments of

10-20 mL/h every 4-8 hours as tolerated. Conservative initiation and advancement rates are recommended for patients who are critically ill, those who have not been fed for a prolonged period, and those who are receiving high-osmolality or calorie-dense formula. In such patients, a starting rate of 10 mL/h yields the trophic benefit of enteral feeds without unduly stressing the GI tract. Patients with gastrostomy tubes may be able to transition to a bolus feeding schedule to allow for a more physiologic and convenient feeding schedule. For example, providing 400 mL of enteral formulas as a bolus three or four times a day. Patients who require long-term EN (eg, head and neck cancer patients) may go home on this type of feeding regimen. It is important to note that bolus feedings are not appropriate for jejunostomy tubes, as the jejunum does not have the same reservoir capacity to accept bolus feedings as the stomach. Bolus feeding into the jejunum may cause patients to experience nausea, vomiting, and/or diarrhea if this is attempted. For patients with a feeding jejunostomy who require long-term EN may have their EN infusion cycled at night to allow the patient to disconnect from the pump during the day to allow for activities of daily living.

D. Early EN

Initiation of EN early in the postoperative period, typically defined as between 12 and 72 hours after surgery, may be beneficial. Enteral nutrition, even at low (trophic) rates of 10-30 mL/h, can maintain gut integrity by promoting blood flow to the gut, stimulating release of trophic endogenous agents, and maintaining tight junctions between intraepithelial cells. In addition, EN promotes maintenance of the gut-associated lymphoid tissue, which plays an important role in host immunity. Meta-analysis of early EN studies have demonstrated decreased incidence of infectious complications (including pneumonia and sepsis), decreased hospital length of stay, and decreased mortality. Traditionally, early EN in surgical patients has been through small-bowel feeding, either with a post-pyloric nasoenteric tube or through a surgical jejunostomy. Early gastric feeding could be considered in select patients as well.

E. Immunonutrition

Specialized EN formulas are available that contain immune-enhancing nutrients, generally a combination of arginine, glutamine, omega-3 fatty acids, and/or nucleotides. These nutrients are thought to enhance immune function through a variety of complementary mechanisms.

Arginine is considered a conditionally essential amino acid, with increased demand during times of metabolic stress. It is a substrate for the urea cycle and nitric oxide production and a secretagogue for growth hormone, prolactin, and insulin. Arginine has been identified as the sole precursor of nitric oxide (endothelial-derived relaxing factor). The effects of arginine on T-cells may be very important in maintaining the gut barrier. Formulas supplemented with arginine have been shown to improve nitrogen balance and wound healing, promote T-cell proliferation, enhance neutrophil phagocytosis, and reduce production of inflammatory mediators and infectious complications.

Glutamine is also considered a conditionally essential amino acid. As the respiratory fuel for enterocytes, it plays an important role in the metabolically stressed patient. Intracellular glutamine stores may be depleted by over 50% and plasma levels may decrease by 25% following injury and other catabolic events. The decline of glutamine associated with injury or stress exceeds that of any other amino acid and persists during recovery after the concentrations of other amino acid have normalized. Supplementation with glutamine maintains intestinal cell integrity, villous height, and mucosal DNA activity and helps minimize reduction in numbers of T- and B-cells during stress. Research evaluating glutamine supplementation has been mixed, with parenteral glutamine showing more effectiveness than enteral glutamine. Parenteral glutamine has limited availability in the United States. Routine supplementation of enteral glutamine is not recommended in critically ill patients as a recent review of five randomized controlled trials demonstrated no significant improvement in infectious complications, hospital length of stay, or mortality.

Omega-3 fatty acids are known to modulate leukocyte activity, affect lipid mediator generation, and change cytokine release. These fatty acids are incorporated into cell membrane, replacing omega-6 fatty acids. Once incorporated into the cell membrane, cytokines with a lower inflammatory profile are produced in response to metabolic stress. Little research has been conducted on the use of omega-3 fatty acids alone, but primarily in conjunction with other immunomodulating nutrients.

Nucleotides are precursors of DNA and RNA and are not normally considered essential for human growth and development. The need for dietary nucleotides increases in severe stress and critical illness. Nucleotides are formed from purines and pyrimidines, and their abundance is especially important for rapidly dividing cells such as enterocytes and immune cells. Immunosuppression has been reported in renal transplant patients being maintained on nucleotide-free diets. Dietary nucleotides are necessary for helper-inducer T-lymphocyte activity. Diets supplemented with RNA or the pyrimidine uracil have been shown to restore delayed hypersensitivity and augment both the lymphoproliferative response and IL-2 receptor expression. Nucleotides may facilitate recovery from infection. These substrates are often incorporated into enteral formulas as potential immunomodulators.

Research evaluating immunomodulating nutrients have evaluated enteral formulas containing a combination of the above nutrients, so it is difficult to determine if a single nutrient is most beneficial, or if there is synergistic effect of a particular combination. Immunonutrition seems to be most beneficial in surgical ICU patients, severe trauma patients, GI surgery patients, and traumatic brain injury patients. The Society of Critical Care Medicine (SSM) and ASPEN recommend avoiding the use of immunomodulating products for medical ICU patients and in septic patients.

F. Specialized Formulas

There are a variety of specialized EN formulas available that are tailored for specific disease states. These include specific formulas for diabetes, neurologic disorders, pulmonary disease, liver disease, and renal disease. Formulas are also available for very specific metabolic disorders that are identified in childhood (eg, phenylketonuria). The literature to support the use of most of these formulas has demonstrated little benefit to support the cost of these formulas, except for (1) those formulas designed for genetic-metabolic disorders and (2) renal specific formulas. Renal-specific formulas are volume and electrolyte restricted, and are particularly important to use in patients with hyperkalemia, which can be fatal. In general, specialty formulas should otherwise be avoided, as they are costlier and do not improve outcome.

G. Monitoring EN Tolerance

Assessing GI tolerance to EN includes monitoring for abdominal discomfort, nausea and vomiting, abdominal distention, and stool output. A major change in monitoring tolerance to EN is the approach to monitoring gastric residual volumes (GRVs). Traditionally, GRVs have been used to monitor gastric emptying to determine risk of aspiration pneumonia. Two large randomized trials in critically ill patients were conducted to determine the effectiveness of monitoring residuals. One study randomized 329 patients to holding EN for a GRV of 200 mL or greater (standard practice), and the other, only holding for a GRV of 500 mL. There were no significant differences in ICU acquired pneumonia, days on mechanical ventilation, ICU length of stay, or hospital mortality. The study group received more enteral formula over the course of the ICU admission. A second study randomized 449 patients to GRV monitoring 6 times/day and holding EN if the GRV was greater than 250 mL (standard practice) versus no residual checking. There were no significant differences in ventilator-associated pneumonia, other ICU-acquired infections, mechanical ventilation days, ICU length of stay, and mortality; the study group received significantly more patients receiving their full EN prescription.

Based on these and other data, ASPEN recommends no longer checking GRVs, but if a clinical scenario prompts GRV monitoring, EN should not be withheld unless the GRV is greater than 500 mL.

H. EN Complications

Technical complications occur in about 5% of patients receiving EN. These complications include clogging of the tube; esophageal, tracheal, bronchial, or duodenal perforation; and tracheobronchial intubation with tube feeding aspiration. Patients with decreased consciousness or impaired gag reflexes or those who have undergone endotracheal intubation are at increased risk for technical complications. The tip of the feeding tube must be positioned and verified radiographically. Other methods to evaluate tube placement (eg, air auscultation, pH monitoring) are not consistently reliable. Generally, the wire stylet used for positioning should not be reinserted once removed. The incidence of tube clogging can be reduced by periodic water flushes and avoiding administration of syrup-based medications through the tube.

Functional complications occur in up to 25% of tube-fed patients, and include nausea, vomiting, abdominal distention, constipation, and diarrhea. Feeding the small bowel instead of the stomach can diminish abdominal symptoms. In the critically injured patient, diarrhea is typically multifactorial; it results from polypharmacy (eg, multiple antibiotics), mechanical gut dysfunction (eg, partial small bowel obstruction), intestinal bacterial overgrowth (eg, *Clostridium difficile*), and protein content or osmolarity of the EN formula. Treatment consists of stopping any unnecessary medications, changing enteral formulation (eg, intact protein versus amino acid or polypeptide formula), or reducing the osmolarity of the formula. In some circumstances, adding highly fermentable or viscous soluble fibers, such as guar gum, psyllium, or pectin, has been shown to decrease diarrhea more than using fiber containing enteral formulas. Administering antidiarrheal agents can be beneficial after establishing that infection is not the source of diarrhea.

In the surgical population, *C. difficile* is a common cause of diarrhea due to the routine use of perioperative antibiotics. The diagnosis of pseudomembranous colitis is confirmed by *C. difficile* polymerase chain reaction or toxin assay, or sigmoidoscopy. The primary treatment is stopping unnecessary antibiotics. Additionally, either oral or intravenous (IV) metronidazole or vancomycin (oral or retention enema) can be started. Antimotility agents should be avoided.

Abnormalities in serum electrolytes, calcium, magnesium, and phosphorus can be minimized through vigilant monitoring. Hyperosmolarity with hypernatremia may lead to mental lethargy or obtundation. The treatment of hypernatremia includes the administration of free water by giving either D_5W intravenously or additional water flushes. Volume overload and subsequent congestive heart failure may occur because of excess sodium administration and is typically observed in patients with impaired ventricular function or valvular heart disease. Hyperglycemia may occur in any patient, but is particularly common in individuals with preexisting diabetes or sepsis. The serum glucose level should be monitored frequently (eg, every 6 hours) and regular insulin administered accordingly.

▶ Parenteral Nutrition

A. Central Versus Peripheral Parenteral Nutrition

Parenteral nutrition is composed of crystalline amino acids, dextrose, lipid, electrolytes, vitamins, and trace minerals. There are two types of PN, peripheral and central. Peripheral PN is a low-osmolarity solution, restricted to 900 mOsm/L or less, so it can be infused through a peripheral vein without causing injury. Infusing a higher osmolarity solution peripherally increases the risk of thrombophlebitis. The low osmolarity of peripheral PN relative to central PN protects the peripheral veins, but requires the solution to be very low in amino acids and dextrose. A typical peripheral PN solution may contain only 4% amino acids and < 10% dextrose, with most calories coming from lipid. This dilution requires a large volume of peripheral PN to provide maintenance energy and protein requirements due to the decreased concentration of protein and dextrose per liter. As a result, it is very difficult to meet high-energy requirements with peripheral PN. Patients with poor peripheral venous access (eg, the elderly) may be poor candidates for peripheral PN. Peripheral PN admixtures are typically a strictly defined admixture to avoid exceeding the osmolarity cutoff, which could be harmful to the patient. There are limited indications for peripheral PN due to these issues. If a patient cannot meet caloric needs via enteral nourishment, they will most likely need central PN.

Central PN requires central venous access, as it is a much more concentrated admixture, with an osmolarity well above 900 mOsm/L. Central PN is appropriate for patients with high-energy requirements, need for volume restriction, or poor peripheral venous access who would not be able to tolerate a peripheral infusion. In addition, central PN admixtures can be more easily customized compared to peripheral PN admixtures, primarily because of the limits placed on peripheral PN to ensure that the osmolarity is less than 900 mOsm/L. Central PN admixtures can be customized for a patient's specific energy and protein requirements. Commercial premixed PN products, with defined concentrations of amino acids, dextrose, lipids, and electrolytes are also available and may be appropriate for smaller institutions that may not have the ability to custom prepare PN for individual patients.

B. Home Parenteral Nutrition

Patients with prolonged GI dysfunction may be candidates to go home on PN. The PN admixture infusion is cycled to a goal of a 10- or 12-hour infusion to allow the patient to infuse PN overnight and for activities of daily living during the day. A patient must demonstrate metabolic stability while on PN (including appropriate glucose control as the PN is cycled) to ensure safe administration at home. Since home PN is a complex therapy, the patient and/or care partner must demonstrate ability to manage the therapy safely at home, including appropriate infection risk reduction interventions, to be a candidate for safe discharge on this therapy.

C. Parenteral Access Devices

Peripheral PN can be infused through a standard peripheral venous access device. The duration of peripheral PN therapy is typically 10-14 days. Research evaluating peripheral PN has shown that it is very difficult to maintain peripheral venous access after about 10 days of peripheral PN therapy.

There are many central venous access options for central PN. The peripherally inserted central catheter (PICC) has become a very popular central venous access device given its ease of placement at the bedside. Although inserted through a peripheral vein, the tip ends in the central venous system and hence PICCs are in fact a type of central venous catheter. Other catheters include percutaneously placed central venous access devices, tunneled catheters, and totally implantable ports. Table 10–16 reviews the characteristics of venous access devices.

In general, a lumen on the patient's central line should be designated for PN. This will minimize the manipulation of the lumen, which may decrease the risk of infection. Some practitioners prefer an "inviolate" lumen for parenteral nutrition, meaning a lumen on a central venous catheter that has not been used and will only be used for PN. The literature to support this was conducted during a time when central line insertion bundles were not used, energy delivery was excessive, and blood glucose levels up to 220 mg/dL were tolerated. With the advent of strict protocols for central line insertion, avoidance of overfeeding, and tighter glucose control, the risk of central line infection has decreased dramatically. The most recent Centers for Disease Control and Prevention (CDC) guidelines no longer recommend a dedicated lumen for PN, stating that this is an unresolved issue. Recent ASPEN guidelines suggest the use of a dedicated (but not necessarily "inviolate") lumen for PN, but it is

Table 10–16. Venous access devices.

Device	Typical Duration of Insertion
Peripheral venous catheter	3-4 days
Percutaneously placed central venous catheter	10-14 days
Peripherally inserted central catheter (PICC)	8-12 weeks
Tunneled catheter	Years
Totally implantable port	Years

Table 10–17. Fluid requirements.

Age (y)	Typical Fluid Requirements (mL/kg)
18-34	30-40
55-65	30
> 65	25

Note: Ranges may be increased or decreased based on clinical condition or medical history.

not a requirement. For percutaneously placed central venous catheters, the subclavian vein carries the lowest risk of infection compared to the internal jugular or femoral veins. Femoral vein catheterization has the highest infectious rate and should be avoided for PN, if possible.

D. PN Initiation, Advancement, and Monitoring

Before initiating PN, the patient must be hemodynamically stable and electrolyte abnormalities corrected. Once stable, the patient is safe to start PN. A PN goal is calculated based on the patient's individual calorie and protein needs (Tables 10–11, 10–13, and 10–17) and a goal PN order is calculated (Table 10–18). In general, a patient is started with 100-200 g

Table 10–18. Steps for calculating a PN prescription.

1. Determine energy, protein, and fluid requirements.
2. Calculate calories from protein.
3. Calculate calories from lipid (generally 20%-30% of total energy requirements).
4. Subtract calories from protein plus lipid from total energy requirements; divide that number by 3.4 to determine grams of dextrose to provide.
5. Check glucose infusion rate by converting grams of dextrose to milligrams, dividing by the patient's weight in kg and by the minutes in the day; this number should not be > 5 mg/kg/min. If it is, provide more calories from fat and/or protein to reduce energy delivery from dextrose.
6. Conduct a safety check to ensure appropriate minimum concentrations of amino acids, dextrose, and lipid.
   a. Convert volume of PN to deciliters.
   b. Divide grams of amino acids by volume in dL to determine amino acid concentration.
   c. Divide grams of dextrose by volume in dL to determine dextrose concentration.
   d. Lipid concentration requires more steps:
      i. Divide calories from lipid by 2 kcal/mL (for 20% lipid emulsion) to determine lipid volume.
      ii. Multiply volume of lipid by 0.2 to determine grams of lipid.
      iii. Divide grams of lipid by volume in dL to determine lipid concentration.

For a stable three-in-one PN admixture, amino acid concentration must be ≥ 4%; dextrose concentration must be ≥ 10%; lipid concentration must be ≥ 2%.

of dextrose on the first day of therapy; malnourished patients may start on the lower end because of the risk of refeeding syndrome. Amino acids and lipids are also typically started below the calculated target amounts. As patient stability is established, the PN admixture is generally advanced over the course of 2-3 days until the calculated goal is reached.

Patients receiving PN must be closely monitored during the initiation and advancement process. At a minimum, electrolytes—including calcium, magnesium, and phosphorus—should be monitored daily during the initial initiation and advancement phase and corrected as appropriate. The PN may not be advanced if the patient experiences significant electrolyte abnormalities. These should be corrected prior to advancing the PN toward the goal. For home PN, electrolyte monitoring can be reduced to weekly if the patient demonstrates appropriate stability. Table 10–19 includes typical electrolyte requirements. All patients require IV multivitamins and trace elements.

Glucose control is essential for patients receiving PN, as hyperglycemia is a major risk factor for infection. For ambulatory patients, an appropriate glucose target is less than 180 mg/dL; for critically ill patients, an appropriate glucose target is less than 150 mg/dL. For at-risk patients (eg, those with diabetes, suffering from metabolic stress, or receiving steroid therapy), glucose monitoring should occur every 6 hours, with regular insulin coverage if needed. Regular insulin can be added to the PN admixture; other types of insulin are not compatible. Typically, one-half to two-thirds of the prior day's insulin is added to the PN admixture. Patients with diabetes may need insulin added on the first day of starting PN.

E. PN Complications

PN complications can be divided into three broad categories: mechanical, infectious, and metabolic. Mechanical complications are those associated with the venous access device. For patients receiving peripheral PN or who have a PICC, thrombophlebitis is the most frequent complication.

Table 10–19. Typical electrolyte requirements in PN.

Electrolyte	Requirement
Sodium	1-2 mEq/kg
Potassium	1-2 mEq/kg
Magnesium	8-20 mEq/d
Phosphorus	20-40 mmol/d
Calcium	10-15 mEq/d
Chloride	Based on acid–base balance needs
Acetate	Based on acid–base balance needs

Insertion of a central venous access device for central PN poses more risks than insertion of a peripheral venous catheter or PICC. Arterial puncture (more common in internal jugular or femoral attempts) can occur in up to 10% of patients, while pneumothorax (predominantly during subclavian insertion) can develop in 2%-5% of patients. The risk for injury increases dramatically after three failed insertion attempts at the same site.

Air embolism occurs when negative intrathoracic pressure draws air into a catheter or needle into a central vein. This is most likely in those who have a jugular or subclavian approach and is highly unlikely with PICC insertions. This is particularly serious in the presence of pulmonary–systemic shunts (eg, patients with a patent foramen ovale). It is characterized by sudden, severe respiratory distress, hypotension, and a cogwheel cardiac murmur. To reduce this risk, the patient should be placed in the Trendelenburg position (head down) during line insertion. When suspicion of air embolism is high, treatment involves placing the patient in the Durant position (Trendelenburg and left lateral decubitus) to direct the embolus to the apex of the right ventricle. Catheter-based aspiration can then be attempted.

The growing popularity of the PICC has reduced the risk of some of these major, life-threatening complications. These catheters can be easily inserted in the upper extremity at the bedside with or without ultrasound guidance. Because of the location of the insertion site, the risk of pneumothorax is eliminated. Although arterial puncture and air embolism remain risks, it significantly reduced with PICC insertion compared to other type of central venous access devices. Phlebitis is a risk with PICCs because of the peripheral insertion site.

Infectious complications are a risk of any venous access device (peripheral or central), given the direct access to the bloodstream. Bloodstream infections related to peripheral venous access devices happen rarely; soft-tissue infection (often seen in conjunction with phlebitis) is a more common risk. Daily inspection of the peripheral venous access device is necessary to identify early signs of infection to allow for prompt removal of the device and appropriate intervention to treat infection.

Central venous access devices (including PICCs) carry a higher risk of infectious complications compared to peripheral venous access devices. The CDC makes a distinction between catheter-related bloodstream infection (CRBSI) and central line-associated bloodstream infection (CLABSI). Clinically, CRBSI refers to infection that identifies the catheter as the source of bloodstream infection. This term is not used for formal infection control surveillance because of the challenges in determining if the catheter is truly the cause of the infection. The National Healthcare Safety Network (a division of the CDC) uses the term CLABSI, which is a bloodstream infection in a patient who had a central line within the 48-hour period before the development of the bloodstream infection and is not related to an infection at any other known site.

Patients should be monitored for signs and symptoms of infection including elevated white blood cell count, fever, chills, nausea, vomiting, hypotension, and tachycardia. Headache and backache may also be signs of line infection. The line insertion site should also be inspected for signs and symptoms of infection including erythema, swelling, tenderness, and purulent exudate.

Central venous catheter infection can occur in up to 15% of patients with an indwelling catheter. There may be a slight increase in infectious risk with multilumen catheters, as each lumen can be a potential source of infection. The use of antibiotic-impregnated catheters has been shown to significantly reduce bloodstream infections. As noted previously, insertion in the subclavian vein reduces the risk of infection. The most common offending organisms are skin flora (*Staphylococcus aureus, Staphylococcus epidermidis*), although gram-negative rods can also colonize an indwelling catheter. An infected catheter should be removed in most cases, but in some cases, catheter salvage may be appropriate. Attempts to salvage a catheter may be done by treating with ethanol lock therapy (silicone catheters only) or antibiotic lock therapy in addition to systemic antibiotics. Ethanol and antibiotic locks consist of instilling a low volume of a concentrated antimicrobial solution into the catheter and allowing it to dwell for 12-24 hours before removing. This method would be appropriate in patients with limited central venous access options.

The refeeding syndrome was first described in prisoners freed from concentration camps after World War II. Similar pathophysiology may develop when initiating total parenteral nutrition (TPN) in patients with severe malnutrition. In starvation, energy is derived principally from fat metabolism. With initiation of nutrition support (PN or EN), there is a shift from fat to glucose as the predominant fuel, and rapid anabolism increases the production of phosphorylated intermediates of glycolysis. These intermediates trap phosphate, producing profound hypophosphatemia. Hypokalemia and hypomagnesemia also occur. The lack of phosphate and potassium lead to a relative adenosine triphosphate (ATP) deficiency, resulting in the insidious onset of respiratory failure and reduced cardiac stroke volume. In its most severe forms, refeeding syndrome can result in sudden death. Because of these risks, the rate of PN administration in a severely malnourished patient should be slowly increased over several days. Twice-daily monitoring of electrolytes is also indicated, with repletion as appropriate. Supplemental folic acid and thiamin should be provided to support DNA synthesis and to meet demand for carbohydrate metabolism and prevent Wernicke's encephalopathy, respectively.

Hepatic dysfunction is a common manifestation of long-term parenteral nutrition support, particularly in the pediatric population. The exact etiology is unclear. However, PN-induced hepatic dysfunction is in part related to the initial bypassing of the portal circulation. The form of lipid may also play a role in hepatic dysfunction; a new lipid emulsion comprised of a blend of soybean, medium-chain triglycerides, olive oil, and fish oil may be beneficial in long-term PN patients. Severe hepatic steatosis may progress to cirrhosis. Acalculous cholecystitis can also occur in these patients, likely from biliary stasis and lack of gallbladder contraction. Patients on PN need weekly liver function tests and lipid panels.

Monitoring Adequacy of Nutrition Support

Monitoring for adequacy and response to nutrition support is challenging, as traditional measures of nutritional status are not reliable in acutely ill patients.

Weight trends must be interpreted carefully in the acute care setting. Many patients require volume resuscitation in the early phase of their hospital stay, leading to weight gain that can be attributed to fluid accumulation alone. Patients who experience the refeeding syndrome often experience massive volume overload in the early phase of initiation of nutrition support and may require diuresis back to their prior "dry" weight.

A reasonable weight-gain target is 8 ounces-1 lb per week. Adequate nutrition therapy, as well as appropriate physical activity to promote accretion of lean body mass, are necessary to support healthy weight gain. A reasonable early surrogate to monitor response to nutrition therapy is improvement in strength and endurance as well as adequacy of wound healing. Many patients experience improvements in these areas before experiencing weight gain. Work with a physical therapist with objective measurement of improvements in strength and endurance is an important part of monitoring response to nutrition support.

Albumin and prealbumin are often used as part of the nutrition assessment process, but are unreliable, as previously discussed. Albumin is a negative acute-phase protein and will not improve until underlying inflammation is resolved. Its long half-life (21 days) also leads to a lag in response to aggressive nutrition therapy, and it may take months to see an improvement in albumin levels. In addition, strategies to correct hypoalbuminemia acutely with albumin infusions do little to improve outcome.

Prealbumin has a much shorter half-life than albumin, at only 2-3 days. Because of this, it may show a more rapid response to nutrition intervention. However, prealbumin is also a negative acute-phase protein and is very sensitive to inflammation. Measuring C-reactive protein (CRP) at the same time as prealbumin may help in the interpretation of a low level. If a patient has a significantly elevated CRP with a low prealbumin, inflammation, rather than inadequate nutrition support, is the likely cause of the low level. Serial measurements of CRP and prealbumin over the course of

Table 10–20. Nitrogen balance study.

$$Nitrogen_{(balance)} = Nitrogen_{(intake)} - Nitrogen_{(output)}$$
$$Nitrogen_{(intake)} = g\ protein_{(intake)}/6.25$$
$$Nitrogen_{(output)} = (UUN \times Vol) + 3$$

UUN, urine area nitrogen; vol, volume of urine produced over the time of measurement.

illness may provide more useful information about nutritional status compared to a single measurement.

A way to determine net protein synthesis or breakdown is to conduct a nitrogen balance study (Table 10–20). A protein intake of 6.25 g is equivalent to 1 g of nitrogen. Nitrogen intake is the sum of all of the nitrogen from EN, PN, and/or oral diet. Nitrogen output is the sum of nitrogen excreted in the urine and stool, as well as other losses (eg, exudative wounds, fistula). Urea nitrogen losses are determined from a 24-hour urine collection. Fecal nitrogen loss is difficult to determine; thus an estimate of 1 g/d is used. Non-urea nitrogen losses (eg, ammonia in the urine) are also estimated, at approximately 2-3 g/d. A nitrogen balance of positive 2-3 g/d suggests anabolism. However, it is difficult to achieve positive nitrogen balance in critically ill patients given their high catabolic rates. Therefore a more reasonable target is to minimize nitrogen losses, as it may be difficult to achieve anabolism until the acute illness and inflammation are resolved and the patient transitions into the rehabilitation phase of care.

In general, the need to estimate all sources of nitrogen loss from stool, urine, wounds, and drainage from other areas can make nitrogen balance studies inaccurate. Patients with large insensible losses of nitrogen (eg, severe diarrhea, protein-losing enteropathy, high-output fistulae, chyle leaks, or large burns) are particularly prone to inaccurate nitrogen balance studies because of the difficulty in estimating these losses. Any nitrogen balance study conducted should be interpreted with caution because of these issues. Serial nitrogen balance studies (rather than a single study) may help to improve the accuracy of the measurements and to guide nutrition therapy.

DISEASE-SPECIFIC NUTRITION-SUPPORT ISSUES

Discussion of the nutrition management of all the diseases found in surgical patients is beyond the scope of this review. However, a few of the more commonly encountered conditions are briefly presented.

Burns

Thermal injury has a tremendous impact on metabolism because of prolonged, intense neuroendocrine stimulation.

Extensive burns can double or triple the REE and urinary nitrogen losses, producing a nitrogen loss of 20-25 g/m^2 TBSA/d. If left unattended, lethal cachexia becomes imminent in less than 30 days. The increase in metabolic demands following thermal injury is proportional to the extent of ungrafted body surface. The principal mediators of burn hypermetabolism are catecholamines, corticosteroids, and inflammatory cytokines, which return to baseline only after skin coverage is complete. Decreasing the intensity of neuroendocrine stimulation by providing adequate analgesia and a thermoneutral environment lowers the accelerated metabolic rate and helps to decrease catabolic protein loss until the burned surface can be grafted. Burned patients are prone to infection, and the cytokines activated by sepsis further augment catabolism.

The preferred route of feeding in burn patients is EN, ideally started within the first 6-12 hours post-burn to attenuate the hypermetabolic response and improve post-burn survival. Gastric ileus can be avoided using a nasojejunal tube. Protocols exist to allow for continued feeding during operative procedures to avoid significant interruptions in EN delivery.

Patients with burns have increased energy requirements, and the gold standard for determining energy requirements in this population is indirect calorimetry, as discussed previously. Energy expenditure should be measured at least once/week to guide adjustments in nutrition therapy. As patients recover from their injuries, measured REE should decrease over time. In the absence of indirect calorimetry, predictive equations may be used, applying appropriate stress factors to meet the overwhelming metabolic demand of this injury. Protein requirements are also significantly increased from maintenance requirements. Close monitoring and adjustment of nutrition delivery is required to adjust the nutrition plan based on the patient's response to nutrition therapy and clinical course. Supplemental glutamine should be provided, as it has been shown to reduce mortality in the burn population. Anabolic agents such as oxandrolone may be used to accelerate wound healing in those receiving adequate nutrition.

Renal Failure

Nutrition intervention for patients with acute kidney injury (AKI), chronic kidney disease (CKD), and end-stage renal disease (ESRD) will vary based on other concurrent clinical conditions. Depending on the type, cause, and severity of renal impairment, the nutrition intervention will vary. Most patients will require fluid restriction and may also require restriction in potassium, phosphorus, and magnesium. Patients receiving renal replacement therapies should receive supplemental water-soluble vitamins to replace what is lost in the dialysate. A protein restriction is rarely appropriate, as some incorrectly advocate for avoiding dialysis; and in many cases, particularly after surgery, protein requirements are increased. Protein restriction under these circumstances limits the supply of protein needed to recover from critical illness and increases degradation of endogenous sources of protein from the lean body mass.

Hepatic Failure

Most patients with hepatic failure present with acute decompensation superimposed on chronic hepatic insufficiency. There is a high prevalence of protein–calorie malnutrition in this population. Inadequate oral intake contributes to the chronic depletion of protein, vitamins, and trace elements. Water-soluble vitamins—including folic acid, ascorbic acid, niacin, thiamin, and riboflavin—are especially likely to be deficient. Fat malabsorption can lead to a critical loss of calories in the stool. Fat-soluble vitamin deficiency may be a result of malabsorption due to bile acid insufficiency (vitamins A, D, E, and K), deficient storage (vitamin A), inefficient utilization (vitamin K), or failure of conversion to active metabolites (vitamin D). Hepatic iron stores may be depleted either from poor intake or because of gastrointestinal blood loss. Total body zinc is decreased owing to the above factors plus increased urinary excretion.

Indirect calorimetry is the best choice to determine energy requirements for patients with liver disease. These patients often have significant volume overload due to ascites, with concurrent fat and muscle wasting in the extremities, making it difficult to determine a true dry weight. Use of predictive equations may lead to overfeeding if the volume-overloaded weight is used to calculate energy needs. The use of branched-chain amino-acid (BCAA)-enriched amino acid formulations for EN and PN in patients with liver disease is controversial because the results of controlled trials are inconclusive. The efficacy of BCAA-enriched amino acid formulations for nutrition support therapy in patients with hepatic encephalopathy has been studied in numerous controlled trials, which had contradicting results. Meta-analysis of these studies demonstrated an improvement in mental state by the BCAA-enriched solutions. However, there was no definite benefit in survival. Protein restriction should be avoided except in the short term for patients with grade III or IV hepatic encephalopathy. Standard, concentrated EN formulas or concentrated PN admixtures are appropriate, depending on GI function.

Cardiac Disease

Malnutrition is associated with myocardial dysfunction, particularly in the late stages, and fatal cardiac failure can develop in extreme cachexia. Cardiac muscle uses free fatty acids and BCAAs as preferred metabolic fuels instead of glucose. During starvation, the heart rate slows, cardiac size decreases, and the stroke volume and cardiac output decrease. As starvation progresses, cardiac failure ensues, along with chamber enlargement and anasarca.

The profound nutritional depletion that may accompany chronic heart failure, particularly in valvular disease, results from anorexia of chronic disease, passive congestion of the liver, malabsorption due to venous engorgement of the small bowel mucosa, and enhanced peripheral proteolysis due to chronic neuroendocrine secretion. Attempts at aggressive nutritional repletion in patients with cardiac cachexia have produced inconclusive results. When planning a nutrition support regimen, use of a concentrated EN formula would be the first choice, but for patients with bowel edema, malabsorption may present a challenge. In that case, a concentrated PN admixture may be appropriate.

Pulmonary

High-fat, low-carbohydrate EN formulations used to be recommended for patients with chronic obstructive pulmonary disease (COPD), particularly those requiring mechanical ventilation with difficulty weaning from the ventilator. However, large, randomized controlled trials have not shown benefit with this feeding regimen. Overfeeding energy is much more detrimental to patients with COPD; avoiding overfeeding is a much more important intervention. Indirect calorimetry is the best way to determine energy requirements in this population.

For critically ill patients with acute respiratory distress syndrome (ARDS), a specialized formula that is high in fat, and enriched with fish and borage oils and additional antioxidant micronutrients, initially showed promise in reducing mortality in this population. However, other studies showed no significant benefit with use of this specialized formula. The current SCCM and ASPEN Critical Care Guidelines do not recommend use of this formula at this time in the management of ARDS patients. Volume overload is a major problem in ARDS, so a concentrated EN formula (or in the case of EN intolerance, a concentrated PN admixture) is recommended as well as optimization of serum phosphorus levels to optimize respiratory muscle function and oxygen exchange.

Intestinal Failure

Inadequate intestinal absorptive surface leads to malabsorption, excessive water loss, electrolyte derangements, and malnutrition. The absorptive capacity of the small intestine is highly redundant, and resection of up to half its functional length is reasonably well tolerated. Traditionally, the term "short-bowel syndrome" has been used to describe patients with less than 200 cm of anatomic small bowel remaining.

However, the clinical picture characteristic of short-bowel syndrome is multifactorial and includes several elements in addition to remaining bowel length. This includes the presence or absence of an ileocecal valve; whether the colon is present and in continuity with the small bowel; what portion of bowel has been removed (jejunum versus ileum); and whether the remaining bowel is free of diseases such as radiation enteritis and inflammatory bowel disease. Recognizing the multiple factors that contribute to a patient's ability to achieve nutritional autonomy from PN when GI function is impaired, the term "short bowel syndrome" is being abandoned in favor of the term "intestinal failure."

The optimal nutritional therapy for a patient with intestinal failure must be tailored individually and depends upon the underlying disease process and the remaining anatomy. Following resection, the remaining bowel undergoes long-term adaptation, with observed increases in villous height, luminal diameter, and mucosal thickness. Adaptation to intestinal dysfunction after bowel resection occurs over time, and initial management should be directed at avoiding electrolyte imbalance and dehydration while providing daily caloric requirements through PN.

It should be noted that inhibiting enteral nourishment may inhibit the adaptive response. Hence, when clinically stable and after the primary disease process has been controlled, patients should be encouraged to supplement PN with oral intake. In these patients, dietary management includes consuming frequent small meals, avoiding hyperosmolar foods, and limiting consumption of foods high in oxalate (which precipitates nephrolithiasis). Hydration should be achieved with an appropriate oral rehydration solution containing appropriate amounts of glucose and sodium. The intestines have a sodium glucose transporter that improves absorption of water. Drinking plain water may limit fluid absorption and exacerbate diarrhea.

Pancreatitis

The concept of pancreatic rest has evolved in recent years. Ranson criteria can serve as a rough estimate of the need for nutritional support. Patients with acute pancreatitis who present with three or fewer Ranson criteria should be treated with fluid replacement, pain control, and brief bowel rest. Most of these patients can rapidly resume an oral diet and do not benefit from PN or EN. Those with more than three Ranson criteria should receive nutritional support. Recent data document the successful use of enteral feeding into the stomach or jejunum. Data also suggest that when PN is indicated (eg, for gastric outlet obstruction symptoms), it should be avoided for the first 7-10 days. PN may exacerbate inflammation and worsen outcomes in patients with severe acute pancreatitis who receive PN within the first 7-10 days of hospitalization.

SUMMARY AND CONCLUSION

The metabolic response to traumatic injury and critical illness leads to rapid depletion of endogenous glucose and protein if left unchecked. The response is driven by both neuroendocrine and inflammatory mediators, which makes it distinct from the metabolic response to simple starvation. The key to limiting degradation of lean body mass in the critically ill surgical patient—and the associated morbidity and mortality risk that goes along with such degradation—is an aggressive and comprehensive nutrition management plan. All patients who are malnourished or at risk for malnourishment should be identified and undergo formal evaluation by a nutrition expert who can develop the appropriate nutrition plan. Nutrition support with EN or PN is indicated in those who go without oral intake for more than 7-10 days. Although nutrition support is an afterthought for some caregivers, a comprehensive nutrition plan should be considered an integral component of the overall treatment plan for all patients, as it may improve outcomes.

▶ References

Almeida AI, et al. Nutritional risk screening in surgery: Valid, feasible, easy! Clin Nutr. 2012;31(2):206-211.

Ayers P, et al. A.S.P.E.N. parenteral nutrition safety consensus recommendations. JPEN J Parenter Enteral Nutr. 2014;38:296-333.

Boullata JI, et al. A.S.P.E.N. clinical guidelines: Parenteral nutrition ordering, order review, compounding, labeling, and dispensing. JPEN J Parenter Enteral Nutr. 2014;38:334-377.

Boullata JI, et al. ASPEN safe practices for enteral nutrition therapy. JPEN J Parenter Enteral Nutr. 2017;41:15-103.

Cuthbertson DP. The disturbance of metabolism produced by bony and non-bony injury, with notes on certain abnormal conditions of bone. Biochem J. 1930;24:1244-1263.

Doig GS, et al. Early parenteral nutrition in critically ill patients with short-term relative contraindications to early enteral nutrition. A randomized controlled trial. JAMA. 2013;309:2130-2138.

Duggal S, et al. HIV and malnutrition: Effects on immune system. Clin Dev Immunol. 2012;2012:784740.

Harvey SE, et al. Trial of the route of early nutritional support in critically ill adults. N Engl J Med. 2014;371:1673-1684.

Heidegger CP, et al. Optimization of energy provision with supplemental parenteral nutrition in critically ill patients: A randomized controlled clinical trial. Lancet. 2013;381:385-393.

Kim S, et al. Hypoalbuminemia and clinical outcomes: What is the mechanism behind the relationship? Am Surg. 2017;83:1220-1227.

Langer G, et al. Nutritional interventions for liver-transplanted patients. Cochrane Database Syst Rev. 2012;8:CD007605.

Manzanares W, et al. Antioxidant micronutrients in the critically ill: A systematic review and meta-analysis. Crit Care. 2012;16:R66.

Mattox EA. Complications of peripheral venous access devices: Prevention, detection and recovery strategies. Crit Care Nurse. 2017;37:e1-e14.

McClave SA, et al. Guidelines for the provision and assessment of nutrition support therapy in the adult critically ill patient: Society of Critical Care Medicine (SCCM) and American Society for Parenteral and Enteral Nutrition (A.S.P.E.N.). JPEN J Parenter Enteral Nutr. 2016;40:159-211.

Metheny NA, et al. Monitoring for intolerance to gastric tube feedings: A national survey. Am J Crit Care. 2012;21(2):e33-e40.

Mirtallo JM, et al. International consensus guidelines for nutrition therapy in pancreatitis. JPEN J Parenter Enteral Nutr. 2012;36(3):284-291.

Morris CR, et al. Acquired amino acid deficiencies: A focus on arginine and glutamine. Nutr Clin Pract. 2017;32:30S-47S.

Owers CE, et al. Perioperative optimization of patients undergoing bariatric surgery. J Obes. 2012;2012:781546.

Rahman A, et al. Identifying critically ill patients who will benefit most from nutritional therapy: Further validation of the "Modified NUTRIC" nutritional risk assessment tool. Clin Nutr. 2016;35:158-162.

Weimann A. ESPEN guideline: Clinical nutrition in surgery. Clin Nutr. 2017;36:623-650.

White JV, et al. Consensus statement: Academy of Nutrition and Dietetics and American Society for Parenteral and Enteral Nutrition: Characteristics recommended for the identification and documentation of adult malnutrition (undernutrition). JPEN J Parenter Enteral Nutr. 2012;36:275-283.

Worthington P, et al. Parenteral nutrition: Risks, complications, and management. J Infus Nurs. 2012;35(1):52-64.

Worthington P, et al. When is parenteral nutrition appropriate? JPEN J Parenter Enteral Nutr. 2017;34:41:324-377.

Zhang Y, et al. Perioperative immunonutrition for gastrointestinal cancer: A systematic review of randomized controlled trials. Surg Oncol. 2012;21(2):e87-e95.

MULTIPLE-CHOICE QUESTIONS

1. Which of the following is *not* an indicator of malnutrition?

   A. Unintentional weight loss.
   B. Prolonged inadequate energy intake.
   C. Albumin.
   D. Fat wasting.

2. Which of the following stressors results in the greatest increase in energy expenditure above basal metabolic needs?

   A. Sepsis.
   B. Trauma.
   C. Elective operations.
   D. Burns.

3. Which of the following is true?

   A. Gastric residuals should routinely be checked when administering tube feeds, as this has been shown to reduce aspiration risk.
   B. Gastric residuals of 100 mL should prompt holding of tube feeds.
   C. When gastric residuals are checked, tube feeds should only be held if the residual volume is greater than 500 mL.
   D. Enteral nutrition carries a technical complication rate of 10%.

4. The most appropriate central venous access device for short-term (3-4 weeks) PN is:

   A. Tunneled catheter.
   B. Port.
   C. PICC.
   D. Percutaneously placed central catheter.

5. Indirect calorimetry may be inaccurate in which patient population?

   A. 90% TBSA burn.
   B. Multiple chest tubes with air leaks.
   C. Amputee.
   D. Morbid obesity.

Anesthesia

Theodore J. Sanford Jr, MD
Gerard M. Doherty, MD

Anesthesiology is a "team sport." Providing the best and safest care for patients depends on all members of the team—surgeons, nurses, and anesthesia providers—communicating in a timely, efficient, and patient-focused manner. Anesthesiologists today not only provide patient care in the operating room but also have patient responsibilities in other areas, including preoperative anesthesia clinics (PACs), postanesthesia care units (PACUs), obstetrics, ambulatory surgery centers, endoscopy suites, postoperative pain management, critical care units, and chronic pain management.

Anesthesia is a term derived from the Greek meaning "without sensation" and is commonly used to indicate the condition that allows patients to undergo a variety of surgical or nonsurgical procedures without the pain or distress they would otherwise experience. More importantly, this blocking of pain and/or awareness is reversible. **Anesthesiology** is the medical practice of providing anesthesia to patients and is most commonly provided by a medical doctor, an **anesthesiologist,** either alone or in conjunction with a certified registered nurse anesthetist (CRNA), anesthesia assistant, or resident physician. Anesthesia is most often described as being a **general anesthetic,** ie, a drug-induced loss of consciousness during which patients are not arousable even by noxious stimulus and often require a controlled airway. Anesthesia can also be provided without inducing unconsciousness by utilizing **regional blockade, local anesthesia with monitored anesthesia care (MAC),** or **conscious sedation**.

HISTORY OF ANESTHESIA

One of modern medicine's most important discoveries was that the application of diethyl ether (ether) could provide the classic requirements of anesthesia: analgesia, amnesia, and muscle relaxation in a reversible and safe manner. Crawford Long was the first to use ether in 1842, and William Morton's successful 1846 public demonstration of

ether as an anesthetic in the "Ether Dome" of Massachusetts General Hospital ushered in the modern day of anesthesia and surgery. Chloroform was used by Sir James Y. Simpson to provide analgesia to Queen Victoria in 1853 during the birth of Prince Leopold. This royal approval of inhalation agents led to the wide acceptance of their use as surgical anesthesia. Ether (flammability, solubility) and chloroform (liver toxicity) each had significant drawbacks, and over time, inhalation agents were developed with similar anesthetic effects but much safer physiologic and metabolic properties.

Cocaine's ability to produce topical anesthesia for ophthalmic surgery was discovered in the late 1800s. The hypodermic needle was introduced in 1890 and facilitated the injection of cocaine to produce reversible nerve blockade and later the injection of cocaine via a lumbar puncture to produce a spinal anesthetic and the first spinal headache. The chemical properties of cocaine were soon determined and manipulated to synthesize numerous other local anesthetic agents used to achieve what became known as regional anesthesia, which lacks the unconsciousness and amnesia of the general anesthetics but does produce analgesia and lack of motor movement in the "blocked" region.

Underwood EA. Before and after Morton. A historical survey of anaesthesia. *Br Med J.* 1946;2:525.

OVERALL RISK OF ANESTHESIA

Anesthesia is performed over 70 million times per year in the United States and is remarkably safe. The number of anesthesia-related deaths has decreased dramatically over the past four decades. The realization that most problems are related to airway compromise has led to advanced respiratory monitoring utilizing pulse oximetry and capnography for every patient undergoing anesthesia. Overall, the risk of anesthesia-related death in the healthy patient is estimated to be as low as 1:100,000-200,000 anesthetics.

The combination of amnesia, with or without unconsciousness, analgesia, and muscle relaxation is purposely induced by an anesthetic caregiver and is achieved either by administering inhalation agents in appropriate doses to affect the central nervous system (CNS) or by using specific intravenous pharmacologic agents to produce the same effects as inhaled vapors. These agents include amnestics, such as benzodiazepines (midazolam or diazepam); analgesics, such as the opioids morphine and fentanyl derivatives; the neuromuscular blocking drugs succinylcholine, pancuronium, or vecuronium; and sedative hypnotics, such as sodium pentothal and propofol. All of the agents have adverse physiologic consequences, including respiratory depression, cardiovascular depression, and loss of consciousness. Furthermore, some of these agents may induce allergic reactions. Some have also been known to trigger malignant hyperpyrexia.

The most common problems associated with adverse outcomes still relate to airway compromise, medication errors, and central venous cannulation. Other concerns are postoperative neurologic complications (eg, nerve injury), ischemic optic neuropathy, coronary ischemia, anesthesia in remote locations (eg, interventional radiology sites), and probably most importantly, inadequate preoperative evaluation and preparation.

The anesthesia provider must be able to (1) achieve a state of anesthesia quickly and safely by choosing the appropriate techniques and agents, taking into consideration the patient's medical condition; (2) maintain and monitor a state of anesthesia throughout the surgical procedure while compensating for the effects of varying degrees of surgical stimulation and blood and fluid losses; (3) reverse the muscle relaxation and amnesia as necessary; and (4) return the patient to physiologic homeostasis while maintaining sufficient analgesia to minimize postprocedure pain.

PREOPERATIVE EVALUATION

A preoperative evaluation is a responsibility of the anesthesiologist and is a basic element of anesthesia care (Table 11–1). This evaluation consists of information gathered from multiple sources, including the patient's medical record, history and physical examinations, and findings from medical tests and consults or other evaluations performed prior to the patient being seen by the anesthesiologist. Improved patient outcomes and satisfaction are the result of an adequate, structured, formal presurgical or preprocedure evaluation and preparation performed on all patients.

▷ Timing

The timing of the preoperative evaluation depends primarily on the degree of planned surgical invasiveness. For high surgical invasiveness, the initial assessment should be done, at a minimum, the day before the planned procedure by the anesthesia staff. Patients undergoing medium surgical invasive

Table 11–1. Preoperative evaluation.

Goals
    Optimize patient condition
    Understand and control comorbidities and drug therapy
    Ensure patient's questions are answered
Timing
    High surgical invasiveness: at least 1 day prior
    Medium invasiveness: day before or day of surgery
    Low invasiveness: day of surgery
Content
    Review medical records
    Directed history and physical examination: airway, heart, and lungs
    Indicated laboratory or additional consultations

procedures can be evaluated the day before or even on the day of surgery, and for low surgical invasiveness, the initial assessment may be done the day of surgery. Time must be allotted to follow up on conditions discovered during the preoperative visit and to answer patient questions. Perioperative complications and deaths are most often a combination of patient comorbidities, surgical complexity, and anesthesia effects. The physical status classification of the American Society of Anesthesiologists is the best known of many perioperative classification schemes (Table 11–2). This classification system does not assign risk but is a common language used to describe patients' preoperative physical status. The system is an alert to the anesthesia practitioner and all members of the patient care team.

Patients should ideally be seen in a PAC staffed by personnel who evaluate patients from the anesthetic and postoperative recovery perspective and who look for physical conditions (airway) and controlled, uncontrolled, or unrecognized medical conditions that can lead to perioperative morbidity and mortality. There must be adequate communication between anesthesiology and surgical teams such that any conditions that may result in patient compromise are addressed. Prior to referring patients to the PAC, the surgeon

Table 11–2. American Society of Anesthesiologists (ASA) physical status (PS) classification.

ASA 1 (PS 1): A normal healthy patient
ASA 2 (PS 2): A patient with mild systemic disease
ASA 3 (PS 3): A patient with severe systemic disease
ASA 4 (PS 4): A patient with severe systemic disease that is a constant threat to life
ASA 5 (PS 5): A moribund patient who is not expected to survive without the operation
ASA 6 (PS 6): A declared brain-dead patient whose organs are being removed for donor purposes
E: Emergency

Adapted with permission from American Society of Anesthesiologists.

should have already ordered the necessary preoperative labs and, in many instances, will have already detected uncontrolled medical conditions that require consultations from other specialties in order to recommend management strategies and, in some instances, improve a patient's status.

The optimal preoperative evaluation has the following two elements: (1) **content**—readily accessible medical records, patient interview, a directed preanesthesia examination, indicated preoperative laboratory tests, and additional consultations when indicated; the minimum acceptable examination includes an assessment of the airway, heart, and lungs well in advance of the planned date of surgery; and (2) **preoperative tests**—only as indicated by comorbidities and never as a screen, these tests should be specifically aimed at helping the anesthesiologist formulate an anesthetic plan.

> Practice advisory for preanesthesia evaluation: a report by the American Society of Anesthesiologists Task Force on Preanesthesia Evaluation. *Anesthesiology.* 2012;116:1-17.

History & Physical Examination

The anesthesiologist should specifically ask the patient about previous operations, anesthetic type, and any complications, such as allergic reactions, abnormal bleeding, delayed emergence, prolonged paralysis, difficult airway management, awareness, or jaundice. Each of these describes a possible specific anesthetic morbidity that must be further investigated either by history or specific testing. Medical conditions detected as decreased exercise tolerance, shortness of breath, orthopnea, kidney or liver disease, and metabolic abnormalities, such as diabetes or thyroid disease, should be ascertained. A comprehensive history seeks to identify serious cardiac conditions, such as unstable coronary syndromes, angina, myocardial infarctions either recent or past, decompensated congestive heart failure, significant arrhythmias, or severe valvular disease. Any recent changes in cardiac symptoms or other associated diseases, such as diabetes, renal disease, or cerebrovascular disease symptoms, should be identified.

Any family history of adverse responses to anesthetics (malignant hyperthermia) and social history of smoking, drug use, and alcohol consumption are important. Finally, a comprehensive review of concurrent medications including antihypertensives, insulin, bronchodilators, or any other medications that can interact with anesthetic agents should be documented. Certain medications may result in increased or decreased anesthetic requirements, prolongation of muscle relaxants, abnormal responses to sympathomimetics, delayed or enhanced metabolism of anesthetics, and/or augmentation of the depressant effects of anesthetics. The patient's use of herbal medicines can have an adverse reaction with some anesthetics, and these should be discontinued 2-3 weeks before surgery.

Airway Examination & Classification

After the vital signs are obtained, the physical examination begins with the upper airway. Ability to control the airway is mandatory. The focus of the examination is to assess those factors that would make airway control (eg, endotracheal intubation) difficult or impossible. Seven keys to the upper airway examination should be documented:

1. Range of motion of the cervical spine: Patients should be asked to extend and flex their neck to the full range of possible motion so the anesthesiologist may look for any limitations.

2. Thyroid cartilage to mentum distance: ideal is greater than 6 cm.

3. Mouth opening: ideal is greater than 3 cm.

4. Dentition: dentures, loose teeth, poor conservation.

5. Jaw protrusion: ability to protrude the lower incisors past the upper incisors.

6. Presence of a beard.

7. Examination and classification of the upper airway based on the size of patient's tongue and the pharyngeal structures visible on mouth opening with the patient sitting looking forward. This visual description of the airway structures is known as the Mallampati score (Figure 11–1):

> Grade I: The soft palate, anterior and posterior tonsillar pillars, and uvula are visible—suggests easy airway intubation.
>
> Grade II: Tonsillar pillars and part of the uvula obscured by the tongue.
>
> Grade III: Only soft palate and hard palate visible.
>
> Grade IV: Only the hard palate is visible—suggests challenging airway.

The physical examination then focuses on heart and lungs, potential intravenous catheter sites, and potential sites for regional anesthesia. Range of motion of limbs must also be noted because this may affect positioning in the operating room. Finally, any neurologic abnormalities must be noted.

When a metabolic or physical finding or symptom is discovered during this visit, the anesthesiologist may believe that a specialty consultation is necessary to suggest ways to optimize the patient for surgery and anesthesia. If this is the case, the anesthesiologist should communicate with the surgeon in order to prevent unnecessary or unexpected delays in the surgical schedule. It is imperative that any consults ordered be completed and the results be available by the day of surgery.

The anesthesiologist can then advise the patient on appropriate options for general anesthesia versus regional techniques based on the patient's history, physical examination, and type of surgery. Although some surgical procedures

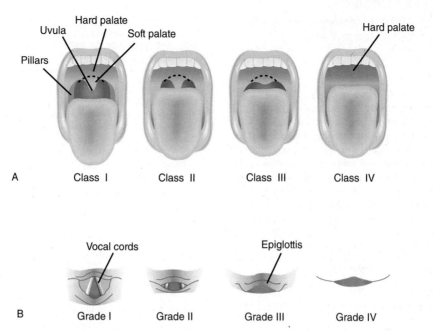

▲ Figure 11–1. Mallampati airway classification of oral opening. (Reproduced with permission from Mallampati SR: Clinical sign to predict difficult tracheal intubation (hypothesis), *Can Anaesth Soc J.* 1983 May;30(3 Pt 1):316-317.)

must always be performed under general anesthesia, the anesthesiology and surgical teams may discuss other options with the patient.

Mallampati SR et al. A clinical sign to predict difficult tracheal intubation: a prospective study. *Can Anaesth Soc J.* 1985;32:429.

Preoperative Fasting

The perioperative process must make the requirements for preprocedure fasting and the management of medications clear to the patient. Current guidelines for routine patients are as follows: (1) Clear liquids, including those prescribed as a part of an Enhanced Recovery After Surgery (ERAS) protocol are permissible up to 2 hours prior to surgery. (2) A light solid meal or nonhuman breast milk should not be consumed less than 6 hours prior to surgery. Fried or fatty foods or a heavy meal should not be consumed less than 8 hours prior to surgery. (3) Pediatric fasting guidelines vary among institutions, so practitioners should consult with their particular pediatric anesthesia group.

American Society of Anesthesiologists. Practice guidelines for preoperative fasting and the use of pharmacologic agents to reduce the risk of pulmonary aspiration: application to healthy patients undergoing elective procedures. *Anesthesiology.* 2011; 114:495-511.

Drugs to Continue Preoperatively

In the perioperative period, patients should continue taking beta-blocking agents, statin medications, and antihypertensives except the angiotensin II receptor blockers (ARBs) and angiotensin-converting enzyme (ACE) inhibitors. Patients taking ARBs or ACE inhibitors can experience marked hypotension with the induction of general anesthesia and respond poorly to common vasopressors. Patients taking anticoagulants such as warfarin, clopidogrel, and dabigatran (Pradaxa) should stop these medications prior to most operations, as directed by the surgical team. The timing and bridging of cessation of these anticoagulants are the responsibility of the surgical service. Continuation of low-dose aspirin for patients with coronary stents or atrial fibrillation is recommended. Oral antihyperglycemic agents should not be taken the day of surgery. Insulin-dependent patients should receive instructions during the preanesthesia visit as to the management of their insulin. Other medications should be discussed with the patient and surgery team at the time of the preoperative anesthesia visit.

Comorbidities

Comorbidities should be well controlled in the preoperative period to avoid postprocedure morbidity and even mortality.

▶ Cardiovascular Disease (Hypertension, Coronary Artery Disease, Congestive Heart Failure)

A. Hypertension

Hypertension is the most common preexisting medical disease identified preoperatively and is a major risk factor for renal, cerebrovascular, or peripheral vascular disease; cardiac ischemia or infarction; and congestive heart failure. The triad of lipid disorders, diabetes, and obesity is classically found in patients with hypertension and should alert the clinician that further evaluation for these conditions is needed. Hypertension has an association with coronary artery disease, and the preoperative evaluation is a unique opportunity to identify and treat the nonessential causes of hypertension. The literature strongly supports the notion that all hypertensive patients should be treated medically to be as close to normotension as possible before any planned surgical procedure. Diastolic pressures of 110 mm Hg or higher result in a higher incidence of intraoperative hypotension and myocardial ischemia. However, the literature does not support delaying surgery if the delay would be detrimental to the patient. The introduction of perioperative selective beta-blocking drugs provides a marked benefit in reducing the incidence of significant myocardial ischemia during the perioperative period. Although somewhat controversial, starting patients on beta-blockers immediately preoperatively may have some risk, but any patient already taking beta-blockers should continue taking the drug preoperatively.

B. Coronary Artery Disease

Ischemic heart disease is a leading cause of death in the United States and is the leading cause of morbidity and mortality in the perioperative period. About 25% of patients who present for surgery each year have coronary artery disease, and thus, much of the preoperative evaluation focuses on detecting the presence and degree of ischemic heart disease and determining whether it is likely to impact anesthesia and surgery. A major goal of preoperative assessment of cardiac status is to determine what, if any, interventions (eg, coronary artery bypass graft [CABG] or percutaneous coronary intervention [PCI]) would benefit patients undergoing noncardiac surgery. In general, preoperative cardiac tests are recommended only if the information obtained will lead to changes in patient management. However, certain active clinical conditions (Table 11–3) demand evaluation and treatment before noncardiac surgery. Determining which patient characteristics indicate high perioperative risk is very difficult, but the Revised Cardiac Risk Index (RCRI) factors of (1) ischemic heart disease, (2) heart failure, (3) high-risk surgery, (4) diabetes mellitus, (5) renal insufficiency, and (6) cerebral vascular diseases are a validated set of independent predictors of cardiac risk for

Table 11–3. Active cardiac conditions for which the patient should undergo evaluation and treatment before noncardiac surgery.

Condition	Examples
Unstable coronary syndromes	Unstable or severe angina Recent myocardial infarction (> 7 but < 30 days ago)
Decompensated heart failure (New York Heart Association class IV): worsening or new onset Significant arrhythmias	High-grade atrioventricular block Mobitz II atrioventricular block Third-degree atrioventricular block Symptomatic ventricular arrhythmias Supraventricular arrhythmias (including atrial fibrillation with uncontrolled ventricular rate [> 100] at rest) Symptomatic bradycardia Newly recognized ventricular tachycardia
Severe valvular disease	Severe aortic stenosis (mean pressure gradient > 40 mm Hg or aortic valve area < 1.0 cm^2 or symptomatic) Symptomatic mitral stenosis (progressive dyspnea on exertion, exertional syncope, or heart failure)

patients. The practitioner in a preoperative clinic should screen for these factors and recommend further studies based on the presence or absence of RCRI factors. Patients with no RCRI factors have a very low (0.4%) cardiac risk, whereas patients with three or more risk factors have 5.4% risk of an adverse cardiac event and warrant further testing. A simple exercise tolerance description of the functional capacity of the patient (eg, ability to climb two flights of stairs without stopping) is a practical screening for cardiopulmonary function. This initial history by the surgeon or anesthesiologist may be the first cardiac assessment the patient has ever had. The assessment of functional capacity may be the first indication of the need for further evaluation of potential cardiac pathology.

The American Heart Association (AHA) developed a useful algorithm for all providers (Figure 11–2). This algorithm, updated in 2014, no longer focuses on stress testing but recommends testing only if the results could have an impact on surgery or anesthesia and lead to changes in patient management. The AHA guidelines state that most patients who have asymptomatic heart disease can safely undergo elective noncardiac surgery without performing invasive or even noninvasive cardiac testing.

Fleisher LA et al. 2014 ACC/AHA guideline on perioperative cardiovascular evaluation and management of patients undergoing noncardiac surgery. *J Am Coll Cardiol.* 2014;64(22):e79-e137.

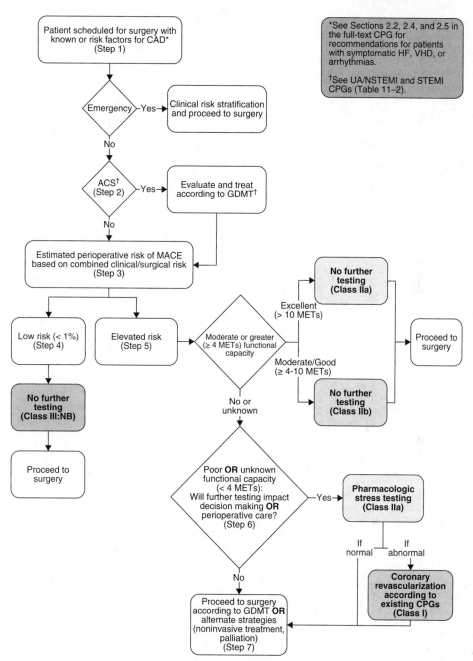

▲ **Figure 11–2.** Summary of the American College of Cardiology (ACC)/American Heart Association (AHA) 2014 perioperative guideline algorithm on cardiovascular evaluation and care for noncardiac surgery based on active clinical conditions, known cardiovascular disease, or cardiac risk factors for patients age 50 years or older. ACS = acute coronary syndrome; CAD = coronary artery disease; CPG = clinical practice guideline; GDMT = guideline-directed medical therapy; MACE = major adverse cardiac event; MET = metabolic equivalent. (Reproduced with permission from Fleisher LA, Fleischmann KE, Auerbach AD, et al: 2014 ACC/AHA guideline on perioperative cardiovascular evaluation and management of patients undergoing noncardiac surgery: a report of the American College of Cardiology/American Heart Association Task Force on practice guidelines, *J Am Coll Cardiol*. 2014 Dec 9;64(22):e77-e137.)

C. Patients With Prior Percutaneous Coronary Intervention (Angioplasty & Stents)

There is much controversy about the best treatment for patients who have had a PCI procedure, angioplasty without stents, or angioplasty with either a bare metal or drug-eluting stent. Because of the risk for thrombosis at the site of intervention, patients are usually placed on dual antiplatelet therapy of aspirin and clopidogrel for 2-4 weeks following angioplasty, 4-6 weeks for bare metal stents, and 1 year for drug-eluting stents. Stopping these antiplatelet drugs for a surgical intervention that falls in the therapy period presents a risk for perioperative cardiac events if stent thrombosis occurs. The AHA guidelines recommend that if the procedure is elective, then the operation should be postponed until the case can be done with aspirin as the only antiplatelet drug. If the operation is urgent, then consideration must be given to the timing of the surgery and the risk of surgical bleeding. If the risk of bleeding is low, then a PCI with a stent should be considered and the patient placed on dual antiplatelet therapy. If the bleeding risk is high, the AHA recommends customizing the timing of the PCI and operation, recognizing the balanced risks of surgical bleeding and coronary thrombosis.

The AHA guidelines recommend several other measures. Perioperative beta-blockade is indicated for patients previously on beta-blockers and may be reasonable to start in patients undergoing major vascular surgery and in patients undergoing intermediate-risk surgery or those with three or more RCRI factors present. Beta-blockade may be started several days to weeks before planned surgery in order to produce a consistent targeted heart rate between 65 and 70 beats/min. The addition of statin class agents, alpha-2 agonists, and calcium channel blockers may also be reasonable to continue if ongoing and to start if risk is intermediate or higher. Left ventricular function should be assessed preoperatively for patients with unexplained dyspnea or who have active or a history of compensated heart failure with changing symptoms.

Levine GN et al. 2016 ACC/AHA guideline focused update on duration of dual antiplatelet therapy in patients with coronary artery disease. *J Am Coll Cardiol.* 2016;68(10):1082-1115.

D. Pulmonary Disease

The presence of significant pulmonary disease is suspected or confirmed by the history and physical examination. Poor functional capacity may be the first indication that further workup may be necessary. The presence of either obstructive or restrictive lung disease always puts the patient at risk for perioperative complications, such as pneumonia and prolonged difficulty weaning from the ventilator. In some instances, arterial blood gas analysis or pulmonary function tests are necessary to determine responsiveness to bronchodilators. Asthmatic patients should be asked about the severity of their disease, hospitalizations, responsiveness to inhalers, and steroid usage. There is no value for routine preoperative chest x-rays. Surgical history and physical examination may be the first indication of significant pulmonary disease, and workup may be initiated before sending the patient to the PAC. Optimally, patients who smoke should stop smoking at least 8 weeks before scheduled surgery. Recent cessation of cigarette smoking may pose a greater risk of pulmonary complication because of the commonly observed increase in cough and sputum production. Patients should abstain from smoking for as long as possible both before and after surgery.

E. Obesity

The national epidemic of obesity poses particular problems for surgery and anesthesia. The body mass index (BMI), the ratio of weight (kg)/height (meters)^2, gives an idea of the degree of obesity. Normal BMI is about 21.6 kg/m^2, overweight is 25-30 kg/m^2, obese is 30-35 kg/m^2, and extreme obesity is more than 35 kg/m^2. Extreme obesity patients have a variety of perioperative issues and should be evaluated in a PAC. Particular attention should include the upper airway and evaluation of cardiovascular, respiratory, metabolic, and gastrointestinal systems. Abnormal BMI patients have cardiovascular issues with venous access, hypertension, cardiomegaly, decreased left ventricular function, and cor pulmonale, and they have twice the incidence of ischemic heart disease than patients at normal weight. Extreme obesity is associated with significant pulmonary problems, including restrictive lung volumes, obstructive sleep apnea, hypoxemia, increased PaCO$_2$, increased hematocrit, and right heart failure. The extremely obese patient's airway is often difficult to maintain with mask ventilation secondary to decreased neck mobility and adiposity and requires careful preoperative evaluation. Almost all the major endocrine problems with extreme obesity involve the effects of diabetes mellitus and require preoperative assessment of glycemic control. Obesity also leads to abnormal fatty deposits in the liver that cause increased metabolism of inhalation anesthetics. Morbidly obese patients may have a higher risk of gastric aspiration and development of aspiration pneumonia. Finally, postoperative pain management must be considered.

F. Diabetes Mellitus

The most common metabolic abnormality is diabetes mellitus, and its presence should cause a high index of suspicion for cardiac problems. Patients on insulin therapy are at higher risk for cardiac morbidity and mortality, including myocardial infarction and heart failure. Glucose control may be very difficult to maintain in the perioperative period, and preoperative assessment of control should always be ascertained through history or laboratory testing. Tight glucose control may reduce infections postoperatively, but it is controversial whether intensive insulin therapy decreases mortality, perioperative hypoglycemia, or cardiac events. Anesthesia providers are responsible for glucose control during the procedure, and the surgical service is typically responsible for this care in the postoperative period.

Hua J et al. Intensive intraoperative insulin therapy versus conventional insulin therapy during cardiac surgery: a meta-analysis. *J Cardiothoracic Vasc Anesth.* 2012;26(5):829-834.

G. Patients on Low-Molecular-Weight Heparin

Patients taking low-molecular-weight (LMWH) for deep venous thrombosis prophylaxis present an unusual problem for both surgeon and anesthesiologist. The current guidelines dictate that unless absolutely indicated, neuraxial anesthesia (spinal, epidural) should not be performed unless LMWH has been stopped for at least 12 hours and preferably 24 hours. That means that a substitute anticoagulant should be initiated if neuraxial anesthesia is to be done, or this approach is avoided.

H. Renal Impairment

Acute renal failure (ARF) occurs in approximately 1%-5% of all hospitalized patients and is responsible for increased length of stay and mortality. The preoperative visit can help to identify patient risk factors for ARF in those with previously normal renal function undergoing noncardiac surgery. The perioperative onset of ARF in patients with previously normal renal function is associated with increased postoperative mortality, especially significant within 1 year after surgery. BMI higher than 32 kg/m^2, age, emergency surgery, liver disease, high-risk surgery (intrathoracic, intraperitoneal, suprainguinal vascular, large blood loss), peripheral vascular occlusive disease, and chronic obstructive pulmonary disease necessitating chronic bronchodilator therapy place patients at increased risk for perioperative renal impairment.

▶ Preoperative Medications

The use of preoperative medications is hampered by the fact that most patients are not in the medical facility until the day of surgery. Most premedications now consist of an anxiolytic agent (eg, midazolam) and an opiate (eg, fentanyl) given in the immediate preanesthesia period. These premedications are often given because patients have a preconceived notion that they need something to relax. Alternatively, a thorough explanation of what the patient can expect in terms of surgery and anesthesia has a significant calming effect comparable to that of medications given to relieve anxiety. Administration of premedication to prevent pulmonary aspiration syndrome is often considered with the use of agents that increase gastric pH (H$_2$ blockers, proton pump inhibitors, antacids) or agents that lower gastric volume.

▶ Informed Consent

Many institutions and practices obtain a signed informed consent from patients for anesthesia, whereas other institutions include the anesthesia consent in the surgical consent. Regardless of the particular facility requirements, the anesthesiologist should write a note in the patient chart indicating that the patient has been informed of the issues surrounding anesthesia and understands the risks and complications as described. The informed consent for anesthesia should include a discussion of what to expect from the administration of anesthesia and possible adverse effects and risks. A number of issues should be discussed routinely, including timing of surgery, premedication, risks of dental injury, cardiac risks, sequence of events prior to anesthesia induction, awakening from anesthesia, presence of catheters, duration of time in the PACU, anticipated return to a hospital bed or discharge, postoperative pain management, and the likelihood of nausea and vomiting. Patients may have questions concerning perioperative awareness. Rather than cause undue worry, clinical judgment should dictate how detailed a description of each of these issues should be for each patient.

▶ Choice of Anesthesia

Considerations in choosing an anesthetic technique include the planned surgical procedure, positioning requirements, patient preferences, surgeon preferences, the urgency of the operation, postoperative pain management, and potential for admission to a critical care unit. Some procedures (eg, thoracotomy) cannot be performed under a regional anesthetic or neuraxial blockade and necessitate a general anesthetic. Other procedures (eg, extremity surgery) can be performed under regional, neuraxial, or general anesthesia. Sometimes a combination of an epidural and a general anesthetic may be chosen with continuation of the epidural for postoperative pain management. Emergency surgery for patients with a full stomach may necessitate a rapid-sequence general anesthetic to protect from pulmonary aspiration. Regional anesthesia may provide anesthesia for hip surgery but may not provide much in the way of patient comfort because of the position requirements of a fracture table. Patient age and preference must also be included in the decision of choice of anesthetic technique. However, some regional anesthesia may be contraindicated for patients with the peripheral neuropathy of diabetes. Notation of the proposed type of anesthesia must be entered into record of the preanesthesia evaluation.

▶ Holding Room & Operating Room

The nurse, surgeon, and anesthesiologist have many tasks to perform, starting in the holding area, before the surgery can begin. The nurse checks the patient in and records vital signs, checks for a signed consent, and starts an intravenous line if needed. The surgeon should confirm and mark the site of surgery. The anesthesiologist should confirm the preoperative evaluation and type of anesthetic selected.

Wrong Site Surgery

In July 2004, The Joint Commission instituted a patient safety mandate known as the Universal Protocol for Preventing Wrong Site, Wrong Procedure, Wrong Person Surgery. All members of the care team must be familiar with and always participate in and perform the following three steps of this Universal Protocol.

Step 1: Initial verification of the intended patient, procedure, and site of the procedure. This step begins at the time the procedure is scheduled and again at the time of admission into the medical facility, anytime care responsibility is transferred to another caregiver, and before the patient leaves the preoperative area for the operating room.

Step 2: Marking the operative site. An unambiguous mark must be made using a marker that is sufficiently permanent to be visible after surgical prep and draping on or near the intended surgical incision site. This mark should not be an X, as in "X marks the spot," but rather a word or line representing the proposed incision. This mark must be made by a member of the surgical team performing the procedure. If possible, the patient should participate when the site is marked.

Step 3: The time out immediately before starting the procedure. A time out must be conducted in the location where the surgical procedure will be done, and all members of the care team—surgeon, nurses, anesthesiologists—must *actively* participate in verification of correct patient identity, correct side and site of surgery, agreement on the scheduled procedure, and assurance that all of the necessary implants and special equipment are immediately available. This time out must take place before incision.

The Operating Room

The anesthesiologist must check the equipment in the operating room before helping to transport the patient. Once in the operating room, the patient is transferred to the operating table with the assistance of the nurses and anesthesiologist. It is standard anesthesia practice to apply monitors to measure arterial blood pressure (a-line, blood pressure cuff), heart rate, oxygenation (pulse oximeter), and ventilation (capnography) before induction of anesthesia (Table 11–4).

The anesthesiologist must be certain that the surgical team is available for the operation before beginning induction. The final time out should then be performed, confirming site, patient, procedure, and surgical personnel.

Table 11–4. Standards for basic anesthesia monitoring.

Parameter	Equipment
Oxygenation: Ensure patient concentration in inspired gas and blood during all anesthetics	*Oxygen analyzer:* Part of anesthesia machine *Pulse oximeter:* Continuously audible variable pitch pulse tone
Ventilation: Ensure adequate patient ventilation	*Capnography:* Continuous monitoring for the presence of end-tidal carbon dioxide
Circulation: Ensure adequacy of patient circulatory function	*Electrocardiogram (ECG):* Continuously displayed from the beginning until leaving the room *Arterial blood pressure monitor:* Measured at least every 5 minutes *Measurement of patient heart rate:* Usually from ECG or pulse oximeter
Temperature: Aid in maintenance of appropriate patient temperature	Oral, skin, nasal, or bladder temperature probe

General Anesthesia Management

Patients are preoxygenated before induction of a general anesthetic by having them breathe supplemental oxygen through a facemask. This affords more time for tracheal intubation before blood hemoglobin desaturation occurs. General anesthesia is commonly induced by administration of intravenous drugs (eg, propofol or thiopental) and, in cases when cardiovascular status is compromised, etomidate or ketamine. Patients receiving propofol may complain of discomfort at the intravenous sites, and patients receiving etomidate may have some athetoid movements that appear seizure-like. Almost all anesthetics are preceded by the administration of an opiate (eg, fentanyl) in a dose that is not intended to induce an anesthetic but that helps reduce the amount of induction agent. Most general anesthetics then include a muscle relaxant to facilitate endotracheal intubation. Tracheal intubation is almost always performed during general anesthesia and is especially important for patients presenting for emergent surgery with presumed full stomach or when positive-pressure ventilation is required. The laryngeal mask airway can also be used to maintain a patent airway. To minimize the time that the trachea is unprotected, a rapid-sequence induction of anesthesia using rapid administration of induction agent and rapid-acting muscle relaxant (eg, succinylcholine) can be utilized. The "crash induction" is a modification of this rapid-sequence technique with the application of cricoid pressure by a caregiver other than the inducing anesthesia personnel.

General anesthesia may also be induced by mask using an inhalation anesthetic (eg, isoflurane or sevoflurane). This method is commonly used for children. Once adequate depth of anesthesia is assured, a muscle relaxant may be administered to help facilitate endotracheal intubation. Inhalation induction takes longer than rapid-sequence induction, and the airway may be unprotected for a longer time. A combination of inhalation agent and intravenous agent can also be used to induce general anesthesia.

Once an adequate depth of anesthesia and adequate muscle relaxation are attained, the trachea is intubated. Ease of endotracheal intubation can usually be predicted from the careful preoperative airway evaluation.

However, the anesthesiologist occasionally encounters an unexpected difficult intubation, and additional maneuvers may be necessary: these can include cricoid manipulation, adjustment of the patient's head position, or use of a long, stiff catheter (eg, a bougie) or a fiberoptic bronchoscope. The American Society of Anesthesiologists provides an algorithm for the management of the difficult airway. If another provider is placing cricoid pressure, the anesthesiologist must directly state what maneuver would be the most helpful. If the airway cannot be secured after multiple attempts, patients can be awakened and a decision made to proceed with an awake fiberoptic intubation or to cancel the anesthetic until further workup can be performed. The most serious complication of endotracheal intubation, and the most common cause of serious anesthesia morbidity and mortality, is the failure to secure the airway. Other common complications are dental injuries, soft tissue injury to the lips, hypertension and tachycardia, and laryngospasm on extubation.

Following anesthetic induction, the patient must be properly positioned for the procedure. It is the responsibility of both the surgical and nursing teams and the anesthesiologist to assure that the patient is positioned to avoid physical or physiologic complications. The American Society of Anesthesiologists Closed Claims study notes that nerve damage from malpositioning during surgery is the second most common anesthetic complication. Careful attention must be paid to adequately protect all potential pressure and vulnerable areas such as elbows, knees, heels, and eyes. The ulnar nerve is particularly susceptible to injury, as is the brachial plexus when patient's arms are abducted too far. Hemodynamics may also be compromised by position changes that may result in decreased venous return and resultant hypotension.

Maintenance of General Anesthesia

Once the airway is safely secured, anesthesiologists commonly maintain the anesthetic with a combination of an inhalation agent, nitrous oxide, opiate, and muscle relaxant. This "balanced anesthetic" allows for titration of agents to maintain the requirements of anesthesia: analgesia, amnesia (unconsciousness), skeletal muscle relaxation, and control of the hemodynamic responses to surgical stimulation. Drugs with specific pharmacologic profiles are chosen to help satisfy the anesthetic requirements. Analgesia is provided by opiates and inhalational agents; amnesia is provided by benzodiazepines, nitrous oxide, and inhalation agents; and muscle relaxation is provided by neuromuscular blocking drugs, inhaled agents, or local anesthetics. The provision of the right amount of muscle relaxation to facilitate the procedure but not too much to obscure a clinical sign of anesthetic depth or to result in prolonged relaxation postoperatively presents a challenge to the anesthesiologist. A peripheral nerve stimulator can monitor muscle relaxation such that the relaxant is reversible at the end of the case to allow for safe extubation.

Regional Anesthesia for Surgery

Many operations require no general anesthetic. These include almost any procedure done below the waist, on lower abdomen, and on the upper extremities. Spinal or epidural anesthesia provides excellent muscle relaxation, profound analgesia, and avoidance of airway manipulation, and allows the patient to be conscious. Spinal or epidural anesthesia has additional advantages: decreased blood loss during orthopedic procedures, fewer thrombotic complications, less pulmonary compromise, maintenance of vasodilatation for postoperative vascular surgeries, earlier hospital discharge, and avoidance of immune response compromise.

A. Spinal Anesthesia

Most spinal anesthetics are performed in either the lateral position or with the patient sitting on the operating table. Following sterile prep and local skin anesthetic, a small 25- to 27-gauge spinal needle is introduced in the lower lumbar spine, and the subdural space is identified by the presence of cerebrospinal fluid (CSF). Depending on the planned length of surgery, either lidocaine or bupivacaine (with or without epinephrine or an opiate) is injected. Lidocaine spinal anesthesia provides at most 2 hours of anesthesia, whereas bupivacaine provides up to 5 hours of anesthesia. However, due to patient discomfort from tourniquet breakthrough pain, the use of orthopedic tourniquets limits the usefulness of spinal anesthesia no matter which local anesthetic is used to no more than 2 hours. Once the local agent is injected, patients are placed in the supine position for 5-10 minutes to allow for proper spread of the local anesthetic. During this time, blood pressure and heart rate are monitored; both hypotension and bradycardia can be induced by a sympathectomy due to the cephalad spread of the local. During this 5- to 10-minute period, patient movement should be limited. Once the block has stabilized, the surgical preparation and positioning can proceed. The anesthesiologist monitors the patient in the same manner as for general anesthesia and administers sedation as needed.

Other than expected hemodynamic changes, the most common complication of spinal anesthesia is postspinal headaches. The incidence is very low when smaller gauge spinal needles are used, and these headaches are more common in young women. The spinal headache is almost always positional and abates when the patient is recumbent. Severe headaches can result in diplopia as a result of stretching of the sixth cranial nerve as the brain sinks from loss of CSF. Patients usually complain of the headache a day or two following the operation. Conservative treatment involves maintenance of adequate hydration, remaining recumbent, and an analgesic such as acetaminophen. Severe headache may require a "blood patch" to plug the leak of CSF.

B. Epidural Anesthesia

Epidural anesthesia has several distinct differences from spinal anesthesia. The epidural space is between the ligamentum flavum and the dural structures; in placing an epidural, the subdural space is not entered, and so no CSF leak is created with the potential for a spinal headache. The epidural anesthetic may be continued by insertion of a small catheter into the epidural space. Additional local anesthetic can be added to move the block to higher spinal levels or to maintain the selected level of anesthesia. This continuous epidural technique can be used for postoperative pain control. The catheter can be placed at spinal levels in the midthoracic region for thoracotomy or lower thoracic or lumbar region for abdominal operations or lower extremity procedures. Epidural anesthesia requires the administration of high volumes of local anesthetics. There is the potential for intravascular injection with resultant cardiovascular compromise or high block. There is also the potential for misplacement of the catheter or epidural needle in the subarachnoid space. Instillation of larger volumes of local anesthetic in the subarachnoid space can result in a total spinal or high block with resultant cardiovascular collapse. Therefore, small test doses of local anesthetic are administered to evaluate for signs of intravenous injection or high block. Another potential disadvantage of epidural anesthesia is that the onset is much slower than with spinal anesthesia. The same hemodynamic changes observed with epidural anesthesia can occur with spinal anesthesia.

A common complication of both spinal and epidural anesthesia is prolonged blockade of parasympathetic fibers that innervate the bladder with resultant urinary retention and the need for a urinary bladder catheter.

C. Peripheral Nerve Block

True regional anesthesia is useful for procedures on the extremities. Useful anesthesia of the upper extremity can be obtained by blockade of the brachial plexus using an interscalene approach, a supraclavicular approach, or an axillary approach. Lower extremity surgery may be performed utilizing blockade of the lumbar plexus and its major branches: femoral nerve, sciatic nerve, lateral femoral cutaneous nerve, obturator nerve, and popliteal nerve. In some instances, a catheter can be placed near the nerve or plexus to allow for continuous blockade and postoperative pain control. The usefulness of these blocks for extremity surgery is limited in time by the use of tourniquets if the patient is to remain awake during the procedure. These blocks are very useful if avoidance of a general anesthetic is desired. Additional advantages of peripheral nerve blocks include earlier discharge from recovery areas and return to home, lack of administration of large doses of opiates, less nausea and vomiting, no instrumentation of patient airway, and earlier ambulation. Intraoperative sedation may be provided, and the anesthesiologist monitors the patient in the standard manner.

▶ Monitored Anesthesia Care

MAC was previously termed *local anesthesia with standby*. The "standby" is an anesthesia caregiver who monitors the patient's status while the surgeon performs a procedure under local anesthesia. The anesthesiologist can also provide sedation and analgesia as needed for the patient. This type of anesthesia is usually requested by the surgeon for patients who may be especially frail in health; it provides the option to convert to a general anesthetic if necessary.

▶ Completion of Surgery

At the end of the procedure, most often patients who have been intubated for the surgery have their muscle relaxation reversed and the anesthetic depth decreased to allow them to return to consciousness. Once the return of muscle function has been assured and the patient is able to respond to commands, the endotracheal tube can be removed and the patient closely observed to ensure adequate ventilation. Patients are then transferred to a stretcher and transported to the PACU, accompanied by a member of the anesthesia care team who monitors the patient's condition during transport. Many institutions require that a member of the surgical team also accompany the patient to the PACU along with the anesthesiologist. Some critically ill patients are transported directly to the intensive care unit (ICU), still intubated, sedated, and ventilated.

▶ Postanesthesia Recovery Room

The PACU, most commonly known as the recovery room, is where most patients are transferred after surgery. The PACU is the designated area in which patients receive postanesthesia monitoring of vital signs as well as the beginning of the nursing care for their surgical recovery. Once in the PACU, a verbal report is provided to the responsible PACU nurse by a member of the anesthesia care team who is familiar with and who accompanied the patient during transport. The surgeon can also give a report as to the surgical issues that may impact on the patient's recovery.

The PACU is equipped with essentially the same monitors as the operating room and with the drugs and equipment needed for emergency resuscitation. The PACU is a specialized, short-stay ICU. PACUs are staffed with specially trained nurses to monitor patients who are recovering from the anesthetic. Patients are continually monitored in the PACU for approximately 1 hour or until they fulfill specific objective criteria. Discharge from the PACU requires the clinical judgment of the PACU team. Particular attention is focused on the monitoring of oxygenation, ventilation, circulation, level of consciousness, and temperature.

Most PACUs use a discharge scoring system (eg, the Aldrete score) describing objective criteria that must be fulfilled before the patient can be discharged from the PACU. These criteria include quantitative analysis of a patient's ability to move extremities in response to verbal commands, adequacy of ventilation (pulse oximetry), circulation (stable vital signs), level of consciousness, and pain control. After outpatient surgery, patients must have an adult to escort them home. Most institutions have policies requiring that anesthesiologists, in conjunction with the PACU nursing team, discharge patients from the PACU.

Aldrete JA, Kroulik D. A postanesthetic recovery score. *Anesth Analg.* 1970;49:924.
Awad JT, Chung F. Factors affecting recovery and discharge following ambulatory surgery. *Can J Anaesth.* 2006;53:858.

COMMON POSTOPERATIVE PROBLEMS

There are many reasons why patients may experience a stay in the PACU that is other than routine. The three most common PACU problems are hypothermia, nausea and vomiting, and pain control. Hypotension/hypertension, hypoxemia, hypercapnia/hypoventilation, and agitation can also occur.

▶ Hypothermia

A very common complication of anesthesia and surgery is hypothermia. Every effort should be made in the operating room to avoid hypothermia in patients, even if this requires that the operating room temperature is maintained at a warmer than comfortable level. Patients who are admitted to the PACU and are hypothermic must be rewarmed to avoid the adverse consequence of shivering (ie, increased oxygen consumption). Hypothermia may also have an adverse effect on coagulation parameters and may delay recovery from anesthesia due to decreased drug metabolism. The most effective methods of rewarming are forced-air warming devices or water-jacket devices. Shivering can be actively treated with small doses of meperidine.

▶ Postoperative Nausea & Vomiting

According to the Society of Ambulatory Anesthesia (SAMBA), untreated, postoperative nausea and vomiting (PONV) occurs in 20%-30% of the general surgical population and up to 70%-80% of the high-risk surgical population.

The increased PACU stays and sometimes hospital admission to control PONV add to patient discomfort and morbidity and add a financial burden to the healthcare system. SAMBA's Seven Guidelines have been adopted by many healthcare facilities for the prevention and treatment of PONV.

1. Identify patients at high risk for PONV. The most consistent independent predictors for PONV are female gender, nonsmoking status, and a history of PONV or motion sickness, coupled with the anesthesia-related factors of general anesthesia with volatile anesthetics, nitrous oxide, and postoperative opioids.

2. Reduce baseline risk factors for PONV. The most reliable strategy is to use regional anesthesia when possible. Otherwise, propofol used for induction; minimization of intraoperative volatile agents, opioids, and nitrous oxide; and epidurals for postoperative pain management may be the best strategy to reduce PONV.

3. Administer PONV prophylaxis using one or two interventions in adults at moderate risk for PONV. The 5-HT$_3$ receptor antagonists (ondansetron, dolasetron, granisetron), dexamethasone, and low-dose droperidol are among the most effective first-line antiemetics for PONV prophylaxis. Each independently reduces PONV by 25%. It is recommended that adults who present with moderate risk for PONV receive a combination therapy for prophylaxis with drugs from different classes and with different mechanisms.

4. For patients at high risk for PONV, SAMBA recommends a multimodal approach to prophylaxis that includes using two or more interventions and trying to reduce the baseline factors (eg, anxiolysis), minimizing the anesthetic agents chosen, and using the pharmacologic interventions mentioned earlier.

5. Administer prophylactic antiemetics to children at high risk for PONV. Use the same combination therapy as in adults.

6. Some patients have no risk factors for PONV and therefore receive no prophylaxis but develop PONV postoperatively. Recommended treatment is to begin with a low-dose 5-HT$_3$ antagonist, which is the only class of drugs that has been adequately studied to be effective for the treatment of existing PONV.

7. If rescue therapy for patients who have received prophylaxis is required, it is recommended that the antiemetic(s) chosen should be from a different therapeutic class than the drugs used for prophylaxis.

Apfelbaum JL et al. Practice guidelines for postanesthetic care: an updated report by the American Society of Anesthesiologists Task Force on Postanesthetic Care. *Anesthesiology.* 2013;118:291-307.

Postoperative Acute Pain Management

The management of postoperative surgical pain is the responsibility of both the anesthesiology and surgery services. Other than PONV, inadequate postoperative pain control is a primary cause of unanticipated hospital admission for outpatient surgery. The severity of the pain is usually site dependent (upper abdominal procedures tend to be more painful than lower abdominal procedures; ie, appendectomy is more painful than inguinal hernia surgery, which is more painful than minor chest wall surgery), but the individual patient's responses to the pain and to the efforts to treat it vary widely. What may appear to be a minor incision to some may be very painful to others. The clinical challenge of providing adequate postoperative pain management is also a major mandate by The Joint Commission and the national media. Thus, almost every anesthesia department has an acute pain management team that can help with the management of patients in the PACU and later in the surgical intensive care or general care unit.

Morphine has been the historical postoperative analgesic, administered either intramuscularly or intravenously. Patient response to a standardized administration protocol is variable, however, and can fail to control pain or cause symptoms of overdosage. Every patient is different in the required serum concentration of drug that results in adequate pain control.

There are four common modalities or approaches to postoperative pain management:

Oral medications. For minor procedures, such as excision of skin lesions, nonsteroidal analgesics may be sufficient. For more intense levels of pain, oral narcotics in combination with acetaminophen are often effective.

Intravenous opioids. Occasionally, one or two intravenous doses of morphine, hydromorphone, or fentanyl may be sufficient to control postoperative pain. However, a more reliable method is the administration of small doses of narcotic given on demand by the patient. Patient-controlled analgesia (PCA) uses the same or even less total narcotic to control pain and is as safe as intramuscular medications. Patients are instructed on how to use the PCA device to administer narcotic on demand. PCA has widespread acceptance by patients, physicians, and nurses because it provides pain control in a timely manner that more closely matches the patient's requirements. Caution must be used when pain control appears to be inadequate and house staff covering the patient are tempted to give an intravenous "boost" of narcotic.

Epidural opiate analgesia. The application of opioids or narcotics at the neuraxial receptor sites via an epidural catheter is probably the modality of choice for severe acute postoperative pain control. An epidural catheter is preferably placed preoperatively at a spinal dermatome level close to the site of incision: midthoracic level for thoracic surgeries, lower thoracic for upper abdominal surgeries, or lumbar for lower abdominal incisions or lower extremity surgeries. This technique utilizes a continuous infusion of a combined solution of a low concentration of local anesthetic (bupivacaine 0.125 mg/mL) and an opioid (morphine, hydromorphone, or fentanyl). This modality does not require patient cooperation but can be used in a PCA mode. Epidural analgesia can be continued for multiple days; it has beneficial effects for maintaining peripheral vasodilatation after vascular procedures and improving respiratory mechanics due to reduced pain when patients are breathing on their own. Patients must be monitored for respiratory depression while receiving epidural analgesia, because respiratory depression is the major complication from this pain control therapy.

Specific nerve or plexus block. Local anesthesia block of single nerves or continuous catheter infusion of local anesthetic around major nerve plexuses is becoming more popular. Examples include single injection or placement of a continuous catheter around the femoral nerve for controlling pain from knee surgery and continuous catheters around the brachial plexus (usually supraclavicular) for controlling pain from upper extremity surgery.

Complications of Anesthesia

No matter how well patients are prepared for anesthesia and surgery, there is always the possibility of a complication from the delivery of anesthesia. These complications can be minor in nature (eg, intravenous infiltration, hypothermia, or minor ocular injury) or major issues (eg, an unanticipated difficult airway that may result in significant morbidity or death). Many complications are preventable with good preoperative preparation, but some are not preventable (unexpected drug reactions or metabolic crisis, eg, malignant hyperthermia). Four common complications are anesthesia awareness, peripheral nerve injury, malignant hyperthermia, and visual loss.

Awareness

Many patients are concerned about being aware during the surgical procedure. Intraoperative awareness under general anesthesia is rare, with a reported incidence of 0.1%-0.2%. Intraoperative awareness does occur and can lead to significant psychological sequelae and extended disability for the patient. Certain types of surgery have a higher incidence of intraoperative awareness, including cardiac surgery, major trauma, and obstetrics. All are associated with critical or life-threatening situations of hemodynamic compromise that make awareness unavoidable if the caregiver is to achieve other critical anesthetic goals of maintaining cardiac, respiratory, and vascular homeostasis. The Practice Advisory from the American Board of Anesthesiologists defines intraoperative awareness as follows: "When a patient becomes conscious when a surgical procedure is performed under a general anesthetic and subsequently has (explicit) recall of these events." The Advisory notes that the recall does not include the time before the general anesthetic is induced or the time of intentional emergence and return to consciousness.

Strategies suggested to lessen or eliminate the risk of intraoperative awareness include the following:

1. Preoperative evaluation. Patients with a history of previous intraoperative awareness, substance abuse, chronic use of opioids for pain control, and limited hemodynamic reserve have increased risk for intraoperative awareness. Such patients undergoing high-risk operations should be informed of the potential for awareness. There is no consensus that informing all patients about the possibility of intraoperative awareness leads to higher incidence of awareness.

2. Preanesthesia preparation. A strict preoperative equipment checklist involving the anesthesia machine and its components (eg, the volatile anesthesia vaporizer agent levels) is mandatory. Although this strategy does not prevent human errors, it does provide the anesthesiologist with a constant reminder that there are preventable components to the complication of awareness.

3a. Intraoperative monitoring. The currently accepted strategy is to use all the standard anesthesia patient monitors (electrocardiogram, blood pressure measurements, heart rate monitors, continuous agent analyzers, and capnography) and to intermittently assess for purposeful or reflex movement to detect intraoperative consciousness. There are instances in which there were no reported changes in vital signs in patients who have reported recall.

3b. Monitoring brain electrical activity. Several monitoring devices are claimed to be able to interpret data from the processed, raw electroencephalogram of patients and correlate it to the depth of anesthesia and thus help prevent recall under general anesthesia. The most common device currently available is known as the bispectral index monitor (BIS; Aspect Medical Systems, Natick, MA). Currently, the use of BIS for patients undergoing general anesthesia has not been shown to offer any advantage over a protocol that uses end-tidal anesthetic agent concentrations in decreasing the incidence of intraoperative awareness.

In conclusion, when awareness occurs, either reported spontaneously by the patient in the postoperative period or elicited during the postoperative visit by the anesthesiologist, the patient's report must be taken seriously. Some patients will require significant counseling and treatment postoperatively, and caregivers should be sensitive to the potential issue and offer any help requested.

Avidan MS et al. Prevention of intraoperative awareness in a high-risk surgical population. *N Engl J Med.* 2011;365:591-600.

Peripheral Nerve Injury

Peripheral nerve injury is a known complication of anesthesia and can occur under general anesthesia or a regional technique. These injuries are almost always due to patient positioning and the patient's inability to report and respond to abnormal pressure points or awkward position of an extremity. The ulnar nerve at the elbow is the most common injury and occurs even if the patient has had what was felt to be adequate padding provided for protection. Other peripheral nerves that are less commonly injured include the peroneal nerve at the knee and the radial nerve as it passes through the spiral groove of the humerus. The peroneal nerve is typically injured by abnormal position against a lithotomy stirrup, and the radial nerve is injured by a blood pressure cuff or abnormal pressure from surgical towels. Patients usually report numbness along the course of the nerve, but some motor weakness may also occur. These injuries usually resolve in a short time period. Abnormal stretching of the brachial plexus from extreme abduction of the arms, improperly placed shoulder braces, or chest wall retractors during cardiac surgery may result in more serious injuries, including not only sensory but also motor loss that may not recover as rapidly or completely as the ulnar, radial, or peroneal nerves. More severe injuries that involve motor loss need to have a baseline examination established and therapy started. Because most of these peripheral nerve injuries are due to malpositioning during surgery, it is the responsibility of surgeons, nurses, and anesthesiologists to adequately position patients and provide sufficient padding or other protection.

Malignant Hyperthermia

Malignant hyperthermia is a rare, genetically inherited disease characterized by intense muscle contraction. It results from an uncontrolled release of calcium from the sarcoplasmic reticulum and massive increase of intracellular calcium in skeletal muscle due to the inability of the calcium to be reabsorbed. This intense muscle contraction leads to a hypermetabolic state manifested by hyperthermia, hypercapnia, tachycardia, and metabolic acidosis. It is fatal if untreated. Malignant hyperthermia is commonly triggered by the administration of anesthetic agents or administration of the depolarizing muscle relaxant succinylcholine alone or in conjunction with a volatile agent. The more modern anesthetic vapors sevoflurane and desflurane are less frequently implicated as triggers. Early clinical manifestations of malignant hyperthermia include unexplained tachycardia and metabolic acidosis, but temperature elevation may be a late finding. Although not always reliable, the earliest sign of malignant hyperthermia is sometimes masseter spasm following the administration of succinylcholine during induction. Careful monitoring must always ensue. Relying on temperature elevation alone is dangerous, and arterial blood gases must be monitored for unexplained metabolic acidosis. In some patients, malignant hyperthermia develops insidiously during the surgery, and temperature elevation can be the first manifestation.

Malignant hyperthermia is treatable and preventable. The treatment of choice is intravenous dantrolene. Every operating room must have a malignant hyperthermia protocol and a kit that includes multiple doses of dantrolene. Dantrolene is supplied as a powder and requires several minutes to mix it into a useable intravenous solution. Malignant hyperthermia is a true anesthesia emergency, and the anesthesiologist will require assistance from the operative team. The surgical procedure may have to be postponed. Successful treatment of malignant hyperthermia is the usual outcome. Patients should be monitored in a critical care unit for 24 hours or until stable and referred for confirmatory testing.

Malignant hyperthermic reactions can be prevented. Any patient with a personal or family history of malignant hyperthermia should be administered a completely nontriggering anesthetic without relying on succinylcholine or volatile agents.

Larach MG et al. Succinylcholine use and dantrolene availability for malignant hyperthermia treatment: database analyses and systematic review. *Anesthesiology.* 2019;130:41-54.

▶ Perioperative Visual Loss

A recently described complication of prolonged (> 6.5 hours) spinal surgical procedures performed in the prone position, associated with large blood losses, is partial or complete visual loss. Vision loss seems to be associated with an ischemic optic neuropathy without any known etiology. There does not seem to be any identifiable preoperative patient characteristic. Intraoperative management for patients undergoing prolonged procedures involving substantial blood loss includes continuous blood pressure monitoring and central venous pressure monitoring. There is no consensus on lower limits of hematocrit, limits of vasopressors, or prone positioning. There is no known treatment. The risk of visual loss should be discussed with patients in the preoperative phase of surgery and anesthesia for those operations that require prone positioning.

Apfelbaum JL et al. Practice advisory for perioperative visual loss associated with spine surgery. An updated report by the American Society of Anesthesiologists Task Force on Perioperative Visual Loss. *Anesthesiology.* 2012;116:274-285.

MULTIPLE CHOICE QUESTIONS

1. Many patients take over-the-counter herbal remedies. In the perioperative period, patients should be advised to

   A. Continue taking their usual herbal remedies
   B. Stop only those remedies that have been approved by their physician
   C. Continue taking only those remedies that have been approved by the US Food and Drug Administration (FDA)
   D. Stop all over-the-counter herbal remedies

2. Which of the following is true regarding the timing of the preoperative anesthesia workup for patients scheduled for a surgical procedure?

   A. The initial assessment can be done the day of surgery for healthy patients undergoing procedures of high surgical invasiveness.
   B. The initial assessment should be done at a minimum the day before surgery for patients undergoing procedures of high surgical invasiveness.
   C. Preoperative assessment of healthy patients by an anesthesiologist is not required.
   D. A note from the patient's primary care physician stating that the patient is "cleared for anesthesia and surgery" will suffice as the preoperative assessment.

3. Which of the following is true regarding patients who have had a recent drug-eluting stent placed and are scheduled for an elective surgical procedure with a high risk of bleeding?

   A. Surgery may be performed within 4 weeks of stent placement as long as the patient continues taking aspirin and clopidogrel.
   B. Surgery may be performed within 4 weeks of stent placement with the patient stopping the clopidogrel and continuing on low-dose aspirin.
   C. Patients should have the surgical procedure delayed until the procedure can be performed with patients only taking low-dose aspirin.
   D. Surgery should be delayed for 1 year.

4. Strategies to prevent intraoperative awareness include which of the following?

   A. Strict monitoring of intraoperative vital signs by the anesthesiologist to detect intraoperative awareness
   B. Informing patients during the preoperative workup of the possibility of awareness
   C. Monitoring brain electrical activity with the bispectral index monitor (BIS) monitor
   D. None of the above

5. The preoperative assessment by an anesthesiologist includes an assessment of a patient's risk for an intraoperative cardiac event. The Revised Cardiac Risk Index factors include all of the following except

   A. A history of ischemic heart disease
   B. Diabetes mellitus
   C. Obesity
   D. Renal insufficiency
   E. High-risk surgery
   F. Heart failure

Shock in Surgical Patients

Anupamaa Seshadri, MD

Joaquim M. Havens, MD

INITIAL TREATMENT OF SHOCK

Cardiovascular failure, or shock, can be caused by (1) depletion of intravascular volume, (2) compression of the heart or great veins, (3) intrinsic failure of the heart itself or failure arising from excessive hindrance to ventricular ejection, (4) loss of autonomic control of the vasculature, (5) severe untreated systemic inflammation, and (6) severe but partially compensated systemic inflammation. If the shock is decompensated, the mean arterial pressure or the cardiac output (more precisely, the product of the pressure and output) will be inadequate for peripheral perfusion; in compensated shock, perfusion will be adequate but at the expense of excessive demands on the heart. Depending on the type and severity of cardiovascular failure and on response to treatment, shock can go on to compromise other organ systems. This chapter discusses the cardiovascular and pulmonary disorders associated with shock.

HYPOVOLEMIC SHOCK

▶ Diagnosis

Hypovolemic shock (shock caused by inadequate circulating blood volume) is most often caused by bleeding but may also be a consequence of protracted vomiting or diarrhea, sequestration of fluid in the gut lumen (eg, bowel obstruction), or loss of plasma into injured or burned tissues. Regardless of the etiology, the compensatory responses, mediated primarily by the adrenergic nervous system, are the same: (1) constriction of the venules and small veins in the skin, fat, skeletal muscle, and viscera with displacement of blood from the peripheral capacitance vessels to the heart; (2) constriction of arterioles in the skin, skeletal muscle, gut, pancreas, spleen, and liver (but not the brain or heart); (3) improved cardiac performance through an increase in heart rate and contractility; and (4) increased sodium and water reabsorption through the renin–angiotensin–aldosterone axis as well

as vasopressin release. The result is improved cardiac filling, increased cardiac output (both directly by the increase in contractility and indirectly through increased end-diastolic volumes), and increased blood flow to organs with no or limited tolerance for ischemia (brain and heart).

The symptoms and signs of hypovolemic shock are many and can be caused either by the inadequate blood volume or by the compensatory responses. Some signs manifest themselves early, in mild forms of shock. Some present late and only in severe forms of shock. The goal is to recognize the early signs to prevent morbidity and mortality.

The most sensitive of the early signs of hypovolemic shock is diminished blood flow to the skin and subcutaneous tissues. This can be noted on casual assessment by noting difficulty with peripheral intravenous (IV) access or skin coolness, but is objectively assessed by documentation of capillary refill. This is best performed in the skin on the plantar surface of the foot, an area without pigmentation, with the color determined solely by the blood contained in the tissues. One begins by compressing the skin over the plantar surface of a toe with intense pressure, followed by milking of the blood contained in the compressed area proximally, to the skin over the metatarsal phalangeal joint. The compression is then suddenly released. The previously compressed area will be profoundly pale, but will fill quickly, within a few seconds, if the patient is not in shock (and does not have peripheral vascular disease). In a hypovolemic patient, the refill takes longer. The test is usually done with the foot at the level of the heart, but if the patient is reasonably stable and if the lower extremities are not injured, it is more sensitive if it can be done with the foot raised above the level of the heart, to a height of perhaps 30 cm. Although the toe is usually used, one can also use the skin over the heel. The heel affords a larger surface for observation but requires different criteria for assessment. If the toe is used, color should begin to return within 4 seconds; if the heel is used, color should return in 2 seconds.

Orthostatic hypotension—defined as a fall in the systolic blood pressure of more than 20 mm Hg or diastolic blood pressure of more than 10 mm Hg within 3 minutes of standing—can be a sign of early or mild shock. It is very useful in patients who are suspected of being hypovolemic from either dehydration or occult internal blood loss (eg, in a patient who might have gastrointestinal bleeding). It cannot be used, however, in very ill patients and in injured patients, who might not tolerate changes in position.

Low filling pressures in the right atrium are always present in hypovolemic shock, even in cases of mild shock, assuming there is no accompanying cardiac compression. Filling pressures high enough to distend the neck veins when the patient's head, neck, and torso are elevated 30 degrees, in the absence of cardiac compression, rule out hypovolemic shock. Failure to see the veins suggests, but is not diagnostic of, hypovolemia.

Oliguria is a consistent sensitive and specific finding in early shock, in the absence of a hyperosmolar-induced diuresis. A bladder catheter should be inserted in any patient suspected of being hypovolemic. Urine output is considered to be inadequate if it is less than 0.5 mL/kg/h in an adult, less than 1 mL/kg/h in a child, or less than 2 mL/kg/h in an infant.

The hematocrit will fall within minutes in the bleeding patient, even when the blood loss is mild, if the patient has been given asanguineous fluids. In the absence of fluid administration, however, the fall can take hours—restitution of the intravascular volume from interstitial albumin and water and electrolytes takes time. One can make an estimate of the blood loss, if the patient has been given asanguineous fluids, by the magnitude of the fall in the hematocrit. A hematocrit fall of 3%-4% indicates that the blood volume was depleted by about 10%; a fall of 6%-8% indicates a depletion of about 20% (or 1 L in an average adult). These calculations assume that the patient has been given enough fluid to correct the hypovolemia. They also assume that the patient was not dehydrated prior to the hemorrhage, and that the patient did not have large loses of plasma into the extravascular spaces, as in a patient with large burns prior to a possible hemorrhage. The hematocrit in these patients can be normal in the face of even substantial bleeding.

Hypovolemic shock is easier to recognize when it becomes more severe. In moderate cases (a deficit of 20%-30% of the blood volume), the patient can be thirsty. Hypotension can be present, even in the supine position. A metabolic acidemia, usually with a compensatory rapid respiratory rate, can develop after initial resuscitation. (The acidemia is usually not present before resuscitation. The products of anaerobic metabolism in the ischemic tissues are only flushed into the circulating blood volume once some degree of reperfusion has been achieved.)

In profound hypovolemic shock (a deficit of more than 30% of blood volume), the blood pressure will always be low, even in the supine position. Cerebral and cardiac perfusion can become inadequate. Signs of the former include changes in mental status, restlessness, agitation, confusion, lethargy, or the appearance of inebriation; signs of the latter include an irregular heartbeat or electrocardiographic evidence of myocardial ischemia, such as ST–T segment depression and, over time, the appearance of Q-waves. A metabolic acidemia will always be present after initial resuscitation.

There are many pitfalls in making the diagnosis of hypovolemic shock. In some patients, especially children and young adults, strong compensatory mechanisms can maintain the blood pressure at normal levels in the setting of mild to moderate shock. In other patients, one might not know if the observed pressure is abnormally low—a young patient might normally have systolic pressures in the low 100s; the same pressure in a chronically hypertensive patient might precede catastrophe. Pain-producing injuries in the absence of blood loss should produce hypertension; a normal pressure in a patient with a pain-producing injury suggests hypovolemia. Administration of a sedative or narcotic in the face of hypovolemia can produce hypotension but usually has no effect on the pressure in a normovolemic subject; one should not ascribe hypotension to sedatives or narcotics until the possibility of hypovolemia has been ruled out.

The heart rate is notoriously unreliable as a sign of hypovolemic shock. Although it increases in response to graded hemorrhage in anesthetized animals, the correlation between hypovolemia and heart rate in unanesthetized human beings is poor. Unanesthetized hypovolemic human beings often have normal heart rates. Severe hypovolemia can even produce bradycardia, as the cardiovascular system makes a last attempt to allow filling of the ventricles during diastole. A normal heart rate provides no assurance that the patient is not in shock. (A rapid heart rate, however, must be taken seriously, as it might be the only indication of shock. The pitfall is in the assumption that a normal heart rate rules out shock.)

There are at least three other pitfalls that can lead to missing the diagnosis of shock: (1) the cutaneous vasoconstriction of hypovolemic shock can be ablated by the vasodilation induced by alcohol or other pharmacologic agents, both therapeutic and recreational; the patient might have well-perfused skin even when hypovolemic. (2) The oliguria of shock can be overcome by an osmotic diuresis induced by high blood alcohol or glucose levels. And finally (3), shock can cause alterations in mental status that resemble intoxication with drug use or inebriation. If so, the patient might be in a preterminal state, in which the shock is so severe that cerebral blood flow becomes inadequate. The diagnosis of drug or alcohol use, as the cause of the mental abnormalities, should only be made after shock has been ruled out.

▶ Treatment

A. Airway and Ventilation

Resuscitation of patients in hypovolemic shock, either hemorrhagic or nonhemorrhagic, begins with ensuring adequacy of the airway. In many patients in shock, especially severe shock, this means preemptive intubation and mechanical ventilation. The physician cannot let uncertainty about the airway interfere with evaluation and resuscitation of other problems in the often-confusing picture of shock. A patient who later turns out to need no support for the airway or ventilation can typically easily be extubated; failure to intubate a patient who later loses control of an airway or who can no longer ventilate means, at the least, an emergency intubation under difficult conditions and, at the worse, anoxic brain damage or death.

If the patient requires mechanical ventilation (and almost all patients intubated for shock do), volume-control ventilation, or some variant thereof, is preferable in the initial phases of resuscitation (in the latter phases, pressure-modulated ventilation is typically used—see the section in this chapter on treatment of acute pulmonary failure).

Airway management is critically important and cannot be delayed. However, it is important for the clinician to know that a patient in profound hemorrhagic shock can suddenly deteriorate, to the point of losing his vital signs, with intubation and initiation of positive-pressure ventilation. Positive-pressure ventilation can have negative effects on the cardiovascular system in the face of hypovolemia. The positive pressure compresses the superior and inferior venae cavae, increasing the time needed to fill the right atrium and right ventricle during diastole. (Normal negative pressure ventilation, spontaneous ventilation, decreases the time needed.) Positive pressure squeezes the thin-walled chambers of the heart (the atria and the right ventricle), making it harder for the chambers to fill during diastole. (Negative pressure ventilation makes it easier for the chambers to fill.) Positive pressure squeezes the pulmonary arteries, pulmonary microvasculature, and pulmonary veins, making it hard for the right ventricle to transmit its generated energy into the pulmonary arteries. (Negative pressure makes it easier to transmit the energy.) Positive-pressure ventilation also compresses the pulmonary veins, mandating longer times for the left atrium to fill during diastole. (Negative pressure allows for quicker filling.)

In an ideal situation, if the patient loses his vital signs in the operating room with intubation, the surgeon and anesthesiologist would be situated to deal definitively with the underlying problems of hemorrhage and airway management. However, in cases where a patient must be intubated in the emergency department, the team needs to be aware of the potential for cardiovascular collapse and should both discuss and prepare for this event prior to intubation.

B. Bleeding

Direct pressure should be the first maneuver in controlling external bleeding from any part of the body. Commercially available tourniquets or improvised pneumatic tourniquets can be used for bleeding from extremities. They are easy to apply and are usually safe for up to 2 hours, with the caveat that bleeding should be controlled quickly to minimize tourniquet time. Several commercially available, FDA-approved hemostatic agents are available for temporary control of external bleeding. They have been proven to be effective in prehospital and combat environments and can be effective in the hospital setting as well. Blood in the pleural cavities should be drained with a chest tube. Expansion of the lung will decrease further bleeding from the pulmonary parenchyma through apposition of the visceral and parietal pleurae and will reestablish ventilation through the compressed lung. The tube will also allow monitoring for ongoing bleeding, providing key information that can prompt early operative intervention. Bleeding from open book pelvic fractures may require temporary pelvic binder placement, with plan for more definitive control using angiographic embolization or surgical control. Major long-bone fractures should be immobilized. Any unstable patient with intra-abdominal or intrathoracic bleeding should immediately proceed to the operating room.

Blind clamping without direct visualization in the emergency room should not be attempted in the initial control of external bleeding. It can result in worsened target vessel injury or adjacent venous laceration with increased bleeding.

C. Initial Fluid Resuscitation

Vascular access is best obtained with percutaneously placed, large-bore (ideally 16-gauge or larger) venous catheters. The catheters can be placed in superficial veins in the upper extremities, in central veins at the thoracic outlet, or in the femoral veins. Catheters can also be placed in the saphenous veins by cutdown, or directly into interosseus sites (sternum, tibia, or humerus) using specially designed needle introducer systems (FAST-1, EZ IO). The major advantage of the intraosseous introducer devices is that minimal training is required to achieve successful access. Choice of access depends on severity of the shock, pattern of injury, provider experience, and consequences of a complication with the access. Gaining central venous access should be done carefully and with ultrasound guidance whenever possible, as patients in hypovolemic shock will frequently have collapsed central veins, making placement more difficult.

Initial fluid resuscitation begins with a warmed crystalloid solution. Either normal saline or lactated Ringer's solution can be used. Use of lactate in the resuscitative fluid is reasonable if the shock seems to be severe and if the arterial pH is likely to be less than 7.20. The lactate will buffer the hydrogen ions that are released into the central circulation with the initiation of resuscitation. The resultant lactic acid is then oxidized in the liver to carbon dioxide and water, which are excreted by the lungs and kidneys.

If the arterial pH is not likely to be excessively low, normal saline can be used as the initial resuscitative fluid. A modest hyperchloremic acidemia in the immediate post-resuscitative state might favorably change the conformation of albumin molecules, decreasing movement of plasma into the interstitium. The acidemia might also increase myocardial contractility.

Blood flow to the liver is not a factor in deciding on lactated Ringer's versus normal saline. Even minimal flow, as in severe shock, will be enough to deliver the buffered hydrogen ion to the liver parenchyma. Lactated Ringer's should not be used, however, if the patient has preexisting liver disease. Adequate oxidation requires functioning liver cells.

The rate at which the initial crystalloid resuscitation should be given depends on two factors: the severity of the shock and the presence of uncontrolled bleeding. When bleeding has been controlled, resuscitation to normovolemia is the goal. Advanced Trauma Life Support (ATLS) guidelines recommend 1-2 L of initial fluid bolus in the bleeding patient. If the patient does not hemodynamically respond to this initial crystalloid challenge, blood transfusion should be initiated; blood transfusion can also be considered earlier in a patient who you suspect may need massive transfusion.

D. Blood Products

Transfusion therapy can be lifesaving, but it is not without risk. Transfusion reactions, transmission of blood-borne pathogens, acute lung injury, and immunomodulation can all arise from the administration of blood products. In the acutely bleeding patient, allogeneic packed red cells should be used when the estimated blood loss exceeds 1.5 L (30% of the blood volume), and possibly earlier if there is the potential for ongoing bleeding or if the patient is at risk for having coronary artery disease (see Table 12–1).

In urgent settings, type-O blood should be given to restore circulating blood volume. Rh-positive blood can be given to men and women who are beyond childbearing age; Rh-negative blood must be used in women of childbearing age. The patient's blood type can be determined within 10 minutes in most hospitals, and type-specific, cross-matched red cells should be used when they become available (except in the case of massive casualties, when type O, Rh-negative universal donor cells should be used, to minimize the chance of giving the wrong type of blood to a misidentified patient). Type specific cells should also be used in the setting of massive transfusion, when cross-matching becomes impossible because of the heterogeneous origin of the circulating cells following rapid blood volume replacement.

If resuscitation is ongoing and if it appears that the transfusion requirement is likely to equal or exceed 6 units of packed red blood cells (PRBCs), plasma and platelets should be given in amounts sufficient to approximate a 1:1:1 ratio. This should be determined as early as possible to avoid dilutional coagulopathy. "Massive transfusion protocols" can maximize efficient use of blood products through the utilization of predetermined component ratios, bedside

Table 12–1. Hematocrit triggers for transfusion: Influence of Coronary Artery Disease (CAD), environment in which patient is being treated (emergency department versus intensive care unit), and likelihood of bleeding.

Coronary Artery Disease (CAD)	Environment	Likelihood of Bleeding	Desired Hematocrit (%)
No	ICU	Unlikely	21
No	ICU	Possible	21
No	ED	Unlikely	24
No	ED	Possible	27
Yes	ICU	Unlikely	27[1]
Yes	ICU	Possible	30[2]
Yes	ED	Unlikely	33[2]
Yes	ED	Possible	36[2]

[1]Hematocrit values less than 27% may be sufficient in some patients with treated CAD when there is no risk of bleeding.
[2]Hematocrit values greater than 30% generally serve as a buffer for unanticipated or unmeasurable bleeding. They are not necessary in all patients with CAD.

refrigeration, and in some cases, protocol-driven laboratory monitoring. Crystalloid infusion can be restricted in the case of massive transfusions.

E. Goals of Fluid Resuscitation

Giving excessive amounts of fluids to restore the blood pressure to normal or supranormal levels will create edema. Edema in the gut can create an abdominal compartment syndrome, with compression of the inferior vena cava (IVC), displacement of the diaphragm into the chest, and compression of the heart and lungs. Edema in the liver can lead to compression of biliary ductules and inability to excrete bilirubin into the gut. Edema in the lungs can hinder ventilation and oxygenation. Edema in wounded tissues can impede healing and the ability to fight off infection. Unnecessarily high blood pressures can also potentially exacerbate bleeding. On the other hand, inadequate resuscitation can leave the patient exposed to the many adverse late effects of prolonged shock, such as multiorgan failure.

The primary goal in fluid resuscitation for all forms of shock is the same: restoration of adequate end-organ perfusion, the product of the mean pressure perfusing the organ and the blood flow to the organ. Resuscitating to a brachial systolic pressure of 80 mm Hg or a radial pulse in the bleeding patient is reasonable until hemorrhage has been controlled. (The treating physician will not know the cardiac output or organ blood flow in the early phases of resuscitation, but he or she can use clinical criteria, such as skin perfusion, urine output, and mental status, in managing the patient, along with the blood pressure.) After the bleeding is controlled, a systolic pressure of 90 mm Hg might be reasonable. In the very old, the blood pressure goal should be higher to ensure a cushion of perfusion for the brain, heart, and other viscera that might be supplied by arteries obstructed by atherosclerosis.

One must keep in mind during the resuscitation, however, that using the blood pressure to define severity of shock or to assess the adequacy of resuscitation can be hazardous. Most patients in hypovolemic shock will be able to constrict the arterioles in their skin, muscle, and visceral organs in response to the hypovolemia (the exception being inebriated patients). They can often maintain a normal pressure even in the face of continued shock. One must consider many variables in assessing adequacy of resuscitation, including peripheral perfusion, urine output, mental status, acid–base balance, and resolution of any signs of myocardial ischemia.

F. Correction of Coagulation Abnormalities

After severe trauma or major sepsis, many patients will demonstrate signs of intravascular coagulation, with prolonged clotting times, low platelet counts, decreased fibrinogen levels, and production of fibrin degradation products or fibrin monomers. Correction requires administration of plasma and platelets, especially to patients who continue to bleed and to those with severe head injuries with intracranial hemorrhage.

Traditional replacement of coagulation factors has been done with thawed frozen plasma. The advantages of frozen plasma are logistic; the disadvantage is that it must be thawed prior to use, which may take from 30 to 60 minutes. Increasingly, trauma centers are using either pre-thawed plasma or "liquid" plasma that has never been frozen. The advantage of the former is that the product does not have to be thawed; the major disadvantage is the potential for waste. "Liquid" plasma has the potential advantage of increased factor activity with the disadvantage of waste. Finally, there has been interest in developing freeze-dried plasma (FDP), particularly by the military. Although the Europeans have extensive experience with the product (it is approved for use in Europe), there is currently no FDA-approved formulation in the United States.

Recently there has been discussion of not only providing red blood cells in the prehospital setting, but also using prehospital plasma. In the PAMPER trial, there was approximately a 10% improvement in mortality in injured patients at risk for hemorrhagic shock who received thawed plasma in the prehospital setting.

Over the last decade, pharmacologic therapy for hemorrhage-related coagulopathy has become a standard adjunct in the setting of hemorrhagic shock. Kcentra, or prothrombin complex concentrate (PCC), is a four-factor concentrate of factors II, VII, IX, and X, as well as protein C and protein S. It can be given to patients on warfarin requiring urgent reversal, including in massive hemorrhage or intracranial bleeding, who cannot wait for the infusion time of FFP or cannot tolerate the volume of FFP.

Tranexamic acid (TXA) is an antifibrinolytic agent that is being used with increasing frequency in civilian settings. The impetus for use in trauma originated from a large prospective international trial (CRASH-2) as well as a large retrospective cohort of combat casualties, demonstrating some improvement in mortality when patients received TXA within 3 hours of injury. The benefits of thromboelastography (TEG) monitoring in the use of TXA is currently being investigated to evaluate outcomes when patients with hyperfibrinolytic profiles are specifically targeted and treated.

If the patient is not bleeding and is not at risk for a devastating consequence of rebleeding, one should not give procoagulant factors—they will only fuel the fire of systemic inflammation and coagulation. As with any intervention, the benefit-to-risk ratio should be individualized.

G. Hypothermia: Prevention and Treatment

Maintenance of normothermia is critical in the setting of hemorrhagic shock. Patients who have significant blood loss may lose the ability to increase metabolic heat production. In addition, initial fluid replacement is often done using room temperature or cold solutions such as crystalloid administered in the field by paramedics or unwarmed blood products in the hospital. The added stress of environmental or surgical exposure can make it difficult to maintain normothermia. The impact cannot be overstated: the adverse effects of hypothermia on coagulopathy can be profound.

For these reasons, hypothermia prevention and treatment should be an immediate and ongoing management priority during resuscitation from hemorrhagic shock. At the very least, one should keep the environment warm, infuse fluids through warmers, and keep the patient covered as much as possible. These efforts should commence as soon as possible after the injury or after the onset of illness.

H. Modalities to be Avoided

There is no role for using colloid solutions in the setting of hypovolemic shock except when size and weight of the crystalloid solutions limit their availability, as in treating mass casualties or under wartime conditions. Under these circumstances, solutions containing hetastarch or hypertonic saline and dextran (HSD) can be used. Otherwise, colloids provide no benefit over crystalloid solutions, and they add to cost. Vasopressors should not be used in resuscitating neurologically intact hypovolemic patients, except in desperate situations for short periods while the vascular volume is reexpanded. Patients given vasopressors for hemorrhagic shock are at risk for ischemic gangrene of the limbs, gut necrosis, liver failure, and acute tubular necrosis.

American College of Surgeons. *ATLS: Advanced Trauma Life Support Student Manual.* 10th ed. American College of Surgeons; 2018.

CRASH-2 trial collaborators; Shakur H, Roberts I, Bautista R, et al. Effects of tranexamic acid on death, vascular occlusive events, and blood transfusion in trauma patients with significant haemorrhage (CRASH-2): A randomized, placebo-controlled trial. *Lancet.* 2010;376:23-32.

Holcomb JB, de Junco DJ, Fox EE, et al. The Prospective, Observational, Multicenter, Major Trauma Transfusion (PROMMTT) study. *JAMA Surg.* 2013;148:127-136.

Sperry JL, Guyette FX, Brown JB, et al. Prehospital plasma during air medical transport in trauma patients at risk for hemorrhagic shock. *N Engl J Med.* 2018;379(4):315-326.

CARDIAC COMPRESSIVE SHOCK

Diagnosis

Cardiac compressive shock can arise from any condition that compresses the heart or great veins, including pericardial tamponade, tension pneumothorax, massive hemothorax, rupture of the diaphragm with encroachment of abdominal viscera into the chest, and distention of the abdomen with compression of the intra-abdominal great veins and elevation of the diaphragm into the chest. All of these conditions are worsened if the patient has to be mechanically ventilated.

The signs of compressive shock are similar to those of hypovolemic shock—postural hypotension, poor cutaneous perfusion, oliguria, hypotension in the supine position, mental status changes, electrocardiographic signs of myocardial ischemia, metabolic acidemia, and hyperventilation—combined with distended neck veins. The only other type of shock that can produce the combination of poor perfusion associated with distended neck veins is cardiogenic shock, which rarely poses a problem in differential diagnosis. Cardiogenic shock usually develops against a background of evident disease that predisposes to primary myocardial dysfunction. Cardiac compression usually follows trauma or occurs in a setting where mechanical compromise of the heart or great veins can arise from imposition of external pressure (as in a possible pericardial tamponade).

The so-called paradoxic pulse is occasionally helpful in diagnosis. A spontaneous breath in a normovolemic subject without cardiac compression produces little effect on systemic blood pressure. If the heart is compressed, the systolic pressure can fall by more than 10 mm Hg. (In contrast, a fall in the blood pressure with positive-pressure ventilation is common and nonspecific, especially in hypovolemic patients; the concept of a paradoxic pulse applies only to patients who are breathing on their own.)

Treatment

Infusion of fluid can transiently overcome some of the ill effects of cardiac compression, but the cause of shock in these patients is mechanical, and definitive treatment must correct the mechanical abnormality. Treatment of compressive shock caused by large-volume, high-pressure mechanical ventilation is discussed later in this chapter in the section on mechanical ventilation.

CARDIOGENIC SHOCK

Diagnosis

Cardiogenic shock can arise from several causes, including arrhythmias, ischemia-induced myocardial failure, valvular or septal defects, systemic or pulmonary hypertension, myocarditis, and myocardiopathies. Of all the forms of shock, it can be the most resistant to treatment. If the heart cannot pump, there may be nothing that can be done. On the other hand, in less severe cases, it is possible to improve the efficiency of the pumping capability that remains.

The diagnosis of cardiogenic shock usually depends on recognizing an underlying medical condition predisposing the heart to dysfunction in conjunction with an abnormal electrocardiogram (ECG). Given the relative oxygen demands of the left and right ventricles, shock caused by left ventricular failure is much more common in patients with ischemic heart disease, and typically presents with chest pain, a third heart sound, rales, ST segment elevation on a 12-lead electrocardiogram, and, on chest film, an enlarged heart or pulmonary edema. Cardiogenic shock may be associated with distended neck veins if the right ventricle has failed, unless the patient is also hypovolemic, as in a bleeding patient with a recent myocardial infarction. In many cases, patients with recent shock or trauma may have mild to moderate forms of right ventricular dysfunction related primarily to the heart's response to systemic inflammation or elevated ventilator pressures. Right-sided dysfunction can be associated with peripheral edema, an enlarged and tender liver, and, on chest film, an enlarged heart. The diagnosis is usually easy, but two common situations may pose a problem.

The first is a ruptured abdominal aortic aneurysm in a patient with coronary artery disease. The patient might have lower chest pain consistent with a myocardial infarction and electrocardiographic signs of ischemia—the ischemia being caused by hypovolemia and shock. The key is to observe the neck veins.

The second is to ascribe shock to myocardial contusion in a patient who has just suffered a blunt injury to the chest. Although blunt chest trauma can damage the heart, the damage is usually either fatal, with death at the scene of the injury, or, more often, of no clinical significance. A contusion that produces failure but not death is rare. Shock after blunt trauma in a patient who survives to reach the hospital is almost never caused by contusion—it is far more likely to be caused by hypovolemia or by a mechanical problem.

Treatment

A. Initial Management of Dysrhythmias

In the initial treatment of acute dysrhythmias, we use the approach described by Ursic and Harken. A bradydysrhythmia in a hypotensive patient with a heart rate less than 50 beats/min deserves treatment, even if the ventricular contractions are well coordinated. One should begin with intravenous (IV) administration of atropine, at a dose of 0.5 mg, repeated at 2-minute intervals for a maximum dose of 2 mg. If the rate remains slow and if the patient is still unstable, the heart should be paced by transvenous or external means.

A tachydysrhythmia can put a patient at risk for myocardial ischemia regardless of origin (sinus vs. nonsinus) or etiology (hypovolemic or cardiogenic shock). Thus one has to decide if the rate is so rapid that it threatens the patient's myocardium. As a first approximation, the goal for most patients should be a ventricular rate between 50 and 100. However, the goal can be different for different patient populations. The maximal ventricular rate, the rate that can be sustained for perhaps 5 minutes, but not longer, declines with age (220 – age in years). The maximal aerobic rate, a rate that can be maintained indefinitely, but with strain, is 60%-90% of this value depending on the physical condition of the patient and the presence or absence of ischemic heart disease. For example, a healthy 20-year-old man in good condition should be able to tolerate and sustain a heart rate of 160 (80% of 200) without difficulty (although one should search for the cause of the tachycardia). On the other hand, a 65-year-old man with known coronary stenosis may have a myocardial aerobic threshold of 93 beats/min: (220 – 65) × 0.6. Rates exceeding these limits should be treated.

A *moribund* patient with a tachydysrhythmia should undergo electrical cardioversion, an intervention that results in full cardiac function with normal blood supply to the brain in a matter of seconds. No other treatment has this potential. Electrical cardioversion is the treatment of choice for coarse ventricular fibrillation, ventricular tachycardia, and for supraventricular dysrhythmias with unsustainably rapid ventricular responses. It is not the treatment of choice for asystole or fine ventricular fibrillation.

One hundred joules should be used initially, with rapid escalation to 360 J, as needed. The cardioversion takes precedence over securing the airway, and it takes precedence over obtaining vascular access; it even takes precedence over making a diagnosis of the arrhythmia. Once converted, the patient should be given a single 100-mg dose of lidocaine. Serum electrolytes should be measured and corrected, if needed. One to two grams of magnesium sulfate should be given intravenously over 15 minutes, regardless of initial plasma concentrations. More should be given later if the values are low.

Treatment of any *non-moribund* patient with a tachydysrhythmia begins with ensuring euvolemia and treating other possible extracardiac causes of a tachycardia (such as fever, stress, pain, and anxiety). Dangerously rapid tachydysrhythmias associated with *abnormal ventricular conduction* should be electrically cardioverted, followed by lidocaine, electrolyte correction, and administration of a single dose of magnesium. In the non-moribund patient with a dangerously rapid tachydysrhythmia and *normal ventricular conduction*, the initial goal is to slow the rate. The first-line medication for narrow-complex tachydysrhythmia is adenosine if thought to be caused by atrioventricular nodal reentrant tachycardia (AVNRT), or a β-blocker or calcium channel blocker if thought to be other atrial tachycardia. Electrolytes, again, should be corrected; magnesium should be supplemented.

If more than one drug must be used, the patient will need to be in a monitored setting. Complete heart block is a potentially disastrous side effect with all of these drugs, especially when used in combination.

B. Opioids

Opioids can be especially effective in treating cardiac failure after myocardial infarction. They relieve pain, provide sedation, block adrenergic discharge to the arterioles, block discharge to the venules and small veins, redistribute the blood from the atria and ventricles to the venous capacitance vessels in the periphery, and decrease myocardial oxygen requirements.

C. Diuretics

Diuretics are the keystone of therapy in congestive heart failure with large ventricular end-diastolic volumes. By decreasing vascular volume, diuretics decrease atrial pressures and mobilize peripheral and pulmonary edema. Pulmonary vascular pressures and volumes decrease; effectiveness of right ventricular contraction increases. Coronary blood flow increases as coronary sinus pressure drops. Decreasing pressures in the ventricles during diastole, when the ventricular muscle receives its nutrient blood flow, alleviates compression of the coronary vasculature in the endocardium. Decreasing pressures in the right atrium decreases the stiffness of the coronary vasculature, which decreases the stiffness of the ventricles during diastole (the garden hose effect). The ventricular end-diastolic volumes potentially can increase without much of an associated increase in the end-diastolic pressures.

D. Beta-Blockers

Almost all patients in cardiac failure with ischemia and a rapid heart rate will benefit from a beta-adrenergic blocking agent (eg, esmolol or metoprolol). Decreasing the rate and reducing ventricular stiffness during systole decreases myocardial oxygen requirements. Increasing time in diastole and decreasing ventricular stiffness during diastole augments ventricular filling and increases efficiency of ventricular contraction. All of these effects reduce myocardial oxygen consumption and potentially salvage marginal myocardium. In many patients, the reduced oxygen requirements can be achieved with only minimal loss of energy output from the ventricles. The only contraindication to the use of beta-blockers, beyond the rare development of bronchospasm with administration of the drugs, is hypotension. This latter problem is easily monitored.

E. Vasodilators

Hypertension is unusual but not unheard of in patients with cardiogenic shock. The hypertension is usually associated with inefficient delivery of energy into the aortic root. Treatment should begin with opioids, if the patient is in pain, and then diuresis, if the ventricular end-diastolic volumes are large. Nitroprusside and nitroglycerin are the most useful short-term vasodilators in surgical patients in heart failure (besides opioids). Both drugs act quickly and are easy to monitor; both dilate the systemic arterioles, and nitroglycerin also dilates the systemic venules and small veins. For long-term control of pressure, angiotensin-converting enzyme (ACE) inhibitors and calcium channel blockers should be used in place of the nitrates. If the patient has a tachycardia or if the patient is at risk for having coronary artery disease or myocardial ischemia, beta-blockade can be used.

Beneficial consequences of controlling the pressure include mobilization of edema, both pulmonary and systemic; enhanced perfusion of the myocardium; and reduction of ventricular work and oxygen requirements and, consequently, relief of myocardial ischemia. On the other hand, excessive venous dilation can decrease cardiac filling enough so that stroke volumes and blood pressures fall; excessive arteriolar dilation can make the pressures fall further.

F. Inotropic Agents

Inotropic agents, such as dobutamine or milrinone, can increase cardiac output in some, but not all, patients in cardiogenic shock. Inotropic agents almost always result in increased myocardial oxygen requirements, but this is not usually a problem. Patients receiving the agents should be monitored in an ICU. Development of chest pain or ischemic electrocardiogram changes suggests that oxygen demand is exceeding supply. Systemic arterial pressures, atrial filling pressures, and cardiac output should be determined at different infusion rates. If any question remains about the adequacy of volume resuscitation, cardiovascular parameters should be measured before and after a fluid bolus is given.

Digitalis compounds should not be used in acute cardiac failure except to control ventricular rates in patients with supraventricular tachydysrhythmias. Toxicity may develop, especially when pH and electrolyte changes are unpredictable. The inotropic actions of digitalis are no different from those of dopamine and milrinone.

G. Chronotropic Agents

Although uncommon in the surgical setting, patients with cardiac failure and a low heart rate (< 70) may temporarily benefit from the administration of a chronotropic agent, such as dopamine. When using dopamine, the heart rate should be increased only to levels that can be tolerated comfortably. A 60-year-old patient with normal coronary arteries gains little with a heart rate that exceeds 120 beats/min; the limit is about 90 beats/min in the presence of coronary artery disease. In most cases, however, the price to be paid for using a chronotropic agent exceeds the potential benefit. Chronotropic agents increase myocardial work and oxygen requirements and shorten the time during diastole for coronary blood flow and ventricular filling. They should be used only as a temporary expedient. The goal of therapy is a normal or slightly supranormal cardiac output that provides adequate end-organ perfusion and reverses shock. Trying to achieve more than that only increases the risk of myocardial ischemia.

H. Vasoconstrictors

A vasoconstrictor is occasionally useful to increase coronary perfusion pressure in the setting of coronary stenoses. To be effective, the agent must increase aortic pressure enough so that the increased myocardial perfusion compensates for the increase in the myocardial oxygen requirements.

The major untoward effect of these agents is ischemic necrosis of noncardiac organs, such as the extremities or intestine. They will not increase perfusion to the brain in the setting of cardiogenic shock, assuming that the carotid arteries are open and that the patient has a functioning adrenergic nervous system. The endogenous adrenergic nervous system is ideally suited for ensuring adequate blood flow to the brain. Constrictors should be used only when absolutely necessary.

I. Transaortic Balloon Pump

The transaortic balloon pump decreases the afterload that the left ventricle faces when it ejects its blood into the aortic root, and can be very effective in resuscitating selected patients with severe reversible left ventricular dysfunction (eg, after cardiopulmonary bypass or acute myocardial infarction). It also allows for improved coronary perfusion as the balloon is inflated during diastole.

J. Extracorporeal Membrane Oxygenation

Extracorporeal membrane oxygenation is most often used in conditions in which one can expect cardiac function to recover within a matter of days to weeks. Bleeding complications make it impractical for periods exceeding that time.

K. Ventricular Assist Devices

Ventricular assist devices (VADs) are implantable mechanical circulatory support devices that support the right ventricle, the left ventricle, or both. They are often used in chronic heart failure as a bridge to transplantation. The ISAR-SHOCK study supports the use of VADs in acute cardiogenic shock in that they provided better hemodynamic results than an intra-aortic balloon pump (IABP), but the data have yet to support improvement in survival using VADs.

L. Operative Correction

Although listed last, surgically correctable cardiac conditions should be identified and corrected early, prior to the development of irreversible organ dysfunction. Ruptured valves, occluded arteries, aneurysmal ventricular walls, and certain arrhythmias are examples of potentially correctable lesions. In these cases, early cardiac surgical consultation should be the rule.

Chan PS, et al; American Heart Association National Registry of Cardiopulmonary Resuscitation Investigators. Delayed time to defibrillation after in-hospital cardiac arrest. *N Engl J Med.* 2008;358:9.

Seyfarth M, Sibbing D, Bauer I, et al. A randomized clinical trial to evaluate the safety and efficacy of a percutaneous left ventricular assist device versus intra-aortic balloon pumping for treatment of cardiogenic shock caused by myocardial infarction. *J Am Coll Cardiol.* 2008;52(19):1584-1588.

Unverzagt S, Buerke M, de Waha A, et al. Intra-aortic balloon pump counterpulsation (IABP) for myocardial infarction complicated by cardiogenic shock. *Cochrane Database Syst Rev.* 2015;3:CD007398.

NEUROGENIC SHOCK

▶ Diagnosis

Shock caused by failure of the autonomic nervous system can arise from regional or general anesthetics, injuries to the spinal cord, or administration of autonomic blocking agents. The venules and small veins lose tone, worsened by paralysis of surrounding skeletal muscles. Blood pools in the periphery, ventricular end-diastolic volumes decrease, and stroke volumes and blood pressure fall. Loss of arteriolar tone in the denervated areas makes the pressure fall further. If the lesion is below the midthoracic sympathetic outflow (approximately T3), activation of the cardiac adrenergic nerves will increase the heart rate and augment ventricular systolic function; if the lesion is more cephalad, the heart will not be able to compensate. Cardiovascular decompensation in neurogenic shock can be profound.

The diagnosis rests on knowledge of the circumstances preceding the onset of shock and on the physical examination. The patient will always be hypotensive, and the skin will be warm and flushed in the denervated areas. The cause is usually obvious.

Nonfatal head injury—in contrast to spinal cord injury—does not produce neurogenic or any other kind of shock. In fact, increased intracranial pressure typically increases blood pressure and slows the heart rate (Cushing reflex). Hypotension and tachycardia should never be attributed to head injury—even severe head injury with cerebral dysfunction—until hypovolemia has been ruled out.

▶ Treatment

The Trendelenburg position, if it does not complicate other aspects of care, is useful. Intravenous fluids to fill the dilated venules and small veins should be given. Vasoconstrictors should be used if fluids and Trendelenburg position are not enough. Norepinephrine and phenylephrine are good choices if the heart rate is rapid. Dopamine is a good choice if the heart rate is slow.

The primary purpose of vasoconstricting agents in this setting is to restore tone in the venules and small veins; a secondary goal is to constrict dilated arterioles. The blood pressure should be increased to the point that coronary perfusion is sustained—as judged by normal ST–T segments on electrocardiography and absence of chest pain—and to the point that perfusion to the brain and spinal cord is supported. The pressure also has to be high enough to perfuse organs with preexisting obstructing proximal arterial lesions. These patients should be placed in the ICU for both neurologic and hemodynamic monitoring.

Mallek JT, Inaba K, Branco BC, et al. The incidence of neurogenic shock after spinal cord injury in patients admitted to a high-volume level I trauma center. *Am Surg.* 2012;78(5):623-626.

LOW-OUTPUT INFLAMMATORY SHOCK

▶ Diagnosis

Bowel perforation, intestinal necrosis, abscesses, gangrene, and soft-tissue infections can produce low-output inflammatory shock, as can ischemia–reperfusion and inadequate resuscitation of massive injuries or large burns. The cytokinemia arising from the systemic inflammation can disrupt the microvascular endothelium and prompt the loss of plasma into the interstitium. The shock mimics the clinical picture of severe hypovolemic shock, with signs of adrenergic discharge, oliguria, obtundation, and metabolic acidemia. The ECG may show signs of ischemia. Hyperthermia or hypothermia may be present.

▶ Treatment

Treatment consists of administration of IV fluids and antibiotics when appropriate, as well as treatment of the underlying cause, including correction of gastrointestinal leaks, debridement of dead tissue, and drainage of pus. The patient should be transferred to an ICU. Vasoconstrictors can be used adjunctively to support perfusion while resuscitation is ongoing, but are not a replacement for volume expansion.

HIGH-OUTPUT INFLAMMATORY SHOCK

Diagnosis

High-output inflammatory shock can precede low-output inflammatory shock or can be the result of successful treatment of low-output shock. The shock usually, but not always, is associated with a fever. The patient is hypotensive with warm, well-perfused extremities, as the body attempts to control its core temperature by off-loading heat to the environment. Cardiac output will remain high, occasionally as high as twice normal, as long as the inflammatory state persists. The oxygen consumption may be increased by a factor of 1.5.

Treatment

Treatment consists of control of the underlying cause and fluid administration. Inotropes may be useful. If large amounts of fluids are necessary for the resuscitation and if inotropes are being considered, an assessment of ventricular end-diastolic volume should be made to ensure the heart is adequately filling and to assess the impact of the intervention. This can be performed by measurement of central venous pressure (CVP) and serial echocardiography. The goal is to perfuse the inflamed tissues with adequate power so that the product of the cardiac output and the mean arterial pressure is normal. In many patients, the result will be a cardiac output that is increased by a factor of 1.5 with a blood pressure that is decreased to a value that is two-thirds of normal. As in other forms of shock, the pressure has to be high enough to perfuse the heart and brain and organs with potentially obstructed arteries, but it does not have to be normal. Vasoconstrictors can be dangerous, potentially leading to necrosis of the limbs, the gut, and the kidneys, especially if there is any degree of hypovolemia. They should not be used unless the clinician is positive that both the right and left ventricular end-diastolic volumes are normally expanded.

TREATMENT OF THE MORE CHALLENGING PATIENT

This discussion of shock in the surgical patient has concentrated on making a clinical diagnosis and directing treatment on the basis of that diagnosis. This approach works well in many patients, but in some it is not sufficient. Effective treatment in the more seriously ill patient frequently has to take into account the underlying physiologic abnormalities if the treatment is to work. With this approach, the clinical

diagnosis becomes less important. Dealing with the underlying physiologic problem becomes paramount.

Common Physiologic Responses to Severe Shock

The body responds to the shock state with compensatory responses. These responses help the patient deal with the initial abnormalities of the shock but can contribute to the later consequences of cardiac and pulmonary failure. Understanding these responses can help the physician in managing the consequences.

Neurohumoral Responses

The neurohumoral responses to shock include discharge of the cardiovascular nerves and release of vasoactive, metabolically active, and volume-conserving hormones. The responses can be lifesaving before therapy begins and serve to maintain homeostasis once therapy has started.

Adrenergic discharge constricts the arterioles, venules, and small veins in all parts of the body except the brain and heart, and augments myocardial systolic function. The result is increased cardiac output and blood pressure and diversion of flow to the brain and heart.

The vasoactive hormones angiotensin II and vasopressin act in concert with discharge of the cardiovascular adrenergic nerves. Angiotensin II constricts the vasculature in the skin, kidneys, and splanchnic organs and diverts blood flow to the heart and brain. It also stimulates the adrenal medulla to release aldosterone, resulting in reabsorption of sodium ions from the glomerular filtrate. Vasopressin, like adrenergic discharge and angiotensin II, constricts the vascular sphincters in the skin and splanchnic organs (it does not constrict the renal vasculature) and diverts blood flow to the heart and brain. It also stimulates reabsorption of water from the distal tubules.

Metabolic Responses

In all severe shock states, intracellular hydrogen ion concentrations increase. To compensate, extracellular sodium flows down its electrochemical gradient into the cells, along with chloride and water, in exchange for intracellular hydrogen ion. Intracellular pH increases back toward normal, but the cells swell, with perhaps an increase of 3 L in the intracellular volume.

Hypovolemia, hypotension, pain, and other stresses of critical illness stimulate the release of cortisol, glucagon, and epinephrine—all of which increase extracellular glucose concentrations. Thus, glucose should not be used in the initial fluid resuscitation of the patient in shock—it is not necessary and can even induce an osmotic diuresis, worsening hypovolemia and confusing the clinical picture. Glucose-containing solutions should be reserved for those patients who might be in insulin shock.

On the other hand, the endogenously produced glucose generated by the physiologic release of the counterregulatory hormones provides fuel for nervous system function, metabolism of blood cells, and wound healing. The modest increase in extracellular osmolality also helps to replenish vascular volume by drawing water out of the cells and by increasing the interstitial hydrostatic pressure. The increased pressure drives interstitial protein into the lymphatics and from there into the vascular space. Interstitial oncotic pressure falls, and plasma oncotic pressure rises. The augmented oncotic gradient between the vascular and interstitial spaces draws water, sodium, and chloride into the vascular space from the interstitial space. This replenishment of vascular volume will continue as long as interstitial hydrostatic pressures are maintained and as long as interstitial protein stores, which constitute more than half of the total extracellular protein content, can be recruited. A certain degree of hyperglycemia might be beneficial in the post-resuscitative phase. Once the patient has recovered, however, it appears that it is best to keep the blood glucose levels lower, at 180 mg/dL or less.

Other hormones with potential metabolic actions, including insulin and growth hormone, are also released during critical illnesses. They have little effect, however, compared with cortisol, glucagon, and epinephrine. Indeed, infusion of cortisol, glucagon, and epinephrine in normal subjects can produce most of the metabolic changes of critical illness.

Microvascular Responses

In severely ill patients, three responses—dilation of systemic arterioles, failure of cell membrane function, and disruption of the vascular endothelium—serve to worsen the patient's condition. In decompensated shock, the systemic arterioles lose their ability to constrict, while the postcapillary sphincters remain constricted. Microvascular hydrostatic pressure rises. Water, sodium, and chloride are driven out of the vascular space and into the interstitium. The process is limited, however, because the oncotic gradient—which increases as fluid is lost from plasma— prevents further fluid losses.

Trauma and sepsis activate coagulation and inflammation, which can disrupt microvascular endothelial integrity in severely ill patients. Platelet and white cell microaggregates that form in injured or infected tissues embolize to the lungs or liver, where they lodge in the microvasculature. The microaggregates, endothelium, and plasma in the regions of embolization release kinins, platelet-activating factors, fibrin degradation products, thromboxanes, prostacyclin, prostaglandins, complement, leukotrienes, lysosomal enzymes, oxygen radicals, and other toxic factors, which damage the endothelium and dilate the vasculature in the region of the emboli and distally. Protein, water, sodium, and chloride extravasate into the interstitium. The amount of extravasation is limited by the increases in interstitial hydrostatic pressure that arise from interstitial flooding and by dilution of interstitial protein concentrations. The edema that results can be massive and can involve any tissue in the body.

Ultrasound as Adjunct to Evaluate Resuscitation

In the past, several invasive measures were used to help diagnose the underlying source of shock and direct resuscitation in critically ill patients. These procedures included central line placement to evaluate central venous pressures (CVP), as well as Swan–Ganz catheters to measure pulmonary wedge pressures and to sample mixed-venous O_2. In the modern era, the field of critical care is moving away from these invasive monitoring techniques as noninvasive methods are coming more to the forefront; these methods provide important information that can help guide diagnosis and resuscitation without the complications associated with invasive monitoring.

The method most commonly used currently in the trauma resuscitation bay and the ICU is the use of ultrasound imaging to help diagnose the source of a patient's shock. An extended focused assessment with sonography for trauma (eFAST) is often performed immediately in trauma patients to determine whether there is free fluid in any of the dependent portions of the abdomen (the hepatorenal space, the splenorenal space, or the pelvis), any pericardial effusion, or evidence of pneumothorax, to rapidly diagnose reasons for shock.

In a nontrauma patient or a trauma patient who has been ruled out from having hemorrhagic shock, a cardiac examination with ultrasound can be performed to evaluate the cardiac contractility of the left ventricle and right ventricle (RV) dilation. IVC measurements can also be performed to determine whether the IVC appears dilated, collapsed, or normal to assess intravascular volume. Finally, the costophrenic angles can be assessed to look for pleural effusions. While a cardiologist or highly skilled ultrasound technician may be necessary to evaluate for more subtle findings such as valvular disease or vegetations, the findings described above such as gross cardiac dysfunction, intra-abdominal free fluid, pericardial effusion, and IVC filling can be assessed quite readily by the ICU clinician after some experience. These findings can have a major impact on the ongoing management of the critically ill patient.

American College of Surgeons. *ATLS: Advanced Trauma Life Support Student Manual.* 10th ed. American College of Surgeons; 2018.

Monnet X, Marik PE, Teboul JL. Prediction of fluid responsiveness: An update. *Ann Intens Care.* 2016;6(1):111.

Saranteas T, Mavrogenis AF, Mandila C, et al. Ultrasound in cardiac trauma. *J Crit Care.* 2017;38:144-151.

RISK ASSESSMENT

Predicting the likelihood of survival in critically ill surgical patients is best accomplished by evaluating clinical and laboratory findings. Computation of a severity of illness score is usually unnecessary. Nonetheless, several scoring systems have been developed with the intention of increasing the precision of the estimate. All such systems assign a mathematical probability for survival in groups of patients, and many are useful for research purposes because they allow comparisons of patients among different institutions. None of them, however, are accurate enough to predict survival for an individual patient, though some are still clinically useful for assessing the effects of therapy.

Currently, the most commonly used risk stratification score used to identify patients at high risk for mortality from critical illness and/or sepsis is the Sequential Organ Failure Assessment (SOFA) score, published in 1996. This score predicts mortality by evaluating dysfunction of the respiratory, coagulation, hepatic, cardiovascular, central nervous, and renal systems, by evaluation of PaO_2/FiO_2 ratio, platelet count, bilirubin, blood pressure, Glasgow Coma Scale (GCS), and creatinine. For ease of clinical use, the quick SOFA (qSOFA) score was developed, which evaluates GCS, respiratory rate, and systolic blood pressure to determine whether patients are or are not at high risk for in-hospital mortality. These scoring systems merely direct the clinician to evaluate the patient in a multisystem fashion to determine whether they have systemic symptoms of serious illness, but provide a common language to discuss the severity of a patient's disease between clinicians.

▶ References

Angus DC, Seymour CW, Coopersmith CM, et al. A framework for the development and interpretation of different sepsis definitions and clinical criteria. *Crit Care Med.* 2016;44(3):e113-121.

Vincent JL, Moreno R, Takala J, et al. The SOFA (Sepsis-related Organ Failure Assessment) score to describe organ dysfunction/failure. *Intens Care Med.* 1996;22(7):707-710.

MULTIPLE-CHOICE QUESTIONS

1. Shock can be caused by:

    A. Depletion of intravascular volume.
    B. Loss of autonomic control of the vasculature.
    C. Severe untreated systemic inflammation.
    D. Both A and C.
    E. A, B, and C.

2. Hypothermia in hemorrhagic shock:

    A. Is of limited risk in the initial 24 hours after injury.
    B. Can contribute to coagulopathy.
    C. Is unusual in the trauma population outside of cold-weather or water immersion injuries.
    D. Is best treated by warming the ambient room temperature.
    E. Is a secondary concern that can be addressed after the care of injuries.

3. Cardiac or great vessel compressive shock:

    A. Can be caused by pericardial tamponade.
    B. May accompany tension pneumothorax.
    C. Is worsened by the need for positive pressure ventilation.
    D. Cannot be caused by intraabdominal injury.
    E. A, B, and C.

4. Neurogenic shock is characterized by:

    A. Hypertension and warm skin.
    B. Hypotension and warm skin.
    C. Hypertension and cool skin.
    D. Hypotension and cool skin.

5. Ultrasound use in the ICU for evaluation of a patient in shock includes:

    A. E-FAST.
    B. IVC evaluation as assessment of intravascular volume.
    C. Echocardiogram to evaluate for cardiac function.
    D. All of the above.

Acute Pulmonary Failure in Surgical Patients

Anupamaa Seshadri, MD

Joaquim M. Havens, MD

▼ INITIAL TREATMENT OF ACUTE PULMONARY FAILURE

DIAGNOSIS OF PULMONARY FAILURE IN SURGICAL PATIENTS

Most causes of pulmonary failure in the surgical patient can be ascribed to one or more of nine causes: the pulmonary failure of shock, trauma, and sepsis; mechanical failure caused by deranged respiratory system mechanics; atelectasis; aspiration; pulmonary contusion; pneumonia; pulmonary embolism; cardiogenic pulmonary edema; and, rarely, neurogenic pulmonary edema.

The pulmonary failure of shock, trauma, and sepsis arises from extrapulmonary trauma, infection, or ischemia–reperfusion in the setting of shock. Products of coagulation and inflammation are carried intravascularly from the damaged tissues and carried to the lungs (or to the liver, in the case of the splanchnic circulation, and from there to the lungs), where they set up an acute inflammatory reaction. The extrapulmonary causes are many and range from necrotizing infections to noninfective inflammatory responses (such as pancreatitis) to reperfusion of ischemic limbs to soft-tissue injury.

The concept of pulmonary failure secondary to extrapulmonary ischemia–reperfusion, coagulation, and inflammation, which is common in surgical patients, can be subsumed into a broader category of pulmonary failure known as the **acute respiratory distress syndrome** (ARDS). ARDS is defined by the Berlin criteria as the acute onset of hypoxemia with bilateral infiltrates on chest x-ray or CT scan as well as a Pao_2:Fio_2 ratio less than 300, not fully explained by cardiac failure or fluid overload.

The causes of ARDS include those that are responsible for the pulmonary failure of shock, trauma, and sepsis, and also include severe pneumonia and aspiration. The end result in all of these conditions is activation of macrophages and other inflammatory cells in the lungs. The mediators disrupt the microvascular endothelium, increasing its permeability. Plasma extravasates into the interstitium and, in the case of the lungs, into the alveoli. The resultant pulmonary edema impairs both ventilation and oxygenation; microembolization to the lungs impairs perfusion. Arterial oxygen saturation decreases and carbon dioxide content increases, assuming that no compensatory mechanisms come into play. Lastly, to make things worse, the inflammatory process in the lungs releases mediators into the systemic circulation that can lead to inflammation and dysfunction in the liver, gut, and kidneys.

A number of different mediators of coagulation and inflammation have been implicated as causes of the increased permeability. Proteases, kinins, complement, oxygen radicals, prostaglandins, thromboxanes, leukotrienes, lysosomal enzymes, and other mediators are released from aggregates of platelets and white cells or from the endothelium or plasma because of the interaction between the aggregates and vessel wall. Some of these substances are chemoattractants of more platelets and white blood cells, and a vicious cycle of inflammation develops that worsens the disruption of the vascular endothelium.

Pathologically, ARDS (and the pulmonary failure of shock, trauma, and sepsis) is characterized by diffuse alveolar damage and a nonspecific inflammatory reaction, with the loss of alveolar epithelium and hyaline membrane formation. Monocytes and neutrophils invade the interstitium. Edema appears within a few hours, alveolar flooding is florid within 1 day, and fibrosis begins in 1-2 weeks. If the process is unchecked, the lungs become sodden and resemble liver tissue on gross inspection; scar tissue appears within a week, and function-limiting fibrosis begins to develop within 2 weeks. If early treatment is effective, the lungs return to normal, both grossly and microscopically.

Mechanical failure can arise from chest-wall trauma, pain and weakness after surgery and anesthesia, debility caused by the catabolic metabolism of long-term illness, or bronchopleural fistula. Massive trauma to the chest with multiple fractures of multiple ribs or bilateral disruption of the costochondral junctions can result in a free-floating segment of chest wall known as a flail chest. Expansion and relaxation of the chest wall during spontaneous breathing results in paradoxic motion of the free segment in response to changes in intrathoracic pressure; ventilation becomes compromised, and the partial pressure of arterial carbon dioxide ($PaCO_2$) increases. In addition, hypoventilation leads to progressive atelectasis and hypoxemia. Lesser degrees of chest-wall injury can lead to hypoventilation secondary to pain with similar results. Prolonged mechanical ventilation with loss of muscle mass and power in the diaphragm and the accessory muscles of respiration can require ventilatory support until muscle function returns to normal. A bronchopleural fistula—a communication from the airway to the pleural cavity to the atmosphere, either through a chest tube or through a hole in the chest wall—can develop after pulmonary surgery, trauma, or infection. Large air leaks can compromise ventilation to the uninvolved lung as well as to the diseased side because inhaled air preferentially goes to the side with the fistula.

Atelectasis—localized collapse of alveoli—can develop with prolonged immobilization, as during anesthesia or in association with bed rest. The problem is usually full-blown within a few hours after the initiating event. Only mechanical failure (to which it is related), aspiration, cardiogenic pulmonary edema, and pulmonary embolism can produce equivalent levels of hypoxemia so soon, and no other cause of hypoxemia can respond so quickly to therapy. The diagnosis is supported by auscultation of bronchial breath sounds at dependent portions of the lung and occasionally, if severe enough, by x-ray confirmation of plate-like collapse of pulmonary parenchyma. The most reliable confirmation of the diagnosis, however, comes with response to therapy, which can include pain control when necessary and encouragement of deep breathing, coughing, and ambulation when practical. When the hypoxia is severe and refractory to conservative measures, noninvasive positive-pressure ventilation or intubation and mechanical ventilation may be necessary, particularly if the underlying etiology (pain, immobility) cannot be reversed easily (eg, high spinal cord injury). Rarely, flexible bronchoscopy may be useful if the lung parenchymal volume loss is due to proximal bronchial obstruction. In general, most forms of atelectasis respond within a few hours to conservative therapy.

Aspiration of gastric contents or blood can occur in any patient who cannot protect the airway. Shock, severe brain injury, or pharmacologic depression (anesthesia, narcotics, or benzodiazepines) can result in a depressed level of consciousness and loss of airway protective reflexes. Gastric acid or particulate matter in the airways leads to disruption of the alveolar and microvascular membranes, causing interstitial and alveolar edema. The resultant hypoxemia is usually evident within a few hours and is associated with a localized infiltrate on x-ray. Recovery of gastric contents by suctioning from the endotracheal tree confirms the diagnosis.

Pulmonary contusion arises from direct trauma to the chest wall and the underlying lung parenchyma. Hypoxemia associated with a localized infiltrate on x-ray develops over 24 hours as the injured lung becomes edematous.

Pneumonia can arise primarily or may be superimposed on aspiration, pulmonary contusion, or the pulmonary failure of shock, trauma, and sepsis. The diagnosis is made by recovery of bacteria and purulent material from the endotracheal tree, hypoxemia, signs of systemic inflammation, and a localized infiltrate on x-ray. The Clinical Pulmonary Infection Score (CPIS), which is derived from these parameters, can be used to quantify the clinical, radiographic, and laboratory findings of pneumonia. It is useful both for diagnosis and for determining length of treatment. Bronchoalveolar lavage and quantitative culture may occasionally be used to assist in distinguishing pneumonia from ARDS and other causes of pulmonary inflammation.

Pulmonary embolism typically presents with sudden deterioration of pulmonary function after an event—such as an operation, injury, or the beginning of immobilization—that can stimulate deposition of clot in a large systemic vein. Patients with cancer are at particularly high risk, and in any patient, the greater the magnitude of operation or injury, the greater the chance of venous thrombosis and embolization. Clot emboli must be organized to be clinically significant; embolism to the lung of fresh soft clot rarely causes any difficulty. The pulmonary endothelium contains potent fibrinolysins that can break up any poorly organized embolus.

The chest film is usually nonspecific. A definite diagnosis can be made by high-definition contrast-enhanced computed tomograms of the pulmonary vasculature. Modern imaging is extremely sensitive. A negative study rules out an embolism. The CT can also identify atelectasis, infiltrates, and effusions that may not be readily apparent using a standard anterior–posterior radiograph done in the intensive care unit (ICU). The major risk involves the physical movement of the patient to the radiology suite. The risk of contrast nephropathy is very low in a euvolemic patient, even in the setting of mild baseline renal disease. Once diagnosed, pulmonary embolism is typically treated with systemic anticoagulation in patients who are hemodynamically stable.

Pulmonary arteriography, with right heart catheterization, can also be used to make the diagnosis of embolism but is seldom used nowadays, with one exception. The study can be very useful in hemodynamically unstable patients in whom a large "saddle embolus" is suspected. The catheter can be left in place, if an embolus is found, and used for catheter-directed thrombolysis. A massive saddle embolus may also require pulmonary embolectomy if not amenable to catheter-directed lytic therapy.

Cardiogenic pulmonary edema arises from high left atrial and pulmonary microvascular hydrostatic pressures.

Patients who have suffered an acute myocardial infarction can present this way, as can patients with underlying myocardial or coronary artery disease when faced with fluid shifts and surgical stress. Occasionally, the rapid administration of intravenous (IV) fluid—especially in elderly patients with poor myocardial performance—will outstrip the heart's ability to pump, and pulmonary edema will result. Acute valvular disease, though rare after injury or cardiac surgery, is another possible cause of inability of the left heart to pump effectively. The diagnosis is made based on hypoxemia, rales, a third heart sound, perihilar infiltrates, Kerley lines, and cephalization of blood vessels on x-ray.

Neurogenic pulmonary edema is associated both experimentally and clinically with head injury and increased intracranial pressure. The exact mechanism by which this occurs is unknown, but it is probably related to sympathetic discharge with postmicrovascular vasoconstriction in the lungs and a resultant increase in pulmonary microvascular hydrostatic pressure. This form of pulmonary edema and oxygenation defect is rare. In the great majority of patients with a head injury and pulmonary edema, the edema will be caused by some other mechanism, such as ARDS.

INDICATIONS FOR INTUBATION & USE OF MECHANICAL VENTILATION

The indications for intubation and mechanical ventilation are related but often assessed separately. Patients who have primary airway compromise—caused by stridor, maxillofacial trauma, facial and airway burns with edema, or a depressed mental status—may need intubation to protect the airway. In these cases, early intervention is the rule, as rapid clinical deterioration can convert a semi-urgent procedure into an emergency. In some cases, intubation should be performed before the patient shows evidence of airway compromise. In severe cases, such as massive facial edema, fiberoptic intubation can be attempted, but one should prepare for potential cricothyroidotomy during the intubation attempt.

Intubation of the airway is also indicated if mechanical ventilation is needed for the treatment of established pulmonary failure or for prophylaxis against impending failure. The decision to intubate and initiate mechanical ventilation should be made on the basis of clinical criteria. A respiratory rate exceeding 36 breaths/min, labored ventilation, use of accessory muscles of ventilation, and significant hypercarbia are all indications for intervention. Finally, intubation and mechanical ventilation should be considered in anticipation of treatment that can compromise the airway or worsen the pulmonary status. These include the need for excessive sedation or narcotics (eg, in patients requiring prolonged and painful dressing changes for burns), massive fluid resuscitation, and the manipulation of fractures.

Arterial blood gas (ABG) measurements are of no value in making decisions about intubation and mechanical ventilation in patients in extremis—if the patient cannot protect his or her airway or is in florid respiratory failure, there is no indication to wait for an ABG result prior to intubation. ABG measurements, however, can assist in the decision to intubate less severely stressed patients. In the setting of hypoxemia, intubation should be considered if the Pao_2 is less than 60 mm Hg and the patient's supplemental oxygen exceeds an O_2 concentration of 50%. For hypercapneic patients, a $PaCO_2$ greater than 45 mm Hg in the setting of acidemia should prompt intubation, especially if serial measurements demonstrate a worsening respiratory acidosis. Regardless of the laboratory values, these guidelines should always be put in the clinical context. A $PaCO_2$ of 40 mm Hg in a patient breathing 40 breaths/min is as alarming as a $PaCO_2$ of 60 mm Hg in a patient with a respiratory rate of 10 breaths/min. A Pao_2 of 60 mm Hg on room air in a patient with chronic lung disease may be acceptable; the same value in a patient who is tensing the sternocleidomastoid and intercostal muscles with each breath, making excessive or discoordinated use of the abdominal musculature, and who seems to be struggling to draw in enough air, mandates immediate intubation.

The indications for intubation should be more liberal for a surgical patient than for a medical patient. The medical patient with an exacerbation of chronic obstructive lung disease can be poorly served by placement of a foreign body in the trachea. Airway resistance increases, coughing becomes less effective, and opportunistic organisms obtain a foothold on and near the tube. The benefit from intubation may be minimal, and noninvasive ventilation techniques, such as bilevel positive airway pressure (BiPAP), may be all that is needed. This support can be given simultaneously with other treatments—such as administration of bronchodilators, antibiotics, and diuretics—in order to avoid intubation and its potential complications.

Circumstances for the seriously ill surgical patient are usually different. The patient who has multiple injuries, for example, can temporarily tolerate the increased airway resistance, loss of cough, and increased likelihood of tracheobronchial infection. What cannot be tolerated is respiratory arrest during trauma resuscitation or during preparation for an operation.

The indications for intubation in the patient with a suspected or known injury to the cervical spine are the same as those in patients with no likelihood of injury. Under no circumstances should concern about the cervical spine lead to procrastination about securing the airway; methods of intubation that protect the stability of the cervical spine can be employed.

▶ Types of Intubation

The trachea can be intubated via the mouth, the nose, the cricothyroid membrane (cricothyroidotomy), or directly (tracheostomy). The tubes used for intubation used to come with either high-pressure cuffs or low-pressure cuffs. Because of problems with compromise of tracheal blood supply, and the subsequent problems of tracheomalacia, erosion into the innominate artery or the esophagus, and tracheal stenosis, the high-pressure cuffs are no longer used. All modern tubes come with low-pressure cuffs.

Of the four methods available for intubation, the orotracheal route is usually the easiest. Nasotracheal intubation requires the presence of spontaneous ventilation in order to guide tube placement; cricothyroidotomy and tracheotomy require surgical exposure. Orotracheal intubation allows for passage of a larger tube than the nasotracheal route and avoids the problems of sinusitis and necrosis of the nares, which can occur with nasotracheal intubation. On the other hand, nasotracheal intubation can be accomplished in the awake patient with minimal sedation, and some patients seem to find long-term presence of a nasotracheal tube more comfortable than that of an orotracheal tube. Neither nasotracheal nor orotracheal intubation requires neck flexion or axial rotation. Either approach can be used in patients with suspected injuries to the cervical spine, assuming that axial traction is maintained during the intubation.

Cricothyroidotomy is indicated when an urgent surgical airway is needed. Extensive maxillofacial trauma can make intubation by the orotracheal or nasotracheal route impossible. Translaryngeal intubation can also be difficult because of poor patient cooperation, altered anatomy, or airway or laryngeal swelling. If the patient is in extremis and respiratory collapse is imminent, attempts at orotracheal or nasotracheal intubation should not be prolonged. As a rule, if translaryngeal intubation is not successful after one or two attempts, cricothyroidotomy should be done. The cricothyroid membrane in the midline is bounded superiorly by the lower border of the thyroid cartilage. It is located by palpation and is incised by a stab incision. After the hole has been enlarged with the knife handle, a size 6 or 6.5 endotracheal tube should be inserted. After the airway is secured, the tube can be trimmed (without cutting the balloon tubing) to prevent accidental dislodgement. Alternatively, a no. 4 or no. 6 tracheostomy tube can be used if available.

There are several advantages to using the endotracheal tube during an urgent cricothyroidotomy. These include increased tube compliance, which facilitates insertion; and perhaps most importantly, universal availability. They are typically found in every airway kit or crash cart. A 6.5 tube will usually accommodate a bougie introducer, which may facilitate insertion, particularly when the anatomy is difficult (obese or short neck) and the field is bloody. Larger endotracheal or tracheostomy tubes should not be used, as they may not always pass easily through the cricothyroid space. In the short term, these smaller tubes are more than adequate as a rescue treatment and can easily be changed under more controlled circumstances.

Once the airway is secured and the patient stable, a more definitive airway can be planned as needed. The need to convert to a tracheotomy is not absolute. In some cases, the patient may no longer require airway protection. In others, endotracheal intubation may be a reasonable option. In the past, concerns over subglottic stenosis necessitated conversion of the cricothyroidotomy within several days. This has not been uniformly supported by the literature and should be individualized based on anticipated continued need for airway protection and mechanical ventilation.

Conversion of either an endotracheal airway or cricothyroidotomy to a tracheostomy should be done under controlled conditions. A transverse incision overlying the upper trachea is developed by separating the strap muscles of the neck in the midline. Often the thyroid isthmus must be either displaced or divided to allow for adequate exposure of the anterior surface of the trachea. The tracheostomy tube is placed through the second or third tracheal ring.

Tracheostomy placement is frequently performed for patients who require long-term mechanical ventilation. There are advantages and disadvantages to both the endotracheal tube and the tracheostomy. As a result, there are few absolute diagnostic or time standards for conversion beyond airway control.

One of the theoretical advantages of continued endotracheal intubation is the ease of tube repositioning, which allows distributing pressure on the tracheal mucosa over a larger area, compared with the balloon on the end of a tracheostomy tube, which is fixed in place. The result is a much lower incidence of late tracheal stenosis and tracheoinnominate artery and tracheoesophageal fistulas, compared with a tracheostomy. In addition, because the opening of a translaryngeal tube is well away from the neck and chest, IV catheters in these areas can be kept sterile. Finally, the cuffs on translaryngeal tubes usually lie in a more axial position in the trachea than those on a tracheostomy tube and are better able to maintain a seal in patients with poor pulmonary compliance and high inspiratory pressures.

On the other hand, for long-term care, airway resistance with a tracheostomy is lower, nursing care is simpler, suctioning is more direct, and the tubes do not damage the vocal cords or larynx. In addition and perhaps most importantly, accidental extubation is less serious—a well-established tracheostomy tract can be easily reintubated while the patient continues to breathe through the stoma. Tracheostomy is also of benefit when weaning from mechanical ventilation is slow and the patient has failed extubation on multiple occasions. The presence of a tracheostomy allows for prolonged periods off the ventilator without the need for reintubation. If the patient develops respiratory distress off the ventilator and a tracheostomy is present, the ventilator can simply be reconnected to the tracheostomy tube. This allows for ease in lightening of sedation and earlier mobilization of the patient, as well as potentially avoiding a more prolonged length of stay.

The timing of conversion from a translaryngeal intubation to a tracheostomy is controversial. Recommendations

Table 13–1. Characteristics of five commonly used modes of mechanical ventilation.

Mode	Trigger	Limit	Cycle	Notes
Intermittent mandatory ventilation (IMV)	Time (machine)	Flow (volume) or pressure	Time	Volume control IMV or pressure control IMV. Can be synchronized to patient's effort (SIMV) and/or used in conjunction with pressure support.
Assist control (AC)	Patient and/or time	Flow (volume) or pressure	Time	Assist control volume control (AC VC) or assist control pressure control (AC PC).
Pressure support (PS)	Patient	Pressure	Flow	Purely spontaneous mode and often referred to as a form of continuous positive airway pressure (CPAP) on the ventilator controls.
Inverse ratio	Time	Pressure	Time	PC IMV mode with prolonged inspiratory phase to increase mean airway pressure and functional residual capacity.
Pressure-regulated volume control	Patient and/or time	Pressure	Time	Variation of pressure control that limits pressure but adjusts between breaths to ensure preset tidal volume.

as short as 3 days have been made, but historically, large numbers of patients have been intubated for months by the orotracheal or nasotracheal route without serious sequelae. Patients should be converted when airway protection, pulmonary toilet, or any of the other indications outlined above are present. If, in addition, the need for more than 2-3 weeks of intubation is obvious, the threshold for performing tracheostomy should be lowered.

▶ Modes of Mechanical Ventilation

Once the airway is controlled, the ventilator should be set up beginning with the mode of ventilation. There are three primary variables used to describe the mode of mechanical ventilation: trigger, limit, and cycle (see Table 13–1). The **trigger** can be patient or time triggered, with the latter often referred to as "machine triggered." This is the variable that determines when a patient receives a breath (starts inspiration). The second is the **limit** variable, and refers to the setting that, when reached, is maintained constant throughout the inspiratory cycle (ie, the "upper limit"). Limit variables are either pressure or flow. When flow is the limit variable, the ventilator is said to be in **volume control** or **volume limited** because of the relationship *flow × time = volume*. Finally, the **cycle** variable is that which, once reached, terminates the inspiratory cycle and allows passive expiration. Using these three variables, different modes of ventilation have been created. Some are mostly of historical interest, and others are newer, combination modes designed to maximize patient physiology, safety, and comfort.

Machine triggers are time functions based on the set rate, inspiratory time, and inspiratory to expiratory ratio (I:E ratio). Two of the three can be set, and the third is determined. A rate of 20 breaths/min and an inspiratory time of

1 second results in an I:E ratio of 1:2 (1 s inspiration + 2 s expiration = 3 s for a complete cycle; 20 cycles/min).

Patient triggers for delivery of an assisted breath can be either pressure-based or "flow by" depending on the ventilator model. A pressure trigger requires the patient to generate negative pressure at the onset of inspiration—the pressure in the ventilator tubing falls below a preset value and the ventilator detects this fall in pressure and responds by delivering a breath. The time involved in generating and delivering the breath to the patient, however, can make this form of breathing uncomfortable for the patient. Modern ventilators avoid this problem of triggering by using a flow-by circuit. The ventilator delivers a constant flow of air through the ventilator tubing during expiration, usually at a low level of approximately 5 L/min. The ventilator compares the expiratory and inspiratory flow rates. If the patient is making no inspiratory effort, the flow rates will be the same. If the patient begins to take a breath, the expiratory rate will fall below the inspiratory rate. The ventilator is programmed to trigger a breath when the difference in the flow rates reaches a preset value, usually around 2 L/min, or when the expiratory flow rate falls to 3 L/min. The patient is rewarded with the free flow of at least some air as soon as the effort is initiated. The great majority of patients prefer flow-by over pressure triggering.

A. Volume Control Ventilation

Volume control ventilation is most often used today in situations in which the ventilation needs to be kept simple and the efforts made by the patient need to be minimized, as in the acutely injured or ill patient. The assist-control (AC) mode is the most commonly used mode of volume ventilation. It is designed to assist any ventilatory effort made by the patient by delivering a machine breath. Whenever the patient begins to inspire, the ventilator is triggered and the preset machine tidal volume is given. A machine backup rate is also set to ensure a minimal number of machine breaths in the absence of spontaneous ventilatory efforts.

B. Pressure Control Ventilation and Pressure Support Ventilation

In **pressure control (PC) ventilation,** the inspiratory pressure, inspiratory time, and I:E ratio are selected, and the ventilator automatically adjusts the gas flow rate to maintain a constant pressure during inspiration. The main advantage of this over volume control is that gas flow more closely matches the change in lung compliance that occurs during inspiration. This has the theoretical benefit of a more even distribution of inspired gas and possibly a lower risk of regional alveolar overdistention. It is also more comfortable for the awake patient. Although this can be achieved through manipulating the flow pattern in more advanced volume control ventilators, it is automatic in pressure control ventilation. Physiologic inspiratory times and I:E ratios are usually chosen to improve patient comfort. An inspiratory time of 1 second with an expiratory time of 2 or 3 seconds is typical. Longer inspiratory times with shorter expiratory times (**inverse ratio ventilation**) can be used if the physiologic times prove inadequate to provide enough support. The long inspiratory times, along with the short expiratory times, result in air trapping and increase the mean airway pressure. The net result is an increase in functional residual capacity (FRC), similar to that accomplished with high positive end-expiratory pressure (PEEP) levels.

Pressure support ventilation is also a pressure-limited form of ventilation and in most cases, can be considered a distinct mode of ventilation (see Table 13–1). It differs from pressure control in that it is always patient triggered, and the inspiratory time is determined by the patient and not set by the ventilator. As in pressure control ventilation, the ventilator adjusts the flow to maintain a constant pressure during inspiration. The inspiratory time, however, is determined by the interaction of the gas flow with the patient's inspiratory effort. To do this, the ventilator measures the peak inspiratory flow rate during inspiration. The flow rate usually reaches a maximum value early in the inspiration and then tapers off as the patient's inspiratory effort decreases. When the flow rate decreases to a predetermined fraction of the maximal flow (generally 25% of maximum), gas flow is terminated, and the patient is allowed to exhale. Pressure support can also be used in conjunction with the intermittent mandatory ventilation (IMV) mode (see next section).

The level of the pressure support (PS) is set so that the patient breathes comfortably at a reasonable rate, usually less than 24 breaths/min. The goal of the support is to ensure adequate oxygenation and a pH greater than 7.30. The tidal volume generated under these circumstances is generally unimportant.

The mode has many advantages. It is usually comfortable for the patient. It overcomes resistance to inspiratory flow in the endotracheal tube and in the ventilatory apparatus and decreases the work of breathing. It makes it impossible for the ventilator to deliver excessively high pressures. The flow is maintained for as long as the patient continues to make an inspiratory effort, so the patient can sigh at will. This minimizes the development of atelectasis. It is also ideally suited for preparing the patient for weaning and extubation.

C. Intermittent Mandatory Ventilation and Assist Control Ventilation

With **intermittent mandatory ventilation** (IMV), all aspects of breathing are controlled including the rate, inspiratory time, and expiratory time (and as a result, I:E ratio). The limit variable can be either pressure (PC IMV) or volume (VC IMV). The breaths are generally synchronized (SIMV) if the patient has spontaneous respiratory effort. In this mode, any attempt to breathe at a greater frequency than the set rate is unsupported unless additional pressure support is added. In this case, the patient receives two different modes during mechanical ventilation. The first is the mandatory, machine-triggered breath at the set rate and inspiratory time. The second is a spontaneous, patient-triggered breath at a rate equal to the total minus the set rate with an inspiratory time determined by the patient (see previous discussion of pressure support ventilation). These two breaths will have different waveform characteristics on the ventilator display.

Assist control mode was originally set up to "assist" the patient's spontaneous effort with a completely supported mechanical breath. It can be used with a volume or pressure limit (VC or PC) and set up with a backup rate when spontaneous effort is minimal or absent. The main distinction from SIMV is that all of the patient's inspiratory efforts are completely supported (not just those at the set rate). This has the small disadvantage of air trapping when the patient's respiratory rate is excessively high (> 30-35 breaths/min) and should be used with caution in patients at risk for hyperinflation (severe emphysema). There is no role for pressure support ventilation in this mode as all breaths are completely assisted.

D. Hybrid Modes

Over the past 15 years, it has become possible to ventilate patients with even more sophisticated hybrid modes. Some ventilators can be set up to deliver constant pressure during the inspiration in such a way that the tidal volume delivered falls in a preset range (**pressure-regulated volume control, PRVC**). Some ventilators can be set up to deliver a preset tidal volume but without exceeding a preset pressure. Some ventilators can be set up with gradually decreasing ventilatory support with algorithms built into the system to minimize the need for physician adjustment of the ventilator during weaning.

Setting Up the Ventilator

After choosing the mode (AC, SIMV, or PS; PC or VC), five parameters remain to be determined: the backup ventilatory rate, the goal tidal volume of the machine-delivered breaths, the inspiratory time, the inspired oxygen concentration (FIO_2), and the PEEP level. The first two of these parameters determine ventilation; the latter three are important in determining oxygenation.

Ventilation has three components: minute ventilation (V_E), alveolar ventilation (V_A), and dead space ventilation (V_D). Although V_A is most closely related to $PaCO_2$, at steady state, the relationship with V_E and V_D is roughly constant, and therefore V_E, which is easily quantified, can be used as a surrogate. In patients with uncomplicated pulmonary failure, the respiratory rate can be set at 12-15 breaths/min and the tidal volume set to 7 mL/kg IBW. This produces a V_E of 6-7.5 L/min and a V_A of 4-5 L/min (assuming V_D of 33% in a 70-kg patient). In the absence of significant pulmonary dysfunction, this will result in a $PaCO_2$ of approximately 40 mm Hg and is a good starting point from which adjustments can be made.

If the $PaCO_2$ is elevated, increases in the respiratory rate will often correct the problem. Although this is less efficient than increasing the tidal volume (due to the increased dead space ventilation that occurs with higher respiratory rates), it is a reasonable first step when the respiratory rate is less than 25. Excessively high respiratory rates (> 30 breaths/min) can result in air trapping, especially in patients with expiratory air flow obstruction (chronic obstructive pulmonary disease or severe asthma). On the other hand, excessively high volumes may be associated with elevated airway pressures and can result in barotrauma (pneumothorax), volutrauma (alveolar overdistention), or both. Except in certain circumstances (intracranial hypertension), it is better to accept a mild respiratory acidosis than to ventilate the patient using excessively large tidal volumes (greater than 10 mL/kg IBW) or excessively high airway pressures (plateau pressure greater than 30 cm H_2O). When the pH is less than 7.20, very high rates or volumes may be necessary until the pH can be brought into the normal range either through renal compensatory mechanisms or administered bicarbonate. Very high rates or volumes may also be necessary when a bronchopleural fistula is present, to compensate for the volume lost through the fistula.

The inspired oxygen concentration should be kept high enough so that, in most cases, the oxygen saturation of arterial blood exceeds 92%. Patients with chronic obstructive pulmonary disease and long-standing CO_2 retention are an exception. Such patients have lost the ability to increase their respiratory rate in response to increases in $PaCO_2$ and rely instead on their response to hypoxemia. Increasing the arterial oxygen saturation by adding exogenous oxygen takes away this hypoxic ventilatory stimulus and makes weaning from ventilatory support more difficult.

All of the non-oxygen volume of ventilator gas is made up of nitrogen, which, unlike oxygen, is not absorbed from alveoli. Nitrogen can be of great value in stenting open the alveoli. When it is replaced by increasing concentrations of oxygen, increased atelectasis caused by oxygen absorption can occur. In addition, high concentrations of oxygen can cause chronic pulmonary fibrosis. Ideally, the inspired oxygen concentration should be kept at 0.50 or less.

Keeping the inspired oxygen levels at acceptably low levels is frequently facilitated by the use of PEEP. The pressure is generated by closure of a valve in the expiratory circuit of the ventilator to keep the airway pressure above a preset level during expiration and to minimize alveolar collapse. Placement of an endotracheal tube bypasses the normal physiologic PEEP present during spontaneous ventilation from closure of the glottis at the end of expiration. In addition, supine patients may have a lower functional residual capacity due to increased intra-abdominal pressure and cephalad displacement of the diaphragm into the chest. This can be overcome through the use of low levels of "physiologic" PEEP (5 cm H_2O). Increasing the PEEP should be considered when the respiratory system compliance is low or when adequate oxygenation requires an FIO_2 that exceeds 0.50.

Low levels of PEEP (< 10 cm H_2O) are well tolerated by most patients. The consequences of excessive PEEP are barotrauma and decreased cardiac output. First, the high pressure can compress the superior and inferior vena cava and the pulmonary veins, compromising diastolic filling of the ventricles (in contrast with a spontaneous inspiration, which augments filling). Second, the high pressures can compress the thin-walled atria and right ventricle, further compromising end-diastolic volumes (also in contrast with a spontaneous inspiration). Finally, the high pressures can compress the pulmonary microvasculature, making it difficult for the right ventricle to push blood through the pulmonary vasculature. The remedy for the decreased cardiac output is usually fluid infusion. The potential problem with this remedy is worsening of the pulmonary failure that prompted the use of the PEEP in the first place. Titrating to the optimal oxygen delivery, and not arterial PaO_2, will ensure a balance between the risks and benefits of high PEEP levels. Even with invasive monitoring, PEEP levels greater than 15-20 cm H_2O are rarely of benefit.

Ventilator Safety & Alarms

As can be inferred, modern ventilators are complex, and they should, in general, be used only in the setting of continuous cardiopulmonary monitoring to include electrocardiography and pulse oximetry. In addition, the ventilators themselves have alarms for early warning of apnea, changes in tidal volume or minute ventilation, and excessive inspiratory pressures. These should be individualized to each patient so that nurses, respiratory therapists, and physicians are notified early in the course of the physiologic derangement. In many cases, the ventilator alarm will precede changes in the pulse oximeter or electrocardiogram. All personnel taking care of the patient should be knowledgeable with both the equipment and the mode of ventilation.

Discontinuing Mechanical Ventilation

Patients who seem to be doing well and who have required mechanical ventilation for less than 24 hours can frequently be extubated quickly after undergoing a trial of spontaneous ventilation. Patients must be able to maintain their own airway, and their acute illness should be resolving. They should be able to maintain adequate oxygenation with an inspired oxygen concentration of 0.40 or less and with a PEEP of 8 cm H_2O or less.

The majority of ventilated patients are most effectively weaned with daily spontaneous breathing trials (SBT). The breathing trial can be given with T-piece ventilation in which the endotracheal tube is attached to a length of tubing connected to a blow-by oxygen source. Alternatively, the trial can be accomplished with a low level (typically 5 cm H_2O) of pressure support with PEEP or with PEEP alone. In either case, the patient is asked to support his or her own breathing for 30 minutes. If the patient is breathing comfortably at the end of the trial, the patient can be extubated. If a question arises as to the degree of comfort, arterial blood should be drawn for gases, and the patient should be put back on the ventilator while waiting for the results of the blood gas analysis. If the patient was reasonably comfortable at the end of the 30-minute trial and if the pH comes back at a normal value, the patient can be extubated. Note that at the conclusion of the 30-minute trial, full ventilator support should be resumed pending the laboratory results. The patient needs to be well rested when the endotracheal tube is removed. If the patient fails the 30-minute trial, full support is resumed for the remainder of the day, and the trial is repeated the following day. In some cases, the duration of the breathing trial can be extended to up to 2 hours. Although the ability to predict successful extubation is not significantly different, the increased duration may be appropriate for patients who have already required reintubation following completion of a 30-minute SBT. There is generally no role for breathing trials of longer duration when the patient is endotracheally intubated. In fact, this may serve to unnecessarily fatigue the patient, making successful extubation less likely.

Weaning from mechanical ventilation can also be achieved with IMV. Although generally inferior to the once-daily spontaneous breathing trial, patients who are severely debilitated and have required mechanical ventilation for prolonged periods (> 2-3 weeks) can be successfully weaned using this technique when combined with a gradual reduction in pressure support. The IMV rate is gradually decreased, requiring the patient to contribute increasingly

to the maintenance of adequate minute ventilation. The patient's overall clinical status, respiratory rate, and arterial Pco_2 are used as guidelines to determine the rate of weaning. When an IMV of 4/min or less is well tolerated for long periods, the patient is placed on pressure support, which is weaned daily until mechanical support is no longer needed. As noted above, patients with an endotracheal tube in place (vs tracheostomy) should only undergo brief periods where the pressure support is below 5-8 cm H_2O (30-120 minutes). This amount of PS is required to mitigate the increased resistance of the endotracheal tube. Patients who repeatedly fail extubation or are severely deconditioned benefit from a more deliberate and gradual weaning of the ventilator. Frequently, these patients benefit from tracheostomy and optimization of nutritional status as adjuncts to weaning. Factors that increase the work of breathing—such as reactive airway disease, large pleural effusions, and chest wall or visceral edema—should be treated and minimized.

Extubation

The decision to extubate the patient depends both on the assessment for the need for airway protection as well as the need for mechanical ventilation. As mentioned previously, the latter can be determined based on the result of a 30-minute trial of spontaneous breathing. The former should be based on several factors, including the patient's level of consciousness, the presence of airway injury or edema, the need for ongoing endotracheal suctioning, and the possible need for further operative procedures within the next 24 hours. Finally, a subjective determination of a patient's ability to tolerate extubation and spontaneous ventilation should be made. An alert and communicative patient who can lift her head off the pillow is a good candidate for extubation; a lethargic, diaphoretic patient is not. For patients who require continued airway protection but no longer require mechanical ventilatory support, a tracheostomy should be considered.

ADJUVANT DIAGNOSTIC & THERAPEUTIC MEASURES

Chest Radiographs

Chest x-rays should be obtained daily in patients being treated with mechanical ventilation. A review of the film should confirm the placement of all lines and tubes, including the endotracheal tube, central venous catheters, pleural tubes (thoracostomies), and naso/orogastric or naso/oroenteric tubes. A search for specific pulmonary and pleural processes should be performed. Local infiltrates such as pneumonia or patchy/diffuse processes such as the acute respiratory distress syndrome should be identified.

In addition to a daily chest radiograph, a STAT chest x-ray should be obtained whenever a patient's cardiopulmonary status rapidly deteriorates. Tubes or lines might be displaced; new problems with a reversible etiology—such a pneumothorax, a lobar collapse, or a new infiltrate suggesting aspiration—might be identified.

▶ Sedation, Muscle Relaxants, & Other Adjuncts

Mechanically ventilated patients frequently require sedatives and/or analgesia to ameliorate the agitation and pain associated with their disease and treatment. Narcotic analgesia in the form of intermittent or continuous opiate infusion may be sufficient. Narcotics, however, should not be used to treat agitation and anxiety that is thought to be caused by the ventilator. Sedating agents, including propofol and benzodiazepines, should be used instead. In addition, haloperidol and risperidone may be useful adjuncts, either alone or in combination with benzodiazepines. As a general rule, intermittent dosing is preferred to continuous infusions. When the latter is used, the agent should be stopped at least once daily—giving the patient a so-called sedation holiday—to assess neurologic status and determine the need for continuing sedation.

Neuromuscular blocking agents such as cisatracurium add an additional level of patient control and can greatly simplify ventilatory management in patients with severe pulmonary insufficiency. These agents should be reserved for severe patient–ventilator dyssynchrony, a situation in which the patient's spontaneous respiratory efforts result in discoordinated and inadequate ventilation by the mechanical ventilator.

Nonphysiologic ventilatory methods, such as inverse ratio or high-frequency oscillatory ventilation, may also require the use of neuromuscular blocking agents. Major side effects include a potential increased risk of ventilator-associated pneumonia (VAP), through loss of cough mechanism, and an association with late polyneuromyopathy of critical illness. As a result, they should be used only when absolutely necessary and for the shortest possible time.

In severe ARDS, prone positioning should be considered. Although prone positioning has not been found to decrease time to extubation or ICU length of stay, it has been found to significantly decrease mortality in patients with severe ARDS as compared to supine positioning alone. This is thought to be secondary to prone positioning improving alveolar recruitment and reducing overdistention of the lung. It is important that prone positioning be performed by a coordinated team as adverse events directly related to repositioning, such as endotracheal tube dislodgement, can be life threatening.

▶ Antibiotics

VAP is the most common nosocomial infection in the intensive care unit. The risk of acquiring VAP is directly related to the duration of mechanical ventilation. There is no gold standard for VAP diagnosis. Possible criteria include a new or progressive infiltrate on chest radiograph, worsening hypoxemia, increased sputum quantity, new onset of purulent sputum associated with abundant white cells and organisms on Gram-stained smears, or positive sputum cultures with known pathogenic organisms. Signs of systemic sepsis with increased temperature, leukocytosis, increasing fluid requirements, and glucose intolerance are also common findings in VAP.

If all of these are present, antibiotics should be started. If only one or two are present, antibiotics are probably best withheld to avoid overgrowth of resistant organisms that could later cause fatal pneumonia. Exceptions to this approach include older, severely debilitated patients, immunocompromised patients, and those who are critically ill in whom delayed antibiotic therapy might result in irretrievable deterioration. Thus, an 80-year-old patient with flail chest and a new infiltrate should probably be given antibiotics early; a 20-year-old patient who was hospitalized for a gunshot wound involving the colon and who develops questionable pneumonia 2 weeks later is more likely to tolerate a delay in the initiation of antibiotics until the diagnosis is more definite. In addition, the latter patient may have an alternative explanation for his fever and leukocytosis, such as an intra-abdominal abscess. In this case, the wrong diagnosis might delay appropriate source control (abscess drainage). The CPIS can be useful to guide the diagnosis. The goal is to avoid overtreatment with the risk of antimicrobial resistance and superinfection. Antibiotics can safely be discontinued in patients empirically started on antibiotics for suspected pneumonia who have a CPIS value of 6 or less at 72 hours.

Most importantly, VAP can be mitigated by the use of a VAP-prevention bundle, as recommended by the Institute of Healthcare Improvement. These bundles typically consist of five elements: oral care with chlorhexidine, head of bed elevation, stress ulcer prophylaxis with H2 blockers or proton pump inhibitors (PPI), deep vein thrombosis (DVT) prophylaxis, and daily sedation assessments and spontaneous breathing trials as appropriate. Although these elements do not decrease time to extubation or time in the ICU, they have been shown to decrease VAP rates. Of course, this bundle is only as effective as the compliance of the healthcare staff in implementing the elements, and this should be emphasized to both ordering physicians and nursing care staff.

Barr J, Fraser GL, Puntillo K, et al. Clinical practice guidelines for the management of pain, agitation, and delirium in adult patients in the intensive care unit. *Crit Care Med.* 2013;41:263-306.

Graham DB, Eastman AL, Aldy KN, et al. Outcomes and long term follow up after emergent cricothyroidotomy: Is routine conversion to tracheostomy necessary? *Am Surg.* 2011;77:1707-1711.

Institute for Healthcare Improvement. *How-to Guide: Prevent Ventilator-Associated Pneumonia.* Cambridge, MA: Institute for Healthcare Improvement; 2012.

King DR. Emergent cricothyroidotomy in the morbidly obese: A safe, no-visualization technique. *J Trauma.* 2011;71:1873-1874.

Schweickert WD, Pohlman MC, Pohlman AS, et al. Early physical and occupational therapy in mechanically ventilated, critically ill patients: A randomized controlled trial. *Lancet.* 2009; 373:1874-1882.

▼ TREATMENT OF THE MORE CHALLENGING PATIENT

OXYHEMOGLOBIN DISSOCIATION

The amount of oxygen contained in the blood and the amount of oxygen available to be delivered to the tissues can be expressed as a concentration, a saturation, or a partial pressure. All three have their values. Understanding their relationships can help in understanding the cardiac and pulmonary pathophysiology of the critically ill surgical patient.

The concentration of oxygen in the blood, or oxygen content, is expressed as milliliters of O_2/dL of blood, or vol%. The oxygen content can be measured directly, but the measurement is time-consuming, and the content is usually calculated on the basis of the other two measures of blood oxygenation: the oxygen saturation (So_2) and the Po_2. The oxygen content is related to these other quantities by the following formula:

$$Co_2 = 1.34 \times [Hb] \times So_2 + 0.0031 \times Po_2 \qquad (1)$$

where [Hb] is expressed as g/dL and the Po_2 as mm Hg. Thus, for example, the oxygen content of a blood specimen with a [Hb] of 12 g/dL, an So_2 of 90%, and a Po_2 of 60 mm Hg is 14.7 vol%.

The first term in the equation represents the O_2 carried by the hemoglobin molecule; the second, the O_2 dissolved in the blood water. This second term is small compared with the first as long as the [Hb] is greater than, say, 7 g/dL and the Po_2 is less than, say, 100 mm Hg. Omitting the second term then simplifies the formula to read as follows:

$$Co_2 = 1.34 \times [Hb] \times So_2 \qquad (2)$$

For the previous set of blood gases, this would give a Co_2 of 14.5 vol%.

The formula can be made even simpler by substituting the fraction 4/3 for the decimal 1.34:

$$CO_2 = 4/3 \times [Hb] \times SO_2 \qquad (3)$$

Because [Hb] and the So_2 can usually be approximated by integers with little loss of accuracy, the calculation frequently allows cancellation of the 3 and can be done mentally. For the previous example, the oxygen content would be 14.4 vol%.

▲ **Figure 13–1.** Oxyhemoglobin dissociation curve for human blood at 37°C with a Pco_2 of 40 mm Hg, a pH of 0.40, and a normal 2,3-DPG red cell concentration. Approximate values from Table 13–3 fall close to the idealized curve.

Calculation of the oxygen content requires knowledge of the So_2. Most laboratories will calculate the So_2 from the Po_2. This calculation is frequently inaccurate for mixed venous specimens but is usually accurate for arterial blood. The calculation is made from equations that are based on the oxyhemoglobin dissociation curve (Figure 13–1), an empirically derived relationship between the So_2 of nonfetal human blood and its Po_2. The saturation for a given Po_2 depends on blood temperature, [H+], and Pco_2 and on the red cell concentration of 2,3-diphosphoglycerate (2,3-DPG). The laboratory should be told the temperature, and it will measure the [H+] and Pco_2. It will then calculate the So_2 from the Po_2 with the assumption that the 2,3-DPG concentration is normal.

It is helpful, however, to have some guidelines for converting back and forth between So_2 and Po_2. Five approximations for points on the dissociation curve for a patient with normal temperature, [H+], Pco_2, and 2, 3-DPG levels are given in Table 13–2. The P_{50} of human hemoglobin—the Po_2 at which the molecule is half-saturated—is 27 mm Hg (approximated as 25 mm Hg in the table). The Po_2 and So_2 for mixed venous blood in a person with a [Hb] of 15 g/dL and a normal O_2 consumption and cardiac output are 40 mm Hg and 75%, respectively. A Po_2 of 60 mm Hg—a value that should be exceeded by most patients in an intensive care unit—corresponds to a So_2 of 90%. A Po_2 of 80 mm Hg corresponds to a So_2 of 95%. Remembering the values in the table allows construction of a dissociation curve and facilitates conversion from one measure of oxygenation to the other. For example, in a patient with a normal temperature, [H+], Pco_2, and 2,3-DPG, and a [Hb] of 10 g/dL, a Po_2 of 60 mm Hg in the systemic arterial blood would create an

Table 13–2. Approximate correlations for partial pressures of oxygen and oxygen saturation (in blood at 37°C with a pH of 7.4, a P_{CO_2} of 40 mm Hg, and a normal 2,3-DPG red cell concentration).

P_{O_2}	S_{O_2}
0 mm Hg	0%
25 mm Hg	50%
40 mm Hg	75%
60 mm Hg	90%
80 mm Hg	95%

oxygen content of 12 vol% (from Equation 1), a value that would be adequate if the patient had normal coronary arteries and a good heart. Such a value would be inadequate, however, in the face of underlying heart disease.

CAUSES OF ELEVATED PaCO$_2$

The patient in pulmonary failure will frequently have an elevated arterial carbon dioxide tension. The arterial P_{CO_2} is proportionate to CO_2 production divided by alveolar ventilation—defined as the volume of air exchanged per unit time in functioning alveoli. Since CO_2 production is usually fairly constant in adequately perfused patients, the PaCO$_2$ comes to be inversely proportionate to alveolar ventilation. An elevated PaCO$_2$ in the presence of normal CO_2 production means inadequate alveolar ventilation. Ventilation should be assessed with respect to how much work is required to generate the PaCO$_2$. In the case of spontaneous ventilation, this assessment involves the frequency and depth of breathing; in the case of mechanical ventilation, the frequency of the machine-generated breaths and the tidal volume of those breaths.

The PaCO$_2$ also gives an indication of dead space ventilation—the ventilation of nonperfused airways. Since minute or total ventilation is dead space ventilation plus alveolar ventilation, a normal PaCO$_2$ combined with a normal minute ventilation implies a normal dead space ventilation. A normal PaCO$_2$ that must be generated by a supranormal minute ventilation implies increased dead space ventilation. Normal dead space ventilation is one-third of total ventilation, but many critically ill surgical patients will have dead space ventilation that is up to two-thirds of total ventilation. Increased dead space ventilation can be caused by hypovolemia with poor perfusion of nondependent alveoli, ARDS, pulmonary emboli, pulmonary vasoconstriction, and mechanical ventilation-induced compression of the pulmonary vasculature. Hypovolemia should be treated by expansion of the vascular volume. Emboli should be treated by anticoagulation or by elimination of their source. Dead space generated by mechanical ventilation should be minimized by adjustment

of the ventilator, usually by decreasing tidal volumes or end-expiratory pressures, while at the same time maintaining enough mechanical support to generate a normal P_{CO_2} and alveolar ventilation.

CAUSES OF LOW Pao$_2$

Almost all surgical patients with pulmonary failure will have systemic arterial hypoxemia. There are five physiologic causes: low inspired O_2 concentration, diffusion block between alveolar gas and capillary blood, subnormal alveolar ventilation, shunting of blood through completely nonventilated portions of the lung or bypassing of blood past the lung, and perfusion of parts of the lung that have low ventilation/perfusion ratios. In addition, any process that decreases the mixed venous oxygen content in the presence of any of the above can lower the arterial P_{O_2} even further. Low mixed venous oxygen content can be caused by a low arterial oxygen content, low cardiac output, or high O_2 consumption.

Arterial hypoxemia in the surgical patient is usually caused by shunting, low ventilation/perfusion ratios, low mixed venous oxygen content, or a combination of these factors. Low inspired O_2 concentrations at sea level are impossible so long as the ventilator is functioning properly. (This must be checked, however, as the first step in diagnosing and correcting the cause of a low Pao$_2$.) Diffusion block is exceedingly rare in surgical patients. Subnormal alveolar ventilation can be ruled out with a normal arterial P_{CO_2} assuming CO_2 production is not depressed. Thus, shunting and areas of low ventilation/perfusion ratios, along with low mixed venous oxygen content, remain as causes for almost all cases of hypoxemia in the surgical patient. Shunting and low ventilation/perfusion ratios do not need to be distinguished from each other very often, but the distinction can be made by increasing the inspired O_2 concentration to 100%: Hypoxemia caused by areas of low ventilation/perfusion ratios will be at least partially corrected by 100% O_2; hypoxemia caused by shunting will not.

ACID–BASE BALANCE

Acid–base abnormalities can arise from the hypoventilation of pulmonary insufficiency or from the metabolic abnormalities of shock. The former has already been discussed. The latter can become more involved.

The hydrogen ion, carbon dioxide gas, and bicarbonate equilibrate with one another in the plasma water, and if two of the quantities are known, the third can be calculated. In practice, the P_{CO_2} and [H$^+$], which are measured directly with the blood gas apparatus, will be known. The [HCO$_3^-$] can then be calculated by the Henderson–Hasselbach equation, which can be written in the following form:

$$[HCO_3^-] = \frac{24 \times P_{CO_2}}{[H^+]} \tag{4}$$

Table 13–3. Conversion of pH to hydrogen ion concentration.

pH	Hydrogen Ion Concentration (nmol/L)
7.0	100
7.1	$100 \times 0.8 = 80$
7.2	$80 \times 0.8 = 63$
7.3	$63 \times 0.8 = 50$
7.4	$50 \times 0.8 = 40$
7.5	$40 \times 0.8 = 32$
7.6	$32 \times 0.8 = 25$

Values not indicated in the table can be derived by interpolation. For example, a pH of 7.35 corresponds to a hydrogen ion concentration of approximately 45.

where $[HCO_3^-]$ is expressed as mmol/L, Pco_2 as mm Hg, and $[H^+]$ as nmol/L. This form of the equation requires conversion of pH, the more common expression of $[H^+]$, into nmol/L, the more logical expression, but the conversion is not difficult (Table 13–3). The values in the table are easy to remember if one notes that each value in the column under $[H^+]$ is 80% of the value immediately above, with the exception of 80 and 63, which are off by 1. Thus, by Equation 4, if the Pco_2 is 60 mm Hg and the pH is 7.30, the $[HCO_3^-]$ is 29 mmol/L.

The $[HCO_3^-]$ calculated by this equation is the amount of bicarbonate ion dissolved in the plasma water and can be obtained only from a specimen of blood that is obtained and processed without exposure to the atmosphere. The "Co_2 combining power" that is typically measured along with electrolyte concentrations in blood that is not processed anaerobically includes not only the $[HCO_3^-]$ but any Co_2 gas and carbonic acid that is dissolved in the plasma as well. The Co_2 combining power is usually about 2 mmol/L greater than the calculated (and actual) $[HCO_3^-]$.

The base deficit or excess is determined by comparing the calculated $[HCO_3^-]$ with the $[HCO_3^-]$ that might be expected in a patient with a given Pco_2 and $[H^+]$. These expected values have been determined by analyzing blood obtained from patients with a wide variety of pulmonary disorders. For example, the kidneys in a patient with chronic respiratory acidemia can usually compensate to the extent that a chronic elevation in Pco_2 of 10 mm Hg will generate an increase in $[HCO_3^-]$ of 3 mmol/L. A patient with chronic obstructive lung disease and a chronically elevated Pco_2 of 60 mm Hg would be expected to have a $[HCO_3^-]$ of 30 mmol/L—6 mmol/L more than a normal value of 24. If such a patient had a pH of 7.30, the actual $[HCO_3^-]$ would be 29 mmol/L (from Equation 4; see the example in the

preceding paragraph). That is, the observed value would be 1 mmol/L less than predicted, and the patient would be said to have a base deficit of 1 mmol/L.

The difficulty with the concept of base deficit and excess is that it rests on historically determined values, which may not be applicable to the patient at hand. For example, if a surgical patient with previously normal lungs lost his or her airway after an operation and began to hypoventilate, one would expect the $[HCO_3^-]$ to be normal—24 mmol/L—because the kidneys would not have had time to compensate for the hypercapnia. If the Pco_2 was 60 mm Hg and the pH 7.30, the physician should be concerned because the $[HCO_3^-]$ is 29 mmol/L (these values are the same as in the preceding paragraphs). A value of 29 mmol/L should alert the physician to the fact that the $[HCO_3^-]$ is too high, perhaps because $NaHCO_3$ had been given unnecessarily. The base deficit, however, would be 1 mmol/L, suggesting that the patient's $[HCO_3^-]$ was appropriate. The base deficit would be misleading.

The use of base deficit and excess is ensconced in the literature, and the terms are used in this chapter. However, the concept of $[HCO_3^-]$ may be preferable. Errors in patient evaluation are more likely to be minimized if the physician interprets that value in the light of a particular patient's situation. If a chronically ill patient in the intensive care unit has severe ARDS and a Pco_2 of 60 mm Hg with a pH of 7.30, no attempt should be made to change the accompanying $[HCO_3^-]$ of 29 mmol/L—that value represents the expected renal compensation for such a chronic hypercapnia (though the impaired alveolar ventilation should be of concern). Alternatively, if the patient's Pco_2 is 60 mm Hg and the pH is 7.45, the patient has an inappropriately high $[HCO_3^-]$ of approximately 40 mmol/L (calculated from Equation 4), perhaps because of unreplaced losses of hydrogen ion from the stomach, chronic use of a loop diuretic, or administration of excessive amounts of acetate in the patient's parenteral nutrition. In this situation, the $[HCO_3^-]$ should be brought down into the low 30s. The excessively high $[HCO_3^-]$ and its resultant alkalemia may be blunting the patient's ventilatory drive.

Thus, in dealing with acid–base disorders, the calculation of the bicarbonate concentration in arterial plasma can be taken from the blood gas laboratory or calculated by the clinician. In the case of a metabolic acidemia, the underlying abnormality should be corrected and then, if the pH remains less than 7.20, sodium bicarbonate can be used, but only after resuscitation has been initiated and only with the intent of bringing the pH up to a modestly higher level, such as 7.30. The bicarbonate produces carbon dioxide and water locally, in the interstitial fluid at the sites where the hydrogen ions are being produced. In the absence of resuscitation, the locally generated carbon dioxide can cross back into the cell, worsening intracellular acidosis. There is no problem with bicarbonate if it is given after some local flow has been achieved. The generated carbon dioxide will be washed centrally into the pulmonary vasculature, where it will be eliminated by the lungs.

Metabolic alkalemia in the surgical patient is usually easy to recognize and treat. Contraction alkalemia is treated with fluid expansion. Hypokalemic, hypochloremic metabolic alkalemia caused by unreplaced loss of gastric fluid (continuous nasogastric suction or protracted vomiting) is treated with normal saline supplemented with potassium chloride. Hypokalemic hypochloremic alkalemia caused by use of loop diuretics is treated by withholding diuresis. In situations where continued diuresis is warranted, the addition of acetazolamide to the diuretic regimen is helpful. Although the administration of 0.1 N hydrochloric acid can reverse severe alkalemia, it is rarely necessary and should only be given as a slow central intravenous drip over a period of 48 hours. The amount of acid to be given is calculated on the basis of the presumed extracellular chloride deficit, with the assumption that the interstitial chloride concentration is the same as the plasma concentration—that is, with the assumption that the Donnan factor for chloride is 1.

MULTIPLE-CHOICE QUESTIONS

1. The pulmonary failure of shock, trauma, and sepsis:
   A. Can be related to products of coagulation and inflammation that are washed out from the damaged tissues.
   B. Can be effectively treated with a combination of antibiotics and corticosteroids.
   C. Is always related to systemic infection.
   D. Is caused by a decrease in pulmonary vascular permeability.
   E. Both A and C .

2. All of the following are true about pressure support ventilation, *except:*
   A. PSV is a pressure-limited ventilator mode.
   B. PSV includes a set inspiratory time.
   C. PSV breaths are patient-triggered.
   D. Inspiratory flow is adjusted to maintain airway pressure.
   E. PSV can be combined with intermittent mandatory ventilation.

3. The Berlin criteria for ARDS include all of the following *except:*
   A. Acute onset of hypoxemia.
   B. Positive sputum cultures.
   C. Bilateral infiltrates on CXR or CT scan.
   D. Pao_2:Fio_2 less than 300.

4. Indication for intubation include the following except:
   A. Significant hypercarbia.
   B. Tachypnea with significant work of breathing and use of accessory muscles.
   C. Need for excessive sedation as in prolonged and painful burn dressings.
   D. GCS < 14.

5. Which of the following is *not* an element of a typical ventilator-associated pneumonia prevention bundle?
   A. Oral care with chlorhexidine.
   B. Prophylactic antibiotics.
   C. Head of bed elevation.
   D. Stress ulcer prophylaxis with H2 blockers or PPI.
   E. Daily sedation assessments and spontaneous breathing trials as appropriate.

Management of the Injured Patient

Mark R. Hemmila, MD

EPIDEMIOLOGY OF TRAUMA

As a "disease," trauma is a major public health problem. In the United States, it is the leading cause of death among people aged 1-45. For younger persons, trauma is responsible for more deaths than all other diseases combined, and results in the loss of more working years than all other causes of death. The prevalence of injury in the elderly population is also significant; 6% of Medicare inpatient admissions have traumatic injury as their primary diagnosis. The presence of alcohol is a significant contributor to trauma fatalities, and one-third of all traffic deaths are alcohol related. The financial costs of injury are substantial, exceeding $671 billion annually (fatal inquiries, $214 billion; nonfatal injuries, $457 billion). Regrettably, nearly 40% of all trauma deaths could be avoided by injury-prevention measures, alcohol cessation, and by the establishment of regional trauma systems that would expedite the evaluation and treatment of seriously injured patients.

Trauma deaths have classically been described as having a trimodal distribution (Figure 14–1a), with peaks that correspond to the types of intervention that would be most effective in reducing mortality. However, with advancements in care and maturation of trauma systems, the trimodal concept no longer applies. The incidence of late deaths has declined from 20% to 7%–8% of all deaths, and early deaths have shifted toward the left, creating a bimodal distribution (Figure 14–1b). Early deaths still predominate, with the remainder dying at a slow rate over many days. **Immediate deaths** represent patients who die of their injuries before reaching the hospital. The injuries accounting for these deaths include major brain or spinal cord trauma and those resulting in rapid exsanguination. Few of these patients would have any chance of survival even with access to immediate care, because almost 60% of these deaths occur at the same time as the injury. Prevention remains the major strategy to reduce these deaths.

Early deaths are those that occur within the first few hours after injury. Half are caused by internal hemorrhage, and the other half by central nervous system injuries. Almost all of these injuries are potentially treatable. However, in most cases, salvage requires prompt and definitive care of the sort available at a trauma center, which is a specialized institution that can provide immediate resuscitation, identification of injuries, and access to a ready operating room 24 hours a day. Development of well-organized trauma systems with rapid transport and protocol-driven care can reduce the mortality in this time period by 30%.

Late deaths consist of patients who die days or weeks after injury. Fewer deaths overall are occurring during this period. Development of trauma systems has changed the epidemiology of these deaths. During the first week, refractory intracranial hypertension following severe head injury is now responsible for a significant number of these deaths. Improvements in critical care management continue to be essential in reducing deaths during this phase, which are largely attributed to infection and multiple-organ failure. It is paramount that surgeons caring for trauma patients have genuine expertise in surgical critical care.

TRAUMA SYSTEMS

The terrorist attacks of September 11, 2001 and ongoing mass shooting and bombing incidents highlight the need for national and state trauma systems that can handle both routine events and mass casualty situations. The Zero Preventable Deaths Campaign for trauma care has identified the pragmatic, rapid model for learning "focused empiricism" developed and employed by the Joint Trauma System of the U.S. military as evidence of a learning healthcare system that improves patient outcomes and reduces preventable mortality. A learning healthcare system, as defined by the Institute of Medicine, is characterized by a consistent emphasis on a collaborative approach that shares data and

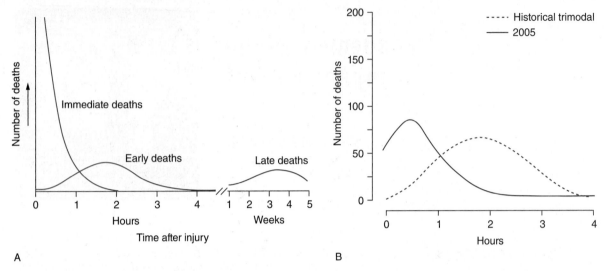

▲ **Figure 14–1.** Mortality timing: Periods of peak mortality after injury. *A:* Historical. *B:* Current. (Modified with permission from Greenfield LJ, Mulholland MW, Oldham KT, et al: *Surgery, Scientific Principles and Practice*, 3rd ed. Philadelphia, PA: Lippincott Williams & Wilkins; 2001.)

insights across boundaries to drive better, more efficient medical practice and patient care. A regional collaborative quality-improvement model provides the optimal framework to deliver improved patient outcomes while promoting compliance with processes of care for trauma patients.

The purpose of a trauma system is to provide timely, organized care in order to minimize preventable morbidity and mortality following injury. The system includes prehospital care designed to identify, triage, treat, and transport victims with serious injuries. Criteria for staging patients with major trauma consist of standardized scoring systems based on readily discernible anatomic and physiologic variables. These criteria are designed to identify not only the more severe and complex single injuries but also combinations of injuries that require tertiary care. Trauma centers that are part of a larger trauma system are already organized to respond to unexpected multiple-casualty events. Regional trauma centers have established links with emergency medical service providers and participate in systemwide patient triage and quality improvement. Gaps remain, however, in areas of the country not served by trauma systems, and a wide range in the degree of disaster preparedness exists at all levels of trauma care.

The American College of Surgeons (ACS) defines four levels of institutional trauma care. **Level I** is the highest designation a trauma center can receive. It indicates that the hospital has committed itself to the care of trauma patients and offers the highest level of skill available in trauma care. A Level I trauma center is directed by a board-certified surgeon specializing in trauma care and is staffed by a team of board-certified trauma care specialists available 24 hours a day—including emergency room physicians, trauma surgeons, neurosurgeons and neurologists, orthopedic surgeons, plastic surgeons, anesthesiologists, and radiologists. **Level II** trauma centers provide 24-hour care by in-hospital and on-call physicians. They can deliver the same quality of care as a level I center but without the same teaching and research obligations. **Level III** trauma center provides prompt assessment, resuscitation, and stabilization followed by surgical treatment or interhospital transfer as appropriate. Level III centers serve a valuable function in less populated areas where resuscitation and stabilization before transport may be lifesaving. **Level IV** centers are designed to provide advanced trauma life support prior to patient transfer in remote areas in which no higher level of care is available.

Determining if a patient requires care at a trauma center is a decision for emergency medical responders. The Centers for Disease Control and Prevention (CDC) has sponsored research and policy making aimed at providing guidance to answer this question. It is established that care at a Level I trauma center reduces the risk of death by 25% for severely injured patients, when compared to treatment at a hospital that does not have verified trauma center resources. The CDC has published guidelines based on research and expert panel findings for the field triage of injured patients. The published guidelines for the field triage of injured patients provides a rapid, easily understood algorithm that allows for determination of where to triage trauma patients based upon findings at the scene, taking into account assessment of vital signs/level of consciousness, anatomic evidence of injury, and mechanism of injury with regard to the level of energy involved (Figure 14–2).

2011 guidelines for field triage of injured patients

▲ **Figure 14–2.** CDC 2011 Guidelines for field triage of injured patients.

PREHOSPITAL CARE & IMMEDIATE MEASURES AT AN INCIDENT SITE

At first glance, the trauma victim may not appear to be badly injured. Sometimes there may be little external evidence of injury; however, when the mechanism of trauma is sufficient to produce severe injury, the victim must be handled as if a severe injury has occurred. It is critical at the scene that the injured person be protected from further trauma; likewise, rescue personnel need to take precautions to avoid injury to themselves. First aid at the scene of an accident should be administered by trained personnel whenever possible.

Whether the patient is first seen on the battlefield, beside a road, in the emergency ward, or in the hospital, the basic principles of initial management are the same:

1. Is the victim breathing? If not, provide an airway and establish bag-mask ventilation.

2. Is there a pulse or heartbeat? If not, begin closed-chest compression.

3. Is there gross external bleeding? If so, elevate the part if possible and apply enough external pressure to stop the bleeding. A tourniquet when utilized by trained providers is acceptable in circumstances of extreme bleeding.

4. Is there any question of injury to the spine? If so, protect the neck and spine before moving the patient.

5. Splint obvious fractures.

As soon as these steps have been taken, the patient can be safely transported.

The Stop the Bleed Program was born in the aftermath of the active shooter disaster on December 14, 2012 at Sandy Hook Elementary School in Newtown, Connecticut. In April 2013, a group known as the Joint Committee to Create a National Policy to Enhance Survivability from Active Shooter Events and Intentional Mass Casualty, was convened by the ACS in collaboration with others in the medical community and representatives from the federal government. The committee's recommendations are called the Hartford Consensus. Massive bleeding from any cause, but particularly from an active shooter or explosive event where a response is delayed, can result in death. Similar to how the general public learns and performs cardiopulmonary resuscitation, the public must learn proper bleeding-control techniques, including how to use their hands, dressings, and tourniquets. Victims can quickly die from uncontrolled bleeding, within 5-10 minutes. However, anyone at the scene can act as an immediate responder and save lives if they know what to do. BleedingControl.org is an initiative to educate and train the public on bleeding control measures that anyone can perform at the scene to save a life.

EVALUATION OF THE TRAUMA PATIENT

In most situations, a brief history is obtained from prehospital personnel via radio communication or when the patient arrives at the hospital. In the case of motor vehicle crashes, for example, it is important to determine the circumstances of the injury, including the speed of impact, the condition of the vehicle, the position of the patient at the scene, type of restraint systems present, evidence of blood loss, and the condition of other passengers. The time that the injury occurred and the treatment rendered while en route are recorded. Knowing the mechanism of injury often gives a clue to concealed trauma. Information regarding serious underlying medical problems should be sought from Medic Alert bracelets or wallet cards. If the patient is conscious and stable, the examiner should obtain a complete history and use this information to direct the examination in order to avoid unnecessary tests.

Trauma victims require a precise, rapid, systematic approach to initial evaluation in order to ensure their survival. The Advanced Trauma Life Support (ATLS) system developed by the ACS Committee on Trauma represents the best current approach to the severely injured patient. The sequence of evaluation includes primary survey, resuscitation, secondary survey, and definitive management. The primary survey attempts to identify and treat immediate life-threatening conditions. Resuscitation is performed, and the response to therapy is evaluated. The secondary survey includes a comprehensive physical examination designed to detect all injuries and establish a treatment priority for potentially life-threatening and/or limb-threatening ones. During the primary and secondary surveys, appropriate laboratory and imaging studies are performed to aid in the identification of injuries and prepare the patient for definitive care.

1. PRIMARY SURVEY

The ATLS 10th edition manual and provider course published by the ACS Committee on Trauma is the accepted guideline for the primary survey. The primary survey is a rapid assessment to detect life-threatening injuries following the ABCDE algorithm: airway, breathing, circulation, disability, and exposure/environment.

AIRWAY

The establishment of an adequate airway has the highest priority in the primary survey. Oxygen by high-flow nasal cannula (10–12 L/min), 100% nonrebreather mask, or bag-mask ventilation with pulse oximetry should be started if not already in place. Maneuvers used in the trauma patient to establish an airway must consider a possible cervical spine injury. Any patient with multisystem trauma, especially those with an altered level of consciousness or blunt trauma above

▲ **Figure 14–3.** Relief of airway obstruction.

▲ **Figure 14–4.** *Top:* Nasotracheal intubation. *Bottom:* Orotracheal intubation.

the clavicles, should be assumed to have a cervical spine injury. The rapid assessment for signs of airway obstruction should include inspection for foreign bodies and facial, jaw, or tracheal/laryngeal fractures that may result in acute loss of airway patency. Techniques that can be used to establish a patent airway while protecting the cervical spine include the chin lift or jaw thrust maneuvers (Figure 14–3).

Patients who can speak without difficulty are unlikely to have an impaired airway. Repeated assessment of airway patency is always prudent. Those patients with a severe head injury, altered level of consciousness, or Glasgow coma scale (GCS) score of 8 or less usually require placement of a definitive airway. Orotracheal or nasotracheal intubation can be attempted with cervical spine precautions if a second person maintains axial immobilization of the head to prevent destabilization of the spine (Figure 14–4). If ventilatory failure occurs and an adequate airway cannot be obtained readily by orotracheal or nasotracheal intubation, surgical cricothyroidotomy should be performed as rapidly as possible (Figure 14–5).

BREATHING

Once the airway has been established, it is necessary to ensure that oxygenation and ventilation are adequate. Examine the patient to determine the degree of chest expansion, breath sounds, tachypnea, crepitus from rib fractures, subcutaneous emphysema, and the presence of penetrating or open wounds. Immediately life-threatening pulmonary injuries that must be detected and treated promptly include tension pneumothorax, open pneumothorax, flail chest, and massive hemothorax. Chest injury has the second-highest case-fatality rate in the trauma patient. The following are examples of life-threatening pulmonary injuries and their treatment.

1. Tension pneumothorax—This condition occurs when air becomes trapped in the pleural space under pressure. The harmful effects result primarily from shift of the mediastinum, impairment of venous return, and potential occlusion of the airway. Tension pneumothorax is difficult to diagnose even when the patient reaches the hospital. The clinical findings consist of hypotension in the presence of distended neck veins, decreased or absent breath sounds on the affected side, hyperresonance to percussion, and tracheal shift away from the affected side. These signs may be difficult to detect in a hypovolemic patient with a cervical collar in place. Cyanosis may be a late manifestation. Emergency treatment consists of insertion of a large-bore needle or plastic intravenous cannula (angiocath) through the chest wall into the pleural space in the second intercostal space along the midclavicular line to relieve the pressure and convert the tension pneumothorax to a simple pneumothorax. The needle or cannula should be left in place until a thoracostomy tube is inserted for definitive management (Figure 14–6).

A	B	C

▲ **Figure 14–5.** Surgical cricothyroidotomy.

▲ **Figure 14–6.** Relief of pneumothorax. Tension pneumothorax must be immediately decompressed by a needle introduced through the second anterior intercostal space. A chest tube is usually inserted in the midaxillary line at the level of the nipple and is directed posteriorly and superiorly toward the apex of the thorax. The tube is attached to a "three-bottle" suction device, and the rate of escape of air is indicated by the appearance of bubbles in the second of the three bottles. Cessation of bubbling suggests that the air leak has become sealed.

2. Open pneumothorax—This condition results from an open wound of the chest wall with free communication between the pleural space and the atmosphere. The resulting impairment of the thoracic bellows and its ability to expand the lung results in inadequate ventilation. With chest expansion during a breath, air moves in and out of the chest wall opening instead of through the trachea, producing hypoventilation that can be rapidly fatal. Emergency treatment consists of sealing the wound with an occlusive sterile dressing taped on three sides to act as a flutter-type valve, or with any material if nothing sterile is available. Definitive treatment requires placement of a chest tube to reexpand the lung and surgical closure of the defect. Airway intubation with positive-pressure mechanical ventilation can be helpful in massive open pneumothorax.

3. Flail chest—Multiple rib fractures resulting in a free-floating segment of chest wall may produce paradoxical motion that impairs lung expansion (Figure 14–7). In patients with flail chest, injury-associated pulmonary contusion is common and is often the major cause of respiratory failure. The injury is identified by careful inspection and palpation during physical examination. Patients with large flail segments will almost always require endotracheal intubation and mechanical ventilation both to stabilize the flail segment and to optimize gas exchange. Smaller flail segments may be well tolerated if supplemental oxygen and adequate analgesia are provided. The work of breathing is increased considerably, and many patients who initially appear to be compensating well may suddenly deteriorate a few hours later. Therefore, most patients with flail chest require monitoring in an intensive care unit.

▲ **Figure 14–7.** Flail chest.

CIRCULATION

▶ Hemorrhage

Free hemorrhage from accessible surface wounds is usually obvious and can be controlled in most cases by local pressure and elevation of the bleeding point. Firm and precise pressure on the major artery in the axilla, antecubital space, wrist, groin, popliteal space, or at the ankle may suffice for temporary control of arterial hemorrhage distal to these points. When all other measures have failed, a tourniquet may be necessary to control major hemorrhage from extensive wounds or major vessels in an extremity. Failure to manage a tourniquet properly may cause irreparable vascular or neurologic damage. For this reason, the tourniquet should be used only when necessary and must be kept exposed and loosened at least every 20 minutes for 1 or 2 minutes while the patient is in transit. Transport to definitive care where the tourniquet can be safely removed and treatment rendered should be a top priority. It is wise to write the time of tourniquet application in military time on the patient's forehead with a skin-marking pen or on adhesive tape.

▶ Vascular Access and Resuscitation

All patients with significant trauma should have large-caliber peripheral intravenous catheters inserted immediately for administration of resuscitation fluids as needed. If any degree of shock is present, at least two 14-16 gauge peripheral intravenous lines should be established usually in the antecubital fossa. If venous access cannot be obtained by percutaneous peripheral or central venous cannulation, an intraosseous line in the tibia, humerus, or other uninjured site should be placed. A venous cutdown of the saphenous vein at the ankle

using an angiocath or intravenous extension tubing with the tip cut off can be performed but is a difficult procedure in the field. A blood sample for type and cross-match should be sent from the venous line, if not already drawn.

As soon as the first intravenous line is inserted, an initial crystalloid infusion should begin. Adult patients should be given 1 L of Ringer's lactate or normal saline. For children, the initial administered crystalloid volume should be 20 mL/kg. Large-volume crystalloid fluid resuscitation is not recommended for patients with evidence of active hemorrhage, and infusion of more than 1.5 L of crystalloid has been associated with increased mortality. Patients in hemorrhagic shock for whom there is no improvement in blood pressure from initial crystalloid infusion, or who transiently respond, should be switched to resuscitation with blood products. Beyond the administration of the first two units of packed red blood cells (PRBCs), it is important to also administer fresh plasma or thawed fresh frozen plasma (FFP) to avoid coagulopathy in the massively transfused patient. Massive transfusion is defined as more than 10 units of PRBC in 24 hours or more than 4 units in 4 hours. The exact ratio of FFP to PRBC is still under active investigation, but a target range between 1:1 and 1:2 is considered acceptable. Military data have shown that the early use of plasma can reduce mortality by up to 50% in the massively transfused trauma patient. Giving platelets as part of the massive transfusion protocol is also supported by military data demonstrating a 20% reduction in mortality for patients who received platelets as fresh whole blood or apheresis platelets in conjunction with PRBC. The exact platelet-to-PRBC ratio for optimal treatment of the hemorrhaging trauma patient is not known, but giving 1 unit of pooled platelets for every 5 units of PRBC is a reasonable ratio (a unit of platelets contains pooled platelets from four to six donors). Type O, Rh-negative PRBC should be immediately available in the emergency department for any patient with impending cardiac arrest or massive hemorrhage. Some high-volume trauma centers now also stock fresh or "pre-thawed" AB plasma as well. Type-specific blood should be available within 15–20 minutes of patient arrival to the hospital.

Tranexamic acid is an antifibrinolytic agent that inhibits the breakdown of clotted blood. It does not promote new blood clot formation. Two large clinical trials, one in the military setting and another in the civilian population, have demonstrated the efficacy of tranexamic acid when utilized as part of a blood product resuscitation strategy in patients with traumatic hemorrhage. The survival benefit is greatest in patients who received massive transfusion and those in whom early treatment was accomplished (≤1 hour after injury). Tranexamic acid started more than 3 hours after injury increased the risk of death due to bleeding and is likely ineffective. Dosing is typically 1 g intravenously over 10 minutes, followed by a drip infusion of an additional 1 g over 8 hours.

Transfusion of blood products is not without risk. Despite rigorous screening programs, transmission of viral bloodborne diseases can occur. The current incidence of bloodborne pathogen transmission following red blood cell transfusion are hepatitis B, 1:350,000; hepatitis C, 1:400,000; and HIV, 1:2 million. Transfusion of blood products is also associated with transfusion-related immunomodulation and transfusion-related acute lung injury. Both of these problems can increase morbidity and mortality. The storage age of blood transfused can also contribute to problems. Transfusion of a patient with older units of PRBC has been shown to cause generation of systemic proinflammatory mediators and increase the risk of wound infection.

► Monitoring

As intravenous access is obtained, electrocardiogram leads for continuous cardiac monitoring should be placed. Noninvasive blood pressure measurements should be acquired with a time-cycled blood pressure cuff. Pulse oximetry is valuable in ensuring that adequate hemoglobin oxygen saturation is present in the injured patient. Temperature is a crucial vital sign, and it should be measured and recorded along with the first pulse and blood pressure in the emergency department.

NEUROLOGIC DISABILITY

A brief neurologic examination should be documented to assess patients' degree of neurologic impairment. Many factors may contribute to altered levels of consciousness and should be considered in addition to central nervous system injury in all trauma patients. Other than the direct trauma, the most common contributing causes of altered mental status for trauma patients are alcohol intoxication, other central nervous system stimulants or depressants, diabetic ketoacidosis, cerebrovascular accident, and hypovolemic shock. Less common causes are epilepsy, eclampsia, electrolyte imbalances associated with metabolic and systemic diseases, anaphylaxis, heavy metal poisoning, electric shock, tumors, severe systemic infections, hypercalcemia, asphyxia, heat stroke, severe heart failure, and hysteria. These uncommon causes of coma or diminished mental status should be considered if routine testing such as blood alcohol and glucose level, urine toxicology, and head computed tomography (CT) scanning are unrevealing as to the etiology of mental impairment. In such cases, further laboratory and diagnostic testing may be warranted.

The differential diagnosis depends upon a careful history and complete physical examination, with particular attention to the neurologic examination with documentation of the patient's GCS score (Table 14–1), and an urgent head CT scan. The GCS score is useful in monitoring acute changes in neurologic function and is used for prognosticating outcomes after severe head injury. The motor component of the GCS score is the most accurate for predicting outcome and has a linear relationship with mortality. Lateralizing signs may also suggest evidence of an intracranial mass effect or

Table 14–1. Glasgow coma scale score (structured assessment)

Structured Assessment Steps
1. Check for factors interfering with communication, ability to respond, and other injuries.
2. Observe eye opening, content of speech, and movements of right and left sides.
3. Stimulate. Sound: Spoken or shouted request. Physical: Pressure on fingertip, trapezius, or supraorbital notch.
4. Assign rate according to highest response observed.

Eye Opening

Criterion	Rating	Score
Open before stimulus	Spontaneous	4
After spoken or shouted request	To sound	3
After fingertip stimulus	To pressure	2
No opening at any time, no interfering factor	None	1
Closed by local factor	Not testable	NT

Verbal Response

Criterion	Rating	Score
Correctly gives name, place, and date	Oriented	5
Not oriented but communicates coherently	Confused	4
Intelligible single words	Words	3
Only moans/groans	Sounds	2
No audible response, no interfering factor	None	1
Factor interfering with communication	Not testable	NT

Best Motor Response

Criterion	Rating	Score
Obeys two-part request	Obeys commands	6
Brings hand above clavicle to stimulus on head neck	Localizing	5
Bends arm at elbow rapidly but features not predominantly abnormal	Normal flexion	4
Bends arm at elbow, features clearly predominantly abnormal	Abnormal flexion	3
Extends arm at elbow	Extension	2
No movement in arms/legs, no interfering factor	None	1
Paralyzed or other limiting factor	Not testable	NT

Adapted with permission from Royal College of Physicians and Surgeons of Glasgow: The Glasgow Structured Approach to Assessment of the Glasgow Coma Scale. https://www.glasgowcomascale.org/

carotid or vertebral artery injury, while loss of distal motor and/or sensory function may help localize potential spinal cord injuries.

EXPOSURE/ENVIRONMENT

All clothing should be removed (cut off with trauma shears, usually) from the seriously injured patient, with care taken to avoid unnecessary movement. The removal of helmets or other protective clothing may require additional personnel to stabilize the patient and prevent further injury. All skin surfaces should be examined to identify occult injuries that may not be readily apparent, such as posterior penetrating trauma or open fractures. After inspecting all surfaces, warm blankets or warming devices should be placed to avoid hypothermia in the seriously injured patient.

EMERGENCY ROOM THORACOTOMY

Certain injuries are so critical that operative treatment must be undertaken as soon as the diagnosis is made. In these cases, resuscitation is continued as the patient is being operated on. For cardiopulmonary arrest that occurs in the emergency room as a direct result of trauma, external cardiac compression is rarely successful in maintaining effective perfusion of vital organs. An emergency left anterolateral thoracotomy should be performed in the fourth or fifth intercostal space, and the pericardium should be opened anterior to the phrenic nerve (Figure 14–8). Open cardiac massage, cross-clamping of the descending thoracic aorta, repair of cardiac injuries, and internal defibrillation can be performed as appropriate. Wounds of the lung producing severe hemorrhage or systemic air embolus may require pulmonary hilar cross-clamping.

▲ **Figure 14–8.** Emergency thoracotomy and open cardiac massage.

Emergency room thoracotomy is most useful for cardiac arrest due to penetrating thoracic trauma, particularly in patients with pericardial tamponade from stab wounds. This extreme procedure is ineffective for most patients with cardiac arrest due to blunt trauma and for all patients who have no detectable vital signs in the field (<1% survival). If vital signs are present in the emergency room but arrest appears imminent, the patient should be transferred rapidly to the operating room if at all possible, since conditions in the operating room are optimal for surgical intervention. Resuscitative thoracotomy in the ED can be considered futile care when prehospital CPR exceeds 10 minutes after blunt trauma without a response, prehospital CPR exceeds 15 minutes after penetrating trauma without a response, and asystole is the presenting rhythm and there is no pericardial tamponade.

Resuscitative endovascular balloon occlusion of the aorta (REBOA) is a new technique for patients with hemorrhagic shock that can be used for temporary aortic occlusion similar to resuscitative thoracotomy with aortic cross-clamping (Figure 14–9). It supports proximal aortic pressure and minimizes ongoing hemorrhage until definitive hemorrhage control and hemostasis measures can be deployed. REBOA can also be performed in a proactive manner in the presence of refractory hemorrhagic shock. This allows it to function as a bridge to definitive therapy. The advantage of REBOA is that it is a potentially a less invasive and morbid procedure as compared to resuscitative thoracotomy. The exact indications for and clinical results of REBOA usage are the focus of current trauma research.

RESUSCITATION PHASE

▶ Shock

Shock is defined as inadequate end-organ tissue perfusion. Some degree of shock accompanies most severe injuries and is manifested initially by pallor, cold sweat, weakness, lightheadedness, tachycardia, hypotension, thirst, air hunger, and eventually, loss of consciousness. Patients with any of these signs should be presumed to be in shock and evaluated thoroughly. All patients determined to be in any degree of shock should be reexamined at regular intervals. The degree of shock has been categorized to guide resuscitation and help caregivers recognize the severity of symptoms (Table 14–2).

A. Hypovolemic Shock

Hypovolemic shock is due to loss of whole blood or plasma. Blood pressure may be maintained initially by vasoconstriction. Tissue hypoxia increases when hypotension ensues, and shock may become irreversible if irreparable damage occurs to the vital organs. Massive or prolonged hemorrhage, severe crush injuries, major fractures, and extensive burns are the most common causes. The presence of any of these conditions is an indication for prompt intravenous fluid infusion.

ER-REBOA™ Catheter

US and Foreign Patents Pending

▲ **Figure 14–9.** *Top:* Example of 6F REBOA catheter. (Reproduced with permission from Prytime Medical Devices, Inc.) *Bottom:* Aortic zones in which REBOA balloon can be deployed. Zone I extends from the origin of the left subclavian artery to the celiac artery and is a potential zone of occlusion. Zone II extends from the celiac artery to the lowest renal artery and is a no-occlusion zone. Zone III exists from the lowest renal artery to the aortic bifurcation. (Adapted with permission from Stannard A, Eliason JL, Rasmussen TE: Resuscitative endovascular balloon occlusion of the aorta (REBOA) as an adjunct for hemorrhagic shock. *J Trauma.* 2011 Dec;71(6):1869-1872.)

In mild or class 1 shock (<15% blood volume loss), compensatory mechanisms may preserve adequate perfusion, and no skin or physiologic changes may be apparent. In moderate or class 2 shock (15%-30% blood loss), the skin on the extremities becomes pale, cool, and moist as a result of vasoconstriction and release of epinephrine. Systolic blood pressure is often maintained at near-normal levels, but urine output will usually decrease. With severe or class 3 shock (30%-40% blood volume loss), these changes—particularly diaphoresis—become more marked, and urine output declines significantly. Hypotension ensues. In addition, changes in cerebral function become evident, consisting chiefly of agitation, disorientation, and memory loss. A common error is to attribute uncooperative behavior to intoxication, drug use, or brain injury when in fact it may be due to cerebral ischemia from blood loss. With class 4 shock (>40% blood volume loss), profound hypotension is typically accompanied by loss of consciousness and anuria. In this situation, rapid resuscitation with crystalloid and blood products is necessary to prevent imminent death.

In the case of class 3 or 4 shock due to hemorrhage, early resuscitation with blood and blood products is recommended.

Table 14–2. Classification of hypovolemic shock.

	Class I	Class II	Class III	Class IV
Blood loss (mL)	Up to 750	750-1500	1500-2000	> 2000
Blood loss (% BV)	Up to 15%	15%-30%	30%-40%	> 40%
Pulse rate (beats/min)	< 100	> 100	> 120	> 140
Blood pressure	Normal	Minimal decrease	Decreased	Significantly decreased
Pulse pressure	Normal	Narrowed	Narrowed	Unobtainable or very narrow
Hourly urine output	≥ 0.5 mL/kg	≥ 0.5 mL/kg	< 0.5 cc/kg	Minimal
CNS/mental status	Slightly anxious	Mildly anxious	Anxious and confused	Confused or lethargic

Resuscitation should continue until hemorrhage is controlled, the signs of shock abate, and urine output returns to normal. If shock appears to be due to blood loss, blood transfusion should be given, starting with 2 units of uncross-matched O-negative blood if cross-matched blood is unavailable. Additional resuscitation with blood products is guided by massive transfusion protocols. Modifications of the specific blood products transfused along with blood during a resuscitation can be based upon information from viscoelastic hemostatic assays such as thromboelastography (TEG) or rotational thromboelastometry (ROTEM). Successful resuscitation is indicated by warm, dry, well-perfused skin, a urine output of 30-60 mL/h, and an alert sensorium. Improvement in pH toward normal, correction of lactic acidosis, and minimization of base deficit as measured on an arterial blood gas sample are also indicators of successful resuscitation.

As a general principle, measurements of blood pressure and pulse are less reliable than changes in urine output in assessing the severity of shock. Young and athletic older patients may have compensatory mechanisms that maintain adequate blood pressure even with moderate volume loss. Older patients and those taking cardiac or blood pressure medications often do not exhibit tachycardia even with extreme volume loss. Therefore, a Foley catheter should be inserted into the bladder to monitor urine output in any patient with major injuries or shock. Oliguria is the most reliable sign of moderate shock, and successful resuscitation is indicated by a return of urine output to 0.5-1 mL/kg/h. Absence of oliguria is an unreliable index of the absence of shock if the patient has an osmotic diuresis due to alcohol, glucose, mannitol, or intravenous contrast material.

B. Neurogenic Shock

Neurogenic shock is due to the pooling of blood in autonomically denervated venules and small veins and is usually due to spinal cord injury. Neurogenic shock is not caused by an isolated head injury, and in those patients, other causes of shock should be sought. A patient exhibiting signs of neurogenic shock (warm and well-perfused distal extremities in the presence of hypotension) should be given a 2-L crystalloid fluid bolus—followed by an additional bolus if the response is suboptimal. If neurogenic shock persists with fluid resuscitation, phenylephrine or another vasopressor should be given as a drip with the dosage adjusted until the blood pressure is maintained at a satisfactory level. If the patient does not improve quickly, other kinds of shock must be considered. Patients with neurogenic shock may require central venous pressure monitoring to ensure an optimal volume status.

C. Cardiac Compressive Shock

Cardiac compressive shock is caused by compression of the thin-walled chambers of the heart—the atria and the right ventricle—or by compression or distortion of the great veins entering the heart. The usual causes of this type of shock in the trauma patient are pericardial tamponade, tension pneumothorax, massive hemothorax, diaphragmatic rupture with herniation of abdominal contents into the chest, and an elevated diaphragm from massive abdominal hemorrhage. Treatment consists of urgent decompression depending on the specific cause. In severe cases, emergency thoracotomy may be necessary to restore adequate cardiac function.

D. Cardiogenic Shock

Cardiogenic shock is caused by decreased myocardial contractility and is most commonly caused by myocardial infarction or arrhythmia. Older trauma patients may develop a myocardial infarction as a complication of their injuries. On occasion an acute myocardial infarction may precede a traumatic event and be a cause of injury or loss of consciousness. Rarely, a severe myocardial contusion may lead to cardiogenic shock. Treatment is supportive, with volume replacement guided by hemodynamic monitoring and administration of inotropic agents to augment cardiac output as necessary to maintain adequate end-organ perfusion.

Unfortunately, patients with traumatic injuries are not usually candidates for anticoagulant or lytic therapy, and treatment of their acute myocardial ischemia is sometimes hindered by concerns about bleeding. Echocardiography is helpful for assessment of wall-motion abnormalities from severe cardiac contusion.

Laboratory Studies

Immediately after intravenous catheters are placed, a blood sample should be drawn for blood typing and cross-matching. If the patient has a history of renal, hepatic, or cardiac disease or is taking diuretics or anticoagulants, serum electrolytes and coagulation parameters should be measured. In most patients with serious injuries, an arterial blood gas provides rapid data about acidosis and base deficit, both of which are markers of under-resuscitation in addition to oxygenation (Pao_2) and ventilation ($Paco_2$). Gross blood in the urine indicates the need for further diagnostic testing with abdominal CT scan or, in selected cases, a cystogram and urethrogram. Patients with obvious severe head injury, where intracranial pressure monitoring may be indicated, should have coagulation studies and a platelet count performed. Measurement of blood alcohol level and urine toxicology screen may be useful in patients with altered mental status.

Imaging Studies

Radiographic plain films of the chest and pelvis are required in all major injuries. Lateral C-spine films have been supplanted by formal CT scanning of the neck in patients with suspicion of or mechanism for cervical spine injury. Bedside focused assessment with sonography for trauma (FAST) is the preferred triage method for determining the presence of hemoperitoneum in blunt trauma patients or cardiac tamponade in blunt and penetrating trauma patients. The presence of hemoperitoneum in an unstable patient on FAST may be an indication for exploratory laparotomy. Presence of hemoperitoneum in a stable patient, or a negative FAST in a patient with abdominal pain, is an indication for further evaluation with abdominal CT scan.

Patients who have an abnormal chest radiograph with a mechanism for blunt aortic injury should undergo further screening with either helical chest CT done at the time of abdominal imaging or with aortography, if necessary. Cervical spine CT scans should be obtained for patients who are unconscious, have pain in the cervical region, have neurologic deficits, or have painful or distracting injuries. CT scanning of the head should be performed in all patients with loss of consciousness or more serious neurologic impairment. Radiographs of the long bones and noncervical spine can usually be deferred until the more critical injuries of the thorax and abdomen have been delineated and stabilized.

2. SECONDARY SURVEY & PATTERNS OF INJURY

A rapid and complete history and physical examination are essential for patients with serious or multiple injuries. Progressive changes in clinical findings are often the key to correct diagnosis, and negative findings that change to positive may be of great importance in revising an initial clinical evaluation. This is particularly true in the case of abdominal, thoracic, and intracranial injuries, which frequently do not become manifest until hours after the trauma.

Recognition of injury patterns is also important in identifying all injuries. For example, fractures of the calcaneus resulting from a fall from a great height are often associated with central dislocation of the hip and fractures of the spine and of the skull base. A crushed pelvis is often combined with laceration of the posterior urethra or bladder, vagina, or rectum. Crush injuries of the chest are often associated with lacerations or rupture of the spleen, liver, or diaphragm. Penetrating wounds of the chest may involve not only the thoracic contents but also the abdominal viscera. These combinations occur frequently and should always be suspected.

TREATMENT PRIORITIES

In all cases of patients with multiple injuries, there must be a "captain of the team" who directs the resuscitation, decides which x-rays or special diagnostic tests should be obtained, and establishes priority for care by continuous consultation with other surgical specialists and anesthesiologists. A trauma surgeon or a general surgeon experienced in the care of injured patients usually has this role.

After controlling the airway if necessary, resuscitation and blood volume replacement have first priority. Deepening stupor in patients under observation should arouse suspicion of an expanding intracranial lesion requiring serial neurologic examinations and head CT. Too often, obvious signs of acute alcohol intoxication have been assumed to be the cause of unconsciousness, and intracranial hemorrhage has been overlooked.

Cerebral injuries take precedence in care when there is rapidly deepening coma. Extradural bleeding is a critical emergency, requiring operation for control of bleeding and cerebral decompression. Subdural bleeding may produce a similar emergency. If the patient's condition permits, CT scanning should be performed for localization of the bleeding within the cranium prior to other operative interventions being initiated. In many cases of combined cerebral and abdominal injury with massive bleeding, laparotomy and craniotomy should be performed simultaneously.

Most urologic injuries are managed at the same time as associated intra-abdominal injuries. Pelvic fractures present special problems and are discussed in Chapter 40. Unless there is associated vascular injury with threatened ischemia of the limb, fractures of the long bones can be splinted and treated on an urgent basis. Open contaminated fractures should be cleansed and debrided as soon as possible. Injuries of the hand run the risk of infection that may result in a lifelong handicap without early effective treatment. Early treatment of the hand at the same time as treatment of any life-threatening injuries avoids infection and preserves the means of livelihood. Tetanus prophylaxis should be given in all instances of open contaminated wounds, puncture wounds, and burns.

Patients with a severe burden of trauma and shock may not be candidates for definitive treatment of all injuries in the immediate setting. Three physiologic derangements comprise the "lethal triad" in the trauma literature: hypothermia, acidosis, and coagulopathy. These are boundaries of a patient's physiologic envelope beyond which the patient will develop irreversible shock and eventual death. Bailing out of the abdomen with damage-control maneuvers in a patient headed for the lethal triad is not a sign of defeat; instead it is usually the intelligent option. Early warning signs of physiologic compromise that could lead to the lethal triad are edema of the small bowel, midgut distension, dusky serosal surfaces, tissue that is cool to the touch, noncompliant swollen abdominal wall, diffuse oozing from surgical or raw surfaces, and lack of obvious clot formation. Successful packing relies on clot formation, so employing a strategy of early packing is recommended rather than turning to it as a last resort.

Details of definitive management of injuries are discussed in the sections on trauma that follow and in the various organ system chapters of this book.

American College of Surgeons Committee on Trauma: ACS TQIP Best Practices Guidelines in Imaging. https://www.facs.org/~/media/files/quality%20programs/trauma/tqip/best_practices_in_imaging.ashx. Accessed Nov. 30, 2018.

American College of Surgeons Committee on Trauma: *Advanced Trauma Life Support for Doctors Student Manual*, 10th ed. Chicago: American College of Surgeons; 2018.

American College of Surgeons Committee on Trauma: Stop the Bleed. https://www.bleedingcontrol.org/. Accessed Nov. 26, 2018.

Bardes JM et al: The contemporary timing of trauma deaths. *J Trauma Acute Care Surg.* 2018;84:893.

Brenner M et al: Joint statement from the American College of Surgeons Committee on Trauma (ACS COT) and the American College of Emergency Physicians (ACEP) regarding the clinical use of resuscitative endovascular balloon occlusion of the aorta (REBOA). *Trauma Surg Acute Care Open* 2018;3:1.

Cannon JW et al: Damage control resuscitation in patients with severe traumatic hemorrhage: A practice management guideline from the Eastern Association for the Surgery of Trauma. *J Trauma Acute Care Surg.* 2017;82:605.

Centers for Disease Control and Prevention: Costs of injury and violence in the United States. https://www.cdc.gov/injury/wisqars/overview/cost_of_injury.html. Accessed Oct. 4, 2018.

Centers for Disease Control and Prevention: Injury prevention and control: Field triage. https://www.cdc.gov/mmwr/preview/mmwrhtml/rr5801a1.htm. Accessed Nov. 26, 2018.

Committee on Military Trauma Care's Learning Health System and Its Translation to the Civilian Sector, Board on Health Sciences Policy, Board on the Health of Select Populations, Health and Medicine Division, National Academies of Sciences, Engineering, and Medicine; Berwick D, Downey A, Cornett E, eds: *A National Trauma Care System: Integrating Military and Civilian Trauma Systems to Achieve Zero Preventable Deaths After Injury.* Washington, DC: National Academies Press; 2016.

Cotton BA et al: Damage control resuscitation is associated with a reduction in resuscitation volumes and improvement in survival in 390 damage control laparotomy patients. *Ann Surg.* 2011; 254:598.

CRASH-2 collaborators et al: Effects of tranexamic acid on death, vascular occlusive events, and blood transfusion in trauma patients with significant haemorrhage (CRASH-2): A randomised, placebo-controlled trial. *Lancet.* 2010;376:23.

CRASH-2 collaborators et al: The importance of early treatment with tranexamic acid in bleeding trauma patients: An exploratory analysis of the CRASH-2 randomised controlled trial. *Lancet.* 2011;377:1096.

Haas B et al: The mortality benefit of direct trauma center transport in a regional trauma system: A population-based analysis. *J Trauma Acute Care Surg.* 2012;72:1510.

Holcomb JB et al: Transfusion of plasma, platelets, and red blood cells in a 1:1:1 vs. a 1:1:2 ratio and mortality in patients with severe trauma: The PROPPR randomized clinical trial. *JAMA.* 2015; 313:471.

McKenzie EJ et al: A national evaluation of the effect of trauma-center care on mortality. *N Engl J Med.* 2006;354:366.

Moore EE et al: Defining the limits of resuscitative emergency department thoracotomy: A contemporary Western Trauma Association perspective. *J Trauma.* 2011;70:334.

Stannard A et al: Resuscitative endovascular balloon occlusion of the aorta (REBOA) as an adjunct for hemorrhagic shock. *J Trauma Acute Care Surg.* 2011;71:1869.

NECK INJURIES

All injuries to the neck are potentially life threatening because of the many vital structures in this area. Injuries to the neck are classified as blunt or penetrating, and the treatment is different for each. The patient must be examined closely for associated head and chest injuries. The initial level of consciousness is of paramount importance; progressive depression of the sensorium may signify intracranial bleeding or cerebral ischemia and requires neurosurgical evaluation. Trauma to the base of the neck may lacerate major blood vessels or have associated pneumothorax. Hemorrhage into the pleural cavity may occur suddenly as contained hematomas rupture.

▶ Clinical Findings

Injuries to the larynx and trachea can be asymptomatic or may cause hoarseness, laryngeal stridor, or dyspnea secondary to airway compression or aspiration of blood. Subcutaneous emphysema in the neck can be present if the wall of the larynx or trachea has been disrupted.

Esophageal injuries are rarely isolated and by themselves may not cause immediate symptoms. Severe chest pain and dysphagia are characteristic of esophageal perforation. Hours later, as mediastinitis develops, progressive sepsis may occur. Mediastinitis results because the deep cervical space is in direct continuity with the mediastinum. Esophageal injuries can be recognized promptly if the surgeon is alert to the possibility and seeks out early diagnosis. Exploration of the neck, radiographic examination of the esophagus with contrast medium, and in selected cases flexible esophagoscopy confirms the diagnosis.

Cervical spine fractures and spinal cord injuries should always be suspected in deceleration injuries or following direct trauma to the neck. If the patient complains of cervical pain or tenderness or if the level of consciousness is depressed, the head and neck should be immobilized (eg, with a rigid cervical collar or sandbags) until cervical radiologic imaging can be performed to rule out a cervical fracture or ligamentous injury.

Injury to the great vessels (subclavian, common carotid, internal carotid, and external carotid arteries; subclavian, internal jugular, and external jugular veins) may follow blunt or penetrating trauma. Fractures of the clavicle or first rib may lacerate the subclavian artery and vein. With vascular injuries, the patient typically presents with visible external blood loss, neck hematoma formation, and in varying degrees of shock. Occasionally, bleeding may be contained and the injury may go undetected for a short time. Auscultation may reveal bruits that suggest arterial injury.

▶ Types of Injuries

A. Penetrating Neck Injuries

Penetrating injuries of the neck are divided into three anatomic zones (Figure 14–10). Zone I injuries occur at the

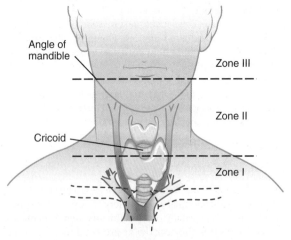

▲ **Figure 14–10.** Zones of the neck.

Angle of mandible

Zone III

Zone II

Cricoid

Zone I

thoracic outlet, which extends from the level of the cricoid cartilage to the clavicles. Included in this area are the proximal carotid arteries, the subclavian vessels, and the major vessels of the chest. Proximal control of injuries to vascular structures in this zone often requires a thoracotomy or sternotomy. Zone II injuries occur in the area between the cricoid and the angle of the mandible. Injuries here are the easiest to expose and evaluate. Zone III injuries are between the angle of the mandible and the base of the skull. Exposure is much more difficult in this zone and in some cases may require disarticulation of the mandible. High injuries can be inaccessible, and control of hemorrhage may require ligation of major proximal vessels or angiographic embolization.

Penetrating trauma to the posterior neck may injure the vertebral column, the cervical spinal cord, the interosseous portion of the vertebral artery, and the neck musculature. Penetrating trauma to the anterior and lateral neck may injure the larynx, trachea, esophagus, thyroid, carotid arteries, subclavian arteries, jugular veins, subclavian veins, phrenic and vagus nerves, and thoracic duct.

With any penetrating cervical trauma, the likelihood of significant injury is high because there are so many vital structures in such a small space. Any patient with shock, expanding hematoma, or uncontrolled hemorrhage should be taken to the operating room for emergency exploration. The location of the injury suggests which structures may be involved. Vascular injuries at the base of the neck require thoracotomy or sternotomy to obtain proximal control of injured blood vessels before the site of probable injury is exposed. If the patient is stable after resuscitation, additional diagnostic testing may be considered.

Computed tomography angiography is usually recommended for patients with stable injuries in zones I and III because precise identification of the location and extent of injury may alter the operative approach. If possible, angiography should be performed before exploration of any injury in which blood vessels may be damaged below the level of the cricoid cartilage or above a line connecting the mastoid process with the angle of the jaw. Arterial injuries above this line are practically inaccessible. If injury to the carotid artery at the base of the skull is confirmed by angiography, repair may not be possible and ligation may be required to control bleeding, or endovascular intervention may be required. Injured carotid arteries that have produced a neurologic deficit should be repaired if possible. The morbidity and mortality of patients undergoing carotid artery repair are significantly lower than those who have ligation of the carotid artery (15% vs 50%). Carotid artery ligation is indicated in the patient who presents with uncontrollable hemorrhage or coma with no prograde flow in the carotid artery.

Since exposure of injuries in zone II is relatively easy to obtain, a policy of mandatory exploration was the traditional recommendation for all injuries penetrating the platysma muscle. Although this approach is safe, reliable, and time-tested, studies have demonstrated that a selective approach is as safe provided that diagnostic testing does not detect a major injury and the patient is stable. High-resolution CT scanning of the neck can also be used to guide surgical decision making in penetrating injuries. Invasive studies such as endoscopy and conventional angiography can often be eliminated if CT demonstrates a trajectory remote from vital structures such as blood vessels or the aerodigestive tract.

In the absence of an obvious vascular injury on clinical examination, ultrasound with color-flow Doppler has been demonstrated to be reliable in ruling out carotid artery injuries. Computed tomography angiography can also be used in this setting, and may offer the advantage of identifying an unsuspected vertebral artery injury. Vertebral artery injuries should also be suspected when bleeding from a posterior or lateral neck wound cannot be controlled by pressure on the carotid artery or when there is bleeding from a posterolateral wound associated with fracture of a cervical transverse process. Flexible or rigid endoscopy can be used to evaluate the trachea and esophagus. A contrast study of the upper esophagus should be performed to identify esophageal injuries that might not be readily apparent on endoscopy. These injuries can be difficult to detect and are occasionally missed on surgical exploration. In either case, repeated, careful examinations should be performed.

B. Blunt Neck Injuries

The most important injuries resulting from blunt cervical trauma are (1) cervical fracture, (2) cervical spinal cord injury, (3) vascular injury, and (4) laryngeal and tracheal injury. Radiographic examination of the cervical spine and soft tissues is essential. Careful neurologic examination can differentiate between injuries to the spinal cord, brachial plexus, and brain.

The diagnosis of a cervical spine fracture is reliant on the history, physical examination, and confirmatory studies. The use of plain radiographs has been supplanted by non-contrast CT of the cervical spine. Awake, unimpaired patients with a negative physical exam are unlikely to have a clinically significant cervical spine injury. Obtunded patients with a negative CT scan and no clinical signs of cervical spine injury are also unlikely to have an injury. Following a negative CT scan, the cervical collar is typically removed once the patient is no longer obtunded and the exam can be repeated, or immediately if the patient is likely to remain obtunded/intubated in the ICU. The pediatric patient with an unreliable physical exam often requires additional imaging to clear the spine. Adult patients with a negative CT scan and pain often require an MRI to rule out ligamentous injury. Cervical fractures are often managed with external immobilization using rigid collars or a halo/vest apparatus. In some cases, unstable cervical spine fractures require reduction and internal fixation.

Table 14–3. NEXUS criteria for cervical spine imaging.

- Radiologic imaging of the cervical spine is indicated if any of these findings are present:
- Focal neurologic deficit
- Midline spinal tenderness
- Altered level of consciousness
- Intoxication
- Distracting injury

Data from Hoffman JR, Mower WR, Wolfson AB, et al: Validity of a set of clinical criteria to rule out injury to the cervical spine in patients with blunt trauma. National Emergency X-Radiography Utilization Study Group, *N Engl J Med.* 2000 Jul 13;343(2):94-99.

Algorithms and clinical decision rules have been developed for clearance of the cervical spine. The National Emergency X-Radiography Utilization Study (NEXUS) criteria (Table 14–3) or Canadian Cervical Rules (CCR) can guide imaging decisions for cervical spine evaluation in awake and stable trauma patients where cervical spine injury is a concern. However, both the NEXUS and CCR criteria are not applicable in pediatric patients or older adult patients (≥55 years). The Eastern Association for the Surgery of Trauma (EAST) guidelines recommend removal of the cervical collar after a normal cervical spine CT scan in an unconscious adult patient. The limitation of this practice is that while pragmatic and low risk, at this time, this recommendation is based on very-low-quality evidence. Until better evidence is published in the literature, the recommendation is for trauma centers to develop a policy and PI process regarding cervical collar removal and when to perform additional studies (MRI) in the obtunded patient.

Vascular injuries may occur in cases of severe or localized blunt neck trauma. The common or internal carotid arteries can be torn or sustain intimal disruption and require intervention. Imaging of the cervical vessels is recommended in blunt trauma patients with lateralizing neurologic symptoms or GCS less than 8 with head CT findings that do not explain the neurologic symptoms. Screening should also be considered in patients with mandible or facial fractures, complex skull fractures, traumatic brain injury with thoracic injuries, scalp degloving, and thoracic vascular injuries. A dedicated cervical CT angiogram or MR angiogram are the preferred screening tools for injury. Formal arteriograms are reserved for patients who may have injuries amenable to angiographic intervention or if the diagnosis cannot be made by other means and would alter treatment. Most blunt carotid injuries are not amenable to operative intervention due to the location or extent of injury. The use of endovascular stent techniques to repair or control blunt carotid artery injuries is also an option. Patients with blunt carotid or vertebral artery injuries should be considered for anticoagulation or antiplatelet therapy. The value of anticoagulation continues to be debated due to associated bleeding complications, and antiplatelet therapy is a reasonable alternative to full systemic anticoagulation.

Complications

The complications of untreated neck trauma are related to the individual structures injured. Injuries to the larynx and trachea can result in acute airway obstruction, late tracheal stenosis, and sepsis. Cervicomediastinal sepsis can result from esophageal injuries. Carotid artery injuries can produce death from hemorrhage, stroke or cerebral ischemia, and arteriovenous fistula with cardiac decompensation. Major venous injury can result in exsanguination, air embolism, and arteriovenous fistula formation if there is concomitant arterial injury. Cervical fracture can result in paraplegia, quadriplegia, or death.

Prevention of these complications depends upon immediate resuscitation by intubation of the airway, prompt control of external hemorrhage and blood replacement, protection of the head and neck when cervical fracture is possible, accurate and rapid diagnosis, and prompt operative treatment when indicated.

Treatment

Control of the airway with early intubation is the first key maneuver to successful management of severe neck injuries. Any wound of the neck that penetrates the platysma requires prompt surgical exploration or diagnostic work-up to rule out major vascular injury. In patients with zone II injuries, color-flow Doppler imaging may provide a reliable way to assess for vascular injury and can be a safe alternative to contrast angiography. Arteries damaged by high-velocity missiles require debridement. End-to-end anastomosis of the mobilized vessels is preferred, but if a significant segment is lost, an autogenous vein graft can be used. Vertebral artery injury presents a formidable technical problem because of the interosseous course of the artery shortly after it arises from the subclavian artery. Although unilateral vertebral artery ligation has been followed by fatal midbrain or cerebellar necrosis, because of inadequate communication to the basilar artery, only 3% of patients with left vertebral ligation and 2% of patients with right vertebral ligation develop these complications. Therefore, in the face of massive hemorrhage from a partially severed vertebral artery, ligation with surgical clips applied to the vessel between the transverse processes above and below the laceration is accepted.

Subclavian artery injuries are best approached through a combined cervicothoracic incision. Proper exposure is the key to success in the management of these difficult and too-often fatal injuries. Ligation of the subclavian artery is relatively safe, but primary repair is preferable. Care should be taken to avoid phrenic nerve and thoracic duct injury when operating in this region of the neck. If the patient is stable

and a subclavian injury is identified at arteriography, an endovascular stent is another therapeutic option.

Venous injuries are best managed by ligation. The possibility of air embolism must be kept constantly in mind. A simple means of preventing this complication is to lower the patient's head using the Trendelenburg position until bleeding is controlled.

Esophageal injuries should be sutured closed primarily and drained. Use of muscle flaps using omohyoid or sternocleidomastoid muscles to cover the repair can be helpful. Drainage is the mainstay of treatment. Extensive injury to the esophagus is often immediately fatal because of associated injuries to the spinal cord. Systemic antibiotics should be administered routinely to patients with esophageal injuries.

Minor laryngeal and tracheal injuries do not require treatment, but immediate tracheostomy should be performed when airway obstruction exists. If there has been significant injury to the thyroid cartilage, a temporary laryngeal stent (Silastic) should be employed to provide support. Mucosal lacerations should be approximated before insertion of the stent. Conveniently located small perforations of the trachea can be utilized for tracheostomy. Otherwise, the wounds can be closed after they are debrided and a distal tracheostomy performed. Extensive circumferential tracheal injuries may require resection and anastomosis or reconstruction using synthetic materials.

Cervical spinal cord injury should be managed in such a way as to prevent further damage. When there is cervical cord compression from hematoma, vertebral fractures, or foreign bodies, decompression laminectomy is necessary.

Prognosis

Severe laceration of the cervical spinal cord often results in paralysis. Injuries to the soft tissues of the neck, trachea, and esophagus have a good to excellent prognosis if promptly treated. Major vascular injuries have a good prognosis if promptly treated before the onset of irreversible shock or neurologic deficit. The overall death rate for major cervical injuries is about 10%.

Bromberg WJ et al: Blunt cerebrovascular injury practice management guidelines: Eastern Association for the Surgery of Trauma. *J Trauma.* 2010;68:471.

Burlew CC et al: Blunt cerebrovascular injuries: Redefining screening criteria in the era of noninvasive diagnosis. *J Trauma Acute Care Surg.* 2012;72:330.

Chung S et al: Trauma Association of Canada Pediatric Subcommittee National Pediatric Cervical Spine Evaluation Pathway: Consensus guidelines. *J Trauma.* 2011;70:873.

Como JJ et al: Computed tomography alone may clear the cervical spine in obtunded blunt trauma patients: A prospective evaluation of a revised protocol. *J Trauma.* 2011;70:345.

DiCocco JM et al: Optimal outcomes for patients with blunt cerebrovascular injury (BCVI): Tailoring treatment to the lesion. *J Am Coll Surg.* 2011;212:549.

Emmett KP et al: Improving the screening criteria for blunt cerebrovascular injury: The appropriate role for computed tomography angiography. *J Trauma.* 2011;70:1058.

Hennessy D et al: Cervical spine clearance in obtunded blunt trauma patients: A prospective study. *J Trauma.* 2010;68:576.

Hoffman JR et al: Validity of a set of clinical criteria to rule out injury to the cervical spine in patients with blunt trauma. National Emergency X-Radiography Utilization Study Group. *N Engl J Med.* 2000;343:94.

Inaba K et al: Evaluation of multidetector computed tomography for penetrating neck injury: A prospective multicenter study. *J Trauma Acute Care Surg.* 2012;72:576.

Inaba K et al; WTA C-Spine Study Group: Cervical spinal clearance: A prospective Western Trauma Association multi-institutional trial. *J Trauma Acute Care Surg.* 2016;81:1122.

Patel MB et al.: Cervical spine collar clearance in the obtunded adult blunt trauma patient: A systematic review and practice management guideline from the Eastern Association for the Surgery of Trauma. *J Trauma Acute Care Surg.* 2015;78:430.

Stiell IG et al: The Canadian C-spine rule for radiography in alert and stable trauma patients. *JAMA.* 2001;286:1848.

Wang AC et al: Evaluating the use and utility of noninvasive angiography in diagnosing traumatic blunt cerebrovascular injury. *J Trauma Acute Care Surg.* 2012;72:1601.

THORACIC INJURIES

Thoracic trauma accounts directly for or is a contributing factor in 50% of deaths from trauma. Early deaths are commonly due to (1) airway obstruction, (2) flail chest, (3) open pneumothorax, (4) massive hemothorax, (5) tension pneumothorax, and (6) cardiac tamponade. Later deaths are due to respiratory failure, sepsis, and unrecognized injuries/complications. The majority of blunt thoracic injuries are the result of automobile accidents. Even what appears to be a minor blunt thoracic injury leading to rib fractures and pulmonary contusions can have a profound effect on patients. Near-side collisions are responsible for a higher incidence of blunt aortic injury among older adults and are associated with lower delta V forces compared to those in younger patients. Penetrating chest injuries from knives, bullets, and so on, are deadly and can result in complex patterns of injury. The mortality rate in hospitalized patients with isolated chest injury is 4%–8%; it is 10%–15% when one other organ system is involved, and rises to 35% if multiple additional organs are injured.

Combined injuries of multiple intrathoracic structures are typical. There are often other injuries to the abdomen, head, or skeletal system. When performing an operation on the chest for trauma, it is often necessary to operate on the abdomen as well. Therefore, when trauma patients are brought to the operating room for a laparotomy or thoracotomy, both body regions should be prepped into the operative field. Eighty-five percent of chest injuries do not require open thoracotomy, but immediate use of lifesaving measures is often necessary and should be within the competence of all surgeons.

A rapid estimate of cardiorespiratory status and possible associated injuries from the physical examination gives the physician a valuable overview of a patient who has sustained thoracic injuries. For example, patients with upper airway obstruction appear cyanotic, ashen, or gray; examination reveals stridor or gurgling sounds, ineffective respiratory excursion, constriction of cervical muscles, and retraction of the suprasternal, supraclavicular, intercostal, or epigastric regions. The character of chest wall excursions and the presence or absence of penetrating wounds should be observed. If respiratory excursions are not visible, ventilation is probably inadequate. Severe paradoxic chest wall movement in flail chest is usually located anteriorly and can be seen immediately. Sucking wounds of the chest wall should be obvious. A large hemothorax may be detected by percussion, and subcutaneous emphysema is easily detected on palpation as crepitus. Both massive hemothorax and tension pneumothorax may produce absent or diminished breath sounds and a shift of the trachea to the opposite side, but in massive hemothorax the neck veins are usually collapsed. If the patient has a thready or absent pulse and distended neck veins, the main differential diagnosis is between cardiac tamponade and tension pneumothorax.

In moribund patients, diagnosis must be immediate, and treatment may require chest tube placement, pericardiocentesis, or thoracotomy in the emergency room. The first priority of management should be to provide an airway and restore circulation. One can then reassess the patient and outline definitive measures. A cuffed endotracheal tube and assisted ventilation are required for apnea, ineffectual breathing, severe shock, deep coma, airway obstruction, flail chest, or open sucking chest wounds. Persistent shock or hypoxia due to thoracic trauma may be caused by any of the following: massive hemopneumothorax, cardiac tamponade, tension pneumothorax or massive air leak, or air embolism. If hemorrhagic shock is not explained readily by findings on chest x-ray or external losses, it is almost certainly due to intra-abdominal bleeding.

► Tube Thoracostomy

If time permits, the chest is prepared and draped in a sterile fashion. In awake patients, local anesthetic (1% lidocaine) is injected in the skin and surrounding tissues at the planned site of tube insertion. In an unconscious patient, this step is usually unnecessary. The location of the chest tube insertion site is the interspace between the fourth and fifth ribs in the midaxillary line. A 2- to 3-cm skin incision is created with a #10 scalpel and carried down into the subcutaneous tissue. Using a large hemostat, a soft-tissue tunnel is created just superior to the cephalad edge of the fifth rib. A finger or blunt clamp is used to penetrate the parietal pleura and enter the pleural space. The wound is explored with an index finger to confirm entry into the pleural cavity and check for pulmonary adhesions.

A 36F straight thoracostomy tube is inserted and directed posteriorly toward the apex of the lung. The tube is anchored to the skin with stitches and connected to a Pleur-Evac device set at 20 cm H_2O suction with a water seal. An emerging alternative to a large thoracostomy tube is the Wayne pneumothorax catheter kit, which contains a 14F thoracostomy tube that can be placed using the Seldinger technique.

▶ Types of Injuries

A. Chest Wall

Rib fracture, the most common chest injury, varies across a spectrum from simple fracture to fracture with hemopneumothorax to severe multiple fractures with flail chest, pulmonary contusion, and internal injuries. With simple fractures, pain on inspiration is the principal symptom; treatment consists of providing adequate analgesia. In cases of multiple fractures, intercostal nerve blocks or epidural analgesia may be required to ensure adequate ventilation. Multiple fractures can be associated with decreased ventilation and subsequent pneumonia, particularly in the elderly patient.

Flail chest occurs when a portion of the chest wall becomes isolated by multiple fractures and paradoxically moves in and out with inspiration and expiration with a potentially severe reduction in ventilatory efficiency. The magnitude of the effect is determined by the size of the flail segment and the amount of pain with breathing. The rib fractures are usually anterior, and there are at least two fractures of the same rib. Bilateral costochondral separation and sternal fractures can also cause a flail segment. An associated lung contusion may produce a decrease in lung compliance not fully manifest until 12-48 hours after injury. Increased negative intrapleural pressure is then required for ventilation, and chest wall instability becomes apparent. If ventilation becomes inadequate, atelectasis, hypercapnia, hypoxia, accumulation of secretions, and ineffective cough occur. Arterial Pao_2 is often low before clinical findings appear. Serial blood gas analysis is the best way to determine if a treatment regimen is adequate. For less severe cases, intercostal nerve block or continuous epidural analgesia may be adequate treatment. However, more severe cases require ventilatory assistance for variable periods of time with a cuffed endotracheal tube and a mechanical ventilator.

Most rib or sternal fractures will heal without treatment. In selected patients, internal fixation may be useful; however, determining the patient population that would most benefit is still under investigation. Commercially produced, implantable rib and sternal fracture plating systems are now available. A system with bioabsorbable plates has been described that allows fixation of fragments during the healing process and metabolism by the body within 24 months. Patients who would potentially benefit from an open reduction internal fixation procedure are those with nonunion, severely displaced rib fractures with overriding fragments, severe pain with respiratory compromise (eg, difficulty in being weaned off the mechanical ventilator), multiple unstable rib fractures, and those undergoing thoracotomy for another intrathoracic indication. Because of the peristomal bacterial burden associated with a tracheostomy, this procedure should be used with caution in patients with a prior tracheostomy and need for a surgical incision high on the chest wall.

B. Trachea and Bronchus

Blunt tracheobronchial injuries are often due to compression of the airway between the sternum and the vertebral column in decelerating or high-velocity crush accidents. The distal trachea or mainstem bronchi are usually involved, and 80% of all injuries are located within 2.5 cm from the carina. Penetrating tracheobronchial injuries may occur at any location. Most patients have pneumothorax, subcutaneous emphysema, pneumomediastinum, and hemoptysis. Cervicofacial emphysema may be dramatic. Tracheobronchial injury should be suspected when there is a massive air leak or when the lung does not readily reexpand after chest tube placement. In penetrating injuries of the trachea or mainstem bronchi, there is usually massive hemorrhage and hemoptysis. Systemic air embolism resulting in cardiopulmonary arrest may occur if a bronchovenous fistula is present. If air embolism is suspected, emergency thoracotomy should be performed with cross-clamping of the pulmonary hilum on the affected side. The diagnosis is confirmed by aspiration of air from the heart. In blunt injuries, the tracheobronchial injury may not be obvious and may be suspected only after major atelectasis develops several days later. Diagnosis may require flexible or rigid bronchoscopy. Immediate primary repair with absorbable sutures is indicated for all tracheobronchial lacerations.

C. Pleural Space

Hemothorax (blood within the pleural cavity) is classified according to the amount of blood: minimal, 350 mL; moderate, 350-1500 mL; or massive, 1500 mL or more. The rate of bleeding after evacuation of the hemothorax is clinically even more important. If air is also present, the condition is called *hemopneumothorax.*

Hemothorax should be suspected with penetrating or severe blunt thoracic injury. There may be decreased breath sounds and dullness to percussion, and a chest x-ray should be promptly obtained. In experienced hands, ultrasound can diagnose pneumothorax and hemothorax, but this technique is not widely employed at this time. Tube thoracostomy should be performed expeditiously for all hemothoraces. In 85% of cases, tube thoracostomy is the only treatment required. If bleeding is persistent, as noted by continued output from the chest tubes, it is more likely to be from the chest wall and an intercostal artery rather than a pulmonary artery. The use of positive end-expiratory pressure (PEEP) can help tamponade pulmonary parenchymal bleeding in trauma patients who are intubated. When the rate of bleeding shows a steady trend of greater than 200 mL/h, or the total hemorrhagic output exceeds 1500 mL, thoracoscopy or thoracotomy should usually be performed. The trend and rate of thoracic bleeding is probably more important than the absolute numbers in deciding to perform surgical intervention. Thoracoscopy has been shown to be effective in controlling chest tube bleeding in 82% of cases. This technique has also been shown to be 90% effective in evacuating retained hemothoraces. Retained hemothoraces less than 300 mL can often be observed. Retained hemothoraces greater than 900 mL often require thoracoscopy or thoracotomy evacuation. In most of these cases, the chest wall is the source of hemorrhage. Thoracotomy is required for management of injuries to the lungs, heart, pericardium, and great vessels.

Pneumothorax occurs in lacerations of the lung or chest wall following penetrating or blunt chest trauma. Hyperinflation (eg, blast injuries, diving accidents) can also rupture the lungs. After penetrating injury, 80% of patients with pneumothorax also have blood in the pleural cavity. Most cases of pneumothorax are readily diagnosed on chest x-ray. In some cases, an occult pneumothorax will be identified on a chest or abdominal CT scan. Pneumothorax or hemothorax may be identified on the lateral scans performed as part of the FAST examination of the abdomen for trauma (see section on abdominal trauma). Most cases of traumatic pneumothorax should be treated with immediate tube thoracostomy; however, small occult pneumothoraces in stable patients can be observed.

Tension pneumothorax develops when a flap-valve leak allows air to enter the pleural space but prevents its escape; intrapleural pressure rises, causing total collapse of the lung and a shift of the mediastinal viscera to the opposite side, interfering with venous return to the heart. It must be relieved immediately to avoid impairment of cardiac function. Immediate treatment involves placement of a large-bore needle or plastic angiocath in the pleural space, with care being taken to avoid injury to the intercostal vessels. After this emergency measure has been instituted, tension pneumothorax should be treated definitively by tube thoracostomy.

Sucking chest wounds, which allow air to pass in and out of the pleural cavity, should be promptly treated by a three-sided occlusive dressing and tube thoracostomy. The pathologic physiology resembles flail chest except that the extent of associated lung injury is usually less. Definitive management includes surgical closure of the defect in the chest wall.

D. Lung Injury

Pulmonary contusion due to sudden parenchymal concussion occurs after blunt trauma or wounding with a high-velocity missile. Pulmonary contusion happens in 75% of patients with flail chest but can also occur following blunt trauma without rib fracture. Alveolar rupture with fluid transudation and extravasation of blood are early findings. Fluid and blood from ruptured alveoli enter alveolar spaces and bronchi and produce localized airway obstruction and atelectasis. Increased mucous secretions and overzealous intravenous fluid therapy may combine to produce copious secretions and further atelectasis. The patient's ability to cough and clear secretions effectively is weakened because of chest wall pain or mechanical inefficiency from fractures. Elasticity of the lungs is decreased, resistance to air flow increases, and as the work of breathing increases, blood oxygenation and pH drop and $Paco_2$ rises. The cardiac compensatory response may be compromised, because as many as 35% of these patients have an associated myocardial contusion.

Treatment is often delayed because clinical and x-ray findings may not appear until 12-48 hours after injury. The clinical findings are copious, thin, blood-tinged secretions; chest pain; restlessness; apprehensiveness; and labored respirations. Eventually, dyspnea, cyanosis, tachypnea, and tachycardia develop. X-ray changes consist of patchy parenchymal opacification or diffuse linear peribronchial densities that may progress to diffuse opacification ("white-out") characteristic of acute respiratory distress syndrome.

Mechanical ventilatory support permits adequate alveolar ventilation and reduces the work of breathing. Blood gases should be monitored and arterial saturation adequately maintained. There is some controversy over the best regimen for fluid management, but excessive hydration or blood transfusion should be avoided. Serial measurement of central venous pressure, mixed venous oxygen saturation, and cardiac output help to avoid over- or under-resuscitation. Despite optimal therapy, about 15% of patients with pulmonary contusion die. Use of protective mechanical ventilator strategies is essential in these patients to avoid progressive ventilator-induced lung injury. Use of low-tidal volumes (6 mL/kg) and avoidance of plateau pressures greater than 35 cm H_2O are recommended.

Most lung lacerations are caused by penetrating injuries, and hemopneumothorax is usually present. Tube thoracostomy is indicated to evacuate pleural air or blood and to monitor continuing leaks. Since expansion of the lung tamponades the laceration, most lung lacerations do not produce massive hemorrhage or persistent air leaks. Should a pulmonary laceration require operative intervention, lung-sparing techniques rather than formal anatomic lung resection should be employed when feasible to reduce morbidity and mortality.

Lung hematomas are the result of local parenchymal destruction and hemorrhage. The x-ray appearance is initially a poorly defined density that becomes more circumscribed a few days to 2 weeks after injury. Cystic cavities occasionally develop if damage is extensive. Most hematomas resolve adequately with expectant treatment.

E. Heart and Pericardium

Blunt injury to the heart occurs most often from compression against the steering wheel in automobile accidents. This injury is in decline with the increasing prevalence of airbag technology in motor vehicles. The injury varies from localized contusion to cardiac rupture. Autopsy studies of victims of immediately fatal accidents show that as many as 65% have rupture of one or more cardiac chambers, and 45% have pericardial lacerations. The incidence of blunt myocardial injury in patients who reach the hospital is unknown but is probably higher than generally suspected. The clinical relevance of this diagnosis is widely debated. Most trauma surgeons advocate the diagnosis and treatment of the actual clinical problem such as acute heart failure, valvular injury, cardiac rupture, or dysrhythmia.

Early clinical findings include friction rubs, chest pain, tachycardia, murmurs, dysrhythmias, or signs of low cardiac output. Patients with risk factors for blunt myocardial injury should undergo evaluation with a 12-lead electrocardiogram (ECG). If the ECG is normal and the patient is asymptomatic, the work-up is complete. An abnormal ECG should prompt further evaluation with an echocardiogram. Patients with proven injury on echocardiogram and/or hemodynamic instability should be admitted to the intensive care unit and managed appropriately for the diagnosed injury. Normal admission and 8-hour ECG and troponin I rules out blunt cardiac injury. An abnormal ECG with a normal echocardiogram merits at least 24 hours of monitoring in a telemetry unit and daily repeat ECGs until stable or the dysrhythmia resolves. If the patient is suspected of having a myocardial infarction or acute myocardial ischemia, then cardiac enzymes should be obtained and a cardiology consultation arranged.

Management of symptomatic blunt myocardial injury should be the same as for acute myocardial infarction. Hemopericardium may occur without tamponade and can be treated by pericardiocentesis. Tamponade in blunt cardiac trauma is often due to myocardial rupture or coronary artery laceration. Tamponade produces distended neck veins, shock, and cyanosis. Immediate thoracotomy and control of the injury are indicated. If cardiopulmonary arrest occurs before the patient can be transported to the operating room, emergency room thoracotomy with relief of tamponade should be performed. Treatment of injuries to the valves, papillary muscles, and septum must be individualized; and when tolerated, delayed repair is usually recommended.

Pericardial lacerations from stab wounds tend to seal and cause tamponade, whereas gunshot wounds frequently leave a sufficient pericardial opening for drainage. Gunshot wounds produce more extensive myocardial damage, multiple perforations, and massive bleeding into the pleural space. Hemothorax, shock, and exsanguination occur in nearly all cases of cardiac gunshot wounds. The clinical findings are those of tamponade or acute blood loss. Use of ultrasound and the FAST examination technique can reveal the presence of clinically significant blood in the pericardial space.

Treatment of penetrating cardiac injuries requires prompt thoracotomy, pericardial decompression, and control of hemorrhage. Most patients do not require cardiopulmonary bypass. The standard approach has been to repair the laceration using mattress sutures with pledgets while controlling hemorrhage with a finger on the heart. Suture control of cardiac lacerations may be technically difficult when working with a beating heart or in patients with large or multiple lacerations. Several studies have demonstrated that in most cases, emergency temporary control of hemorrhage from cardiac lacerations can be achieved with the use of a skin stapler (Figure 14–11). Following stabilization of the patient, the staples can be removed after definitive suture repair is performed in the operating room. Hemostatic sealants such as FloSeal offer significant promise as additional tools in the surgical armamentarium when dealing with lacerations to the heart or great vessels. Regardless of the approach utilized, care must be taken to avoid injury to the coronary arteries.

Pericardiocentesis or creation of a pericardial window is reserved for selected cases when the diagnosis is uncertain

▲ **Figure 14–11.** Technique of cardiac stapling. Finger pressure (not shown) is used to maintain hemostasis during stapling. (Reproduced, with permission, from Macho JR, Markison RE, Schecter WP: Cardiac stapling in the management of penetrating injuries of the heart: rapid control of hemorrhage and decreased risk of personal contamination, *J Trauma.* 1993;May;34(5):711-715.)

or in preparation for thoracotomy. In approximately 75% of cases of stab wounds and 35% of cases of gunshot cardiac wounds, the patient survives the operation. However, it is estimated that 80%-90% of patients with gunshot wounds of the heart do not reach the hospital.

F. Esophagus

Anatomically, the esophagus is well protected, and perforation from external penetrating trauma is relatively infrequent. Blunt injuries are exceedingly rare. The most common symptom of esophageal perforation is pain; fever develops within hours in most patients. Hematemesis, hoarseness, dysphagia, or respiratory distress may also be present. Physical findings include shock, local tenderness, subcutaneous emphysema, or Hamman sign (pericardial or mediastinal "crunch" synchronous with cardiac sounds). Leukocytosis occurs soon after injury. X-ray findings on plain chest films include evidence of a foreign body or missile and mediastinal air or widening. Pleural effusion or hydropneumothorax is frequently seen, usually on the left side. Contrast x-rays of the esophagus should be performed but are positive in only about 70% of proven perforations.

A nasogastric tube should be passed to evacuate gastric contents. If recognized within 24-48 hours after injury, the esophageal perforation should be closed and pleural drainage instituted with large-bore catheters. Repair of these perforations requires special techniques that include buttressing of the esophageal closure with pleural or pericardial flaps; pedicles of intercostal, diaphragmatic, or cervical strap muscles; and serosal patches from stomach or jejunum. Illness and death are due to mediastinal and pleural infection.

G. Thoracic Duct

Chylothorax and chylopericardium are rare complications of trauma but are difficult to manage when they occur. Penetrating injuries of the neck, thorax, or upper abdomen can injure the thoracic duct or its major tributaries.

Symptoms are due to mechanical effects of the accumulations (eg, shortness of breath from lung collapse or low cardiac output from tamponade). The diagnosis is established when the fluid is shown to have characteristics of chyle.

The patient should be maintained on a fat-free, high-carbohydrate, high-protein diet and the effusion aspirated. Chest tube drainage should be instituted if the effusion recurs. Lipid-free total parenteral nutrition with no oral intake may be effective in treating persistent leaks. Conservative treatment for 3-4 weeks is usually curative. If daily chyle loss exceeds 1500 mL for 5 successive days, or persists after 2-3 weeks of conservative treatment, the thoracic duct should be ligated via a right thoracotomy. Intraoperative identification of the leak may be facilitated by preoperative administration of a fat-containing lipophilic dye.

H. Diaphragm

Penetrating injuries of the diaphragm outnumber blunt diaphragmatic injuries by a ratio of at least 6:1. Diaphragmatic lacerations occur in 10%-15% of cases of penetrating wounds to the chest and in as many as 40% of cases of penetrating trauma to the left chest. Injuries to the right diaphragm are more common than previously thought. The injury is rarely obvious. Wounds of the diaphragm must not be overlooked because they rarely heal spontaneously and because herniation of abdominal viscera into the chest can occur with catastrophic complications either immediately or years after the injuries.

Associated injuries are usually present, and as many as 25% of patients are in shock when first seen. There may be abdominal tenderness, dyspnea, shoulder pain, or unilateral breath sounds. The diagnosis is often missed. Although chest radiography is a sensitive diagnostic tool, it may be entirely normal in 40% of cases. The most common finding is ipsilateral hemothorax, which is present in about 50% of patients. Occasionally, a distended, herniated stomach is confused with a pneumothorax. Passage of a nasogastric tube before x-rays will help to identify an intrathoracic stomach. CT scan or contrast x-rays may be necessary to establish the diagnosis in some cases. Newer generation helical CT scanners that allow sagittal reformatting can be helpful in definitively diagnosing diaphragmatic injury. Laparoscopy is a useful but invasive technique for detecting occult diaphragmatic injuries in patients who have no other indications for formal laparotomy.

Once the diagnosis is made, a transabdominal surgical approach should be used in cases of acute rupture. Laparoscopic suturing for repair of the injury may be possible in selected cases. The diaphragm should be reapproximated and closed with interrupted or running nonabsorbable sutures. Chronic herniation is associated with adhesions of the affected viscera to the thoracic structures and should be approached via thoracotomy, with the addition of a separate laparotomy when indicated. These cases can be quite challenging and appropriate preoperative planning is recommended.

Bhatnagar A et al: Rib fracture fixation for flail chest: What is the benefit? *J Am Coll Surg.* 2012;215:201–205.

Cook CC et al: Great vessel and cardiac trauma. *Surg Clin North Am.* 2009;89:797.

DuBose J et al: Management of post-traumatic retained hemothorax: A prospective, observational, multicenter AAST study. *J Trauma Acute Care Surg.* 2012;72:11.

Kaiser M et al: The clinical significance of occult thoracic injury in blunt trauma patients. *Am Surg.* 2010;76:1063.

Marasco SF et al: Prospective randomized controlled trial of operative rib fixation in traumatic flail chest. *J Am Coll Surg.* 2013; 216:924.

Nagarsheth K et al: Ultrasound detection of pneumothorax compared with chest x-ray and computed tomography scan. *Am Surg.* 2011;77:480.

Neschis DG et al: Blunt aortic injury. *N Engl J Med.* 2008;359:1708.

Nirula R et al: Rib fracture fixation: Controversies and technical challenges. *Am Surg.* 2010;76:793.

O'Connor J et al: Penetrating cardiac injury. *J R Army Med Corps.* 2009;155:185.

Pieracci FM et al: A multicenter evaluation of the optimal timing of surgical stabilization of rib fractures. *J Trauma Acute Care Surg.* 2018;84:1.

Salim A et al: Clinically significant blunt cardiac trauma: Role of serum troponin levels combined with electrocardiographic findings. *J Trauma.* 2001;50:237.

Seamon MJ et al: An evidence-based approach to patient selection for emergency department thoracotomy: A practice management guideline from the Eastern Association for the Surgery of Trauma. *J Trauma Acute Care Surg.* 2015;79:159.

ABDOMINAL INJURIES

The specific type of abdominal injury varies according to whether the trauma is penetrating or blunt. Blunt injuries predominate in rural areas, while penetrating injuries are more common in urban areas. The mechanism of injury in blunt trauma is rapid deceleration, and noncompliant organs such as the liver, spleen, pancreas, and kidneys are at greater risk of injury due to parenchymal fracture. Occasionally, hollow viscous organs may be injured, with the duodenum and urinary bladder being particularly susceptible. The small bowel occupies a large portion of the total abdominal volume and is more likely to be injured by penetrating trauma. Most blunt abdominal injuries are related to motor vehicle accidents. Although the use of restraints has been associated with a decrease in the incidence of head, chest, and solid organ injuries, their use may be associated with pancreatic, mesenteric, and intestinal injuries due to organ compression against the spinal column. These injuries should be considered in patients who have signs of seat belt–related contusions of the abdominal wall. Internal abdominal injury may be present in as many as 30% of these cases. In any abdominal trauma, hemoperitoneum may not manifest clinical signs of peritoneal irritation, particularly in patients with other distracting injuries or depressed mental status. Retroperitoneal injury may be more subtle and difficult to diagnose during the initial evaluation.

Deaths from abdominal trauma result largely from early severe hemorrhage and coagulopathy or from later sepsis. Most deaths from abdominal trauma are preventable. Patients at risk of abdominal injury should undergo prompt and thorough evaluation. In most trauma centers, after physical examination, the initial diagnostic evaluation includes bedside FAST and portable radiographs of the pelvis and chest to assess for other potential sites of bleeding. In unstable patients who cannot be adequately evaluated with FAST due to size, technical problems, or subcutaneous air, diagnostic peritoneal lavage is warranted. After the initial FAST exam, patients who are stable or who respond to initial fluid resuscitation should have a CT scan of the abdomen and pelvis to evaluate for intra-abdominal and retroperitoneal injuries. Patients with persistent hypotension requiring fluid and blood resuscitation in the face of a positive FAST exam should be transported to the operating room emergently for exploratory laparotomy.

In some cases, dramatic physical findings may be due to abdominal wall injury in the absence of intraperitoneal injury. If the results of diagnostic studies are equivocal, diagnostic laparoscopy or exploratory laparotomy should be considered, since they may be lifesaving if serious injuries are identified early. Evaluation always includes a comprehensive physical examination with pelvic and rectal examinations included and may require specific laboratory and radiologic tests (eg, retrograde urethrogram or cystogram, rigid sigmoidoscopy, abdominal CT). Serial physical examinations may be necessary to detect subtle findings.

▶ Types of Injuries

A. Penetrating Trauma

Penetrating injuries to the abdomen that present with shock or ongoing resuscitation require prompt exploration. Lacerations of major blood vessels or the liver can cause severe and early shock. Penetrating injuries of the spleen, pancreas, or kidneys usually do not bleed massively unless a major vessel to the organ (eg, the renal artery) is damaged. Bleeding must be controlled promptly with packing and appropriate clamping for vascular control. A patient in shock with a penetrating injury of the abdomen who does not respond to 1 L of crystalloid fluid resuscitation should be operated on immediately following chest x-ray and switched to blood product resuscitation.

Patients with hollow visceral injuries may have very few physical signs initially but will progress to sepsis if the injuries are not recognized. Increasing abdominal tenderness demands surgical exploration. White blood cell count elevations, and fever appearing several hours following injury, are keys to early diagnosis.

The treatment of hemodynamically stable patients with penetrating injuries to the lower chest or abdomen varies. All surgeons agree that patients with signs of peritonitis or hypovolemia should undergo surgical exploration, but operative treatment is less certain for patients with no signs of peritonitis or sepsis who are cardiovascularly stable.

Most stab wounds of the lower chest or abdomen should be explored, since a delay in treatment of a hollow viscous perforation can result in severe sepsis. Some surgeons recommend a selective policy in the management of these patients. When the depth of injury is in doubt, local wound exploration may rule out peritoneal penetration. Laparoscopy has a role in the evaluation of penetrating injuries in experienced hands, but requires considerable diligence to avoid missed injuries. All gunshot wounds of the lower chest and abdomen should be explored, unless there is a likely superficial scything wound, because the incidence of injury to major intra-abdominal structures exceeds 90% in such cases.

B. Blunt Trauma

A major advance in management of blunt trauma has been the FAST examination. Ultrasound has proven to be an ideal modality in the immediate evaluation of the trauma patient because it is rapid and accurate for the detection of intra-abdominal fluid or blood and is readily repeatable. It provides valuable information that augments the surgeon's diagnostic capabilities. Since its introduction in North America in 1989, ultrasonography has become commonplace, and a recent survey reports that 78% of U.S. trauma centers routinely use the FAST examination in the evaluation of patients.

The goal of the FAST examination is the identification of abnormal collections of blood or fluid. In this regard, it obviates the need for diagnostic peritoneal lavage. The primary focus is on the peritoneal cavity, but attention is also directed to the pericardium and to the pleural space. Unclotted blood or fluid allows transmission of ultrasound waves without echoes and thus appears black (Figure 14–12). In the standard FAST examination, four areas are scanned: the right upper quadrant, the subxiphoid area, the left upper quadrant, and the pelvis (Figure 14–13). Most surgeons recommend scanning initially in the right upper quadrant because more than half of the positive tests will reveal blood or fluid in this area. Unstable patients with a positive FAST examination should undergo urgent exploratory laparotomy.

The other diagnostic procedures most commonly used in patients without obvious indications for immediate laparotomy include CT scanning and diagnostic laparoscopy.

▶ Computed Tomography

CT is noninvasive, qualitative, sensitive, and accurate for the diagnosis of intra-abdominal and retroperitoneal injuries. Modern multi-slice spiral scanners have greatly decreased the time required for obtaining high-quality images. However, CT scanning remains expensive, involves the use of intravenous contrast administration, exposes the patient to radiation, and requires an experienced radiologist for proper interpretation of the scans. CT scanning also involves transport from the acute care area and should not be attempted in the unstable patient.

CT scanning has a primary role in defining the location and magnitude of intra-abdominal injuries related to blunt trauma. It has the advantage of detecting most retroperitoneal injuries, but it may not identify all gastrointestinal injuries. The information provided on the magnitude of injury allows for potential nonoperative management of patients with solid organ injuries. Nonsurgical therapy is now used in more than 80% of blunt liver and spleen injuries. Detection of high-grade solid organ injuries or bleeding pelvic fractures by CT in relatively stable patients can

▲ **Figure 14–12.** *Top:* Normal ultrasound of the right upper quadrant. *Bottom:* Right upper quadrant ultrasound revealing blood between the liver and the kidney and between the liver and the diaphragm. (Used with permission from San Francisco General Hospital.)

also lead to other minimally invasive interventions, such as angiographic embolization, which increases the success of nonoperative management. Table 14–4 compares the time, costs, advantages, and disadvantages of nonoperative methods used for evaluation of the injured abdomen.

▶ Diagnostic Laparoscopy

Laparoscopy has an important diagnostic role in stable patients with penetrating abdominal trauma. It can quickly establish whether peritoneal penetration has occurred, and thus reduce the number of negative and nontherapeutic trauma laparotomies performed. In selected patients, therapeutic laparoscopy has been used to repair injuries to the bowel and diaphragm. This approach offers all the

▲ **Figure 14–13.** Transducer positions for FAST. Pericardial area, right and left upper quadrants, and pelvis. (Reproduced with permission from Rozycki GS et al. Surgeon-performed ultrasound for the assessment of truncal injuries: lessons learned from 1540 patients, *Ann Surg* 1998;Oct;228(4):557-567.)

Table 14–4. Comparison of diagnostic methods for abdominal trauma.

Methods	Time/Cost	Advantages/Disadvantages
Physical examination	Quick/no cost	Useful for serial examinations, very limited by other injuries, coma, drug intoxication, poor sensitivity and specificity.
Diagnostic peritoneal lavage (DPL)	Quick/ inexpensive	Rapid results in unstable patient but invasive and may be overly sensitive for blood and not specific for site of injury; requires experience and may be limited if previous surgery.
Focused assessment with sonography for trauma (FAST)	Quick/ inexpensive	Rapid detection of intraabdominal fluid and pericardial tamponade; may be limited by operator experience, large body habitus, subcutaneous air; poor for detection of bowel injury. Fairly sensitive but not highly specific.
Helical computed abdominal tomography (CT)	Slower/ expensive	Most specific for site of injury and can evaluate retroperitoneum; very good sensitivity but may miss bowel injury; risk of reaction to contrast dye.

advantages and disadvantages of minimally invasive surgery. Laparoscopy has also been applied safely and effectively as a screening tool in stable patients with blunt abdominal trauma. However, its use in this context requires further study. Concerns regarding the use of laparoscopy in trauma include the possibility of missed injuries, air embolism, hemodynamic instability related to the pneumoperitoneum, and complications related to trocar placement.

▶ **Exploratory Laparotomy**

The three main indications for exploration of the abdomen following blunt trauma are peritonitis, ongoing intra-abdominal hemorrhage, and the presence of other injuries known to be frequently associated with intra-abdominal injuries. Peritonitis after blunt abdominal trauma is rare and can arise from rupture of a hollow organ, such as the duodenum, bladder, intestine, or gallbladder; from pancreatic injury; or occasionally from the presence of retroperitoneal blood.

Emergency abdominal exploration should be considered for patients with profound hypovolemic shock and a normal chest x-ray unless extra-abdominal blood loss is sufficient to account for the hypovolemia. In most cases, a rapidly performed FAST examination or peritoneal lavage will confirm the diagnosis of intraperitoneal hemorrhage. Patients with blunt trauma and hypovolemia should be examined first for intra-abdominal bleeding even if there is no overt evidence of abdominal trauma. For example, hypovolemia may be due to loss of blood from a large scalp laceration, but it may also be due to unsuspected rupture of the spleen. Hemoperitoneum may present with no signs except hypovolemia. The abdomen may be flat and nontender. Patients whose extra-abdominal bleeding has been controlled should respond to initial fluid resuscitation with an adequate urine output and stabilization of vital signs. If signs of hypovolemia (tachycardia, hypotension, low urine output, metabolic acidosis) recur, intra-abdominal bleeding must be considered to be the cause.

Other injuries frequently associated with abdominal trauma are rib fractures, pelvic fractures, abdominal wall injuries, and fractures of the thoracolumbar spine (eg, 20% of patients with fractures of the left lower ribs have a splenic laceration).

▶ Treatment

A. Splenic Injuries

The spleen is the most commonly injured organ in cases of blunt abdominal trauma. Splenic injuries in children are typically managed without surgery. Currently, 50%-88% of adults with blunt splenic injuries are also treated nonoperatively. Patients must be monitored closely, and immediate availability of an operating room is essential. Patients should be evaluated frequently for the possibility of other missed injuries or recurrent bleeding. Stable patients who have high-grade splenic injuries on CT scan or have evidence of ongoing bleeding on CT scan may be candidates for angiographic embolization. Unstable patients with splenic injuries should undergo splenectomy or attempts at splenic repair if appropriate.

Associated injuries are uncommon for patients in whom nonoperative management is attempted. In unstable patients, emergent celiotomy should be performed. Splenic salvage procedures such as splenorrhaphy, partial resection, wrapping with Vicryl mesh, or topical therapy with hemostatic agents should be attempted if the patient's condition permits and there are a limited number of concomitant abdominal injuries. In the face of multiple injuries, ongoing cardiovascular compromise, or vascular avulsion of the spleen, total splenectomy is indicated. Following splenectomy, immunizations against *Pneumococcus* species, *Meningococcus* species, and *Haemophilus influenzae* are recommended postoperatively to reduce the risk of overwhelming postsplenectomy sepsis.

B. Liver Injuries

Approximately 85% of all patients with blunt hepatic trauma are stable following resuscitation. In this group, nonoperative management has been proven to be superior to open operation in avoiding complications and decreasing mortality. The primary requirement for nonoperative therapy is continued hemodynamic stability. Patients are monitored in the intensive care unit with frequent assessment of vital signs and serial hematocrits. If transfusion with more than two units of PRBC is required, arteriography with possible embolization of bleeding vessels should be considered.

Nonoperative management of blunt hepatic trauma is successful in more than 90% of cases. With more severe injuries, repeat CT scanning may be necessary to evaluate for possible complications such as parenchymal infarction, hematoma, or biloma. Extrahepatic bile collections should generally be drained percutaneously. Intrahepatic collections of blood and bile usually resolve spontaneously over the course of several months. Patients with high-grade liver injuries have up to a 40% chance of developing bile leaks from the injured liver bed. Nuclear medicine scanning to delineate biliary flow with derivatives of iminodiacetic acid is useful in detection of bile leaks, and should be done in the first few days after injury to reduce complications. Laparoscopic washout and placement of drains is an option for patients found to have evidence of extrahepatic bile leakage on HIDA scan. In addition, 1%-4% of patients with blunt liver injury will have injuries to other abdominal organs, which should prompt the clinician to consider the possibility of missed injury in patients who develop abdominal sepsis after injury.

Severe liver injury may result in exsanguinating hemorrhage with hypotension that does not respond to fluid resuscitation. For these patients, operative exploration is warranted. At laparotomy, immediate efforts should be directed to control of hemorrhage and stabilization of the patient by restoration of circulating blood volume. The initial techniques for the control of hepatic hemorrhage include manual compression, perihepatic packing, and the Pringle maneuver. Manual compression or perihepatic packing with laparotomy pads will control hemorrhage in most cases. The Pringle maneuver—clamping of the hepatic pedicle—should be performed when life-threatening hemorrhage is unresponsive to packing; it will control all hepatic bleeding except that from the hepatic veins or the intrahepatic vena cava. In most cases, the Pringle maneuver should not be maintained for more than 1 hour in order to prevent ischemic damage to the liver. Hepatic bleeding can be controlled by suture ligation or application of surgical clips directly to the bleeding vessels. Electrocautery or the argon beam coagulator can be used to control bleeding from raw surfaces of the liver. Microfibrillar collagen or hemostatic gelatin foam sponges soaked in thrombin can be applied to bleeding areas with pressure to control diffuse capillary bleeding. Fibrin glue has been used in treating both superficial and deep lacerations and appears to be the most effective topical agent, but reports of fatal anaphylactic reactions have limited its use. When injury has already resulted in massive blood loss, packing of the abdomen with laparotomy pads and planned reexploration should be considered. Avoidance of the lethal triad of hypothermia, acidosis, and coagulopathy is paramount to successful surgical treatment of a major liver injury and may require further resuscitation in the intensive care unit prior to return to the operating room. At the time of reexploration in 24 to 48 hours, hemorrhage is usually well controlled and can be managed with individual vessel ligation and debridement. Evidence of persistent hemorrhage should prompt earlier reexploration. Angiographic embolization may be a useful adjunct to surgical packing if arterial hemorrhage is still present or not well controlled. Rarely, selective hepatic artery ligation, resectional debridement, or hepatic lobectomy may be required to control hemorrhage. The raw surface of the liver may then be covered with omentum. Drains should always be used. Decompression of the biliary system is contraindicated, though sutures or clips should be used to control intraparenchymal bile ducts.

Hepatic vein injuries frequently bleed massively. Hepatic venous or intrahepatic vena caval injury should be suspected immediately when the Pringle maneuver fails to control bleeding. Several techniques have been described for isolation of the intrahepatic cava prior to attempted repair of these injuries. Unfortunately, even with the use of these techniques, mortality remains very high.

C. Biliary Tract Injuries

Biliary tract injuries are relatively uncommon, particularly for blunt trauma. Injury to the gallbladder should be treated in most cases by cholecystectomy. Minor injuries to the common bile duct can be treated by suture closure and insertion of a T-tube. Avulsion of the common bile duct, or in combination with duodenal or ampullary trauma, may require choledochojejunostomy in conjunction with total or partial pancreatectomy, duodenectomy, or other diversion procedures. Segmental loss of the common bile duct is best treated by choledochojejunostomy and drainage.

D. Pancreatic Injuries

Pancreatic injuries may present with few clinical manifestations. Injury should be suspected whenever the upper abdomen has been traumatized, especially when serum amylase and lipase levels remain persistently elevated. The best diagnostic study for pancreatic injury (other than exploratory celiotomy) is CT scan of the abdomen. Peritoneal lavage is usually not helpful. Upper gastrointestinal studies with water-soluble contrast material may suggest pancreatic injury by demonstrating widening of the duodenal C-loop. Endoscopic retrograde cholangiopancreatography may be used in selected cases to evaluate for injuries to the major ducts.

The treatment of pancreatic injury depends on its grade and extent. Minor injuries not involving a major duct may be treated nonoperatively. Moderate injuries usually require operative exploration, debridement, and the placement of external drains. More severe injuries, including those with major duct injury or transection of the gland, may require distal resection or external drainage. Traumatic injuries to the head of the pancreas often include associated vascular injuries and carry a high mortality rate. Efforts should be directed at controlling hemorrhage, and drains can be placed in the area of the pancreatic injury. In most cases, pancreaticoduodenectomy should not be attempted in the setting of an unstable patient with multiple injuries.

The late complications of pancreatic injuries include pseudocyst, pancreatic fistula, and pancreatic abscess. Patients treated without resection may require reoperation for resection or Roux-en-Y internal gastrointestinal drainage.

E. Gastrointestinal Tract Injuries

Most injuries of the stomach can be repaired. Large injuries, such as those from shotgun blasts, may require subtotal or total resection. Failure to identify posterior stomach wall injuries by opening the lesser space is a pitfall to guard against.

Duodenal injuries may not be evident from the initial physical examination or x-ray studies. Abdominal films will reveal retroperitoneal gas within 6 hours after injury in most patients. CT performed with a contrast agent will frequently identify the site of perforation. Most duodenal injuries can be treated with lateral repair. Some may require resection with end-to-end anastomosis. Occasionally, pancreaticoduodenectomy or duodenal diversion with gastrojejunostomy and pyloric closure is required to manage a severe injury. A duodenostomy tube is useful in decompressing the duodenum and can be used to control a fistula caused by an injury. Jejunal or omental patches may also aid in preventing a suture line leak. A distal jejunostomy feeding tube is helpful in the long-term recovery from these injuries.

Duodenal hematomas causing high-grade obstruction usually resolve with nonoperative management. Patients may require total parenteral nutrition. In some cases, a small-bore enteral feeding tube can be passed beyond the area of obstruction utilizing interventional radiology techniques. Large hematomas may require operative evacuation, particularly when the obstruction lasts for more than 10-14 days and a persistent hematoma is seen on CT scan.

Most small-bowel injuries can be treated with a two-layer sutured closure, though mesenteric injuries leading to devascularized segments of small bowel will require resection. The underlying principle is to preserve as much small bowel as possible.

For injuries to the colon, the past approach has been to divert the fecal stream or exteriorize the injury. However, more recent studies have shown a higher complication rate with colostomy formation than with primary repair. Wounds should be considered for primary repair if the blood supply is not compromised. Primary repair is more likely to be associated with complications in patients with ongoing shock, in those requiring multiple transfusions, if more than 6 hours elapsed between injury and operation, or if there is gross contamination or peritonitis. Small, clean rectal injuries may be closed primarily if conditions are favorable. The treatment of larger rectal wounds involving pelvic fracture should include proximal diversion. Insertion of presacral drains is optional. In this latter case, direct repair of the rectal injury is not mandatory but should be performed if it can be readily exposed. Irrigation of the distal stump should be performed in most cases unless it would further contaminate the pelvic space.

F. Abdominal Wall Injuries

Abdominal wall injuries from blunt trauma are most often due to shear forces, such as being run over by the wheels of a tractor or bus. The shearing often devitalizes the subcutaneous tissue and skin, and if debridement is delayed, a serious necrotizing anaerobic infection may develop.

The management of penetrating abdominal wall injuries is usually straightforward. Debridement and irrigation are appropriate surgical treatment. Every effort must be made to remove foreign material, shreds of clothing, necrotic muscle, and soft tissue. Abdominal wall defects may require insertion of absorbable mesh or coverage with a myocutaneous flap.

G. Genitourinary Tract Injuries

The most commonly injured genitourinary tract organs are the male genitalia, uterus, urethra, bladder, ureters, and kidneys. The work-up for these injuries consists primarily of radiologic examinations, which may include abdominal CT scan, cystogram, or retrograde urethrogram. In unstable patients with associated injuries, it may not be possible to obtain these studies prior to emergency laparotomy. In these patients, an intraoperative single-shot intravenous urogram is safe and of high quality in most cases. This study often provides important information that facilitates rapid and accurate decision making. It can confirm function in the noninjured kidney and help in identifying blunt renal injuries that may be safely observed.

1. Bladder injuries—Rupture of the bladder, like urethral disruption, is frequently associated with pelvic fractures. Seventy-five percent of ruptures are extraperitoneal and 25% intraperitoneal. Intraperitoneal bladder ruptures should be repaired through a midline abdominal incision. Rupture of the anterior wall of the bladder can be repaired by direct suture; rupture of the posterior wall can be repaired from inside the bladder after an opening has been made in the anterior wall. Care should be taken to avoid entering a pelvic hematoma. Retroperitoneal injuries can often be treated with urinary drainage, depending on the size of injury. Postoperatively, urine should be diverted for at least 7 days.

2. Urethral injuries—Membranous prostatic urethral disruption is often associated with pelvic fractures or deceleration injuries. Blood at the urethral meatus associated with scrotal hematoma and high-riding prostate on digital rectal examination are the classic signs of injury to the male urethra. The prostate may be elevated superiorly by the pelvic hematoma and will be free-riding and high on rectal examination. If these signs are present, a retrograde urethrogram should be performed before attempts at catheter placement, which may convert an incomplete injury to a complete disruption. If an injury is present, urethrography will demonstrate free extravasation of contrast from the urethra into the preperitoneal space.

Penetrating injuries are best treated with primary repair. Suprapubic bladder drainage and delayed reconstruction of blunt urethral disruption injuries are safe and effective in most cases. Immediate realignment with cystourethroscopy and placement of a urethral catheter is an attractive, minimally invasive alternative. In cases of partial disruption, it has been shown to result in stricture-free outcomes.

Major injuries to the bulbous or penile urethra should be managed by suprapubic urinary diversion. A voiding cystourethrogram may later reveal a stricture, but operative correction or dilation is usually not necessary.

3. Renal injuries—Advances in the imaging and staging of renal trauma as well as in treatment strategies have decreased the need for operation and increased renal preservation. More than half of renal injuries can be treated nonoperatively. Management criteria are based on radiographic, laboratory, and clinical findings. Nonoperative treatment of penetrating renal lacerations is appropriate in hemodynamically stable patients without other injuries. Small to moderate injuries can be treated nonoperatively, but severe injuries are associated with a significant risk of delayed bleeding if treated expectantly. Stable patients may be candidates for angiographic procedures to control bleeding, revascularize a dissection, or injuries leading to vessel thrombosis. Renal exploration should be considered if laparotomy is indicated for associated injuries. A midline transabdominal approach is preferred. The renal artery and vein are secured before the Gerota fascia is opened. The injury should be managed by suture repair, partial nephrectomy, or rarely, total nephrectomy. Pedicle grafts of omentum or free peritoneal patch grafts can be used to cover defects. Renal vascular injuries require immediate operation to save the kidney. Meticulous attention to reconstructive techniques in renal exploration can ensure an excellent renal salvage rate. Adherence to the principles of early proximal vascular control, debridement of devitalized tissue, hemostasis, closure of the collecting system, and coverage of the defect will maximize the salvage of renal function while minimizing potential complications.

Perirenal hematomas found incidentally at celiotomy should be explored if they are expanding, pulsatile, or not contained by retroperitoneal tissues, or if a preexploration urogram shows extensive urinary extravasation.

4. Injuries to the male genitalia—Injuries to the male genitalia usually result in skin loss only; the penis, penile urethra, and testes are usually spared. Skin loss from the penis should be treated with a primary skin graft. Scrotal skin loss should be treated by delayed reconstruction; an exposed testis can be temporarily protected by placing it in a subcutaneous tissue pocket in the thigh.

5. Uterine injuries—Injuries of the female reproductive organs are infrequent except in combination with genitourinary or rectal trauma. Injuries to the uterine fundus usually can be repaired with absorbable sutures; drainage is not necessary. In more extensive injuries, hysterectomy may be preferable. The vaginal cuff may be left open for drainage, particularly if there is an associated urinary tract or rectal injury.

Injuries involving the uterus in a pregnant woman usually result in death of the fetus. Bleeding may be massive in such patients, particularly in women approaching parturition. Cesarean section plus hysterectomy may be the only alternative.

6. Ureteral injuries—Ureteral injuries are easily missed because urinalysis and imaging studies can be unreliable. Most such injuries can be successfully reconstructed by primary repair over stents, ureteral reimplantations, or ureteroureterostomy depending on the level of injury.

Bhullar IS et al: Age does not affect outcomes of nonoperative management of blunt splenic trauma. *J Am Coll Surg*. 2012; 214:958.

Bhullar IS et al: Selective angiographic embolization of blunt splenic traumatic injuries in adults decreases failure rate of nonoperative management. *J Trauma Acute Care Surg*. 2012;72:1127.

Biffl WL et al: Validating the Western Trauma Association algorithm for managing patients with anterior abdominal stab wounds: A Western Trauma Association multicenter trial. *J Trauma*. 2011;71:1494.

Bjurlin MA et al: Comparison of nonoperative management with renorrhaphy and nephrectomy in penetrating renal injuries. *J Trauma*. 2011;71:554.

Burlew CC et al: Sew it up! A Western Trauma Association multi-institutional study of enteric injury management in the postinjury open abdomen. *J Trauma*. 2011;70:273.

Dabbs DN et al: Treatment of major hepatic necrosis: Lobectomy versus serial debridement. *J Trauma*. 2012;69:562.

Miller PR et al: Prospective trial of angiography and embolization for all grade III to V blunt splenic injuries: Nonoperative management success rate is significantly improved. *J Am Coll Surg*. 2014;218:644.

Natarajan B et al: FAST scan: Is it worth doing in hemodynamically stable blunt trauma patients? *Surgery*. 2010;148:695.

Peitzman AB et al: Surgical treatment of injuries to the solid abdominal organs: A 50-year perspective from the Journal of Trauma. *J Trauma*. 2010;69:1011.

Piper GL and Peitzman AB: Current management of hepatic trauma. *Surg Clin North Am*. 2010;90:775.

Sharp JP et al: Adherence to a simplified management algorithm reduces morbidity and mortality after penetrating colon injuries: A 15-year experience. *J Am Coll Surg*. 2012;214:591.

Sharp JP et al: Impact of a defined management algorithm on outcome after traumatic pancreatic injury. *J Trauma Acute Care Surg*. 2012;72:100.

VASCULAR INJURIES

Historical Perspective

Much of our knowledge of blood vessel injuries was developed during the course of military conflicts in the 20th century. Although techniques for the management of vascular injuries were in use prior to World War I, arterial ligation to save a life rather than arterial repair to salvage a limb was generally employed, and amputation frequently resulted after vascular injury.

The current mortality rate for lower extremity arterial injury is low in both civilian and recent military series: 2%-6%. Limb salvage rates in civilian series are 85%-90%, with best results obtained for interposition vein grafts. Ligation, need for reoperation, and failed revascularization are associated with worse outcomes and higher amputation rates. Low mortality and improved limb salvage is a result of more rapid transport of injured people, improved blood volume replacement, selective use of arteriography and shunts, and better operative techniques.

The Epidemiology of Vascular Trauma

The epidemiology of vascular trauma has been studied in three different settings: military conflicts, large urban locations, and to a lesser extent, rural areas. The types of injuries seen in civilian vascular trauma, once much different from those in military settings, are now more similar to military wounds. The incidence is increasing as a result of the rise in urban violence, motor vehicle crashes, and iatrogenic injuries owing to more frequent use of minimally invasive diagnostic and therapeutic procedures.

Peripheral vascular trauma typically occurs in young men between the ages of 20 and 40 years. In both urban and rural environments, penetrating mechanisms dominate, accounting for 50%-90% of vascular injuries. Because many vascular injuries of the head, neck, and torso are immediately fatal, most patients with vascular injuries surviving transport have extremity trauma. This is especially true in the military experience, where extremity vascular injuries account for approximately 90% of all arterial trauma. In the urban civilian experience, extremity vascular injuries comprise about 50% of arterial injuries. In rural vascular trauma, blunt injuries occur more frequently than in urban populations.

Mortality and utilization of medical resources is higher among patients with vascular injuries than among patients who do not have blood vessel injuries. Vascular injuries from automobile accidents or falls from heights and crush injuries account for up to half of all non-iatrogenic vascular injuries in U.S. hospitals. The likelihood of vascular injury after blunt trauma correlates with the overall severity of the injury and the presence of specific orthopedic injuries. For example, up to 45% of patients with posterior knee dislocations or severe instability from high-velocity blunt trauma sustain popliteal artery injury.

The number of iatrogenic vascular injuries has risen dramatically in recent decades. Most involve diagnostic and therapeutic procedures utilizing the femoral (less frequently the brachial or axillary) vessels, which serve as percutaneous access routes. In order of decreasing frequency, injuries include hemorrhage and hematoma, pseudoaneurysm, arteriovenous fistula formation, vessel thrombosis, and embolization. Rates of injury range from 0.5% for diagnostic procedures to as high as 10% for therapeutic procedures involving large catheters. Increasing age, female gender, use of anticoagulation, and the presence of atherosclerosis increase the risk of these complications. Complications remote from the puncture site include vessel rupture and dissection. Operative procedures (especially hepatic and pancreaticobiliary surgery) are associated with iatrogenic vascular trauma. In addition, anterior and retroperitoneal approaches to the lumbar spine and other orthopedic procedures such as total joint replacement and arthroscopy can produce vascular injuries.

▶ Types of Injuries

A. Penetrating Trauma

The local and regional effects of penetrating wounds are determined by the mechanism of vessel injury. Stab wounds, low-velocity (<2000 ft/s) bullet wounds, iatrogenic injuries from percutaneous catheterization, and inadvertent intra-arterial injection of drugs produce less soft-tissue injury and disrupt collateral circulation less than injuries from sources with greater kinetic energy. The high-velocity missiles responsible for war wounds produce more extensive vascular injuries, which involve massive destruction and contamination of surrounding tissues. The temporary cavitational effect of high-velocity missiles causes additional trauma to the ends of severed arteries and may produce arterial thrombosis due to disrupted intima even when the artery has not been directly hit. This blast effect can also draw material such as clothing, dirt, or pieces of skin along the wound tract, which contributes to the risk of infection. Associated injuries are often major determinants of the eventual outcome.

Shotgun blasts present special problems. Although muzzle velocity is low (about 1200 ft/s), the multiple pellets produce widespread damage, and shotgun wadding entering the wound enhances the likelihood of infection. Similar to high-velocity injuries, the damage is often much greater than might be anticipated from inspection of the entry wound. Moreover, the multiplicity of potential sites of arterial damage often mandates diagnostic arteriography even in the presence of obvious arterial insufficiency.

B. Blunt Trauma

Motor vehicle accidents are a major cause of blunt vascular trauma. Multiple injuries include fractures and dislocations; and while direct vascular injury may occur, in most instances the damage is indirect due to fractures. This is especially likely to occur with fractures near joints, where vessels are relatively fixed and vulnerable to shear forces. For example, the popliteal artery and vein are frequently injured in association with posterior dislocation of the knee. Fractures of large heavy bones such as the femur or tibia transmit forces that have cavitation effects similar to those caused by high-velocity bullets. There is extensive damage to soft tissues and neurovascular structures, and edema formation interferes with evaluation of pulses. Delay in diagnosis and the presence of associated injuries decrease the chances of limb

Table 14–5. Clinical features of traumatic aortic rupture.

History of high-speed deceleration injury
Flail chest
Fractured sternum
Superior vena cava syndrome
Multiple or first or second rib fractures
Upper extremity hypertension or pulse deficits
Hematoma in the carotid sheaths
Interscapular bruits
Hoarseness with normal larynx

salvage. Contusions or crush injuries may result in complete or partial disruption of arteries, producing intimal flaps or intramural hematomas that impede blood flow.

Blunt thoracic aortic injury (BTAI) is a serious traumatic injury that continues to have a high initial mortality and is associated with modern high-speed methods of transportation or significant falls. Autopsy data from cases of fatal BTAI demonstrated that 57% of patients were dead at the scene or on arrival to the hospital, 37% died during the first 4 hours at the hospital, and only 6% died after 4 hours in the hospital. The disruption generally occurs at the aortic isthmus (between the left subclavian artery and the ligamentum arteriosum) due to a deceleration injury in which the heart, the ascending aorta, and the transverse arch continue to move forward while movement of the isthmus and the descending aorta is limited by their posterior attachments. Clinical findings associated with traumatic rupture of the thoracic aorta are listed in Table 14–5 and radiographic findings in Table 14–6. Blunt traumatic injury to the abdominal aorta is uncommon, but it has been reported from lap seat belt trauma.

Almost any vessel can be injured by blunt trauma, including the extracranial cerebral and visceral arteries. Blunt carotid arterial injuries are associated with mortality rates of 20% to 30%, with over 50% of survivors having permanent,

Table 14–6. Radiographic features of traumatic aortic rupture.

Widening of mediastinum
Fractured sternum
Multiple or first rib or second rib fractures
Esophageal deviation to the right
Tracheal deviation to the right
Apical cap
Depression of left main stem bronchus
Obliteration of the aortic knob
Obliteration of the descending aorta
Obliteration of the aortopulmonary window
Obliteration of the medial left upper lobe
Widened paravertebral stripe

severe neurologic deficits. Whereas in the past vertebral artery injuries were considered innocuous, recent studies have reported devastating complications related to these injuries, including a 70% incidence of coexistent cervical spine injuries. Traumatic injury to the superior mesenteric artery is associated with a 50% mortality rate. The brachial and popliteal arteries, which cross joints and are exposed to direct trauma, are particularly susceptible to injury as a result of fractures and dislocations.

▶ Clinical Findings

A. Hemorrhage

When pulsatile external hemorrhage is present, the diagnosis of arterial injury is obvious; but when blood accumulates in deep tissues of the extremity, the thorax, abdomen, or retroperitoneum, the only manifestation may be shock. Peripheral vasoconstriction may make evaluation of peripheral pulses difficult until blood volume is restored. If the artery is completely severed, thrombus may form at the contracted vessel ends and a major vascular injury may not be suspected. The presence of arterial pulses distal to a penetrating wound does not preclude arterial injury; as many as 20% of patients with injuries of major arteries in an extremity have palpable pulses distal to the injury, either because the vessel has not thrombosed or because pulse waves are transmitted through soft clot. Conversely, the absence of a palpable pulse in an adequately resuscitated patient is a sensitive indicator of arterial injury.

B. Ischemia

Acute arterial insufficiency must be diagnosed promptly to prevent tissue loss. Ischemia should be suspected when the patient has one or more of the "five Ps": pain, pallor, paralysis, paresthesia, or pulselessness. The susceptibility of different cells to hypoxia varies (eg, sudden occlusion of the carotid artery results in brain damage within minutes unless collateral circulation can maintain adequate perfusion, but a kidney can survive severe ischemia for up to an hour). Peripheral nerves are quite vulnerable to ischemia because they have a high basal energy requirement to maintain ion gradients over large membrane surfaces and because they have few glycogen stores. Hence, interruption of arterial flow for relatively short periods can result in nerve damage due to interrupted substrate delivery. In contrast, skeletal muscle is more tolerant of decreased arterial flow. Muscle can be ischemic for up to 4 hours without developing histologic changes. In general, complete interruption of all arterial inflow (including collateral blood supply) results in neuromuscular ischemic damage after 4-6 hours. Restoration of flow can actually worsen this damage as part of the reperfusion syndrome and can increase the severity of the original ischemic insult.

Prolonged ischemia can produce muscle necrosis and rhabdomyolysis, which releases potassium and myoglobin into the circulation. Myoglobin is an oxygen-transporting protein similar in structure to hemoglobin; it is innocuous unless it dissociates into hematin, which is nephrotoxic in an acidic milieu. Precipitation of hematin pigment also occurs when urine flow is reduced by hypotension or hypovolemia, obstructing renal tubules and worsening nephrotoxicity. Myoglobinemia can lead to acute tubular necrosis and renal failure, hyperkalemia, and a risk of life-threatening arrhythmias. Thus, in addition to limb loss, acute arterial ischemia can produce organ failure and death.

C. False Aneurysm

Disruption of an arterial wall as a result of trauma may lead to formation of a false aneurysm. The wall of a false aneurysm is composed primarily of fibrous tissue derived from nearby tissues, not arterial tissue. Because blood continues to flow past the fistulous opening, the extremity is seldom ischemic. False aneurysms may rupture at any time. They continue to expand because they lack vascular wall integrity. Spontaneous resolution of pseudoaneurysms larger than 3 cm is unlikely, and operative repair becomes increasingly difficult as the aneurysms increase in size and complexity with time. Symptoms gradually appear as a result of compression of adjacent nerves or collateral vessels or from rupture of the aneurysm—or as a result of thrombosis with ischemic symptoms. Iatrogenic false aneurysms after arterial puncture thrombose spontaneously within 4 weeks when they are less than 3 cm in diameter. Simple ultrasound follow-up rather than operative therapy is indicated. Color-flow duplex-guided compression of iatrogenic pseudoaneurysms is successful in 70%-90% of attempts, but the procedure is uncomfortable and may take hours of probe pressure. Ultrasound-guided thrombin injection has been effective for thrombosis of large false aneurysms in a matter of seconds, but distal arterial thrombosis has also been described using this technique.

D. Arteriovenous Fistula

With simultaneous injury of an adjacent artery and vein, a fistula may form that allows blood from the artery to enter the vein. Because venous pressure is lower than arterial pressure, flow through an arteriovenous fistula is continuous; accentuation of the bruit and thrill can be detected over the fistula during systole. Traumatic arteriovenous fistulas may occur as operative complications (eg, aortocaval fistula following removal of a herniated intervertebral disk). Iatrogenic femoral arteriovenous fistulas after arteriograms and cardiac catheterization are seen with increasing frequency. Long-standing large arteriovenous fistulas may result in high-output cardiac failure. Similar to iatrogenic pseudoaneurysms occurring after arteriography, spontaneous resolution of acute arteriovenous fistulas usually occurs.

Diagnosis

Arterial injury must be considered in any injured patient. Patients who present in shock following penetrating injury or blunt trauma should be assumed to have vascular injury until proven otherwise. Any injury near a major artery should arouse suspicion. A plain film may be helpful in demonstrating a fracture whose fragments could jeopardize an adjacent vessel or a bullet fragment that could have passed near to a major vessel. Before the x-ray is taken, entrance and exit wounds should be marked with radiopaque objects such as a paper clip.

Diagnosis is usually established on the basis of physical examination looking for signs of injury (Table 14–7). In addition to checking for obvious hemorrhage and the five Ps, the physician should listen for a bruit, palpate for a thrill (eg, of an arteriovenous fistula), and look for an expanding hematoma (eg, of a false aneurysm). Secondary hemorrhage from a wound is an ominous sign that may herald massive hemorrhage. The finding of these "hard" signs reliably reflects the presence of a vascular injury; hard signs mandate immediate exploration in most instances. The presence of "soft" signs (history of bleeding, diminished but palpable pulse, injury in proximity to a major artery, neurapraxia) requires further tests or serial observation.

Doppler flow studies have gained importance in the diagnosis of arterial trauma. An ankle brachial index (ABI), determined by dividing the systolic pressure in the injured limb by the systolic pressure in an uninjured arm, is highly reliable for excluding arterial injury after both blunt and penetrating trauma. An ABI less than 0.9 has sensitivity of 95%, specificity of 97%, and negative predictive value of 99% for determining the presence of clinically significant arterial injury. Thus, only patients with soft signs and an ABI less than 0.9 require arteriography.

Color-flow duplex ultrasonography combines real-time B mode (brightness modulation) ultrasound imaging with a steerable pulsed Doppler flow detector. This technology can provide images of vessels and velocity spectral analysis. Color-flow duplex scanning of an area of injury is noninvasive, painless, portable, and easily repeated for follow-up examinations. When compared with arteriography and performed by experienced examiners, duplex ultrasound identifies nearly all major injuries that require treatment, potentially at considerable cost savings. In addition to screening for arterial trauma, duplex scanning has been used to detect pseudoaneurysms, arteriovenous fistulas, and intimal flaps. However, potential logistical and resource problems exist. The technology is sophisticated and requires skill in operation and interpretation, which is not always immediately available.

Arteriography is the most accurate diagnostic procedure for identifying vascular injuries (Figure 14–14). Arteriography to exclude vascular injury for soft signs results in a negative exploration rate of 20% to 35% and an arteriography-related complication rate of 2% to 4%. Proximity as the sole indication for arteriography has an extremely low yield, ranging from 0% to 10%. Patients with unequivocal signs of arterial injury on physical examination or plain films should have urgent operation. The false-negative rate of arteriography is low, and a normal arteriogram precludes the need for surgical exploration. Virtually all arteriographic errors are due to false-positives, which occur in 2% to 8% of patients. Technical considerations in performing arteriography include the following: (1) entrance and exit wounds should be marked with a radiopaque marker; (2) the injection site should not be near the suspected injury; (3) an area 10 to 15 cm proximal and distal to the suspected injury should be included in the arteriographic field; (4) sequential films should be obtained to detect early venous filling; (5) any abnormality should be considered an indication of arterial injury unless it is obviously the result of preexisting disease; and (6) two different projections should be obtained.

Emergency-center arteriography using micropuncture Seldinger technique or cannulating the artery to be studied with an 18-gauge catheter (antegrade in the lower extremity and prograde in the upper extremity arteries) is quick and

Table 14–7. Signs of extremity vascular injury.

Hard signs
Expanding or pulsatile hematoma
Limb ischemia
Bruit or thrill
Absence of distal pulse
Soft signs
History of hemorrhage at scene, now stopped
Deficit of nerve associated with vessel
Stable, nonexpanding hematoma
Proximity of wound to major extremity blood vessel
Ankle brachial index < 0.9

▲ **Figure 14–14.** Arteriogram showing traumatic pseudoaneurysm of subclavian/axillary artery from penetrating injury.

accurate. The use of fluoroscopy, especially if equipped with subtraction capability, simplifies the timing of contrast injection and x-ray exposure. Fluoroscopy is particularly helpful to visualize distal arteries and minimize the amount of contrast media needed. Arteriography may be particularly useful in differentiating arterial injury from spasm. In general, it is risky to attribute abnormal physical findings in an injured patient to arterial spasm; an arteriogram is indicated in such patients.

Arteriography is also valuable when arterial injuries may have occurred at multiple sites or to localize an injury when a long parallel penetration makes this determination difficult. Complications of arteriography include groin hematomas, iatrogenic pseudoaneurysms, arteriovenous fistulas, embolic occlusions, and delays in diagnosis that may lead to irreversible ischemia in marginally perfused limbs. The availability of CT angiograms with latest-generation multidetector contrast-enhanced spiral scanners is a viable alternative to traditional angiography. CT angiograms can diagnose intimal dissections, pseudoaneurysms, arteriovenous fistulas, thrombosis or occlusion, and active bleeding. Metallic foreign bodies can create artifacts that interfere with generation of optimal CT angiogram studies.

For patients suspected of having BTAI based on mechanism of injury, the chest x-ray is a good screening tool to determine the need for further investigation. The most significant radiographic findings for possible BTAI include widened mediastinum, obscured aortic knob, deviation of the left mainstem bronchus or nasogastric tube, and opacification of the aortopulmonary window. Helical chest CT scanning is a useful diagnostic tool for screening and diagnosis of BTAI (Figure 14–15). A negative chest CT scan can obviate the need for further evaluation with a contrast aortogram. Patients with indeterminate CT scans or positive scans should have confirmation and delineation of the

▲ **Figure 14–15.** Computed tomography scan of the chest showing traumatic disruption of the aorta from blunt injury.

extent of BTAI with arteriography or a CT angiogram. In selected instances, cardiothoracic and/or trauma surgeons may consider helical CT scanning alone to be an adequate and complete work-up for BTAI. In addition, a helical CT angiogram with 3D reconstruction guides potential endovascular approach for treatment of BTAI. The use of either transesophageal echocardiography or intraluminal ultrasound in the diagnosis of BTAI continues to evolve, but they are not considered standard diagnostic modalities.

▶ Management

A. Initial Treatment

A rapid but thorough examination should be performed to determine the complete extent of injury. The physician must establish the priority of arterial injury in the overall management of the patient, and should remember that delay in arterial repair decreases chances of a favorable outcome. When repair is performed within 12 hours after injury, amputation is rarely necessary; if repair is performed later, the incidence of amputation is about 50%. Depending on the degree of ischemia, delay in arterial repair will lead to lasting neuromuscular damage after as short a period as 4 to 6 hours.

Restoration of blood volume and control of hemorrhage are done simultaneously. If exsanguinating hemorrhage precludes resuscitation in the emergency room, the patient should be moved directly to the operating room. External bleeding is best controlled by firm direct pressure or packing. Probes or fingers should not be inserted into the wound because a clot may be dislodged, causing profuse bleeding. Tourniquets occlude venous return, disturb collateral flow, and further compromise circulation and should not be employed unless exsanguinating hemorrhage cannot be controlled by other means. Atraumatic vascular clamps may be applied to accessible vessels by trained surgeons, but blind clamping can increase damage and injure adjacent nerves and veins.

After hemorrhage has been controlled and general resuscitation accomplished, further assessment is possible. The extent of associated injuries is determined and a plan of management made. Large-bore intravenous catheters should be placed in extremities with no potential venous injuries. It is prudent to preserve the saphenous or cephalic vein in an uninjured extremity for use as a venous autograft for vascular repair.

B. Nonoperative Treatment

Some arterial injuries remain asymptomatic and heal. Data supporting the practice of observation of small or asymptomatic arterial injuries have emerged from experimental animal studies and clinical reports showing resolution, improvement, or stabilization of arterial injuries. In well-defined settings, this strategy has proved safe in follow-up reports covering periods of up to 10 years. Thus, a nonoperative approach may be appropriate for compliant patients willing to return for follow-up who have (1) no active hemorrhage, (2) low-velocity injuries (particularly stab wounds or iatrogenic punctures), (3) minimal arterial wall disruptions (<5 mm), (4) small (<5 mm) intimal defects, and (5) intact distal circulation.

Follow-up must include frequent physical examinations and carefully performed noninvasive studies, and patients should be asymptomatic—and the strategy must be reconsidered if symptoms develop. Adjuvant therapy with antiplatelet agents is usually recommended to improve patency in patients with intimal flaps.

Endovascular management has assumed a greater role in the treatment of arterial trauma in recent years. Transcatheter embolization with coils or balloons has been successful in managing selected arterial injuries such as pseudoaneurysms, arteriovenous fistulas, and active bleeding from nonessential arteries. Coils are made of stainless steel with wool or polyester tufts. They are extruded at the site of vessel injury through 5F or 7F catheters. After deployment, the coils expand and lodge at the extrusion site and the tufts promote thrombosis. Catheter-based intra-arterial infusion of vasodilators has also been used to treat vasospasm in small distal arteries.

The recent popularity of endovascular grafting in elective vascular surgery (see Chapter 34) has been applied to the treatment of arterial trauma. A fixation device such as a stent is attached to a graft, and the stent graft is inserted endoluminally from a remote site and deployed at the site of injury to repair false aneurysms or arteriovenous fistulas. The indications for endovascular grafting are likely to change as technology advances, but the most frequent application currently is in stable patients with delayed presentations who have complex false aneurysms or arteriovenous fistulas. Use of stent grafts in the acute setting requires the availability of a wide variety of sizes and lengths of grafts and advanced catheter skills.

Endovascular repair of BTAI can be performed either electively or even emergently (Figure 14–16). In an American Association for the Surgery of Trauma (AAST) multicenter study, two-thirds of patients underwent endovascular stent graph repair as compared to one-third who underwent traditional open repair. When adjusted for confounding variables, the endovascular approach was associated with reduced mortality (odds ratio 8.42, 95% confidence interval 2.76-25.69) and fewer blood transfusions. Further study is needed to determine the long-term outcome using endovascular techniques to repair BTAI. Commercial grafts have yielded better results than the noncommercial "homemade" grafts. Thoracic aorta lacerations of more than 1.5 cm resulting in graft apposition length less than 2 cm, or those near or in the curvature of the aortic arch, are associated with an increased risk of endoleak. Endoleak occurred in 14% of the AAST BTAI trial patients, with half being successfully managed with the deployment of additional stent grafts.

▲ **Figure 14–16.** Aortogram and placement of aortic stent graft to repair a blunt aortic disruption.

In selected cases of BTAI repair, whether it is operative or endovascular, treatment is delayed because treatment and recovery from other more life-threatening injuries has priority (eg, severe pulmonary contusion, brain injury). This is acceptable, and the incidence of aortic rupture after 4 hours in the hospital is low. Systemic blood pressure and heart rate should be controlled with a beta-blocker and other pharmacologic agents as necessary to minimize the risk of rupture while waiting for definitive repair of the injured aorta.

C. Operative Treatment

General anesthesia is preferable to spinal or regional anesthesia. When vascular injuries involve the neck or thoracic outlet, endotracheal intubation must be performed carefully to avoid dislodging a clot and to protect the airway. Moreover, care is necessary to avoid neurologic damage in patients with associated cervical spine injuries. At least one uninjured extremity should also be prepared for surgery so that saphenous or cephalic vein conduit may be obtained if a vein graft is required. Provision should also be made for operative arteriography.

Incisions should be generous and parallel to the injured vessel. Meticulous care in handling incisions is essential to avoid secondary infections; all undamaged tissue should be conserved for use in covering repaired vessels. Preservation of all arterial branches is important in order to maintain collateral circulation. Atraumatic control of the vessel should be achieved proximal and distal to the injury so that the injured area may be dissected free of other tissues and inspected without risk of further bleeding. When large hematomas and multiple wounds make exposure and clamping of vessels difficult, it is wise to place a sterile orthopedic tourniquet proximal to the injury that can be inflated temporarily if needed.

The extent of arterial injury must be accurately determined. Arterial spasm generally responds to gentle hydraulic or mechanical dilation. Local application of warm saline or drugs such as papaverine, tolazoline, lidocaine, or nitroglycerin is occasionally effective in relieving spasm. Intra-arterial injection of nitroglycerin or papaverine is also very effective in alleviating spasm. If spasm persists, however, it is best to assume that it is caused by an intramural injury, and the vessel should be opened for direct inspection. An old adage is that spasm is spelled "c-l-o-t."

All devitalized tissue, including damaged portions of the artery, must be debrided. One should resect only the grossly injured portion of the vessel. The method of reconstruction depends on the degree of arterial damage. In selected instances, the ends of injured vessels can be approximated and an end-to-end anastomosis created. If the vessels cannot be mobilized well enough to provide a tension-free anastomosis, an interposition graft should be used. Early experience with prosthetic interposition grafts was disappointing since postoperative infection, thrombosis, and anastomotic disruption were common. These problems have decreased considerably with the use of grafts made of expanded polytetrafluoroethylene (PTFE). Proponents of synthetic graphs focus on the fact that they fail well (eg, infected pseudoaneurysm), whereas a vein graft will disintegrate and result in a sudden blow-out type hemorrhage. Nevertheless, most surgeons still prefer to use an autogenous graft (ie, vein or artery) in severely contaminated wounds. Saphenous vein grafts should be obtained from the *noninjured* leg to avoid impairment of venous return on the side of the injury. Patch angioplasty using saphenous vein is performed when closure of a partially transected vessel would result in narrowing. Suturing should be done with fine 5-0 or 6-0 monofilament material.

In the unusual circumstance of isolated vascular injury, 5000-10,000 units of intravenous heparin can be given to prevent thrombosis. Otherwise, a small amount of dilute heparin solution (100 units/mL) may be gently injected into the proximal and distal lumen of the injured vessel before clamps are applied. Proximal and distal thrombi are removed with a Fogarty embolectomy catheter. Back-bleeding from the distal artery is not a sure indication that thrombus is absent. A completion operative arteriogram is indicated to determine distal patency and to check on the adequacy of the reconstruction—even when distal pulses are palpable.

It was formerly taught that fractures should be stabilized before vascular injuries were repaired so that manipulation of bones would not jeopardize vascular repair. The disadvantages of this dictum were delay in restoration of flow to ischemic tissue and interference with vascular reconstruction and subsequent arteriographic study of the completed repair by the fixation device. It is currently recommended that vascular repair be performed first, followed by careful application of external traction devices that allow easy access to the wound for observation and dressing changes. Another alternative is to place an intraluminal shunt temporarily across the vascular injury to decrease ischemia while fractures or other injuries are treated. Once the fracture is stabilized, the temporary shunt can be removed and definitive vascular repair completed. Improved outcomes similar to civilian lower extremity vascular trauma have been attributed to the use of temporary vascular shunts and damage-control techniques in the current Iraq War.

Repaired vessels must be covered with healthy tissue. If left exposed, they invariably desiccate and rupture. Skin alone is inadequate, because subsequent necrosis of the skin would leave the vessels exposed, greatly endangering the reconstruction. Generally, an adjacent muscle (eg, sartorius muscle for coverage of the common femoral artery) can be mobilized and placed over the repair. Musculocutaneous flaps can be constructed by plastic surgeons to cover almost any site. In an extensive or severely contaminated wound, a remote bypass may be routed through clean tissue planes to circumvent difficult soft-tissue coverage problems.

D. Venous Injuries

Venous injuries commonly accompany arterial injuries. In order of decreasing frequency, the most common extremity venous injuries are the superficial femoral vein, the popliteal vein, and the common femoral vein. The relative importance and timing of venous repair in an injured extremity is controversial. Advocates of routine venous repair contend that ligation is associated with significant postoperative morbidity, including more frequent failure of arterial repairs due to compromised outflow, venous insufficiency, compartment syndrome, and limb loss. Proponents of venous ligation argue that venous repairs are difficult (requiring interposition, compilation, and spiral grafting), time consuming (dangerous in the multiply-injured patient), and likely to cause occlusion (patency rates are only about 50%). The presence of postoperative edema after combined arterial and venous injuries is not reliably reduced by attempted venous repair. It seems reasonable to recommend repair of venous injuries when the repair is not too technically difficult (lateral venorrhaphy) and the patient is hemodynamically stable. Complex repair with autologous vein or ringed PTFE can yield good short-term patency in experienced hands (77% primary repair, 67% vein graft, 74% PTFE). Thus, the decision to repair the vein depends on the condition of the patient and the condition of the vein. When venous ligation is necessary, postoperative edema can be controlled by elevation of the extremity and use of compression stockings or wraps. In patients undergoing venous repair, patency should be monitored using duplex scanning. If thrombosis of the repair is detected and there are no contraindications, anticoagulation should be instituted and maintained for at least 3 months postoperatively.

E. Fasciotomy

Fasciotomy is an important adjunctive treatment in many cases of arterial trauma. Indications include the following: (1) combined arterial and venous injury, (2) massive soft-tissue damage, (3) delay between injury and repair (4-6 hours), (4) prolonged hypotension, and (5) excessive swelling or high tissue pressure measured by one of several techniques. Whenever compartment pressures (measured with a needle and manometer) approach 25-30 mm Hg, fasciotomy should be considered. Fasciotomies must be performed through adequate skin incisions because when edema is massive, the skin envelope itself can compromise neurovascular function.

Fasciotomies are not benign procedures. They create large open wounds, and chronic venous insufficiency is a recognized late complication even in the absence of venous reflux or obstruction. The chronic swelling is thought to be related to loss of integrity of the ensheathing fascia of the calf muscles, reducing the efficiency of the calf muscle pump. Thus, some authorities recommend against routine use of fasciotomies at the initial operation. This approach is dependent on the ability to conduct frequent serial physical examinations and the ready availability of an operating room should problems arise. In the postoperative period, compartmental pressures can be measured using a handheld solid-state transducer as often as clinically indicated. Normal intracompartmental pressure is less than 10 mm Hg. In general, a pressure of 25-30 mm Hg requires either fasciotomy or continuous monitoring. When the pressure exceeds 30 mm Hg, fasciotomy is mandatory. In patients who are obtunded or who cannot cooperate with serial physical examination, earlier fasciotomy should be considered.

F. Immediate Amputation

High-energy or crush injuries of the extremities are associated with high morbidity and a poor prognosis for useful limb function—there is a high late amputation rate despite initial limb salvage. Vascular injuries are now repaired with a high rate of success, but associated orthopedic, soft-tissue, and nerve injuries are the critical factors that determine long-term function. A number of scoring systems or indices have been proposed to help determine when to amputate immediately and thus reduce the number of protracted reconstructive procedures that ultimately fail. Management of the mangled extremity is particularly difficult, and none of the scoring systems are universally accepted. Evaluation and management of these patients should be multidisciplinary, and the decision to amputate emergently should be made by two independent surgeons whenever possible.

▶ References

Avery LE et al: Evolving role of endovascular techniques for traumatic vascular injury: A changing landscape? *J Trauma Acute Care Surg.* 2012;72:41.

Brenner M et al: Long-term outcomes of thoracic endovascular aortic repair: A single institution's 11-year experience. *J Trauma Acute Care Surg.* 2017;82:687.

Demetriades D et al and the American Association for the Surgery of Trauma Thoracic Aortic Injury Study Group: Operative repair or endovascular stent graft in blunt traumatic thoracic aortic injuries. Results of an American Association for the Surgery of Trauma Multicenter Study. *J Trauma.* 2008;64:561.

Feliciano DV and Shackford SR: Vascular injury: Fiftieth anniversary year review article of the *Journal of Trauma. J Trauma* 2010;68:1009.

Fox CJ et al: Damage control resuscitation for vascular surgery in a combat support hospital. *J Trauma.* 2008;65:1.

Karmy-Jones R et al: Endovascular repair compared with operative repair of traumatic rupture of the thoracic aorta: A nonsystemic review and a plea for trauma-specific reporting guidelines. *J Trauma.* 2011;71:1059.

Patterson BO et al: Imaging vascular trauma. *Br J Surg.* 2012;99:494.

Paul JS et al: Minimal aortic injury after blunt trauma: Selective nonoperative management is safe. *J Trauma.* 2011;71:1519.

Rasmussen TE et al: Tourniquets, vascular shunts, and endovascular technologies: Esoteric or essential? A report from the 2011 AAST military liaison panel. *J Trauma Acute Care Surg.* 2012; 73:282.

Sepehripour AH et al: Management of the left subclavian artery during endovascular stent grafting for traumatic aortic injury: A systematic review. *Eur J Vasc Endovasc Surg.* 2011;41:758.

Sohn VY et al: Demographics, treatment, and early outcomes in penetrating vascular combat trauma. *Arch Surg.* 2008;143:783.

Subramanian A et al: A decade's experience with temporary intravascular shunts at a civilian level I trauma center. *J Trauma.* 2008;65:316.

Woodward EB et al: Penetrating femoropopliteal injury during modern warfare: Experience of the Balad Vascular Registry. *J Vasc Surg.* 2008;47:1259.

MULTIPLE-CHOICE QUESTIONS

1. A 31-year-old man with a stab wound to the left neck over the sternocleidomastoid at the level of the lower pole of the thyroid gland

   A. Has a wound in an area that is easily explored in the operating room as most injuries here can be identified and controlled directly.
   B. Has a penetrating injury in zone 3.
   C. Should have an initial assessment including airway, breathing and circulation.
   D. Should be taken to angiography if unstable.
   E. Has little risk of vascular injury.

2. All of the following are correct about a patient with a systolic blood pressure of 75 torr after a rollover automobile accident that resulted in the death of another passenger except

   A. Should be transported to a trauma center as expediently as possible.
   B. Can have shock due to hypovolemia, cardiac failure, or neurogenic causes.
   C. Should have an algorithmic approach to his care in the prehospital and trauma resuscitation phases of care.
   D. Should bypass the trauma room and go directly to the operating room.
   E. Has a mechanism of injury that places him at substantial risk of being severely injured.

3. Thoracic injuries

   A. Are unusually contributors to the death of a trauma patient.
   B. Can cause late deaths due to respiratory failure or sepsis.
   C. Can include acceleration/deceleration as common mechanism of a severe aortic injury.
   D. Carry a similar mortality in older and younger patients.
   E. A, B, and C are all correct.

4. Abdominal injuries

   A. Can only be reliably assessed by CT scan or laparotomy.
   B. Require laparotomy and repair for all identified liver parenchyma injuries.
   C. Can routinely be evaluated by laparoscopy.
   D. Can be definitively repaired when the patient is hypotensive and hypothermic.
   E. From gunshot wounds below the nipple line typically require laparotomy for evaluation and management.

5. Peripheral vascular injuries

   A. Are common in young men.
   B. Are more likely from penetrating than blunt injury.
   C. Are not often evaluated by CT scan.
   D. Can commonly be iatrogenic from medical procedures.
   E. All are correct.

Burns & Other Thermal Injuries

Stephanie Nitzschke, MD

▼ BURNS

A severe thermal injury is one of the most devastating physical and psychological injuries a person can suffer. The overall incidence of burn injuries has been declining over the past decade, with 500,000 burn injuries per year and only 3250 deaths. This trend is due in large part to public health initiatives to improve fire safety as well as advancements in critical care. Most burn injuries are due to flame burns, but scald burns follow closely as the second most common type of injury. Most burns are less than 10% total body surface area (TBSA), but for patients who suffer large TBSA burns, the hospital length of stay can last months, with much of that time in the intensive care unit (ICU). These patients frequently require lifelong care due to the physical and psychological effects of the injury and the suffering endured from repeated surgeries and wound care.

ANATOMY & PHYSIOLOGY OF THE SKIN

The skin is the largest organ of the body, ranging in area from 0.25 m^2 in the newborn to 1.8 m^2 in the adult. It consists of three layers: the epidermis, the dermis (corium), and the hypodermis. The outermost cells of the epidermis are dead cornified cells that act as a tough protective barrier against the environment, including bacterial invasion and chemical exposure. These cells vary in thickness in different parts of the body and are thickest on the palms of the hand and soles of the feet. The inner cells of the epidermis are metabolically active, producing compounds such as growth factor, which help the ongoing replication process every 2 weeks, and contain melanocytes, which are specialized cells of the epidermis that produce melanin. Most humans have a similar number of melanocytes but vary in the amount melanin produced.

The second layer, the dermis (0.06-0.12 mm), is composed chiefly of fibrous connective tissue. The dermis contains the blood vessels and nerves to the skin and the epithelial appendages of specialized function such as sweat glands. The dermis is a barrier that prevents loss of body fluids by evaporation and loss of excess body heat. Sweat glands help maintain body temperature by controlling the amount of water that evaporates. Some other important functions can be found within the dermis, which is interlaced with sensory nerve endings that mediate the sensations of touch, pressure, pain, heat, and cold. This is a protective mechanism that allows an individual to adapt to changes in the physical environment. The skin produces vitamin D, which is synthesized by the action of sunlight on certain intradermal cholesterol compounds.

The hypodermis is made mostly of fatty tissues that attach the dermis to the underlying tissue of muscle and bones. It provides a pathway for nerves and blood vessels and provides insulation to assist with thermoregulation.

DEPTH OF BURNS

The depth of a burn (Figure 15–1) significantly affects all subsequent clinical events. The depth may be difficult to determine and, in some cases, is not known until after spontaneous healing has occurred or when the eschar is surgically removed or separates, exposing the wound bed.

Traditionally, burns have been classified as first-, second-, or third-degree burns. However, the current emphasis on burn healing has led to classification as partial-thickness burns (subclassified as superficial or deep partial-thickness burns), which can heal spontaneously, and full-thickness burns, which require skin grafting, although deep partial-thickness burns are usually excised and grafted as well.

A **first-degree burn** involves only the epidermis and is characterized by erythema and minor microscopic changes; tissue damage is minimal, protective functions of the skin are intact, skin edema is minimal, and systemic effects are rare. Pain, the chief symptom, usually resolves in 48-72 hours, and healing takes place without scarring in 5-10 days. The most common causes of first-degree burns are overexposure to sunlight and brief scalding.

▲ **Figure 15–1.** Layers of the skin showing depth of first-degree, second-degree, and third-degree burns.

Second-degree or partial-thickness burns are deeper, involving all of the epidermis and some of the corium or dermis. The systemic severity of the burn and the quality of subsequent healing are directly related to the amount of undamaged dermis. Superficial burns are often characterized by blister formation, a pink and weepy wound bed that blanches when touched and is painful. Complications from superficial second-degree burns are mainly pain related. These burns usually heal with minimal scarring in 10-14 days unless they become infected.

Deep dermal burns heal over a period of 4-8 weeks with epithelial cells that migrate over the injured wound bed from the residual uninjured epithelium of the deep dermal sweat glands and hair follicles. Severe hypertrophic scarring occurs when such an injury heals; the resulting new epithelial cells are more fragile and are prone to blistering and breakdown and increased evaporative losses due to the loss of the dermis. Infection of partial-thickness burn wounds can cause loss of tissue that creates a wound more similar to a full-thickness injury. Skin grafting of deep dermal burns, when feasible, improves the appearance of the wound and provides timely wound closure, thereby decreasing the risk of infection.

Full-thickness (third-degree) burns have a characteristic white, dry, waxy appearance and may be difficult to discern from unburned skin. These burns can involve fat and underlying tissue, which may be brown, dark red, or black. The diagnostic findings of full-thickness burns are lack of sensation in the burned skin, lack of capillary refill, and a dry leathery texture that is unlike normal skin. All dermal epithelial elements are destroyed, leaving no potential for reepithelialization from within the wound. The epithelium is repopulated from the edges of the burn wound, which leads to lengthy wound healing times and significant scarring.

DETERMINATION OF SEVERITY OF INJURY

Burn injury severity and mortality are related to the size (TBSA) and depth of the burn, patient age, medical comorbidities, and the severity of associated injuries, particularly lung injuries caused by smoke inhalation.

The TBSA involved in the burn is most accurately determined by using the age-related charts designed by Lund and Browder (Figure 15–2). A set of these charts should be filled out for every burn patient on admission and when resuscitation is begun. However, these charts are imperfect because they are two-dimensional images of a three-dimensional person, and thus, accurate prediction of the TBSA can be difficult.

A careful calculation of the percentage of total body burned is useful for several reasons. As stated previously, prognosis is directly related to both the extent of injury and the depth. Ryan and colleagues published a paper showing that mortality was affected by age, TBSA, and inhalation injury. The impact of age was nonlinear, with patients at the extremes of age (pediatric and elderly) having higher mortality rates.

Patients under age 2 years have a significantly higher death rate for any given extent of burn. The higher death rate in infants results from a number of factors. First, the body surface area in children relative to body weight is much greater than in adults. Therefore, a burn of comparable surface area has a greater physiologic impact on a child. Second, immature kidneys and liver do not allow for removal of a high solute load from injured tissue or the rapid restoration of adequate nutritional support. Third, the incompletely developed immune system increases susceptibility to infection.

Elderly patients are at increased risk of mortality due to complex medical comorbidities but also due to the concept of frailty (lack of physiologic reserve). Therefore, these patients are prone to complications from a prolonged hospital stay that may involve the ICU or multiple operations.

Burns involving the hands, face, feet, or perineum are at risk for severe complications if not properly treated. Patients with such burns should be referred to a burn center for the consideration for admission to the hospital. Chemical and electrical burns or those involving the respiratory tract are invariably far more extensive than is evident on initial inspection and require expertise in management of potential complications from specific chemicals or sequela from electrical injury. The American Burn Association has created a list of criteria for transfer of patients to a burn center for specialty care to mitigate potential excess morbidity and mortality. See Table 15–1 for a complete list of transfer criteria.

PATHOLOGY & PATHOPHYSIOLOGY OF THERMAL INJURIES

The microscopic pathologic feature of the burn wound is principally surface coagulation necrosis. Burned tissue has three distinct zones. The first is the zone of "coagulation," or necrosis with irreversible cell death and no capillary blood flow. Surrounding this is a zone of injury or stasis, characterized by sluggish capillary blood flow and injured cells. Although damaged, the tissue is still viable.

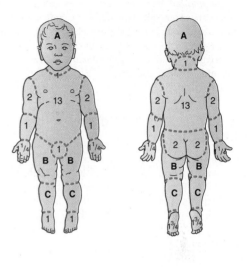

Relative percentages of areas affected by growth

Area	Age		
	10	15	Adult
A = half of head	5 1/2	4 1/2	3 1/2
B = half of one thigh	4 1/4	4 1/2	4 3/4
C = half of one leg	3	3 1/4	3 1/2

Relative percentages of areas affected by growth

Area	Age		
	0	1	5
A = half of head	9 1/2	8 1/2	6 1/2
B = half of one thigh	2 3/4	3 1/4	4
C = half of one leg	2 1/2	2 1/2	2 3/4

▲ **Figure 15–2.** Table for estimating extent of burns. In adults, a reasonable system for calculating the percentage of body surface burned is the "rule of nines": Each arm equals 9%, the head equals 9%, the anterior and posterior trunk each equal 18%, and each leg equals 18%; the sum of these percentages is 99%.

Further tissue injury can be caused by products of inflammation such as oxidants and vasoconstrictor mediators. Environmental insults such as hypoperfusion, desiccation, or infection can also cause the injured tissue to become

Table 15–1. American Burn Association burn transfer criteria.

1. Partial-thickness burns > 10% total body surface area
2. Burns that involve the face, hands, feet, genitalia, perineum, or major joints
3. Third-degree burns in any age group
4. Electrical burns, including lightning injury
5. Chemical burns
6. Inhalation burns
7. Burn injury in older patients or patients with complex medical disorders that could affect mortality or recovery
8. Any patient with burns or concomitant trauma
9. Burned children should go to hospitals qualified to care for children
10. Burn injury in patients who require special social, emotional, or rehabilitative interventions

necrotic. The third zone is that of "hyperemia," which is the usual inflammatory response of healthy tissue to nonlethal injury. Vasodilatation and increased capillary permeability are typically present.

Burn shock is a time-limited phenomenon that occurs in patients who have burns that cover greater than 20% TBSA. Burn shock occurs during the first 24 hours after injury and results in a marked release of inflammatory mediators. The physiologic response to injury includes systemic vasodilation, decrease in cardiac output, and widespread capillary leakage in burned and unburned tissue. Rapid loss of intravascular fluid and protein occurs through the heat-injured capillaries. The volume loss is greatest in the first 6-8 hours, with capillary integrity returning toward normal by 36-48 hours. A transient increase in vascular permeability also occurs in nonburned tissues, probably as a result of the initial release of vasoactive mediators. The edema that develops in nonburned tissues appears to be due in large part to the marked hypoproteinemia caused by protein loss into the burn itself. A systemic inflammatory response occurs in response to a large body burn, resulting in the release of oxidants and other inflammatory mediators into unburned tissues. A generalized decrease in cell energy and membrane potential occurs as a result. This leads to a shift of extracellular sodium and water into the intracellular space. Smoke inhalation markedly increases the hemodynamic instability, fluid requirements, and mortality rates by adding another source of intense inflammation, leading to local lung and systemic tissue damage.

METABOLIC RESPONSE TO BURNS & METABOLIC SUPPORT

The initial metabolic response appears to be activated by proinflammatory cytokines with high levels of interleukin (IL)-1 and IL-6. The secretion of catecholamines, cortisol, glucagon, renin-angiotensin, antidiuretic hormone, and aldosterone is also increased. Early in the response, energy is supplied by the breakdown of stored glycogen and by the process of anaerobic glycolysis.

Profound hypermetabolism and catabolism are characterized by an increase in metabolic rate that approaches 1.5-2 times the resting energy expenditure as compared to non-burned controls. This hypermetabolic response is persistent and lasts well after the burn wounds have healed. The degree of response is proportionate to the degree of injury, with a plateau occurring when the burn involves about 40%-60% TBSA. The initiating and perpetuating factors are the mediators of inflammation, especially the cytokines and endotoxin. Added environmental stresses such as pain, difficulties with thermoregulation, and sepsis syndrome can increase hypermetabolism and catabolism.

During the first postburn week, the hypermetabolic response is characterized by several changes in metabolism. Patients experience insulin resistance due to increased gluconeogenesis from the liver, as well as lipolysis and skeletal muscle proteolysis, leading to increased glucose production. Skeletal muscle becomes the major source of glucose production during burn injury and contributes to the significant loss of lean body mass.

The evaporative water loss from the wound may reach 300 mL/m^2/h (normal is about 15 mL/m^2/h). This produces a heat loss of about 580 kcal/L of water evaporated. Covering the burn with an impermeable membrane, such as skin substitute, reduces the heat loss. Similarly, placing the burn patient in a warm environment, where convection and radiant loss of heat are minimized, also modestly reduces the heat loss and the metabolic rate.

Aggressive nutritional support, along with rapid wound closure and control of pain, stress, and sepsis, will help control the hypermetabolic catabolic state. Medications have been used to help mitigate the body's catabolic response to the burn injury. Use of a beta-blocker, specifically propranolol, has been shown to decrease catabolism and overall blunt the effects of the catecholamine surge, leading to

increased protein synthesis and decreased lipolysis. Oxandrolone, a testosterone analog, has been shown to decrease protein muscle catabolism, leading to improved outcomes for patients such as decreased hospital length of stay and improved wound healing.

IMMUNOLOGIC FACTORS IN BURNS

Burn patients are predisposed to infections due to loss of the skin barrier to the environment but also because of alterations in their immune function. Serum IgA, IgM, and IgG levels are decreased, reflecting depressed B-cell function. Cell-mediated immunity or T-cell function is also impaired, as demonstrated by prolonged survival of allografts and xenografts.

Polymorphonuclear (PMN) chemotactic activity is suppressed. A decrease in chemotaxis predates evidence of clinical sepsis by several days. Decreased oxygen consumption and impaired bacterial killing have also been demonstrated in PMNs. Depressed killing is probably due to decreased production of hydrogen peroxide and superoxide; this has been demonstrated by decreased PMN chemiluminescent activity in burn patients.

▼ BURN MANAGEMENT

ACUTE RESUSCITATION

The burn patient should be assessed and treated like any patient with major trauma. Life-threatening traumatic injuries will need to be evaluated and stabilized as part of the resuscitation for the burn injury. As for all trauma and burn patients, the first priority is to ensure an adequate airway. If there is a possibility that smoke inhalation has occurred—as suggested by exposure to a fire in an enclosed space or burns of the face, nares, or upper torso—arterial blood gases and arterial oxygen saturation of hemoglobin and carboxyhemoglobin levels should be measured, and 100% oxygen should be administered. If carboxyhemoglobin is elevated, 100% oxygen should be administered until levels return to normal.

Endotracheal intubation is indicated if the patient has a depressed Glasgow Coma Scale (GCS) score, typically less than 8; has deep burns to the face and neck; or is otherwise critically injured. Intubation should be done early in cases where there is clinical concern for airway loss, because delayed intubation will be difficult to achieve in cases associated with facial and pharyngeal edema or upper airway injury. Otherwise, an emergency tracheostomy may become necessary later under difficult circumstances.

If the burn exceeds 20% TBSA, which is the extent of injury that creates the burn shock state, a urinary catheter should be inserted to monitor urine output. Two large-bore intravenous catheters should be inserted, preferably into a large peripheral vein. These interventions are critical because the severely burned patient will need to undergo a fluid resuscitation over the next 24-48 hours.

Severe burns are characterized by large losses of intravascular fluid, which are greatest during the first 8-12 hours. Fluid loss occurs as a result of the altered capillary permeability, severe hypoproteinemia, and shift of sodium into the cells. These fluid shifts diminish significantly by 24 hours postburn. An isotonic crystalloid salt solution, typically lactated Ringer's solution, is infused to counterbalance the loss of plasma volume into the extravascular space and the further loss of extracellular fluid into the intracellular space.

The resuscitation goals are to provide enough fluid for organ perfusion without causing complications from hypervolemia. Traditional resuscitation guidelines used formulas, such as the Parkland formula (4 mL × weight [kg] × TBSA burned [%]) or the modified Brooke formula (2 mL × weight [kg] × TBSA burned [%]). For each of these formulas, half of the fluid is given in the first 8 hours after the burn and the remaining half is given over the next 16 hours. However, resuscitation strategies have changed to give a more streamlined approach to fluid where the fluid rate is adjusted hourly based on the clinician's assessment of the patient's volume status. These patients are typically admitted to the ICU, where routine lab work and vital signs are monitored and the fluid rates are titrated up or down by 20% of the lactated Ringer's volume to ensure the patient receives only the fluid that is needed and not more.

Patient management during the first 24 hours after the burn is critical. Patients require specialty burn care and should be referred to a burn care center. The labs should be monitored every 4-6 hours and could include arterial blood gas, lactate, basic metabolic panel, complete blood count, and central venous oxygen saturation. These patients are at high risk of developing acute kidney injury and other organ dysfunction due to the high-volume fluid shifts. These patients also sometimes require vasopressors to augment the fluid resuscitation due to the known effects of burn injury to cause suppression of cardiac output and systemic vasodilation. Urine output remains a main goal of the resuscitation strategy, with a target urine output of 30-50 mL/h.

Although the importance of restoring colloid osmotic pressure and plasma proteins is well recognized, the timing of colloid infusion can be used to augment crystalloid infusion, especially in patients who require high volumes of fluid during their fluid resuscitation. The addition of a protein infusion to the treatment regimen has been shown to decrease the fluid requirements and helps to mitigate some of the consequences of hypervolemia.

After intravenous fluids are started and vital signs stabilized, the wound should be debrided of all loose skin and debris. To avoid severe hypothermia, debridement is best done by completing one body area before exposing a second. Wounds are cleaned and then covered with dressings that have some antimicrobial properties to help with infection and to help mitigate hypothermia. Controlling pain is a significant part of burn care, and for those with larger surface burns, intravenous narcotics are frequently used. Tetanus toxoid, 0.5 mL, should be administered to patients with any significant burn injury.

POSTRESUSCITATION PERIOD

Treatment should aim to decrease excessive catecholamine stimulation and provide enough calories to offset the effects of the hypermetabolism. Hypothermia, pain, and anxiety all need to be aggressively controlled. Hypovolemia should be prevented by giving enough fluid to make up for the body losses. The overall critical care should focus on mitigating complications and evaluation for infection because ventilator-associated pneumonia is the most common cause of death in a burn patient in the postresuscitation period, followed by bacteremia and wound infection.

Nutritional support should begin as early as possible in the postburn period to maximize wound healing and minimize immune deficiency. Patients with moderate body burns may be able to meet nutritional needs by voluntary oral intake. Patients with large burns invariably require calorie and protein supplementation to reach a daily caloric goal of 25 kcal/kg body weight and protein goal of 1.5-2 g/kg body weight. The majority of calories delivered are carbohydrates because they are a major source of glucose and prevent protein breakdown. This can usually be accomplished by administering a formula diet through a small-bore feeding tube. Parenteral nutrition is also occasionally required, but the intestinal route is preferred if needs can be met this way. Early restoration of gut function will also decrease gut bacterial translocation and endotoxin leak. Monitoring for overfeeding is important because this can cause increased carbon dioxide production, leading to difficulty with ventilation. In addition, too much protein can cause an elevated blood urea nitrogen level and hyperglycemia.

Patients with larger surface burns also need supplementation of their micronutrients. Vitamins A, E, C, and D and zinc should be given until the burn wound is closed. Many of these micronutrients are involved in wound healing, specifically with collagen formation. Selenium is also supplemented, and levels can be checked and followed. Selenium plays a role in cell-mediated immunity, and levels are frequently low in patients with large surface area burns.

CARE OF THE BURN WOUND

The management of superficial partial-thickness or second-degree burns, an aseptic environment is important to prevent infection. Daily wound care is undertaken to ensure a clean wound bed and is usually accompanied by some type of cleansing process, either in a shower or washing at the bedside. Occlusive dressings are used to minimize exposure to air, increase the rate of reepithelialization, and decrease pain. The exception is the face, which can be treated open with an antibacterial ointment. If there is no infection, superficial burns will heal spontaneously.

The goals in managing deep partial-thickness or full-thickness (third-degree) burns are to prevent invasive infection (ie, burn wound sepsis), to remove dead tissue, and to cover the wound with skin or skin substitutes as soon as possible. All topical antibiotics are especially useful for deep second- or third-degree burns or wounds, which have a high risk of infection. Burns covering more than 20% TBSA that have a full-thickness component are surgically excised within 72 hours of the burn wound to expedite burn wound healing and, importantly, to mitigate the inflammatory response and lessen infectious complications. The wound is covered with a skin graft, a temporary dermal substitute, or some type of an occlusive dressing (eg, negative-pressure wound therapy).

Topical Antibacterial Agents

Topical agents have definitely advanced the care of burn patients. Although burn wound sepsis is still a major problem, the incidence is lower, and the death rate has been markedly reduced, particularly in burns of less than 50% TBSA. There are many different products available, and the evaluation of the wound should guide your choice in management because there are strengths and weaknesses for all of them. The majority of superficial partial-thickness wounds are covered with some type of antimicrobial ointment and a nonadherent gauze with a subsequent protective dressing, but there are many other options available.

Silver sulfadiazine is a cream that is effective against a wide spectrum of gram-positive and gram-negative organisms but is only moderately effective in penetrating the burn eschar. A transient leukopenia secondary to bone marrow suppression often occurs with use of silver sulfadiazine in large burns, but the process is usually self-limiting, and the agent does not have to be discontinued. This medication cannot be used on patients with a sulfur allergy.

Mafenide acetate (Sulfamylon) is available as a 5% solution or 8.5% cream. It has broad-spectrum coverage but poor antifungal properties. It is a carbonic anhydrase inhibitor and can cause a metabolic acidosis when used over large surface areas. It can penetrate an eschar and cartilage, so it is preferred on the nose and ears.

Silver dressings come in many different forms, and the mechanism of action depends on the deposition of silver ions that bind to proteins and disrupt cellular functions. They have a fairly broad spectrum of action and have little detrimental effect on the healing burn wound.

Temporary Skin Substitutes

Skin substitutes are another alternative to topical agents for partial-thickness burns or for wounds that need temporary coverage after surgical excision. A number of synthetic and biologically active temporary skin substitutes are in use. The benefits of these temporary skin substitutes include maturation of the wound, management of fluid losses, and improvement in pain at the wound site. **Allografts (human skin)** work better for this purpose on large excised wounds but are expensive. **Xenografts (porcine skin substitute)** are available for similar indications as the homograft but at much less of the cost. Both the xenograft and homograft will engraft into the wound bed but will eventually be rejected due to host immune system and will either fall off or be removed at a subsequent surgery.

Hydrotherapy

The use of immersion hydrotherapy for wound management has substantially decreased. A few studies have shown that the infection rate is actually increased when patients are immersed in a tub because of the generalized inoculation of burn wounds with bacteria from what was previously a localized infection. Hydrotherapy, on a slant board, is a very useful approach once the wounds are in the process of being debrided and closed. Showering is also effective for wound cleansing in the more stable patient.

Debridement & Grafting

Burn wound inflammation, even in the absence of infection, can result in multiple organ dysfunction and perpetuation of the hypermetabolic catabolic state. Early wound closure is the ultimate goal for these patients because this will mitigate the hypermetabolic response. Surgical excision of the burn wound should be done within 72 hours of the burn. More rapid closure of burn wounds clearly decreases the rate of sepsis and significantly decreases the mortality rate. The approach to operative debridement varies from an extensive burn excision and grafting within several days of injury to a more moderate approach of limiting each debridement to less than 15% of the burned area. Excision can be carried down to fascia or to viable remaining dermis or fat. Excision to fascia is more commonly used when the burn extends well into the fat. Excision to viable tissue, referred to as tangential excision, is advantageous because it provides a vascular base for grafting while preserving remaining viable tissue, especially dermis. Surgeons and anesthesiologists should be prepared to transfuse patients who undergo large burn excisions due to the vascularity of the injured wound bed.

A number of **permanent skin substitutes** could further facilitate wound closure, particularly in large burns with insufficient donor sites. Autologous cultures of epithelium have been applied with some success. Permanent skin substitutes composed of both dermis and epidermis have been designed to maintain coverage and improve skin function.

Maintenance of Function

The maintenance of functional motion during evolution of the burn wound is necessary to avoid loss of motion at joints. If wounds are kept immobile due to pain or for healing of a graft, contracture of the scar, muscles, and tendons across a joint causes loss of motion. Early mobility is key tenet for burn patients to ensure maximal function recovery of joints.

The scar is a metabolically active tissue, continually undergoing reorganization. The extensive scarring that frequently occurs after burns can lead to disfiguring and disabling contractures, but these may be avoided using splints and elevation to maintain a functional position. Following application of the skin graft, maintenance of proper positioning with splints is indicated, along with active motion exercises.

If reinjury does not occur, the amount of collagen in the scar tends to decrease with time (usually over a year). Stiff collagen becomes softer, and on flat surfaces of the body, where reinjury and inflammation are prevented, remodeling may eliminate contracture. However, around joints or the neck, contractures can persist, and surgical reconstruction may be necessary. The sooner the burn wound can be covered with skin grafts, the less likely is contracture formation.

MANAGEMENT OF COMPLICATIONS

Infection is a major cause of complications in the severely injured burn patient. The large open wound is always colonized with bacteria and, with excellent wound care, rarely becomes infected. The most common source of infection for burn patients in the ICU is ventilator-associated pneumonia, followed by bacteremia. Burn wounds are the third most common source of infection. Signs of burn wound infection are loss of the temporary coverage of the wound, changes in wound appearance, erythema of the uninjured tissue surrounding the wound, and systemic signs of infection. Patients with a burn wound infection have a wound that is purulent in appearance as well as one of the signs listed above. Table 15–2 lists the common pathogens in burn wounds. Burn wounds can also become infected with a fungus or mold. This is a dreaded complication because it is associated with a high mortality rate.

Table 15–3. American Burn Association Burn Consensus Conference for the definition of sepsis.

Sepsis should be considered if three of the following criteria are met:
1. Temperature > 39°C or < 36.5°C
2. Progressive tachycardia: > 110 beats/min
3. Progressive tachypnea: > 25 breaths/min for unventilated patients or > 12 L/min ventilation for ventilated patients
4. Thrombocytopenia
5. New hyperglycemia
6. Intolerance of tube feeding

Sepsis syndrome frequently occurs in patients with major burns, and the critical care team should constantly evaluate patients for signs and symptoms. Fever, hypermetabolism, catabolism, and leukocytosis are typical characteristics of critically injured burn patients. These findings are due to the intense inflammatory response stimulated by the burn, and it can be difficult to discern patients with sepsis from those with severe inflammation. There is little evidence to guide the clinician in trying to diagnose sepsis in the burn patient; thus, the American Burn Association has developed consensus criteria to help define sepsis (Table 15–3). However, these criteria are neither very sensitive nor specific and should be used in conjunction with good clinical judgment.

Eschar syndrome occurs with circumferential burns of an extremity or of the trunk and poses special problems. Swelling beneath the unyielding eschar may act as a tourniquet to blood and lymph flow, and the distal extremity may become swollen and tense. More extensive swelling may compromise the arterial supply. Escharotomy, or excision of the eschar, may be required. To avoid permanent damage, escharotomy must be performed before arterial ischemia develops. Constriction involving the chest or abdomen may severely restrict ventilation and may require longitudinal escharotomies. Anesthetics are rarely required, and the procedure can usually be performed in the patient's room.

Table 15–2. Most common pathogens in burn infections.

	Staphylococcus aureus	*Pseudomonas aeruginosa*	*Candida albicans*
Wound appearance	Loss of wound granulation	Surface necrosis; patchy, black	Minimal exudate
Course	Slow onset over 2-5 days	Rapid onset over 12-36 hours	Slow (days)
Central nervous system signs	Disorientation	Modest changes	Often no change
Temperature	Marked increase	High or low	Modest changes
White blood count	Marked increase	High or low	Modest changes
Hypotension	Modest	Often severe	Minimal change
Mortality rate	5%	20%-30%	30%-50%

Table 15–4. Carbon monoxide poisoning.

Carboxyhemoglobin Level	Severity	Symptoms
< 20%	Mild	Headache, mild dyspnea, visual changes, confusion
20%-40%	Moderate	Irritability, diminished judgment, dim vision, nausea, easy fatigability
40%-60%	Severe	Hallucinations, confusion, ataxia, collapse, coma
> 60%	Fatal	

Gastrointestinal bleeding from acute gastroduodenal (Curling) ulcers were at one time a frequent complication of severe burns, but the incidence is now extremely low, largely as a result of the early and routine institution of proton pump inhibitors or histamine receptor antagonists, along with nutritional therapy and the overall improvement of critical care over the past decade.

RESPIRATORY INJURY IN BURNS

Today, the major cause of death after burns is respiratory failure or complications in the respiratory tract. The problems include inhalation injury, aspiration in unconscious patients, bacterial pneumonia, pulmonary edema, and post-traumatic pulmonary insufficiency. Smoke inhalation markedly increases mortality from burn injury.

Smoke inhalation injuries, which are caused by incomplete products of combustion and which predispose to other complications, are divided into three categories: carbon monoxide poisoning (Table 15–4), upper airways injury, and inhalation of noxious compounds in the lower airways (Table 15–5).

Table 15–5. Sources of toxic chemicals in smoke.

Wood, cotton	Aldehydes (acrolein), nitrogen dioxide, carbon monoxide (CO)
Polyvinylchloride	Hydrochloric acid, phosgene, CO
Rubber	Sulfur dioxide, hydrogen sulfide, CO
Polystyrene	Copious black smoke and soot—carbon dioxide, water, and some CO
Acrylonitrile, polyurethane, nitrogenous compounds	Hydrogen cyanide
Fire retardants may produce toxic fumes	Halogens (F_2, Cl_2, Br_2), ammonia, hydrogen cyanide, CO

Carbon monoxide poisoning must be considered in every patient suspected of having inhalation injury based on having been burned in a closed space and physical evidence of inhalation. Arterial blood gases and carboxyhemoglobin levels must be determined. Levels of carboxyhemoglobin above 5% in nonsmokers and above 10% in smokers indicate carbon monoxide poisoning. Carbon monoxide has an affinity for hemoglobin 200 times that of oxygen. The molecule displaces oxygen and produces a leftward shift in the oxyhemoglobin dissociation curve (P_{50}, the oxygen tension at which half the hemoglobin is saturated with oxygen, is lowered). Calculations of oxyhemoglobin saturation may be misleading because the hemoglobin combined with carbon monoxide is not detected and the percentage saturation of oxyhemoglobin may appear normal.

Mild carbon monoxide poisoning (< 20% carboxyhemoglobin) is manifested by headache, slight dyspnea, mild confusion, and diminished visual acuity. Moderate poisoning (20%-40% carboxyhemoglobin) leads to irritability, impairment of judgment, dim vision, nausea, and fatigability. Severe poisoning (40%-60% carboxyhemoglobin) produces hallucinations, confusion, ataxia, collapse, and coma. Levels in excess of 60% carboxyhemoglobin are usually fatal.

Various **toxic chemicals** in inspired smoke produce tracheobronchial respiratory injuries. Inhalation of kerosene smoke, for example, is relatively innocuous. Smoke from a wood fire is extremely irritating because it contains aldehyde gases, particularly acrolein. Direct inhalation of acrolein, even in low concentrations, irritates mucous membranes and causes severe airway damage. Smoke from some plastic compounds, such as polyurethane, is the most serious kind of toxic irritant, and some plastics give off poisonous gases such as chlorine, sulfuric acid, and cyanides.

Cyanide absorption can be lethal because it binds to ferric ion in the electron transport chain, which stops the production of adenosine triphosphate (ATP). This leads to tissue hypoxia at the cellular level, which manifests as an unexplained lactic acidosis. For most hospitals, the cyanide level is a send-out test, and so treatment needs to be empiric based on clinical suspicion and not the cyanide level. The treatment modality of choice is hydroxocobalamin (typical dose is 5 g), which directly binds the cyanide molecule, is rapid acting, and is secreted in the urine. Carbon monoxide poisoning and cyanide poisoning frequently occur in the same clinical scenarios; therefore, clinicians should have a high clinical suspicion for cyanide poisoning and institute empiric treatment as needed.

Inhalation injury below the glottis causes severe mucosal edema followed soon by sloughing of the mucosa. The destroyed mucosa in the larger airways is replaced by a mucopurulent membrane. The edema fluid enters the airway and, when mixed with the cellular debris in the lumen, may form casts and plugs in the smaller bronchioles. The distal airways, the terminal bronchioles and alveoli, contain the carbonaceous material, which causes direct mucosal injury or airway compromise. These patients are at high risk of developing acute bronchiolitis and bronchopneumonia within a few days after admission. Airway clearance is impeded due to ciliary damage and denuded airways coupled with alteration of normal oropharyngeal flora due to colonization by pathogens, which then leads to bronchopneumonia.

When inhalation injury is suspected, early endoscopic examination of the airway with fiberoptic bronchoscopy is helpful in determining the area of injury (ie, the extent of upper and lower airway involvement). Unfortunately, the severity of the injury cannot be accurately quantified by bronchoscopy—it can only be shown that an injury is present. Direct laryngoscopy probably gives as much information. Other clinical signs of airway injury can be unexplained hypoxia, hoarseness, swelling of the vocal cords or surrounding tissue on laryngoscopy, and the detection of soot in the airways.

▶ **Treatment**

Management of a burn patient in whom there is concern for inhalation injury should include frequent evaluation of the lungs throughout the hospital course. All patients who initially have evidence of smoke inhalation should receive humidified oxygen in high concentrations. If carbon monoxide poisoning has occurred, 100% oxygen should be given until the carboxyhemoglobin content returns to normal levels and symptoms of carbon monoxide toxicity resolve. With severe exposures, carbon monoxide may still be bound to the cytochrome enzymes, leading to cell hypoxia even after carboxyhemoglobin levels have returned to near normal. Continued oxygen administration will also reverse this process. Hyperbaric oxygen is not indicated and has not been shown to improve outcomes. Bronchodilators may help if wheezing is due to the reflex bronchospasm typically present. Chest physical therapy can also help to mobilize secretions.

Mechanical ventilation should be instituted early if a significant pulmonary injury is anticipated. A large body burn with chest wall involvement will result in decreased chest wall compliance, increased work of breathing, and subsequent atelectasis. Tracheobronchial injury from inhaled chemicals is accentuated by the presence of a body burn, with a resultant increase in the potential for atelectasis and infection. Controlled ventilation along with sedation will diminish the degree of injury and also conserve energy expenditure. Early excision of the deep chest wall burn will help remove the constricting component. Wound closure, in turn, will decrease the excessive carbon dioxide production caused by the hypermetabolic state.

REHABILITATION OF THE BURNED PATIENT

Plastic surgery consultation for revision of scars is often necessary after the initial grafting, particularly to release contractures over joints to improve function and, especially for burns on the face, for cosmetic reasons. This typically occurs in the outpatient setting after the patient has begun to recover from the initial injury. The physician must be realistic in defining an acceptable result, and the patient should be told that it may take years to achieve. Burn scars are often unsightly, and although hope should be extended that improvement can be made, total resolution is not possible in many cases.

Skin expansion techniques using subdermal implants that are gradually expanded over time have greatly improved scar revision management. The ability to enlarge the available skin to be used for replacement of scar improves both cosmetic appearance and function. Advances in microvascular flap surgery have also resulted in substantial improvements in outcomes.

The patient must take special care of the skin of the burn scar, especially for scars on the hands and face. Hypertrophic scars and keloids are particularly bothersome and can be diminished with the use of pressure garments, which must be worn until the scar matures, which takes approximately 12 months. Because the skin appendages are often destroyed by full-thickness burns, creams and lotions are required to prevent drying and cracking and to reduce itching. Substances such as lanolin, vitamin A and D ointment, and Eucerin cream are all effective.

Brown D: Propranolol dosing practices in adult burn patients: implication for safety and efficacy. *J Burn Care Res.* 2016;37(3):e218.

Caruso D: Monitoring end points of burn resuscitation. *Crit Care Med.* 2016;32:525.

Chung K: Simple derivation of the initial fluid rate for the resuscitation of severely burned adult combat casualties: in silico validation of the rule of 10. *J Trauma.* 2010;69:S49.

Jeschke M: Effect of insulin on the inflammatory and acute phase response after burn injury. *Crit Care Med.* 2007;9:519.

Palmieri T: Inhalation injury research progress and needs. *J Burn Care.* 2007;4:594.

Rowan M: Burn wound healing and treatment: review and advancements. *Crit Care.* 2015;19:243.

Rubino C: Total upper and low eyelid replacement following thermal injury using an ALT flap. *J Plast Reconstruct Aesthet Surg.* 2007;20:215.

Tenenhaus M: Burn surgery. *Clin Plast Surg.* 2007;34:697.

Wascak J: Early versus later internal nutritional support in adults with burn injury: a systemic review. *J Hum Nutr Diet.* 2007;20:25.

▼ ELECTRICAL INJURY

There are three kinds of electrical injuries: electrical current injury, electrothermal burns from arcing current, and flame burns caused by ignition of clothing. Occasionally, all three are present in the same patient.

Electrical current injury, or "hidden injury," results from the passage of electrical current through the body. Flash or arc burns are thermal injuries to the skin caused by a high-tension electrical current creating local heat and damaging skin. The thermal injury to the skin is intense and deep, because the electrical arc has a temperature of about 2500°C (high enough to melt bone). Flame burns from ignited clothing are often the most serious part of the injury. Treatment is the same as for any thermal injury.

Once current enters the body, its pathway depends on the resistances it encounters in the various organs. The following are listed in descending order of resistance: bone, fat, tendon, skin, muscle, blood, and nerve. The pathway of the current determines immediate survival; for example, if the current passes through the heart or the brainstem, death may be immediate from ventricular fibrillation or apnea. Current passing through muscles may cause spasms severe enough to produce long-bone fractures or dislocations.

The type of current is also related to the severity of injury with low-voltage (150 V) current. The usual 60-cycle alternating current that causes most injuries in the home is particularly severe. Alternating current causes tetanic contractions, and the victim may become "locked" to the contact. Cardiac arrest is common from contact with low-voltage house current.

High-voltage electrical current injuries are more than just burns. Focal deep burns occur at the points of entrance and exit through the skin. These burns often extend through local muscle, resulting in fourth-degree burn. Once inside the body, the current travels through muscles, causing an injury more like a crush than a thermal burn. This leads to blood and fluid extravasation, increasing interstitial pressure in the muscle compartments. A fasciotomy is often necessary, opening all the muscle compartments involved. Early action is necessary to avoid severe vascular insufficiency or nerve damage. Thrombosis frequently occurs in vessels deep in an extremity, causing a greater depth of tissue necrosis than is evident at the initial examination. The greatest muscle injury is usually closest to the bone, where the highest heat of resistance is generated. The treatment of electrical injuries depends on the extent of deep muscle and nerve destruction more than on any other factor.

Severe myoglobinuria may develop with the risk of acute tubular necrosis as the muscle pigment is released from muscle and precipitates in renal tubules. The urine output must be kept two to three times normal with intravenous fluids. Alkalinization of the urine and osmotic diuretics may be indicated if myoglobinuria is present to more rapidly clear the pigment.

A rapid drop in hematocrit sometimes follows as sudden destruction of red blood cells by the electrical energy occurs. Bleeding into deep tissues may occur as a result of disruption of blood vessels and tissue planes. In some cases, thrombosed vessels disintegrate later and cause massive interstitial hemorrhage. Increased fluid infusion is required for initial resuscitation compared to extent of external thermal burns alone.

The skin burn at the entrance and exit sites is usually a depressed gray or yellow area of full-thickness destruction surrounded by a sharply defined zone of hyperemia. Charring may be present. The lesion should be debrided to underlying healthy tissue. Frequently, there is deep destruction not initially evident, especially to muscles beneath the skin surface. This dead and devitalized tissue must also be excised as soon as possible. Amputation rate for extremity involved is still high but decreasing. A second debridement is usually indicated 24-48 hours after the injury because the necrosis is found to be more extensive than originally thought. The strategy of obtaining skin covering for these burns can tax ingenuity because of the extent and depth of the wounds. Microvascular flaps are now used routinely to replace large tissue losses.

In general, the treatment of electrical injuries is complex at every step, and these patients are referred to specialized centers. There are no formulas for determining severity and outcome of high-voltage electrical injuries.

Edlich R: Modern concepts of treatment and prevention of electrical burns. *J Long Term Eff Med Implants.* 2005;15:511.

Moughsoudi H: Electrical and lightning injuries. *J Burn Care Res.* 2007;28:255.

▼ HEAT STROKE & RELATED INJURIES

Heat stroke occurs when core body temperature exceeds 40°C and produces severe central nervous system dysfunction. Two related syndromes induced by exposure to heat are heat cramps and heat exhaustion.

In humans, heat is dissipated from the skin by radiation, conduction, convection, and evaporation. When the ambient temperature rises, heat loss by the first three is impaired; loss by evaporation is hindered by a high relative humidity. Predisposing factors to heat accumulation are dermatitis; use of phenothiazines, beta-blockers, diuretics, or anticholinergics; intercurrent fever from other disease; obesity; alcoholism; and heavy clothing. Cocaine and amphetamines may increase metabolic heat production.

Heat cramps—muscle pain after exertion in a hot environment—are usually attributed to salt deficit. It is probable, however, that many cases are real examples of **exertional rhabdomyolysis**. This condition, which may also be a complicating factor in heat stroke, involves acute muscle injury due to severe exertional efforts beyond the limits for which the individual has trained. It often produces myoglobinuria, which rarely affects kidney function except when it occurs in patients also suffering from heat stroke. Complete recovery is the rule after uncomplicated heat cramps.

Heat exhaustion consists of fatigue, muscular weakness, tachycardia, postural syncope, nausea, vomiting, and an urge to defecate caused by dehydration and hypovolemia from heat stress. Temperature usually exceeds 39°C. Although body temperature is normal in heat exhaustion, there is a continuum between this syndrome and heat stroke.

Heat stroke, a result of imbalance between heat production and heat dissipation, kills about 4000 persons yearly in the United States. Exercise-induced heat stroke most often affects young people (eg, athletes, military recruits, laborers) who are exercising strenuously in a hot environment, usually without adequate training. Heat production exceeds the ability to dissipate the heat; core temperature then rises, and hypovolemia is evident. Sedentary heat stroke is a disease of elderly or infirm people whose cardiovascular systems are unable to adapt to the stress of a hot environment and release sufficient heat such that body temperature rises. Epidemics of heat stroke in elderly people can be predicted when the ambient temperature surpasses 32.2°C and the relative humidity reaches 50%-76%.

The mechanism of injury is direct damage by heat to the parenchyma and vasculature of the organs. In addition, there is a marked cytokine-induced activation of inflammation similar to sepsis, leading to inflammation-induced organ damage. The central nervous system is particularly vulnerable, and cellular necrosis is found in the brains of those who die of heat stroke. Hepatocellular and renal tubular damage are apparent in severe cases. Subendocardial damage and occasionally transmural infarcts are discovered in fatal cases, even in young persons without previous cardiac disease. Disseminated intravascular coagulation may develop, aggravating injury in all organ systems and predisposing to bleeding complications.

▶ **Clinical Findings**

A. Symptoms and Signs

Heat stroke should be suspected in anyone who develops sudden neurologic changes in a hot environment. If the patient's temperature is above 40°C (range: 40-43°C), the diagnosis of heat stroke is definitive. Measurements of body temperature must be made rectally. A prodrome including dizziness, headache, nausea, chills, and goose-flesh of the chest and arms is seen occasionally but is not common. In most cases, the patient recalls having experienced no warning symptoms except weakness, tiredness, or dizziness. Confusion, belligerent behavior, or stupor may precede coma. Convulsions may occur.

The skin is pink or ashen and sometimes, paradoxically, dry and hot; dry skin in the presence of hyperpyrexia is virtually pathognomonic of heat stroke. Profuse sweating is usually present in runners and other athletes who have heat stroke. The heart rate ranges from 140 beats/min to 170 beats/min; central venous or pulmonary wedge pressure is high; and in some cases, the blood pressure is low. Hyperventilation may reach 60 breaths/min and may give rise to respiratory alkalosis. Pulmonary edema and bloody sputum may develop in severe cases. Jaundice is frequent within the first few days after onset of symptoms.

Dehydration, which may produce the same central nervous system symptoms as heat stroke, is an aggravating factor in about 50% of cases.

B. Laboratory Findings

There is no characteristic pattern to the electrolyte changes. The serum sodium concentration may be normal or high, and the potassium concentration is usually low on admission or at some point during resuscitation. In the first few days, the aspartate aminotransferase (AST), lactate dehydrogenase (LDH), and creatine kinase (CK) may be elevated, especially in exertional heat stroke. Proteinuria and granular and red cell casts are seen in urine specimens collected immediately after diagnosis. If the urine is dark red or brown, it probably contains myoglobin. The blood urea nitrogen and serum creatinine rise transiently in most patients and continue to climb if renal failure develops. Hematologic findings may be normal or may be typical of disseminated intravascular coagulation (ie, low fibrinogen, increased fibrin split products, slow prothrombin and partial thromboplastin times, and decreased platelet count).

C. Prevention

For the most part, heat stroke in military recruits and athletes in training is preventable by adhering to a graduated schedule of increasing performance requirements that allows acclimatization over 2-3 weeks and increasing fluid replacement using water and some electrolytes, especially sodium. Heat produced by exercise is dissipated by increased cardiac output, vasodilation in the skin, and increased sweating. With acclimatization, there is increased efficiency for muscular work, increased myocardial performance, expanded extracellular fluid volume if hydration is maintained, greater output of sweat for a given amount of work (releasing more heat), a lower salt content of sweat, and a lower central temperature for a given amount of work.

Access to drinking water should be unrestricted during vigorous physical activity in a hot environment. Free water is preferable to electrolyte-containing solutions. Clothing and protective gear should be lightened as heat production and air temperature rise, and heavy exercise should not be scheduled at the hottest times of day, especially at the beginning of a training schedule.

▶ **Treatment**

The patient should be cooled rapidly. The most efficient method is to induce evaporative heat loss by spraying the patient with water at 15°C and fanning with cool air. Immersion in an ice water bath or use of ice packs is also effective but causes cutaneous vasoconstriction and shivering and makes patient monitoring more difficult. Monitor the rectal temperature frequently. To avoid overshooting the end point, vigorous cooling should be stopped when the temperature reaches 38.9°C. Shivering should be controlled with parenteral phenothiazines. Oxygen should be administered, and if the Pao_2 drops below 65 mm Hg, tracheal intubation should be performed to control ventilation.

Fluid, electrolyte, and acid–base balance must be controlled by frequent monitoring. Intravenous fluid administration should be based on the central venous or pulmonary artery wedge pressure, blood pressure, and urine output; overhydration must be avoided. Intravenous mannitol (12.5 g) may be given early if myoglobinuria is present to avoid renal dysfunction. Disseminated intravascular coagulation may require treatment with heparin. Occasionally, inotropic agents (eg, isoproterenol, dopamine) may be indicated for cardiac insufficiency, which should be suspected if hypotension persists after hypovolemia has been corrected.

Prognosis

Bad prognostic signs are temperature of 42.2°C or greater, coma lasting more than 2 hours, shock, hyperkalemia, and an AST greater than 1000 units/L during the first 24 hours. The death rate is about 10% in patients who are correctly diagnosed and treated promptly. Deaths in the first few days are usually due to cerebral damage; later deaths may be from bleeding or may be due to cardiac, renal, or hepatic failure.

Jardine DS: Heat illness and heat stroke. *Pediatr Rev.* 2007;28:249.
Leon LR: Heat stroke and cytokines. *Prog Brain Res.* 2007;162:481.

FROSTBITE

Frostbite involves freezing of tissues. Ice crystals form between and in the cells and grow at the expense of intracellular water. The resulting ischemia due to vasoconstriction and increased blood viscosity is the mechanism of tissue injury. Skin and muscle are considerably more susceptible than tendons and bones to freezing damage due to a lower oxygen requirement, which explains why the patient may still be able to move severely frostbitten digits.

Frostbite is caused by cold exposure, the effects of which can be magnified by moisture or wind. For example, the chilling effects on skin are the same with an air temperature of 6.7°C and a 40-mph wind as with an air temperature of −40°C and only a 2-mph wind. Contact with metal or gasoline in very cold weather can cause virtually instantaneous freezing; skin will often stick to metal and be lost. The risk of frostbite is increased by generalized hypothermia, which produces peripheral vasoconstriction as part of the mechanism for preservation of core body temperature.

Two related injuries, trench foot and immersion foot, involve prolonged exposure to wet cold above freezing (eg, 10°C). The resulting tissue damage is produced by tissue ischemia.

Clinical Findings

Frostnip, a minor variant of this syndrome, is a transient blanching and numbness of exposed parts that may progress to frostbite if not immediately detected and treated. It often appears on the tips of fingers, ears, nose, chin, or cheeks and should be managed by rewarming through contact with warm parts of the body or warm air.

Frostbitten parts are numb, painless, and of a white or waxy appearance. With **superficial frostbite,** only the skin and subcutaneous tissues are frozen, so the tissues beneath are still compressible with pressure. **Deep frostbite** involves freezing of underlying tissues, which imparts a wooden consistency to the extremity.

After rewarming, the frostbitten area becomes mottled blue or purple and painful and tender. Blisters appear that may take several weeks to resolve. The part becomes edematous and to a varying degree painful.

Treatment

The frostbitten part should be rewarmed (thawed) in a water bath at 40-42.2°C for 20-30 minutes. Thawing should not be attempted until the victim can be kept permanently warm and at rest. It is far better to continue walking on frostbitten feet even for many hours than to thaw them in a remote cold area where definitive care cannot be provided. If a thermometer is unavailable, the temperature of the water should be adjusted to be warm but not hot to a normal hand. Never use the frozen part to test the water temperature or expose it to a source of direct heat such as a fire. The risk of seriously compounding the injury is great with any method of thawing other than immersion in warm water.

After thawing has been completed, the patient should be kept recumbent and the injured part left open to the air, protected from direct contact with sheets, clothing, or other material. Blisters should be left intact and the skin gently debrided by immersing the part in a whirlpool bath for about 20 minutes twice daily. No scrubbing or massaging of the injured part should be allowed, and topical ointments, antiseptics, and so on are of no value. Vasodilating agents and surgical sympathectomy do not appear to improve healing.

The tissue will heal gradually, and any dead tissue will become demarcated and usually slough spontaneously. Early in the course, it is nearly impossible, even for someone with considerable experience in the treatment of frostbite, to judge the depth of injury; most early assessments tend to overestimate the extent of permanent damage. Therefore, expectant treatment is the rule, and surgical debridement should be avoided even if evolution of the injury requires many months. Surgery may be indicated to release constricting circumferential eschars, but rarely should the process of spontaneous separation of gangrenous tissue be surgically facilitated. Even in severe injuries, amputation is rarely indicated before 2 months unless invasive infection supervenes. Nuclear scans may be useful to delineate tissue viability.

Concomitant fractures or dislocations create challenging and complex problems. Dislocations should be reduced immediately after thawing. Open fractures require operative reduction, but closed fractures should be managed with a posterior plastic splint. Anterior tibial compartment syndrome, which may develop in patients with associated fractures, may be diagnosed by arteriography and treated by fasciotomy.

After the eschar separates, the skin is noted to be thin, shiny, tender, and sensitive to cold; occasionally it exhibits a tendency to perspire more readily. Gradually, it returns toward normal, but pain on exposure to cold may persist indefinitely.

Prognosis

The prognosis for normal function is excellent if appropriate treatment is provided. Individuals who have recovered from frostbite have increased susceptibility to another frostbite injury on exposure to cold.

Affleck DG et al: Assessment of tissue viability in complex extremity injuries: utility of the pyrophosphate nuclear scan. *J Trauma.* 2001;50:263.

Gonzage T: Use of intra-arterial thrombolytic therapy for acute treatment of frostbite in 62 patients with review of thrombolytic therapy in frostbite. *J Burn Care Res.* 2016;37:e323.

Murphy JV et al: Frostbite: pathogenesis and treatment. *J Trauma.* 2000;48:171.

ACCIDENTAL HYPOTHERMIA

Accidental hypothermia consists of the uncontrolled lowering of core body temperature below 35°C by exposure to cold. The syndrome may be seen, for example, in elderly people living alone in inadequately heated homes, in alcoholics exposed to the cold during a binge, in those engaged in winter sports, and in people who become lost in cold weather. Alcohol facilitates the induction of hypothermia by producing sedation (inhibiting shivering) and cutaneous dilation. Other sedatives, tranquilizers, and antidepressants are occasionally implicated. Diseases that predispose to hypothermia include myxedema, hypopituitarism, adrenal insufficiency, cerebral vascular insufficiency, mental impairment, and cardiovascular disorders.

The heart is the organ most sensitive to cooling and is subject to ventricular fibrillation or asystole when the temperature drops to 21-24°C. Hypothermia affects the oxyhemoglobin dissociation curve, so less oxygen is released to the tissues. Cardiac standstill may cause death in less than 1 hour in shipwreck victims immersed in cold water (6.7°C). Increased capillary permeability, manifested by generalized edema and pulmonary, hepatic, and renal dysfunction, may develop as the patient is rewarmed. Coagulopathies and disseminated intravascular coagulation are seen occasionally. Pancreatitis and acute renal failure are common in patients whose temperature on admission is below 32°C.

Clinical Findings

A. Symptoms and Signs

The patient is mentally depressed (somnolent, stuporous, or comatose), cold, and pale to cyanotic. The clinical findings are not always striking and may be mistaken for the effects of alcohol. The core temperature ranges from 21°C to 35°C. Shivering is absent when the temperature is below 32°C. Respirations are slow and shallow. The blood pressure is usually normal and the heart rate slow. When the core temperature drops below 32°C, the patient may appear to be dead. The extremities may be frostbitten or frozen.

B. Laboratory Findings

Dehydration may increase the concentration of various blood constituents. Severe hypoglycemia is common, and unless detected and treated immediately, it may become dangerously worse as rewarming produces shivering. The serum amylase is elevated in about half of cases, but autopsy studies show that it does not always reflect pancreatitis. Diabetic ketoacidosis becomes a management problem in some patients whose amylase values are elevated on entry. The AST, LDH, and CK enzymes are usually elevated but are of no predictive significance. The electrocardiogram shows lengthening of the PR interval, delay in interventricular conduction, and a pathognomonic J wave at the junction of the QRS complex and ST segment.

Treatment

Hypothermic patients should never be considered dead until all measures for resuscitation have failed, because cardiopulmonary arrest in severe hypothermia is still compatible with some recovery.

Mild hypothermia (body temperature 32-35°C) can be treated in most cases by passive rewarming (heavy clothing and blankets in a warm environment) for a few hours, especially when the patient is shivering. The patient's temperature should be continuously monitored with a rectal or esophageal probe until body temperature reaches normal. Because the volume of intravenous fluids required for resuscitation is often substantial, their temperature can affect the outcome. Consequently, intravenous fluids should be warmed with a heat exchanger during administration.

Active rewarming is indicated for temperatures below 32°C, cardiovascular instability, or failure of passive rewarming. The methods include immersion in a warm water bath, inhalation of heated air, pleural lavage, and blood warming with an extracorporeal bypass machine. Active external rewarming is most often performed by immersion in a warm (40-42°C) water bath, which will raise body temperature at a rate of 1-2 degrees per hour. A disadvantage of this method is that the core temperature may continue to decline after initiation of the rewarming efforts (known as afterdrop), which is associated with worsening cardiovascular function.

Closed pleural irrigation should be performed by flushing the right hemithorax with warm (40-42°C) saline solution through two large thoracostomy tubes, one anterior and the other posterior. Rewarming by peritoneal lavage involves giving warm (40-45°C) crystalloid solutions, 6 L/h, which raises core temperature by 2-4 degrees per hour.

Active core rewarming with partial cardiopulmonary bypass, the most efficient technique, is indicated for patients with ventricular fibrillation and severe hypothermia or those with frozen extremities. At a flow rate of 6-7 L/min, core temperature can be raised by 1-2°C every 3-5 minutes.

In severe cases, endotracheal intubation should be used for better management of ventilation and protection against aspiration, a common lethal complication. Arterial blood gases should be monitored frequently. Bretylium tosylate in an initial dose of 10 mg/kg is the best drug for ventricular fibrillation. Antibiotics are often indicated for coexisting pneumonitis. Serious infections are often unsuspected upon admission, and delay in appropriate therapy may contribute to the severity of the illness. Hypoglycemia calls for intravenous administration of 50% glucose solution. Fluid administration must be gauged by central venous or pulmonary artery wedge pressures, urine output, and other circulatory parameters. Increased capillary permeability following rewarming predisposes to the development of pulmonary edema and compartment syndromes in the extremities. To minimize these complications, the central venous or wedge pressure should be kept below 12-14 cm water. Drugs should not be injected into peripheral tissues, because absorption will not take place while the patient is cold and because drugs may accumulate to produce serious toxicity as rewarming occurs.

As rewarming proceeds, the patient should be continually reassessed for signs of concomitant disease that may have been masked by hypothermia, especially myxedema and hypoglycemia. Any inexplicable failure to respond should suggest adrenal insufficiency.

▶ Prognosis

Survival can be expected in only 50% of patients whose core temperature drops below 32.2°C. Coexisting diseases (eg, stroke, neoplasm, myocardial infarction) are common and increase the death rate to 75% or more. Survival does not correlate closely with the lowest absolute temperature reached. Death may result from brain damage pneumonitis, heart failure, or renal insufficiency.

MULTIPLE CHOICE QUESTIONS

1. Burn severity can be informed by each of the following except

   A. Fraction of body surface area affected
   B. Patient age
   C. Presence of medical conditions
   D. Inhalation injury
   E. All of the above

2. Hypermetabolism after burn injuries

   A. Can last for 24 hours after the burn
   B. Causes an increase in muscle formation
   C. Can cause an increase in glycolysis and insulin production
   D. Can be slowed with beta-adrenergic blockade
   E. Is not catabolic and can be limited by decreased caloric intake

3. Care of the burn wound may include which of the following?

   A. Closed method occlusive dressings with twice-daily dressing changes
   B. Excision of eschar from areas of deep burn injury
   C. Exposure therapy with topical agents applied to uncovered areas of the face
   D. Temporary coverage with a skin substitute
   E. All of the above

4. Maintenance of functional motion during burn wound healing

   A. Benefits from early consideration with functional position splinting and active motion
   B. Is benefitted, in general, by the tendency of the wounds to contract
   C. Suffers after early skin grafting due to promotion of wound contracture
   D. Is easier to maintain around joints due to increased natural motion
   E. A and C

5. Respiratory compromise after burn wounds is commonly due to

   A. Early pulmonary emboli (12-36 hours after injury)
   B. Inhalational injury
   C. Cardiogenic pulmonary edema
   D. Fungal bronchitis
   E. Viral pneumonitis

Otolaryngology: Head and Neck Surgery

Joseph Zenga, MD

Michael S. Harris, MD

INTRODUCTION

From hearing loss or nasal hemorrhage to expert management of acute airway emergencies, otolaryngology–head and neck surgery is a surgical subspecialty that focuses on the management of a wide range of disorders of the head and neck. Even at the anatomical boundaries of the head and neck, otolaryngologists are frequently involved in surgical management of both benign and malignant conditions in collaborative efforts with thoracic surgeons in the cervical esophagus or superior mediastinum, ophthalmologists or oculoplastic surgeons in orbital pathology, and neurosurgeons at the skull base. The limits inherent to a single book chapter preclude covering such a broad field comprehensively. Therefore, this chapter will present an overview of selected disease processes in otolaryngology that are of importance to the general surgeon in training. Each section will focus on a specific anatomic subsite of the head and neck because each has a particular anatomy, physiology, and disease processes that make workup and management unique to that head and neck subsite. These sections will address the differential diagnosis of the most common presenting complaints seen in practice. Treatment will focus on both common disorders and urgencies and emergencies that must be recognized early and managed appropriately. Through a targeted history and physical examination, an understanding of the basic anatomy and possible differential diagnoses, and appropriate laboratory or imaging investigations, these common presenting complaints or emergent situations may be logically and efficient distilled to the underlying cause and treated appropriately. Although malignant etiologies may occur in each head and neck subsite and must often be included in the differential diagnosis, for a consistent and comprehensive discussion, the staging and management of malignant head and neck tumors are addressed separately in the final section of this chapter.

DISORDERS OF THE EAR, AUDITORY, VESTIBULAR SYSTEMS, AND TEMPORAL BONE

▶ Anatomy and Physiology

The ear consists of three anatomically distinct and functionally unique components: the external ear, the middle ear, and the inner ear. The external ear includes the auricle or pinna and the external auditory canal (EAC). The auricle's height is generally twice its width, and it projects from the lateral aspect of the head at an average of 30 degrees. The auricle is composed of elastic cartilage with tightly adherent perichondrium and overlying skin. The exception is the lobule, which lacks a cartilaginous framework. Functionally, the pinna is important for sound source amplification and localization, most notably in the vertical plane.

The EAC is a curvilinear tubal structure immediately posterior to the temporomandibular joint. The EAC is cartilaginous in its lateral third and bony in its medial two-thirds. The lateral third features hair follicles, sebaceous glands, and ceruminous glands that produce cerumen, or ear wax. Cerumen is a slightly acidic (average pH 6.1) substance with antimicrobial properties that serves to cleanse, lubricate, and protect the EAC from insects and microbial infection. Rarely, sebaceous and ceruminous glands can derive benign or malignant neoplasia. The cartilaginous portion of the anterior EAC often features subcutaneous clefts within the cartilage, known as the fissures of Santorini, representing potential paths of least resistance for spread of infection or neoplasia to or from the parotid gland. The medial two-thirds of the EAC is virtually devoid of subcutaneous tissue with skin resting directly over the underlying bone and, thus, vulnerable to trauma from instrumentation.

The tympanic membrane separates the EAC from the middle ear. The tympanic membrane is a trilaminar structure obliquely oriented with an outer squamous layer, an intermediate fibrous layer, and an inner mucosal layer. The malleus, the outermost part of the ossicles, or middle ear bones, is attached directly to the tympanic membrane, most densely at the umbo.

The middle ear, or tympanum, is a bony cleft bound laterally by the tympanic membrane, medially by the inner ear, posteriorly and inferiorly by the mastoid portion of the temporal bone, and anteriorly by the petrous portion of the internal carotid artery and the Eustachian tube orifice. The middle ear is in communication with the nasopharynx via the functionally dynamic Eustachian tube, which serves to equalize pressure between the tympanum and the external environment. Posteriorly, the middle ear communicates with the mastoid cavity via the aditus ad antrum. The middle ear contains the ossicular chain: the malleus, the incus, and the stapes, from lateral to medial. Neurovascular structures in this space, which may be variably exposed or dehiscent, include the chorda tympani nerve, conveying taste sensation from the anterior two-thirds of the ipsilateral tongue; the tympanic segment of the facial nerve (cranial nerve VII); the petrous portion of the internal carotid artery; and the jugular bulb. The middle ear is also home to the two smallest skeletal muscles in the body, the stapedius and the tensor tympani muscles.

The ear is the peripheral headquarters for the sensation of hearing and vestibular function. The conversion of rarified and condensed sounds waves in the air to liquid waves within the cochlea of the inner ear presents a unique acoustic challenge: the vast majority of energy in this transfer is lost due to the higher impedance of liquid. The external and middle ear have evolved a complex set of strategies to address this problem. Functioning as resonant amplifiers of sound energy, the concha of the auricle (Figure 16–1) has a resonance frequency—the frequency at which the response amplitude is at its relative maximum—of approximately 5 kHz, and the EAC has a resonance frequency of approximately 3.5 kHz. Combined, the external ear amplifies sound by approximately 10-15 dB in the 2- to 5-kHz range.

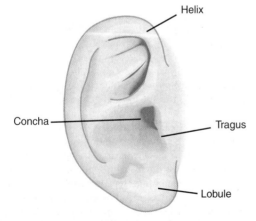

▲ **Figure 16–1.** Normal external ear anatomy.

Helix

Concha

Tragus

Lobule

The middle ear plays the most important role in the process of compensating for the impedance mismatch associated with transducing energy from air to liquid media. The mechanics of the middle ear further amplify sound energy using two predominant methods. First, the tympanic membrane is approximately 17 times larger than the footplate of the stapes, the medial interface between the ossicular chain and the inner ear; this results in proportionally greater sound pressure (ie, force per unit area) delivered to the inner ear than was initially presented to the tympanic membrane. Second, the ossicles working in concert act as a lever, providing a mechanical advantage of 1:1.3 from the tympanic membrane to the oval window. Combined, these two mechanisms result in a 25- to 30-dB gain in amplification.

The inner ear consists of the cochlea and the vestibular apparatus, the combined auditory and vestibular sensory organ. The vestibular system senses both linear acceleration (gravity) and angular acceleration (rotation). The cochlea is a coiled tube with an average of 2.5 turns that physically resembles a snail shell. Divided into three separate chambers, the scala vestibuli and the scala tympani are filled with perilymph (similar in composition to extracellular fluid), whereas the scala media is filled with endolymph (similar in composition to intracellular fluid). The endolymph composition is maintained by Na^+/K^+ ATPase pumps within the stria vascularis located on the lateral walls of the scala media. These different chambers have different electrolyte compositions, establishing a critical electrical gradient between the compartments.

Sound energy, once transferred through the ossicles to the oval window of the cochlea, is coupled directly to the perilymph of the scala vestibuli. Minute movements of the stapes footplate into the vestibule set into motion a traveling perilymph wave. The mechanical energy of the traveling wave is then converted to electrical (neural) impulses within the scala media by the organ of Corti. The organ of Corti consists of one row of inner hair cells (which are the sensory cells), three rows of outer hair cells (which function as modulators of the inner hair cells), support cells, and the tectorial membrane. The cochlea is organized tonotopically such that low-frequency sounds are transmitted from cochlear hair cells close to the base and high-frequency sounds are transmitted from hair cells close to the apex. The nerve impulses produced by the inner hair cells are transmitted to the brainstem by the acoustic portion of the eighth cranial nerve, which travels from the cochlea through the internal auditory canal.

The peripheral vestibular system consists of the utricle, saccule, and the three semicircular canals. Enveloped within the endolymphatic membrane, these structures are surrounded by perilymph and encased in a portion of the temporal bone known as the otic capsule, the hardest bone in the human body. The utricle detects horizontal acceleration, whereas the saccule detects vertical acceleration. Three semicircular canals, situated orthogonally to each other and paired with a semicircular canal on the opposite side of the head, detect angular acceleration. Linear or angular motion causes their respective sensory cells to deflect and the sensory cell bodies to depolarize. Depending on the direction, each vestibular apparatus will either increase or decrease its discharge rate relative to a basal rate, providing both direction and speed of acceleration. Vestibular information is transmitted to the brainstem by the vestibular branch of the eighth cranial nerve.

▶ Workup and Differential Diagnosis

A. Hearing Loss

There are three basic categories of hearing loss: sensorineural, conductive, and mixed. Sensorineural hearing loss is related to dysfunction or impairment of transmission of the neural impulse that is initially converted from a fluid wave within the cochlea and ultimately delivered to the brain. Common causes of sensorineural hearing loss include a host of genetic causes, noise exposure, ototoxicity, and age-related changes, or presbycusis. Conductive hearing loss describes hearing loss due to dysfunction of the mechanics of sound transmission and transduction from sound waves to the cochlea. Common examples include cerumen impaction, tympanic membrane perforation or severe tympanic membrane scarring, middle ear effusion, cholesteatoma, ossicular chain dislocation or erosion, and fixation or immobility of the stapes, known as otosclerosis. Mixed hearing loss is a combination of sensorineural hearing loss and conductive hearing loss.

History and physical examination of the patient with hearing loss provide some important indications of the type of hearing loss a patient is experiencing. The provider should inquire about prior otologic surgery or trauma, recent upper respiratory infection, and family history of hearing loss. Critically, the onset and duration of hearing loss must be well characterized because these factors have a strong bearing on diagnosis and management. Handheld otoscopy or otomicroscopy, pneumatoscopy, and tuning fork examination using a 512-Hz fork are essential components of the physical exam of a patient with hearing loss. The Weber and Rinne tests together help discern a conductive hearing loss from a sensorineural loss. The Rinne test is performed by tapping the tines of the tuning fork on a surface such as the examiner's elbow and placing the stem of the fork firmly on the mastoid process behind the ear (testing bone conduction). The patient is asked to indicate when the tone is no longer audible in this position, and then the fork is moved off of the mastoid and the tines are held lateral to the EAC (testing air conduction); if the tone is still audible in this position, then the patient is hearing better through air conduction. The Weber test involves placing the stem of the tuning fork on the forehead or the nasal bones and asking the patient to indicate whether the tone is louder in one ear than the other or if they are equal. If the Weber lateralizes to the side that the Rinne indicated heard better or equally through bone conduction, a conductive hearing loss is indicated; if the Weber lateralizes to the side where air conduction was greater than bone conduction, a sensorineural hearing loss on the opposite side is indicated.

Air and bone conduction audiometry and speech discrimination testing are objective measures of hearing status performed by an audiologist. An audiogram reflects a patient's type of hearing loss (ie, sensorineural, conductive, or mixed) and its configuration (ie, high frequency, low frequency, pan-frequency, or a "cookie bite" pattern, often suggestive of congenital sensorineural hearing loss), symmetry, and overall severity. When available, it is imperative to compare prior audiograms to current assessments to characterize hearing loss of any type as stable, improved, progressive, or fluctuant.

As noted, establishing the time frame of hearing loss is essential because this often dictates workup and management. The sudden onset of unilateral, or less commonly bilateral, sensorineural hearing loss is a phenomenon reported to occur at an annual incidence of 5-20 cases per 100,000 persons. Sudden sensorineural hearing loss (SSHL) is a uniquely unsettling experience for patients, who are generally completely unequipped and unprepared for such a deficit (ie, no alternative communication strategies or experience with hearing loss). Current guidelines define SSHL as greater than or equal to a 30-dB hearing loss occurring over 3 days or less. The prevailing understanding of SSHL relates to microvascular compromise and inflammatory changes of the cochlea or the cochlear nerve associated with viral infection (particularly herpes family viruses), trauma, thromboembolic phenomena or vasospasm, autoimmune disease, or ototoxicity (eg, chemotherapy, antibiotics, or salicylates).

Early recognition of SSHL is imperative because timely onset of treatment maximizes prognosis for recovery of hearing. Because of the multitude of potential mechanisms, a careful history should be elicited. Details such as intense antecedent noise exposure, recent upper respiratory infection, or thromboembolic phenomenon may suggest an underlying etiology. Often, however, a clear cause or inciting factor is not apparent. Patients should be questioned about coincident tinnitus (ie, ringing in the ears) and imbalance or vertiginous symptoms, which are indicative of vestibular as well as auditory pathology.

Workup and evaluation of SSHL begins with puretone audiometry and speech discrimination testing. If the patient reports vestibular or balance symptoms, investigation of the vestibular system should be performed. The Dix-Hallpike maneuver and the head thrust test are two brief, easy-to-perform bedside tests for vertigo that evaluate for positional vestibulopathy and the integrity of the vestibulo-ocular reflex, respectively. Simple tests of the auditory system

Table 16–1. Weber and Rinne tuning fork tests.

Condition	Weber	Rinne
Left sensorineural hearing loss	Louder on *right*	A > B bilaterally
Left conductive hearing loss	Louder on *left*	A > B on right A = B or A < B on left
Normal hearing	Midline/no difference	A > B bilaterally

In the **Weber** test, the tuning fork is struck and applied in the midline to the skull or teeth. This stimulates both cochlea by direct bone conduction. The patient is asked whether he or she hears the sound the same on both sides or whether it is louder on one side.

In the **Rinne** test, a tuning fork is struck and held by the auricle (condition "A," air conduction). Sound is conducted through the ossicular chain and to the cochlea. The fork is then applied to the mastoid tip, and acoustic energy is transmitted to the cochlea by direct bone conduction (condition "B," bone conduction). The patient is then asked which is louder, A or B. In a normal-hearing ear, A (air) is greater than B (bone). In sensorineural hearing loss, A will still be greater than B. In conductive hearing loss, A = B or even B > A.

(Weber and Rinne tests) can also be performed at the bedside using a 512-Hz tuning fork and help differentiate conductive from sensorineural hearing loss (Table 16–1).

Diagnostic workup for SSHL should include evaluation for a vestibular schwannoma (discussed in detail later), because this represents approximately 1%-3% of the SSHL. The gold standard evaluation for a vestibular schwannoma is gadolinium-enhanced magnetic resonance imaging (MRI) of the internal auditory canal. If there is a family history of sudden hearing loss, a computed tomography (CT) scan looking for an enlarged vestibular aqueduct should be obtained. Current guidelines on SSHL recommend against routinely obtaining laboratory studies in the setting of SSHL. If other historical elements or physical exam findings raise specific suspicion, complete blood count (CBC) with differential, erythrocyte sedimentation rate (ESR), prothrombin time/partial thromboplastin time, syphilis testing (either microhemagglutination *Treponema pallidum* [MHA-TP] or fluorescent treponemal antibody absorption [FTA-Abs]), or thyroid function tests may be useful.

Current guidelines strongly recommend empirically beginning high-dose corticosteroid therapy as the first-line treatment for SSHL. Oral prednisolone and prednisone are the best studied regimens, with the preponderance of data supporting high-dose (60 mg daily) treatment for 7-14 days followed by a taper over 5 days. In patients unable to take oral steroids (eg, labile diabetics or patients who poorly tolerated steroids in the past), intratympanic injection of buffered dexamethasone may be provided, whereby steroid delivered into the middle ear through the tympanic membrane diffuses into the inner ear through the round window membrane.

With the prevailing understanding that SSHL is related to a viral insult, coadministration of antiviral medications such as acyclovir has been studied, and some studies suggest an added benefit when given alongside high-dose steroids. Guidelines recommend against antivirals, however, as stand-alone therapy.

The prognosis for spontaneous recovery of function in SSHL is hopeful because approximately 60% of patients will recover full or partial hearing. Although the time frame is not well understood, recovery usually occurs within a month of onset. With corticosteroid treatment, the recovery rate may increase to 80%, according to some studies. Even in the context of fully salvaged hearing, with or without therapy, an MRI to rule out a vestibular schwannoma is strongly recommended because recovery does not preclude the possibility of retrocochlear pathology (ie, vestibular schwannoma). In situations where hearing loss persists or recovery is incomplete, hearing rehabilitation strategies may include acoustic amplification using conventional hearing aids, strategies for single-sided deafness such as contralateral routing of signal (CROS) systems, or cochlear implantation, depending on the degree of debility.

B. Facial Nerve Weakness

The seventh cranial nerve (facial nerve) innervates the muscles of facial expression as well as special motor afferents to the parotid and lacrimal glands. A careful history will help define the onset of paralysis (eg, acute deterioration over less than 2-3 days versus gradual decline). Antecedent events such as temporal bone trauma or recent acute otitis media (AOM), hearing loss or imbalance, or viral illness should be elicited and can help guide further workup and management.

Potential causes of acute facial nerve paralysis are numerous; however, over 50% are idiopathic and termed *Bell palsy*. Note that Bell palsy is a diagnosis of exclusion, and therefore, a focused but complete workup must be performed. Fully 20% of facial nerve paralyses are caused by trauma. Other common causes (but by no means an exhaustive list) include herpes zoster oticus (Ramsey Hunt syndrome), complications from otitis media and mastoiditis, Lyme disease, cholesteatoma, and neoplasm.

A complete physical examination with emphasis on the neurologic system and cranial nerves is critical. A distinction should be made between weakness (paresis) as opposed to complete lack of motion (paralysis). Several grading systems have been proposed to track recovery and facilitate communication among providers; the House-Brackmann scale is the most widely used and is presented in Table 16–2. Using this scheme, facial nerve function is graded from I (normal) to VI (total paralysis) for each side.

It is imperative to note and address ipsilateral eyelid function. Facial paresis or paralysis leads to inability to close the upper eyelid (opening of the eyelid is performed by the third

Table 16–2. House-Brackmann facial nerve paralysis scale.

Grade	Characteristics
I (Normal)	Normal function in all branches
II (Mild dysfunction)	Slight weakness to visual inspection Normal symmetry and tone at rest Forehead: moderate to good function Eye: complete closure, minimal effort Mouth: slight asymmetry
III (Moderate dysfunction)	Mild difference to gross inspection between sides Normal symmetry and tone at rest Forehead: slight to moderate movement Eye: compete closure, requires effort Mouth: slightly weak, requires effort
IV (Moderately severe dysfunction)	Obvious weakness to gross inspection between sides Normal symmetry and tone at rest Forehead: no motion even with effort Eye: incomplete closure even with effort Mouth: asymmetric with maximum effort
V (Severe dysfunction)	Only barely perceptible motion to gross inspection Asymmetry at rest Forehead: no motion even with effort Eye: incomplete closure even with effort Mouth: slight movement even with maximum effort
VI (total paralysis)	No movement

cranial nerve), impaired tear production, and an incomplete Bell phenomenon or palpebral oculogyric reflex (upward and outward rotation of the eyeball with eyelid closure). Impairment of these functions may lead to corneal drying, exposure keratitis, and irreversible vision loss. Frequent administration of artificial tear drops throughout waking hours, hydrating ophthalmic ointment at bedtime, and upper eyelid taping or use of a humidification chamber are strategies to protect the cornea when it is exposed. The care provider should inquire about foreign body sensation, eye pain, and vision loss and have a low threshold for referral to ophthalmology.

Another important consideration in evaluating the patient with acute facial nerve paralysis is distinguishing between central and peripheral lesions. In central lesions, associated with cerebrovascular accident (CVA), there is sparing of forehead elevation on the affected side due to decussating fibers from the contralateral side. In peripheral lesions, the fibers have already crossed, and there is no forehead sparing. The presence of other neurologic impairments, ipsilateral extremity weakness, and speech changes also raises suspicion for CVA over idiopathic acute facial paralysis.

Current guidelines for the workup and evaluation of Bell palsy recommend against routine laboratory testing or neuroimaging if the history and physical exam are not otherwise suggestive of an alternative process. In the presence of history or findings indicative of other etiologies, laboratory studies may include CBC with differential, ESR, C-reactive protein, autoimmune serologies, or Lyme titers. The natural history of Bell palsy is recovery of facial function within 3 or 4 months. If weakness or paralysis does not improve within this time frame or if there is relapse or progression of weakness, imaging is indicated. This may include MRI capturing the entire course of the facial nerve from its origin at the pontomedullary junction, through its circuitous course within the temporal bone, to its point of exit from the skull base at the stylomastoid foramen and into the substance of the ipsilateral parotid gland. In other clinical contexts featuring acute facial paralysis, high-resolution CT of the temporal bone may be the imaging study of choice for evaluating bony changes (ie, from mastoiditis, temporal bone trauma, cholesteatoma, or neoplasm).

If facial nerve paralysis is caused by traumatic injury, management depends on the onset of paralysis; immediate and complete paralysis will often benefit from surgical decompression. In delayed or partial dysfunction, spontaneous recovery is likely and surgical intervention may not be beneficial. For idiopathic paralysis (Bell palsy), initial medical therapy is targeted to reducing inflammation and targeting a possible viral etiology. A corticosteroid course should be initiated, either prednisone or prednisolone. Similar to SSHL, guidelines on the management of acute idiopathic facial paralysis recommend against antivirals as monotherapy but list combination therapy with high-dose steroids and antivirals as an option.

Some surgeons offer surgical decompression for appropriately selected Bell palsy patients. The best-known protocol for facial nerve decompression selects for patient with a complete facial paralysis who present within an early time frame (days 3 to 14) and meet certain electrophysiologic test criteria using electroneurography (ENoG) and electromyography (EMG). Greater than 90% degeneration on ENoG and absence of voluntary motor potentials on EMG portend a poor prognosis for recovery. Therefore, some surgeons offer patients fitting this profile the option of facial nerve decompression via a middle cranial fossa approach in addition to medical therapy. Appropriate surgical expertise must be available, and the patient must be appropriately apprised of the associated surgical risks and natural history of Bell palsy.

C. Ear Drainage

Ear drainage, or otorrhea, may be a feature of several otologic conditions. The differential diagnosis may include otitis externa, otitis media with a tympanic membrane perforation, cholesteatoma, EAC or middle ear malignancy, or cerebrospinal fluid leakage. The duration of otorrhea, recent head trauma or surgery, and appearance of the drainage, including its color, odor, and consistency, are important to consider, in addition to the presence of other infectious signs or symptoms.

Otitis externa (OE) is diffuse infection of the EAC that features otorrhea. It may be acute or chronic (≥ 3 months in duration). The most commonly isolated bacterial species in acute OE are *Pseudomonas aeruginosa* and *Staphylococcus aureus*, with a broader host of microbes implicated in chronic OE, including *Klebsiella, Streptococcus, Enterobacter,* and fungal species, in particular *Aspergillus* and *Candida.*

Evaluation and management of patients with suspected OE include a complete history and physical examination with emphasis on the otologic assessment. Patients will often give a history of recent water exposure, such as from swimming. Hearing aid use is another common predisposing factor because an occluded EAC traps moisture and impairs normal cerumen egress. Inquiry should be made into dermatologic disorders, allergic reactions, and inflammatory skin conditions. History of such often leads to pruritis and EAC instrumentation (eg, aggressive scratching or cotton swab use) that predispose to canal trauma, infection, or poor wound healing.

Examination of the patient with OE begins with inspection and palpation. Gentle manipulation of the pinna and tragus usually elicits exquisite pain. In otitis media, by contrast, this maneuver should not elicit pain. Otoscopy will reveal the canal wall as diffusely erythematous and edematous, often severe enough to preclude visualization of the tympanic membrane. In this case, insertion of a lubricated otowick is necessary to deliver ototopical medications the length of the EAC past the obstructed site.

Treatment of OE in severe cases may require frequent suction debridement under microscopic visualization. Patients should be placed on ototopical antibiotic drops containing a topical corticosteroid, such as ciprofloxacin 0.3%/dexamethasone 0.1% suspension (Ciprodex). Some physicians allow the use of hydrocortisone 1%/polymyxin/neomycin (Cortisporin) as an alternative. This is not recommended for several reasons. First, several authors have demonstrated up to 10% risk of contact dermatitis with polymyxin/neomycin ototopical drops. Second, if a possibility of tympanic membrane perforation exists, these drops carry the possibility of ototoxicity, according to laboratory studies in animals; they are not approved for use in the middle ear (unlike fluoroquinolones). In addition, some studies have demonstrated faster pain relief with Ciprodex compared to Cortisporin. It is essential to note that failure to respond to appropriate therapy within 48-72 hours should prompt the clinician to reassess the patient to confirm a diagnosis of OE.

Malignant OE is severe form of OE, most often seen in elderly patients with poorly controlled diabetes mellitus or other forms of immunosuppression or compromise. *P aeruginosa* predominates in malignant OE. Otalgia and otorrhea, recalcitrant to initial ototopical therapy, are often reported. Otoscopic exam frequently reveals copious granulation tissue along the floor of the EAC at the bony cartilaginous junction. This tissue should be biopsied in intractable cases to rule out an EAC malignancy, most commonly squamous cell carcinoma. Treatment for malignant OE will usually involve combination therapy with an ototopical fluoroquinolone, ototopical corticosteroid, and oral or intravenous (IV) fluoroquinolone therapy. Engagement of internal medicine colleagues is often helpful to bring comorbidities and predisposing factors (ie, hyperglycemia) under strict control. Frequent cleaning and debridement in the clinic or bedside are a cornerstone of management of malignant OE, but surgical intervention is rarely required.

Otomycosis is OE due to a fungal infection, usually due to *Aspergillus* or *Candida* species. On otoscopy, there is usually far less edema and erythema than with bacterial infection. Spores or fungal elements are often readily apparent. The use of ototopical antibiotic solutions will not improve the condition in these patients and usually worsens their condition. Otomycosis can be notoriously difficult to treat, but many cases do respond to serial suction debridement followed by acidic eardrops to reestablish the acid-base milieu. A commonly used topical preparation is acetic acid 2% with hydrocortisone 1% (Vosol HC). Alternative ototopicals include treatment with gentian violet and corticosteroids. Topical antifungals such as nystatin or amphotericin B are also available, but use of these should be reserved for difficult cases.

▶ Treatment

A. Foreign Bodies in the External Auditory Canal

The majority of cases of foreign bodies in the EAC occur in children or mentally impaired adults. Many otologic foreign bodies, if carefully selected, are amenable to removal under direct visualization in an emergency department or primary care office setting. In a large series of over 600 cases of ear foreign bodies, Shulze and colleagues found an overall 77% success rate for the removal under direct visualization by emergency physicians. It is important to note that the majority of those foreign bodies successfully removed in this manner fit the category of "soft, irregular" material, such as paper or cotton, and "pliable or rubber-like" material, such as silly putty or erasers. Success with hard objects and especially spherical objects, such as plastic beads, was markedly lower. Thus, an argument can be made for a single attempt by the pediatrician or emergency physician under direct visualization, if the object meets the former criteria. This should be tempered, however, with the understanding that complication rates are much higher with removal under direct vision. Complications of foreign body removal most commonly include canal wall lacerations (47%), with tympanic membrane perforations being less common (4%). When initial foreign body removal is performed instead by the otolaryngologist using binocular otomicroscopy, either in the office or operative setting, the complication rate is quite low (6.3%).

Foreign body removal using binocular otomicroscopy is the primary method used by most otolaryngologists. Specific techniques depend on the characteristics of the foreign body. Objects with sharp edges can often be grasped with alligator or duck-bill forceps. Soft objects are often amenable to removal with otologic suction. Removal of spherical and hard, irregular objects requires more finesse. In these cases, a 90-degree probe is invaluable. The probe is carefully guided behind the object under binocular otomicroscopic visualization. Then the probe is rotated along its axis to bring the end behind the object, and it is guided out of the EAC.

Extraction of insects, notably cockroaches, from the EAC poses a unique challenge. This can be quite alarming to the patient if the insect is still alive and its movement is audible. The proximity of the insect to the tympanic membrane translates movement of the insect to distressingly loud perceived sound levels. In such cases, the EAC can be gently irrigated with either mineral oil or lidocaine to suffocate the insect, followed by prompt extraction.

Some non-otolaryngologist providers advocate the use of gentle irrigation to attempt dislodgement of EAC foreign bodies. This technique can be used successfully but requires caution. First, if there is any suspicion of tympanic membrane perforation, irrigation is contraindicated because it could flush debris into the middle ear space and is likely to induce vertigo. Second, if the foreign body is composed of vegetable material (eg, a popcorn kernel), irrigation should be avoided. If the object is not successfully flushed out, subsequent swelling of the vegetable foreign body can result in extreme pain as the EAC skin is compressed against the bony canal. Removal once this occurs can be problematic and may require general anesthesia and the use of an operating microscope. For this reason, otologic medications are also contraindicated in vegetable material otologic foreign bodies. The third condition where irrigation (and otologic medications) is specifically contraindicated is in the case of button batteries in the EAC.

Although the previously described foreign bodies can be managed on an outpatient basis, the finding of a button battery in the EAC is considered an emergent situation, requiring immediate removal by an otolaryngologist. If left in place for any length of time, batteries in the EAC can result in severe complications. In an early description of this problem by Kavanagh and coauthors, 100% of patients experienced multiple, serious sequelae. These included tympanic membrane perforation or total destruction (75%), marked dermal destruction with bone exposure (88%), impairment of hearing (38%), ossicular chain erosion (25%), and even facial nerve paralysis (13%). Both leakage of corrosive battery acid and electrical current discharge resulting in chlorine gas and sodium hydroxide by electrolysis have been hypothesized

to contribute to the destructive effects of button batteries. Removal is accomplished under binocular otomicroscopy in the operating room and sometimes requires piecemeal removal of the battery. Following removal of the battery, the EAC should be flushed with copious amounts of saline, and careful inspection of the external canal and tympanic membrane should be performed.

A cholesteatoma is a cyst-like, expansile lesion of the temporal bone consisting of stratified squamous epithelium and trapped desquamated keratin. It occurs in the pneumatized temporal bone, most commonly the middle ear and mastoid (Figure 16–2). There are two types of cholesteatoma, acquired and congenital, with the former being the most common. Acquired cholesteatomas arise from either retraction pockets within the tympanic membrane or secondarily from a tympanic membrane perforation. Congenital cholesteatomas are thought to arise from epithelial cell rests that fail to undergo apoptosis during development. Whatever the origin, once formed, cholesteatomas behave in a locally destructive manner. Bone erosion is common, especially of the ossicular chain, but also potentially the bone surrounding the inner ear (the otic capsule). If left untreated, cholesteatomas can even invade intracranially through erosion of the tegmen tympani or tegmen mastoideum.

▲ **Figure 16–2.** Cholesteatoma of the left middle ear. Large arrowhead indicates the external ear canal. Note the soft tissue density (cholesteatoma) in the middle ear space and the absence of any visible ossicular chain. Part of the bony covering of the inner ear semicircular canal (the otic capsule) has also been eroded.

Early cholesteatomas have few, if any, symptoms and usually start with a slowly progressive conductive hearing loss. If an infection develops in a cholesteatoma, foul otorrhea will develop, which is often the presenting symptom. If a cholesteatoma is suspected, careful inspection under binocular otomicroscopy is essential. All debris must be removed to allow a full visualization of the entire visible portion of the tympanic membrane. Cholesteatomas will appear as a whitish keratin mass. A pneumatic otoscopy test is essential; if vertigo is elicited, the surgeon must suspect erosion into the inner ear structures.

The treatment for cholesteatoma is surgery, usually involving removal of the mastoid air cell septations by otologic drill, exposing the middle ear space. This accomplishes two goals—providing safe visualization and access and removal of all cholesteatoma tissue. This procedure is performed under careful microscopic visualization because as many important structures (eg, the facial nerve and the inner ear) should be preserved as possible. The primary goal of surgery is creation of a safe, dry ear. All other considerations, including preservation of hearing, take second place.

B. Otitis Media

A collection of common infectious and noninfectious middle ear pathologies include the root term *otitis media*. A tremendous healthcare and societal burden is imposed by this group of conditions, in large part associated with missed school and work. AOM represents what is commonly referred to as a "middle ear infection." The typical patient is a young child, with history of upper respiratory tract symptoms, fever, and fussiness. Otoscopy will reveal a bulging, erythematous tympanic membrane. Distension of the intact tympanic membrane accounts for the pain associated with AOM. Unlike OE (discussed earlier), there is no pain with manipulation of the auricle or tragus. The predominant pathogens responsible for AOM include the bacteria *Streptococcus*, *Haemophilus*, and *Moraxella*.

Current guidelines developed by the American Academy of Otolaryngology and the American Academy of Pediatrics guide management of AOM in children ages 6 months to 12 years. A strong recommendation is issued for immediate treatment of pain associated with AOM, primarily using nonsteroidal anti-inflammatory drug (NSAID) therapy. Either oral antibiotic therapy or an initial period of observation may be offered in cases of nonsevere unilateral AOM in children age 6 months to 23 months or in cases of nonsevere, unilateral or bilateral AOM in children age 24 months or older. The caveat in electing for a period of observation is that a mechanism must exist to ensure follow-up within 48 to 72 hours should symptoms persist or progress. Upfront oral antibiotic therapy is recommended for bilateral AOM without severe signs or symptoms in children age 6 months through 23 months. Likewise, oral antibiotic therapy is recommended for bilateral or unilateral AOM in children age 6 months and

older with a temperature of 39°C (102.2°F) or higher or moderate or severe otalgia or otalgia persisting beyond 48 hours. Amoxicillin is the recommended first-line therapy, with amoxicillin/clavulanic acid (Augmentin) serving as the initial escalation therapy. Exceptions to first-line therapy include if the patient has taken amoxicillin in the past 30 days, if there is history of an allergic reaction to this class of medications, or if there is a history of AOM recalcitrant to amoxicillin. Finally, a recommendation is provided against routine prophylactic antibiotics to reduce the frequency of episodes of AOM, even in the setting of recurrent AOM. Otolaryngologists may consider offering myringotomy with tympanostomy tube placement for recurrent AOM, defined as three episodes in 6 months or four episodes in 1 year with one episode in the preceding 6 months. Once tympanostomy tubes are in place, future episodes of AOM can be treated with ototopical drops instead of systemic oral antibiotic therapy.

Otitis media with effusion (OME) is defined as fluid in the middle ear without signs of infection. OME commonly results from Eustachian tube dysfunction in both children and adults. Impaired equalization of pressure in the tympanum with the external environment leads to generation of negative pressure in this closed space, thus promoting transudation of fluid from surrounding mucosa and, when more severe, retraction of the tympanic membrane into the middle ear. OME is especially common in young children, with a prevalence approaching 30% according to some reports. Patients with OME may present with complaints of muffled or decreased hearing, aural fullness, and using a softer than normal voice, because this attenuates the reverberant quality of one's own voice (in contrast to sensorineural hearing loss, where patients compensate with a louder than normal voice). Otoscopy reveals serous fluid in the middle ear cleft. Chronic serous otitis media results when middle ear fluid after an episode of AOM fails to clear after a 4- to 6-weeks period.

Management of OME in children is also supported by a set of guidelines developed by the American Academy of Otolaryngology. Pneumatic otoscopy, which involves introducing a puff of air into the EAC via a modified otoscope, is recommended as the initial diagnostic maneuver for OME. When motion of the tympanic membrane is not visualized (the normal response), tympanometry, an audiometric assessment of middle ear pressure and tympanic membrane motion, is recommended. Children with OME who are at risk for speech, language, or learning problems associated with comorbid conditions with sensory, physical, or cognitive sequelae should be promptly evaluated for hearing, speech, and language delays and deficits. An initial 3-month period of observation is recommended for children with OME who are not at increased risk for speech, language, or learning problems. Hearing testing should be performed in the setting of OME lasting 3 months or longer or at any time if language delay, learning problems, or a significant hearing loss is suspected. Follow-up should be ensured at 3- to 6-months intervals until the effusion is resolved, significant hearing loss is identified, or structural abnormalities of the eardrum or middle ear are suspected. Presence of any of these features is an indication for myringotomy with tympanostomy tube placement by an otolaryngologist. Oral antibiotics, decongestants, and antihistamines are not recommended in the management of OME.

C. Vestibular Schwannoma

Vestibular schwannoma (historically referred to by the misnomer *acoustic neuroma*) is a nonmalignant neoplastic proliferation of Schwann cells ensheathing the vestibular components of the eighth cranial nerve. Vestibular schwannoma represents nearly 10% of all intracranial tumors and approximately 90% of tumors of the internal auditory canal and cerebellopontine angle (CPA). Vestibular schwannomas most often present with unilateral high-frequency sensorineural hearing loss, asymmetric nonpulsatile tinnitus, and/ or dysequilibrium (vertigo, or room-spinning dizziness, is far less common). Asymmetric speech discrimination out of proportion to the degree of asymmetric hearing loss indicated by pure-tone audiometry is a hallmark finding of vestibular schwannoma. As noted earlier in the discussion of SSHL, approximately 1%-3% of patients with this entity will have a vestibular schwannoma; conversely, 10%-20% of patient with vestibular schwannomas will present with SSHL. Therefore, neuroimaging is imperative in this context. In the case of larger tumors, patients can sometimes present with facial numbness or paresthesia (from impingement on the fifth cranial nerve), weakness of facial muscles (from seventh nerve involvement), or headache (from ventricular effacement, obstructive hydrocephalus, and brainstem compression).

When tracked longitudinally for 1 year from the time of initial presentation, approximately 50% of vestibular schwannomas demonstrate no growth. The majority of the remaining 50% demonstrate growth on the order of 1 mm over this interval. A smaller proportion of the subset will grow more rapidly. One important syndrome associated with vestibular schwannomas is neurofibromatosis type 2 (NF2). NF2 is transmitted in an autosomal dominant fashion and is linked to mutations in the *NF2* gene located at 22q12.2 of chromosome 22. Bilateral vestibular schwannomas are pathognomonic for NF2. Other common lesions associated with NF2 include intracranial and spinal meningiomas, gliomas, neurofibromas, and posterior subcapsular lenticular opacities and cataracts.

Presumptive diagnosis of vestibular schwannoma is made by MRI with gadolinium contrast of the internal auditory canal and CPA. Schwannomas enhance avidly on T1- or T2-weighted images with gadolinium. The differential diagnosis for vestibular schwannomas of the internal auditory canal and CPA includes meningiomas, epidermoid tumors, arachnoid cyst lesions, and metastases; neuroimaging characteristics and clinical presentation usually readily differentiate these entities from each other. All patients with suspected vestibular schwannomas should have audiometric testing (pure-tone averages and speech discrimination scores) to characterize the degree to which they need or may benefit from hearing rehabilitation strategies because this will strongly influence management decisions.

Multiple factors are considered in the management of vestibular schwannomas. These include tumor factors, such as tumor location and size (eg, confined to the internal auditory canal, extending into the CPA, or displacing the brainstem); patient factors (personal predilections, age, overall health, and comorbidities); and degree and type of symptomatology (eg, hearing status, vestibular status, headache). The conventional armamentarium for vestibular schwannomas includes observation with serial neuroimaging and audiometry, stereotactic radiosurgery (eg, Gamma Knife, CyberKnife), and microsurgical resection. Many authors advocate that small schwannomas confined to the internal auditory canal can be successfully watched via serial imaging performed between 6 and 12 months after initial identification. Tumors demonstrating no growth (< 2 mm) can continue to be watched, whereas most authors would argue for intervention if growth greater than 2 mm occurs. A considerable amount of practice center variability and controversy exists around the issue of when microsurgical resection versus stereotactic radiosurgery is most appropriate. The authors advocate for a collaborative approach among otolaryngologists, neurosurgeons, and radiation oncologists in the care of patients with vestibular schwannoma. Observation, microsurgical resection, and stereotactic radiosurgery are all associated with significant risks including facial nerve weakness or paralysis (temporary or permanent), hearing loss (partial or complete), vertigo (typically transient with some long-term disequilibrium), tumor recurrence, headache, and, with large tumors, lower cranial neuropathies. Modern multidisciplinary teams weigh the likelihood of these risks in the specific context of their patient to maximize potential for tumor resection or control and to minimize the probability of associated morbidity and long-term functional debility.

D. Vertigo and Dizziness

Dizziness is an extremely common phenomenon with a tremendous impact on quality of life. An important distinction should be made between various sensations commonly described by patients as "dizziness." For patients describing dizziness symptoms, an attempt to elicit a more accurate description should always be sought. Vertigo is specifically defined as the illusion of rotation. This should be distinguished from sensations of imbalance or unsteadiness or of almost losing consciousness (presyncope). Regardless of the descriptor, it is important to be mindful of the fact that vertigo, dizziness, and disequilibrium are symptoms, rather than diagnoses, and an attempt should be made to identify an underlying etiology. It is also critical to acknowledge that one's sense of balance is informed by three streams of information to the brain: vision, proprioception, and the peripheral vestibular apparatuses. Comorbid conditions affecting visual acuity or depth perception, lower extremity joint disease or peripheral neuropathy, and cervical spine issues affecting coordinated neck motion can contribute or complicate dizziness related to any etiology. Finally, recognizing and minimizing the risk of falls in patients with dizziness are paramount because falls constitute a major source of associated morbidity.

Benign paroxysmal positional vertigo (BPPV) is the most common cause of acute-onset vertigo. Patients will describe sudden onset of intense vertigo lasting seconds rather than minutes, usually brought on by changes in head or body position relative to gravity. Co-occurring otologic symptoms such as aural fullness, hearing loss, tinnitus, or otalgia are features of BPPV. There is sometimes an associated history of head trauma or labyrinthitis. The etiology of BPPV is thought to be due to dislocation of microcrystals of calcium hydroxyapatite (otoconia) from the vestibule into the semicircular canals, most often the posterior canal. Certain head movements cause the otoconia to abnormally trigger deflection of the cupula, the neurosensory bundle that sends neural impulses to the vestibular nerve, eliciting imbalanced vestibular input to the brainstem and thus triggering intense vertigo.

Diagnosis of posterior canal BPPV is made by bedside positional testing, most commonly the Dix-Hallpike maneuver. In this test, the patient's head is turned to one side and the patient is laid into a recumbent position with the head maintained in the rotated position. Elicitation of vertigo, often accompanied by the expected rotatory nystagmus, essentially confirms the diagnosis.

Guidelines on management of BPPV through the American Academy of Otolaryngology strongly support the use of particle-repositioning techniques such as the Epley maneuver. These maneuvers are designed to rotate the otoconia through the semicircular canal, depositing them back in a more physiologic location within the vestibule. Often several treatments are required, and patients can be instructed in the self-application of these maneuvers. A strong recommendation is made against routine use of vestibular suppressants including first-generation antihistamines, benzodiazepines, or anticholinergics for BPPV, because these medications are unlikely to help and do serve as an independent risk factor for falls.

Ménière disease is characterized by waxing and waning monaural sensorineural hearing loss (typically low frequency more than high), intense episodes of vertigo, sensation of unilateral aural fullness, and roaring tinnitus in the same ear. Hearing loss typically follows an episodic but slowly progressive course, with times of worse hearing followed by partial recovery. The hearing loss (and vestibular dysfunction) is most commonly unilateral, although bilateral disease can develop. The vertigo attacks associated with Ménière disease can be debilitating and are often accompanied by nausea,

vomiting, and inability to perform normal activities. Diagnosis of Ménière disease is made based on clinical presence of the tetrad of symptoms, combined with audiometric evidence of hearing loss. The episodic nature of the disease is an important characteristic; a single episode of hearing loss and vertigo does not constitute a diagnosis of Ménière disease.

The pathogenesis of Ménière disease remains incompletely understood. The prevailing theory relates to dilation of the membranous labyrinth, possibly from dysfunction within the endolymphatic sac. Anatomic cadaver studies have demonstrated endolymphatic hydrops (swelling of the scala media and endolymphatic sac) in patients with Ménière disease. Unfortunately, these anatomic changes have also been demonstrated in presumably normal (asymptomatic) patients.

The mainstay of treatment for Ménière disease remains medical therapy. Patients are typically begun on a low-sodium diet (target of < 1500 mg/d). Avoidance of caffeine and nicotine and stress reduction are also commonly recommended, although supportive data are limited. In patients who remain symptomatic, hydrochlorothiazide/triamterene (Dyazide, Maxzide) is initiated, typically 37.5/25 mg once per day in the morning. An oral steroid taper is occasionally used to break a cycle of severe attacks. During episodes of vertigo, vestibular suppressants such as meclizine have temporizing utility, but these are not to be taken daily or as preventative measures.

When conservative medication management is inadequate to bring Ménière disease under control, more invasive interventions are discussed. Many authors advocate unilateral chemical ablation of the vestibular system. This can be accomplished nonsurgically by transtympanic injection of gentamicin. Although gentamicin injection is efficacious for vertigo resolution, it is associated with sensorineural hearing loss in up to 25% of patients. For patients with intact hearing, many experts feel endolymphatic sac decompression and shunting can offer significant relief with preservation of hearing, although this remains unproven in randomized controlled trials. An alternative technique for patients with intact hearing is vestibular neurectomy. Vestibular neurectomy involves selective sectioning of the vestibular branch of the eighth cranial nerve and is accomplished by accessing the nerves via a middle cranial fossa craniotomy or retrolabyrinthine approach. For patients with severe hearing loss and vertigo, a total transmastoid labyrinthectomy relieves vertigo in over 90% of patients, at the cost of complete hearing loss on the affected side.

DISORDERS OF THE NOSE AND PARANASAL SINUSES

▶ Anatomy and Physiology

The nose and paranasal sinuses serve to warm, filter, and humidify inspired air; to modulate vocalizations and speech; and to provide for the sense of smell. The external nose

▲ **Figure 16–3.** Sinonasal anatomy. In this coronal plane CT scan, several key sinonasal landmarks can be seen. M, maxillary sinus; IT, inferior turbinate; MT, middle turbinate; im, inferior meatus; mm, middle meatus; arrowhead indicates nasal septum.

consists of soft tissue and skin resting on a largely cartilaginous framework. The internal nose (nasal cavity) begins at the nasal vestibule anteriorly and extends posteriorly to the choana (which forms the boundary between the nasal cavity and the nasopharynx).

The nasal cavity (Figure 16–3) is divided in the sagittal plane in largely symmetric halves by the nasal septum. These cavities are partially filled by the three turbinates (superior, middle, and inferior, and occasionally a fourth supreme turbinate), which arise from the lateral nasal wall. The spaces below each turbinate are called meati (eg, superior meatus, middle meatus, and inferior meatus). These meati are important for localizing the outflow tracts of the various paranasal sinuses, which drain in a characteristic pattern. The nasolacrimal duct drains into the inferior meatus. The maxillary, frontal, and anterior ethmoid sinuses all drain into the middle meatus. The sphenoid sinus and posterior ethmoids drain into the superior meatus. Additionally, the olfactory nerve endings (the end organ for the sense of smell) are located on the superior nasal septum and superior turbinate mucosa.

The paranasal sinuses consist of hollow cavities that derive from pneumatization into the frontal, ethmoid, sphenoid, and maxillary bones of the craniofacial skeleton. They are lined with respiratory epithelium (pseudostratified ciliated columnar epithelium), which serves to circulate and drain mucus along with entrapped particulate matter. They are normally air filled but can become fluid filled if the ostia become obstructed by inflammation, anatomic abnormalities, or disease processes.

▶ Workup and Differential Diagnosis

A. Epistaxis

Epistaxis is hemorrhage from the nasal cavity or paranasal sinuses, which may drain anteriorly out the nose or posteriorly through the nasopharynx into the pharynx. The nasal cavity has two main blood supplies, the sphenopalatine artery posteriorly and the Kiesselbach plexus anteriorly, and either may be the source of hemorrhage. Important elements of the history include duration and severity of bleeding, a predominant side, and whether blood runs from the nose or is expectorated from the mouth. Past medical history is often essential in diagnosis, including hypertension, antiplatelet or anticoagulant use, and thrombocytopenia. A history of a prior nasal or skull base surgery should be determined. The intranasal mucosa should be inspected for the site of bleeding to help determine an anterior or posterior source and guide treatment. In uncomplicated cases, with no signs or symptoms of a concerning underlying etiology, CT and MRI are not indicated and may be contraindicated in patients with continued active or intermittent bleeding.

However, although most common episodes of epistaxis are multifactorial and related to mucosal dryness in combination with other risk factors for hemorrhage, rare and more serious causes are possible. Patients with hereditary hemorrhagic telangiectasia (HHT) will demonstrate small friable telangiectasias over the nasal mucosa and often the oral cavity and oropharyngeal mucosa as well. Patients with an autoimmune etiology will often have associated symptoms of a vasculitis or granulomatous disease including fever, fatigue, joint pain, or rash. Finally, malignant disease of the skull base may lead to epistaxis and is commonly associated with cranial neuropathy, particularly changes in vision or facial sensation, which must be investigated carefully.

B. Nasal Congestion and Rhinorrhea

Nasal congestion and rhinorrhea are often interrelated presenting complaints and may represent a wide range of underlying pathophysiology. A detailed history should focus on the duration, severity, and quality of symptoms. An acute process, with associated pain and fever, suggests a sinonasal infectious etiology. Attention should be directed to the past medical history and current state of health. Immunocompromise, whether through immunosuppressive drugs, hematologic malignancy, or severe diabetes, can predispose patients to developing an invasive fungal sinusitis. These infections, characterized by anesthesia of the affected area

Table 16–3. Major and minor criteria for diagnosis of rhinosinusitis.

Major Criteria	Minor Criteria
Facial pain or pressure	Headache
Nasal obstruction	Fever (for chronic rhinosinusitis)
Nasal discharge or purulence	Halitosis
Purulence in nasal cavity	Fatigue
Anosmia or hyposmia	Dental pain
Fever (for acute rhinosinusitis)	Cough
	Ear pain/pressure/fullness

Adapted with permission from Lanza DC, Kennedy DW: *Adult rhinosinusitis defined, Otolaryngol Head Neck Surg.* 1997 Sep;117(3 Pt 2): S1-7.

and soft tissue necrosis, are life-threatening emergencies and must be diagnosed and managed efficiently. Prolonged processes marked by facial pain, congestion, and purulent rhinorrhea are most often related to chronic rhinosinusitis, with or without sinonasal polyps, a common inflammatory disorder of the sinonasal mucosa. A set of diagnostic symptoms for rhinosinusitis have been established. Patients must have two major or one major and two minor criteria. These criteria are outlined in Table 16–3.

In rare cases, however, such symptoms may be a manifestation of a systemic autoimmune condition, including sarcoidosis or granulomatosis with polyangiitis. These are often associated with other signs of systemic inflammation such as fever and weight loss.

Isolated nasal congestion or clear rhinorrhea is most commonly allergic in nature and may be perennial or seasonal depending on the allergen. Patients often have associated pruritis, epiphora, and sneezing. Underlying anatomical abnormalities, such as septal deviation, may exacerbate the sensation of congestion. Medication history is important to ascertain, however, because overuse of oxymetazoline (Afrin) spray may cause rebound congestion, leading patients to develop a dependence on the medication. Finally, a rare but important diagnosis to recognize is cerebrospinal fluid (CSF) rhinorrhea. Patients can develop a CSF leak after recent anterior skull base surgery, but it may also occur spontaneously. In these cases, the rhinorrhea is intensified by bending over and straining and may be associated with positional headaches.

▶ Treatment

A. Epistaxis

The first concern in a patient with epistaxis is to determine hemodynamic stability and the safety of the airway. Patients in distress may need immediate treatment with nasal packing or even intubation if in an emergency setting. It is important to gain critical aspects of the history when possible, even in urgent situations, as these can guide the safety and direction of treatment. In patients with recent skull base surgery or trauma, ill-placed nasal packs may lead to iatrogenic intracranial injury. In patients with severe thrombocytopenia or skull base malignancy or those with HHT, a dry or poorly placed nasal pack may worsen bleeding.

In patients with slow bleeding from a clear anterior septal source, holding pressure for 20 to 30 minutes by squeezing the nasal alae against the septum is the first and often most successful therapy. Light cautery may also be performed but should only be done unilaterally to avoid risk of septal perforation. In those requiring more substantial intervention, hemostatic gelatins or foams can work well, especially in cases where manipulation of the mucosa may worsen bleeding (eg, HHT, thrombocytopenia). When greater force is required, inflatable nasal packs are the next usual intervention. These must be adequately lubricated prior to insertion and must be placed along and parallel to the nasal floor (in an axial plane, perpendicular to the face). If early resistance is felt, this is often the pack encountering the head of the inferior turbinate, and gentle pressure medially can typically guide the pack into the appropriate position. All patients with intranasal packing should be placed on antistaphylococcal antibiotics to prevent possible toxic shock syndrome. Patients who bleed through well-placed nasal packs may require surgical management or embolization.

Chronic medical management of patients predisposed to epistaxis includes management of hypertension, minimizing antiplatelet and anticoagulant therapy if possible, and promoting moist nasal mucosa. Patients are commonly placed on three times daily application of nasal saline spray and topical petroleum jelly or antibiotic ointment to the anterior septum. Patients with severe, recurrent epistaxis should be evaluated for possible systemic disease, such as HHT or an autoimmune condition, and malignancies must be ruled out.

B. Nasal Foreign Body

Similar to foreign bodies of the external ear, nasal foreign bodies are most commonly encountered in children. Typical presentation is a young child with a several-day history of unilateral purulent rhinorrhea. Often the offending foreign body was inserted days to weeks before symptom onset, and the patient or parents may not recall a specific event precipitating the symptoms.

Unlike external ear foreign bodies, nasal foreign bodies should always be treated as relative urgencies regardless of the type of object present. If a nasal foreign body becomes dislodged, it can easily become an airway foreign body (a true emergency). For this reason, many otolaryngologists recommend removal of all but the most anteriorly placed nasal foreign bodies under general anesthesia using endoscopic visualization. The threshold for performing retrieval under sedation should likewise be low. In our practice, nasal foreign bodies confined to the nasal vestibule or easily visible by anterior rhinoscopy can be safely removed without sedation in a cooperative patient. Young children, superior or posterior location, and difficult visualization are all indications for removal in the operating room with endoscopic visualization. Another advantage to removing nasal foreign bodies in this manner is that postremoval inspection of the nasal cavity is easily performed. The nasal mucosa is often significantly inflamed, and placement of absorbable material can prevent unwanted adhesions between opposing mucosal surfaces.

Nasal button batteries present a similar situation to external ear button batteries. The potential for extensive tissue damage from leakage of acid and electrical current discharge usually necessitates removal under general anesthesia. Following removal, extensive flushing with normal saline and careful inspection of the nasal cavity should be performed.

C. Fungal Sinusitis

Invasive fungal sinusitis is almost always encountered in immunocompromised patients, most often those undergoing chemotherapy for malignancy or in poorly controlled diabetics, and is a surgical emergency. It is caused by uncontrolled infiltrative growth of usually nonpathogenic fungal organisms. Offending agents are ubiquitous in the environment and are commonly found in the nasal secretions of healthy normal patients. The most common fungi are *Aspergillus, Fusarium,* and the Mucorales. The latter is an order of fungi including several genera that cause clinically aggressive infections, such as the *Mucor* and *Rhizopus* species, and such infections are termed mucormycosis. The Mucorales tend to preferentially grow in acidic environments and are thus found more often in the setting of diabetic ketoacidosis. Even with early diagnosis, maximal surgical therapy, and modern antifungal agents, the disease still carries a significant mortality rate. This varies depending on causative agent and reversibility of immunosuppression, from approximately 10% (*Aspergillus*, correctable diabetes) to well over 30% (mucormycosis, uncontrolled hematologic malignancy).

The index of suspicion for invasive fungal sinusitis must, therefore, be high for any immunocompromised patient, because the symptoms can be subtle and the disease rapidly progressive. Patients are usually ill appearing and complain of facial pain, headache, and nasal discharge; in addition, patients may have mental status changes. Careful inspection of the face, oral cavity, and nasal cavity is mandatory. Dark ulcers (Figure 16–4) may be noted on the anterior face of the middle turbinate, inferior turbinate, lateral nasal wall, septum, or palate, and these are often without sensation on examination. Specific cranial nerve deficits may be noted in later stages of the disease.

If invasive fungal sinusitis is suspected, biopsies should be taken of the suspicious areas and sent for immediate pathologic examination. The pathologist should be alerted

▲ **Figure 16–4.** Invasive fungal sinusitis. In this patient with invasive fungal sinusitis, the initial finding was a dark area (arrowhead) on the inferior face of the middle turbinate found on bedside nasal endoscopy.

that invasive fungal sinusitis is suspected, so that specific fungal stains can be performed. A worrisome finding is lack of bleeding at the biopsy site, because this may signify retrograde tissue infarction secondary to angioinvasive fungus.

Once invasive fungal sinusitis is confirmed, therapy consists of rapid reversal of immunosuppression when possible followed by aggressive surgical debridement of all necrotic tissue and systemic antifungal therapy. Amphotericin B provides the broadest coverage and is usually the initial agent of choice. Voriconazole may also be used and is particularly effective against *Aspergillus* species, but is generally ineffective against mucormycosis. A newer agent, which can be dosed IV or orally, is isavuconazole, which has activity against both classes of pathogen. In addition to broad antifungal coverage, in most cases, multiple surgical debridements are required to achieve disease clearance. However, regardless of the extent of debridement, cure is often not possible without reversal of underlying immunosuppression. A multidisciplinary team including otolaryngology, hematology/oncology, and infectious disease specialists should closely follow these patients.

Invasive fungal sinusitis should not be confused with other forms of fungal disease of the paranasal sinuses, including mycetoma (fungal ball) and allergic fungal sinusitis. In mycetoma, obstructed sinonasal outflow results in trapped secretions and can lead to colonization and growth of fungal elements, filling a sinus cavity. CT often shows characteristic hyperdensities within the mycetoma and surrounding bony sclerosis. This does not represent an invasive infection, and surgical removal is typically curative. Allergic fungal sinusitis is a chronic allergic inflammatory response to noninvasive colonizing fungal elements and results in thick eosinophilic mucin, nasal polyps, and bony remodeling. These patients will generally require functional endoscopic sinus surgery (FESS) to remove mucoid secretions and open the sinonasal tracts as well as long-term oral and topical glucocorticoid therapy.

D. Acute Rhinosinusitis

Rhinosinusitis refers to inflammation of the mucosal lining of the nose and paranasal sinuses. Acute rhinosinusitis is present for less than 4 weeks and is usually precipitated by a viral upper respiratory tract infection. It is important to emphasize that only a minority of cases of acute rhinosinusitis are a result of a bacterial infection (< 2%). Similarly, change in color of nasal discharge is not a specific sign of bacterial rhinosinusitis. Acute bacterial rhinosinusitis should be suspected if symptoms persist after 10 days or worsen within 10 days after an initial improvement. Physical examination may reveal purulent nasal secretions, nasal mucosal erythema, and tenderness overlying the sinuses. Nasal endoscopy (with middle meatal cultures) can be very useful, and visualization of purulent secretions emanating from the osteomeatal complex should increase suspicion for bacterial rhinosinusitis.

Treatment of acute rhinosinusitis is largely conservative in nature, and axial imaging, such as maxillofacial CT, is reserved only for cases refractory to initial empiric therapy. Nasal saline lavage helps to eliminate excess mucus and inflammatory mediators and restore mucociliary clearance. Mucolytics such as guaifenesin can help thin mucous secretions, allowing easier mucociliary transport. The only therapy validated by placebo-controlled trials, however, is intranasal topical glucocorticoids. These have demonstrated reduced time to symptom resolution, both for bacterial and viral acute rhinosinusitis. Importantly, topical decongestants (eg, oxymetazoline) are generally discouraged because they are of unproven benefit and patients quickly develop tachyphylaxis. With 3 or more days of use, patients can develop rebound nasal congestion and chronic dependence on these topical decongestants. Antihistamines also have no proven benefit in acute rhinosinusitis and may actually cause symptom exacerbation by drying mucous secretions.

Antibiotic therapy should be reserved only for patients suspected of having acute bacterial rhinosinusitis. With emerging resistance patterns, initial recommended antibiotic therapy is currently amoxicillin/clavulanic acid. Alternatives for penicillin-allergic patients include doxycycline and clindamycin or third-generation oral cephalosporins for patients who can tolerate them. Fluoroquinolones are reserved only as second-line agents in the case of recalcitrant disease because recent concerns have emerged regarding

serious adverse reactions of these drugs, including tendon rupture, hepatotoxicity, QT prolongation, and arrythmia.

Patients experiencing multiple episodes of acute rhinosinusitis should be evaluated carefully for predisposing conditions. These may include anatomic obstruction (which may be relieved by septoplasty and/or FESS), underlying impairment of mucociliary clearance (eg, from immotile cilia/Kartagener syndrome or cystic fibrosis), or immune system dysfunction. Complications of acute bacterial rhinosinusitis are exceedingly rare but can include orbital infection, meningitis, and even cavernous sinus thrombosis. Patients developing high fever, vision change, severe headache, or altered mental status must be evaluated and imaged immediately.

E. Chronic Rhinosinusitis

Chronic rhinosinusitis (CRS) is common, affecting up to 15% of people in the United States. It is defined as the presence of rhinosinusitis symptoms for greater than 12 weeks (Table 16–3) combined with evidence of inflammation on either endoscopy or axial imaging. Endoscopic findings can include purulent mucus in the middle meatus or ethmoid region, nasal polyps, or polypoid degeneration of the nasal mucosa. Radiographic findings can include diffuse mucosal thickening, chronic bony remodeling, and sinus opacification (Figure 16–5).

Current understanding of the pathogenesis of CRS considers it fundamentally a chronic inflammatory disorder of the sinonasal mucosa marked by intermittent exacerbations and secondary bacterial infections. The etiology of CRS is

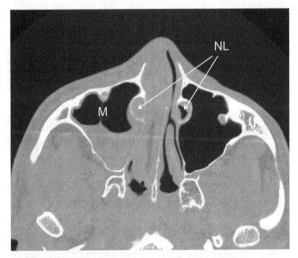

▲ **Figure 16–5.** Chronic sinusitis. In this axial plane CT of a patient with chronic sinusitis, radiographic evidence of inflammation can be seen. The right nasolacrimal duct (NL) mucosa is edematous. There is an air-fluid level and opacification of the right maxillary sinus (M).

not fully elucidated, and there are no current treatments that target the underlying pathobiology. Most otolaryngologists feel that there are several disease processes currently described together under the generic heading CRS. The goals of therapy, therefore, are to control symptoms and stabilize the inflammatory process. The mainstays of management are nasal saline irrigations and topical nasal glucocorticoids. Burst oral steroids are often prescribed in cases of severe mucosal inflammation or in patients with a large polyp burden. In cases where symptoms persist despite maximal medical therapy, a maxillofacial CT scan is useful to evaluate disease burden and to assess for any anatomic abnormalities that may be amenable to surgical correction. Surgery is aimed at removing the obstruction to natural mucus flow from the paranasal sinuses, and most patients will continue to require topical medications after surgery to prevent return of symptoms.

F. Rhinitis

Rhinitis, or isolated inflammation of the nasal cavity leading to sneezing, nasal drainage, and nasal congestion, can be allergic or nonallergic in etiology. Allergic rhinitis is most commonly seen in children and is often associated with asthma. Treatment options including allergen avoidance, pharmacotherapy, and immunotherapy. The mainstay of treatment in most patients is a topical nasal glucocorticoid, with nasal saline irrigations, oral and nasal antihistamines, leukotriene receptor antagonists, and mast cell stabilizers as adjunctive therapies. Nonallergic rhinitis is a group of related syndromes with an overall unclear pathogenesis but that are unresponsive to oral antihistamine therapy. These patients are managed with topical glucocorticoids, and for those with significant rhinorrhea, nasal ipratropium can be very effective. Finally, as mentioned earlier, extended use of topical nasal decongestants (eg, oxymetazoline) or other vasoconstrictors (eg, intranasal cocaine) can lead to tachyphylaxis and mucosal dependence. This resulting syndrome of severe rebound mucosal edema and nasal obstruction is termed *rhinitis medicamentosa*. Patients will report daily topical vasoconstrictor/decongestant use and absolute dependence on these medications for any appreciable nasal airflow. Treatment requires cessation of the offending agent, and patients should be managed with nasal saline lavage and topical nasal glucocorticoids. Oral decongestants and a course of oral corticosteroids may help hasten symptom resolution and increase patient compliance.

G. Cerebrospinal Fluid Leak

CSF rhinorrhea may occur in patients with prior skull base surgery but may also arise spontaneously and should not be confused with allergic or nonallergic rhinorrhea. Patients with CSF leaks have worsening symptoms when bending over and straining and lack associated sneezing, itching, and congestion. A high index of suspicion should be maintained in any patient with persistent clear rhinorrhea because untreated CSF leakage may lead to intracranial infection. Diagnosis can be made by testing nasal drainage for beta-2 transferrin. Localization of the leak is confirmed through high-resolution CT of the skull base, and often, intrathecal fluorescein is used for direct visualization. Repair is generally performed through an endoscopic approach.

DISORDERS OF THE ORAL CAVITY AND PHARYNX

▶ Anatomy and Physiology

The oral cavity is bounded anteriorly by the vermilion border of the lips and posteriorly by the anterior tonsillar pillars, hard-soft palate junction, and circumvallate papilla of the tongue. The superior aspect of the oral cavity includes the hard palate and maxillary dentition, and the inferior aspect includes the floor of mouth mucosa, the anterior two-thirds of the tongue, and the mandibular dentition.

The pharynx connects the nasal and oral cavities to the esophagus and larynx. It consists of three segments—the nasopharynx, the oropharynx, and the hypopharynx (Figure 16–6). The nasopharynx begins as an extension from the posterior aspect of the nasal cavity and extends from the nasal choanae to the soft palate. The oropharynx extends from the soft palate to the level of the hyoid bone. It includes the base of tongue, lateral and posterior pharyngeal walls, and tonsillar fossae. The hypopharynx extends from the level of the hyoid bone to the inferior aspect of the cricoid cartilage, and includes the pyriform sinuses, postcricoid region, and posterior hypopharyngeal wall.

The primary functions of the oral cavity are related to chewing and swallowing (mastication and deglutition) and shaping of phonatory vibrations to produce intelligible speech. Taste buds on the dorsum of the tongue are responsible for basic taste perception—savory, sweet, salty, bitter, and sour. This sensory information is transmitted to the facial nerve via the chorda tympani nerve for the anterior two-thirds of the tongue. General sensation of the tongue is carried by the lingual nerve. All sensory information from the posterior one-third of the tongue is carried by the glossopharyngeal nerve. Complex nuances of taste are mediated by olfactory receptors in the superior-most aspect of the nasal cavity and are not directly related to the tongue or oral cavity.

The tongue has four pairs of intrinsic muscles, which interdigitate throughout the tongue. These muscles act to lengthen or shorten the tongue, curl the apex and edges, and flatten or round the dorsal surface. The intrinsic tongue muscles originate and insert within the tongue itself. Extrinsic tongue muscles (genioglossus, hyoglossus, styloglossus, and palatoglossus) also act to protrude, depress, elevate, and retract the tongue. All motor function of the tongue is mediated by cranial nerve XII (the hypoglossal nerve).

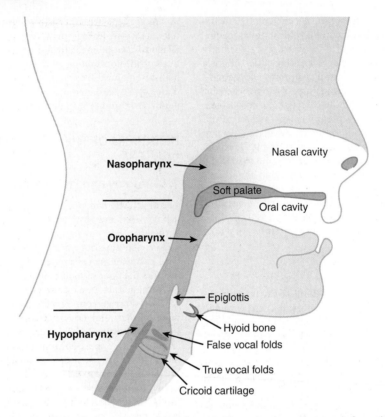

▲ **Figure 16–6.** Relationship of the three sections of the pharynx. The nasopharynx extends from the nasal choanae to the soft palate. The oropharynx then extends from the soft palate to the level of the hyoid bone. The hypopharynx extends from the level of the hyoid bone to the level of the cricoid cartilage.

The act of swallowing is complex and consists of three main phases—oral, pharyngeal, and esophageal. The oral phase is under voluntary control, whereas the remaining phases proceed under reflex control. The oral phase of swallowing consists of preparation of the food bolus by mastication to soften and shape the bolus. Following this, oral transport ensues and the food bolus is transported to the posterior tongue. The anterior tongue then elevates against the hard palate and contracts and propels the bolus to the oropharynx. Simultaneously, the nasopharynx is sealed off by the soft palate, preventing nasal regurgitation. In the pharyngeal phase, several complex actions occur that elevate the larynx, temporarily halt respirations and protect the airway from aspiration, and relax the cricopharyngeus muscle to allow passage of the food bolus. The esophageal phase then propels the food bolus distally by means of sequential peristaltic contractions. Alteration of the timing or execution of any of these phases can result in dysphagia, or difficulty swallowing.

▶ **Workup and Differential Diagnosis**

A. Odynophagia and Dysphagia

Odynophagia (pain with swallowing) and dysphagia (difficulty swallowing) may represent a broad range of pathologic conditions and should never be dismissed as part of the aging process in the elderly patient. Acute sudden-onset dysphagia is almost always the result of an impacted esophageal food bolus or foreign body and should be addressed urgently. Such esophageal impactions cause great discomfort and risk esophageal perforation or uncontrolled regurgitation of the bolus and subsequent aspiration. These are best managed in the endoscopy suite with a controlled airway.

Subacute or chronic dysphagia has many more potential etiologies, and the initial step in diagnosis is determining whether the location of the obstruction is oropharyngeal or esophageal. Oropharyngeal dysphagia includes difficulty or pain with the act of swallowing and may be accompanied by velopharyngeal insufficiency or symptoms of aspiration.

Esophageal obstruction is felt lower in the chest and is more commonly associated with the sensation of slowed bolus transit or delayed regurgitation.

The causes of oropharyngeal dysphagia are varied and may be diagnosed by careful upper airway examination. A mucosal disorder of the upper aerodigestive tract is a common cause, as seen in patients with infectious or inflammatory mucositis or those with xerostomia. Infectious processes typically present over the course of days to weeks and are associated with significant pain and often systemic symptoms. Oropharyngeal angioedema may present over the course of hours and must be addressed urgently because it can lead rapidly to upper airway obstruction. Oropharyngeal lesions that cause a mass effect on the pharynx can also cause dysphagia. Such lesions generally present in a chronic insidious fashion and may represent benign tumors, large cervical osteophytes, or malignancy. Finally, neuromuscular disorders affecting function of the pharyngeal constrictors can lead to dysphagia; these disorders include stroke, neurodegenerative disorders, hypothyroidism, and cricopharyngeal dysfunction.

All patients with a new presentation of oropharyngeal dysphagia or odynophagia should undergo a full upper aerodigestive tract examination including flexible laryngoscopy. Laboratory evaluation should be targeted and based on history and physical examination findings. Modified barium swallow is often an excellent adjunct diagnostic test and can further characterize the nature and cause of dysphagia as well as evaluate for objective signs of aspiration. Axial imaging with CT scan is generally reserved for patients with an infectious presentation when concerned for deep neck space abscess or for patients with a suspected neoplasm.

B. Oral Cavity Lesions

Although oral cavity lesions are common, many clinicians are unfamiliar with the oral examination and the range of possible diagnoses. It is essential, however, to be able to formulate an appropriate differential diagnosis and be able to triage those patients with urgent conditions requiring immediate referral. Oral lesions may be structural, infectious, inflammatory, or neoplastic in etiology. In general, asymptomatic lesions that have been present and stable for long periods of time are rarely urgencies. A common example is a large torus, a bony exostosis found either in the midline of the hard palate or the lingual aspect of the mandible with normal overlying mucosa. Despite their often impressive appearance, these rarely cause symptoms or require treatment. Other common examples of long-standing benign lesions include mucoceles and ranulas, which are related to impaired or obstructed salivary gland flow.

Lesions that are painful or changing rapidly in size or shape are more concerning. Many of these are infectious or inflammatory in nature. Aphthous stomatitis (canker sores) is the most common cause of oral ulceration and is thought to be autoimmune in etiology. Common infectious causes include candidiasis, which may be seen as friable white patches or painful erythematous lesions, and herpes simplex virus, painful sores occurring most commonly on the lips. Although most infectious or inflammatory oral lesions are benign in nature and locally treatable, patients with extensive or severe lesions should undergo evaluation for an underlying systemic autoimmune or immunodeficiency condition such as inflammatory bowel disease, systemic lupus erythematosus, Behçet syndrome, or human immunodeficiency virus (HIV). When mucosal ulceration is particularly severe and progressive, autoimmune blistering diseases should be considered, including pemphigus vulgaris or other pemphigoid syndromes.

Several oral lesions are premalignant in nature and should be recognized and diagnosed appropriately. Squamous cell carcinoma (SCC) is the most common malignancy of the oral cavity and is discussed in a later section in this chapter. Patients present with nonhealing irregular ulcerations or polypoid lesions that are often painful and require tissue biopsy for diagnosis. Oral SCC carries a poor prognosis in later stages, and it is important to diagnosis early in its progression or in a premalignant stage. Leukoplakia is an asymptomatic white plaque of the mucosa that cannot be scraped off and has been associated with a malignant transformation rate of approximately 5%. Its prevalence has been estimated to be as high as 5% of the population and is often related to tobacco exposure or mechanical trauma. The rates of dysplasia are highest for lesions found on the floor of the mouth, ventral tongue, lips, and retromolar trigone. Erythroplakia is a velvety red plaque that cannot be removed, and although it is less common than traditional white leukoplakia, it is associated with a higher degree of premalignant dysplasia, with over half of cases having in situ or overtly invasive SCC on histologic examination.

C. Snoring

Although isolated snoring may be a benign symptom of elongated or collapsible upper airway anatomy and is present in over 30% of adults, it may also indicate the presence of obstructive sleep apnea (OSA). OSA is an intrinsic dyssomnia that affects roughly 15-20 million people in the United States. It is classically described as the presence of hypopneic episodes, apneic episodes, and respiratory effort–related arousals that occur during sleep. An apneic event requires 10 or more seconds of cessation of airflow, followed by arousal with restoration of normal ventilation. The definition of hypopnea varies between sleep laboratories, but generally, it refers to an episode of decreased airflow (> 50% reduction) for greater than 10 seconds that is associated with decreased oxygen saturation or arousal. Patients usually present with nighttime snoring, daytime hypersomnolence, irritability, morning headaches, cognitive impairment, and often witnessed apneic events with cessation of airflow followed by choking or gasping. When taking a history, it is important to confer with the patient's bed partner, as the patient may be unaware of his or her nighttime symptoms. Cardiovascular disease, hypertension, metabolic dysfunction, respiratory failure, and right-heart failure are among the serious long-term effects of OSA.

Obstructive sleep apnea is more common in men, and the overall incidence appears to increase with age. Important risk factors include obesity, smoking, diabetes mellitus, alcohol consumption, hypothyroidism, and anatomic abnormalities including macroglossia, adenotonsillar hypertrophy, elongation of the soft palate, and retrognathia. A thorough head and neck examination should be performed to fully assess airway patency. Oral cavity examination may reveal tonsillar hyperplasia. Flexible fiberoptic endoscopy can assess for nasal obstruction secondary to a deviated nasal septum, polyp disease, or turbinate hyperplasia and can evaluate for lingual tonsillar hypertrophy or mass lesions of the pharynx.

Polysomnography remains the gold standard in diagnosing OSA, which can be defined by either the apnea-hypopnea index (AHI) or the respiratory disturbance index (RDI). The AHI includes the number of hypopneas and apneas that occur per hour of sleep, whereas the RDI is the number of hypopneas, apneas, and respiratory effort–related arousals per hour of sleep. The generally accepted guidelines for diagnosis of OSA are an AHI of 15 or greater in an asymptomatic patient or an AHI of greater than 5 in a symptomatic patient. Imaging studies are usually not required to diagnose OSA, although they may help assess for upper airway anatomic abnormalities.

▶ Treatment

A. Acute Angioedema

Acute angioedema is characterized by localized swelling of subcutaneous and submucosal tissue of the head and neck. The swelling may begin with mild facial involvement but may progress to involve the oral cavity, tongue, pharynx, and larynx. It is often self-limited but may present as a medical emergency. Tongue or laryngeal involvement may rapidly lead to airway obstruction and asphyxiation. Angioedema has a rapid onset and, with proper medical treatment, usually resolves within 24-48 hours. The underlying pathophysiology of angioedema involves vasoactive mediators such as bradykinin and histamine, causing interstitial edema through endothelial-mediated vasodilation of arterioles with subsequent capillary and venule leakage. The three major etiologies are drug-induced, hereditary, and allergic angioedema. Drug-induced and hereditary angioedema appear to

be mediated by the kallikrein-kinin system, whereas allergic angioedema appears to be mast cell mediated.

Initial management of acute angioedema is focused on airway maintenance. Depending on clinical presentation, this may include nebulized epinephrine inhalation, intubation (either oral or transnasal fiberoptic), or tracheotomy. Due to the potentially rapid progression of this disease process, there should be a low threshold for securing an airway by the latter two methods. Many authors advocate the use of glucocorticoids (10 mg dexamethasone IV every 8 hours) combined with histamine receptor antagonists (both an H_1 antagonist, such as diphenhydramine [Benadryl] 25 mg IV every 6 hours, and an H_2 antagonist such as ranitidine 50 mg IV every 6 hours) for 24 hours. Recent evidence has shown that these therapies may not be beneficial in drug-induced or hereditary angioedema. Rapid differentiation of the exact subtype of angioedema, however, may not be as practical as empiric therapy given the relatively benign nature of these medications compared to the potential threat of airway obstruction. There are also several recently developed first-line medications specifically for the treatment of drug-induced or hereditary angioedema. These include C1 inhibitors (plasma-derived or recombinant), ecallantide (Kalbitor, a kallikrein inhibitor), and icatibant (Firazyr, a bradykinin-B2-receptor antagonist).

Drug-induced angioedema has classically been associated with the use of angiotensin-converting enzyme (ACE) inhibitors, although many other medications can also less commonly cause this phenomenon. The incidence of angioedema secondary to ACE inhibitor use is less than 1%. The pathophysiology of ACE inhibitor–induced angioedema appears to be secondary to a localized increase in bradykinin levels related to the inhibition of ACE. Studies have shown that one-half of all cases of ACE inhibitor–induced angioedema occur within the first week of initiating treatment. However, some patients undergo years of ACE inhibitor therapy without incident before their first attack of acute angioedema. Treatment should again begin with emergent airway maintenance and with discontinuation of any possible offending drugs. Studies involving angiotensin II receptor antagonists (ARBs) have revealed a decreased incidence of angioedema in comparison to ACE inhibitors therapy. However, clinicians should still use caution when initiating an ARB in a patient with known ACE inhibitor–induced angioedema.

Hereditary angioedema is an autosomal dominant deficiency or dysfunction of the C1 inhibitor, which leads to increased levels of vasoactive bradykinin. Clinically, hereditary angioedema often presents with recurrent episodes of facial and oral swelling, as well as abdominal pain secondary to intestinal wall edema. Certain drugs (eg, estrogen, ACE inhibitors, ARBs), surgery, and infections may elicit acute angioedema attacks in hereditary angioedema patients.

Allergic angioedema is mast cell mediated, and histamine plays the major role in its pathophysiology. In contrast to drug-induced and hereditary angioedema, skin changes including urticaria and pruritis are commonly seen in allergic angioedema. This form of angioedema is frequently seen in patients who also suffer from atopic dermatitis, allergic rhinitis, and asthma. Triggers of acute attacks of allergic angioedema include certain drugs, infections, food, and plant products.

B. Ludwig Angina

Ludwig angina is an uncommon life-threatening condition characterized by cellulitis involving the submental, sublingual, and submandibular spaces. The source of the infection is typically odontogenic, and infection spreads rapidly. The infection is usually polymicrobial, with aerobic and anaerobic gram-positive cocci and gram-negative rods. Clinically, patients present with painful neck swelling and edema of the floor of mouth, often leading to elevation and displacement of the tongue. The most common cause of death in these patients is airway compromise, and therefore, primary treatment should be centered on airway maintenance with early involvement of anesthesiology and otolaryngology physicians. Intubation is often anatomically difficult, and awake nasal fiberoptic intubation or tracheotomy under local anesthesia are often the preferred methods of ensuring a patent airway. Airway observation in an intensive care unit may be an option for less severe cases. After the airway has been secured, proper systemic antibiotic therapy should be initiated immediately followed by incision and drainage for most cases. Major complications include extension of the infection posteriorly to involve the parapharyngeal and retropharyngeal spaces as well as the superior mediastinum. The diagnosis is clinical, but CT may be used to assess for deep fluid collection or retropharyngeal extension of the infection.

C. Tonsillitis

Tonsillitis is one of the most common problems encountered by the otolaryngologist. In general, tonsillitis refers to inflammation of the palatine tonsils located on the lateral walls of the oropharynx between the palatoglossal and palatopharyngeal folds. Acute tonsillitis is primarily a pediatric disease that tends to affect children age 5 to 15 years. It is most commonly caused by group A β-hemolytic streptococcal species, although anaerobes, *Haemophilus influenzae*, and viruses can also be causative agents. Patients usually present with fever, painful sore throat, halitosis, and dysphagia. It is important to note the distinction in clinical presentation between acute tonsillitis, viral pharyngitis, and infectious mononucleosis (caused by the Epstein-Barr virus). Viral pharyngitis commonly presents with associated symptoms including cough, nasal congestion or drainage, or conjunctivitis, whereas patients with mononucleosis typically present with weeks of anterior and posterior cervical lymphadenopathy, odynophagia, and a grayish tonsillar exudate. On physical examination, the acute tonsillitis patient has erythematous tonsils, purulent tonsillar exudate, and anterior cervical lymphadenopathy.

The diagnosis of acute tonsillitis is clinical, although many practitioners rely on a positive streptococcal test or culture. The mainstay in treatment of acute tonsillitis continues to be a 10-day course of penicillin or a comparable cephalosporin. However, it is now estimated that failure with penicillin therapy occurs in up to 30% of cases. Following up culture results and adjusting the antibiotic therapy have therefore become important steps in management. Complications from acute tonsillitis include the formation of peritonsillar or deep neck space abscess. Antibiotic use has greatly decreased the incidence of rare systemic complications such as poststreptococcal glomerulonephritis and rheumatic fever.

Many patients have a solitary episode of acute tonsillitis, which responds favorably to antibiotic treatment, whereas some patients have recurrent acute tonsillitis with multiple infections over the course of years. Chronic tonsillitis is a state of persistent tonsillar inflammation for greater than 3 months following an episode of acute infection. It is characterized by chronic sore throat and odynophagia with tonsillar enlargement, tonsillolithic debris, and cervical lymphadenitis present on physical examination. Recent studies have suggested that polymicrobial infections, drug-resistant organisms, *H influenzae*, *S aureus*, anaerobes, and actinomycetes may all play a role in chronic tonsillar disease. Treatment of chronic tonsillitis, therefore, should begin with the use of broader spectrum antibiotics such as amoxicillin/clavulanate or clindamycin, which may target these offending organisms. Although medical management with antibiotics is always the first-line therapy for tonsillitis, certain patients with recurrent acute or chronic tonsillitis may benefit from tonsillectomy. Tonsillectomy during acute episodes, however, substantially increases the technical difficulty and bleeding risk of the procedure and is only considered when complications such as deep neck space abscess or acute airway obstruction are concurrently present.

D. Peritonsillar Abscess

Peritonsillar abscess (PTA) is a common infection of the peritonsillar space between the palatine tonsil, tonsillar pillars, and the superior pharyngeal constrictor muscle. Its prevalence in the United Stated has been estimated at 30 per 100,000 people annually. The infection is suppurative in nature and thought to be secondary to either extension of adjacent acute tonsillitis or obstruction of Weber glands (minor salivary glands) at the tonsillar pole. The typical patient presents complaining of sore throat and fever for several days, with worsening trismus, odynophagia, dysphagia, and inability to tolerate secretions. PTA should be managed acutely, because the infection may progress and spread to the deep neck tissue or compromise the airway.

The diagnosis of PTA is made by physical examination, which reveals bulging soft tissue of the lateral pharyngeal wall and soft palate, tonsillar erythema and exudate, and uvular deviation. CT may be necessary in patients with severe trismus and can aid in differentiating PTA from retropharyngeal abscess.

The management of PTA is dependent on the patient characteristics. Needle aspiration can be performed quickly, is relatively safe, and can be both diagnostic and therapeutic. Incision and drainage should only be performed by physicians with an understanding of the relevant pharyngeal anatomy, because multiple vital structures including cranial nerves and the carotid artery potentially lie within the surgical field. In cooperative adults, it can usually be performed using local anesthesia, but patients with severe trismus may require general anesthesia. In our practice (for adult patients), preprocedure administration of 3 g of ampicillin/sulbactam, 10 mg of dexamethasone, IV fluid hydration, and IV morphine for analgesia can greatly facilitate the procedure by reducing trismus and promoting patient comfort and cooperation. After instillation of local anesthetic, a needle aspiration can be used to confirm the site of incision. A limited mucosal incision is made with a scalpel, taking care not to penetrate the underlying muscular layer. Blunt dissection is then used to penetrate the abscess cavity. Oral suction should be in place before penetration of the abscess cavity to prevent possible aspiration of purulence. Studies have shown both needle aspiration and incision and drainage to be greater than 90% effective, but both carry a 10%-15% risk of recurrent PTA. The pediatric patient usually will not tolerate either needle aspiration or incision and drainage under local anesthesia, and general anesthesia is often necessary. Antibiotic therapy against *Streptococcus pyogenes* and oral anaerobes with either amoxicillin/clavulanic acid or clindamycin should follow abscess drainage. Most patients with PTA can be treated as outpatients. If needle aspiration or incision and drainage of a PTA is performed, it is important to counsel the patient that future risk of PTA is increased. Many otolaryngologists recommend an elective tonsillectomy be performed 2-3 months following a recurrent PTA.

E. Deep Neck Space Infections

Although greatly decreased in incidence since the advent of modern antibiotics, deep neck space infections remain a potentially life-threatening condition and require immediate recognition and treatment. The source of deep neck space infection is most commonly odontogenic. Other sources of infection include adjacent tonsillar, upper respiratory, and salivary infections as well as instrumentation and foreign bodies. These infections are usually polymicrobial, composed predominantly of anaerobes mixed with various streptococcal and staphylococcal species. Symptoms depend on the exact location of the abscess, but patients commonly present with fever, decreased neck range of motion, dysphagia, and odynophagia. Physical examination can reveal trismus, a toxic appearance with facial or neck edema, cervical lymphadenopathy, and purulent oral secretions. It is not uncommon for patients to present several days after being discharged on antibiotics for a less severe, local infection. It is important to note that patients on antibiotic or immunosuppression therapy may have more subtle signs of infection and systemic toxicity may be masked.

A thorough understanding of the anatomy of the cervical fascia and deep spaces of the neck is essential in diagnosing and managing these rapidly spreading infections. The cervical fascia is divided into superficial and deep layers. The deep cervical fascia is further divided into three separate layers—superficial, middle, and deep layers. Furthermore, the middle layer of deep cervical fascia is subdivided into muscular and visceral divisions, and the deep layer of deep cervical fascia is subdivided into the alar and prevertebral layers. These divisions of the deep cervical fascia separate the neck into numerous potential spaces, and infection with a specific compartment is associated with specific symptoms and appropriate management options. Spread of infection often occurs contiguously, and many clinical situations involve infection of multiple deep neck space compartments.

Parapharyngeal abscess must be differentiated from PTA, because the former may require external drainage, whereas the latter is best drained intraorally. Retropharyngeal abscesses are most commonly seen in children and are located deep to the pharyngeal constrictor between the visceral layer and the alar layer of deep cervical fascia. Retropharyngeal abscess represents a potential source of airway obstruction and should be managed accordingly. The danger space is the region between the alar and prevertebral layers, which extends from the base of the skull to the diaphragm. Infection of the danger space usually arises from contiguous spread from retropharyngeal, prevertebral, or pharyngomaxillary infections. The lack of definitive anatomic barriers in the danger space offers very little resistance to spread of infection. The prevertebral space is directly posterior to the danger space between the prevertebral division of deep cervical fascia and the paravertebral fascia. Infection of the prevertebral space is usually secondary to penetrating trauma or vertebral disc space infection.

Initial treatment should focus on ensuring a secure airway. IV antibiotics are started immediately and should cover both aerobic and anaerobic organisms. Ampicillin/sulbactam is an excellent first-line choice, and if methicillin-resistant *S aureus* is suspected, vancomycin should also be initiated. Early operative intervention is essential for deep neck abscesses confirmed by axial imaging. This may be performed either transorally or transcervically depending on the location. Major complications of deep neck space infections include mediastinitis, osteomyelitis, cranial nerve deficits, and progression to necrotizing fasciitis. Involvement of the carotid sheath may also lead to suppurative jugular thrombophlebitis (Lemierre syndrome). Early diagnosis and proper treatment may help limit these serious complications.

F. Oral Cavity Lesions

The management of oral cavity lesions is tailored to the underlying etiology. Patients with oral manifestations of systemic autoimmune disease require immunosuppressive therapy for regression of their oral lesions. Viral ulcerations, such as with herpes simplex virus infection, may be managed with systemic antiviral therapy. Candidiasis typically responds well to topical antifungal agents. Recurrent aphthous ulcers are managed symptomatically, and many patients obtain relief with topical glucocorticoid formulations. Patients with leukoplakia may also be treated with a trial of oral topical glucocorticoids. Nonresponding lesions must be followed closely for malignant transformation, and repeated in-office biopsies are usually required. Recent studies have also suggested that chemopreventive agents may be useful, particularly retinoid compounds.

G. Ranula

A ranula is caused by sublingual gland secretions that have extravasated into the soft tissues of the floor of mouth. This leads to a soft submucosal fullness of the floor of mouth that can occasionally be large in size and extend into the neck. An inflammatory fibrous pseudocapsule forms around this mucus collection and slowly expands as sublingual secretions continue. The definitive treatment for a ranula, regardless of size or extent, is transoral resection of the ipsilateral sublingual gland. Because the pseudocystic capsule is nonsecretory, it does not need to be included in the resection.

H. Obstructive Sleep Apnea

Treatment of OSA should begin with the identification and prevention of risk factors. Behavior modifications such as weight loss, smoking and alcohol cessation, and discontinuation of any central nervous system depressants may help improve the patient's apneic index. Safety precautions related to daytime hypersomnolence need to be discussed for high-risk patients such as pilots and commercial truck drivers.

Continuous positive airway pressure (CPAP) is considered first-line therapy after behavioral modifications. Positive pressure helps keep the airway patent and has been shown to be highly effective in reducing OSA symptoms. Some patients have trouble tolerating CPAP therapy, because breathing against the positive-pressure airflow can be difficult to adjust to. Bilevel positive airway pressure (BiPAP) is another system that employs a higher inspiratory pressure with a lower expiratory pressure to allow for easier expiration. There are numerous oral appliances that may help adjust the airway during sleep to improve patency, although studies have shown these appliances to be less effective than CPAP in improving the apneic index.

Several surgical options are available for patients who do not respond well to initial treatment. Routine adenoidectomy and tonsillectomy have been shown to be effective in pediatric

patients with isolated adenotonsillar hypertrophy contributing to their OSA symptoms. For adult patients, more extensive surgery is usually required. Uvulopalatopharyngoplasty (UP3) is the first-line surgical therapy in which the uvula, a small amount of soft palate, and the palatine tonsils are removed. The concept of multilevel sleep surgery is important, because UP3 alone is associated with a significant (> 50%) failure rate. Most commonly, UP3 is combined with additional procedures to address other areas of obstruction. Septoplasty and inferior turbinate reduction can improve nasal airflow. The tongue base can be advanced by suture suspension, hyoid suspension, or genioglossus advancement. Other more invasive surgical interventions include maxillomandibular advancement. Some authors have advocated less invasive therapy including palatal stiffening implants and radiofrequency ablation, but the long-term data are lacking. Life-threatening OSA that does not respond to CPAP/BiPAP or surgical intervention may require permanent tracheostomy. A repeat polysomnogram should be performed in surgical patients 1-3 months postoperatively to monitor for improvements.

DISORDERS OF THE LARYNX AND TRACHEA

▶ Anatomy and Physiology

The anatomy of the larynx (Figures 16–7 and 16–8) is best understood in the context of its three core functions: laryngeal protection, respiration, and speech. The primary function of the larynx is to protect the airway from aspiration during swallowing. The epiglottis and aryepiglottic folds help

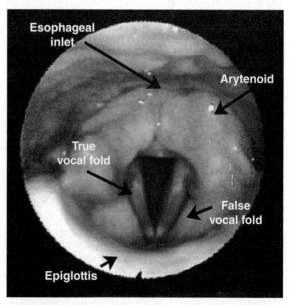

▲ **Figure 16–7.** Internal anatomy of the larynx as seen on endoscopy.

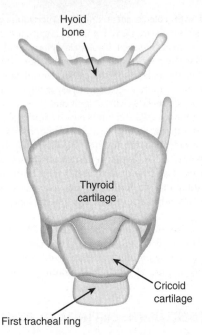

Hyoid
bone

Thyroid
cartilage

Cricoid
cartilage

First tracheal ring

▲ **Figure 16–8.** Cartilaginous and bony laryngeal
framework.

direct food and liquids laterally into the pyriform sinuses and
away from the midline laryngeal inlet. The paired arytenoid
cartilages act as attachment points for most of the intrinsic muscles of the larynx, serving to move the vocal folds
together (adduction) and apart (abduction). The false vocal
folds and true vocal folds adduct during swallow to prevent
entry of food or liquids into the airway. Conversely, reflex
pathways in the brainstem lead to glottic opening just prior
to inspiration for effortless unobstructed breathing. Phonation, unlike laryngeal protection and respiration, is voluntary and achieved through vibration of the free edge of the

true vocal folds during exhalation. Changing the tension
within the vocal fold changes the pitch at which the vocal
fold vibrates.

Several cartilages compose the framework of the larynx
(see Figure 16–8). The thyroid cartilage is the largest laryngeal cartilage. This shield-shaped cartilage is responsible for
the anterior neck prominence, and it provides protection to
the internal components of the larynx. The cricoid cartilage
lies inferior to the thyroid cartilage and is the only complete cartilaginous ring within the upper airway, serving as
the major support mechanism for the larynx. Internally, the
paired arytenoid cartilages articulate with the cricoid cartilage and attach to the vocal folds. Rotational movement of
the cricoarytenoid joint results in abduction or adduction of
the vocal folds. The epiglottis is a flexible cartilage located
above the larynx. It is not involved in structural support of
the larynx but serves to assist in protecting the airway during
swallowing.

Innervation to the larynx is provided by the vagus
nerve. The vagus exits the skull base through the jugular
foramen and descends in the neck at the posterior aspect
of the carotid sheath. The superior laryngeal nerve arises
directly from the vagus and has an internal and external
branch. The internal superior laryngeal nerve enters the
larynx through the thyrohyoid membrane and supplies
sensation to the laryngeal mucosa above the true vocal
cords. The external superior laryngeal nerve provides
motor innervation to the cricothyroid muscle. The right
recurrent laryngeal nerve arises from the vagus and loops
around the subclavian artery. The left recurrent laryngeal
nerve arises more distally in the thorax and loops around
the aortic arch. Both recurrent laryngeal nerves then ascend
in the tracheoesophageal grooves and enter the larynx near
the cricothyroid joint. The recurrent laryngeal nerves provide motor innervation to all of the intrinsic muscles of the
larynx except the cricothyroid. A summary of the laryngeal
muscles is provided in Table 16–4.

Table 16–4. Major muscles of the larynx.

Muscle	Function	Innervation	Key Point
Posterior cricoarytenoid	Abducts vocal folds, tenses vocal folds	Recurrent laryngeal nerve	ONLY abductor of vocal folds
Lateral cricoarytenoid	Adducts true vocal folds	Recurrent laryngeal nerve	
Interarytenoid	Adducts posterior glottis	Recurrent laryngeal nerve	ONLY laryngeal muscle receiving bilateral innervation
Oblique arytenoids	Closes laryngeal inlet during swallowing	Recurrent laryngeal nerve	
Thyroarytenoid	Adducts, tenses vocal fold	Recurrent laryngeal nerve	
Cricothyroid	Increases vocal fold tension, especially at higher pitches	External branch of superior laryngeal nerve	ONLY muscle not innervated by recurrent laryngeal nerve

Workup and Differential Diagnosis

A. Stridor

The rapid and accurate evaluation of a patient in respiratory distress is one of the most critical skills of an otolaryngologist. Noisy breathing and respiratory distress have multiple etiologies, and the clinician must rapidly differentiation between acute emergencies and chronic conditions. It is essential to recognize that not all noisy breathing is stridor.

True stridor may represent an impending airway failure and thus must be distinguished from other upper airway noises that are sometimes mistakenly referred to as stridor. Airway obstruction at the level of the nasopharynx produces snoring sounds, or stertor. Stridor specifically refers to the noise that is produced by air movement through a partially obstructed airway. Inspiratory stridor usually signifies an obstruction above or at the level of the vocal cords, whereas expiratory stridor most often occurs with tracheal obstruction or primary lung pathology. Biphasic stridor can also occur with an obstruction at the level of the vocal cords or subglottis. Although these guidelines are helpful, patients may present with atypical stridor, and any patient with noisy breathing should have a full airway evaluation. Importantly, in patients with impending airway obstruction, oxygen saturation is one of the last objective measures to be affected and should not be used as a marker for a safe airway.

Directed history and physical examination should be performed as time allows. An accurate diagnosis of the etiology of the patient's dyspnea leads to more informed and successful decision making about airway management. History is often critical and can help quickly differentiate between likely infectious, inflammatory, structural, or neoplastic etiologies. Additionally, an early flexible fiberoptic examination of the airway can quickly demonstrate any supraglottic or glottic pathology. This may not be possible in the pediatric patient, however, as an invasive examination may exacerbate a potentially unstable airway.

Stridor may be acute, occurring over minutes or hours; subacute, progressing over days; or chronic, extending for weeks or more. Acute stridor is commonly infectious in etiology. Bacterial tracheitis and epiglottis are more frequently seen in children, and patients are often toxic in appearance and febrile and have difficulty managing their own secretions. A bacterial infection of an underlying laryngocele (a dilation of the laryngeal saccule) may also occur, termed a *laryngopyocele*, leading to dysphagia and often rapid airway distress. Acute stridor may also be inflammatory in etiology, such as with upper airway angioedema as discussed earlier, or due to foreign body aspiration.

Subacute stridor is also commonly caused by an infectious process. In children, laryngotracheitis, or croup, is a frequent viral upper airway infection that produces a wheezy, often biphasic stridor and barking cough. Deep neck space infections, such as peritonsillar, parapharyngeal, and retropharyngeal abscesses, can also lead to subacute airway distress when not managed in their early stages. Primary pulmonary pathology, such as asthma or exacerbation of chronic obstructive pulmonary disease, may lead to expiratory wheezing that can be easily mistaken for true stridor.

Chronic or slowly progressive stridor is generally due to anatomic structural insufficiency or expanding mass lesions. Laryngomalacia and bronchomalacia are common in infants and can produce characteristic inspiratory and expiratory stridor, respectively. Subglottic stenosis, which may be congenital or acquired, is often related to prior intubations and may be subacute or chronic in presentation. Bilateral vocal cord immobility can lead to a fixed median or paramedian position of the cords, substantially narrowing the airway and causing progressive inspiratory stridor. Laryngeal mass lesions in children are most often benign and include subglottic hemangioma or respiratory papillomatosis. Laryngeal masses leading to progressive airway obstruction in adults should be considered malignant until proven otherwise.

B. Hoarseness

Hoarseness, or dysphonia, is defined as an alteration in the quality or character of phonation. Patients may describe their voice as being breathy, harsh, or rough. Patients should be questioned about onset, frequency, and nature of the hoarseness. As previously discussed, the larynx is an essential part of swallowing, and any history of coughing or choking after eating should be elicited. Likewise, the patient should be questioned about recurrent episodes of pneumonia. Any history of intubation, head and neck trauma, or previous head and neck or thoracic surgery should be sought. Patients should be questioned about smoking and alcohol use.

A full head and neck physical examination is required with visualization of the larynx. Methods of visualization include indirect mirror examination, rigid endoscopy, or transnasal flexible fiberoptic laryngoscopy. Videostroboscopy offers invaluable information about vocal fold motion and can identify adynamic segments and altered areas of mucosal wave propagation.

Hoarseness may be infectious, inflammatory, neurogenic, or due to a laryngeal mass lesion. Laryngopharyngeal reflux (LPR) is a common cause of hoarseness and results from inflammation caused by spillover of refluxate into the larynx. Its symptoms are separate and distinct from classic gastroesophageal reflux disease (GERD). Patients with LPR typically present with frequent throat clearing, globus sensation, cough, and hoarseness (as opposed to postprandial heartburn with GERD). Several laryngeal findings are common in patients with LPR and include vocal cord granuloma, laryngeal edema and erythema, and cobblestoning of the laryngeal mucosa. Viral laryngitis may also present with laryngeal edema and erythema, but findings are more acute and often associated with significant voice change.

The most common neurogenic cause of hoarseness is vocal cord paralysis. Importantly, vocal cord immobility or paralysis is a sign of pathology and is not itself a diagnosis. Vocal cord mobility problems represent a wide range of etiologies characterized by diverse patient presentation and prognostic outcomes. The distinction between unilateral and bilateral paralysis and between paretic (hypomobile) and paralyzed cords is imperative. Patients with unilateral vocal cord paralysis may be asymptomatic but often present with a hoarse, breathy voice. Patients often have difficulty with aspiration, especially of liquids, because the paralyzed vocal cord leads to a glottic gap. The vocal cords derive their innervation from the vagus nerve, and any injury along the course of this nerve may result in vocal cord paralysis. This may result from neurodegenerative processes, stroke, or thoracic, skull base, or thyroid malignancy. Iatrogenic surgical injury, however, is common, including nonthyroid surgical procedures such as cardiac or thoracic surgery, anterior approaches to the cervical spine, and carotid endarterectomy. Table 16–5 summarizes the most common causes of vocal fold paralysis. It should be noted that laryngeal manifestations of autoimmune disease, such as rheumatoid arthritis, can rarely mimic vocal cord paralysis, although the underlying problem in such cases is vocal cord immobility secondary to fixation of the arytenoid cartilages.

Table 16–5. Most common causes of vocal cord paralysis.

Unilateral vocal cord paralysis	
Surgical injury	37%
Cardiovascular, anterior cervical spine procedures	(51%)
Thyroid surgery	(33%)
Idiopathic (viral, inflammatory)	19%
Malignancy	18%
Intubation-related injury	6%
Trauma	6%
Bilateral vocal cord paralysis	
Surgical injury	37%
Cardiovascular, anterior cervical spine procedures	(10%)
Thyroid/parathyroid surgery	(90%)
Malignancy	14%
Intubation	13%
Idiopathic (viral, inflammatory)	11%
Neurologic (Wallenberg syndrome, Parkinson, multiple sclerosis, Guillain-Barré, others)	11%
Trauma	7%

Often, however, the cause of vocal cord immobility is not identifiable, and the vocal cord paralysis is deemed idiopathic. A thorough workup should nonetheless be performed. Diagnostic testing should include axial imaging following the entire course of the vagus nerve (from skull base to the mid chest). Laryngeal EMG can also provide useful information regarding the degree and likely site of injury as well as the potential for spontaneous recovery.

Laryngeal mass lesions are also a common cause of hoarseness. Vocal polyps, nodules, and granulomas are benign vocal cord lesions that are usually traumatic or inflammatory in etiology. Hoarseness, however, can also be the presenting symptom for laryngeal cancer. Symptoms from early lesions are often subtle, and patients have little more than voice change. Advanced lesions may be associated with weight loss, dysphagia, and hemoptysis. Although early-stage laryngeal cancer is highly curable, advanced-stage disease carries a dramatically reduced prognosis. For this reason, any patient with hoarseness lasting longer than 2 weeks should be evaluated by an otolaryngologist and undergo fiberoptic visualization of the larynx.

C. Laryngeal Trauma

Laryngeal trauma is rare, representing one out of every approximately 30,000 emergency department visits. Quick recognition of laryngeal trauma is essential because it can rapidly lead to acute airway obstruction. Up to one-third of laryngeal trauma victims die prior to arrival to a hospital setting.

Laryngeal trauma can be classified as blunt or penetrating. Blunt laryngeal trauma is caused by crushing of the laryngeal framework against the cervical spine and usually results from motor vehicle accidents. Other common etiologies include strangulation-type and clothesline injuries. Penetrating laryngeal trauma usually results from projectile injury, such as a gunshot or knife wound to the neck.

Every patient with neck trauma should be evaluated for potential laryngeal injury. Patients may report dyspnea, hoarseness, or aphonia. Other less common symptoms include dysphagia, anterior neck pain, and odynophagia. Evaluation should begin with a comprehensive trauma workup, including assessment of airway, breathing, and circulation. Physical findings common in patients with laryngeal trauma include stridor, subcutaneous crepitus (emphysema), bruising or edema to the anterior neck, loss of palpable landmarks, and hemoptysis. As outlined previously, the type of stridor can often give an indication of the site of airflow obstruction.

Further evaluation of laryngeal trauma is dictated by the patient's condition. If an adult patient's airway is unstable, most experts would advocate awake tracheostomy or cricothyrotomy under local anesthesia, because endotracheal intubation in the setting of laryngeal trauma can lead to further laryngeal injury. For unstable pediatric laryngeal trauma, inhalational anesthetic followed by rigid endoscopic intubation is recommended by many experts. Once a stable airway has been determined or secured, evaluation can proceed.

Flexible fiberoptic laryngoscopy is advocated for awake, stable patients. The airway should be evaluated for vocal cord mobility, edema, laryngeal lacerations, and hematomas. Because the underlying mechanism of injury often results in damage to other adjacent structures, laryngeal trauma patients should undergo complete cervical spine radiography, and evaluation for esophageal or vascular injury should be considered. Some authors recommend fine-cut CT imaging of the larynx to help guide treatment planning. It should be emphasized that CT scanning rarely provides useful information regarding the immediate airway management for patients suspected of having laryngeal trauma, but it often provides helpful information regarding surgical planning for repair.

▶ Treatment

A. Pediatric Airway Obstruction

One of the most common causes of pediatric stridor is laryngotracheobronchitis, or croup. This is an acute viral illness, most commonly caused by the parainfluenza virus. The typical patient is an infant or young child with low-grade fever, barking cough, and occasionally biphasic stridor. The classic radiographic finding is a "steeple sign" visible on anteroposterior views, indicative of the characteristic narrowed subglottic airway from edema. The typical course for most patients is resolution over several days, and few patients require hospitalization. Signs of respiratory distress, including tachypnea, retractions, and cyanosis, may necessitate closer observation such as hospitalization. For these more severe cases, treatment with humidified air, nebulized racemic epinephrine, and systemic steroids may be indicated. Manipulation of the airway may exacerbate the clinical situation and should be avoided unless clearly indicated.

Epiglottitis is fortunately becoming extremely rare in most industrialized countries due to nearly universal vaccination of children against *H influenzae* type B. If recognized and managed appropriately, with early airway control, outcomes are usually excellent. If managed conservatively, without early airway intervention, epiglottitis is associated with up to a 10% mortality rate. Patients present with high fever, drooling, and odynophagia and are usually toxic in appearance. Epiglottitis can progress rapidly, and patients can decompensate clinically in a matter of hours. Therefore, evaluation and treatment ideally consist of immediate control of the airway in the operating room under general inhalational anesthesia. An inflamed edematous epiglottis will be visible on endoscopic examination. Pharyngeal and blood cultures should be obtained, and the child should be started on broad-spectrum IV antibiotics such as ceftriaxone. Once

definitive identification of the culprit organism is made, antibiotic selection can be narrowed appropriately. Children are left intubated until air leak around the endotracheal tube is evident.

Chronic pediatric stridor is most often due to laryngomalacia. Parents will usually report onset of symptoms shortly after birth. It often worsens initially, but in the vast majority of cases, it resolves without the need for intervention, usually by 12-18 months. A variety of factors have been hypothesized to contribute to laryngomalacia, including neurologic, muscular, and reflux-induced inflammation. The stridor is worsened while crying or in an excited state and is usually relieved by placement in the prone position. Flexible fiberoptic laryngoscopy reveals collapse of floppy supraglottic structures such as the epiglottis and aryepiglottic folds. There is a strong association of laryngomalacia with reflux, and presumptive treatment with an acid-blocking medication (eg, ranitidine) may be beneficial. Surgical treatment of the supraglottis is reserved for severe cases such as patients with cyanosis or failure to thrive. The most common procedure is aryepiglottoplasty, where cold knife or carbon dioxide laser is used to excise redundant mucosa over the arytenoid cartilages or release the aryepiglottic folds to improve airway patency. Rarely, tracheostomy may be necessary.

Subglottic stenosis is the second most common cause of chronic pediatric stridor. Causes include both congenital conditions and acquired stenosis (most often from prolonged intubation). Typically, patients have recurrent episodes similar to laryngotracheitis during periods of inflammation and edema of the narrowed subglottis along with biphasic stridor. If present in older children, the patient may only become symptomatic periodically, in association with upper respiratory tract infections. Diagnosis requires endoscopic evaluation and can be defined as a subglottic airway diameter of less than 4 mm in full-term infants and less than 3 mm in premature infants. Pediatric subglottic stenosis is traditionally graded according to the Cotton scale (Table 16-6). Tracheotomy may be required in moderate to severe cases. Treatment of subglottic stenosis can consist of tracheal dilatation (either by rigid serial dilation or controlled radial balloon expansion), debridement by microdebrider or carbon dioxide laser, cricoid split, or laryngotracheoplasty.

Table 16–6. Summary of the Cotton grading system for subglottic stenosis.

Grade	Degree of Subglottic Obstruction
Grade 1	< 50% obstruction
Grade 2	50%-70% obstruction
Grade 3	71%-99% obstruction
Grade 4	100% obstruction

B. Foreign Body Aspiration

Foreign body aspiration typically involves children between 1 and 4 years of age, but can occur in any age group. Children in this age range tend to place objects in their mouths and lack molars for grinding of food. Objects can range from peanuts (most common) to coins, marbles, and toy products. Adult foreign body aspiration is usually associated with food ingestion. Foreign body aspiration is potentially life threatening, and it is recognized as the fifth most common cause of unintentional injury-related mortality in the United States. Pharyngeal foreign body (most commonly in the vallecula) represents a potential impending airway foreign body and should be treated as such.

The clinical presentation of patients with an airway foreign body depends on the anatomic location. Patients with pharyngeal or hypopharyngeal foreign bodies typically present with dysphagia, odynophagia, and occasionally drooling from inability to tolerate secretions. If large objects become lodged in the larynx, patients may present with pain, dysphonia, inspiratory stridor, and dyspnea. Tracheal foreign bodies produce both inspiratory and expiratory stridor. Distally located foreign bodies (Figure 16–9) often lodge in the right lung due to the less acute angle of the right mainstem bronchus. Distal foreign bodies typically produce unilateral

▲ **Figure 16–9.** Airway foreign body in a 4-year-old child. The patient in question had a history of brief choking while eating dinner three nights earlier, followed by intermittent nonproductive cough. He had a normal chest x-ray and slight wheezing heard on one side only. On rigid bronchoscopy, a soft green bean was found in a right distal bronchus.

wheezing and decreased breath sounds. A history of acute choking episode is commonly associated with foreign body aspiration.

Acute management of airway foreign body is dictated by patient condition. Patients unable to move air require immediate intervention. The Heimlich maneuver can be performed as three manual abdominal thrusts to compress the lungs and potentially produce enough airway pressure to dislodge the foreign body. If unsuccessful, immediate cricothyrotomy should be performed. For patients without impending loss of airway, anteroposterior and lateral radiographs of the neck and chest can be helpful. Although only radio-opaque foreign bodies can be visualized, radiographs may demonstrate obstructive emphysema, atelectasis, or consolidation. Additionally, they can provide a baseline study for future comparison.

Definitive removal of an airway foreign body requires general anesthesia and direct laryngoscopy. Distally located foreign bodies are best addressed with rigid bronchoscopy for removal. A clear history consistent with aspiration often should prompt operative evaluation, even if specific symptoms (stridor, unilateral wheezing, decreased breath sounds) are lacking, because these may be absent in up to 40% of cases. Suspected nut aspiration (common in children) should be treated aggressively. Local tissue reactions to the nut oils and proteins are common and can be robust. After removal, patients with peanut aspiration may require intensive care unit observation and ventilatory support while the inflammatory reaction resolves.

C. Laryngopharyngeal Reflux

Treatment for LPR currently consists of H_2 blockers or proton pump inhibitors (PPIs) as a first-line therapy, with surgery (eg, Nissen fundoplication) for selected treatment failures. Although multiple uncontrolled studies have demonstrated benefit of PPIs for the treatment of LPR, most randomized controlled trials have failed to confirm this finding. Possible confounding factors include lack of clear gold standard for the diagnosis of LPR and differing treatment regimens. Our current practice is to place patients with LPR on once-daily PPI therapy for a 3- to 6-month period, after which response to treatment is assessed. The extended length of time is critical, as studies have shown that resolution of laryngeal findings can take up to 6 months once PPI therapy is initiated. If there is no response to once-daily PPI therapy, the patient can be advanced to twice-daily PPI therapy.

D. Vocal Cord Immobility

Initial therapy for unilateral vocal cord paralysis consists of observation and speech therapy. Often the opposing vocal cord can compensate by crossing the midline and closing the glottal gap. This can produce an acceptable vocal quality, usually occurring within a 3- to 6-month time span. Patients with unsatisfactory results from conservative measures or those with symptoms significant affecting quality of life can be treated by a variety of surgical interventions. The goal of surgical treatment for unilateral vocal cord paralysis is medialization of the affected cord. This reduces the glottic gap and allows the opposing, innervated cord to contact the other vocal fold with less effort. Treatment selection for unilateral vocal cord paralysis depends on the potential for recovery. In cases such as iatrogenic surgical injury with little chance of spontaneous recovery, definitive therapy can be initiated early. For idiopathic causes, a more conservative approach is usually advocated with short-acting injectable fillers. Overall, up to 60% of patients with idiopathic unilateral vocal cord paralysis will recover to a near-normal voice within 8-12 months. Thus, most experts would recommend waiting at least 1 year before proceeding with definitive therapy. Clear indications for earlier intervention include significant dysphagia and aspiration from glottic incompetence.

Definitive surgical procedures for unilateral vocal fold paralysis include laryngeal framework surgery, injection of longer lasting material, and reinnervation techniques. The thyroplasty technique (a laryngeal framework surgical procedure) is performed through an external skin incision. After exposing the thyroid cartilage, a window is cut in the thyroid ala overlying the position of the vocal fold on the affected side. An implant is then placed in a subperichondrial window, thus pushing the vocal fold toward the midline. Implants can include Silastic, autologous cartilage, and Gore-Tex. Most laryngologists perform this procedure with the patient lightly sedated. A flexible fiberoptic laryngoscope can be suspended in position, and the patient is asked to phonate periodically so that the surgical effects can be evaluated in real time and adjusted accordingly.

Another common surgical intervention is injection medialization. This can be performed as an office-based procedure using only local anesthesia or in the operating room under general anesthesia. In either case, a variety of injectable materials are placed within the vocal fold lateral to the vocal process to medialize the cord. In the past, Teflon was commonly used for this purpose, but it has now fallen out of favor secondary to a high rate of complications. An alternative, long-lasting (but not permanent) injectable is calcium hydroxyapatite microspheres in methylcarboxycellulose carrier gel (Radiesse Voice). Temporary injectables include gelfoam paste, hyaluronic acid, micronized cadaveric dermis (Cymetra), cross-linked collagen (Zyderm), and methylcarboxycellulose gel (Radiesse Voice Gel).

Surgical reinnervation for unilateral vocal cord paralysis is gaining popularity. Approaches can include nerve-muscle pedicle (using the omohyoid and ansa hypoglossi nerve) and direct nerve-nerve reinnervation (ansa cervicalis to recurrent laryngeal nerve). Results from these techniques are generally good but can take 6 months or longer to be realized. For this reason, many surgeons combine reinnervation with injection medialization using a temporary substance.

For bilateral vocal cord paralysis, treatment approaches have a different perspective. Whereas restoration of voice is the primary goal for unilateral paralysis, resolution of potential or actual airway compromise is of greatest importance in cases of bilateral paralysis. Most patients are initially treated with a tracheotomy to bypass the glottic obstruction. One common surgical procedure is lateralization of the vocal folds by arytenoidectomy. Although this usually provides a patent airway and allows decannulation (reversal of the tracheotomy), the patient's vocal quality usually suffers significantly, and swallowing can be severely affected. Another surgical approach, partial posterior cordectomy, can often preserve vocal quality to some degree, while providing an improved airway. This approach uses a laser through a surgical laryngoscope to remove a C-shaped wedge from the posterior portion of one vocal cord. This preserves a bilateral vibratory margin anteriorly while providing an airway posteriorly. The technique is often best performed as multiple less aggressive procedures to fine-tune vocal quality versus airway, rather than as a single definitive procedure. Ultimately, management of patients with bilateral vocal cord paralysis is a delicate balance of maintaining vocal quality, stabilizing the airway, and preventing aspiration.

E. Vocal Cord Lesions

Polypoid corditis, also known as Reinke edema, is an accumulation of gelatinous extracellular material in the Reinke space along the bilateral true vocal cords. This condition is almost entirely related to irritation and inflammation from smoking and causes a deepening in pitch and hoarseness of the voice. Vocal polyps are due to local tissue inflammation and often result from vocal strain or prior vocal hemorrhage. Vocal nodules are, similarly, due to vocal overuse but are distinct from polyps and always occur symmetrically bilaterally. Vocal fold granulomas are usually due to prior intubation, laryngeal trauma, or extraesophageal acid reflux damage related to LPR.

Initial treatment of most vocal cord lesions is conservative including speech therapy, smoking cessation, and preventing vocal strain. Vocal nodules, in particular, are best treated conservatively and very rarely require intervention. Polyps or other benign vocal cord lesions that are considerably bulky, risk airway compromise, or have any concern for an underlying malignant process are best treated with microlaryngoscopy and excision.

F. Recurrent Respiratory Papillomatosis

Recurrent respiratory papillomatosis (RRP) is caused by the human papillomavirus (HPV), specifically types 6 and 11. HPV is a small nonenveloped virus that infects the nuclei of host cells for replication. Papillomaviruses show a preference for infection of epithelial tissues and are very common in humans. HPV is responsible for a variety of diseases, including skin warts, RRP, and invasive cancers such as cervical or oropharyngeal carcinoma. Transmission is hypothesized to occur during childbirth. Maternal presence of condylomata during the perinatal period confers a 200-fold increase in relative risk for developing respiratory papillomatosis.

RRP is characterized by recurrent hyperplastic growth of benign tissue in the upper aerodigestive tract. It has a bimodal age distribution, with incidence peaks in children (infants to 12 years old) and adults (30-40 years of age). Patients typically present with dysphonia or aphonia, although advanced disease can cause stridor from impending airway obstruction.

The primary site affected is the larynx, with the glottis being the most common area, followed by the supraglottic larynx (Figure 16–10). RRP generally remains confined to the larynx but can spread distally to affect the trachea, bronchi, and lungs. Disease recurrence is frequent, and most cases require multiple surgical procedures for disease control.

The primary therapy for RRP remains surgical debulking, primarily by microdebrider or carbon dioxide laser ablation. Adjuvant medical treatments include cidofovir, indole-3-carbinol, ribavirin, mumps vaccine, and photodynamic therapy. The role for these adjuvant therapies in the treatment of RRP is still being elucidated. Many otolaryngologists advocate avoidance of tracheotomy if possible, because this has been epidemiologically associated with increased risk of spread of papilloma to the lower respiratory tract. It is possible that this is because patients with inherently more

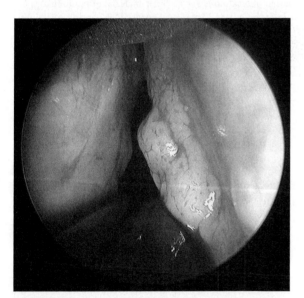

▲ **Figure 16–10.** Adult recurrent respiratory papillomatosis. The right true vocal fold is involved with respiratory papillomatosis. In this patient, the disease was confined mostly to the single true vocal fold, although some disease was also present in the anterior portion of the contralateral vocal fold.

aggressive disease are also those who are more likely to require tracheostomy.

G. Traumatic Laryngeal Injury

Management of the patient with laryngeal trauma depends on the severity of injury. Patients with small laryngeal hematomas, small lacerations not involving the vocal fold edge or anterior commissure, and nondisplaced stable thyroid cartilage fractures can often be managed without tracheostomy. Most such patients should be hospitalized for 24 hours of airway observation and placed on systemic steroids, humidified air, and PPI therapy. If mucosal disruption is present, antibiotics should be initiated.

More severe laryngeal traumas place the patient at risk for airway compromise and often require awake tracheostomy. Patients with displaced laryngeal cartilage fractures require direct laryngoscopy and open laryngeal exploration and repair. This should ideally be performed within 24 hours of the initial injury. Open laryngeal exploration is performed via a midline approach. A horizontal skin incision is made at the level of the cricothyroid membrane. Subplatysmal flaps are elevated, and the strap muscles are divided at the midline. The laryngeal cartilages are reapproximated and can be sutured or plated into place. The larynx is simultaneously exposed transorally by a co-surgeon to assure appropriate placement and stability of the vocal cords. If endolaryngeal repairs must be made, the airway is entered in the midline of the cricothyroid membrane, and a vertical incision through the midline thyroid cartilage is made and extended superiorly. Care must be taken to avoid injury to the anterior commissure during thyrotomy. Once the endolarynx is exposed, mucosal lacerations can be closed and the anterior commissure can be replaced in the appropriate position. A laryngeal stent may be needed to prevent anterior glottic webbing, although placement of a stent itself leads to some degree of laryngeal injury. If placed, stents should be removed as soon as possible, usually around 2 weeks.

Outcomes for laryngeal trauma patients are good once initial control of the airway is obtained. Most patients usually achieve a stable airway, and those requiring tracheostomy are eventually decannulated, which may take up to 6 months or longer depending on the extent of injury. Overall, up to 90% of patients can recover a satisfactory vocal quality if managed appropriately.

DISORDERS OF THE NECK AND LYMPHATIC COMPARTMENTS

▶ Anatomy and Physiology

The lymphatic compartments of the neck are traditionally divided into levels based on lymphatic drainage patterns. Level 1 is composed of the submental and submandibular space above the hyoid bone and digastric muscles and primarily drains the oral cavity and lower face. The lymphatics of the lateral neck are divided into levels 2 through 4 and are located between the sternocleidomastoid muscle, scalene musculature, and the carotid sheath. These lymphatics primarily drain the upper aerodigestive tract, although cervical skin and thyroid pathology may drain to these regions as well. Level 2 is located high in the neck, above the hyoid bone; level 3 is located in the mid-neck between the hyoid bone and cricoid cartilage; and level 4 is located in the low neck between the cricoid cartilage and clavicle. Level 5 is considered the posterior triangle of the neck and is located between the posterior aspect of the sternocleidomastoid muscle, the anterior aspect of the trapezius muscle, and the clavicle. Level 5 lymphatics generally drain posterior structures including the nasopharynx as well as posterior scalp and cervical skin. Finally, level 6 lymphatics are located in the central neck between the left and right carotid sheaths and are the primary lymphatic basin for anterior neck structures including the thyroid gland.

In addition to the location of lymphatics, it is essential to understand the basic anatomy of major neurovascular structures in the neck. The plane of the styloid process delineates an important distinction in anatomic territory of structures either posterior (poststyloid) or anterior (prestyloid) to this plane. The poststyloid space contains critical neurovascular elements including the carotid artery, jugular vein, and vagus and sympathetic nerves. The prestyloid space mainly contains salivary gland tissue, adipose tissue, and sensory nerves.

▶ Workup and Differential Diagnosis of a Neck Mass

A thorough history and physical examination should be performed with attention to patient demographics as well as the location and characteristics of the mass. Younger patients are more likely to have congenital, infectious, or inflammatory processes, whereas older patients and those with significant tobacco or alcohol exposure have a higher likelihood of an underlying malignancy. The time course should be ascertained, because malignant disease generally enlarges progressively, whereas infectious or inflammatory disorders often follow a fluctuating course. The location of the mass is also of critical importance and the differential diagnosis can be formulated from an understanding of the anatomy. Axial imaging with CT scan is an excellent initial diagnostic modality and can delineate the extent of the neck mass and its relationship to surrounding structures. MRI can be useful if further soft tissue refinement is necessary, such as for masses of the salivary glands or parapharyngeal space. If a thyroidal mass is suspected, ultrasound is generally the preferred modality. The next step in diagnosis for most neck masses will be a fine-needle aspiration biopsy to obtain a histologic diagnosis. These procedures do not lead to spillage or seeding if the mass is malignant and are highly accurate

and minimally invasive. Excisional or incisional biopsies, however, are discouraged because these can lead to tumor seeding and, in rare cases, such as a carotid body tumor or vagal paraganglioma, can lead to catastrophic hemorrhage or cranial nerve injury.

▶ Treatment

A. Congenital

There are several common congenital masses of the neck. Branchial cleft cysts most commonly present as a lateral cystic neck mass in younger patients who often have a history of repeated infection. Definitive treatment is surgical resection. However, prior to treatment, it is of critical importance to rule out malignancy in these cases. A common presentation of HPV-associated oropharyngeal cancer is a cystic neck mass, which can be easily mistaken for a branchial cleft cyst. Such patients are often younger adults without the common tobacco- and alcohol-related risk factors. In these patients, the primary tumor is often asymptomatic, is located in the tonsil or base of tongue, and has metastasized to a regional lymph node, resulting in the cystic neck mass (see later section on head and neck cancer).

Thyroglossal duct cysts are cystic remnants of the thyroid gland's embryonic descent from the tongue base to its position anterior to the trachea. These present as midline anterior cystic neck masses that move with tongue protrusion. These masses are often intimately associated with the central hyoid bone, which should be resected in continuity with the mass (Sistrunk procedure).

B. Infectious

Neck masses of infectious etiology may follow either an acute or prolonged time course. Acute infectious neck masses are generally enlarged draining lymph nodes related to a viral or bacterial process of the upper aerodigestive tract, mucosa, teeth, or salivary glands. Acute suppurative sialadenitis occurs most commonly in dehydrated patients who are postoperative or elderly or those on diuretic therapy. The parotid gland is affected in most cases due to the diminished bacteriostatic activity of its serous saliva. Salivary stasis, ductal obstruction, and decreased saliva production appear to be predisposing conditions to acute sialadenitis. Patients usually present with fever, systemic toxicity, and tender swelling and enlargement of the affected glands. Treatment involves hydration, warm facial compresses, and sialagogues to stimulate saliva secretion in the affected gland. Antibiotics targeted against S aureus should be started immediately and continued for 7-10 days. CT may be necessary to rule out abscess formation or stone (sialolithiasis) in patients who do not improve clinically after several days of appropriate therapy.

In patients with immunocompromise or unusual environmental exposures, consideration should be given to more uncommon conditions, such as cat-scratch disease, tuberculosis, tularemia, or brucellosis. In the pediatric population, an atypical mycobacterial infection can present as a neck mass overlying the submandibular or parotid regions. These patients typically have overlying skin changes, including induration and a violaceous hue. Although the majority of infectious neck masses are treated with antibiotic therapy, patients with purulent collections or those with atypical mycobacterial infections will usually require some form of incision and drainage.

C. Inflammatory

Inflammatory neck masses are most commonly autoimmune in etiology, and patients will often exhibit associated signs and symptoms related to the underlying diagnosis. Sjögren syndrome leads to salivary gland swelling, which may present as a neck mass. Such patients will also complain of dry eye and dry mouth. Treatment is primarily symptomatic in nature, including meticulous dental hygiene and ocular lubrication. Sarcoidosis is a systemic granulomatous disease that can present with enlargement of cervical lymph nodes or salivary glands. Patients generally exhibit weight loss and fatigue and are managed with immunosuppressive therapy. Immunoglobulin G (IgG)-4–related sialadenitis is a chronic autoimmune condition marked by swelling and sclerosis primarily of the submandibular glands. IgG-4–related processes are highly responsive to corticosteroid therapy.

D. Benign Neoplasms

There are several benign neoplasms of the neck that are essential to be aware of, primarily to prevent a catastrophic complication from inappropriate excisional or incisional biopsy. Paragangliomas are highly vascular tumors that occur most commonly at the carotid body or along the cervical course of the vagus nerve. Open biopsy in these cases can result in severe bleeding or vagal nerve injury. Schwannomas are tumors of neural origin that can arise from several nerves in the head and neck, commonly the vagus nerve or sympathetic trunk, and biopsy can result in inadvertent cranial nerve injury. Finally, parapharyngeal or periparotid masses may represent pleomorphic adenomas, a common benign tumor of salivary gland origin. Open biopsy of such tumors may result in tumor spillage and diffuse tumor seeding of the soft tissues of the neck.

E. Sialolithiasis

Sialolithiasis may occur in the setting of acute or chronic sialadenitis, or it may be an incidental finding on routine imaging studies. Salivary calculi affect males more than females and are seen most frequently between ages 30 and 60 years. In contrast to sialadenitis, sialolithiasis preferentially affects the submandibular glands because of their alkaline, high-calcium, mucus-rich environment. Large, solitary, radio-opaque stones are usually found in the submandibular glands, whereas the parotid glands are more likely to have multiple smaller, radiolucent stones. Calculus formation is believed to be secondary to partial obstruction of the salivary duct combined with calcium-rich stagnant saliva. Salts composed of calcium phosphate, magnesium, ammonium, and carbonate precipitate in this environment. Contributing factors to the development of salivary calculi include underlying acute or chronic sialadenitis, dehydration, and anticholinergic medications. Uric acid salivary calculi may also be seen in the setting of gout.

Patients with sialolithiasis frequently present with pain and swelling of the affected gland, although many patients have asymptomatic calculi discovered incidentally. Eating usually exacerbates the pain. Physical examination may reveal the location of the calculi by simple palpation. Obstruction of the flow of saliva can be analyzed by massaging the gland. CT is the preferred method of imaging if sialolithiasis is suspected but a calculus is unable to be palpated on physical examination. CT has a 10-fold greater sensitivity than plain films in detecting salivary calculi.

Treatment of sialolithiasis should begin conservatively with hydration, salivary gland massage, warm compresses, and sialagogues. Anticholinergic medications should be discontinued, and antibiotics should be initiated if there is concern for acute suppurative sialadenitis. There are several options for more invasive therapy for patients who do not respond to conservative management. Transoral removal of submandibular stones, lithotripsy, and sialoendoscopy have all been shown to be effective in the appropriate patient. Sialoadenectomy may ultimately be necessary in patients who fail conservative and minimally invasive management.

HEAD AND NECK CANCER

▶ Pathophysiology of Head and Neck Squamous Cell Carcinoma

Excluding skin cancer, the majority of head and neck malignancies are SCCs. Head and neck SCC (HNSCC) is the sixth most common malignancy, and over 500,000 patients worldwide are diagnosed with HNSCC each year. HNSCC is a highly curable malignancy when diagnosed at an early stage. Unfortunately, patients often present with locally advanced disease. Overall, the prognosis is poor in this latter group of patients. For those with advanced disease, over 30% may develop locoregional recurrence within 2 years.

Despite numerous advances in our understanding of this disease and in development of improved medical and surgical therapies, mortality rates have only modestly improved over the past two decades. Additionally, current therapies (both surgical and nonsurgical) carry a high level of treatment-related morbidity. Patients with advanced-stage disease often suffer significant speech and swallowing impairment following treatment.

Development of HNSCC is traditionally attributed to the synergistic carcinogenic effects of tobacco and alcohol. Other factors, such as poor oral dentition, gastroesophageal reflux, betel nut chewing, and viral infection, are also important contributors. It is now accepted that high-risk types (eg, 16, 18, and 31) of HPV are causal agents in the development of some SCCs of the oropharynx. Currently, as many as 70% of oropharyngeal cancers are HPV associated. In HPV-mediated transformation, oncoproteins (primarily E6 and E7) encoded by the HPV genome are transcribed by infected human epithelial cells, resulting in the degradation and inactivation of host tumor suppressor genes *p53* and *Rb*. This is thought to allow unchecked cell cycle progression and development of genetic instability. Most importantly, HPV-associated oropharyngeal cancers have a significantly improved prognosis over HPV-negative, smoking-related disease.

Head and neck cancers are thought to progress through characteristic stages of premalignancy (dysplasia and carcinoma in situ), until finally reaching invasive carcinoma. This progression reflects the accumulation of multiple genetic changes from mutation, gene silencing (via methylation), chromosomal rearrangements, deletions, and duplications. Importantly, most HNSCCs are thought to arise in areas of field cancerization. According to this theory, first described in the 1950s, the entire mucosa of the upper aerodigestive tract is exposed to similar carcinogenic insults. Thus, premalignant changes occur in a wide field, not just at the site of the original cancer. Even if that cancer is successfully treated, the patient remains at high risk for developing subsequent malignancies throughout the upper aerodigestive tract. Recent molecular-based investigations have provided strong support for this concept, and multiple studies have demonstrated genetic alterations in histologically normal tissue from high-risk individuals. For this reason, patients with a history of HNSCC should be closely followed with yearly screening examinations for life.

▶ Evaluation of the Patient with Head and Neck Cancer

A. History and Physical Examination

Any patient with a significant history of alcohol and tobacco use who presents with complaints related to the upper aerodigestive system should be evaluated with an index of suspicion for HNSCC. Mechanical obstruction and dysfunction from a tumor mass can produce dysphagia and odynophagia. Referred pain from the oral cavity or pharynx can also result in otalgia, as can cancers arising in the nasopharynx or those affecting the EAC. Cancers of the true vocal cords often produce significant hoarseness early during disease progression. Other symptoms can include hemoptysis, globus sensation, trismus, and weight loss. Sometimes the presenting symptom is a neck mass representing nodal metastases from an asymptomatic primary source.

Patients should be asked about family history of cancers and personal risk factors such as alcohol use and use of all forms of tobacco. Certain ethnic populations (specifically emigrants from India) may give a history of betel nut chewing. This nut has been found, like tobacco, to have synergistic carcinogenic risk when present in combination with alcohol consumption.

Physical examination should include a comprehensive evaluation of all sites of the head and neck. Unilateral serous fluid in the middle ear space in an adult should raise suspicion for a nasopharyngeal lesion. The entire oral cavity should be evaluated, including each gingivobuccal sulcus. The floor of mouth and base of tongue should be manually palpated for induration, pain on palpation, and asymmetry. Evaluation of the larynx and base of tongue can be performed by headlamp and mirror examination (indirect laryngoscopy). Flexible fiberoptic evaluation often provides additional detail and visualization not possible with the former method. Additionally, the nasal cavity and nasopharynx can easily be evaluated during the same procedure. A complete evaluation of the cranial nerves should be performed. This can often give insight into nerves affected by tumor mass effect (compression) or direct nerve invasion (perineural spread). The neck should be carefully palpated for cervical lymphadenopathy. The pads of the fingers and thumbs are the most sensitive parts of the hands and should be used instead of the tips of the digits.

B. Imaging

Imaging is an important part of the diagnostic evaluation of a patient with head and neck cancer. Goals of imaging include preoperative identification of site and extent of tumor infiltration, presence of suspicious lymph nodes, and presence of anatomic variations. The imaging modality of choice for most suspected head and neck tumors is CT scan with intravenous contrast. This allows adequate soft tissue and bony detail. Most head and neck cancers will demonstrate enhancement with IV contrast administration. Contrast MRI may offer additional information in evaluation of the skull base, parapharyngeal space and orbit, and cranial nerves for evidence of perineural spread.

Increasingly, evaluation of HNSCC patients for distant metastases and monitoring for posttreatment disease recurrence or persistence involves the use of tumor imaging by ^{18}F-fluorodeoxyglucose positron emission tomography (FDG-PET) (Figure 16–11). The use of FDG-PET and combined PET/CT modalities is extremely important because early identification of persistent or recurrent disease has the potential to impact survival. Although CT and MRI rely on contrast enhancement patterns and differences in tissue attenuation, FDG becomes concentrated in cells with elevated glucose utilization. Because changes in tumor metabolism often precede changes discernable on clinical examination, FDG-PET is valuable in discovering clinically

▲ **Figure 16–11.** Positron emission tomography (PET) scan. PET scan showing uptake in the original primary site (palate, indicated by large arrowhead) as well as new mediastinal uptake indicative of nodal metastases (thin arrow). Note the normal physiologic uptake in the liver (moderate intensity) and heart and brain (high intensity), demonstrating the relatively high glucose utilization of these organs.

nondetectable tumor spread or recurrence. PET-CT results are generally reported as standardized uptake values (SUV). This is the ratio of tissue FDG uptake normalized to injected dose of FDG, patient body weight, and serum glucose levels. Higher SUV values indicate increased FDG uptake. In addition to malignancy, multiple tissue metabolic changes can lead to increased FDG uptake, including inflammation, infection, and radiation response.

C. Staging of Head and Neck Squamous Cell Carcinoma

Staging for HNSCC in the United States uses the tumor-node-metastasis (TNM) system published by the American Joint Committee on Cancer, currently in its eighth edition.

Staging allows estimation of prognosis, treatment planning, and expected response to treatment. The TNM system classifies cancers by primary tumor size, locoregional nodal metastases, and distant metastatic spread. The rules for classification vary by subsite within the head and neck. In general, cancers of subsites that can be seen directly (eg, oral cavity, oropharynx) are T (tumor) staged by size. By comparison, cancers of subsites not visible directly (eg, larynx, hypopharynx, sinonasal) are T staged by anatomic spread of disease.

Initial evaluation of the primary site and T staging is best accomplished by operative direct laryngoscopy and esophagoscopy. This allows examination of the primary site and evaluation of the entire upper aerodigestive tract for simultaneous second primary tumors and biopsy of suspicious areas.

N (nodal) stage is determined by the presence of clinically evident regional lymph node metastases on both physical examination and imaging. Radiologic findings suspicious for malignant lymph node metastases include lymph nodes that are round, heterogeneously enhancing, and larger than 1 cm. Important prognostic features that have recently changed the staging criteria include extranodal extension of disease and HPV association. The current criteria for N staging (for subsites other than the nasopharynx) are summarized in Tables 16–7 and 16–8.

M (metastasis) stage is determined by the presence of distant metastatic disease. The most common sites of metastases for HNSCC are the liver and the lungs. Therefore, part of the initial staging workup for a patient with head and neck cancer includes some method of evaluating these structures. This most commonly consists of chest CT or whole-body CT-PET scanning. M stage is reported as Mx (cannot be determined), M0 (no distant metastases), or M1 (distant metastatic disease). Overall staging is achieved by combining the T, N, and M stages to yield four broad stages (stages I to IV, with I carrying the best prognosis and IV the worst). The specific definitions of such staging and related prognoses are highly dependent on disease subsite and other factors such as HPV association.

Table 16–7. Determination of N stage for cancers of the oral cavity, oropharynx, hypopharynx, and larynx.

Nx	Regional lymph nodes cannot be assessed
N0	No regional lymph node metastases
N1	Metastases in a single ipsilateral lymph node, 3 cm or less
N2	
N2a	Metastases in a single ipsilateral lymph node, > 3 cm but not > 6 cm
N2b	Metastases in multiple ipsilateral lymph nodes < 6 cm
N2c	Metastases in bilateral or contralateral lymph nodes < 6 cm
N3	Metastases in lymph node(s) > 6 cm

Table 16–8. Summary of TNM staging for cancers of the oral cavity, oropharynx, hypopharynx, and larynx.

Stage	T Stage	N Stage	M Stage
Stage 0	T-is (in situ)	N0	M0
Stage I	T1	N0	M0
Stage II	T2	N0	M0
Stage III	T3 T1-T3	N0 N1	M0
Stage IVA	T4a T1-T4a	N0-N1 N2	M0
Stage IVB	T4b Any T	N0-N2 N3	M0
Stage IVC	Any T	Any N	M1

Table 16–9. T stage for cancers of the oral cavity.

T1	Tumor of 2 cm or less in greatest dimension
T2	Tumor > 2 cm, but not > 4 cm, in greatest dimension
T3	Tumor > 4 cm in greatest dimension
T4	
T4a	Tumor invades through adjacent structures
	Lip: cortical bone, floor of mouth, facial skin of chin or nose Oral cavity proper: cortical bone, deep muscles of tongue (genioglossus, palatoglossus, hyoglossus, styloglossus), skin
T4b	Tumor invades masticator space, pterygoid plates, or skull base and/or encases carotid artery

D. Overview of Treatment

Traditional therapy for HNSCC depends on the stage of the cancer and varies by subsite. Simplified, early-stage cancers are usually treated with single-modality therapy, either surgical excision or radiation therapy. Advanced-stage (stages III and IV) cancers are best treated by combined-modality therapy, either surgery and postoperative adjuvant therapy or definitive chemoradiation. The specific treatment paradigm depends greatly on disease subsite, pretreatment functional status, and patient preferences.

Patients with distant metastatic disease or recurrent unresectable cancer are generally managed with systemic therapy. A combination of 5-fluorouracil, cisplatin, and cetuximab has been demonstrated in a randomized trial to provide the best first-line therapy for such patients. Traditional chemotherapy in those with recurrent or metastatic disease may provide symptom control but offers little chance of long-term cure. Newer immuno-oncology agents, such as programmed cell death 1 (PD-1) or programmed death ligand 1 (PD-L1) inhibitors, have shown promise in recent randomized trials. Although response rates to these drugs are modest in patients with heavy prior treatment, long-term durable responses have been reported.

▶ Treatment for Specific Head and Neck Sites

A. Cancers of the Oral Cavity

Patients with oral cavity cancer typically present with a painful mass of the tongue, buccal mucosa, floor of mouth, or alveolar ridge. Although most cancers have either an ulcerative or an exophytic appearance, many can have only subtle visually detectable changes. On palpation, the involved area is usually firm and indurated. The mass should be manipulated to discern mobility. Oral cavity cancers can invade the mandible quite readily, and immobility should raise concern for bone invasion.

As with other head and neck subsites where the primary tumor can be directly visualized, T staging is assessed by tumor size (summarized in Table 16–9). Cancers that invade adjacent structures are, in general, upstaged to T4 regardless of size.

The nodal drainage patterns of oral cavity cancers are of particular concern, because the incidence of occult metastases can approach 30% depending on T stage and depth of invasion. When planning treatment of occult metastases, it is important to remember that midline cancers of the oral cavity often drain bilaterally.

Treatment for oral cavity cancer is primarily surgical. Cancers of the lip can often be addressed with simple wedge excision, with 5-mm borders of surrounding normal tissue. If less than one-third of the lip is excised, a reasonable result can be obtained with simple closure. Larger excisions require a reconstructive procedure, often involving transfer of lip tissue from the contralateral lip. Cancers of the tongue, floor of mouth, and buccal mucosa are excised with a 1-cm margin of normal-appearing tissue. Often primary closure, with or without a split-thickness skin graft, will provide acceptable functional outcomes. Large resections usually require a flap reconstruction, either soft tissue only or including an osseous component for resections of the mandible or maxilla. Such reconstructions, either pedicled or free flaps, use vascularized tissue from regional or distant body sites to reconstruct complex wounds in the head and neck. These procedures are generally performed by otolaryngologists or plastic surgeons with additional formal training in complex head and neck reconstruction. Pedicled flaps (eg, the pectoralis major flap) are isolated on their vascular pedicle and rotated into the head and neck defect. Free flaps (eg, radial forearm, anterolateral thigh, or fibular free flaps) are isolated on their vascular pedicles, which are then divided and transferred up to the head and neck wound (Figure 16–12). A donor artery and vein are identified in the neck and used to provide a feeding

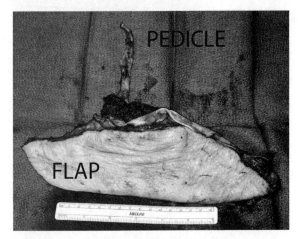

▲ **Figure 16–12.** Free anterolateral thigh flap in preparation for reconstruction of a complex glossectomy defect. The vascular pedicle (the descending branches of the lateral circumflex femoral artery and vein) has been isolated, and a small cuff of vastus lateralis muscle has been harvested around the vascular perforators entering the skin flap.

and draining blood supply to the flap. The arterial anastomosis is typically performed with 9-0 suture, and the venous anastomosis is most commonly done with a coupling device in which the veins are loaded onto silicone rings brought together in end-to-end fashion (Figure 16–13).

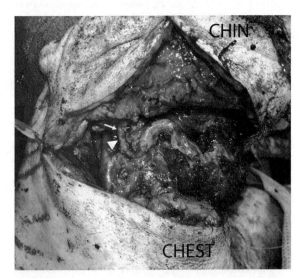

▲ **Figure 16–13.** Microvascular inset of the anterolateral thigh flap from Figure 16–12. The facial artery (arrow) has been anastomosed to the flap artery (arrowhead) with 9-0 suture. The silicone disc of the venous coupler can be seen just above the arterial anastomosis.

With appropriate treatment, outcomes for patients with oral cavity cancer are generally good. The prognosis for SCC of the lip is excellent, with 5-year survival of over 90% for stage I to II and over 80% for stage III to IVa. SCC of the oral cavity proper carries a reduced, yet still relatively good prognosis, with 5-year survival rates of over 70% for stage I to II disease. Advanced-stage disease carries a worse prognosis, however, with 5-year survival rates of less than 60% for most subsites.

B. Cancers of the Oropharynx

The single most important development in oropharyngeal cancer in the past several decades is the understanding that a subset of oropharyngeal SCC is associated with HPV. Such tumors carry a significantly improved prognosis over those unrelated to HPV, which are most commonly due to tobacco and alcohol exposure.

As is the case for oral cavity cancer, T staging for SCC of the oropharynx is generally determined by tumor size (summarized in Table 16–10). Again, invasion of adjacent structures results in classification as T4 regardless of size. Nodal metastases from oropharyngeal cancers are common, with 70% of patients with oropharyngeal cancer having ipsilateral cervical nodal metastases at the time of presentation. Bilateral cervical nodal metastases are also relatively common, up to 30%, depending on size and subsite of the primary tumor.

Oropharyngeal cancer, particularly that of the tongue base and tonsil, may be treated with either a surgical or nonsurgical treatment paradigm. In the modern era, primary surgery for oropharyngeal cancer is performed transorally, either with a carbon dioxide laser or robotic assistance. Management decisions are generally based on tumor location, clinician experience, comorbidities, and patient preference. Both surgical and nonsurgical strategies appear to have similar oncologic outcomes, and the differences in functional outcomes between these options remain an area of active investigation. Survival for HPV-negative oropharyngeal cancer is poor and mirrors advanced-stage oral cavity cancer.

Table 16–10. T stage for cancers of the oropharynx.

T1		Tumor of 2 cm or less in greatest dimension
T2		Tumor > 2 cm, but not > 4 cm, in greatest dimension
T3		Tumor > 4 cm in greatest dimension
T4		
	T4a	Tumor invades through adjacent structures (larynx; deep muscles of tongue, such as genioglossus, palatoglossus, hyoglossus, styloglossus; medial pterygoid, hard palate, mandible)
	T4b	Tumor invades masticator space, pterygoid plates, lateral nasopharynx, or skull base and/or encases carotid artery

Survival for HPV-related disease, however, is excellent, and even for advanced disease, a 5-year survival rate of greater than 70% can be expected.

C. Cancers of the Larynx

Laryngeal cancer was a relatively rare disease until the 20th century. Mass production of cigarettes was associated with a dramatic rise in the incidence of laryngeal cancer. Tobacco exposure is now accepted as the primary etiologic agent responsible for laryngeal cancer. Other possible additive factors include laryngopharyngeal reflux and possibly certain viruses, such as herpes simplex virus or HPV.

Laryngeal cancers can arise from above the true vocal folds (supraglottic region), below the true vocal folds (subglottic region), or directly from the true vocal folds (glottic region). The latter represents greater than 75% of all laryngeal cancers. For patients with glottic laryngeal cancer, dysphonia (hoarseness) is the most common presenting symptom. Any hoarseness that persists longer than 2 weeks, especially in a patient with associated risk factors of tobacco or alcohol use, should undergo laryngeal examination. Patients with hoarseness, however, are more likely to have a nonmalignant cause for their symptoms than to have laryngeal cancer.

Laryngeal cancers arising from the subglottis or supraglottis usually present at a later stage than do glottic cancers, because hoarseness does not develop until late in the disease process. Often, the presenting symptom can be life-threatening stridor from an obstructive mass. Emergent awake tracheotomy is sometimes required to secure a stable patent airway in these cases. Other symptoms can include globus sensation ("lump in the throat") and dysphagia. Evaluation for pre-existing swallowing dysfunction is emerging as an essential part of the diagnostic workup for laryngeal cancers. Because of the emphasis on organ-preservation strategies, identification of patients likely to end up with a nonfunctioning larynx may alter treatment planning. Currently, this is an area of active investigation.

Unlike oral cavity and oropharyngeal cancer (T staged by tumor size), cancers of the larynx are T staged by anatomic spread of disease (Table 16–11). One important factor is determination of vocal cord fixation. This can be reliably determined with in-office flexible fiberoptic evaluation. Laryngeal cancer N staging follows the convention for other head and neck subsites (except nasopharynx).

Therapy for early (T1-T2) glottic cancer is single-modality therapy, either transoral laser surgery or definitive radiation therapy. Again, the choice depends on tumor location, clinician experience, comorbidities, and patient preference. Radiation therapy generally results in improved voice quality over surgery. However, in cases of recurrence, patients with prior radiation generally require an open surgical approach, most commonly a total laryngectomy. Those who experience recurrence after surgery alone are often candidates for further transoral surgery as well as definitive (chemo)radiotherapy.

Table 16–11. T stage for cancers of the larynx.

Supraglottis	
T1	Tumor limited to one subsite of the supraglottis. Normal vocal cord mobility.
T2	Tumor invades mucosa of more than one subsite of the supraglottis, glottis, or adjacent structure (tongue base, vallecula, medial wall of pyriform). Normal vocal cord mobility.
T3	Tumor limited to the larynx but presence of vocal cord fixation, and/or invades postcricoid, pre-epiglottic tissues, or paraglottic space, or inner cortex only invasion of thyroid cartilage.
T4	
T4a	Tumor invades through thyroid cartilage and/or extends to other tissues beyond the larynx (eg, trachea, deep extrinsic tongue muscles, strap muscles, thyroid, esophagus).
T4b	Tumor invades prevertebral space, encases carotid artery, or invades mediastinal structures.
Glottis	
T1	
T1a	Tumor limited to unilateral true vocal cord with normal mobility (may involve anterior or posterior commissure).
T1b	Tumor limited to bilateral true vocal cords with normal mobility (may involve anterior or posterior commissure).
T2	Tumor extends to supraglottis and/or subglottis and/or impaired vocal cord mobility.
T3	Tumor limited to larynx with vocal cord fixation and/or invades paraglottic space, and/or minor thyroid cartilage invasion (inner cortex only).
T4	
T4a	Tumor invades through the thyroid cartilage and/or invades tissues beyond the larynx (trachea, soft tissues of the neck including deep extrinsic tongue muscles, strap muscles, thyroid, esophagus).
T4b	Tumor invades prevertebral space, encases carotid artery, or invades mediastinal structures.
Subglottis	
T1	Tumor limited to subglottis.
T2	Tumor extends to true vocal cord(s) with normal or impaired mobility (but no fixation).
T3	Tumor limited to larynx, with vocal cord fixation.
T4	
T4a	Tumor invades cricoid or thyroid cartilage and/or invades tissues beyond larynx (trachea, soft tissues of the neck including deep extrinsic tongue muscles, strap muscles, thyroid, esophagus).
T4b	Tumor invades prevertebral space, encases carotid artery, or invades mediastinal structures.

The goal of organ preservation (ie, preserving a functional ability to phonate and protect the airway during deglutition) should be kept in mind when planning treatment options for patients with advanced laryngeal cancer. Patients who present with a functioning larynx, primarily the ability to swallow prior to treatment, are often best served with primary nonsurgical management with definitive chemoradiotherapy. A randomized trial performed in the Veterans Affairs (VA) population demonstrated similar oncologic outcomes between total laryngectomy and nonsurgical management for such patients. However, patients who present with significant tumor invasion of laryngeal cartilages or those with tracheostomy and gastrostomy dependence prior to treatment are often best managed with total laryngectomy for both optimal oncologic and long-term functional outcomes. Although patients with total laryngectomy are obligate neck breathers, because the trachea is sewn to the neck skin in this operation, the pharyngoesophageal tract is surgically separated from the airway and patients can no longer aspirate. Additionally, modern rehabilitation with tracheoesophageal prostheses can allow motivated patients to regain intelligible pulmonary-driven speech.

Surgical options for organ-preservation strategies in patients with advanced disease include transoral endoscopic excision or open partial laryngeal procedures. Both options often require substantial swallowing rehabilitation and are generally only performed for select recurrent tumors at institutions with significant experience using these techniques.

Outcomes for patients with laryngeal cancer can be excellent. For early stage I glottic carcinoma (tumor limited to the true vocal folds), 5-year overall survival rates of 90% can be expected. With invasion of adjacent structures characteristic of stage III to IVB disease, however, 5-year survival decreases to less than 60%.

D. Cancers of the Hypopharynx

The hypopharynx is a continuation of the oropharynx and extends superiorly from the level of the hyoid bone to the level of the inferior aspect of the cricoid cartilage. It consists of the pyriform sinuses (the most common subsite for hypopharyngeal cancer), the posterior pharyngeal wall, and postcricoid regions. The hypopharynx is lined with stratified squamous epithelium and is invested with an abundant lymphatic drainage network. Patients with hypopharyngeal cancer typically present with advanced-stage disease, because small lesions in this region are often asymptomatic. Typical presenting symptoms can include referred otalgia, odynophagia, and dysphagia. Other symptoms can include a neck mass (from nodal metastases), hoarseness (due to laryngeal involvement), and weight loss. Like laryngeal cancer, hypopharyngeal cancer is chiefly related to excessive alcohol and tobacco exposure. There is also some evidence for a possible contribution of GERD to hypopharyngeal cancer. This may explain the increased likelihood for patients with Plummer-Vinson syndrome to develop hypopharyngeal cancer, regardless of

Table 16–12. T stage for cancers of the hypopharynx.

T1	Tumor limited to one subsite and 2 cm or less in greatest dimension
T2	No fixation of hemilarynx, and tumor: • Invades more than subsite or an adjacent area (larynx, oropharynx) and/or • Is > 2 cm, but not > 4 cm, in greatest dimension
T3	Tumor > 4 cm in greatest dimension or fixation of hemilarynx
T4	
T4a	Tumor invades through adjacent structures (thyroid/cricoid cartilage, hyoid bone, thyroid gland, esophagus, central compartment)
T4b	Tumor involves prevertebral fascia or mediastinal structures and/or encases carotid artery

tobacco or alcohol exposure. In Plummer-Vinson syndrome, patients develop esophageal webs, and chronic acid exposure above the site of webbing is thought to possibly result in chronic inflammation predisposing to malignancy.

Hypopharyngeal cancer T staging is a combination of tumor size (as for oral cavity and oropharyngeal tumors) and anatomic spread (as for laryngeal cancer). The T-staging criteria for hypopharyngeal cancer are summarized in Table 16–12. N staging and M staging are the same as for the majority of head and neck sites (except nasopharynx).

Early-stage (T1-T2 tumors) hypopharyngeal cancer is often treated with primary radiotherapy. Alternatively, transoral laryngeal conservation surgery may be a reasonable option for some of these early-stage cancers. More advanced (T3-T4) tumors can be treated by surgical resection with postoperative adjuvant therapy or definitive chemoradiotherapy. As for advanced laryngeal cancer, a similar randomized trial has demonstrated equivalent oncologic outcomes for total laryngectomy and nonsurgical management of advanced hypopharyngeal cancer. In that way, management decisions are based on preoperative functional status and tumor extent. Those with preoperative tracheostomy and gastrostomy dependence and those with tumors causing destruction of laryngeal cartilages are best served with total laryngectomy, whereas those with good preoperative function may be candidates for nonsurgical organ-preservation strategies. Again, as for laryngeal cancer, surgical organ preservation options for advanced-stage disease include transoral or open partial pharyngolaryngeal procedures. Such operations are complex, often involve advanced reconstruction, and are generally only performed at select centers with a significant volume of experience.

Hypopharyngeal cancer carries the worst prognosis of any head and neck subsite. The underlying reasons for this are unclear, but several hypotheses have been suggested.

A distinctive pathologic feature of hypopharyngeal cancer is the propensity for submucosal spread of disease, often resulting in clinically understaging disease extent. The abundant lymphatic drainage of the hypopharynx may also predispose the patient to early nodal metastases, and many patients eventually develop distant metastases. Five-year survival for stage I to II hypopharyngeal cancer is approximately 50%, whereas 5-years survival for stage III to IVB is generally less than 40%.

E. Salivary Gland Neoplasms

Neoplasms (both benign and malignant) of the salivary glands are relatively uncommon, representing a small proportion of all head and neck neoplasms. Major salivary glands include the parotid, submandibular, and sublingual glands. The minor salivary glands are scattered mainly throughout the mucosa of the lips and oral cavity and, to a lesser extent, the entire upper aerodigestive tract. The parotid gland accounts for 80% of all neoplasms, whereas 15% arise from the submandibular glands and 5% from the sublingual and minor salivary glands. For any given tumor, however, the incidence of malignancy is 20% for parotid tumors, 60% for submandibular tumors, and 80% for sublingual and minor salivary gland tumors. Unlike SCC, tobacco and alcohol exposure does not appear to play an etiologic role in salivary gland malignancy. It should be noted that the parotid gland contains lymph nodes that drain the preauricular and temporal skin. Any parotid mass should raise suspicion for a skin cancer with intraparotid nodal metastases, and a complete examination of the scalp and preauricular skin is indicated.

The most common benign salivary gland tumor is pleomorphic adenoma (also called benign mixed tumor), representing 60% of all salivary gland neoplasms. Patients typically present with a slowly enlarging, painless, firm mass (most often in the parotid gland). Facial nerve paralysis is exceedingly rare, even with very large tumors, due to the slow-growing nature of these neoplasms. Malignant transformation of pleomorphic adenoma is rare but does occur, and the resultant malignancy is highly aggressive. Treatment for pleomorphic adenoma is complete surgical excision, including a surrounding margin of normal tissue. Due to microscopic transcapsular tumor infiltration, simple enucleation is insufficient for these benign neoplasms.

The second most common benign salivary neoplasm is papillary cystadenoma lymphomatosum (also known as Warthin tumor). This benign tumor is responsible for 10% of parotid neoplasms but is rare outside of the parotid gland. Bilateral tumors are present in up to 10% of patients, so careful palpation and imaging of both parotid beds are important if this tumor is suspected. Patients typically present with a slowly enlarging parotid mass, which is painless and rubbery upon palpation. Standard treatment is complete surgical excision (eg, superficial parotidectomy with facial nerve preservation), although some authors advocate that enucleation of these tumors may be adequate therapy.

The most common salivary gland malignancy is mucoepidermoid carcinoma. Despite the propensity of the smaller salivary gland neoplasms to be malignant, the most common site for mucoepidermoid carcinoma is still the parotid gland. Approximately 45% to 70% of mucoepidermoid carcinomas arise from the parotid gland, whereas 20% occur in minor salivary glands of the palate. Typical symptoms at presentation can be quite like those of benign salivary neoplasms, with a painless enlarging mass. Symptoms such as pain or facial paralysis are uncommon, but when present, they should raise suspicion for an aggressive high-grade lesion. Mucoepidermoid cancers are graded as low grade (mostly mucous cells), intermediate grade, and high grade (characterized by a hypercellular solid tumor). The latter can be difficult to distinguish from SCC without immunohistochemical staining. Treatment is tailored to the extent of disease, tumor grade, and location. Localized disease is usually amenable to surgical excision (parotidectomy with facial nerve preservation, submandibular gland excision, or wide local excision for minor salivary gland origin). Advanced disease requires extensive resection, often combined with neck dissection and postoperative radiotherapy.

The second most common salivary gland malignancy is adenoid cystic carcinoma. It is most common in the submandibular, sublingual, and minor salivary glands. Of all parotid neoplasms, adenoid cystic carcinoma is more likely to present with pain or paresthesia, although an asymptomatic mass is still the most common presentation. Adenoid cystic carcinoma is characterized by a propensity for perineural spread. Thus, preoperative imaging with gadolinium-enhanced MRI is often helpful in therapeutic planning. Treatment consists of complete surgical resection (sometimes requiring facial nerve sacrifice) and postoperative radiation therapy. Adenoid cystic carcinoma rarely spreads to cervical lymphatics, so neck dissection is not routinely advocated. It does, however, have a propensity for distant metastases, particularly to the lung. The disease is also characterized by frequent local recurrence (up to 40%) even after adequate local excision. Because of the relatively slow-growing nature of this disease, survival for adenoid cystic carcinoma at 5 years is favorable (approximately 65% for all stages). Due to the propensities for local recurrence and distant metastases, however, this statistic decreases to less than 30% at 15 years.

As mentioned earlier, malignant degeneration of pleomorphic adenomas can occur, although it is uncommon. Some authors have estimated the risk of malignant degeneration at 1.5% for the first 5 years, increasing to 9.5% by 15 years or longer. The resulting malignant tumor is termed *carcinoma ex pleomorphic adenoma* and is characterized by an aggressive natural history and poor clinical outcome. The most common presentation is sudden rapid growth of a previously stable parotid mass. Histologically, the malignant cells can take the form of any epithelial malignancy except acinic cell. Carcinoma ex pleomorphic adenoma is

Table 16–13. T stage for major salivary gland cancer.

T1	Tumor of 2 cm or less in greatest dimension, no extraparenchymal extension
T2	Tumor > 2 cm, but not > 4 cm, in greatest dimension; no extraparenchymal extension
T3	Tumor > 4 cm in greatest dimension and/or extraparenchymal extension
T4	
T4a	Tumor invades through adjacent structures (skin, mandible, external auditory canal, and/or facial nerve involvement)
T4b	Tumor invades skull base or pterygoid plates and/or encases carotid artery

characterized by frequent lymph node metastases, and up to 25% of patients will have clinically evident cervical lymphadenopathy on presentation. Treatment includes radical surgical resection, often combined with neck dissection and postoperative radiotherapy.

The prognosis of salivary gland malignancies varies according to histologic type, location, extent of disease, and grade. The criteria for T staging are similar to other head and neck sites with directly measurable tumor size and are summarized in Table 16–13. Overall, early stage (stage I-II) salivary gland cancers carry an excellent prognosis (> 80% at 5 years). Advanced (stage III-IV) salivary gland cancers, on the other hand, have overall 5-year survival rates ranging from 20% to 60% depending heavily on type and grade.

▶ References

Carter KB, Jr., Loehrl TA, Poetker DM: Granulocyte transfusions in fulminant invasive fungal sinusitis. *Am J Otolaryngol.* 2012;33(6):663-666.

Hamilos DL: Chronic rhinosinusitis: epidemiology and medical management. *J Allergy Clin Immunol.* 2011;128(4):693-707; quiz 708-699.

Oosthuizen JC: Paediatric blunt laryngeal trauma: a review. *Int J Otolaryngol.* 2011;2011:183047.

Pullens B, van Benthem PP: Intratympanic gentamicin for Meniere's disease or syndrome. *Cochrane Database Sys Rev.* 2011;3:CD008234.

MULTIPLE CHOICE QUESTIONS

1. You are asked to evaluate a 6-year-old child with nasal pain. She is on the pediatric hematology-oncology service and is undergoing chemotherapy for acute lymphoblastic leukemia. She has no other pertinent medical history. The pain has been present for 12 hours. On examination, you note no abnormalities in the oral cavity, oropharynx, or external head and neck examination. Her pulse is regular, and her respirations are nonlabored. On nasal examination, you note a slight duskiness to the anterior face of the left middle turbinate. An appropriate response would be to

   A. Reassure the child and her parents that she is most likely fine, and schedule a follow-up visit for the following day
   B. Take her to the operating room immediately for an emergent biopsy
   C. Order contrasted magnetic resonance imaging (MRI) of the nose/face/orbits and a complete blood count (CBC) with differential
   D. Start her on nasal decongestant spray (oxymetazoline) twice daily, nasal saline irrigations, and an oral antihistamine once daily

2. You are asked to evaluate a patient in the emergency department with rapid onset of lip and tongue swelling. He develops shortness of breath and stridor during your examination. Following an emergent tracheotomy to establish his airway, you do a thorough review of his medication history. Which of the following drug classes is/are known to be associated with acute angioedema?

   A. Angiotensin-converting enzyme (ACE) inhibitors (eg, lisinopril)
   B. Angiotensin II receptor blockers (ARBs; eg, losartan)
   C. Recombinant tissue plasminogen activators (r-tPAs; eg, alteplase)
   D. Anticoagulant direct thrombin inhibitors (eg, lepirudin)
   E. All of the above

3. A 34-year-old woman is seen in the emergency department with submandibular swelling, fever, and pain. She is unable to open her mouth more than a few millimeters. One hour later, she collapses, and she has only minimal air movement with bag-mask ventilation. Attempts at oral intubation are unsuccessful. Fortunately, you are standing nearby and offer to perform an emergency cricothyrotomy. Where is the best place to rapidly create an airway inferior to the vocal cords with a minimum danger of hemorrhage?

   A. Immediately superior to the cricoid cartilage
   B. Immediately superior to the hyoid bone
   C. Immediately superior to the jugular notch
   D. Immediately superior to the third tracheal ring
   E. Immediately superior to the thyroid cartilage

4. A 25-year-old man undergoes thyroidectomy with right recurrent laryngeal nerve sacrifice due to encasement by papillary thyroid carcinoma. The ansa cervicalis is then anastomosed to the cut distal end of the recurrent laryngeal nerve. The patient has vocal hoarseness initially, which improves over several months. At 6 months postoperatively, a transnasal endoscopy is performed and the right vocal fold is found to be immobile but in a median position, allowing the left vocal fold to make midline contact with the paralyzed side. Reinnervation of which of the following muscle groups is most likely responsible for the vocal fold position noted?

A. Adductor musculature only
B. Abductor musculature only
C. Both adductor and abductor synkinesis
D. Cricothyroid muscle
E. Vocalis muscle

5. You perform an excisional biopsy of a lateral tongue lesion, which returns as squamous cell carcinoma extending to the margins of resection with a depth of invasion of 10 mm. You see the patient back in clinic after 1 week, and this area is healing well with no obvious disease. You should

A. Watch the patient closely in follow-up for recurrent disease and order a neck computed tomography (CT) scan in 3 months
B. Plan for definitive radiotherapy
C. Plan for a definitive resection of the primary site and order a neck CT scan in 3 months
D. Plan for a definitive resection of the primary site with ipsilateral neck dissection and possible adjuvant radiotherapy after resection depending on pathologic results

Thyroid & Parathyroid

Lindsay E. Kuo, MD, MBA
Nancy L. Cho, MD

▼ THE THYROID GLAND

EMBRYOLOGY & ANATOMY

The thyroid gland develops as a median endodermal downgrowth from the first and second pharyngeal pouches (Figure 17–1). During its caudal migration, it contacts the ultimobranchial bodies developing from the fourth pharyngeal pouches. When it reaches the position it occupies in the adult, with the isthmus situated just below the cricoid cartilage, the thyroid divides into two lobes. The site from which it originated persists as the foramen cecum at the base of the tongue. The path the gland follows may result in thyroglossal remnants (cysts) or ectopic thyroid tissue (lingual thyroid). A pyramidal lobe, extending cranially from the isthmus, is frequently present. Agenesis of one thyroid lobe, almost always the left, may occur.

The normal thyroid weighs 15-25 g and is attached to the trachea by loose connective tissue. It is a highly vascularized organ that derives its blood supply principally from the superior and inferior thyroid arteries. A thyroid ima artery may also be present. Venous drainage is via the superior, middle, and inferior thyroid veins.

PHYSIOLOGY

The function of the thyroid gland is to synthesize, store, and secrete the hormones thyroxine (T_4) and triiodothyronine (T_3). Iodide is absorbed from the gastrointestinal tract and actively trapped by the acinar cells of the thyroid gland. It is then oxidized and combined with tyrosine in thyroglobulin to form monoiodotyrosine (MIT) and diiodotyrosine (DIT). These are coupled to form the active hormones T_4 and T_3, which initially are stored in the colloid of the gland. Following hydrolysis of the thyroglobulin, T_4 and T_3 are secreted into the plasma, becoming almost instantaneously bound to plasma proteins. T_4 is the dominant hormone secreted by the thyroid, and extrathyroidal conversion of T_4 to T_3 accounts for the majority of circulating T_3.

Thyroid function is regulated by a feedback mechanism that involves the hypothalamus and pituitary. Thyrotropin-releasing factor (TRF) is formed in the hypothalamus and stimulates the release of the thyroid-stimulating hormone (TSH) thyrotropin from the pituitary. Thyrotropin binds to TSH receptors on the thyroid plasma membrane, stimulating thyroid cellular function and thyroid growth.

EVALUATION OF THE THYROID

In a patient presenting with thyroid disease, a thorough history and physical examination of the gland are critical and are complemented by appropriate laboratory tests and imaging. The history should question both systemic and local symptoms. Family history of thyroid dysfunction or malignancy is also important. Physical palpation of the gland determines the contour, consistency, nodularity, and fixation of the gland, and examines for displacement of the trachea or palpable cervical lymph nodes.

Thyroid function is assessed with a highly sensitive TSH assay that differentiates among patients with hypothyroidism (increased TSH levels), euthyroidism, and hyperthyroidism (decreased TSH levels). In most cases, therefore, serum T_3, T_4, and other variables need not be measured to diagnose thyroid function. A free T_4 level, which measures T_4 that is not bound to plasma proteins, is helpful in monitoring patients during treatment for Graves disease. A free T_3 level can be useful to diagnose the severity of the hyperthyroidism.

The thyroid is most often imaged with either an ultrasound or a radioactive iodine uptake scan, depending on the indication. The ultrasound provides a clear picture of thyroid anatomy, its relationship to surrounding structures, and the presence of nodularity. It also evaluates for cervical lymph node abnormalities. The radioactive iodine uptake scan measures thyroid activity and localizes the site of the hyperfunctioning tissue.

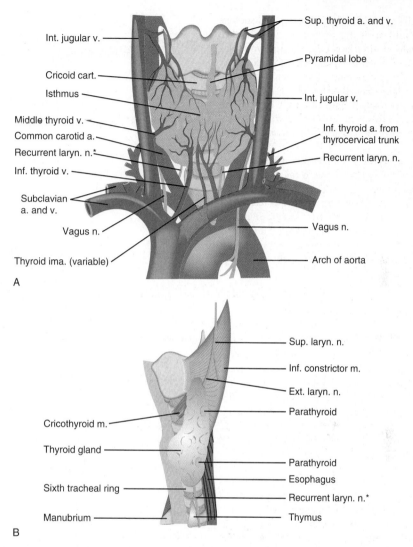

Int. jugular v.
Cricoid cart.
Isthmus
Middle thyroid v.
Common carotid a.
Recurrent laryn. n.*
Inf. thyroid v.
Subclavian a. and v.
Vagus n.
Thyroid ima. (variable)

Sup. thyroid a. and v.
Pyramidal lobe
Int. jugular v.
Inf. thyroid a. from thyrocervical trunk
Recurrent laryn. n.
Vagus n.
Arch of aorta

A

Sup. laryn. n.
Inf. constrictor m.
Ext. laryn. n.
Parathyroid
Cricothyroid m.
Thyroid gland
Parathyroid
Esophagus
Sixth tracheal ring
Recurrent laryn. n.*
Manubrium
Thymus

B

▲ **Figure 17–1.** Thyroid anatomy. The recurrent laryngeal nerve runs in the tracheoesophageal groove on the left and has a slightly more oblique course on the right before it enters the larynx just posterior to the cricothyroid muscle at the level of the cricoid cartilage.

DISEASES OF THE THYROID

HYPERTHYROIDISM (THYROTOXICOSIS)

ESSENTIALS OF DIAGNOSIS

▸ Nervousness, weight loss with increased appetite, heat intolerance, increased sweating, muscular weakness and fatigue, increased bowel frequency, polyuria, menstrual irregularities, infertility

▸ Goiter, tachycardia, atrial fibrillation, warm moist skin, thyroid thrill and bruit, cardiac flow murmur, gynecomastia

▸ Eye signs: stare, lid lag, exophthalmos

▸ TSH low or absent; thyroid-stimulating immunoglobulin, iodine uptake, T_3, and T_4 increased; T_3 suppression test abnormal (failure to suppress radioiodine uptake)

General Considerations

Hyperthyroidism is caused by the increased secretion of thyroid hormone. Specific primary causes include Graves disease, toxic nodular goiter (Plummer disease), and solitary toxic nodule. Graves disease is an autoimmune disease, often with a familial predisposition. Secondary hyperthyroidism may be due to amiodarone toxicity, pregnancy, TSH-secreting pituitary tumors, human chorionic gonadotropin–secreting tumors, or iodine induced (Jod-Basedow effect). Most cases of hyperthyroidism are easily diagnosed on the basis of the signs and symptoms, while subclinical hyperthyroidism may be recognized only with laboratory testing revealing a suppressed TSH level.

In all forms, the symptoms of hyperthyroidism are due to increased levels of thyroid hormone in the bloodstream. The clinical manifestations of thyrotoxicosis may be subtle or marked and tend to go through periods of exacerbation and remission. Some patients ultimately develop hypothyroidism, either spontaneously (~ 15%) or as a result of treatment. If left untreated, thyrotoxicosis may cause progressive and profound catabolic disturbances and cardiac damage. Death may occur in thyroid storm or because of heart failure or severe cachexia.

▶ Clinical Findings

A. Symptoms and Signs

The clinical findings are those of hyperthyroidism as well as those related to the underlying cause (Table 17–1). Nervousness, increased diaphoresis, heat intolerance, tachycardia, palpitations, fatigue, and weight loss in association with a nodular, multinodular, or diffuse goiter are the classic findings in hyperthyroidism. The patient may have a flushed and staring appearance. The skin is warm, thin, and moist, and the hair is fine. The Achilles reflex time is shortened in hyperthyroidism and prolonged in hypothyroidism. The patient on the verge of thyroid storm has accentuated symptoms and signs of thyrotoxicosis: hyperpyrexia, tachycardia, cardiac failure, neuromuscular excitation, delirium, or jaundice.

In Graves disease, there may be exophthalmos (in which the eye bulges anteriorly), pretibial myxedema, or vitiligo. These signs are virtually never seen in multinodular toxic goiter or solitary toxic nodule.

B. Laboratory Findings

Laboratory tests reveal a suppressed TSH and an elevation of T_3 and free T_4. A history of medications is important, since certain drugs and organic iodinated compounds affect some thyroid function tests. In mild forms of hyperthyroidism, the usual diagnostic laboratory tests are likely to be only slightly abnormal. In these difficult-to-diagnose cases, two additional tests are helpful: the T_3 suppression test and the thyrotropin-releasing hormone (TRH) test. In the T_3 suppression test, hyperthyroid patients fail to suppress the thyroidal uptake of radioiodine when given exogenous T_3. In the TRH test, serum TSH levels fail to rise in response to administration of TRH in hyperthyroid patients.

Table 17–1. Clinical findings in thyrotoxicosis.

Clinical Manifestations	Frequency
Tachycardia	Nearly all
Nervousness	Nearly all
Goiter	Nearly all
Skin changes	Nearly all
Tremor	Nearly all
Increased sweating	Majority
Hypersensitivity to heat	Majority
Palpitations	Majority
Fatigue	Majority
Weight loss	Majority
Bruit over thyroid	Majority
Dyspnea	Majority
Eye signs	Majority
Weakness	Majority
Increased appetite	Majority
Eye complaints	Majority
Leg swelling	Some
Hyperdefecation (without diarrhea)	Some
Diarrhea	Some
Atrial fibrillation	Some
Splenomegaly	Few
Gynecomastia	Few
Anorexia	Few
Liver palms	Few
Constipation	Few
Weight gain	Few

Graves disease is diagnosed by testing for thyrotropin-receptor antibodies (thyroid-stimulating immunoglobulin), in addition to the patient's clinical appearance.

C. Radiologic Findings

A thyroid uptake scan can help determine the cause of hyperthyroidism. Either a technetium Tc-99m pertechnetate or radioactive iodine (^{123}I) uptake scan is performed, and uptake of the radiolabeled isotope in the thyroid tissue is measured. Homogenous diffuse uptake is consistent with Graves disease, whereas multiple areas of increased uptake are seen in Plummer disease. A single site of uptake in contrast with a suppressed gland is diagnostic of a solitary toxic nodule.

Differential Diagnosis

Anxiety, heart disease, anemia, gastrointestinal disease, cirrhosis, tuberculosis, myasthenia and other muscular disorders, pheochromocytoma, primary ophthalmopathy, and thyrotoxicosis factitia may be clinically difficult to differentiate from hyperthyroidism. Differentiation is especially difficult when the thyrotoxic patient presents with minimal or no thyroid enlargement. Patients may also have painless or spontaneously resolving thyroiditis and are hyperthyroid because of increased release of thyroid hormone from the thyroid gland. This condition, however, is self-limited, and treatment is rarely necessary.

Anxiety is perhaps the condition most frequently confused with hyperthyroidism. Anxiety is characterized by persistent fatigue usually unrelieved by rest, clammy palms, a normal sleeping pulse rate, and normal laboratory tests of thyroid function. The fatigue of hyperthyroidism is often relieved by rest, the palms are warm and moist, tachycardia persists during sleep, and thyroid function tests are abnormal.

Organic disease of nonthyroidal origin that may be confused with hyperthyroidism must be differentiated largely on the basis of evidence of specific organ system involvement and normal thyroid function tests. Other causes of exophthalmos (eg, orbital tumors) or ophthalmoplegia (eg, myasthenia) must be ruled out by ophthalmologic, ultrasonographic, computed tomography (CT) or magnetic resonance imaging (MRI), and neurologic examinations.

Treatment

Hyperthyroidism may be effectively treated by antithyroid drugs, radioactive iodine ablation, or thyroidectomy. Treatment must be individualized and depends on the underlying pathologic process, symptoms, comorbid conditions, and the patient's ability to obtain follow-up care.

A. Antithyroid Drugs

The principal antithyroid drug used in the United States is methimazole (MMI), 30-100 mg orally daily; propylthiouracil (PTU), 300-1000 mg orally daily, has become an infrequent choice due to side effects but is preferred in pregnant patients. These agents decrease hormone synthesis by interfering with organic binding of iodine and coupling of iodotyrosines in the thyroid gland. PTU also inhibits peripheral conversion of T_4 to T_3. One advantage of these medications is that they inhibit the function of the gland without destroying tissue; therefore, there is a lower incidence of subsequent hypothyroidism. These medications are often employed as a first-line treatment to control the disease. Reliable patients with small goiters are good candidates for this regimen. A prolonged remission after 18 months of treatment occurs in 30% of patients, some of whom eventually become hypothyroid. Patients who fail to achieve long-term remission should then consider radioactive iodine treatment or surgical resection.

Up to 25% of patients on MMI or PTU experience minor side effects, such as pruritis. Side effects of PTU include rashes and fever (3%-4%), agranulocytosis (0.1%-0.4%), and, rarely, liver failure. Patients must be warned to immediately stop the drug, see a physician, and have a white blood cell count checked if sore throat or fever develops. Patients on MMI or PTU should be closely monitored.

B. Radioactive Iodine

Radioactive iodine (^{131}I) is indicated for patients with recurrent hyperthyroidism, patients with hyperthyroidism that has not gone into remission, or patients who are poor surgical candidates. Patients take a single dose of a liquid or a pill, which can be done as an outpatient. The radioiodine is taken up by thyroid follicular cells and subsequently causes tissue necrosis over a period of 6-18 weeks. Patients receiving radioiodine can become hypothyroid. Other side effects include dry mouth and radiation thyroiditis, due to release of thyroid hormone by necrotic thyroid tissue.

Radioactive iodine treatment at doses necessary to treat hyperthyroidism does not appear to increase the risk of leukemia or congenital anomalies. In young patients, the radiation hazard is certainly increased, and the chance of developing hypothyroidism is virtually 100%. Therefore, hyperthyroid children should not be treated with radioiodine. Because radioiodine crosses the placenta and is secreted in breast milk, pregnant or lactating women should also not receive radioiodine. Patients taking radioactive iodine should avoid contact with these populations for a short time.

C. Surgery

1. Indications for Thyroidectomy—The main advantage of thyroidectomy is definitive, curative treatment. Surgery is often the preferred treatment (1) in the presence of a large goiter or a multinodular goiter with relatively low radioactive iodine uptake, (2) if there is a suspicious or malignant thyroid nodule, (3) for patients with ophthalmopathy, (4) for the treatment of pregnant patients or children, (5) for the treatment of women who wish to become pregnant within 1 year after treatment, and (6) for patients with amiodarone-induced hyperthyroidism.

2. Preparation for Surgery—The risks of thyroidectomy for toxic goiter are small due to the combined preoperative use of iodides and antithyroid drugs. An antithyroid drug is administered until the patient becomes euthyroid and is continued until the time of operation. Potassium iodide or

Lugol's iodine solution is also given for about 5-7 days before surgery because this may decrease the friability and vascularity of the thyroid, thereby technically facilitating thyroidectomy. Rebound hyperthyroidism may occur in some patients following prolonged treatment with iodide solution, so prompt thyroidectomy should be planned within 1-2 weeks to avoid this phenomenon.

An occasional untreated or inadequately treated hyperthyroid patient may require an emergency operation for some unrelated problem such as acute appendicitis and thus require immediate control of the hyperthyroidism. Such a patient should be treated in a manner similar to one in thyroid storm, since **thyroid storm** or hyperthyroid crises may be precipitated by surgical stress or trauma. Treatment of hyperthyroid patients requiring an emergency operation or those in thyroid storm is as follows: Prevent release of preformed thyroid hormone by administration of Lugol's iodine solution; give β-adrenergic blocking agents to antagonize the peripheral manifestations of thyrotoxicosis; and decrease thyroid hormone production and extrathyroidal conversion of T_4 to T_3 by giving PTU, MMI, or steroids. Other important considerations are to treat precipitating causes (eg, infection, drug reactions); to support vital functions by giving oxygen, sedatives, intravenous fluids, and corticosteroids; and to reduce fever. Benzodiazepines may be useful in the patient in whom anxiety is a prominent symptom, and a cooling blanket should be used in patients, if needed, for temperature control.

3. Thyroidectomy—The treatment of hyperthyroidism by subtotal, near-total, or total thyroidectomy eliminates both the hyperthyroidism and the goiter. As a rule, nearly all of the thyroid gland is removed, sparing the parathyroid glands and the recurrent laryngeal nerves. Patients with a solitary toxic nodule may be treated with lobectomy alone.

The mortality associated with these procedures is extremely low—less than 0.1%. Thyroidectomy thus provides safe and rapid correction of the thyrotoxic state. The frequency of recurrent hyperthyroidism and hypothyroidism depends on the amount of thyroid remaining and on the natural history of the hyperthyroidism. Given an accomplished surgeon and good preoperative preparation, injuries to the recurrent laryngeal nerves and parathyroid glands occur in less than 2% of cases. Adequate exposure and avoidance of injury to the recurrent laryngeal nerves and parathyroid glands are essential.

▶ Ocular Manifestations of Graves Disease

The pathogenesis of the ocular problems in Graves disease relates to circulating autoantibodies that cross-react against eye tissues to cause inflammation and edema in varying degrees. Smoking can worsen the severity of disease as well as increase the incidence of afflicted patients.

The eye changes of Graves disease vary from no signs or symptoms to loss of sight. Mild cases are characterized by upper lid retraction and stare with or without lid lag or proptosis. These cases present only minor cosmetic problems and usually require no treatment unless the eyes are dry. In more severe disease, proptosis, extraocular muscle involvement, and finally optic nerve involvement occur due to retroorbital soft tissue inflammation caused by the stimulation of thyrotropin receptors in these tissues. Some cases may have marked chemosis, periorbital edema, conjunctivitis, keratitis, diplopia, ophthalmoplegia, and impaired vision. Ophthalmologic consultation is required.

Symptoms may begin before there is any evidence of thyroid dysfunction or after the hyperthyroidism has been appropriately treated. Usually, however, the ocular manifestations develop concomitantly with the hyperthyroidism. Relief of the eye problems is often difficult to accomplish until coexisting hyperthyroidism or hypothyroidism is controlled.

Treatment of the ocular problems of Graves disease includes maintaining the patient in a euthyroid state without increase in TSH secretion, protecting the eyes from light and dust with dark glasses and eye shields, elevating the head of the bed, using diuretics to decrease periorbital and retrobulbar edema, and giving methylcellulose or guanethidine eye drops. Smokers should be counseled to stop smoking, which can worsen symptoms and render treatments less effective. High doses of glucocorticoids are beneficial in certain patients, but their effectiveness is variable and unpredictable. If exophthalmos progresses despite medical treatment, lateral tarsorrhaphy, retrobulbar irradiation, or surgical decompression of the orbit may be necessary.

Total thyroidectomy is the treatment of choice when it can be done with a low risk of complications. Some patients enjoy a halt in the progression, or even improvement, of their eye symptoms corresponding to a decrease in the level of circulating autoantibodies following surgery. Graves disease is more likely to worsen after radioiodine treatment than after thyroidectomy, and antithyroid medications have no effect. It is important that patients with ophthalmopathy understand the natural history of the disease and also that they be kept euthyroid, since hyperthyroidism and hypothyroidism may produce visual deterioration. Operations to correct diplopia should be deferred until after the ophthalmopathy has stabilized.

Ross DS et al: 2016 American Thyroid Association guidelines for diagnosis and management of hyperthyroidism and other causes of thyrotoxicosis. *Thyroid*. 2016;26:1343-1421.

EVALUATION OF THYROID NODULES & GOITERS

▶ Thyroid Nodules

Thyroid nodules are very common, but only 10% of nodules are cancerous. The differential diagnosis includes benign goiter, intrathyroidal cysts, thyroiditis, benign and malignant tumors, and, rarely, metastatic tumors to the thyroid.

Some nodules are discovered on physical examination or incidentally on imaging performed for another reason, whereas other nodules have associated symptoms. The history should specifically emphasize the duration of swelling, recent growth, local symptoms (dysphagia, pain, shortness of breath, choking sensation, or voice changes), and systemic symptoms (hyperthyroidism, hypothyroidism, or those from possible tumors metastatic to the thyroid). The patient's age, gender, place of birth, family history, and history of radiation to the neck are most important. Low-dose therapeutic radiation (6.5–2000 cGy) in infancy or childhood is associated with an increased incidence of benign goiter (~ 35%) or thyroid cancer (~ 13%) in later life. A thyroid nodule is more likely to be a cancer in a man than in a woman and in young (under 20 years) and older (over 60 years) patients. Thyroid cancer is familial in about 25% of patients with medullary thyroid cancer (familial medullary thyroid cancer, multiple endocrine neoplasia [MEN] types 2A and 2B) and in about 7% of patients with papillary or Hürthle cell cancer. Papillary thyroid cancer occurs more often in patients with Cowden syndrome, Gardner syndrome, or Carney syndrome.

The clinician must systematically palpate the thyroid to evaluate the consistency and mobility of any nodules and to examine for palpable lymph nodes. A solitary hard thyroid nodule is likely to be malignant, whereas most multinodular goiters are benign. Ultrasound evaluation helps document the number of nodules, whether a nodule is suspicious for cancer, and whether there are coexistent suspicious lymph nodes. Radioiodine scanning can be used selectively in hyperthyroid patients to determine whether a follicular neoplasm by cytologic examination is functioning (warm or hot) or nonfunctioning (cold). Hot solitary thyroid nodules may cause hyperthyroidism but are rarely malignant. Thyroid nodules incidentally discovered by CT, MRI, or positron emission tomography (PET) scans should be evaluated by dedicated ultrasound.

Based on ultrasound appearance, some nodules are concerning for malignancy and require biopsy. This is performed via percutaneous needle biopsy, also known as fine-needle aspiration. Cytologic results are classified using the Bethesda criteria, which categorizes each result into one of six groupings (Table 17–2). Each classification has an associated risk of malignancy and a recommended next step in diagnosis or treatment. If the specimen is reported as inadequate, biopsy should be repeated. Genetic testing, such as the Afirma gene expression classifier or Thyroseq, may be helpful in these patients. False-positive diagnoses of cancer are rare, but false-negative diagnoses are slightly more common, especially in nodules > 3 cm because there is increased risk of sampling error. Needle biopsy is not as helpful in patients with a history of irradiation to the neck because radiation-induced tumors are often multifocal, and a negative biopsy may therefore be unreliable. Furthermore, approximately 40% of previously irradiated patients will have thyroid cancer.

Table 17–2. Bethesda classification for thyroid cytology.

Cytology Result	Likelihood of Malignancy	Usual Management
Nondiagnostic	1%–4%	Repeat US-guided FNA
Benign	0%–3%	Surveillance
Atypia or follicular lesion of undetermined significance	5%–15%	Surveillance versus repeat FNA with molecular/genetic testing versus surgery
Follicular or Hürthle cell neoplasm	20%–30%	Repeat FNA with molecular/genetic testing versus surgery
Suspicious for malignancy	60%–75%	Generally treat as for malignancy
Malignant	98%–99%	Treat for malignancy (total thyroidectomy versus thyroid lobectomy)

FNA, fine-needle aspiration; US, ultrasound.

Thyroid carcinoma is uncommon (~ 3%) in multinodular goiters, but any nodule that meets criteria for biopsy on ultrasound should be tested. Abnormal lymph nodes seen on ultrasound can also be biopsied. CT or MRI scans are usually not necessary for the evaluation of thyroid nodules but are helpful when the limits of the tumor or gland cannot be defined, such as in patients with large, invasive, or substernal goiters or tumors.

The principal indications for surgical removal of a nodular goiter are (1) suspicion of or documented cancer, (2) inability to rule out cancer in a suspicious nodule, (3) compressive symptoms, (4) hyperthyroidism, (5) substernal extension, and (6) cosmetic deformity. Nonoperative treatment is appropriate in asymptomatic patients with small or moderately sized multinodular goiters and Hashimoto thyroiditis, unless there is a clinically suspicious or enlarging nodule, if the patient was exposed to radiation, or if the patient has a family history of thyroid carcinoma.

▶ Simple or Nontoxic Goiter (Diffuse & Multinodular Goiter)

The term *goiter* refers to an enlargement of the thyroid gland. Simple nontoxic (not hyperfunctional) goiter may be physiologic, occurring during puberty or pregnancy. Simple goiter may also occur in patients from endemic (iodine-poor) regions or as a result of prolonged exposure to goitrogenic foods or drugs. Goiters may also occur early in life as a consequence of a congenital defect in thyroid hormone production or in patients with Hashimoto thyroiditis. It is generally assumed that nontoxic goiter represents a compensatory response to inadequate thyroid hormone production, although thyroid growth immunoglobulins may also be important.

In diffuse goiter, the thyroid is symmetrically enlarged and has a smooth surface. As the goiter persists, there is a tendency to form nodules, and most patients have multinodular glands by the time they seek medical care. Thyroid function is usually normal, although TSH may be suppressed and the radioiodine uptake increased. Symptoms caused by goiters include neck pressure, dyspnea, dysphagia, or symptoms caused by interference with venous obstruction. Surgery is indicated to relieve the pressure symptoms of a large goiter for substernal goiter or to rule out cancer when there are localized areas of hardness, rapid growth, or suspicious nodules. Fine-needle aspiration biopsy is helpful in these patients.

Alexander EK et al: Preoperative diagnosis of benign thyroid nodules with indeterminate cytology. *N Engl J Med.* 2012;367(8):705-715.
Cibas ES et al: The 2017 Bethesda system for reporting thyroid cytopathology. *Thyroid.* 2017;27(11):1341-1346.

INFLAMMATORY THYROID DISEASE

The inflammatory diseases of the thyroid are termed acute, subacute, or chronic thyroiditis, which can be either suppurative or nonsuppurative.

Acute suppurative thyroiditis is uncommon and is characterized by the sudden onset of severe neck pain accompanied by dysphagia, fever, and chills. It usually follows an acute upper respiratory tract infection; can be diagnosed by percutaneous aspiration, smear, and culture; and is treated by surgical drainage. The organisms are most often streptococci, staphylococci, pneumococci, or coliforms. It may also be associated with a piriform sinus fistula. A barium swallow is therefore recommended in persistent or recurrent cases.

Subacute thyroiditis, a noninfectious disorder, is characterized by thyroid swelling, head and chest pain, fever, weakness, malaise, palpitations, and weight loss. Some patients with subacute thyroiditis have no pain (silent thyroiditis), in which case the condition must be distinguished from Graves disease. In subacute thyroiditis, the erythrocyte sedimentation rate and serum gamma globulin are almost always elevated, and radioiodine uptake is very low or absent with increased or normal thyroid hormone levels. The illness is usually self-limited, and aspirin and corticosteroids relieve symptoms. Most of these patients eventually become euthyroid.

Hashimoto thyroiditis, the most common form of thyroiditis, is usually characterized by enlargement of the thyroid with or without pain and tenderness. It is much more common in women (~ 15% of U.S. women) and occasionally causes dysphagia, neck tightness, or hypothyroidism.

Hashimoto thyroiditis is an autoimmune disease. Serum titers of antimicrosomal and antithyroglobulin antibodies are elevated. Appropriate treatment for most patients consists of giving small doses of thyroid hormone. Surgery is indicated for marked pressure symptoms, suspected malignant tumor, and cosmetic reasons. If the thyroid is large or asymmetric, contains a discrete nodule, or grows rapidly, percutaneous needle biopsy is recommended. Thyroid lymphoma can rarely occur in patients with Hashimoto thyroiditis.

Riedel thyroiditis is a rare condition that presents as a hard, woody mass in the thyroid region with marked fibrosis and chronic inflammation in and around the gland. The inflammatory process infiltrates muscles and causes symptoms of tracheal compression. Hypothyroidism is usually present, and hypoparathyroidism may develop. Surgical treatment is required to relieve tracheal or esophageal obstruction.

BENIGN TUMORS OF THE THYROID

Benign thyroid tumors are adenomas, cysts, or localized thyroiditis. Most adenomas are of the follicular type. Adenomas are usually solitary and encapsulated and compress the adjacent thyroid. The major reasons for removal are a suspicion of cancer, functional overactivity producing hyperthyroidism, and cosmetic disfigurement.

MALIGNANT TUMORS OF THE THYROID

 ESSENTIALS OF DIAGNOSIS

▶ History of irradiation to the neck in some patients

▶ Painless or enlarging nodule, dysphagia, or hoarseness

▶ Firm or hard, fixed thyroid nodule; ipsilateral cervical lymphadenopathy

▶ Normal thyroid function; solid nodule stippled with microcalcifications (ultrasound), cold (radioiodine scan); positive or suspicious cytology

▶ Family history of thyroid cancer

▶ General Considerations

An appreciation of the classification of malignant tumors of the thyroid is important, because thyroid tumors demonstrate a wide range of growth and malignant behavior. At one end of the spectrum is **papillary carcinoma,** which usually occurs in young adults, grows very slowly, metastasizes through lymphatics, and is compatible with long life even in the presence of metastases (Table 17–3). At the other extreme is **anaplastic carcinoma,** which appears late in life and is nonencapsulated and invasive, forming large

Table 17–3. Five-year survival rate by carcinoma type.

Stage	Papillary	Follicular	Medullary	Anaplastic
I	Near 100%	Near 100%	Near 100%	
II	Near 100%	Near 100%	98%	
III	93%	71%	81%	
IV	51%	50%	28%	7%
Overall	96%	91%	85%	7%

Data from the American College of Surgeons. Amin MB, Edge SB, Greene FL, et al. (Eds.) *AJCC Cancer Staging Manual*, 8th Ed. Springer New York, 2017.

infiltrating tumors composed of small or large anaplastic cells. Most patients with anaplastic thyroid carcinoma succumb within 6 months as a consequence of local recurrence, pulmonary metastasis, or both. Between these two extremes are follicular, Hürthle cell, and medullary carcinomas, sarcomas, lymphomas, and metastatic tumors. The prognosis depends on the histologic pattern, the age and gender of the patient, the extent of tumor spread at the time of diagnosis, whether the tumor takes up radioiodine, and other factors. On average, 5% of patients with papillary, 10% of those with follicular, 15% of those with Hürthle cell, and 20% of those with medullary thyroid cancer will die within 10 years from these tumors.

The cause of most cases of thyroid carcinoma is unknown, although patients who received low-dose (6.5-2000 cGy) therapeutic radiation to the thymus, tonsils, scalp, and skin in infancy, childhood, or adolescence have an increased risk of developing thyroid tumors. Children are most susceptible to radiation exposure such as occurred with the Chernobyl nuclear accident, but adults up to 50 years of age who were exposed to the atomic blast at Hiroshima had an increased incidence of benign and malignant thyroid tumors. The incidence of thyroid cancer increases for at least 30 years after irradiation. *RET/PTC* rearrangements occur in about 80% of radiation-associated papillary thyroid cancers.

Types of Thyroid Cancer

A. Papillary Carcinoma

Papillary carcinoma accounts for 85% of cancers of the thyroid gland. The tumor usually appears in early adult life and presents as a solitary nodule. It then spreads via intraglandular lymphatics within the thyroid gland and then to the subcapsular and pericapsular lymph nodes. Fifty percent of children and 20% of adults present with palpable lymph nodes. The tumor may metastasize to lungs or bone. Microscopically, it is composed of papillary projections of columnar epithelium. Psammoma bodies are present in about 60%

of cases. Mixed papillary-follicular or follicular variants of papillary carcinoma and more aggressive variants, including tall cell, diffuse sclerosing, and columnar cell papillary thyroid carcinomas, are sometimes found. The rate of growth may be stimulated by TSH. A *BRAF* mutation is the most common mutation in papillary thyroid carcinoma and is associated with lymph node metastases and a higher recurrence rate.

Recently, a nomenclature change was introduced to reflect the indolent nature of the encapsulated follicular variant of papillary thyroid carcinoma. Previously considered a malignancy treated with surgical resection and radioactive iodine, these lesions are now termed *noninvasive follicular thyroid neoplasms with papillary-like nuclear features* (NIFTPs) and can be treated as an indolent tumors, albeit still with surgery. Because of the relatively recent introduction of NIFTP, ongoing evaluation of its impact on patient care, mortality rates, and long-term follow-up will be important to validate the indolent behavior of this neoplasm.

B. Follicular Carcinoma

Follicular carcinoma accounts for approximately 10% of malignant thyroid tumors. It appears later in life than the papillary form and may be rubbery or even soft on palpation. Follicular tumors are encapsulated. Microscopically, follicular carcinoma may be difficult to distinguish from normal thyroid tissue. Capsular invasion (through the tumor capsule) and vascular invasion distinguish follicular carcinoma from follicular adenoma. Follicular thyroid cancers only occasionally (~ 5%) metastasize to the regional lymph nodes, but they have a greater tendency to spread hematogenously to the lungs, the skeleton, and, rarely, the liver. Metastases from this tumor often demonstrate an avidity for radioactive iodine after total thyroidectomy. Skeletal metastases may appear years after resection of the primary lesion.

Hürthle cell carcinoma is considered a clinical variant of follicular carcinoma. It is more likely to be multifocal and involve lymph nodes than follicular carcinoma. Like follicular carcinoma, it makes thyroglobulin; however, it does not usually take up radioiodine. Both follicular and Hürthle cell carcinomas have a poorer prognosis than papillary carcinoma.

C. Medullary Carcinoma

Medullary thyroid carcinoma (MTC) accounts for approximately 7% of malignant tumors of the thyroid and 15% of thyroid cancer deaths. It contains amyloid and is a solid, hard, nodular tumor that secretes calcitonin and does not take up radioiodine. Medullary carcinomas arise from parafollicular cells of the ultimobranchial bodies or C cells. Serum calcitonin and carcinoembryonic antigen (CEA) levels should be drawn in all patients.

Familial MTC occurs in about 25% of patients. It may be isolated or occur with pheochromocytomas (often bilateral),

Table 17–4. Multiple endocrine neoplasia (MEN) syndromes.

Syndrome	Major Clinical Components	Associated Clinical Components	Site of Genetic Abnormality
MEN 1	• Hyperparathyroidism • Duodenopancreatic neuroendocrine tumors • Pituitary adenomas	• Thyroid adenoma • Adrenal adenoma • Thymic carcinoid tumor • Subcutaneous lipoma • Cutaneous collagenomas and angiofibromas	• *Menin*—tumor suppressor gene • Mutation eliminates function from one allele
MEN 2A	• Medullary thyroid cancer • Hyperparathyroidism • Pheochromocytoma	• Lichen planus	• *Ret*—protooncogene • Mutation causes constitutive receptor activation
MEN 2B	• Medullary thyroid cancer • Pheochromocytoma • Neurofibromas of lips and tongue • Marfanoid habitus	• Colonic dysfunction similar to Hirschsprung disease	
Familial medullary thyroid cancer	• Medullary thyroid cancer		

lichen planus amyloidosis, and hyperparathyroidism (MEN 2A; Table 17–4). It may also occur with or without pheochromocytomas (usually bilateral), marfanoid habitus, multiple neuromas, and ganglioneuromatosis (MEN 2B). Hirschsprung disease occurs more frequently in patients with familial medullary cancer. Isolated familial MTC is the least aggressive form, whereas this cancer is most aggressive in MEN 2B patients.

All patients with MTC should be screened for a *RET* mutation on chromosome 10 because 1%-7% of patients with presumed sporadic MTC have germline *RET* mutations, and these patients should be evaluated for pheochromocytomas and hyperparathyroidism. First-degree relatives of patients with hereditary MTC should also receive *RET* mutation testing and genetic counseling. For patients detected by family genetic screening, most experts recommend prophylactic total thyroidectomy at an age determined by the risk associated with the specific mutation.

D. Anaplastic Carcinoma

This rapidly growing tumor occurs principally beyond middle life and accounts for 1% of all thyroid cancers. This tumor usually evolves from a papillary or follicular neoplasm. It is a solid, quickly enlarging, hard, irregular mass diffusely involving the gland and often invades the trachea, muscles, and neurovascular structures. The tumor may be painful and somewhat tender, may be fixed on swallowing, and may cause laryngeal or esophageal obstructive symptoms. Microscopically, there are three major types: giant cell, spindle cell, and small cell. Mitoses are frequent. Cervical lymphadenopathy and pulmonary metastases are common.

Surgical intervention to debulk may palliate patients, but many patients are not candidates for resection due to direct invasion of surrounding structures. Combination treatment with external radiation therapy, chemotherapy, and surgery offers palliation to some patients but is rarely curative.

▶ Treatment

The treatment of **differentiated thyroid carcinoma** (which does not include anaplastic or medullary thyroid carcinoma) is resection. For microcarcinomas, which measure < 1.0 cm, thyroid lobectomy is sufficient. Selected patients with microcarcinomas may consider surveillance instead. For carcinomas > 4 cm, acceptable operations are near-total or total thyroidectomy. Historically, carcinomas measuring 1-4 cm were treated with total thyroidectomy, which treats potential multiple foci of tumors and allows for radioactive iodine ablation, as well as easier assessment for recurrence by serum thyroglobulin assay and neck ultrasounds during follow-up examinations. However, recent studies have indicated that there is no difference in overall survival between patients treated with lobectomy or thyroidectomy, although the risk of local recurrence may be slightly higher. Total thyroidectomy is also associated with a higher complication rate and requires postoperative lifelong thyroid hormone replacement. Therefore, thyroid lobectomy is an acceptable alternative to total thyroidectomy for select patients with differentiated thyroid carcinoma between 1 and 4 cm.

Preoperative ultrasound is essential in patients with thyroid cancer to evaluate the tumor as well as potential lymph node metastases. A central neck dissection, which involves clearing the lymph nodes between the carotid sheath and the trachea, should be performed for all patients with central node metastases. Whether an ipsilateral prophylactic central neck dissection should be done is controversial. A functional modified radical ("lateral") neck dissection preserving the jugular vein, sternocleidomastoid muscle, spinal accessory nerve, and sensory nerves is performed if lymph nodes in the lateral neck are clinically involved.

Isolated distant metastatic deposits of differentiated thyroid carcinoma should be removed surgically if possible and treated with radioactive iodine after thyroidectomy. All patients with differentiated thyroid cancer should be maintained indefinitely on suppressive doses of thyroid hormone (mild suppression for low-risk patients). For follow-up, it is helpful to measure basal and TSH-stimulated serum levels of thyroglobulin (a tumor marker for differentiated thyroid cancer), which are usually increased (> 2 ng/mL) in patients with residual tumor after total thyroidectomy.

MTC is associated with such a high incidence of nodal involvement that a bilateral central neck dissection should be considered in all patients at the time of total thyroidectomy. Concomitant ipsilateral and contralateral modified radical neck dissection is indicated when suspicious lateral nodes are visualized on preoperative imaging and may be indicated when the central neck nodes are involved or if the calcitonin level is extremely elevated. When serum calcitonin or CEA levels remain elevated after thyroidectomy, ultrasound or cross-sectional imaging of the neck and mediastinum should be performed. Laparoscopic evaluation of the liver for the presence of miliary metastases is recommended for patients with markedly elevated calcitonin levels. If there is no metastatic disease in the liver, then central neck dissection and bilateral functional neck dissections should be done, if not already done, including removal of nodes from the superior mediastinum. Patients with MTC should receive a physical examination, neck ultrasound, serum calcitonin, and CEA tests every 6-12 months.

For **anaplastic carcinoma, malignant lymphoma,** or **sarcoma,** the tumor should be excised as completely as possible and then treated by radiation and chemotherapy. It is common that no operation beyond a diagnostic biopsy is useful for these patients, as they may be locally inoperable with a course dictated by the systemic disease. For lymphoma, diagnostic biopsy is usually sufficient because many thyroid lymphomas will respond to systemic therapy alone.

Adam MA et al: Extent of surgery for papillary thyroid cancer is not associated with survival: an analysis of 61,775 patients. *Ann Surg.* 2015;260:601-605.

Haugen BR et al: 2015 American Thyroid Association management guidelines for adult patients with thyroid nodules and differentiated thyroid cancer. *Thyroid.* 2016;26(1):1-133.

Wells Jr SA et al: Revised American Thyroid Association guidelines for the management of medullary thyroid carcinoma. *Thyroid.* 2015;25:567-610.

▼ THE PARATHYROID GLANDS

EMBRYOLOGY & ANATOMY

The parathyroid glands arise from pharyngeal pouches III and IV and descend during development to the posterior capsule of the thyroid gland. Four parathyroid glands are present in 85% of the population, whereas approximately 15% of people have more than four glands. The glands are usually located on the posterior lateral aspect of the thyroid gland: the two superior glands, arising from the fourth pharyngeal pouch, generally reside at the level of the cricoid posterior to the recurrent laryngeal nerve; the two inferior glands, arising from the third pharyngeal pouch, are located more inferior and anterior to the recurrent laryngeal nerve. Occasionally one or more glands may be incorporated into the thyroid gland (intrathyroid) or thymus (intrathymic). The inferior parathyroid glands are more likely to be ectopic because the thymus, which also descends from the third pharyngeal pouch, can pull the glands into the chest. The upper parathyroids may be loosely attached by a long vascular pedicle and migrate caudally in the trachea-esophageal groove. Either superior or inferior glands may have an arrested descent and may lie as high as the hyoid bone. However, about 85% of parathyroid glands lie within 1 cm of where the inferior thyroid artery and recurrent laryngeal nerve cross.

The normal parathyroid gland has a distinct yellowish-brown color; is ovoid, tongue-shaped, polypoid, or spherical; and averages $2 \times 3 \times 7$ mm. The total mean weight of four normal parathyroid glands is about 150 mg. These encapsulated glands are usually supplied by a branch of the inferior thyroid artery but may be supplied by the superior thyroid artery. The vessels can be seen entering the gland at a hilum-like structure, a feature that differentiates parathyroid glands from fat. Parathyroid glands consist of two types of cells, oxyphil cells and chief cells, which are responsible for parathyroid hormone (PTH) synthesis and secretion.

PHYSIOLOGY

PTH, vitamin D, and calcitonin play vital roles in calcium and phosphorus metabolism in bone, kidney, and the gut. PTH and calcitonin work in concert to modulate fluctuations in plasma levels of ionized calcium. When the ionized calcium level falls, the parathyroid glands secrete more PTH, and the parafollicular cells within the thyroid secrete less calcitonin. The rise in PTH and fall in calcitonin produce increased bone resorption and increased resorption of calcium in the renal tubules. More calcium enters the blood, and ionized calcium levels return to normal.

Because PTH levels rise in normal subjects if ionized calcium levels are low, calcium and PTH must be determined from samples drawn simultaneously to diagnose hyperparathyroidism. The combination of increased PTH levels and hypercalcemia without hypocalciuria is almost always diagnostic of hyperparathyroidism. Measurement of intact PTH by immunoassay is best for screening for hyperparathyroidism and for selective venous catheterization to localize the source of PTH production. PTH-related peptide that is secreted by nonparathyroid malignant tumors does not cross-react with intact PTH assays.

DISEASES OF THE PARATHYROIDS

PRIMARY HYPERPARATHYROIDISM

ESSENTIALS OF DIAGNOSIS

- ▸ Increased fatigue, depression, weakness, arthralgias, nausea, vomiting, dyspepsia, constipation, polydipsia, polyuria, nocturia, psychiatric disturbances, renal colic, bone pain, and joint pain. ("Stones, bones, abdominal groans, psychic moans, and fatigue overtones.") Some patients are asymptomatic.
- ▸ Nephrolithiasis and nephrocalcinosis, osteopenia, osteoporosis, osteitis fibrosa cystica, peptic ulcer disease, renal dysfunction, gout, pseudogout, chondrocalcinosis, pancreatitis
- ▸ Hypertension, band keratopathy, neck masses
- ▸ Serum calcium, PTH, and chloride usually increased; serum phosphate low or normal; uric acid and alkaline phosphatase sometimes increased; urine calcium increased, normal or, rarely, decreased; urine phosphate increased; tubular reabsorption of phosphate decreased; osteocalcin and deoxypyridinoline cross-links increased
- ▸ X-rays: subperiosteal resorption of phalanges, demineralization of the skeleton (osteopenia or osteoporosis), bone cysts, and nephrocalcinosis or nephrolithiasis

▶ General Considerations

Primary hyperparathyroidism (pHPT) is due to excess or nonsuppressed PTH secretion from a single parathyroid adenoma (83%), multiple adenomas (6%), hyperplasia (10%), or carcinoma (1%). Once thought to be rare, pHPT is now found in 0.1%-0.3% of the general population, although this may be underreported, and is the most common cause of hypercalcemia in unselected patients. pHPT is uncommon before puberty; its peak incidence is between the third and fifth decades, and it is two to three times more common in women than in men.

Overproduction of PTH despite upper normal or elevated serum levels of calcium results in mobilization of calcium from bone and inhibition of the renal reabsorption of

phosphate, thereby producing hypercalcemia and hypophosphatemia. This causes a wasting of calcium and phosphorus, with osseous mineral loss and osteopenia or **osteoporosis.** Other associated or related conditions that offer clues to the diagnosis of hyperparathyroidism are nephrolithiasis, nephrocalcinosis, osteitis fibrosa cystica, peptic ulcer, pancreatitis, hypertension, and gout or pseudogout. Hyperparathyroidism also occurs in both MEN 1, known as **Wermer syndrome**, and MEN 2, known as **Sipple syndrome** (Table 17–4). The former is characterized by tumors of the parathyroid, pituitary, and pancreas (hyperparathyroidism, pituitary tumors, and functioning or nonfunctioning islet cell pancreatic tumors) that may cause Zollinger-Ellison syndrome (gastrinoma), hypoglycemia (insulinoma), glucagonoma, somatostatinoma, and pancreatic polypeptide tumors (PPomas). Other tumors in MEN 1 syndrome include adrenocortical tumors, carcinoid tumors, multiple lipomas, and cutaneous angiomas. MEN 2A consists of hyperparathyroidism (20%) in association with MTC (98%), pheochromocytoma (50%), and lichen planus amyloidosis. MEN 2B patients have a marfanoid habitus, multiple neuromas, and pheochromocytomas but rarely have hyperparathyroidism. Familial hyperparathyroidism can also occur alone or in the presence of jaw tumor syndrome.

Parathyroid adenomas range in weight from 65 mg to > 35 g, and the size usually parallels the degree of hypercalcemia. Microscopically, these tumors are generally the chief cell type. Multigland hyperplasia involves all four of the parathyroid glands. Microscopically, there are two types: chief cell hyperplasia and water-clear cell (wasserhelle) hyperplasia. Hyperplastic glands vary considerably in size but are usually larger than normal (65 mg). Double adenomas are rare (~ 5%) and are seen more often in older patients; they appear to be separate entities from single adenomas and multigland hyperplasia because removal of two diseased glands results in durable cure rates similar to those seen following surgery for single-gland disease.

Parathyroid carcinoma is rare (1%) but is more common in patients with profound hypercalcemia and in patients with familial hyperparathyroidism and jaw tumor syndrome. Parathyroid cancers are palpable in half of patients and should be suspected during surgery when the parathyroid gland is hard, has a whitish or irregular capsule, or is invasive into surrounding structures. Parathyromatosis is a rare condition causing hypercalcemia due to multiple embryologic rests or, more commonly, due to seeding when a parathyroid tumor has ruptured or the tumor capsule has been disrupted.

▶ Clinical Findings

A. Symptoms and Signs

Historically, the clinical manifestations of hyperparathyroidism have changed. Forty years ago, the diagnosis was based on bone pain and deformity (osteitis fibrosa cystica), and in later years on the renal complications (nephrolithiasis and nephrocalcinosis) of the disease. Presently, over two-thirds of patients are detected by routine screening or because of osteopenia or osteoporosis. Many patients are asymptomatic. Patients with even mild pHPT are predisposed to cardiovascular events and fractures. After successful surgical treatment, many patients thought to be asymptomatic become aware of improvement in unrecognized preoperative symptoms such as fatigue, mild depression, weakness, constipation, polydipsia, polyuria, and bone and joint pain. Hyperparathyroidism should be suspected in all patients with hypercalcemia and the above symptoms, especially if associated with nephrolithiasis, nephrocalcinosis, hypertension, left ventricular hypertrophy, peptic ulcer, pancreatitis, or gout. Patients with pHPT appear to have a shortened life expectancy that improves after successful parathyroidectomy. Younger patients and those with less severe hypercalcemia after parathyroidectomy have the best prognosis.

B. History, Laboratory Findings, Imaging Studies, and Differential Diagnosis (Approach to the Hypercalcemic Patient)

1. History—Together, hyperparathyroidism and humoral hypercalcemia of malignancy (nonparathyroid cancer) are responsible for about 90% of all cases of hypercalcemia. Hyperparathyroidism is the most common cause of hypercalcemia detected by undirected methods such as routine screening, whereas cancer is the most common cause of hypercalcemia in hospitalized patients. Other causes of hypercalcemia are listed in Table 17–5. In many patients, the diagnosis is obvious, whereas in others, it may be challenging. At times, more than one reason for hypercalcemia may exist in the same patient, such as cancer or sarcoidosis plus hyperparathyroidism. A careful history must be obtained documenting (1) the duration of any symptoms related to hypercalcemia; (2) symptoms related to malignant disease; (3) conditions associated with hyperparathyroidism such as renal colic, peptic ulcer disease, pancreatitis, hypertension, or gout; and (4) possible excess use of milk products, antacids, baking soda, or vitamins. In patients with a recent cough, wheeze, or hemoptysis, epidermoid carcinoma of the lung should be considered. Hematuria might suggest hypernephroma, bladder tumor, or renal lithiasis. A long history of renal stones or peptic ulcer disease suggests that hyperparathyroidism is possible.

2. Laboratory Findings—The most important tests for the evaluation of hypercalcemia are serum calcium and PTH (Table 17–6).

Measurement of **serum PTH** has its greatest value in this situation, since the PTH level is low or nil in patients with hypercalcemia due to *all* causes other than pHPT or familial hypocalciuric hypercalcemia. Even patients with high normal PTH in conjunction with elevated calcium levels should raise suspicion for pHPT as the PTH is inappropriately elevated in this setting. In general, serum PTH levels should be

Table 17–5. Causes of hypercalcemia.

	Approximate Frequency
Cancer Metastatic breast cancer PTH-related peptide secreting (lung, kidney) Multiple myeloma Leukemia Other metastatic cancer	Common
Endocrine disorders Hyperparathyroidism Hyperthyroidism Addison disease, pheochromocytoma Hypothyroidism, VIPoma	Common
Increased calcium or vitamin intake and drugs Milk-alkali syndrome Vitamin D and A overdosage Thiazide diuretics, lithium	Uncommon
Granulomatous diseases Sarcoidosis Tuberculosis	Uncommon
Benign familial hypocalciuric hypercalcemia and other disorders Paget disease Immobilization Idiopathic hypercalcemia of infancy Aluminum intoxication Dysproteinemias Rhabdomyolysis	Rare

measured in all patients with persistent hypercalcemia without an obvious cause and in normocalcemic patients who are suspected of having hyperparathyroidism. Determination of intact serum PTH levels is sensitive and is not influenced by tumors that secrete parathyroid-related peptide. Nonparathyroid tumors that secrete pure PTH are extremely rare.

High serum calcium and low serum phosphate suggest hyperparathyroidism, but about half of patients with hyperparathyroidism have normal serum phosphate concentrations. Patients with vitamin D intoxication, sarcoidosis, malignant disease without metastasis, and hyperthyroidism may also be hypophosphatemic, but patients with breast cancer and hypercalcemia are only rarely so. In fact, if hypophosphatemia and hypercalcemia are present in association with breast cancer, concomitant hyperparathyroidism is possible.

An elevated serum chloride concentration is a useful diagnostic clue found in about 40% of hyperparathyroid patients. PTH acts directly on the proximal renal tubule to decrease the resorption of bicarbonate, which leads to increased resorption of chloride and mild hyperchloremic renal tubular acidosis. An increased serum chloride is not found in other causes of hypercalcemia. Calculation of

Table 17–6. Laboratory evaluation of hypercalcemia.

Essential	Selective
Blood tests	
Calcium	Creatine and blood urea nitrogen

PTH (intact or two-site assay)	Phosphate
	Chloride
	Alkaline phosphatase
	Uric acid
	pH
	Protein electrophoresis or albumin:
	   globulin ratio
	25-Dihydroxyvitamin D and
	   1,25-dihydroxyvitamin D

Radiographic or nuclear medicine procedures	
Neck ultrasound	Sestamibi scan of neck or four-dimensional computed tomography (4DCT)

Bone density (hip, lumbar
   spine, wrist)
	Chest x-ray, abdominal plain films, kidney
	   ultrasound

Urine tests	
24-hour urinary calcium[1]	Urinalysis Deoxypyridinoline cross-links Osteocalcin

[1]When urine calcium is < 100 mg/24 h, a diagnosis of benign familial hypocalciuric hypercalcemia must be considered.

the **serum chloride–to–phosphate ratio** takes advantage of slight increases in serum chloride and slight decreases in serum phosphate concentrations. A ratio > 33 suggests hyperparathyroidism; this was a more clinically useful observation before the availability of rapid and accurate PTH measurement.

A 24-hour urine calcium level is helpful for diagnosing hypercalcemic patients who have low urinary calcium levels resulting from benign familial hypocalciuric hypercalcemia (BFHH) and for patients with marked hypercalciuria (> 400 mg/24 h). Patients with BFHH do not benefit from parathyroidectomy. Measurement of 25-hydroxy and 1,25-hydroxy vitamin D levels is helpful in selected patients when other tests are equivocal. Many patients with hyperparathyroidism will have concurrent vitamin D deficiency, so it is important to rule this out as a secondary cause.

Serum protein electrophoretic patterns are helpful for diagnosis of multiple myeloma and sarcoidosis. Hypergammaglobulinemia is rare in hyperparathyroidism but is not uncommon in patients with multiple myeloma and sarcoidosis. Roentgenograms of the skull or site of bone pain in patients with elevated alkaline phosphatase levels will often

reveal typical "punched-out" bony lesions, and the diagnosis of myeloma can be firmly established by bone marrow examination. Sarcoidosis can be difficult to diagnose, because it may exist for years with limited clinical findings. A chest x-ray revealing a diffuse fibronodular infiltrate and prominent hilar adenopathy is suggestive, and the demonstration of noncaseating granuloma in lymph nodes is diagnostic.

Serum alkaline phosphate levels are elevated in about 10% of patients with pHPT and may also be increased in patients with Paget disease and cancer. When the serum alkaline phosphatase level is elevated, serum 5′-nucleotidase, which parallels liver alkaline phosphatase, should be measured to determine if the increase is from bone, which suggests parathyroid disease, or liver.

3. Bone Studies—Bone densitometry and radiographic examination of bone frequently reveal osteopenia (1 standard deviation below normal density) or osteoporosis (2.5 standard deviations below normal). Overt skeletal changes, such as subperiosteal resorption or brown tumors, are found in < 10% of patients with hyperparathyroidism. Bone changes of osteitis fibrosa cystica are rare on x-ray unless the serum alkaline phosphatase concentration is increased. Primary and secondary hyperparathyroidism can produce subperiosteal resorption of the phalanges and bone cysts (Figure 17–2). A ground-glass appearance of the skull with loss of definition of the tables and demineralization of the outer aspects of the clavicles are less frequently seen. In patients with markedly elevated serum alkaline phosphatase levels without

▲ **Figure 17–2.** Subperiosteal resorption of radial side of second phalanges.

subperiosteal resorption on x-ray, Paget disease or cancer must be suspected. A 24-hour urine test for deoxypyridinoline cross-link assay or osteocalcin detects increased bone loss.

4. Differential Diagnosis—The differentiation between hyperparathyroidism due to primary parathyroid disease and that due to humoral hypercalcemia of malignancy can now almost always be determined by **measuring intact PTH,** which is increased in pHPT but suppressed in humoral hypercalcemia of malignancy. The most common tumors causing humoral hypercalcemia of malignancy are squamous cell carcinoma of the lung, renal cell carcinoma, and bladder cancer. Less commonly, it is due to hepatoma or to cancer of the ovary, stomach, pancreas, parotid gland, or colon. Recent onset of symptoms, increased sedimentation rate, anemia, serum calcium > 14 mg/dL, and increased alkaline phosphatase activity without osteitis fibrosa cystica suggest **humoral hypercalcemia of malignancy;** mild hypercalcemia with a long history of nephrolithiasis or peptic ulcer suggests pHPT. Documented hypercalcemia of 6 months or longer essentially rules out malignancy-associated hypercalcemia.

In **milk-alkali syndrome,** a history of excessive ingestion of milk products, calcium-containing antacids, and baking soda is often obtained. These patients become normocalcemic after discontinuing these habits. Patients with milk-alkali syndrome usually have renal insufficiency and low urinary calcium concentrations and are usually alkalotic rather than acidotic. Because of the high incidence of ulcer disease in hyperparathyroidism, milk-alkali syndrome may occasionally coexist with that disorder. This is very infrequent now that acid-suppressing medications, such as proton pump inhibitors, are available to manage peptic ulcer disease.

Hyperthyroidism, another cause of hypercalcemia and hypercalciuria, can usually be differentiated because hyperthyroid symptoms rather than hypercalcemia bring the patient to the physician. Thyroid function tests, including TSH, should be evaluated in hypercalcemic patients whose PTH levels are not increased. Treatment of hyperthyroidism with antithyroid medications causes serum calcium to normalize within 8 weeks.

Patients taking **thiazide diuretics** may develop a transient increase in serum calcium levels, usually < 1 mg/dL. Larger rises in serum calcium induced by thiazides have been reported in patients with pHPT and idiopathic juvenile osteoporosis. Most patients who have hypercalcemia while taking thiazides have another reason for the increase. The best way to evaluate these patients is to switch them to a nonthiazide antihypertensive agent or diuretic and to measure the PTH level after several months. Thiazide-induced hypercalcemia is not associated with increased serum PTH in patients without hyperparathyroidism.

Benign familial hypocalciuric hypercalcemia is one of the few conditions that causes chronic hypercalcemia and mildly elevated PTH levels. It can be difficult to distinguish from mild pHPT. The best way to diagnose this disorder is to document a low urinary calcium (< 100 mg/24 h) and a family history of hypercalcemia, especially in children.

Other miscellaneous causes of hypercalcemia include Paget disease, immobilization, dysproteinemias, idiopathic hypercalcemia of infancy, aluminum intoxication, and rhabdomyolysis (Table 17–5).

C. Approach to the Normocalcemic Patient With Possible Hyperparathyroidism

Renal failure, hypoalbuminemia, pancreatitis, vitamin D or magnesium deficiency, and excess phosphate intake may cause serum calcium levels to be normal in hyperparathyroidism. Correction of these disorders results in hypercalcemia if hyperparathyroidism is present. Determination of serum ionized calcium is also sometimes revealing, because it may be increased in patients with normal total serum calcium levels. If a patient has elevated serum levels of ionized calcium and PTH, the diagnosis of normocalcemic hyperparathyroidism has been confirmed.

There are three major causes of hypercalciuria and nephrolithiasis: (1) increased absorption of calcium from the gastrointestinal tract (absorptive hypercalciuria), (2) increased renal leakage of calcium (renal hypercalciuria), and (3) pHPT. Patients with absorptive hypercalcemia absorb too much calcium from the gastrointestinal tract and therefore have low serum PTH levels. Patients with renal hypercalciuria lose calcium from leaky renal tubules and have increased PTH levels. They can be distinguished from patients with normocalcemic hyperparathyroidism by their response to treatment with thiazides. In renal leak hypercalcemia, serum PTH levels become normal because thiazides correct the excessive loss of calcium, whereas in pHPT, increased serum PTH levels persist and the patient often becomes hypercalcemic.

▶ Natural History of Untreated & Treated Hyperparathyroidism

Most patients with hyperparathyroidism—even those with normocalcemic hyperparathyroidism—have symptoms and associated conditions. In 80% of patients, these clinical manifestations improve or disappear after parathyroidectomy. Bone marrow density also improves following parathyroidectomy, although this can take several years. Without treatment, hyperparathyroidism becomes more severe, and patients may experience one or more complications of the disease, including hypertension, nephrolithiasis, osteopenia, peptic ulcer disease, gout, renal dysfunction, and pancreatitis.

Patients with untreated hyperparathyroidism have an increased risk of premature death, mainly from cardiovascular and malignant disease. There is decreased respiratory muscular capacity and increased frequency of hypertrophic cardiomyopathy with left ventricular hypertrophy and decreased vascular compliance even in hyperparathyroid patients without hypertension. After successful parathyroidectomy, previously hyperparathyroid patients still have an increased risk of premature death; however, younger patients and those with less severe disease return to a normal survival curve sooner than do older patients or those with more severe hyperparathyroidism.

▶ Treatment

The only curative treatment for pHPT is parathyroidectomy. There are no convincing data to support a plan of medical observation, whereas considerable data support a surgical approach. Once associated conditions such as hypertension and renal dysfunction become well established, they seem to progress despite correction of the pHPT. Thus, it appears optimal to intervene early while it is still possible to correct these problems. Parathyroidectomy should be discussed with all symptomatic patients, except when surgical risks outweigh the benefits of surgical intervention. Patients choosing nonsurgical care should be monitored with annual calcium checks and bone density scans.

Asymptomatic patients often report improved quality of life following parathyroidectomy. The criteria for intervention in asymptomatic patients have been revised several times over three decades (Table 17–7) but have always included the option for correction of the abnormality based on individual patient and physician judgments. Indications for intervention in asymptomatic patients include calcium > 1 mg/dL above normal, renal involvement (nephrolithiasis, hypercalciuria > 400 mg/dL for 24 hours, glomerular filtration rate < 60 mL/min), osteoporosis, fragility fracture or vertebral compression fracture, and age < 50 years old.

A. Marked Hypercalcemia (Hypercalcemic Crisis)

The initial treatment in patients with marked hypercalcemia and acute symptoms is hydration and correction of hypokalemia and hyponatremia. While the patient is being hydrated, assessment of the underlying problem is essential so that more specific therapy may be started. Milk and alkaline products, estrogens, thiazides, and vitamins A and D should be immediately discontinued. Furosemide is useful to increase calcium excretion in the rehydrated patient. Etidronate, plicamycin, and calcitonin are usually effective for short periods in treating hypercalcemia regardless of cause. Glucocorticoids are very effective in vitamin D intoxication, hyperthyroidism, and sarcoidosis and in many patients with cancer, including those with peptide-secreting tumors, but are less effective when there is extensive bone disease. As mentioned previously, hyperparathyroid patients only occasionally respond to glucocorticoid administration. Hypercalcemia of malignancy is often responsive to bisphosphonates, including clodronate, pamidronate, and ibandronate. If renal function is significantly impaired, hemodialysis may be indicated.

In patients with marked hypercalcemia, once the diagnosis of hyperparathyroidism is established, localization studies, cervical exploration, and parathyroidectomy should be performed in a vigorously hydrated patient, since this is the most rapid and effective method of normalizing the serum calcium.

B. Localization

Preoperative localization of parathyroid tumors can now be accomplished in about 80%-90% of patients (Figure 17–3). An experienced surgeon can identify the tumors in about 95% of patients who have not undergone previous parathyroid or thyroid surgery without preoperative tests, so **preoperative localization is not a requirement for surgery**. However, preoperative knowledge of the location of the abnormal glands can simplify the operation.

Cervical ultrasound both localizes parathyroid abnormalities and examines for thyroid nodular disease and should be performed in all patients prior to surgery. Technetium (Tc-99m) sestamibi scans measure relative uptake and

Table 17–7. Indications for parathyroidectomy in asymptomatic primary hyperparathyroidism.

Criterion	1990	2002	2008	2016
Hypercalcemia	Serum calcium > 1.5 mg/dL above normal	Serum calcium > 1 mg/dL above normal	Serum calcium > 1 mg/dL above normal	Serum calcium > 1 mg/dL above normal
Hypercalciuria	24-h urine calcium > 400 mg	24-h urine calcium > 400 mg	Not included	24-hr urine calcium >400mg/dL
Renal insufficiency	Reduced by 30%	Reduced by 30%	GFR < 60 mL/min	GFR < 60 mL/min
Osteoporosis	Z-score < 2	T-score < 2.5	T-score < 2.5 or history of fragility fracture	T-score < 2.5, history of fragility fracture, or vertebral compression fracture
Age	< 50 y	< 50 y	< 50 y	< 50 y

GFR, glomerular filtration rate.

▲ **Figure 17–3.** Parathyroid adenomas. **A:** Sestamibi scan of right lower parathyroid adenoma. **B:** Sagittal ultrasound scan of left lower parathyroid adenoma. **C:** Transverse ultrasound scan of left lower parathyroid adenoma.

washout of the radioisotope by the thyroid and parathyroid glands and are therefore less sensitive for multigland disease. Four-dimensional CT (4DCT) scans involve timed injection of contrast and are often informative in the reoperative setting.

For patients who have had prior neck operations, including thyroid and parathyroid procedures, preoperative localization is especially important. 4DCT scan and selective venous catheterization with PTH immunoassay are often helpful. The surgeon must carefully evaluate these cases prior to exploration to optimize the opportunity for a successful operation.

C. Operation

Three approaches are now acceptable for patients with sporadic pHPT. **Bilateral neck exploration** (exposing all four parathyroid glands) is safe and does not depend on preoperative tests or intraoperative PTH testing for success. A smaller incision is used in a **minimally invasive parathyroidectomy**, which refers to a variety of targeted operations. A **unilateral approach** can be elected when one or more localization tests lateralize a solitary parathyroid tumor. At operation, a normal and abnormal parathyroid should be identified on the side of the localized tumor to minimize the chance of multigland disease. A **focused approach** can also be performed in similarly localized patients and the operation completed when the abnormal gland is resected and the intraoperative PTH level decreases appropriately. When two separate imaging studies concordantly identify the same tumor, a successful operation occurs in approximately 96% of patients.

In > 80% of cases, the parathyroid tumor is found attached to the posterior capsule of the thyroid gland. The parathyroid glands are usually symmetrically placed, and lower parathyroid glands are situated anterior to the recurrent laryngeal nerve, whereas the upper parathyroid glands lie posterior to the recurrent laryngeal nerve, where it enters the cricothyroid muscle. Parathyroid tumors may also lie cephalad to the superior pole of the thyroid gland, along the great vessels of the neck in the tracheoesophageal area, in thymic tissue, in the thyroid gland itself, or in the mediastinum. Care must be taken to avoid bleeding because color is useful in distinguishing parathyroid glands from surrounding thyroid, thymus, lymph nodes, and fat. Furthermore, rupture of the parathyroid gland may result in parathyromatosis (seeding of parathyroid tissue) and possible recurrent hyperparathyroidism.

Two helpful maneuvers for localizing parathyroid tumors during surgery are (1) following the course of a branch of the inferior thyroid artery and (2) looking for the fat that is usually associated with the parathyroid glands. One should attempt to identify four parathyroid glands when a bilateral approach is elected, although there may be more or fewer than four.

In a unilateral or focused parathyroidectomy, if a probable parathyroid adenoma is found, it is removed, and the diagnosis of adenoma confirmed by a decrease in PTH of > 50% from baseline and into the normal range. If the intraoperative PTH does not fall appropriately, then further exploration to identify additional abnormal parathyroid tissue should be undertaken immediately. If normal glands are identified, they should be carefully documented. If two adenomas are found, both are removed, and successful resection of all adenomas can be confirmed with additional PTH levels. All normal glands can be biopsied for confirmation but should not be removed.

The presence of a completely normal parathyroid gland at operation indicates that the tumor removed is adenomatous rather than hyperplastic, since in hyperplasia all the parathyroid glands are involved. However, the variation in the appearance of normal parathyroid glands and the subtlety of hyperplastic glands can make this distinction challenging.

When all parathyroid glands are hyperplastic, the most normal gland should be partially resected, leaving a 50-mg remnant, and confirmed to be well vascularized prior to removal of the remaining glands. The upper thymus and perithymic tract should be removed in patients with hyperplasia, because a fifth parathyroid gland is present in 15% of cases.

If exploration fails to reveal a parathyroid tumor, a missing lower gland is often in the thymus (anterior mediastinum), whereas a missing upper gland is usually paraesophageal (or in the posterior mediastinum). One should therefore perform a careful and thorough exploration of the areas in which ectopic parathyroid tissue is likely to reside.

The recurrence rate of hyperparathyroidism after the removal of a single adenoma in patients with sporadic hyperparathyroidism is 2% or less. In patients with MEN and familial hyperparathyroidism, recurrent hyperparathyroidism is expected as long as they have residual parathyroid tissue. Thus, the plan for management of these patients over their lifetime should be to limit both the complications from hyperparathyroidism and the number and complexity of operations required to manage their disease.

D. Postoperative Care

Following removal of a parathyroid adenoma or hyperplastic glands, the serum calcium concentration falls to normal or below normal in 24-48 hours. Patients with severe skeletal depletion ("hungry bones"), long-standing hyperparathyroidism, vitamin D deficiency, or high preoperative serum calcium levels may develop profound hypocalcemia with paresthesias, carpopedal spasm, or even seizures. For most patients, oral calcium supplementation is sufficient to manage symptoms over several weeks. When marked symptoms develop, it can be necessary to administer intravenous calcium gluconate. If the response is not rapid, the serum magnesium concentration should be determined and replenished. Treatment with calcitriol is sometimes required (see section on hypoparathyroidism).

Outpatient parathyroidectomy is appropriate for most patients. An overnight hospital stay may be indicated for patients with significant comorbid disease or potential medication nonadherence. Cure is defined as a normal calcium level for at least 6 months. Patients with normocalcemic hyperparathyroidism should also have a normal PTH level. Ongoing PTH elevation should prompt evaluation for secondary disease, although it may take several years after successful surgery for PTH levels to normalize. Persistent hyperparathyroidism is defined as the failure to achieve a normal calcium level within 6 months after surgery, whereas recurrent hyperparathyroidism is the recurrence of elevated calcium levels after a period of normal calcium at least 6 months postoperatively.

E. Reoperation

Treatment of persistent or recurrent hyperparathyroidism requires careful evaluation and planning. First the diagnosis must be reestablished, and the rationale for correcting the hyperparathyroidism must be specifically confirmed. If operation is planned, then preoperative localization is mandatory. Most surgeons perform noninvasive localization tests (eg, ultrasound, sestamibi scan, 4DCT scan) initially. If the localization is not clear, then invasive testing follows (selective venous catheterization with PTH measurement and rarely angiography). Most patients have a parathyroid tumor that can be removed through a cervical incision, making mediastinal exploration unnecessary. The success rate for patients requiring reoperation is about 90%, and the complication rate is higher depending on the nature of the prior operation(s) and the location of the abnormal gland. The success rate is lower in patients with negative or equivocal localization tests and in patients with parathyromatosis and parathyroid cancer.

Bilezikian JP: Primary hyperparathyroidism. *Endocr Pract.* 2012,18: 781-790.

Wilhelm SM et al: The American Association of Endocrine Surgeons guidelines for the management of primary hyperparathyroidism. *JAMA Surg.* 2016,151:959-968.

SECONDARY & TERTIARY HYPERPARATHYROIDISM

In secondary hyperparathyroidism, there is an increase in PTH secretion in response to low plasma concentrations of ionized calcium, usually due to renal disease or vitamin D deficiency, or malabsorption. This results in chief cell hyperplasia. When secondary hyperparathyroidism occurs as a complication of renal disease, the serum phosphorus level is usually high, whereas in malabsorption, osteomalacia, or rickets, it is frequently low or normal. Secondary

hyperparathyroidism with renal osteodystrophy is a frequent complication of hemodialysis and peritoneal dialysis. Factors that play a role in renal osteodystrophy are (1) phosphate retention secondary to a decrease in the number of nephrons; (2) failure of the diseased or absent kidneys to hydroxylate 25-dihydroxyvitamin D to the biologically active metabolite 1,25-dihydroxyvitamin D, with decreased intestinal absorption of calcium; (3) resistance of the bone to the action of PTH; and (4) increased serum calcitonin concentrations. The resulting skeletal changes are identical with those of pHPT but are often more severe.

Most patients with secondary hyperparathyroidism are treated medically. Maintaining relatively normal serum concentrations of calcium and phosphorus during hemodialysis and treatment with calcitriol (orally or intravenously) have decreased the incidence of bone disease.

Indications for operation in patients with secondary hyperparathyroidism include (1) a calcium × phosphate product > 70, (2) severe bone disease and pain, (3) pruritus, (4) extensive soft tissue calcification with tumoral calcinosis, and (5) calciphylaxis. Most patients with secondary hyperparathyroidism requiring parathyroidectomy have very high serum PTH levels. In the patient with secondary hyperparathyroidism in whom subtotal parathyroidectomy or total parathyroidectomy with autotransplantation is indicated, all but about 50 mg of the most normal parathyroid gland should be removed. Total parathyroidectomy with autotransplantation consists of removing all parathyroid glands from the neck and reimplanting several 1-mm slices of parathyroid tissue into a muscle pocket in the forearm or sternocleidomastoid.

Following parathyroidectomy, patients usually respond with dramatic relief of bone and joint pain and pruritus. Profound hypocalcemia frequently results, both because of "hungry bones" and because of decreased PTH secretion. Hypocalcemia due to hungry bones can be anticipated in patients with markedly elevated alkaline phosphatase levels and hand films documenting subperiosteal resorption. Patients are usually hospitalized for several days and may receive several doses of intravenous calcium.

In most secondary hyperparathyroidism patients after successful renal transplantation, the serum calcium concentration returns to normal, and the hyperplastic parathyroid glands regress. In some patients, however, profound hypercalcemia develops (**tertiary hyperparathyroidism**) due to the development of autonomous hyperplastic parathyroid glands. In general, surgical therapy for so-called tertiary HPT should be delayed until all medical approaches, including treatment with vitamin D, calcium supplementation, and phosphate binders, have been exhausted; if the condition persists beyond 1 year after transplant or if the hypercalcemia is severe, then operation for tertiary disease should be considered.

Kasiske BL et al: KDIGO clinical practice guideline for the care of kidney transplant recipients: a summary. *Kidney Int.* 2010; 77(4):299-311.

Kidney Disease: Improving Global Outcomes (KDIGO) CKD-MBD Work Group: KDIGO clinical practice guideline for the diagnosis, evaluation, prevention, and treatment of chronic kidney disease-mineral and bone disorder (CKD-MBD). *Kidney Int Suppl.* 2009;113:S1-130.

Kovacevic B et al: Parathyroidectomy for the attainment of NKF-K/DOQI™ and KDIGO recommended values for bone and mineral metabolism in dialysis patients with uncontrollable secondary hyperparathyroidism. *Langenbeck Arch Surg.* 2012;397:413.

HYPOPARATHYROIDISM

 ESSENTIALS OF DIAGNOSIS

- ▶ Paresthesias, muscle cramps, carpopedal spasm, laryngeal stridor, convulsions, malaise, muscle and abdominal cramps, tetany, urinary frequency, lethargy, anxiety, psychoneurosis, depression, and psychosis

- ▶ Surgical neck scar; positive Chvostek and Trousseau signs

- ▶ Brittle and atrophied nails, defective teeth, cataracts

- ▶ Hypocalcemia and hyperphosphatemia, low or absent urinary calcium, low or absent circulating PTH

- ▶ Calcification of basal ganglia, cartilage, and arteries as seen on x-ray

▶ General Considerations

Hypoparathyroidism, although uncommon, occurs most often as a complication of thyroidectomy, especially when performed for carcinoma or recurrent goiter. Idiopathic hypoparathyroidism, an autoimmune process associated with autoimmune adrenocortical insufficiency, is also unusual, and hypoparathyroidism after ^{131}I therapy for Graves disease is rare. Neonatal tetany may be associated with maternal hyperparathyroidism. Hypothyroidism, as well as hypoparathyroidism, may occur in patients with Riedel struma.

▶ Clinical Findings

A. Symptoms and Signs

The manifestations of acute hypoparathyroidism are due to hypocalcemia. Low serum calcium levels precipitate tetany. Initial manifestations include paresthesias, circumoral numbness, muscle cramps, irritability, carpopedal spasm, convulsions, opisthotonos, and marked anxiety. Chronically dry skin, brittleness of the nails, and spotty alopecia including loss of the eyebrows are common. Latent tetany may be indicated by mild or moderate paresthesias with a positive Chvostek or Trousseau sign. Because primary hypoparathyroidism is rare, a history of thyroidectomy is almost always present. Generally speaking, the sooner the clinical manifestations appear postoperatively, the more serious the prognosis. After many years, some patients become adapted to a low serum calcium concentration, so that tetany is no longer evident.

B. Laboratory Findings

Hypocalcemia and hyperphosphatemia are demonstrable. The urine phosphate is low or absent, tubular resorption of phosphate is high, and the urine calcium is low.

C. Imaging Studies

In chronic hypoparathyroidism, x-rays may show calcification of the basal ganglia, arteries, and external ear.

▶ Differential Diagnosis

A good history is most important in the differential diagnosis of hypocalcemic tetany. Symptomatic hypocalcemia occurring after thyroid or parathyroid surgery is due to parathyroid removal or injury or is secondary to hungry bones. Occasionally, tetany occurs with alkalosis and hyperventilation. Other major causes of hypocalcemic tetany are intestinal malabsorption and renal insufficiency. These conditions may also be suggested by a history of diarrhea, pancreatitis, steatorrhea, or renal disease. Laboratory abnormalities include decreased concentrations of serum proteins, cholesterol, and carotene and increased concentrations of stool fat in malabsorption and an increased blood urea nitrogen and creatinine in renal failure.

Serum PTH concentrations are low in hypocalcemia secondary to idiopathic or iatrogenic hypoparathyroidism. In hypocalcemia secondary to malabsorption and renal failure, serum PTH concentrations are elevated and the serum alkaline phosphatase concentration is normal or increased.

▶ Treatment

The aim of treatment is to raise the serum calcium concentration in order to bring the patient out of tetany and to lower the serum phosphate level so as to prevent metastatic calcification. Most postoperative hypocalcemia is transient; if it requires supplementation with calcium or calcitriol for longer than 6 months, the hypoparathyroidism may be permanent.

A. Acute Hypoparathyroid Tetany

Acute hypoparathyroid tetany requires emergency treatment. Make certain an adequate airway exists. Reassure the anxious patient to avoid hyperventilation and resulting alkalosis, which exacerbates the hypocalcemia. Intravenous calcium gluconate, 10-20 mL of 10% solution administered slowly, resolves the tetany. Fifty milliliters of 10% calcium gluconate may then be added to 500 mL of 5% dextrose solution and administered by intravenous drip at a rate of 1 mL/kg/h. Adjust the rate of infusion so that hourly determinations of serum calcium are normal.

To make the transition to oral supplements to support the serum calcium level, calcitriol (1,25-dihydroxyvitamin D), 0.25-0.5 μg twice daily, is very helpful and takes effect within 48-72 hours. This enables the gastrointestinal tract to absorb increased amounts of calcium. Oral calcium supplements of up to 6 g daily will generally resolve the hypocalcemia even in patients with permanent, severe hypoparathyroidism. Hypomagnesemia is present in some cases of tetany that is unresponsive to calcium treatment. In such cases, magnesium (as magnesium sulfate) should be given in a dosage of 4-8 g/d intramuscularly or 2-4 g/d intravenously.

B. Chronic Hypoparathyroidism

Once tetany has responded to intravenous calcium, change to oral calcium (citrate, gluconate, lactate, or carbonate) three times daily or as necessary. The management of the hypoparathyroid patient is difficult to avoid vitamin D toxicity. Episodes of hypercalcemia in treated patients are often unpredictable and may occur in the absence of symptoms. Vitamin D intoxication may develop after months or years of good control on a given therapeutic regimen. Dihydrotachysterol is useful in the exceptional case to supplement treatment with calcium and 1,25-dihydroxyvitamin D, when the usual measures fail to treat the hypocalcemia. Frequent serum calcium determinations are necessary to regulate the proper dosage of vitamin D and to avoid vitamin D intoxication. Phosphorus should also be limited in the diet; in most patients, simple elimination of dairy products is sufficient. In some patients, aluminum hydroxide gel may be necessary to bind phosphorus in the gut to increase fecal losses.

Exogenous PTH analogs may be helpful in the long-term management of bone disease in patients with hypoparathyroidism. The optimal strategies are under development.

Cusano NE et al: The effect of PTH(1-84) on quality of life in hypoparathyroidism. *J Clin Endocrinol Metab*. 2013;98(6):2356-2361.
Sikjaer T et al: PTH (1-84) replacement therapy in hypoparathyroidism: a randomized controlled trial on pharmacokinetic and dynamic effects following 6 months of treatment. *J Bone Miner Res*. 2013;28(10):2232-2243.

MULTIPLE CHOICE QUESTIONS

1. The best test to assess the thyroid function status of a patient who does not have known pituitary disease is

    A. Free T_4
    B. T_3
    C. T_4
    D. TSH
    E. T_4/T_3 ratio

2. Indications for surgery to correct hyperthyroidism include

    A. Pregnancy
    B. Age over 50 years
    C. Large goiter with low radioiodine uptake
    D. Both A and C
    E. None of the above

3. Follicular thyroid cancer

    A. Is separated from papillary thyroid cancer because it develops from the follicular cells of the thyroid
    B. Is less likely to spread to lymph nodes than is papillary thyroid cancer
    C. Is commonly inoperable because of local invasion and encompassment of surrounding structures
    D. Commonly makes thyroid hormone producing hyperthyroidism
    E. Is best treated with radioiodine therapy, followed by thyroidectomy

4. The differential diagnosis of hypercalcemia includes

    A. Vitamin A toxicity
    B. Vigorous exercise
    C. Hypothyroidism
    D. Myasthenia gravis
    E. None of the above

5. Which patient characteristic would meet current indications for surgery to correct asymptomatic hyperparathyroidism?

    A. Renal insufficiency with a glomerular filtration rate of 72 mL/min
    B. Age of 57 years
    C. Positive localization tests with concordant ultrasound and sestamibi scans
    D. Osteoporosis with a T-score of 2.8
    E. A serum calcium level of 10.8 mg/dL with an upper limit of normal of 10.3 mg/dL

Breast Disorders

Armando E. Giuliano, MD
Sara A. Hurvitz, MD

BENIGN BREAST DISORDERS

FIBROCYSTIC CONDITION

ESSENTIALS OF DIAGNOSIS

- ► Painful breast masses; often multiple and bilateral.
- ► Rapid fluctuation in mass size is common.
- ► Pain often worsens during premenstrual phase of cycle.
- ► Most common age is 30-50. Rare in postmenopausal women not receiving hormonal replacement.

General Considerations

Fibrocystic condition is the most frequent lesion of the breast. Although commonly referred to as "fibrocystic disease," it does not, in fact, represent a pathologic or anatomic disorder. It is common in women 30-50 years of age but rare in postmenopausal women who are not taking hormonal replacement. Estrogen is considered a causative factor. There may be an increased risk in women who drink alcohol, especially women between 18 and 22 years of age. Fibrocystic condition encompasses a wide variety of benign histologic changes in the breast epithelium, some of which are found so commonly in normal breasts that they are probably variants of normal but have nonetheless been termed a "condition" or "disease."

The microscopic findings of fibrocystic condition include cysts (gross and microscopic), papillomatosis, adenosis, fibrosis, and ductal epithelial hyperplasia. Although fibrocystic condition has generally been considered to increase the risk of subsequent breast cancer, *only the variants with a component of epithelial proliferation (especially with atypia), papillomatosis, or increased breast density on mammogram represent true risk factors.*

Clinical Findings

A. Symptoms and Signs

Fibrocystic condition may produce an asymptomatic mass in the breast that is discovered by accident, but pain or tenderness often calls attention to it. Discomfort often occurs or worsens during the premenstrual phase of the cycle, at which time the cysts tend to enlarge. Fluctuations in size and rapid appearance or disappearance of a breast mass are common with this condition, as are multiple or bilateral masses and serous nipple discharge. Patients will give a history of a transient lump in the breast or cyclic breast pain.

B. Diagnostic Tests

Mammography and ultrasonography should be used to evaluate a mass in a patient with fibrocystic condition. Ultrasonography alone may be used in women under 30 years of age. Because a mass due to fibrocystic condition is difficult to distinguish from carcinoma on the basis of clinical findings, *suspicious lesions should be biopsied.* Core needle biopsy, rather than fine-needle aspiration (FNA), is the preferred technique. Excisional biopsy is rarely necessary but should be done for lesions with atypia or where imaging and biopsy results are discordant. Surgery should be conservative, since the primary objective is to exclude cancer. Occasionally, FNA cytology will suffice. Simple mastectomy or extensive removal of breast tissue is rarely, if ever, indicated for fibrocystic condition.

Differential Diagnosis

Pain, fluctuation in size, and multiplicity of lesions are the features most helpful in differentiating fibrocystic condition from carcinoma. If a dominant mass is present, the diagnosis of cancer should be assumed until disproven by biopsy. Mammography may be helpful, but the breast tissue in young women is usually too radiodense to permit a worthwhile study. Sonography is useful in differentiating a cystic mass from a solid mass, especially in women with dense breasts. Final diagnosis, however, depends on analysis of a biopsy specimen.

Treatment

When the diagnosis of fibrocystic condition has been established by previous biopsy or is likely because the history is classic, aspiration of a discrete mass suggestive of a cyst is indicated to alleviate pain and, more importantly, to confirm the cystic nature of the mass. The patient is reexamined at intervals thereafter. If no fluid is obtained by aspiration, if fluid is bloody, if a mass persists after aspiration, or if at any time during follow-up a persistent or recurrent mass is noted, biopsy should be performed.

Breast pain associated with generalized fibrocystic condition is best treated by avoiding trauma and by wearing a good supportive brassiere during the night and day. Hormone therapy is not advisable because it does not cure the condition and has undesirable side effects. Danazol (100-200 mg orally twice daily), a synthetic androgen, is the only treatment approved by the U.S. Food and Drug Administration (FDA) for patients with severe pain. This treatment suppresses pituitary gonadotropins, but androgenic effects (acne, edema, hirsutism) usually make this treatment intolerable; in practice, it is rarely used. Similarly, tamoxifen reduces some symptoms of fibrocystic condition, but because of its side effects, it is not useful for young women unless it is given to reduce the risk of cancer. Postmenopausal women receiving hormone replacement therapy may stop or change doses of hormones to reduce pain. Oil of evening primrose, a natural form of gamolenic acid, has been shown to decrease pain in 44%-58% of users. The dosage of gamolenic acid is six capsules of 500 mg orally twice daily. Studies have also demonstrated a low-fat diet or decreasing dietary fat intake may reduce the painful symptoms associated with fibrocystic condition. Topical treatments such as nonsteroidal anti-inflammatory drugs are rarely of value.

The role of caffeine consumption in the development and treatment of fibrocystic condition is controversial. Some studies suggest that eliminating caffeine from the diet is associated with improvement, while other studies refute the benefit entirely. Many patients are aware of these studies and report relief of symptoms after giving up coffee, tea, and chocolate. Similarly, many women find vitamin E (400 international units daily) helpful; however, these observations remain anecdotal.

Prognosis

Exacerbations of pain, tenderness, and cyst formation may occur at any time until menopause, when symptoms usually subside, except in patients receiving hormonal replacement. The patient should be advised to examine her own breasts regularly just after menstruation and to inform her clinician if a mass appears. The risk of breast cancer developing in women with fibrocystic condition with a proliferative or atypical epithelial hyperplasia or papillomatosis is higher than that of the general population. These women should be monitored carefully with physical examinations and imaging studies.

Chetlen AL, et al: Mastalgia: imaging work-up appropriateness. *Acad Radiol.* 2017;24:345-349.

Groen JW, et al: Cyclic and non-cyclic breast pain: a systematic review on pain reduction, side effects, and quality of life for various treatments. *Eur J Obstet Gynecol Reprod Biol.* 2017;219:74-93.

Neal L, et al: Diagnosis and management of benign, atypical, and indeterminate breast lesions detected on core needle biopsy. *Mayo Clin Proc.* 2014;89(4):536-547.

Tice JA, et al: Benign breast disease, mammographic breast density, and the risk of breast cancer. *J Natl Cancer Inst.* 2013;105(14):1043-1049.

FIBROADENOMA OF THE BREAST

This common benign neoplasm occurs most frequently in young women, usually within 20 years after puberty. It is somewhat more frequent and tends to occur at an earlier age in black women. Multiple tumors are found in 10%-15% of patients.

The typical **fibroadenoma** is a round or ovoid, rubbery, discrete, relatively movable, nontender mass 1-5 cm in diameter. It is usually discovered accidentally. Clinical diagnosis in young patients is generally not difficult. In women over 30 years, fibrocystic condition of the breast and carcinoma of the breast must be considered. Cysts can be identified by aspiration or ultrasonography. Fibroadenoma does not normally occur after menopause but may occasionally develop after administration of hormones.

No treatment is usually necessary if the diagnosis can be made by core needle biopsy. Excision with pathologic examination of the specimen is performed if the diagnosis is uncertain or the lesion grows significantly. Cryoablation, or freezing of the fibroadenoma, appears to be a safe procedure if the lesion is a biopsy-proven fibroadenoma prior to ablation. Cryoablation is not appropriate for all fibroadenomas because some are too large to freeze or the diagnosis may not be certain. There is no obvious clinical advantage to cryoablation of a histologically proven fibroadenoma except that some patients may feel relief that a mass is gone. However, at times, a mass of scar or fat necrosis replaces the mass of the fibroadenoma. Reassurance seems preferable. It is usually not possible to distinguish a large fibroadenoma from a phyllodes tumor on the basis of needle biopsy results or imaging alone, and histology is usually required. Presumed fibroadenomas larger than 3-4 cm should be excised to rule out phyllodes tumors.

Phyllodes tumor is a fibroadenoma-like tumor with cellular stroma that grows rapidly. It may reach a large size and, if inadequately excised, will recur locally. The lesion can be benign or malignant. If benign, phyllodes tumor is treated by local excision. The treatment of malignant phyllodes tumor is more controversial, but complete removal of the tumor with a margin of normal tissue avoids recurrence. Because these tumors may be large, total mastectomy is sometimes necessary. Lymph node dissection is not performed, since the sarcomatous portion of the tumor metastasizes to the lungs and not the lymph nodes.

Co M, et al: Mammary phyllodes tumour: a 15-year multicentre clinical review. *J Clin Pathol.* 2018;71(6):493-497.

Koh VCY, et al: Size and heterologous elements predict metastases in malignant phyllodes tumours of the breast. *Virchows Arch.* 2018;472(4):615-621.

Krings G, et al: Fibroepithelial lesions; the WHO spectrum. *Semin Diagn Pathol.* 2017;34(5):438-452.

Lightner AL, et al: A single-center experience and review of the literature: 64 cases of phyllodes tumors to better understand risk factors and disease management. *Am Surg.* 2015;81(3):309-315.

NIPPLE DISCHARGE

In order of decreasing frequency, the following are the most common causes of nipple discharge in the nonlactating breast: duct ectasia, intraductal papilloma, and carcinoma. The important characteristics of the discharge and some other factors to be evaluated by history and physical examination are listed in Table 18–1.

Spontaneous, unilateral, serous or serosanguineous discharge from a single duct is usually caused by an ectatic duct or an intraductal papilloma or, rarely, by an intraductal cancer. A mass may not be palpable. The involved duct may be identified by pressure at different sites around the nipple at the margin of the areola. Bloody discharge is suggestive of cancer but is more often caused by a benign papilloma in the duct. Cytologic examination may identify malignant cells, but negative findings do not rule out cancer, which is more likely in women over age 50 years. In any case, the involved bloody duct—and a mass if present—should be excised. A ductogram (a mammogram of a duct after radiopaque dye has been injected), like cytology, is of limited value since excision of the suspicious ductal system is indicated regardless of findings. Ductoscopy, evaluation of the ductal system with a small scope inserted through the nipple, has been attempted but is not effective management.

In premenopausal women, spontaneous multiple duct discharge, unilateral or bilateral, most noticeable just before menstruation, is often due to fibrocystic condition. Discharge

Table 18–1. Characteristics of nipple discharge in the nonpregnant, nonlactating woman.

Finding	Significance
Serous	Most likely benign FCC, ie, duct ectasia
Bloody	More likely neoplastic—papilloma, carcinoma
Associated mass	More likely neoplastic
Unilateral	Either neoplastic or nonneoplastic
Bilateral	Most likely nonneoplastic
Single duct	More likely neoplastic
Multiple ducts	More likely FCC
Milky	Endocrine disorders, medications
Spontaneous	Either neoplastic or nonneoplastic
Produced by pressure at single site	Either neoplastic or nonneoplastic
Persistent	Either neoplastic or nonneoplastic
Intermittent	Either neoplastic or nonneoplastic
Related to menses	More likely FCC
Premenopausal	More likely FCC
Taking hormones	More likely FCC

FCC, fibrocystic condition.
Reproduced with permission from Papadakis MA, McPhee SJ, Rabow MW: *Current Medical Diagnosis & Treatment* 2020. New York, NY: McGraw-Hill Education; 2020..

may be green or brownish. Papillomatosis and ductal ectasia are usually detected only by biopsy. If a mass is present, it should be removed.

A milky discharge from multiple ducts in the nonlactating breast may occur from hyperprolactinemia. Serum prolactin levels should be obtained to search for a pituitary tumor. Thyroid-stimulating hormone (TSH) helps exclude causative hypothyroidism. Numerous antipsychotic medications and other medications may also cause a milky discharge that ceases on discontinuance of the medication.

Oral contraceptive agents or estrogen replacement therapy may cause clear, serous, or milky discharge from a single duct, but multiple duct discharge is more common. In the premenopausal woman, the discharge is more evident just before menstruation and disappears on stopping the medication. If it does not stop, is from a single duct, and is copious, exploration should be performed since this may be a sign of cancer.

A purulent discharge may originate in a subareolar abscess and require removal of the abscess and the related lactiferous sinus.

When localization is not possible, no mass is palpable, and the discharge is nonbloody, the patient should be reexamined every 3 or 4 months for a year, and a mammogram and an ultrasound should be performed. Although most discharge is from a benign process, patients may find it annoying or disconcerting. To eliminate the discharge, proximal duct excision can be performed both for treatment and diagnosis.

Castellano I, et al: The impact of malignant nipple discharge cytology (NDc) in surgical management of breast cancer patients. *PLoS One.* 2017;12(8):e0182073.

de Paula IB, et al: Breast imaging in patients with nipple discharge. *Radiol Bras.* 2017;50(6):383-388.

Li GZ, et al: Evaluating the risk of underlying malignancy in patients with pathologic nipple discharge. *Breast J.* 2018;24(4):624-627.

FAT NECROSIS

Fat necrosis is a rare lesion of the breast but is of clinical importance because it produces a mass (often accompanied by skin or nipple retraction) that is usually indistinguishable from carcinoma even with imaging studies. In the past, most fat necrosis has been seen after trauma, but now fat necrosis is commonly seen after fat injections to augment breast size or fill defects after breast surgery. The resultant mass may be confused with cancer. If untreated, the mass gradually disappears. If imaging is not typical of fat necrosis, the safest course is to obtain a biopsy. Core needle biopsy is usually adequate. Fat necrosis is also common after segmental resection, radiation therapy, or flap reconstruction after mastectomy.

Nakada H, et al: Fat necrosis after breast-conserving oncoplastic surgery. *Breast Cancer.* 2019;26(1):125-130.

BREAST ABSCESS

During nursing, an area of redness, tenderness, and induration may develop in the breast. The organism most commonly found in these abscesses is *Staphylococcus aureus.*

Infection in the nonlactating breast is rare. A subareolar abscess may develop in young or middle-aged women who are not lactating. These infections tend to recur after incision and drainage unless the area is explored during a quiescent interval, with excision of the involved lactiferous duct or ducts at the base of the nipple. In the nonlactating breast, inflammatory carcinoma must always be considered. Thus, incision and biopsy of any indurated tissue with a small piece of erythematous skin is indicated when suspected abscess or cellulitis in the nonlactating breast does not resolve promptly with antibiotics. Often needle or catheter drainage is adequate to treat an abscess, but surgical incision and drainage may be necessary.

Barron AU, et al: Do acute-care surgeons follow best practices for breast abscess management? A single-institution analysis of 325 consecutive cases. *J Surg Res.* 2017;216:169-171.

Berens PD: Breast pain: engorgement, nipple pain, and mastitis. *Clin Obstet Gynecol.* 2015;58(4):902-914.

Dixon JM: Breast infection. *BMJ.* 2013;347:f3291.

Kasales CJ, et al: Nonpuerperal mastitis and subareolar abscess of the breast. *AJR Am J Roentgenol.* 2014;202(2):W133-W139.

Lam E, et al: Breast abscess: evidence based management recommendations. *Expert Rev Anti Infect Ther.* 2014;12(7):753-762.

Mahoney MC, et al: Breast emergencies: types, imaging features, and management. *AJR Am J Roentgenol.* 2014;202(4):W390-W399.

Saboo A, et al: Trends in non-lactation breast abscesses in a tertiary hospital setting. *ANZ J Surg.* 2018;88(7-8):739-744.

Taffurelli M, et al: Recurrent periductal mastitis: surgical treatment. *Surgery.* 2016;160(6):1689-1692.

DISORDERS OF THE AUGMENTED BREAST

At least 4 million American women have had breast implants. Breast augmentation is performed by placing implants under the pectoralis muscle or, less desirably, in the subcutaneous tissue of the breast. Most implants are made of an outer silicone shell filled with a silicone gel, saline, or some combination of the two. Capsule contraction or scarring around the implant develops in about 15%-25% of patients, leading to a firmness and distortion of the breast that can be painful. Some require removal of the implant and surrounding capsule.

Implant rupture may occur in as many as 5%-10% of women, and bleeding of gel through the capsule is noted even more commonly. Although silicone gel may be an immunologic stimulant, there is *no increase* in autoimmune disorders in patients with such implants. The FDA has advised symptomatic women with ruptured silicone implants to discuss possible surgical removal with their clinicians. However, women who are asymptomatic and have no evidence of rupture of a silicone gel prosthesis should probably not undergo removal of the implant. Women with symptoms of autoimmune illnesses often undergo removal, but no benefit has been shown.

Studies have failed to show any association between implants and an increased incidence of breast cancer. However, breast cancer may develop in a patient with an augmentation prosthesis, as it does in women without them. Detection in patients with implants may be more difficult because mammography is less able to detect early lesions. Mammography is better if the implant is subpectoral rather than subcutaneous. Prostheses should be placed retropectorally after mastectomy to facilitate detection of a local recurrence of cancer, which is usually cutaneous or subcutaneous and is easily detected by palpation. Rarely, lymphoma of the breast with silicone implants has been reported.

If a cancer develops in a patient with implants, it should be treated in the same manner as in women without implants.

Such women should be offered the option of mastectomy or breast-conserving therapy, which may require removal or replacement of the implant. Radiotherapy of the augmented breast often results in marked capsular contracture. Adjuvant treatments should be given for the same indications as for women who have no implants.

Clemens MW, et al: NCCN consensus guidelines for the diagnosis and management of breast implant-associated anaplastic large cell lymphoma. *Aesthet Surg J.* 2017;37(3):285-289.

Doren EL, et al: U.S. epidemiology of breast implant-associated anaplastic large cell lymphoma. *Plast Reconstr Surg.* 2017; 139(5):1042-1050.

Elston JB, et al: Complications and recurrence in implant-sparing oncologic breast surgery. *Ann Plast Surg.* 2017;78(6S Suppl 5): S269-S274.

Gidengil CA, et al: Breast implant-associated anaplastic large cell lymphoma: a systematic review. *Plast Reconstr Surg.* 2015;135(3):713-720.

Jewell ML: Silicone gel breast implants at 50: the state of the science. *Aesthet Surg J.* 2012;32(8):1031-1034.

Mango VL, et al: Breast carcinoma in augmented breasts: MRI findings. *AJR Am J Roentgenol.* 2015;204(5):W599-W604.

Nanayakkara PW, et al: Silicone gel breast implants: what we know about safety after all these years. *Ann Intern Med.* 2016;164(3):199-200.

Rohrich RJ, et al: Working toward a solution: the unanswered questions about silicone gel breast implants. *Ann Intern Med.* 2016;164(3):201-202.

Rupani A, et al: Lymphomas associated with breast implants: a review of the literature. *Aesthet Surg J.* 2015;35(5):533-544.

▼ CARCINOMA OF THE FEMALE BREAST

 ESSENTIALS OF DIAGNOSIS

▸ Risk factors: Age, nulliparity, childbirth after age 30, family history of breast cancer or genetic mutations (*BRCA1*, *BRCA2*), and personal history of breast cancer or some types of proliferative conditions.

▸ Early findings: Single, nontender, firm to hard mass with ill-defined margins; mammographic abnormalities and no palpable mass.

▸ Later findings: Skin or nipple retraction; axillary lymphadenopathy; breast enlargement, erythema, edema, pain; fixation of mass to skin or chest wall.

▷ Incidence & Risk Factors

Breast cancer will develop in *one of eight* American women. Next to skin cancer, breast cancer is the most common cancer in women; it is second only to lung cancer as a cause of death. In 2018, there were approximately 268,670 new cases and 41,400 deaths from breast cancer in the United States. Worldwide, breast cancer is diagnosed in approximately 2.1 million women, and about 626,679 die of breast cancer each year, with the highest rates of diagnosis in Australia/New Zealand, Europe, and North America and lowest rates in Eastern/Middle Africa and South Central Asia. The highest rates of death are in black women in the United States, and the lowest rates are in Korean women. These regional differences in incidence are likely due to the variable availability of screening mammography as well as differences in reproductive, nutrition, and hormonal factors. In Western countries, incidence rates decreased with a reduced use of postmenopausal hormone therapy and mortality declined with increased use of screening and improved treatments. In contrast, incidence and mortality from breast cancer in many African and Asian countries have increased as reproductive factors have changed (eg, childbirth after age 30) and as the incidence of obesity has risen.

The most significant risk factor for the development of breast cancer is age. A woman's risk of breast cancer rises rapidly until her early 60s, peaks in her 70s, and then declines. A significant family history of breast or ovarian cancer may also indicate a high risk of developing breast cancer. Germline mutations in the *BRCA* family of tumor suppressor genes or other breast cancer susceptibility genes account for approximately 5%-10% of breast cancer diagnoses and tend to cluster in certain ethnic groups, including women of Ashkenazi Jewish descent. Women with a mutation in the *BRCA1* gene, located on chromosome 17, have an estimated 85% chance of developing breast cancer in their lifetime. Other genes associated with an increased risk of breast and other cancers include *BRCA2* (associated with a gene on chromosome 13), ataxia-telangiectasia mutation (*ATM*), *BARD1*, *CHEK2*, *PALB2*, and *RAD51D*, and mutation of the tumor suppressor gene *p53*. If a woman has a compelling family history (eg, breast cancer diagnosed in two first-degree relatives, especially if diagnosed younger than age 50; ovarian cancer; male breast cancer; or a first-degree relative with bilateral breast cancer), genetic testing may be appropriate. In general, it is best for a woman who has a strong family history to meet with a genetics counselor to undergo a risk assessment and decide whether genetic testing is indicated.

Even when genetic testing fails to reveal a predisposing genetic mutation, women with a strong family history of breast cancer are at higher risk for development of breast cancer. Compared with a woman with no affected family members, a woman who has one first-degree relative with breast cancer has double the risk of developing breast cancer, and a woman with two first-degree relatives with breast cancer has triple the risk of developing breast cancer. The risk is further increased for a woman whose affected family member was premenopausal at the time of diagnosis or had bilateral breast cancer. Lifestyle and reproductive factors also contribute to risk of breast cancer. Nulliparous women and women whose first full-term pregnancy occurred after the age of 30 have an elevated risk. Early menarche (under age 12) and late natural menopause (after age 55) are associated with an increase in risk, especially for hormone receptor–positive breast cancer. Combined oral contraceptive pills also appear to increase the risk of breast cancer, with longer use associated with higher risk. Several studies show that concomitant administration of progesterone and estrogen to postmenopausal women may increase the incidence of breast cancer, compared with the use of estrogen alone or with no hormone replacement treatment. The Women's Health Initiative prospective randomized study of hormone replacement therapy stopped treatment with estrogen and progesterone early because of an increased risk of breast cancer compared with untreated women or women treated with estrogen alone. Alcohol consumption, high dietary intake of fat, and lack of exercise may also increase the risk of breast cancer. Fibrocystic breast condition is also associated with an increased incidence of cancer when it is accompanied by proliferative changes, papillomatosis, atypical epithelial hyperplasia, and increased breast density on mammogram. A woman who had cancer in one breast is at increased risk for cancer developing in the other breast. In these women, a contralateral cancer develops at a rate of 1% or 2% per year. Women with cancer of the uterine corpus have a risk of breast cancer significantly higher than that of the general population, and women with breast cancer have a comparably increased risk of endometrial cancer. Socioeconomic and racial factors have also been associated with breast cancer risk. Breast cancer tends to be diagnosed more frequently in women of higher socioeconomic status.

Women at greater than average risk for developing breast cancer (Table 18–2) should be identified by their clinicians and monitored carefully. Several risk assessment models have been validated (most extensively the Gail 2 model) to evaluate a woman's risk of developing cancer. Those with an exceptional family history should be counseled about the option of genetic testing. Some of these high-risk women may consider prophylactic mastectomy, oophorectomy, tamoxifen, or an aromatase inhibitor (AI). The Prevention and Observation of Surgical Endpoints (PROSE) consortium monitored women with deleterious *BRCA1/2* mutations from 1974 to 2008 and reported that 15% of women with a known *BRCA* mutation underwent bilateral prophylactic mastectomy, and none of them developed breast cancer during the 3 years of follow-up. In contrast, subsequent breast cancer developed in 98 (7%) of the 1372 women who did not have surgery. Moreover, women who underwent prophylactic salpingo-oophorectomy had a lower risk of ovarian cancer, all-cause mortality, as well as breast cancer– and ovarian cancer–specific mortality.

Women with genetic mutations in whom breast cancer develops may be treated in the same way as women who do not have mutations (ie, lumpectomy), although there is an increased risk of ipsilateral and contralateral breast cancer after lumpectomy for these women. One study showed that of patients with a diagnosis of breast cancer who were found to be carriers of a *BRCA* mutation, approximately 50% chose to undergo bilateral mastectomy.

Table 18–2. Factors associated with increased risk of breast cancer (listed in alphabetical order).

Age	Older
Family history	Breast cancer in parent, sibling, or child (especially bilateral or premenopausal)
Genetics	*BRCA1, BRCA2,* or other unknown mutations
Menstrual history	Early menarche (under age 12) Late menopause (after age 50)
Previous medical history	Endometrial cancer Proliferative forms of fibrocystic disease Cancer in other breast
Race	White
Reproductive history	Nulliparous or late first pregnancy

Reproduced with permission from Papadakis MA, McPhee SJ, Rabow MW: *Current Medical Diagnosis & Treatment* 2020. New York, NY: McGraw-Hill Education; 2020.

Bray F, et al: Global cancer statistics 2018: GLOBOCAN estimates of incidence and mortality worldwide for 36 cancers in 185 countries. *CA Cancer J Clin.* 2018;68(6):394-424.

Brouckaert O, et al: Reproductive profiles and risk of breast cancer subtypes: a multi-center case-only study. *Breast Cancer Res.* 2017;19(1):119.

Couch FJ, et al: Associations between cancer predisposition testing panel genes and breast cancer. *JAMA Oncol.* 2017;3(9):1190-1196.

Day FR, et al: Genomic analyses identify hundreds of variants associated with age at menarche and support a role for puberty timing in cancer risk. *Nat Genet.* 2017;49(6):834-841.

Frey MK, et al: Prevalence of nonfounder *BRCA1/2* mutations in Ashkenazi Jewish patients presenting for genetic testing at a hereditary breast and ovarian cancer center. *Cancer.* 2019; 125(5):690-697.

Ginsburg O, et al: The global burden of women's cancers: a grand challenge in global health. *Lancet.* 2017;389(10071):847-860.

Hardefeldt PJ, et al: Physical activity and weight loss reduce the risk of breast cancer: a meta-analysis of 139 prospective and retrospective studies. *Clin Breast Cancer.* 2018;18(4):e601-e612.

Ma H, et al: Reproductive factors and the risk of triple-negative breast cancer in white women and African-American women: a pooled analysis. *Breast Cancer Res.* 2017;19(1):6.

Michailidou K, et al: Association analysis identifies 65 new breast cancer risk loci. *Nature.* 2017;551(7678):92-94.

Mørch LS, et al: Contemporary hormonal contraception and the risk of breast cancer. *N Engl J Med.* 2017;377(23):2228-2239.

Schwartz MD, et al: Long-term outcomes of *BRCA1/BRCA2* testing: risk reduction and surveillance. *Cancer.* 2012;118(2):510-517.

Sefton P: JAMA patient page. Testing for *BRCA1/2* mutations. *JAMA.* 2017;318(20):2054.

Siegel RL, et al: Cancer statistics, 2018. *CA Cancer J Clin.* 2018;68(1): 7-30.

Toss A, et al: The impact of reproductive life on breast cancer risk in women with family history or BRCA mutation. *Oncotarget.* 2017;8(6):9144-9154.

Prevention

Several clinical trials have evaluated the use of **selective estrogen receptor modulators (SERMs)**, including tamoxifen and raloxifene, for prevention of breast cancer in women with no personal history of breast cancer but at high risk for developing the disease. A meta-analysis of nine of these studies including 83,399 women with a median follow-up of 65 months demonstrated a 38% reduction in breast cancer incidence (hazard ratio [HR], 0.62; 95% confidence interval [CI], 0.56-0.69) with a 10-year cumulative incidence of 6.3% in control groups and 4.2% in SERM-treated groups. An increased risk of endometrial cancer, cataracts, and venous thromboembolic events but a reduced risk of vertebral fractures was seen in SERM groups. Although SERMs have been shown to be effective at reducing the risk of breast cancer and saving costs, the use of this intervention by women has been relatively low, possibly due to the perceived risks and side effects of therapy. A cost-effectiveness study based on a meta-analysis of four randomized prevention trials showed that tamoxifen reduced costs and improved life expectancy when higher risk (Gail 5-year risk at least 1.66%) women under the age of 55 years were treated.

Similar to SERMs, AIs, such as exemestane and anastrozole, have shown success in preventing breast cancer with a lower risk of uterine cancer and thromboembolic events, although bone loss is a significant side effect of this treatment. In one study, 4560 postmenopausal women at high risk for breast cancer were randomly assigned to receive exemestane or placebo for 5 years. With a median follow-up of 35 months, there was a 65% relative risk reduction in the annual risk of invasive breast cancer (0.19% vs 0.55%; HR, 0.35; 95% CI, 0.18-0.70; $P = 0.002$) for patients who received exemestane. Although exemestane use was associated with a higher rate of adverse events (88% vs 85%; $P = 0.003$), there were no significant differences between the groups in terms of skeletal fractures or cardiovascular events, although longer follow-up is needed to accurately assess these outcomes. The IBIS-II study randomized 3864 postmenopausal women at high risk for breast cancer to receive placebo or anastrozole for 5 years and demonstrated a 53% risk reduction in the anastrozole group (HR, 0.47; 95% CI, 0.32-0.68; $P < 0.0001$). Based on these data, exemestane and anastrozole are reasonable risk-reducing options for postmenopausal women at higher risk for breast cancer.

Colditz GA, et al: Priorities for the primary prevention of breast cancer. *CA Cancer J Clin.* 2014;64(3):186-194.

Cuzick J et al; IBIS-II Investigators: Anastrozole for prevention of breast cancer in high-risk postmenopausal women (IBIS-II): an international, double-blind, randomised placebo-controlled trial. *Lancet.* 2014;383(9922):1041-1048.

Cuzick J et al; SERM Chemoprevention of Breast Cancer Overview Group: Selective oestrogen receptor modulators in prevention of breast cancer: an updated meta-analysis of individual participant data. *Lancet.* 2013;381(9880):1827-1834.

Cuzick J, et al: Tamoxifen for prevention of breast cancer: extended long-term follow-up of the IBIS-I breast cancer prevention trial. *Lancet Oncol.* 2015;16(1):67-75.

Goss PE, et al; CTG MAP.3 Study Investigators: Exemestane for breast-cancer prevention in postmenopausal women. *N Engl J Med.* 2011;364(25):2381-2391.

Meads C, et al: A systematic review of breast cancer incidence risk prediction models with meta-analysis of their performance. *Breast Cancer Res Treat.* 2012;132(2):365-377.

Nelson HD, et al: Use of medications to reduce risk for primary breast cancer: a systematic review for the U.S. Preventive Services Task Force. *Ann Intern Med.* 2013;158(8):604-614.

Early Detection of Breast Cancer

A. Screening Programs

A number of large screening programs, consisting of physical and mammographic examination of asymptomatic women, have been conducted over the years. On average, these programs identify 10 cancers per 1000 women over the age of 50 and 2 cancers per 1000 women under the age of 50. Screening detects breast cancer before it has spread to the lymph nodes in about 80% of the women evaluated. This increases the chance of survival to about 85% at 5 years.

Substantial evidence supports the use of **routine screening mammography;** however, recommendations relating to timing and frequency vary by different agencies and countries. About one-third of the abnormalities detected on screening mammograms will be found to be malignant when biopsy is performed. The probability of cancer on a screening mammogram is directly related to the Breast Imaging Reporting and Data System (BIRADS) assessment, and workup should be performed based on this classification. The sensitivity of mammography varies from approximately 60% to 90%. This sensitivity depends on several factors, including patient age, breast density, tumor size, tumor histology (lobular vs ductal), location, and mammographic appearance. In young women with dense breasts, mammography is less sensitive than in older women with fatty breasts, in whom mammography can detect at least 90% of malignancies. Smaller tumors, particularly those without calcifications, are more difficult to detect, especially in dense breasts. The lack of sensitivity and the low incidence of breast cancer in young women have led to questions concerning the value of mammography for screening in women 40-50 years of age. The specificity of mammography in women under 50 years varies from about 30% to 40% for nonpalpable mammographic abnormalities to 85%

to 90% for clinically evident malignancies. Guidelines from at least six separate organizations exist in the United States, and each differs slightly, making it somewhat complex for clinicians and patients to navigate. Although the American College of Radiology, American Medical Association, and National Comprehensive Cancer Network (NCCN) recommend starting mammography screening at age 40, the US Preventive Services Task Force (USPSTF) recommends starting screening at age 50. Most guidelines recommend annual screening; however, the American Cancer Society recommends decreasing the frequency of screening to every 1-2 years starting at age 55 years, and the USPSTF recommends routine mammography be done no more than every 2 years beginning at age 50 years. It is generally agreed that mammography should continue until life expectancy is shorter than 7-10 years, although the USPSTF recommends stopping screening after age 74 years regardless of life expectancy. Thus, clinicians should have an informed discussion with patients about screening mammography regarding its potential risks (eg, false positives, overdiagnosis, radiation exposure) and benefits (eg, early diagnosis), taking into consideration a patient's individual risk factors.

B. Imaging

1. Mammography—Mammography is the most reliable means of detecting breast cancer before a mass can be palpated. Most slowly growing cancers can be identified by mammography at least 2 years before reaching a size detectable by palpation.

Indications for mammography are as follows: (1) screening at regular intervals asymptomatic women at risk for developing breast cancer; (2) evaluating each breast when a diagnosis of potentially curable breast cancer has been made and at regular intervals thereafter; (3) evaluating a questionable or ill-defined breast mass or other suspicious change in the breast; (4) searching for an occult breast cancer in women with metastatic disease in axillary nodes or elsewhere from an unknown primary; (5) screening women prior to cosmetic operations or prior to biopsy of a mass, to examine for an unsuspected cancer; (6) monitoring women with breast cancer who have been treated with breast-conserving surgery and radiation; and (7) monitoring the contralateral breast in women with breast cancer treated with mastectomy.

Film screen mammography has largely been replaced by digital mammography. Although full-field digital mammography provides an easier method to maintain and review mammograms and may improve image quality, it has not been proven to improve overall cancer detection and is less economical. It may offer screening benefits to women younger than age 50 years and to women with dense breasts. Although computer-assisted detection may increase the sensitivity of mammography, it has not been shown to improve mortality rates. Tomosynthesis creates tomographic "slices" of the breast volume with a single acquisition. This technique may improve the sensitivity of mammogram, especially in patients with dense breast tissue, and reduces the number of callbacks but has not yet been shown in prospective studies to improve long-term patient outcomes.

Calcifications are the most easily recognized mammographic abnormality. The most common findings associated with carcinoma of the breast are clustered pleomorphic microcalcifications. Such calcifications are usually at least five to eight in number, are aggregated in one part of the breast, and differ from each other in size and shape, often including branched or V- or Y-shaped configurations. There may be an associated mammographic mass density or, at times, only a mass density with no calcifications. Such a density usually has irregular or ill-defined borders and may lead to architectural distortion within the breast but may be subtle and difficult to detect.

Patients with a dominant or suspicious mass on examination must undergo biopsy despite mammographic findings. The mammogram should be obtained prior to biopsy so that other suspicious areas can be noted and the contralateral breast can be evaluated. *Mammography is never a substitute for biopsy* because it may not reveal clinical cancer, especially in a very dense breast.

Communication and documentation among the patient, the referring clinician, and the interpreting physician are critical for high-quality screening and diagnostic mammography. The patient should be told about *how* she will receive timely results of her mammogram; that mammography does not "rule out" cancer; and that she may receive a correlative examination such as ultrasound at the mammography facility if referred for a suspicious lesion. She should also be aware of the technique and need for breast compression and that this may be uncomfortable. The mammography facility should be informed in writing by the clinician of abnormal physical examination findings. The Agency for Health Care Policy and Research Clinical Practice Guidelines strongly recommends that all mammography reports be communicated in writing to the patient and referring clinician. Legislation has been passed in a number of U.S. states that requires imaging facilities to report to patients the density of their breasts. This may prompt women with dense breasts to discuss with their clinician whether or not additional screening options would be appropriate in addition to mammogram.

2. Other imaging—Magnetic resonance imaging (MRI) and ultrasound may be useful screening modalities in women who are at high risk for breast cancer but not for the general population. The *sensitivity* of MRI is much higher than mammography; however, the *specificity* is significantly lower, and this results in multiple unnecessary biopsies. The increased sensitivity despite decreased specificity may be considered a reasonable trade-off for those at increased risk for developing breast cancer but not for the normal-risk population.

The NCCN guidelines recommend MRI in addition to screening mammography for high-risk women, including those with *BRCA1/2* mutations, those who have a lifetime risk of breast cancer of at least 20%, and those with a personal history of lobular carcinoma in situ. Women who received radiation therapy to the chest in their teens or twenties are also known to be at high risk for developing breast cancer, and screening MRI may be considered in addition to mammography. MRI is useful in women with breast implants to determine the character of a lesion present in the breast and to search for implant rupture, and at times, it is also helpful in patients with prior lumpectomy and radiation.

C. Clinical Breast Examination and Self-Examination

Breast self-examination has *not* been shown to improve survival. Because of the lack of strong evidence demonstrating value, the American Cancer Society no longer recommends monthly breast self-examination. Although breast self-examination is not a recommended practice, patients should recognize and report any breast changes to their clinicians as it remains an important facet of proactive care.

Bleyer A, et al: Effect of three decades of screening mammography on breast-cancer incidence. *N Engl J Med.* 2012;367(21):1998-2005.

Fuller MS, et al: Breast cancer screening: an evidence-based update. *Med Clin North Am.* 2015;99(3):451-468.

Gross CP, et al: The cost of breast cancer screening in the Medicare population. *JAMA Intern Med.* 2013;173(3):220-226.

Independent UK Panel on Breast Cancer Screening: The benefits and harms of breast cancer screening: an independent review. *Lancet.* 2012;380(9855):1778-1786.

Miller AB, et al: Twenty five year follow-up for breast cancer incidence and mortality of the Canadian National Breast Screening Study: randomised screening trial. *BMJ.* 2014;348:g366.

Morrow M, et al: MRI for breast cancer screening, diagnosis, and treatment. *Lancet.* 2011;378(9805):1804-1811.

Onega T, et al: Breast cancer screening in an era of personalized regimens: a conceptual model and National Cancer Institute initiative for risk-based and preference-based approaches at a population level. *Cancer.* 2014;120(19):2955-2964.

Pace LE, et al: A systematic assessment of benefits and risks to guide breast cancer screening decisions. *JAMA.* 2014;311(13):1327-1335.

Plescia M, et al: The National Prevention Strategy and breast cancer screening: scientific evidence for public health action. *Am J Public Health.* 2013;103(9):1545-1548.

Powell JL, et al: Impact of the addition of digital breast tomosynthesis (dbt) to standard 2d digital screening mammography on the rates of patient recall, cancer detection, and recommendations for short-term follow-up. *Acad Radiol.* 2017;24(3):302-307.

Walter LC, et al: Screening mammography in older women: a review. *JAMA.* 2014;311(13):1336-1347.

Welch HG, et al: Breast-cancer tumor size, overdiagnosis, and mammography screening effectiveness. *N Engl J Med.* 2016;375(15):1438-1447.

▶ Clinical Findings Associated With Early Detection of Breast Cancer

A. Symptoms and Signs

The presenting complaint in about 70% of patients with breast cancer is a lump (usually painless) in the breast. About 90% of these breast masses are discovered by the patient. Less frequent symptoms are breast pain; nipple discharge; erosion, retraction, enlargement, or itching of the nipple; and redness, generalized hardness, enlargement, or shrinking of the breast. Rarely, an axillary mass or swelling of the arm may be the first symptom. Back or bone pain, jaundice, or weight loss may be the result of systemic metastases, but these symptoms are rarely seen on initial presentation.

The relative frequency of carcinoma in various anatomic sites in the breast is shown in Figure 18–1.

Inspection of the breast is the first step in physical examination and should be carried out with the patient sitting, arms at her sides and then overhead. Abnormal variations in breast size and contour, minimal nipple retraction, and slight edema, redness, or retraction of the skin can be identified (Figure 18–2). Asymmetry of the breasts and retraction or dimpling of the skin can often be accentuated by having the patient raise her arms overhead or press her hands on her hips to contract the pectoralis muscles. Axillary and supraclavicular areas should be thoroughly palpated for enlarged

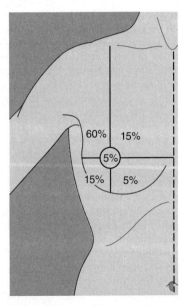

▲ **Figure 18–1.** Frequency of breast carcinoma at various anatomic sites. (Reproduced with permission from Papadakis MA, McPhee SJ, Rabow MW: *Current Medical Diagnosis & Treatment* 2020. New York, NY: McGraw-Hill Education; 2020.)

▲ **Figure 18–2.** Skin dimpling. (Used with permission from Armando E. Giuliano, MD.)

▲ **Figure 18–4.** Paget disease. (Used with permission from Armando E. Giuliano, MD.)

nodes with the patient sitting (Figure 18–3). Palpation of the breast for masses or other changes should be performed with the patient both seated and supine with the arm abducted. Palpation with a rotary motion of the examiner's fingers as well as a horizontal stripping motion has been recommended.

Breast cancer usually consists of a nontender, firm or hard mass with poorly delineated margins (caused by local infiltration). Very small (1-2 mm) erosions of the nipple epithelium may be the only manifestation of Paget disease of the breast (Figure 18–4). Watery, serous, or bloody discharge

▲ **Figure 18–3.** Palpation of axillary region for enlarged lymph nodes. (Reproduced with permission from Papadakis MA, McPhee SJ, Rabow MW: *Current Medical Diagnosis & Treatment* 2020. New York, NY: McGraw-Hill Education; 2020.)

from the nipple is an occasional early sign but is more often associated with benign disease.

A lesion smaller than 1 cm in diameter may be difficult or impossible for the examiner to feel but may be discovered by the patient. She or he should always be asked to demonstrate the location of the mass; if the clinician fails to confirm the patient's suspicions and imaging studies are normal, the examination should be repeated in 2-3 months, preferably 1-2 weeks after the onset of menses. During the premenstrual phase of the cycle, increased innocuous nodularity may suggest neoplasm or may obscure an underlying lesion. If there is any question regarding the nature of an abnormality under these circumstances, the patient should be asked to return after her menses.

Metastases tend to involve regional lymph nodes, which may be palpable. One or two movable, nontender, not particularly firm axillary lymph nodes 5 mm or less in diameter are frequently present and are generally of no significance. Firm or hard nodes larger than 1 cm are typical of metastases. Axillary nodes that are matted or fixed to skin or deep structures indicate advanced disease (at least stage III). On the other hand, if the examiner thinks that the axillary nodes are involved, that impression will be borne out by histologic section in about 85% of cases. The incidence of positive axillary nodes increases with the size of the primary tumor. Noninvasive cancers (in situ) do not metastasize. Metastases are present in about 30% of patients with clinically negative nodes.

In most cases, no nodes are palpable in the supraclavicular fossa. Firm or hard nodes of any size in this location or just beneath the clavicle should be biopsied. Ipsilateral supraclavicular or infraclavicular nodes containing cancer indicate that the tumor is in an advanced stage (stage III or IV). Edema of the ipsilateral arm, commonly caused by metastatic infiltration of regional lymphatics, is also a sign of advanced cancer.

B. Laboratory Findings

Liver or bone metastases may be associated with elevation of serum alkaline phosphatase. Hypercalcemia is an occasional important finding in advanced cancer of the breast. Serum tumor markers such as carcinoembryonic antigen (CEA) and CA 15-3 or CA 27-29 are not recommended for diagnosis of early lesions or for routine surveillance for recurrence after a breast cancer diagnosis.

C. Imaging

1. For lesions felt only by the patient—Ultrasound is often valuable and mammography essential when an area is felt by the patient to be abnormal but the clinician feels no mass. MRI should not be used to rule out cancer because MRI has a false-negative rate of about 3%-5%. Although lower than mammography, this false-negative rate cannot permit safe elimination of the possibility of cancer. False-negative results are more likely seen in infiltrating lobular carcinomas and ductal carcinoma in situ (DCIS) than invasive ductal carcinoma.

2. For metastatic lesions—For patients with suspicious symptoms or signs (bone pain, abdominal symptoms, elevated liver biochemical tests) or locally advanced disease (clinically abnormal lymph nodes or large primary tumors), staging scans are indicated prior to surgery or systemic therapy. Chest imaging with CT or radiographs may be done to evaluate for pulmonary metastases. Abdominal imaging with CT or ultrasound may be obtained to evaluate for liver metastases. Bone scans using ^{99m}Tc-labeled phosphates or phosphonates are more sensitive than skeletal radiographs in detecting metastatic breast cancer. Bone scanning has not proved to be of clinical value as a routine preoperative test in the absence of symptoms, physical findings, or abnormal alkaline phosphatase or calcium levels. The frequency of abnormal findings on bone scan parallels the status of the axillary lymph nodes on pathologic examination. Positron emission tomography (PET) scanning alone or combined with computed tomography (PET-CT) may also be used for detecting soft tissue or visceral metastases in patients with symptoms or signs of metastatic disease.

D. Diagnostic Tests

1. Biopsy—The diagnosis of breast cancer depends ultimately on examination of tissue or cells removed by biopsy. Treatment should never be undertaken without an unequivocal histologic or cytologic diagnosis of cancer. **The safest course is biopsy examination of all suspicious lesions found on physical examination or imaging, or both.** About 60% of lesions clinically thought to be cancer prove on biopsy to be benign, while about 30% of clinically benign lesions are found to be malignant. These findings demonstrate the fallibility of clinical judgment and the necessity for biopsy.

All breast masses require a histologic diagnosis by biopsy with one probable exception: a nonsuspicious, presumably fibrocystic mass, in a premenopausal woman. Rather, these masses can be observed through one or two menstrual cycles. However, if the mass is not cystic and does not completely resolve during this time, it must be biopsied. Figures 18–5 and 18–6 present algorithms for management of breast masses in premenopausal and postmenopausal patients.

The simplest biopsy method is needle biopsy, either by aspiration of tumor cells (FNA cytology) or by obtaining a small core of tissue with a hollow needle (core needle biopsy).

Large-needle (core) biopsy removes a core of tissue with a large cutting needle and *is the diagnostic procedure of choice* for both palpable and image-detected abnormalities. Handheld biopsy devices make large-core needle (14-gauge) biopsy of a palpable mass easy and cost effective in the office with local anesthesia. As in the case of any needle biopsy, the main problem is sampling error due to improper positioning of the needle, giving rise to a false-negative test result. This is extremely unusual with image-guided biopsies. Core biopsy allows the tumor to be tested for the expression of biological markers, such as estrogen receptor (ER), progesterone receptor (PR), and *HER2*.

FNA cytology is a technique whereby cells are aspirated with a small needle and examined cytologically. This technique can be performed easily with virtually no morbidity and is much less expensive than excisional or open biopsy. The main disadvantages are that it requires a pathologist skilled in the cytologic diagnosis of breast cancer and it is subject to sampling problems. Furthermore, noninvasive cancers usually cannot be distinguished from invasive cancers and immunohistochemical tests to determine expression of hormone receptors, and the amplification of the *HER2* oncogene cannot be reliably performed on FNA biopsies. The incidence of false-positive diagnoses is extremely low, perhaps 1%-2%. The false-negative rate is as high as 10%. Most experienced clinicians would not leave a suspicious dominant mass in the breast even when FNA cytology is negative unless the clinical diagnosis, breast imaging studies, and cytologic studies were all in agreement, such as a fibrocystic lesion or fibroadenoma. Given the stated limitations, *FNA is not the modality of choice for sampling an abnormal breast mass and has been largely replaced by core needle biopsy.*

Open biopsy under local anesthesia as a separate procedure prior to deciding upon definitive treatment has become less common with the increased use of core needle biopsy. Needle biopsy, when positive, offers a more rapid approach with less expense and morbidity, but when nondiagnostic, it must be followed by open biopsy. It generally consists of an excisional biopsy, which is done through an incision with the

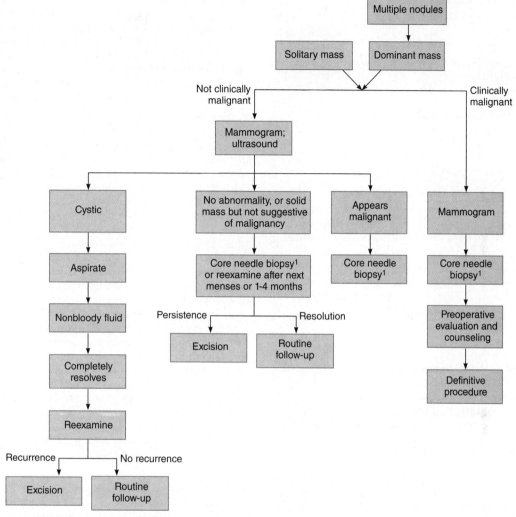

▲ **Figure 18–5.** Evaluation of breast masses in premenopausal women. (Reproduced with permission from Berek JS, Hacker NF: *Practical Gynecologic Oncology,* 4th ed. Philadelphia, PA: Lippincott Williams & Wilkins; 2004.)
[1]Lesions that are atypical but not malignant should be excised.

intent to remove the entire abnormality, not simply a sample. Intraoperative frozen section examination of a breast biopsy has generally been abandoned unless there is a high clinical suspicion of malignancy in a patient well prepared for the diagnosis of cancer and its treatment options.

In general, the two-step approach—outpatient large-needle core biopsy followed by definitive operation at a later date—is preferred in the diagnosis and treatment of breast cancer because patients can be given time to adjust to the diagnosis of cancer, can consider alternative forms of

therapy, and can seek a second opinion if they wish. *There is no adverse effect on the cancer from the few weeks' delay of the two-step procedure.*

2. Biopsy with ultrasound guidance—Ultrasonography is performed primarily to differentiate cystic from solid lesions but may show signs suggestive of carcinoma. Ultrasonography may show an irregular mass within a cyst in the rare case of intracystic carcinoma. If a tumor is palpable and feels like a cyst, an 18-gauge needle can be used to aspirate the

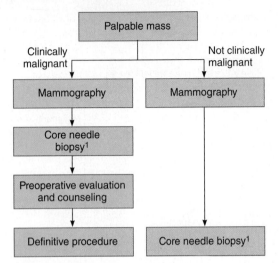

▲ Figure 18–6. Evaluation of breast masses in postmenopausal women. (Adapted with permission from Berek JS, Hacker NF: *Practical Gynecologic Oncology*, 4th ed. Philadelphia, PA: Lippincott Williams & Wilkins; 2004.

[1]Lesions that are atypical but not malignant should be excised.

fluid and make the diagnosis of cyst. If a cyst is aspirated and the fluid is nonbloody, it does not have to be examined cytologically. If the mass does not recur, no further diagnostic test is necessary. Nonpalpable mammographic densities that appear benign should be investigated with ultrasound to determine whether the lesion is cystic or solid. These may even be needle biopsied with ultrasound guidance.

3. Biopsy with mammographic guidance ("stereotactic biopsy")—When a suspicious abnormality is identified by mammography alone and cannot be palpated by the clinician, the lesion should be biopsied under mammographic guidance. In the **computerized stereotactic guided core needle** technique, a biopsy needle is inserted into the lesion with mammographic guidance, and a core of tissue for histologic examination can then be examined. Vacuum assistance increases the amount of tissue obtained and improves diagnosis.

    Mammographic localization biopsy is performed by obtaining a mammogram in two perpendicular views and placing a needle, hook-wire, or radioactive or radar-detectable seed localizer near the abnormality so that the surgeon can locate the lesion intraoperatively. After mammography confirms the position of the localizer in relation to the lesion, an incision is made and the localizer is identified. Often, the abnormality cannot even be palpated through the incision—as is the case with microcalcifications—and thus it is essential to obtain a mammogram of the specimen to document that the lesion was excised. At that time, a

second marker needle can further localize the lesion for the pathologist. Image-guided core needle biopsies have proved equivalent to mammographic localization biopsies. Core biopsy is preferable to mammographic localization for accessible lesions since an operation can be avoided. A metal clip should be placed after any image-guided core biopsy to facilitate finding the site of the lesion if subsequent treatment is necessary.

4. Other imaging modalities—Other modalities of breast imaging have been investigated for diagnostic purposes. Automated breast ultrasonography is useful in distinguishing cystic from solid lesions but should be used only as a supplement to physical examination and mammography. Ductography may be useful to define the site of a lesion causing a bloody discharge, but since biopsy is almost always indicated, ductography may be omitted and the blood-filled nipple system excised. Ductoscopy has shown some promise in identifying intraductal lesions, especially in the case of pathologic nipple discharge, but in practice, this technique is rarely used. MRI is highly sensitive but not specific and should not be used for screening except in highly selective cases. For example, MRI is useful in differentiating scar from recurrence after lumpectomy and may be valuable to screen high-risk women (eg, women with *BRCA* mutations). It may also be of value to examine for multicentricity when there is a known primary cancer; to examine the contralateral breast in women with cancer; to examine the extent of cancer, especially lobular carcinomas; or to determine the response to neoadjuvant chemotherapy. Moreover, MRI-detected suspicious findings that are not seen on mammogram or ultrasound may be biopsied under MRI guidance. PET scanning does not appear useful in evaluating the breast itself but is useful to examine for distant metastases.

5. Cytology—Cytologic examination of nipple discharge or cyst fluid may be helpful on rare occasions. As a rule, mammography (or ductography) and breast biopsy are required when nipple discharge or cyst fluid is bloody or cytologically questionable.

▶ Differential Diagnosis

The lesions to be considered most often in the differential diagnosis of breast cancer are the following, in descending order of frequency: fibrocystic condition of the breast, fibroadenoma, intraductal papilloma, lipoma, and fat necrosis.

▶ Staging

The American Joint Committee on Cancer and the International Union Against Cancer have a joint TNM (tumor, regional lymph nodes, distant metastases) staging system for breast cancer. Using the TNM staging system (www.cancer-staging.org) enhances communication between researchers

Table 18–3. Histologic types of breast cancer.

Type	Frequency of Occurrence
Infiltrating ductal (not otherwise specified)	80%–90%
Medullary	5%–8%
Colloid (mucinous)	2%–4%
Tubular	1%–2%
Papillary	1%–2%
Invasive lobular	6%–8%
Noninvasive	4%–6%
Intraductal	2%–3%
Lobular in situ	2%–3%
Rare cancers	< 1%
Juvenile (secretory)	
Adenoid cystic	
Epidermoid	
Sudoriferous	

Reproduced with permission from Papadakis MA, McPhee SJ, Rabow MW: *Current Medical Diagnosis & Treatment* 2020. New York, NY: McGraw-Hill Education; 2020.

and clinicians. The eighth edition is a landmark change in the TNM staging system because it adds biologic markers to modify the anatomic staging.

Pathologic Types

Numerous pathologic subtypes of breast cancer can be identified histologically (Table 18–3).

Except for the in situ cancers, the histologic subtypes have only a slight bearing on prognosis when outcomes are compared after accurate staging. The noninvasive cancers by definition are confined by the basement membrane of the ducts and lack the ability to spread. Histologic parameters for invasive cancers, including lymphovascular invasion and tumor grade, have been shown to be of prognostic value. Immunohistochemical analysis for expression of hormone receptors and for overexpression of HER2 in the primary tumor offers prognostic and therapeutic information.

Special Clinical Forms of Breast Cancer

A. Paget Carcinoma

Paget carcinoma is not common (about 1% of all breast cancers). Over 85% of cases are associated with an underlying invasive or noninvasive cancer, usually a well-differentiated infiltrating ductal carcinoma or a DCIS. The ducts of the nipple epithelium are infiltrated, but gross nipple changes are often minimal, and a tumor mass may not be palpable.

Because the nipple changes appear innocuous, the diagnosis is frequently missed. The first symptom is often itching or burning of the nipple, with superficial erosion or ulceration. These are often diagnosed and treated as dermatitis or bacterial infection, leading to delay or failure in detection. The diagnosis is established by biopsy of the area of erosion. When the lesion consists of nipple changes only, the incidence of axillary metastases is less than 5%, and the prognosis is excellent. When a breast mass is also present, the incidence of axillary metastases rises, with an associated marked decrease in prospects for cure by surgical or other treatment.

B. Inflammatory Carcinoma

This is the most malignant form of breast cancer and constitutes less than 3% of all cases. The clinical findings consist of a rapidly growing, sometimes painful mass that enlarges the breast. The overlying skin becomes erythematous, edematous, and warm. Often there is no distinct mass, since the tumor infiltrates the involved breast diffusely. The inflammatory changes, often mistaken for an infection, are caused by carcinomatous invasion of the subdermal lymphatics, with resulting edema and hyperemia. If the clinician suspects infection but the lesion does not respond rapidly (1-2 weeks) to antibiotics, biopsy should be performed. The diagnosis should be made when the redness involves more than one-third of the skin over the breast and biopsy shows infiltrating carcinoma with invasion of the subdermal lymphatics. Metastases tend to occur early and widely, and for this reason, inflammatory carcinoma is rarely curable. Radiation, hormone therapy (if hormone receptor positive), anti-HER2 therapy (if HER2 overexpressing or amplified), and chemotherapy are the measures most likely to be of value initially rather than operation. Mastectomy is indicated when chemotherapy and radiation have resulted in clinical remission with no evidence of distant metastases. In these cases, residual disease in the breast may be eradicated.

Breast Cancer Occurring During Pregnancy or Lactation

Breast cancer complicates up to 1 in 3000 pregnancies. The diagnosis is frequently delayed, because physiologic changes in the breast may obscure the lesion and screening mammography is not done in young or pregnant women. Data are insufficient to determine whether interruption of pregnancy improves the prognosis of patients who are identified to have potentially curable breast cancer and who receive definitive treatment during pregnancy. Theoretically, the high levels of estrogen produced by the placenta as the pregnancy progresses could be detrimental to the patient with occult metastases of hormone-sensitive breast cancer. The decision regarding whether or not to terminate the pregnancy must be made on an individual basis, taking into account the patient's clinical stage of the cancer and overall prognosis, the gestational age of the fetus, the potential for premature ovarian failure in the future with systemic therapy, and the patient's wishes.

It is important for primary care and reproductive specialists to aggressively work up any breast abnormality discovered in a pregnant woman. Pregnancy (or lactation) is not a contraindication to operation or treatment, and therapy should be based on the stage of the disease as in the nonpregnant (or nonlactating) woman. Women with early-stage gestational breast cancer who choose to continue their pregnancy should undergo surgery to remove the tumor and systemic therapy if indicated. Retrospective reviews of patients treated with anthracycline-containing regimens for gestational cancers (including leukemia and lymphomas) have established the relative safety of these regimens during pregnancy for both the patient and the fetus. Taxane-based and trastuzumab-based regimens have not been evaluated extensively, however. Radiation therapy should be delayed until after delivery. Overall survival rates have improved, since cancers are now diagnosed in pregnant women earlier than in the past and treatment has improved.

Bilateral Breast Cancer

Bilateral breast cancer occurs in less than 5% of cases, but there is as high as a 20%-25% incidence of later occurrence of cancer in the second breast. Bilaterality occurs more often in familial breast cancer, in women under age 50 years, and when the tumor in the primary breast is lobular. The incidence of second breast cancers increases directly with the length of time the patient is alive after her first cancer—about 1%-2% per year.

In patients with breast cancer, mammography should be performed before primary treatment and at regular intervals thereafter to search for occult cancer in the opposite breast or conserved ipsilateral breast.

Noninvasive Cancer

Noninvasive cancer can occur within the ducts (**DCIS**) or lobules (lobular carcinoma in situ [**LCIS**]). DCIS tends to be unilateral and most often progresses to invasive cancer if untreated. In approximately 40%-60% of women who have DCIS treated with biopsy alone, invasive cancer develops within the same breast. LCIS is generally agreed to be a marker of an increased risk of breast cancer rather than a direct precursor of breast cancer itself. The probability of breast cancer (DCIS or invasive in either breast) in a woman in whom LCIS has been diagnosed is estimated to be 1% per year. If LCIS is detected on core needle biopsy, an excisional biopsy without lymph node sampling should be performed to rule out DCIS or invasive cancer since these are found in

10%-20% of patients. The incidence of LCIS is rising, likely due to increased use of screening mammography. In addition, the rate of mastectomy after the diagnosis of LCIS is increasing despite the fact that mastectomy is only recommended in those patients who otherwise have an increased risk of breast cancer through family history, genetic mutation, or past exposure to thoracic radiation. Pleomorphic LCIS may behave more like DCIS and may be associated with invasive carcinoma. For this reason, pleomorphic LCIS should be surgically removed with clear margins.

The treatment of intraductal lesions is controversial. DCIS can be treated by wide excision with or without radiation therapy or with total mastectomy. Conservative management is advised in patients with small lesions amenable to lumpectomy. Patients in whom LCIS is diagnosed or who have received lumpectomy for DCIS may discuss chemoprevention (with hormonal blockade therapy) with their clinician, which is effective in reducing the risk of invasive breast cancer in DCIS that has been completely excised by breast-conserving surgery and in LCIS. Axillary metastases from in situ cancers should not occur unless there is an occult invasive cancer. Because one cannot perform a sentinel lymph node biopsy after mastectomy, one might consider performing a sentinel node biopsy in a patient undergoing mastectomy for DCIS in case an invasive component is discovered.

Adepoju L, et al: The evaluation of national time trends, quality of care, and factors affecting the use of minimally invasive breast biopsy and open biopsy for diagnosis of breast lesions. *Am J Surg.* 2014;208(3):382-390.

Case AS: Pregnancy-associated breast cancer. *Clin Obstet Gynecol.* 2016;59(4):779-788.

Colfry AJ 3rd: Miscellaneous syndromes and their management: occult breast cancer, breast cancer in pregnancy, male breast cancer, surgery in stage IV disease. *Surg Clin North Am.* 2013;93(2):519-531.

Genin AS, et al: Association with pregnancy increases the risk of local recurrence but does not impact overall survival in breast cancer: a case-control study of 87 cases. *Breast.* 2016;30:222-227.

Hartman EK, et al: The prognosis of women diagnosed with breast cancer before, during and after pregnancy: a meta-analysis. *Breast Cancer Res Treat.* 2016;160(2):347-360.

Portschy PR, et al: Trends in incidence and management of lobular carcinoma in situ: a population-based analysis. *Ann Surg Oncol.* 2013;20(10):3240-3246.

Robertson FM, et al: Inflammatory breast cancer: the disease, the biology, the treatment. *CA Cancer J Clin.* 2010;60(6):351-375.

Vapiwala N, et al: No impact of breast magnetic resonance imaging on 15-year outcomes in patients with ductal carcinoma in situ or early-stage invasive breast cancer managed with breast conservation therapy. *Cancer.* 2017;123(8):1324-1332.

Biomarkers & Gene Expression Profiling

Determining the **ER, PR,** and **HER2** status of the tumor at the time of diagnosis of early breast cancer and, if possible, at the time of recurrence is critical, both to gauge a patient's prognosis and to determine the best treatment regimen. In addition to ER status and PR status, the rate at which the tumor divides (assessed by an immunohistochemical stain for **Ki67**) and the grade and differentiation of the cells are also important prognostic factors. These markers may be obtained on core biopsy or surgical specimens, but not reliably on FNA cytology. Patients whose tumors are hormone receptor positive tend to have a more indolent disease course than those whose tumors are receptor negative. Moreover, treatment with an antihormonal agent is an essential component of therapy for hormone receptor–positive breast cancer at any stage. Although up to 60% of patients with metastatic breast cancer will respond to hormonal manipulation if their tumors are ER positive, less than 5% of patients with metastatic, ER-negative tumors will respond.

Another key element in determining treatment and prognosis is the amount of the *HER2* oncogene present in the cancer. HER2 overexpression (*HER2* oncogene–positive breast cancer) is generally more aggressive than breast cancer with normal HER2 expression (*HER2*-negative breast cancer). HER2 expression is measured by an immunohistochemical assay that is scored using a numerical system: 0 and 1+ are considered negative for overexpression, 2+ is borderline/indeterminate, and 3+ is overexpression. In the case of 2+ expression, fluorescence in situ hybridization (FISH) is recommended to more accurately assess *HER2* amplification. Guidelines for the interpretation of *HER2* results by immunohistochemistry and FISH are published by American Society of Clinical Oncology (ASCO)/College of American Pathologists. According to these guidelines, a tumor is positive for *HER2* amplification if dual-probe *HER2/CEP17* ratio is 2.0 or more and average HER2 copy number is at least 4.0. It is negative if dual-probe *HER2/CEP17* ratio is less than 2.0 and average HER2 copy number is less than 4.0. Additional workup is required for those with *HER2/CEP17* ratio at least 2.0 but average *HER2* copy number less than 4.0 and *HER2/CEP17* ratio less than 2.0 but average *HER2* copy number of 4.0 or greater. The presence of *HER2* amplification and overexpression is of prognostic significance and predicts the response to trastuzumab. Occasionally, a tumor has an indeterminate *HER2* result by both immunohistochemistry and FISH testing. The College of American Pathologists guidelines provide direction for further analysis in this situation. Individually, these biomarkers are predictive and thus provide insight to guide appropriate therapy. Moreover, when combined, they provide useful information regarding risk of recurrence and prognosis. In general, tumors that lack expression of HER2, ER, and PR ("**triple negative**") have a higher risk of early recurrence and metastases and are associated with a worse survival compared with other types. Neither endocrine therapy nor HER2-targeted agents are useful for this type of breast cancer, leaving chemotherapy as the only treatment option. In contrast, patients with early-stage, hormone receptor–positive breast cancer may not benefit from the addition of chemotherapy to hormonally targeted treatments.

Several molecular tests have been developed to assess risk of recurrence and to predict which patients are most likely to benefit from chemotherapy. **Oncotype DX** (Genomic Health) evaluates the expression of 21 genes relating to ER, HER2, and proliferation in a tumor specimen and categorizes a patient's risk of recurrence (recurrence score) as high, intermediate, or low risk. In addition to providing prognostic information, the test also has predictive value. For example, studies have shown that patients in the high-risk category are most likely to respond to chemotherapy. This test is primarily indicated for ER-positive, lymph node–negative tumors, but an ongoing study (RxPONDER; ClinicalTrials.gov identifier: NCT01272037) is addressing its predictive value in lymph node–positive, ER-positive breast cancer in a prospective manner. **MammaPrint** (Agendia) is an FDA-approved, 70-gene signature assay that is available for evaluating prognosis. This test classifies patients into good and poor prognostic groups to predict clinical outcome and may be used on patients with hormone receptor–positive or –negative breast cancer. ASCO guidelines indicate this assay may be best used to help determine whether chemotherapy may be safely withheld in patients with hormone receptor–negative, HER2-negative, node-positive breast cancer at high clinical risk. ASCO does not recommend using this assay in hormone receptor–negative or HER2-positive breast cancer. Several other assays are in development to better classify risk of relapse, including EndoPredict, PAM50, and Breast Cancer Index.

Barcenas CH, et al: Outcomes in patients with early-stage breast cancer who underwent a 21-gene expression assay. *Cancer.* 2017;123(13):2422-2431.

Cardoso F, et al; MINDACT Investigators: 70-Gene signature as an aid to treatment decisions in early-stage breast cancer. *N Engl J Med.* 2016;375(8):717-729.

Dowsett M, et al: Comparison of PAM50 risk of recurrence score with oncotype DX and IHC4 for predicting risk of distant recurrence after endocrine therapy. *J Clin Oncol.* 2013;31(22):2783-2790.

Dubsky P, et al; Austrian Breast and Colorectal Cancer Study Group (ABCSG): The EndoPredict score provides prognostic information on late distant metastases in ER+/HER2- breast cancer patients. *Br J Cancer.* 2013;109(12):2959-2964.

Esserman LJ, et al: Use of molecular tools to identify patients with indolent breast cancers with ultralow risk over 2 decades. *JAMA Oncol.* 2017;3(11):1503-1510.

Gluz O, et al: West German Study Group Phase III PlanB Trial: first prospective outcome data for the 21-gene recurrence score assay and concordance of prognostic markers by central and local pathology assessment. *J Clin Oncol.* 2016;34(20):2341-2349.

Ibraheem AF, et al: Community clinical practice patterns and mortality in patients with intermediate Oncotype DX recurrence scores: who benefits from chemotherapy. *Cancer.* 2019;125(2):213-222.

Krop I, et al: Use of biomarkers to guide decisions on adjuvant systemic therapy for women with early-stage invasive breast cancer: American Society of Clinical Oncology clinical practice guideline focused update. *J Clin Oncol.* 2017;35(24):2838-2847.

Mamounas EP, et al: 21-gene recurrence score and locore-gional recurrence in node-positive/ER-positive breast cancer treated with chemo-endocrine therapy. *J Natl Cancer Inst.* 2017;109(4):djw259.

Press MF, et al: Assessment of ERBB2/HER2 status in HER2-equiv-ocal breast cancers by FISH and 2013/2014 ASCO-CAP guide-lines. *JAMA Oncol.* 2019;5(3):366-375.

Press MF, et al: HER2 gene amplification testing by fluorescent in situ hybridization (FISH): comparison of the ASCO-College of American Pathologists Guidelines with FISH Scores used for enrollment in Breast Cancer International Research Group clini-cal trials. *J Clin Oncol.* 2016;34(29):3518-3528.

Sgroi DC, et al: Prediction of late distant recurrence in patients with oestrogen-receptor-positive breast cancer: a prospective compar-ison of the breast-cancer index (BCI) assay, 21-gene recurrence score, and IHC 4 in the TransATAC study population. *Lancet Oncol.* 2013;14(11):1067-1076.

Sparano JA, et al: Adjuvant chemotherapy guided by a 21-gene expression assay in breast cancer. *N Engl J Med.* 2018;379(2):111-121.

Sparano JA, et al: Prospective validation of a 21-gene expression assay in breast cancer. *N Engl J Med.* 2015;373(21):2005-2014.

Tsai M, et al: Association of 70-gene signature assay findings with physicians' treatment guidance for patients with early breast can-cer classified as intermediate risk by the 21-gene assay. *JAMA Oncol.* 2017;26:e173470.

Wolff AC, et al: Human epidermal growth factor receptor 2 testing in breast cancer: American Society of Clinical Oncology/College of American Pathologists Clinical Practice Guideline focused update. *Arch Pathol Lab Med.* 2018;142(11):1364-1382.

Curative Treatment

Not all breast cancer is systemic at the time of diagnosis, and a pessimistic attitude concerning the management of breast cancer is unwarranted. Most patients with early breast cancer can be cured. Treatment with a curative intent is advised for clinical stage I, II, and III disease. Patients with locally advanced (T3, T4) and even inflammatory tumors may be cured with multimodality therapy, but metastatic disease will be diagnosed in most patients, and at that point, palliation becomes the goal of therapy. Treatment with palliative intent is appropriate for all patients with stage IV disease and for patients with unresectable local cancers.

A. Choice and Timing of Primary Therapy

The extent of disease and its biologic aggressiveness are the principal determinants of the outcome of primary therapy. Clinical and pathologic staging help in assessing extent of disease, but each is to some extent imprecise. Other factors such as tumor grade, hormone receptor assays, and *HER2* oncogene amplification are of prognostic value and are key to determining systemic therapy but are not as relevant in determining the type of local therapy.

Controversy has surrounded the choice of primary ther-apy of stage I, II, and III breast carcinoma. Currently, the standard of care for stage I, stage II, and most stage III cancer

is surgical resection followed by adjuvant radiation or sys-temic therapy, or both, when indicated. Neoadjuvant therapy has become popular since large tumors may be shrunk by chemotherapy prior to surgery, making some patients who require mastectomy candidates for lumpectomy. It is impor-tant for patients to understand all of the surgical options, including reconstructive options, prior to having surgery. Patients with large primary tumors, inflammatory cancer, or palpably enlarged lymph nodes should have staging scans performed to rule out distant metastatic disease prior to definitive surgery. In general, adjuvant systemic therapy is started when the breast has adequately healed, ideally within 4-8 weeks after surgery. While no prospective studies have defined the appropriate timing of adjuvant chemotherapy, a single-institution study of over 6800 patients suggests that *systemic therapy should be started within 60 days of surgery,* especially in women with stage II or III breast cancer, triple-negative breast cancer, or HER2-positive disease.

B. Surgical Resection

1. Breast-conserving therapy—Multiple, large, random-ized studies including the Milan and National Surgical Adjuvant Breast and Bowel Project (NSABP) trials show that disease-free and overall survival rates are similar for patients with stage I and stage II breast cancer treated with partial mastectomy (breast-conserving lumpectomy or "breast conservation") plus axillary dissection followed by radiation therapy and for patients treated by modified radical mastectomy (total mastectomy plus axillary dissection).

Tumor size is a major consideration in determining the feasibility of breast conservation. The NSABP lumpectomy trial randomized patients with tumors as large as 4 cm. To achieve an acceptable cosmetic result, the patient must have a breast of sufficient size to enable excision of a 4-cm tumor without considerable deformity. Therefore, large tumor size is only a relative contraindication. Subareolar tumors, also difficult to excise without deformity, are not contraindica-tions to breast conservation. Clinically detectable multi-focality is a relative contraindication to breast-conserving surgery, as is fixation to the chest wall or skin or involve-ment of the nipple or overlying skin. The patient—not the surgeon—should be the judge of what is cosmetically accept-able. Given the relatively high risk of poor outcome after radiation, concomitant scleroderma is a contraindication to breast-conserving surgery. A history of prior therapeutic radiation to the ipsilateral breast or chest wall (or both) is also generally a contraindication for breast conservation.

Axillary dissection is primarily used to properly stage cancer and plan radiation and systemic therapy. Intraop-erative lymphatic mapping and sentinel node biopsy iden-tify lymph nodes most likely to harbor metastases if present (Figure 18–7). **Sentinel node biopsy** is a proven alternative to axillary dissection in patients without clinical evidence of axillary lymph node metastases. If sentinel node biopsy

▲ **Figure 18–7.** Sentinel node. (Used with permission from Armando E. Giuliano, MD.)

reveals no evidence of axillary metastases, it is highly likely that the remaining lymph nodes are free of disease and axillary dissection may be omitted. An important study from the American College of Surgeons Oncology Group randomized women with sentinel node metastases to undergo completion of axillary dissection or to receive no further axillary-specific treatment after lumpectomy; no difference in 10-year survival was found. *Omission of axillary dissection is acceptable for women with tumor-free sentinel nodes or those with involvement of one or two sentinel nodes who are treated with lumpectomy, whole breast irradiation, and adjuvant systemic therapy.*

Breast-conserving surgery with sentinel node biopsy and radiation is the preferred form of treatment for patients with early-stage breast cancer. Despite the numerous randomized trials showing no survival benefit of mastectomy over breast-conserving partial mastectomy with irradiation or of axillary dissection over sentinel node biopsy, these conservative procedures appear to be underutilized.

2. Mastectomy—Modified radical mastectomy was the standard therapy for most patients with early-stage breast cancer. This operation removes the entire breast, overlying skin, nipple, and areolar complex usually with underlying pectoralis fascia with the axillary lymph nodes in continuity. The major advantage of modified radical mastectomy is that radiation therapy may not be necessary, although radiation may be used when lymph nodes are involved with cancer or when the primary tumor is 5 cm or larger. The disadvantage of mastectomy is the cosmetic and psychological impact associated with breast loss. Radical mastectomy, which removes the underlying pectoralis muscle, should be performed rarely, if at all. Axillary node dissection is not indicated for noninvasive cancers because nodal metastases are rarely present. Skin-sparing and nipple-sparing mastectomy is available but is not appropriate for all patients. Breast reconstruction, immediate or delayed, should be discussed with patients who choose or require mastectomy. Patients should have an interview with a reconstructive plastic surgeon to discuss options prior to making a decision regarding reconstruction. Time is well spent preoperatively in educating the patient and family about these matters.

C. Radiotherapy

Radiotherapy after partial mastectomy consists of 5-7 weeks of five daily fractions to a total dose of 5000-6000 cGy. Most radiation oncologists use a boost dose to the cancer location. Shorter fractionation schedules may be reasonable for women over the age of 50 with early stage, lymph node–negative breast cancer. Accelerated partial breast irradiation, in which only the portion of the breast from which the tumor was resected is irradiated for 1-2 weeks, appears effective in achieving local control for selected patients; however, the prospective randomized NSABP B-39/Radiation Therapy Oncology Group (RTOG) 0413 trial failed to demonstrate noninferiority of partial breast irradiation compared to whole breast irradiation. With 4216 patients randomized and treated on this study, ipsilateral breast tumor recurrences at 10 years were slightly higher in the partial breast irradiation arm (4.8% vs 4.1%) and the 10-year relapse-free interval was significantly in favor of whole breast irradiation (93.4% vs 91.9%). Toxicity also tended to favor whole breast irradiation. In women over the age of 70 with small (< 2 cm), lymph node–negative, hormone receptor–positive cancers, radiation therapy may be avoided. The recurrence rates after intraoperative radiation, while low, appear significantly higher than postoperative whole breast radiation therapy. However, in all of these situations, a balanced discussion with a radiation oncologist to weigh the risks and benefits of each approach is warranted.

Current studies suggest that radiotherapy after mastectomy may improve recurrence rates and survival in younger patients and those with tumors 5 cm or larger or positive lymph nodes. The AMAROS study randomized women with sentinel node metastases to axillary lymph node dissection or nodal irradiation and found no significant difference in survival but lower lymphedema rates after radiation. An American College of Surgeons Oncology Group (ACOSOG) study (Z0010) and large NSABP trial (B-32) showed no adverse impact of micrometastases on survival and support no alteration in treatment when found. A Canadian trial (MA20) of postoperative nodal irradiation after lumpectomy and axillary dissection showed improved disease-free survival but not overall survival with nodal irradiation.

Donker M, et al: Radiotherapy or surgery of the axilla after a positive sentinel node in breast cancer (EORTC 10981-22023 AMAROS): a randomized, multi-centre, open-label, phase 3 non-inferiority trial. *Lancet Oncol.* 2014;15(12):1303-1310.

Giuliano AE, et al: Effect of axillary dissection vs no axillary dissection on 10-year overall survival among women with invasive breast cancer and sentinel node metastasis: The ACOSOG Z0011 (Alliance) Randomized Clinical Trial. *JAMA.* 2017;318(10):918-926.

Giuliano AE, et al: Locoregional recurrence after sentinel lymph node dissection with or without axillary dissection in patients with sentinel lymph node metastases: long-term follow-up from the American College of Surgeons Oncology Group (Alliance) ACOSOG Z0011 Randomized Trial. *Ann Surg.* 2016;264(3):413-420.

Grover S, et al: Survival after breast-conserving surgery with whole breast or partial breast irradiation in women with early stage breast cancer: a SEER data-base analysis. *Breast J.* 2017;23(3):292-298.

Hughes KS, et al: Lumpectomy plus tamoxifen with or without irradiation in women age 70 years or older with early breast cancer: long-term follow-up of CALGB 9343. *J Clin Oncol.* 2013;31(19):2382-2387.

Jagsi R, et al: Progress and controversies: radiation therapy for invasive breast cancer. *CA Cancer J Clin.* 2014;64(2):135-152.

Lyman GH, et al: Sentinel lymph node biopsy for patients with early-stage breast cancer: American Society of Clinical Oncology clinical practice guideline update. *J Clin Oncol.* 2017;35(5):561-564.

Poortmans PM, et al; EORTC Radiation Oncology and Breast Cancer Groups: Internal mammary and medial supraclavicular irradiation in breast cancer. *N Engl J Med.* 2015;373(4):317-327.

Whelan TJ et al; MA.20 Study Investigators: Regional nodal irradiation in early-stage breast cancer. *N Engl J Med.* 2015;373(4):307-316.

D. Adjuvant Systemic Therapy

The goal of systemic therapy, including hormone-modulating medications (endocrine therapy), cytotoxic chemotherapy, and HER2-targeted agents such as trastuzumab, is to kill cancer cells that have escaped the breast and axillary lymph nodes as *micro*metastases before they become *macro*metastases (ie, stage IV cancer). Systemic therapy improves survival and is advocated for most patients with curable breast cancer. In practice, most medical oncologists use adjuvant chemotherapy for patients with either node-positive or higher-risk (eg, hormone receptor–negative or HER2-positive) node-negative breast cancer and use endocrine therapy for all hormone receptor–positive invasive breast cancer unless contraindicated. Prognostic factors other than nodal status that are used to determine the patient's risks of recurrence are tumor size, ER and PR status, nuclear grade, histologic type, proliferative rate, oncogene expression (Table 18–4), and patient's age and menopausal status. In general, systemic chemotherapy decreases the chance of recurrence by about 30%, hormonal modulation decreases the relative risk of recurrence by 40%-50% (for hormone receptor–positive cancer), and HER2-targeted therapy decreases the relative risk of recurrence by approximately 40% (for HER2-positive cancer). Systemic chemotherapy is usually given sequentially, rather than concurrently with radiation. In terms of

Table 18–4. Prognostic factors in node-negative breast cancer.

Prognostic Factors	Increased Recurrence	Decreased Recurrence
Size	T3, T2	T1, T0
Hormone receptors (estrogen receptor, progesterone receptor)	Negative	Positive
Histologic grade	High	Low
S phase fraction	> 5%	< 5%
Lymphatic or vascular invasion	Present	Absent
HER2 oncogene amplification	High	Low
Epidermal growth factor receptor	High	Low
High Oncotype DX recurrence score or other genomic prognostic assays	High score	Low score

Reproduced with permission from Papadakis MA, McPhee SJ, Rabow MW: *Current Medical Diagnosis & Treatment* 2020. New York, NY: McGraw-Hill Education; 2020.

sequencing, typically chemotherapy is given before radiation and endocrine therapy is started concurrent with or after radiation therapy.

The long-term advantage of systemic therapy is well established. All patients with invasive hormone receptor–positive tumors should consider the use of hormone-modulating therapy. Most patients with HER2-positive tumors should receive trastuzumab-containing chemotherapy regimens. In general, adjuvant systemic chemotherapy should not be given to women who have small node-negative breast cancers with favorable histologic findings and tumor biomarkers. The ability to predict more accurately which patients with HER2-negative, hormone receptor–positive, lymph node–negative tumors should receive chemotherapy is improving with the advent of prognostic tools, such as Oncotype DX and MammaPrint (see previous section, Biomarkers and Gene Expression Profiling). In the MINDACT study, the 5-year distant metastasis–free survival improved by 1.5% in women with high clinical risk but low-risk gene expression as assessed by MammaPrint if they did *not* receive chemotherapy. In the TAILORx study, patients with an intermediate Oncotype DX recurrence score (11-25) were randomized to receive chemotherapy followed by endocrine therapy or endocrine therapy alone. This study demonstrated no significant benefit associated with adjuvant chemotherapy for patients with a recurrence score of less than 26, although some benefit was observed for women age 50 years or younger with a recurrence score of 16-25. These tests are thus validated tools to enable clinicians to better select patients who can safely omit chemotherapy.

1. Chemotherapy—The Early Breast Cancer Trialists' Collaborative Group (EBCTCG) meta-analysis involving over 28,000 women enrolled in 60 trials of adjuvant polychemotherapy versus no chemotherapy demonstrated a significant beneficial impact of chemotherapy on clinical outcome in non–stage IV breast cancer. This study showed that *adjuvant chemotherapy reduces the risk of recurrence and breast cancer–specific mortality in all women and also showed that women under the age of 50 derive the greatest benefit.*

A. ANTHRACYCLINE- AND CYCLOPHOSPHAMIDE-CONTAINING REGIMENS—On the basis of the superiority of anthracycline-containing regimens in metastatic breast cancer, both doxorubicin and epirubicin have been studied extensively in the adjuvant setting. Studies comparing Adriamycin (doxorubicin) and cyclophosphamide (AC) or epirubicin and cyclophosphamide (EC) to cyclophosphamide-methotrexate-fluorouracil (CMF) have shown that treatments with anthracycline-containing regimens are at least as effective as treatment with CMF. The EBCTCG analysis including over 14,000 patients enrolled in trials comparing anthracycline-based regimens to CMF showed a small but statistically significant improved disease-free and overall survival with the use of anthracycline-based regimens. It should be noted, however, that most of these studies included a mixed population of patients with HER2-positive and HER2-negative breast cancer and were performed before the introduction of trastuzumab. Retrospective analyses of a number of these studies suggest that anthracyclines may be primarily effective in tumors with HER2 overexpression or alteration in the expression of topoisomerase IIa (the target of anthracyclines and close to the *HER2* gene). Given this, for HER2-negative, node-negative breast cancer, four cycles of AC or six cycles of CMF are probably equally effective.

B. TAXANES—When taxanes (paclitaxel and docetaxel) emerged in the 1990s, multiple trials were conducted to evaluate their use in combination with anthracycline-based regimens. The majority of these trials showed an improvement in disease-free survival, and at least one showed an improvement in overall survival with the taxane-based regimen. A meta-analysis of taxane versus nontaxane anthracycline-based regimen trials showed an improvement in disease-free and overall survival for the taxane-based regimens. Several regimens have been reported, including AC followed by paclitaxel (AC-P) or docetaxel (Taxotere) (AC-T), docetaxel concurrent with AC (TAC), fluorouracil-epirubicine-cyclophosphamide (FEC)-docetaxel, and FEC-paclitaxel.

The US Oncology 9735 trial compared four cycles of AC with four cycles of docetaxel (Taxotere) and cyclophosphamide (TC). With a median of 7 years of follow-up, this study showed a statistically significantly improved disease-free survival and overall survival in the patients who received TC. Until this trial, no trial had compared a nonanthracycline, taxane-based regimen to an anthracycline-based regimen.

Subsequently, substudy results from the phase III MIND-ACT trial were presented in which 1301 patients with operable tumors were randomized 1:1 to standard anthracycline/cyclophosphamide-based therapy (with taxane in the 30% of patients with node-positive disease) or docetaxel plus capecitabine (DC). The 5-year disease-free survival was similar for the anthracycline arm (88.8%) and DC arm (90.7%) ($P = 0.263$), and 5-year overall survival was also similar (96.2% anthracycline vs 96.3% DC, $P = 0.722$).

The three Anthracyclines in Early Breast Cancer (ABC) (USOR 06-090, NSABP B-46, and NSABP B-49) trials (total N = 4242) each compared the TC regimen to anthracycline/taxane-based chemotherapy regimens (TaxAC) in HER2-negative early-stage breast cancer. An interim joint analysis showed that the invasive disease-free survival at 4 years was improved by 2.5% with the addition of an anthracycline ($P = 0.04$) but that the benefit of an anthracycline was primarily seen in triple-negative disease (HR, 1.42; 95% CI, 1.04-1.94). No survival difference was observed at the time of interim reporting. In contrast, the West German Study Group phase III PlanB study compared six cycles of adjuvant TC to four cycles of EC followed by four cycles of docetaxel (EC-D) in 2449 patients with intermediate- to high-risk, HER2-negative breast cancer. Dose reductions were higher in the anthracycline arm (19.7% vs 6.6%, $P < 0.001$), and grade ¾ toxicities were consistently and significantly higher in the anthracycline arm. TC demonstrated noninferiority to EC-D, with a 5-year disease-free survival of 90% for each arm (HR TC vs EC-D = 0.996; 95% CI, 0.77-1.29). In contrast to the ABC study, subset analysis indicated a similar disease-free survival in each treatment arm regardless of recurrence score, nodal status, Ki67 reactivity, grade, or triple-negative subtype. A Danish phase III study was conducted to compare six cycles of TC to six cycles of EC-D in 2012 high-risk patients with *TOP2A* normal breast cancer. The 5-year disease-free survival was 87.9% for EC-D versus 88.3% for DC (HR, 1.00; $P = 1.00$). Although it is generally agreed that *taxanes should be used for most patients receiving chemotherapy for early breast cancer, data relating to the benefits of anthracyclines are conflicting;* thus, a balanced discussion regarding the potential risks versus benefits of the addition of anthracyclines is warranted.

C. DURATION AND DOSE OF CHEMOTHERAPY—The ideal duration of adjuvant chemotherapy still remains uncertain. However, based on the meta-analysis performed in the Oxford Overview (EBCTCG), the current recommendation is for 3-6 months of the commonly used regimens. Data suggest that the timing and sequencing of anthracycline/taxane-based chemotherapy may be important. Multiple trials beginning in the 1980s sought to demonstrate whether dose-intensification of adjuvant chemotherapy, by shortening the intervals between cycles ("dose-dense") or by giving chemotherapy at full dose sequentially rather than concurrently at reduced doses, is associated with better outcomes.

The EBCTCG meta-analysis included 37,298 patients treated on 26 trials and showed a significant 3.4% absolute decrease and 14% relative risk reduction in breast cancer recurrences with dose-intensification. Moreover, the absolute 10-year breast cancer mortality was improved by 2.4%. While impressive, the benefit of dose-intensification appeared to be strongest in node-positive disease. Its benefit, if any, in HER2-positive disease in the era of HER2-targeted therapy has not been validated. Additionally, the use of dose-intensification in (nonanthracycline) taxane-based regimens has not been evaluated.

D. Chemotherapy side effects—Chemotherapy side effects are generally well controlled. Nausea and vomiting are abated with medications that directly affect the central nervous system, such as ondansetron and granisetron. Infertility and premature ovarian failure are common side effects of chemotherapy and should be discussed with patients prior to starting treatment. The risk of life-threatening neutropenia associated with chemotherapy can be reduced by use of growth factors such as pegfilgrastim and filgrastim (granulocyte colony-stimulating factor), which stimulate proliferation and differentiation of hematopoietic cells. Long-term toxicities from chemotherapy, including cardiomyopathy (anthracyclines), peripheral neuropathy (taxanes), and leukemia/myelodysplasia (anthracyclines and alkylating agents), remain a small but significant risk.

2. Targeted therapy—Targeted therapy refers to agents that are directed specifically against a protein or molecule expressed uniquely on tumor cells or in the tumor microenvironment.

A. HER2 overexpression—Approximately 20% of breast cancers are characterized by amplification of the *HER2* oncogene, leading to overexpression of the HER2 oncoprotein. The poor prognosis associated with HER2 overexpression has been drastically improved with the development of HER2-targeted therapy. Trastuzumab (Herceptin [H]), a monoclonal antibody that binds to HER2, is effective in combination with chemotherapy in patients with HER2-overexpressing metastatic and early breast cancer. In the adjuvant setting, the first and most commonly studied chemotherapy backbone used with trastuzumab is AC-T. Subsequently, the BCIRG006 study showed similar efficacy for AC-TH and a non–anthracycline-containing regimen, TCH (docetaxel, carboplatin, trastuzumab). Both were significantly better than AC-T in terms of disease-free and overall survival, and TCH had a lower risk of cardiac and bone marrow (leukemia/myelodysplasia) toxicity. Both AC-TH and TCH are FDA approved for nonmetastatic, HER2-positive breast cancer. In these regimens, trastuzumab is given with chemotherapy and then continues beyond the course of chemotherapy with a goal, in general, to complete a full year. Seven comparative trials (HERA, FinHER, SOLD,

ShortHER, PHARE, Hellenic Oncology study, and PERSE-PHONE) have evaluated the ideal length (2 years, 1 year, 6 months, or 9 weeks) of adjuvant trastuzumab. All but one of these studies confirmed that 1 year is the ideal length of trastuzumab, although the PERSEPHONE study presented at the ASCO 2018 annual meeting demonstrated noninferiority of 6 months of trastuzumab compared to 12 months, indicating that for selected patients with lower-risk disease, a shorter duration of trastuzumab may be adequate. At least one study (N9831) suggests that concurrent, rather than sequential, delivery of trastuzumab with chemotherapy may be more beneficial. Neoadjuvant chemotherapy plus dual *HER2*-targeted therapy with trastuzumab and pertuzumab (also a HER2-targeted monoclonal antibody that prevents dimerization of HER2 with HER3 and has been shown to be synergistic in combination with trastuzumab) is a standard-of-care option available to patients with stage II/III HER2-positive breast cancer (see Neoadjuvant Therapy). The phase III, randomized, placebo-controlled, adjuvant APHINITY study, reported in 2017, evaluated 1 year of adjuvant pertuzumab in combination with trastuzumab and showed a small but statistically significant reduction in recurrence of disease with pertuzumab (7.1% vs 8.7%; HR, 0.81; $P = 0.045$). The improved disease-free survival is most pronounced in patients with node-positive disease. Neratinib, an orally bioavailable dual HER1 (EGFR) and HER2 tyrosine kinase inhibitor, is FDA approved as adjuvant therapy. The phase III placebo-controlled EXTENET study demonstrated that neratinib improves invasive disease-free survival when given for 1 year after completion of a year of standard adjuvant trastuzumab-based therapy (median follow-up, 5.2 years; stratified HR, 0.73; 95% CI, 0.57-0.92, $P = 0.0083$). Neratinib is associated with gastrointestinal toxicity, most notably moderate to severe diarrhea in approximately 40% of patients who did not use antidiarrheal prophylaxis. Measures to mitigate this side effect are being evaluated in the CONTROL clinical trial (ClinicalTrials.gov identifier: NCT02400476). Pending those final results, patients should be treated with upfront prophylaxis with loperamide.

Patients who undergo neoadjuvant trastuzumab-based chemotherapy and have residual disease remaining at the time of surgery have a comparatively poor outcome compared to those who achieve a pathologic complete response. In the phase III randomized KATHERINE trial, 1486 patients with residual disease after standard neoadjuvant trastuzumab/taxane-based therapy (18% of whom also received neoadjuvant pertuzumab) were randomized to receive the antibody-drug conjugate trastuzumab emtansine or standard trastuzumab for 14 cycles after surgery. Patients treated with trastuzumab emtansine had a statistically significantly improved 3-year invasive disease-free survival (88% vs 77%), associated with a 50% relative risk reduction. These data may lead to the FDA approval of trastuzumab emtansine in the adjuvant setting.

Retrospective studies have shown that even small (stage T1a,b) *HER2*-positive tumors have a worse prognosis compared with same-sized *HER2*-negative tumors and may thus be appropriate for trastuzumab-based regimens. The NSABP B43 study is ongoing to evaluate whether the addition of trastuzumab to radiation therapy is warranted for DCIS.

Cardiomyopathy develops in a small but significant percentage (0.4%-4%) of patients who receive trastuzumab-based regimens. For this reason, anthracyclines and trastuzumab are rarely given concurrently, and cardiac function is monitored periodically throughout therapy.

B. Endocrine therapy—Adjuvant hormone modulation therapy is highly effective in decreasing relative risk of recurrence by 40%-50% and mortality by 25% in women with hormone receptor–positive tumors regardless of menopausal status.

(1) Tamoxifen—The traditional regimen had been 5 years of the ER antagonist/agonist tamoxifen until the 2012 reporting of the Adjuvant Tamoxifen Longer Against Shorter (ATLAS) trial in which 5 versus 10 years of adjuvant tamoxifen were compared. In this study, disease-free and overall survival were significantly improved in women who received 10 years of tamoxifen, particularly after year 10. The Adjuvant Tamoxifen (aTTom) study confirmed these results. Although these results are impressive, the clinical application of long-term tamoxifen use must be discussed with patients individually, taking into consideration risks of tamoxifen (eg, secondary uterine cancers, venous thromboembolic events, and side effects that impact quality of life). Ovarian suppression in addition to tamoxifen was shown to significantly improve 8-year disease-free survival (83.2% vs 78.9%) and 8-year overall survival (93.3% vs 91.5%) compared to tamoxifen alone in the randomized Suppression of Ovarian Function Trial [SOFT], although the benefits appeared to be seen primarily in chemotherapy-treated patients with higher-risk disease.

(2) Aromatase inhibitors—AIs, including anastrozole, letrozole, and exemestane, reduce estrogen production and are also effective in the adjuvant setting for postmenopausal women. AIs should not be used in a patient with functioning (premenopausal) ovaries since *they do not block ovarian production of estrogen*. At least seven large randomized trials enrolling more than 24,000 postmenopausal patients with hormone receptor–positive nonmetastatic breast cancer have compared the use of AIs with tamoxifen or placebo as adjuvant therapy. All of these studies have shown small but statistically significant improvements in disease-free survival (absolute benefits of 2%-6%) with the use of AIs. In addition, AIs have been shown to reduce the risk of contralateral breast cancers and to have fewer associated serious side effects (eg, endometrial cancers and thromboembolic events) than tamoxifen. However, they are associated with accelerated bone loss and an increased risk of fractures as well as

a musculoskeletal syndrome characterized by arthralgias or myalgias (or both) in the majority of patients. ASCO and the NCCN have recommended that *postmenopausal* women with hormone receptor–positive breast cancer be offered an AI either initially or after tamoxifen therapy. HER2 status should not affect the use or choice of hormone therapy. Until recently, the use of AIs was restricted to postmenopausal women whose ovaries were not producing estrogen. A combined analysis of the SOFT and Tamoxifen and Exemestane Trial (TEXT) studies showed for the first time that exemestane plus ovarian suppression with triptorelin was associated with a reduced risk of relapse compared to tamoxifen, making this a viable adjuvant therapy option for *premenopausal* women with high-risk ER-positive breast cancers.

3. Bisphosphonates—Multiple randomized studies have evaluated the use of adjuvant bisphosphonates in addition to standard local and systemic therapy for early-stage breast cancer and have shown, in addition to improvement in bone density, a consistent reduction in the risk of metastatic recurrence in postmenopausal patients. A meta-analysis evaluating more than 18,000 women with early-stage breast cancer treated with bisphosphonates or placebo showed that bisphosphonates reduce the risk of cancer recurrence (especially in bone) and improve breast cancer–specific survival primarily in postmenopausal women. Side effects associated with bisphosphonate therapy include bone pain, fever, osteonecrosis of the jaw (rare, < 1%), esophagitis or ulcers (for oral bisphosphonates), and kidney injury. Although the FDA has not yet approved the adjuvant use of bisphosphonates to reduce the risk of breast cancer recurrence, the 2017 jointly published guidelines of Cancer Care Ontario and ASCO recommend that bisphosphonate use (zoledronic acid or clodronate) be considered in the adjuvant therapy plan for postmenopausal breast cancer patients. In addition, denosumab (another bone-stabilizing medication), which is an antibody directed against receptor activator of nuclear factor-kappa B ligand (RANK-L), was evaluated in the phase III adjuvant D-CARE study, in which patients with early-stage breast cancer (all biologic subtypes) were randomized to receive denosumab or placebo. This study, reported by ASCO in 2018, failed to demonstrate a reduction in breast cancer recurrences or deaths with RANK inhibition. It is speculated that one possible reason for this negative result may be due to the fact that premenopausal patients (who do not have a demonstrated metastatic recurrence benefit from bisphosphonates) were included in the study.

4. Adjuvant therapy in older women—Data relating to the optimal use of adjuvant systemic treatment for women over the age of 65 are limited. Results from the EBCTCG overview indicate that although adjuvant chemotherapy yields a smaller benefit for older women compared with younger women, it still improves clinical outcomes. Moreover, individual studies do show that older women with higher-risk disease derive benefits from chemotherapy. One study compared the use of oral chemotherapy (capecitabine) to standard chemotherapy in older women and concluded that standard chemotherapy is preferred. Another study (USO TC vs AC) showed that women over the age of 65 derive similar benefits from the taxane-based regimen as women who are younger. The benefits of endocrine therapy for hormone receptor–positive disease appear to be independent of age. In general, decisions relating to the use of systemic therapy should take into account a patient's comorbidities and physiologic age, more so than chronologic age.

E. Neoadjuvant Therapy

The use of systemic therapy prior to resection of the primary tumor (neoadjuvant) is a standard option that in many cases should be discussed with patients prior to surgery. This enables the assessment of in vivo sensitivity of the tumor to the selected systemic therapy. Patients with hormone receptor–negative, triple-negative, or HER2-positive breast cancer are more likely to have a pathologic complete response (meaning no residual invasive cancer at the time of surgery) to neoadjuvant chemotherapy than those with hormone receptor–positive breast cancer. A complete pathologic response at the time of surgery, especially in hormone receptor–negative tumors, is associated with improvement in event-free and overall survival. Neoadjuvant chemotherapy also increases the chance of breast conservation by shrinking the primary tumor in women who would otherwise need mastectomy for local control. Survival after neoadjuvant chemotherapy is similar to that seen with postoperative adjuvant chemotherapy.

1. HER2-positive breast cancer—Dual targeting of HER2 with two monoclonal antibodies, trastuzumab and pertuzumab, showed positive results in two clinical trials in the neoadjuvant setting, the TRYPHAENA and the NEOSPHERE studies. TRYPHAENA was a phase II, open-label study in which 225 patients with operable HER2-positive breast cancer were randomly assigned to six neoadjuvant cycles every 3 weeks of either fluorouracil, epirubicin, and cyclophosphamide (FEC) plus trastuzumab (H) and pertuzumab (P) for three cycles followed by docetaxel (T) plus HP for three cycles (arm A) or FEC for three cycles followed by THP for three cycles (arm B) or TCHP for six cycles (arm C). Pathologic complete response (in breast and lymph nodes) was seen in 50.7% of patients in arm A, 45.3% in arm B, and 51.9% in arm C. Symptomatic left ventricular systolic dysfunction developed in two patients in this study, both in arm B. Declines in left ventricular ejection fraction of 10% or more from baseline to less than 50% were observed in four patients in arm A (5.6%), four patients in arm B (5.3%), and three patients in arm C (3.9%).

The NEOSPHERE study randomly assigned 417 patients with HER2-positive breast cancer to four cycles of trastuzumab (H) plus docetaxel (T) (group A), pertuzumab (P) plus TH (group B), PH (group C), or PT (group D). Pathologic complete response in the breast and lymph nodes was seen in 21.5% of patients in group A, 39.3% in group B, 11.2% in group C, and 17.7% in group D. In 2013, given the results of these two studies, the FDA granted accelerated approval for neoadjuvant pertuzumab. This is the first medication to receive regulatory approval in the neoadjuvant setting for breast cancer.

Based on these clinical trials, three regimens are FDA approved in the HER2-positive neoadjuvant setting: docetaxel, cyclophosphamide, trastuzumab, and pertuzumab (TCHP) for six cycles; FEC for three cycles followed by docetaxel, trastuzumab, and pertuzumab (THP) for three cycles; or THP for four cycles (followed by three cycles of postoperative FEC). After completing surgery, patients should resume trastuzumab to complete a full year. Dual HER2-targeted therapy without standard cytotoxic chemotherapy has been evaluated in the neoadjuvant setting as well. The phase III KRISTINE study evaluated the antibody-medication conjugate trastuzumab emtansine (T-DM1, Kadcyla) in combination with pertuzumab (T-DM1/P) compared to standard TCHP treatment. Although the T-DM1/P arm was well tolerated and yielded a pathologic complete response in 44% of patients, TCHP performed significantly better, with a pathologic complete response rate of 56%. Thus, the use of T-DM1 in the neoadjuvant setting outside of a clinical trial is not recommended.

2. Hormone receptor–positive, HER2-negative breast cancer—Patients with hormone receptor–positive breast cancer have a lower chance of achieving a pathologic complete response with neoadjuvant therapy than patients with triple-negative or HER2-positive breast cancers. Studies indicate similar response rates with neoadjuvant endocrine therapy compared to neoadjuvant chemotherapy. Typically, responses are not appreciated unless 4-6 or more months of therapy are given. Outside of the clinical trial setting, the use of neoadjuvant hormonal therapy is generally restricted to postmenopausal patients who are unable or unwilling to tolerate chemotherapy.

3. Triple-negative breast cancer—No targeted therapy has been identified for patients with breast cancer that is lacking in HER2 amplification or hormone receptor expression. Neoadjuvant chemotherapy leads to pathologic complete response in up to 40%-50% of patients with triple-negative breast cancer. Patients who achieve a pathologic complete response seem to have a similar prognosis to other breast cancer subtypes with pathologic complete response. However, patients with residual disease at the time of surgery have a poor prognosis. Based on the theory that triple-negative breast cancers may be more vulnerable to DNA-damaging agents, several studies have evaluated whether the addition of platinum salts to a neoadjuvant chemotherapy regimen is beneficial in this disease subtype, several of which have shown improved outcomes (pathologic complete response and disease-free survival) with platinum use. A randomized phase II trial (GeparSixto) randomly assigned 595 patients with triple-negative or HER2-positive breast cancer to weekly paclitaxel plus weekly liposomal doxorubicin (18 weeks) alone or with weekly carboplatin. Patients with triple-negative disease also received bevacizumab. Patients with triple-negative disease who received carboplatin had a pathologic complete response rate of 53.2% compared to those who did not receive carboplatin (36.9%; $P = 0.005$). The 3-year disease-free survival data were presented in 2015; the addition of carboplatin improved disease-free survival from 76.1% to 85.8% (HR, 0.56; 95% CI, 0.33-0.96; $P = 0.0350$). Similarly designed phase II studies including the Cancer and Leukemia Group B (CALGB) 40603 trial and the Adjuvant Dynamic Marker-Adjusted Personalized Therapy (ADAPT) triple-negative trial showed improved pathologic complete response rates with platinum-based neoadjuvant therapy. Other studies are ongoing to evaluate the pathologic complete response rates and long-term outcomes associated with incorporating platinums into standard chemotherapy regimens.

4. Timing of sentinel lymph node biopsy in neoadjuvant setting—There is considerable concern about the timing of sentinel lymph node biopsy, since the chemotherapy may affect cancer present in the lymph nodes. Several studies have shown that sentinel node biopsy can be done after neoadjuvant therapy. However, a large multicenter study, ACOSOG 1071, demonstrated a false-negative rate of 10.7%, well above the false-negative rate outside the neoadjuvant setting (< 1%-5%). If three nodes are removed and isotope and dye are used, the false-negative rate falls to an acceptable level. Some physicians recommend performing sentinel lymph node biopsy before administering the chemotherapy in order to avoid a false-negative result and to aid in planning subsequent radiation therapy. Others prefer to perform sentinel lymph node biopsy after neoadjuvant therapy to avoid a second operation and assess postchemotherapy nodal status. If a complete dissection is desired, this can be performed at the time of the definitive breast surgery. The SENTINA trial showed similarly poor results for sentinel node biopsy after neoadjuvant therapy. No study has evaluated the survival impact of no axillary treatment for node-positive patients who become node negative after neoadjuvant therapy. Important questions remain to be answered involving the use of neoadjuvant therapy, including which neoadjuvant agents to use, duration of treatment, and additional postoperative therapy.

Boughey JC, et al: Sentinel lymph node surgery after neoadjuvant chemotherapy in patients with node-positive breast cancer: the ACOSOG Z1071 (Alliance) clinical trial. *JAMA.* 2013;310(14):1455-1461.

Early Breast Cancer Trialists' Collaborative Group (EBCTCG): Long-term outcomes for neoadjuvant versus adjuvant chemotherapy in early breast cancer: meta-analysis of individual patient data from ten randomised trials. *Lancet Oncol.* 2018;19(1):27-39.

Kuehn T, et al: Sentinel-lymph-node biopsy in patients with breast cancer before and after neoadjuvant chemotherapy (SENTINA): a prospective, multicentre cohort study. *Lancet Oncol.* 2013;14(7):609-618.

Kümmel S, et al: Surgical treatment of primary breast cancer in the neoadjuvant setting. *Br J Surg.* 2014;101(8):912-924.

▶ Palliative Treatment

Palliative treatments are aimed to manage symptoms, improve quality of life, and even prolong survival, without the expectation of achieving cure. In the United States, it is uncommon to have distant metastases at the time of diagnosis (de novo metastases). However, most patients who have a breast cancer recurrence after initial local and adjuvant therapy have metastatic rather than local (in breast) disease. Breast cancer most commonly metastasizes to the liver, lungs, and bone, causing symptoms such as fatigue, change in appetite, abdominal pain, cough, dyspnea, or bone pain. Headaches, imbalance, vision changes, vertigo, and other neurologic symptoms may be signs of brain metastases. Triple-negative (ER-, PR-, and HER2-negative) and HER2-positive tumors have a higher rate of brain metastases than hormone receptor–positive, HER2-negative tumors.

A. Radiotherapy and Bisphosphonates

Palliative radiotherapy may be advised for primary treatment of locally advanced cancers with distant metastases to control ulceration, pain, and other manifestations in the breast and regional nodes. Irradiation of the breast and chest wall and the axillary, internal mammary, and supraclavicular nodes should be undertaken in an attempt to cure locally advanced and inoperable lesions when there is no evidence of distant metastases. A small number of patients in this group are cured despite extensive breast and regional node involvement.

Palliative irradiation is of value also in the treatment of certain bone or soft tissue metastases to control pain or avoid fracture. Radiotherapy is especially useful in the treatment of isolated bony metastases, chest wall recurrences, and brain metastases, and, sometimes, in lieu of the preferred option of orthopedic surgery for acute spinal cord compression.

In addition to radiotherapy, bisphosphonate therapy has shown excellent results in delaying and reducing skeletal events in women with bony metastases. Pamidronate and zoledronic acid are FDA-approved intravenous bisphosphonates given for bone metastases or hypercalcemia of malignancy from breast cancer. Denosumab, a fully human monoclonal antibody that targets RANK ligand, is FDA approved for the treatment of bone metastases from breast cancer, with data showing that it reduced the time to first skeletal-related event (eg, pathologic fracture) compared to zoledronic acid.

Caution should be exercised when combining radiation therapy with chemotherapy because toxicity of either or both may be augmented by their concurrent administration. In general, only one type of therapy should be given at a time unless it is necessary to irradiate a destructive lesion of weight-bearing bone while the patient is receiving chemotherapy. Systemic therapy should be changed only if the disease is clearly progressing. This is especially difficult to determine for patients with destructive bone metastases, since changes in the status of these lesions are difficult to determine radiographically.

B. Targeted Therapy

1. Hormonally based therapy for metastatic disease—The first targeted therapy for cancer was the use of antiestrogen therapy in hormone receptor–positive breast cancer. The following therapies have all been shown to be effective in hormone receptor–positive metastatic breast cancer: administration of medications that block or downregulate ERs (eg, tamoxifen or fulvestrant, respectively) or medications that block the synthesis of hormones (such as AIs); ablation of the ovaries, adrenals, or pituitary; and the administration of hormones (eg, estrogens, androgens, progestins); see Table 18–5. Because only 5%-10% of women with ER-negative tumors respond, they should not receive endocrine therapy. The rate of response is nearly equal in premenopausal and

postmenopausal women with ER-positive tumors. A favorable response to hormonal manipulation occurs in about one-third of patients with metastatic breast cancer. Of those whose tumors contain ER, the response is about 60% and perhaps as high as 80% for patients whose tumors contain PR as well. Women within 1 year of their last menstrual period are arbitrarily considered to be premenopausal and should have surgical (bilateral oophorectomy) or chemical ovarian ablation (using a gonadotropin-releasing hormone [GnRH] analog such as leuprolide [Lupron], goserelin [Zoladex], or tritorelin). Premenopausal women who have had chemical or surgical ovarian ablation are then eligible to receive the same hormonally targeted therapies that are available to postmenopausal women. Current guidelines indicate that sequential hormonal therapy is the preferred treatment for hormone receptor–positive metastatic breast cancer except in the rare case when disease is immediately threatening visceral organs.

A. First-line treatment options

(1) Hormonally targeted agents—Single-agent hormonally targeted therapy options include fulvestrant (500 mg intramuscularly on days 1 and 15, then every month), tamoxifen (20 mg orally daily), or an AI (anastrozole, letrozole, or exemestane). The average time to progression associated with single-agent first-line tamoxifen is 5-8 months, and with AI,

Table 18–5. Hormonal agents commonly used for management of metastatic breast cancer (listed in alphabetical order).

Medications	Action	Dose, Route, Frequency	Major Side Effects
Anastrozole (Arimidex)	AI	1 mg orally daily	Hot flushes, skin rashes, nausea and vomiting, bone loss
Exemestane (Aromasin)	AI	25 mg orally daily	Hot flushes, increased arthralgia/arthritis, myalgia, bone loss
Fulvestrant (Faslodex)	Steroidal estrogen receptor antagonist	500 mg intramuscularly days 1, 15, 29 and then monthly	Gastrointestinal upset, headache, back pain, hot flushes, pharyngitis, injection site pain
Goserelin (Zoladex)	Synthetic luteinizing hormone–releasing hormone analog	3.6 mg subcutaneously monthly	Arthralgias, blood pressure changes, hot flushes, headaches, vaginal dryness, bone loss
Letrozole (Femara)	AI	2.5 mg orally daily	Hot flushes, arthralgia/arthritis, myalgia, bone loss
Leuprolide (Lupron)	Synthetic luteinizing hormone–releasing hormone analog	3.75 or 7.5 mg subcutaneously monthly	Arthralgias, blood pressure changes, hot flushes, headaches, vaginal dryness, bone loss
Megestrol acetate (Megace)	Progestin	40 mg orally four times daily	Fluid retention; venous thromboembolic events; rarely used except in very late stage, treatment-refractory disease
Tamoxifen citrate (Nolvadex)	SERM	20 mg orally daily	Hot flushes, uterine bleeding, thrombophlebitis, rash
Toremifene citrate (Fareston)	SERM	60 mg orally daily	Hot flushes, sweating, nausea, vaginal discharge, dry eyes, dizziness

AI, aromatase inhibitor; SERM, selective estrogen receptor modulator.
Reproduced with permission from Papadakis MA, McPhee SJ, Rabow MW: *Current Medical Diagnosis & Treatment* 2020. New York, NY: McGraw-Hill Education; 2020.

it is approximately 8-12 months. The side effect profile of AIs differs from tamoxifen. The main side effects of tamoxifen are nausea, skin rash, and hot flushes. Rarely, tamoxifen induces hypercalcemia in patients with bony metastases. Tamoxifen also increases the risk of venous thromboembolic events and uterine hyperplasia and cancer. The main side effects of AIs include hot flushes, vaginal dryness, and joint stiffness; however, osteoporosis and bone fractures are significantly higher than with tamoxifen. Results from the phase III FALCON study (comparing first-line treatment with the pure estrogen antagonist fulvestrant to anastrozole) confirmed that the use of first-line fulvestrant improves progression-free survival by almost 3 months (HR, 0.79; 95% CI, 0.637-0.999; P = 0.0486) with the largest treatment effect observed in patients without visceral disease. Overall survival data are needed. The combination of fulvestrant plus anastrozole may also be more effective than anastrozole alone, although two studies evaluating this question have yielded conflicting results.

(2) Hormonally targeted therapy plus cyclin-dependent kinase inhibition—Hormonally driven breast cancer may be particularly sensitive to inhibition of cell cycle regulatory proteins, called cyclin-dependent kinases (CDK). A phase II randomized study evaluating letrozole with or without an oral CDK 4/6 inhibitor (palbociclib) for the first-line treatment of postmenopausal women with hormone receptor–positive advanced breast cancer demonstrated a striking and highly significant doubling of progression-free survival with palbociclib compared to the control arm. A phase III, randomized, placebo-controlled study (PALOMA-2) of letrozole plus an oral CDK4/6 inhibitor (palbociclib) for the first-line treatment of postmenopausal women with hormone receptor–positive advanced breast cancer demonstrated a striking and highly significant 10-month improvement in progression-free survival associated with the use of palbociclib. Two additional CDK4/6 inhibitors, ribociclib and abemaciclib, were also evaluated in placebo-controlled phase III trials (MONALEESA-2 and MONARCH-3, respectively) in the same disease setting and demonstrated a similar improvement in progression-free survival when added to an AI. These three studies all demonstrated a median progression-free survival of over 2 years, which is the longest median progression-free survival reported in metastatic ER-positive breast cancer to date, leading many to consider the use of a **CDK4/6 inhibitor plus AI the gold standard treatment in the first-line setting**. Importantly, these therapies yield objective response rates as good as or better than those seen with chemotherapy. All three agents are FDA approved in the first-line setting in combination with an AI. Overall survival results are not yet mature. Similar progression-free survival benefits were achieved with ribociclib in younger women in the phase III randomized trial (MONALEESA-7) that exclusively enrolled premenopausal women (treated with goserelin to suppress ovarian function in combination

with endocrine therapy). In general, CDK4/6 inhibitors are well tolerated, although monitoring patients for grade 3/4 neutropenia (especially with ribociclib and palbociclib) and management of diarrhea (especially with abemaciclib) are necessary. Febrile neutropenia and infections are rare, and use of growth factors is not required; however, palbociclib and ribociclib are given for 3 consecutive weeks, stopping for 1 week to allow white cell count to recover. Abemaciclib is given twice daily continuously (28-day cycles).

B. TREATMENT OPTIONS WHEN DISEASE PROGRESSES AFTER HORMONAL-BASED THERAPY

(1) Secondary or tertiary hormonal therapy—Patients who have disease progression following first-line hormonal therapy may be offered a different form of endocrine therapy. For example, if a patient has been treated with an AI as first-line therapy, fulvestrant or tamoxifen should be considered at the time of disease progression as second-line therapy. Androgens (eg, testosterone) have many toxicities and should be used infrequently. Neither hypophysectomy nor adrenalectomy should be performed. Estrogen therapy has also paradoxically been shown to induce responses in advanced breast cancer. A study that evaluated the use of low-dose (6 mg) versus high-dose (30 mg) estradiol daily orally for postmenopausal women with metastatic AI-resistant breast cancer showed that the two doses yielded similar clinical benefit rates (29% and 28%, respectively), and as expected, the higher dose was associated with more adverse events than the low dose.

(2) Fulvestrant plus CDK4/6 inhibitor—All three CDK4/6 inhibitors have also been evaluated in phase III trials (PALOMA-3, MONALEESA-3, MONARCH-2) in patients whose disease has progressed on prior endocrine therapy, and all have shown a significant improvement in median progression-free survival with the addition of CDK4/6 inhibitor to fulvestrant compared to placebo plus fulvestrant. Palbociclib (125 mg orally daily) and abemaciclib (150 mg orally twice daily) are both FDA approved in combination with fulvestrant for this indication. Abemaciclib is also FDA approved as a single agent (200 mg orally twice daily) for patients with advanced ER-positive breast cancer who have received prior endocrine therapy and chemotherapy. It should be noted that there is no evidence to date that use of a CDK4/6 inhibitor benefits patients whose disease has progressed despite therapy with a CDK4/6 inhibitor. Thus, at this time, use of any CDK4/6 inhibitor after disease progression on a CDK4/6 inhibitor is not appropriate outside of a clinical trial.

(3) Everolimus plus endocrine therapy—Everolimus (Afinitor) is an oral inhibitor of the mammalian target of rapamycin (MTOR)—a protein whose activation has been associated with the development of endocrine resistance. A phase III, placebo-controlled trial (BOLERO-2) evaluated the AI exemestane

with or without everolimus in 724 patients with AI-resistant, hormone receptor–positive metastatic breast cancer and found that patients treated with everolimus had a significantly improved progression-free survival (7.8 months vs 3.2 months; HR, 0.45; 95% CI, 0.38-0.54; $P < 0.0001$) but no significant difference in overall survival. Everolimus has also been evaluated in combination with fulvestrant and shown to have similar improvements in progression-free survival compared to single-agent fulvestrant. The main side effect of everolimus is stomatitis (mouth sores). This can be avoided, almost completely, by the prophylactic use of oral steroid mouthwash starting with cycle 1.

(4) Phosphatidylinositol-3-kinase (PI3K) inhibitors plus endocrine therapy—Approximately 40% of hormone receptor–positive breast cancers have activation of the PI3K-AKT-mTOR pathway, most commonly due to an activating mutation of PI3K on the *PIK3CA* gene. Taselisib and alpelisib are both oral alpha-isoform selective inhibitors of PI3K with clinical activity in *PIK3CA*-mutated breast cancer. Both were evaluated in randomized phase III clinical trials (fulvestrant with or without a PI3K inhibitor) in patients with hormone receptor–positive breast cancer who had been previously treated with an AI. In SANDPIPER, presented at the ASCO meeting in 2018, the addition of taselisib to fulvestrant was associated with a 2-month improvement (7.4 vs 5.4 months) in *PIK3CA*-mutant tumors. The SOLAR-1 study presented at the European Society of Medical Oncology meeting in 2018 demonstrated over a 5-month improvement in median progression-free survival (11.0 vs 5.7 months) associated with the addition of alpelisib to fulvestrant in patients with tumor *PIK3CA* mutations. Benefits with these PI3K inhibitors were not observed in wild-type tumors. Side effects of PI3K inhibitors include hyperglycemia, diarrhea, rash, and transaminitis.

2. HER2-targeted agents—For patients with HER2-positive tumors, trastuzumab plus chemotherapy significantly improves clinical outcomes, including survival compared to chemotherapy alone. **Pertuzumab** is an FDA-approved monoclonal antibody that targets the extracellular domain of HER2 at a different epitope than targeted by trastuzumab and inhibits receptor dimerization. A phase III placebo-controlled randomized study (CLEOPATRA) showed that patients treated with the combination of pertuzumab, trastuzumab, and docetaxel had a significantly longer progression-free survival (18.5 vs 12.4 months; HR, 0.62; 95% CI, 0.51-0.75; $P < 0.001$) compared with patients treated with docetaxel and trastuzumab. Longer follow-up revealed a significant overall survival benefit associated with pertuzumab as well.

Lapatinib, an oral targeted medication that inhibits the intracellular tyrosine kinases of the epidermal growth factor and HER2 receptors, is FDA approved for the treatment of trastuzumab-resistant HER2-positive metastatic breast cancer in combination with capecitabine, thus, a completely oral regimen. The combination of trastuzumab plus lapatinib has been shown to be more effective than lapatinib alone for trastuzumab-resistant metastatic breast cancer. Moreover, several trials have shown a significant clinical benefit for continuing HER2-targeted agents beyond progression. T-DM1 ado-trastuzumab emtansine (Kadcyla) is an FDA-approved novel antibody-drug conjugate in which trastuzumab is stably linked to a derivative of maytansine, enabling targeted delivery of the cytotoxic chemotherapy to HER2-overexpressing cells. T-DM1 is associated with an improved progression-free and overall survival compared to lapatinib plus capecitabine in patients with HER2-positive, trastuzumab-pretreated, advanced disease (EMILIA). T-DM1 with or without pertuzumab was compared to trastuzumab plus a taxane for the first-line treatment of HER2-positive advanced breast cancer in the phase III MARIANNE study. This study showed that the two ado-trastuzumab–containing arms were noninferior (but not superior) to the trastuzumab plus taxane arm. Thus, for the time being, ado-trastuzumab is primarily used in the second-line setting and beyond. Several other medications targeting HER2 and its associated signaling pathways are in development, including neratinib, tucatinib (ONT-380), trastuzumab deruxtecan (DS-8201), margetuximab, pyrotinib, and HER2-targeted vaccines.

3. Targeting triple-negative breast cancer—Breast cancers lacking expression of the hormone receptors ER, PR, and HER2 behave more aggressively and have traditionally been amenable only to therapy with cytotoxic chemotherapy, although emerging clinical trial data may lead to approval of new agents for this type of cancer. A phase II placebo-controlled randomized trial (LOTUS) demonstrated a significantly improved progression-free survival (6.2 vs 4.9 months; stratified HR, 0.60; $P = 0.037$) by adding the oral AKT inhibitor ipatasertib to first-line paclitaxel. These results need to be confirmed in a larger phase III study but are the first promising results of an AKT inhibitor for triple-negative breast cancer. Early-phase clinical trials showed promise for immune checkpoint inhibitors (eg, monoclonal antibodies that target PDL-1 or PD-1). Results from the first phase III randomized trial of immune therapy for triple-negative metastatic breast cancer (IMPASSION) were presented and published in 2018 and demonstrated that the anti-PD-L1 antibody atezolizumab added to nab-paclitaxel significantly improved the median progression-free survival in the intent-to-treat population (7.2 vs 5.5 months) and in the population with PD-L1–positive tumors (7.5 vs 5.0 months) compared to nab-paclitaxel plus placebo. While median overall survival was not significantly improved in the intent-to-treat population, there was almost a 10-month improvement in overall survival in patients with PD-L1–positive tumors (25.0 vs 15.5 months). **These are the first results to demonstrate effectiveness of immune modulation therapy in breast cancer and will likely prove to be practice changing.**

Another therapy garnering attention for triple-negative disease is sacituzumab govitecan, an antibody-drug conjugate that delivers SN-38 (active metabolite of the chemotherapy irinotecan) to Trop-2–overexpressing breast cancer cells. This antibody-drug conjugate has demonstrated significant clinical activity in heavily pretreated triple-negative breast cancer, leading to its priority review designation by the FDA. An ongoing phase III trial, ASCENT, is underway.

4. Targeting PARP in *BRCA1/2* mutation–associated breast cancer—Poly (adenosine diphosphate-ribose) polymerase (PARP) is an enzyme important in single-strand DNA repair. Patients who carry germline mutations in *BRCA1* or *BRCA2* have tumors with deficient double-strand DNA repair mechanisms. Experts have theorized that inhibiting PARP selectively kills *BRCA1/2*-mutated cancers. A phase III clinical trial (OlympiAD) that compared olaparib (an oral PARP inhibitor) to treatment of physician's choice (single-agent chemotherapy) demonstrated a significantly improved progression-free survival (7.0 vs 4.2 months; HR, 0.58; $P < 0.001$), an improved response rate, and a lower rate of adverse events than standard therapy. Talazoparib, a second PARP inhibitor, has also been shown to improve outcomes similarly in the phase III EMBRACA study. Other studies of PARP inhibitors are ongoing for this indication. Both olaparib and talazoparib are FDA approved for *BRCA*-mutated metastatic breast cancer as single agents.

C. Palliative Chemotherapy

Cytotoxic medications should be considered for the treatment of metastatic breast cancer (1) if life- or organ-threatening visceral metastases are present (especially brain, liver, or lymphangitic pulmonary), (2) if hormonal treatment is unsuccessful or the disease has progressed after an initial response to hormonal manipulation (for hormone receptor–positive breast cancer), or (3) if the tumor is ER negative or HER2 positive. Prior adjuvant chemotherapy does not seem to alter response rates in patients who relapse. A number of chemotherapy medications (including vinorelbine, paclitaxel, docetaxel, gemcitabine, ixabepilone, carboplatin, cisplatin, capecitabine, albumin-bound paclitaxel, eribulin, and liposomal doxorubicin) may be used as single agents with first-line objective response rates ranging from 30% to 50%.

Combination chemotherapy yields statistically significantly higher response rates and progression-free survival rates but has not been conclusively shown to improve overall survival rates compared with sequential single-agent therapy. Combinations that have been tested in phase III studies and have proven efficacy compared with single-agent therapy include capecitabine/docetaxel, gemcitabine/paclitaxel, and capecitabine/ixabepilone. Various other combinations of medications have been tested in phase II studies, and a number of clinical trials are ongoing to identify effective combinations. Patients should be encouraged to participate in clinical trials

given the number of promising targeted therapies in development. It is generally appropriate to treat willing patients with multiple sequential lines of therapy as long as they tolerate the treatment and as long as their performance status is good (eg, at least ambulatory and able to care for self, up out of bed more than 50% of waking hours).

Amiri-Kordestani L, et al: First FDA approval of neoadjuvant therapy for breast cancer: pertuzumab for the treatment of patients with *HER2*-positive breast cancer. *Clin Cancer Res.* 2014;20(21):5359-5364.

Bardia A: Efficacy and safety of anti-Trop 2 antibody drug conjugate sacituzumab govitecan (IMMU-132) in heavily pretreated patients with metastatic triple negative breast cancer. *J Clin Oncol.* 2017;35(19):2141-2148.

Baselga J, et al; CLEOPATRA Study Group: Pertuzumab plus trastuzumab plus docetaxel for metastatic breast cancer. *N Engl J Med.* 2012;366(2):109-119.

Blum JL, et al: Anthracyclines in early breast cancer: the ABC Trials-USOR 06-090, NSABP B-46-I/USOR 07132, and NSABP B-49 (NRG Oncology). *J Clin Oncol.* 2017;35(23):2647-2655.

Cameron D, et al; Herceptin Adjuvant (HERA) Trial Study Team: 11 years' follow-up of trastuzumab after adjuvant chemotherapy in HER2-positive early breast cancer: final analysis of the HERceptin Adjuvant (HERA) trial. *Lancet.* 2017;389(10075):1195-2205.

Cardoso F, et al; MINDACT Investigators: 70-gene signature as an aid to treatment decisions in early-stage breast cancer. *N Engl J Med.* 2016;375(8):717-729.

Cardoso F, et al: Standard anthracycline-based vs. docetaxel-capecitabine in early breast cancer: results from the chemotherapy randomization (R-C) of EORTC 10041/BIG 3-04 MINDACT phase III trial. *J Clin Oncol.* 2017;35(suppl):abstr 516.

Chavez-MacGregor M, et al: Delayed initiation of adjuvant chemotherapy among patients with breast cancer. *JAMA Oncol.* 2016;2(3):322-329.

Cortazar P, et al: Pathological complete response and long-term clinical benefit in breast cancer: the CTNeoBC pooled analysis. *Lancet.* 2014;384(9938):164-172.

Dhesy-Thind S, et al: Use of adjuvant bisphosphonates and other bone-modifying agents in breast cancer: a Cancer Care Ontario and American Society of Clinical Oncology clinical practice guideline. *J Clin Oncol.* 2017;35(18):2062-2081.

Doi T, et al: Safety, pharmacokinetics, and antitumour activity of trastuzumab deruxtecan (DS-8201), a HER2-targeting antibody-drug conjugate, in patients with advanced breast and gastric or gastro-oesophageal tumours: a phase 1 dose-escalation study. *Lancet Oncol.* 2017;18(11):1512-1522.

Early Breast Cancer Trialists' Collaborative Group: Adjuvant bisphosphonate treatment in early breast cancer: meta-analyses of individual patient data from randomized trials. *Lancet.* 2015;386(10001):1353-1361.

Diéras V, et al: Trastuzumab emtansine versus capecitabine plus lapatinib in patients with previously treated HER2-positive advanced breast cancer (EMILIA): a descriptive analysis of final overall survival results from a randomised, open-label, phase 3 trial. *Lancet Oncol.* 2017;18(6):732-742.

Early Breast Cancer Trialists' Collaborative Group (EBCTCG). Long-term outcomes for neoadjuvant versus adjuvant chemotherapy in early breast cancer: meta-analysis of individual patient data from ten randomised trials. *Lancet Oncol.* 2018;19(1):27-39.

Ejlertsen B, et al: Adjuvant cyclophosphamide and docetaxel with or without epirubicin for early TOP2A-normal breast cancer: DBCG 07-READ, an open-label, phase III, randomized trial. *J Clin Oncol.* 2017;35(23):2639-2646.

Ellis MJ, et al: Fulvestrant 500 mg versus anastrozole 1 mg for the first-line treatment of advanced breast cancer: overall survival analysis from the phase II FIRST study. *J Clin Oncol.* 2015;33(32):3781-3787.

Finn RS, et al: Palbociclib and letrozole in advanced breast cancer. *N Engl J Med.* 2016;375(20):1925-1936.

Finn RS, et al: The cyclin-dependent kinase 4/6 inhibitor palbociclib in combination with letrozole versus letrozole alone as first-line treatment of oestrogen receptor-positive, HER2-negative, advanced breast cancer (PALOMA-1/TRIO-18): a randomised phase 2 study. *Lancet Oncol.* 2015;16(1):25-35.

Francis PA, et al; SOFT and TEXT Investigators and the International Breast Cancer Study Group: Tailoring adjuvant endocrine therapy for premenopausal breast cancer. *N Engl J Med.* 2018;379(2):122-137.

Gagliato Dde M, et al: Clinical impact of delaying initiation of adjuvant chemotherapy in patients with breast cancer. *J Clin Oncol.* 2014;32(8):735-744.

Gluz O, et al: Comparison of neoadjuvant nab-paclitaxel+carboplatin vs nab-paclitaxel+gemcitabine in triple-negative breast cancer: randomized WSG-ADAPT-TN trial results. *J Natl Cancer Inst.* 2018;110(6):628-637.

Goetz MP, et al: MONARCH 3: abemaciclib as initial therapy for advanced breast cancer. *J Clin Oncol.* 2017;35(32):3638-3646.

Harbeck N, et al: De-escalation strategies in human epidermal growth factor receptor 2 (HER2)-positive early breast cancer (BC): final analysis of the West German Study Group Adjuvant Dynamic Marker-Adjusted Personalized Therapy trial optimizing risk assessment and therapy response prediction in early BC HER2- and hormone receptor-positive phase II randomized trial-efficacy, safety, and predictive markers for 12 weeks of neoadjuvant trastuzumab emtansine with or without endocrine therapy (ET) versus trastuzumab plus ET. *J Clin Oncol.* 2017;35(26):3046-3054.

Harbeck N, et al: Prospective WSG phase III PlanB trial: final analysis of adjuvant 4xEC→4x doc vs. 6x docetaxel/cyclophosphamide in patients with high clinical risk and intermediate-to-high genomic risk HER2-negative, early breast cancer. *J Clin Oncol.* 2017;35(suppl):abstr 504.

Hortobagyi GN, et al: Ribociclib as first-line therapy for HR-positive, advanced breast cancer. *N Engl J Med.* 2016;375(18):1738-1748.

Hurvitz SA, et al: Neoadjuvant trastuzumab, pertuzumab, and chemotherapy versus trastuzumab emtansine plus pertuzumab in patients with HER2-positive breast cancer (KRISTINE): a randomised, open-label, multicentre, phase 3 trial. *Lancet Oncol.* 2018;19(1):115-126.

Kim SB, et al; LOTUS Investigators: Ipatasertib plus paclitaxel versus placebo plus paclitaxel as first-line therapy for metastatic triple-negative breast cancer (LOTUS): a multicentre, randomised, double-blind, placebo-controlled, phase 2 trial. *Lancet Oncol.* 2017;18(10):1360-1372.

Litton J, et al: Talazoparib in patients with advanced breast cancer and a germline BRCA mutation. *N Engl J Med.* 2018;379(8):753-763.

Ma F, et al: Phase I study and biomarker analysis of pyrotinib, a novel irreversible pan-ErbB receptor tyrosine kinase inhibitor, in patients with human epidermal growth factor receptor 2-positive metastatic breast cancer. *J Clin Oncol.* 2017;35(27):3105-3112.

Martin M, et al; ExteNET Study Group: Neratinib after trastuzumab-based adjuvant therapy in HER2-positive breast cancer (ExteNET): 5-year analysis of a randomised, double-blind, placebo-controlled, phase 3 trial. *Lancet Oncol.* 2017;18(12):1688-1700.

Moore HC, et al; POEMS/S0230 Investigators: Goserelin for ovarian protection during breast cancer adjuvant chemotherapy. *N Engl J Med.* 2015;372(10):923-932.

National Comprehensive Cancer Network: NCCN guidelines: breast cancer. http://www.nccn.org/professionals/physician_gls/f_guidelines.asp

Perez EA, et al: Sequential versus concurrent trastuzumab in adjuvant chemotherapy for breast cancer. *J Clin Oncol.* 2011;29(34):4491-4497.

Perez EA, et al: Trastuzumab emtansine with or without pertuzumab versus trastuzumab plus taxane for human epidermal growth factor receptor 2-positive, advanced breast cancer: primary results from the phase III MARIANNE Study. *J Clin Oncol.* 2017;35(2):141-148.

Perez EA, et al: Trastuzumab plus adjuvant chemotherapy for human epidermal growth factor receptor 2-positive breast cancer: planned joint analysis of overall survival from NSABP B-31 and NCCTG N9831. *J Clin Oncol.* 2014;32(33):3744-3752.

Pivot X, et al; PHARE Trial Investigators: 6 months versus 12 months of adjuvant trastuzumab for patients with HER2-positive early breast cancer (PHARE): a randomised phase 3 trial. *Lancet Oncol.* 2013;14(8):741-748.

Robertson JF, et al: Fulvestrant 500 mg versus anastrozole 1 mg for hormone receptor-positive advanced breast cancer (FALCON): an international, randomised, double-blind, phase 3 trial. *Lancet.* 2016;388(10063):2997-3005.

Robson M, et al: Olaparib for metastatic breast cancer in patients with a germline BRCA mutation. *N Engl J Med.* 2017;377(6):523-533. Erratum in: *N Engl J Med.* 2017;377(17):1700.

Rugo HS, et al: Prevention of everolimus-related stomatitis in women with hormone receptor-positive, HER2-negative metastatic breast cancer using dexamethasone mouthwash (SWISH): a single-arm, phase 2 trial. *Lancet Oncol.* 2017;18(5):654-662.

Rugo HS, et al: Endocrine therapy for hormone receptor-positive metastatic breast cancer: American Society of Clinical Oncology guideline. *J Clin Oncol.* 2016;34(25):3069-3103.

Schmid P, et al: Atezolizumab and nab-paclitaxel in advanced triple negative breast cancer. *N Engl J Med.* 2018;379(22):2108-2121.

Schneeweiss A, et al: Pertuzumab plus trastuzumab in combination with standard neoadjuvant anthracycline-containing and anthracycline-free chemotherapy regimens in patients with HER2-positive early breast cancer: a randomized phase II cardiac safety study (TRYPHAENA). *Ann Oncol.* 2013;24(9):2278-2284.

Sikov WM, et al: Impact of the addition of carboplatin and/or bevacizumab to neoadjuvant once-per-week paclitaxel followed by dose-dense doxorubicin and cyclophosphamide on pathologic complete response rates in stage II to III triple-negative breast cancer: CALGB 40603 (Alliance). *J Clin Oncol.* 2015;33(1):13-21.

Slamon D, et al; Breast Cancer International Research Group: Adjuvant trastuzumab in HER2-positive breast cancer. *N Engl J Med.* 2011;365(14):1273-1283.

Sledge GW Jr, et al: MONARCH 2: abemaciclib in combination with fulvestrant in women with HR+/HER2- advanced breast cancer who had progressed while receiving endocrine therapy. *J Clin Oncol.* 2017;35(25):2875-2884.

Tolaney SM, et al: Adjuvant paclitaxel and trastuzumab for node-negative, HER2-positive breast cancer. *N Engl J Med.* 2015;372(2):134-141. Erratum in: *N Engl J Med.* 2015;373(20):1989.

Tripathy D, et al: Ribociclib plus endocrine therapy for premenopausal women with hormone-receptor-positive advanced breast cancer (MONALEESA-7): a randomised phase 3 trial. *Lancet Oncol.* 2018;19(7):904-915.

Turner NC, et al; PALOMA3 Study Group: Palbociclib in hormone-receptor-positive advanced breast cancer. *N Engl J Med.* 2015;373(3):209-219.

Urruticoechea A, et al: Randomized phase III trial of trastuzumab plus capecitabine with or without pertuzumab in patients with human epidermal growth factor receptor 2-positive metastatic breast cancer who experienced disease progression during or after trastuzumab-based therapy. *J Clin Oncol.* 2017;35(26):3030-3038.

von Minckwitz G, et al; APHINITY Steering Committee and Investigators: Adjuvant pertuzumab and trastuzumab in early HER2-positive breast cancer. *N Engl J Med.* 2017;377(2):122-131. Erratum in: *N Engl J Med.* 2017;377(7):702.

von Minckwitz G, et al; KATHERINE Investigators: Trastuzumab emtansine for residual invasive HER2-positive breast cancer. *N Engl J Med.* 2019;380(7):617-628.

von Minckwitz G, et al: Neoadjuvant carboplatin in patients with triple-negative and *HER2*-positive early breast cancer (GeparSixto; GBG 66): a randomised phase 2 trial. *Lancet Oncol.* 2014;15(7):747-756.

▶ Prognosis

Stage of breast cancer is the most reliable indicator of prognosis (Table 18–6). Axillary lymph node status is the best-analyzed prognostic factor and correlates with survival at all tumor sizes. When cancer is localized to the breast with no evidence of regional spread after pathologic examination, the clinical cure rate with most accepted methods of therapy is 75% to more than 90%. In fact, patients with small mammographically detected, biologically favorable tumors and no evidence of axillary spread have a 5-year survival rate greater than 95%. When the axillary lymph nodes are involved with tumor, the survival rate drops to 50%-70% at 5 years and probably around 25%-40% at 10 years. The use of biologic markers, such as ER, PR, grade, and HER2, helps identify high-risk tumor types as well as direct treatment used (see Biomarkers & Gene Expression Profiling). Gene analysis studies can predict disease-free survival for some subsets of patients. The American Joint Committee on Cancer Cancer Staging Manual (8th edition) has incorporated these factors into staging.

Five-year statistics do not accurately reflect the final outcome of therapy. The mortality rate of breast cancer patients exceeds that of age-matched normal controls for nearly 20 years. Thereafter, the mortality rates are equal, although deaths that occur among breast cancer patients are often directly the result of tumor.

In general, breast cancer appears to be somewhat more aggressive and associated with worse outcomes in younger than in older women, and this may be related to the fact that fewer younger women have ER-positive tumors. Disparities in treatment outcome for different racial and ethnic backgrounds have been reported by several studies. These differences appear to be not only due to different socioeconomic factors (and a resulting difference in access to healthcare) but also due to differences in the subtype of breast cancer diagnosed.

For patients whose disease progresses despite treatment, some studies suggest supportive group therapy may improve survival. As they approach the end of life, such patients will require meticulous palliative care (see Chapter 5).

Table 18–6. Approximate survival of patients with breast cancer by TNM stage.

TNM Stage	5 Years	10 Years
0	95%	90%
I	85%	70%
IIA	70%	50%
IIB	60%	40%
IIIA	55%	30%
IIIB	30%	20%
IV	5%-10%	2%
All	65%	30%

TNM, tumor, node, metastasis.
Reproduced with permission from Papadakis MA, McPhee SJ, Rabow MW: *Current Medical Diagnosis & Treatment* 2020. New York, NY: McGraw-Hill Education; 2020.

DeSantis CE, et al: Breast cancer statistics, 2017, racial disparity in mortality by state. *CA Cancer J Clin.* 2017;67(6):439-448.

Giuliano AE, et al: Eighth edition of the AJCC Cancer Staging Manual: Breast Cancer. *Ann Surg Oncol.* 2018;25(7):1783-1785.

Manson JE, et al: Menopausal hormone therapy and health outcomes during the intervention and extended poststopping phases of the Women's Health Initiative randomized trials. *JAMA.* 2013;310(13):1353-1368.

Miller JW, et al: Disparities in breast cancer survival in the United States (2001-2009): findings from the CONCORD-2 study. *Cancer.* 2017;(123 Suppl 24):5100-5118.

Miller KD, et al: Cancer statistics for hispanics/latinos, 2018. *CA Cancer J Clin.* 2018;68(6):425-445.

Pan H, et al; EBCTCG: 20-year risks of breast-cancer recurrence after stopping endocrine therapy at 5 years. *N Engl J Med.* 2017;377(19):1836-1846.

Parmeshwar R, et al: Patient surveillance after initial breast cancer therapy: variation by physician specialty. *Am J Surg.* 2013;206(2):218-222.

▶ Follow-Up Care

After primary therapy, patients with breast cancer should be monitored long term in order to detect recurrences and to observe the opposite breast for a second primary carcinoma. Local and distant recurrences occur most frequently within the first 2-5 years. During the first 2 years, most patients should be examined every 6 months, then annually thereafter. Special attention is paid to the contralateral breast because a new primary breast malignancy will develop in 20%-25% of patients. In some cases, especially in hormone receptor–positive breast cancer, metastases are dormant for long periods and may appear 15 years or longer after removal of the primary tumor. Although studies have failed to show an adverse effect of hormonal replacement in disease-free patients, it is rarely used after breast cancer treatment, particularly if the tumor was hormone receptor positive. Even pregnancy has not been associated with shortened survival of patients rendered disease free—yet many oncologists are reluctant to advise a young patient with breast cancer that it is safe to become pregnant. The use of estrogen replacement for conditions such as osteoporosis, vaginal dryness, and hot flushes may be considered for a woman with a history of breast cancer after discussion of the benefits and risks; however, it is not routinely recommended, especially given the availability of nonhormonal agents for these conditions (eg, bisphosphonates and denosumab for osteoporosis). Topical vaginal estrogen is frequently used to treat vaginal atrophy with no obvious ill effects.

A. Local Recurrence

The incidence of local recurrence correlates with tumor size, the presence and number of involved axillary nodes, the histologic type of tumor, the presence of skin edema or skin and fascia fixation with the primary tumor, and the type of definitive surgery and local irradiation. Local recurrence on the chest wall after total mastectomy and axillary dissection develops in as many as 8% of patients. When the axillary nodes are not involved, the local recurrence rate is less than 5%, but the rate is as high as 25% when they are heavily involved. A similar difference in local recurrence rate was noted between small and large tumors. Factors such as multifocal cancer, in situ tumors, lymphovascular invasion, positive resection margins, chemotherapy, and radiotherapy have an effect on local recurrence in patients treated with breast-conserving surgery. Adjuvant systemic therapy greatly decreases the rate of local recurrence.

Chest wall recurrences usually appear within the first several years but may occur as late as 15 or more years after mastectomy. All suspicious nodules and skin lesions should be biopsied. Local excision or localized radiotherapy may be feasible if an isolated nodule is present. If lesions are multiple or accompanied by evidence of regional involvement in the internal mammary or supraclavicular nodes, the disease is best managed by radiation treatment of the entire chest wall including the parasternal, supraclavicular, and axillary areas as well as systemic therapy.

Local recurrence after mastectomy usually signals the presence of widespread disease and is an indication for studies to search for metastases. Distant metastases will develop within a few years in most patients with locally recurrent tumor after mastectomy. When there is no evidence of metastases beyond the chest wall and regional nodes, irradiation for cure after complete local excision should be attempted. After partial mastectomy, local recurrence does not have as serious a prognostic significance as after mastectomy. However, patients in whom a recurrence develops have a worse prognosis than those who do not have recurrence. It is speculated that the ability of a cancer to recur locally after radiotherapy is a sign of aggressiveness and resistance to therapy. Completion of the mastectomy should be done for local recurrence after partial mastectomy; some of these patients will survive for prolonged periods, especially if the breast recurrence is DCIS or occurs more than 5 years after initial treatment. Systemic chemotherapy or hormonal treatment should be used for women in whom disseminated disease develops or those in whom local recurrence occurs.

B. Breast Cancer Survivorship Issues

Given that most women with nonmetastatic breast cancer will be cured, a significant number of women face survivorship issues stemming from either the diagnosis or the treatment of the breast cancer, or both. These challenges include psychological struggles, upper extremity lymphedema, weight management problems, cardiovascular issues, bone loss, postmenopausal side effects, and fatigue. One randomized study reported that survivors who received psychological intervention from the time of diagnosis had a lower risk of recurrence and breast cancer–related mortality. A randomized study in older, overweight cancer survivors showed that diet and exercise reduced the rate of self-reported functional decline compared with no intervention. Cognitive dysfunction (also called "chemo brain") is a commonly reported symptom experienced by women who have undergone systemic treatment for early breast cancer. An interesting study reported that 200 mg of modafinil daily improved speed and quality of memory as well as attention for breast cancer survivors dealing with cognitive dysfunction. This promising study requires validation in a larger clinical trial.

1. Edema of the arm—Significant edema of the arm occurs in about 10%-30% of patients after axillary dissection with or without mastectomy. It occurs more commonly in obese women, in women who had radiotherapy, and in women who had postoperative infection. Partial mastectomy with radiation to the axillary lymph nodes is followed by chronic edema of the arm in 10%-20% of patients. Sentinel lymph node dissection has proved to be an accurate form of axillary staging without the side effects of edema or infection.

Judicious use of radiotherapy, with treatment fields carefully planned to spare the axilla as much as possible, can greatly diminish the incidence of edema, which will occur in only 5% of patients if no radiotherapy is given to the axilla after a partial mastectomy and lymph node dissection.

Late or secondary edema of the arm may develop years after treatment, as a result of axillary recurrence or infection in the hand or arm, with obliteration of lymphatic channels. When edema develops, a careful examination of the axilla for recurrence or infection is performed. Infection in the arm or hand on the dissected side should be treated with antibiotics, rest, and elevation. If there is no sign of recurrence or infection, the swollen extremity should be treated with rest and elevation. A mild diuretic may be helpful. If there is no improvement, a compressor pump or manual compression decreases the swelling, and the patient is then fitted with an elastic glove or sleeve. Most patients are not bothered enough by mild edema to wear an uncomfortable glove or sleeve and will treat themselves with elevation or manual compression alone. Benzo-pyrones have been reported to decrease lymphedema but are not approved for this use in the United States. Rarely, edema may be severe enough to interfere with use of the limb. A prospective randomized study has shown that twice-weekly progressive weight lifting improves lymphedema symptoms and exacerbations and improves extremity strength.

2. Breast reconstruction—Breast reconstruction is usually feasible after total or modified radical mastectomy. Reconstruction should be discussed with patients prior to mastectomy, because it offers an important psychological focal point for recovery. Reconstruction is not an obstacle to the diagnosis of recurrent cancer. The most common breast reconstruction has been implantation of a silicone gel or saline prosthesis in the subpectoral plane between the pectoralis minor and pectoralis major muscles. Alternatively, autologous tissue can be used for reconstruction.

Autologous tissue flaps have the advantage of not feeling like a foreign body to the patient. The most popular autologous technique currently is reconstruction using abdominal tissue flaps. This includes the deep inferior epigastric perforator (**DIEP**) flap and the more traditional transrectus abdominis muscle (**TRAM**) flap. The free TRAM flap is done by completely removing a small portion of the rectus with overlying fat and skin and using microvascular surgical techniques to reconstruct the vascular supply on the chest wall. A latissimus dorsi flap can be swung from the back but offers less volume than the TRAM flap and thus often requires supplementation with an implant. Reconstruction may be performed immediately (at the time of initial mastectomy) or may be delayed until later, usually when the patient has completed adjuvant therapy. When considering reconstructive options, concomitant illnesses should be considered, since the ability of an autologous flap to survive depends on medical comorbidities. In addition, the need for radiotherapy may affect the choice of reconstruction as radiation may increase fibrosis around an implant or decrease the volume of a flap.

3. Risks of pregnancy—Clinicians are often asked to advise patients regarding the potential risk of future pregnancy after definitive treatment for early-stage breast cancer. **To date, no adverse effect of pregnancy on survival of women who have had breast cancer has been demonstrated.** When counseling patients, oncologists must take into consideration the patients' overall prognosis, age, comorbidities, and life goals.

In patients with inoperable or metastatic cancer (stage IV disease), induced abortion may be advisable because of the possible adverse effects of hormonal treatment, radiotherapy, or chemotherapy upon the fetus in addition to the expectant mother's poor prognosis.

Asdourian MS, et al: Association between precautionary behaviors and breast cancer-related lymphedema in patients undergoing bilateral surgery. *J Clin Oncol.* 2017;35(35):3934-3941.

Berger AM, et al: Cancer-related fatigue: implications for breast cancer survivors. *Cancer.* 2012;118(8 Suppl):2261-2269.

Carroll JE, et al: Cognitive performance in survivors of breast cancer and markers of biological aging. *Cancer.* 2019;125(2):298-306.

Coughlin SS, et al: Survivorship issues in older breast cancer survivors. *Breast Cancer Res Treat.* 2019;174(1):47-53.

Dieli-Conwright CM, et al: Hispanic ethnicity as a moderator of the effects of aerobic and resistance exercise in survivors of breast cancer. *Cancer.* 2019;125(6):910-920.

Fong DY, et al: Physical activity for cancer survivors: meta-analysis of randomized controlled trials. *BMJ.* 2012;344:e70.

Gerstl B, et al: Pregnancy outcomes after a breast cancer diagnosis: a systematic review and meta-analysis. *Clin Breast Cancer.* 2018;18(1):e79-88.

Hartnett KP, et al: Pregnancy after cancer: does timing of conception affect infant health? *Cancer.* 2018;124(22):4401-4407.

Hermelink K: Acute and late onset cognitive dysfunction associated with chemotherapy in women with breast cancer. *Cancer.* 2011;117(5):1103.

Hummel SB, et al: Efficacy of internet-based cognitive behavioral therapy in improving sexual functioning of breast cancer survivors: results of a randomized controlled trial. *J Clin Oncol.* 2017;35(12):1328-1340.

Janelsins MC, et al: Cognitive complaints in survivors of breast cancer after chemotherapy compared with age-matched controls: an analysis from a nationwide, multicenter, prospective longitudinal study. *J Clin Oncol.* 2017;35(5):506-514.

Lambertini M, et al: Long-term safety of pregnancy following breast cancer according to estrogen receptor status. *J Natl Cancer Inst.* 2018;110(4):426-429.

Mandelblatt JS, et al: Cancer-related cognitive outcomes among older breast cancer survivors in the thinking and living with cancer study. *J Clin Oncol.* October 3, 2018; JCO1800140. [Epub ahead of print]

Van Dyk K, et al: The cognitive effects of endocrine therapy in survivors of breast cancer: a prospective longitudinal study up to 6 years after treatment. *Cancer.* 2019;125(5):681-689.

CARCINOMA OF THE MALE BREAST

ESSENTIALS OF DIAGNOSIS

- ► A painless lump beneath the areola in a man usually over 50 years of age.
- ► Nipple discharge, retraction, or ulceration may be present.
- ► Generally poorer prognosis than in women.

General Considerations

Breast cancer in men is a rare disease; the incidence is only about 1% of all breast cancer diagnoses. The average age at occurrence is about 70 years, and there may be an increased incidence of breast cancer in men with prostate cancer. As in women, hormonal influences are probably related to the development of male breast cancer. There is a high incidence of both breast cancer and gynecomastia in Bantu men, theoretically owing to failure of estrogen inactivation by associated liver disease. It is important to note that first-degree relatives of men with breast cancer are considered to be at high risk. This risk should be taken into account when discussing options with the patient and family. In addition, BRCA2 mutations are common in men with breast cancer. Men with breast cancer, especially with a history of prostate cancer, should receive genetic counseling. The prognosis, even in stage I cases, is worse in men than in women.

Clinical Findings

A painless lump, occasionally associated with nipple discharge, retraction, erosion, or ulceration, is the primary complaint. Examination usually shows a hard, ill-defined, nontender mass beneath the nipple or areola. Gynecomastia not uncommonly precedes or accompanies breast cancer in men. Nipple discharge is an uncommon presentation for breast cancer in men but is an ominous finding associated with carcinoma in nearly 75% of cases.

Breast cancer staging is the same in men as in women. Gynecomastia and metastatic cancer from another site (eg, prostate) must be considered in the differential diagnosis. Benign tumors are rare, and biopsy should be performed on all males with a defined breast mass.

Treatment

Treatment consists of modified radical mastectomy in operable patients, who should be chosen by the same criteria as women with the disease. Breast-conserving therapy is rarely performed. Irradiation is the first step in treating localized metastases in the skin, lymph nodes, or skeleton that are causing symptoms. Examination of the cancer for hormone receptors and HER2 overexpression is of value in determining adjuvant therapy. Over 95% of men have ER-positive tumors, and less than 10% have overexpression of HER2. Androgen receptor is also commonly overexpressed in male breast cancer. Adjuvant systemic therapy and radiation are used for the same indications as in breast cancer in women.

Because breast cancer in men is frequently a disseminated disease, endocrine therapy is of considerable importance in its management. Tamoxifen is the main medication for management of advanced breast cancer in men. Tamoxifen (20 mg orally daily) should be the initial treatment. There are few data regarding the use of AIs in men. Castration in advanced breast cancer is a successful measure and more beneficial than the same procedure in women but is rarely used. Objective evidence of regression may be seen in 60%-70% of men with endocrine therapy for metastatic disease—approximately twice the proportion in women. Bone is the most frequent site of metastases from breast cancer in men (as in women), and endocrine therapy relieves bone pain in most patients so treated. The longer the interval between mastectomy and recurrence, the longer is the remission following treatment. Corticosteroid therapy alone has been considered to be efficacious but probably has no value when compared with major endocrine ablation.

Chemotherapy should be administered for the same indications and using the same dosage schedules as for women with metastatic disease or for adjuvant treatment.

Prognosis

A large, population-based, international study reported that after adjustment for prognostic features (age, stage, treatment), men have a significantly improved relative survival from breast cancer compared to women. For node-positive disease, 5-year survival is approximately 69%, and for node-negative disease, it is 88%. A practice-patterns database study reported that based on NCCN guidelines, only 59% of patients received the recommended chemotherapy, 82% received the recommended hormonal therapy, and 71% received the recommended postmastectomy radiation, indicating a *relatively low adherence to NCCN guidelines for men.*

For patients whose disease progresses despite treatment, meticulous efforts at palliative care are essential.

Giordano SH: Breast cancer in men. *N Engl J Med.* 2018;378(24): 2311-2320.

Javidiparsijani S, et al: Male breast carcinoma: a clinical and pathological review. *Int J Surg Pathol.* 2017;25(3):200-205.

MULTIPLE CHOICE QUESTIONS

1. Fibrocystic condition of the breast is

   A. Communicable disease
   B. Common in postmenopausal women
   C. Caused at least in part by estrogen stimulation of breast tissue
   D. Carries a threefold increased risk of breast cancer
   E. Does not actually include any cysts on histology

2. Risk factors for breast cancer include

   A. Early childbearing
   B. Iodine deficiency
   C. BRCA1 mutation only in families of Ashkenazi Jewish descent
   D. A personal history of breast cancer
   E. None of the above

3. Breast cancer screening in asymptomatic women

   A. Identifies about 2 cancers per 1000 women over age 50 years
   B. Identifies cancer without node involvement in about 80% of detected cases
   C. Includes a history, physical examination, bilateral mammogram and ultrasound for women between ages 40 and 50 years
   D. Is followed by a 5-year survival of 95% for women diagnosed through screening
   E. Should include all women yearly after the age of 30 years

4. The clinical findings at breast cancer presentation most commonly include

   A. A painless mass identified by the patient
   B. A new mass discovered during a clinician physical examination (60% of cases)
   C. Nipple discharge (60% of cases)
   D. An axillary mass due to metastatic lymph nodes (40% of cases)
   E. None of the above

5. Axillary lymph node metastases from breast cancer

   A. Are not important for predicting patient survival in women with breast cancer
   B. Are generally palpable if present
   C. Can be reliably detected by sestamibi scintigraphy
   D. Can be reliably detected by sentinel lymph node biopsy in women with clinically uninvolved axillary lymph nodes
   E. Are frequently present in residual lymph nodes when sentinel lymph node biopsy shows no evidence of disease

19

Thoracic Wall, Pleura, Mediastinum, & Lung

William B. Weir, MD
Andrew C. Chang, MD

▼ ANATOMY & PHYSIOLOGY

ANATOMY OF THE CHEST WALL & PLEURA

The physiology of respiration and the anatomy of the chest wall are intricately connected. The chest wall is an airtight, expandable, cone-shaped cage comprised of a vast array of skin, fat, muscle, bone, and vital organs. This design serves to facilitate protection of the vital organs as well as ventilation and gas exchange. Normal ventilation occurs when expansion of the rib cage and simultaneous diaphragmatic excursion create negative intrathoracic pressure, allowing inward flow of air.

The function of the chest wall is made possible by its segmentally arranged anatomy. The ventral wall of the bony thorax extends from the suprasternal notch to the xiphoid, approximately 18 cm in the adult. It is formed by the manubrium, sternum, and xiphoid process. The remainder of the anterior wall and the lateral walls are formed by 12 ribs. The first seven pairs of ribs articulate directly with the sternum, the next three pairs connect to the lower border of the preceding rib, and the last two terminate in the wall of the abdomen. The sides of the chest wall consist of the upper 10 ribs, which slope obliquely downward from their posterior attachments. The posterior chest wall is formed by the 12 thoracic vertebrae, their transverse processes, and the 12 ribs (Figure 19–1). The upper ventral portion of the thoracic cage is covered by the clavicle and the subclavian vessels. Laterally, it is covered by the shoulder girdle and axillary nerves and vessels; dorsally, it is covered in part by the scapula.

The superior aperture of the thorax (also called the thoracic inlet or the thoracic outlet) is a downwardly slanted 5- to 10-cm kidney-shaped opening bounded by the first costal cartilages and ribs laterally, the manubrium anteriorly, and the body of the first thoracic vertebra posteriorly. The inferior aperture is bounded by the 12th vertebra and ribs posteriorly and the cartilages of the 7th to 10th ribs and the

xiphisternal joint anteriorly. The diaphragm comprises a large portion of the lower thoracic cavity.

The blood supply and innervation of the chest wall are via the intercostal vessels and nerves (Figures 19–2 and 19–3). The upper thorax also receives vessels and nerves from the cervical and axillary regions. Blood supply to the underside of the sternum arises from bilateral internal thoracic artery branches, which arise from the intercostal vessels laterally.

The entirety of the thoracic cavity is lined by a pleural membrane. The parietal pleura is the innermost lining of the chest wall and is divided into four parts: the cervical pleura (cupola or cupula), costal pleura, mediastinal pleura, and diaphragmatic pleura. The visceral pleura is a mesodermal layer investing the lungs and is continuous with the parietal pleura, joining it at the hilum of the lung. The potential pleural space is a capillary gap that normally contains only a few drops of serous fluid. However, this space may be enlarged when fluid (hydrothorax), blood (hemothorax), pus (pyothorax or empyema), lymphatic fluid (chylothorax), or air (pneumothorax) fill this cavity.

PHYSIOLOGY OF THE CHEST WALL & PLEURA

▶ Mechanics of Respiration

Ventilation is the process of moving gas through the airways, to and from the alveoli. This is facilitated when elevation of the rib cage and descent of the diaphragm cause an increase in thoracic volume and generate negative intrathoracic pressure. Furthermore, accessory muscles of respiration contribute to the conformational change in the thoracic cage during periods of intense exercise or respiratory distress (Figure 19–4). However, in infants, the ribs have not yet assumed their oblique contour and ventilation depends largely on diaphragmatic breathing.

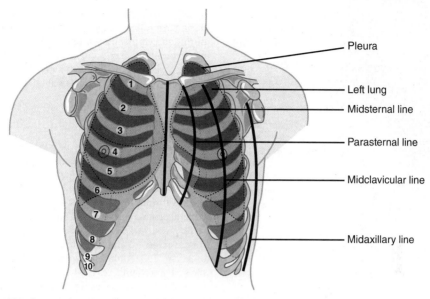

▲ **Figure 19–1.** The thorax, showing rib cage, pleura, and lung fields.

Expiration is mainly passive, resulting from elastic recoil of the lungs. An exception to this is deep breathing, or forced expirations, when the abdominal musculature contracts, pulling the rib cage downward and simultaneously elevating the diaphragm by compressing the abdominal viscera against it.

▶ **Physiology of the Pleural Space**

A. Pressure

The pleural cavity pressure is normally negative, owing to the opposing forces of elastic recoil of the lung and active expansion of the space by the chest wall. During quiet respiration,

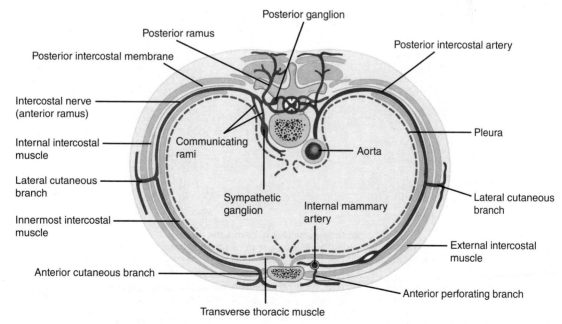

▲ **Figure 19–2.** Transverse section of thorax.

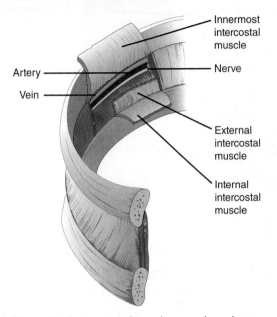

▲ Figure 19–3. Intercostal muscles, vessels, and nerves.

it varies from −15 cm H_2O with inspiration up to 2 cm H_2O during expiration. Larger pressure changes (eg, −60 cm H_2O during forced inspiration up to +30 cm H_2O during vigorous expiration) may occur with deep breathing. Because of gravity, pleural pressure at the apex is more negative when the body is upright and changes about 0.2 cm H_2O per centimeter of vertical height.

B. Fluid Formation and Reabsorption

The formation (transudation) and reabsorption of fluid within the pleural space depends on hydrostatic, colloid, and tissue pressures (the Starling equation), in addition to permeability of the pleural membrane. Absent any pathology, fluid is formed by the parietal pleura and absorbed by the visceral pleura (Figure 19–5). Since systemic capillary hydrostatic pressure is 30 cm H_2O, and intrapleural negative pressure averages −5 cm H_2O there is a net *hydrostatic* pressure of 35 cm H_2O. Additionally, the colloid osmotic pressure of the systemic capillaries is 34 cm H_2O and an opposing 8 cm H_2O of pleural space osmotic pressure. Thus, a net 26 cm H_2O *osmotic* pressure draws fluid back into systemic capillaries. Since systemic hydrostatic pressure (35 cm H_2O)

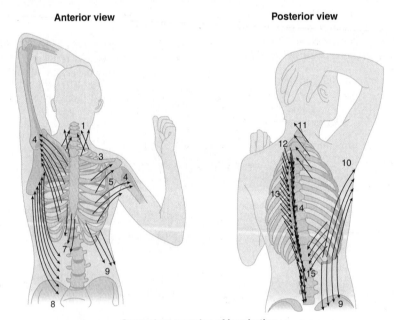

Anterior view   **Posterior view**

Secondary muscles of inspiration
(1) sternocleidomastoideus (3) scalenes (4) pectoralis major (5) pectoralis minor
(10) serratus anterior (11) serratus posterior superior (12) upper iliocostalis

Secondary muscles of expiration
(8) external oblique (9) internal oblique (7) rectus abdominus (13) lower iliocostalis
(14) lower longissimus (15) serratus posterior inferior

▲ Figure 19–4. Accessory muscles of respiration. (Reproduced with permission from Kapandji IA: The Physiology of the Joints: Vol. 3. *The Trunk and the Vertebral Column.* Philadelphia, PA: Churchill Livingstone; 1974.)

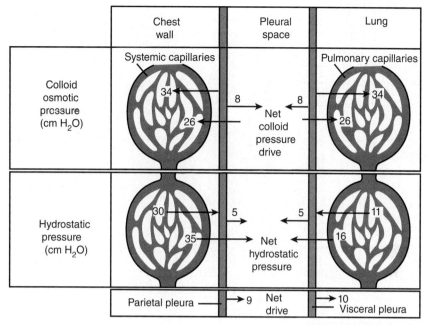

▲ **Figure 19–5.** Movement of fluid across the pleural space, showing production and absorption of pleural fluid.

exceeds osmotic capillary pressure (26 cm H_2O) by 9 cm H_2O, there is a 9 cm H_2O net drive of fluid into the pleural space by systemic capillaries in the chest wall. Similar calculations for the visceral pleura involving the low-pressure pulmonary circulation will show that there is a resulting net drive of 10 cm H_2O that attracts pleural fluid into pulmonary capillaries. Thus there is normally a balance favoring neither loss nor gain of fluid in this space.

Ordinarily pleural fluid is low in protein (<100 mg/dL). When it increases in disease to about 1 g/dL, the net colloid osmotic pressure of the visceral pleural capillaries is equaled and pleural fluid reabsorption becomes dependent on lymphatic drainage. Thus, abnormal amounts of pleural fluid may accumulate (1) when hydrostatic pressure is increased, such as in heart failure; (2) when capillary permeability is increased, as in inflammatory or neoplastic disease; or (3) when colloid osmotic pressure is decreased.

ANATOMY OF THE MEDIASTINUM

The mediastinum is the anatomic compartment between the pleural cavities. Anteriorly, it extends from the suprasternal notch to the xiphoid process and posteriorly from the 1st to the 11th thoracic vertebrae. Superiorly, fascial planes in the neck are in direct communication; inferiorly, the mediastinum is bounded by the diaphragm. Extending through the inferior aspect of the mediastinum are the aorta, inferior vena cava, esophagus, and vagus nerve.

The mediastinum may be divided into a number of compartments in several ways. Classically, it may be divided into the superior, anterior, middle, and posterior compartments. The superior compartment contains all structures above a line that is drawn from the fourth thoracic vertebra to the sternomanubrial junction (angle of Louis). In the three-compartment Burkell classification (Figure 19–6), the anterior mediastinum contains the thymus gland, lymph nodes, the ascending aorta and transverse aorta, the great vessels, and areolar tissue. The middle mediastinum contains the heart, the pericardium, the trachea, both hila of the lungs, the phrenic nerves, lymph nodes, and areolar tissue. The posterior mediastinum contains the sympathetic chains, the vagus nerves, the esophagus, the thoracic duct, lymph nodes, and the descending aorta.

Displacement of the mediastinum can occur from masses or from accumulations of air, fluid, blood, or chyle interfering with vital functions. Tracheal compression, vena caval obstruction, and esophageal obstructions cause clinical symptoms. The mediastinum can also be displaced laterally when pathologic processes of one hemithorax cause mediastinal shift. Fibrosis and lung volume loss can shift the mediastinum toward the affected side. Open pneumothorax and massive hemothorax shift the mediastinum away from the affected side. Open pneumothorax produces alternating paradoxical mediastinal shifts with respiration. This pathologic deviation from normal physiology adversely affects ventilation. Acute mediastinal displacement may produce hypoxia or reduced venous return and cause dysrhythmias, hypotension, or cardiac arrest.

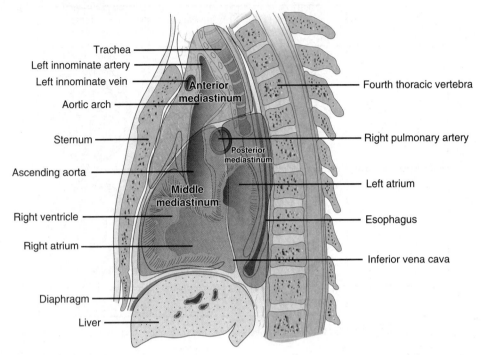

▲ **Figure 19–6.** Divisions of the mediastinum (Burkell classification). Light screening: anterior mediastinum; lower dark screening: middle mediastinum; gray oblong area at right: posterior mediastinum.

Congenital abnormalities within the mediastinum are numerous. A defect in the anterior mediastinal pleura with communication of the right and left hemithorax is rare. This retrosternal part of the anterior mediastinum is normally thin, and overexpansion of one pleural space may cause "mediastinal herniation" or a bulge of mediastinal pleura toward the opposite side.

ANATOMY OF THE LUNG

The fundamental unit of lung anatomy is a bronchopulmonary segment (Figure 19–7). The right lung has three lobes: upper, middle, and lower. The left lung consists of two lobes: upper and lower. On the left, the lingular segments of the upper lobe are the homolog of the right middle lobe. Two fissures of varying completeness separate the lobes on the right side. The major, or oblique, fissure divides the upper and middle lobes from the lower lobe. The minor, or horizontal, fissure separates the middle from the upper lobe. On the left side, the single oblique fissure separates the upper and lower lobes. The parenchymal anatomy can be seen by studying the sequential division of the bronchopulmonary tree. The trachea and mainstem bronchi and their branches contain a posterior membranous area and are prevented from collapsing by horseshoe-shaped anterior segments made of cartilage. The cartilaginous reinforcement of the airway gradually becomes less complete as the branches become smaller, and reinforcement ceases with bronchi measuring 1-2 mm. The bronchopulmonary segmental anatomy is designated by numbers (Boyden) or by name (Jackson and Huber). There are typically 18 bronchopulmonary segments (three right upper, two right middle, five right lower, four left upper, four left lower) as shown. The segmental bronchial anatomy is for the most part constant with the pulmonary vascular structures showing more variability.

Knowledge of the blood supply is crucial to surgery. The lungs have a dual blood supply: the pulmonary and the bronchial arterial systems. The pulmonary arteries transmit deoxygenated blood from the right ventricle for oxygenation. They closely accompany the bronchi. The bronchial arteries usually arise directly from the aorta or nearby intercostal arteries and are variable in number. They transmit oxygenated blood to the bronchial wall up to the level of the terminal bronchioles. The pulmonary veins travel in the interlobar septa and do not correspond to the distribution of the bronchi or the pulmonary arteries.

THE LYMPHATIC SYSTEM

The lymphatics travel in intersegmental septa centrally as well as to the parenchymal surface to form subpleural networks. Drainage continues toward the hilum in channels that

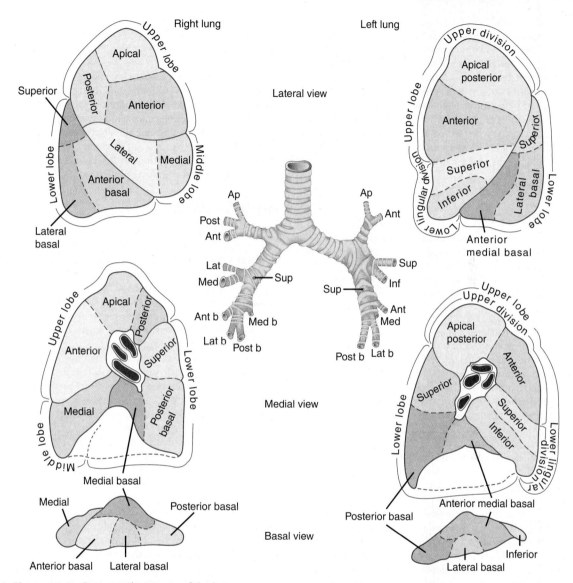

▲ **Figure 19–7.** Segmental anatomy of the lungs.

follow the bronchi and pulmonary arteries. The lymphatics eventually enter lymph nodes in the major fissures of the lungs, the hilum, and the paratracheal regions.

The direction of lymphatic drainage—irrespective of the primary site—is cephalad and ipsilateral, but contralateral flow may occur from any lobe. The usual sequence of lymphatic spread of pulmonary cancer is first to the regional parabronchial nodes and then to the ipsilateral paratracheal, subcarinal, scalene, or inferior deep cervical nodes. The lymphatics from the left lower lobe may be almost equally distributed to the left and right. From the left upper lobe, distribution is often to the anterior mediastinal group (A-P window and paraaortic lymph nodes).

▼ DIAGNOSTIC STUDIES

SKIN TESTS

Skin tests are used in the diagnosis of tuberculosis (TB), histoplasmosis, and coccidioidomycosis. Tuberculin testing is usually done with purified protein derivative (PPD) injected intradermally. Intermediate-strength PPD should be used in patients who seem likely to have active disease. Induration of 10 mm or more at the injection site after 48-72 hours is positive and indicates either active or arrested disease. Because false-negative reactions are rare, a negative test often reliably rules out tuberculosis. Mumps antigen can be placed on the opposite forearm to test for anergy in those patients suspected of being incapable of mounting a reaction to an intradermal antigen. Skin tests for histoplasmosis and coccidioidomycosis are performed in a similar way, but skin tests for fungal infections are often unreliable and serologic tests should be performed instead.

ENDOSCOPY

▶ Laryngoscopy

Indirect laryngoscopy is used to assess vocal cord mobility in patients suspected of having lung carcinoma when there has been a voice change. It can also be performed to search for an otherwise occult source for malignant cells in sputum or metastases in cervical lymph nodes.

▶ Bronchoscopy

Roentgenographic evidence of bronchial obstruction, unresolved pneumonia, foreign body, suspected carcinoma, hemoptysis, aspiration pneumonia, and lung abscess are only a few of the indications for bronchoscopy. Depending on the indication, either flexible or rigid bronchoscopy may be performed. Rigid bronchoscopy must be done under general anesthesia and is most often used for clearing major airways of bulky obstructing lesions such as tumor, foreign bodies, or blood clots. Tumor ablation may be done via multiple techniques, including use of the Nd: YAG (neodymium-doped yttritium aluminum garnet) laser.

Flexible bronchoscopy is a highly effective diagnostic and therapeutic tool that any surgical provider should become familiar with. It can be performed under local and/or intravenous sedation. Washings are usually obtained for bacterial or fungal culture and cytologic examination. Visible lesions are biopsied directly and brush biopsies are obtained from specific bronchopulmonary segments in question. Occasionally, transcarinal needle biopsy of a subcarinal node is obtained.

Bronchoscopically, 30%-50% of lung tumors are visible. Brushing, random biopsies, and sputum cytology may still yield a positive diagnosis of cancer or tuberculosis in the absence of a visible lesion. The yield is influenced by size, location, and histologic cell type of the lesion.

Additional techniques available during bronchoscopy include the use of endobronchial ultrasound (EBUS) and electromagnetic navigational bronchoscopy (ENB). Endobronchial ultrasound enables visualization of masses and lymph nodes from the central airways, and facilitates fine-needle aspiration of these lesions for proper staging. In workup of lung malignancy EBUS biopsy is often the first test of choice if there are available, experienced clinicians. Sensitivity by EBUS has been reported as 45%-100% in experienced hands who are ideally able to get three passes per lymph node.

ENB combines the use of cross-sectional imaging (usually computed tomography [CT] scan) and simulated virtual bronchoscopy to create a three-dimensional roadmap. The operator can then access lesions deep within the lung parenchyma by using electromagnetic localization technology, which helps calibrate the system to the patient's anatomy. This is useful for previously unreachable peripheral lesions or for positioning and marking for further interventional or surgical procedures.

MEDIASTINOSCOPY

Cervical mediastinoscopy remains a mainstay of evaluation of the mediastinum despite rapid advances in imaging. Guidelines recommend that a thorough mediastinoscopy sample nodes from five stations, ideally including ipsilateral and contralateral paratracheal levels 2 and 4 and subcarinal station 7 (systematic sampling). A standard cervical mediastinoscopy is performed through a 3- to 4-cm incision one fingerbreadth above the sternal notch. Dissection proceeds immediately beneath the pretracheal fascia, allowing safe access to mediastinal nodes and avoiding major vascular structures. After palpation, the mediastinoscope can be inserted and nodes biopsied under direct vision. Unclear structures are aspirated prior to attempted biopsy.

Enlarged lymph nodes in the aorticopulmonary window are technically inaccessible by means of a standard cervical mediastinoscopy. In this setting, consideration can be given to performing a Chamberlain procedure. However, transcervical extended mediastinal lymphadenectomy (TEMLA) has become more widely practiced and allows access to the aorticopulmonary window nodes. It is performed through the same neck incision as standard mediastinoscopy, except the dissection is carried laterally beside the left carotid artery toward and then over the aorta into the aorticopulmonary space. In the setting of a left upper lobe pathology the ability to access station 5 and 6 lymph nodes is better served by TEMLA over the other new staging option, video-assisted mediastinal lymphadenectomy (VAMLA). Because of the surrounding structures, TEMLA carries significant risks and is contraindicated in patients with aortic pathology or previous cardiac operations.

The complications of mediastinoscopy are minimal (<1%-2%). Major bleeding complications requiring sternotomy or thoracotomy for repair are infrequent (1%-2%). However, the surgeon must take care and plan for these complications. Other possible complications include pneumothorax, recurrent nerve injury, infection, and esophageal injury.

Mediastinoscopy is almost invariably accurate in the diagnosis of sarcoidosis. It is also useful to diagnose tuberculosis, histoplasmosis, Castleman silicosis, metastatic carcinoma, lymphoma, and carcinoma of the esophagus. It should not be used in the investigation of primary mediastinal tumors, as those lesions should have a more definitive, excisional biopsy.

CHAMBERLAIN PROCEDURE

Anterior mediastinotomy (the Chamberlain procedure) is used to sample nodes and biopsy tissue in the anterior mediastinum, most commonly in the aortopulmonary window. A small (3- to 4-cm) incision is made over the second or third interspace on the appropriate side of the lesion. Alternatively, the procedure can be performed with videoscopic guidance (video-assisted thoracoscopic surgery [VATS]). The mediastinum is approached through the interspace directly or after excising the costochondral cartilage using either the mediastinoscope or open technique. Careful attention is paid to preserving the mammary vessels encountered in the dissection. The mediastinum is approached extrapleurally unless lesions specifically within the thorax (effusions or tumors invading the hilum or chest wall) need to be investigated. Furthermore, if additional access is required to facilitate the dissection or to treat a complication, the incision can be converted to a larger anterior thoracotomy. Complications from anterior mediastinotomy can include damage to the recurrent laryngeal nerve, bleeding, and infection. In experienced hands, major morbidity is less than 1%-2%.

VIDEO-ASSISTED THORACOSCOPIC SURGERY

Video-assisted thoracoscopic surgery (VATS) plays an important role in the diagnosis and staging of thoracic malignancies, as well as in the resection of isolated peripheral pulmonary nodules and bullous lung disease. Furthermore, it has been a welcome advance for lung biopsy and pleurodesis procedures. Although some oncologic concerns persist, thoracoscopic procedures are the standard of care for many resections. As instruments and techniques have evolved, complications from VATS procedures (persistent air leaks, hemorrhage, tumor seeding, etc) have decreased. Overall, major complication rates of 1%-2% are reported. Faster patient recovery, shorter hospital stays, and decreased pain are major advantages of VATS, although long-term differences between videoscopic-assisted thoracic surgery and thoracotomy using muscle-sparing incisions are yet to be demonstrated.

PLEURAL BIOPSY

Biopsies of the pleura can be performed using percutaneous needle techniques, VATS, or open surgical approaches. Common indications for pleural biopsy include workup of pleural effusion where fluid analysis has been unrevealing, tuberculosis, or pleural based malignancies. A definitive diagnosis can be obtained in 60%-80% of cases of tuberculosis or cancer. The principal complication is pneumothorax. Biopsy of the pleura can be performed via videoscopic or open technique with minimal morbidity, providing the pathologist with a specimen superior to that of needle biopsy. However, 5%-10% of biopsy specimens are inadequate for diagnosis even among experienced surgeons.

Detterbeck F, et al. Classification of the thoroughness of mediastinal staging of lung cancer. *Chest.* 2010;137(2):436-442.

Khan K, et al. Navigational bronchoscopy for early lung cancer: A road to therapy. *Adv Ther.* 2016;33:580-596.

Kużdżał J, et al. Current evidence on transcervical mediastinal lymph nodes dissection. *Eur J Cardiothorac Surg.* 2011; 40(6):1470.

Yasufuku K, et al. A prospective controlled trial of endobronchial ultrasound-guided transbronchial needle aspiration compared with mediastinoscopy for mediastinal lymph node staging of lung cancer. *J Thorac Cardiovasc Surg.* 2011;142(6):1393.

Yendamuri S, et al. Transcervical extended mediastinal lymphadenectomy: Experience from a North American cancer center. *Ann Thorac Surg.* 2017;104(5):1644-1649.

LUNG BIOPSY

▶ Needle Biopsy

The most common indication for the use of transthoracic needle biopsy of the lung is the evaluation of a solitary pulmonary nodule. It may also be used to confirm the presence of metastatic disease. Lung biopsy may also be indicated in diffuse parenchymal disease and in some patients with localized lesions. Most commonly, lung biopsies are now performed under CT guidance with a diagnostic yield of approximately 60%. Complications following percutaneous needle biopsy include pneumothorax (5%-30%), hemothorax, hemoptysis, and air embolism; several deaths have been reported. Pulmonary hypertension or cysts and bullae are contraindications as large cysts or bullae predispose the patient to pneumothorax. Additionally, there is controversy concerning the risks of spreading the tumor by needle biopsy in localized disease.

▶ Surgical Biopsy

Thoracoscopy is the standard approach for open-lung biopsy in patients who can tolerate single-lung ventilation. Techniques for port placement vary, but all allow introduction of a stapler and operating thoracoscope. In addition to allowing smaller incisions, thoracoscopy allows for the visualization of multiple segments and taking multiple biopsies in diffuse diseases. For open biopsies, a limited intercostal or anterior parasternal incision is used to remove a 3- to 4-cm wedge of lung tissue in diffuse parenchymal lung disease. The site of incision is selected based on accessibility and potential diagnostic value. The incision is generally made at the fifth interspace in the right anterior axillary line to allow for access to all three lobes for biopsy. The middle lobe and lingula are selected in specific cases when pathology exists only in these areas, as they generally yield results of the poorest quality. The surgeon must be cognizant of the other visceral and vascular structures coursing in the left chest. Additionally, open-lung biopsy is associated with a lower death rate, fewer complications, and greater diagnostic yield than needle biopsy. It is especially useful in critically ill, immunosuppressed patients for differentiation of infectious, infiltrative lesions from neoplastic, infiltrative lesions. Peripheral lesions are totally excised by wedge or segmental resection, and deeply placed lesions are removed by lobectomy in suitable candidates.

SPUTUM ANALYSIS

Sputum cytology can be valuable for detecting lung cancer. Specimens are obtained by deep coughing or by abrasion with a brush, or bronchial washings are obtained by bronchoscopic washing techniques. Specimens should be collected in the morning and delivered to the laboratory promptly. Centrifugation or filtration can be used to concentrate the cellular elements.

In primary lung cancer, sputum cytology is positive in 30%-60% of cases. Repeated sputum examination improves the diagnostic return, as does the combination with bronchoalveolar lavage. Examination of the first bronchoscopic washing material yields a diagnosis in 60% of cases. Postbronchoscopy sputum analysis should always be made at 6-12 and 24 hours, as findings may be positive at these times when previous tests were negative. Cytologic analysis using immunohistochemistry to molecular markers (cytokeratins, hnRNP, etc) has improved accuracy and sensitivity and the ability to detect premalignant lesions.

ADVANCED IMAGING

Computed tomography (CT) is a cornerstone of evaluation of chest pathology. CT scanning is critical in the staging of thoracic cancer, evaluating the extent of metastatic disease, and in post-interventional surveillance.

Although the major value of magnetic resonance imaging (MRI) in the thorax has been in cardiovascular imaging, it can also show invasion of lung cancer into the chest wall, vertebrae, and spinal cord as well as mediastinal structures. MRI has a particular niche in the evaluation of superior sulcus (Pancoast) tumors to establish involvement of the brachial plexus, subclavian vessel, or bony chest wall.

Positron emission tomography (PET) is an important tool in staging and workup of the cancer patient and is widely available. PET scanning may identify unsuspected regional or distant disease in up to 20%-30% of patients with lung cancer or esophageal cancer compared with conventional imaging methods (CT, bone scan). PET scanning is more accurate than CT scan in detection of cancer spread to mediastinal lymph nodes. Because of the high negative predictive value of PET scanning, a negative PET scan in

the mediastinum permits direct progression to surgery. The presence of a positive PET scan in the mediastinum mandates either mediastinoscopy or, more recently, endoscopic evaluation of mediastinal lymph nodes because of false-positive PET scan results.

Combined PET/CT is highly accurate (>90%), but PET by itself has a 10%-20% false-positive rate in the mediastinum. Therefore, interpretations of PET results must be accepted with caution and must be confirmed by surgical staging when inconsistent with the overall clinical picture.

▼ DISEASES OF THE CHEST WALL

LUNG HERNIA

A lung hernia resulting from a defect in the chest wall may be congenital or acquired as the result of trauma or a surgical operation. Most lung hernias are thoracic in location, but cervical (defects of Sibson fascia) or diaphragmatic herniation may occur occasionally. Lung hernias may present as a tender subcutaneous mass that enlarges with cough or valsalva. Other than this mass, they are usually asymptomatic. Once diagnosed, these hernias should be repaired, with repair of the skeletal defect and prosthetic mesh reinforcement as an open or thoracoscopic procedure.

CHEST WALL INFECTIONS

Infections of the chest wall or pleural spaces may pose complex challenges in medical management. Infections that appear to involve only the skin and soft tissues may actually represent outward extensions of deeper infection of the ribs, cartilage, sternum, or even the pleural space (empyema necessitatis). Inadequate drainage of superficial infection can lead to inward extension into the pleural space, causing an empyema.

Subpectoral abscess is caused by suppurative adenitis of the axillary lymph nodes, rib or pleural infection, or posterior extension of a breast abscess. It may also occur as a complication of chest wall surgery (eg, mastectomy, pacemaker placement). Symptoms include erythema, induration of the pectoral region, and obliteration of the normal infraclavicular depression and may progress to systemic sepsis. Shoulder movement is painful. Organisms most commonly involved include hemolytic streptococci and *Staphylococcus aureus.* Treatment involves incisional drainage along the lateral border of the pectoralis major muscle and administration of systemic antibiotics.

Subscapular abscess may arise from osteomyelitis of the scapula but most commonly follows thoracic operations such as thoracotomy or thoracoplasty. Winging of the scapula or paravertebral induration of the trapezius muscle is usually present. A pleural communication is suggested if a cough impulse is present or if the size of the mass varies with position or direct pressure. The diagnosis is established by needle aspiration. Open drainage is indicated for pyogenic infections not involving the pleural space. Extrapulmonary, tubercular lesions should be treated with antimicrobials therapy and needle aspiration, if possible, as chest wall tuberculosis can arise from an initial pulmonary source and bronchopleural fistula (BPF).

Osteomyelitis of the Ribs

In the past, osteomyelitis of the ribs was often caused by typhoid fever and tuberculosis. Except in children, hematogenous osteomyelitis occurs rarely in the modern era; and when encountered, is likely the result of a thoracotomy incision.

Sternal Osteomyelitis

Infection of the sternum most commonly follows median sternotomy incisions, particularly in diabetics. It presents as a postoperative wound infection or mediastinitis with drainage, fever, leukocytosis, and instability of the sternal closure. Treatment consists of control of systemic sepsis with appropriate antibiotics, open drainage, and resection or debridement of the involved sternum. Finally, there must be definitive reconstruction of the defect with pectoralis muscle, serratus muscle, or omental coverage. Occasionally, sternal osteomyelitis will be due to tuberculosis.

Infection of the Costal Cartilages & Xiphoid

Costal cartilage infections are relatively unresponsive to antibiotic therapy. Once devascularized, perichondral tissue necroses and acts as a foreign body to perpetuate the infection and favor sinus tract formation. The most common cause is direct extension of other surgical infections (eg, wound infection, subphrenic abscess). Surgical division of costal cartilages, as in a thoracoabdominal incision, may predispose to cartilage infection postoperatively if local sepsis develops. A wide variety of organisms have been implicated.

Erythema and induration with fluctuance and often spontaneous drainage can occur. The course can be fulminant or may be indolent over months or years, with periodic exacerbations. Associated osteomyelitis of the sternum, ribs, or clavicle may occur.

The treatment of choice includes resection of the involved cartilage and adjacent involved bony structures. Recurrence is due to underestimation of the extent of disease and inadequate resection.

Reconstruction of the Chest Wall

Chest wall reconstruction may be necessary following trauma, surgical resection, or infection resulting in destruction of chest wall structures. Rigid reconstruction of the chest wall is generally recommended for defects greater than 5 cm, although posterior resections covered by the scapula will not necessarily need rigid mesh reconstruction. Advances in the use of musculocutaneous flaps and the supportive use of methyl methacrylate and Marlex mesh to produce solidity below these muscular flaps have facilitated repairs. In massive chest wall defects, vascularization of the area is essential and can be accomplished by use of omental flaps as well as pectoralis, latissimus dorsi, and rectus flaps. Microsurgical techniques for repair of such defects have greatly expanded the ability of plastic surgeons to deal with extensive resectional and infective processes.

Harati K, et al. Thoracic wall reconstruction after tumor resection. *Front Oncol.* 2015;5:247.

Madeo J, et al. Tuberculous empyema presenting as a persistent chest wall mass: Case report. *Germs.* 2013;3(1):21-25.

Mahabir RC, Butler CE. Stabilization of the chest wall: Autologous and alloplastic reconstructions. *Semin Plast Surg.* 2011; 25:34-42.

TIETZE SYNDROME (COSTOCHONDRITIS)

Tietze syndrome (costochondritis) is a painful, nonsuppurative inflammation of the costochondral cartilages and is of unknown cause. Evidence suggests that costochondritis may represent a manifestation of seronegative rheumatic disease. Local swelling and tenderness are the only symptoms; they usually disappear without therapy although the syndrome may recur.

Several reports have suggested the use of bone scintigraphy and chest CT for diagnosis of infected costochondritis. Bone scanning was effective in localizing and identifying inflamed costochondral junctions. Treatment is symptomatic and may include analgesics (NSAIDs) and local or systemic corticosteroids. When symptoms persist longer than 3 weeks and tumefaction suggests neoplasm, excision of the involved cartilage may be indicated and is usually curative.

Gologorsky R, et al. Surgical management of medically refractory Tietze syndrome. *Ann Thorac Surg.* 2017;104(6):e443-e445.

Winzenberg T, et al. Musculoskeletal chest wall pain. *Aust Fam Physician.* 2015;44(8):540-544.

MONDOR DISEASE (THROMBOPHLEBITIS OF THE THORACOEPIGASTRIC VEIN)

Mondor disease consists of localized thrombophlebitis of the anterolateral chest wall and at times, the breast tissue. It is more prominent in women than in men and occasionally follows mastectomy. There are few symptoms other than the presence of a localized tender, cordlike structure in the subcutaneous tissues of the abdomen, thorax, or axilla. The disease is self-limited and does not pose a risk of thromboembolism. However, the possibility of an infective origin or stasis of the interrupted venous return due to neoplasm must be ruled out.

PECTUS EXCAVATUM

Pectus excavatum is a commonly encountered, congenital chest wall malformation comprising nearly 90% of chest wall deformities and characterized by a concave (or caved in) appearance of the chest. Occasionally, this condition can be present with others such as Marfan syndrome and scoliosis. A majority of patients are diagnosed in early childhood, although the defect often progresses through development and puberty. Patients can present with asymmetry of the chest, shortness of breath (due to a restrictive type lung pathology), and chest pain. However, many may be asymptomatic. Physical exam must include auscultation as mitral valve prolapse has been reported in patients with pectus excavatum.

Although cosmetically troubling for many patients, most patients do not require treatment and the condition does not necessitate intervention unless certain criteria are met. Nevertheless, the psychologic impact on the adolescent should not be minimized. Standard preoperative workup includes chest CT allowing anatomic evaluation including evaluation of displacement of the heart. CT also allows for calculation of the Haller Index by dividing the transverse diameter of the chest by the AP diameter. Classically, a Haller Index of 3.2 or greater warrants surgical consideration.

Historically, pectus excavatum was treated by an open Ravitch operation which involves creation of muscle and skin flaps, sternal osteotomy, and then resection of the involved cartilage. This allows the sternum to move anteriorly into a more anatomically correct position. More current treatment also includes a minimally invasive option, the Nuss procedure. The minimally invasive approach entails inserting a metal bar posterior to the ribs and advancing it anterior to the pericardium with thoracoscopic guidance, yielding excellent results.

CHEST WALL TUMORS

Chest wall tumors may be imitated by enlarged costal cartilages, chest wall infection, fractures, rickets, scurvy, hyperparathyroidism, and other conditions. Most commonly, chest wall lesions present as a mass with localized or referred pain; fewer than 25% are asymptomatic. These tumors demand attention as approximately 60% of all chest wall masses prove to be malignant. Lesions arise from one of the three components of the chest wall: soft tissues (muscle, nerve, fascia), bone, or cartilage.

The majority of these tumors arise from either bone or cartilage. Rib involvement is more common than sternal presentation. Often, chest wall sarcomas are associated with pulmonary metastasis. On initial workup, simple chest x-rays may initially identify a mass, especially if it is calcified. Chest CT offers the most information for diagnosis, and staging and bone scans should be obtained to complete evaluation.

Initial diagnosis is obtained by limited incisional biopsy (transverse) if the mass is large (> 4 cm). Smaller lesions are excised en bloc, ensuring negative margins, with full knowledge that a malignancy is present in many cases. Classic teaching has been used to perform en bloc wide local excisions with immediate reconstruction for all lesions at initial presentations. However, progress with adjuvant multimodality therapy, for tumors such as rhabdomyosarcomas and Ewing sarcoma, supports the use of initial limited biopsy for tissue diagnosis to guide treatment planning.

▶ Specific Neoplasms

A. Benign Soft-Tissue Tumors

1. Lipomas—Lipomas are the most common benign tumors of the chest wall. Occasionally, they are very large and lobulated, and they may have dumbbell-shaped extensions that indent the endothoracic fascia beneath the sternum through an intercostal space. They may communicate with a large mediastinal or supraclavicular component. Often, full excision is paramount to prevent recurrence.

2. Neurogenic tumors—These may arise from intercostal or superficial nerves. Solitary neurofibromas are most common, followed by neurolemmomas.

3. Cavernous hemangiomas—Hemangiomas of the thoracic wall are usually painful and occur in children. Tumors may be isolated or may involve other tissues (eg, lung), as in Rendu–Osler–Weber syndrome. Percutaneous or incisional biopsy should be avoided given the risk for bleeding. Local excision is diagnostic as well as therapeutic.

4. Lymphangiomas—These rare lesions are seen most often in children. They may have poorly defined borders that make complete excision difficult. Multidisciplinary team input is crucial in this pediatric lesion.

B. Malignant Soft-Tissue Tumors

Roughly 50% of all chest wall masses are sarcomas, yet overall they represent only a small percentage (5%) of all malignant soft-tissue sarcomas. Survival is determined by the histologic grade, the completeness of resection, and the presence and development of metastases (synchronous or metachronous). Low-grade tumors have 5-year and 10-year survival rates approaching 90% and 82%, respectively. With high-grade lesions, however, 5-year survival rates are only 30%-50%, and the development of metastasis greatly reduces the chances of survival.

Proper evaluation includes MRI to identify soft-tissue planes and degree of infiltration into surrounding neurovascular structures. Treatment is directed at complete resection with emphasis on achieving negative margins (at least 1-2 cm). En bloc resection techniques include raising skin flaps and chest wall reconstruction with soft-tissue flaps or prosthetic options such as Marlex mesh with methyl methacrylate to correct chest wall deformity and prevent paradoxic chest movement. Chest wall resection for soft-tissue sarcoma is relatively safe with a low morbidity and mortality rate (~1%) in patients without radiation-induced sarcoma.

There are many histologic subtypes of soft-tissue sarcoma. Typically, low-grade sarcomas include desmoids or liposarcomas with low-grade features. Next most frequently seen are malignant fibrosarcoma, rhabdomyosarcoma, and malignant fibrous histiocytoma, which are usually high-grade lesions.

Individual histologic subtype is not by itself a significant prognostic variable, but histologic grade is very significant. Metastases—either synchronous or metachronous—occur most commonly to the lungs (75%) and must be ruled out with chest CT prior to surgery. If present, these should be resected if negative margins can be achieved and adequate lung function preserved. Therapy for low-grade lesions should consist of complete resection. Incompletely resected lesions should be treated with external beam radiation therapy. High-grade lesions should be resected and patients enrolled into clinical trials evaluating the efficacy of systemic adjuvant chemotherapy. Postoperative radiotherapy is often helpful in the setting of close margins or tumor spillage. Notable histologic subtypes include the following.

1. Fibrosarcomas—Fibrosarcoma is the most common primary soft-tissue cancer of the chest wall. It occurs most frequently in young adults. A subtype of this tumor is neurofibrosarcoma, which involves the thoracic wall almost twice as often as other parts of the body. Also referred to as malignant peripheral nerve sheath tumors or malignant schwannomas, they often occur in patients with neurofibromatosis and usually originate from intercostal nerves. Treatment is neoadjuvant chemotherapy followed by resection.

2. Malignant fibrous histiocytoma/high-grade pleomorphic sarcoma—Malignant fibrous histiocytoma has a bimodal distribution, with peaks between 20 and 30 years of age and between 50 and 60 years of age. Although they are the most common soft-tissue sarcoma of adults, they rarely rise from the chest wall. Treatment is neoadjuvant chemotherapy followed by resection, followed by additional adjuvant chemotherapy.

3. Rhabdomyosarcoma—Rhabdomyosarcoma is an uncommon tumor in adults but is the second most common chest wall tumor in children. Treatment is neoadjuvant chemoradiation, surgical resection, and then ongoing chemotherapy and radiation. These tumors are aggressive and often unresectable.

4. Liposarcomas—These tumors account for approximately one-third of all primary cancers of the chest wall and have many subtypes. They occur more often in men. In general, those that are encapsulated carry a better surgical prognosis. Treatment is wide local excision and chest wall reconstruction. Adjuvant therapy should be considered, although it remains controversial.

C. Benign Skeletal Tumors

1. Chondromas, osteochondromas, and myxochondromas—The combined frequency of these three cartilaginous tumors is about 30%-45% of all benign skeletal tumors. Cartilaginous tumors are usually single and occur with equal frequency in males and females between childhood and the fourth decade. The tumors are usually painless and tend to occur anteriorly along the costal margin or in the parasternal area. A key to management is differentiating the benign chondroma from the malignant chondrosarcoma. Often wide local excision is curative.

2. Fibrous dysplasia—Fibrous dysplasia (bone cyst, osteofibroma, fibrous osteoma, fibrosis ossificans) accounts for one-third or more of benign skeletal tumors of the chest wall. This cystic bone tumor can occur in any portion of the skeletal system, but approximately half involve the ribs. The differential diagnosis includes cystic bone lesions associated with hyperparathyroidism. The tumor is usually single and may be related to previous trauma. Some patients experience swelling, tenderness, or vague discomfort, but the lesion is usually silent and is detected on routine chest x-ray. Treatment consists of local excision.

3. Eosinophilic granuloma—Eosinophilic granuloma may occur in the clavicle, the scapula, or (rarely) the sternum. Coexisting infiltrates of the lung are often present. This condition often represents a more benign form of Langerhans cell histiocytosis or Hand–Schüller–Christian disease. Fever, malaise, leukocytosis, eosinophilia, or bone pain may be present. Rib involvement presents as a swelling with cortical bone destruction and new periosteal growth. The clinical picture can resemble osteomyelitis or Ewing sarcoma. When the disease is localized, excision will result in cure.

4. Hemangioma—Cavernous hemangioma of the ribs presents as a painful mass in infancy or childhood. The tumor appears on chest x-ray either as multiple radiolucent areas or as a single trabeculated cyst.

5. Miscellaneous—Fibromas, lipomas, osteomas, and aneurysmal bone cysts are all relatively rare lesions of the chest wall. The diagnosis is established after excisional biopsy. Given their relative infrequent nature, providers are encouraged to seek multidisciplinary guidance.

D. Malignant Skeletal Tumors

1. Chondrosarcomas—Chondrosarcomas are the most common primary malignant tumor of the chest wall (20%-40%). They most commonly develop from the costochondral junctions of the first four ribs but can involve the sternum. About 15%-20% of all skeletal chondrosarcomas occur in the ribs or sternum. Most appear in patients 20-40 years of age. Local involvement of pleura, adjacent ribs, muscle, diaphragm, or other soft tissue may develop. Pain is uncommon and most patients complain only of the mass. Chest x-ray shows destroyed cortical bone, usually with diffuse mottled calcification, and the border of the tumor is indistinct. Successful treatment necessitates wide local excision and en bloc resection to achieve negative margins. Incomplete excision carries a significantly worse prognosis. Overall survival, as in all soft-tissue sarcomas, is heavily dependent on the histologic grade. Completely resected low-grade chondrosarcoma has a 60%-80% 5-year survival rate. Patients with high-grade lesions who subsequently develop distant metastasis have only a 20%-30% 5-year survival.

Although complete resection can often be curative, local recurrence portends future metastatic disease and poor survival. Therefore, even in the setting of large tumors (>15-20 cm), resection should be considered even if it necessitates removal of more than eight ribs. With epidural pain control and immediate reconstruction techniques, most patients will do well. Despite large chest wall resections, most patients can be immediately extubated and will not suffer drastic changes in pulmonary function or chest wall dynamics.

2. Ewing sarcoma (hemangioendothelioma, endothelioma)—

Ewing sarcoma is a small, round cell-type tumor which most commonly occurs in a single rib. It accounts for 10%-15% of all primary chest wall tumors, although its presentation as a primary chest lesion is not common (<15%). Typically, Ewing sarcoma presents as a large, warm, painful soft-tissue mass usually associated with a pleural effusion. Systemic symptoms such as fever, malaise, and weight loss are common. Radiologic studies demonstrate the classic "onion skin" appearance caused by widening and sclerosis of the cortex as multiple layers of new bone are produced.

Diagnosis can usually be made by fine-needle aspirate or incisional biopsy. Histologically, these tumors are unique and consist of broad sheets of small polyhedral cells with pale cytoplasm and small hyperchromatic nuclei. They stain periodic acid-Schiff-positive.

Ewing sarcoma is commonly a disease of childhood and adolescence. The most important prognostic indicator for survival is development of distant metastases. Current therapy consists of neoadjuvant chemotherapy (including cyclophosphamide, dactinomycin, doxorubicin, and vincristine) and surgical resection if the tumor is well demarcated and can be completely resected. Radiotherapy may be indicated as postoperative adjuvant treatment, or in the case of tumors that are not completely resectable. Overall, 5-year survival rates range from 15% to 70%. Long-term survival (10 years) is achievable in patients who do not develop metastases, and approaches 50% in those receiving multiagent chemotherapy in addition to local resection.

3. Osteogenic sarcoma (osteosarcoma)—

Osteosarcoma occurs in the second and third decades, and 60% of cases occur in men. It is more aggressive than chondrosarcoma. X-ray findings consist of bone destruction and recalcification at right angles to the bony cortex, which gives the characteristic "sunburst" appearance. Osteogenic sarcoma most commonly presents as an extremity lesion, with only a small percentage of cases being chest wall primaries. Overall, less than 5% of all osteogenic sarcomas arise in the chest wall. Osteogenic sarcoma occurs in the second to fourth decades of life, half-again more commonly in men than in women. It is associated with environmental triggers, as well as with mutations in the retinoblastoma gene (RB1, 500-1000 times the risk) and Li–Fraumeni syndrome (p53, 15 times the risk). Typically, it is a more aggressive tumor with a propensity for early metastasis to lung and bone.

Osteogenic sarcoma differs from chondrosarcoma in that it is usually sensitive to chemotherapy. It is relatively unresponsive to radiation. They are treated with neoadjuvant chemotherapy followed by surgical resection. Even with neoadjuvant treatment, however, overall 5-year survival rate after complete resection and postoperative chemotherapy may only be 15%.

4. Myeloma (solitary plasmacytoma)—

Solitary plasmacytomas of the chest wall are comparatively rare lesions. They constitute 5%-20% of all chest wall tumors. Radiologically, they present as classic "punched-out" lytic lesions in the ribs and sternum without evidence of new bone formation. They are more common in men than in women and typically present in the fifth to seventh decades of life. Over 75% of the time, solitary chest wall plasmacytomas are associated with diffuse multiple myeloma. Survival is based on the development of systemic disease. Local control and relief of pain are achieved with radiation therapy (usually 3000-4600 cGy). Once progressive, systemic disease is diagnosed, treatment consists of chemotherapy. Overall, 5-year and 10-year survivals for solitary plasmacytomas of the chest wall are 35%-40% and 15%-20%, respectively. Typical median survival rates after treatment with radiation therapy and chemotherapy average 56 months.

E. Metastatic Chest Wall Tumors

Metastases to bones of the thorax are often multiple and are usually from tumors of the kidney, thyroid, lung, breast, prostate, stomach, uterus, or colon. Renal cell and thyroid malignancies have a high propensity for metastasizing to the sternum. Occasionally, they present as a pulsatile mass due to the excessive vascularity of the metastasis. An aneurysm of the ascending thoracic aorta, while rare, must be considered in the differential diagnosis and ruled out with imaging modalities prior to attempts at excisional biopsy. Involvement by direct extension occurs in carcinoma of the breast and lung. Primary lung cancer with direct extension to chest wall without nodal involvement (T3 N0) carries a reasonable 5-year survival (40%-50%) when treated with radical en bloc resection. Lung metastasis with direct chest wall extension should be treated with radical en bloc resection of the chest wall and underlying lung.

Ferraro P, et al. Principles of chest wall resection and reconstruction. *Thorac Surg Clin*. 2010;20(4):465.

Hemmati SH, et al. The prognostic factors of chest wall metastasis resection. *Eur J Cardiothorac Surg*. 2011;40(2):328.

Smith SE, Keshavjee S. Primary chest wall tumors. *Thoracic Surg Clin*. 2010;20(4):495.

Stelzer P, Gay WA Jr. Tumors of the chest wall. *Surg Clin North Am*, 1980;60:779-791.

Van Geel AN, et al. Chest wall resection for adult soft tissue sarcomas and chondrosarcomas: Analysis of prognostic factors. *World J Surg*. 2011;35(1):63-69.

▼ DISEASES OF THE PLEURA

Diseases of the pleura may be benign or malignant, and may represent primary pleural processes, localized extrapleural disease, or systemic illness. The most common pleural problem is the presence of air (pneumothorax) within the pleural space. Pleural effusions—accumulations of fluid—result from benign sterile fluid, malignant fluid, pus, chyle, or blood. Primary pleural tumors are uncommon, but involvement of the pleura with metastatic cancer is common.

The most common symptoms of pleural disease are pain and dyspnea. The pain is sharp, and it is characteristically worsened by respiratory movements, often inhibiting inspiration. Pleural pain is mediated through somatic intercostal nerves of the chest wall (cervical and costal pleura) and through the phrenic nerve (diaphragmatic and mediastinal pleura), causing chest wall or back pain and pain referred to the shoulder, respectively. The visceral pleura contains only sympathetic and parasympathetic nerve fibers and therefore is insensate; however, extension of visceral processes to involve the parietal pleura can produce typical pleuritic chest pain.

PLEURAL EFFUSION

Pleural effusion is the presence of fluid within the pleural space. More specific terminology may be used when the nature of the fluid is known. Hydrothorax is a collection of serous (most often transudative but also exudative) fluid, while pus in the pleural cavity is referred to as a pyothorax or empyema. Additional terms are used for blood (hemothorax) and chyle (chylothorax). Abnormal pleural fluid accumulates as a result of one or more of the following mechanisms: (1) increase in the pulmonary vascular hydrostatic pressure (congestive heart failure, mitral stenosis); (2) decrease in the vascular colloid oncotic pressure (hypoproteinemia); (3) increase in the capillary permeability due to inflammation (pneumonia, pancreatitis, sepsis); (4) decrease in the

intrapleural pressure (atelectasis); (5) decrease in lymphatic drainage (carcinomatosis); (6) transdiaphragmatic movement of abdominal fluid through lymphatics or physical defects (ascites, pancreatic pseudocyst rupture); and (7) rupture of a vascular or lymphatic structure (traumatic injury).

Signs of a pleural effusion include decreased respiratory excursion, diminished breath sounds, dullness to percussion, or a pleural friction rub. With long-standing and advanced disease, contraction of the hemithorax with narrowed intercostal spaces and localized bulging, swelling, or redness may occur. Chest radiographs demonstrate varying degrees of opacification of the ipsilateral hemithorax. Accumulation of 300-500 mL of fluid causes blunting of the costophrenic angle on x-ray. If the entire hemithorax is opacified, 2000-2500 mL may be present. The mediastinum may be shifted to the contralateral side in the presence of a large effusion, or it may remain in the midline—particularly if proximal bronchial obstruction results in lobar or total lung atelectasis, if the mediastinum is fixed from fibrosis or tumor infiltration, if the ipsilateral lung is infiltrated with tumor, or if malignant mesothelioma is present. CT scanning may be required to evaluate complex, loculated, or recurrent pleural fluid collections. Interventional radiology services are useful for loculated pleural effusions that may be best managed by CT-guided percutaneous drain placement.

Generally, serous effusions are separated into two broad categories—transudates and exudates—based on the physical and cellular characteristics of the pleural fluid. Identification of the specific type of effusion aids in determination of the cause and most often depends on examination of at least 20 mL of fluid obtained by thoracentesis. Basic tests should include total protein, lactate dehydrogenase (LDH), total and differential cell counts, glucose, pH, cytology, and Gram stain with culture. Furthermore, simultaneous serum total protein, LDH, and glucose should be measured to calculate Light's criteria for exudative effusions. Effusions with total protein content less than 3 g/dL (or a fluid–serum ratio lower than 0.5), an LDH level less than 200 units/dL (or a fluid–serum ratio lower than 0.6), and a specific gravity below 1.016 represent transudates, while all other effusions are classified as exudates. The results of these basic tests frequently allow the underlying pathologic process to be elucidated (see Table 19–1).

1. Hydrothorax

▶ Malignancy

More than 25% of all pleural effusions are secondary to cancer, and 35% of patients with lung cancer, 23% of patients with breast cancer, and 10% of patients with lymphoma develop malignant pleural effusions during the course of their disease. Approximately 10% of malignant effusions are secondary to primary pleural tumors, mostly mesothelioma. The mechanism is primarily through lymphatic obstruction

Table 19–1. Differential diagnosis of pleural effusions.

	Tuberculosis	Cancer	Congestive Heart Failure	Pneumonia and Other Nontuberculous Infections	Rheumatoid Arthritis and Collagen Disease	Pulmonary Embolism
Clinical context	Younger patient with history of exposure to tuberculosis.	Older patient in poor general health.	Presence of congestive heart failure.	Presence of respiratory infection.	History of joint involvement; subcutaneous nodules.	Postoperative immobilized, or venous disease.
Gross appearance	Usually serous; often sanguineous.	Often sanguineous.	Serous.	Serous.	Turbid or yellow-green.	Often sanguineous.
Microscopic examination	May be positive for acid-fast bacilli; cholesterol crystals.	Cytology positive in 50%.	—	May be positive for bacilli.	—	—
Cell count	Few have >10,000 erythrocytes; most have >1000 leukocytes, mostly lymphocytes.	Two-thirds bloody; 40% >1000 leukocytes, mostly lymphocytes.	Few have >10,000 erythrocytes or >1000 leukocytes.	Polymorphonuclears predominate.	Lymphocytes predominate.	Erythrocytes predominate.
Culture	May have positive pleural effusion; few have positive sputum or gastric washings.	—	—	May be positive.	—	—
Specific gravity	Most >1.016.	Most >1.016.	Most >1.016.	>1.016.	>1.016.	>1.016.
Protein	90% 3 g/dL or more.	90% 3 g/dL or more.	75% >3 g/dL.	3 g/dL or more.	3 g/dL or more.	3 g/dL or more.
Sugar	60% <60 mg/dL.	Rarely <60 mg/dL.	—	Occasionally <60 mg/dL.	5-17 g/dL (rheumatoid arthritis).	—
Other	No mesothelial cells on cytology. Tuberculin test usually positive. Pleural biopsy positive.	If hemorrhagic fluid, 65% will be due to tumor; tends to recur after removal.	Right-sided in 55%-70%.	Associated with infiltrate on x-ray.	Rapid clotting time; LE cell or rheumatoid factor may be present.	Source of emboli may be noted.

Other exudates: Specific gravity > 1.016.
Fungal infection: Exposure in endemic area. Source fluid. Microscopy and culture may be positive for fungi. Protein 3 g/dL or more. Skin and serologic tests may be helpful.
Trauma: Serosanguineous fluid. Protein 3 g/dL or more.
Chylothorax: History of procedure, injury, or cancer. Chylous fluid with no protein but with fat droplets.

Modified with permission from Therapy of pleural effusion. A statement by the Committee on Therapy, *Am Rev Respir Dis* 1968;Mar;97(3):479-483.

in either the peripheral lung or central lymph node channels of the mediastinum. Malignant pleural effusions can be serous, serosanguineous, or bloody and are diagnosed primarily by demonstrating malignant cells in the fluid. Cytologic confirmation is successful 50%, 65%, and 70% of the time after one, two, or three thoracenteses, respectively. Closed pleural biopsy alone is successful in only 50% of cases, but coupled with thoracentesis it can increase the diagnostic yield to 80%. Thoracoscopy with direct pleural biopsy, however, is successful in 97% of patients and should be considered in any patient with a suspicious effusion after two negative thoracenteses.

Treatment of malignant effusions is strictly palliative. As most patients die within 3-6 months of developing a malignant pleural effusion, prompt diagnosis and therapy are essential. The goals of treatment are lung reexpansion and pleural symphysis. This is most readily accomplished with placement of a chest tube (20-28F) and closed-tube drainage for 24-48 hours. Generally, no more than 1 L is allowed to drain initially. Subsequently, 200-500 mL is allowed to drain every 1-2 hours until the effusion is fully drained. This controlled draining avoids the rare complication of reexpansion pulmonary edema. Once full lung expansion is obtained, pleurodesis should be performed with an appropriate agent before loculations have formed. Different chemical, radioactive, and infectious agents have been used in the past with varying success rates, but most commonly used are talc (87%-100% insufflation; 83%-100% slurry), or doxycycline. Finally, mechanical pleurectomy without chemical instillation can control pleural effusions in over 99% of patients, but this requires an operative procedure. Talc is inexpensive, highly effective, and easily administered either as a powder insufflated into the open chest or as a slurry instilled through a chest tube.

Complications following pleurodesis include pneumothorax, loculated hydrothorax, fever, infection (empyema), acute respiratory distress syndrome (ARDS, particularly following bilateral simultaneous pleurodeses, which for this reason alone are contraindicated), and recurrence. Problems are uncommon, and most patients can have their chest tubes removed within 48-72 hours following talc pleurodesis. Among patients who are not candidates for pleuordesis, palliative options can include placement of a long-term, indwelling tunneled pleural catheter.

Cardiovascular Disease

Pleural effusions are common findings in patients with moderate to severe congestive heart failure. Heart failure may be secondary to ischemia, valvular heart disease, viral myocarditis, congenital heart disease, or other less common lesions. The effusion may be bilateral or unilateral. Although bilateral effusions occur more frequently, when unilateral, the right hemithorax is most often affected. Fluid frequently involves the interlobar fissures (most commonly the minor fissure on the right) and can form localized collections simulating mass lesions known as "pseudotumors." Other cardiovascular causes of pleural effusions include constrictive pericarditis and pulmonary venous obstruction.

Renal Disease

Hydronephrosis, nephrotic syndrome, and acute glomerulonephritis are on occasion associated with pleural effusions. Rupture of the collecting system into the pleural space can also produce a hydrothorax. In this latter case, the pleural fluid creatinine will be elevated (fluid–serum creatinine ratio significantly greater than 1.0).

Pancreatitis

Moderate to severe pancreatitis is associated with a pleural effusion that characteristically occurs on the left and contains fluid with an amylase concentration substantially higher than that in the serum. Rarely pseudocysts of the capsule of the pancreas may communicate with the pleural space, resulting in *high-volume* pleural effusions.

Cirrhosis

Approximately 5% of patients with cirrhosis and ascites will develop a pleural effusion. In contrast to pancreatitis, nearly all of these effusions occur on the right side.

Thromboembolism

Pulmonary thromboemboli are sometimes accompanied by a pleural effusion. These effusions are typically serosanguineous and small, but they may be frankly bloody and massive. Characteristic x-ray findings are almost always present in the lung. Since the fluid is usually reabsorbed in a short period of time, drainage is seldom necessary.

2. Thoracic Empyema

Pyothorax (empyema thoracis) is the accumulation of pus within the pleural cavity. The pus is usually thick, creamy, and malodorous. If empyema occurs in the setting of underlying suppurative lung disease (ie, pneumonia, lung abscess, or bronchiectasis), it is referred to as a parapneumonic empyema (60% of cases). Other causes of thoracic empyema are surgery (20%), trauma (10%), esophageal rupture, other chest wall or mediastinal infections, bronchopleural fistula, extension of a subphrenic or hepatic abscess, instrumentation of the pleural space (thoracentesis, chest tube placement, etc), and rarely, hematogenous seeding from a distant site of infection.

Empyemas are divided into three phases based on their natural history: acute exudative, fibrinopurulent, and chronic organizing. The *acute exudative phase* is characterized by the outpouring of sterile pleural fluid (incited by pleural inflammation), with a low viscosity, white blood cell count, and LDH concentration as well as normal glucose level and normal pH. The pleura remains mobile during this phase. The *fibrinopurulent phase* develops at approximately 2-7 days, marked by an increase in the turbidity, white blood cell count, and LDH levels in the fluid. Glucose levels and pH of the fluid decrease and fibrin is deposited on pleural surfaces, limiting the empyema but also fixing (trapping) the lung. The chronic organizing phase begins 7-28 days after the onset of the disease and is characterized by a pleural fluid glucose level less than 40 mg/dL and a pH less than 7.0. The pleural exudate becomes thick, and the pleural fibrin deposits thicken and begin to organize, further immobilizing the lung. In patients with inadequately treated chronic

Table 19–2. Incidence of various complications of staphylococcal pneumonia in adults and children (in %).

	Adults	Children
Abscess	25	50
Empyema	15	15
Pneumatocele	1	35
Effusion	30	55
Bronchopleural fistula	2	5

empyema, erosion through the chest wall (empyema necessitatis), chondritis, osteomyelitis of the ribs or vertebral bodies, pericarditis, and mediastinal abscesses may occur.

The bacteriology of thoracic empyema has evolved over the years. Prior to the discovery of penicillin in the 1940s, most empyemas were caused by pneumococci and streptococci. With modern antibiotics and improved anaerobic culture techniques, however, the most common isolates from adult empyemas are now anaerobic bacteria, particularly *Bacteroides* species as well as *Fusobacterium* and *Peptococcus* species.

Staphylococcus is the most common organism causing empyema (92% in children under 2 years old), and staphylococcal empyema is one of the most common complications of staphylococcal pneumonias in both adults and children (Table 19–2). Gram-negative bacteria also continue to be significant pathogens, particularly in parapneumonic empyemas. *Escherichia coli* and pseudomonas species account for 66% of aerobic gram-negative empyemas, and other organisms include *Klebsiella pneumoniae, Proteus* species, *Enterobacter aerogenes,* and *Salmonella.* Rarely, fungi (*Aspergillus, Coccidioides immitis, Blastomyces,* and *Histoplasma capsulatum*) and parasites such as *Entamoeba histolytica* can cause empyemas. In a review, empyemas were found to contain anaerobic bacteria in only 35% of cases, aerobic bacteria in only 24%, and a combination in 41%. In addition, the average number of bacterial species isolated was 3.2 per patient.

Aspiration of oropharyngeal flora may represent a source of polymicrobial infection.

Although patients may rarely be completely asymptomatic, most patients with thoracic empyemas present with varying symptoms depending on the underlying disease process, the extent of the pleural involvement, and the immunologic state of the patient. Patients typically complain of fever, pleuritic chest pain or a sense of chest heaviness, dyspnea, hemoptysis, and a cough usually productive of purulent sputum. Signs of thoracic empyema include anemia, tachycardia, tachypnea, diminished breath sounds with dullness to percussion on the involved side, clubbing of fingertips, and occasionally pulmonary osteoarthropathy.

Although the medical history and physical examination often suggest the presence of thoracic empyema, the plain chest radiograph is the most important noninvasive diagnostic test. Empyema may be associated with an underlying pneumonia, lung abscess, or pleural effusion and appear as posterolateral D-shaped densities on x-ray. In large empyemas, the mediastinum may be shifted away from the affected side. Bronchoscopy should be performed on all patients to exclude the presence of endobronchial obstruction. CT scanning provides critical anatomic detail regarding loculations and can assist in differentiation of empyema from lung abscess.

Thoracentesis is the procedure of choice for the diagnosis of thoracic empyema. Aspiration of pus establishes the diagnosis, permitting identification of the offending organisms. In early empyemas—particularly those partially treated with antibiotics—the pleural fluid may not be frankly purulent. In these cases, a pleural fluid pH less than 7.0, glucose less than 40 mg/dL, and an LDH level greater than 1000 units/L strongly suggest an evolving empyema even if Gram stain and cultures fail to identify organisms.

Goals for the treatment of thoracic empyemas include (1) control of the infection, (2) removal of the purulent material with obliteration and sterilization of the pleural space and reexpansion of the lung, and (3) elimination of the underlying disease process.

Options for treatment include repeated thoracentesis, closed tube thoracostomy, rib resection and open drainage, decortication and empyemectomy, thoracoplasty, and muscle flap closure. Adjunctive maneuvers reported to aid in the disruption and drainage of loculated empyemas include instillation of fibrinolytic enzymes (such as tPA) and video-assisted thoracoscopic debridement. A rational approach to empyema management is outlined in Figure 19–8. Initially, an intercostal catheter of adequate size is carefully inserted into the most dependent portion of the empyema cavity. If after 24-72 hours sepsis persists—or if there is any question as to the adequacy of drainage—a CT scan should be obtained. If, on the other hand, complete drainage and reexpansion of the lung are achieved, no further drainage procedures are necessary.

Patients with residual spaces that are inadequately drained, patients with continued sepsis, and patients thought to require prolonged tube drainage are candidates for open drainage procedures. These can usually be safely performed 10-14 days after closed-tube drainage, since the pleurae fuse by that time and the risk of pneumothorax and lung collapse is eliminated. Options for open drainage include simple rib resection and open flap drainage (Eloesser procedure). Simple rib resection involves the removal of short segments (3-6 cm) of one, two, or three ribs at the most dependent portion of the empyema cavity (at or anterior to the posterior axillary line). A tube can be placed through this opening and effective drainage established. A second approach involves

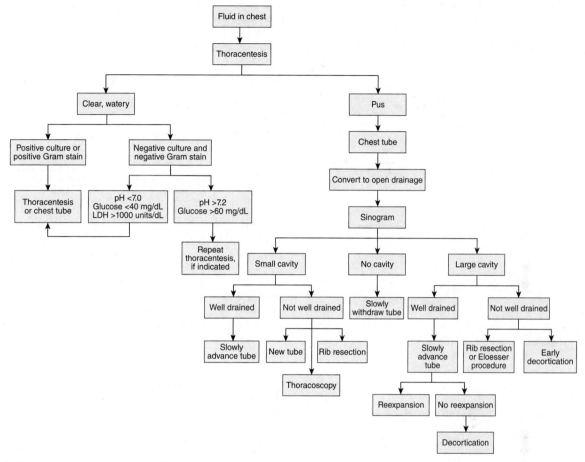

▲ **Figure 19–8.** Management of empyema. (Modified with permission from Shields TW: *General Thoracic Surgery*, 3rd ed. Philadelphia, PA: Williams & Wilkins; 1989.)

the creation of a U-shaped flap of chest wall that is sewn to the parietal pleura after resection of short segments (3-6 cm) of one, two, or three ribs. This creates an epithelialized tract for long-term tubeless drainage of empyema cavities. This type of open drainage allows the empyema cavity to drain reliably and to be easily debrided, irrigated, and cleaned. Ultimately, through lung reexpansion, wound contraction, and granulation, the cavity often completely disappears.

Another option is early decortication and empyemectomy. This is especially useful for good-risk patients with early loculated empyemas and inadequate tube drainage or lung expansion. Furthermore, if performed early in the course of the process, resection of both parietal and visceral pleural peels (decortication) can be performed as a thoracoscopic procedure. More advanced or chronic disease involves a thoracotomy with decortication with resection of the intact empyema itself (empyemectomy), if possible. The best results with this approach are obtained when the underlying

lung is entirely normal and reexpands fully. Posttraumatic empyema, in particular, has been amenable to this treatment.

Empyemas that occur following pulmonary resection may be difficult to manage. If residual lung is present (resections less than pneumonectomy), the general principles outlined above still apply, although a complicating bronchopleural fistula is often present (Figure 19–9). Simple tube drainage is instituted initially followed by open drainage if necessary. Empyemas following pneumonectomy, however, pose a special problem because there is no longer any lung to obliterate the infected space. In addition, postpneumonectomy empyemas frequently are associated with bronchopleural fistulas. In these patients, specific surgical procedures designed to obliterate residual intrathoracic spaces and in many cases close remaining bronchopleural fistulas may be required (Figure 19–10). In the absence of a bronchopleural fistula, sterilization and closure of a postpneumonectomy space (without obliteration) may be attempted using an

▲ **Figure 19–9. Postlobectomy empyema.** (Modified with permission from Shields TW: *General Thoracic Surgery*, 3rd ed. Philadelphia, PA: Williams & Wilkins; 1989.)

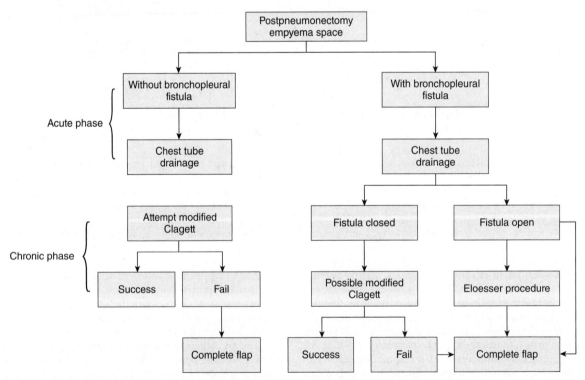

▲ **Figure 19–10. Postpneumonectomy empyema.** (Modified with permission from Shields TW: *General Thoracic Surgery*, 3rd ed. Philadelphia, PA: Williams & Wilkins; 1989.)

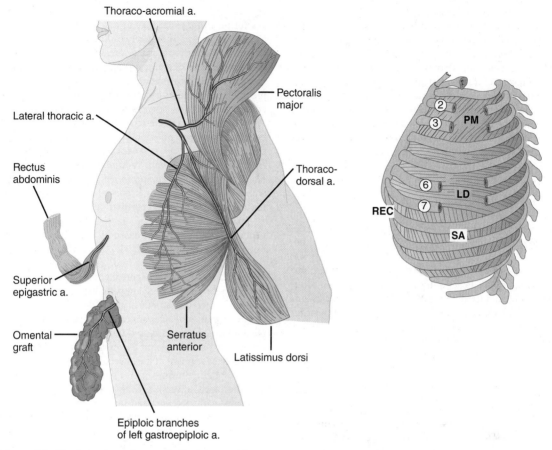

▲ Figure 19–11. Extrathoracic muscle flap closure of a postpneumonectomy empyema cavity.

irrigation catheter inserted into the apex of the chest cavity. An antibiotic solution specific for the organisms present is then infused into the chest. The solution is allowed to drain through a dependent tube or opening created by simple rib resection. After 2-8 weeks, the catheters are removed and the cavity is closed. The success rate with this technique is quite variable ranging in the literature from 20% to 88%. For patients who fail this approach and for those patients with bronchopleural fistulas, the main goal of therapy is to obliterate the residual space and close any bronchopleural fistulas. This is most readily accomplished by the transposition of muscle with or without omentum into the empyema cavity. Multiple muscles may be required, including pectoralis major, latissimus dorsi, serratus anterior, intercostal muscle, and rectus abdominis (Figure 19–11). Use of these muscles is highly successful in closing any remaining bronchopleural fistulas and in completely obliterating the remaining intrathoracic space. The success of muscle flap closure of empyema spaces has made thoracoplasty (once a common procedure for reducing empyema spaces) a rare operation.

Antibiotics are an important adjunct in the treatment of empyemas, but it must be emphasized that source control via drainage is the primary treatment modality. Although antibiotic therapy is always instituted early in the course of therapy when signs of systemic infection generally are present, they need not be continued once effective drainage is established. In fact, overuse of antibiotics may lead to the generation of resistant bacteria and therefore compromise the success of any subsequent procedures designed to obliterate residual intrathoracic space.

Krassas A, et al. Current indications and results for thoracoplasty and intrathoracic muscle transposition. *Eur J Cardiothorac Surg.* 2010;37(5):1215.

3. Hemothorax

Blood in the pleural space usually occurs secondary to trauma, surgery, diagnostic or therapeutic procedures, neoplasms, pulmonary infarction, and infections (tuberculosis). Most hemothoraces can be treated effectively with large-bore (28-36F) closed chest tube drainage, particularly since small amounts of blood (occupying less than one-third of the hemithorax) are readily reabsorbed by the body. However, if significant blood clot has formed (occupying more than one-third of the hemithorax) or if secondary infection occurs, further measures must be taken to avoid the development of an empyema or fibrothorax with pulmonary compromise. Many hemothoraces requiring more than simple tube drainage can be managed with VATS procedures. Rarely, open thoracotomy may be required for complete decortication and evacuation.

4. Chylothorax

Accumulation of chyle within the pleural space is most often due to surgical procedures, particularly cardiothoracic and esophageal operations. Trauma, malignancy, central venous catheterization, congenital lymphatic malformations, thoracic aortic aneurysms, filariasis, and cirrhosis may also rarely cause chylothorax (from chylous ascites passing transdiaphragmatically). Penetrating thoracic trauma can lacerate the thoracic duct at any level, but blunt thoracic trauma usually causes a shearing of the duct at the right crus of the diaphragm. This may also occur with violent coughing or hyperextension of the spine. The initial treatment of chylothorax is similar to that of a malignant pleural effusion. Closed chest tube drainage is instituted; the lung is fully reexpanded; and a low-fat diet is started. In some cases, intravenous hyperalimentation (either peripheral or central) may greatly improve the patient's condition. Some evidence supports the use of somatostatin to decrease the output from chylous effusions. The irritating nature of chyle promotes pleurodesis, and in half of patients the leak will stop spontaneously. The instillation of sclerosing agents (see section on pleural effusion, above) has also been advocated to increase the chances of success. If chyle continues to drain for more than 7 days or if significant drainage continues for even a shorter period of time, serious consideration should be given to operation since patients quickly become malnourished from the large associated protein losses. Video-assisted thoracoscopic techniques are usually ideal, making open thoracotomy rarely necessary. The standard approach is via the right chest, where the thoracic duct may be identified as it emerges from beneath the diaphragm between the aorta and the azygos vein. Ligation of the tissues in this area is usually all that is needed. Recently, treatment including lymphangiography with percutaneous thoracic duct embolization has become a viable option in centers with an experienced interventional radiology team.

PNEUMOTHORAX

Air in the pleural space (pneumothorax) can occur as a result of a breach in either the parietal (trauma, esophageal perforation, surgery, etc) or visceral pleura (bulla, fine-needle aspirations, etc). Rarely, infections of the pleural space with gas-forming organisms may produce a pneumothorax. Since a chest radiograph is only a two-dimensional representation of a three-dimensional space, a relatively small separation of the pleural surfaces (eg, 1 cm) on a chest x-ray can translate into a relatively large pneumothorax. A large amount of intrapleural air that causes a shift of the mediastinum toward the contralateral lung is referred to as a tension pneumothorax. A pneumothorax associated with an open chest wound may be termed an open pneumothorax or sometimes a "sucking chest wound." *Tension and open pneumothoraces are surgical emergencies because both ventilation and venous return of blood to the heart are compromised.* Intrapleural air may mix with blood, as frequently occurs after trauma (hemopneumothorax) or esophageal perforation (pyopneumothorax).

Pneumothoraces usually are classified as either spontaneous or acquired (those caused by a specific event such as trauma, invasive procedures, etc). Spontaneous pneumothoraces sometimes are divided into "primary" and "secondary" categories; however, all spontaneous pneumothoraces are secondary to some underlying pathologic process, and such a division is therefore strictly artificial. Most commonly, spontaneous pneumothoraces are caused by rupture of small subpleural blebs due to increased transpulmonary pressure most pronounced at the apex of the lung (apex of the upper lobe and superior segment of the lower lobe). Coughing, rapid falls in atmospheric pressure (>10 millibars/24 h), rapid decompression (scuba divers), and high altitudes (jet pilots) all are associated with increased transpulmonary pressures and spontaneous pneumothorax. In addition, normal transpulmonary pressures can cause rupture of blebs in patients with connective tissue disorders such as Marfan syndrome. Other causes of spontaneous pneumothorax include apical bullae (patients with COPD), *Pneumocystis* pneumonia (patients with AIDS), metastatic cancer (particularly sarcomas), lymphangioleiomyomatosis, eosinophilic granuloma, rupture of the esophagus or of a lung abscess, cystic fibrosis (CF), and menstruation (catamenial pneumothorax). Classically, however, spontaneous pneumothoraces occur in tall, slender males (male-to-female ratio 6:1) between the ages of 16 and 24, often with a history of smoking. The true incidence is unknown, since up to 20% of patients remain asymptomatic and do not seek medical attention.

Patients with pneumothoraces complain of pleuritic chest pain and dyspnea. If severe underlying cardiopulmonary disease exists or if a tension pneumothorax develops, symptoms become much more dramatic and include diaphoresis, cyanosis, weakness, and symptoms of hypotension and cardiovascular collapse. Physical examination reveals tachypnea, tachycardia, deviation of the trachea away from the involved side (tension pneumothorax), decreased breath sounds, hyperresonance, and diminished vocal fremitus on the involved side. Arterial blood gases may demonstrate hypoxia and occasionally hypocapnia from hyperventilation, and the ECG may show axis deviations, nonspecific ST segment changes, and T-wave inversion. The standard test for the diagnosis of pneumothoraces is the posteroanterior (PA) and lateral chest radiograph. Exhalation accentuates the contrast between the collapsed lung and the intrapleural air as well as the magnitude of the collapse. Rarely, a CT scan may be necessary to differentiate a pneumothorax from a large bulla in patients with severe emphysema. In 5%-10% of patients, a small pleural effusion may be present and can be hemorrhagic.

The treatment of spontaneous pneumothoraces varies depending on the patient's symptoms and condition, the degree of collapse, the cause, and the estimate of the chance of recurrence. Small (<20%-25%), stable, asymptomatic pneumothoraces in otherwise healthy patients can be followed (often on an outpatient basis) with the expectation of complete resolution within several weeks, since air is normally reabsorbed at a rate of 1%-1.25% per day. Larger asymptomatic pneumothoraces taking longer than 2-3 weeks to resolve place the patient at risk for developing trapped lung as a result of deposition of fibrin on the visceral pleura. These patients—as well as patients with symptoms, increasing pneumothoraces, or pneumothoraces associated with pleural effusions—should have them evacuated. In highly selected patients, this can be accomplished with simple aspiration as long as the immediate and 2-hour delayed chest radiographs document reexpansion. It should be emphasized, however, that some small breaks in the visceral pleural seal once the lung collapses and can reopen with reexpansion. The chance of recurrence is 20%-50% with this method, and follow-up x-ray is therefore mandatory after 24 hours.

Most patients with significant pneumothoraces (>30%) require placement of a closed-chest catheter (8-20F) for acceptable reexpansion, which is the gold standard treatment. This catheter then can be placed either to underwater suction drainage or to a Heimlich (one-way) valve. If a Heimlich valve maintains full expansion, the patient may be treated as an outpatient; however, if a Heimlich valve fails to reexpand the lung fully or if the patient's condition is not optimal, admission to hospital and underwater chest tube suction drainage is required. Unless some contraindication exists, chest tubes should be placed in the midaxillary line at the level of the fifth intercostal space (nipple line). Placement with the use of blunt clamp dissection avoids the dangers of trocar insertion and should almost always be used. Following resolution of any air leakage, the tube may be taken off suction (water seal) and removed if the lung remains fully inflated. In patients with classic spontaneous pneumothoraces, the chance of recurrence increases with each episode. Following a single episode, the risk of a recurrent pneumothorax is 40%-50%. After two episodes, the risk increases to 50%-75%, and with three previous episodes, the risk is in excess of 80%. Currently, most first-time patients are treated initially with simple chest tube drainage; however, with subsequent recurrences, additional therapy generally

is indicated including such measures as surgical exploration and pleurodesis. Furthermore, with the development of VATS, some feel that a more aggressive approach should be taken even for first-time pneumothoraces.

Patients with air leaks lasting longer than 7 days, patients who do not fully reexpand their lungs, patients in high-risk occupations (scuba divers, airline pilots, etc), patients with large bullae or poor pulmonary function, and patients with bilateral or recurrent pneumothoraces are candidates for additional medical (pleurodesis) or surgical intervention. Furthermore, patients who frequently travel to places distant from medical care are offered early surgical intervention. Previously, tetracycline pleurodesis was used to decrease the incidence of recurrent pneumothoraces. The use of this substance, however, was associated with significant pain and controversy. It is currently no longer available. The use of talc slurry or powder in this setting is also controversial due to the potential for long-term fibrothorax and restrictive lung disease, but has been shown to reduce the recurrence rate to as low as 2%. Many other chemical agents have been used in the past, including mechlorethamine, doxycycline, bleomycin, minocycline, iodoform, guaiacol, urea, and hypertonic glucose, with varying success rates. Pleurodesis can make subsequent surgical procedures more difficult, and should be considered with surgical consultation.

Medically fit patients who are candidates for bedside pleurodesis are also candidates for operation. The procedures used to prevent recurrent pneumothoraces include (1) axillary thoracotomy with apical bullectomy, mechanical pleurodesis, and partial pleurectomy; and (2) complete parietal pleurectomy. Both procedures can be performed with either open or VATS techniques. Complete parietal pleurectomy generally is avoided, since some patients may require future thoracic surgical procedures that are extremely difficult in the face of total parietal pleurectomy. Apical bullectomy, mechanical pleurodesis, and partial apical pleurectomy have been shown to reduce the recurrence rate to near zero. In addition, this procedure is easily accomplished either with VATS techniques or through a small transaxillary thoracotomy, both of which are well tolerated.

Several special situations exist that require particular expertise in treatment decisions. Patients with cystic fibrosis and severe chronic obstructive pulmonary disease (COPD) may be candidates for lung transplantation, and both pleurodesis and operation may make subsequent transplantation more dangerous. Therefore, consultation with a transplant surgeon is advisable prior to considering these therapies. AIDS patients with *Pneumocystis* pneumonia and pneumothorax are extremely difficult to manage, having a high rate of persistent bronchopleural fistula, treatment failure, and death. For optimal management, the surgeon should have extensive experience in the management of chest catheters.

PRIMARY PLEURAL TUMORS

Primary pleural tumors are uncommon neoplasms of two main types: diffuse malignant pleural mesotheliomas and localized fibrous tumors of the pleura (previously referred to as localized mesotheliomas). Although diffuse malignant pleural mesothelioma is the most common primary pleural tumor, involvement of the pleura with metastatic disease is more frequent and represents the most likely cause of any newly diagnosed pleural malignancy.

1. Localized Fibrous Tumors of the Pleura

Localized fibrous tumors of the pleura arise from subpleural fibroblasts that produce an array of lesions varying from peripheral pulmonary nodules to sessile subpleural masses to the more typical large pedunculated neoplasms. The visceral pleura is involved more often than the parietal pleura, and both benign (70%) and malignant (30%) variations exist. Histologically, benign tumors can exhibit three patterns—fibrous, cellular, and mixed—while malignant ones also have three distinct appearances: tubulopapillary, fibrous, and dimorphic. These tumors behave more like sarcomas of the pleura than diffuse malignant mesotheliomas. Most localized fibrous tumors of the pleura are asymptomatic, discovered only incidentally on chest radiography. Extremely large tumors, however, may produce symptoms of bronchial compression with dyspnea, cough, and chest heaviness—and, rarely, symptoms of hypoglycemia from the production of an insulinlike peptide (4% of patients). On physical examination, signs of clubbing and hypertrophic pulmonary osteoarthropathy (20%-35%) may be present. Chest radiography most often demonstrates a well-circumscribed mass that may move with changes in position if the tumor is pedunculated. A pleural effusion is present in 15% of cases and can be bloody, although this does not indicate unresectability. Fine-needle aspiration cytology may be suggestive; however, the diagnosis generally can be established with certainty only at surgery.

The treatment of these lesions is complete resection. Although full lobectomy is usually not required for lesions involving the visceral pleura, wedge resection of the pulmonary parenchyma in the area of the tumor is recommended. For neoplasms arising from the parietal pleura, chest wall resection is prudent. Following complete surgical excision, no further therapy is indicated and the prognosis is good, with some patients surviving for over 10 years without recurrence; however, if the resection is incomplete, radiation therapy should be considered because the prognosis is poor, with a median survival of only 7 to 9 months.

2. Diffuse Malignant Pleural Mesothelioma

Diffuse malignant pleural mesothelioma is the most common primary tumor of the pleura. Since 1960, the disorder has been strongly linked to the use of asbestos. Thick serpentine asbestos fibers (chrysotile) generally are deposited in the proximal airways and are easily cleared with less risk of the development of tumors; however, thin needlelike amphibole fibers (crocidolite, amosite, actinolite, anthophyllite, and tremolite) and the soil silicate zeolite, found in the Anatolia region of Turkey, usually lodge in the terminal airways and migrate to the pleura, thereby increasing the risk of diffuse malignant pleural mesothelioma to more than 300 times that of the general population. The increased incidence of mesothelioma in shipbuilders exposed to asbestos-laden insulation from World War II–era ships further implicates asbestosis in the pathophysiology of the disease. The latency period after exposure ranges from 15 years to 50 years. Research suggests that the generation of free radicals (including nitric oxide), depression of the immune system (both cellular and humoral), induction of cytokines (tumor necrosis factor [TNF]-α, interleukin [IL]-1α, IL-1β, and IL-6), and the production of genetic defects, such as abnormalities of chromosomes 1, 3, 4, 6, 7, 9, 11, 17 (p53), and 22 (involves c-*sis,* which encodes for one chain of platelet-derived growth factor) all may play a role in the mechanism of asbestos-related disease.

Histologically, diffuse malignant pleural mesotheliomas are divided into four categories: (1) epithelial or tubopapillary (35%-40%), which are associated with pleural effusions and a slightly better prognosis; (2) fibrosarcomatous or mesenchymal (20%), which are often "dry" mesotheliomas; (3) mixed (35%-40%); and (4) undifferentiated (5%-10%). The right hemithorax (60%) is affected more often than the left (35%), and 5% are bilateral.

Most patients with diffuse malignant pleural mesotheliomas complain of dyspnea on exertion and chest wall discomfort, but other symptoms also occur, such as cough, fever (paraneoplastic), malaise, weight loss, and dysphagia. Complaints of severe chest wall pain, abdominal distention, pericardial tamponade, and superior vena cava syndrome all suggest advanced disease. Although most patients develop distant metastases at some time during the course of their disease, these lesions rarely become symptomatic. Chest radiographs are distinctly abnormal, showing pleural thickening, effusion (75%), and narrowing of intercostal spaces. CT often suggests the diagnosis because of diffuse irregular pleural thickening. The diagnosis generally requires substantial tissue samples and is not generally obtainable from fine-needle aspiration cytology. Tissue can be easily acquired with VATS techniques.

Immunohistochemical stains for carcinoembryonic antigen (CEA), LeuM1, B72.3, MOC-31, and BerEP4 are usually negative, while those for vimentin and keratin are generally positive. Calretinin stain, which is specific for cells of mesothelial origin, has become available. This immunohistochemical marker can with near certainty determine whether an epithelial malignant tumor is either metastatic to pleura—for example, an adenocarcinoma (calretinin-negative)—or a primary malignant mesothelioma (calretinin-positive). This stain has become an important clinical tool and should be performed on all suspected cases of diffuse malignant pleural mesothelioma. Electron microscopy may also be helpful in distinguishing this disorder from metastatic adenocarcinoma, with which it is often confused. Pathologic staging of diffuse malignant pleural mesothelioma, like its treatment (see below), has been controversial. The original Butchart staging system and a more recently promulgated tumor, node, metastases (TNM) staging system are set forth in the Table 19–3; however, neither is widely accepted or utilized.

The treatment of diffuse malignant pleural mesothelioma also remains variable. Owing to the low incidence of this disease, its natural history has not been carefully defined with regard to various prognostic factors, and few randomized trials have been conducted to compare treatment strategies. The reported median survival for all patients ranges from 8 to 14 months. Recent randomized prospective trials have demonstrated benefit of platinum-based chemotherapy in combination with the antifolates pemetrexed or raltitrexed, which have become standard of care. Vogelzang and coworkers randomized 448 patients with unresectable pleural mesothelioma to receive cisplatin versus cisplatin in combination with pemetrexed. Patients treated with pemetrexed in addition to cisplatin demonstrated improved median survival (12.1 versus 9.3 months) and progression-free survival. The improved survival came at a cost of increased bone marrow–related toxicity (neutropenia and leukopenia). Van Meerbeeck and coworkers demonstrated similar findings in a randomized sample of patients comparing cisplatin and combination cisplatin and raltitrexed. Mean survival in the cohort receiving combination cisplatinum and raltitrexed was 11.2 months versus 8.8 months in patients receiving cisplatin alone. Newer chemotherapeutic agents under active investigation include Rampirinase, intrapleural IL-2, and vascular endothelial-derived growth factor antagonists (bevacizumab).

Surgery alone has also been used in attempts to improve survival, and two major approaches have been utilized: radical extrapleural pneumonectomy (EPP) or parietal pleurectomy with decortication. The initial experience with EPP demonstrated greater associated morbidity without improved long-term survival when compared to parietal pleurectomy and decortication. When combined with postoperative chest wall irradiation, the latter procedure results in a median survival of up to 25 months. Other approaches have combined preoperative chemotherapy (MD Anderson), intraoperative and postoperative chemotherapy (Lung Cancer Study Group, Cleveland Clinic), photodynamic therapy (NCI), and immunotherapy with TNF-α as well as interferon (IFN)-α and IFN-γ (NCI, SWOG) with limited success. Currently, the use of intraoperative radiation therapy (UCSF, MSKCC) and gene therapy are also being investigated. Although the general impression is that multimodality therapy is superior to any one therapy alone, the exact combination of treatment options for this disease remains a key question, as does the degree to which a microscopically negative resection with extrapleural pneumonectomy is possible.

Bibby A, et al. Malignant pleural mesothelioma: An update on investigation, diagnosis and treatment. *Eur Respir Rev.* 2016; 25:472-486.

Kondola S, et al. Malignant pleural mesothelioma: An update on diagnosis and treatment options. *Ther Adv Respir Dis.* 2016; 10(3):275-288.

Rusch V, et al. The role of surgical cytoreduction in the treatment of malignant pleural mesothelioma: Meeting summary of the International Mesothelioma Interest Group Congress, September 11-14, 2012, Boston, Mass. *J Thorac Cardiovasc Surg.* 2013; 145(4):909.

▼ DISEASES OF THE MEDIASTINUM

MEDIASTINITIS

Mediastinitis may be acute or chronic. There are four sources of mediastinal infection: direct contamination, hematogenous or lymphatic spread, extension of infection from the neck or retroperitoneum, and extension from the lung or pleura. The most common direct contamination is esophageal perforation. Acute mediastinitis may follow esophageal, cardiac, and other mediastinal operations. Rarely, the mediastinum is directly infected by suppurative conditions involving the ribs or vertebrae. Most direct mediastinal infections are caused by pyogenic organisms. Most mediastinal infections that invade via the hematogenous and lymphatic routes are granulomatous. Contiguous involvement of the mediastinum along fascial planes from cervical infection is frequent; this occurs less commonly from the retroperitoneum because of the influence of the diaphragm. Empyema often loculates to form a paramediastinal abscess, but extension to form a true mediastinal abscess is uncommon. Extension of mediastinal infections to involve the pleura however, is common.

1. Acute Mediastinitis

Esophageal perforation, the source of 90% of acute mediastinal infections, can be caused by vomiting (Boerhaave syndrome), iatrogenic trauma (endoscopy, dilation, operation), external trauma (penetrating or blunt), cuffed endotracheal tubes, ingestion of corrosives, carcinoma, or other esophageal disease. Mediastinal infection secondary to cervical disease may follow oral surgery; cellulitis; external trauma involving the pharynx, esophagus, or trachea; and cervical operative procedures such as tracheostomy, mediastinoscopy, and thyroidectomy.

Table 19–3. Staging systems for malignant mesothelioma.

BUTCHART STAGING SYSTEM

Stage I: Tumor is confined within the "capsule" of the parietal pleura—ie, involving the ipsilateral pleura, lung, diaphragm, and external surface of the pericardium within the pleural reflection only.

Stage II: Tumor invades the chest wall or mediastinum (esophagus, trachea, or great vessels). Alternatively, lymph nodes within the chest are involved with metastatic disease.

Stage III: Tumor penetrates the diaphragmatic muscle to involve the peritoneum or retroperitoneum, the pericardium to involve the internal surface or heart, and the mediastinum to involve the contralateral pleura. Alternatively, lymph nodes outside the chest are involved with metastatic disease.

Stage IV: Distant hematogenous metastatic (bone, brain, liver).

BRIGHAM STAGING SYSTEM

Stage I: Tumor is confined to the pleura without lymph node involvement.

Stage II: Tumor confined to the pleura with ipsilateral lymph node involvement (intraparenchymal or mediastinal).

Stage III: Local tumor metastasis (chest wall, diaphragm, mediastinum) with or without involvement of contralateral lymph nodes.

Stage IV: Distant tumor metastasis

TNM STAGING SYSTEM

Tumor Stage

TX: Primary tumor cannot be assessed

T0: No evidence of primary tumor

T1: Tumor limited to the ipsilateral parietal pleura with or without involvement of
- visceral pleura
- mediastinal pleura
- diaphragmatic pleura

T2: Tumor involving each of the ipsilateral pleural surfaces (parietal, mediastinal, diaphragmatic, and visceral pleura) with at least one of the following features:
- involvement of diaphragmatic muscle
- extension of tumor from visceral pleura into the underlying pulmonary parenchyma

T3: Describes locally advanced but **potentially resectable** tumor.
Tumor involving all the ipsilateral pleural surfaces (parietal, mediastinal, diaphragmatic, and visceral pleura) with at least one of the following features:
- involvement of the endothoracic fascia
- extension into the mediastinal fat
- solitary, completely resectable focus of tumor extending into the soft tissues of the chest wall
- nontransmural involvement of the pericardium

T4: Describes locally advanced **technically unresectable** tumor. Tumor involving all the ipsilateral pleural surfaces (parietal, mediastinal, diaphragmatic, and visceral pleura) with at least one of the following features:
- diffuse extension or multifocal masses of tumor in the chest wall, with or without associated rib destruction
- direct transdiaphragmatic extension of tumor to the peritoneum
- direct extension of tumor to the contralateral pleura
- direct extension of tumor to mediastinal organs
- direct extension of tumor into the spine
- tumor extending through to the internal surface of the pericardium with or without a pericardial effusion; or tumor involving the myocardium

Lymph Node Stage

NX: Regional lymph nodes cannot be assessed

N0: No regional lymph node metastases

N1: Metastases in the ipsilateral bronchopulmonary, hilar, or mediastinal (including the internal mammary, peridiaphragmatic, pericardial fat pad, or intercostal) lymph nodes

N2: Metastases in the contralateral mediastinal, ipsilateral, or contralateral supraclavicular lymph nodes

Metastic Stage

M0: No distant metastasis

M1: Distant metastasis present

STAGE GROUPS

When T is...	And N is...	And M is...	Then the stage group is...
T1	N0	M0	IA
T2 or T3	N0	M0	IB
T1	N1	M0	II
T2	N1	M0	II
T3	N1	M0	IIIA
T1-3	N2	M0	IIIB
T4	Any N	M0	IIIB
Any T	Any N	M1	IV

Used with the permission of the American College of Surgeons. Amin MB, Edge SB, Greene FL, et al. (Eds.) *AJCC Cancer Staging Manual,* 8th Ed. Springer New York, 2017.

Clinical Findings

Emetogenic esophageal perforation (Boerhaave syndrome) is usually associated with a history of vomiting but in some cases is insidious in onset. Severe boring pain located in the substernal, left or right chest, or epigastric regions is the chief complaint in over 90% of cases. One-third of patients have radiation to the back, and in some cases pain in the back may predominate. Low thoracic mediastinitis can sometimes be confused with acute abdominal diseases or pericarditis. Acute mediastinitis is often associated with chills, fever, or shock. If pleural extension develops, breathing may aggravate the pain or cause radiation to the shoulder. Swallowing increases the pain, and dysphagia may be present. The patient is febrile, and tachycardia is noted. About 60% of patients have subcutaneous emphysema or pneumomediastinum. A pericardial crunching sound with systole (Hamman sign) is often a late sign. Almost half of patients with esophageal perforation have pleural effusion or hydropneumothorax. Pneumomediastinum or pneumothorax following esophageal endoscopy are highly concerning for esophageal perforation. Neck tenderness and crepitation are more often found in higher, cervical perforations.

The diagnosis may be confirmed by contrast x-ray examination of the esophagus, preferably using thin barium. If no esophageal leak is evident then the study is completed using standard concentration barium. The use of water-soluble media is to be avoided to prevent consequences of water-soluble contrast aspiration in this population that is at increased risk for respiratory complication. Endoscopic visualization of the perforation is not recommended as an initial diagnostic maneuver as this may inadvertently extend the perforation. Chest CT scan with oral and intravenous contrast is helpful in determining the level of the perforation and the degree of mediastinal soilage as well as possible underlying esophageal or pulmonary pathology. The patient, however, must be clinically stable to be subjected to the rigors of these tests. For more critically ill patients, simple oral administration (or administration through a proximally placed nasogastric tube) of contrast and a simultaneous portable chest x-ray in an intensive care setting can often confirm the diagnosis. Myocardial infarction is sometimes mistakenly diagnosed in patients with esophageal perforation when a predisposing cause of pneumomediastinum is not apparent.

Treatment

Surgical management of intrathoracic esophageal perforation depends on the underlying cause (iatrogenic, tumor, stricture, etc) and the amount of elapsed time from leak to diagnosis. All intrathoracic leaks should be surgically explored. Initial management includes immediate drainage of associated pleural contamination by large-bore chest tubes and decompression of the occasional pneumothorax. Broad-spectrum antibiotics must be initiated to cover GI tract flora,

including antifungal therapy, as fungi such as *Candida* colonize nearly 25% of the population. Failure to include appropriate antifungal therapy can increase mortality by up to 30% in this critically ill population, and early goal directed therapy with fluid administration is strongly advised.

Surgically, a right thoracotomy offers the most access to the intrathoracic (middle) esophagus and should be used through the sixth interspace. A left thoracotomy is appropriate when a perforated esophagus from a distal esophageal stricture is encountered.

Treatment of an immediately recognized (<24 hours) iatrogenic esophageal perforation in an otherwise normal esophagus includes primary two-layer closure with careful attention to complete mucosal closure by interrupted absorbable sutures or surgical staplers. Esophageal muscle is then closed over the mucosal injury and buttressed with a flap of parietal pleura, diaphragm, or intercostal muscle. Copious irrigation and wide drainage is performed. Occasionally, closure over a T-tube drain has been successful.

Esophageal perforations more than 48 hours old are widely drained and the esophagus either defunctionalized or resected. This depends on the degree of mediastinal soilage discovered upon exploration, the extent of sepsis, and the patient's performance status. When perforation occurs secondary to esophageal cancer or manipulation for severe reflux stricture, achalasia, or an otherwise abnormal esophagus, different surgical options exist. If the perforation is recognized immediately and the patient is not floridly septic, esophageal resection is preferred. Reconstruction (usually using a gastric conduit) can be done at the same setting but only if the patient is stable and the degree of contamination minimal. Otherwise, the patient is left in discontinuity and reconstruction is performed at a later date when the patient has fully recovered from the septic event. Esophageal stent placement and adequate drainage of the mediastinal and pleural spaces also can be considered.

The mortality associated with esophageal perforation remains high (30%-60%) despite advances in critical care, nutritional support, and operative management. The specific surgical approach—repair, resection, or endoscopic —must be tailored to the individual circumstances (mechanism of perforation, underlying pathology, time to diagnosis, and patient performance status) in order to achieve optimal results.

2. Chronic Mediastinitis

Chronic mediastinitis usually involves specific granulomatous processes with associated mediastinal fibrosis and chronic abscesses. Histoplasmosis, tuberculosis, actinomycosis, nocardiosis, blastomycosis, and syphilis have been implicated. Amebic abscesses and parasitic disease such as echinococcal cysts are rare causes. The infectious process is usually due to histoplasmosis or tuberculosis and involves the mediastinal lymph nodes. Esophageal obstructions may occur. Adjacent mediastinal structures may become secondarily infected. Granulomatous mediastinitis and fibrosing mediastinitis are different manifestations of the same disease. Mediastinal fibrosis is a term used synonymously with idiopathic, fibrous, collagenous, or sclerosing mediastinitis. Eighty or more cases of mediastinal fibrosis have been reported, but the cause has been determined in only 16%, and of these the overwhelming majority were due to histoplasmosis or tuberculosis. In only 25% of 103 cases of granulomatous mediastinitis has the cause been identified. Histoplasmosis was the most common known cause (60%) and tuberculosis the second-most common (25%).

About 85% of patients with mediastinal fibrosis have symptoms from entrapment of mediastinal structures as follows: superior vena caval obstruction in 82%; tracheobronchial obstruction, 9%; pulmonary vein obstruction, 6%; pulmonary artery occlusion, 6%; and esophageal obstruction, 3%. Rarely, inferior vena caval obstruction or involvement of the thoracic duct, atrium, recurrent laryngeal nerve, or stellate ganglion is found. Multiple structures may be simultaneously involved.

Seventy-five percent of patients with granulomatous mediastinitis have no symptoms, and disease is discovered by chest x-ray, which shows a mediastinal mass. The mass is in the right paratracheal region in 75% of cases. In the 25% of patients with symptoms, about half have superior vena caval obstruction and one-third have esophageal obstruction. Occasional patients have bronchial obstruction, bronchoesophageal fistula, or pulmonary venous obstruction.

A mediastinal tuberculous or fungal abscess occasionally dissects long distances to present on the chest wall paravertebrally or parasternally. Secondary rib or costal cartilage infections with multiple draining sinus tracts occur.

► Clinical Findings

A. Symptoms and Signs

Granulomatous and fibrosing mediastinitis affects women two to three times more commonly than men. Women aged 20-30 years are most typically affected, though the disorder may present in the fourth to fifth decades. Esophageal involvement results in dysphagia or hematemesis. Tracheobronchial involvement may cause severe cough, hemoptysis, dyspnea, wheezing, and episodes of obstructive pneumonitis. Pulmonary vein obstruction—the most common serious manifestation—produces congestive heart failure resembling advanced mitral stenosis and is usually fatal. Although not diagnostic, the respective skin tests in cases due to histoplasmosis or tuberculosis are strongly positive.

B. Imaging Studies

X-ray findings demonstrate a right paratracheal or anterior mediastinal mass. There may be spotty or subcapsular calcifications. Classically, histoplasmosis presents with hilar node calcification or so-called popcorn granuloma appearance. Calcification can also occur in thymoma or teratoma located in the anterior mediastinum. Chest CT (with intravenous and oral contrast) is most effective in defining the extent of mediastinal fibrosis and impingement on vital structures.

► Treatment

Specific antimicrobial therapy is indicated when an infecting organism is identified. Patients with symptomatic mediastinal masses and fibrosis can require palliative resection for relief of obstruction.

► Prognosis

The prognosis following surgical excision of granulomatous mediastinal masses is good. Operative procedures do not appear to activate fibrosing mediastinitis, but success in treatment has been unpredictable. Most patients with fibrosing mediastinitis—whether treated or not—survive but have persistent symptoms.

Abu-Omar Y, et al. European Association for Cardiothoracic Surgery Expert Consensus Statement on the Prevention and Management of Mediastinitis. *Eur J Cardiothorac Surg.* 2017; 51:10-29.

Kieser T, et al. Toward zero: Deep sternal wound infection after 1001 consecutive coronary artery bypass procedures using arterial grafts. Implications for diabetic patients. *J Thorac Cardiovasc Surg.* 2014;148(5):1887-1895.

Van Wingerden JJ, et al. Poststernotomy mediastinitis: A classification to initiate and evaluate reconstructive management based on evidence from a structured review. *J Cardiothorac Surg.* 2014; 19:179.

SUPERIOR VENA CAVAL SYNDROME

Superior vena caval obstruction produces a distinctive clinical syndrome. Malignant tumors are the cause in 80%-90% of cases; lung cancer accounts for about 90%. The incidence of superior vena caval syndrome in lung cancer patients is 3%-5%. The male-to-female ratio is about 5:1. Other primary mediastinal tumors that may cause superior vena caval obstruction include thymoma, Hodgkin disease, and lymphosarcoma. Metastatic tumors from the breast or thyroid or from melanoma also occasionally cause superior vena caval obstruction. Benign tumors are an unusual cause, but substernal goiter, any large benign mediastinal masses, and atrial myxoma have been implicated. Thrombotic conditions, either idiopathic or associated with polycythemia, mediastinal infection, or indwelling catheters, are unusual causes. The association of superior vena caval obstruction with chronic mediastinitis is discussed in the preceding section. Trauma may produce acute venous obstruction (eg, traumatic asphyxia, mediastinal hematoma).

The clinical manifestations depend on the abruptness of onset, the location of the obstruction, the completeness of occlusion, and the availability of collateral pathways.

Venous pressure measured in the arms or head varies from 200 to 500 mm H_2O, and severity of symptoms is correlated with the pressure. Fatal cerebral edema can occur within minutes of an acute complete obstruction, whereas a slowly evolving one permits development of collaterals and may be only mildly symptomatic. Symptoms are milder when the azygos vein is patent. Azygous blood flow—normally about 11% of the total venous return—can increase to 35% of the venous return from the head, neck, and upper extremities. Thus, the most severe cases occur when occlusion is complete and the azygos vein is involved. The thrombus may propagate proximally to occlude the innominate and axillary veins.

Clinical Findings

Symptoms include puffiness of the face, arms, and shoulders and a blue or purple discoloration of the skin. Central nervous system symptoms include headache, nausea, dizziness, vomiting, distortion of vision, drowsiness, stupor, and convulsions. Respiratory symptoms include cough, hoarseness, and dyspnea, often due to edema of the vocal cords or trachea. Nasal congestion is often an early presenting symptom. These symptoms are made worse when the patient lies flat or bends over. In long-standing cases, esophageal varices may develop and produce gastrointestinal (GI) bleeding. The veins of the neck and upper extremities are visibly distended, and in long-standing cases there are marked collateral venous channels over the anterior chest and abdomen. Chronic pleural effusions may develop as a result of impaired lymphatic drainage. Onset of symptoms in fibrosing mediastinitis may be insidious, consisting initially of early morning edema of the face and hands. Occasionally, symptoms and findings are localized to one side when the level of obstruction is above the vena cava and only the innominate vein is blocked. In this situation, symptoms are mild because communicating veins in the neck usually decompress the affected side.

The diagnosis can be confirmed by measuring upper extremity venous pressure; in patients with severe symptoms, a pressure of 350 mm H_2O or more is usual. Of patients with malignant vena caval obstruction studied by venography, 35% have thrombosis involving the innominate or axillary veins, 15% have complete caval obstruction without thrombosis, and 50% have partial superior vena caval obstruction. Chest x-ray may show a right upper lobe lung lesion or right paratracheal mass. Aortography is occasionally required to exclude aortic aneurysm. CT or magnetic resonance imaging (MRI) scan with contrast enhancement provides sufficient anatomic detail, supplanting the need for arteriography or venography as a diagnostic modality for this syndrome. The differential diagnosis may include angioneurotic edema,

congestive heart failure, constrictive pericarditis, and fibrosing mediastinitis. Effort thrombosis of the axillary vein and innominate vein obstruction from elongation and buckling of the innominate artery can be considered in unilateral cases.

Complications

In patients with partial superior vena caval obstruction, thrombosis may suddenly change mild symptoms to marked venous distention, cyanotic swelling, vocal cord edema, and impaired neurologic function. Bleeding from esophageal varices is rare except in severe long-standing cases.

Treatment

Superior vena caval obstruction caused by cancer should be treated with diuretics, restriction, avoidance of upper extremity intravenous lines, head elevation, and prompt palliative radiation therapy. Cases of superior vena cava obstruction due to tumor begin to subside by 7-10 days of treatment. Because of the possibility of thrombosis in malignant cases, the use of fibrinolytic agents has been suggested. Caution must be advised in using anticoagulants, however, because many patients have advanced disease and may harbor occult cerebral metastases. Therefore, before starting therapy, patients should undergo CT or MRI brain scanning to prevent the occurrence of intracerebral hemorrhage. Recently, the use of intravascular expansile stents has been pioneered. Limited early experience suggests that the lumen can be reopened and that good venous drainage and decompression can be achieved by minimally invasive interventional radiologic techniques. Disadvantages include the need for anticoagulation to prevent recurrent thrombosis.

Chemotherapy is sometimes used alone or with radiotherapy. Most cases of malignant superior vena caval obstruction are not remediable by operation. Tissue diagnosis is important for diagnosis and for guiding therapy. Invasive procedures, however, must be tailored to the individual patient and the severity of the caval obstruction. Patients with new, severe, or rapidly progressive symptoms should receive immediate palliative radiation therapy. Patients with subacute presentations can better tolerate the time required to make the diagnosis.

Fine-needle aspiration, bronchoscopy, cervical mediastinoscopy, and anterior mediastinotomy—and even, occasionally, thoracotomy—offer possible approaches for obtaining tissue. Caution must be advised, however, in the setting of acute fulminant superior vena caval obstruction because any invasive procedure will carry a significantly higher morbidity due to bleeding from venous obstruction. In this case, attempts at invasive techniques for tissue diagnosis should be avoided. Most frequently, the disease process has been previously histologically confirmed because superior vena caval obstruction presents typically as a complication of locally advanced disease. In benign incomplete superior vena caval obstruction, surgical excision of the compressing mass can provide an excellent result. In total obstruction, such as occurs in fibrosing mediastinitis, most patients will gradually improve without treatment. There are numerous surgical procedures designed to bypass caval obstruction, replace the superior vena cava, or recanalize the vena caval lumen. These procedures have been dramatically effective in some cases, but only recently have they been sufficiently successful to warrant consideration.

Prognosis

Radiotherapy is most effective when superior vena caval obstruction is incomplete. Mean survival of patients with malignant caval obstruction from lung cancer is 6-8 months. The death rate from causes related to the vena caval obstruction itself is only 1%-2%.

Rachapalli V, Boucher LM. Superior vena cava syndrome: Role of the interventionalist. *Can Assoc Radiol J*. 2014;65(2):168-176.

MEDIASTINAL MASS LESIONS

Lesions within the mediastinum include a variety of masses, both malignant and benign, that arise from the diverse organs and tissues that occupy the central thorax. Overall, the incidence of all mediastinal masses is low, especially compared with the frequency of lesions arising within the lung (bronchogenic cancer, etc). Mediastinal malignancies constitute less than 20% of all thoracic tumors.

Mediastinal masses arise from specific structures that reside in relatively constant anatomic arrangement. The mediastinum itself is defined laterally by the mediastinal pleura of each lung; superiorly and inferiorly by the thoracic inlet and diaphragm, respectively; anteriorly by the sternum; and posteriorly by the vertebral bodies. For purposes of definition, the mediastinum is divided loosely into three main compartments: anterior (or anterosuperior), middle, and posterior. The anterior mediastinum contains the thymus, fat, and lymph nodes while the middle mediastinum contains the heart, pericardium, ascending and transverse aorta, brachiocephalic veins, trachea, bronchi, and lymph nodes. The posterior mediastinum consists of the descending thoracic aorta, esophagus, azygous vein, autonomic ganglia and nerves, lymph nodes, and fat. This has important implications for diagnosing suspected masses. The likelihood of malignancy is influenced primarily by three main factors: anatomic location, age, and the presence or absence of symptoms. Although two-thirds of mediastinal tumors are benign, masses in the anterior compartment are more likely to be malignant. Age is an important predictor as well, with many lymphomas and germ-cell tumors (GCTs) presenting between the second and fourth decades of life. Symptomatic patients are more likely to have a malignancy. Although classically in

adults the majority of mediastinal masses tend to be benign (cysts, neurogenic tumors, etc), recent series have demonstrated a shift toward malignant processes being more prevalent.

An anterior mediastinal mass can indicate the following: thymoma (the most common), thymic hyperplasia, thymolipoma, thymic cyst, thymic carcinoid, thymic carcinoma, germ-cell tumor (teratoma, seminoma, nonseminomatous germ-cell tumor), lymphoma, parathyroid adenoma, substernal thyroid, and lymphangioma. A middle mediastinal mass can include lymphoma, pericardial cyst, bronchogenic cyst, aneurysm, and lymphadenopathy. A posterior mediastinal mass can include neurogenic tumor, enteric cyst, bronchogenic cyst, meningocele, diaphragmatic or hiatus hernia, and paravertebral abscess. The most common mediastinal masses in children are neurogenic tumors (50%-60%). In young children (<4 years of age), they are invariably malignant (neuroblastomas). In the adults, a neurogenic tumor is the most common mediastinal mass. This arises in the posterior compartment (typically from a peripheral nerve sheath) and is usually benign, occasionally calcified, and well circumscribed.

An extensive workup of a mediastinal lesion is usually not required for diagnosis, since surgery is usually required both to establish the diagnosis and provide effective treatment. Standard posteroanterior and especially lateral chest films will often provide much useful information; however, contrast CT scanning has become the preferred diagnostic test. MRI, while helpful for assessing vascular or spinal cord extension, has not proved to be more effective than dynamic CT scanning but can be vital for operative planning in those masses abutting vital organs and vascular structures.

Fluoroscopy may show pulsation or variation of shape or location with change of position and respiration. Tomography may reveal calcification or air–fluid levels. Barium swallow is used to evaluate intrinsic esophageal lesions or esophageal displacement by extrinsic masses. Contrast studies of the intestinal tract may reveal the stomach, colon, or small bowel in a hernia. Myelography can be of crucial importance in neurogenic tumors to explain symptoms or to plan operative management. CT angiography can identify aneurysms or displacement. Pulmonary arteriography may be useful to distinguish mediastinal and pulmonary tumors.

Scintigraphy scanning is important in evaluating possible substernal goiter in anterior mediastinal lesions, since goiters can generally be removed by the standard cervical approach. Skin tests and serologic studies may be used in suspected granulomatous disease. Bone marrow examination, hormone assays, and serum tumor markers (α-fetoprotein [AFP], β-human chorionic gonadotropin [β-HCG], LDH) are important adjuncts to evaluate a suspected germ-cell tumor.

Bronchoscopy and esophagoscopy are occasionally useful to identify primary lung lesions or lesions of the esophagus.

Mediastinoscopy and mediastinal biopsy must be used cautiously in mediastinal tumors that are potentially curable. Excisional biopsy is imperative in lesions (eg, thymomas) that are histologically difficult to evaluate since a curable but locally invasive malignancy might be dispersed. Mediastinoscopy is useful for the diagnosis of sarcoidosis, Castleman disease, or disseminated lymphoma.

▶ **Clinical Findings**

Symptoms are more frequent among patients with malignant rather than benign lesions. About one-third of patients have no symptoms. Those patients who become symptomatic can present with cough (60%); chest pain (30%); fevers/chills (20%); or dyspnea (16%). Hemoptysis and, rarely, expectoration of cyst contents may occur. Weight loss and dysphagia are found each in about 10% of patients. Myasthenia gravis (MG, 15%-20% with thymoma), fever, and superior vena caval obstruction are found each in about 5% of patients.

Symptoms can be categorized into two groups: localizing symptoms and systemic symptoms. Localizing symptoms are secondary to tumor invasion and include respiratory compromise; dysphagia; paralysis of the limbs, diaphragm, and vocal cords; Horner syndrome; and superior vena cava syndrome. These findings are concerning for a malignant process. Malignant tumors, especially lymphomas, may produce chylothorax. Systemic symptoms are typically due to the release of excess hormones, antibodies, or cytokines. Thymoma has been associated with myasthenia, hypogammaglobulinemia, Whipple disease, red blood cell aplasia, and Cushing disease. Hypoglycemia is a rare complication of mesothelioma, teratoma, and fibroma. Hypertension and diarrhea occur with pheochromocytoma and ganglioneuroma. Neurogenic tumors may produce specific neurologic findings from cord pressure or may be associated with hypertrophic osteoarthropathy and peptic ulcer disease.

A. Neurogenic Tumors

Neurogenic tumors are derived from tissue of the neural crest, including cells of the peripheral, autonomic, and paraganglionic nervous systems. Neurogenic tumors almost always occur in the posterior mediastinum—often the superior portion—arising from intercostal or sympathetic nerves. Rarely, the vagus or phrenic nerve is involved. Seventy to eighty percent of all neurogenic tumors are benign. The most common tumor (40%-65%) arises from the nerve sheath (schwannoma and neurofibroma) and is usually benign. Malignant tumors occur more frequently in children. Most malignant tumors (neuroblastoma, etc) arise from the nerve cells. Neurogenic tumors may be multiple or dumbbell in type, with widening of the intervertebral foramen. In these cases, MRI is necessary to determine if the mass extends within the spinal canal. Dumbbell tumors have

been removed in the past by a two-stage approach, though a single-stage approach is now more widespread. [123]I metaiodobenzylguanidine scintigraphy can be applicable particularly for patients with middle metastatic tumor suspected to be a pheochromocytoma.

B. Mediastinal Cystic Lesions

Cysts of the mediastinum may arise from the pericardium, bronchi, esophagus, or thymus. Pericardial cysts are also called "springwater" or mesothelial cysts. Seventy-five percent are located near the cardiophrenic angles, and 75% of these are on the right side. Ten percent are actually diverticula of the pericardial sac that communicate with the pericardial space. Bronchogenic cysts arise close to the mainstem bronchus or trachea, often just below the carina. Histologically, these contain elements found in bronchi, such as cartilage, and are lined by respiratory epithelium. Enterogenous cysts are known by several names, including esophageal cyst, enteric cyst, or duplication of the alimentary tract. They arise along the surface of the esophagus and may be embedded within its wall. They may be lined by squamous epithelium similar to the esophagus or gastric mucosa. Enterogenous cysts are occasionally associated with congenital abnormalities of the vertebrae. About 10% of cysts in the mediastinum are nonspecific, without a recognizable lining.

C. Germ-Cell Tumors

Germ-cell tumors (GCTs) are common mass lesions found in young adults and represent 15% of anterior mediastinal mass lesions. Malignant germ-cell tumors are more common in men (>90%). Historically, they are both solid and cystic, and the more differentiated tumors can contain hair or teeth. Microscopically, ectodermal, endodermal, and mesodermal elements are present. These tumors occasionally rupture into the pleural space, lung, pericardium, or vascular structures. Most germ-cell tumors of the mediastinum are metastatic and present with concomitant retroperitoneal disease.

Primary mediastinal extragonadal germ-cell malignancies are rare, representing fewer than 5% of all mediastinal germ-cell cancers and less than 5% of all primary mediastinal tumors. As pluripotent cells, GCTs can give rise to several histologically distinct malignancies, including seminoma (40%), embryonal carcinomas and nongestational choriocarcinomas (20%), and yolk sac tumors (20%). Teratomas (20%) can have both benign and malignant components. Almost all such tumors (>90%) produce tumor markers, including β-HCG and AFP. LDH—a nonspecific tumor marker—is produced by most bulky mediastinal GCTs and is often an effective indicator of tumor burden.

Much progress in treating these tumors has been made with multimodality therapy (surgery, radiation therapy, and chemotherapy). Currently, only a 40%-45% 5-year survival is achievable for nonseminomatous GCTs, and over 90%

5-year survival is typical for seminomatous mediastinal GCTs. Patients should be screened and followed with AFP, β-HCG, and LDH markers. Resection should be offered after combination chemotherapy has been administered and only after all elevated tumor markers have normalized.

Residual mediastinal masses following chemotherapy and normalization of tumor markers should be resected. At surgery, approximately 40% will be mature teratomas (with the potential for malignant degeneration), 40% necrotic tumors, and 20% residual tumors (requiring postoperative salvage chemotherapy). Rarely is palliative debulking surgery indicated if tumor markers remain elevated after several cycles of chemotherapy. Instead, alternative chemotherapy or investigational therapy should be offered.

D. Lymphoma

Lymphoma is usually associated with disseminated disease metastatic to the mediastinum. It is typically identified in the anterior compartment but can present anywhere through the mediastinum. This is the second-most common mass in the anterior mediastinum. Occasionally, lymphosarcoma, Hodgkin disease, or reticulum cell sarcoma arises as a primary mediastinal lesion.

► Treatment

Treatment is tailored to the specific disease process causing the mediastinal mass. In almost all cases, tissue diagnosis is imperative for guiding appropriate therapy. Minimally invasive techniques (fine-needle aspiration or core-needle biopsy) or mediastinoscopy and mediastinotomy are appropriate for diagnosis of a mediastinal mass that is secondary to metastatic disease (eg, lymphomas, germ-cell tumors). Mediastinal masses that represent primary malignancies (thymoma, neurogenic tumors, etc) are treated usually with initial resection. Percutaneous biopsy of primary malignancies should be reserved for patients with locally advanced disease, considered either unresectable or suitable for preoperative systemic therapy and/or radiation therapy prior to attempted resection.

Surgical approaches include median sternotomy (anterior masses), posterolateral thoracotomy (posterior and middle mediastinal masses) as well as VATS or bilateral anterior thoracotomy (all mediastinal compartments). Adjuvant chemotherapy is important for malignant germ cell lesions, malignant neurogenic tumors, and bulky or advanced thymomas. Postoperative radiation therapy decreases local recurrence in higher-stage thymoma and in other incompletely resected lesions. Radiation and chemotherapy constitutes the principal therapy for primary mediastinal lymphoma.

Complete resection is the treatment of choice for all neurogenic tumors. A standard posterolateral thoracotomy offers optimal exposure; however, more limited incisions, including thoracoscopy, can be effective for resection of

clinically benign small (<6 cm) lesions. "Dumbbell lesions" involving the spinal canal warrant a neurosurgical consultation for a combined approach. For lesions that cannot be completely excised, postoperative radiation may decrease local recurrence and symptoms. Incompletely excised or especially large or infiltrative neuroblastomas should receive combination radiation and chemotherapy in conjunction with surgery.

► Prognosis

Overall, the outlook for patients with mediastinal masses has improved, with advances in combined chemotherapy and multimodality therapy. Surgical morbidity and mortality remain low (1%-4%). Patients with benign mediastinal lesions do significantly better (>95% cure rates) than those who have malignant mediastinal masses (<50% overall survival).

Albany C, et al. Extragonadal germ cell tumors: Clinical presentation and management. *Curr Opin Oncol.* 2013;225(3):261-265.
Busch J, et al. Male extragonadal germ cell tumors of the adult. *Oncol Res Treat.* 2016;39:140-144.

TUMORS OF THE THYMUS & MYASTHENIA GRAVIS

The thymic gland is the site of a variety of neoplasms that include thymoma, lymphoma (eg, Hodgkin's disease), granuloma, and other less common tumors. Cell types of the thymus include epithelial cells, myoid cells, thymic lymphocytes, and B-lymphocytes. Tumors of the thymus can arise from any of these cell types with thymic epithelial tumors (thymoma, thymic carcinoma, and neuroendocrine tumor) being the most common. Lymphoid or hematopoietic neoplasms and mesenchymal tumors occur less frequently. Thymoma is a primary neoplasm of the thymus gland arising from thymic epithelial cells without cytologic or histologic signs of malignancy. A well-differentiated thymic carcinoma has some cytologic features of atypia, and thymic cancer cells are cytologically malignant. Thymoma is the most common tumor of the anterior mediastinum composing approximately 50% of all tumors of the anterior mediastinum and nearly 20% of all mediastinal tumors.

Thymoma may be classified according to predominant cell type into lymphocytic (25%), epithelial (25%), and lymphoepithelial (50%) varieties. Spindle-cell tumor, which is sometimes associated with red cell aplasia, is considered among the epithelial tumors. The histologic subtypes have not been associated with prognostic significance. The World Health Organization (WHO) consensus guidelines provide a histologic classification system for thymoma and thymic carcinoma based on both morphology and lymphocyte-to-epithelial cell ratio. The WHO classification system classifies thymoma and thymic carcinoma in categories ranging from type A (bland spindle cells and limited lymphocytes) to type C (grossly atypical cells that are indicative of thymic carcinoma). The identification of a single pathologic subtype is difficult however, since there is considerable histologic heterogeneity. The Masaoka staging system, originally described in 1981 and revised in 1994, is the most frequently used staging method of thymoma and thymic carcinoma. This staging system classifies thymoma into four stages based on the presence of invasion and anatomic extent of involvement observed both clinically and histopathologically. The Masaoka staging system has been shown to be a significant independent factor for survival, with 5-year survival rates by stage approaching 86%-100% for stage I and II disease, 69% in stage III disease, and 70%-52% for patients with stages IVa and IVb, respectively. The WHO classification system as well as the modified Masaoka staging system is set forth in Table 19–4. Classification of thymoma has undergone a paradigm shift in considering all such tumors along a continuum of increasing malignancy.

Myasthenia gravis is a neuromuscular disorder characterized by weakness and fatigability of voluntary muscles owing to decreased numbers of available acetylcholine receptors at neuromuscular junctions. These receptors are blocked by autoantibodies to the neuromuscular junction. Because of the high incidence of thymic abnormalities, improvement after thymectomy, association with other autoimmune disorders, and presence in the serum of 90% of patients of an antibody against acetylcholine receptors, myasthenia gravis is thought to be of autoimmune etiology. Nearly 50% of patients with thymoma have myasthenia gravis (MG), and about 15%-20% of patients with myasthenia develop a thymoma. Thymic carcinoma, which carries a worse prognosis than other thymomas, is rarely associated with MG. About 85% of patients with MG have thymic abnormalities consisting of germinal center formation in 70% and thymoma in 15%. Myasthenia gravis can occur in association with tumors of any cell type but is more common with the lymphocytic variety. The mean age of patients with thymoma-associated MG is between 44 and 49 years of age without significant differences between males and females. Patients with thymoma-associated MG tend to be younger than those with non-MG thymoma.

▶ Clinical Findings

Fifty percent of thymomas are first identified in an asymptomatic patient on a chest x-ray obtained for another purpose. Symptomatic patients may present with chest pain, dysphagia, myesthenic symptoms, dyspnea, or superior vena caval syndrome. Paraneoplastic symptoms are fairly common in the setting of thymoma and account for approximately 60% of all presentations of thymoma.

Computed tomography (CT) with intravenous contrast of the chest provides information on the size, density, and relationship of the tumor to the surrounding intrathoracic organs and vessels. It may also reveal any pleural metastases. MRI is occasionally helpful to assess vascular invasion.

The diagnosis of myasthenia gravis can be made from the patient's history of easy fatigability and associated decremental response in muscular contraction to repeated stimulation of the motor nerve or from improvement in these abnormalities in response to edrophonium (Tensilon), a short-acting anticholinesterase drug.

Level of clinical suspicion for thymoma may dictate the need for biopsy prior to resection. In patients with a high likelihood of thymoma, excision without biopsy may be both diagnostic and therapeutic. CT-guided core needle biopsy is a useful and less invasive technique for determining histology of an anterior mediastinal mass, but should be considered only if there is evidence for local invasion such that a greater extent of resection might be necessary. Definitive diagnosis of thymoma is based on histologic study of a tissue sample usually after excisional biopsy or complete resection has been performed. Small, well-encapsulated anterior mediastinal masses should not be biopsied, as the procedure penetrates the tumor capsule and can lead to tumor seeding and recurrence, thus jeopardizing the opportunity for cure of an early-stage thymoma.

▶ Treatment

The surgical approaches to thymectomy are varied and reflect the balance between complete, curative resection and the magnitude and morbidity of a procedure. Important

Table 19–4. Staging system for malignant thymoma.

Masaoka Stage	Description
I	Macroscopically, completely encapsulated; microscopically, no capsular invasion.
IIa	Macroscopic invasion into surrounding fatty tissues or mediastinal pleura (without microscopic invasion).
IIb	Microscopic evidence of capsular invasion or microscopic invasion of surrounding fatty tissues or mediastinal pleura.
III	Macroscopic invasion into a neighboring organ (pericardium, great vessels, or lung).
IVa	Pleural or pericardial dissemination.
IVb	Lymphatic or hematogenous distant metastases.

WHO Classification	Description
A	Medullary thymoma
AB	Mixed
B1	Predominantly cortical
B2	Cortical thymoma
B3	Well differentiated carcinoma; atypical thymoma; squamous type thymoma; epithelial thymoma
C	Thymic carcinoma

principles for operative planning include patient factors (such as BMI) as well as anatomic considerations including thymic size. All approaches enable complete resection of the capsular thymus, with the extent of peri-thymic mediastinal and cervical tissue resection distinguishing each of the procedures. The goal of the operation is total thymectomy as the overall recurrence rate of thymic neoplasm is 30%. Transsternal thymectomy with en bloc resection of the anterior mediastinal fat tissue from phrenic to phrenic laterally and the diaphragm to the thyroid gland is considered the standard, classical operative approach. Alternative approaches include transcervical thymectomy and minimally invasive approaches such as VATS thymectomy and robotic-assisted thymectomy. VATS thymectomy allows for adequate visualization and should be considered in patients without a high BMI and in those with a thymus at or below 3.5 cm. Recently, in Asia a subxiphoid approach has been employed for thymectomy, although this remains controversial for removal of malignant thymoma.

Despite a paucity of randomized controlled trials, summary treatment guidelines for each stage of the disease have been established by consensus in the literature. Multidisciplinary discussion is encouraged to assure appropriate therapy is recommended and provided. For disease stages I and II, complete resection alone is the standard of care. Radiotherapy may be considered for patients at risk for recurrence. Risk factors for recurrence include invasion through the capsule, close surgical margins, WHO grade B type, and a tumor adherent to the pericardium. Patients presenting with resectable or potentially resectable stage III disease should be evaluated for multimodal therapy. Surgical resection can be considered either initially or following neoadjuvant therapy if complete resection is not initially feasible. Neoadjuvant or induction chemotherapy may decrease the volume of the tumor, thereby facilitating complete resection after restaging. If resection is not appropriate, then chemotherapy—either concurrent or sequential—with radiotherapy can be considered. For patients with stage IVa disease, surgery can be offered only if pleural or pericardial metastases are resectable.

Anticholinesterase drugs (eg, neostigmine bromide) are given as initial treatment to patients with myasthenia gravis. Corticosteroids may be given in selected cases, but a high incidence of side effects makes them unsuitable for more liberal use. Early thymectomy is now recommended for all patients with symptomatic myasthenia gravis whether or not a thymoma is suspected. The course of the disease is usually improved, and subsequent development of a malignant thymoma is eliminated. Thymectomy can be postponed in the occasional patient with mild disease well controlled by anticholinesterase therapy.

Following thymectomy, about 75% of patients with myasthenia gravis are improved and 30% achieve complete remission. Younger patients benefit more from thymectomy than do those over age 40 years, but a positive effect also accrues to the latter group. Recently, minimally invasive approaches to thymectomy for myasthenia patients has resulted in reduced length of stay, decreased blood loss, and decreased pain in comparison with more traditional partial sternal splitting procedures.

▶ Prognosis

The rates of complication and death with thymectomy are low except in the setting of locally advanced disease. Respiratory care of patients with myasthenia gravis in the immediate postoperative period now presents little difficulty because of the availability of anticholinesterase drugs. Evidence including a retrospective review by Okereke and associates suggests that neither myasthenia gravis nor paraneoplastic syndromes are associated with a poor prognosis, and there are no differences in survival between those with and without myasthenia gravis.

The Masaoka staging system has been widely accepted as the best predictor of survival in thymoma patients. Although in general, WHO histologic classification of thymoma has been considered reproducible, issues have been raised regarding interobserver variability that may impact its prognostic ability. Completeness of resection has been shown to be one of the most important independent predictors of survival.

Overall survival rates are extremely good for early-stage thymomas, and 10-year survival rates are excellent. Stage I lesions approach 100% 10-year survival rates. Stage II tumors with resection and postoperative radiation therapy have approximately 75% 10-year survival rates. Patients with locally advanced stage III thymomas, however, have long-term survival rates of less than 25%. Outcomes with multimodality therapy (neoadjuvant chemotherapy, surgery followed by chemotherapy and radiation therapy) are improving, as marked by significant tumor responses and enhanced resectability rates. Long-term disease-specific survival can be expected not only after surgery for early-stage thymoma but also after surgery for advanced disease, including select patients with pleural metastases. However, patients who undergo surgery for stage IVa disease have reduced disease-free survival.

THYMIC CARACINOMA

This tumor is a rare variant (<15%) of thymic lesions and is histologically and biologically quite different from invasive or malignant thymoma. A large number of histologic types of thymic carcinoma have been described and range from low-grade, well-differentiated neoplasms to high-grade, poorly differentiated malignancies. The most common type of thymic carcinoma in Western patients is poorly differentiated, nonkeratinizing squamous-cell carcinoma. Thymic carcinomas tend to be very invasive and difficult to resect completely. Unfortunately, even in the setting of complete resection, recurrence is common both locally and at distant sites. Still, when at all possible, an aggressive combined-modality approach (induction chemotherapy, resection, and postoperative chemoradiotherapy) should be employed. Typically, these are young men (age <50 years) with an otherwise excellent performance status. Although a good response to induction therapy and complete resection will provide a significant disease-free interval, long-term survival is still unlikely. Better systemic agents and a molecular understanding of this cancer hold hope for significant improvements in cure rates.

Friedant AJ, et al. Minimally invasive versus open thymectomy for thymic malignancies: Systematic review and meta-analysis. *J Thorac Oncol.* 2016;11(1):30-38.

Okereke IC, et al. Prognostic indicators after surgery for thymoma. *Ann Thorac Surg.* 2010;89(4):1071.

Scorsetti M, et al. Thymoma and thymic carcinomas. *Crit Rev Oncol Hematol.* 2016;99:332-350.

▼ DISEASES OF THE LUNGS

CONGENITAL CYSTIC ANOMALIES OF THE LUNG

Congenital lesions of the lung include primarily tracheobronchial atresia, bronchogenic cysts, pulmonary dysplasia, pulmonary sequestration, congenital cystic adenomatoid malformations (CCAM), and congenital lobar emphysema (CLE). Although many of these lesions present early in life with dramatic symptoms and physical findings, most remain occult until late childhood and even into adult life. These uncommon lesions arise from aberrations in normal aerodigestive tract development, which begins during the fourth week of fetal life when the lung bud forms at the caudal end of a groove in the primordial pharynx. Thus an understanding of normal development is important to appreciate pathologic development. An initial phase of sequential airway branching occurs until as many as 20-25 generations are reached by the 16th week of fetal life. These branches are divided into three zones: a proximal conductive zone (branches 1-16), an intermediate transitional zone (branches 17-19), and a distal respiratory zone (branches 20-25). A second canalicular phase is then entered as capillaries develop in the distal air passages. Finally, the alveolar phase begins at approximately 26 weeks of fetal life as prototype alveolar air sacs appear complete with both type I and type II pneumocytes. The number and size of alveoli continue to increase through the postnatal period until the total alveolar surface reaches the adult size of nearly 100 m^2.

A. Tracheobronchial Atresia

Atresia of the tracheobronchial tree can occur at any level and may involve an isolated segment or multiple diffuse areas of the airway. Tracheal atresia is associated with polyhydramnios, prematurity, esophageal atresia, and tracheoesophageal fistula. Typically, neonates present with intractable cyanosis and despite a normal-appearing larynx are unable to be intubated. Emergency tracheostomy can be life-sustaining in babies with isolated subglottic atresia; in other infants with more diffuse disease, mask ventilation can achieve some palliation through anomalous esophagobronchial connections. Diffuse airway involvement, however, is invariably fatal.

Isolated bronchial atresia results in a bronchus that ends in a blind pouch. A mucocele develops distal to the obstruction and, as a result of compression of neighboring normal bronchial structures, causes emphysematous changes in the surrounding lung. Because children frequently develop wheezing, stridor, and pulmonary infections in the involved segments, resection is almost always indicated. Much like bronchial atresia, true congenital bronchial stenosis is rare, although right mainstem bronchial stenosis occurs not infrequently from iatrogenic airway trauma in chronically ventilated patients.

Related anomalies of the tracheobronchial tree include anomalous tracheal or esophageal bronchi and tracheal diverticula. These rare lesions often present with symptoms of bronchial obstruction, and in many cases require resection of involved lung tissue due to chronic infection and the development of bronchiectasis (see "Bronchiectasis" later in the chapter). Similar to pulmonary sequestration, these lesions can have a dominant systemic arterial blood supply that must be kept in mind if operation is contemplated.

B. Bronchogenic Cysts

Bronchogenic cysts are the most common cystic lesions of the mediastinum and arise from abnormal budding of the foregut during development. The cyst wall consists of fibroelastic tissue, smooth muscle, and cartilage, whereas the cyst itself is lined with respiratory tract epithelia. It may also contain mucus-producing cuboidal cells, which contribute to enlargement of the cyst with mucus. They may occur anywhere along the tracheobronchial tree, but occur most commonly in the vicinity of the right pulmonary hilum and subcarinal region. Less frequently, they present in the neck, lower lobes of the lung, pleura, pericardium, or below the diaphragm. As they enlarge, cysts can compress surrounding vital structures, including the aerodigestive tract causing dysphagia, pneumothorax, cough, or hemoptysis or become infected. The diagnosis is confirmed by CT as a spherical fluid- or mucus-filled non-enhancing mass. An air–fluid level may be present thus suggesting communication with the airway. Cysts within the pulmonary parenchyma more commonly communicate with a bronchus, as opposed to those in the mediastinum. In general, mediastinal bronchogenic cysts present with airway compression and parenchymal cysts are manifested by pulmonary infection. Some cysts have been noted to enlarge rapidly and rupture into the pleural space, causing tension pneumothorax. Rare cases of malignant transformation have been reported. All bronchogenic cysts—regardless of location—are best treated with either simple or segmental resection by video-assisted thoracic surgery (VATS) due to their predisposition to become infected. Rarely, lobectomy is required.

C. Bronchopulmonary Dysplasia

Bronchopulmonary dysplasia (BPD) is a form of chronic lung disease that occurs in infants, usually in preterm infants receiving respiratory support with mechanical ventilation or prolonged oxygen supplementation. With the introduction of positive pressure ventilation in newborn infants, Northway and colleagues originally described a pattern of lung injury characterized by airway injury, inflammation, and parenchymal fibrosis in preterm infants who had received mechanical ventilation. Since the introduction and implementation of antenatal corticosteroids and postnatal surfactant replacement, BPD now more commonly affects those of extremely low birthweight and born at less than 26 weeks of gestation. BPD nowadays is fundamentally viewed as the result of abnormal reparative processes in response to injury and inflammation occurring in an immature lung of a genetically susceptible infant. The pathogenesis of BPD begins with a very immature lung complicated by iatrogenic damage from therapy with oxygen and volume ventilation, with superimposed infection and inflammation as well as pulmonary edema complicated by poor nutrition. Treatment is supportive, combining new approaches to ventilation (nasal CPAP and inhaled nitric oxide) with vitamin A. The American Thoracic Society has provided a position paper on the care of the child with chronic lung disease of infancy and childhood that addresses many of these issues.

D. Pulmonary Aplasia and Agenesis

Pulmonary hypoplasia is a relatively common abnormality of lung development and is defined pathologically as an abnormally low radial alveolus count and low ratio of lung weight to body weight. Pulmonary hypoplasia is termed primary pulmonary hypoplasia when no inciting cause is identified and is likely caused by abnormalities of the transcription factors that regulate early lung morphogenesis. These neonates present with tachypnea and hypoxemia resistant to administration of supplemental oxygen due to abnormal thickening of the pulmonary arteriolar wall. Persistent fetal circulation, hypoxemia, hypercapnia, and acidosis lead to early death in over 75% of patients. Secondary pulmonary hypoplasia is associated with a restriction of lung growth or the absence of fetal breathing. Any reduction of the chest cavity by a mass, effusion, or external compression can negatively impact lung growth. The most common of these abnormalities is congenital diaphragmatic hernia (see Chapter 43). Other conditions associated with secondary pulmonary hypoplasia include those that produce oligohydramnios and direct chest compression (eg, bilateral renal agenesis [Potter syndrome], renal dysplasia, and amniotic fluid leaks); those with

abnormal bone development and small rigid chest walls (eg, achondroplasia, chondrodystrophia fetalis calcificans, osteogenesis imperfecta, and spondyloepiphyseal dysplasia); those with decreased fetal respiratory movements (eg, phrenic nerve agenesis, abdominal masses or ascites with elevation of the diaphragm, arthrogryposis multiplex congenita, camptodactyly, and congenial myotonic dystrophy); those with intrathoracic mass lesions (eg, congenital cystic adenomatoid malformation, cystic hygroma, and esophageal duplication cysts); and those with pulmonary vascular abnormalities (eg, scimitar syndrome and pulmonary artery agenesis).

Unilateral pulmonary agenesis occurs when one lung and the associated vascular structures fail to develop. Neonates with pulmonary agenesis may present with tachypnea and cyanosis, particularly if associated cardiac anomalies exist (50% of cases). Some patients, however, remain asymptomatic until childhood, when they complain of dyspnea and wheezing suggestive of asthma. Physical examination in these patients reveals marked tracheal deviation toward the side of the agenesis, and chest x-ray, barium esophagography, and chest CT may be required to exclude other diagnostic possibilities such as total lung atelectasis from foreign body aspiration, total lung sequestration, and esophageal bronchus.

E. Pulmonary Sequestration

Pulmonary sequestration describes a mass of lung parenchyma that arises through abnormal budding of the caudal embryonic foregut and consequently has *no bronchial communication* with the otherwise normal tracheobronchial tree. Sequestration may occur either within normal lung tissue, termed intralobar sequestration; or as separate masses with their own visceral pleura, referred to as extralobar sequestration. The majority (85%) of sequestrations are of the intralobar type. Intralobar sequestrations receive their blood supply from the aorta and/orsplenic artery and their venous drainage from the pulmonary veins. In some cases this may be associated with anomalous venous drainage of the normal lung. Intralobar sequestrations are most commonly found on the left side in the lower lobe. Meanwhile, extralobar sequestrations are less common and receive their blood supply from the thoracic or abdominal aorta and the venous drainage via the systemic veins such as the azygos, hemiazygos, or inferior vena cava. Both are associated with foregut communications but more commonly in extralobar sequestrations.

Intralobar sequestrations are usually diagnosed later in childhood or adolescence after multiple episodes of pneumonia. Common symptoms include a chronic or recurrent cough. Extralobar sequestrations usually present in infancy with respiratory distress and chronic cough or manifest as gastrointestinal symptoms if a communication with the gastrointestinal tract exists. In rare instances, patients may present with hemoptysis or congestive heart failure from large left-to-right shunts through the sequestration. The diagnosis is usually suspected on chest x-ray and confirmed with a

CT scan of the chest delineating the arterial and venous drainage. Angiography can be used to confirm the diagnosis and elucidate aberrant vascular anatomy. Treatment consists of segmental resection or, if necessary, lobectomy via a thoracoscopic approach. Extreme attention must be given to understanding the arterial and venous anatomy of the malformation to avoid exsanguinating hemorrhage from division of an unrecognized systemic artery or venous infarction of the normal lung from ligation of the common draining vein. Following successful resection, the prognosis is favorable.

F. Congenital Cystic Adenomatoid Malformation

Congenital cystic adenomatoid malformation (CCAM) is the second most common cause of newborn respiratory distress, secondary to structural problems. CCAM is a discrete, space-occupying intrapulmonary mass that contain variable-sized cysts. These lesions do not function in normal gas exchange yet airspaces within these masses communicate with the tracheobronchial tree. Histologically, CCAM is distinguished from other lesions and normal lung by polypoid projections of the mucosa, an increase in smooth muscle and elastic tissue within cyst walls, an absence of cartilage, the presence of mucus-secreting cells, and the absence of inflammation. The classification system described by Stocker organizes these lesions on pathologic appearance and clinical outcome. Class I consists of large cysts >2 cm; class II consists of small cysts <2 cm; class III consists of solid lesions without cysts. Children will present either at birth or in early childhood with recurrent respiratory infections. The growth of CCAMs usually plateaus between 25 and 28 weeks, at which time the fetus appears to grow around the lesion. The vast majority of small- to moderate-sized CCAMs remain asymptomatic during fetal life. Approximately 15% of CCAMs will shrink significantly before birth. However, large lesions represent 5%-10% of CCAMs and may produce significant mass effect, which can lead to pulmonary hypoplasia, impaired fetal swallowing, polyhydramnios, impaired venous return, and heart failure. Fetal hydrops can result and appears to depend on the mass size, growth rate, and result from compression of the superior vena cava and impaired venous return. As therapeutic fetal interventions have become feasible, the ability to predict which infants will progress to hydrops has become critical. High-resolution fetal magnetic resonance imaging can calculate a cyst volume ratio which is useful in predicting progression to hydrops. Fetal interventions including a short course of maternal betamethasone for microcystic CCAM and minimally invasive in utero thoracoamniotic shunting for macrocystic CCAM have been shown to be successful. If fetal development is uncomplicated, early delivery is not encouraged. At birth, the infants are stratified based on symptoms. Critically ill infants require immediate resection of the involved lobe. However, an asymptomatic neonate should be initially evaluated with chest radiography.

Although surgery can be delayed in those patients with small lesions, any patient with known CCAM should undergo elective resection due to possible future complications including pneumonia and malignant transformation.

G. Congenital Lobar Emphysema

Congenital lobar emphysema (CLE) is the cause of half of the episodes of newborn respiratory distress due to structural abnormalities and is defined as an overdistended lobe resulting from the obstruction of a lobar bronchus. Obstruction can arise from abnormal cartilage development or an ischemic event during bronchial development. CLE also can develop as the result of meconium aspiration, lobar torsion, or an extrinsic cause such as obstructing lymph nodes. The left upper lobe is most commonly involved, followed by the right middle lobe. In addition, neonates who require prolonged mechanical ventilation can develop lobar emphysema from a combination of suction catheter trauma and barotrauma. The right lower lobe is most frequently affected in such patients.

Most infants present within the first 6 months of life with respiratory distress. In some patients, severe respiratory distress may occur in the neonatal period, requiring emergency evaluation and treatment. Common presentations include tracheal and mediastinal deviation away from the affected side, hyperresonance and decreased breath sounds on the affected side, and a chest radiograph demonstrating hyperlucency in the area of the affected lobe with compression of adjacent lung. Often a chest radiograph is sufficient for diagnosis and operative planning. Yet some (often older) children may require chest CT to exclude other pathology (eg, bronchogenic cysts, anomalous pulmonary vessels, and hilar lymphadenopathy). Bronchoscopy also may be necessary to rule out the presence of a foreign body causing ball-valve airway obstruction.

Successful therapy in all patients requires pulmonary resection, almost uniformly a lobectomy. Attention to airway management is paramount as during induction, positive-pressure ventilation can cause progressive mediastinal shift. If such a situation arises, an emergent thoracotomy should be performed to allow the affected lobe to herniate through the incision, thereby decompressing the mediastinum and restoring venous return and hemodynamic stability. Long term, these patients may have bronchomalacia and a predisposition to bronchospasm.

Correia-Pinto J, et al. Congenital lung lesions: Underlying molecular mechanisms. *Semin Pediatr Surg*. 2010;19(3):171.

Moyer J, et al. Thoracoscopic lobectomy for congenital lung lesions. *Clin Perinatol*. 2017;44(4):781-794.

Puligandla PS, Laberge J. Congenital lung lesions. *Clin Perinatol*. 2012;39(2):331-347.

Statement on the care of the child with chronic lung disease of infancy and childhood. *Am J Respir Crit Care Med*. 2003; 168(3):356-396.

CONGENITAL VASCULAR LESIONS OF THE LUNG

Vascular diseases of the lung include two main processes: arteriovenous malformations and vascular rings. Arteriovenous malformations are uncommon congenital lesions that develop as a result of abnormal capillary formation during the canalicular phase of development. Most arise from the pulmonary artery, but occasionally a systemic arterial source can be involved similar to that in pulmonary sequestration. Rarely, an arteriovenous malformation can arise from a coronary artery, with the right coronary artery involved 55% of the time. Coronary arteriovenous fistulas drain into the right ventricle (40%), right atrium (25%), pulmonary artery (20%), coronary sinus (7%), superior vena cava (1%), or left-sided heart chambers (7%). Patients are either asymptomatic or develop signs of congestive heart failure. Myocardial infarction is rare. A continuous murmur and signs of reduced left ventricular afterload may be present. Although the diagnosis often can be established with echocardiography and color Doppler imaging, the definitive diagnosis, shunt fraction, and complete preoperative planning require catheterization and angiography. Operation is indicated for symptomatic patients and for those asymptomatic patients with large shunts.

Vascular rings occur from abnormal development of the aortic arches and major branches, with resulting compression of the trachea and esophagus. In normal fetal development, a dual system of six aortic arches regresses in such a way that the left fourth arch becomes the main left-sided aorta, the left sixth arch develops as the ductus arteriosus, and the right fourth arch persists as the right innominate artery and subclavian artery. Most vascular rings, however, are associated with a right-sided aortic arch and are classified as complete vascular rings or incomplete rings (arterial slings). Complete vascular rings include a double aortic arch (67%, the most common complete ring), a right aortic arch with a left subclavian and left ductus arteriosus (30%), a right aortic arch with mirror-image branching and a left ductus arteriosus (rare), and a left aortic arch with an aberrant right subclavian and right ductus arteriosus (very rare). Incomplete rings consist of an aberrant right subclavian artery that originates on the left side and passes posterior to the esophagus (most common incomplete ring) and an anomalous left pulmonary artery arising from the right pulmonary artery and passing between the trachea and the esophagus (pulmonary artery sling).

Most patients present with symptoms of tracheal or esophageal compression. Patients with an anomalous right subclavian artery may present later in life with obstructive symptoms (dysphagia lusoria), while those with complete vascular rings and pulmonary artery slings typically present early in life (within 6 months) with symptoms of respiratory distress (often frank stridor), particularly with neck flexion and poor feeding. The diagnosis is often suggested by characteristic findings on barium esophagogram. Bilateral indentations imply double aortic arch. A posterior indentation suggests an aberrant right subclavian artery, large right-sided indentations suggest complete rings associated with a right aortic arch, and an anterior impression is typical of a pulmonary artery sling. Often, the diagnosis can be confirmed by echocardiography. MRI/MRA often provides useful anatomic details. Surgical repair of these lesions is indicated once the diagnosis is established and is accomplished by dividing the vascular ring usually through a left thoracotomy. With double aortic arches, the smaller of the two arches is divided distal to the subclavian artery, while other complete rings generally are treated by division of the ligamentum arteriosum. Aberrant right subclavian arteries may be simply divided or, if necessary, divided and transposed to the right side. Pulmonary artery slings require reimplantation of the left pulmonary artery and often resection of the compressed trachea, which often has severe tracheomalacia and stenosis from impaired development. Rarely, tracheomalacia secondary to vascular ring compression necessitates suspension of the aortic arch from the sternum.

SUPPURATIVE DISEASES OF THE LUNG

1. Lung Abscess

A lung abscess usually begins as a necrotizing pneumonia progressing to liquefactive necrosis of the lung parenchyma. The liquefied necrotic material eventually empties into a draining bronchus, forming a necrotic cavity of pus containing an air–fluid level. With rupture, the infection can extend into the pleural space, producing an empyema. Arbitrarily, abscesses are termed acute if the duration is less than 6 weeks and chronic if more than 6 weeks. Although the incidence of lung abscesses fell dramatically following the introduction of effective antibiotics in the 1940s and 1950s, a recent increase in the number of immunocompromised individuals secondary to organ transplantation, chemotherapy, and HIV has resulted in a resurgence in the numbers of lung abscesses requiring treatment.

Lung abscesses can be divided into two major categories based on etiology: primary and secondary. Lung abscesses are termed primary when they arise in a previously healthy individual, or secondary to an underlying cause. Most commonly a primary abscess occurs as a result of aspiration owing to impaired consciousness or swallowing dysfunction due to neuromuscular or esophageal diseases. Sixty to seventy percent of lung abscesses present in the right lung in the dependent posterior segment of the right upper lobe and superior segment of the lower lobe. They are most commonly polymicrobial, with a predominance of anaerobic organisms including *Peptostreptococcus*, *Bacteroides fragilis*, and *Fusobacterium*. Conditions that predispose to aspiration include anesthesia (both general and monitored), neurologic disorders (cerebrovascular accidents, seizures, diabetic coma, head trauma, etc), drug ingestion (alcohol, narcotics, etc), normal sleep, poor oral hygiene (increases bacterial load), and esophageal disease (gastroesophageal reflux, achalasia, cancer, tracheoesophageal fistula). Secondary causes include bronchial obstruction (tumor, foreign body, hilar lymphadenopathy), necrotizing pneumonia (*Staphylococcus auerus*, *Klebsiella pneumoniae*), chronic pneumonia (due to fungi, tubercle bacilli), and opportunistic infection in an immunodeficient host. Over the years, the incidence of secondary lung abscess arising in the setting of an immunocompromised state has increased. As a result, virulent aerobic species such as *Klebsiella*, *Pseudomonas*, *Proteus*, *Enterobacter*, and *Staphylococcus aureus* now comprise the majority of these infections as opposed to anaerobic species. Gram-negative lung abscess occurs in elderly and immunocompromised patients with nosocomial pneumonia. Cavitating lesions may arise in the setting of a malignancy or pulmonary infarct. Direct extension of a localized infection such as amebiasis or subphrenic abscess may also progress to a secondary lung abscess. Bloodborne infections can give rise to multiple lung abscesses in the periphery of the lung and are the result of septic emboli from bacteria, endocarditis, septic thrombophlebitis, or subphrenic infection. It should be noted that secondary infections of congenital or acquired cystic lesions, such as bronchogenic cysts, bullae, tuberculous cavities, and hydatid cysts, are not true pulmonary abscesses because they occur in a preformed space.

▶ Clinical Findings & Diagnosis

Patients with lung abscesses typically report symptoms of cough, fevers, putrid sputum, hemoptysis, dyspnea, pleuritic chest pain, and weight loss. Symptoms are often insidious in onset and associated with malaise and weight loss if chronic. Complications include rupture into a bronchus, with initial hemoptysis followed by the production of foul-smelling, purulent sputum (and the potential for life-threatening pneumonia from aspiration of pus into normal lung); and rupture into the pleural space with resulting pyopneumothorax, sepsis, and possibly empyema necessitatis. On physical examination, signs of lobar consolidation predominate; but clubbing, signs of pleural effusion, cachexia, and rarely a draining chest wound (empyema necessitatis) can be present. Laboratory studies should include a white blood cell count and sputum culture. Chest radiography and CT scan of the thorax are usually sufficient to aid diagnosis and differentiate between empyema and abscess. Cavitation is generally apparent on chest radiographs 2 weeks after the onset of symptoms. Radiologic resolution lags behind clinical and biochemical improvement, taking up to 3 months to resolve in nearly 70% of patients. In cases of suspected bronchial obstruction or in all patients with unexplained lung abscesses, bronchoscopy is indicated. Fine-needle aspiration

of the abscess cavity for diagnostic culture has been shown to isolate the offending pathogens in 94% of patients compared with only 11% and 3% from sputum culture and bronchoalveolar lavage, respectively. Early fine-needle aspiration can prompt a change of the antibiotic regimen and can be lifesaving in immunocompromised patients with unusual organisms.

▶ Treatment

As these patients can present with florid sepsis, antibiotic administration has been the mainstay of therapy following general resuscitation measures. First-line treatment should include aerobic and anaerobic coverage for a period of 4-6 weeks. Once the acute sepsis subsides (after up to 2 weeks), therapy can frequently be changed to an oral outpatient regimen and continued until complete resolution of the abscess occurs (3-5 months). Important adjuncts to antibiotic administration include chest physiotherapy, postural drainage, bronchoscopy (may require repeated examinations to maintain bronchial drainage), and health maintenance measures (general nutrition, dental hygiene, etc).

In patients who do not respond to this initial regimen and who do not have surgical indications (see below), early percutaneous drainage has been shown to be a safe and effective procedure (mortality rate, 1.5%; morbidity rate, 10%). In patients unresponsive to antimicrobials, source control is of the utmost importance. Specific proposed indications for percutaneous drainage include (1) an abscess under tension as evidenced by mediastinal shift, displacement of fissures, or downward displacement of the diaphragm; (2) radiographic verification of contralateral lung contamination; (3) unremitting signs of sepsis after 72 hours of adequate antibiotic therapy; (4) abscess size larger than 4 cm or increasing abscess size; (5) rising fluid level; and (6) persistent ventilatory dependency.

In addition to drainage, intervention permits microbiologic analysis of the aspirate. In nearly half of patients, initial antibiotic regimens require adjustment based on microbial speciation and sensitivity analyses. Tube thoracostomy is cautioned against because of the risk of parenchymal injury with resulting chronic air leak and/or bronchopleural fistula (BPF). Operative intervention is rarely indicated in the management of lung abscess, but should be considered in patients with failure of clinical or radiologic improvement after 4-6 weeks of antibiotic therapy, abscesses larger than 6 cm, massive or life-threatening hemoptysis (4%), empyema or BPF (4%), or bronchial obstruction (particularly if secondary to resectable cancer). Furthermore, acute rupture into the pleural space (pyopneumothorax) is still a surgical emergency. When surgery is indicated, either thoracoscopic or open lobectomy generally is the preferred procedure and can be accomplished with low morbidity and mortality (0%-2%). Routine buttressing of the bronchial stump with a vascularized pedicle (intercostal muscle or pericardial fat) is recommended to prevent BPF. Double-lumen intubation should be performed in order to protect the airway and limit abscess spillage into the contralateral lung.

▶ Prognosis

Antibiotics given over 4-6 weeks alongside percutaneous drainage is effective in 85%-95% of patients. Mortality for lung abscess has decreased from 30% to 40% in the preantibiotic era to 10% in the present era, but remains greater for elderly individuals; immunocompromised patients; or those who have abscess larger than 6 cm, bronchial obstruction, multiple abscesses, necrotizing pneumonia, or gram-negative pneumonia.

Agasthian T. Results of surgery for bronchiectasis and pulmonary abscesses. *Thorac Surg Clin.* 2012;22:333.

2. Bronchiectasis

Bronchiectasis is defined as irreversible dilation of the peripheral airways secondary to damage of the structural components of the bronchial wall (elastin, muscles, and cartilage). Mechanisms of damage include bronchial wall injury, bronchial lumen obstruction, and traction from adjacent fibrosis seen in end-stage lung fibrosis. Cole's "vicious cycle" hypothesizes that initial infection, in a background of genetic susceptibility of impaired mucosal clearance, results in retention of microorganisms in the bronchial tree. Overproduction of thick inflammatory mucus in the setting of persistent microbial colonization of dilated airways, together with impairment of mucociliary clearance mechanisms, causes a vicious cycle of repeated and prolonged episodes of chronic inflammation resulting in progressive airway and lung damage.

The clinical syndrome manifests as chronic dilation of bronchi, a paroxysmal cough that produces variable amounts of fetid, mucopurulent sputum, and recurrent pulmonary infections. Aspirated foreign bodies, endobronchial neoplasms, and hilar lymphadenopathy (see "Middle Lobe Syndrome" later in the chapter) also can cause retention of secretions, infections, and progressive bronchiectasis. The presence of true established bronchiectasis, however, must be distinguished from pseudobronchiectasis, which is a cylindric bronchial dilation that is associated with acute bronchopneumonia. When left untreated, true bronchiectasis progresses, while pseudobronchiectasis reverses completely after weeks to months.

Most cases are related to acquired disorders and are caused by two factors: infection and bronchial obstruction. Acquired viral and bacterial infections in infancy and childhood—eg, pertussis, measles, influenza, tuberculosis, and bronchopneumonia—were common predisposing conditions that led to bronchiectasis in the past and are still common in developing countries. With the reemergence of

tuberculosis, postinfectious bronchiectasis is also becoming more prevalent, and is seen 11% of such patients. In developed countries, more common causes are immune deficiency syndromes (hypogammaglobulinemia and leukocyte dysfunction), metabolic defects (cystic fibrosis, α_1-antitrypsin deficiency), ultrastructural defects (primary ciliary dyskinesia, Young syndrome, Kartagener syndrome, congenital defects of cartilage), and pulmonary sequestration.

Reid has categorized bronchiectasis into three main types based on pathologic appearance: (1) tubular or cylindrical, characterized by smooth dilation of the bronchi; (2) varicose, in which the bronchi are dilated with multiple indentations; and (3) cystic or saccular, in which dilated bronchi terminate in blind ending sacs of pus with no communication with the rest of the lung. Saccular bronchiectasis follows severe infections and cases of bronchial obstruction, while the cylindrical variant is associated with tuberculosis and immune disorders. Varicose consists of alternating areas of cylindrical and saccular types.

Bronchiectasis can be classified also as perfused or nonperfused types according to functional hemodynamic perfusion studies as described by Ashour. The perfused type has cylindrical bronchiectatic changes with intact pulmonary artery flow, whereas the nonperfused type involves cystic bronchiectasis with absent pulmonary artery flow and retrograde filling of the pulmonary artery through the systemic circulation.

Taken together, tubular or cylindric bronchiectasis tends to have better prognosis than cystic/varicose varieties, as the lung areas affected by the former tend to have good function and perfusion. Cystic bronchiectasis tends to indicate a completely destroyed, nonfunctional, and nonperfused lung. Additionally, all parameters of respiratory function are worse in the saccular type as compared with the tubular type. Saccular type bronchiectasis also is associated with higher bacterial loads with virulent strains, such as *Pseudomonas*.

In general, bronchiectasis involves the second- to fourth-order branches of the segmental bronchi, and its distribution is largely characteristic of the underlying pathology. The left lung tends to be more involved than the right lung in 55%-80% of cases. This may be because the left mainstem bronchus is narrower and longer than the right and subject to greater compression pressures, especially by the aortic arch. The lower lobes are commonly affected owing to gravity-dependent retention of infected secretions. Congenital disorders, for example, are associated with diffuse bilateral bronchiectasis, while tuberculosis and granulomatous diseases are characterized by unilateral or bilateral disease, most commonly limited to the upper lobes and superior segments of the lower lobes. Furthermore, bronchiectasis following pyogenic and viral pneumonias usually involves only the lower lobes, middle lobe, and lingula, and postobstructive bronchiectasis is generally limited to the obstructed segments (see also "Middle Lobe Syndrome" later in the chapter). Common pathogens in patients with bronchiectasis include *H. influenzae, S. aureus, K. pneumoniae, E. coli,* and, in the chronic setting, *Pseudomonas* species. Mycobacteria, fungi, and *Legionella* also should be considered.

Clinical Findings & Diagnosis

Patients often have a history of recurrent febrile episodes and complain of a chronic or intermittent cough that produces variable amounts of foul-smelling sputum (up to 500 mL/d). Hemoptysis occurs in 41%-66% of patients, but is rarely massive. Bronchiectasis associated with granulomatous disease may not be associated with a productive cough at all (so-called dry bronchiectasis). Exacerbations and advanced disease are manifested by increased sputum production, fever, dyspnea, anorexia, fatigue, and weight loss. A history of sinus problems, infertility, or a family history of similar problems suggests the presence of an inherited disorder associated with bronchiectasis. Physical examination may reveal cyanosis, clubbing, pulmonary osteoarthropathy, evidence of malnutrition, and in advanced disease, signs of cor pulmonale.

Although bronchiectasis is suspected, an imaging study is usually required for confirmation. Bronchograms were at one time required, but high-resolution chest computed tomography (CT) scans are now the imaging procedure of choice to document bronchial dilation, particularly with saccular disease. Even with the diagnosis of bronchiectasis, however, endobronchial neoplasm or foreign body must be excluded by flexible fiberoptic bronchoscopy.

Treatment

In nearly all patients, conservative medical therapy is indicated and generally is sufficient. This includes broad-spectrum antibiotics, bronchodilators, humidification, expectorants, mucolytics, and effective chest PT and routine postural drainage. In patients with continued infection, bronchoscopy with bronchoalveolar lavage should be considered to obtain more accurate culture results. Other adjunctive therapies include influenza and pneumococcal vaccines and, in patients with multiple yearly exacerbations, chronic "prophylactic" antibiotics with amoxicillin, doxycycline, or preferably a macrolide (erythromycin or azithromycin). A medical advance in controlling underlying bacterial (especially *Pseudomonas*) infection and symptoms associated with bronchiectasis has been the use of inhaled antibiotics and suppressive macrolide usage. In the cystic fibrosis and chronic bronchiectasis population, nebulized tobramycin or gentamicin has proven effective in controlling infection, sputum production, and symptoms in a significant proportion of patients.

Patients who fail intensive medical therapy may be candidates for surgical resection if the following criteria are met: (1) the disease must be localized and completely resectable, (2) pulmonary reserve must be adequate, (3) the process must be irreversible (ie, not pseudobronchiectasis, bronchial stricture, foreign body, etc), and (4) significant symptoms must persist. Preoperative assessment requires a high-resolution chest CT scan. Pulmonary function studies generally are not necessary, since the involved segments do not function.

The goals of surgery are to remove all active disease and to preserve as much functioning lung parenchyma as possible. The surgical approach includes complete segmental resection of the involved areas. Partial resection almost always ends in recurrence. Resection most commonly involves all basal segments (unilaterally or bilaterally) along with the middle lobe or lingula. With tuberculosis, however, removal of the upper lobe or lobes with or without the superior segment of the lower lobes is more likely. During operation, meticulous maintenance of a clear airway devoid of mucopurulent secretions and blood is essential. Careful dissection of the bronchovascular structures is difficult in patients with chronic inflammation and scarring but is essential to avoid complications. In those cases where the degree of anatomic resection would create prohibitive risk, lung transplantation should be considered.

Prognosis

Although most patients are successfully treated with medical therapy, some require operation. The results of pulmonary resection depend on the cause and type of parenchymal involvement. Success with elimination of symptoms occurs in up to 80% of patients with limited localized disease but only 36% of those with diffuse disease. Prognostic factors include (1) unilateral disease restricted to the basal segments, (2) young age, (3) absence of sinusitis and rhinitis, (4) history of pneumonia, and (5) no major airway obstruction. Overall morbidity and mortality rates are surprisingly low at 3%-5%, and less than 1%, respectively.

Polverino E, et al. European respiratory society guidelines for the management of adult bronchiectasis. *Eur Respir J.* 2017;50(3).

3. Middle Lobe Syndrome

Middle lobe syndrome (MLS) is characterized by recurrent or chronic collapse of the middle lobe of the right lung, but can also involve the lingula of the left lung. There are two forms of MLS: obstructive and nonobstructive. Obstructive MLS occurs as a result of an endobronchial lesion or extrinsic compression of the middle lobe bronchus from hilar lymphadenopathy or tumor causing postobstructive atelectasis and pneumonitis. The most common cause of extrinsic compression of the right middle lobe bronchus is enlargement of peribronchial lymph nodes due to fungal infections such as histoplasmosis or atypical mycobacterial infections. Adenopathy due to sarcoidosis or lymph node metastases has also been described in obstructive MLS. Less common causes include aspirated foreign objects, broncholiths, inspissated mucus (associated with cystic fibrosis), and endoluminal granulomas associated with sarcoidosis.

Nonobstructive MLS is characterized by the absence of a mechanical obstruction of the middle lobe bronchus on bronchoscopy and/or CT of the chest. Though poorly understood, the narrow diameter and long length of the middle lobe bronchus, combined with an acute angle at its origin, create poor conditions for adequate drainage. This form of MLS is the most common cause of MLS and commonly occurs in adults and children with recurrent pneumonia and is often related to asthma, bronchitis, and cystic fibrosis.

The diagnosis of MLS should be entertained in a patient with repeated episodes of right-sided pneumonia, only after other causes of obstruction (bronchogenic cancer, foreign body, etc) have been ruled out. Evaluation includes chest radiography, bronchoscopy, and CT of the chest. Most patients respond to intensive medical therapy including bronchodilators, mucolytics, and broad-spectrum antibiotics in addition to therapeutic bronchoscopy. Those who do not respond should be offered resection of the right middle lobe and/or debulking lymphadenopathy, which is associated with a low mortality rate and favorable outcome. Other indications for surgery include bronchiectasis, fibrosis (bronchial stenosis), abscess, unresolved or intractable recurrent pneumonia, hemoptysis, and suspicion of neoplasm.

Gudbjartsson T, et al. Middle lobe syndrome: A review of clinic pathological features, diagnosis and treatment. *Respiration.* 2012;84:80.

4. Broncholithiasis

Broncholithiasis is defined as the presence of calculi (broncholiths) within the tracheobronchial tree. In most cases, a broncholith is formed by erosion and extrusion of a calcified adjacent lymph node into the bronchial lumen and is usually associated with long-standing foci of necrotizing granulomatous lymphadenitis. Calcified lymph nodes can remain attached to the bronchial wall, lodge in a bronchus, or be expectorated (lithoptysis). The most common cause of broncholithiasis in the United States is histoplasmosis. Tuberculosis is another frequent cause in some parts of the world.

Patients with broncholithiasis often complain of hemoptysis, lithoptysis (30%), cough, sputum production, fever, chills, and pleuritic chest pain. The hemoptysis is characteristically sudden and self-limited, though rarely it may be massive. Symptoms of pneumonia may indicate bronchial obstruction from an impacted broncholith. Signs suggesting broncholithiasis include localized wheezing on physical examination, evidence of hilar calcifications or segmental atelectasis and pneumonia on chest x-ray, and bronchoscopic evidence of peribronchial disease. The diagnosis is confirmed by documentation of lithoptysis or the presence of an endobronchial "lung stone."

The complications of broncholithiasis include hemoptysis, which on occasion can be massive and life-threatening; suppurative lung diseases (eg, pneumonia and bronchiectasis); midesophageal traction diverticula; and, rarely, tracheobronchoesophageal fistula.

In addition to instituting appropriate therapy for underlying pulmonary diseases, treatment is primarily directed at removal of endobronchial stones. This can be accomplished at the time of bronchoscopy if the broncholith is freely floating within the tracheobronchial tree or if it extends well into the bronchial lumen and can be removed without excessive force or traction (20% of cases). The main danger of transbronchoscopic removal of broncholiths is the risk for massive hemorrhage. This results during inappropriate removal of broncholiths that remain substantially attached to the parabronchial tissues. Because of intense peribronchial fibrosis in this situation, the broncholith not infrequently becomes adherent to vascular structures such as the pulmonary artery, which may be torn with vigorous attempts at broncholith removal.

Nearly 80% of patients with broncholiths that remain in situ require surgical removal. The goal of surgery in this disease is preservation of lung function. The broncholith may be removed safely with bronchotomy; however, most patients require segmentectomy or lobectomy, particularly if destruction of lung parenchyma has occurred from postobstruction suppurative lung disease. Fistulas between the airway and the esophagus should be repaired with interposition of normal tissue (intercostal muscle flap, etc) between the two structures to prevent recurrence. Following surgery, the prognosis is excellent.

Cerfolio R, et al. Rigid bronchoscopy and surgical resection for broncholithiasis and calcified mediastinal lymph nodes. *J Thorac Cardiovasc Surg.* 2008;136:186.
Lim S, et al. Classification of broncholiths and clinical outcomes. *Respirology.* 2013;18(4):637-642.

5. Cystic Fibrosis and Mucoid Impaction of the Bronchi

Cystic fibrosis is an autosomal recessive multisystem congenital disorder that is characterized by chronic airway obstruction and infection and by exocrine pancreatic insufficiency and gastrointestinal tract dysfunction with consequent effects on nutrition, growth, and maturation. The disorder is the result of several characterized mutations in the cystic fibrosis transmembrane regulator (CFTR) gene, most commonly the ΔF508 mutation. Such mutations cause abnormalities of chloride and likely sodium transport, leading to abnormal regulation and reduction of airway surface liquid volume. The result is a viscous and tenacious mucus that adheres to the airway surface epithelium resulting in airflow obstruction and bacterial infection (S. aureus,

P. aeruginosa, and *Burkholderia cepacia).* Once established, infection of the CF lung is rarely eradicated. Pulmonary manifestations of the disorder include mucoid impaction, bronchitis, bronchiectasis, pulmonary fibrosis, emphysema, and lung abscess. Mucoid plugs are rubbery, semisolid, gray to greenish-yellow in color, and round, oval, or elongated in shape. There is often a history of recurrent upper respiratory infection, fever, and chest pain. Expectoration of hard mucus plugs or hemoptysis may occur.

The earliest manifestation of CF lung disease is a cough that progressively worsens to becoming a daily event and productive. It often becomes paroxymal and associated with gagging and emesis. Sputum is usually tenacious, purulent, and often green, reflecting bacterial infection. Hyperinflation of the lungs due to airway obstruction is noted early in the progression of lung disease. Asthmatic or bronchiolitic-type wheezing is common. CF patients typically have mild bronchitis symptoms for long periods of time punctuated by increasingly frequent acute exacerbations of symptoms that include increased intensity of cough, tachypnea, shortness of breath, decreased activity and appetite, and weight loss. Intense antibiotic therapy and assistance with clearance of mucus are usually required to reduce lung symptoms and improve lung function. End-stage lung disease is characterized by substantial hypoxemia, pulmonary hypertension, cor pulmonale, and death.

The primary objectives of CF treatment are to control infection, promote mucus clearance, and improve nutrition. Therapy includes postural drainage with chest percussion, expectorants, bronchodilators, antibiotics, and aerosol inhalation. More novel therapies include (1) inhaled hypertonic saline, which osmotically draws water onto the airway surface, thereby "rehydrating" the airway mucus and allowing for easier expectoration; (2) aerosolized rhDNase, which lyses the viscous DNA contained within airway mucus; and (3) ibuprofen, which has been shown to slow the decline in lung function. Surgery including partial lung resection is indicated for apparently localized disease (lung abscess and bronchiectasis) and recurrent severe exacerbations. Lobectomy is occasionally indicated for massive hemoptysis that is refractory to bronchial artery embolization.

Double lung transplantation has become an accepted therapy for respiratory failure secondary to CF. Patients should be referred when their prognosis is about equal to the waiting time for donor lungs, currently about 2 years after acceptance as a lung transplant candidate. Relative contra-indications to transplant include severe malnutrition (ideal body weight <70%), chronic steroid use greater than 20 mg of prednisone daily, and mechanical ventilation (center dependent). Multi-resistant *P. aeruginosa* infection is not a contraindication for transplantation, although pan-resistant *P. aeruginosa* is considered, at some centers, to be a contraindication. *Burkholderia cepacia* is viewed by some to be a contraindication to lung transplantation. The transplanted lungs remain free of CF, but are subject to secondary infection, acute rejection, and chronic rejection (bronchiolitis obliterans syndrome). The 5-year survival following lung transplantation is 48%. The median survival in all CF patients now exceeds 31 years.

Savant AP, McColley SA. Cystic fibrosis year in review 2017. *Pediatr Pulmonol.* 2018;53(9):1307-1317.

6. Tuberculosis

Tuberculosis markedly declined as a cause of death between 1953 and 1984, but since 1985 this disease has experienced resurgence due to increased immigration of infected individuals and patients who are immunocompromised. A reservoir of about 5000-8000 clinical cases exists, and an additional 25,000 new cases occur annually. Multidrug-resistant tuberculosis (MDR-TB) and, most recently, extensively drug-resistant tuberculosis (XDR-TB) have emerged over the last 20 years. MDR-TB is defined as those strains resistant to at least isoniazid and rifampicin. XDR-TB strains are defined as those resistant to rifampicin, isoniazid, fluroquinolones, and any of capreomycin, kanamycin, or amikacin. Resistance to these antitubercular drugs is the result of spontaneous mutations in the genome and is due to a number of factors, most commonly inadequate treatment of active pulmonary tuberculosis. Less than 20% of the United States population is tuberculin-positive, but tuberculosis remains a common infectious cause of death worldwide. It is estimated that there are 440,000 new MDR-TB cases indentified each year worldwide, many of these arising in previously treated patients. Nearly 50% of cases occur in India and China. The prognosis of treatment of MDR-TB or XDR-TB is significantly worse than for drug-susceptible disease.

Several species of the genus *Mycobacterium* may cause lung disease, but 95% of cases of lung disease are due to *M. tuberculosis.* Several "atypical" species of mycobacterium, such as *M. bovis* and *M. avium,* that are chiefly soil-dwellers have become clinically more important in recent years because they are less responsive to preventive and therapeutic measures. Mycobacteria are nonmotile, nonsporulating, weakly gram-positive rods classified in the order *Actinomycetales.* Dormant organisms remain alive for the life of the host.

The initial infection often involves pulmonary parenchyma in the midzone of the lungs. When hypersensitivity develops after several weeks, the typical caseation appears. Regional hilar lymph nodes become enlarged. Most cases arrest spontaneously at this stage. However, should the infection progress, caseation necrosis develops and giant cells produce a typical tubercle. A cause of latent disease in the elderly or debilitated patient is dormant reactivation tubercles. Sites in the apical and posterior segments of the upper lobes and superior segments of the lower lobes are the usual areas of infection.

▶ Clinical Findings

A. Symptoms and Signs

Patients may present with minimal symptoms, including fever, cough, anorexia, weight loss, night sweats, excessive perspiration, chest pain, lethargy, and dyspnea. Extrapulmonary disease may be associated with more severe symptoms, such as involvement of the pericardium, bones, joints, urinary tract, meninges, lymph nodes, or pleural space. Erythema nodosum is occasionally seen in patients with active disease.

B. Laboratory Findings

False-negative tests with intermediate-strength PPD are usually due to anergy, improper testing, or outdated tuberculin. Anergy is sometimes associated with disseminated tuberculosis, measles, sarcoidosis, lymphomas, or recent vaccination with live viruses (eg, poliomyelitis, measles, rubella, mumps, influenza, or yellow fever). Immunosuppressive drugs (eg, corticosteroids, azathioprine) and disease states (eg, AIDS, organ transplantation) may also cause false-negative responses. Culture of sputum, gastric aspirates, and tracheal washings as well as pleural fluid and pleural and lung biopsies may establish the diagnosis.

C. Imaging Studies

Radiographic findings include involvement of the apical and posterior segments of the upper lobes (85%) or the superior segments of the lower lobes (10%). Seldom is the anterior segment of the upper lobe solely involved, as in other granulomatous diseases such as histoplasmosis. Involvement of the basal segments of the lower lobes is uncommon but occurs occasionally in women, African Americans, and diabetics, but endobronchial disease usually involves the lower lobes, producing atelectasis or consolidation. Differing x-ray patterns correspond to the pathologic variations of the disease: the local exudative lesion, the local productive lesion, cavitation, acute tuberculous pneumonia, miliary tuberculosis, Rasmussen aneurysm, bronchiectasis, bronchostenosis, and tuberculoma.

D. Differential Diagnosis

It is critical to distinguish the x-ray findings from bronchogenic carcinoma, particularly when there is tuberculoma without calcification.

▶ Treatment

A. Medical Treatment

Active disease should be treated with one of the antibiotic regimens that have recently been shown to shorten the period of treatment while maintaining their potency. Such drugs include isoniazid, streptomycin, rifampin, and ethambutol;

and recent recommendations advise using combination formulations to aid in medication adherence.

Treatment of MDR-TB and XDR-TB is less well defined. The World Health Organization (WHO) recently updated and put forth recommendations for treating drug susceptible TB and MDR-TB. This includes:

Rapid drug-susceptibility testing of at least rifampicin should be performed at the initial diagnosis of tuberculosis.

The use of sputum microscopy and culture should be used instead of microscopy alone.

The treatment of MDR-TB should include at least pyrazinamide as well as four core second-line TB medications: (1) a fluoroquinolone; (2) a parenteral agent (kanamycin, amikacin, streptomycin, or capreomycin); (3) ethionamide; and (4) linezolid, cycloserine, or clofazimine. Strengthening the regimen with high-dose isoniazid and/or ethambutol is recommended.

An intensive treatment of at least 6-months duration is recommended, and those with MDR-TB should undergo a minimum of 9-12 months of treatment.

The success of MDR-TB therapy is approximately 55% with a mortality rate of 16%.

B. Surgical Treatment

The role of surgery in treatment of tuberculosis has diminished dramatically since antimicrobials became available. It is now confined to the following indications: (1) failure of chemotherapy, (2) performance of diagnostic procedures, (3) destroyed lung, (4) postsurgical complications, (5) persistent bronchopleural fistula, and (6) intractable hemorrhage. The most common parenchymal resection includes lobectomy or wedge resection, followed by pneumonectomy, although the latter has fallen out of favor. Muscle flap coverage is strongly recommended. The infectious process often involves the pleural space and it is useful to perform an extrapleural dissection to minimize contamination or bacterial superinfection of the resection cavity.

Pulmonary resection is adjunctive to medication. The rationale for lung resection of parenchyma affected by MDR-TB is to remove a large focal burden of organisms present in destroyed nonviable lung tissue. The destroyed lung parenchyma and associated cavities are an ideal environment for the bacillus to grow due to its isolation from the circulation and therefore the host's defenses. Surgery is recommended in MDR-TB patients with extensive drug resistance—those with localized disease amenable to resection and those with high drug activity. Pretreatment with antibiotic regimens for at least 2 months is required before operation to reduce the bacterial burden, followed by 12-24 months of treatment after surgery. Those patients who have been treated long enough to have culture conversion of disease tend to respond better to wedge resection or lobectomy (not pneumonectomy).

Diagnostic lung resection may be necessary to rule out other diseases, such as cancer, or to obtain material for cultures. Patients with destroyed lobes or cavitary tuberculosis of the right upper lobe containing large infected foci may sometimes be candidates for resection to help with source control.

The disease can become reactivated in some patients who have had thoracoplasty, plombage, or resection, and a few will require reoperation. The most common indications for surgery after plombage therapy are pleural infection (pyogenic or tuberculous) and migration of the plombage material, causing pain or compression of other organs. Following pulmonary resection, tuberculous empyema may develop in the postpneumonectomy space, sometimes associated with a bronchopleural fistula or bony sequestration. Persistent bronchopleural fistula after chemotherapy and closed tube drainage may require direct operative closure. Use of muscle flaps (intercostal, etc) is highly recommended to cover any bronchial stumps, especially in the setting of pneumonectomy.

Tuberculous empyema poses unique problems of management. Treatment depends upon whether the empyema is (1) associated with parenchymal disease, (2) mixed tuberculous and pyogenic or purely tuberculous, and (3) associated with bronchopleural fistula. The ultimate objective is complete expansion of the lung and obliteration of the empyema space. Pulmonary decortication or resection may be used for tuberculosis, but open or closed drainage is necessary when the process is complicated by pyogenic infection or bronchopleural fistula.

▶ Prognosis

The prognosis is excellent in most drug-susceptible cases treated medically; the death rate decreased from 25% in 1945 to less than 10% currently. Perioperative mortality for pulmonary resections for tuberculosis ranges from 10% for pneumonectomy to 3% for lobectomy and 1% for segmentectomy and subsegmental resections. Debate is ongoing as to the improved outcomes in patients undergoing surgery and medical treatment compared to medication alone.

The morbidity of surgical resection ranges from 12% to 39%, with the most common complications being bleeding, empyema, wound complications, and bronchopleural fistula. Factors leading to poorer outcomes include retreatment cases, XDR-TB, bilateral disease, and low body mass index.

Guidelines for treatment of drug-susceptible tuberculosis and patient care, 2017 update. Geneva: World Health Organization; 2017. License: CC BY-NC-SA 3.0 IGO.

Harris RC, et al. The effect of surgery on the outcome of treatment for multidrug-resistant tuberculosis: A systematic review and meta-analysis. *BMC Infect Dis.* 2016;16(1).

Kempker RR, et al. Surgical treatment of drug-resistant tuberculosis. *Lancet Infect Dis.* 2012;12(2):157-166.

Massard G, et al. Surgery for the sequelae of postprimary tuberculosis. *Thorac Surg Clin.* 2012;22(3):287-300.

WHO Treatment Guidelines for Drug-resistant Tuberculosis, 2016 Update. Geneva: World Health Organization; 2016.

FUNGAL INFECTIONS OF THE LUNG

Pulmonary fungal infections are increasing due to the widespread use of broad-spectrum antibiotics, the use of corticosteroids and other immunosuppressive drugs, and the spread of HIV infection. However, infection can occur in immunocompetent hosts. Fungal infections frequently involve the respiratory tract and include histoplasmosis, coccidioidomycosis, blastomycosis, cryptococcosis, aspergillosis, mucormycosis, and candidiasis. Fungal infections, though ubiquitous, are notable for several characteristic endemic areas. Candidiasis rarely if ever requires operative treatment and thus will not be discussed here.

1. Histoplasmosis

Histoplasma capsulatum is a dimorphic fungus found in soil enriched by the nitrogen contained in bird and bat guano. Abandoned buildings, attics, lofts, and areas under trees that serve as bird and bat roosts and caves are especially likely to contain high concentrations. In endemic areas, exposure is common, and most infections are sporadic. Outbreaks have been traced to spelunking, demolition of buildings, and activities that disrupt contaminated soil. This organism is found primarily in the Ohio and Mississippi River valleys and in Central America. Mammals, including humans, inhale the organism, and macrophages engulf the fungus. It then transforms into the budding yeast form, causing activation of inflammatory cytokines. Over several months the ongoing inflammation causes granuloma formation in lymph nodes with resulting caseation, necrosis, fibrosis, and calcification. The diagnosis of histoplasmosis is made definitively by growth of the organism from sputum, BAL fluid, lung tissue, or mediastinal lymph nodes—though incubation periods of 4-6 weeks are required and yield is higher in chronic disease. Serology also plays an important role in the diagnosis. Both complement fixation and immunodiffusion tests should be ordered. Serology is not useful in immunosuppressed patients who are unable to mount an antibody response. The *Histoplasma* EIA has been developed as a diagnostic aid and detects the galactomannan component of the cell wall of *H. capsulatum*. The original assay was marked by poor sensitivity; however, with modifications its sensitivity has increased, and when combined with EIA for antibodies, the sensitivity is superior to complement fixation tests.

Infections are classified as acute, chronic, or disseminated, and most infections in immunocompetent individuals are asymptomatic. Acute infections are manifested (1) as a flulike syndrome with fever, chills, dry cough, headache, retrosternal discomfort, arthralgias, and a rash suggesting erythema nodosum; (2) with symptoms similar to a flulike syndrome but limited to the lungs and occasionally accompanied by a productive cough; or (3) as an acute diffuse nodular disease with mild symptoms. Radiographic findings in these three acute syndromes typically demonstrate ill-defined upper lobe nonsegmental opacities; nonsegmental areas of consolidation that tend to change; and diffuse, discrete 3- to 4-mm nodules, respectively. Hilar adenopathy on chest x-ray is common. Physical examination can be normal or may reveal signs of pneumonia.

In contrast, chronic infections include (1) an asymptomatic solitary, discrete nodule less than 3 cm in diameter known as a histoplasmoma (most common), often with central and concentric calcifications ("target lesion") and frequently located in the lower lobes; (2) chronic cavitary histoplasmosis, which typically occurs in patients with underlying obstructive disease, characteristically mild symptoms, fibronodular upper lobe infiltrates, and centrilobular emphysematous spaces; (3) mediastinal granulomas that may result in broncholithiasis, esophageal traction diverticula, superior vena cava compression, and tracheobronchoesophageal fistulas; and (4) fibrosing mediastinitis, which can produce compression of the superior vena cava, tracheobronchial tree, or esophagus.

Disseminated disease includes an acute, subacute, and chronic form. These infections occur in children (acute and subacute) as well as adults (subacute and chronic). Fever and abdominal pain are common. Other findings include hepatosplenomegaly, pancytopenia, meningitis, endocarditis, adrenocortical insufficiency, and oropharyngeal ulceration (chronic form).

Radiographic imaging in disseminated disease may demonstrate diffuse interstitial pneumonitis (25%) or minimal findings. The symptoms and roentgenographic findings of histoplasmosis resemble those of tuberculosis, although the disease appears to progress more slowly. Yet as many as 30% of cases coexist with tuberculosis. There may be cough, malaise, hemoptysis, low-grade fever, and weight loss. Pulmonary fibrosis, bulla formation, and pulmonary insufficiency occur in advanced cases of histoplasmosis. Mediastinal involvement is quite frequent and may take the form of granuloma formation, or dysphagia. Furthermore, mediastinal fibrosis is among the most common benign causes of superior vena caval syndrome (discussed earlier in the chapter). Erosion of inflammatory lymph nodes into bronchi may cause expectoration of broncholiths, hemoptysis, wheezing, or bronchiectasis. Traction diverticula of the esophagus may lead to development of tracheoesophageal fistula.

In lesions that present as solitary pulmonary nodules, histoplasmosis is diagnosed in about 15%-20% of cases. Radiologically, early infections appear as diffuse mottled parenchymal infiltrations surrounding the hila, with enlargement of hilar lymph nodes. Cavitation indicates advanced infection and is the complication about which the surgeon is most often consulted. The diagnosis rests upon finding a positive skin test or complement fixation test and culturing the fungus from sputum or a bronchial aspirate.

Medical therapy of histoplasmosis is indicated only in cavitary and severe disease and for most infections in immunocompromised hosts. Azoles are recommended as first-line treatment for patients who have mild to moderate pulmonary histoplasmosis. Itraconazole is the drug of choice for mild to moderate cavitary disease, while amphotericin B is reserved for patients with more serious infections and infections in immunocompromised patients. In those who cannot tolerate itraconazole, fluconazole may be substituted. Reflecting increasing use of corticosteroids for ARDS in the last decade, the current American Thoracic Society Guidelines recommend the use of intravenous methylprednisilone as adjunctive therapy for severe acute pulmonary histoplasmosis. Operative intervention is reserved for treatment of complications and to rule out neoplastic disease in the case of suspicious pulmonary nodules. Broncholithectomy via rigid bronchoscopy with or without pulmonary resection, repair of tracheobronchoesophageal fistulas, decompression of mediastinal granulomas, and spiral saphenous vein bypass of severe symptomatic superior vena cava obstruction are typical surgical consultations. As pericardial involvement may occur, the Infectious Diseases Society of America recommends pericardiectomy for recurrent pericardial effusions. In cases of vascular fibrosis of the superior vena cava and pulmonary vessels, percutaneous intravascular dilation and stenting is recommended as first-line treatment.

2. Coccidioidomycosis

Coccidioides immitis is a dimorphic soil fungus endemic to the Sonoran life zone (Utah, Arizona, California, Nevada, and New Mexico) and is associated with creosote brush. Because of its endemic territory, the fungus—also known as "San Joaquin Valley Fever"—proliferates in dry heat with brief intense rain, and is spread by strong winds. Infection occurs through inhalation of as few as 1-10 arthrospores, which then germinate as parasitic spherules. Spherules have a double refractile cell wall and produce endospores that cause the spherule to rupture, spreading the infection into the surrounding tissues. Caseation, suppuration, abscess formation, and fibrosis follow. The diagnosis of coccidioidomycosis relies on the detection of acutely elevated titers of immunoglobulin M (IgM) antibodies (by latex agglutination and confirmed by immunodiffusion tube precipitin tests) or rising serum immunoglobulin G (IgG) antibody complement fixation titers (seroconversion or fourfold rise) in the appropriate clinical context. The coccidioidin and Spherulin skin tests, which become positive 3-21 days following infection, are generally useful only for epidemiologic studies and not for the diagnosis of acute disease. Identification of the spherules in tissue, lavage samples, and fine-needle aspirates are helpful in making the diagnosis in some patients. Although many stains can be used, including routine fungal (potassium hydroxide, KOH) preparations, Pap staining is most sensitive. Gram stains, however, fail to demonstrate the spherules.

Primary infection is asymptomatic in 60% of patients, while most others develop a constellation of symptoms known as desert fever: with fever, productive cough, pleuritic chest pain, pneumonitis, and a rash typical of erythema nodosum or erythema multiforme. Disease that includes arthralgias is known as desert rheumatism. Radiographic findings demonstrate segmental or nonsegmental, homogeneous or mottled infiltrates with a predilection for the lower lobes. Physical examination is often unrevealing, but rales and rhonchi may be present. Other findings include eosinophilia (66%), hilar adenopathy (20%), and small, exudative pleural effusions (2%-20%). Symptomatic persistent infection associated with chest x-ray findings 6-8 weeks after primary infection is classified as one of five types: persistent pneumonia, chronic progressive pneumonia, miliary coccidioidomycosis, coccidioidal nodules, or pulmonary cavities. Persistent pneumonia manifests with symptoms of fever, productive cough, and pleuritic chest pain in association with protracted infiltrates and consolidation on chest x-ray, and generally resolves within 8 months. Patients with chronic progressive pneumonia complain of fever, cough, dyspnea, hemoptysis, and weight loss, with bilateral apical nodular densities and multiple cavities lasting years. This presentation closely resembles tuberculosis and chronic histoplasmosis. Miliary coccidioidomycosis occurs early and rapidly, associated with bilateral diffuse infiltrates. This form of disease implies the presence of impaired immunity and has an associated mortality rate of 50%. Nearly half of patients with coccidioidal nodules are asymptomatic. These nodular densities (coccidiomas) appear in the middle and upper lung fields, often within 5 cm of the hilum; range from 1 to 4 cm in size; and do not calcify, making it hard to distinguish them from malignancy. In endemic areas, 30%-50% of all nodules are coccidiomas. Patients develop pulmonary cavities in 10%-15% of cases of coccidioidomycosis. Typically, these are solitary (90%), thin-walled, located in the upper lobes (70%), less than 6 cm in size (90%), and close spontaneously within 2 years (50%). Some cavities, however, cross fissures; cause hemoptysis (25%-50%), usually mild; rupture, producing a pyopneumothorax with a bronchopleural fistula; or later become infected with *Aspergillus*. Uncommonly, dissemination can occur, particularly in immunocompromised individuals, in pregnancy (third trimester), and in non-Caucasian individuals. Although pulmonary symptoms in disseminated disease are mild, meningeal involvement is common and the mortality rate is high (50%).

Medical therapy is not indicated in asymptomatic, immunocompetent individuals. Patients with persistent or chronic pneumonia, miliary disease, and those at risk for dissemination should be treated with antifungal therapy. Initial therapy consists of fluconazole or itraconazole. Amphotericin B is now considered the treatment of choice for severe cases of coccidioidal pneumonia due to risk of toxicity. Surgery is reserved for patients with coccidiomas when cancer is a concern and in patients with cavities that have an associated radiographic abnormality suggesting carcinoma (ie, thick wall) or that develop a complication (eg, hemoptysis and pyopneumothorax from rupture). Resection should include all diseased tissue and most often requires lobectomy.

3. Blastomycosis

Blastomyces dermatitidis is a dimorphic soil fungus found in warm, wet, nitrogen-rich soil in an endemic area that extends east of a line from the Texas Gulf coast to the border between Minnesota and North Dakota (except Florida and New England). Infection occurs characteristically in males (male-to-female ratio 6:1 to 15:1) from 30 to 60 years of age through inhalation of conidia (asexual spores). At 37°C, the conidia germinate as yeasts, producing caseation in a manner similar to tuberculosis. Rarely, infection may develop through direct skin inoculation. Risk factors include poor hygiene, exposure to dust and wood, manual labor, and poor housing conditions. Since no accurate skin or serologic tests exist, the diagnosis depends on culture or histologic identification of the yeast form. *B dermatitidis* grows as white to tan colonies of septate hyphae at room temperature but changes to budding yeast at 37°C. The yeast form can be found in sputum (33%), bronchoalveolar lavage specimens (38%), lung biopsies (21%), and fine-needle aspirates (7%), and can be demonstrated with standard KOH preparations or many other histologic stains (but not Gram stain). The yeast, however, does not have a large capsule (which distinguishes it from *Cryptococcus neoformans*) and does not grow intracellularly (which differentiates it from *Histoplasma capsulatum*).

Manifestations of blastomycosis can occur in many organ systems, including the lungs, skin, bone, genitourinary tract (prostatitis and epididymoorchitis), and central nervous system. Pulmonary infection can be asymptomatic or may present with flulike symptoms, evidence of pneumonia, or pleurisy. Cough (36%), weight loss (20%), pleuritic pain (26%), fever (23%), hemoptysis (21%), erythema nodosum, and ulcerative bronchitis are common. Radiographic findings include homogeneous or patchy consolidation in a nonsegmental distribution with pleural effusions, thickening, or cavitation (15%-35%). In some patients, the appearance of pulmonary masses may mimic carcinoma. A predilection for the upper lobes has been noted; however, unlike histoplasmosis and coccidioidomycosis, in blastomycosis, hilar and mediastinal adenopathy is unusual.

Disease confined to the lungs in an asymptomatic immunocompetent patient generally does not require treatment.

However, for extrapulmonary or worsening disease, pregnant women, or the immunocompromised, treatment with amphotericin B is indicated. In disease not involving the central nervous system, itraconazole may be used. Surgical resection is rarely necessary except for unclear diagnosis or when the possibility of malignancy cannot be excluded.

4. Cryptococcosis

Cryptococcus neoformans is an encapsulated yeast like budding fungus. It is a saprophyte existing on the skin, nasopharynx, gastrointestinal tract, and vagina of humans as well as in pigeon excreta, grasses, trees, plants, fruits, bees, wasps, insects (cockroaches), birds, milk products, pickle brine, and soil. Cryptococcal infection generally indicates the presence of an underlying debilitating disease in an immunocompromised host. Infection occurs from inhalation of the yeast form. The diagnosis can be established by the detection of serum antigen (via complement fixation tests) in patients with appropriate clinical and radiographic findings. More commonly, however, histologic identification with India ink stains is used; routine cultures are not performed because they are extremely time-consuming and require multiple biochemical tests for differentiation of cryptococcus from other fungi. No accurate skin test exists for cryptococcosis.

The most common sites of infection are the lungs and central nervous system. Pulmonary infection may remain asymptomatic, or patients may complain of cough, pleuritic chest pain, and fever. Radiographically, cryptococcus can appear as a localized, well-defined 3- to 10-cm pleural-based mass without smooth borders; as single or multiple areas of consolidation, usually within one lobe but in nonsegmental distribution; or as a disseminated miliary nodular infiltrate. A predilection for the lower lobes has been noted. Central nervous system infection usually follows an asymptomatic pulmonary infection. Central nervous system symptoms are highly variable, since many patients are severely immunocompromised and do not manifest the usual signs and symptoms of meningitis or cerebritis.

Medical therapy is indicated in most cases of pulmonary infection except for rare cases of limited localized disease. Azole compounds (eg, fluconazole, itraconazole, and voriconazole) have been used with increasing frequency as first-line therapy both as single agents and in combination. In immunocompromised patients or those with extrapulmonary disease, treatment consists of induction therapy with both amphotericin B and flucytosine for a minimum of 2 weeks, before switching to maintenance treatment with fluconazole. Surgery is rarely indicated, and is useful only to exclude the possibility of malignancy or to determine the etiology of an undiagnosed diffuse pulmonary infiltrate. Very rarely has surgery been utilized to resect an isolated area of parenchyma not responding to conventional treatment.

5. Aspergillosis

Aspergillus species are ubiquitous dimorphic fungi found in soil and decaying organic matter. The most common pathogenic species include *A. fumigatus* (most common), *A. niger, A. flavus,* and *A. glaucus.* In culture, these fungi resemble an aspergillum, which is a brush used to sprinkle holy water. Aspergillosis represents the second-most common (after candidiasis) opportunistic fungal infection in immunocompromised hosts, and the third-most common systemic fungal infection requiring hospital care. Infection occurs almost exclusively through inhalation of conidia into areas of lung with impaired mucociliary function (eg, tuberculous cavities). Although the diagnosis is supported by demonstrating immediate and delayed-type hypersensitivity skin reactions, by culturing uniform septate hyphae with dichotomous branching at 45 degrees, and by detecting specific IgG and IgE antibodies, a definitive diagnosis requires demonstration of hyphal tissue invasion or documentation of hyphae on methenamine silver stain in a suspected aspergilloma. Galactomannan enzyme-linked immunosorbent assays can serve as a sensitive serum measure of invasive infection.

Infection with *Aspergillus* species usually takes one of three forms: allergic bronchopulmonary aspergillosis, invasive aspergillosis, or aspergilloma. Allergic bronchopulmonary aspergillosis occurs in patients who are atopic (asthmatics) and in patients with cystic fibrosis. Endobronchial fungal growth leads to dilated airways filled with mucus and fungus. Continuous exposure to fungal antigens results in precipitating antibodies, increased IgE levels (which correlate with disease activity), and both immediate and delayed-type hypersensitivity. Patients complain of cough, fever, wheezing, dyspnea, pleuritic pain, and hemoptysis. Chest x-ray shows homogeneous densities in a "gloved-finger," inverted Y, or "cluster of grapes" pattern. Five stages have been defined, depending on disease activity and steroid dependency. Stage 1 includes acute infection with characteristic x-ray and laboratory evidence of disease; stage 2 occurs with steroid-induced remission; stage 3 is characterized by asymptomatic exacerbations of laboratory and x-ray findings; steroid-dependent asthma with worsening laboratory tests (total IgE, precipitins, etc) is indicative of stage 4 disease; and end-stage fibrosis, bronchiectasis, and obstruction define stage 5.

Invasive aspergillosis is found exclusively in immunocompromised patients, particularly in patients with leukemia (50%-70% of cases). Dissemination occurs frequently, and three types of pulmonary disease have been described: tracheobronchitis (uncommon), necrotizing bronchopneumonia, and hemorrhagic infarction (most common). In tracheobronchitis, disease is usually limited to the larger airways (bronchus moreso than trachea) with little parenchymal involvement. Focal or diffuse mucosal ulceration, pseudomembranes, and intraluminal fungal plugs are common. Patients often present with cough, dyspnea, wheezing, and hemoptysis. Occasionally, patchy areas of atelectasis secondary to bronchial obstruction can be seen on chest x-ray. Necrotizing bronchopneumonia should be suspected in patients with unremitting fever, dyspnea, tachypnea, radiologic evidence of bronchopneumonia, and a poor response to standard antibiotic therapy. Finally, hemorrhagic infarction due to vascular permeation with nonthrombotic occlusion of small- to medium-sized arteries and necrosis typically results in either a well-defined nodule or a wedge-shaped, pleura-based density. Symptoms are nonspecific and include fever, dyspnea, dry cough, pleuritic chest pain, and hemoptysis. Cavitation is common, and radiologic examination may reveal "round" pneumonia or "air crescents" of a mycotic lung sequestrum.

Aspergillomas ("fungus balls" or mycetomas) are divided into two types: (1) simple, thin-walled cysts lined with ciliated epithelium and surrounded by normal parenchyma; and (2) complex cavities associated with markedly abnormal surrounding lung tissue. Aspergillomas most often occur in the upper lobes and in the superior segments of the lower lobes. Although they may be multiple (22%), calcification and air–fluid levels are rare. Most aspergillomas—particularly complex ones—are associated with cavitary lung disease, ie, tuberculosis (most common), histoplasmosis, sarcoidosis, bronchiectasis, and others. Hemoptysis occurs in 50%-80% and can present with frequent minor episodes (30% subsequently have massive bleeding), repeated moderate episodes, or a single episode of massive hemoptysis. Chest x-ray may reveal a 3- to 6-cm round, mobile density with a crescent of air.

Corticosteroids are indicated in patients with allergic bronchopulmonary aspergillosis in addition to measures to relieve bronchospasm (inhaled β-agonists or anticholinergics). In invasive aspergillosis, treatment regimens remain debated but standard choices include voriconazole with or without the addition of an echinocandin. Traditional treatment choices also still include amphotericin B.

In addition, some patients with complex aspergillomas and severe pulmonary disease are not candidates for surgical resection, and intracavitary amphotericin has been used with modest success. Surgery is indicated for complications of aspergillus infection such as hemoptysis. Furthermore, hemoptysis associated with localized invasive aspergillosis (particularly once cavitation has occurred) can be treated by resection and amphotericin B. Generally, wide excision (lobectomy) is required; yet in some high-risk patients with aspergillomas, cavernostomy and muscle flap closure is an alternative.

6. Mucormycosis

Infection with *Rhizopus arrhizus*, *Absidia* species, and *Rhizomucor* species of the class Zygomycetes and the order Mucorales occurs in certain distinct immunosuppressed patient populations: people with poorly controlled diabetes and leukemia patients. These fungi are ubiquitous organisms that are found in decaying fruit, vegetable matter, soil, and manure. Infection occurs following inhalation of sporangiospores, which germinate in a hyphal form. The diagnosis is made by demonstrating the organism in symptomatic patients. No accurate skin or serologic tests exist. Although the fungi do grow in culture as broad, irregular nonseptate hyphae that branch at angles up to 90 degrees (occasionally being confused with *Aspergillus* species), most commonly the diagnosis is made on histologic examination. The sine qua non for mucormycosis is hyphal vascular invasion between the internal elastic membrane and the media of blood vessels, causing thrombosis, infarction, and necrosis.

In addition to pulmonary infections, mucormycosis manifests as distinct clinical syndromes such as rhinocerebral infection (direct extension into the central nervous system from paranasal sinus infection), cutaneous infection (burn patients), gastrointestinal infection (children with protein–calorie malnutrition), and disseminated infection (uremic patients receiving deferoxamine therapy). Patients with pulmonary infection complain of fever, cough, pleuritic chest pain, and hemoptysis. Frequently, this type of infection occurs in immunocompromised hosts and follows a fulminant course. Three patterns of infection are noted on chest x-ray: limited disease with involvement of a single lobe or segment, diffuse or disseminated disease with involvement of both lungs and the mediastinum, and endobronchial disease with bronchial obstruction and secondary bacterial infection. Characteristic CT findings include a halo sign (area of low attenuation around a dense infiltrate), ring enhancement, and an air-crescent sign (area of contrast between normal lung and a radiodense cavitating lesion). Amphotericin B is standard treatment. In nonneutropenic patients, the newer azole compounds may be useful; however, infection with these fungi remains highly lethal, with a mortality of 90%. The cause of death in these patients is often fungal sepsis, progressive pulmonary dysfunction, and hemoptysis. In the small group of patients with limited disease, aggressive surgical resection in combination with amphotericin B has lowered the mortality to only 50%. In contrast, the endobronchial form can be effectively treated with transbronchoscopic resection (using the Nd: YAG laser) in a large proportion of patients.

7. Pneumocystosis

Pneumocystis carinii is a fungal organism that has been found in the lungs of a variety of domesticated and wild mammals and is distributed worldwide in humans. Pulmonary involvement leads to progressive pneumonia and respiratory insufficiency. Disease has been seen with increasing frequency in recipients of organ transplants who are undergoing immunosuppressive therapy. Diagnosis is made by lung biopsy. Without treatment with trimethoprim-sulfamethoxazole, pentamidine, or inhaled antimicrobial therapy, the course is one of relentless progression. However, with improved antiviral therapy for HIV infections, the incidence of pneumocystosis has been declining.

LoCicero J, et al. Surgery for other pulmonary fungal infections, *Actinomyces*, and *Nocardia*. *Thorac Surg Clin*. 2012;22:363-374.
Smith JA, et al. Pulmonary fungal infections. *Respirology*. 2012; 17:913-926.

SARCOIDOSIS (BOECK SARCOID, BENIGN LYMPHOGRANULOMATOSIS)

Sarcoidosis is a noncaseating granulomatous disease of unknown cause involving the lungs, liver, spleen, lymph nodes, skin, and bones. The highest incidence is reported in Scandinavia, England, and the United States. The incidence in those of African ancestry is 10-17 times above the incidence in Caucasians. Half of patients diagnosed are between ages 20 and 40 years, with women more frequently affected than men.

▶ Clinical Findings

A. Symptoms and Signs

Sarcoidosis may present with symptoms of pulmonary infection, but usually these are insidious and nonspecific. Erythema nodosum may herald the onset, and weight loss, fatigue, weakness, and malaise may appear later. Fever occurs in approximately 15% of cases. Pulmonary symptoms occur in 20%-30% and include dry cough and dyspnea. Hemoptysis is rare. One fifth of patients with sarcoidosis have myocardial involvement, and heart block or failure may occur. Peripheral lymph nodes are enlarged in 75%, scalene lymph nodes are microscopically involved in 80% and mediastinal nodes in 90%, and cutaneous involvement is present in 30%. Hepatic and splenic involvement can be shown by biopsy in 70% of cases. There may be migratory or persistent polyarthritis, and central nervous involvement occurs in a few patients.

B. Imaging Studies

The x-ray findings in sarcoidosis are classified into five descriptive categories or stages (Table 19–5). Pulmonary

Table 19–5. Radiographic stages of sarcoidosis.

Stage 0: No x-ray abnormality.
Stage 1: Hilar and mediastinal lymph node enlargement without pulmonary abnormalities.
Stage 2: Hilar and mediastinal lymph node enlargement with pulmonary abnormalities.
Stage 3: Diffuse pulmonary disease without adenopathy.
Stage 4: Pulmonary fibrosis.

disease can manifest as a reticulonodular infiltrate, an acinar pattern of opacities, or large nodules with or without mediastinal adenopathy. Mediastinal lymph node involvement characteristically includes bilateral, symmetric hilar and paratracheal lymphadenopathy. Anterior or posterior mediastinal adenopathy or asymmetric hilar involvement should prompt a suspicion of other diseases, such as lymphoma. Pleural effusions and cavitation are rare and, if present, necessitate an evaluation for tuberculosis, congestive heart failure, and coincidental pneumonia.

C. Diagnosis

Although no single test exists to confirm absolutely the diagnosis of sarcoidosis (the diagnosis remains one of exclusion), it may be suggested by the characteristic radiographic appearance of bilateral hilar and mediastinal lymphadenopathy, by gallium 67 scanning, and by elevated serum and bronchoalveolar fluid levels of angiotensin-converting enzyme (ACE) and lysozyme. However, ACE serum testing has poor sensitivity. Pathologic documentation of noncaseating granulomas should normally be obtained either via transbronchial biopsy, mediastinoscopy, or VATS biopsy (more reliable, with >95% success rate). Culture for mycobacteria, fungi, and other atypical infections must also be negative.

D. Treatment

Asymptomatic patients and those with minimal clinical disease may require no therapy. Corticosteroids, calcineurin inhibitors, and antimetabolites have been used in symptomatic patients with stage 2 and higher disease with some success. Despite the indolent nature of the disease and steroid therapy, long-term mortality is reported as high as 10%. Lung transplantation has been utilized with success in patients refractory to medical management.

▼ NEOPLASMS OF THE LUNG

PRIMARY LUNG CANCER

Lung cancer is the most common cause of cancer-related death in both men and women in the United States. In 2018, it is estimated for this country that 234,030 new cases and 154,050 deaths occurred due to lung cancer. This represents 14% of all new cancer cases and 27% of all cancer-related deaths. Tobacco smoking accounts for nearly 85% of all lung cancer cases. The effect is greatest for cigarettes and least for pipe smoking, and is directly related to the amount of tobacco smoked. Following 5-6 years of smoking cessation, the risk exponentially declines, and after 15 years approaches, but never reaches, that of nonsmokers. "Passive" exposure to cigarette smoke, on the other hand, increases the risk in nonsmokers by two to three times. Exposure to all forms of asbestos (amosite, chrysotile, and crocidolite) has been implicated in as many as 23% of lung cancers, accounting for the high incidence among shipyard workers, insulators, cement makers, truck drivers, and plumbers. The effect is particularly pronounced in smokers and is most commonly associated with squamous-cell and small-cell carcinoma. Exposure to radon and its alpha-emitting daughter isotopes have been implicated in the increased incidence of lung cancer in both uranium miners and populations living in geographic areas naturally contaminated with high levels of radon gas. Although it has been known for some time that people with high activity of 4-debrisoquine hydroxylase, the so-called debrisoquine metabolic phenotype, have a 10-fold increased risk of lung cancer, only recently has the role of genetic factors been appreciated.

Chromosome deletions (particularly 11p, 13q, 17p, and 3p), tumor suppressor gene mutations (p53, Hap-1, ErbAb, etc), and constitutive, high-level expression of both growth factor genes (insulin-like and transferrin-like growth factors), epidermal growth factor receptors (HER2/*neu, EGFR1*, etc), and protooncogenes (c-, N- and L-*myc*; H-, N-, and K-*ras*; and c-*myb*) have all been implicated in the pathogenesis of lung cancer. Other factors such as vitamin A deficiency; air pollution; exposure to arsenic, cadmium, chromium, ether, and formaldehyde; and employment as bakers, cooks, construction workers, cosmetologists, leather workers, pitchblende miners, printers, rubber workers, and pottery workers have also been incriminated. Finally, certain diseases (eg, progressive systemic sclerosis [scleroderma]) have a defined predisposition for the development of lung cancer. Silencing of genes by aberrant promoter hypermethylation is viewed as a crucial component in lung cancer pathobiology. High-throughput genomic analysis has identified scores of genes and metabolic pathways that appear to be associated with the progression of lung cancer.

▶ **Pathology**

Lung cancer occurs more commonly in the right lung than the left, and the upper lobes are involved more commonly than the lower lobes or the right middle lobe. Synchronous primary lung cancers occur in up to 7% of patients, and 10% of patients will develop a metachronous new tumor (2% per year risk postresection of early-stage disease). Furthermore, patients with lung cancer are at higher risk of developing cancers of the upper respiratory tract, oral cavity, esophagus, bladder, and kidney, presumably related to the "field effect" of smoking. Lung cancers typically spread by local extension to involve the visceral and parietal pleura, chest wall, great vessels, pericardium, diaphragm, esophagus, and vertebral column. Common sites of metastatic involvement include the ipsilateral pulmonary and hilar lymph nodes; the mediastinal lymph nodes; and the lung, liver, bone, brain, adrenal glands, pancreas, kidney, soft tissues, and myocardium. The exact pathologic classification of lung

Table 19–6. Location of lung cancer by histologic type.

Histology	Central (%)	Peripheral (%)
Squamous-cell carcinoma	64-81	19-36
Adenocarcinoma	5-29	71-95
Large-cell carcinoma	42-49	51-58
Small-cell carcinoma	74-83	17-26
Overall	63	37

Reproduced with permission from Cameron RB: *Pracitcal Oncology.* New York, NY: McGraw-Hill Education; 1994.

cancer has not been uniform despite attempts at standardization by the World Health Organization. Functionally, however, squamous-cell carcinoma, large-cell carcinoma, and adenocarcinoma are grouped together under the designation of non–small-cell carcinomas and constitute 80%-85% of all lung tumors. Small-cell carcinoma represents 15%-20%, while bronchial gland adenomas, including carcinoids, comprise approximately the remaining 5%. The differential locations of some of these neoplasms are summarized in Table 19–6.

A. Squamous-Cell Carcinoma

The major pathologic features of squamous-cell carcinoma are keratinization, cellular stratification, and intercellular bridges. Squamous-cell carcinomas account for about 20% of all cases of lung cancer and 70% of non–small-cell tumors. Two-thirds are located centrally near the hilum and one-third peripherally. The growth rate and the rate of metastasis tend to be slower than those of other lung tumors.

B. Adenocarcinoma

Adenocarcinomas, which constitute 30% of lung cancers and 60% of non–small-cell tumors, are characterized as acinar, papillary, lepidic (formerly nonmucinous bronchioloalveolar [BAC] with >5 mm invasion), micropapillary and solid, as well as pre-invasive lesions including atypical adenomatous hyperplasia and adenocarcinoma in situ (≤3 cm, formerly BAC) and minimally invasive (≤3 cm lepidic predominant tumor with ≤5 mm invasion). Acinar adenocarcinoma is composed of glands lined by columnar cells that secrete mucin. Lepidic carcinoma is characterized by intraluminal papillary fragments that appear in alveoli or small bronchioles. The incidence of adenocarcinoma of the lung is increasing relative to squamous-cell carcinoma, perhaps as a consequence of the rise in lung cancer among women, although the exact cause remains unclear.

C. Small-Cell Carcinoma

Small-cell (oat cell) carcinomas have small, round nuclei with nuclear chromatin and cytoplasm. They are biologically and clinically distinct from all other cell types such that the term non–small-cell lung cancer (NSCLC) often is applied to all other cell types. Small-cell carcinomas comprise 15%-20% of all lung cancers. They occur centrally, and metastasize early, but also can exhibit significant partial response to combined-modality treatment, albeit with limited 5-year survival.

D. Large-Cell Carcinoma

Large-cell carcinomas are composed of large polygonal spindle or oval cells arranged in sheets, nests, or clusters. Multinucleated giant cells, intracellular hyalin droplets, glycogen, and acidophilic nuclear inclusions may be present. These tumors are seen peripherally and are less common.

E. Adenosquamous Tumors

Adenosquamous tumors show both cellular features and are more biologically aggressive than other non–small-cell lung cancers. Survival percentages of patients with adenosquamous tumors are significantly lower than what is reported for adenocarcinoma or squamous-cell cancer.

F. Bronchial Gland Adenomas

Bronchial gland adenoma is a misnomer, since the vast majority of these tumors are malignant. Included in this group are carcinoid tumors, adenoid cystic carcinomas, mucoepidermoid carcinoma, mixed tumors of the salivary gland type, and mucous gland adenoma. Carcinoid tumors are derived from Kulchitsky cells, have a vascular stroma, and tend to be located centrally in proximal airways. Although they are slow-growing, they can metastasize widely. Carcinoid syndrome is rarely associated with bronchial carcinoids, as opposed to intestinal carcinoids that metastasize to the liver. Adenoid cystic carcinomas—also referred to as cylindromas—feature groups of epithelial cells that form ductlike structures interspersed with cystic spaces. These neoplasms are locally aggressive and often extend beyond apparent gross pathologic margins. Metastases from adenoid cystic carcinomas often involve the lung, are slow growing, and are amenable to surgical excision. Mucoepidermoid carcinomas are rare tumors characterized by the presence of squamous cells, mucus-secreting cells, and an intermediate cell type. The cells are bland and less aggressive than those of adenosquamous carcinomas. Mixed tumors of the salivary type are extremely rare infiltrating tumors that are curable with wide local excision. Finally, mucus gland adenomas (papillary or bronchial cyst adenomas) are the only true benign "adenomas" of this group with no metastatic potential. These neoplasms are rare tumors of the major bronchi and consist of numerous mucus-filled cysts lined by a well-differentiated epithelium. Generally, bronchoscopic removal can be accomplished in this specific case and results in long-term cure.

▶ Clinical Presentation

Nearly 94% of patients present with symptoms from the effects of the primary tumor, regional spread, or metastatic disease. Local effects of the primary tumor account for 27% of presenting symptoms and vary depending on the location of the tumor. Central tumors are associated with cough, hemoptysis, respiratory difficulty (wheezing, stridor, or dyspnea), pain, and pneumonia. Peripheral tumors can cause cough, chest wall pain, pleural effusions, pulmonary abscess, Horner syndrome (ipsilateral miosis, ptosis, and anhidrosis), and Pancoast syndrome (ipsilateral shoulder and arm pain in the C8–T1 nerve root distribution, Horner syndrome, and a superior sulcus—usually squamous—lung cancer). Symptoms due to the effect of regional spread include hoarseness from recurrent nerve paralysis, dyspnea due to phrenic nerve paralysis, dysphagia from compression of the esophagus, superior vena cava syndrome from compression or invasion of the superior vena cava, and pericardial tamponade from invasion of the pericardium. Metastatic disease may present with symptoms of systemic illness (anorexia, weight loss, night sweats, weakness, and malaise), local manifestations of distant metastases (jaundice, abdominal mass, bony pain or fracture, neurologic deficits, mental status changes, seizures, and soft-tissue masses). A number of paraneoplastic syndromes associated with lung cancer have been identified (Table 19–7).

▶ Diagnosis & Evaluation

Lung cancer is usually suspected from abnormal findings on a chest x-ray obtained in the course of a routine physical examination or, more commonly, after a complaint of pulmonary symptoms (see previous discussion). Findings vary from a small peripheral nodule to an unresolving infiltrate or even total lung atelectasis. Occasionally, the location of the abnormality may suggest certain cell types (Table 19–6). Once the diagnosis of lung cancer is suspected, a definitive diagnosis can be obtained in over 90% of patients with either bronchoscopy for proximal lesions or fine-needle aspiration cytology for peripheral lesions.

CT scanning is an integral part of the assessment of patients with lung cancer. Chest CT scans should also include the upper abdomen to assess two of the most common sites of metastases (liver and adrenal glands). Injection of IV contrast while the scan is obtained facilitates evaluation of the mediastinum. Additional radiographic evaluation includes tests to evaluate other common sites of metastases, such as bone and brain. A serum alkaline phosphatase is essential, and a bone scan and brain CT

Table 19–7. Paraneoplastic syndromes associated with lung cancer.

Cardiovascular
Thrombophlebitis
Nonbacterial thrombotic endocarditis
Neuromuscular
Subacute cerebellar degeneration
Dementia
Limbic encephalitis
Optic neuritis, retinopathy
Subacute necrotic myelopathy
Autonomic neuropathy (small cell)
Myasthenic (Eaton–Lambert) syndrome (small cell)
Polymyositis
Gastrointestinal
Carcinoid syndrome (carcinoid and small cell)
Anorexia, cachexia
Hematologic
Erythrocytosis
Leukocytosis
Metabolic
Inappropriate adrenocorticotropic hormone (ACTH) (small cell)
Inappropriate antidiuretic hormone (ADH) (small cell)
Hypercalcemia (squamous-cell carcinoma)
Inappropriate gonadotropins
Dermatologic
Acanthosis nigricans (adenocarcinoma)
Dermatomyositis
Erythema gyratum
Ichthyosis
Other
Hypertrophic pulmonary osteoarthropathy (squamous cell, large cell, and adenocarcinoma)
Nephrotic syndrome
Fever

scan (or preferably MRI) should be obtained if indicated by neurologic symptoms, elevated alkaline phosphatase levels, or if advanced-stage disease (stage III or beyond) is present. Fluorodeoxyglucose (FDG) PET has evolved into a critical staging test. It is most effective as a tool for assessing for distant occult disease. It can be helpful for predicting mediastinal node involvement, but it is not definitive. False-positive rates as high as 15%-20% have been reported, and reliance on PET varies institution to institution. Furthermore, nodules less than 1 cm in diameter generally are not imaged reliably by PET scanning. Combination high-resolution CT scan and PET scan assessment permits improved correlation of abnormal CT findings with FDG uptake suggestive of tumor.

Thoracentesis or thoracoscopy (or both) should be performed in any patient with evidence of a pleural effusion to exclude diffuse involvement of the pleura (M1 or stage IV disease) that indicates metastatic disease. Despite increasing reliance on PET scan to stage the mediastinum, patients with non–small-cell lung cancer but without metastatic disease should be evaluated with endobronchial ultrasound-guided fine-needle aspiration (FNA), cervical mediastinoscopy, or parasternal mediastinotomy (Chamberlain) if necessary to document the status of the mediastinal nodes in equivocal cases. PET scanning is informative but tissue confirmation typically is necessary. For small-cell lung cancer staging should be directed at assessing the presence of extrathoracic disease, to confirm limited-stage tumor extent. The use of CT scans alone is inaccurate in 40%-60% of patients with enlarged lymph nodes over 1 cm (false positive) and 15% of patients without "significant" lymphadenopathy (false negative).

Once all the information from these staging procedures is in hand, the patient with non–small-cell lung cancer can be classified into one of three categories: (1) early lung cancer without mediastinal involvement, ie, stage I/II (see next section); (2) locally advanced lung cancer, ie, stage IIIA/B; and (3) metastatic lung cancer, or stage IV. Therapy is determined by disease stage. Patients with small-cell lung cancer usually are grouped into two categories: (1) disease limited to the ipsilateral hemithorax, including supraclavicular nodes (limited disease); or (2) disease extending beyond the thorax (extensive disease, eg, below the diaphragm or brain metastases).

Several recent analyses indicate that lung cancer screening by either regular routine chest radiography or sputum cytology is not an adequate form of screening. In fact, when directly compared in the National Lung Screening Trial (NLST), there was a 20% reduction in mortality when screening was performed by CT scan compared with chest radiograph alone. Utility of screening with low-dose chest CT was further evaluated by the NELSON trial, which demonstrated that CT screening of high-risk patients reduced mortality by 26% in men and up to 61% in women. Thus, low-dose screening chest CT should be considered, but only among select individuals in the context of multidisciplinary comprehensive care that includes not only screening but also image interpretation, evaluation, management, and appropriate treatment of findings. Currently, the U.S. Preventive Services Task Force recommends screening for lung cancer using annual low-dose CT scanning in patients meeting the following criteria: (1) age 55-80 years old, (2) current smokers or those having quit in the last 15 years, and (3) those with at least a 30-pack-year smoking history.

► Staging

By 1987, the American Joint Committee on Cancer (AJCC) and the Union Internationale Contre le Cancer (UICC) had developed a joint staging system for lung carcinoma based on data gathered primarily by Clifford Mountain of the MD Anderson Cancer Center. The most recent iteration (eighth edition) of the lung cancer staging system, published in 2017, is based on the tumor (T), the status of regional lymph nodes (N), and the presence or absence of distant metastases (M), as outlined in Table 19–8.

Table 19–8. TNM stage groupings.

Primary Tumor	
T Category	**T Criteria**
TX	Primary tumor cannot be assessed, or tumor proven by the presence of malignant cells in sputum or bronchial washings but not visualized by imaging or bronchoscopy
T0	No evidence of primary tumor
Tis	Carcinoma *in situ*
	Squamous cell carcinoma *in situ* (SCIS)
	Adenocarcinoma *in situ* (AIS): adenocareinoma with pure lepidlc pattern, ≤3 cm in greatest dimension
T1	Tumor ≤3 cm in greatest dimension, surrounded by lung or visceral pleura, without bronchoscopic evidence of invasion more proximal than the lobar bronchus (i.e., not in the main bronchus)
T1mi	Minimally invasive adenocarcinoma: adenocarcinoma (≤3 cm in greatest dimension) with a predominantly lepidic pattern and ≤5 mm invasion in greatest dimension
T1a	Tumor ≤1 cm in greatest dimension. A superficial, spreading tumor of any size whose invasive component is limited to the bronchial wall and may extend proximal to the main bronchus also is classified as T1a, but these tumors are uncommon.
T1b	Tumor > 1 cm but ≤2 cm in greatest dimension
T1c	Tumor >2 cm but ≤3 cm in greatest dimension
T2	Tumor >3 cm but ≤5 cm or having any of the following features.
	• Involves the main bronchus regardless of distance to the carina, but without involvement of the carina
	• Invades visceral pleura (PL1 or PL2)
	• Associated with atelectasis or obstructive pneumonitis that extends to the hilar region, involving part or all of the lung
	T2 tumors with these features are classified as
	T2a if ≤4 cm or if the size cannot be determined and T2b if >4 cm but ≤5 cm.
T2a	Tumor >3 cm but ≤4 cm in greatest dimension
T2b	Tumor >4 cm but ≤5 cm in greatest dimension
T3	Tumor >5 cm but ≤7 cm in greatest dimension or directly invading any of the following: parietal pleura (PL3), chest wall (including superior sulcus tumors), phrenic nerve, parietal pericardium; or separate tumor nodule(s) in the same lobe as the primary
T4	Tumor >7 cm or tumor of any size invading one or more of the following: diaphragm, mediastinum, heart, great vessels, trachea, recurrent laryngeal nerve, esophagus; vertebral body, or carina; separate tumor nodule(s) in an ipsilateral lobe different from that of the primary

Regional Lymph Node (N Stage)	
N Category	**N Criteria**
NX	Regional lymph nodes cannot be assessed
N0	No regional lymph node metastasis
N1	Metastasis in ipsilateral peribronchial and/or ipsilateral hilar lymph nodes and intrapulmonary nodes, including involvement by direct extension
N2	Metastasis in ipsilateral mediastinal and/or subcarinal lymph node(s)
N3	Metastasis in contralateral mediastinal, contralateral hilar, ipsilateral or contralateral scalene, or supraclavicular lymph node(s)

Distant Metastasis (M Stage)	
M Category	**M Criteria**
M0	No distant metastasis
M1	Distant metastasis
M1a	Separate tumor nodule{s) in a contralateral lobe; tumor with pleural or pericardial nodules or malignant pleural or pericardia! effusion: Most pleural (pericardial) effusions with lung cancer are a result of the tumor. In a few patients, however, multiple microscopic examinations of pleural (pericardial) fluid are negative for tumor, and the fluid is nonbloody and not an exudate. If these elements and clinical judgment dictate that the effusion is not related to the tumor. the effusion should be excluded as a staging descriptor.
M1b	Single extrathoracic metastasis in a single organ (including involvement of a single nonregional node)
M1c	Multiple extrathoracic metastases in a single organ or in multiple organs

(Continued)

Table 19–8. TNM stage groupings. (*Continued*)

Stage Groups

When T is...	And N is...	And M is...	Then the stage group is...
TX	N0	M0	Occult carcinoma
Tis	N0	M0	0
T1mi	N0	M0	IA1
T1a	N0	M0	IA1
T1a	N1	M0	IIB
T1a	N2	M0	IIIA
T1a	N3	M0	IIIB
T1b	N0	M0	IA2
T1b	N1	M0	IIB
T1b	N2	M0	IIIA
T1b	N3	M0	IIIB
T1c	N0	M0	IA3
T1c	N1	M0	IIB
T1c	N2	M0	IIIA
T1c	N3	M0	IIIB
T2a	N0	M0	IB
T2a	N1	M0	IIB
T2a	N2	M0	IIIA
T2a	N3	M0	IIIB
T2b	N0	M0	IIA
T2b	N1	M0	IIB
T2b	N2	M0	IIIA
T2b	N3	M0	IIIB
T3	N0	M0	IIB
T3	N1	M0	IIIA
T3	N2	M0	IIIB
T3	N3	M0	IIIC
T4	N0	M0	IIIA
T4	N1	M0	IIIA
T4	N2	M0	IIIB
T4	N3	M0	IIIC
Any T	Any N	M1a	IVA
Any T	Any N	M1B	IVA
Any T	Any N	M1C	IVB

Used with the permission of the American College of Surgeons. Amin MB, Edge SB, Greene FL, et al. (Eds.) *AJCC Cancer Staging Manual*, 8th Ed. Springer New York, 2017.

▶ Treatment

Treatment for small-cell carcinoma consists primarily of chemotherapy and radiation, although recent data indicate that for early disease (T1–T2 lesions without hilar adenopathy) resection may improve local control and result in increased long-term survival (as high as 50%), particularly when combined with postoperative chemotherapy.

Treatment for non–small-cell lung cancer varies with stage. Early-stage disease (stage I/II) had historically been treated with surgery alone as long as pathology confirms negative margins. Several randomized prospective trials have demonstrated a statistically significant increase in survival among patients treated with adjuvant chemotherapy for early-stage (stages II and III) non–small-cell lung cancer.

Combined-modality therapy utilizing induction chemotherapy or chemoradiotherapy appears to confer a survival advantage for patients with potentially resectable stage IIIA disease, although overall survival was not improved compared with patients receiving chemotherapy with definitive-dose radiation therapy. Locally advanced and surgically unresectable disease (stage IIIB) is best managed with concurrent platinum-based chemotherapy and fractionated radiation therapy. Among patients with metastatic disease (stage IV), chemotherapy is best for palliation of symptoms. Radiotherapy in this case also is reserved primarily for symptomatic lesions. Combined-agent chemotherapy offers 2-3 months (20%) survival extension to advanced-stage patients. It has been shown to be cost-effective and improve quality of life and is generally well tolerated by patients with reasonable performance status. New biologic agents—so-called targeted therapies—are showing activity in clinical trials and should improve overall survival statistics. It is hoped that with advances in targeted and conventional therapies, the current overall survival (18% at 5 years) of patients with lung cancer can continue to improve.

► Induction Chemotherapy

Recently completed clinical trials and several ongoing studies suggest survival benefit of treatment with platinum-based chemotherapy prior to resection. Induction chemotherapy has been standard for locally advanced surgically resectable disease, but evidence is accumulating to support induction therapy in early-stage non–small-cell lung cancer.

A. Surgical Treatment

1. Surgical Staging—As noted earlier, almost all patients with non–small-cell lung cancer limited to the thorax should undergo cervical mediastinoscopy or EBUS-FNA to exclude involvement of N2 mediastinal lymph nodes (N2 or N3 disease). A possible exception is a small peripheral (T1) nodule, especially of squamous-cell histology without any evidence for mediastinal adenopathy on chest CT scan. PET scan is used with increasing frequency to stage the mediastinum and depending on practice patterns may influence the decision to perform a mediastinoscopy in early-stage disease. However, surgical staging with cervical mediastinoscopy remains the most accurate staging maneuver. Adenocarcinomas with negative mediastinal nodes by CT have an 18%-25% false-negative rate. For left-sided lesions, left parasternal mediastinotomy (Chamberlain) may be required to assess the status of the aorticopulmonary lymph nodes. Without pathologic confirmation of the status of mediastinal lymph nodes, CT scans have been associated with high false-positive and false-negative rates. A surgical assessment of the proximal airways is also required even if this means repeating this invasive procedure, often previously performed by the pulmonologist. Because treatment decisions are based on accurate staging, and treatment of early-stage disease (stage I/II) differs significantly from locally advanced disease (stage IIIA/B), these procedures are essential to high-quality surgical oncology. The importance of accurate staging for patients with non–small-cell lung cancer cannot be overstated.

2. Indications and Preoperative Assessment—Pulmonary resection is indicated for early-stage lung cancer (stage I/II) and in combination with chemotherapy and radiation in locally advanced resectable disease (stage IIIA or resectable T4, IIIb). In addition, resection may be indicated for patients with a single site of metastatic disease, such as a solitary brain or adrenal gland metastasis. Both relative and absolute contraindications to surgical resection are listed in Table 19–9.

Table 19–9. Medical and surgical contraindications to pulmonary resection.

Absolute	Relative
Myocardial infarction within previous 3 months	Myocardial infarction within previous 6 months
SVC syndrome (due to metastatic tumor)	SVC syndrome (due to primary tumor)
Bilateral endobronchial tumor	Recurrent laryngeal nerve paralysis (due to primary tumor in aorticopulmonary window)
Contralateral lymph node metastases (N3)	Horner syndrome
Malignant pleural effusion	Small-cell histology
Distant metastases (except solitary brain and adrenal metastases)	Metastases higher than the midtracheal lymph nodes
	Pericardial involvement
	FEV_1 <0.8 L (<50%)
	FEV_1 0.9-2.4 and insufficient pulmonary reserve for planned resection
	Main pulmonary artery involvement

Preoperative assessment is directed towards evaluating both cardiopulmonary reserve and overall patient fitness. The patient's general performance status or functional classification is probably the most accurate factor in predicting a successful outcome following operation. Advanced age alone is not a contraindication to resection, especially when assessment of physiologic age (eg, morphomics) is considered. A thorough cardiac evaluation is also necessary since lung cancer and cardiovascular disease share common risk factors (eg, smoking). Patients with cardiac symptoms, an abnormal ECG, or other findings suggestive of ischemic heart disease should be screened by a stress test (exercise treadmill, dipyridamole- or adenosine-thallium study, or dobutamine echocardiogram). Significant coronary artery disease should be treated with coronary artery bypass or catheter-based intervention as indicated, prior to any contemplated pulmonary resection. Furthermore, significant pulmonary hypertension and myocardial infarction within 3 months have been associated with up to 20% perioperative mortality and constitute absolute contraindications to standard resection. Other high-risk findings include myocardial infarction within 6 months, ventricular arrhythmias, and heart block, particularly left posterior fascicular hemiblock. Finally, the patient's pulmonary function and predicted ability to tolerate the required pulmonary resection should be assessed. This is accomplished with pulmonary function tests (spirometry, diffusing capacity of the lungs for carbon monoxide, exercise oximetry) and with differential (quantitative) ventilation–perfusion scanning when appropriate.

In a 70-kg patient, the following preoperative studies suggest high risk for perioperative morbidity and are relative contraindications to resection: forced expiratory volume in 1 second (FEV_1) below 0.8 L, a predicted postoperative FEV_1 below 0.8 L, a predicted maximum voluntary ventilation under 50%, a $PaCO_2$ higher than 45 mm Hg, and a Pao_2 less than 50 mm Hg. A diffusion limitation capacity of carbon monoxide (DLCO) under 60% predicted is correlated with an increase in perioperative mortality. Generally, for patients whose predicted postoperative values for forced vital capacity (FVC), forced expiratory volume in 1 second (FEV_1), or DLCO are projected to be less than 40% predicted, further assessment of functional status and operability are recommended.

3. Pulmonary Resection

A. EARLY AND LOCALLY ADVANCED NON–SMALL-CELL LUNG CANCER—The extent of pulmonary resection is dictated by the location of the primary tumor and the presence or absence of involved hilar (interlobar) lymph nodes. Limited segmental resection for stage I/II non–small-cell lung cancer has been evaluated by the Lung Cancer Study Group and found to result in an increased local recurrence rate (15% versus 3%) and lower overall survival, although more recent cohort studies suggest that sublobar resection, particularly segmentectomy rather than non-anatomic wedge excision, may be considered for smaller lung nodules without evidence for local (N1) lymph node involvement. Factors favoring sublobar resection include peripheral stage IA disease, ground glass nodules, and patients with poor cardiopulmonary reserve. Recent case series have suggested that sublobar resection actually might be adequate in terms of local recurrence and disease-free survival particularly for stage I carcinoma; this is the focus of multiple ongoing multi-center clinical trials within North America and Asia. Nevertheless, until the results of large prospective studies are known, lobectomy remains the standard of care for treatment of early-stage non–small-cell lung cancer in the patient with adequate cardiopulmonary reserve, although considerable debate continues.

Preoperative or intraoperative lymph-node sampling dictates the degree of anatomical resection required. Samples of interlobar (hilar) lymph nodes are submitted for immediate pathologic examination to exclude involvement that would require more invasive resections such as a pneumonectomy. Depending on anatomic location of the lesion, a "sleeve" resection of mainstem bronchus can also be utilized in order to obtain clear surgical margins while preserving the remaining lung parenchyma. Pneumonectomy may be necessary for proximal lesions involving the mainstem bronchus or the interlobar (hilar) lymph nodes, although bronchial and/or vascular sleeve resections should be considered. In addition, techniques are available for more extensive resection, such as intrapericardial pneumonectomy and tracheal sleeve pneumonectomy.

The overall mortality rates following segmental resection, lobectomy, and pneumonectomy are 1.4%, 2.9%, and 6.2%, respectively, in centers with large experience. Complications following pulmonary resection include cardiac arrhythmias, hemorrhage, infection (empyema), bronchopleural fistula, respiratory insufficiency, and pulmonary embolism.

B. ADVANCED (METASTATIC) NON–SMALL-CELL LUNG CANCER—Patients with solitary brain and adrenal metastases, especially if metachronous, are still candidates for resection and have benefited by prolonged survival in a few small retrospective studies in comparison with historical controls. Systemic preoperative (induction) chemotherapy and radiotherapy, however, should be administered initially. In addition, transbronchial Nd: YAG laser resection of tumors obstructing the proximal airways can provide satisfactory palliation for selected patients. Improvements in the design and deployment techniques of expansile stents have been a significant advance for palliation of cancer causing proximal airway obstruction. Finally, photodynamic laser therapy with photosensitizers can alleviate airway obstruction from tumors, albeit not as quickly as Nd: YAG laser ablation.

C. SMALL-CELL LUNG CANCER—Resection for small peripheral tumors followed by aggressive postoperative chemotherapy may increase the local control rate and potentially the overall survival rate in the early small-cell lung cancer. Although survival rates as high as 50% with this approach have been reported, the majority of patients diagnosed with small-cell lung cancer present with advanced disease, and surgical management therefore is rare.

B. Radiation Therapy

1. Non–small-cell lung cancer—Radiation therapy can be administered with curative intent in stage I/II disease in patients who refuse or are not medically suitable candidates for surgery. The 5-year survival rate with this approach, however, is only 22%-33%. With locally advanced disease (stage IIIA/B), radiation therapy (5500-6000 cGy) until recently has been the treatment of choice. Although local or nodal recurrence rates are less than 30%, long-term survival is less than 10% in these patients, and the type of fractionation scheme has not altered the outcome. Stereotactic radiation techniques appear to have early efficacy in terms of tumor control and overall survival, particularly for medically inoperable patients.

Adjuvant radiation therapy following resection has been extensively studied by the Lung Cancer Study Group and has been found to decrease local or nodal recurrence but not to prolong overall survival. A much-disputed meta-analysis (the PORT study) showed a decrease in survival for stage I/II patients treated with postoperative radiation. Differences in radiotherapy techniques within the analysis may account for the worse outcomes. Preoperative radiation has been used with T3 lesions, particularly Pancoast tumors, with improved survival; however, there is no objective evidence that radiation must be given preoperatively. A multicenter intergroup trial (SWOG) has shown a significant survival advantage for combined chemoradiotherapy (etoposide, platinum, and 4500 cGy) prior to resection for Pancoast (superior sulcus) tumors that were N1 or less. Complete resection rates were improved, 20%-25% complete pathologic responses were achieved, and survival was significantly improved (45%-50% at 3 years) over surgery alone or preoperative radiotherapy and surgery. Among patients with metastatic disease, therapeutic radiation is indicated in patients with symptoms of pain, neurologic symptoms, and symptoms of superior vena cava compression.

2. Small-cell lung cancer—Multiple randomized trials have been conducted comparing the combination of radiation and chemotherapy to chemotherapy alone in limited-stage small-cell lung cancer. The majority show improved local control and modest (3–4 months) prolonged survival with the combination. This was at the cost of increased morbidity, however. In extensive disease, no benefit has been demonstrated for radiation therapy other than for palliative radiation of symptomatic metastases. Prophylactic cranial irradiation may be beneficial in those limited-stage patients who respond to initial treatment, but can cause significant cognitive deficits.

C. Chemotherapy

1. Non–small-cell lung cancer—Although chemotherapy alone has not generally been used in the treatment of early or locally advanced non–small-cell lung cancer, combinations of chemotherapy and radiotherapy have been evaluated in locally advanced unresectable disease. In some instances, no benefit to the combination was demonstrated, particularly when only single agents were used; however, a threefold to fourfold increase in 5-year survival with concurrent radiation and combined-agent chemotherapy has been documented. In the presence of metastatic disease, multiple trials of combination chemotherapy have demonstrated a modest improvement in overall survival (14 weeks, or 25% improved survival) but not without some toxicity. Even so, quality-of-life assessments and cost analyses support the use of outpatient combined-agent chemotherapy over palliative care alone.

A. Postoperative adjuvant therapy—A progressive trend in lung cancer therapy has evolved in favor of far more widespread use of adjuvant chemotherapy. Three large multicenter randomized trials in Europe and North America have served as a basis for the increased application of postoperative platinum-based chemotherapy (Italian stage IB, the International Adjuvant Lung Cancer Trial [IALT], Cancer and Leukemia Group B [CALGB] 9633, and National Cancer Institute of Canada [NCIC] BR10). Although the absolute gold standard regimen of combined chemotherapy has not been clearly defined, the commonly used regimens include either carboplatin and paclitaxel or cisplatin and etoposide alongside concurrent adjuvant radiation. The benefit of chemotherapy appears to vary based on patient selection but is estimated to be an increase of 5%-15% survival measured at 5 years from diagnosis (Table 19–10).

2. Small-cell lung cancer—Research has shown combination chemotherapy to have superior outcomes to single drugs, currently producing 80%-100% and 60%-80% response rates in limited-stage and extensive-stage disease, respectively. Furthermore, median survival is 15-20 months and 8-12 months in each group. Platinum-based agents and etoposide (or teniposide) have become common first-line regimens

Table 19–10. Adjuvant trials favoring use of chemotherapy in completely resected non–small-cell lung cancer.

Study	CT Regimen	Radiation Therapy	5-year Survival CT vs Control (%)
Italian Stage IB Study	Cis/Etoposide × 6	No	59 vs 30
IALT	Various platinum	Yes ±	44.5 vs 40.4
CALGB 9633	Carbo/Taxol × 4	No	60 vs 58[1]
JBR.10	Vin/P × 4	No	69 vs 54
ANITA	Vin/P × 4	Yes ±	+8.6

CT, Carbo/Taxol, carboplatin paclitaxel; Vin/P, vinorelbine cisplatin; Cis, cisplatin.
[1]No significant difference.

and standard of care based on their side-effect profiles. Furthermore, the monoclonal antibody drug, atezolizumab has gained traction as a third additive agent. The optimal duration of therapy has not been defined, but the majority of the effect appears to occur within the first four to six cycles.

D. Immunotherapy

Immunotherapy for non–small-cell lung cancer using immune checkpoint inhibitors (PD-1, PD-L1, etc) has gained traction among oncologists. Thus the anti-PD-1 antibody agent pembrolizumab has become more common place either as monotherapy or in combination with chemotherapeutic regimens based on the patient's level of PD-L1 expression. Currently, IgG4 monoclonal antibody antagonist (nivolumab) is under investigation for treating NSCLC, as is atezolizumab (anti-PD-L1). In the past, immunotherapy with bacillus Calmette-Guérin (BCG), levamisole, TNF-α, lymphokine-activated killer (LAK) cells, and tumor-infiltrating lymphocytes were attempted but these have not proven to reliably change outcomes. Furthermore, treatment with IL-2, induced killer cells, remains controversial.

However, in extensive-stage small-cell carcinoma, atezolizumab, a PD-L1 (anti-programmed death-ligand) monoclonal antibody drug mentioned above, has become a more frequent addition to chemotherapeutic regimens. Additionally, treatment of small-cell carcinoma with targeted therapy towards CTLA-4, DLL3, and others remain investigational.

E. Targeted Therapies

As part of multimodal therapy, investigation continues into targeted drugs, which by and large are mechanistically different that standard chemotherapy. As the name implies, targeted therapy allows for a specific drug to target specific driver mutations that are expressed by cancer cells. Given the improved median survival when able to use targeted drugs, screening for driver mutations in lung cancer has become commonplace, allowing for treatment planning with targeted therapy prior to chemotherapy, or concomitantly. One promising monoclonal antibody drug, bevacizumab, has been employed to target the vascular endothelial growth factor receptor (VEGF). However, use of bevacizumab with current gold-standard therapy has shown near-prohibitive risk due to toxicity and side effects; and if used, it is only used concurrently with chemotherapy for a short time before stopping an agent. Molecular-based therapies targeting overexpressed growth receptors (EGFR1, HER-2/neu) by monoclonal antibody or small molecules have demonstrated clinical effectiveness among select patient populations but translation to improved outcomes remains contested.

A small percentage of NSCLC will display anaplastic lymphoma kinase (ALK) mutations and can be treated with the targeted drugs: crizotinib, alectinib, certinib, etc. These targeted therapies for ALK mutations have been used with and without standard chemotherapy in late-phase trials and show improved progression-free survival. Yet high-quality data showing improvement in overall survival is still lacking. In the same vein, ROS1 mutations respond similarly to tumors with ALK translocations and treatment can be considered with crizotinib, which has recently shown improvement in progression-free survival.

Additional agents targeting signal transduction pathways (eg, farnesyl transferase inhibitors) for the *ras* pathway as well as antisense oligonucleotide and gene therapies all remain investigational. Lastly, the addition of thalidomide to concurrent chemoradiation has not statistically changed outcomes; and a great deal of research remains on the frontier of targeted therapies.

▶ Prognosis

A. Non–Small-Cell Lung Cancer

By and large, pathologic stage is the best predictor of patient survival in non–small-cell lung cancer. Overall, according to compiled data and the American Cancer Society, the 5-year survival rate of patients with stages I, II, IIIA, IIIB, IIIC, and IV is 68%-92%, 53%-60%, 36%, 26%, 13%, and <1%-10%, respectively (Table 19–11). Improved survival will likely depend on earlier diagnosis and further coordinated

Table 19–11. Survival in non–small-cell lung cancer.

Stage	TNM Description	Five-Year Survival (%)
I		68-92
A1	T1a, N0	92
A2	T1b, N0	83
A3	T1c, N0	77
B	T2a, N0	68
II		53-60
A	T2b, N0	60
B	T1-2, N1 or T3, N0	53
III		
A	T1-2, N2 or T3 N1, or T4 N0-1	36
B	T3-4, N2 or T1-2, N3	26
C	T3-4 N3	13
IV		
A	M1a-b	10
B	M1c	<1
Overall		18

efforts among surgeons, medical oncologists, and radiation oncologists.

B. Small-Cell Lung Cancer

Patients with limited-stage disease achieve a median survival rate of 15-20 months with an approximately 10% 5-year survival rate. Conversely, those with extensive-stage disease have a median survival rate of only 8-12 months, with only 1%-2% surviving 5 years.

De Koning H, et al. Effects of volume CT lung cancer screening: Mortality results of the NELSON randomised-controlled population based trial. 19th World Conference on Lung Cancer. Abstract PL02.05, presented September 25, 2018.

Detterbeck FC, et al. Screening for lung cancer: Diagnosis and management of lung cancer, 3rd ed. American College of Chest Physicians Evidence-Based Clinical Practice Guidelines. *Chest.* 2013;143(5 suppl):e78S-e92S. doi:10.1378/chest.12-2350.

Jett JR, et al. Treatment of small cell lung cancer: Diagnosis and management of lung cancer, 3rd ed. American College of Chest Physicians Evidence-Based Clinical Practice Guidelines. *Chest.* 2013;143(5 suppl):e400S-e419S. doi:10.1378/chest.12-2363.

Lin J, Fernandez F. Indications for invasive mediastinal staging for non-small cell lung cancer. *J Thorac Cardiovasc Surg.* 2018: 156(6):2319-2324.

The National Lung Screening Trial Research Team. Reduced lung-cancer mortality with low-dose computed tomographic screening. *N Engl J Med.* 2011;365(5):395-409.

Noone AM, et al, eds. *SEER Cancer Statistics Review, 1975-2015.* Bethesda: National Cancer Institute. https://seer.cancer.gov/csr/1975_2015/. Based on November 2017 SEER data submission, posted to the SEER website, April 2018.

Shah A, et al. Cost-effectiveness of stereotactic body radiation therapy versus surgical resection for stage I non-small cell lung cancer. *Cancer.* Online publication May 29, 2013.

Wood DE, et al. Lung cancer screening, version 3.2018, NCCN clinical practice guidelines in oncology. *J Natl Compr Canc Netw.* 2018;16:412-441.

Zhang L, et al. Comparison of the oncologic outcomes of anatomic segmentectomy and lobectomy for early-stage non-small cell lung cancer. *Ann Thorac Surg.* 2015;99:728-737.

UNUSUAL PULMONARY NEOPLASMS

▶ Malignant Neoplasms

Bronchial adenomas are a group of low-grade malignancies arising from the bronchial tree. Carcinoid tumors constitute 85%-90% of these neoplasms, with adenoid cystic carcinoma (10%) and mucoepidermoid carcinoma (<5%) accounting for most of the remainder. Carcinoid tumors are classified as either typical or atypical, with markedly different histologic characteristics (Table 19–12). Adenoid cystic carcinomas occur in the lower trachea; infiltrate locally along submucosal

Table 19–12. Characteristics of typical and atypical carcinoid tumors.

	Typical (%)	Atypical (%)
Incidence	90	10
Central location	80	50
Peripheral location	20	50
Metastases	10-15	??

and perineural tissue planes, often far beyond the boundaries of gross tumor; and metastasize late. Mucoepidermoid carcinomas resemble salivary tumors, with varying numbers of three distinct cell types: mucous, squamous, and intermediate. Patients with bronchial adenomas complain of cough, recurrent pulmonary infections, hemoptysis, pain, and wheezing. Only 15% of patients are completely asymptomatic. Carcinoid syndrome is rare with pulmonary carcinoid tumors. Most bronchial adenomas are diagnosed with a combination of plain chest radiography, CT, and bronchoscopy. Biopsy at the time of bronchoscopy can be associated with significant bleeding, and measures to control this must be readily available.

Lung resection is indicated for these tumors, with lobectomy being the most common procedure. Sleeve and bronchoplastic resections are particularly useful to preserve pulmonary function in these patients and make standard pneumonectomy rare. Removal of adenoid cystic carcinomas requires generous margins and frozen-section examination of the margins at the time of surgery. This is achieved owing to the fact that up to 8 cm of trachea can be removed and still reconstructed primarily. When wide margins are not feasible, postoperative radiation may be indicated. With the possible exception of atypical carcinoid, chemotherapy is generally not indicated in the treatment of these neoplasms.

Overall, the long-term outlook is good even for those patients with metastatic disease. Even patients with adenoid cystic carcinoma and distant metastases may do well for extended periods due to the slow-growing nature of this malignancy; however, lymph node and distant metastases in patients with carcinoid tumors generally carry a poor prognosis.

▶ Benign Neoplasms

Benign neoplasms of the lung are uncommon, accounting for less than 1% of all pulmonary tumors. Most are hamartomas, but fibromas, leiomyomas, neurofibromas, myoblastomas, and benign metastasizing leiomyomas also occur. Most lesions are peripheral and asymptomatic; however, central lesions can produce the usual symptoms of cough, wheezing, hemoptysis, and recurrent pneumonia. Typically, the lesions are discovered on routine chest radiographs and appear as a 1- to 2-cm well-circumscribed, bosselated lower lung nodule with calcifications in 10%-30%. Central lesions may require bronchoscopy for diagnosis, but a pathologic diagnosis is most often obtained by fine-needle aspiration biopsy or surgery. Prognosis is quite good following surgery and resection usually only requires limited to wedge excision unless the lesion occupies the proximal bronchial airway and is associated with recurrent distal infections or bronchiectasis. Lobectomy is usually only indicated in such an occasion. Following resection, the prognosis is excellent.

SPECIAL PROBLEM: THE SOLITARY PULMONARY NODULE

With the frequent use of chest radiography, solitary pulmonary nodules ("coin lesions") are frequently found in patients without pulmonary symptoms. These lesions pose a diagnostic problem for clinicians because they may represent something as benign as a nipple shadow or as malignant as lung cancer. The overall incidence of cancer in coin lesions is as low as 10%. Other diagnostic possibilities include (1) infections due to mycobacteria (tuberculosis), fungi (histoplasmosis, coccidioidomycosis), and helminths (echinococcosis); (2) inflammatory nodules from rheumatoid arthritis, focal pneumonitis, and Wegener granulomatosis; (3) congenital anomalies, such as bronchogenic cysts and arteriovenous malformations; (4) benign neoplasms such as hamartomas, hemangiomas, papillary tumors, fibrous tumors of the pleura; (5) malignant neoplasms of the lung; and (6) miscellaneous processes such as hematomas, pulmonary infarcts, pleural plaques, loculated effusions, chest-wall masses, and mucoid impaction. Although certain radiographic findings may suggest malignancy or benignity, solid pathologic proof that the nodule does not represent a malignancy rests with the clinician. In general, malignant neoplasms are larger and grow rapidly, appear spiculated, often with surface umbilication or notching and eccentric excavation. In addition, cancers often occur in smokers (or former smokers) over the age of 40 with negative skin tests for tuberculosis, histoplasmosis, or coccidioidomycosis (although positive tests do not exclude cancer), and in nodules that lack calcium (CT Hounsfield units <175). In contrast, benign lesions are small (<1 cm), stable (>2 years), and calcified ("target" or "popcorn" distribution; CT Hounsfield units >175) and are associated with positive skin tests in 70%-90% of patients.

Evaluation of these patients usually includes chest CT scan, but sputum cytology, cultures, bronchoscopy, and mediastinoscopy are sometimes helpful. FDG-PET scanning plays an important role in the evaluation of tumors that are suspicious for malignancy. PET scan can often differentiate among lesions suspicious for malignancy.

With the advent of spiral CT scanning, and increasing support for lung cancer screening, the incidence of asymptomatic pulmonary nodules can vary from 25% to 70%. The vast majority of these lesions now identified are smaller than 1 cm and often as small as 2-3 mm. In one series, the incidence of lung cancer in the asymptomatic 10-pack-year smoking history population over the age of 50 years was 27% of all lesions identified, followed, and treated.

Ultimately, a pathologic diagnosis must be made. In some instances, fine-needle aspiration cytology may be helpful, particularly if a tissue diagnosis of hamartoma can be made or if cultures demonstrating infectious organisms are obtained. The vast majority of solitary pulmonary nodules require excisional biopsy to exclude the possibility of malignancy. Currently, this is accomplished with video-assisted techniques in most patients, particularly if the lesion is in the periphery of the lung. If a benign lesion is encountered, nothing further is warranted; but if a lung cancer is diagnosed, immediate lobectomy is indicated. The prognosis following resection of a coin lesion that turns out to be a bronchogenic carcinoma is good, with a 5-year survival of as high as 80%-90% for lesions smaller than 1 cm.

SECONDARY LUNG CANCER

Autopsy studies have demonstrated that 30% of all patients with malignancies develop pulmonary metastases, and 12% have been shown to have isolated lung disease that is totally resectable. In addition, 10% of these latter patients (1.2% of all patients) have solitary lung metastases. Most pulmonary metastases occur through hematogenous spread from the primary site; lymphatic or transbronchial spread is extremely rare. Secondary metastatic spread to the pulmonary and mediastinal lymph nodes, however, can also occur. In patients with known extrathoracic primary cancers, multiple pulmonary lesions almost always represent metastatic disease. Solitary lesions, however, may be due to benign disease (18%) or new primary lung cancer (18%) as well as metastatic disease (64%). Most patients with pulmonary metastases are asymptomatic even with extensive disease. If symptoms do develop, cough, hemoptysis, fever, dyspnea, and pain are common. The diagnosis is generally initially suggested by routine chest radiography, and CT of the chest should always be ordered to assess the lungs for other nodules. Although CT scans are more sensitive, detecting nodules as small as 1-3 mm, they are also less specific (false-positive rate of 55%) than plain x-rays. Pathologic confirmation of the diagnosis is essential and usually is obtained at the time of resection. For patients who are not surgical candidates, fine-needle aspiration cytology is useful for peripheral lesions, while central lesions may require bronchoscopy for tissue diagnosis.

Medically fit patients with resectable disease are surgical candidates as long as the following criteria are fulfilled: (1) the primary tumor must be controlled or imminently controllable, (2) no other sites of disease may exist, (3) no other therapy can offer comparable results, and (4) the operative risk must be low. Since adenocarcinomas (especially breast cancer) commonly involve multiple organs, it is imperative that with this histology a full evaluation be performed, including bone scan and head CT or MRI. Solitary squamous-cell nodules, even in the presence of a previous squamous-cell carcinoma (eg, head and neck tumors), should be considered a new primary (lung) cancer.

Pulmonary resection can be accomplished through a standard posterolateral thoracotomy, median sternotomy, or bilateral anterior thoracotomies. The latter approach is particularly beneficial for bilateral disease involving the lower lobes. Video-assisted thoracoscopy is increasingly applied to metastatic disease in an attempt to reduce the morbidity of multiple resections. On occasion, during open operations for metastatic disease, several unsuspected nodules are found by direct palpation that might be missed with thoracoscopy. Wedge resection is the treatment of choice unless the lesion is a solitary squamous-cell carcinoma or adenocarcinoma. These latter lesions cannot be distinguished from primary lung cancer on frozen section pathologic examination, and they must therefore be treated as primary lung cancers with lobectomy and mediastinal lymph node dissection. Occasionally, other malignant tumors identified by histologic examination may require lobectomy or, rarely, even pneumonectomy because of involvement of the proximal pulmonary artery or bronchus.

The success rate with surgical removal of pulmonary metastases has been greatest with testicular (51% 5-year survival) and head–neck cancers (47% 5-year survival). Other types of tumors, such as osteogenic and soft-tissue sarcomas, renal cell carcinoma, and colon carcinoma, are all associated with prolonged survival in 20%-35% of patients. Results of resection for melanoma are less favorable (10%-15% survival benefit). Isolated, resectable pulmonary metastases from rectal cancer can have as high as a 55% 5-year survival rate with metastasectomy alone.

Furthermore, multiple thoracotomies over periods in excess of 10 years are not unusual with the sarcomas. Numerous studies have been conducted in attempts to identify prognostic factors that could aid in the selection of patients for resection. Adverse prognostic factors have included (1) multiple or bilateral lesions, (2) more than four lesions seen on CT scan, (3) tumor doubling time less than 40 days, (4) a short disease-free interval, and (5) advanced age.

Although no consensus has developed regarding the selection of candidates for surgical exploration, it is generally agreed that no single criterion should be used to exclude patients from surgical resection. In all series, long-term benefit and survival hinges on complete resection. If complete resection is not deemed possible, resection should not be offered.

References

Chudgar NP, et al. Pulmonary metastasectomy with therapeutic intent for soft tissue sarcoma. *J Thorac Cardiovasac Surg.* 2017; 154(1):319-330.e1.

Kikano GE, et al. Evaluation of the solitary pulmonary nodule. *Am Fam Physician.* 2015;92(12):1084A-1091A.

Lou F, Huang J, Sima CS, et al. Patterns of recurrence and second primary lung cancer in early-stage lung cancer survivors followed with routine computed tomography surveillance. *J Thorac Cardiovasc Surg.* 2013;145(1):75.

Petrella F, et al. Pulmonary metastasectomy: An overview. *J Thorac Dis.* 2017;9:S1291-S1298.

von Meyenfeldt EM, Wouters MW, Fat NL, et al. Local treatment of pulmonary metastases: From open resection to minimally invasive approach? Less morbidity, comparable local control. *Surg Endosc.* 2012;26(8):2312.

MULTIPLE-CHOICE QUESTIONS

1. Chest wall masses:

   A. Are nearly always benign.
   B. Are common in postmenopausal women.
   C. Mostly arise from bone or cartilage.
   D. Most commonly arise from muscle, nerve, or fascia.
   E. Are rarely resectable.

2. Risk factors for lung cancer include all of the following *except*:

   A. Exposure to asbestos.
   B. Tobacco smoking.
   C. Vitamin A deficiency.
   D. Iodine deficiency.
   E. Exposure to arsenic.

3. Pleural effusion, the presence of fluid within the pleural space, can collect through all of the following mechanisms *except*:

   A. Increase in the pulmonary vascular hydrostatic pressure (congestive heart failure, mitral stenosis).
   B. Ureteral obstruction with transdiaphragmatic urine leak.
   C. Decrease in the vascular colloid oncotic pressure (hypoproteinemia).
   D. Increase in the capillary permeability due to inflammation (pneumonia, pancreatitis, sepsis).
   E. Pancreatic pseudocyst rupture with transdiaphragmatic movement of abdominal fluid.

4. The four sources of mediastinal infection include all of the following *except:*

   A. Spontaneous bacterial mediastinitis of sarcoidosis.
   B. Direct contamination.
   C. Hematogenous or lymphatic spread.
   D. Extension of infection from the neck or retroperitoneum.
   E. Extension from the lung or pleura.

5. Cystic fibrosis is all of the following *except:*

   A. An autosomal recessive multisystem congenital disorder.
   B. Characterized by chronic airway obstruction and infection.
   C. The result of mutation in the cystic fibrosis transmembrane regulator gene.
   D. Effectively cured by double lung transplantation with a 10-year graft survival rate exceeding 85%.
   E. A predisposing factor for chronic lung infection.

Acquired Cardiac Disease

Jonathan W. Haft, MD

Gerard M. Doherty, MD

CORONARY ARTERY DISEASE

▶ Pathophysiology

The heart has the highest metabolic demands when compared to other organs. The vast majority of the energy substrate utilization is expended during unrelenting periodic contraction of the myocardium. Blood flow is delivered at a rate of 1 mL per gram of cardiac tissue per minute at rest. Increases in myocardial oxygen consumption, via adenosine diphosphate and adenosine-mediated arteriolar vasodilation, can result in a reciprocal increase in blood flow, up to five times normal. This increased blood flow is accommodated by recruitment of an extensive capillary bed within the myocardium, with nearly one capillary per myocyte. Between 70% and 80% of available oxygen is extracted from coronary blood flow at rest. Thus, the metabolic needs of the heart are tightly coupled to the availability of coronary blood flow, since additional extraction is limited. In addition, blood flow through the left ventricular epicardial arteries is phasic. During myocardial contraction, extravascular compression of intramyocardial capillaries prevents forward flow during systole, limiting flow to the diastolic phase of the cardiac cycle. This is even more pronounced in the subendocardial region where myocardial oxygen demands are greatest as a result of increased wall tension and greater sarcomere shortening. Because of the elevated and insistent myocardial oxygen consumption, the restriction of blood flow to diastole, and the high basal level of oxygen consumption, the heart is particularly susceptible to ischemic injury related to stenosis of the epicardial coronary arteries.

The heart receives its blood supply from the left and right coronary arteries (Figure 20–1). These epicardial vessels originate as the first branches off of the aortic root, in their respective sinuses of Valsalva. The coronary circulation is traditionally divided into three territories or regions: the left anterior descending and the circumflex (arising from the left coronary artery) and the right (from the right coronary artery). The dominance of the heart refers to which major artery terminates as the posterior descending branch. Ninety percent of individuals are right dominant, as the right coronary artery supplies the posterior descending artery. The remaining 10% are left dominant, as the terminal branch of the circumflex artery supplies the posterior descending artery.

The left coronary artery is referred to as the left main coronary artery. After its origin in the left sinus of Valsalva, it courses between the left atrial appendage and the pulmonary artery. The left main coronary artery varies in length but is typically less than 2 cm long. It terminates in two branches: the left anterior descending (LAD) and the circumflex coronary arteries. In less than 1% of patients, the left main artery is absent, with the LAD and circumflex originating as separate ostia from the left sinus of Valsalva.

The LAD, or anterior interventricular artery, courses anteriorly and inferiorly in the interventricular groove toward the apex of the heart. Several branches of the LAD travel along the anterolateral surface of the left ventricle and are known as diagonal arteries. Their number and size are highly variable. Branches to the interventricular septum take off perpendicularly, the first of which is often sizable. The LAD is the most prominent of the three coronary territories and carries approximately 50% of myocardial blood flow.

After arising from the left main, the circumflex coronary artery dives posteriorly along the atrioventricular groove. Several obtuse marginal branches supply the lateral wall of the left ventricle; these branches vary in both size and number. In 10% of patients, the circumflex continues posteriorly and gives rise in its terminal branch to the posterior descending coronary artery, running from the posterior atrioventricular groove toward the posterior apex in the interventricular groove. Some patients have a third branch of the left main referred to as the ramus intermedius. If present, this branch is often large and supplies the anterolateral wall of the left ventricle.

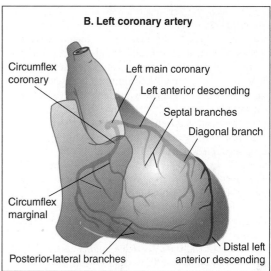

A. Right coronary artery

SA nodal artery
Right coronary
Conus artery
Anterior ventricular branches
Acute marginal
Atrial branches
AV nodal artery
Posterior-lateral branch
Posterior descending

B. Left coronary artery

Circumflex coronary
Left main coronary
Left anterior descending
Septal branches
Diagonal branch
Circumflex marginal
Posterior-lateral branches
Distal left anterior descending

▲ **Figure 20–1.** Anatomy of the coronary circulation. AV, atrioventricular; SA, sinoatrial.

The right coronary artery originates from the right sinus of Valsalva in the aortic root. It courses anteriorly and rightward until reaching the right atrioventricular groove. The vessel then descends around the acute margin of the heart, giving rise to one or more branches supplying the right ventricle. In 90% of patients, the right coronary artery continues posteriorly, terminating as the posterior descending coronary artery and the posterolateral artery.

Atherosclerosis, a progressive multifocal disease of medium and large muscular arteries of the systemic circulation, tends to occur predominantly at vessel bifurcations, sharp curvatures, and other regions, creating pressure wave reflections and recirculation. Because of these flow-related considerations, atherosclerotic stenotic lesions are generally restricted to the proximal regions of the large epicardial coronary arteries. In particular, stenosis found in the LAD and circumflex vessels is frequently isolated, short, and in the proximal segments. The right coronary artery, however, develops diffuse obstructions, although it rarely extends into the posterior descending or intramural branches.

The pathologic mechanism of coronary atheroma formation is identical to the lesions found elsewhere in the vascular tree. Endothelial injury from cigarette smoke, hypercholesterolemia, hyperglycemia, hypertension, or other causes of inflammation initiate a cascade of events. These include endothelial dysfunction with reduced nitric oxide production, monocyte adhesion and migration, lipid accumulation, and smooth muscle cell proliferation. The end result is an enlarging plaque encroaching on the arterial lumen, separated from the bloodstream by a collagen-rich fibrous plaque. The lesion can cause flow limitations, particularly when the luminal cross-sectional area is reduced by at least 75%. With this degree of obstruction, the vasodilatory reserve required during increased myocardial demand is restricted, resulting in transient myocardial ischemia until demand returns to baseline. The atherosclerotic plaque also causes coronary ischemia when the lesion becomes unstable. The fibrous plaque can fracture, causing rupture of the plaque contents and complete epicardial thrombosis, the presumed mechanism of ST-segment elevation myocardial infarction (STEMI). Additionally, subtotal plaque disruption can cause vasoconstriction, platelet activation, and embolization, resulting in ischemia without total occlusion of the epicardial vessel. This is the presumed mechanism of unstable angina and non–ST-segment elevation myocardial infarction (NSTEMI).

▶ **Patient Presentation**

Patients with coronary atherosclerosis can present with a variety of symptoms depending on the severity and nature of their occlusive lesions as well as on their other medical comorbidities. Chronic stable angina is the most frequent complaint of the patient with coronary artery disease. At rest, coronary blood flow is adequate to meet myocardial demand, and patients are without symptoms. However, during exercise or stress, as myocardial oxygen demand increases, autoregulatory mechanisms vasodilate to increase myocardial blood flow fivefold to sixfold. Stable coronary obstructions become flow limiting, resulting in an imbalance of oxygen demand and supply. Chest pain develops rapidly and is typically described as tightness, squeezing, constricting, or aching. It is usually midsternal and radiates to the left shoulder, arm, or neck. The classically described Levine sign with a clenched fist over the sternum is a common finding. Some patients, however, describe symptoms that are collectively referred to as "anginal equivalents." These include dyspnea, diaphoresis, nausea, heartburn, and dizziness or presyncope. Although the clinical manifestations of angina are variable, the pathognomonic feature of chronic stable angina is that the symptoms occur predictably with exertion and are always relieved with rest.

Acute coronary syndrome (ACS) encompasses a spectrum of conditions related to coronary occlusive disease, including unstable angina, NSTEMI, and STEMI. Patients with unstable angina experience chest pain or an anginal equivalent that is new, occurs at rest, or occurs with increasing severity from their baseline chronic stable symptoms, also called crescendo angina. Patients who develop NSTEMI have evidence of myocardial injury with elevated blood levels of myocardial enzymes (troponin and the myoglobin [Mb] fraction of creatine kinase). Unstable angina and NSTEMI are important prognostic indicators, as 10% of patients will die of cardiovascular causes within 6 months.

STEMI represents the consequences of large epicardial vessel occlusion typically associated with plaque rupture. Patients usually describe severe retrosternal chest pain that persists for more than 30 minutes. Patients with previous chronic stable angina will report that the current pain does not resolve with rest or nitroglycerine and is more intense in quality. Patients often describe additional symptoms such as diaphoresis, nausea, and dizziness. Although improvements in health systems have drastically increased survival from myocardial infarction, mortality for STEMI remains near 10%.

Diagnostic Evaluation

Patients with suspected coronary artery disease should undergo a resting electrocardiogram. Although most patients with chronic stable angina have a normal electrocardiogram pattern, evidence of previous myocardial infarctions may be identified with the presence of either Q waves or conduction abnormalities. The most widely used diagnostic test to evaluate for coronary artery disease is exercise electrocardiography. Using standardized protocols, patients are exercised on a treadmill or bicycle ergometer while a 12-lead electrocardiogram is continuously recorded. The test is continued until the patient's symptoms are noted or until the development of significant ST-segment shifts suggesting myocardial ischemia. The diagnostic accuracy of exercise stress electrocardiogram testing can be enhanced with myocardial perfusion imaging. Several radioactive tracers are used clinically, the most frequent of which is thallium-201. Because of its similarities to potassium ions, it is taken up preferentially by the viable cardiac myocytes. Its distribution within the myocardium is proportional to the rate of perfusion. In some cases, patients are unable to exercise because of additional physical or psychological limitations. Pharmacologic agents can substitute for exercise by increasing myocardial oxygen demand (dobutamine) or by directly vasodilating coronary arteries (adenosine), thus demonstrating regions with fixed restrictions in myocardial blood flow. Echocardiography can be used as an alternative to nuclear perfusion imaging to increase the accuracy of exercise electrocardiogram testing. Echocardiography demonstrates regional changes in wall motion that can be observed during myocardial ischemia. It can also identify valvular abnormalities or other conditions that may influence treatment choices.

Coronary angiography, also known as cardiac catheterization, is indicated in symptomatic patients with suspected coronary occlusive lesions. After percutaneous access is obtained in the arterial system, preformed catheters of varying sizes are advanced fluoroscopically to selectively engage the ostia of the left and right coronary arteries. Radiopaque contrast is injected with imaging of the opacified coronary artery. Standardized views are obtained of both the right and left coronary systems to provide different projections to clearly define the vascular anatomy and to quantify the severity of occlusive lesions (Figure 20–2). Additionally, catheters can be inserted across the aortic valve into the left ventricular cavity. Contrast injection for ventriculography can provide information about ventricular systolic function, cavity size, and the presence of left-sided valvular abnormalities. During cardiac catheterization, stenotic lesions in the epicardial vessels can be treated using percutaneous techniques, described in the section on percutaneous intervention. Newer imaging techniques using high-resolution multislice computed tomography (CT) scanning with three-dimensional reconstruction and magnetic resonance imaging (MRI) are increasingly used. These noninvasive approaches have the potential to improve the safety and convenience of coronary imaging; however, resolution remains inferior to standard coronary angiography.

Medical Treatment

Medical therapy of coronary artery disease begins with controlling risk factors that contribute to formation and destabilization of the atherosclerotic plaque. The most important intervention is cessation of cigarette smoking. Other interventions include control of hypertension, diabetes, and hypercholesterolemia. Dietary modifications and exercise can improve all of these conditions, but pharmacologic treatment is often necessary.

Statins can improve cholesterol levels and improve the ratio of low-density to high-density lipoproteins, and they have been demonstrated to reduce rates of myocardial infarction and death. Angiotensin-converting inhibitors have been shown to reduce mortality and myocardial infarction in patients with coronary artery disease coupled with hypertension, diabetes, or left ventricular dysfunction. Aspirin, by inhibiting platelet activity, reduces death and myocardial

▲ **Figure 20–2. A:** Left anterior oblique (LAO) view of the left coronary artery. **B:** Right anterior oblique (RAO) view of the left coronary artery. **C:** LAO view of the right coronary artery. Cx, circumflex; LAD, left anterior descending; LM, left main; OM, obtuse marginal; RCA, right coronary artery.

infarctions in patients with coronary artery disease and should be prescribed to all patients unless significant contraindications exist. Beta-blocking agents reduce myocardial oxygen consumption by reducing heart rate and wall tension, and they increase oxygen delivery by increasing the diastolic phase and thus subendocardial perfusion. Despite these perceived benefits, beta-blockers have not been shown to reduce cardiovascular mortality or morbidity in patients without left ventricular dysfunction or hypertension. Nitrates also decrease myocardial oxygen consumption via venodilation, reducing cardiac preload and wall tension, and vasodilation, reducing afterload. Some epicardial vasodilation will occur, improving coronary blood flow. Nitrates can control symptoms, either immediately when given sublingually or prophylactically when used as an oral long-acting agent. Headaches are notable side effects, and the vasodilatory properties of nitrates can be exaggerated by phosphodiesterase inhibitors frequently used for the treatment of erectile dysfunction. Medical treatment alone is appropriate for patients with coronary artery disease affecting one or two epicardial vessel territories and satisfactory symptom control.

▶ Percutaneous Intervention

In 1977, Dr. Andreas Gruentzig performed the first percutaneous intervention with balloon angioplasty on a stenotic lesion in the LAD. This pioneer laid the foundation for a revolution in the treatment of coronary artery disease worldwide. Percutaneous coronary intervention is one of the most frequently performed medical procedures in the world, and its use continues to expand. These interventions include balloon angioplasty, intracoronary stent implantation, and rotational and laser atherectomies. Using the same techniques described for cardiac catheterization, small, highly flexible, and steerable guidewires can be advanced percutaneously down the lumen of stenotic epicardial coronary arteries. Over this guidewire, balloon-tipped catheters can be advanced across the stenosis and inflated to supraatmospheric pressures. This stretches and dilates the affected vessel, restoring the lumen to its predisease dimensions. Restenosis with balloon angioplasty was common, occurring in nearly 40% of patients. The use of nitinol scaffolding stents has greatly reduced restenosis rates to nearly 15%, and they are now used in nearly 90% of percutaneous procedures in the United States. The latest addition in the armamentarium of percutaneous coronary interventions is the drug-eluting stent. The drugs impregnated into the walls of the stent are antiproliferative, similar to agents used to prevent replication of immune cells in transplant recipients. The sirolimus-eluting and paclitaxel-eluting stents have further reduced the rate of target vessel restenosis and the need for repeat interventions. However, reports of late stent thrombosis have raised concerns, and indefinite use of antiplatelet regimens has been recommended.

▶ Surgical Treatment

Although alternative surgical approaches to myocardial ischemia had been attempted previously, René Favaloro is credited with creation of the coronary bypass procedure from his work at the Cleveland Clinic. Since its inception in 1967, coronary artery bypass grafting (CABG) has been among the most frequent, successful, and well-studied procedures performed in medicine.

A. Indications

Three large, prospective, multicenter, randomized clinical trials evaluating CABG versus medical therapy are widely quoted and should be understood when considering the indications for coronary bypass grafting. Despite the historical nature of these studies and the evolution in both surgical technique and medical treatment, these trials continue to provide important information about the benefits of surgical revascularization in patients with advanced coronary atherosclerosis.

The Veterans Administration Cooperative Study enrolled 1000 patients between 1970 and 1974. Patients had chronic anginal complaints and were free of myocardial infarction within 6 months. Medical treatment consisted largely of nitrates and aspirin, and surgical mortality was extremely high when compared to contemporary results. A statistically significant survival advantage was seen in the surgical group versus the medical group at 7 years (77% vs 72%), despite 38% of medical patients crossing over to surgical treatment. Subgroup analysis demonstrated more pronounced survival advantages for patients with three-vessel disease, patients with left ventricular dysfunction, and patients with significant stenosis of the left main coronary artery.

The European Coronary Surgery Study recruited 767 men with chronic angina from 1973 to 1976. Only patients with preserved left ventricular function were included. A survival advantage for the surgical group was seen in the overall cohort, but particularly in patients with three-vessel disease and those with proximal LAD stenosis. There were also advantages demonstrated in reduction of angina and exercise capacity.

The Coronary Artery Surgery Study enrolled patients from a nonrandomized registry of patients who underwent coronary angiography from 1974 to 1979 at 15 centers. Patients with mild angina were randomized to medical treatment and CABG. There was no survival advantage in the 790 randomized patients; however, the cohort with left ventricular dysfunction had better survival with surgery, particularly those with left ventricular dysfunction and three-vessel disease. Evaluation of the nonrandomized patients in the registry also found survival advantages for surgically treated patients with left main stenosis or left main equivalent stenosis.

Although these three landmark studies are over 40 years old, some important principles continue to apply: patients with more advanced coronary atherosclerosis, particularly those with left ventricular dysfunction, stand to achieve the most benefit from surgical revascularization. Numerous clinical trials have more recently compared CABG with percutaneous interventions. The Randomized Intervention Treatment of Angina (RITA) trial compared balloon angioplasty with CABG for patients with single-vessel and multivessel disease. There was no difference in survival, but repeat intervention was required five times more frequently in the angioplasty group. The Bypass Angioplasty Revascularization Investigation (BARI) enrolled 1829 patients with chronic or unstable angina from 1988 to 1991. There was no survival advantage at 5 years; however, 31% of the patients in the percutaneous group crossed over for CABG. The need for repeat revascularization was again five times higher in the percutaneous group, and the subgroup of patients with diabetes had improved survival at 5 years (81% vs 66%).

A comparison between patients with multivessel coronary disease treated with PCI versus CABG was performed using Medicare claims data as well as the Society of Thoracic Surgeons Database and the American College of Cardiology Foundation PCI Data Registry. Adjusted and unadjusted survival rates were superior for those undergoing CABG at 4 years. As technology and pharmacology continue to evolve, additional studies will be required. However, CABG offers survival and quality-of-life advantages in selected patients with coronary artery disease.

B. Techniques

The principles of coronary bypass surgery are to restore normal myocardial perfusion by creating alternative routes for blood to reach the jeopardized territories. This strategy has several advantages, including the large-caliber conduits, their extramyocardial location in avoiding the compressive forces during systole, and their attachment at strategic locations to maximize return of normal blood flow. The most important aspect of the procedure is construction of a technically sound and strategically well-created bypass graft.

A variety of conduits may be chosen; the most traditional and still most frequently utilized is the saphenous vein. The vessel is easily harvested with minimal morbidity, and it is technically easy to create the precise anastomosis. Minimally invasive approaches using endoscopic techniques now reduce the impact on the patient. Limitations of the saphenous vein are primarily based on its tendency to develop accelerated atherosclerotic lesions. The vein graft plaque is more frequently circumferential and diffuse, with a weaker fibrous cap and a higher predilection for distal embolization. Patency of saphenous vein grafts is approximately 50% at 10 years. In addition, suitable vein conduit may not be available, either harvested for previous coronary or peripheral bypass procedures or unusable from varicosities or sclerosis.

The left internal mammary artery can be mobilized from its pedicle on the left subclavian artery and anastomosed to the anterior or lateral epicardial vessels of the heart, most frequently to the LAD. This strategy has several well-described advantages owing to the improved patency rate of the internal mammary graft when compared to saphenous vein grafts. The right internal mammary artery can also serve as a bypass conduit; however, harvesting of both internal mammary vessels increases the risk of sternal ischemia and surgical wound-healing complications. Because of the improved patency of arterial grafts as compared to saphenous vein grafts, the radial and gastroepiploic arteries have been explored as alternatives to vein grafts. However, improved long-term patency has not been reliably established, and morbidity from harvesting has slowed widespread adoption of this approach.

The standard approach for coronary bypass grafting is via the median sternotomy, where the sternum is divided longitudinally, exposing the heart and great vessels. The left thoracotomy could be alternatively used, particularly after previous heart surgery where sternal reentry could hazard injury to adhesed cardiac structures or patent grafts. Preparation is then made to institute cardiopulmonary bypass (CPB). Anticoagulation with 300 IU of heparin per kilogram is infused to achieve an activated clotting time of greater than 400 seconds. Typically, the ascending aorta is used for arterial inflow, and venous return is accomplished via a cannula in the right atrial appendage (Figure 20–3). CPB is commenced, evacuating venous blood into the cardiotomy reservoir. Mechanical ventilation can be discontinued. Using a heat exchanger, the blood is actively cooled to 28-32°C to reduce tissue oxygen requirements and organ injury. Shed mediastinal blood can be scavenged and returned to the CPB system, reducing blood loss during the anticoagulation period. Cardioplegic arrest is then initiated by cross-clamping the ascending aorta and infusing cold blood cardioplegia solution into the aortic root. The makeup of cardioplegia solutions differs among centers and even among surgeons; however, most centers combine autologous blood obtained from the CPB system with crystalloid solution cooled to 12°C containing citrate to bind ionic calcium, dextrose, pH buffers, and potassium (approximately 30 mM/L) to arrest all cardiac activity. Cardioplegia is administered intermittently to maintain myocardial temperature and diastolic arrest during the cross-clamp period.

With the arrested heart, a dry and motionless surgical field is created, allowing creation of precise surgical anastomoses on even the smallest of epicardial coronary arteries. The targets are identified on the epicardial surface, and the sites for anastomotic reconstruction are determined on the basis of information from the preoperative cardiac catheterization and suitability of the native vessel. An arteriotomy is created on the exposed vessel, and it is extended for approximately 5 mm. The conduit is fashioned with an appropriately sized bevel or spatulation, and the anastomosis is created, typically in running fashion with fine polypropylene suture. The conduits are tested for patency and hemostasis, and they are cut to the appropriate size, avoiding tension or kinking. Saphenous vein or free arterial conduits are typically connected to the ascending aorta. A 4- to 5-mm punch device

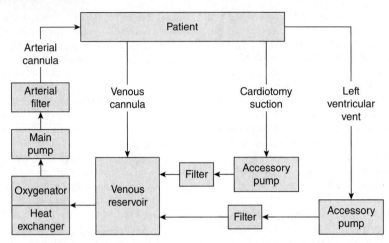

▲ **Figure 20–3.** Schematic of cardiopulmonary bypass (CPB). (Reproduced with permission from Morgan GE, Mikhail MS, Murray MJ. *Clinical Anesthesiology*, 4th ed. New York, NY: McGraw-Hill Education; 2006.)

is used to create a circular aortotomy. The anastomoses are constructed in running fashion with polypropylene suture. If conduit length is limited, the proximal anastomoses can be created as Y grafts off of other vein grafts or off of the pedicled internal mammary artery graft.

After completion of all anastomoses, weaning from CPB is prepared. The patient is warmed to normothermia. As the heart begins to warm, ventricular fibrillation often occurs, requiring electrical defibrillation. Temporary conduction abnormalities may require epicardial pacing, but it is often transient. Mechanical ventilation is resumed, and the patient is gradually weaned from CPB. Pharmacologic inotropic support may be required but is often unnecessary if ventricular function was preserved preoperatively. An appropriate dose of protamine is infused to reverse the effects of heparin, and cannulae for bypass are removed. Once hemostasis is adequate, chest closure is performed with stainless steel wires. The pericardium is typically left open to avoid constriction of the atria or kinking of the bypass grafts. The pedicled left internal mammary artery graft is positioned posterior to the anterior surface of the left lung to protect it from injury should sternal reentry be required in the future.

Recently, attempts to reduce the invasive nature of CABG and the potential complications of CPB have been introduced. Techniques to perform bypass grafting without CPB have improved and are promoted by its advocates. Off-pump coronary bypass grafting (OPCAB) has potential advantages in reducing neurologic complications associated with air and atheroemboli, as well as reducing blood transfusion requirements and cost. The procedure involves manipulation and stabilization of the beating heart to expose the epicardial targets. Particularly for vessels on the posterior and posterolateral surfaces, hemodynamic instability can result while the heart is elevated and rotated for optimal exposure.

The anesthesiologist must be capable of responding to these rapid changes, and the surgeon must have the judgment and ability to immediately abandon off-pump attempts and institute CPB before significant organ injury occurs. The anastomoses are more challenging, with blood in the moving operative field. Although several single-center reports have demonstrated satisfactory short-term results and mid-term graft patency rates, multicenter randomized and observation studies have suggested that OPCAB techniques may offer some benefits but at the expense of reduced graft patency rates and increased incomplete revascularization. As a result, OPCAB penetrance has not markedly increased over the past several years.

C. Results

Since the creation of the Society of Thoracic Surgeons voluntary reporting database in 1989, short-term outcomes of coronary bypass grafting are widely available to the public, providing information for patients, referring physicians, and practicing surgeons to compare their results to national averages. The Society of Thoracic Surgeons also provides a validated risk assessment scoring system, creating mortality estimates based on an individual patient's clinical data. Overall, risk of perioperative death is 1%-3%. Multivariate predictors of death include advanced age, recent myocardial infarction, decreased ventricular function, renal insufficiency, and female gender. Conduit patency is determined from clinical trials that included angiographic assessments at varying time intervals in the absence of symptoms. Data are largely historical and are subject to biases of patient selection but are largely considered to be reliable. Saphenous vein grafts occlude 20%-30% by 1 year. Early graft loss is felt to be attributable to anastomotic imperfections or graft kinking, endothelial injury during harvest, limited native coronary runoff, or progression of native occlusive disease. Late failures appear to occur at a rate of 5% per year, with 10-year patency rates of approximately 40%-50%. Late failures are primarily attributed to accelerated atherosclerosis of the vein conduit. The pedicled internal mammary artery has far superior patency, particularly when anastomosed to the LAD. With adequate target vessel runoff, 10-year patency rates of 90%-95% have been reported in multiple independent studies. Radial arteries and free mammary artery conduits appear to have patency rates intermediate to saphenous vein and pedicled mammary arteries and are more frequently utilized in younger patients.

Afilalo J, et al: Off-pump vs. on-pump coronary artery bypass surgery: an updated meta-analysis and meta-regression of randomized trials. *Eur Heart J.* 2012;33:1257.

Kelbaek H, et al: Drug-eluting versus bare metal stents in patients with st-segment-elevation myocardial infarction: eight-month follow-up in the Drug Elution and Distal Protection in Acute Myocardial Infarction (DEDICATION) trial. DEDICATION Investigators. *Circulation.* 2008;118:1155.

Lamy A, et al: Off-pump or on-pump coronary-artery bypass grafting at 30 days. *N Engl J Med.* 2012;366:1489.

Stone GW, et al, for the EXCEL Trial Investigators: Everolimus-eluting stents or bypass surgery for left main coronary artery disease. *N Engl J Med.* 2016;375(23):2223-2235.

Taggart DP, et al, for the Arterial Revascularization Trial Investigators: Bilateral versus single internal-thoracic-artery grafts at 10 years. *N Engl J Med.* 2019;380(5):437-446.

Weintraub WS, et al: Comparative effectiveness of revascularization strategies. *N Engl J Med.* 2012;366:1467.

▼ VALVULAR HEART DISEASE

MITRAL REGURGITATION

▶ Pathophysiology

A. Anatomy

The mitral valve separates the left atrium from the left ventricle. It should be considered as the sum of its three components: the leaflets, the annulus to which the leaflets attach, and the subvalvar apparatus, consisting of the cords and papillary muscles. The mitral valve has two leaflets, anterior and posterior (Figure 20–4). The anterior leaflet is larger in surface area, but its attachment to the annulus represents only one-third of the circumference. The anterior portion of the mitral valve annulus is in direct continuity with the annulus of the left and noncoronary cusps of the aortic valve, also known as the aortomitral continuity. The posterior leaflet is shorter, but its annular attachments cover two-thirds of the circumference. The posterior leaflet often can be separated into three distinct scallops, although the prominence of these separations varies among individuals.

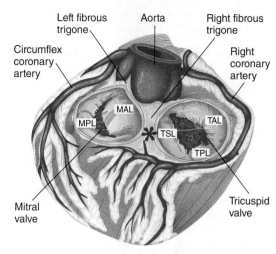

▲ **Figure 20–4.** Anatomy of the mitral and tricuspid valves. MAL, mitral anterior leaflet; MPL, mitral posterior leaflet; TAL, tricuspid anterior leaflet; TPL, tricuspid posterior leaflet; TSL, tricuspid septal leaflet.

The anterior and posterior leaflets are separated from each other by the anterolateral and posteromedial commissures, which mark the location of the right and left fibrous trigones respectively. The trigones are dense collagenous structures within the annulus representing a portion of the fibrous skeleton of the heart. The mitral annulus is elliptical in shape, and its dimensions change dynamically during cardiac contraction, reducing its cross-sectional area by as much as 40%. The anterolateral and posteromedial papillary muscles are vertically oriented bundles of cardiac myocytes. Chordae tendineae originate from the heads of the papillary muscles and span the distance to both the anterior and posterior mitral valve leaflets. Chords are designated as primary if they attach to the leading edge of the leaflet, secondary if they attach to the ventricular surface of the leaflets, or tertiary if they attach to the ventricular surface of the mitral annulus. The chords play an important role in preventing leaflet prolapse. The posteromedial papillary muscle is prone to ischemic injury, since it relies on a single right coronary artery for circulation. In contrast, the anterolateral papillary muscle gains its blood supply from the LAD and circumflex branches and tends to be more resistant to ischemic injury.

B. Classification of Mitral Regurgitation

Regurgitation through the mitral valve can result from a variety of pathologic conditions. Alain Carpentier developed a simplified classification scheme based on leaflet motion (Table 20–1) to organize the different disease processes that can cause mitral regurgitation. In Carpentier type I mitral regurgitation, the leaflet motion is normal. The regurgitation

Table 20–1. Carpentier classification of mitral regurgitation.

I	Normal leaflet motion *Annular dilation, leaflet perforation*
II	Excessive leaflet motion *Prolapsed or myxomatous leaflet, ruptured chord*
III	Restricted leaflet motion *Rheumatic disease, ischemic mitral regurgitation*

is a result of either dilation of the annulus, as can be seen in cardiomyopathy with progressive ventricular enlargement, or of leaflet perforation, as can be seen with destructive endocarditis. Type II is associated with excessive leaflet motion. Patients with type II mitral regurgitation have ruptured chordae or papillary muscles from ischemia or endocarditis, or they have with pathologically redundant mitral leaflet tissue. Redundant, prolapsing, or myxomatous mitral leaflets can be either acquired from fibroelastic deficiency or hereditary from weak connective tissue. In either case, the excessive leaflet motion prevents proper coaptation of the anterior and posterior leaflets. Patients with type III have restricted leaflet motion. Type III is often associated with rheumatic heart disease, where leaflets can become calcified, and the chords are thickened and foreshortened. The leaflets do not adequately rise in systole, and coaptation is impaired. Alternatively, some patients develop severe mitral regurgitation owing to ischemic injury. Typically, a previous myocardial infarction has resulted in ventricular remodeling, resulting in dilation and retraction of the papillary muscles. As a result, the leaflets are tethered into the ventricle, limiting mobility and preventing proper coaptation.

Mitral regurgitation is always pathologic but can be tolerated surprisingly well when the onset is gradual, allowing for a series of physiologic adaptations. On the other hand, acute mitral regurgitation, as can be associated with infective endocarditis or ischemic papillary muscle rupture, results in immediate pulmonary congestion because the unprepared left atrium is incapable of handling the additional volume load. Several compensatory mechanisms occur as mitral regurgitation develops and progressively worsens. The left atrium and pulmonary venous system gradually dilates, thus increasing compliance to better accommodate the excess volume. The backward flow of mitral regurgitation reduces ventricular afterload, reducing myocardial wall tension. The reduction in forward flow is accounted for by increased diastolic filling, increasing preload. This maintains cardiac output and can delay onset of symptoms for significant time. Gradually, left ventricular end diastolic volume continues to rise, resulting in pathologic remodeling, creating a dilated and more spherical ventricular

cavity. Systolic function is progressively and inexorably impaired as a result of both mechanical considerations owing to the altered shape and molecular mechanisms, both intracellular and extracellular. A vicious cycle ensues, with deteriorating systolic function and rising end-diastolic volume promoting further ventricular remodeling and dilation and worsening mitral regurgitation. Longstanding mitral regurgitation will result in sustained elevation in left atrial pressure and volume, resulting in pulmonary vascular changes, pulmonary hypertension, and eventually, right ventricular dysfunction.

C. Symptoms

Acute mitral regurgitation is poorly tolerated and is typically associated with pulmonary congestion and low cardiac output. Patients describe dyspnea, poor exercise tolerance, and fatigue. Often, the etiology of the mitral regurgitation is more dominant in the clinical presentation. Patients with acute endocarditis may have fever, shaking chills, and manifestations of septic embolization such as stroke and intestinal or extremity ischemia. Patients suffering from acute myocardial infarction with a ruptured papillary muscle complain of chest pain and diaphoresis.

Chronic mitral regurgitation can be asymptomatic for many years as a result of progressive atrial and ventricular adaptation. Eventually, patients develop symptoms of heart failure, including dyspnea, fatigue, and lower extremity edema. When left atrial dilation results in atrial fibrillation, patients may describe heart palpitations. Often, the onset of atrial fibrillation is the initial presentation of symptoms, as rapid ventricular response decreases diastolic filling time and creates a sudden reduction in cardiac output. As ventricular function deteriorates and pulmonary vascular changes occur, signs of right-sided heart failure develop, such as lower extremity edema and ascites.

▶ Diagnostic Testing

The physical findings of mitral regurgitation vary depending on the duration and the degree of compensation. For patients with longstanding mitral regurgitation, ventricular dilation displaces the point of maximal impulse laterally. On auscultation, an S_3 gallop is often heard, resulting from increased diastolic flow. The systolic murmur is characteristically described as blowing, best heard over the cardiac apex and radiating to the axilla. In acute mitral regurgitation, the murmur tends to be limited to early in systole. With more chronicity, the murmur is progressively holosystolic.

The chest radiograph often demonstrates cardiomegaly from ventricular dilation. With severe uncompensated heart failure, pulmonary edema may be evident; however, this is more commonly seen with acute mitral regurgitation. The electrocardiogram is often nonspecific but may demonstrate evidence of previous myocardial infarction and will confirm the presence of atrial fibrillation.

Echocardiography is the mainstay in the diagnosis of mitral regurgitation; it provides information about the mechanism of the disease, which is essential in planning surgical intervention. Images of the leaflets can determine if the leaflet motion is normal, restricted, or excessive. Information about annular size and mobility can be obtained. Using color Doppler, the size and direction of the regurgitant jet can quantify the severity and give clues as to the mechanism (Figure 20–5). The severity of the regurgitation is determined by the width and length of the regurgitant jet or the presence of reversed flow within the pulmonary veins. Echocardiography also provides information about the chronicity of the disease and can document progressive adaptation such as left atrial and ventricular dilation. This information is often used in determining timing of surgical intervention, particularly in asymptomatic patients. Echocardiography is usually performed transthoracic. However, in some patients, the views are obscured by body habitus or emphysema, limiting the image quality. Transesophageal echocardiography (TEE) can improve the resolution of images and better clarify the severity and mechanism of the mitral valve pathology.

Cardiac catheterization is an important adjunctive tool, helping to identify additional cardiac pathology, and can determine the adequacy of preoperative medical optimization. Coronary angiography is performed to identify coronary arterial occlusive lesions that may require bypass grafting at the time of mitral valve repair or replacement.

Although contrast ventriculography can demonstrate the regurgitant jet, it is no longer necessarily used to quantify the regurgitant volume, since echocardiography has become the standard technique. Right heart catheterization will demonstrate intravascular volume overload and low cardiac output. It may also be helpful in diagnosing pulmonary vascular changes in patients who deny symptoms.

▶ Surgical Treatment

A. Indications

The indications for operation on the mitral valve depend on the specific pathology as well as clinical symptoms. In addition, the indications have evolved in recent years owing to improved outcomes related to better surgical techniques, anesthetic considerations, myocardial protection, and postoperative care. Furthermore, intervention on the mitral valve may be performed for less severe disease if operation is indicated for coronary artery disease or aortic valve pathology.

Certainly, among patients who represent reasonable operative risks, those with severe mitral regurgitation and heart failure symptoms should be offered an operation. In addition, those with severe mitral regurgitation and signs of left ventricular dysfunction should undergo operation because myocardial decompensation can progress rapidly without corrective action. There is insufficient evidence that operative intervention for asymptomatic severe mitral regurgitation and normal ventricular function improves

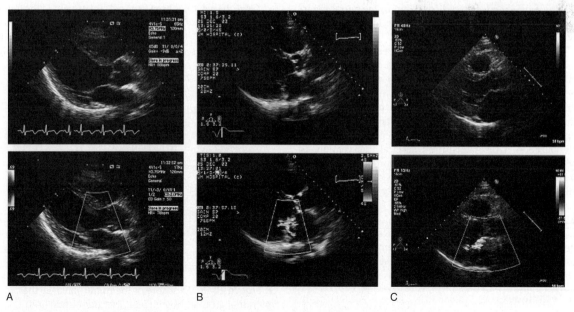

▲ **Figure 20–5.** Echocardiographic view of the mitral valve. **A:** Normal valve. **B:** Dilated annulus with central regurgitation. **C:** Prolapsing posterior leaflet with eccentric regurgitation.

survival. Historically, these patients were observed with close clinical follow-up and serial echocardiography. Signs of left ventricular dilation, dysfunction, or new-onset symptoms prompted surgical referral. Some have argued that the presence of pulmonary hypertension or atrial fibrillation represents maladaptive changes and suggests surgical correction.

Surgical techniques of addressing the mitral valve have changed dramatically in recent years. Increasingly, operations have focused on repair rather than prosthetic replacement of the mitral valve. Valve preservation has several advantages. The interaction of the mitral valve and the left ventricle goes beyond just competence and the handling of blood volume. A complex interdependence exists between ventricle and valve, and long-term ventricular function depends on its relationship with the mitral annulus, papillary muscles, and chordae tendineae. Surgical techniques to correct mitral regurgitation that preserve these relationships are more likely to maintain normal ventricular function. In addition to the effects on ventricular function, prosthetic mitral valves carry limitations. Bioprosthetic devices (porcine or bovine) have limited durability because of structural valvular degeneration. The rate of bioprosthetic valve failure is proportional to age, with faster deterioration in younger patients. Mechanical valves are more durable but require lifelong systemic anticoagulation with warfarin. Because of the limitations imposed by prosthetic valves (durability and anticoagulation), surgical referral for mitral regurgitation is often delayed if there is a high likelihood of valve replacement. If valve repair is expected because of mitral pathology and surgeon experience, earlier operation for mitral regurgitation is often considered, particularly in the absence of symptoms or ventricular dilation.

Surgical indications for operation in endocarditis of the mitral valve are different than for other pathologies. Certainly, valvular destruction with severe mitral regurgitation, heart failure, and ventricular dilation requires operative intervention. However, there are other specific indications for valve replacement. A history of systemic embolization or the presence of large, highly mobile vegetations at risk of embolization necessitates urgent surgical intervention. In addition, ongoing bacteremia despite appropriate antibiotic treatment coverage mandates early operation. The presence of certain organisms, such as highly resistant bacteria or fungal endocarditis, warrants surgical treatment. Surgery is required for the presence of mitral annular abscess with incipient cardiac conduction abnormalities or creation of an intracardiac fistula. Prior to surgery, attempts at controlling the original source of infection should be made, including dental extractions and drainage of abscesses.

B. Techniques

Approach to the mitral valve is best accomplished via a median sternotomy. Although the mitral valve can be exposed via a right or left thoracotomy, the median sternotomy offers the best access for initiation of CPB as well as the ability to perform other cardiac procedures if necessary, such as coronary bypass grafting or aortic valve replacement. CPB is initiated, typically draining the superior and inferior vena cavae separately and infusing into the ascending aorta. The heart is arrested using cold cardioplegia delivered into the aortic root. The left ventricle is vented, typically using the right superior pulmonary vein.

A variety of incisions can be used to expose the mitral valve, and the quality of exposure is essential in obtaining a good surgical result. The most frequent approach is by an incision directly into the left atrium. The interatrial groove of Sondergaard can be developed using sharp technique, lifting the right atrium anteriorly off of the left atrium (Figure 20–6). A vertical incision is made in the left atrium, just medial to the confluence of the right-sided pulmonary veins. Self-retaining retractors are available to elevate the atriotomy and provide visualization. Often, rotation of the table to the left away from the surgeon improves the exposure. Alternatively, an approach across the interatrial septum can be chosen. The superior and inferior vena cavae are controlled with snares, and the right atrium is opened. The fossa ovalis is identified and incised vertically. This incision is extended superiorly toward the superior vena cava through the muscular portion of the interatrial septum. The septal incision can also be extended medially along the dome of the left atrium, the so-called superior septal approach. While exposure of the mitral valve is excellent, there is a risk of injury to the sinus node, requiring implantation of a permanent pacemaker.

Once the valve has been exposed, assessment of the mitral valve is performed to determine the mechanism of mitral regurgitation and the technique for repair or replacement. Injection of cold saline into the left ventricle will identify the

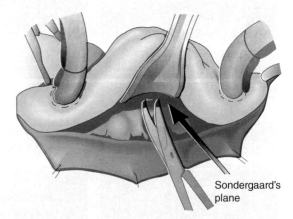

Sondergaard's plane

▲ **Figure 20–6.** Exposure of the mitral valve via the interatrial groove. (Reproduced with permission from Cohn LH. *Cardiac Surgery in the Adult*, 3rd ed. New York, NY: McGraw-Hill Education; 2007.)

▲ **Figure 20–7.** Panels **A–E** represent atrial views of posterior leaflet reconstruction for isolated posterior leaflet prolapse and insertion of an annuloplasty ring.

location of regurgitation and the presence of flail or significantly prolapsed leaflets. The leaflets are inspected for their mobility and the presence of calcifications or perforations. The annulus is inspected for dilation and calcium. Once the mechanism of regurgitation is clear, a plan is made for repair or replacement. The strategy used depends on the pathologic mechanism (Figure 20–7).

When the mitral regurgitation is purely a result of annular dilation or posterior leaflet restriction from a previous myocardial infarction, mitral annuloplasty alone often adequately alleviates the leak. Horizontal sutures are placed along the mitral annulus, including the fibrous trigones. Care must be taken to avoid injury to underlying structures, such as the circumflex coronary artery, the coronary sinus, and the atrioventricular node. Annuloplasty is typically performed with the assistance of prosthetic rings or bands of varying degrees of rigidity. Some of the rings completely encircle the entire annulus, and some are incomplete, designed to extend posteriorly from trigone to trigone (Figure 20–8). The annular mattress sutures are brought up through the sewing cuff of the ring and tied down. The size of the ring is selected to match the area of the anterior leaflet and the distance between the trigones. Competence is tested with saline injection, and the cardiac chambers are closed.

After weaning from CPB, the valve is inspected using TEE. An adequate repair must demonstrate both competence and low resistance, as evidenced by low pressure gradients across the valve.

▲ **Figure 20–8.** Operative photograph of a mitral ring annuloplasty for ischemic mitral regurgitation. The ring plicates the posterior annulus to restore leaflet coaptation.

Myxomatous degeneration of the mitral valve typically involves the posterior leaflet, particularly the P2 scallop. This lesion can be reproducibly repaired using techniques with the potential for indefinite durability. After exposure of the mitral valve, the point of prolapse is identified.

A quadrangular portion of the prolapsing section is excised to the annulus. The gap is bridged by undercutting the annular attachments of the adjacent portion of the posterior leaflet. The mobilized edge of the posterior leaflet is sewn back to the annulus with running suture (Figure 20–9), reducing

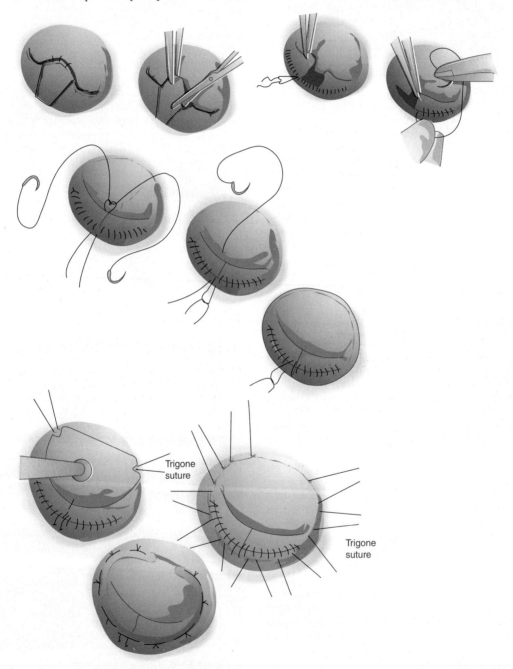

▲ **Figure 20–9.** Quadrangular resection and sliding annuloplasty for prolapse of the posterior mitral valve leaflet.
(Reproduced with permission from Cohn LH. *Cardiac Surgery in the Adult*, 3rd ed. New York, NY: McGraw-Hill Education; 2007.)

its effective height. An annuloplasty can be performed to address any annular dilation as well as to provide reinforcement to the posterior annular reconstruction.

When prolapse or chordal rupture involves the anterior leaflet, repair is more difficult. A variety of approaches have been described, but the likelihood of durable repair is far less when compared to the more common posterior leaflet prolapse. One approach involves the creation of artificial cords. Typically, polytetrafluoroethylene is used to create neochords from the papillary muscle to the edge of the leaflet. The challenge is to create the precise length to allow coaptation without prolapse. Alternatively, the flail anterior segment can be removed and is replaced with a resected portion of the posterior leaflet, including its attached chords. A simpler approach is the edge-to-edge technique, in which the opposing edges of the anterior and posterior leaflets are sewn together with a single suture, creating a double-orifice mitral valve. Popularized by Alfieri and colleagues, this approach has been applied using catheter-based techniques, obviating the need for open surgery (Figure 20–10).

Often, the regurgitant mitral valve cannot be repaired, such as when there is severe valvular destruction from infective endocarditis or extensive calcifications, as can be seen with rheumatic mitral valve disease. The mitral valve is exposed, and the leaflets are excised. Attempts are made to preserve chordal attachments to the annulus, and portions of the posterior leaflet can be plicated to the annulus to preserve secondary chords. This is typically not possible with rheumatic disease because the calcified annulus will require extensive debridement. Annular mattress sutures with felt or Teflon pledgets are placed circumferentially. For mechanical prostheses, the pledgets are oriented on the atrial side to avoid interference with the actuation of the disk. For bioprosthetic implants, the pledgets can be placed on the ventricular side, which allows for a slightly larger prosthetic (Figure 20–11). After sutures are placed, the annulus is sized and an appropriate prosthetic is chosen. The sutures are driven through the sewing ring of the valve and tied down. After weaning from CPB, the valve is carefully inspected using TEE for signs of paravalvular leak, normal motion of the leaflets or disks, and a low pressure gradient across the valve.

A

B

▲ **Figure 20–11. A:** Edwards mitral bovine pericardial bioprosthetic. (Reproduced with permission from Edwards Lifesciences, Irvine, California.) **B:** St. Jude Medical bileaflet mechanical valve. (Reproduced with permission from St. Jude Medical, St. Paul, Minnesota.)

▲ **Figure 20–10.** Percutaneous clip device for mitral valve repair. (Reproduced with permission from Abbott Laboratories, Abbott Park, Illinois.)

C. Results

Repair or replacement of the mitral valve for regurgitation preserves ventricular function and allows some remodeling by eliminating the volume overload and its associated incipient changes. However, loss of myocardial contractility, as a result of longstanding mitral regurgitation or otherwise, typically does not recover. Only its progressive decline can be halted. This reinforces the need to intervene before severe ventricular dilation has occurred, even in asymptomatic patients.

Mitral regurgitation associated with prolapsing myxomatous leaflets carries low perioperative mortality, and the freedom from degeneration of a repaired valve is greater than 90% at 10 years. Some of the low periprocedural mortality is related to the young age and low incidence of comorbidities in this patient population. Mitral valve repair associated with coronary bypass grafting carries a perioperative mortality of approximately 5%, with ejection fraction, renal function, and age being independent predictors of death. Although mortality after coronary bypass grafting is associated with the severity of preoperative mitral regurgitation, there is no evidence that mitral repair reduces this mortality. Repairing the mitral valve, however, is associated with improved long-term survival, as compared to replacing the valve.

MITRAL VALVE STENOSIS

▶ Pathophysiology

Rheumatic heart disease is the most common cause of mitral valve stenosis. Although nearly 20 million people are affected with rheumatic fever in underdeveloped countries, the incidence in the United States and Western Europe has declined markedly, largely a result of advanced medical care and use of antibiotics to treat infections caused by group A streptococci. Untreated infection results in an immunologic response to bacterial antigens that resemble cardiac tissue. The degree of the immunologic response and the severity of ongoing valvular destruction appear to be related to genetic factors. Although the damage can affect the entire endocardium and even the pericardium, the mitral valve is the most commonly involved, with 40% of patients having only mitral valve disease. Mitral and aortic valve disease is also frequently seen, and rarely patients will have isolated aortic valve involvement. It remains unclear why right-sided valves are rarely affected.

The characteristic features of rheumatic mitral valve disease include leaflet and chordal thickening and retraction. Commissural fusion is also apparent, and a late feature is dense calcification of the annulus and leaflets. Turbulence created by impaired leaflet mobility exacerbates the valve destruction, accelerating further fibrosis and calcification.

Mitral valve stenosis can also be caused by mitral annular calcification, which can become quite bulky, protruding into the valve orifice. The posterior leaflet can become contracted and fixed, while the anterior leaflet thickens and becomes less mobile. Structural valvular degeneration of bioprosthetic mitral valves can cause mitral valve stenosis as well as thrombosis or pannus formation in mechanical prostheses. Advanced endocarditis can result in effective mitral valve stenosis, as bulky vegetations obstruct the inflow path. Congenital abnormalities, such as the parachute mitral valve with a single papillary muscle, can become stenotic, requiring intervention.

The stenotic mitral valve results in a pressure gradient between the left atrium and ventricle. This fixed resistance increases the left atrial pressure even further during exercise, as cardiac output increases, but resistance across the valve is unchanged. Severe mitral valve stenosis is associated with a mean transvalvular gradient of 10-15 mm Hg at rest. Cardiac output is dependent on ventricular filling, and left ventricular end-diastolic pressure and volume are typically low. Exercise-induced tachycardia decreases diastolic filling time, producing a paradoxical reduction in cardiac output. Left ventricular function is typically normal or hyperdynamic, but some patients have combined mitral valve stenosis and mitral regurgitation, as well as significant aortic valve insufficiency, and will develop chronic left ventricular volume overload and dysfunction. Thus, the hemodynamic consequences of mitral valve stenosis depend to a certain degree on the presence of mitral regurgitation and other associated valvular pathology.

As the mitral transvalvular gradient worsens, the left atrial wall hypertrophies. The a-wave on the atrial pressure tracing is accentuated during atrial contraction. Progressively, the left atrium dilates, creating disorganized electrical conduction pathways. Reentry pathways lead to frequent premature atrial contractions and eventually to atrial fibrillation. The onset of atrial fibrillation often is the inciting clinical event, with the reduced diastolic filling time from rapid ventricular response and the loss of atrial contraction both resulting in reduced left ventricular filling and a drop in cardiac output. The sustained elevation in left atrial pressure results in pulmonary vascular changes producing pulmonary hypertension. These changes can lead to right ventricular pressure overload with tricuspid valve insufficiency and to right ventricular volume overload.

Symptoms of mitral valve stenosis often do not develop until the disease is advanced, owing to ventricular and atrial adaptive responses. Patients describe dyspnea from pulmonary congestion or reduced cardiac output, initially limited to exertion. Onset of atrial fibrillation often prompts urgent evaluation, as the loss of atrial contraction and tachycardia cause a precipitous drop in cardiac output and pulmonary congestion. Late findings include signs of right-sided heart failure such as ascites and lower extremity edema. Cerebrovascular events or other thromboembolic complications from an intracardiac thrombus are not uncommon with longstanding mitral valve stenosis, as the dilated left atrium and left atrial appendage have regions of stagnation and thrombus formation, particularly in the setting of atrial fibrillation. Because two-thirds of the patients with mitral valve stenosis are women, symptoms often present during later stages of pregnancy as the increased cardiac output results in higher left atrial pressures and pulmonary congestion.

Diagnostic Evaluation

Because presentation tends to be late, many patients present with signs of longstanding heart failure, including cachexia, ascites, and lower extremity edema. On auscultation, the low diastolic rumble is best heard over the cardiac apex. An opening snap can be heard in the early stages of the disease, and the systolic murmur of tricuspid regurgitation is a late finding, as is a parasternal heave from right ventricular hypertrophy.

The electrocardiogram will diagnose atrial fibrillation, and right axis deviation may be present, suggesting advanced pulmonary hypertension. The chest radiograph is often normal but may demonstrate straightening of the left heart border caused by dilation of the pulmonary arteries. Pulmonary edema may be present on initial evaluation when atrial fibrillation is the inciting event. Cardiac catheterization is important in identifying associated coronary arterial pathology and can confirm the severity of the mitral stenosis using simultaneous left and right heart catheterization with pressure measurements. The degree of pulmonary hypertension and its reversibility with provocative agents may be assistive in determining surgical candidacy in advanced cases.

Echocardiography is the mainstay in diagnosis of mitral valve stenosis. Surface or transthoracic echocardiography is preferred because it is noninvasive and can usually provide images demonstrating the characteristic thickening and restricted mobility of the mitral leaflets. If images are obscured by patient body habitus or obstructive lung disease, a TEE can be performed. The proximity of the esophagus with the left atrium provides excellent visualization and can easily demonstrate the thickened mitral subvalvar apparatus typical of rheumatic disease. Color Doppler can be used to show turbulent flow across the valve orifice, and the pressure gradients can be estimated by measuring the peak and mean velocity of blood through the valve.

Treatment

Medical treatment is limited to control of symptoms. Complications of mitral valve stenosis should be addressed and controlled. Rapid ventricular response to atrial fibrillation can be treated with a number of pharmacologic agents, and attempts at cardioversion should be made once the presence of intracardiac thrombus has been excluded. It is often difficult to maintain sinus rhythm in the mitral valve stenosis patient with a significantly dilated left atrium in whom rate

control alone may be acceptable. Systemic anticoagulation with warfarin should be initiated if there has been a history of atrial fibrillation. Once the patient describes symptoms of heart failure, intervention on the mitral valve should be considered. For symptomatic patients who are not candidates for catheter-based or surgical intervention, diuretics and oral sodium restriction to control heart failure symptoms are all that is available.

Catheter-based balloon mitral valvotomy can reduce the obstructing pressure gradient and improve symptoms in selected patients. Patients with severe mitral valve stenosis and symptoms and asymptomatic patients with severe mitral valve stenosis and pulmonary hypertension are eligible if there is no mitral regurgitation, no left atrial thrombus, and favorable valve morphology, such as absence of extensive subvalvular fibrosis and calcification. The procedure is performed by femoral venous puncture and transseptal access to the mitral valve across the interatrial septum. A 25-mm hourglass Inoue balloon is advanced across the valve orifice and inflated. Significant improvement in hemodynamics is seen immediately, with reduction in transvalvular pressure gradients by as much as 15 mm Hg. The incidence of restenosis in selected patients is approximately 25% at 4 years.

Indications for surgical treatment are the same as for balloon valvuloplasty, including symptomatic patients with moderate or severe mitral valve stenosis and asymptomatic patients with pulmonary hypertension. Valve repair can be performed in carefully selected patients with reasonable long-term results. CPB is initiated in the same manner as for mitral repair for mitral regurgitation. After cardioplegic arrest, the mitral valve is exposed. Any thrombus within the atrium or atrial appendage is removed. The left atrial appendage can be transected and oversewn at its base to remove its future embolic potential. The areas of commissural fusion are cut, and the leaflets are decalcified. Occasionally, fused chords are divided to increase leaflet mobility. In carefully selected patients, recurrent mitral valve stenosis is less than 20% at up to 15 years.

In most cases, however, severe leaflet and subvalvular calcification has made the valve unreconstructable, requiring valve replacement. Overaggressive debridement of the posterior mitral annulus can result in perforation and atrioventricular separation and should be avoided. The selection of valve prosthetic depends on the unique clinical circumstances. Bioprosthetic valves are minimally thrombogenic and do not require lifelong anticoagulation with warfarin. However, they are prone to structural valvular degeneration, resulting in recurrent mitral valve stenosis or mitral regurgitation. Valve prosthetics are improving, and freedom from structural valvular degeneration is as high as 85% at 10 years. Mechanical valves are thrombogenic and require lifelong anticoagulation, such as warfarin, which is associated with a 1%-2% annual incidence of major bleeding complications. They are more durable and reduce the need for reoperation.

In general, patients younger than 60 years of age or those already requiring warfarin for atrial fibrillation should be considered for a mechanical valve.

AORTIC VALVE DISEASE

The aortic valve separates the outflow tract of the left ventricle with the ascending aorta. It is a trileaflet structure, with three semilunar cusps named for the coronary arteries that arise within the underlying sinuses. The left and right coronary arteries originate within these respective sinuses, with no coronary artery arising within the *noncoronary* sinus. The free edges of the cusps are thickened at regions called the nodules of Arantius. The valve leaflets attach to the wall of the aorta at the annulus, and the locations where two adjacent cusps meet are the commissures. Important structures can be identified under these triangular-shaped zones (Figure 20–12). The commissure between the right and noncoronary cusp serves as the superior border to the membranous interventricular septum and the atrioventricular conduction center. The nonleft commissure guards the aortomitral curtain and the center of the anterior leaflet of the mitral valve. The left-right commissure overlies the muscular interventricular septum and the medial border of the right ventricular outflow tract. These intimate intracardiac

relationships are no more apparent than within the left ventricular outflow tract.

The thin-walled aortic valve leaflets easily open and close during the cardiac cycle, purely following the pressure changes and blood flow path. Under normal circumstances, opening offers very little resistance to flow. The aortic sinuses have an important role during valve closure, as the volume of blood within the space between the opened valve cusp and the aortic wall develops vortices as blood velocity falls. These vortices exert central pressure and initiate valve closure. The sudden reversal of flow from deceleration completes the diastolic closure.

AORTIC STENOSIS

▶ Pathophysiology

The most common cause of aortic stenosis is senile calcific aortic stenosis. It is believed to represent degenerative changes at the cellular level, including lipid accumulation and inflammatory infiltrates, similar to atherosclerotic changes seen in the medium-sized arterial tree. Not surprisingly, it is associated with elevated cholesterol, hypertension, cigarette smoking, diabetes, and other risk factors for atherosclerosis. It is most common in the seventh and eighth decades of life

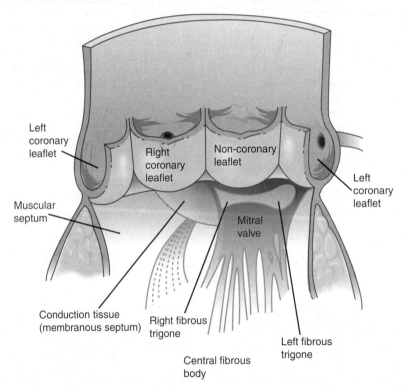

▲ **Figure 20–12.** Anatomic relationships of the aortic root. (Reproduced with permission from Cohn LH. *Cardiac Surgery in the Adult*, 3rd ed. New York, NY: McGraw-Hill Education; 2007.)

and occurs in patients whose valves previously appeared normal. The cusps become progressively immobilized and calcified, starting at the flexion points and extending both along the leaflets and into the wall of the aortic root.

Congenital bicuspid aortic valve represents the most common congenital cardiac lesion, occurring in 2% of the general population. Turbulent flow across the valve causes trauma, leading to fibrosis and calcium deposition, further increasing turbulence, and accelerating the process. Significant stenosis typically occurs in the fifth and sixth decades of life, although it can present earlier. Patients with congenital bicuspid aortic valves often have dilation or aneurysmal degeneration of the ascending aorta. Some evidence suggests a genetic etiology, with presence of abnormal microfibrils causing premature cystic medial necrosis.

Rheumatic heart disease can affect the aortic valve, although it is unusual for the disease to be limited to the aorta, with mitral involvement far more common. As with rheumatic mitral stenosis, fusion of the commissures tends to be the initial feature, followed by progressive thickening and retraction of the leaflets. The reduced leaflet mobility results in a clinical picture of combined aortic valve stenosis and insufficiency.

Aortic stenosis develops gradually, allowing adaptive changes to maintain cardiac output. The left ventricle gradually hypertrophies in response to the severity of the outflow tract obstruction, often resulting in pressure gradients exceeding 100 mm Hg. As a result, patients can remain asymptomatic until severely advanced disease is present. While concentric left ventricular hypertrophy maintains systolic function in the face of severe outflow obstruction, diastolic function of the thickened and noncompliant ventricle is progressively impaired. Diastolic dysfunction can be overcome to a certain degree with atrial hypertrophy and enhanced atrial kick. In addition, as left ventricular end-diastolic pressure rises, intravascular volume status and peripheral vascular resistance adjust to maintain the required preload. Certain triggers can disrupt this delicate balance, including loss of atrial contribution from atrial fibrillation or reduced diastolic filling time from increased heart rate, as might be seen during exercise. These triggers can create sudden clinical decompensation, producing markedly reduced cardiac output and pulmonary edema, even in a previously asymptomatic patient.

The most common clinical presentation in a patient with aortic stenosis is gradual decrease in exercise tolerance. The fixed outflow obstruction prevents an increase in stroke volume typically seen in exercise with elevated circulating catecholamines. Any change in cardiac output is limited to an increase in heart rate, decreasing diastolic filling time for the stiff and noncompliant ventricle. As a result, there is limited boost in cardiac output during exercise, producing premature exertional fatigue and dyspnea. Some patients describe angina, as myocardial oxygen demand exceeds supply. The hypertrophied heart consumes more oxygen without

reciprocal increase in epicardial delivery. In addition, the outflow obstruction prolongs systole, further increasing oxygen demand. Symptoms are typically exertional, as the increased heart rate reduces diastolic coronary perfusion time. Syncope or presyncope is occasionally described in patients with aortic stenosis, presumably related to systemic vasodilation during exercise without a reciprocal increase in cardiac output. Advanced heart failure with symptoms at rest or with minimal activity suggests a decrease in systolic function, likely a result of longstanding disease with alterations within the myocardium at the cellular level.

Diagnostic Evaluation

Physical examination of the patient reveals several findings specific for aortic stenosis. There is a characteristic systolic crescendo/decrescendo murmur heard best over the base of the heart and radiating up the carotid arteries. The murmur becomes harsher and peaks later in systole as the severity worsens. Palpation of the carotid pulses reveals parvus et tardus, or a late-peaking and low-amplitude pulse. A palpable thrill may be felt over the right second intercostal space.

The electrocardiogram demonstrates left ventricular hypertrophy in the majority of patients. Conduction or rhythm abnormalities are identified in some patients. The chest radiograph typically is normal but may demonstrate dilation of the ascending aorta in patients with congenital bicuspid valve. Cardiac catheterization provides important information about associated cardiac pathology, particularly coronary occlusive disease. In addition, hemodynamic assessment can confirm the severity of the aortic valve stenosis and quantify the degree of pulmonary hypertension.

The standard evaluation of patients with suspected aortic stenosis is echocardiography. Images of the valve reveal the severity of the stiffness and calcifications. Images also differentiate bicuspid from tricuspid anatomy and identify associated dilation of the ascending aorta. Ventricular function and additional valvular pathology, particularly in patients with rheumatic heart disease, are essential. Doppler echocardiography can measure the velocity of the aortic jet, allowing reliable estimates of the pressure gradients using the modified Bernoulli equation.

Treatment

A. Medical Therapy

Because aortic stenosis can progress over 10-15 years, patients with mild to moderate disease and without symptoms can be followed without intervention. Serial echocardiography should be performed annually or every other year to assess for disease progression. The most important aspect of medical therapy is education of the patient about potential symptoms. Since symptoms can develop gradually, many patients will unconsciously alter their lifestyles and activity levels without recognizing the presence of limitations. Although there is some suggestion that cholesterol reduction with statins can reduce the calcifications, there is little evidence that medications can adequately palliate the symptomatic patient or can alter the timing of surgical intervention in asymptomatic patients.

B. Indications for Surgery

The indications for surgery on the stenotic aortic valve have been largely determined by the presence of symptoms. Numerous studies have demonstrated reasonably good prognosis in asymptomatic patients managed without surgery. However, symptoms may be equivocal, particularly in the elderly population. Exercise stress testing under the observation of a physician can help elucidate significant limitations that may not be apparent by merely questioning the patient. Surgery is also indicated for patients with moderate to severe aortic stenosis who are undergoing cardiac surgery for other indications, such as coronary bypass grafting or mitral valve replacement.

Handling of the asymptomatic patient with severe aortic stenosis is facing some controversy. The severity of aortic stenosis can be quantified using Doppler echocardiography to estimate the pressure gradient across the aortic valve using the velocity of the outflow jet and the modified Bernoulli equation. Severe aortic stenosis is present when the mean gradient exceeds 40 mm Hg in the normal ventricle. Although some have described an increase in the rate of sudden death in patients with severe aortic stenosis, there remains no evidence to justify aortic valve replacement in the absence of symptoms.

AORTIC INSUFFICIENCY

▶ Pathophysiology

Several conditions can cause incompetence of the aortic valve. Any of the disease processes that cause aortic stenosis can also cause some degree of aortic valve insufficiency, including senile calcific aortic stenosis, degenerated bicuspid aortic valve, and rheumatic aortic valve disease. Aortic valve endocarditis is another common cause of aortic valve insufficiency. The most common cause of incompetence of the aortic valve is related to pathology within the aortic root and ascending aorta. Aneurysmal dilation of the ascending aorta, from congenital conditions such as Marfan disease, from degenerative age-related changes, or from changes associated with a bicuspid aortic valve, can cause aortic valve insufficiency. As the wall of the aorta enlarges, the aortic valve annulus dilates and the leaflets separate, causing incompetence.

As with mitral valve regurgitation, aortic valve insufficiency is best tolerated when it occurs gradually. As the volume of regurgitation worsens, the ventricle adapts by dilating to accommodate the increased preload, and it hypertrophies to maintain the same level of systolic pressure at larger volumes. Despite progressive dilation, ventricular output and systolic function are maintained for long periods of time, leaving many patients asymptomatic for years. While end-diastolic volume is elevated, end-systolic volume is normal. With severe degrees of chronic aortic insufficiency, the heart can require ejecting as much as two to three times the circulating cardiac output, resulting in longstanding volume overload. Eventually, systolic function declines, resulting in a rapid and progressive rise in end-diastolic volume, and heart failure symptoms ensue.

Most patients with chronic aortic insufficiency do not develop symptoms of heart failure until there is severe left ventricular dilation. Some patients describe palpitations or the sensation of ventricular heave, particularly when lying down. Acute aortic valve insufficiency, as can occur with aortic valve endocarditis, can present with cardiogenic shock because the relatively noncompliant ventricle is unprepared for the excess volume during both systole and diastole. There is a combination of high intracardiac filling pressures and low cardiac output. Patients are tachycardic and hypotensive as well as acutely dyspneic at rest. The patient with endocarditis may also be febrile with signs of embolization of vegetations, causing stroke, or ischemia of an extremity or intestines.

▶ Diagnostic Testing

Certain characteristic physical examination findings are pathognomonic for chronic aortic valve insufficiency. The water-hammer pulse can be appreciated, with accentuated systole and abrupt collapse. Patients may have a head bob with each heart beat, or a pulse may be seen in the uvula. A systolic thrill is also described over the femoral artery from the augmented forward flow. The apical impulse is displaced laterally and inferiorly from cardiomegaly, and diastolic blood pressure is low. Auscultation will reveal a high-pitched diastolic murmur heard immediately after the second heart sound. The severity of the valvular lesion usually correlates with the duration of the murmur, not the intensity. The murmur is best heard with the patient leaning forward during a breath hold.

Echocardiography will establish the etiology of the aortic valve insufficiency, visualizing the motion of the leaflets and dilation of the aorta or the presence of vegetations or leaflet perforations. In addition, the ventricular size can be followed, as elevated end-systolic volumes or reduced ejection fraction are indications for surgery. Reversal of flow seen in the descending aorta is a sign of severe aortic valve insufficiency. More sophisticated techniques can quantify the regurgitant volume, such as evaluating the regurgitant jet velocity/time integral.

▶ Treatment

For asymptomatic patients with moderate aortic insufficiency and normal ventricular dimensions, no treatment is necessary. Patients with severe aortic valve insufficiency and normal ventricular size should be followed every 6 months with assessment of symptoms and echocardiography. Some advocate the use of afterload reduction agents to reduce the volume of regurgitant blood, but no evidence demonstrates reduced need for surgery. Symptomatic patients who are not candidates for surgery should be treated with afterload reduction agents, such as calcium channel blockers or inhibitors of angiotensin-converting enzyme. Diuretics and salt restrictions may help in alleviating heart failure symptoms.

For operative candidates, development of heart failure symptoms is an indication for surgery. Asymptomatic patients with decreased left ventricular systolic function or elevated left ventricular end-systolic volumes should also undergo operative treatment. Because ventricular dilation is associated with irreversible changes at the cellular level, intervention is best performed before these permanent changes occur.

Surgical Techniques

As with most other cardiac surgical procedures, median sternotomy is the standard incision used for access to the aortic valve. The pericardium is opened longitudinally, and the reflection is mobilized off of the great vessels. The pulmonary artery and aorta are separated as they emanate from the heart, taking care to avoid injury to the takeoff of the right pulmonary artery or the left main coronary artery. The patient is anticoagulated with 300 IU of heparin, and an activated clotting time of at least 400 seconds is confirmed. Cannulation for CPB is performed, using the distal ascending aorta or the transverse aortic arch to maximize the distance between the aortic cross-clamp and the aortotomy. Venous return is via the right atrial appendage. CPB is initiated, and the left ventricle is vented via a catheter advanced from the right superior pulmonary vein. The patient is cooled systemically to 32°C. An aortic cross-clamp is applied to the distal ascending aorta just proximal to the CPB cannula. The heart is arrested with cold blood cardioplegia solution delivered antegrade down the coronary arteries using a catheter in the aortic root. Cardioplegia solution is also delivered retrograde via a balloon-tipped catheter in the coronary sinus. If severe aortic valve insufficiency is present, only retrograde cardioplegia can be delivered. Once diastolic cardiac arrest is achieved, the ascending aorta is opened transversely approximately 1-2 cm above the takeoff of the right coronary artery. The aortotomy is extended two-thirds of the circumference of the aorta, providing excellent visualization of the valve, the coronary ostia, and the ventricular outflow tract (Figure 20–13).

Excision of the stenotic aortic valve can be time consuming and requires meticulous attention to detail. The extensive calcifications can extend deep into the annulus and up the wall of the aortic root or down along the anterior leaflet of the mitral valve. The calcium buildup must be debrided aggressively enough to allow proper seating of the valve prosthesis without a paravalvular leak while avoiding residual

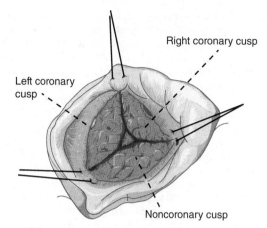

▲ **Figure 20–13.** Surgeon's view of the stenotic trileaflet aortic valve. (Reproduced with permission from Cohn LH. *Cardiac Surgery in the Adult*, 3rd ed. New York, NY: McGraw-Hill Education; 2007.)

outflow tract obstruction. However, overaggressive debridement can result in perforations of the aortic wall, ventricular septal defect, or unhinging of the mitral leaflet with resultant severe mitral regurgitation. In cases of endocarditis, any granulation tissue or residual vegetations must be removed and debrided to avoid recurrent infection of the implanted prosthetic. The outflow tract and aortic root are thoroughly irrigated to ensure removal of loose deposits and debris.

Once the native valve has been removed and the annulus satisfactorily debrided, the outflow tract is sized using tools provided by each manufacturer of valve prostheses. The appropriately sized valve is selected and secured in place. Mechanical valve prosthetics are implanted using a pledgeted mattress technique, leaving the pledgets on the aortic side. This eliminates the likelihood of the bulky pledgets interfering with the disk mechanisms on the ventricular surface. Alternatively, if a bioprosthetic valve is selected, the pledgets can be oriented on the ventricular side of the annulus. This allows supra-annular seating of the bioprosthetic and implantation of a slightly larger valve. The sutures are then placed through the sewing cuff of the prosthetic, and the valve is lowered into the surgical field. The sutures are tied, ensuring that the valve has seated properly to the annulus. The ostia of the coronary arteries should be inspected and clearly free of impingement by the prosthetic valve. The aortotomy is then closed with running polypropylene suture, occasionally reinforced with Teflon felt in the older patient with a thin aortic wall.

The patient is then gradually weaned from CPB, thoroughly deairing with gentle suction applied using the left ventricular vent and the aortic root catheter. The valve is inspected using the TEE for competency and adequacy of the size. There should be no paravalvular leak, and the gradients across the valve should be low. Elevated pulmonary artery pressures or reduced cardiac output should alert the surgeon of the possibility of an unrecognized paravalvular leak.

Aortic valve endocarditis also poses unique surgical challenges. The infective process often results in abscess formation and occasionally intracardiac fistulas. The most important first step in addressing these problems is aggressive debridement of infected and devitalized tissue. Not only will residual infection colonize the implanted prosthetic, but inadequate debridement with securing of the prosthetic to infected and devitalized tissue will lead to dehiscence with need for early reoperation. Abscesses are common within the intervalvular fibrous body. The annular defect should be covered with a pericardial patch. Often, the entire root requires excision, requiring replacement with a valved conduit and reimplantation of the coronary ostia. Results for endocarditis are dependent on the clinical status of the patient at the time of surgery as well as the etiology of the infection. Intravenous drug users carry the worst prognosis, in large part related to recurrence of their addiction with subsequent reinfection.

TRANSCATHETER AORTIC VALVE REPLACEMENT

Recently, aortic valve replacement has been approached without sternotomy using endovascular techniques. Bioprosthetic valves of bovine or porcine pericardium are crimped and loaded onto a metallic frame (Figure 20–14). An 18F to 24F delivery system can be inserted via the femoral vessels and expanded at the level of the left ventricular outflow tract either by balloon or using self-expanding titanium alloys. The native aortic valve is displaced by the prosthetic rather than removed, as is done in surgical aortic valve replacement. The procedure can often be performed under local anesthesia, dramatically reducing perioperative morbidity. Current indications for this approach are patients with severe aortic stenosis and prohibitive surgical risk or as an alternative to surgery in higher risk patients (estimated perioperative mortality of 15%). While the femoral access route is most frequently used, some patients with small peripheral vessels or extensive atherosclerotic disease may not accommodate the large-size delivery systems. Alternative approaches include the iliac artery, axillary artery, ascending aorta, and left ventricular apex. The latter two require mini-thoracotomies for exposure. Paravalvular leaks are common, with moderate to severe regurgitation occurring in 10%-15% of patients. Long term survival is diminished in patients with significant aortic insufficiency. Stroke represents a concern as the large catheters traverse the aortic arch and the calcified aortic valve is dilated, hazarding cerebral embolization. When directly compared to surgery in high-risk patients, the risk of neurologic event was twice as high with transcatheter aortic valve replacement (TAVR) (5.5% vs 2.4%). This risk may be justified in the context of an overall reduction in perioperative mortality for TAVR as compared to surgical aortic

A

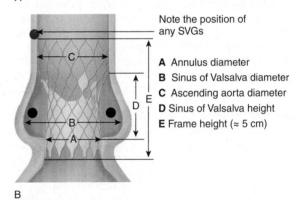

Note the position of any SVGs

A Annulus diameter
B Sinus of Valsalva diameter
C Ascending aorta diameter
D Sinus of Valsalva height
E Frame height (≈ 5 cm)

B

▲ **Figure 20–14. A:** Edwards Sapien percutaneous aortic valve. (Reproduced with permission from Edwards Lifesciences, Irvine, California.) **B:** Medtronic CoreValve. (Reproduced with permission from Medtronic CV Luxembourg SARL.)

valve replacement in these high-risk patients (3.4% vs 6.5%). TAVR is efficacious for high-risk patients with severe aortic stenosis, and the approved indications have been serially extended to lower risk populations.

Kodali SK, et al: Two-year outcomes after transcatheter or surgical aortic valve replacement. *N Engl J Med.* 2012;366:1686.

Mack MJ, et al for the PARTNER 3 Investigators. Transcatheter aortic-valve replacement with a balloon-expandable valve in low-risk patients. *N Engl J Med.* 2019;380(18):1695-1705.

Popma JJ, et al, for the Evolut Low Risk Trial Investigators. Transcatheter aortic-valve replacement with a self-expanding valve in low-risk patients. *N Engl J Med.* 2019;380(18):1706-1715.

Reardon MJ, et al, for the SURTAVI Investigators. Surgical or transcatheter aortic-valve replacement in intermediate-risk patients. *N Engl J Med.* 2017;376(14):1321-1331.

THORACIC AORTA

The ascending aorta represents a continuation of the aortic root at the sinotubular junction. The aortic arch extends from the ascending aorta, traveling posteriorly and to the left as it gives off the three "head vessels" superiorly: the innominate, left carotid, and left subclavian arteries. The thoracic aorta continues from the aortic arch into the descending thoracic aorta beyond the left subclavian artery. The descending thoracic aorta continues until the level of the diaphragm, where it becomes the abdominal aorta. The only branches originating from the descending thoracic aorta are the bronchial and esophageal arteries and multiple intercostal vessels that contribute important sources of blood flow to the spinal cord.

Some common variants are seen in the branch pattern of the thoracic aorta. The most common is the "bovine arch" in which the left carotid originates from the innominate artery. An aberrant right subclavian artery originates from the distal aortic arch on the lesser curvature and travels posterior to the esophagus from left to right. It has been associated with unusual causes of dysphagia from mechanical compression of the esophagus. Other abnormal variants of the aortic arch include a right-sided arch and double ligamentum arteriosum, which can cause tracheal or esophageal compression early in life and are discussed in Chapter 21.

THORACIC AORTIC ANEURYSMS

Pathophysiology

During systole, kinetic energy imparted by ventricular ejection is absorbed in the compliance of the aorta, resulting in transient expansion and recoil. The amount of energy absorption is proportional to the proximity to the left ventricle. As such, the ascending, descending, and abdominal aortae have different cellular features to accommodate their unique fluid-mechanical environments. Elastin fiber content is typically higher in the ascending aorta. These fibers are synthesized and degraded continuously by the smooth muscle cells, and a progressive fragmentation of these fibers is associated with aging, which is the reason for gradual dilation of the ascending aorta in the elderly. However, certain acquired conditions can accelerate the process, producing the pathologically enlarged aorta and resulting in aneurysms. Aortic atherosclerosis is associated with aneurysm formation, predominantly in the descending thoracic aorta. The inflammatory process extends from the intima to the media, causing elastin fiber breakdown. Cystic medial degeneration is the end result of any of the acquired degenerative processes, resulting in elastin fiber fragmentation and loss of smooth muscle cells. The weakened aortic media progressively dilates and can become prone to rupture or dissection. Infection, inflammatory conditions, and trauma can also cause localized medial degeneration and aneurysm formation.

Certain heritable conditions are also associated with aneurysmal disease of the thoracic aorta. Most notable is Marfan syndrome, an autosomal dominant abnormality of fibrillin, an important component in elastin. Patients with Marfan syndrome present with aneurysmal degeneration of the thoracic aorta at any level, most notably in the ascending aorta, in the second and third decades of life. Patients with bicuspid aortic valves are prone to develop aneurysms of the ascending aorta, likely related to abnormalities of their aortic smooth muscle.

The natural history of unresected thoracic aortic aneurysms is dependent on the size and the etiology. The larger the aneurysm, the greater the wall tension and thus the risk of rupture or dissection. Beyond 5.5 cm in maximal diameter, there is a significant increase in the risk of rupture, dissection, or death. Although it varies with age and etiology, there is a reasonably predictable growth rate, estimated at approximately 0.1-0.2 cm per year. Marfan syndrome and other genetic causes of thoracic aortic pathology tend to have a higher likelihood of rupture at smaller aneurysm sizes, and the growth rate is faster than in acquired thoracic aneurysms.

Most patients with thoracic aortic aneurysms are asymptomatic. The diagnosis is often established on screening chest radiograph, CT, or echocardiography performed for other indications. Occasionally, patients with unruptured aneurysms describe chest pain presumably related to rapid enlargement or encroachment on adjacent structures. Unfortunately, many patients are not diagnosed with a thoracic aortic aneurysm until the time of rupture or dissection. Rupture of ascending aneurysms typically presents with crushing chest pain, whereas descending aneurysms cause tearing back or flank pain.

Diagnostic Testing

In a patient presenting with a thoracic aneurysm without rupture, the physical examination is typically unremarkable. Chest radiograph may demonstrate a widened mediastinum. The electrocardiogram is helpful only for associated cardiac pathology. An echocardiogram demonstrates enlargement of the ascending aorta or descending aorta. The aortic arch is typically obscured from view by the trachea and the lungs.

Contrast-enhanced CT scanning is the most widely used test for aneurysms of the thoracic aorta (Figure 20–15). The CT scan can diagnose the aneurysm and accurately describe its size and extent, can be used for direct comparison for patients managed expectantly, and can differentiate isolated aneurysmal disease from an aortic dissection. Three-dimensional reconstruction is helpful in accurately assessing size and location of branch vessels. The limitation of CT scanning is the need for intravenous iodinated contrast, with its inherent nephrotoxic properties.

MRI provides quality resolution similar to CT scanning but can provide dynamic imaging for cardiac assessment and does not require iodinated contrast material. MRI, however, is more time consuming and less available in many centers. Cardiac catheterization and aortography are performed

▲ **Figure 20–15.** Computed tomography scan of a dilated ascending aorta.

only in planning operative intervention to exclude coronary artery disease or pulmonary hypertension.

▶ Surgical Therapy

The most frequent indication for operation on the aneurysmal ascending aorta is incidental to other cardiac pathology. It is generally agreed that an asymptomatic ascending aorta greater than 4.5-5 cm in size should be replaced at the time of aortic valve replacement or coronary bypass surgery, assuming the risk of the procedure would not be significantly altered. Any patient with a symptomatic ascending aneurysm should receive urgent surgery, although it is unusual for patients with ruptured ascending aortas to survive long enough to be given this opportunity. For asymptomatic patients without associated cardiac pathology, the indication for surgery is when the maximal diameter of the ascending aorta is greater than 5.5 cm. For patients with Marfan syndrome, surgery is indicated for lesser degrees of dilation. Additionally, for patients followed with serial CT scans, interval enlargement of the ascending aorta by a least 1 cm warrants consideration for surgical resection.

Sudden rupture or dissection is less frequent in the descending aorta, and thus the indications for operation are less stringent. In general, operation should be considered when the aneurysm reaches 6 cm in maximal diameter or if there is interval enlargement by at least 1 cm over 1 year. Patients with Marfan syndrome require surgery at smaller aortic sizes to prevent catastrophic complications. Increasingly, the descending thoracic aorta is treated using endovascular techniques. Balloon or self-expanding stents are covered with vascular grafts and inserted via peripheral

vessels and deployed creating a seal at the proximal and distal extent of the descending thoracic aneurysm, the so-called "landing zones." Although the aneurysm is not removed, pressurized blood is excluded from the sac, eliminating the risk of rupture (Figure 20–16). Because the procedure does not require thoracotomy and aortic clamping, morbidity

A

B

▲ **Figure 20–16.** Endovascular repair of a descending thoracic aneurysm. **A:** Chest radiograph. **B:** Computed tomography image. Note exclusion of contrast from the old aneurysm sac.

is substantially lower. However, endoleaks are frequent, in which there is failure to completely exclude blood flow into the aneurysm sac. These endoleaks may result in late aneurysm-related complications. Endovascular treatment of descending thoracic aneurysm continues to evolve with experience and refinement of technology.

Medical treatment of small ascending or descending aneurysms involves aggressive blood pressure control using beta-blocking agents to reduce the forceful contraction against the weakened aortic wall, activity restriction to avoid straining, cessation of cigarette smoking, and weight loss. Patients followed with ascending or descending aortic aneurysms should receive repeat imaging for signs of interval growth prompting surgical intervention.

AORTIC DISSECTION

▶ Pathophysiology

Dissection of the thoracic aorta is among the most feared entities in all of medicine because of the exceedingly high mortality and the speed with which its injuries become irreversible. An intimal tear of the aorta allows blood flow to exit the lumen and travel a variable distance within the media. Depending on the location of the intimal tear and the direction in which blood travels, aortic dissections can be categorized using two prominent classification schemes. The DeBakey classification describes the location and the extent, whereas the more simplified Stanford classification looks at location alone. A Stanford type A dissection involves the ascending aorta; a Stanford type B involves the arch or descending aorta (Figure 20–17).

The precise etiology of aortic dissections is unclear, but there is an unambiguous association with a variety of conditions, including aortic aneurysms, hypertension, smoking, pregnancy, and recent intravascular trauma. Once blood enters the medial plane, the intima "floats" within the aortic lumen and has a characteristic appearance on CT scans (Figure 20–18). The blood within the false lumen reenters the true lumen through any number of naturally created fenestrations or holes, either from disruption of the side branches or from reentry at the termination of the false lumen. Blood flow to any of the side branches off of the aorta can be compromised by the intimal flap, causing ischemia, a condition referred to as malperfusion. Malperfusion can involve the coronary arteries, branches of the aortic arch to the brain, the renal arteries, the mesenteric arteries, or branches to the lower extremities or the spinal cord. Blood can also exit the false lumen pathway into the adventitial space, causing free rupture. Rupture is more likely in Stanford type A dissections because of the intrapericardial location of the ascending aorta and the increased mechanical forces related to the proximity to the left ventricular outflow tract. Type B dissections in the descending aorta do not experience the same mechanical

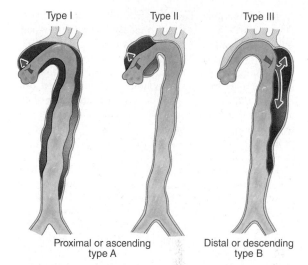

▲ **Figure 20–17.** DeBakey and Stanford classifications of aortic dissection. DeBakey types I and II represent Stanford type A, whereas DeBakey type III is the same as a Stanford type B.

forces, because the more proximal aorta absorbs a significant amount of the kinetic energy. In addition, the extrapleural tissue helps reinforce the weakened adventitia, containing potential ruptures.

▲ **Figure 20–18.** Computed tomography scan of an acute aortic dissection. This Stanford type A dissection involves both the ascending and descending aortae. The large false lumen is nearly obstructing the true lumen.

In addition to the free intrapericardial rupture of type A dissections, there are two other modes of early death responsible for the nearly 50% mortality associated with type A dissections. Malperfusion of the coronary ostia, typically the right coronary artery, causes acute myocardial infarction, resulting in ventricular arrhythmias and myocardial dysfunction with shock. In addition, proximal migration of the dissection flap can disrupt the attachments of the aortic valve to the wall of the aortic root. The unsupported valve tissue prolapses into the ventricle during diastole, producing massive aortic valve insufficiency.

Patients with aortic dissections complain of tearing back pain or crushing chest pain. They are often hypertensive and tachycardic. The diagnosis can often be confused with acute myocardial infarction, ureterolithiasis, cholelithiasis, or pancreatitis. Patients with malperfusion can present with flank or abdominal pain from renal or mesenteric ischemia, lower extremity pain or paresthesias from iliac occlusion, stroke from carotid occlusion, or acute paralysis from occlusion of the multiple branches to the spinal cord. These symptoms of malperfusion can often overwhelm the chest or back pain from the dissection, clouding the diagnostic evaluation. Delay in diagnosis is exceedingly common in acute aortic dissection.

Diagnostic Testing

On physical examination, patients appear acutely ill and are tachycardic and hypertensive. Hypotension should warrant suspicion of pericardial tamponade, myocardial infarction, aortic valve insufficiency, or free rupture. Blood pressure should be assessed in all four extremities to document perfusion abnormalities from the dissection flap. Abdominal pain should prompt evaluation of possible mesenteric or renal malperfusion. Neurologic deficits suggest either cerebral embolization or spinal ischemia.

Chest radiographs are often performed as the initial diagnostic test. They may reveal widening of the mediastinum, a left pleural effusion, or cardiomegaly if pericardial tamponade is present. CT is the standard imaging modality used to diagnose aortic dissection and should be obtained promptly in a patient with new-onset tearing back or chest pain. The CT scan diagnoses the dissection and identifies associated aneurysmal disease as well as organs at risk for malperfusion. TEE has a critical role in patients with aortic dissection. TEE excludes involvement of the ascending aorta in cases that are equivocal on CT scan. In addition, TEE identifies cardiac dysfunction and, most importantly, aortic valve insufficiency from extension of the dissection into the aortic root.

Treatment

A. Medical Therapy

Initial management of the patient with an acute aortic dissection is immediate control of elevated blood pressure. Narcotic agents can be given initially to control pain and reduce the catecholamine surge. Beta-blocking agents are particularly critical not only to reduce blood pressure, but also to lower the force of contraction and the sheer stress directly impacting the weakened aortic tissue. Esmolol is a short-acting agent that can be administered as a continuous infusion to obtain fine control of blood pressure, avoiding excessive bradycardia or hypotension. If high blood pressure persists, an arterial vasodilator can be given, such as nitroprusside, with a goal of maintaining systolic blood pressure of 100-120 mm Hg.

Patients with type B aortic dissections are frequently treated with medical therapy only, consisting of pain and blood pressure control, as well as observation for signs of malperfusion or rupture. Most patients with type B dissections can be safely discharged from the hospital once blood pressure control is adequate and the pain has resolved. They are carefully followed for good antihypertensive control as well as surveillance CT scanning to assess for interval growth in the size of the descending aorta. The indications for operative intervention in an acute type B aortic dissection are ongoing chest pain despite adequate blood pressure control, aneurysmal enlargement of the descending aorta greater than 6 cm, or evidence of impending rupture on CT scanning.

B. Surgical Therapy

1. Indications—Patients with type A aortic dissections should undergo emergency surgery to avoid one of the three fatal complications associated with 95% of patients with untreated dissections. These complications include intrapericardial rupture with tamponade, aortic valve insufficiency, or acute myocardial infarction. Once the diagnosis of a type A dissection has been established, either by CT scan or TEE, the patient should be taken emergently to the operating room in preparation for emergency surgery. The only exception to immediate emergency surgery is when signs of malperfusion of the abdominal viscera exist. Although this strategy remains controversial, some advocate angiographic investigation for signs of malperfusion. Using a combination of contrast fluoroscopy, intravascular ultrasound, and selective cannulation of all branches from the aorta with pressure measurements, the extent of the dissection can be evaluated and areas of definite malperfusion can be identified. If the intimal flap is obstructing blood flow to any of the aortic branches, fenestration using balloon catheters can restore flow from the false to the true lumen, reperfusing ischemic organs. While patients with severe visceral malperfusion can have mortality rates of nearly 80%, more recent series adopting a strategy of initial catheter-based fenestration followed by surgical repair show estimated mortality rates in selected patients of less than 20%. Since catheter-based techniques are becoming more universally available, this strategy of delayed surgical repair may become more widespread.

2. Techniques— Once a patient with a type A dissection has been diagnosed, emergency surgery is usually indicated. The femoral or axillary artery is exposed for arterial cannulation for CPB. A median sternotomy is performed, exposing the dilated and dissected ascending aorta. After administration of 300 IU/kg of heparin, the patient is cannulated for CPB, using the right atrium for venous drainage. The patient is cooled aggressively to 18°C in preparation for hypothermic circulatory arrest. A catheter is placed in the coronary sinus to deliver retrograde cardioplegia for myocardial protection. A left ventricular vent is placed in the right superior pulmonary vein. Once the patient has reached 18°C, CPB is discontinued, and the ascending aorta can be opened. The dissected aorta is removed, typically extending along the lesser curvature of the aortic arch. The remaining arch is carefully inspected for additional intimal tears. An appropriately sized and spatulated Dacron graft is anastomosed to the aortic arch using running polypropylene suture buttressed with Teflon felt. CPB can be reinstituted, flushing air and debris out of the open anastomosis. The aortic cross-clamp can then be applied to the graft material. The proximal ascending aorta is resected to the sino-tubular junction, and the Dacron graft is trimmed to size. The proximal anastomosis is performed in a similar fashion using running polypropylene suture buttressed with felt. A deairing needle is placed in the graft, and the aortic cross-clamp is removed. The patient is rewarmed and weaned from CPB.

Occasionally, the pathology extends proximally into the aortic root, requiring reconstruction or resection. If the root is not significantly enlarged, the dissection flap can be obliterated by inserting Teflon felt into the false lumen and reapproximating the intima to the adventitia using polypropylene suture. The aortic valve commissures can be resuspended to the aortic wall with pledgeted sutures from intima to adventitia. If the aortic root is dilated, the sinuses and valve tissue can be excised and replaced with a mechanical valve conduit, reattaching the coronary ostia using the Bentall technique (Figure 20–19). Under certain scenarios, the entire aortic arch must be removed and replaced with Dacron graft material. When the aortic arch is significantly aneurysmal, if the intimal tear is within the aortic arch, or in a patient with Marfan syndrome, the entire arch should be replaced. Each branch of the arch can be individually reimplanted to the graft, the three vessels can be attached as an island, or a multibranch graft of Dacron with side branches preattached can be anastomosed to the individual arch branches. When the arch is reconstructed, a longer duration of hypothermic circulatory arrest will be required. Cerebral perfusion can be initiated using balloon-tipped catheters inserted directly into the innominate and left carotid arteries. Blood flow at a rate of 600 mL/min at 18°C is generally considered adequate to prevent neurologic compromise.

3. Results— As previously described, the mortality of acute aortic dissection may be as high as 50%, since many patients will rupture before arrival at a qualified hospital. Operative mortality is in the range of 10%-20%, which includes consideration of the selection bias of choosing operative candidates. Cause of death is primarily related to malperfusion syndrome, resulting in neurologic, intestinal, or extremity ischemia. Cerebral injury related to hypothermic circulatory arrest is limited and should result in clinically significant stroke in less than 5% of patients. Long-term survival following repair of acute aortic dissection is good, approximately 50%-60% at 10 years.

Abraha I, et al: Thoracic stent graft versus surgery for thoracic aneurysm. *Cochrane Database Syst Rev.* 2016;6:CD006796.
Goodney PP, et al: Survival after open versus endovascular thoracic aortic aneurysm repair in an observational study of the Medicare population. *Circulation.* 2011;124:2661.

▼ SURGICAL TREATMENT OF HEART FAILURE

HEART TRANSPLANTATION

▶ Indications

The incidence of congestive heart failure (CHF) is steadily rising, owing to the increase in the aging population and the reduced mortality of myocardial infarction. Nearly 5 million Americans live with heart failure, and 500,000 new cases are diagnosed annually. Causes are multifactorial, but by far the most frequent etiology is related to coronary occlusive disease, with repeated ischemic insults and loss of viable myocardial contractility. Chronic ventricular volume overload from conditions such as undiagnosed valvular pathology or intracardiac septal defects can result in cardiomyopathy and advanced heart failure. Other causes of heart failure include viral myocarditis, peripartum cardiomyopathy, and idiopathic dilated cardiomyopathy.

All of these processes lead to the same result: loss of myocardial contractility with decreased cardiac output, elevated diastolic cardiac filling pressures, and pathologic neurohormonal adaptive responses. This leads to increased sympathetic tone, elevated peripheral vascular resistance, and salt and water retention, creating a vicious cycle with further reduction in cardiac output, edema, and pulmonary congestion.

Medical therapy includes reduction in salt intake and modest exercise to reduce sympathetic activation. Diuretics and aldosterone inhibitors counteract the inappropriately activated renin-angiotensin system. Angiotensin-converting enzyme inhibitors decrease peripheral vascular resistance and alter the myocardial intercellular matrix, allowing opportunities for reverse cardiac remodeling. The inotropic properties of digitalis glycosides have been demonstrated to reduce hospital admission for heart failure exacerbations, although at higher levels, they can increase mortality because

▲ **Figure 20–19.** Aortic root replacement with a mechanical valve conduit using the Bentall technique. The aortic valve and root are replaced and the coronary arteries are directly reimplanted. (Reproduced with permission from Cohn LH. *Cardiac Surgery in the Adult*, 3rd ed. New York, NY: McGraw-Hill Education; 2007.)

of their proarrhythmic properties. Beta-blocking agents reduce sympathetic tone, allow upregulation of β-receptors, and significantly reduce mortality in advanced heart failure patients. As the left ventricle dilates, electrical reentry pathways are generated, predisposing to malignant ventricular arrhythmias and sudden cardiac death. Strong evidence now demonstrates that implantation of automated internal cardiac defibrillators reduces mortality, and their use has become standard practice in heart failure management.

In addition, selected patients with conduction system disturbances may benefit from cardiac resynchronization therapy by insertion of biventricular pacemakers that stimulate both the left and right ventricles simultaneously.

The effectiveness of medical therapy is often described by the New York Heart Association (NYHA) classification (Table 20–2). As a patient's NYHA functional class deteriorates despite adequate medical therapy, consideration for transplantation should be made. Because heart transplantation remains

Table 20–2. New York Heart Association classification of heart failure symptoms.

I	No limitations
II	Dyspnea with ordinary activity
III	Dyspnea with less than ordinary activity
IV	Dyspnea

a scarce resource, selection of patients is crucial to maximize outcomes. Exclusion criteria have been established on the basis of solid evidence of increased perioperative or reduced long-term survival; criteria are listed in Table 20–3. The most frequently applied exclusion criteria include advanced age, end-organ injury from diabetes mellitus, chronic renal insufficiency (serum creatinine > 2.5), poor medical compliance or psychosocial instability, and morbid obesity (body mass index > 35).

Creation of concrete inclusion criteria has been more elusive because it is often difficult to predict mortality in this population. Historically, patient selection has relied on exercise stress evaluation and determination of maximal oxygen consumption (VO_2 max). Patients with a VO_2 max of less than 10 mL/kg/min have a definite survival advantage with transplantation, and those with a peak VO_2 of less than 14 mL/kg/min with NYHA class III or IV limitations appear to have a survival advantage. Recently, several scoring models have allowed more accurate risk stratification of mortality for ambulatory patients with advanced heart failure. These models have proven helpful for those patients in whom exercise testing appears intermediate in risk assessment, such as those with peak VO_2 between 10 and 14 mL/kg/min. The Heart Failure Survival Score (HFSS) uses seven independent predictors of mortality and creates high-, medium-, and low-risk groups for 1-year mortality. These variables include peak VO_2, QRS interval, ejection fraction, serum sodium, resting heart rate, ischemic versus nonischemic etiology, and mean blood pressure. Patients with intermediate peak VO_2 scores should be considered for transplantation if scoring models such as the HFSS predict high or medium risk for mortality.

Table 20–3. Heart transplant exclusion criteria.

Severe renal insufficiency
Recent malignancy
Advanced age
Obesity
Elevated pulmonary vascular resistance
Medication noncompliance

Heart transplants are allocated according to a protocol prioritizing based on need and geographic distribution. Organs are allocated using a complex algorithm that considers patient status, size, blood type compatibility, and geography.

▶ **Technique**

Patients are briefly evaluated to ensure that there have been no interval changes in their health status since their transplant evaluation. In particular, anticoagulation status is assessed and reversed if necessary, renal function should be reasonably stable, and a pulmonary artery catheter should be inserted to ensure that pulmonary vascular resistance has not changed appreciably since the most recent evaluation. Potential concerns should be discussed between the transplant surgeon and heart failure cardiologist.

Upon confirmation by the procuring team that the donor heart is visibly suitable, the recipient is anesthetized and prepared. A median sternotomy is performed. In the current era, the majority of recipients have undergone previous cardiac surgery, often including insertion of ventricular assist devices. As such, significant time may be required for dissection and identification of cardiac structures, and appropriate time should be allowed. The patient is heparinized to achieve an activated clotting time of at least 450 seconds. Arterial cannulation is preferred high on the lesser curvature of the aortic arch to allow for significant aortic removal, particularly if the recipient has a ventricular assist device. Venous cannulation is in the superior and inferior vena cavae, and CPB is initiated. The cavae are controlled with snares, and an aortic cross-clamp is applied when the donor heart is within 20–30 minutes of arrival. Recipient cardiectomy is performed initially along the right atrioventricular groove and extending down into the coronary sinus. The aorta is transected just above the coronary arteries, avoiding entry into the dome of the left atrium or injury to the right pulmonary artery. The pulmonary artery is transected at the level of the pulmonary valve. The interatrial septum is opened, and the left atrium is divided along the mitral valve annulus. Once the recipient heart is removed, the left atrium is trimmed, removing the appendage and a portion of the interatrial septum.

The donor heart is carefully inspected for abnormalities, including a patent foramen ovale. The atrial cuff is trimmed to size-match the recipient. The left atrial anastomosis is performed with polypropylene in running fashion, everting the edges to minimize incorporation of epicardial tissue within the atria. Before completion of the anastomosis, the left ventricular vent is inserted via the right superior pulmonary vein through the mitral valve. This facilitates deairing and prevents premature rewarming from pulmonary effluent. The donor and recipient ascending aortas are trimmed appropriately, and the anastomosis is performed with running polypropylene suture. At the completion of this suture line, the aortic cross-clamp can be removed, thus terminating the period of cold ischemia. The ascending aorta and left ventricle are vented of residual air. Spontaneous resumption of cardiac activity typically occurs. The inferior vena cava anastomosis is completed with running polypropylene suture. A flexible cardiotomy suction catheter is placed through the donor superior vena cava and advanced into the coronary sinus to improve visualization. The superior vena cava is anastomosed with running polypropylene suture, and the caval snares can be removed. The pulmonary artery anastomosis is performed with running polypropylene, typically imbricating the posterior wall for greater strength. Care must be taken to avoid excess length and potential kinking of the pulmonary artery. The technique just described is for a *bicaval* implant. With a *biatrial* technique, the recipient cardiectomy preserves the superior and inferior vena caval attachments, instead creating an atriotomy along the lateral wall of the right atrium. The donor superior vena cava is ligated, and an incision in the inferior vena cava is extended several centimeters along the posterolateral atrial wall. This older approach is technically easier but is associated with more tricuspid valve regurgitation and atrial arrhythmias, and thus less desirable.

The patient is rewarmed, ventilated, and then weaned off of CPB. If sinus rhythm is less than 100-110 beats/min, atrial pacing is initiated. Inotropic support is typically required in light of the cold ischemic time, even for young and vigorous donor hearts. Right ventricular dysfunction is the most frequently seen complication, attributed to recipient pulmonary hypertension in the "untrained" heart and the inherent sensitivity of the right ventricle to preservation injury. This can be exacerbated by postoperative bleeding, necessitating blood product transfusions with volume overload and worsening of pulmonary vascular resistance. Judicious volume administration, rapid pacing, and catecholamine infusions can overcome right ventricular dysfunction. Inhaled nitric oxide or prostacycline can selectively reduce pulmonary vascular resistance and improve hemodynamic stability.

Immunosuppression after heart transplantation is similar to that for other solid organs and includes antimetabolite agents such as mycophenolate, calcineurin inhibitors such as cyclosporine or tacrolimus, and corticosteroids. Because of their nephrotoxicity, initiation of calcineurin inhibitors is often delayed during the immediate postoperative period. As an alternative, induction therapy with either monoclonal or polyclonal antibodies against specific immune cells can be administered. Although routine use of induction therapy has not been demonstrated to improve outcomes, selected use for patients with perioperative renal insufficiency may be beneficial.

Outcomes

Despite the absence of any prospective randomized evidence, heart transplantation offers long-term survival advantages over medical therapy for appropriately selected patients with advanced heart failure. Survival rates have improved since the introduction of the procedure in 1967, with 1-year survival is now approximately 85%. Most early deaths are attributable to perioperative complications or severe rejection. After this early period of attrition, there continues to be a linear decrement in survival, at a rate of approximately 3%-4% per year, and this rate has not decreased over the past 20 years. Causes of late mortality include transplant vasculopathy, opportunistic infections, immunosuppression-related malignancies, and rejection. Transplant vasculopathy is an accelerated coronary artery disease unique to the heart transplant recipient and is a result of repetitive vascular injury and sustained inflammatory response. Statins and vitamin supplements appear to slow the progression of vasculopathy, but the diffuse nature makes the disease less amenable to percutaneous or surgical revascularization. Median survival after heart transplant is estimated to be between 10 and 11 years.

MECHANICAL CIRCULATORY SUPPORT

▶ Indications

Although heart transplantation has long been considered the gold standard treatment for advanced heart failure, the limited availability of suitable donors affords support for only a small percentage of those in need. Mechanical circulatory support to assist or replace the failing heart has made enormous progress over the last 40 years. Since the introduction of CPB by Gibbon in 1953, the engineering of mechanical blood pumps has become more sophisticated, allowing treatment of an increasing population of patients on an ambulatory basis with reduced size, better blood biocompatibility, and improved pump durability. As this rapid evolution continues, the indications, techniques, and expected results will change dramatically. More than any other aspect of cardiac surgery, the treatment of today will likely be remarkably different only a few years in the future.

The indications for implantable circulatory support are severe cardiac dysfunction despite maximal medical therapy. However, there are three distinct goals of support that represent vastly different patient populations and clinical scenarios: bridge to recovery, bridge to transplant, and destination therapy. Cardiogenic shock may have reversible causes, such as viral or peripartum cardiomyopathy, acute myocardial infarction, and postcardiotomy shock. Initiation of mechanical circulatory support can restore hemodynamics, unload the ventricle, and allow time for myocardial recovery. Chronic heart failure patients felt to be suitable candidates for heart transplantation can rapidly deteriorate, causing end-organ dysfunction and closing their window of opportunity. Implantable circulatory support can reverse acute organ injury and allow functional rehabilitation, improving their candidacy for and potentially their outcomes after heart transplantation.

Patients with advanced heart failure and contraindications for transplantation, such as older age, chronic renal insufficiency, obesity, or fixed pulmonary hypertension, may benefit from implantable circulatory support as destination therapy.

▶ Pumps

A variety of devices are available for mechanical circulatory support to satisfy each of the goals, and many more are currently in clinical trials or preclinical testing. Device selection depends on the clinical circumstances, with considerations including ease of implantation, adequacy and flexibility of support, patient quality of life, durability, and cost. The available devices are discussed in the context of their most frequently used application.

A. Short-Term Devices

Intra-aortic balloon pumps provide counterpulsation during diastole, increasing coronary perfusion and reducing afterload and myocardial oxygen consumption. They are typically inserted percutaneously via the femoral artery and advanced into the descending thoracic aorta. Balloon timing automatically coincides with the electrocardiogram tracing or the arterial pressure waveform. They can be easily removed and have few complications. Intra-aortic balloon pump support is limited, improving cardiac output only by as much as 20%. Alternatives include pneumatically driven extracorporeal blood pumps capable of up to 6 L/min of blood flow. The devices can be connected to any of the cardiac chambers to provide support for the failing left or right ventricle in a variety of configurations. A pneumatic compressor phasically actuates a diaphragm within the pump, producing pulsatile flow. The rate of actuation varies with the pump chamber filling, thus automatically adjusting output according to the patient's volume status. The Thoratec CentriMag is a centrifugal blood pump with a magnetically levitated rotor to improve biocompatibility. There are no valve sinuses or other zones of stagnation, improving thrombogenicity. It produces continuous flow and requires manual pump speed adjustment under conditions of changing preload. The TandemHeart percutaneous ventricular assist device (VAD) uses a venous drainage cannula inserted from the femoral vein and advanced across the interatrial septum. Blood is drained from the left atrium using a centrifugal pump and infused into a cannula inserted into the femoral artery (Figure 20–20). Because of its femoral access, it requires a supine and immobilized patient. They are also available microaxial blood pumps catheters placed across the aortic valve, draining blood from the left ventricular cavity and infusing into the aortic root. The catheters can be inserted peripherally, such as via the femoral artery, or directly into the ascending aorta. The largest of these catheters can produce up to 5 L/min of flow.

▲ **Figure 20–20.** TandemHeart percutaneous ventricular assist device. (Reproduced with permission from CardiacAssist, Inc, Pittsburgh, Pennsylvania.)

B. Long-Term Devices

Implantable mechanical circulatory support, such as left ventricular assist devices (LVADs), is increasingly used for patients with end-stage irreversible heart failure, either as bridge to heart transplantation or for lifelong support (destination therapy). There have been substantial technologic advances in this field, and the use of implantable circulatory support pumps is increasing at rapid pace.

Early LVADs were large, pulsatile pumps that used either electric or pneumatic force to actuate a diaphragm, producing pulsatile ejection. These devices were limited by their large size and the tendency for the motor bearings to fail after prolonged support.

The current generation of circulatory support devices are valveless continuous-flow pumps that use continuously spinning impellers to generate blood flow. Since there is no displacement chamber to generate the flow pulse, the devices are smaller and silent, allowing support to smaller patients and improved patient satisfaction. In addition, the continuous nature of the mechanical load on a single bearing has the important advantage of improved durability.

The first of these pumps to gain US Food and Drug Administration (FDA) approval was the HeartMate 2 (Figure 20–21), which has now been updated to the HeartMate 3. After median sternotomy and creation of a small preperitoneal pocket, the diaphragm is divided, allowing access to the left ventricular apex. On CPB, the inlet cannula of the HeartMate 2 is inserted into the left ventricular apex. The outflow graft is sutured to the ascending aorta. A percutaneous lead exits the right upper quadrant and is connected to a controller allowing interface with the pump. The controller is connected to a power source, either to a power base unit plugged into standard wall outlets or to wearable batteries that can provide untethered support for up to 10 hours. While median survival of VAD patients continues to improve, complications continue to limit the potential success of VAD therapy. Gastrointestinal bleeding occurs in approximately 30% of patients with continuous-flow VADs, likely related to the combination of the required warfarin anticoagulation and acquired platelet dysfunction from device sheer forces. The incidence of stroke is approximately 8%-10% per year from both primary intracerebral hemorrhage and embolic events. Infections at the driveline insertion site can require debridement, prolonged intravenous antibiotics, and when severe, complete pump exchange.

The next generation of LVADs are continuous-flow pumps with centrifugal design, using magnetically levitated rotors. These LVADs eliminate entirely the need for contacting bearings, creating the potential for indefinite support without mechanical failure. In addition, these devices may have improved blood handling characteristics and could reduce some of the complications seen in prolonged mechanical assistance. The significant technological progress in mechanical circulatory support will likely have an enormous impact on the nature of surgical treatment of heart failure.

Rogers JG, et al: Intrapericardial left ventricular assist device for advanced heart failure. *N Engl J Med.* 2017;376(5):451-460.

MULTIPLE CHOICE QUESTIONS

1. Which of the following does *not* contribute to the susceptibility of coronary ischemia?

   A. High baseline oxygen extraction
   B. Coronary flow limited largely during diastole
   C. Atherosclerosis that tends to occur diffusely in small coronary vessels
   D. Increased myocardial oxygen demand, which requires proportional increase in coronary blood flow

2. Which of the following is true about aortic stenosis?

   A. Senile calcific aortic stenosis is associated with ascending aortic aneurysms.
   B. Rheumatic heart disease affects the aortic valve most commonly, followed by the mitral and tricuspid valves.
   C. Presence of left ventricular hypertrophy is an indication for surgery in patients with aortic stenosis.
   D. Typical symptoms are exertional dyspnea, angina, or syncope.

3. For patients with mitral regurgitation, indications for mitral reconstruction do *not* include

   A. Left ventricular dilation
   B. Dyspnea
   C. Asymptomatic with a prolapsed anterior mitral leaflet
   D. Moderate mitral regurgitation at the time of coronary bypass surgery

▲ **Figure 20–21.** HeartMate 2 left ventricular assist device. (Reproduced with permission from Thoratec, Inc., Pleasanton, CA.)

4. Which of the following is true of the thoracic aorta?

   A. Fibrosis results in contraction of the ascending aorta with age.
   B. The ascending aorta should only be replaced when its maximum diameter exceeds 5.5 cm in the absence of symptoms.
   C. Stanford type B dissections cause early death from intrapericardial rupture, aortic valve insufficiency, or coronary malperfusion.
   D. Malperfusion of the abdominal viscera can occur with either Stanford type A or type B aortic dissections.

5. Which of the following is true regarding advanced heart failure?

   A. Beta-blockers improve survival in heart failure in part by upregulation of beta receptors.
   B. The incidence of heart failure is decreasing because of advances in medical treatment.
   C. The use of mechanical circulatory support does not affect priority status for heart transplantation.
   D. Left ventricular dysfunction is the most frequent early complication following heart transplantation.

21

Congenital Heart Disease

Jennifer C. Hirsch-Romano, MD, MS

Richard G. Ohye, MD

Edward L. Bove, MD

Gerard M. Doherty, MD

DIAGNOSIS

Congenital heart disease encompasses a wide range of anomalies that result from abnormal fetal development of the heart. Defects can range from simple to complex. The age of presentation of these defects depends primarily on the physiologic impact of the anomaly. After birth, patients can present within minutes to hours with profound hypoxemia or hemodynamic collapse. Others may present weeks to months later with evidence of a new murmur or signs of congestive heart failure. Relatively asymptomatic lesions can go undetected until children are school age or adolescents. With current ultrasound imaging, many cardiac anomalies are identified on prenatal examination.

Early and accurate diagnosis of congenital heart disease requires careful identification of signs and symptoms of heart disease. The initial workup begins with a focused history and physical examination. Classification of heart murmurs can be highly suggestive of underlying cardiac anomalies. Early signs of heart disease include cyanosis, tachypnea, unequal pulses, and failure to thrive. Key symptoms of congenital heart disease in the patient's history include feeding difficulties, irritability, and frequent respiratory infections.

Standard diagnostic studies include a chest radiograph (CXR) and electrocardiography (ECG). Some cardiac defects have pathognomonic findings on CXR. Other anomalies may be suspected based on heart size, increased or decreased pulmonary markings, aortic arch sidedness, or situs abnormalities (the heart located in the mid or right chest, rather than the typical location in the left chest). ECG can identify rhythm disturbances, axis deviation, atrial enlargement, and ventricular hypertrophy. Transthoracic echocardiography is often the only diagnostic test needed to provide the anatomic detail required for surgical planning. Cardiac catheterization, cardiac magnetic resonance imaging (cMRI), and computed tomography angiography (CTA) are used as adjunct diagnostic tests when additional information on flow, pressure, resistance, or anatomic detail is required.

PREOPERATIVE MANAGEMENT

The care of congenital heart disease patients requires a collaborative effort of a multidisciplinary team of cardiologists, surgeons, interventionalists, echocardiographers, and radiologists. For the majority of congenital heart defects, surgical correction or catheter-based intervention is necessary for definitive treatment. Careful timing and planning of operative and catheter-based interventions along with highly skilled preoperative and postoperative care are essential to a successful outcome.

Certain defects such as atrial septal defects (ASDs), ventricular septal defects (VSDs), and patent ductus arteriosus (PDA) may resolve spontaneously over the first several years of life. The remaining defects require intervention when the risk of surgery is reasonable, when symptoms can no longer be managed medically, and/or prior to the onset of irreversible complications.

Neonates presenting with ductal-dependent lesions require ductal blood flow to maintain systemic or pulmonary perfusion. Ductal patency is achieved with intravenous prostaglandin E_1 therapy. Supplemental oxygen is supplied only as necessary for cyanosis as newborns tolerate relative cyanosis (oxygen saturations > 70%) quite well. The remainder of therapy is directed toward managing congestive heart failure symptoms with diuretics, afterload reduction, and maximal caloric intake.

OPERATIVE MANAGEMENT

For most congenital heart defects, surgical correction is possible. For more complex defects, staged repair with early palliation and staged palliation remain options. The anticipated somatic growth of the child must be considered when determining the surgical approach. Invasive monitoring lines are essential for monitoring patients during surgery and postoperatively. All patients have arterial and central venous catheters placed along with peripheral intravenous catheters and a Foley catheter. For neonates, the umbilical vessels are the desired venous and arterial access. Avoidance of long-standing and repeated femoral lines is important because patency of these vessels is often essential for diagnostic and interventional catheter procedures later in life. Due to variable blood flow with perfusion techniques and underlying cardiac anomalies, it is possible to have differential cooling and rewarming. Therefore, temperature probes are placed in the nasopharynx, the rectum, and on the skin to allow for accurate monitoring.

Most surgical repairs require cardiopulmonary bypass. This involves drainage of venous blood from the patient via cannulae placed in the superior and inferior vena cava (for intracardiac repairs) or a single cannula in the right atrium. Blood passes through the bypass circuit, which warms or cools the blood to the desired temperature, adds oxygen and removes carbon dioxide, and pumps the blood back into the body via an arterial cannula, usually in the ascending aorta. Hypothermia may be employed to decrease the metabolic demands of the body and heart, which provides additional protection against ischemia. The degree of hypothermia, 18-34°C, depends on the complexity and time needed to complete the procedure. The heart can be arrested with high-potassium cardioplegic solution delivered through the coronary arteries antegrade (through a cannula proximal to an aortic cross-clamp in the aorta) or retrograde (through a cannula placed in the coronary sinus). Arresting the heart allows the surgeon to operate safely with a still and bloodless field. An additional vent can be placed via the right superior pulmonary vein to capture pulmonary venous return and to assist in deairing of the heart.

Hypothermic circulatory arrest is required for complex aortic arch reconstructions. This involves cooling the patient to 18°C for a minimum of 20 minutes to ensure even cooling of the brain and body. The head is packed in ice, the patient's blood is drained into the venous reservoir, and the pump is turned off. The cannulae can then be removed from the field to aid in visualization and repair of the arch. No absolute safe duration of hypothermic circulatory arrest has been determined, but it is generally felt that it should be limited to no more than 45 minutes. Alternative techniques, such as regional cerebral perfusion and intermittent low-flow perfusion, have been employed to minimize the need for hypothermic circulatory arrest. To date, however, there is no literature to support that these techniques have additional benefit without additional risk.

POSTOPERATIVE MANAGEMENT

Patients are brought to the intensive care unit intubated and mechanically ventilated. All patients have temporary pacing wires in place for management of bradyarrhythmias

and tachyarrhythmias. Many patients have additional intracardiac lines in place for pulmonary artery and left atrial pressure monitoring. Drainage catheters are placed within the mediastinum to prevent accumulation of blood and fluid. These are usually removed 2-4 days following surgery. Prophylactic antibiotics are given preoperatively as well as postoperatively when drainage tubes are in place.

Cardiopulmonary bypass produces a significant inflammatory response due to activation of cytokines. Patients exhibit fluid retention and pulmonary dysfunction as a result, requiring aggressive use of diuretics and mechanical ventilation as needed. Bleeding is a common complication following cardiac surgery and infrequently requires surgical exploration (< 2%). Postoperative coagulopathy results from a multitude of factors, including hemodilution, platelet damage, factor consumption, immature hepatic production of clotting factors, and incomplete reversal of heparin with protamine sulfate. Approximately 30% of all patients will have some arrhythmia after surgery, ranging from simple premature ventricular contractions to malignant tachyarrhythmias. The risk for long-term arrhythmias requiring chronic medication or heart block requiring a permanent pacemaker is approximately 1%. Most patients require hemodynamic support with vasopressors along with afterload reduction, as necessary, for ventricular dysfunction. Dopamine, epinephrine, and vasopressin are the first-line vasopressors for pediatric patients. Milrinone is used primarily for afterload reduction. Critically ill neonates may have thyroid and adrenal hypofunction, which can further exacerbate postoperative hemodynamic instability. Profound hemodynamic compromise occasionally requires additional mechanical assistance. Extracorporeal membrane oxygenation (ECMO) is the most widely and acutely available mechanical support for the pediatric population. The survival for congenital heart disease patients requiring ECMO support is approximately 50%. For patients in low cardiac output state, it is essential to rule out residual defects or repair failures that could be readdressed surgically or in the catheterization laboratory.

The pediatric population has highly reactive pulmonary vasculature that is unique from the adult cardiac surgery population. Postoperative pulmonary hypertensive crises can occur in the newborn and infant population. Crises can be initiated with agitation such as endotracheal suctioning. Maneuvers to minimize and treat pulmonary hypertensive crises include high-dose opioid anesthesia with fentanyl, paralysis, respiratory alkalosis, high fraction of inspired oxygen, and inhaled nitric oxide. Chronic agents to treat persistent pulmonary hypertension include phosphodiesterase inhibitors (eg, sildenafil) and prostacyclin (eg, epoprostenol sodium [Flolan]).

CYANOTIC HEART DEFECTS

Cyanotic heart defects result from shunting of deoxygenated blood from the right side of the heart to the oxygenated left side of the heart or inadequate pulmonary blood flow.

The relative mixing of deoxygenated and oxygenated blood produces desaturation of the arterial blood. The majority of cyanotic heart defects are diagnosed within the first few days to months of life. Cyanotic heart defects represent approximately 25% of all congenital heart defects.

The classic 5 T's of cyanotic heart defects—(1) tetralogy of Fallot (TOF); (2) transposition of the great arteries (TGAs); (3) truncus arteriosus; (4) total anomalous pulmonary venous return; and (5) tricuspid atresia are presented in this chapter, along with hypoplastic left heart syndrome (HLHS).

Tetralogy of Fallot

A. General Considerations

TOF is the most common cyanotic congenital heart defect. It occurs in 0.6 per 1000 live births and has a prevalence of about 4% among all patients with congenital heart disease. The pathologic anatomy is frequently described as having four components: VSD, overriding aorta, pulmonary stenosis, and right ventricular (RV) hypertrophy (Figure 21–1). Embryologically, the anatomy of TOF is thought to result from a single defect: anterior malalignment of the infundibular septum. The infundibular septum normally separates the primitive outflow tracts and fuses with the ventricular septum. Anterior malalignment of the infundibular septum creates a VSD due to failure of fusion with the ventricular septum and also displaces the aorta over the VSD and right ventricle. Infundibular malalignment also crowds the RV outflow tract, causing pulmonary stenosis and, secondarily, RV hypertrophy. Prominent muscle bands also extend from

the septal insertion of the infundibular septum to the RV free wall and contribute to the obstruction of the RV outflow tract. The pulmonary valve is usually stenotic and is bicuspid in 58% of cases. Pulmonary atresia occurs in about 7% of cases. The branch pulmonary arteries in TOF may exhibit mild diffuse hypoplasia or discrete stenosis (most frequently of the left pulmonary artery at the site of ductal insertion). Coronary artery anomalies are frequently present. The origin of the left anterior descending artery from the right coronary artery, which occurs in 5% of cases, is clinically important because the vessel crosses the RV infundibulum and is vulnerable to injury at the time of surgery. A right aortic arch is present in 25% of patients. Associated defects include ASD, complete atrioventricular septal defect (AVSD), PDA, or multiple VSDs.

B. Clinical Findings

Patients with TOF develop cyanosis due to right-to-left shunting across the VSD. The degree of cyanosis depends on the severity of obstruction of the RV outflow tract. Frequently, cyanosis is mild at birth and may remain undetected for weeks or months. Neonates with severe infundibular obstruction or pulmonary atresia will develop symptoms shortly after birth and require a prostaglandin infusion to maintain ductal patency to ensure adequate pulmonary blood flow. In other patients, the RV outflow tract obstruction is minor, and the predominant physiology is that of a large VSD with left-to-right shunting and congestive heart failure.

The occurrence of intermittent cyanotic spells is a well-known feature of tetralogy. The etiology of "spelling" is still

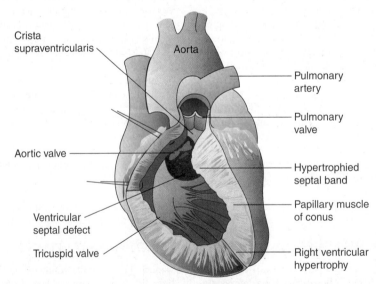

▲ **Figure 21–1.** Tetralogy of Fallot. The aorta overrides the ventricular septum. A large ventricular septal defect is present, and the hypoplastic infundibulum with hypertrophied muscle bands obstructs blood to the pulmonary arteries.

controversial but is clearly related to a transient imbalance between pulmonary and systemic blood flow. A spell may be triggered by hypovolemia or peripheral vasodilation (eg, after a bath or vigorous physical exertion). Spells may occur in neonates but are most frequently reported in infants between the ages of 3 and 18 months. Most spells resolve spontaneously within a few minutes, but some spells may be fatal. Older children have been observed to spontaneously squat to terminate spells. The squatting position is thought to increase systemic vascular resistance, which thereby favors pulmonary blood flow.

Cyanosis is the most frequent physical finding in TOF. Auscultation reveals a normal first heart sound and a single second heart sound. A systolic ejection murmur is present at the left upper sternal border. Older children may develop clubbing of the fingers and toes. Chest radiography typically demonstrates a boot-shaped heart due to elevation of the cardiac apex from RV hypertrophy. Pulmonary vascular markings are usually reduced. A right aortic arch may be present. An ECG shows RV hypertrophy. Echocardiography is definitive, and catheterization is not necessary in most cases.

C. Treatment

The medical management of TOF is directed toward the treatment and prevention of cyanotic spells. The immediate treatment of the spelling patient includes administration of oxygen, narcotics for sedation, and correction of acidosis. Transfusion is indicated for anemic infants. Alpha-agonists are useful for increasing systemic vascular resistance (which favors pulmonary blood flow). Some centers have used beta-blockers as a form of long-term therapy to suppress the incidence of spells. Long-term complications of untreated TOF include clubbing of the fingers and toes, severe dyspnea on exertion, brain abscesses (secondary to right-to-left shunting), paradoxical embolization, and polycythemia (which may lead to cerebral thrombosis). Long-term survival is unlikely for most patients with untreated TOF.

All patients with TOF should undergo surgical repair. Asymptomatic patients should be repaired electively between 4 and 6 months of age. Early repair is indicated for neonates with severe cyanosis and for infants who have had a documented spell or worsening cyanosis.

Classically, the repair of TOF was accomplished in two stages. During the first stage, pulmonary blood flow was augmented by creating a connection (or shunt) between a systemic artery and the pulmonary artery. At the second stage, the shunt was taken down, and a complete repair was performed. The first shunt procedure was the Blalock-Taussig shunt, in which the subclavian artery was mobilized and divided distally and an end-to-side anastomosis was created between the inferiorly deflected subclavian and the ipsilateral pulmonary artery. The modified Blalock-Taussig shunt is the most common type of shunt used today and consists of an interposition graft (polytetrafluoroethylene) between the innominate or subclavian artery and the ipsilateral pulmonary artery. Creation of a shunt may be accomplished with or without the use of cardiopulmonary bypass.

Currently, one-stage repair of TOF is preferred by most centers. Initial palliation with a shunt is still indicated for some patients who present a high risk for complete repair, such as those with multiple congenital anomalies, significant prematurity, severe concurrent illness, or an anomalous coronary artery crossing a hypoplastic infundibulum.

Complete repair of TOF is performed using a median sternotomy and cardiopulmonary bypass with bicaval venous cannulation. By a transatrial approach, the RV outflow tract can be examined through the tricuspid valve. Muscle bundles obstructing the RV outflow tract are divided or resected. The VSD is closed with a patch. Pulmonary valvotomy is performed, when indicated, via a vertical incision in the main pulmonary artery. When the pulmonary valve annulus or infundibulum is severely hypoplastic, a transannular outflow tract patch may be necessary to relieve the obstruction. When an anomalous coronary artery crosses the infundibulum, a transannular incision may be contraindicated. In these cases, and in patients with pulmonary atresia, placement of a conduit (cryopreserved homograft or bioprosthetic heterograft) between the right ventricle (via a separate ventriculotomy) and main pulmonary artery will be necessary. Patients who undergo construction of a transannular patch develop pulmonary insufficiency as a consequence. This is surprisingly well tolerated in most infants, as long as the tricuspid valve is competent.

As these patients grow older, some will develop RV failure due to chronic pulmonary insufficiency, and pulmonary valve replacement may be necessary. Currently, pulmonary valve replacement is indicated for symptomatic patients or those at risk of life-threatening arrhythmias. For asymptomatic patients, it is generally agreed that pulmonary valve replacement should be undertaken before irreversible RV dysfunction occurs. cMRI has evolved as a valuable diagnostic tool for evaluating RV size, function, anatomic detail, and other hemodynamic parameters. An RV size "cutoff" is debated, but recent recommendations suggest considering valve replacement before RV end-diastolic volume index exceeds approximately 160 mL/m^2. Catheter-based pulmonary valve replacement is an option for some patients depending on the RV outflow tract anatomy.

D. Prognosis and Complications

The early mortality following repair of TOF is 1%-5%. The results are worse for patients with TOF and pulmonary atresia. Long-term complications include recurrent obstruction of the RV outflow tract and development of RV dysfunction due to chronic pulmonary insufficiency. Actuarial survival at 20 years is 90% with excellent functional status.

Cheung EW, Wong WH, Cheung YF: Meta-analysis of pulmonary valve replacement after operative repair of tetralogy of Fallot. *Am J Cardiol.* 2010;106:552-557.

Kalfa DM, Serraf AE, Ly M, et al: Tetralogy of Fallot with an abnormal coronary artery: surgical options and prognostic factors. *Eur J Cardiothorac Surg.* 2012;42:e34-39.

Lee C, Kim YM, Lee CH, et al: Outcomes of pulmonary valve replacement in 170 patients with chronic pulmonary regurgitation after relief of right ventricular outflow tract obstruction: implications for optimal timing of pulmonary valve replacement. *JACC.* 2012;60:1005-1014.

Valente AM, Gauvreau K, Assenza GE, et al: Rationale and design of an international multicenter registry of patients with repaired tetralogy of Fallot to define risk factors for late adverse outcomes: the INDICATOR cohort. *Pediatr Cardiol.* 2013;34(1):95-104.

van de Woestijne PC, Mokhles MM, de Jong PL, et al: Right ventricular outflow tract reconstruction with an allograft conduit in patients after tetralogy of Fallot correction: long-term follow-up. *Ann Thorac Surg* 2011;92:161-166.

▶ Transposition of Great Arteries

A. General Considerations

TGA is a congenital cardiac anomaly in which the aorta arises from the right ventricle and the pulmonary artery originates from the left ventricle (Figure 21–2). TGA is divided into *dextro*-looped (d-TGA) and *levo*-looped (l-TGA). The looping refers to the right or left looping of the primitive heart tube during fetal development, which determines whether the atria and ventricles are concordant (right atrium attaches to the right ventricle and left atrium attaches to the left ventricle) or discordant. l-TGA is associated with atrioventricular (AV) discordance (right atrium attaches to the left ventricle and left atrium attaches to the right ventricle) and is also termed congenitally corrected TGA. l-TGA is a rare variant of TGA and is beyond the scope of this chapter, which focuses on d-TGA. The defect can be subdivided into d-TGA with intact ventricular septum (IVS) (55%-60%) and d-TGA with VSD (40%-45%), one-third of which are hemodynamically insignificant. Pulmonic stenosis, causing significant left ventricular outflow tract obstruction, occurs rarely with an IVS and in approximately 10% of d-TGA/VSD.

B. Clinical Findings

d-TGA is a relatively common cardiac anomaly and is the most common form of congenital heart disease presenting as cyanosis in the first week of life. The malformation accounts for approximately 10% of all congenital cardiovascular malformations in infants. The degree of cyanosis depends on the amount of mixing between the pulmonary and systemic circulations. In d-TGA, oxygenated pulmonary venous blood is returned to the lungs, and desaturated systemic blood is returned to the body. Because the two circulations exist in parallel, some mixing between them must occur to allow

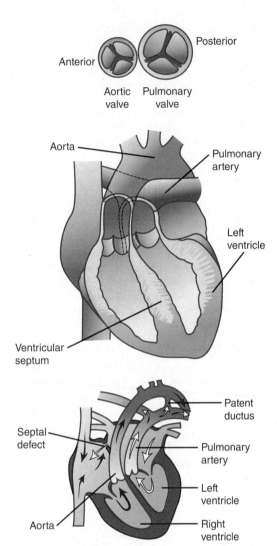

▲ **Figure 21–2.** Typical transposition of the great arteries. The aorta arises from the morphologic right ventricle and is anterior and slightly to the right of the pulmonary artery, which originates from the morphologic left ventricle. Inset at bottom illustrates the independent systemic and pulmonary circulations, which may be connected by a patent ductus arteriosus or atrial septal defect. Inset at top illustrates a common relationship of the two great arteries in typical transposition.

oxygenated blood to reach the systemic circulation and the desaturated blood to reach the lungs. Mixing may occur at a number of levels, most commonly at the atrial level through an ASD or a patent foramen ovale (PFO). Generally, two levels of mixing are necessary to maintain adequate systemic oxygen delivery with a VSD or PDA serving as an additional site for cardiac mixing. In d-TGA, there can be no fixed shunt in one direction without an equal amount of blood passing in the other direction; otherwise, one circulation would eventually empty into the other. Therefore, the amount of desaturated blood reaching the lungs (effective pulmonary blood flow) must equal the amount of saturated blood reaching the aorta (effective systemic blood flow). Clinical characteristics are dependent on the degree of mixing and the amount of pulmonary blood flow. These factors relate to the specific anatomic subtype of d-TGA. Neonates with d-TGA/IVS (or small VSD) have mixing limited to the atrial level and PDA. The ASD may be restrictive, and the PDA generally will close over the first days to week of life. As the degree of mixing decreases, the patient becomes increasingly cyanotic and will eventually suffer cardiovascular collapse. Fortunately, the majority of these neonates will manifest cyanosis early in life, which is recognized by a nurse or physician within the first hour in 56% and in the first day in 92%. In d-TGA with a large VSD, there is additional opportunity for mixing and increased pulmonary blood flow. The neonate with d-TGA/VSD may manifest only mild cyanosis, which may be initially overlooked. However, generally within 2-6 weeks, signs and symptoms of congestive heart failure will emerge. Tachypnea and tachycardia become prominent, while cyanosis may remain mild. Auscultatory findings are consistent with congestive heart failure with increased pulmonary blood flow, including a pansystolic murmur, third heart sound, mid-diastolic rumble, gallop, and narrowly split second heart sound with an increased pulmonary component. Neonates with d-TGA and significant pulmonary stenosis present with severe cyanosis at birth. Lesser degrees of pulmonary stenosis will result in varying levels of cyanosis.

In cases of d-TGA, the ECG is normal at birth, demonstrating the typical pattern of RV dominance. Although the classic chest radiographic appearance of an egg-shaped heart with a narrow superior mediastinum may be seen, this finding is often obscured by an enlarged thymic shadow. The abnormal ventriculoarterial connection is clearly seen on echocardiography, which demonstrates that the posterior great vessel arising from the left ventricle is a pulmonary artery that bifurcates soon after its origin. The anterior great vessel is the aorta and arises from the RV. Associated lesions, including VSD, left ventricular outflow tract obstruction, and coarctation, may also be diagnosed. Although used less frequently for diagnosis, cardiac catheterization may be helpful to improve cardiac mixing by means of balloon atrial septostomy.

C. Treatment

The infant with d-TGA and severe cyanosis requires prompt diagnosis and treatment to improve mixing and increase the arterial oxygen saturation. The first intervention to improve mixing in a cyanotic newborn suspected of having TGA is

to ensure ductal patency by beginning an infusion of prostaglandin E_1. In the presence of a restrictive ASD, a balloon atrial septostomy, a technique developed by William Rashkind in 1966, is performed. The procedure involves inserting a balloon-tipped catheter across the foramen ovale into the left atrium. Inflation and forcible withdrawal of the catheter tears the septum primum and enlarges the ASD. Mixing generally increases immediately, with a substantial increase in arterial oxygen saturation. Without intervention, d-TGA is universally fatal. Untreated, 30% of neonates will die in the first week of life, 50% by the first month, 70% within 6 months, and 90% by 1 year. The definitive surgical treatment of patients with d-TGA has changed dramatically with the advent of the arterial switch operation (ASO). The ASO, first successfully performed by Jatene in 1975, has become the optimal surgical procedure for infants with this condition. Current techniques have reduced the operative mortality to 2%-4%. The operative technique involves transection of both great vessels and direct reanastomosis to reestablish ventriculoarterial concordance. Additionally, the coronary arteries are removed from the anterior aorta and relocated to the posterior great vessel (neoaorta). The extensive experience gained with this procedure has confirmed that any variant of coronary artery anatomy can be successfully repaired, although certain unusual forms impose a higher risk. Because many patients with d-TGA have an IVS, left ventricular pressure falls early in life as pulmonary vascular resistance decreases. In this situation, it is essential that the arterial repair be performed within the first 2-3 weeks of life, while the left ventricle is still able to meet systemic workloads. In patients presenting later, the left ventricle can be retrained with a preliminary pulmonary artery band and aortopulmonary shunt followed by the definitive arterial repair. Although patients with large VSDs do not require early repair because of their decreased left ventricular pressure, experience has indicated that even in this subgroup, the operation is best performed within the first month of life, before secondary complications such as pulmonary hypertension, congestive heart failure, or infection develop.

Patients with fixed left ventricular outflow tract obstruction are not candidates for the arterial repair because correction would result in systemic ventricular outflow tract obstruction. Most of these patients also have large VSDs. Palliation early in life with systemic-to-pulmonary artery shunting is an option, with definitive repair postponed until somatic growth results in cyanosis as the shunt is outgrown. At that time, the Rastelli procedure is performed, in which left ventricular blood is redirected through the VSD to the anterior aorta by placement of an intraventricular patch. The pulmonary artery is ligated, and right ventricle-to-distal pulmonary artery continuity is reestablished with a valve-bearing conduit. An increasing number of experienced centers currently recommend early complete repair in the neonatal period using a Rastelli procedure. Early repair eliminates the interim morbidity and mortality associated with a systemic-to-pulmonary artery shunt and chronic cyanosis.

D. Prognosis

Hospital survival for the ASO is 96.6%-97.2%. Generally, d-TGA/IVS has had a lower mortality than d-TGA/VSD or d-TGA/VSD/pulmonary stenosis. Hospital mortality for d-TGA/IVS is 2.2%, compared to 4.3% for d-TGA/VSD. Long-term survival rates at 5-10 years and 15-20 years are 92.2%-97.9% and 91.6%-96%, respectively. The most common cause for reintervention is supravalvar pulmonary stenosis, occurring in 19.7%-30.3% of patients. A study of 40 patients undergoing a Rastelli operation over a 20-year period revealed a hospital mortality of 0%, with Kaplan-Meier survival of 93% at 5, 10, and 20 years. Freedom from conduit replacement was 86% at 5 years and 59% at 20 years.

Brown JW, Ruzmetov M, Huynh D, et al: Rastelli operation for transposition of the great arteries with ventricular septal defect and pulmonary stenosis. *Ann Thorac Surg*. 2011;91:188-193.

Dodge-Khatami A, Mavroudis C, Mavroudis CD, et al: Past, present, and future of the arterial switch operation: historical review. *Cardiol Young*. 2012;22:724-731.

Fricke TA, d'Udekem Y, Richardson M, et al: Outcomes of the arterial switch operation for transposition of the great arteries: 25 years of experience. *Ann Thorac Surg*. 2012;94:139-145.

Kempny A, Wustmann K, Borgia F, et al: Outcome in adult patients after arterial switch operation for transposition of the great arteries. *Int J Cardiol*. 2013;167(6):2588-93.

Oda S, Nakano T, Suqiura J, et al: Twenty-eight years' experience of arterial switch operation for transposition of the great arteries in a single institution. *Eur J Cardiothoracic Surg*. 2012;42:674-679.

► Truncus Arteriosus

A. General Considerations

Truncus arteriosus is a rare anomaly that accounts for 0.4%-4% of all cases of congenital heart disease. A single arterial vessel arises from the heart, overriding the ventricular septum, and gives rise to the systemic, coronary, and pulmonary circulations. The Collett and Edwards classification of truncus arteriosus focuses on the origin of the pulmonary arteries from the common arterial trunk, as follows:

Type I: Common arterial trunk gives rise to a main pulmonary artery and the aorta.

Type II: Right and left pulmonary arteries arise directly from and in close proximity to the posterior wall of the truncus.

Type III: Right and left pulmonary arteries arise from more widely separated orifices on the posterior truncal wall.

Type IV: Branch pulmonary arteries are absent. Pulmonary blood flow is derived from aortopulmonary collaterals.

Persistent truncus arteriosus is the result of failed development of the aortopulmonary septum and subpulmonary infundibulum (conal septum). Normal septation leads to the development of both pulmonary and systemic outflow tracts, division of the semilunar valves, and formation of the aorta and pulmonary arteries. Failure of septation results in a VSD (absence of the infundibular septum), a single semilunar valve, and a single arterial trunk. Most cases are associated with a VSD with the superior margin of the defect formed by the truncal valve. The truncal valve leaflets are generally dysmorphic and their motion may be restricted. Leaflet number is highly variable, with about 65% tricuspid, 22% quadricuspid, 9% bicuspid, and rarely unicuspid or pentacuspid. As a result of these abnormally developed valve leaflets, a moderate or greater degree of truncal insufficiency is present in 20%-26% of patients. The pulmonary arteries are usually of normal size and most often arise from the left posterolateral aspect of the truncal artery, often in close proximity to the truncal valve and ostium of the left coronary artery.

Other cardiac anomalies are common and include an ASD (9%-20%), an interrupted aortic arch (10%-20%), and coronary ostial abnormalities (37%-49%) with the left coronary artery frequently noted to have a high origin, not uncommonly near the takeoff of the pulmonary arteries. Extracardiac anomalies are reported in approximately 28% of patients with truncus arteriosus. Described abnormalities include skeletal, genitourinary, gastrointestinal, and DiGeorge syndrome (11%).

B. Clinical Findings

The anatomy of truncus arteriosus results in obligatory mixing of systemic and pulmonary venous blood at the level of the VSD and truncal valve, which produces arterial saturations of 85%-90%. The systemic arterial saturation depends on the volume of pulmonary blood flow, which in turn is determined by the pulmonary vascular resistance (PVR). As the resistance begins to fall, excessive pulmonary circulation ensues and leads to pulmonary congestion and signs and symptoms of congestive heart failure. This nonrestrictive left-to-right shunt may cause early development of irreversible pulmonary vascular obstructive disease.

The presence of truncal valve abnormalities poses further hemodynamic burdens. Truncal valve regurgitation leads to ventricular dilation and low diastolic coronary perfusion pressures that can result in myocardial ischemia. Truncal valve stenosis promotes ventricular hypertrophy, increases the myocardial oxygen demand, and limits coronary and systemic perfusion, especially with the large volume of runoff into the pulmonary vascular bed.

Neonates with truncus arteriosus present with signs of congestive heart failure and collapsing peripheral pulses. CXR shows marked cardiomegaly, pulmonary plethora, often with minimal thymus shadow, and a right aortic arch. The ECG most often depicts biventricular hypertrophy. Echocardiography is the diagnostic procedure of choice and can demonstrate the truncal vessel, the structure and function of the truncal valve, associated lesions such as interrupted aortic arch, and often the pulmonary arterial anatomy. Cardiac catheterization is not performed unless the anatomy is unclear, further information is needed about the status of the truncal valve, or the status of the pulmonary vasculature is unclear (ie, infants older than 3 months at diagnosis).

C. Treatment

The natural history of patients born with truncus arteriosus is early demise. Approximately 40% of infants are dead within 1 month, 70% by 3 months, and 90% by 1 year. Early death is caused by congestive heart failure. Survivors may do well for a period of time until the development of pulmonary vascular obstructive disease and Eisenmenger syndrome. The ultimate treatment of truncus arteriosus is surgical correction in the neonatal period. Medical treatment is palliative and directed toward controlling congestive heart failure with fluid restriction, diuretics, and afterload reduction. Complete repair entails separating the pulmonary arteries from the truncus, repairing the resulting defect in the aorta, closing the VSD, and restoring continuity of the RV outflow tract with an extracardiac conduit (Figure 21–3). Severe truncal valve regurgitation requires truncal valve repair or replacement. An associated interrupted aortic arch is repaired by constructing a primary end-to-end anastomosis of the distal ascending aorta with proximal augmentation if necessary.

D. Prognosis

The results of truncus arteriosus repair have improved greatly over the past two decades. Before the importance of early operation to avoid irreversible pulmonary vascular disease was appreciated, patients underwent repair at most institutions at an average age of 2-5 years with high mortality rates. Current hospital mortality for the neonatal repair of truncus arteriosus ranges between 4.3% and 17%, with the majority of deaths occurring in complex truncus arteriosus or in truncus arteriosus with associated severe truncal valve regurgitation. All patients will ultimately require reoperation for replacement of the right ventricle to pulmonary artery conduit, with only 30%-42% being free from reoperation at 10 years. Thirty-year survival is approximately 75%-83%.

de Siena P, Ghorbel M, Chen Q, et al: Common arterial trunk: review of surgical strategies and future research. *Expert Rev Cardiovasc Ther* 2011;12:1527-1538.

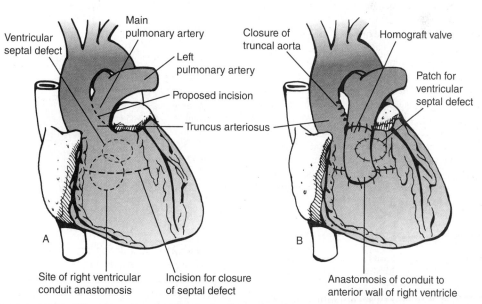

▲ **Figure 21–3.** Type 1 truncus arteriosus. **A:** The main pulmonary artery arises from the truncus arteriosus downstream to the truncal valve. A ventricular septal defect is present. **B:** The main pulmonary artery is incised from the truncus. The ventricular septal defect is closed with a patch. A valved conduit is sutured to the anterior wall of the right ventricle and the distal pulmonary artery.

► Total Anomalous Pulmonary Venous Connection

A. General Considerations

Total anomalous pulmonary venous connection (TAPVC) is a relatively uncommon congenital defect representing approximately 2% of all congenital heart anomalies. TAPVC encompasses a group of anomalies in which the pulmonary veins connect directly to the systemic venous circulation via persistent splanchnic connections. This abnormality results from failed transfer, in the normal developmental sequence, of pulmonary venous drainage from the splanchnic plexus to the left atrium. The most common classification system consists of four types: supracardiac (type 1), cardiac (type 2), infracardiac (type 3), and mixed (Figure 21–4). Partial anomalous pulmonary venous connection defines patients in whom some but not all venous drainage enters the left atrium, while the remaining veins connect to one or more persistent splanchnic veins.

TAPVC can also be classified by the presence of obstruction. Impingement from surrounding structures or inadequate caliber of the draining pulmonary vein(s) can result in varying degrees of obstruction. Obstruction in supracardiac TAPVC can occur by compression of the ascending vertical vein between the left main stem bronchus and left pulmonary artery or by narrowing at the insertion of the vertical vein into the innominate vein. Obstruction is always present in the infracardiac type because the pulmonary venous blood must pass through the sinusoids of the liver. Obstruction is uncommon in the cardiac type.

Supracardiac occurs in approximately 45% of patients. The common pulmonary vein drains superiorly into the innominate vein, superior vena cava, or azygous vein via an ascending vertical vein. Cardiac TAPVC occurs in approximately 25% of patients. The pulmonary venous confluence drains into the coronary sinus, or on rare occasions, individual pulmonary veins will connect directly into the right atrium. Infracardiac TAPVC occurs in approximately 25% of patients. The pulmonary venous confluence drains into a descending vertical vein through the diaphragm into the portal vein or ductus venosus. Finally, a mixed type of TAPVC occurs in approximately 5% of patients and can involve any or all components of the previous three types.

B. Clinical Findings

TAPVC produces a mixing lesion because oxygenated blood from the pulmonary system drains back into the systemic venous circulation. The size of the ASD dictates the distribution of blood flow. Most patients with unobstructed TAPVC have few or no symptoms in infancy and present with signs and symptoms similar to an ASD. In the neonate with obstructed TAPVC, venous drainage from the pulmonary vasculature is impaired, leading to pulmonary venous

Type 1

Type 2

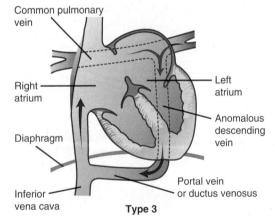

Type 3

▲ **Figure 21–4.** Common types of total anomalous pulmonary venous connection. Type 1: The pulmonary veins connect to a persistent left vertical vein, the innominate vein, and the right superior vena cava. Type 2: The pulmonary veins connect to the coronary sinus and the right atrium. Type 3: The pulmonary veins connect to an anomalous descending vein, a portal vein or persistent ductus venosus, and eventually enter the inferior vena cava.

hypertension and pulmonary edema. In severe cases, this increased pressure will lead to reflexive vasoconstriction of the pulmonary vasculature with pulmonary hypertension. Patients with obstruction present early in life with profound cyanosis from pulmonary edema.

The diagnosis can be made with echocardiographic identification of the anomalous connection of the pulmonary venous confluence to the systemic venous system. The ASD and other associated anomalies can be delineated. Cardiac catheterization is rarely necessary unless accurate measurement of PVR is needed.

The management of TAPVC is surgical repair. In patients with obstruction, medical management for stabilization may be employed but is often unsuccessful and should not delay surgical intervention.

C. Treatment

The principle of operative repair is to establish an unobstructed communication between the pulmonary venous confluence and the left atrium, interrupt the connections with the systemic venous circulation, and close the ASD. The specific repair is dependent on the type of anomalous connection.

1. **Supracardiac TAPVC:** The repair of supracardiac TAPVC may be performed with moderate hypothermia (28-32°C) and bicaval cannulation or with a brief period of hypothermic (18°C) circulatory arrest. The optimal approach is to retract the ascending aorta to the left and the superior vena cava to the right to expose the pulmonary venous confluence. This approach provides excellent exposure without distortion of the heart or venous structures. The vertical vein can be identified and ligated (just prior to opening the confluence) outside the pericardium at the level of the innominate vein. A transverse incision is made in the pulmonary venous confluence, and a parallel incision is placed in the dome of the left atrium beginning at the base of the left atrial appendage. The common pulmonary vein is then anastomosed to the left atrium, taking care to construct an unrestrictive connection. A right atriotomy is made to close the ASD.

2. **Cardiac TAPVC:** The repair of cardiac TAPVC can be performed with bicaval cannulation and moderate hypothermia with the use of a vent or a cardiotomy sucker to capture the pulmonary venous return. A right atriotomy is performed with identification of the ASD and the orifice of the coronary sinus. The roof of the coronary sinus is excised into the left atrium. A patch of pericardium or prosthetic material is then placed to close the enlarged ASD, effectively channeling the pulmonary venous and coronary sinus return into the left atrium. The conduction system travels in proximity to the coronary sinus, and care must be taken while suturing the patch in this area to avoid heart block.

3. **Infracardiac TAPVC:** For infracardiac connections, a brief period of hypothermic circulatory arrest is often required. The heart is rotated superiorly. The descending vertical vein is identified by opening the posterior pericardium. The connection to the descending vertical vein is ligated at the level of the diaphragm. An incision is made along the length of the pulmonary venous confluence with a parallel incision on the posterior wall of the left atrium. The pulmonary venous confluence is then anastomosed to the left atrium, taking care not to narrow the connection. Tissue from the descending vertical vein can be used in the anastomosis. A right atriotomy is performed through which the ASD is closed.

4. **Recurrent pulmonary venous obstruction:** The approach to recurrent pulmonary venous obstruction is dependent on the level of obstruction. Obstruction can develop at the anastomosis or within the individual pulmonary veins. The latter may initially present as an anastomotic constriction, as the true extent of obstruction is not always apparent at first. Isolated narrowing of the anastomosis between the common pulmonary vein and left atrium often can be repaired with revision or patch augmentation of the anastomosis.

Obstruction of the individual pulmonary venous ostia is the greater challenge. Although the obstruction may initially appear to be limited to the ostium, progressive narrowing along the entire length of the vein into the hilum of the lung may occur with time. Repair of this lesion is technically challenging, and recurrent early obstruction is common. A new approach to recurrent pulmonary vein stenosis employs a "sutureless" technique utilizing in situ pericardium to create a neoatrium. The theory behind this repair is based on the concept that pulmonary venous obstruction results from inflammation induced locally by suture placement. Repair involves wide unroofing of the narrowed portion of each involved pulmonary vein from the left atrial anastomosis to the hilum. A wide flap of pericardium is then elevated with care taken to avoid disruption of posterior adhesions and injury to the phrenic nerve. This flap of pericardium is rotated over the unroofed pulmonary veins and sutured to the left atrial wall away from the venous ostia. A large neoatrium is then created into which pulmonary venous return can drain.

D. Prognosis

Early mortality in patients undergoing repair of TAPVC is associated with the initial degree of obstruction present. Early diagnosis and repair as well as optimal postoperative management, including aggressive treatment of pulmonary hypertension, have resulted in a dramatic reduction in operative risk. For patients surviving the perioperative period, the long-term survival and functional status are excellent.

Recurrent venous obstruction develops in 5%-17.5% of patients. Results following balloon angioplasty and/or stent insertion have been disappointing, and recurrent stenoses are the rules. Individual patch angioplasty of the ostia has also been used with poor long-term results. Lung transplantation has been considered in severe cases of extensive, bilateral disease. The mortality associated with reoperation for obstruction can be up to 59% when bilateral stenoses are present. The use of the sutureless technique for recurrent pulmonary vein obstruction has demonstrated improved survival and decreased recurrence.

Aquirre J, Mavroudis C, Jacobs M, et al: Direct operating room triage of neonates with total anomalous pulmonary venous connection. *Pediatr Cardiol.* 2013;34(8):1874-1876.

Hammel JM, Hunt PW, Abdullah I, et al: "Closed-vein" technique for primary sutureless repair of anomalous pulmonary venous connection. *Ann Thorac Surg.* 2012;94:1021-1022.

Hickey EJ, Caldarone CA: Surgical management of post-repair pulmonary vein stenosis. *Semin Thorac Cardiovasc Surg Pediatr Card Surg Annu.* 2011;14:101-108.

Seale AN, Uemura H, Webber SA, et al: Total anomalous pulmonary venous connection: outcome of postoperative pulmonary venous obstruction. *J Thorac Cardiovasc Surg.* 2013; 145(5):1255-1262.

Yoshimura N, Fukahara K, Yamashita A, et al: Management of pulmonary venous obstruction. *Gen Thorac Cardiovasc Surg.* 2012;60(12):785-791.

Tricuspid Atresia

A. General Considerations

Tricuspid atresia refers to single-ventricle hearts that lack a communication between the right atrium and right ventricle. The only outlet for the right atrium is the ASD. If present, aneurysmal tissue of the septum primum may prolapse into the left atrium. The left atrium is normal in morphology but is often dilated. A normal communication with a mitral valve between the left atrium and left ventricle is present. The right ventricle is diminutive in size without an inlet portion. It is connected to the left ventricle by a VSD surrounded completely by muscle. The anatomic subtypes of tricuspid atresia are based on the relationship of the great arteries. Type I defects (70%) have normally related great vessels, type II (30%) have transposed great arteries, and type III (rare) have congenitally corrected TGAs. These types are further subclassified by the degree of obstruction to pulmonary blood flow, which is present in 45%-75% of patients. Aortic valve (10%) and aortic arch (25%) obstruction may also be present. Patients with tricuspid atresia are at increased risk for Wolff-Parkinson-White syndrome due to congenital and surgically acquired pathways.

B. Clinical Findings

The clinical presentation depends on the relationship of the great vessels and degree of restriction at the level of the atrial

and ventricular septum. Most infants present with some degree of cyanosis. Systemic output is usually unobstructed. Prostaglandins may be necessary to maintain ductal patency in infants with severe obstruction to pulmonary blood flow.

C. Treatment

The initial palliation for most patients is the placement of a modified Blalock-Taussig shunt to maintain adequate pulmonary blood flow. A more complex initial palliation with a Norwood procedure may be necessary in the case of transposed great vessels. The remainder of the palliation involves a hemi-Fontan and Fontan procedure (discussed in the section on hypoplastic left heart syndrome).

D. Prognosis

The overall survival for tricuspid atresia is similar to that reported for other single-ventricle lesions palliated with a Fontan procedure. The survival is 83% at 1 year, 70% at 10 years, and 60% at 20 years.

Abdul-Sater Z, Yehya A, Beresian J, et al: Two heterozygous mutations in NFATC1 in a patient with tricuspid atresia. *PLoS One.* 2012;7:e49532.

Berg C, Lachmann R, Kaiser C, et al: Prenatal diagnosis of tricuspid atresia: intrauterine course and outcome. *Ultrasound Obstet Gynecol.* 2010;35:183-190.

Ho PK, Lai CT, Wong SJ, et al: Three-dimensional mechanical dyssynchrony and myocardial deformation of the left ventricle in patients with tricuspid atresia after Fontan procedure. *J Am Soc Echocardiogr.* 2012;25:393-400.

Hypoplastic Left Heart Syndrome

A. General Considerations

A variety of congenital cardiovascular malformations may result in a functional single-ventricle anatomy, most commonly tricuspid atresia, pulmonary atresia, unbalanced AVSD, and HLHS. The most common lesion is HLHS. Approximately 1000 infants with HLHS are born in the United States each year. It is the most common severe congenital heart defect, comprising 7%-9% of all anomalies diagnosed within the first year of life. All single-ventricle lesions share the common physiology of only a single ventricle capable of supporting cardiac output. HLHS refers to a constellation of congenital cardiac anomalies characterized by marked hypoplasia or absence of the left ventricle and severe hypoplasia of the ascending aorta. The systemic circulation is dependent on the right ventricle via a PDA, and there is obligatory mixing of pulmonary and systemic venous blood in the right atrium. There is associated aortic valve stenosis or atresia and mitral valve stenosis or atresia. The descending aorta is essentially a continuation of the ductus arteriosus, and the ascending aorta and aortic arch represents a diminutive branch of this vessel. Initial management includes a prostaglandin infusion to maintain ductal patency and correction of metabolic acidosis. The patient may require intubation and ventilator adjustment to reduce supplemental oxygen and maintain a $PaCO_2$ of about 40 mm Hg to avoid excessive pulmonary flow.

B. Treatment

Surgical approaches to the treatment of this problem include cardiac transplantation and staged reconstruction. In the context of improving results for staged reconstruction, risks of immunosuppression, and limited donor availability, competing risk analysis favors staged repair, and most centers pursue this option as primary therapy for HLHS. Transplantation is generally reserved for very high-risk patients, such as those with depressed RV function, severe tricuspid regurgitation, or significant coronary sinusoids.

The first successful palliation of HLHS was reported by Norwood on a series of infants operated on between 1979 and 1981. This procedure has been technically refined over the years, but three essential components remain: atrial septectomy, anastomosis of the proximal pulmonary artery to the aorta with homograft augmentation of the aortic arch, and aortopulmonary shunt. A "hybrid Norwood" procedure is an alternate form of stage I palliation. This procedure involves bilateral pulmonary artery bands and PDA stenting with or without concomitant balloon atrial septostomy. The ultimate goal of surgical palliation in patients with a univentricular heart is the total diversion of all vena caval blood directly into the pulmonary arteries. The Fontan procedure was first successfully performed in a patient with tricuspid atresia but has since evolved as an excellent way to establish physiologic repair for patients with more complex forms of univentricular heart. The superior vena caval blood returns directly via an end-to-side anastomosis with the pulmonary artery (bidirectional Glenn) or through a right atrial-pulmonary artery connection (hemi-Fontan) performed at 4-6 months of age. The inferior vena caval flow is directed to the pulmonary artery with an intra-atrial baffle (lateral tunnel technique) or an extracardiac conduit at 2-4 years of age. All oxygenated pulmonary venous flow empties into the ventricular chamber through the AV valves to be ejected to the systemic circulation, while superior and inferior vena caval blood flows directly to the lungs to acquire oxygen prior to returning to the heart. For the Fontan procedure to be performed with a low operative mortality and an acceptable functional result, certain criteria must be met. Normal pulmonary artery pressure (< 20 mm Hg) and PVR (< 2 Woods units·m²) are the most important prerequisites. Additionally, it is essential that ventricular function and AV valve function be normal. Although the Fontan procedure cannot be considered a truly corrective operation, it offers benefits that cannot be equaled by those of any of the other palliative procedures. The major advantages include restoration of normal systemic oxygen saturation and reduction of ventricular volume overload.

C. Prognosis

Universally fatal only three decades ago, tremendous strides have been made in improving the outcomes for patients with HLHS. Of the three stages, the highest-risk stage of the repair remains the Norwood operation. During the 1990s, the hospital survival for the Norwood procedure across the United States was approximately 40%. A recent Society of Thoracic Surgeons Congenital Heart Surgery Database study reported an 81% hospital survival rate for more than 2000 Norwood operations performed in 2009. Currently, interstage (time between the Norwood and hemi-Fontan operation) mortality is about 12%. Reported survivals for the hemi-Fontan and Fontan procedures have also been excellent at 98% for both operations. Overall, 75% of patients diagnosed with HLHS will survive through the Fontan procedure.

The current results for the Fontan procedure are excellent, with hospital mortality ranging from 2% to 9%. The condition of survivors is generally good, and most attain a functional status of New York Heart Association class I or II. The long-term results have been reported, with a 93% 5-year survival rate and a 91% 10-year survival rate. Although long-term results are encouraging, late complications may be seen. Continued surveillance for arrhythmias, congenital heart failure, protein-losing enteropathy, and hepatic dysfunction remains important.

Ghanayem NS, Allen KR, Tabbutt S, et al: Interstage mortality after the Norwood procedure: results of the multicenter single ventricle reconstruction trial. *J Thorac Cardiovasc Surg.* 2012;144:896-906.

Hornik CP, He X, Jacobs JP, et al: Complications after the Norwood operation: an analysis of the Society of Thoracic Surgeons Congenital Heart Surgery Database. *Ann Thorac Surg.* 2011;92:1734-1740.

Lee TM, Aiyagari R, Hirsch JC, et al: Risk factor analysis for second-stage palliation of single ventricle anatomy. *Ann Thorac Surg.* 2012;93:614-618.

Lowry AW: Resuscitation and perioperative management of the high-risk single ventricle patient: first-stage palliation. *Congen Heart Dis.* 2012;7:466-478.

Tabbutt S, Ghanayem N, Ravishankar C, et al: Risk factors for hospital morbidity and mortality after the Norwood procedure: a report from the Pediatric Heart Network Single Ventricle Reconstruction trial. *J Thorac Cardiovasc Surg.* 2012; 144:882-895.

ACYANOTIC HEART DEFECTS

1. Left-to-Right Shunting

▶ Atrial Septal Defect

A. General Considerations

Cardiac septation occurs between the third and sixth weeks of fetal development. The septum primum, which arises from the roof of the common atrium and descends inferiorly, initially divides the common atrium. The ostium primum is the opening below the inferior edge of the septum primum, which is obliterated as the septum primum fuses with the endocardial cushions. The ostium secundum forms in the midportion of the septum primum prior to closure of the ostium primum. The septum secundum also arises from the roof of the atrium and descends along the right side of the septum primum and covers the ostium secundum. This creates a flap valve whereby blood from the inferior vena cava may preferentially stream beneath the edge of the septum secundum and through the ostium secundum into the left atrium. After birth, the increase in left atrial pressure usually closes this pathway.

An ASD is a hole in the atrial septum (Figure 21–5). ASDs are the third most common congenital heart defect, occurring in 1 out of 1000 live births and representing 10% of congenital heart defects. The most common ASD is the secundum defect, which occurs when the ostium secundum is too large for complete coverage by the septum secundum. Ostium secundum defects account for about 80% of ASDs. An ostium primum ASD, representing 10% of ASDs, occurs as a result of failure of fusion of the septum primum with the endocardial cushions (ostium primum defect is discussed later in the section on AVSD). A third type of ASD is the sinus venosus defect, seen in about 10% of cases. Sinus venosus ASDs are caused by abnormal fusion of the venous pathways with the atrium and are characterized by defects high in the atrial septum near the orifice of the superior vena cava or, less commonly, low in the atrial septum near the inferior vena cava. Sinus venosus defects are frequently associated with partial anomalous pulmonary venous connection, usually with the right upper pulmonary vein draining into the superior vena cava near the cavoatrial junction. The rarest type of ASD is the unroofed coronary sinus septal defect. This occurs when there is loss of the common wall between the coronary sinus and the left atrium adjacent to the atrial septum. This unroofing of the coronary sinus leads to a communication between the right and left atria at the site of the coronary sinus.

Failure of postnatal fusion of the septum secundum to the septum primum results in a persistent slit-like communication known as a PFO. PFOs are extremely common in the general population, and autopsy studies have demonstrated a prevalence of 27%. PFOs are generally considered separate from other ASDs because of the absence of significant shunting, but they remain important clinically because of the occurrence of paradoxical embolization. A paradoxical embolus is usually a blood clot arising from a systemic vein, which would normally pass to the lungs, but in the presence of a septal defect may instead cross into the systemic circulation.

B. Clinical Findings

ASDs lead to increased pulmonary blood flow secondary to left-to-right shunting. Shunting at the atrial level is determined by the size of the defect and by the relative ventricular compliance (ie, blood preferentially fills the more compliant ventricle). At birth, both chambers are equally compliant, but as PVR falls, the right ventricle remodels and becomes more compliant. Shunting across the atrial septum causes a volume load on the right heart. A volume load is created by additional venous return to a chamber during diastole.

The volume overload from an ASD is usually well tolerated, and patients are frequently asymptomatic. Symptoms tend to develop when the ratio of pulmonary to systemic blood flow (Q_p/Q_s) exceeds 2. The most common symptoms are fatigue, shortness of breath, exercise intolerance, and recurrent respiratory infections. Older patients with untreated ASDs tend to develop atrial dysrhythmias, and adults may develop congestive heart failure and RV dysfunction. Pulmonary vascular obstructive disease may develop rarely as a late complication of untreated ASD. Paradoxical embolization is also an important potential complication of ASD.

The classic physical findings in patients with ASDs include fixed splitting of the second heart sound and a systolic ejection murmur at the left upper sternal border due to increased flow across a normal pulmonary valve. A diastolic flow murmur across the tricuspid valve is occasionally audible. A prominent RV lift and increased intensity of the pulmonary component of the second heart sound may occur

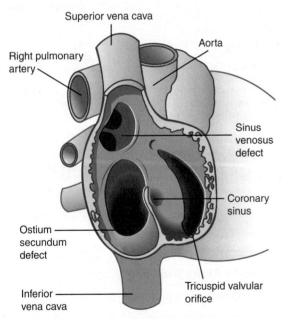

Superior vena cava

Aorta

Right pulmonary artery

Sinus venosus defect

Coronary sinus

Ostium secundum defect

Inferior vena cava

Tricuspid valvular orifice

▲ **Figure 21–5.** Sinus venosus and ostium secundum defects in the atrial septum as viewed from the opened right atrium.

with pulmonary hypertension. CXR shows cardiomegaly, with enlargement of the right atrium, right ventricle, and pulmonary artery. ECG frequently demonstrates right axis deviation and an incomplete right bundle branch block. When right bundle branch block occurs with a leftward or superior axis, the diagnosis of AVSD should be considered. Echocardiography confirms the diagnosis of ASD and defines the anatomy. Cardiac catheterization is important in selected cases to assess PVR in older patients, but it is used more frequently with therapeutic intent for device closure of ASDs.

C. Treatment

Because of the long-term complications associated with ASD, repair is recommended for all patients with symptomatic defects and in asymptomatic patients in whom the Q_p/Q_s is greater than 1.5. Repair is usually performed in children prior to school age. Closure of ASDs may be performed surgically or using a device deployed in the cardiac catheterization lab.

Surgical repair is usually recommended for large secundum defects and for most other types of ASDs. The heart is usually exposed by median sternotomy. Other surgical approaches have been proposed, including minimally invasive techniques, but there are technical drawbacks associated with each of the alternative approaches. In most cases, a limited midline incision with a partial lower sternal split provides adequate exposure and a cosmetically acceptable scar. The atrial septum is exposed through a right atriotomy. Small secundum defects or PFOs may sometimes be closed primarily by suturing the edge of the septum primum to the edge of the septum secundum. More commonly, larger defects are closed using a patch (polytetrafluoroethylene or autologous pericardium) and a running polypropylene suture. When anomalous pulmonary venous drainage is present, a baffle is created to redirect the flow across the ASD. In all cases, care is taken to de-air the left atrium to avoid the complication of air embolization.

The first transcatheter device closure of an ASD was performed in 1976. A number of devices are currently available for percutaneous closure of a secundum ASD, and success rates for device deployment are greater than 90%. Device closure has the advantages of fewer complications and a shorter hospitalization. Device closure of small to moderate secundum ASDs and PFOs has now become the standard of care at most large centers.

Occasionally, adults will present with a newly diagnosed ASD. Many studies have confirmed that ASD closure in adults over the age of 40 increases survival and limits the development of heart failure. When the Q_p/Q_s is less than 1.5 and the ratio of pulmonary to systemic vascular resistance (R_p/R_s) is greater than 0.7, significant pulmonary vascular obstructive disease is usually present. A PVR in excess of 10-12 Woods units·m² represents a contraindication to ASD closure.

D. Prognosis

Operative mortality for ASD repair is close to 0%. Atrial arrhythmias (1.2%) and postpericardiotomy syndrome (4.7%) are the most common postoperative complications. The long-term survival for patients undergoing ASD repair in childhood is normal. The major long-term complication following surgical closure of ASD is the development of supraventricular arrhythmias, although the risk is lowered when the ASD is closed in childhood. The persistence of this risk despite relief of right-sided volume overload is thought to be related to incomplete atrial remodeling or due to the presence of the atriotomy scar. Longer follow-up is required to determine whether device closure alters the risk of atrial dysrhythmias.

Butera G, Biondi-Zoccai G, Sangiorgi G, et al: Percutaneous versus surgical closure of secundum atrial septal defects: a systematic review and meta-analysis of currently available clinical evidence. *EuroIntervention.* 2011;7:377-385.

Irwin B, Ray S: Patent foramen ovale—assessment and treatment. *Cardiovasc Ther.* 2012;30:e128-e135.

Nyboe C, Fenger-Grøn M, Nielsen-Kudsk JE, et al: Closure of secundum atrial septal defects in the adult and elderly patients. *Eur J Cardiothorac Surg.* 2013;43(4):752-757.

Saito T, Ohta K, Nakayama Y, et al: Natural history of medium-sized atrial septal defect in pediatric cases. *J Cardiol.* 2012;60: 248-251.

▶ Ventricular Septal Defect

A. General Considerations

Ventricular septation is a complex process that requires accurate development and alignment of a number of structures including the muscular interventricular septum, the AV septum (arising from the endocardial cushions), and the infundibular septum (which divides the outflow tracts of the right and left ventricles). The membranous septum is a fibrous portion of the ventricular septum, which is adjacent to the central fibrous body (where the mitral, tricuspid, and aortic valve annuli make contact).

VSDs are the most common congenital heart anomalies (with the exception of bicuspid aortic valve, which occurs in about 1.3% of the population). VSDs are present in about 4 of 1000 live births and represent about 40% of congenital heart defects. VSDs are classified based on their location in the ventricular septum (Figure 21–6). The most common defects are perimembranous (80%), which are located in the area of the membranous septum. Inlet defects (5%) are located beneath the septal leaflet of the tricuspid valve and are sometimes called AV canal-type defects. Defects located high in the ventricular septum are outlet defects (10%).

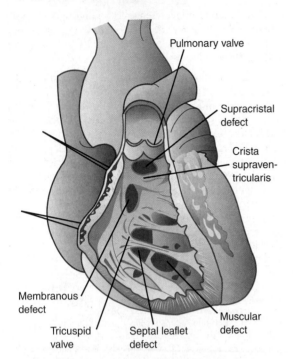

▲ **Figure 21–6.** Anatomic locations of various ventricular septal defects. The wall of the right ventricle has been excised to expose the ventricular septum.

Outlet VSDs are typically adjacent to both the pulmonary and aortic valves. Outlet defects are also known by several other names, including supracristal, infundibular, or doubly committed subarterial. Outlet defects are more common in the Asian population. Muscular (or trabecular) VSDs (5%) are completely bordered by muscle. Muscular VSDs are frequently multiple and may be associated with perimembranous or outlet defects. The size of VSDs varies. By definition, a VSD is nonrestrictive when its size (or the cumulative size of multiple defects) is greater than or equal to the size of the aortic annulus.

B. Clinical Findings

A VSD causes increased pulmonary blood flow due to left-to-right shunting primarily during systole. This creates a volume load on the left heart (the left atrium and ventricle receive the increased venous return during diastole). The right ventricle is not volume loaded (blood is ejected from the left ventricle through the VSD and directly into the pulmonary circulation), but it does experience a pressure load. The volume of shunt flow is determined by the size of the defect and by the ratio of R_p/R_s. After birth, the PVR is still high, and shunting across a VSD is sometimes minimal. Over

the first several weeks of life, shunting tends to increase as the PVR normally falls. Therefore, a patient with a large VSD may be asymptomatic at birth but eventually develop severe congestive heart failure.

The natural history for patients with isolated VSDs is highly variable. Most VSDs are restrictive and tend to close spontaneously during the first year of life. Large VSDs are nonrestrictive, resulting in RV and pulmonary pressures that are systemic or nearly systemic and high pulmonary blood flow with Q_p/Q_s ratios greater than 2.5-3. Moderate VSDs are restrictive, with pulmonary pressures that are one-half systemic (or less) and Q_p/Q_s ratios of 1.5-2.5. Small VSDs are highly restrictive; RV pressures remain normal, and the Q_p/Q_s is less than 1.5. Patients with large VSDs tend to develop symptoms of congestive heart failure by 2 months of age. Untreated, excessive pulmonary blood flow leads to pulmonary vascular obstructive disease by the second year of life. Patients with smaller VSDs may remain asymptomatic. In patients with outlet VSDs, prolapse of the aortic valve may occur, producing aortic insufficiency.

Signs of heart failure in infants with large VSDs include tachypnea, hepatomegaly, poor feeding, and failure to thrive. On physical examination, there is a pansystolic murmur at the left sternal border. Usually, the murmur is louder with smaller defects. The precordium is active. The pulmonary component of the second heart sound is accentuated in the presence of pulmonary hypertension. CXR shows increased pulmonary vascular markings and cardiomegaly. ECG is significant for RV hypertrophy.

Patients with small VSDs have little shunting and are usually asymptomatic, having only a pansystolic murmur. Patients with moderate VSDs manifest symptoms and signs proportional to the degree of shunting.

In patients who have developed significant pulmonary vascular obstructive disease, the volume of left-to-right shunting is decreased, and the murmur may disappear. Eisenmenger physiology results when the shunt flow reverses to right-to-left, creating cyanosis.

The diagnosis of VSD is confirmed by echocardiography, which accurately defines the anatomy and excludes the presence of associated defects. Cardiac catheterization is used selectively in older children and adults in whom elevated PVR is suspected. PVR is calculated by the following formula:

$$PVR = (PA_{mean} - LA)/Q_p$$

where PA_{mean} is the mean pulmonary artery pressure and LA is the left atrial pressure. The units of resistance by this formulation (using pressures in millimeters of mercury and pulmonary flow in liters per minute) are Woods units (which can be expressed in dynes·sec/cm^5 by multiplying by 80). PVR may be fixed or reactive, and at the time of cardiac catheterization, response to various pulmonary vasodilators may be assessed.

C. Treatment

The management of a patient with a VSD depends on the size of the defect, the type of the defect, the shunt volume, and the PVR. In general, patients with large defects who have intractable congestive heart failure or failure to thrive should undergo early surgical repair. If the congestive symptoms can be moderated by medical therapy, then surgery may be deferred until 6 months of age. Patients with moderate VSDs may be safely followed. If closure has not occurred by school age, then surgical closure is indicated. Small VSDs with Q_p/Q_s of less than 1.5 do not require closure. There is a small long-term risk of endocarditis for these patients, but this can be minimized with the appropriate use of prophylactic antibiotics. Patients with outlet VSDs have a significant risk of developing aortic insufficiency due to leaflet prolapse, and therefore, all of these patients should undergo surgical closure. Older children and adults must undergo catheterization to assess the pulmonary circulation. When there is a fixed PVR greater than 8-10 Woods units·m², then surgery is contraindicated.

Exposure of the ventricular septum is most often achieved by making a right atriotomy and retracting the leaflets of the tricuspid valve. This provides access to perimembranous, inlet, and most trabecular VSDs. Outlet VSDs are frequently best exposed via a pulmonary arteriotomy because the defect lies just beneath the valve. Muscular VSDs located near the ventricular apex can be very difficult to expose, and an apical ventriculotomy may be necessary. Once the defect is exposed, it is closed using a polytetrafluoroethylene patch and a running polypropylene suture, although some centers may prefer other patch material or interrupted suture technique. It is important to understand the anatomy of the conduction tissue when closing VSDs. The AV node is an atrial structure that lies at the apex of an anatomic triangle (known as the triangle of Koch) formed by the coronary sinus, the tendon of Todaro (a prominent band leading from the inferior vena cava and inserting in the atrial septum), and the septal attachment of the tricuspid valve. The node then gives rise to the bundle of His, which penetrates the AV junction beneath the membranous septum. The bundle of His then bifurcates into right and left bundle branches, which pass along either side of the muscular ventricular septum. In the presence of a perimembranous VSD, the bundle of His passes along the posterior and inferior rim of the defect, generally on the left ventricular side. In this critical area, sutures must be placed superficially on the RV side a few millimeters from the edge of the defect. The bundle of His tends to run along the posterior and inferior margin of inlet VSDs as well. The conduction tissue is usually remote from outlet and trabecular VSDs.

Pulmonary artery banding is a palliative maneuver used to protect the pulmonary circulation from excessive blood flow. Pulmonary artery banding is currently performed only in patients who are felt to be poor candidates for VSD closure because of either associated illness or anatomic complexity, such as multiple muscular VSDs ("Swiss cheese" septum). A band is placed around the main pulmonary artery and tightened to achieve a distal pulmonary artery pressure of about one-half systemic. The band is secured to the adventitia of the pulmonary artery to prevent its migration. Distal migration may result in narrowing and poor growth of one or both branch pulmonary arteries, while proximal migration can cause deformity of the pulmonary valve. Later, when the patient is a candidate for VSD closure, the band must be removed. Repair of the main pulmonary artery at the band site is usually necessary and can typically be accomplished by scar resection and primary closure or patch repair.

Transcatheter devices allow closure of some VSDs in the cardiac catheterization lab. For specific VSDs, such as muscular, device closure may be preferable. Complications with device closure include complete heart block (3.8%), device embolization (0.01%), and aortic insufficiency (0.03%). For simple perimembranous VSDs, the risk of device closure is in excess of traditional surgical closure.

D. Prognosis

Surgical closure of a VSD is associated with a mortality of less than 1%. Potential complications include injury to the conduction tissue and injury to the tricuspid or aortic valves. Transient heart block may result from tissue swelling or injury from retraction, but permanent heart block occurs in less than 2% of cases. When heart block develops after surgery, patients are usually observed for a period of 7-10 days prior to permanent pacemaker implantation. Tricuspid insufficiency may be precipitated by annular distortion or chordal restriction by the VSD patch or sutures. The aortic valve may also be injured by inaccurate suturing (especially in perimembranous and outlet defects). A residual VSD is seen in about 5% of cases, and reoperation is indicated when significant shunting persists ($Q_p/Q_s > 1.5$) or the residual defect is larger than 2 mm in size. The Q_p/Q_s ratio can be calculated by measuring oxygen saturations and using the following formula derived from the Fick equation:

$$Q_p/Q_s = (Ao - SVC)/(PV - PA)$$

where Ao is the aortic (or systemic) saturation, SVC is the saturation in the superior vena cava, PV is the saturation in the pulmonary veins (which is usually estimated to be 95%-100%), and PA is the saturation in the pulmonary arteries. Intraoperative echocardiography is used routinely to identify residual defects, which can then be repaired before the patient leaves the operating room.

Anderson JB, Czosek RJ, Knilans TK, et al: Postoperative heart block in children with common forms of congenital heart disease: results from the KID database. *J Cardiovasc Electrophysiol.* 2012;23(12):1349-1354.

Liu S, Chen F, Ding X, et al: Comparison of results and economic analysis of surgical and transcatheter closure of perimembranous ventricular septal defect. *Eur J Cardiothoracic Surg.* 2012;42:e157-162.

Oses P, Hugues N, Dahdah N: Treatment of isolated ventricular septal defects in children: Amplatzer versus surgical closure. *Ann Thorac Surg.* 2010;90:1593-1598.

Spicer DE, Anderson RH, Backer CL: Clarifying the surgical morphology of inlet ventricular septal defects. *Ann Thorac Surg.* 2013;95(1):236-241.

Zuo J, Xie J, Yi W, et al: Results of transcatheter closure of perimembranous ventricular septal defect. *Am J Cardiol.* 2010; 106:1034-1037.

Atrioventricular Septal Defect

A. General Considerations

AVSDs represent a group of congenital abnormalities bound by a variable deficiency of the atrioventricular septum immediately above and below the AV valves. Other terms commonly applied to an AVSD include AV canal defects, endocardial cushion defects, and AV communis. Complete AVSDs have a single common AV valve orifice, resulting in a single five-leaflet valve overlying both the right and left ventricles. Incomplete AVSDs have two separate AV valve orifices (tricuspid and mitral) with the mitral valve invariably having a cleft in the anterior leaflet. While most incomplete AVSDs have no ventricular level shunting, the classification of AVSDs as complete and incomplete depends only on the valve anatomy, not on the presence or absence of a VSD. Incomplete defects without associated ventricular level shunting have also been termed ostium primum ASDs, while those with a VSD have been described as intermediate or transitional AVSDs. AVSDs represent approximately 4% of congenital cardiac anomalies and are frequently associated with other cardiac malformations. AVSDs comprise 30%-40% of the cardiac abnormalities seen in patients with Down syndrome.

A complete AVSD is characterized by a common AV orifice, rather than separate mitral and tricuspid orifices, and a deficiency of endocardial cushion tissue, which results in an ASD and an inlet type of VSD (Figure 21–7). AVSDs were subclassified by Rastelli into the following three types according to the morphology of the anterior leaflet of the common AV valve:

Type A: The anterior bridging leaflet is divided and attached to the septum by multiple chordae.

Type B: The anterior bridging leaflet is attached to a papillary muscle in the right ventricle.

Type C: The anterior bridging leaflet is free-floating with no attachments except to the valve annulus.

When both left and right AV valves equally share the common AV valve orifice, the AVSD is termed balanced. Occasionally, the orifice may favor the right AV valve

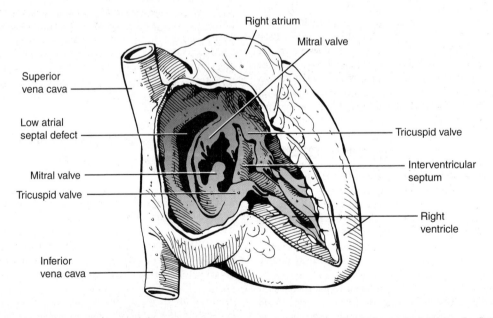

▲ **Figure 21–7.** Complete atrioventricular canal. The most common type has a divided anterior bridging leaflet. Both the left and right valvular components are attached to the interventricular septum with long, nonfused chordae. The left and right components of the posterior bridging leaflet are not separated.

(right dominance) or the left AV valve (left dominance). In marked right dominance, the left AV valve and left ventricle are hypoplastic and frequently coexist with other left-sided abnormalities, including aortic stenosis, hypoplasia of the aorta, and coarctation. Conversely, marked left dominance results in a deficient right AV valve with associated hypoplasia of the right ventricle, pulmonary stenosis or atresia, and TOF. Patients with severe imbalance require staged single-ventricle reconstruction.

The conduction tissue is displaced in an ASVD and is at risk during the surgical repair. The AV node is located posteriorly and inferiorly of its normal position toward the coronary sinus in the triangle of Koch. This triangle is bounded by the coronary sinus, the posterior attachment of the inferior bridging leaflet, and the rim of the ASD. The bundle of His courses posteriorly and inferiorly to run along the leftward aspect of the crest of the VSD, giving off the left bundle branch and continuing as the right bundle branch.

Cardiac anomalies associated with AVSDs include PDA (10%) and TOF (10%). Important abnormalities of the left AV valve include single papillary muscle (parachute mitral valve) (2%-6%) and double orifice mitral valve (8%-14%). A persistent left superior vena cava with or without an unroofed coronary sinus is encountered in 3% of patients with an AVSD. Double-outlet right ventricle (2%) significantly complicates or may even preclude complete surgical correction. As mentioned previously, left ventricular outflow tract obstruction from subaortic stenosis or redundant AV valve tissue occurs in 4%-7%.

B. Clinical Findings

The predominant hemodynamic features of an AVSD are the result of left-to-right shunting at the atrial and ventricular levels. In the absence of ventricular level shunting, the hemodynamics and clinical presentation of a patient with an incomplete AVSD resemble that of a typical secundum ASD with right atrial and RV volume overload. Patients with a complete AVSD with both atrial-level and ventricular-level shunting generally present early in infancy with signs and symptoms of congestive heart failure. In addition, moderate or severe left AV valve regurgitation occurs in approximately 10% of patients, with an AVSD worsening the clinical picture. On physical examination, the precordium is hyperactive, often with a prominent thrill. Auscultatory findings include a systolic murmur along the left sternal border, a high-pitched murmur at the apex from the left AV valve regurgitation, and a middiastolic flow murmur across the common AV valve. In the presence of elevated PVR, there may be a split first heart sound. Significant cardiomegaly and pulmonary overcirculation are found on the CXR. ECG reveals biventricular hypertrophy, atrial enlargement, prolonged PR interval, leftward axis, and counterclockwise frontal plane loop. Echocardiography is diagnostic, defining the atrial and ventricular level

shunting, valvular anatomy, and any associated anomalies. Up to 90% of untreated individuals with a complete AVSD develop pulmonary vascular disease by 1 year of age due to the large left-to-right shunt, potentially exacerbated by the associated AV valve regurgitation. Patients with trisomy 21 tend to develop pulmonary vascular obstructive disease earlier than chromosomally normal infants due to small airway disease, chronic hypoventilation, and elevated $PaCO_2$. Initial aggressive medical management is undertaken to relieve the symptoms of congestive heart failure. Elective surgical correction should be performed by age 3-6 months. Earlier intervention is indicated for failure of medical management.

Cardiac catheterization should be performed for patients over the age of 1 year, for patients with signs or symptoms of increased PVR, or in some cases to further evaluate other associated major cardiac anomalies. If the PVR is high, it is important to remeasure it while the child is breathing 100% oxygen with and without nitric oxide. If the pulmonary resistance falls, it implies that much of the elevated resistance is dynamic and can be managed in the perioperative period by ventilatory manipulation, supplemental oxygen, and nitric oxide. More recently, sildenafil has been shown to decrease elevation in PVR in children with congenital heart disease. Markedly elevated PVR (> 10 Woods units·m²) that does not respond to oxygen administration is generally considered a contraindication to repair.

C. Treatment

Operative treatment is almost always necessary as soon as symptoms are observed to prevent further clinical deterioration. Even in the absence of symptoms, operation is best performed before 6 months of age. Pulmonary artery banding, which permits delaying the repair until the child is larger, is no longer used today except in select complex or single-ventricle cases, extremely low birth weight or prematurity, and very poor clinical condition. This approach exposes the child to the risks of two operations, and the overall mortality exceeds that of primary repair in infancy. Patients with incomplete AVSDs usually require repair within the first few years of life.

Two techniques are widely employed for the repair of complete AVSDs: a one-patch technique and a two-patch technique. Incomplete AVSDs are repaired with the single-patch technique. Regardless of which approach is selected, the goals are to close the ASD and VSD and to separate the common AV valve into two nonstenotic, competent valves. The cleft in the anterior leaflet of the mitral valve is generally closed to lessen the risk of long-term mitral regurgitation. For the two-patch technique, separate patches are used for the ASD and VSD. For the one-patch technique, the superior and inferior bridging leaflets are divided along a line separating them into right and left components. A single patch is used to close both the VSD and ASD. The cut edges of the leaflets are then resuspended to the patch. For defects with a small VSD component, a modified single-patch technique may be employed. For this method, a single patch is sewn directly to the rim of the VSD, sandwiching the bridging leaflets between the patch and the crest of the VSD.

The short-term and long-term success of the operation is highly dependent on the status of the PVR and the surgeon's ability to maintain competence of the mitral valve. In developed countries, it is fortunately relatively uncommon for patients to present late with an AVSD and refractory PVR elevations. Although earlier reports recommend that the cleft in the left AV valve should not be closed and the valve should be treated as a trileaflet structure, most authors now believe that closure of the cleft is an important mechanism in preventing postoperative left AV valve regurgitation. Significant AV valve regurgitation at the conclusion of surgery, severe dysplasia of the left AV valve, and failure to close the cleft of the left AV valve have been identified as important risk factors for reoperation. Significant postoperative left AV valve regurgitation is also a risk factor for operative and long-term mortality. The cleft should not be completely closed in the presence of a single papillary muscle to avoid causing left AV valve stenosis. In the case of a double-orifice valve, the bridging tissue should not be divided to create a single opening in the valve.

D. Prognosis

Operative mortality is related largely to associated cardiac anomalies and left AV valve regurgitation. Mortality for repair of uncomplicated incomplete AVSDs is 0%-1.6%, while the addition of left AV valve regurgitation increases mortality to 4%-6%. For complete AVSDs, the mortality without left AV valve regurgitation is approximately 4%-5%, compared with 13% when significant degrees of regurgitation are present. The difference in operative mortality between patients with and without regurgitation underscores the importance of careful management of the left AV valve.

The majority of reoperations after repair of AVSD are due to left AV valve regurgitation or the development of subaortic stenosis. Significant postoperative AV valve regurgitation occurs in 6%-26% of patients, necessitating reoperation for valve repair or replacement in 3%-12%. The incidence of permanent complete heart block is approximately 1%-2%. Heart block encountered in the immediate postoperative period may be transient due to edema of or trauma to the AV node or bundle of His. However, right bundle branch block is common (22%).

Harmander B, Aydemir NA, Karaci AR, et al: Results for surgical correction of complete atrioventricular septal defect: associations with age, surgical era, and technique. *J Card Surg.* 2012;27:745-753.

Kaza AK, Colan SD, Jaggers J, et al: Surgical interventions for atrioventricular septal defect subtypes: the pediatric heart network experience. *Ann Thorac Surg.* 2011;92:1468-1475.

Stulak JM, Burkhart HM, Dearani JA, et al: Reoperations after repair of partial atrioventricular septal defect: a 45-year single-center experience. *Ann Thorac Surg.* 2010;89:1352-1359.

▶ Patent Ductus Arteriosus

A. General Considerations

The ductus arteriosus is a normal fetal vascular structure that allows blood from the right ventricle to bypass the high-resistance pulmonary vascular bed and pass directly to the systemic circulation. The ductus communicates between the main pulmonary artery (or proximal left pulmonary artery) and the proximal descending thoracic aorta. Histologically, the media of the ductus contains a predominance of smooth muscle cells, while the media of the aorta and pulmonary artery contain well-developed elastic fibers. Vasocontrol of the ductus is mediated by two important mechanisms: oxygen tension and prostaglandin levels. During fetal development, low oxygen tension and high levels of circulating prostaglandin maintain ductal patency. During the final trimester, the ductus becomes less sensitive to prostaglandins and more sensitive to the effects of oxygen tension. Following birth, the rise in oxygen tension and fall in prostaglandins (which were previously supplied principally by the placenta) lead to ductal closure, which is usually complete by 12-24 hours. After closure, the ductus becomes a fibrous cord known as the ligamentum arteriosum. Failure of closure of the ductus leads to the condition called patent ductus arteriosus (PDA), which occurs in about 1 out of 1200 live births and accounts for 7% of congenital heart defect. The incidence is much higher in premature infants (> 20%). This elevated incidence is thought to be related to immaturity of the ductal wall, resulting in impaired sensitivity to oxygen tension.

PDA may occur as an isolated defect, or it may occur in association with a number of other anomalies. Patency of the ductus arteriosus is desirable in a number of defects in which there is either inadequate pulmonary blood flow (eg, pulmonary atresia) or inadequate systemic blood flow (as in severe coarctation of the aorta). The discovery that extrinsic delivery of prostaglandins can maintain ductal patency has played a critical role in improving the survival of these patients.

B. Clinical Findings

The physiologic manifestation of PDA is shunting of blood across the ductus. The shunt volume is determined by the size of the ductus and by the ratio of pulmonary to systemic vascular resistance. At birth, the PVR drops dramatically and continues to decline over the first several weeks of life. As a result, shunting across a PDA is from left to right. Excessive pulmonary blood flow can lead to congestive heart failure. In extreme cases, hypotension and systemic malperfusion may result. Patients with a large PDA who survive infancy tend to develop pulmonary vascular obstructive disease. Eisenmenger physiology results when the PVR exceeds the systemic vascular resistance, producing a reversal of shunting across the ductus to right to left. This leads to cyanosis and, eventually, RV failure. Small PDAs may persist to adulthood without producing any symptoms or physiologic derangement. Endocarditis and endarteritis have been reported as long-term complications of PDA.

In patients with PDA, symptoms are proportional to the shunt volume and the presence of associated defects. Left-to-right shunting produces volume overload of the left heart. Infants with congestive heart failure demonstrate symptoms of tachypnea, tachycardia, and poor feeding. Older children may present with recurrent respiratory infections, fatigue, and failure to thrive. Physical findings include a widened pulse pressure and a continuous "machinery" murmur heard best along the left upper sternal border. CXR shows increased pulmonary vascular markings and left heart enlargement. Left ventricular hypertrophy and left atrial enlargement may be evident on the ECG. Echocardiography is the diagnostic method of choice. Diagnostic cardiac catheterization is performed only in older patients with suspected pulmonary hypertension to evaluate for pulmonary vascular obstructive disease. More frequently, catheterization is used for transcatheter occlusion of the ductus.

C. Treatment

PDA closure is performed for all symptomatic patients. Closure is also recommended for asymptomatic patients due to the risk of heart failure, pulmonary hypertension, and endocarditis. Closure of the ductus may be accomplished by one of three approaches: pharmacologic, surgical, and endovascular. Indomethacin, which is a prostaglandin inhibitor, stimulates PDA closure in premature infants. It is rarely effective in full-term infants. The dosing regimen is 0.1-0.2 mg/kg intravenously at 12- or 24-hour intervals for a total of three doses. This is effective in about 80% of premature babies. Due to its side effects, indomethacin is contraindicated in patients with sepsis, renal insufficiency, intracranial hemorrhage, or bleeding disorders. Failure of indomethacin after two complete courses results in referral for surgical closure.

The surgical approach to PDA is through a left posterolateral thoracotomy via the third or fourth intercostal space. The pleura is incised over the proximal descending thoracic aorta, which allows medial retraction of the vagus nerve. The recurrent laryngeal nerve curves behind the ductus and should be protected throughout the procedure. Dissection is then performed to demonstrate the pertinent anatomy. In many cases, the ductus is the largest vascular structure present, and it must not be confused with the aorta. Ductal tissue is extremely friable, so direct manipulation is minimized. In premature infants, the ductus is controlled with a single surgical clip; this procedure is commonly performed in the neonatal intensive care unit, thereby avoiding problems associated with patient transfer. In older patients, occlusion of the ductus is achieved with simple silk ligature or, preferably, by division between ligatures to minimize recurrence.

Recently, thoracoscopic techniques have been developed to perform PDA ligation. This approach has the potential benefits of decreased pain and quicker recovery. Disadvantages include a substantial learning curve and increased operating time.

A number of endovascular devices have been developed for the purpose of transcatheter occlusion of the PDA. This approach is very successful in older infants, children, and adults with small and moderate-sized PDAs and has become the treatment of choice at many centers. Surgical therapy is reserved for PDAs having a large diameter or very short length.

Rarely, an adult will present with a significant PDA. These patients must be carefully evaluated for the presence of pulmonary vascular obstructive disease prior to ductal closure. If the patient is not a candidate for device closure, surgical closure can be problematic. Calcification of the ductal wall is common in adults, which makes ligation hazardous. In some cases, cardiopulmonary bypass may be required with patch closure of the ductus from within the pulmonary artery.

D. Prognosis

Closure of the ductus by surgical or transcatheter techniques is achieved with a mortality that approaches zero. Potential complications include pneumothorax, recurrent laryngeal nerve injury, and chylothorax (from injury to the thoracic duct). Long-term survival should be normal following PDA ligation in most patients. Survival in premature infants depends primarily on the extent of prematurity with its attendant complications.

Drighil A, Al Jufan M, Al Omrane K, et al: Safety of transcatheter patent ductus arteriosus closure in small weight infants. *J Interv Cardiol.* 2012;4:391-394.

Malviya M, Ohlsson A, Shah S: Surgical versus medical treatment with cyclooxygenase inhibitors for symptomatic patent ductus arteriosus in preterm infants. *Cochrane Database Syst Rev.* 2013;3:CD003951.

Mosalli R, Alfaleh K: Prophylactic surgical ligation of patent ductus arteriosus for prevention of mortality and morbidity in extremely low birth weight infants. *Cochrane Database Syst Rev.* 2008;1:CD006181.

Van der Linde D, Konings EEM, Slager MA, et al: Birth prevalence of congenital heart disease world-wide: a systematic review and meta-analysis. *J Am Coll Cardiol.* 2011;58:2241-2247.

2. Right-Sided Anomalies

Pulmonary Stenosis

A. General Considerations

Isolated pulmonary stenosis occurs in 5%-8% of all congenital cardiac anomalies. The pulmonary valve is usually trileaflet with fusion of the commissures. The valve can appear thickened and domed on echocardiography. Most patients have an associated PFO or a secundum ASD. Pulmonary stenosis may be valvar or subvalvar due to muscular narrowing of the infundibulum (Figure 21–8).

B. Clinical Findings

Young infants with severe pulmonary stenosis present with failure to thrive, right heart failure, and possibly hypoxic

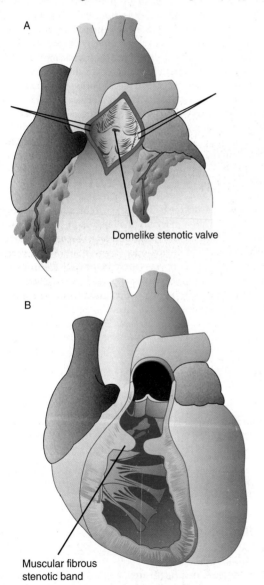

Figure 21–8. Pulmonary stenosis. **A:** Valvular pulmonary stenosis. **B:** Infundibular pulmonary stenosis.

spells. Older children tend to have mild to moderate stenosis that is asymptomatic. They may, however, complain of shortness of breath with exertion or arrhythmias. The murmur of pulmonary stenosis tends to be prominent and therefore is not missed on routine examination. The presence of a systolic ejection murmur should prompt further workup, including an echocardiogram, which is diagnostic. Patients may be followed symptomatically with mild to moderate pulmonary stenosis. Surgical or catheter-based intervention should be considered for a gradient higher than 50 mm Hg, progressive ventricular hypertrophy, or new tricuspid regurgitation.

C. Treatment

Neonates presenting with profound cyanosis from severe pulmonary stenosis need to be placed on prostaglandin E_1 (PGE_1) to maintain ductal patency. The ductus will maintain adequate pulmonary blood flow so that the patient can be stabilized. For isolated pulmonary stenosis, balloon valvuloplasty by an interventional cardiologist is highly successful and has replaced surgical intervention for the majority of patients. Asymptomatic infants with systemic RV pressures from pulmonary stenosis are also excellent candidates for balloon dilation. Surgical valvotomy or a transannular patch for pulmonary stenosis is reserved for patients who have failed balloon dilation, who have a severely hypoplastic valve annulus, or who have other associated anomalies including muscular infundibular narrowing. Older patients with progressive isolated pulmonary stenosis are excellent candidates for elective balloon dilation when they develop elevated RV pressures.

D. Prognosis

Early mortality for patients with critical pulmonary stenosis is 3%-10%. Restenosis occurs in 10%-25% of patients. Once the outflow obstruction is relieved, the RV hypertrophy and tricuspid insufficiency regress. Although overall survival is excellent for isolated pulmonary stenosis, over 50% of patients will require additional interventions, including repeat balloon dilation, pulmonary valve replacement, and ASD closure. Late atrial and ventricular arrhythmias occur in 38% of patients. Twenty-five-year survival is 90%-96%.

Cuypers JA, Witsenburg M, van der Linde D, et al: Pulmonary stenosis: update on diagnosis and therapeutic options. *Heart.* 2013;99(5):339-347.

Harrild DM, Powell AJ, Tran TX, et al: Long-term pulmonary regurgitation following balloon valvuloplasty for pulmonary stenosis risk factors and relationship to exercise capacity and ventricular volume and function. *J Am Coll Cardiol.* 2010;55:1041-1047.

Rigby ML: Severe aortic or pulmonary valve stenosis in premature infants. *Early Hum Dev.* 2012;88:291-294.

Voet A, Rega F, de Bruaene AV, et al: Long-term outcome after treatment of isolated pulmonary valve stenosis. *Int J Cardiol.* 2012;156:11-15.

▶ Ebstein Anomaly

A. General Considerations

Ebstein malformation was first described by Wilhelm Ebstein in 1866 as a constellation of clinical findings resulting from an abnormality of the tricuspid valve. It has become evident over time that the malformation is a disease of the entire right ventricle and the development of the tricuspid valve. It involves a spectrum of anatomical abnormalities of variable severity, which include apical displacement of the septal and mural leaflets of the tricuspid valve, which have failed to delaminate from the underlying myocardium; thinning or atrialization of the inlet component of the right ventricle, with variable dilation; and malformation of the anterosuperior leaflet, with anomalous attachments, redundancy, and fenestrations. Several other cardiac anomalies are often associated with the RV changes, such as ASDs and VSDs, obstruction of the RV outlet, and Wolff-Parkinson-White syndrome. Ebstein malformation can also afflict the left-sided systemic AV valve in the setting of congenitally corrected transposition.

B. Clinical Findings

The malformation is rare, accounting for no more than 1% of all congenital cardiac anomalies. Due to the significant anatomic variability in the abnormalities of the tricuspid valve and right ventricle, the age at presentation and severity of symptoms can also be highly variable. Patients who present in infancy have the poorest prognosis. There is a high rate of fetal death, hydrops, and pulmonary hypoplasia when the diagnosis is made during fetal life. Cyanosis is the most common presentation in infancy. These patients have severe tricuspid regurgitation with a poorly functioning right ventricle in the face of elevated pulmonary arterial resistance. The result is a state of low cardiac output dependent on right-to-left shunting across the fossa ovalis.

With less severe derangements of the tricuspid valve and preserved ventricular function, patients tend to present later in adolescence or early adulthood. Many patients are asymptomatic and present with a murmur noted on physical examination. In symptomatic patients, a common presentation involves the new onset of atrial arrhythmias or reentrant tachycardia. Exercise tolerance may be diminished, with cyanosis during extreme exertion if an ASD is present. Those patients with an intact atrial septum will often progress to congestive heart failure with increasing cardiomegaly.

Echocardiography is usually sufficient for accurate diagnosis and anatomic evaluation. The degree of displacement, tethering, and dysplasia of the valvar leaflets, as well as the amount of regurgitation, can be determined. Ventricular function and the extent of atrialization of the right ventricle can also be evaluated. Additional abnormalities, including the presence and direction of a shunt at the atrial level, can be assessed. ECG findings include incomplete right bundle branch block, right axis deviation, ventricular preexcitation, and atrial arrhythmias. The CXR can vary from normal, in patients with mild anatomic abnormalities, to the classic "wall-to-wall" heart. Cardiac catheterization is rarely necessary.

C. Treatment

As noted previously, neonates often present with profound cyanosis and may require prostaglandins to maintain adequate flow of blood to the lungs during the early neonatal period when pulmonary resistance is high. It is important to distinguish functional from anatomic pulmonary atresia. In patients with functional atresia, it may be possible to wean them from the infusion of prostaglandins while maintaining adequate saturations of oxygen as pulmonary resistance falls. These patients can then be followed for development of further symptoms.

In neonates who cannot be weaned from prostaglandins due to unacceptable levels of hypoxemia or in those with anatomic pulmonary atresia, it is necessary to construct a systemic-to-pulmonary shunt to maintain adequate pulmonary blood flow. For neonates who also develop significant symptoms of congestive heart failure while on prostaglandin, it is necessary to address the underlying valvar pathology. The options include closure of the tricuspid valve, with or without fenestration, along with construction of a modified Blalock-Taussig shunt, repair of the tricuspid valve if ventricular function is reasonable, or cardiac transplantation.

In the older patient with progressive symptoms, a variety of surgical options exist to address the malformed tricuspid valve. Most are based on techniques designed to mobilize the leading edge of the anterosuperior leaflet, aiming to create a competent monocusp valve with or without plication of the atrialized portion of the right ventricle. There is ongoing debate as to the necessity of obliterating the atrialized portion of the right ventricle. Historically, plication of this portion of the ventricle has been an integral part of most repairs; however, no clear physiologic benefit with regard to improved ventricular function has been demonstrated. In addition, the potential exists for injury to the right coronary artery as a result of the plication, which may adversely impact late outcomes and contribute to ventricular arrhythmias.

Replacement of the tricuspid valve is a final option. The late survival free from reoperation, however, has been equivalent to valvar repair. If replacement is required, heterografts are preferred over mechanical valves due to risks of thrombosis. Other options using tissue valves include the insertion of pulmonary autografts, mitral valve homografts, and "top hat" mounted pulmonary or aortic homografts. When replacing the valve, the sutures should be brought around the coronary sinus, leaving it to drain into the right ventricle so as to minimize potential injury to the AV node.

An open antiarrhythmia procedure is frequently performed concomitantly.

D. Prognosis

Ebstein malformation is a rare but challenging congenital cardiac defect. The high degree of anatomic variability makes it difficult to have a standardized approach to these children. The symptomatic neonate carries a very grave prognosis. The presence of associated cardiac and other congenital anomalies often makes survival impossible. Surgical options are limited at this age and often still result in a poor outcome. Medical management, if possible, is the best, as surgical success improves with age. If surgery is required, conversion to functional tricuspid atresia often offers the best survival, as the ventricle in the severely symptomatic neonate functions poorly. Transplantation remains an option, but the availability of organs limits its utility.

Patients who are not symptomatic in the neonatal period will often remain free from symptoms well into adolescence. Electrophysiologic symptoms usually precede symptoms of congestive heart failure. Indications for repair at these ages include symptoms, cyanosis, and progressive cardiomegaly.

Dearani JA, Said SM, O'Leary PW, et al: Anatomic repair of Ebstein's malformation: lessons learned with cone reconstruction. *Ann Thorac Surg.* 2013;95:220-228.

Shinkawa T, Polimenakos AC, Gomez-Fifer CA, et al: Management and long-term outcome of neonatal Ebstein anomaly. *J Thorac Cardiovasc Surg.* 2010;139:354-358.

3. Left-Sided Anomalies

▶ Aortic Stenosis

A. General Considerations

Aortic stenosis is a form of left ventricular outflow tract obstruction that may occur at a valvar (70%), subvalvar (25%), or supravalvar (5%) level. Aortic stenosis occurs in about 4% of patients with congenital heart disease. The severity of aortic stenosis may be graded as mild (peak pressure gradient < 50 mm Hg), moderate (50-75 mm Hg), or severe (> 75 mm Hg).

Valvar aortic stenosis occurs secondary to maldevelopment of the aortic valve. Most commonly, a bicuspid valve is present, although tricuspid and unicuspid valves are also represented. In valvar aortic stenosis, the leaflets are thickened and frequently dysmorphic, and there is a variable degree of leaflet fusion along the commissures. The aortic annulus may be hypoplastic. In 20% of cases, valvar aortic stenosis is associated with other cardiac defects, most commonly coarctation of the aorta, PDA, VSD, or mitral stenosis. Men with valvar aortic stenosis outnumber women by a ratio of 4:1. There is a wide spectrum of clinical presentations of valvar aortic stenosis, but patients tend to present in one of two groups. Neonates and infants with severe aortic stenosis develop symptoms of rapidly progressive congestive heart failure, while older children generally have less severe obstruction and a more slowly progressive course.

Subvalvar aortic stenosis occurs below the level of the aortic valve and may be discrete (80%) or diffuse (20%). Discrete (or membranous) subaortic stenosis is rarely seen in infants and tends to progress over time. This lesion consists of a crescent or circumferential fibrous or fibromuscular membrane that protrudes into the left ventricular outflow tract. The pathogenesis of discrete subaortic stenosis is unknown, but it is thought to be an acquired lesion that develops secondary to a congenital abnormality of the left ventricular outflow tract in which abnormal flow patterns lead to endocardial injury with resultant fibrosis. Although the aortic valve leaflets are usually normal in discrete subaortic stenosis, the turbulent flow created by the obstruction can cause leaflet thickening and progressive aortic insufficiency. Diffuse subaortic stenosis is a more severe form of stenosis that creates a long, tunnel-like obstruction. Diffuse subaortic stenosis should be distinguished from hypertrophic cardiomyopathy. Both forms of subaortic stenosis are associated with a high risk of endocarditis.

Supravalvar aortic stenosis is characterized by thickening of the wall of the ascending aorta. The lesion may be localized (80%) to the region of the sinotubular ridge (at the level of the valve commissures), creating an hourglass deformity, or it may be more diffuse (20%), extending into the aortic arch and its branches. In both varieties, the aortic valve leaflets may be abnormal. The free edges of the aortic valve leaflets may adhere to the aortic wall in the region of intraluminal thickening, and this may lead to reduced coronary blood flow during diastole. Aortic wall thickening may also extend into the coronary ostia and further impair coronary blood flow. Associated cardiac lesions are common, particularly branch pulmonary artery stenoses. A genetic basis for supravalvar aortic stenosis has been established. About 50% of cases of supravalvar aortic stenosis are associated with Williams syndrome, in which a partial deletion of chromosome 7 (including the elastin gene) leads to the triad of supravalvar stenosis, mental retardation, and a characteristic "elfin" facies. Isolated mutations in the elastin gene have also been shown to produce familial supravalvar aortic stenosis with an autosomal dominant pattern of transmission. There is a significant incidence of endocarditis in patients with supravalvar aortic stenosis. Sudden death is frequently reported and is probably related to coronary obstruction.

B. Clinical Findings

Severe aortic stenosis is usually well-tolerated during fetal development. Although left ventricular output and antegrade flow across the aortic valve are decreased, the right ventricle compensates with increased output, and systemic perfusion is maintained by flow across the ductus. After birth, there is increased venous return to the left heart, and this exacerbates the pressure load created by the stenotic aortic valve, leading to left ventricular dysfunction. As the ductus closes during postnatal life, systemic malperfusion may develop with resulting hypotension, acidosis, and oliguria. Coronary perfusion is also impaired due to the combination of systemic hypotension and elevated left ventricular end-diastolic pressures. Patients with critical aortic stenosis typically exhibit severe left ventricular dysfunction. These patients usually show signs of distress soon after birth. On examination, there is impaired distal perfusion with poor capillary refill and diminished, thready pulses. A systolic ejection murmur may be absent if the cardiac output is severely diminished. Differential cyanosis may be observed due to perfusion of the lower body with desaturated blood shunting through the ductus. The ECG shows left ventricular hypertrophy, and the CXR displays cardiomegaly and pulmonary congestion. Echocardiography establishes the diagnosis.

In contrast to infants with critical aortic stenosis, older children with valvar aortic stenosis usually present with less severe stenosis (mild or moderate), and most are asymptomatic. Symptoms of angina, syncope, and congestive heart failure are not commonly reported. Congenital valvar aortic stenosis is a progressive lesion, however, and survival is dependent on the severity of stenosis and its rate of progression. Sudden cardiac death is the most common cause of mortality. Endocarditis occurs in less than 1% of patients. The diagnosis of valvar aortic stenosis in older children can frequently be made on physical examination. There is a classic systolic crescendo-decrescendo murmur at the upper sternal border, which radiates to the neck. An ejection click is often present. A visible apical impulse is suggestive of significant left ventricular hypertrophy. In severe cases, the pulse may be weak and delayed (pulsus tardus et parvus). The ECG shows left ventricular hypertrophy. The CXR is usually normal. Echocardiography accurately defines the level of stenosis and its severity. Using Doppler techniques, the pressure gradient across the stenotic valve may be estimated using a simplified form of the Bernoulli equation $P = 4V^2$, where P is the pressure gradient and V is the peak flow velocity. Cardiac catheterization is generally reserved for therapeutic intervention.

The clinical findings in subvalvar aortic stenosis are similar to those for valvar stenosis. The signs and symptoms of supravalvar aortic stenosis are similar to those in other forms of left ventricular outflow tract obstruction. The diagnosis is made by echocardiography, but cardiac catheterization or cMRI is essential to define the aortic, coronary, and pulmonary arterial anatomy prior to surgical intervention.

C. Treatment

The neonate or infant with critical aortic stenosis represents a true emergency. Endotracheal intubation and inotropic support are routine. Ductal patency is maintained with prostaglandins, and acidosis is corrected. All patients with critical aortic stenosis require some form of urgent intervention. The approach is determined by the valve morphology and by the presence of associated defects. In its most extreme form, critical aortic stenosis may be associated with underdeveloped left-sided cardiac chambers and therefore may represent a form of HLHS. In these cases, single-ventricle palliation must be undertaken. For patients with adequate left-sided chambers, relief of aortic stenosis may be achieved by one of the following three approaches: percutaneous balloon valvuloplasty, surgical valvotomy, or aortic valve replacement. Balloon valvuloplasty is generally considered the procedure of choice when the aortic valve annulus is adequate and there are no associated cardiac defects. Alternatively, surgical valvotomy may be accomplished by closed or open techniques. The closed approach is performed using cardiopulmonary bypass without aortic cross-clamping. Dilators of increasing size are passed through a ventriculotomy in the left ventricular apex and advanced across the aortic valve. Some centers prefer open surgical valvotomy, which allows a precise valvotomy under direct vision, although aortic cross-clamping with cardioplegia is necessary. In all cases, the goal of therapy is to relieve stenosis without creating excessive aortic insufficiency. Dramatic clinical improvement is expected following balloon or surgical valve valvotomy, and early survivals of greater than 80% have been reported. The incidence of aortic insufficiency is slightly higher following balloon valvotomy. In most cases, however, stenosis will recur, and repeat valvotomy or aortic valve replacement will eventually be required. Aortic valve replacement is problematic in the neonate due to small patient size. In these cases, many consider the best valve replacement to be a pulmonary autograft (Ross procedure) with enlargement of the aortic annulus (Konno aortoventriculoplasty). The Ross-Konno procedure has been used successfully for neonates with critical aortic stenosis in whom the aortic annulus is hypoplastic and for selected patients in whom valvuloplasty was unsuccessful. Survival following the Ross-Konno procedure in infants has been shown to be excellent. Growth of the pulmonary autograft has been documented, thereby making it an ideal valve replacement for children. Unfortunately, as part of the Ross procedure, the pulmonary valve must be replaced using a cryopreserved homograft, which does not grow, and homograft replacement must be anticipated at intervals as the patient grows.

All patients with severe valvar aortic stenosis should undergo intervention, as should all symptomatic patients with moderate stenosis. Asymptomatic patients with mild or moderate stenosis are generally observed. As described for critical aortic stenosis, the techniques used to relieve aortic stenosis in older patients include percutaneous balloon valvuloplasty, surgical valvulotomy, and valve replacement. Balloon valvuloplasty is usually performed as the primary intervention and is associated with a success rate of nearly 90% and a mortality of less than 1%. Open surgical valvotomy is an alternative approach with similar results. For valves that are severely dysplastic, develop restenosis after intervention, or become insufficient as a result of prior intervention, valve replacement may be necessary. For older children, there are more options for valve replacement. The choices include mechanical prostheses, bioprosthetic valves, and tissue substitutes, such as porcine xenografts, cryopreserved human allografts, and pulmonary autografts (Ross procedure). The mechanical valves are the most durable but require chronic anticoagulation. The bioprosthetic and tissue valves do not require long-term anticoagulation but tend to deteriorate over time (with the exception of the pulmonary autograft). The pulmonary autograft has the potential advantage of growth, but the homograft used to replace the pulmonary valve will require replacement. Selection of the appropriate replacement valve is a complex decision requiring input from all involved parties.

Intervention for discrete subvalvar stenosis is usually undertaken when the gradient exceeds 30-50 mm Hg or when aortic insufficiency is present. In these patients, resection of the membrane is readily performed by a transaortic approach. In order to reduce the incidence of restenosis, many centers advocate concurrent performance of a septal myomectomy to alter the geometry of the left ventricular outflow tract.

When diffuse subaortic stenosis is associated with hypoplasia of the aortic annulus, repair is best achieved with a Konno aortoventriculoplasty, whereby an incision is carried across the aortic annulus and subjacent ventricular septum, the opening patched, and an aortic valve implanted. Patients with an adequate aortic annulus may undergo a septoplasty (modified Konno), in which the septal incision is confined to the immediate subvalvar area and a patch is used to widen the left ventricular outflow tract without replacing the aortic valve.

Operative intervention is indicated for patients with supravalvar aortic stenosis in whom the gradient exceeds 50 mm Hg. A number of operations have been proposed for the treatment of localized supravalvar stenosis. The classical repair involves a longitudinal incision across the obstruction in the ascending aorta, which is extended into the noncoronary sinus. The thickened, hypertrophic ridge is resected by endarterectomy, and the aortotomy is augmented with an elliptical patch. A variation of this repair involves creation of an inverted-Y aortotomy with one limb of the Y extended into the noncoronary sinus and the other into the right coronary sinus. A Y-shaped patch is then used to augment the aortotomy. Finally, the Brom repair is performed

by transection of the ascending aorta beyond the supravalvar ridge. Separate incisions are then made through the supravalvar ridge into each sinus of Valsalva. Triangular patches are placed to augment each of these incisions, thereby relieving the supravalvar obstruction. Reconnection of the aortic root to the ascending aorta completes the repair. The repair of the diffuse type of supravalvar stenosis is performed under circulatory arrest with extensive patching of the ascending aorta, transverse arch, and involved arch arteries. Branch pulmonary stenoses are best managed using transcatheter techniques.

D. Prognosis

Operative mortality approaches zero for resection of discrete subaortic stenosis. The recurrence rate of discrete stenosis following membrane resection and myomectomy has been reported to be as low as 4%. Despite the technical complexity of repair of diffuse subaortic stenosis, excellent results have been reported with high survival and freedom from reoperation. The results of surgery for localized supravalvar aortic stenosis are generally good with low operative mortality and excellent long-term survival. The diffuse form is more difficult to treat, and recurrence is more likely. Overall results are much worse when severe bilateral pulmonary artery stenoses are present. The mortality for aortic valve replacement regardless of valve choice is 2%-5%. The need for reoperation is dependent on valve choice and patient size. Early and late ventricular arrhythmias may occur commonly in patients with significant left ventricular hypertrophy.

Brown JW, Rodefeld MD, Ruzmetov M, et al: Surgical valvuloplasty versus balloon aortic dilation for congenital aortic stenosis: are evidence-based outcomes relevant? *Ann Thorac Surg.* 2012;94:146-153.

Coskun KO, Popov AF, Tirilomis T, et al: Aortic valve surgery in congenital heart disease: a single-center experience. *Artif Organs.* 2010;34:E85-E90.

Hickey EJ, Caldarone CA, Blackstone EH, et al: Biventricular strategies for neonatal critical aortic stenosis: high mortality associated with early reintervention. *J Thorac Cardiovasc Surg.* 2012;144:409-417.

Maskatia SA, Ing FF, Justino H, et al: Twenty-five year experience with balloon aortic valvuloplasty for congenital aortic stenosis. *Am J Cardiol.* 2011;108:1024-1028.

▶ Aortic Coarctation

A. General Considerations

Coarctation of the aorta is a narrowing of the proximal descending thoracic aorta distal to the origin of the left subclavian artery, near the insertion of the ductus arteriosus (or ligamentum arteriosum). The severity of luminal narrowing and the length of the aorta affected are variable. Coarctation is thought to occur as a result of ectopic tissue from the ductus arteriosus that migrates into the wall of the adjacent aorta. After birth, as the ductus closes, the ectopic tissue in the aorta also constricts. Frequently, a posterior shelf of tissue is present at the point of most severe obstruction. The aortic obstruction caused by coarctation creates a pressure load on the left ventricle.

The incidence of coarctation is about 0.5 per 1000 live births, and its prevalence is about 7% of congenital heart defects. Coarctation is commonly associated with other heart defects, including bicuspid aortic valve (in more than 50% of cases), PDA, and VSD. Other left-sided obstructive lesions may also be present, such as aortic arch hypoplasia, aortic stenosis, mitral stenosis, and left ventricular hypoplasia. Coarctation is also recognized to occur in association with Turner syndrome.

B. Clinical Findings

Patients with severe coarctation present in the newborn period. Aortic obstruction is so significant that perfusion of the lower body is dependent upon flow from the ductus arteriosus. Spontaneous ductal closure typically worsens the aortic obstruction and may lead to malperfusion of tissues distal to the coarctation. The pressure load on the left ventricle may precipitate congestive heart failure. Patients may develop shock with severe acidosis, oliguria, and diminished distal pulses. Infants with severe coarctation will generally not survive without intervention.

Older children with coarctation are usually asymptomatic. The diagnosis is commonly made on the basis of hypertension in the upper extremities with decreased pulses in the lower extremities. Noninvasive blood pressure measurements in all four extremities help to quantify the severity of aortic obstruction. Older patients tend to develop extensive collateral arteries that bypass the obstruction. Life expectancy for these patients is 34 years without operation, typically due to the development of heart failure. Other long-term complications of coarctation include aortic dissection (21%), endocarditis (18%) (frequently involving a bicuspid aortic valve), intracranial hemorrhage (12%) (from Berry aneurysms, which occur more commonly in patients with coarctation), endarteritis (in the poststenotic area of the aorta at the site of the jet of turbulent flow), and aortic aneurysm.

The diagnosis of coarctation can usually be made clinically. The infant with significant coarctation is frequently asymptomatic at birth but, following closure of the ductus, develops signs of heart failure such as irritability, tachypnea, and poor feeding. Lower extremity pulses are absent, and upper extremity pulses may be weak. CXR shows cardiomegaly and pulmonary venous congestion. There is a left ventricular strain pattern on the ECG. Echocardiography is usually diagnostic, demonstrating narrowing of the aorta at the coarctation site with a loss of pulsatility in the descending aorta.

In older children and adults with coarctation, a pressure gradient between the arms and legs usually can be demonstrated by measuring cuff pressures in all four extremities. On CXR, rib notching may be evident, secondary to erosion of the inferior rib borders from the development of large intercostal collateral vessels. Echocardiography usually confirms the diagnosis. Anatomic details may also be clarified with CTA and cMRI. Cardiac catheterization is usually not necessary.

C. Treatment

Generally, all patients with coarctation should undergo surgical repair if the gradient is greater than 20 mm Hg. For neonates, the acute medical management includes initiation of PGE_1 for the purpose of reopening the ductus; this maneuver partially relieves the aortic obstruction and augments perfusion of the lower body due to improved antegrade flow across the arch as well as right-to-left flow across the ductus. Prostaglandins are usually effective for reopening the ductus when initiated within 3-7 days of life but are less successful thereafter.

Surgical repair of coarctation is usually performed through a left posterolateral thoracotomy via the third or fourth intercostal space. The descending thoracic aorta, ductus (or ligamentum), transverse aortic arch, and brachiocephalic vessels are mobilized. Care is taken to preserve the vagus nerve and its recurrent laryngeal branch.

The coarctation is usually evident externally by narrowing or posterior indentation; however, the degree of internal narrowing is usually much more severe. A dose of heparin (100 units/kg) may be given intravenously for patients younger than 2 years. Proximal and distal control of the aorta is achieved using clamps. Usually, the proximal clamp is positioned on the transverse arch between the innominate and left carotid vessels with concomitant occlusion of the left carotid and left subclavian. In infants and children, the preferred surgical approach to coarctation is resection with extended end-to-end repair. A generous resection of the coarctation segment is performed. The proximal aorta is then spatulated along the lesser curvature and the distal aorta along the greater curvature. An extended end-to-end anastomosis is then performed.

In older children and adults, it may not be possible to perform a resection with primary repair without creating excessive tension on the anastomosis, which may lead to hemorrhage or scarring with recurrent coarctation. An alternative strategy is necessary in these cases. Patch aortoplasty may be performed in children in whom further growth is anticipated. The subclavian flap repair augments the narrowed aorta using native arterial tissue. Blood flow to the left arm is maintained by collateral vessels, although long-term studies have demonstrated a slight discrepancy in limb length in some patients. Prosthetic patch material may also be used. By avoiding circumferential prosthetic material, growth potential of the native aorta is preserved.

The disadvantage of patch repair is a high risk of aneurysm formation. In adults, where growth is no longer an issue, resection of the coarctation may be performed with subsequent placement of a prosthetic interposition graft (either Dacron or polytetrafluoroethylene).

One of the principal concerns during coarctation repair is interruption of distal aortic blood flow, especially to the spinal cord. The anterior spinal artery is fed by major radicular branches from intercostal arteries. In patients without well-formed collaterals, ischemia of the spinal cord may be precipitated by aortic cross-clamping, and paraplegia may result. Protective measures include induction of mild hypothermia, maintenance of a high proximal aortic pressure, and minimization of cross-clamp time. In older patients, distal aortic perfusion may be maintained by the technique of left heart bypass, where oxygenated blood is taken from the left atrium and delivered to the femoral artery or distal aorta using a centrifugal pump. Overall, the incidence of paraplegia following coarctation repair is less than 1%.

Transcatheter therapy has been proposed for the primary therapy of coarctation, but this approach is controversial due to the incidence of recurrent coarctation, need for multiple interventions, injury to the femoral vasculature (for access), and aneurysm formation. Improved results have been achieved with balloon angioplasty with concurrent stent placement in older children and adults in whom further aortic growth is not anticipated. Balloon angioplasty is widely accepted for the treatment of recurrent coarctation following surgery, with 88%-94% achieving a gradient of less than 20 mm Hg.

D. Prognosis

The early mortality following repair of coarctation in neonates is 1%-3%, while the risk in older children and adults is about 1%-2%. The incidence of recurrent coarctation following resection and end-to-end repair is about 10%, whereas catheter-based interventions are associated with reintervention rates of 25% for balloon angioplasty and 5%-40% for stent placement. The long-term survival following repair of coarctation is determined by the presence of associated defects and the persistence of hypertension.

Following repair, patients may develop severe hypertension. This can be managed using intravenous beta-blockers (eg, esmolol) or vasodilators (eg, sodium nitroprusside). Uncontrolled hypertension can lead to the complication of mesenteric arteritis. Hypertension usually resolves within days to weeks after repair, although older children and adults may require lifelong antihypertensive therapy. Repair of coarctation during infancy is thought to minimize the risk of late hypertension.

Pádua LM, Garcia LC, Rubira CJ, et al: Stent placement versus surgery for coarctation of the thoracic aorta. *Cochrane Database Syst Rev.* 2012;5:CD008204.

▶ Vascular Rings

A. General Considerations

Vascular rings comprise a spectrum of vascular anomalies of the aortic arch, pulmonary artery, and brachiocephalic vessels. The clinically significant manifestation of these lesions is a varying degree of tracheoesophageal compression. These vascular anomalies can be divided into complete vascular rings and partial vascular rings. Complete vascular rings can be divided into double aortic arch and right aortic arch with left ligamentum arteriosum. These two categories can be further subdivided on the basis of the specific anatomy. Incomplete vascular rings include aberrant right subclavian artery, innominate artery compression, and pulmonary artery sling. Other rare variations that have been described include left aortic arch with right descending aorta and right ligamentum and left aortic arch with aberrant right subclavian artery and right ligamentum. The incidence of clinically significant vascular rings is 1%-2% of all congenital heart defects.

Vascular rings and pulmonary slings have been described in conjunction with other cardiac defects, including TOF, ASD, branch pulmonary artery stenosis, coarctation, AVSD, VSD, interrupted aortic arch, and aortopulmonary window. Significant associated cardiac anomalies occur in 11%-20% of patients with a vascular ring. A right aortic arch is generally associated with a greater incidence of coexisting anomalies.

By the end of the fourth week of embryonic development, the six aortic or branchial arches have formed between the dorsal aortae and ventral roots. Subsequent involution and migration of the arches results in the anatomically normal or abnormal development of the aorta and its branches. The majority of the first, second, and fifth arches regress. The third arch forms the common carotid artery and proximal internal carotid artery. The right fourth arch forms the proximal right subclavian artery. The left fourth arch contributes to the portion of the aortic arch from left carotid to left subclavian arteries. The proximal portion of the right sixth arch becomes the proximal portion of the right pulmonary artery, while the distal segment involutes. Similarly, the proximal left sixth arch contributes to the proximal left pulmonary artery, and the distal sixth arch becomes the ductus arteriosus.

The pulmonary artery is formed from two vascular precursors as well as through a combination of angiogenesis, the de novo development of new blood vessels, and vasculogenesis, the budding and migration of existing vessels. As stated previously, the proximal pulmonary arteries are based on the sixth arches, whereas the primitive lung buds initially derive their blood supply from the splanchnic plexus. Ultimately, these two segments of the pulmonary artery join to form the vascular network of the lung parenchyma.

B. Clinical Findings

Children with a complete vascular ring generally present within the first weeks to months of life. Typically, children with a double aortic arch present earlier in life than those with a right arch and retroesophageal left ligamentum. In the younger age group, respiratory symptoms predominate, as liquids are generally well tolerated. Respiratory symptoms may include stridor, nonproductive cough, apnea, or frequent respiratory infections. The cough is classically described as "seal bark" or "brassy." These symptoms may mimic asthma, respiratory infection, or reflux, and children with vascular rings are often initially misdiagnosed. With the transition to solid food, dysphagia becomes more apparent.

The presentation of a patient with an incomplete vascular ring is variable. Children with innominate artery compression usually present within the first 1-2 years of life with respiratory symptoms. Although aberrant right subclavian artery is the most common arch abnormality, occurring in approximately 0.5%-1% of the population, it rarely causes symptoms. Classically, when symptoms do occur, they present in the seventh and eighth decades, as the aberrant vessel becomes ectatic and calcified, causing dysphagia lusoria due to impingement of the artery on the posterior esophagus. An aberrant right subclavian rarely causes symptoms except when it is of an abnormally large caliber or associated with tracheomalacia.

Children with pulmonary artery slings generally present with respiratory symptoms within the first few weeks to months of life. As with complete rings, respiratory symptoms may include stridor, nonproductive cough, apnea, or frequent respiratory infections and may mimic other conditions, leading to misdiagnosis. Pulmonary artery slings are associated with complete tracheal rings in 30%-40% of patients, leading to focal or diffuse tracheal stenosis.

The methods for diagnosing a vascular ring are multiple because of the variability in presentation and the spectrum of diagnostic tests available. A child with a presumptive diagnosis of asthma or tracheomalacia may be referred to a pulmonologist and a diagnosis of vascular ring made or suspected initially by CXR and bronchoscopy. In some situations, the diagnosis is made by echocardiography during evaluation for concurrent cardiac defects. Regardless, the diagnosis generally begins with a CXR. Complementary studies may include barium esophagogram, CTA, cMRI, and bronchoscopy. Important modalities to define the tracheal anatomy in a patient with a pulmonary artery sling include CTA, cMRI, or bronchoscopy. Echocardiography may be diagnostic and may be used to rule out other cardiac anomalies. Tracheograms and cardiac catheterizations, which have been used extensively in the past, are rarely currently indicated.

C. Treatment

A double aortic arch occurs when the distal portion of the right dorsal aorta fails to regress. The two arches form a complete ring, encircling the trachea and esophagus. The right arch is dominant in the majority of the cases, followed by left dominant, with codominant arches being the least common. The left and right carotid and subclavian arteries generally arise from their respective arches. The ligamentum arteriosum and descending aorta usually remain on the left.

The approach to repair of a double aortic arch is via a left posterolateral thoracotomy. The procedure can easily be accomplished through a limited, muscle-sparing incision through the third or fourth intercostal space. The pleura is incised, after identifying the vagus and phrenic nerves. The ligamentum or ductus arteriosum is divided while preserving the recurrent laryngeal nerve. The nondominant arch is then divided between two vascular clamps at the point where brachiocephalic flow is optimally preserved. If there is concern regarding the location for division, the arches can be temporarily occluded at various points while monitoring pulse and blood pressure in each limb. If there is an atretic segment, the division is done at the point of the atresia. Dissection around the esophagus and trachea in the region of the ligamentum/ductus and nondominant arch allows for retraction of the vascular structures and lysis of any residual obstructing adhesions.

There are three anatomic variations for a right arch with a left ligamentum, which cause a complete vascular ring. If the left fourth arch regresses between the aorta and left subclavian, a right aortic arch with aberrant left subclavian artery results. The ligamentum arteriosum is retroesophageal, bridging the left pulmonary artery and aberrant left subclavian, forming a complete vascular ring. If the left fourth arch regresses after the origin of the left subclavian artery but before the arch reaches the dorsal aorta to communicate with the left sixth arch (which becomes the ductus arteriosum), there is mirror-image branching. The ligamentum arteriosum arises directly from the descending aorta, or from a Kommerell diverticulum off of the descending aorta, forming the complete ring. If communication is maintained between the left fourth and sixth arches, there is mirror-image branching with the ligamentum arising from the anterior, mirror-image left subclavian, and a ring is not formed.

The surgical approach for a right aortic arch with retroesophageal left ligamentum arteriosum is the same as for a double arch. The ligamentum is divided, and any adhesions around the esophagus and trachea are lysed. Rarely, the Kommerell diverticulum has been reported to cause compression even after division of the ligamentum. As such, it may be prudent to resect or suspend the diverticulum posteriorly.

In innominate artery compression syndrome, the aortic arch and ligamentum are in their normal leftward position. However, the innominate artery arises partially or totally to the left of midline. As the artery courses from left to right anterior to the trachea, it causes tracheal compression. The symptoms of innominate artery compression may be mild to severe. With mild symptoms and minimal tracheal compression on bronchoscopy, children can be observed expectantly because the symptoms may resolve with growth. Indications for surgery include apnea, severe respiratory distress, significant stridor, or recurrent respiratory tract infection. Several approaches for the correction of innominate artery compression syndrome have been described. These include simple division, division with reimplantation into the right side of the ascending aorta, and suspension to the overlying sternum.

An aberrant right subclavian artery occurs when there is regression of the right fourth arch between the right common carotid and right subclavian arteries. The right subclavian then arises from the leftward descending aorta, laying posterior to the esophagus as it crosses from left to right. Although the artery can compress the esophagus posteriorly, it is rarely the cause of symptoms in children. Surgical treatment involves simple division via a left posterolateral thoracotomy. Rarely, reimplantation or grafting from the right carotid or aortic arch may be necessary.

Normally, the right and left sixth aortic arches contribute to the proximal portions of their respective pulmonary arteries. If the proximal left sixth arch involutes and the bud from the left lung migrates rightward to meet the right pulmonary artery, a pulmonary artery sling is formed. Pulmonary artery slings are associated with complete tracheal rings and tracheal stenosis in 30%-40% of patients. Origin of the right upper lobe bronchus from the trachea ("pig bronchus" or "bronchus suis") has been reported in frequent association with pulmonary artery sling.

Initial attempts at the repair of a pulmonary artery sling involved reimplantation after division of the left pulmonary artery and translocation of the trachea without cardiopulmonary bypass. These early reports had a high incidence of left pulmonary artery thrombosis. This has led some authors to advocate division of the trachea and translocation of the left pulmonary artery. This approach would seem sensible if the trachea were being divided in the course of tracheal reconstruction. However, currently most authors advocate the reimplantation of the left pulmonary artery, which has resulted in excellent results. The procedure is done via a median sternotomy on cardiopulmonary bypass to ensure optimal visualization of the repair. Aortic cross-clamping is not necessary. The left pulmonary artery is divided off of the right pulmonary artery, translocated anterior to the trachea, and reimplanted into the main pulmonary artery.

Any necessary reconstruction of the trachea for complete tracheal rings is done concurrently with bronchoscopic assistance. Many techniques for tracheal reconstruction have been described, with resection and primary reanastomosis and sliding tracheoplasty offering the most reliable results.

Over 95% of vascular rings without concurrent cardiac defects can be performed through a left thoracotomy. A right thoracotomy is indicated for the rare cases where there is a right ligamentum arteriosum. A right ligamentum occurs in the setting of a left aortic arch with right descending aorta, where the ligamentum bridges from the descending aorta to the right pulmonary artery forming a complete ring. Right ligamentum arteriosum has also been described with a left aortic arch with aberrant right subclavian artery. In this case, the ligamentum may arise from the aberrant subclavian artery, from a diverticulum off of the arch, or directly from the left arch to the right pulmonary artery. In addition, a double aortic arch with an atretic segment proximal to the right carotid artery is more easily divided through a right thoracotomy. The approach to these anomalies is the same as for a left-sided ring division, with the caveat that the right recurrent laryngeal nerve will loop around the right ligamentum.

Repair of vascular rings has been described using video-assisted thoracoscopic surgery (VATS) both with and without robotic assistance. Candidates for thoracoscopic division are limited to patients requiring only the division of non-patent vascular structures. In general, VATS is used for patients weighing more than 15 kg due to current size limitations of the instruments.

D. Prognosis

Hospital mortality for the repair of a vascular ring was 1.6% in a recent series of 183 patients by Ruzmetov and colleagues. Overall survival was 96% at 35 years. Eight patients were repaired using left pulmonary artery division and reimplantation for pulmonary artery sling, three of whom also required cardiopulmonary bypass for tracheal reconstruction. Of the 183 patients there were no operative mortalities and eight late deaths. All deaths were in patients with other complex cardiac anomalies. The major source of morbidity, as well as mortality, in this and other series is related to the tracheal reconstruction.

Dillman JR, Attili AK, Agarwal PP, et al: Common and uncommon vascular rings and slings: a multi-modality review. *Pediatr Radiol.* 2011;41:1440-1454.

Kir M, Saylam GS, Karadas U, et al: Vascular rings: presentation, imaging strategies, treatment, and outcome. *Pediatr Cardiol.* 2012;33:607-617.

Phelan E, Ryan S, Rowley H: Vascular rings and slings: interesting vascular anomalies. *J Laryngol Otol.* 2011;125:1158-1163.

Russell HM, Backer CL: Pediatric thoracic problems: patent ductus arteriosus, vascular rings, congenital tracheal stenosis, and pectus deformities. *Surg Clin North Am.* 2010;90:1091-1113.

▶ Coronary Anomalies

A. General Considerations

Coronary artery anomalies occur in between 0.2% and 1.2% of the population. They can be classified as minor, secondary, or major on the basis of their clinical significance. Minor defects have no functional significance and are usually detected as incidental findings at cardiac catheterization. Secondary defects have no intrinsic significance but alter surgical management when they are present. An example of a secondary defect is an anomalous origin of the left anterior descending from the right coronary artery, which crosses the hypoplastic infundibulum in a patient with TOF. The presence of this vessel may prevent the safe performance of a transannular incision and thereby mandate the use of a conduit. Major defects are the most important form of coronary anomaly because they exert an intrinsically adverse effect on the myocardium. Major anomalies can be subdivided based on anatomy: coronary arteriovenous fistula, anomalous pulmonary origin of a coronary artery, anomalous aortic origin of a coronary artery, myocardial bridging, or coronary artery aneurysm.

Coronary arteriovenous fistula is the most common major coronary anomaly. An abnormal connection exists between a coronary artery (usually the right) and another vascular structure (usually one of the right heart chambers). Most fistulas are isolated and solitary. The fistula leads to left-to-right shunting, which can produce congestive heart failure. Other symptoms include angina, endocarditis, myocardial infarction, arrhythmia, and sudden death. The diagnosis is suggested by echocardiography and confirmed by catheterization.

The second most common major coronary anomaly is the origin of a coronary artery from the pulmonary artery. The most common manifestation is the anomalous left coronary artery arising from the pulmonary artery (ALCAPA). The right coronary (or both coronaries) may also arise anomalously from the pulmonary artery but only in very rare cases. ALCAPA is usually well tolerated during fetal development, but after birth, the pulmonary systolic pressure usually drops (following ductal closure and decline in PVR) and the anomalous coronary is perfused with desaturated blood at low pressure. Collateral vessels develop between the normal right coronary artery and the abnormal left coronary, but the benefit is negated due to the development of coronary steal, whereby the collateral blood shunts left to right by retrograde flow in the anomalous coronary into the low-pressure pulmonary artery. Most patients will present between 6 weeks and 3 months of life. Typical symptoms include irritability, difficulty in feeding, and other signs of congestive heart failure. Untreated, ALCAPA is nearly always fatal. Rarely, patients will survive to adulthood and present with symptoms of angina or sudden death. On examination, patients with ALCAPA frequently have a holosystolic murmur of ischemic mitral regurgitation. The pulmonary component of the second heart sound may be pronounced because of pulmonary hypertension. CXR is significant for cardiomegaly and pulmonary edema. ECG evidence of ischemia and infarction is usually present. Echocardiography is usually diagnostic and is useful for assessing the severity of left ventricular dysfunction and ischemic mitral regurgitation that are commonly present. Catheterization is occasionally necessary to clarify the anatomy, but this technique is used less frequently because of the risk of inducing life-threatening arrhythmias.

Anomalous aortic origins of the coronary arteries are usually minor defects, but a potentially dangerous abnormality exists when the left main coronary artery arises from the right coronary sinus and passes between the pulmonary artery and aorta. This defect has been associated with cardiac symptoms and sudden death, as has the origin of the right coronary artery from the left coronary sinus (usually when the right coronary is dominant). The etiology of ischemia in both defects is thought to be related to the acute angle of origin and slit-like orifice of the anomalous vessel and the extrinsic compression created by the opposing walls of the aorta and pulmonary artery. These defects usually present in older patients. Symptomatic patients are treated surgically by coronary artery bypass.

Myocardial bridging occurs when a segment of an epicardial coronary artery (usually the left anterior descending) takes an intramyocardial course over a short segment. Although this is a common incidental finding at cardiac catheterization, this defect has been associated in some cases with myocardial ischemia. Treatment involves dividing the muscle bridge to free the coronary artery, coronary bypass beyond the bridge, or transcatheter stenting.

Coronary aneurysms occur rarely, usually in conjunction with an inflammatory condition such as Kawasaki syndrome, polyarteritis nodosa, Takayasu arteritis, or syphilis. Coronary aneurysms may thrombose or lead to distal coronary stenosis or embolization. Rupture occurs uncommonly. Treatment ranges from antiplatelet therapy to coronary artery bypass grafting and possible transplantation.

B. Treatment

All symptomatic fistulas should be occluded, either surgically or by transcatheter techniques. In some cases, coronary bypass grafting may be necessary when distal flow is compromised by fistula occlusion. Treatment of asymptomatic fistulas is controversial, but occlusion should probably be undertaken when significant left-to-right shunting is present.

Surgical repair is indicated for all patients with ALCAPA. Historically, the initial surgical approach involved ligation of the proximal left coronary artery. This served to eliminate coronary steal and allow perfusion of the left coronary system by collaterals from the right. Despite the ease of simple ligation, most centers have abandoned this approach in favor of establishment of a two-coronary system, which offers better long-term freedom from ischemia. In older patients, this may be achieved by proximal ligation of the left coronary artery in conjunction with coronary artery bypass, ideally with a left internal mammary graft. Coronary bypass is technically difficult in neonates, and a number of alternative operations have been devised to create a direct connection between the aorta and the anomalous coronary artery. Most commonly, this can be achieved by removing the origin of the left coronary artery (along with a button of adjacent pulmonary artery) and reimplanting the vessel directly into the side of the aorta. Another approach involves creation of a side-to-side connection between the aorta and pulmonary artery with placement of an intrapulmonary baffle to direct flow from this connection to the anomalous left coronary ostium.

C. Prognosis

Survival following surgical repair of ALCAPA has improved over the years. Recent reports have suggested an operative mortality of 0%-6%. Ventricular function tends to normalize after surgery. In most patients, mitral valve function also improves, but for patients with severe mitral regurgitation, concurrent mitral valve repair may be indicated.

Attili A, Hensley AK, Jones FD, et al: Echocardiography and coronary CT angiography imaging of variations in coronary anatomy and coronary abnormalities in athletic children: detection of coronary abnormalities that create a risk for sudden death. *Echocardiography.* 2013;30(2):225-233.

Bartoli CR, Wead WB, Giridharan GA: Mechanism of myocardial ischemia with an anomalous left coronary artery from the right sinus of Valsalva. *J Thorac Cardiovasc Surg.* 2012;144:402-408.

Camarda J, Berger S: Coronary artery abnormalities and sudden cardiac death. *Pediatr Cardiol.* 2012;33:434-438.

Mavroudis C, Dodge-Khatami A, Steward RD, et al: An overview of surgery options for congenital coronary artery anomalies. *Future Cardiol.* 2010;6:627-645.

Sundaram B, Kreml R, Patel S: Imaging of coronary anomalies. *Radiol Clin North Am.* 2010;48:711-727.

MULTIPLE CHOICE QUESTIONS

1. Which of the following statements about ventricular septal defects (VSDs) is *false*?

   A. The most common type of VSD is perimembranous.
   B. Left-to-right shunting through a VSD causes a volume load on the right ventricle.
   C. A patient with a large VSD may be asymptomatic at birth but will eventually develop congestive heart failure due to a drop in pulmonary vascular resistance.
   D. In the presence of a perimembranous VSD, the bundle of His passes along the posterior and inferior rim of the defect, generally on the left ventricular side.

2. Which of the following infants would benefit most from the initiation of prostaglandin E_1 (PGE_1)?

   A. Neonate with prenatal diagnosis of aortic coarctation who develops acidosis, oliguria, and diminished pedal pulses 8 hours after birth.
   B. Two-day-old neonate with prenatal diagnosis of complete atrioventricular canal with oxygen saturation of 80% and poor systemic perfusion.
   C. Six-week-old infant presenting with irritability, poor feeding, and tachypnea who is diagnosed with anomalous left coronary artery arising from the pulmonary artery (ALCAPA) and no patent ductus arteriosus (PDA) is seen on echocardiogram.
   D. One-week-old infant with double aortic arch presenting with increasing respiratory distress.

3. A newborn with dextro-transposition of the great arteries (d-TGA) remains severely cyanotic despite initiation of PGE_1 to maintain ductal patency. What is the recommended next step in management?

   A. Initiate inhaled nitric oxide therapy
   B. Diuresis with intravenous furosemide
   C. Balloon atrial septostomy
   D. Emergent arterial switch operation

4. What is the most common major coronary anomaly?

   A. Left coronary from the pulmonary artery (ALCAPA)
   B. Left anterior descending from the right coronary artery
   C. Coronary arteriovenous fistula
   D. Single coronary

5. In which of the following diagnoses is a *primary* catheter-based approach most likely to be recommended over surgery?

   A. Isolated aortic coarctation in a neonate
   B. Isolated pulmonary stenosis in a neonate
   C. PDA in a 1-kg premature infant with heart failure symptoms
   D. Symptomatic perimembranous VSD in a 6-month-old infant

Esophagus & Diaphragm

Francisco Schlottmann, MD, MPH

Marco G. Patti, MD

THE ESOPHAGUS

ANATOMY

The esophagus is a muscular tube that serves as a conduit for the passage of food and fluids from the pharynx to the stomach. It originates at the level of the sixth cervical vertebra, posterior to the cricoid cartilage. In the thorax, the esophagus passes behind the aortic arch and the left main stem bronchus, enters the abdomen through the esophageal hiatus of the diaphragm, and terminates in the fundus of the stomach. Its muscle fibers originate from the cricoid cartilage and pharynx above and interdigitate with those of the stomach below. About 2-4 cm of esophagus is normally located below the diaphragm. The junction between the esophagus and stomach is maintained in its normal intra-abdominal position by the reflection of the peritoneum onto the stomach and of the phrenoesophageal ligament onto the esophagus. The latter is a fibroelastic membrane that lies beneath the peritoneum, on the inferior surface of the diaphragm. When it reaches the esophageal hiatus, the ligament is reflected in an orad direction onto the lower esophagus, where it inserts into the circular muscle layer above the gastroesophageal sphincter, 2-4 cm above the diaphragm (Figure 22–1).

Three anatomic areas of narrowing occur in the esophagus: (1) at the level of the cricoid cartilage (pharyngoesophageal or upper esophageal sphincter); (2) in the mid thorax, from compression by the aortic arch and the left main stem bronchus; and (3) at the level of the esophageal hiatus of the diaphragm (gastroesophageal or lower esophageal sphincter).

In the adult, the distance as measured from the upper incisor teeth to the cricopharyngeus muscle is 15-20 cm; to the aortic arch, 20-25 cm; to the inferior pulmonary vein, 30-35 cm; and to the gastroesophageal junction, approximately 40-45 cm.

The mucosal lining of the esophagus consists of stratified squamous epithelium that contains scattered mucous glands throughout. The musculature of the pharynx and upper third of the esophagus is skeletal in type (striated muscle); the remainder is smooth muscle. Physiologically, the entire organ behaves as a single functioning unit, so that no distinction can be made between the upper and lower esophagus from the standpoint of propulsive activity. As in the intestinal tract, the muscle fibers are arranged into inner circular and outer longitudinal layers. The esophagus has no serosal layer.

The arterial supply to the esophagus is quite consistent. The upper end is supplied by branches from the inferior thyroid arteries. The thoracic portion receives blood from the bronchial arteries and from esophageal branches originating directly from the aorta. The intercostal arteries may also contribute. The diaphragmatic and abdominal segments are nourished by the left inferior phrenic artery and by the esophageal branches of the left gastric artery. The venous drainage is more complex and variable. The upper and mid portions drain into the hemiazygos and azygos veins. The most important veins are those that drain the lower esophagus. Blood from this region passes into the esophageal branches of the coronary vein, a tributary of the portal vein. This connection constitutes a direct communication between the portal circulation and the venous drainage of the lower esophagus and upper stomach. When there is portal hypertension, as in cirrhosis of the liver, blood is shunted upward through the coronary vein and the esophageal venous plexus to eventually pass by way of the azygos vein into the superior vena cava. The esophageal veins may eventually form varices as they become distended when portal hypertension is present.

PHYSIOLOGY

The coordinated activity of the upper esophageal sphincter (UES), the esophageal body, and the lower esophageal sphincter (LES) is responsible for the motor function of the esophagus.

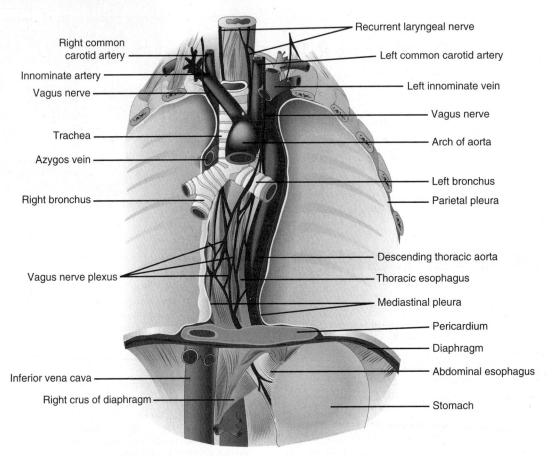

▲ **Figure 22–1.** Anatomy of the esophagus.

1. Upper Esophageal Sphincter

The UES receives motor innervation directly from the brain (nucleus ambiguous). The sphincter is continuously in a state of tonic contraction, with a resting pressure of about 100 mm Hg (anteroposterior axis). The sphincter prevents passage of air from the pharynx into the esophagus and reflux of esophageal contents into the pharynx. During swallowing, a food bolus is moved by the tongue into the pharynx, which contracts while the UES relaxes. After the food bolus has reached the esophagus, the UES regains its resting tone (Figure 22–2).

2. Esophageal Body

When food passes through the UES, a contraction is initiated in the upper esophagus, which progresses distally toward the stomach. The wave initiated by swallowing is referred to as primary peristalsis (Figure 22–2). It travels at a speed of

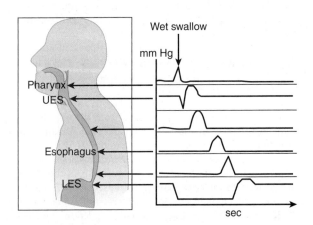

▲ **Figure 22–2.** Swallowing process. Upper esophageal sphincter (UES), esophageal peristalsis, and lower esophageal sphincter (LES) in response to swallowing.

3-4 cm/s and reaches amplitudes of 60-140 mm Hg in the distal esophagus. Local stimulation by distention at any point in the body of the esophagus will elicit a peristaltic wave from the point of stimulus. This is called secondary peristalsis and aids esophageal emptying when the primary wave has failed to clear the lumen of ingested food or when gastric contents reflux from the stomach. Tertiary waves are considered abnormal, but they are frequently seen in elderly subjects who have no symptoms of esophageal disease.

3. Lower Esophageal Sphincter

The LES measures 3-4 cm in length, and its resting pressure ranges between 15 and 24 mm Hg. At the time of swallowing, the LES relaxes for 5 to 10 seconds to allow the food bolus to enter the stomach and then regains its resting tone (Figure 22–2). The LES relaxation is mediated by vasoactive intestinal polypeptide and nitric oxide, both nonadrenergic, noncholinergic neurotransmitters. The resting tone depends mainly on intrinsic myogenic activity. The LES has a tendency to relax periodically at times independent from swallowing. These periodic relaxations are called **transient LES relaxations** to distinguish them from relaxations triggered by swallows. The cause of these transient relaxations is not known, but gastric distention probably plays a role. Transient LES relaxations account for the small amount of physiologic gastroesophageal reflux present in any individual and are also the most common cause of reflux in patients with gastroesophageal reflux disease (GERD). Decrease in length or pressure of the LES (or both) is responsible for abnormal reflux in the remaining patients. Overall, it is thought that although transient LES relaxation is the most common mechanism of reflux in volunteers and patients with either absent or mild esophagitis, the prevalence of a mechanically defective sphincter (hypotensive and short) increases in patients with severe esophagitis, particularly when Barrett metaplasia is present. The crus of the esophageal hiatus of the diaphragm contributes to the resting pressure of the LES. This *pinchcock* action of the diaphragm is particularly important because it protects against reflux caused by sudden increases of intra-abdominal pressure, such as with coughing or bending. This synergistic action of the diaphragm is lost when a sliding hiatal hernia is present, as the gastroesophageal junction is displaced above the diaphragm (Figure 22–3).

DIAGNOSTIC APPROACH TO ESOPHAGEAL DISEASES

▶ Symptomatic Evaluation

Esophageal symptoms can be divided into two groups: (1) *typical,* such as dysphagia, heartburn, and regurgitation; and (2) *atypical,* such as chest pain, cough, and hoarseness.

Peristalsis inefficient

Hernia becomes compartmentalized

Pinchcock does not support LES

▲ **Figure 22–3.** Pathophysiology of hiatal hernia. LES, lower esophageal sphincter.

Dysphagia is a unique symptom because it points to an esophageal disorder, either functional (secondary to abnormalities of esophageal peristalsis or lack of coordination between different parts of the esophagus) or mechanical (secondary to a peptic or malignant stricture or an intraluminal mass). Heartburn can also be caused by nonesophageal disorders such as biliary disease, irritable bowel syndrome, coronary artery disease, and psychiatric diseases.

Upper Gastrointestinal Series

The test is performed by giving the patient barium to swallow. Subsequently, multiple images are taken, including images of the esophagus, the gastroesophageal junction, the stomach, and the duodenum (a barium swallow focuses just on the esophagus and the gastroesophageal junction). This test characterizes a hiatal hernia, an esophageal stricture, an esophageal diverticulum, or an intraluminal mass. A cineesophagram is a dynamic evaluation of the swallowing process, and it is particularly useful in patients with functional dysphagia (secondary to a motility disorder, in the absence of a mechanical cause).

Upper Endoscopy

This test allows visualization of the mucosal surface of the esophagus, stomach, and duodenum. The presence and degree of esophagitis and the presence of an intraluminal mass can be determined, and biopsies taken.

Endoscopic Ultrasound

This test is used in patients with esophageal cancer to define the depth of penetration of the tumor through the esophageal wall (T) and the presence of enlarged periesophageal lymph nodes (N). Fine-needle aspiration of these nodes can be done, and cytologic analysis of the aspirate performed.

Esophageal Manometry

Esophageal manometry allows determination of (1) LES location, length, pressure, and relaxation in response to swallowing; (2) pressure, duration, and velocity of propagation of the peristaltic waves; and (3) location, pressure, relaxation of the UES, and coordination with the pharyngeal contraction.

Ambulatory 24-Hour pH Monitoring

This test measures reflux of acid from the stomach into the esophagus, and it is considered the gold standard for the diagnosis of GERD. By convention, the catheter is placed 5 cm above the upper border of the manometrically determined LES and is kept in place for 24 hours, during which time the patient does not alter the daily activities and diet. In addition to determining whether a pathologic amount of gastroesophageal reflux is present, the test establishes whether there is a temporal correlation between episodes of reflux and symptoms (Figure 22–4). Esophageal impedance

▲ **Figure 22–4.** Ambulatory pH monitoring. The superior plot reports the 24-hour pH recording in the proximal esophagus 20 cm above the upper border of the manometrically determined lower esophageal sphincter (LES). The inferior plot reports the 24-hour pH recording in the distal esophagus 5 cm above the upper border of the manometrically determined LES. A reflux episode occurs when the pH falls below 4 and ends when the pH returns above 4.

is a technique that measures flow of liquids and gas across the gastroesophageal junction, independently of the pH of the gastric refluxate. In association with pH monitoring, impedance is indicated in patients with proton pump inhibitor (PPI)–resistant typical reflux symptoms and chronic unexplained cough.

Gastric Scintigraphy

Gastric scintigraphy is indicated in patients who experience postprandial bloating and fullness to measure the gastric emptying of solids and liquids.

Computed Tomography

A computed tomography (CT) scan is used to assess the presence of metastases (M) (eg, lung, liver, adrenals) in patients with esophageal cancer.

Positron Emission Tomography

A positron emission tomography (PET) scan is used to assess the metastatic spread of esophageal cancer (M). In addition, it might help predict the response of esophageal cancer to neoadjuvant therapy.

Laparoscopy/Thoracoscopy

Laparoscopy or thoracoscopy can be used to stage esophageal cancer, particularly when liver metastasis or extensive lymphadenopathy is suspected.

Akisiniku O et al: High resolution vs conventional esophageal manometry in the assessment of esophageal motor disorders in patients with non-cardiac chest pain. *Neurogastroenterol Motil.* 2018;30(6):e13282.

Patti MG et al: Surgery of the esophagus: anatomy and physiology. *Surg Clin North Am.* 1997;77(5):959-970.

Weber C et al: Current applications of evolving methodologies in gastroesophageal reflux disease testing. *Dig Liver Dis.* 2011;43:353-357.

Winiker M et al: Accuracy of preoperative staging a priori resectable esophageal cancer. *Dis Esophagus.* 2018;31:1-6.

ESOPHAGEAL MOTILITY DISORDERS

The main primary esophageal motility disorder is achalasia. Other disorders include esophagogastric junction outflow obstruction, distal esophageal spasm, hypercontractile esophagus, and absent contractility. These disorders present with a combination of dysphagia, regurgitation, chest pain, and heartburn. Esophageal manometry is the key test that differentiates these disorders.

ACHALASIA

ESSENTIALS OF DIAGNOSIS

- Dysphagia
- Regurgitation
- Absence of esophageal peristalsis and partial or absent relaxation of the LES in response to swallowing on esophageal manometry
- Radiologic evidence of distal esophageal narrowing

General Considerations

Achalasia is a primary esophageal motility disorder characterized by lack of esophageal peristalsis and by partial or absent relaxation of the LES in response to swallowing. Consequently, there is a functional obstruction at the level of the gastroesophageal junction, which determines impairment of the esophageal emptying. The incidence of achalasia is about 1 in 100,000 persons. It occurs with equal frequency in men and women and can occur at any age.

Pathogenesis

The pathophysiology of achalasia involves the selective degeneration of inhibitory neurons of the esophageal myenteric plexus (containing nitric oxide and vasoactive intestinal polypeptide), which are needed for the relaxation of the tonic LES and the adequate peristalsis of the esophageal body. Because the postganglionic cholinergic neurons are spared, there is unopposed cholinergic stimulation, which increases LES resting pressure and decreases LES relaxation. There is no propagation of peristaltic waves in response to swallowing, but rather the presence of simultaneous contractions. The etiology of this degenerative process, however, remains largely unknown. Some viruses such as varicella-zoster, human papilloma, and herpes have been implicated in initiating an inflammatory reaction. An autoimmune etiology has also been suggested, with evidence of antibodies against myenteric neurons in the serum of achalasia patients. Achalasia can also occur in patients with **Chagas disease** (American trypanosomiasis), a condition in which the infective organism destroys parasympathetic ganglion cells throughout the body, including the heart and the gastrointestinal, urinary, and respiratory tracts.

Clinical Findings

A. Symptoms and Signs

Dysphagia is the most common symptom, experienced by about 95% of patients. It is often for both solids and liquids.

Table 22–1. Clinical scoring system for achalasia (Eckardt score).

Score	Weight Loss (kg)	Dysphagia	Retrosternal Pain	Regurgitation
0	None	None	None	None
1	< 5	Occasional	Occasional	Occasional
2	5-10	Daily	Daily	Daily
3	> 10	Each meal	Each meal	Each meal

Most patients adapt with changes in their diet and are able to maintain a stable weight, while other eventually experience some weight loss. Regurgitation of undigested food is the second most common symptom and is present in about 60% of patients. It occurs more often in the supine position and may lead to aspiration. Heartburn is present in about 50% of patients. It is not due to GERD, but rather to stasis and fermentation of undigested food in the distal esophagus. Chest pain also occurs in about 40% of patients, due to esophageal distension, and it is usually experienced at the time of a meal.

The Eckardt score is the grading system most frequently used for the evaluation of symptoms and efficacy of achalasia treatment. It attributes points (0-3 points) to four symptoms of the disease (dysphagia, regurgitation, chest pain, and weight loss), and the score ranges from 0-12 (Table 22–1). Treatment is usually consider successful if it brings the Eckardt score to ≤ 3.

B. Imaging Studies

Endoscopy is usually the first test performed to rule out a mechanical obstruction such as a peptic stricture or cancer. Retained food can be found, and the esophagus can be dilated or tortuous. The esophageal mucosa can be normal or show signs of esophagitis, usually secondary to food stasis or *Candida* infection.

A barium swallow usually shows narrowing at the level of the gastroesophageal junction (so called "bird beak") and slow emptying of contrast (Figure 22–5). A dilated, sigmoid esophagus may be present in patients with longstanding achalasia.

C. Special Tests

Esophageal manometry is the gold standard for the diagnosis of achalasia. Lack of peristalsis and partial or absent relaxation of the LES in response to swallowing are the key criteria for the diagnosis. Although in the past it was thought that the LES was hypertensive in all patients, today it is known that an elevated LES pressure is present in about 50% of patients only.

▲ **Figure 22–5.** Esophageal achalasia. Note dilation of the esophageal body, retained barium, and distal esophageal narrowing (bird's beak).

The Chicago classification divides achalasia into three subtypes (Figure 22–6):

Type I: Incomplete LES relaxation, aperistalsis, and absence of esophageal pressurization

Type II: Incomplete LES relaxation, aperistalsis, and pan-esophageal pressurization in at least 20% of swallows

Type III: Incomplete LES relaxation and premature "spastic" contractions (distal latency < 4.5 seconds) in at least 20% of swallows

▶ Differential Diagnosis

Benign strictures due to GERD and esophageal carcinoma may mimic the clinical presentation of achalasia. Sometimes an infiltrating tumor of the gastroesophageal junction can mimic not only the clinical and radiologic presentation of achalasia, but also the manometric profile. This condition, called **secondary achalasia** or **pseudo-achalasia**, should be suspected in patients older than 60 years with recent onset of dysphagia (< 6 months) and excessive weight loss.

Type I   Type II   Type III

▲ **Figure 22–6.** Chicago classification of esophageal achalasia. Type I: absence of esophageal pressurization; type II: panesophageal pressurization; type III: premature contractions.

Achalasia patients often suffer from heartburn due to food stasis and fermentation. Unfortunately, this symptom is often attributed to GERD, and patients are treated with PPIs with a consequent delay in diagnosis. pH monitoring can help distinguishing between GERD (real reflux) and achalasia (false reflux).

▶ **Complications**

Aspiration of retained and undigested food can cause repeated episodes of pneumonia. Achalasia is also a risk factor for esophageal squamous cell carcinoma, probably due to the continuous irritation of the mucosa by the retained and fermenting food. Adenocarcinoma can occur in patients who develop GERD after pneumatic dilation or myotomy.

▶ **Treatment**

Therapy is palliative, and it is directed toward relief of symptoms by decreasing the outflow resistance caused by the dysfunctional LES. Because peristalsis is absent and does not return after any form of treatment, gravity becomes the key factor that allows emptying of food from the esophagus into the stomach.

▶ **Medical Therapy**

Treatments aimed at relaxing esophageal smooth muscle such as nitrates, calcium channel blockers and antimuscarinic agents may be helpful. However, these drugs have modest effect on the resting LES pressure and do not improve LES relaxation in response to swallowing. Hence, pharmacologic treatment is of marginal clinical value and should be considered only in patients who have contraindications to either pneumatic dilation or to surgery.

A. Endoscopic Treatment

Intrasphincteric injection of botulinum toxin is used to block the release of acetylcholine at the level of the LES, thereby restoring the balance between excitatory and inhibitory neurotransmitters. This treatment, however, is of limited value: Only 60% of treated patients still have relief of dysphagia 6 months after treatment, and this number further decreases to 30% (even after multiple injections) 2.5 years later. In addition, it often causes an inflammatory reaction at the level of the gastroesophageal junction, which makes a subsequent myotomy more difficult. It should be used primarily in patients who are poor candidates for dilatation or surgery.

The goal of **pneumatic dilation (PD)** is to eliminate the functional obstruction at the level of the gastroesophageal junction by disrupting the circular muscle fibers of the LES. The most commonly employed balloon dilator in the United States is the Rigiflex balloon (Boston Scientific Corporation, Marlborough, MA). The first PD session should be performed by using a 30-mm Rigiflex balloon. Larger balloons—35 mm and 40 mm in diameter—should be used 2-4 weeks later if symptoms persist. If dysphagia recurs after a PD with a 40-mm balloon, the response to further PDs is unlikely. The perforation rate is about 2%-5%. If a perforation is suspected, a gastrografin study eventually followed by a barium esophagogram should be performed. Predictors of a favorable outcome are low LES pressure after dilatation, older age, and female gender.

Peroral endoscopic myotomy (POEM) was introduced in 2010 and consists of an endoscopic creation of a submucosal tunnel, which allows performing a myotomy by transection of the circular fibers of the distal esophagus. POEM is a very effective first line of treatment, but it is associated

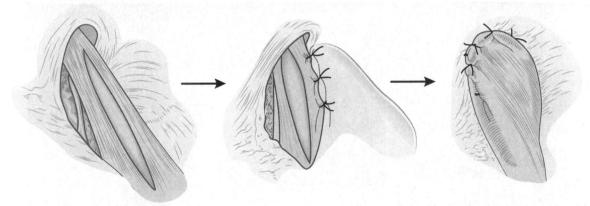

▲ **Figure 22–7.** Laparoscopic Heller myotomy and Dor fundoplication.

with a high incidence of postprocedure gastroesophageal reflux (POEM ablates the LES without any form of antireflux procedure). Data comparing POEM with surgical myotomy are very limited, and to date, there have been no randomized controlled trials comparing these treatment modalities. Schlottmann and colleagues conducted a systematic review and meta-analysis and showed that, at 24 months, improvement in dysphagia for surgical myotomy and POEM was 90.0% and 92.7%, respectively ($P = 0.01$). However, patients undergoing POEM were more likely to develop GERD symptoms (odds ratio [OR] 1.69), GERD evidenced by erosive esophagitis (OR 9.31), and GERD evidenced by pH monitoring (OR 4.30). Studies with longer follow-up are needed to assess the long-term outcomes of POEM.

B. Surgical Treatment

A **laparoscopic Heller myotomy (LHM)** and Dor fundoplication (180 degrees anterior) is an effective and safe procedure, with excellent long-term outcomes. The operation consists of a controlled section of the muscle fibers (myotomy) of the lower esophagus (6 cm) and proximal gastric wall (2-2.5 cm), followed by an anterior partial fundoplication to prevent reflux (Figure 22–7) . Patients spend 24-48 hours in the hospital and return to regular activities in about 2 weeks. The operation effectively relieves symptoms in about 90% of patients. The incidence of postoperative reflux is around 10%, and it is usually controlled by acid-reducing medications. Persistent or recurrent dysphagia after myotomy can be treated with PD or another myotomy.

An esophagectomy should be reserved for patients with severe dysphagia who have failed all other treatment modalities.

OTHER ESOPHAGEAL MOTILITY DISORDERS

Esophagogastric junction outflow obstruction is characterized by an impaired LES relaxation with normal or weak peristalsis. It may be caused by an anatomical abnormality at the cardia (eg, hiatal hernia, diseases of the esophageal wall) or be idiopathic with normal anatomy. Similar to achalasia, treatment is directed toward relief of the obstruction and can be accomplished by botulinum toxin injection, PD, LHM, or POEM.

Distal esophageal spasm (DES) is defined by premature contractions in at least 20% of swallows with a normal LES relaxation. The management of DES remains elusive. Previous reports showed good results in patients with "diffuse esophageal spasm" (Richter classification) who underwent LHM with an extended myotomy. However, scarce data are available after the new classification defined DES.

Hypercontractile esophagus (jackhammer esophagus) is characterized by high-amplitude peristaltic waves (distal contractile interval > 8000 mm Hg/s/cm) in at least 20% of swallows (Figure 22–8). Chest pain is the most common symptom. Patients often come to the attention of gastroenterologists only after a thorough cardiac workup has been performed. About half of the patients complain of dysphagia in addition to chest pain. The results of surgery have been disappointing, as chest pain persists after myotomy in about 50% of patients. Dysphagia, however, is improved in the majority of patients.

Absent contractility is characterized by aperistalsis in the setting of normal LES relaxation. It is mostly diagnosed in patients with connective tissue diseases. There is no specific treatment to restore or improve peristalsis in these patients. Associated GERD is usually the target of therapy.

Boeckxstaens GE et al: Pneumatic dilation versus laparoscopic Heller's myotomy for idiopathic achalasia. *N Engl J Med.* 2011;364:1807-1816.

Inoue H et al: Peroral endoscopic myotomy (POEM) for esophageal achalasia. *Endoscopy.* 2010;42:265-271.

Schlottmann F et al: Laparoscopic Heller myotomy versus peroral endoscopic myotomy (POEM) for achalasia: a systematic review and meta-analysis. *Ann Surg.* 2018;267:451-460.

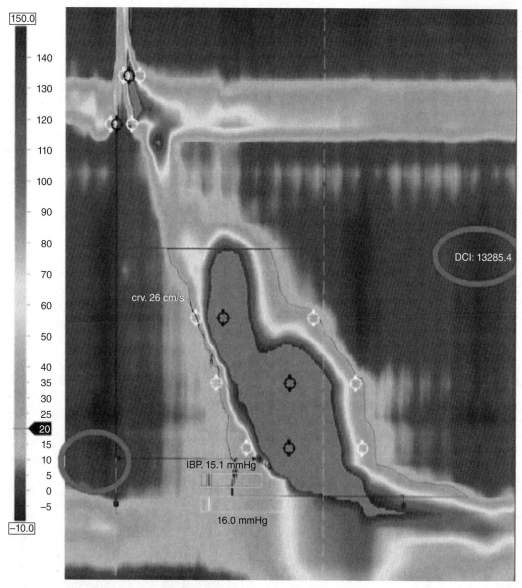

crv. 26 cm/s

DCI: 13285.4

IBP. 15.1 mmHg

16.0 mmHg

▲ **Figure 22–8.** Hypercontractile esophagus (jackhammer esophagus).

Schlottmann F et al: Modern management of esophageal acha-lasia: from pathophysiology to treatment. *Curr Probl Surg.* 2018; 55:10-37.

Schlottmann F et al: Primary esophageal motility disorders: beyond achalasia. *Int J Mol Sci.* 2017;18:7.

Schlottmann F et al: The role of Heller myotomy and POEM for non-achalasia motility disorders. *Dis Esophagus.* 2017;30:1-5.

Schlottmann F et al: Understanding the Chicago Classification: from tracings to patients. *J Neurogastroenterol Motil.* 2017; 23:487-494.

ESOPHAGEAL DIVERTICULA

Esophageal diverticula are rare. They are located above the UES (pharyngoesophageal or Zenker diverticulum) or the LES (epiphrenic diverticulum). They are considered pulsion diverticula and are secondary to abnormalities of the sphincters in terms of resting pressure, relaxation in response to swallowing, and coordination with the segment above the sphincter. As a consequence, mucosa and submucosa protrude through the muscular layers, forming the outpouching.

1. Pharyngoesophageal Diverticulum (Zenker Diverticulum)

ESSENTIALS OF DIAGNOSIS

- ▶ Dysphagia
- ▶ Regurgitation of undigested food (with risk of aspiration)
- ▶ Gurgling sounds in the neck
- ▶ Halitosis

▶ General Considerations

This is the most common of the esophageal diverticula and is three times more frequent in men than in women. Most patients are over age 60. The condition originates from the posterior wall of the esophagus, in a triangular area of weakness (Killian triangle), limited inferiorly by the upper border of the cricopharyngeal muscle and laterally by the oblique fibers of the inferior constrictor muscles of the pharynx. As the diverticulum enlarges, it tends to deviate from the midline, mostly to the left (Figure 22–9).

▶ Pathogenesis

A Zenker diverticulum is due either to lack of coordination between the pharyngeal contraction and the opening time of the UES or to a hypertensive UES. Because of the increased intraluminal pressure, there is progressive herniation of mucosa and submucosa through the Killian triangle. Occasionally, UES dysfunction can occur in the absence of a diverticulum (cricopharyngeal achalasia). A hereditary syndrome called oculopharyngeal muscular dystrophy, consisting of ptosis and dysphagia, has been described in patients of French-Canadian ancestry. The dysphagia is the result of weak pharyngeal musculature in the face of normal UES function; it is considerably improved by UES myotomy. This syndrome also manifests with cervical dysphagia. A chronic cough may develop in some patients from aspiration of saliva and ingested food.

▶ Clinical Findings

A. Symptoms

Dysphagia is the most common symptom and occurs in about 80%-90% of patients. Regurgitation of undigested food from the diverticulum often occurs and can lead to aspiration into the tracheobronchial tree and pneumonia. Patients frequently have halitosis and can hear gurgling sounds in the neck. About 30% of patients have associated GERD.

▲ **Figure 22–9.** Pharyngoesophageal diverticulum (Zenker diverticulum).

B. Imaging Studies

A barium swallow clearly shows the position and size of the diverticulum or a prominent cricopharyngeal bar without diverticulum (Figure 22–9).

C. Special Tests

Esophageal manometry shows a lack of coordination between the pharynx and the cricopharyngeus muscle and often a hypertensive UES. In addition, it can show a hypotensive LES and abnormal esophageal peristalsis. Ambulatory pH monitoring determines if abnormal esophageal acid exposure is present. Endoscopy may be dangerous because the instrument can enter the diverticulum rather than the esophageal lumen and cause a perforation.

▶ Differential Diagnosis

Differential diagnosis includes esophageal stricture, achalasia, and esophageal cancer.

▶ Treatment

The standard treatment consists of eliminating the functional obstruction at the UES level with a myotomy of the cricopharyngeus muscle and the upper 3 cm of the posterior esophageal wall and excision or suspension of the diverticulum. For small diverticula (< 2 cm), the myotomy alone is sufficient.

As an alternative to the conventional surgical treatment, a transoral endoscopic approach (using staplers, laser, or coagulation through an endoscope that ablate the septum between the diverticulum and the cervical esophagus) can be used for diverticula between 3 and 6 cm in size. If present, GERD should be corrected before dividing the UES in order to avoid aspiration. The prognosis is excellent in about 90% of cases. Complications are rare, and the patients are usually able to eat the day after the procedure.

2. Epiphrenic Diverticulum

ESSENTIALS OF DIAGNOSIS

- ▶ Dysphagia
- ▶ Regurgitation
- ▶ Diverticulum evident on barium swallow
- ▶ Esophageal motility disorder shown by esophageal manometry

▶ General Considerations

Epiphrenic diverticulum is located in the distal 10 cm of the esophagus. It is not a primary anatomic abnormality but rather the consequence of an underlying motility disorder of the esophagus that causes an outflow obstruction at the level of the gastroesophageal junction, with consequent increase in intraluminal pressure and progressive herniation of mucosa and submucosa through the esophageal muscle layers.

▶ Clinical Findings

A. Symptoms

The symptoms experienced by the patient are in part due to the underlying motility disorder (dysphagia, chest pain) and in part due to the diverticulum per se (regurgitation with the risk of aspiration). Some diverticula, however, can be asymptomatic.

B. Imaging Studies

A chest radiograph can show an air-fluid level in the posterior mediastinum. A barium swallow clearly shows the position and size of the diverticulum (Figure 22–10). Endoscopy is important to rule out an esophageal malignancy.

C. Special Tests

In the majority of cases, esophageal manometry shows the underlying motility disorder. Sometimes it is difficult to

▲ **Figure 22–10.** Epiphrenic diverticulum.

position the manometry catheter, and endoscopic or fluoroscopic guidance might be necessary.

Differential Diagnosis

A paraesophageal hernia can be confused with an epiphrenic diverticulum. The barium swallow and the endoscopy help in establishing the diagnosis.

Treatment

The treatment is surgical, and the laparoscopic approach is preferred. It consists of (1) resection of the diverticulum; (2) long myotomy (it is performed in the side of the esophagus opposite to where the diverticulum is located, and it extends proximally to the upper border of the neck of the diverticulum and distally for about 2 cm onto the gastric wall); and (3) a partial fundoplication to prevent GERD. A laparoscopic diverticulectomy, with myotomy and fundoplication, is successful in 80%-90% of cases.

Herbella FAM et al: Modern pathophysiology and treatment of esophageal diverticula. *Langenbecks Arch Surg.* 2012;397:29-35.

Koch M et al: Endoscopic laser-assisted diverticulotomy versus open surgical approach in the treatment of Zenker's diverticulum. *Laryngoscope.* 2011;121:2090-2094.

Li L et al: Endoscopic treatment of Zenker's diverticulum: a simplified needle-knife technique. *Gastrointest Endosc.* 2016; 84(6):1050-1051.

Soares R et al: Epiphrenic diverticulum: from pathophysiology to treatment. *J Gastrointest Surg.* 2010;14:2009-2015.

Vicentine FP et al: High resolution manometry findings in patients with esophageal epiphrenic diverticula. *Am Surg.* 2011;77: 1661-1664.

Zaninotto G et al: Therapeutic strategies for epiphrenic diverticula: systematic review. *World J Surg.* 2011;35:1447-1453.

ESOPHAGEAL MANIFESTATIONS IN SCLERODERMA & OTHER SYSTEMIC DISEASES

Scleroderma and several other systemic diseases may involve the esophagus. In scleroderma or progressive systemic sclerosis, there is involvement of the gastrointestinal tract in up to 90% of patients. The most common site of gastrointestinal involvement is the smooth muscle portion of the esophagus, where atrophy and fibrosis occur. The upper esophagus (striated muscle) and the UES are not involved. As a consequence, LES pressure is low and the peristalsis is weak (low amplitude or abnormal propagation of the peristaltic waves). These changes can be followed by an increased amount of GERD with delayed clearance of the refluxed gastric contents. Esophageal symptoms usually appear in patients with the characteristic skin changes and Raynaud syndrome. In addition to heartburn and regurgitation, patients may have respiratory symptoms due to the upward extent of the gastric refluxate and aspiration. Dysphagia may be due to the abnormal peristalsis or to the presence of a peptic stricture. The diagnostic approach is similar to that of patients with GERD:

- A barium swallow may show a hiatal hernia or a stricture.
- Endoscopy shows esophagitis in 50%-60% of patients. Barrett esophagus is present in about 10% of patients.
- Esophageal manometry usually shows a hypotensive LES. Dysmotility is frequent and can progress to complete loss of peristalsis.
- Ambulatory pH monitoring is essential to establish the diagnosis. It can also measure the presence of acid in the proximal esophagus and pharynx in patients with cough or vocal cord problems.
- Gastric scintigraphy is indicated in patients who experience postprandial bloating and fullness to measure the gastric emptying of solids and liquids.

Similar esophageal changes may also occur in rheumatoid arthritis, Sjögren syndrome, Raynaud disease, and systemic lupus erythematosus. Similar motor abnormalities are occasionally seen in alcoholism, diabetes mellitus, myxedema, multiple sclerosis, and amyloidosis.

Medical management should always be tried first. A PPI is the drug of choice. If gastroparesis is present, a prokinetic medication such as metoclopramide should be added. A fundoplication should be considered in patients with regurgitation, cough, or vocal cord problems.

Crowell MD et al: Esophageal motor abnormalities in patients with scleroderma: heterogeneity, risk factors, and effects on quality of life. *Clin Gastroenterol Hepatol.* 2017;15:207-213.

Denaxas K et al: Evaluation and management of esophageal manifestations in systemic sclerosis. *Ann Gastroenterol.* 2018; 31:165-170.

GASTROESOPHAGEAL REFLUX DISEASE

ESSENTIALS OF DIAGNOSIS

▶ Heartburn

▶ Regurgitation

▶ Sliding hiatal hernia on barium swallow

▶ Esophagitis on endoscopy

▶ Abnormal esophageal motility on manometry

▶ Abnormal esophageal exposure on ambulatory pH monitoring

General Considerations

GERD is the most common upper gastrointestinal disorder of the Western world and accounts for about 75% of esophageal diseases. GERD affects approximately 20% of the population in the United States, and its prevalence is increasing worldwide, mostly due to the epidemic of obesity.

Pathogenesis

GERD is caused by the abnormal retrograde flow of gastric contents into the esophagus, resulting in symptoms and mucosal damage. A defective LES is the most common cause of GERD. Transient LES relaxations account for the majority of reflux episodes in patients without mucosal damage or with mild esophagitis, whereas a short and hypotensive LES is more frequently found in patients with more severe esophagitis. In 40%-60% of patients with GERD, abnormalities of esophageal peristalsis are also present. Because esophageal peristalsis is the main determinant of esophageal clearance (the ability of the esophagus to clear gastric contents refluxed through the LES), patients with abnormal esophageal peristalsis have more severe reflux and slower clearance. Therefore, these patients often have more severe mucosal injury and more frequent atypical symptoms such as cough or hoarseness.

A hiatal hernia also contributes to the incompetence of the gastroesophageal junction by altering the anatomic relationship between the esophageal crus and the LES. As the gastroesophageal junction is displaced above the diaphragm, the *pinchcock* action of the esophageal crus is lost. In patients with large hiatal hernias, the LES is usually shorter and weaker, and the amount of reflux is greater.

Clinical Findings

A. Symptoms

Heartburn, regurgitation, and dysphagia are considered *typical* symptoms of GERD. However, a clinical diagnosis of GERD based on these symptoms is correct in only 70% of patients (when compared with the results of pH monitoring). A good response to therapy with PPIs is a good predictor of the presence of abnormal reflux. GERD can also cause *atypical* symptoms such as cough, wheezing, chest pain, hoarseness, and dental erosions. Two mechanisms have been postulated for GERD-induced respiratory symptoms: (1) a vagal reflex arc resulting in bronchoconstriction and (2) microaspiration into the tracheobronchial tree. Hoarseness or dental erosions are instead secondary to the upward extent of the acid with direct damage of the vocal cords or teeth (Table 22-2)

B. Barium Swallow

A barium swallow provides information about the presence and size of a hiatal hernia, the presence and length of a stricture, and the length of the esophagus. This test, however, is not diagnostic of GERD, as a hiatal hernia or reflux of barium can be present in the absence of abnormal reflux.

Table 22–2. Symptoms associated with gastroesophageal reflux disease (GERD).

Clinical Presentation of GERD	
Esophageal	Heartburn Regurgitation Dysphagia
Gastric	Bloating Early satiety Belching Nausea
Pulmonary	Aspiration Asthma Wheezing Cough Dyspnea
Ears, nose, throat	Globus Water brash Hoarseness
Cardiac	Chest pain

C. Endoscopy

Fifty percent of patients with abnormal reflux do not have esophagitis on endoscopy. Therefore, endoscopy is useful for diagnosing complications of GERD such as esophagitis, Barrett esophagus, or a stricture. The Los Angeles (LA) classification is the most validated classification system for esophagitis (Table 22–3).

D. Esophageal Manometry

This test provides information about the LES (resting pressure, length, and relaxation) and the quality of esophageal peristalsis. In addition, manometry is essential for proper

Table 22–3. Los Angeles classification system for esophagitis.

Los Angeles Grading System for Esophagitis.	
Grade A	Mucosal breaks ≤ 5 mm long, none of which extends between the tops of the mucosal folds
Grade B	Mucosal breaks > 5 mm long, none of which extends between the tops of two mucosal folds
Grade C	Mucosal breaks that extend between the tops of two or more mucosal folds but that involve < 75% of the esophageal circumference
Grade D	Mucosal breaks that involve ≥ 75% of the esophageal circumference

placement of the pH probe for ambulatory pH monitoring (5 cm above the upper border of the LES).

E. Ambulatory pH Monitoring

This test has a sensitivity and specificity of about 92%, and is considered the gold standard for diagnosing GERD (Table 22–4). Medications that affect the production of acid by the parietal cells must be stopped 3 days (H_2-blocking agents) to 7 days (PPIs) prior to the study. Diet and exercise are unrestricted during the test in order to mimic a typical day of the patient's life. This test should be performed (1) in patients who do not respond to medical therapy, (2) in patients who relapse after discontinuation of medical therapy, (3) before antireflux surgery, or (4) when evaluating atypical symptoms such as cough, hoarseness, and chest pain. Because fewer than 50% of these patients with atypical symptoms experience heartburn or have esophagitis on endoscopy, a pH monitoring study becomes the only way to determine whether abnormal reflux is present, establishing a temporal link between episodes of reflux and symptoms. A pH probe with two sensors, located 5 cm and 20 cm above the LES, allows determination of the upward extent of the reflux. Tracings are analyzed for a temporal correlation between symptoms and episodes of reflux.

▶ Differential Diagnosis

Heartburn can be the presenting symptom of irritable bowel syndrome, achalasia, cholelithiasis, coronary artery disease, or psychiatric disorders. Esophageal manometry and pH monitoring are essential to determine with certainty whether GERD is present and whether reflux is the cause of the symptoms.

Table 22–4. Normal values for pH monitoring.

Normal Values for Ambulatory 24-Hour pH Monitoring.	
Percentage of total time pH < 4.0	4.5%
Percentage of upright time pH < 4.0	8.4%
Percentage of supine time pH < 4.0	3.5%
Number of episodes of reflux	47
Number of episodes > 5 minutes	3.5
Longest episode (minutes)	20
Composite score[1]	14.7

[1]The composite score indicates the extent to which the patient's values deviate from the normal means of the six variables. It allows one to express in a single figure the degree of the patient's abnormality.

▶ Complications

Esophagitis is the most common complication. Peptic strictures are uncommon, particularly in the era of PPIs. Barrett esophagus is found in about 10%-15% of patients with reflux documented by pH monitoring. Some patients may eventually progress to high-grade dysplasia and adenocarcinoma. Respiratory complications vary from chronic cough to asthma, aspiration pneumonia, and even pulmonary fibrosis. Vocal cord and dental damage can also occur.

▶ Treatment

A. Lifestyle Modifications

Patients should eat frequent small meals during the day (to avoid gastric distention), avoiding fatty foods, spicy foods, and chocolate, as they lower LES pressure. The last meal should be no less than 2 hours before going to bed. To increase the effect of gravity, the head of the bed should be elevated over 4-inch to 6-inch blocks.

B. Medical Therapy

Antacids are useful for patients with mild intermittent heartburn. Acid-suppressing medications are the mainstay of medical therapy. H_2-blocking agents are usually prescribed for patients with mild symptoms or mild esophagitis. PPIs are superior to H_2-blocking agents because they determine a more profound control of the acid secretion, with healing of esophagitis in 80%-90% of patients. However, symptoms and esophagitis tend to recur in the majority of patients after discontinuation of therapy, so most patients need chronic maintenance therapy. In addition, about 50% of patients on maintenance PPIs require increasing doses to maintain healing of esophagitis.

Acid-suppressing medications only alter the pH of the gastric refluxate, but reflux and aspiration can still occur because of an incompetent LES and ineffective esophageal peristalsis. Moreover, medical therapy is largely ineffective for the treatment of the extraesophageal manifestations of GERD due to the upward extension of the refluxate. PPIs can interfere with calcium absorption, causing osteoporosis and fractures. In addition, PPIs can cause *Clostridium difficile* infection, nosocomial and community-acquired pneumonia, kidney disease, and major adverse cardiac events. The latter are mediated by electrolyte abnormalities (hypomagnesemia and hypocalcemia) and reduced activity of nitric oxide synthase. Furthermore, PPIs should not be prescribed for patients who have coronary stents and take clopidogrel bisulfate because they counteract its antiplatelet activity.

C. Surgical Therapy

The ideal patient for antireflux surgery is the one in whom ambulatory pH monitoring shows abnormal GER and whose

Table 22–5. Indications for antireflux surgery.

Symptoms (eg, regurgitation, cough) not controlled by proton pump inhibitor (PPI)
Symptoms and large hiatal hernia
Poor patient's compliance with medical therapy
Cost of medical therapy
Side effects of medications
Symptomatic young patients who refuse lifelong PPI

heartburn is well controlled by PPIs. A careful selection of patients for surgery is mandatory. The operation is indicated in young patients who require chronic therapy with PPIs for control of symptoms, patients in whom regurgitation or respiratory symptoms persist during therapy, patients who do not want to be on long-term medical treatment (compliance or cost), and patients with complications related to PPIs (Table 22–5).

The goal of surgical therapy is to restore the competence of the LES. A laparoscopic Nissen fundoplication (360 degrees) is considered today the procedure of choice (Figure 22–11) because it increases the resting pressure and length of the LES, decreases the number of transient LES relaxations, and improves quality of esophageal peristalsis. The operation is equally safe and effective in young and elderly patients.

The success of the operation is based on the following technical elements:

1. Dissection of the esophagus in the posterior mediastinum to allow 3-4 cm of esophagus to lie without tension below the diaphragm. By bringing the entire stomach and gastroesophageal junction below the diaphragm, a sliding hiatal hernia is reduced.

2. Division of the short gastric vessels in order to create a "floppy" fundoplication using both the anterior and posterior wall of the stomach.

3. Approximation of the right and left pillars of the esophageal crus to decrease the size of the esophageal hiatus, thereby avoiding herniation of the wrap.

4. Construction of a 360-degree fundoplication over a 56-60F bougie.

The hospital stay is short (usually 1-2 days), and the postoperative discomfort is minimal. Most patients return to work within 2-3 weeks. Control of symptoms is obtained in about 80%-90% of patients at 10 years after a fundoplication.

Broeders JA et al: Ten-year outcome of laparoscopic and conventional Nissen fundoplication: randomized clinical trial. *Ann Surg.* 2009;250(5):698-706.
Fisichella PM et al: Gastroesophageal reflux disease and morbid obesity: is there a relation? *World J Surg.* 2009;33:2034-2038.
Galmiche JP et al: LOTUS Trial Collaborators. Laparoscopic antireflux surgery vs esomeprazole treatment for chronic GERD: the LOTUS randomized clinical trial. *JAMA.* 2011;305:1969-1977.
Herbella FA et al: Gastroesophageal reflux disease: from pathophysiology to treatment. *World J Gastroenterol.* 2010;16:3745-3749.
Schlottmann F et al: Antireflux surgery in the USA: influence of surgical volume on perioperative outcomes and costs. Time for centralization? *World J Surg.* 2018;42(7):2183-2189.
Schlottmann F et al: Comparative analysis of perioperative outcomes and costs between laparoscopic and open antireflux surgery. *J Am Coll Surg.* 2017;224:327-333.
Schlottmann F et al: Surgical treatment of gastroesophageal reflux disease. *World J Surg.* 2017;41:1685-1690.
Thijssen AS et al: Cost-effectiveness of proton pump inhibitors versus laparoscopic Nissen fundoplication for patients with gastroesophageal reflux disease: a systematic review of the literature. *Surg Endosc.* 2011;25:3127-3134.
Tutuian R et al: Characteristics of symptomatic reflux episodes on acid suppressive therapy. *Am J Gastroenterol.* 2008;103:1090-1096.

BARRETT ESOPHAGUS

ESSENTIALS OF DIAGNOSIS

▸ GERD symptoms (typical and atypical)
▸ Endoscopic evidence of "salmon pink" epithelium above gastroesophageal junction
▸ Metaplastic columnar epithelium with goblet cells on esophageal biopsy

General Considerations

Barrett esophagus (BE) has been traditionally defined as the presence of at least 1 cm of metaplastic columnar epithelium that replaces the stratified squamous epithelium normally

▲ **Figure 22–11.** Nissen fundoplication (360 degrees).

| Squamous Epithelium | Barrett's Esophagus | Low Grade Dysplasia | High Grade Dysplasia | Adenocarcinoma |

▲ **Figure 22–12.** Pathologic progression from normal esophageal squamous epithelium to adenocarcinoma.

lining the distal esophagus. Currently, the presence of intestinal metaplasia—columnar epithelium with goblet cells—is also needed for the diagnosis of BE. About 10%-15% of patients with GERD will develop BE.

Metaplasia may progress to high-grade dysplasia and eventually adenocarcinoma. Thus, adenocarcinoma represents the final step of a sequence of events in which a benign disease (GERD) evolves into a preneoplastic disease and eventually into cancer (Figure 22–12).

Pathogenesis

BE is due to reflux of gastric contents (acid and duodenal juice) into the esophagus. When compared to patients with GERD with no mucosal injury or less severe esophagitis, patients with BE have a shorter and weaker LES and decreased amplitude of esophageal peristalsis. As a consequence, the amount of reflux is greater and esophageal clearance is slower. In addition, hiatal hernia is more common in patients with Barrett metaplasia.

▶ Clinical Findings

A. Symptoms

Patients with BE typically have a long history of GERD. Although most patients experience both typical and atypical symptoms of GERD, others may become asymptomatic over time due to the decreased sensitivity of the metaplastic epithelium.

B. Imaging Studies

Barium swallow may show ulcerations, a stricture, or a hiatal hernia. Endoscopy shows presence of "salmon pink" epithelium above the gastroesophageal junction, replacing the whitish squamous epithelium (Figure 22–13). The diagnosis is confirmed by pathologic examination of the esophageal mucosa and requires the identification of goblet cells, typical for intestinal epithelium.

C. Special Tests

Esophageal manometry often shows a short and hypotensive LES and abnormal esophageal peristalsis (decreased amplitude of peristaltic waves, simultaneous waves). Ambulatory pH monitoring usually shows a severe amount of acid reflux.

Esophageal exposure to duodenal juice can be quantified by a fiberoptic probe that measures intraluminal bilirubin as a marker for duodenal reflux. In GERD patients, the prevalence of esophageal bilirubin exposure parallels the degree of mucosal injury, being higher in patients with BE. Nonacid reflux can be measured by impedance-pH monitoring.

▶ Treatment

A. Barrett Esophagus: Metaplasia

The treatment options are similar to those of patients with GERD without metaplasia and consist of either PPIs or a fundoplication. A surgical approach might offer an advantage over medical therapy for the following reasons:

1. Successful elimination of reflux symptoms with PPIs does not guarantee control of acid reflux. When pH monitoring is performed in asymptomatic Barrett patients treated with these medications, up to 80% of them still have abnormal acid reflux.

2. PPIs do not eliminate the reflux of bile, a major contributor to the pathogenesis of BE. In contrast, an antireflux operation prevents any form of reflux by restoring the competence of the gastroesophageal junction.

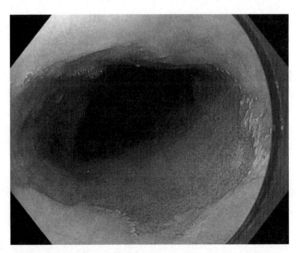

▲ **Figure 22–13.** Endoscopic visualization of Barrett esophagus.

3. A fundoplication may promote regression of the columnar epithelium. Many studies have shown that regression occurs in 15%-50% of patients when the length of the Barrett segment is less than 3 cm. Regardless of the effect of the fundoplication on symptoms, surveillance endoscopy should be performed every 3-5 years.

B. Barrett Esophagus: Low-Grade Dysplasia

In patients with BE and low-grade dysplasia (LGD) endoscopic therapy is the preferred treatment modality. Endoscopic surveillance every 12 months is an acceptable alternative. Radiofrequency ablation (RFA) is currently the preferred ablation method because it has proven to be highly effective for the eradication of intestinal metaplasia and dysplasia. RFA is delivered through either a balloon-based, fully circumferential device or a cap-based focal device. This heat-based technique aims to eliminate the mucosal tissue, while limiting the damage to the muscularis mucosa to prevent stricture formation. Multiple endoscopic treatments may be required depending on the length of the BE segment and the tissue response. Cryoablation is a noncontact method that consists of a directed spray of liquid nitrogen at –196°C onto the Barrett mucosa. Deep freezing and slow thawing cause disruption of cells, vascular ischemia, and thrombosis, resulting in necrosis of the superficial esophageal layers. In contrast to heat-based ablation, cryotherapy leaves the tissue architecture intact and may result in less stricture formation.

C. Barrett Esophagus: High-Grade Dysplasia

For patients with BE and high-grade dysplasia, endoscopic therapy is recommended. Given the safety profile and well-documented efficacy of RFA, this procedure remains the preferred endoscopic modality for most patients with flat dysplastic BE (absence of ulcers or nodules). Patients with discrete visible lesions should undergo endoscopic mucosal resection (EMR) prior to ablation therapy (Table 22–6).

Table 22–6. Management of Barrett esophagus (BE).

BE without dysplasia	Endoscopic surveillance at intervals of 3-5 years
BE indefinite for dysplasia	Repeat endoscopy after optimization of acid suppressive medications for 3-6 months
BE with low-grade dysplasia	Without life-limiting comorbidity, endoscopic therapy (radiofrequency ablation) is the preferred treatment modality; endoscopic surveillance every 12 months is an acceptable alternative
BE with high-grade dysplasia	Endoscopic therapy (radiofrequency ablation) unless life-limiting comorbidity is present

D. Barrett Esophagus: Early Esophageal Adenocarcinoma

The management of superficial adenocarcinoma requires consideration of many factors. Nodal status is one of the most important long-term prognostic factors for esophageal adenocarcinoma. For this reason, although EMR for T1a tumors has gained acceptance (98% 5-year survival), endoscopic resection for T1b cancers remains under debate due to the increased risk of nodal involvement in these tumors. The risk of lymph node metastases for a T1b adenocarcinoma reaches 30%. Therefore, esophagectomy is currently considered the preferred treatment modality for T1b tumors.

Oelschlager BK et al: Clinical and pathologic response of Barrett's esophagus to laparoscopic antireflux surgery. *Ann Surg.* 2003;238(4):458-464.

Pech O et al: Long-term efficacy and safety of endoscopic resection for patients with mucosal adenocarcinoma of the esophagus. *Gastroenterology.* 2014;146(3):652-660.

Schlottmann F et al: Current concepts in treatment of Barrett's esophagus with and without dysplasia. *J Gastrointest Surg.* 2017;21:1354-1360.

Schlottmann F et al: Endoscopic treatment of high-grade dysplasia and early esophageal cancer. *World J Surg.* 2017;41:1705-1711.

Schlottmann F et al: From heartburn to Barrett's esophagus and beyond. *World J Surg.* 2017;41:1698-1704.

Shaheen NJ et al: ACG clinical guideline: diagnosis and management of Barrett's esophagus. *Am J Gastroenterol.* 2016;111:30-50.

Shaheen NJ et al: Durability of radiofrequency ablation in Barrett's esophagus with dysplasia. *Gastroenterology.* 2011;141:460-468.

HIATAL HERNIA

ESSENTIALS OF DIAGNOSIS

▶ May be asymptomatic

▶ Symptoms secondary to mechanical obstruction: dysphagia, epigastric discomfort, anemia

▶ Symptoms secondary to gastroesophageal reflux: heartburn, regurgitation

▶ General Considerations

Obesity, aging, and general weakening of the musculofascial structures set the stage for enlargement of the esophageal hiatus and herniation of the stomach into the posterior mediastinum. Hiatal hernias are divided into sliding hiatal hernias (type 1) and paraesophageal hiatal hernias (types 2, 3, or 4) (Figures 22–14 to 22–17).

The most common (95%) is the type 1 sliding hernia, where the gastroesophageal junction moves above the diaphragm together with some of or the entire stomach.

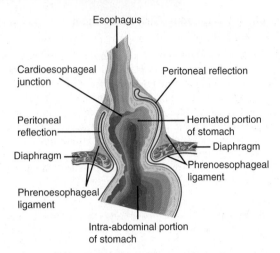

▲ **Figure 22–14.** Sliding esophageal hiatal hernia.

▲ **Figure 22–16.** Paraesophageal hernia.

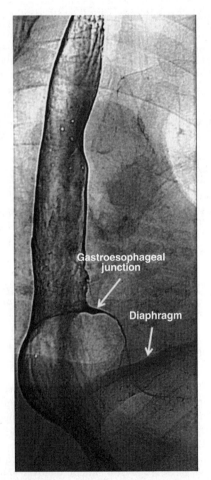

▲ **Figure 22–15.** Large sliding hiatal hernia.

▲ **Figure 22–17.** Paraesophageal hernia. Note that the cardioesophageal junction remains in its normal anatomic position below the diaphragm.

Type 2 hernias are characterized by herniation of the gastric fundus into the mediastinum alongside the esophagus, with the gastroesophageal junction remaining in an intra-abdominal position. Since the gastroesophageal sphincteric mechanism functions normally in most of these cases, reflux of gastric contents is uncommon. Type 3 hernias, also called mixed hernias, involve herniation of the stomach with the gastroesophageal junction into the mediastinum. In types 1 and 3, symptoms due to GERD may occur along with symptoms secondary to the mechanical obstruction.

The rare type 4 hernias are characterized by an intra-thoracic stomach along with associated viscera such as the spleen, colon, small bowel, or pancreas.

Clinical Findings

Small hiatal hernias are in most cases asymptomatic, whereas large hiatal hernias may cause a wide variety of symptoms such as epigastric discomfort, chest pain, postprandial bloating, dysphagia, or respiratory problems (asthma, cough, or dyspnea caused by chronic aspiration). Anemia is secondary to gastric erosions, and it can be the only presenting symptom. In addition, patients may experience symptoms due to GERD.

Diagnosis

A barium swallow will delineate the anatomy and the type of hiatal hernia. Endoscopy is important to determine if gastric or esophageal inflammation is present and to rule out cancer. **Cameron ulcers** are ulcerations of the mucosal folds lining the stomach due to extrinsic compression of the diaphragm on the distal neck of a hiatal hernia. Although typically asymptomatic, they may present as acute, severe upper gastrointestinal bleeding.

Patients with reflux symptoms should also undergo esophageal manometry and pH monitoring.

Complications

The most frequent complications of paraesophageal hernia are hemorrhage, incarceration, obstruction, and strangulation. The herniated portion of the stomach often becomes congested, and bleeding occurs from erosions of the mucosa. Obstruction may occur, most often at the esophagogastric junction as a result of torsion and angulation at this point—especially if a large portion (or all) of the stomach herniates into the chest. In paraesophageal hiatal hernia—in contrast to the sliding type—other viscera such as the small and large intestines and spleen may also enter the mediastinum along with the stomach.

Treatment

Operative repair is indicated in symptomatic patients. The usual method is to return the herniated stomach below the diaphragm into the abdomen, repair the enlarged esophageal hiatus, and then add a fundoplication. In most cases, the operation can be performed laparoscopically. The results of surgical management are excellent in about 90% of patients.

Dallemagne B et al: Laparoscopic repair of paraesophageal hernia. Long-term follow-up reveals good clinical outcome despite high radiological recurrence rate. *Ann Surg.* 2011;253:291-296.

Oelschlager BK et al: Biologic prosthesis to prevent recurrence after laparoscopic paraesophageal hernia repair: long-term follow-up from a multicenter, prospective, randomized trial. *J Am Coll Surg.* 2011;213:461-468.

Schlottmann F et al: Laparoscopic paraesophageal hernia repair: utilization rates of mesh in the USA and short-term outcome analysis. *J Gastrointest Surg.* 2017;21:1571-1576.

Schlottmann F et al: Minimally invasive surgery should be the standard of care for paraesophageal hernia repair. *J Gastrointest Surg.* 2017;21:778-784.

TUMORS OF THE ESOPHAGUS

1. Benign Tumors of the Esophagus

ESSENTIALS OF DIAGNOSIS

- ▶ Dysphagia, epigastric discomfort
- ▶ Radiographic demonstration of a smooth filling defect within the esophageal lumen

General Considerations

Esophageal leiomyomas are the most common benign tumors of the esophagus. They represent 10% of all gastrointestinal leiomyomas. They originate in the smooth muscle layers, mostly in the lower two-thirds of the esophagus, and they narrow the esophageal lumen. These tumors consist of smooth muscle cells surrounded by a capsule of fibrous tissue. The mucosa overlying the tumor is generally intact, but occasionally it may become ulcerated as a result of pressure necrosis by an enlarging lesion. Leiomyomas are not associated with the development of cancer. Other tumors such as fibromas, lipomas, fibromyomas, and myxomas are rare. Congenital cysts or duplications of the esophagus (the second most common benign lesion after leiomyomas) may occur at any level, although they are most common in the lower esophagus.

Clinical Findings

Many benign lesions are asymptomatic and are discovered incidentally during upper gastrointestinal fluoroscopic examination. Benign tumors or cysts grow slowly and become symptomatic only after reaching a size of 5 cm or more. On barium swallow, leiomyomas appear as a smooth

▲ **Figure 22–18.** Leiomyoma of esophagus. Note smooth, rounded density causing extrinsic compression of esophageal lumen.

filling defect within the esophageal lumen (Figure 22–18). An intraluminal mass covered by normal mucosa can be easily recognized during endoscopy, but biopsies should not be taken because they may make subsequent enucleation of the tumor more difficult. Endoscopic ultrasound and chest CT help in the characterization of the tumor and in the differential diagnosis.

▶ **Differential Diagnosis**

Leiomyomas, cysts, and duplications can be distinguished from cancer by their classic radiographic appearance. Intraluminal papillomas, polyps, or granulomas may be indistinguishable radiographically from early carcinoma, so their exact nature must be confirmed histologically.

▶ **Treatment**

Small polypoid intraluminal lesions may be removed endoscopically. The treatment of choice for symptomatic leiomyomas is enucleation. Although in the past a thoracotomy or a laparotomy was used, today enucleation can be accomplished by either a thoracoscopic or a laparoscopic approach or by POEM.

Ha C et al: Benign esophageal tumors. *Surg Clin North Am.* 2015; 95:491-514.
Ko WJ et al: Evaluation and endoscopic management of esophageal submucosal tumor. *Clin Endosc.* 2017;50:250-253.

2. Carcinoma of the Esophagus

ESSENTIALS OF DIAGNOSIS

▶ Progressive dysphagia, initially for solids and later for liquids
▶ Progressive weight loss
▶ Diagnosis established by endoscopy and biopsies
▶ Staging established by endoscopic ultrasound, computed tomography of chest and abdomen, and positron emission tomography; bronchoscopy indicated for cancer of the midthoracic esophagus

▶ **General Considerations**

The epidemiology of esophageal cancer in the United States has changed considerably over the past 30 years. In the 1970s, squamous cell carcinoma was the most common type of esophageal cancer, accounting for about 90% of the total cases. It was located in the thoracic esophagus and affected mostly black men. Over the past three decades, there has been a progressive increase in the incidence of adenocarcinoma of the distal esophagus and gastroesophageal junction, so that today it accounts for more than 70% of all new cases of esophageal cancer. It is more frequent in white men with GERD, and it is linked to BE.

▶ **Pathogenesis**

The most common contributing factors for squamous cell carcinoma are cigarette smoking and chronic alcohol exposure. Chronic ingestion of hot liquids or foods, poor oral hygiene, and nutritional deficiencies may play a role. Certain medical conditions such as achalasia, caustic injuries of the esophagus, and Plummer-Vinson syndrome are associated with an increased incidence of squamous cell cancer.

GERD is the most common predisposing factor for adenocarcinoma of the esophagus, where adenocarcinoma represents the last event of a sequence that starts with GERD and progresses to metaplasia, high-grade dysplasia, and cancer. Increases in the prevalence of overweight and obesity have paralleled rises in the incidence of esophageal adenocarcinoma. Although obesity also favors the development and severity of GERD, it has been shown to act as an independent risk factor for esophageal adenocarcinoma.

Esophageal cancer arises in the mucosa and subsequently invades the submucosa and the muscle layers. Ultimately, structures located next to the esophagus may be infiltrated (tracheobronchial tree, aorta, recurrent laryngeal nerve). At the same time, the tumor tends to metastasize to the lymph nodes (mediastinal, celiac, cervical) and to the liver, lungs, peritoneum, adrenals, and bones.

Clinical Findings

A. Symptoms

Early esophageal cancer may be asymptomatic. As the cancer grows, dysphagia is the most common symptom. It is initially for solids, but eventually it progresses to liquids. Weight loss occurs in more than 50% of patients. Patients can have pain when swallowing. Pain over bony structures may be due to metastases. Hoarseness is usually due to invasion of the right or left recurrent laryngeal nerves with paralysis of the ipsilateral vocal cord. Respiratory symptoms may be due to regurgitation and aspiration of undigested food or to invasion of the tracheobronchial tree, with development of a tracheoesophageal fistula.

B. Imaging Studies

Barium swallow shows the location and the extent of the tumor. Esophageal cancer usually presents as an irregular intraluminal mass or a stricture (Figure 22–19). Endoscopy allows direct visualization and biopsies of the tumor (Figure 22–20).

▲ **Figure 22–20.** Endoscopic visualization of distal esophageal cancer.

For tumors of the upper and mid-esophagus, bronchoscopy is indicated to rule out invasion of the tracheobronchial tree.

C. Special Tests

After the diagnosis is established, it is important to determine the staging of the cancer (Table 22–7). Abdominal and chest CT scans and PET are useful to detect distant metastases and invasion of structures next to the esophagus. Endoscopic ultrasound is the most sensitive test to determine the depth of penetration by the tumor, the presence of enlarged periesophageal lymph nodes, and invasion of structures next to the esophagus. Furthermore, it allows a fine-needle aspiration of enlarged periesophageal lymph nodes. A bone scan is indicated in patients with new onset of bone pain.

Differential Diagnosis

The differential diagnosis includes peptic strictures due to reflux, achalasia, and benign esophageal tumors.

Treatment

Treatment is based on the stage of the cancer. In patients with early esophageal cancer (pT1a), an esophagectomy can be avoided because of the very low risk of lymph node metastasis (0%-3%), and EMR and RFA are very effective. However, patients need to undergo a very strict endoscopic follow-up to detect possible early recurrence.

Patients with T1b/T2 N0 disease should be considered for upfront esophagectomy. An esophagectomy can be performed by using an abdominal and a cervical incision (with blunt dissection of the thoracic esophagus through the esophageal hiatus; *transhiatal esophagectomy*) or by using an abdominal and a right chest incision (*transthoracic esophagectomy*). After removal of the esophagus, continuity of the gastrointestinal

▲ **Figure 22–19.** Barium swallow demonstrating a distal esophageal carcinoma.

Table 22–7. American Joint Committee on Cancer (AJCC) eighth edition staging of esophageal cancer.

T Category	T Criteria
TX	Tumor cannot be assessed
T0	No evidence of primary tumor
Tis	High-grade dysplasia, defined as malignant cells confined to the epithelium by the basement membrane
T1	Tumor invades the lamina propria, muscularis mucosae, or submucosa
T1a	Tumor invades the lamina propria or muscularis mucosae
T1b	Tumor invades the submucosa
T2	Tumor invades the muscularis propria
T3	Tumor invades adventitia
T4	Tumor invades adjacent structures
T4a	Tumor invades the pleura, pericardium, azygos vein, diaphragm, or peritoneum
T4b	Tumor invades other adjacent structures, such as the aorta, vertebral body, or airway
N Category	**N Criteria**
NX	Regional lymph nodes cannot be assessed
N0	No regional lymph node metastasis
N1	Metastasis in one or two regional lymph nodes
N2	Metastasis in three to six regional lymph nodes
N3	Metastasis in seven or more regional lymph nodes
M Category	**M Criteria**
M0	No distant metastasis
M1	Distant metastasis
G	**G Definition**
GX	Grade cannot be assessed
G1	Well differentiated
G2	Moderately differentiated
G3	Poorly differentiated, undifferentiated
Location Category	**Location Category**
X	Location unknown
Upper	Cervical esophagus to lower border of azygos vein
Middle	Lower border of azygos vein to lower border of inferior pulmonary vein
Lower	Lower border of inferior pulmonary vein to stomach, including gastroesophageal junction

Note: Location is defined by the position of the epicenter of the tumor in the esophagus.

SSC

When cT is...	And cN is...	And M is...	Then the stage group is...
Tis	N0	M0	0
T1	N0-1	M0	I
T2	N0-1	M0	II
T3	N0	M0	II
T3	N1	M0	III
T1-3	N2	M0	III
T4	N0-2	M0	IVA
Any T	N3	M0	IVA
Any T	Any N	MI	IVB

(Continued)

Table 22–7. American Joint Committee on Cancer (AJCC) eighth edition staging of esophageal cancer. (Continued)

ADC

When cT is...	And cN is...	And M is...	Then the stage group is...
Tis	N0	M0	0
T1	N0	M0	I
T1	N1	M0	IIA
T2	N0	M0	IIB
T2	N1	M0	III
T3	N0-1	M0	III
T4a	N0-1	M0	III
T1-4a	N2	M0	IVA
T4b	N0-2	M0	IVA
Any T	N3	M0	IVA
Any T	Any N	M1	IVB

ADC, adenocarcinoma; SCC, squamous cell carcinoma.
Used with the permission of the American College of Surgeons. Amin MB, Edge SB, Greene FL, et al. (Eds.) *AJCC Cancer Staging Manual*, 8th Ed. Springer New York, 2017.

tract is reestablished by using either the stomach or the colon. The transhiatal esophagectomy offers the advantage of avoiding the chest incision, with decreased compromise of lung function and decreased postoperative discomfort. The validity of the transhiatal esophagectomy as a cancer operation was initially questioned because part of the operation is not done under direct vision and because of the small number of resected lymph nodes. However, many retrospective studies and prospective randomized trials have shown no difference in survival between the two operations, suggesting that it is not the type of operation that influences survival, but rather the stage of the disease at the time the operation is performed. The morbidity rate of the operation is around 30%, and it is mostly due to respiratory (atelectasis, pneumonia, pleural effusion), cardiac (arrhythmias), and septic complications (anastomotic leak). The mortality rate in specialized and "high-volume" centers is less than 5%. These results are due to the presence of an experienced team composed of surgeons, anesthesiologists, intensivists, cardiologists, radiologists, and nurses.

Over the past 10 years, minimally invasive techniques have been adopted for the esophageal resection with the goal of avoiding a laparotomy and/or a thoracotomy. With experience, the procedure can be performed with excellent patient outcomes, both in terms of perioperative morbidity and oncologic efficacy. Potential oncologic benefits of the minimally invasive approach include improved visualization for more complete lymphadenectomy and less immune dysfunction related to surgical stress and blood transfusion.

The best treatment for patients with locally advanced cancer (T2 N1-3, T3-4 N0-3) is neoadjuvant therapy plus surgery. This treatment modality includes a combination of radiotherapy and chemotherapy used in order to improve local (radiotherapy) and distant control of the disease (chemotherapy), followed by esophagectomy. Overall, it seems that the combination of neoadjuvant therapy followed by surgery offers the best survival benefit. This is particularly true in the subgroup of patients (about 20%) who have a "complete pathologic response" (no tumor found in the specimen).

Nonoperative therapy is reserved for patients who are not candidates for surgery because of local invasion of the tumor to adjacent structures (eg, aorta), distant metastases, or a poor functional status. The goal of therapy in these patients is palliation of the dysphagia. The following treatment modalities are available to achieve this goal:

1. Self-expanding stents can be deployed by endoscopy under fluoroscopic guidance in order to keep the esophageal lumen open. The use of drug-embedded stents has demonstrated promising results. When tracheoesophageal fistulas occur, esophageal stenting alone can divert gut contents and often lead to fistula closure, but in some cases, tracheal stenting may be needed.

2. Intraluminal radiotherapy is often successful in relieving dysphagia.

3. Palliative chemoradiation can be given with the intent of improving quality of life or extending life.

4. Bleeding occurs in up to 10% of patients with advanced malignancy. Treatments to palliate bleeding can include endoscopy, interventional radiologic procedures, or multimodality therapies including radiation or vasoconstricting medications.

▶ Prognosis

The stage of the disease is the most important prognostic factor. The overall 5-year survival rate for esophageal cancer remains approximately 20%.

Allaix ME et al: Hybrid Ivor Lewis esophagectomy for esophageal cancer. *J Laparoendosc Adv Surg Tech*. 2016;26:763-767.

Boshier PR et al: Transthoracic versus transhiatal esophagectomy for the treatment of esophagogastric cancer: a meta-analysis. *Ann Surg*. 2011;254:894-906.

Rice TW et al: 8th edition AJCC/UICC staging of cancers of the esophagus and esophagogastric junction: application to clinical practice. *Ann Cardiothorac Surg*. 2017;6:119-130.

Schlottmann F et al: Esophageal cancer surgery: spontaneous centralization in the US contributed to reduce mortality without causing health disparities. *Ann Surg Oncol*. 2018; 25(6):1580-1587.

Schlottmann F et al: Transhiatal vs. transthoracic esophagectomy: a NSQIP analysis of postoperative outcomes and risk factors for morbidity. *J Gastrointest Surg*. 2017;21:1757-1763.

Straatman J et al: Minimally invasive versus open esophageal resection: three-year follow-up of the previously reported randomized controlled trial: the TIME trial. *Ann Surg*. 2017; 266(2):232-236.

OTHER SURGICAL DISORDERS OF THE ESOPHAGUS

PERFORATION OF THE ESOPHAGUS

ESSENTIALS OF DIAGNOSIS

▶ History of recent instrumentation of the esophagus or severe vomiting

▶ Pain in the neck, chest, or upper abdomen

▶ Signs of mediastinal or thoracic sepsis within 24 hours

▶ Radiographic evidence of an esophageal leak

▶ General Considerations

Esophageal perforations can result from iatrogenic instrumentation (eg, endoscopy, balloon dilation), severe vomiting, external trauma, and other rare causes. The subsequent clinical manifestations are influenced by the site of the perforation (ie, cervical or thoracic) and, in the case of thoracic perforations, whether or not the mediastinal pleura has been ruptured. Morbidity resulting from esophageal perforation is principally due to infection. Immediately after injury, the

tissues are contaminated by esophageal contents, but infection has not become established; surgical closure of the defect will usually prevent the development of serious infection. If more than 24 hours have elapsed since the time of injury, severe contamination has occurred. At this time, the esophageal defect usually breaks down if it is surgically closed, and measures to treat mediastinitis and empyema may not be adequate to avoid a fatal outcome. Although serious infection usually occurs if surgical repair is delayed, a few cases of minor instrumental perforations can be managed by antibiotics without operation.

A. Instrumental Perforations

Medical instrumentation is the most common cause of esophageal perforation (diagnostic or therapeutic endoscopy). Instrumental perforations are most likely to occur in the cervical esophagus. The endoscope may compress the posterior wall of the esophagus against osteoarthritic spurs of the cervical vertebrae, causing contusion or laceration. The cricopharyngeal area is the most common site of injury. Perforations of the thoracic esophagus may occur at any level but are most common at the natural sites of narrowing, at the level of the left main stem bronchus and at the diaphragmatic hiatus. Perforations during PD for achalasia (2%-6%) occur proximal to the gastroesophageal junction.

B. Spontaneous Perforation (Boerhaave Syndrome)

Spontaneous perforation usually occurs in the absence of preexisting esophageal disease, but 10% of patients have reflux esophagitis, esophageal diverticulum, or carcinoma. Most cases follow a bout of heavy eating and drinking. The perforation most frequently occurs in the left posterolateral wall, 3-5 cm above the gastroesophageal junction. The tear results from excessive intraluminal pressure, usually caused by *violent retching and vomiting*. Some cases have also been associated with childbirth, defecation, convulsions, heavy lifting, and forceful swallowing. The overlying pleura is also torn, so both the mediastinum and the pleural cavity are contaminated with esophageal contents. The second most common site of perforation is at the midthoracic esophagus, on the right side at the level of the azygous vein.

▶ Clinical Findings

A. Signs and Symptoms

The principal early manifestation is pain, which is felt in the neck with cervical perforations and in the chest or upper abdomen with perforations of the thoracic esophagus. The pain may radiate to the back. With cervical perforations, pain is followed by crepitus in the neck, dysphagia, and signs of infection. Perforations of the thoracic esophagus, which communicate with the pleural cavity in about 75% of cases, are usually accompanied by tachycardia, tachypnea, dyspnea, and early development of hypotension. With perforation into the chest, pneumothorax is produced, followed by hydrothorax and, if not promptly treated, empyema. The left chest is involved in 70% of cases and the right chest in 20%; involvement is bilateral in 10%. Escape of air into the mediastinum may result in a "mediastinal crunch," which is produced by the heart beating against air-filled tissues (Hamman sign). If the pleura remain intact, mediastinal emphysema appears more rapidly, and pleural effusion is slow to develop.

B. Imaging Studies

X-ray studies are important to demonstrate that perforation has occurred and to locate the site of the injury. In perforations of the cervical esophagus, x-rays show air in the soft tissues, especially along the cervical spine. The trachea may be displaced anteriorly by air and fluid. Later, widening of the superior mediastinum may be seen. With thoracic perforations, mediastinal widening and pleural effusion with or without pneumothorax are the usual findings. An esophagogram using water-soluble contrast medium should be performed promptly in every patient suspected of having an esophageal perforation (Figure 22–21). If a leak is not seen, the examination should be repeated using barium. A CT scan of the chest is also useful to localize the perforation and eventually to drain mediastinal fluid collections.

C. Special Studies

Thoracentesis will reveal cloudy or purulent fluid, depending on how much time has passed since the time of perforation. The amylase content of the fluid is elevated, and serum

▲ **Figure 22–21.** Extravasation of contrast material through instrumental perforation of upper thoracic esophagus. Note loculi of air and fluid anterior to esophagus, indicating that mediastinitis has already developed.

amylase levels may also be high as a result of absorption of amylase from the pleural cavity.

▶ Treatment

Broad-spectrum antibiotics should be given immediately. The infection is usually polymicrobial with *Staphylococcus, Streptococcus, Pseudomonas,* and *Bacteroides.* Nonoperative management consisting of antibiotics alone may be all that is necessary in a few selected cases of instrumental perforation. This approach should be reserved for patients without thoracic involvement (eg, pneumothorax or hydrothorax), whose esophagogram demonstrates no extraluminal extravasation, and who have no systemic signs of sepsis (eg, hypotension and tachypnea).

Patients with just a minimal extraluminal sinus tract without wide mediastinal spread (ie, the contamination is limited) and without signs of sepsis can be managed endoscopically, with stent deployment and over-the-scope clips.

Patients with larger perforations or signs of sepsis should be managed surgically. For lesions treated within 24 hours, the operation should consist of closure of the perforation and external drainage. External drainage alone may suffice for small cervical perforations, which may be difficult to find. Patients with achalasia in whom perforation has resulted from balloon dilation should have the tear in the esophagus repaired and a Heller myotomy performed on the opposite side of the esophagus. Definitive therapy (eg, resection) should also be performed in patients with other surgical conditions, such as esophageal carcinoma.

Primary repair has a high failure rate if the perforation is older than 24 hours. The classic recommendation in this situation has been to isolate the perforation by performing a temporary cervical esophagostomy and placing a feeding jejunostomy for enteral nutrition. Alternatively, the segment of esophagus where the perforation is located can be resected, bringing the proximal end of esophagus out through the neck and closing the distal end. The mediastinum is drained, and a feeding jejunostomy is created. Later, the esophagostomy is taken down, and stomach or colon is interposed to bridge the gap.

The survival rate is 90% when surgical treatment is accomplished within 24 hours. The rate drops to about 50% when treatment is delayed.

Saxena P et al: Endoscopic management of esophageal perforations. Who, when, and how? *Curr Treat Options Gastroenterol.* 2017;15:35-45.
Sdralis EIK et al: Epidemiology, diagnosis, and management of esophageal perforations: systematic review. *Dis Esophagus.* 2017;30:1-6.

INGESTED FOREIGN OBJECTS

Most cases of ingested foreign objects occur in children who swallow coins or other small objects. In adults, the problem most often consists of esophageal meat impaction or, less commonly, lodged bones or toothpicks. Dentures and esophageal disease, such as a benign stricture, are the principal predisposing factors in adults. Prisoners and mentally ill persons occasionally swallow foreign objects intentionally.

About 90% of swallowed foreign objects pass into the stomach and from there into the intestine and are eventually passed without problems. Ten percent stay in the esophagus. If they traverse the esophagus, objects whose dimensions exceed 2-5 cm tend to remain in the stomach.

The patient's history usually defines the problem adequately. The patient with a foreign object in the esophagus may or may not experience dysphagia or chest pain.

▶ **Specific Kinds of Ingested Foreign Objects**

A. Coins

Pennies and dimes usually pass into the stomach, but larger coins will lodge in the esophagus at or just beyond the cricopharyngeus. It is important to know if a swallowed coin has remained in the esophagus, and whether or not the patient has symptoms is an unreliable basis for making the determination. Therefore, anteroposterior and lateral chest x-rays should be obtained to determine whether the coin is in the esophagus or trachea. Small children should be x-rayed from the base of the skull to the anus in order to find any additional coins in the gut.

Coins in the esophagus should be removed promptly, since complications may occur if treatment delay exceeds 24 hours. The procedure is best accomplished with a grasping forceps passed through a flexible endoscope. Sedation is adequate for older children or adults, but general endotracheal anesthesia is required in order to protect the airway of infants and young children. A smooth foreign body too large to grasp with a forceps can be removed by passing a dilating balloon beyond it and then withdrawing the endoscope and balloon as a unit. If the object is small enough (< 20 mm), it may be pushed into the stomach.

Once a coin has passed into the stomach, it can be observed by periodic x-rays for as long as a month before the conclusion is reached that spontaneous elimination is unlikely and endoscopic removal is indicated.

B. Meat Impaction

Meat is the most common foreign object that lodges in the esophagus of adults, and many affected patients have underlying esophageal disease. The site of meat impaction is usually at the cricopharyngeus muscle or in the distal esophagus in patients with achalasia, diffuse esophageal spasm, or a stricture.

No x-rays (especially barium studies) are indicated, because they make the endoscopic task more difficult. If obstruction is complete and the patient cannot handle saliva, endoscopy should be performed as an emergency to prevent aspiration. If the clinical findings are minor, however, endoscopy can be postponed for up to 12 hours to see whether the food will pass spontaneously.

Meat can usually be removed as a single piece using a polypectomy snare passed through a flexible endoscope. In some cases, a meat bolus can be pushed into the stomach, which is safe so long as it passes with minimal pressure. After the esophagus has been cleared, it should be checked endoscopically for underlying disease. An esophageal stricture should be dilated if the esophageal wall is not acutely inflamed as a result of the meat impaction.

C. Sharp and Pointed Objects

Bones, safety pins, hat pins, razor blades, toothpicks, nails, and many other objects constitute this group of foreign objects. The general principles of management are (1) to remove these objects endoscopically by grasping and pulling a blunt side with forceps, (2) to remove a piece of glass or a razor blade by pulling it into the lumen of a rigid esophagoscope, or (3) to operate if neither of these methods appears to be safe. Sharp or pointed objects in the stomach should be removed surgically, since 25% of them will perforate the intestine, usually near the ileocecal valve, if they exit the pylorus.

D. Button Batteries

These small batteries are swallowed by children, just like coins, but unlike coins, they are highly corrosive and should be removed urgently before a serious complication such as an esophagotracheal or esophagoaortic fistula develops.

E. Cocaine Packets

Cocaine smugglers may swallow small packets of cocaine in balloons or condoms. Rupture of just one of these packets can be fatal, so attempts at endoscopic removal are unsafe. If it appears that the packets will pass spontaneously, the patient may be watched; otherwise, surgical removal is indicated.

ASGE Standards of Practice Committee et al: Management of ingested foreign bodies and food impactions. *Gastrointest Endosc.* 2011;73:1085-1091.

Sung SH et al: Factors predictive of risk for complications in patients with oesophageal foreign bodies. *Dig Liver Dis.* 2011; 43:632-635.

CAUSTIC INJURIES OF THE ESOPHAGUS

ESSENTIALS OF DIAGNOSIS

▶ History of ingestion of caustic liquids or solids

▶ Burns of the lips, mouth, tongue, and oropharynx

▶ Chest pain and dysphagia

General Considerations

Ingestion of strong solutions of acid or alkali or of solid substances of similar nature produces extensive chemical burns. The injury usually represents a suicide attempt in adults and accidental ingestion in children. Strong **alkali** produces "liquefaction necrosis," which involves dissolution of protein and collagen, saponification of fats, dehydration of tissues, thrombosis of blood vessels, and deep penetrating injuries. **Acids** produce a "coagulation necrosis" involving eschar formation, which tends to shield the deeper tissues from injury. Depending on the concentration and the length of time the irritant remains in contact with the mucosa, sloughing of the mucous membrane, edema and inflammation of the submucosa, infection, perforation, and mediastinitis may develop.

Ingested lye in solid form tends to adhere to the mucosa of the pharynx and proximal esophagus. Severe acute esophageal necrosis is rare, and the main clinical problems are early edema and late stricture formation, principally of the proximal esophagus. Liquid caustics commonly produce much more extensive esophageal necrosis, and occasionally even tracheoesophageal and esophagoaortic fistulas. If the patient survives the acute phase, a lengthy nondilatable stricture often develops.

Ingestion of strong acid characteristically produces greatest injury to the stomach, with the esophagus remaining intact in over 80% of cases. The result may be immediate gastric necrosis or late antral stenosis.

Nearly all severe injuries are caused by strong alkali. Weak alkali and acid are associated with less extensive lesions.

Clinical Findings

A. Symptoms and Signs

Systemic symptoms roughly parallel the severity of the caustic burn. The most common finding is inflammatory edema of the lips, mouth, tongue, and oropharynx; in the absence of visible injury in this area, severe esophageal damage is rare. Patients with serious esophageal burns often experience chest pain and dysphagia and drooling of large amounts of saliva. Pain on swallowing may be intense. If the damage is severe, the patient often appears toxic, with high fever, prostration, and shock. The absence of toxicity does not rule out severe injury. Tracheobronchitis accompanied by coughing and increased bronchial secretions is frequently noted. Stridor may be present, and in a few patients, respiratory obstruction progresses rapidly and requires tracheostomy for relief. Complete esophageal obstruction due to edema, inflammation, and mucosal sloughing may develop within the first few days.

B. Endoscopy

Endoscopy is the key test in the evaluation of caustic trauma to the esophagus. Determination of the extent of injury by endoscopy contributes substantially to therapeutic decisions.

Table 22–8. Endoscopic grading of corrosive burns of esophagus and stomach.

Grade	Definition	Endoscopic Findings
First degree	Superficial mucosal injury.	Mucosal hyperemia and edema; superficial mucosal desquamation.
Second degree	Full-thickness mucosal involvement. No or partial-thickness muscular injury.	Sloughing of mucosa. Hemorrhage, exudate, ulceration, pseudo-membrane formation, and granulation tissue when examined late.
Third degree	Full-thickness esophageal or gastric injury with extension into adjacent tissues.	Sloughing of tissues with deep ulceration. Complete obliteration of esophageal lumen by edema; charring and eschar formation; full-thickness necrosis; perforation.

Reproduced with permission from Estrera A, Taylor W, Mills LJ, et al: Corrosive burns of the esophagus and stomach: a recommendation for an aggressive surgical approach, *Ann Thorac Surg* 1986 Mar;41(3): 276-283.

Endoscopy should be performed after the initial resuscitation, usually within 24 hours of admission. The scope is inserted far enough to gauge the most serious degree of burn, which is classified as first, second, or third degree, as defined in Table 22–8.

C. Radiology

A chest x-ray should be taken in all patients. It may show signs of esophageal perforation (subcutaneous emphysema, pneumomediastinum, pneumothorax) or aspiration (pulmonary infiltrates). An esophagogram is indicated in the initial evaluation if perforation is suspected and in later stages to detect the presence of a stricture.

Treatment

Patients should be hospitalized, and intravenous fluids and antibiotics should be administered. The use of steroids is still controversial. A nasogastric tube placed under fluoroscopic or endoscopic guidance allows stenting of the esophagus, preventing complete obstruction of the lumen.

Patients with first-degree burns do not require aggressive therapy and may be discharged from the hospital after a short period of observation. Second-degree and minor spotty third-degree injuries are treated by inserting a nasogastric tube. Nutrition can be given through the nasogastric tube or parenterally. Periodic esophagograms are obtained in follow-up to look for stricture formation, which is treated early in its development by dilations and eventually resection.

Third-degree burns involving extensive esophagogastric necrosis require emergency esophagogastrectomy, esophagostomy, and feeding jejunostomy. Esophagectomy is best performed by the blunt technique using a laparotomy and cervical incision. Reconstruction by substernal colon interposition is performed 8-12 weeks later.

Early and proper management of caustic burns provides satisfactory results in most cases. The ingestion of strong acid or alkaline solutions with extensive immediate destruction of the mucosa produces profound pathologic changes that may result in fibrous strictures that require dilations and, in some cases, esophagectomy and colon interposition.

Cabral C et al: Caustic injuries of the upper digestive tract: a population observational study. *Surg Endosc.* 2012;26:214-221.
Chirica M et al: Caustic ingestion. *Lancet.* 2017;389:2041-2052.
Chirica M et al: Late morbidity after colon interposition for corrosive esophageal injury: risk factors, management, and outcome. A 20-years experience. *Ann Surg.* 2010;252:271-280.

ESOPHAGEAL BANDS, WEBS, OR RINGS

A narrow mucosal ring (Schatzki ring) may develop at the lower end of the esophagus. Most patients are relatively free from symptoms. Dysphagia occurs when the ring is less than 12 mm in diameter. In most cases, the ring is located at the squamocolumnar junction and occurs in a patient with GERD. Being confined to the mucosa, it differs from an inflammatory (peptic) stricture, which involves all layers of the esophagus. A barium swallow clearly identifies the problem. Treatment consists of endoscopic dilation of the ring and treatment of the associated reflux (acid-reducing medications or fundoplication).

de Wijkerslooth LR et al: Endoscopic management of difficult or recurrent esophageal strictures. *Am J Gastroenterol.* 2011; 106:2080-2091.
Müller M et al: Is the Schatzki ring a unique esophageal entity? *World J Gastroenterol.* 2011;17:2838-2843.

THE DIAPHRAGM

The diaphragm (Figure 22–22) is a musculotendinous, dome-shaped structure attached posteriorly to the first, second, and third lumbar vertebrae, anteriorly to the lower sternum, and laterally to the costal arches. It separates the abdominal and thoracic cavities. The diaphragm allows the passage of various normal structures through anatomic foramina. The aortic hiatus lies posteriorly at the level of the 12th thoracic vertebra, and through it pass the aorta, the thoracic duct, and the azygos venous system. The esophageal hiatus lies immediately anteriorly and slightly to the left at the level of the tenth thoracic vertebra and is separated from the aortic hiatus by the decussation of the right crus of the diaphragm. Through this hiatus pass the esophagus and the vagus nerves. At the level of the ninth thoracic vertebra and slightly to the right of the esophageal hiatus is the vena caval foramen, which allows passage of the inferior vena cava and small branches of the phrenic nerve.

▲ **Figure 22–22.** Inferior surface of diaphragm.

The phrenic arteries arising directly from the aorta supply the diaphragm along with the lower intercostal arteries and the terminal branches of the internal mammary arteries.

PARASTERNAL OR RETROSTERNAL (FORAMEN OF MORGAGNI) HERNIA & PLEUROPERITONEAL (FORAMEN OF BOCHDALEK) HERNIA

Failure of fusion of the sternal and costal portions of the diaphragm anteriorly in the midline creates a defect (**foramen of Morgagni**) through which hernias can occur. Normally, the diaphragm becomes fused, allowing only the internal mammary arteries and their superior epigastric branches, along with lymphatics, to pass through this area. Posterolaterally, failure of fusion of the pleuroperitoneal canal creates a defect through which viscera may herniate to produce a **foramen of Bochdalek** hernia (Figure 22–23).

Although both types of hernia are congenital, symptoms in the Morgagni hernia usually do not develop until middle life or later. This type of hernia is more frequent in women. These hernias are mostly right-sided and have a hernia sac. The most common contents are the omentum, the colon, and the stomach. Conversely, the Bochdalek hernia occurs more frequently on the left side and may cause severe respiratory distress at birth, requiring an emergent operation. Routine chest films show a retrosternal solid mass, a retrosternal air-filled viscus, or similar findings in the posterolateral thorax if a Bochdalek hernia is present. Chest CT confirms the diagnosis and identifies the contents of the hernia.

Parasternal (Morgagni) hernias

Pleuroperitoneal (Bochdalek) hernias

▲ **Figure 22–23.** Sites of congenital diaphragmatic herniation.

Elective surgical repair is indicated in most instances to prevent complications. An emergent operation may become necessary in the newborn infant who develops progressive cardiorespiratory insufficiency. Repair of the defect by a transabdominal approach is preferable, and the results are excellent. A minimally invasive approach (laparoscopic or thoracoscopic) is feasible and is associated with excellent outcomes.

Putnam LR et al: Minimally invasive vs open congenital diaphragmatic hernia repair: is there a superior approach? *J Am Coll Surg.* 2017;224:416-422.
Ryan JM et al: Technical description of laparoscopic Morgagni hernia repair with primary closure and onlay composite mesh placement. *Hernia.* 2018;22(4):697-705.

TRAUMATIC DIAPHRAGMATIC HERNIA

Traumatic rupture of the diaphragm may occur as a result of penetrating wounds or severe blunt external trauma. Lacerations usually occur in the tendinous portion of the diaphragm, most often on the left side. The liver provides protection to diaphragmatic injury on the right side except from penetrating wounds. Abdominal viscera may immediately herniate through the defect in the diaphragm into the pleural cavity or may gradually insinuate themselves into the thorax over a period of months or years.

▶ Clinical Findings

Diaphragmatic ruptures present in two ways. In the acute form, the patient has recently experienced blunt trauma or a penetrating wound to the chest, abdomen, or back. The clinical manifestations are essentially those of the associated injuries, but occasionally, massive herniation of abdominal viscera through the diaphragm causes respiratory insufficiency. In the chronic form, the diaphragmatic tear is unrecognized at the time of the original injury. Some time later, symptoms (eg, pain, bowel obstruction) appear from herniation of viscera. Respiratory symptoms in such cases are less common.

Plain films of the chest may show a radiopaque area and occasionally an air-fluid level if hollow viscera have herniated. If the stomach has entered the chest, the abnormal path of a nasogastric tube may be diagnostic. Ultrasonography, CT scan, and MRI may demonstrate the diaphragmatic rent. Barium study of the colon may show irregular patches of barium in the colon above the diaphragm or a smooth colonic outline if the colon does not contain feces.

▶ Differential Diagnosis

Traumatic rupture of the diaphragm must be differentiated from atelectasis, space-consuming tumors of the lower pleural space, pleural effusion, and intestinal obstruction due to other causes.

Complications

Hemorrhage and obstruction may occur. If herniation is massive, progressive cardiorespiratory insufficiency may threaten life. The most severe complication is strangulating obstruction of the herniated viscera.

Treatment

For acute ruptures, a transabdominal (most commonly) or transthoracic route is used depending on the procedure required to treat ancillary injuries. When the diaphragmatic tear is the only injury, it is usually fixed by laparotomy. Chronic injuries can be repaired by either approach. Asymptomatic tears of the diaphragm with herniated viscera should be repaired, because the risk of strangulating obstruction is high. Laparoscopy is very useful for both diagnosis and treatment. Surgical repair of the rent in the diaphragm is curative, and the prognosis is excellent. The diaphragm supports sutures well, so recurrences are infrequent.

> Petrone P et al: Diaphragmatic injuries and post-traumatic diaphragmatic hernias. *Curr Probl Surg.* 2017;54:11-32.

TUMORS OF THE DIAPHRAGM

Primary tumors of the diaphragm are not common. The majority are benign lipomas. Pericardial cysts develop in the space between the heart and the diaphragm and are usually unilocular and on the right side.

Benign tumors are usually asymptomatic. Because their benign nature cannot be established except by histology, all lesions of this type should be excised through an appropriate thoracotomy or thoracoabdominal approach. Fibrosarcoma, the most common primary malignant diaphragmatic tumor, is extremely rare.

MULTIPLE CHOICE QUESTIONS

1. Esophageal achalasia is characterized by

    A. Absence of esophageal peristalsis
    B. Heartburn in approximately 80% of the patients
    C. Low intraluminal pH due to gastroesophageal reflux
    D. All of the above

2. Which of the following statements about Zenker diverticulum is incorrect?

    A. It is the most common diverticulum of the esophagus.
    B. It is a consequence of an underlying esophageal motility disorder.
    C. Aspiration of diverticular contents is frequent.
    D. The surgical treatment consists of lower esophageal sphincter (LES) myotomy and resection of the diverticulum or its suspension.

3. Which is the appropriate workup in a patient with suspected gastroesophageal reflux disease?

    A. Upper endoscopy
    B. 24-Hour pH monitoring
    C. Upper endoscopy and 24-hour pH monitoring
    D. Upper endoscopy, esophageal manometry, and 24-hour pH monitoring

4. Barrett esophagus

    A. Becomes more symptomatic over time due to the mucosal inflammation
    B. Is defined as metaplastic columnar epithelium with intestinal metaplasia
    C. Is present in 30%-40% of patients with gastroesophageal reflux disease (GERD)
    D. Is characterized by the presence of fundic-type cells

5. Treatment of esophageal cancer includes

    A. Endoscopic mucosal resection (EMR)/radiofrequency ablation (RFA) for a T1a lesion
    B. Neoadjuvant therapy followed by surgery for locally advanced cancer
    C. Intraesophageal stenting for patients with dysphagia and distant metastases.
    D. All of above

The Acute Abdomen

Sameer Hirji, MD

Reza Askari, MD

23

An "acute abdomen" denotes any sudden, spontaneous, nontraumatic, severe abdominal pain, typically of less than 24 hours in duration. The acute abdomen requires rapid and specific diagnosis because several etiologies demand urgent operative intervention. Because there is frequently a progressive underlying intra-abdominal disorder, undue delay in diagnosis and treatment may adversely affect outcome. Therefore, understanding the clinical presentation, associated laboratory and diagnostic imaging findings, and various facets of preoperative evaluation of acute abdomen is essential.

The approach to a patient with an acute abdomen must be systematic and thorough yet efficient to minimize delay. An acute abdomen should be suspected even in a patient with only mild or atypical presentations. Increasingly, certain patient populations present with atypical complaints, including the immunocompromised, elderly, and bariatric patients. The complete history and physical examination often suggest the probable cause (Table 23–1), allow for timely formation of a differential diagnosis, and guide the choice of appropriate initial diagnostic studies.

Depending on the degree of clinical suspicion and status of the patient, the clinician must then decide if in-hospital observation is warranted, if additional tests are needed, if early operation is indicated, or if nonoperative treatment would be more suitable. If unclear or when in doubt, it is always appropriate to be a little aggressive and pursue additional tests, if needed. This chapter provides important insights and a useful framework to efficiently diagnose and manage a patient with an acute abdomen.

HISTORY

▶ Abdominal Pain

Despite availability of advanced imaging techniques, the fundamental aspect of evaluation is history taking and physical exam. Taking a patient history is an active process whereby a large number of diagnostic possibilities are considered simultaneously and systematically eliminated based on their pretest probability or likelihood of occurrence.

Pain is the most common and predominant presenting feature of an acute abdomen, but as often is the case, it can be variable in nature. Thus, careful consideration of the location, severity, mode of onset and progression, and character of the pain will suggest a preliminary list of diagnoses, which can be further explored.

A. Location of Pain

Determining the location of pain is the initial step but serves only as a rough guide to the diagnosis; "typical" descriptions are reported in only two-thirds of cases. This variability is due to atypical pain patterns, a shift of maximum intensity away from the primary site, advanced or severe disease, or acute on chronic pain. In patients presenting with diffuse peritonitis, generalized pain may completely obscure the precipitating event. Fortunately, some general patterns do emerge that provide clues to diagnosis and narrow the differential of the acute abdomen. Pain confined to either upper quadrant may be evaluated by anatomic consideration of acute conditions affecting underlying organs. The same approach applies to the lower quadrants.

Because of the complex dual visceral and parietal sensory networks innervating the abdominal area, pain is not as precisely localized in the abdomen as in the extremities. Visceral sensation is mediated primarily by afferent C fibers located in the walls of hollow viscera and in the capsules of solid organs. Unlike cutaneous pain, **visceral pain** is elicited by distention, inflammation or ischemia stimulating the receptor neurons, or direct involvement (eg, malignant infiltration) of sensory nerves. Visceral pain is a centrally perceived sensation that is generally slow in onset, dull, poorly localized, and protracted. The pain may be due to increased wall tension or luminal distention or forceful smooth muscle contraction (colic) producing diffuse, deep-seated pain. Visceral pain is most often felt in the midline because of the

Table 23–1. Common causes of the acute abdomen.[1]

Gastrointestinal tract disorders
  Nonspecific abdominal pain
  Appendicitis
  Small and large bowel obstruction
  Perforated peptic ulcer
  Incarcerated hernia
  Bowel perforation
  Meckel diverticulitis
  Boerhaave syndrome
  Diverticulitis
  Inflammatory bowel disorders
  Mallory-Weiss syndrome
  Gastroenteritis
  Acute gastritis
  Mesenteric adenitis
  Parasitic infections
Liver, spleen, and biliary tract disorders
  Acute cholecystitis
  Acute cholangitis
  Hepatic abscess
  Ruptured hepatic tumor
  Spontaneous rupture of the spleen
  Splenic infarct
  Biliary colic
  Acute hepatitis
Pancreatic disorders
  Acute pancreatitis
Urinary tract disorders
  Ureteral or renal colic
  Acute pyelonephritis
  Acute cystitis
  Renal infarct
Gynecologic disorders
  Ruptured ectopic pregnancy
  Twisted ovarian tumor
  Ruptured ovarian follicle cyst
  Acute salpingitis
  Dysmenorrhea
  Endometriosis
Vascular disorders
  Ruptured aortic and visceral aneurysms
  Acute ischemic colitis
  Mesenteric thrombosis
  Portal vein Thrombosis
Peritoneal disorders
  Intra-abdominal abscesses
  Primary peritonitis
  Tuberculous peritonitis
Retroperitoneal disorders
  Retroperitoneal hemorrhage

[1]The most common causes are marked with an asterisk (*). Conditions in italic type often require urgent operation. Please see specific chapters for management.

Table 23–2. Sensory levels associated with visceral structures.

Structures	Nervous System Pathways	Sensory Level
Liver, spleen, and central part of diaphragm	Phrenic nerve	C3-5
Peripheral diaphragm, stomach, pancreas, gallbladder, and small bowel	Celiac plexus and greater splanchnic nerve	T6-9
Appendix, colon, and pelvic viscera	Mesenteric plexus and lesser splanchnic nerve	T10-11
Sigmoid colon, rectum, kidney, ureters, and testes	Lowest splanchnic nerve	T11-L1
Bladder and rectosigmoid	Hypogastric plexus	S2-4

bilateral sensory supply to the spinal cord. Because different visceral structures are associated with different sensory levels in the spine (Table 23–2), visceral pain may be felt in the midepigastrium, periumbilical area, lower abdomen, or flank areas (Figure 23–1) depending on the organ involved.

By contrast, **parietal pain** is mediated by both C and A delta nerve fibers, the latter being responsible for the transmission of more acute, sharper, better localized pain sensation. Direct irritation of the somatically innervated parietal peritoneum by pus, bile, urine, or gastrointestinal secretions leads to a more precisely localized pain. Parietal pain is more easily localized than visceral pain because the somatic afferent fibers are directed to only one side of the nervous system. The cutaneous distribution of parietal pain corresponds to the T6-L1 areas. Abdominal parietal pain is conventionally described as occurring in one of the four abdominal quadrants or in the epigastric or central abdominal area.

Abdominal pain may be referred or may shift to sites removed from the primarily affected organs (Figure 23–2). **Referred pain** denotes noxious (usually cutaneous) sensations perceived at a site distant from that of a strong primary stimulus. Distorted central perception of the site of pain is due to the confluence of afferent nerve fibers from disparate areas within the posterior horn of the spinal cord. For example, pain due to subdiaphragmatic irritation by air, peritoneal fluid, blood, or a mass lesion is referred to the shoulder via the C4-mediated (phrenic) nerve. Pain may also be referred to the shoulder from supradiaphragmatic lesions such as pleurisy or lower lobe pneumonia. Although more often perceived in the right scapular region, referred biliary pain may mimic angina pectoris if it is perceived in the anterior chest or left shoulder areas.

Spreading or shifting pain parallels the course of the underlying condition. The site of pain at onset should be

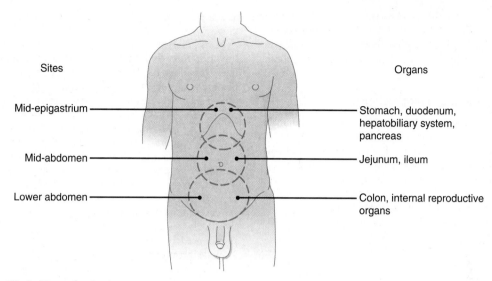

▲ **Figure 23–1.** Visceral pain sites.

distinguished from the site at presentation. The chronology of a patient's pain may be as important as the location itself. For example, in a patient with acute appendicitis, the initial visceral pain begins classically in the epigastric or periumbilical region and then shifts to become sharper parietal pain localized in the right lower quadrant when the overlying peritoneum becomes directly inflamed (Figure 23–2). With a perforated peptic ulcer, pain almost always begins in

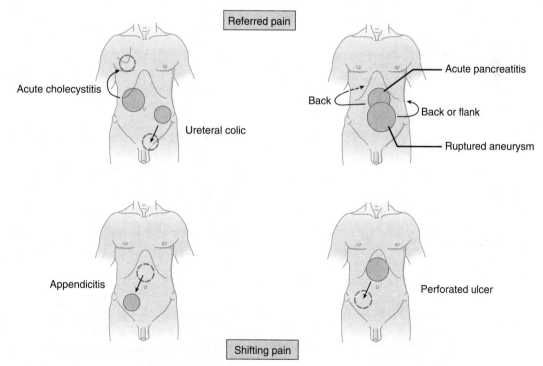

▲ **Figure 23–2.** Referred pain (Top) and shifting pain (Bottom) in the acute abdomen. Solid circles indicate the site of maximum pain; dashed circles indicate sites of lesser pain.

the epigastrium, but as leaked gastric contents track down the right paracolic gutter, pain may descend and become prominent in the right lower quadrant. Thus, localized pain often suggests progression of disease and warrants prompt intervention.

B. Mode of Onset and Progression of Pain

The duration, acuity, and progression of pain should be assessed at initial presentation, and assessment should be repeated as often as necessary. The mode of onset of pain reflects the nature and severity of the underlying process. Onset may be acute (within seconds), rapidly progressive (within 1-2 hours), or insidious (gradually over several hours). One must also determine the time course of the pain (constant, intermittent, decreasing, or increasing) because this will help prioritize the next steps.

For instance, sudden, unheralded, excruciating, increasing generalized pain suggests an ongoing intra-abdominal catastrophe such as a perforated viscus or rupture of an aneurysm, ectopic pregnancy, or abscess. Accompanying systemic signs (tachycardia, sweating, tachypnea, shock) soon supersede the abdominal disturbances and underscore the need for rapid resuscitation and laparotomy. In some cases, portal vein hypertension can progress over time into abdominal pain and distension, and ultimately manifest as acute abdomen if there is sudden obstruction of venous blood flow.

A less dramatic clinical picture is steady, mild pain that becomes intensely localized in a well-defined area within a few (1-2) hours. Any of the above conditions may present in this manner, but this is more typical of acute cholecystitis, acute pancreatitis, strangulated bowel, mesenteric infarction, renal or ureteral colic, and proximal small bowel obstruction.

Finally, some patients initially have slight—at times only vague—abdominal discomfort that is fleetingly present diffusely throughout the abdomen. It may be unclear whether these patients even have an acute abdomen or whether the illness is likely to be a matter for medical rather than surgical attention. Associated gastrointestinal symptoms are infrequent at first, and systemic symptoms are often absent. Eventually, the pain and abdominal findings become more pronounced, become either colicky or steady, and localize to a smaller area. This gradual onset pattern leading to a more localized pain may reflect a slowly developing condition or the body's defensive efforts to cordon off an acute process.

C. Character of Pain

The nature, severity, and periodicity of pain provide useful clues to the underlying pathology (Figure 23–3). Pain may be continual or intermittent. Steady pain is more common and

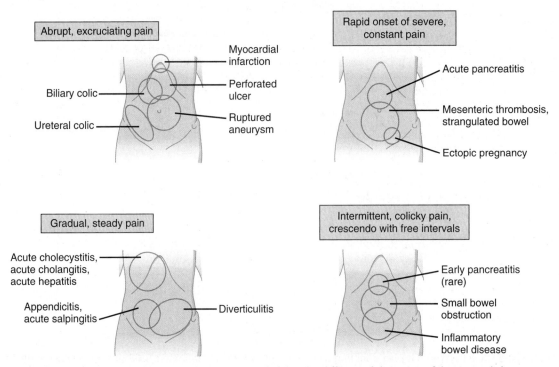

▲ **Figure 23–3.** The location and character of pain are helpful in the differential diagnosis of the acute abdomen.

often indicates a process that will inevitably lead to peritoneal inflammation. It may be constant in severity or fluctuate, but it is always present. Sharp, superficial, constant pain due to peritoneal irritation (often presenting as focal peritonitis) is typical of perforated ulcer or a ruptured appendix, ovarian cyst, or ectopic pregnancy. Intermittent, crampy pain (colic) may occur for short or long periods but is punctuated by pain-free intervals and is most characteristic of obstruction of a hollow viscus. The gripping, mounting pain of small bowel obstruction (and occasionally early pancreatitis) is usually intermittent, vague, deep-seated, and crescendo at first, but becomes sharper, unremitting, and better localized with time. Unlike the disquieting but bearable pain associated with bowel obstruction, pain caused by lesions occluding smaller conduits (bile ducts, uterine tubes, and ureters) rapidly becomes unbearably intense. The pain-free intervals reflect intermittent smooth muscle relaxation. In the strict sense, the term *biliary colic* is a misnomer because biliary pain does not remit because bile ducts do not have peristaltic movements.

The quality of a patient's pain leads to the use of certain descriptors to describe different types of pain and may be typical of certain pathologies. The "aching discomfort" of ulcer pain, the "stabbing, breathtaking" pain of acute pancreatitis and mesenteric infarction, the "gripping" pain of a bowel obstruction, and the "tearing" pain of ruptured aortic aneurysm remain apt descriptions. Despite the use of such descriptive terms, the quality of visceral pain is not a reliable clue to its cause because it is often subjective.

The intensity of a patient's pain may relate to the severity of the insult. Agonizing pain denotes serious or advanced disease. Colicky pain is usually promptly alleviated by analgesics. Ischemic pain due to strangulated bowel or mesenteric thrombosis is only slightly assuaged even by narcotics. Nonspecific abdominal pain is usually mild, but mild pain may also be found with perforated ulcers that have become localized and in mild acute pancreatitis. An occasional patient will deny pain but complain of a vague feeling of abdominal fullness that feels as though it might be relieved by a bowel movement. This visceral sensation (**gas stoppage sign**) is due to reflex ileus induced by an inflammatory lesion walled off from the free peritoneal cavity, as in retrocecal appendicitis. In addition, previous pain episodes and factors that aggravate or relieve pain should be noted. Pain caused by localized peritonitis, especially when it affects upper abdominal organs, tends to be exacerbated by movement or deep breathing.

▶ Other Symptoms Associated With Abdominal Pain

Anorexia, fever, nausea and vomiting, constipation/obstipation, and diarrhea often accompany abdominal pain but are nonspecific symptoms and have limited diagnostic value. However, these symptoms should be managed promptly while the formal diagnosis is sought.

A. Vomiting

When sufficiently stimulated by secondary visceral afferent fibers, the medullary vomiting centers activate efferent fibers to induce reflex vomiting. Hence, pain in the acute surgical abdomen usually *precedes* vomiting, whereas the reverse holds true in medical conditions. Vomiting is a prominent symptom in upper gastrointestinal diseases such as Boerhaave syndrome, Mallory-Weiss syndrome, acute gastritis, and acute pancreatitis. Severe, uncontrollable retching provides temporary pain relief in moderate attacks of pancreatitis. The absence of bile in the vomitus is a feature of pyloric stenosis or gastric outlet obstruction. Where associated findings suggest bowel obstruction, the onset and character of vomiting may indicate the level of the lesion. Recurrent vomiting of bile-stained fluid is typical of proximal small bowel obstruction. In distal small or large bowel obstruction, prolonged nausea precedes vomiting, which may become feculent in late cases. Although vomiting may present in either acute appendicitis or nonspecific abdominal pain, coexisting nausea and anorexia are more suggestive of the former condition.

B. Constipation

Reflex ileus is often induced by visceral afferent fibers stimulating efferent fibers of the sympathetic autonomic nervous system (splanchnic nerves) to reduce intestinal peristalsis. Hence, paralytic ileus undermines the value of constipation in the differential diagnosis of an acute abdomen. Constipation itself is hardly an absolute indicator of intestinal obstruction and often nonspecific. However, **obstipation** (the absence of passage of both stool and flatus) strongly suggests mechanical bowel obstruction if there is progressive painful abdominal distention or repeated vomiting. Clinical history in terms of onset and duration of pain should help provide further clinical context.

C. Diarrhea

Copious watery diarrhea is characteristic of gastroenteritis and other medical causes of an acute abdomen. Blood-stained diarrhea suggests ulcerative colitis, Crohn disease, or bacillary or amebic dysentery. A recent travel or food intake history should be elicited. It is also found with ischemic colitis but often absent in intestinal infarction due to superior mesenteric artery occlusion.

D. Fever

Fever is a marker of inflammation and may be present in a variety of medical and surgical conditions in the abdomen if they are allowed to progress. The sensitivity of this finding is low because the ability of many patient populations to mount a fever is compromised (eg, immunocompromised patients) and, for most diseases leading to acute abdomen, fever is low grade or absent.

E. Other Specific Symptoms

The following findings are extremely helpful if present. Significant weight loss may suggest a chronic condition such as cancer or chronic mesenteric ischemia. **Jaundice** suggests hepatobiliary disorders (both benign and malignant). **Hematochezia** or **hematemesis** may suggest a gastroduodenal lesion or Mallory-Weiss syndrome; **melena** may suggest a lower gastrointestinal bleed or colonic ischemia; and **hematuria** may suggest ureteral colic or cystitis. The passage of blood clots or necrotic mucosal debris may be the sole evidence of advanced intestinal ischemia.

▶ Other Relevant Aspects of the History

A. Past Medical History

A complete past medical history is crucial to identify both medical conditions related to the presentation of the acute abdomen as well as conditions of associated pulmonary, renal, and cardiac systems that may mimic the acute abdomen in their presentation. Many chronic medical conditions complicate the patient's presentation and increase the patient's overall surgical risk. An assessment of the patient's cardiovascular and pulmonary status should always be done before proceeding to the operating room. Particular attention should be paid to elderly and frail patients. Liver disease should be noted because it increases risk for gastrointestinal bleeding and, in severe disease, may be complicated by ascites and spontaneous bacterial peritonitis. In patients with vascular disease or atrial fibrillation, mesenteric ischemia should be included in the differential and correlated with clinical symptoms. Inflammatory bowel disease can cause severe abdominal pain (or "attacks") that is often treated medically but may be complicated by processes requiring more emergent intervention including intraabdominal abscess, stricture, obstruction, or perforation.

A patient should also be asked about any history of recent trauma. This could be either blunt or penetrating trauma. Delayed splenic bleeding is one of the more common examples of traumatic injuries presenting in delayed fashion.

B. Surgical History

Any history of a previous abdominal, groin, vascular, or thoracic operation is relevant to the current illness and must be obtained. Particular attention to the mode of operation (laparoscopic, open, endovascular, transabdominal [eg, biopsies]) and any anatomic reconstructions may clarify aspects of the current complaint. History of foreign implants (eg, meshes, bone implants) should also be taken. If possible within the time constraints imposed by the urgency of the current problem, operative notes and pathology reports should be obtained and reviewed.

C. Gynecologic History

The menstrual history (duration, chronicity, timing) is crucial to the diagnosis of ectopic pregnancy, mittelschmerz (due to a ruptured ovarian follicle), and endometriosis. A history of vaginal discharge or dysmenorrhea may denote pelvic inflammatory disease. A complete sexual history should be performed if indicated, and all women of childbearing age should be evaluated for possibility of pregnancy. If the patient has been previously pregnant, information regarding the nature of delivery (particularly cesarean section) is also relevant.

D. Medication History

In the current era, polypharmacy is increasingly common but equally important to consider when evaluating patients. Medications of interest include anticoagulants, antiplatelets, and immunosuppression medications. For instance, nonsteroidal anti-inflammatory drug (NSAIDs) or aspirin use could explain the etiology of gastric or duodenal ulcer. Anticoagulants have been implicated in retroperitoneal and intramural duodenal and jejunal hematomas. Additionally, patients who are anticoagulated or are on antiplatelet therapy may require correction or further consideration prior to operative management. Oral contraceptives have been implicated in the formation of benign hepatic adenomas and in mesenteric venous infarction. Corticosteroids or other chemotherapeutics and immunosuppressive medications may mask the clinical signs of even advanced peritonitis. Alcohol use should be interrogated because it can be associated with liver disease, ulcers, gastritis, and pancreatitis.

E. Family History

Family history often provides the best information about medical or hereditary causes of an acute abdomen.

F. Travel History

Travel history may raise the possibility of amebic liver abscess or hydatid cyst, malarial spleen, tuberculosis, *Salmonella typhi* infection of the ileocecal area, or dysentery.

▼ FORMING A DIFFERENTIAL DIAGNOSIS LIST

The age, gender, and clinical history of the patient should assist in guiding the development of the differential diagnosis and should be correlated with the history and physical examination. Mesenteric adenitis mimics acute appendicitis in the young, gynecologic disorders complicate the evaluation of abdominal pain in women of childbearing age, and malignant and vascular diseases are more common in the elderly. Knowledge of the common causes of abdominal pain and their incidence in various populations is also helpful. Acute cholecystitis, appendicitis, bowel obstruction, cancer, and vascular conditions are the common causes of a surgical acute abdomen in older patients. In children, appendicitis accounts for one-third of all abdominal pain and nonspecific abdominal pain for much of the remainder. Causes of an acute abdomen reflect disease patterns of the indigenous population, and awareness of common causes within the physician's locale improves diagnostic accuracy.

PHYSICAL EXAMINATION

The tendency to concentrate on the abdomen should be resisted in favor of a methodical and complete physical examination. Examination should begin with an initial assessment of the patient's vital signs, and if hemodynamically unstable or with signs of systemic shock, the patient must be resuscitated aggressively. The patient should be evaluated concurrently with a physical exam in an efficient manner. A more "focused" assessment may be appropriate in time-sensitive situations if it delays a subsequent intervention.

The abdominal exam should be done with the patient in the supine position. A systematic approach to the abdominal examination (Table 23–3) is key to success. The physical exam allows the clinician to search for specific signs that confirm or rule out differential diagnostic possibilities (Table 23–4).

1. **General inspection.** General observation affords a fairly reliable indication of the severity of the clinical situation. Most patients, although uncomfortable, remain calm. The writhing of patients with visceral pain (eg, intestinal or ureteral colic) contrasts with the rigidly motionless bearing of those with parietal pain (eg, acute appendicitis, generalized peritonitis). Diminished responsiveness or an

Table 23–3. Steps in physical examination of the acute abdomen.

1. Global Assessment, Vital Signs
2. Inspection
3. Auscultation
4. Percussion
5. Palpation
   - Guarding or rigidity
   - Local palpation
   - Rebound tenderness
   - Deep tenderness
   - Bump tenderness
   - Masses
6. Special signs
7. External hernias and male genitalia
8. Rectal examination
9. Pelvic examination

Table 23–4. Physical findings in various causes of acute abdomen.

Condition	Helpful Signs
Perforated viscus	Scaphoid, tense abdomen; diminished bowel sounds (late); loss of liver dullness; guarding or rigidity.
Peritonitis	Motionless; absent bowel sounds (late); cough and rebound tenderness; guarding or rigidity.
Inflamed mass or abscess	Tender mass (abdominal, rectal, or pelvic); bump tenderness; special signs (Murphy, psoas, or obturator).
Intestinal obstruction	Distention; visible peristalsis (late); hyperperistalsis (early) or quiet abdomen (late); diffuse pain without rebound tenderness; hernia or rectal mass (some).
Paralytic ileus	Distention; minimal bowel sounds; no localized tenderness.
Ischemic or strangulated bowel	Not distended (until late); bowel sounds variable; severe pain but little tenderness; rectal bleeding (some).
Bleeding	Pallor, shock; distention; pulsatile (aneurysm) or tender (eg, ectopic pregnancy) mass; rectal bleeding (some).

altered sensorium is suggestive of more advance or significant disease and may herald imminent cardiopulmonary collapse.

2. **Assessing systemic signs.** Systemic signs usually accompany rapidly progressive or advanced disorders of the acute abdomen. Extreme pallor, hypotension, hypothermia, tachycardia, tachypnea, and diaphoresis are some of the hard signs suggestive of major intra-abdominal hemorrhage (eg, ruptured aortic aneurysm or tubal pregnancy). These findings warrant immediate attention and rapid diagnostic tests to rule out extra-abdominal pathology. If extra-abdominal pathology is excluded, these are markers of severe or rapidly progressive intra-abdominal pathology and are indications for emergent laparotomy.

3. **Fever.** Constant low-grade fever is common in inflammatory conditions such as diverticulitis, acute cholecystitis, and appendicitis. High fever with lower abdominal tenderness in a young woman without signs of systemic illness suggests acute salpingitis. Disorientation or extreme lethargy combined with a very high fever (> 39°C) or fever with chills and rigors signifies impending septic shock. This is most often due to advanced peritonitis, acute cholangitis, or pyelonephritis. However, fever is often mild or absent in elderly, chronically ill, or immunosuppressed patients despite a serious acute abdomen.

4. **Examination of the acute abdomen**

(a) **Inspection.** The abdomen should be thoughtfully inspected before palpation. One should look for old surgical scars, hernias, evidence of trauma, stigmata of liver disease, obvious masses, distension, and signs of peritonitis. A tensely distended abdomen with an old surgical scar suggests both the presence and the cause (adhesions) of small bowel obstruction. A scaphoid contracted abdomen is seen with perforated ulcer; visible peristalsis occurs in thin patients with advanced bowel obstruction; and soft doughy fullness is seen in early paralytic ileus or mesenteric thrombosis.

(b) **Auscultation.** Auscultation of the abdomen should also precede palpation. Peristaltic rushes synchronous with colic are heard in mid-small bowel obstruction and in early acute pancreatitis. They differ from the high-pitched hyperperistaltic sounds unrelated to the crampy pain of gastroenteritis, dysentery, and fulminant ulcerative colitis. An abdomen that is silent except for infrequent tinkly or squeaky sounds characterizes late bowel obstruction or diffuse peritonitis. Except for these more extreme patterns, the many auscultatory variants heard in abdominal conditions render them largely useless for specific diagnosis.

(c) **Percussion.** Percussion serves several purposes. Tenderness on percussion is akin to eliciting rebound tenderness; both reflect peritoneal irritation and parietal pain. With a perforated viscus, free air accumulating under the diaphragm may efface normal liver dullness. Tympany near the midline in a distended abdomen denotes air trapped within distended bowel loops. Free peritoneal fluid may be detected by demonstrating shifting dullness.

(d) **Palpation.** Palpation is performed with the patient resting in a comfortable supine position. Incisional and periumbilical hernias are noted. Tenderness that connotes localized peritoneal inflammation is the most important finding in patients with an acute abdomen. Its extent and severity are determined first by one- or two-finger palpation, beginning away from the area of cough tenderness and gradually advancing toward it. Tenderness is usually well demarcated in acute cholecystitis, appendicitis, diverticulitis, and acute salpingitis. If there is poorly localized tenderness unaccompanied by guarding, one should suspect gastroenteritis or some other inflammatory intestinal process without peritonitis. Compared with the degree of pain, unexpectedly little or vaguely localized tenderness is elicited in uncomplicated hollow viscus obstruction, walled-off or deep-seated perforations (eg, retrocecal appendicitis or diverticular phlegmons), and very obese patients. In these instances, use of additional imaging may help to localize the source of the problem. Severe pain out of proportion to exam is a hallmark for mesenteric ischemia, but these patients often have concurrent history of atrial fibrillation or stigmata of severe peripheral vascular disease.

Rebound tenderness is elicited by applying deep gentle pressure to the area of concern and then releasing the pressure rapidly. It is a marker of peritoneal inflammation, but its usefulness may be confounded if the patient is startled by the abrupt release and interprets that as pain. Rebound tenderness may also be elicited with a bed bump or by lightly shaking the abdominal wall.

Guarding is assessed by placing both hands over the abdominal muscles and depressing the fingers gently. Properly performed, this maneuver is comforting to the patient. If there is voluntary spasm, the muscle will be felt to relax when the patient inhales deeply through the mouth. With true involuntary spasm, however, the muscle will remain taut and rigid ("boardlike") throughout respiration. Except for rare neurologic disorders—and, for unknown reasons, renal colic—only peritoneal inflammation produces rectus muscle rigidity. Unlike peritonitis, renal colic induces spasm confined to the ipsilateral rectus muscle.

When the patient raises his or her head from the bed, the abdominal muscles will be tensed. Tenderness persists in abdominal wall conditions (eg, rectus hematoma), whereas deeper peritoneal pain due to intraperitoneal disease is lessened (**Carnett test**). Hyperesthesia may be demonstrable in abdominal wall disorders or localized peritonitis, but it is more prominent in herpes zoster, spinal root compression, and other neuromuscular problems. Trigger point sensitivity, lateral costal rib tip tenderness, and pain exacerbated by spinal motion reflect parietal abdominal wall conditions that subside dramatically after infiltration with local anesthetic agents.

Abdominal masses are usually detected by deep palpation. Superficial lesions such as a distended gallbladder or appendiceal abscess are often tender and have discrete borders. Deeper masses may be adherent to the posterior or lateral abdominal wall and are often partially walled off by overlying omentum and small bowel. As a result, their borders are ill-defined, and only dull pain may be elicited by palpation. Examples include pancreatic phlegmon and ruptured aortic aneurysm.

(e) **Maneuvers.** Even if a mass cannot be directly felt, its presence may be inferred by other maneuvers. A large psoas abscess may cause pain when the hip is passively extended or actively flexed against resistance (**iliopsoas sign**). Internal and external rotation of the flexed thigh may exert painful pressure (**obturator sign**) on a loop of the small bowel entrapped within the obturator canal (obturator hernia). **Bump tenderness** over the lower costal ribs indicates an inflammatory condition affecting the diaphragm, liver, spleen, or its adjacent structures. Referred pain to McBurney point from the left lower quadrant (**Rovsing sign**) is associated with acute appendicitis. If one suspects abdominal guarding is masking an acutely inflamed gallbladder, the right subcostal area should be palpated while the patient inhales deeply. Inspiration will be arrested abruptly by pain (**Murphy sign**), or the gallbladder fundus may be felt as it strikes the examining fingers during descent of the diaphragm. Pain in the shoulder indicates irritation of the diaphragm by fluid such as blood, pus, gastric contents, or stool. **Kehr sign** is left shoulder pain associated with hemoperitoneum. **Costovertebral angle tenderness** is common in acute pyelonephritis. Because they are not invariably present, these special signs are helpful in conjunction with a compatible history and related physical findings.

(f) **Inguinal and femoral rings; male genitalia.** The inguinal and femoral rings in both sexes and the genitalia in male patients should be examined as needed, especially if there is suspicion for incarcerated bowel causing an acute abdomen.

(g) **Rectal examination.** A rectal examination should be performed in most patients with an acute abdomen. Diffuse tenderness is nonspecific, but right-sided rectal tenderness accompanied by lower abdominal rebound tenderness is indicative of peritoneal irritation due to pelvic appendicitis or abscess. Other useful findings include a rectal tumor, blood-stained stool, or occult blood (detected by guaiac testing).

(h) **Pelvic examination.** An acute abdomen is incorrectly diagnosed more often in women than in men, particularly in younger age groups. A pelvic examination is vital in women with vaginal discharge, dysmenorrhea, menorrhagia, or left lower quadrant pain. A properly performed pelvic examination is invaluable in differentiating among acute pelvic inflammatory diseases that do not require operation and acute appendicitis, twisted ovarian cyst, or tubo-ovarian abscess. Almost always, these patients undergo additional imaging to further delineate the cause of the pain.

INVESTIGATIVE STUDIES

History and physical examination by themselves remain pivotal in establishing a diagnosis of an acute abdomen. However, adjuncts such as laboratory and diagnostic imaging can help confirm the diagnosis, exclude medical causes not treated by operation, and help in preoperative planning, especially in patients with complex or prior abdominal surgery. In the current era, diagnostic studies can be obtained relatively quickly and improve clinical decision making.

However, the availability and reliability of certain studies vary in different hospitals. When selecting a study, the invasiveness, risk, and cost-effectiveness should be considered. Test results must be interpreted within the clinical context of each case. Basic studies should be obtained in all but the most desperately ill patients, while other less vital tests may be requested later as indicated.

▶ Laboratory Investigations

A. Blood Studies

Hemoglobin, hematocrit, white blood cell, and differential counts taken on admission are highly informative. Both a rising or marked leukocytosis (> 13,000/μL) and leukopenia (< 5000/μL) are indicative of serious infection. The differential counts should be reviewed because the presence of increased neutrophils ("left shift") may suggest the presence of infection, even when the white blood cell count is normal. Additionally, the presence of bands may indicate severe infection.

Serum electrolytes, urea nitrogen, and creatinine are important, especially if hypovolemia is expected (eg, due to shock, copious vomiting or diarrhea, or delay in presentation). Creatinine is considered imperative prior to obtaining radiographic imaging with iodized contrast agents due to potential renal injury. It should also be obtained in patients with existing or prior history of renal disease. Arterial blood gas with lactate should be obtained in patients with hypotension, generalized peritonitis, pancreatitis, possible ischemic bowel, and septicemia. Elevated serum lactate may indicate bowel ischemia due to the correlation with anaerobic metabolism; however, this is nonspecific and may be elevated in other clinical scenarios, such as dehydration, cocaine use, or liver failure. Unsuspected metabolic acidosis may be the first clue to serious disease.

A raised serum amylase or more specifically lipase level corroborates a clinical diagnosis of acute pancreatitis. Moderately elevated amylase values must be interpreted with caution because abnormal levels frequently accompany strangulated or ischemic bowel, twisted ovarian cyst, or perforated ulcer. Lipase is more specific to pancreatitis.

In patients with suspected hepatobiliary disease, liver function tests (serum bilirubin, alkaline phosphatase, aspartate aminotransferase, alanine aminotransferase, albumin, and globulin) are useful to differentiate medical from surgical hepatic disorders and to gauge the severity of underlying parenchymal disease.

Clotting studies (platelet counts, prothrombin time, and partial thromboplastin time) may be obtained in certain patients in anticipation of surgical intervention. They should be evaluated in patients on anticoagulants such as warfarin to ensure therapeutic levels or alert the clinician that correction is needed prior to surgical intervention. Prothrombin time is also a marker of the synthetic function of the liver in those with advanced liver disease. A peripheral blood smear should be considered if the history hints at a hematologic abnormality (eg, cirrhosis, petechiae). The erythrocyte sedimentation rate, often nonspecifically raised in the acute abdomen, is of dubious diagnostic value; a normal value does not exclude serious surgical illness.

A specimen of clotted blood for cross-matching should be sent whenever urgent surgery is anticipated or there is suspicion of hemorrhage. Beta-human chorionic gonadotropin serum testing is routinely performed at many institutions in lieu of urine testing. This should be performed on all women of childbearing age.

B. Urine Tests

Urinalysis is easily performed and may reveal useful information. Dark urine or a raised specific gravity reflects mild dehydration in patients with normal renal function. Hyperbilirubinemia may give rise to tea-colored urine that froths when shaken. Microscopic hematuria or pyuria can confirm ureteral colic or urinary tract infection and obviate a needless operation. Dipstick testing (for albumin, bilirubin, glucose, and ketones) may reveal a medical cause of an acute abdomen. Pregnancy tests must be ordered on all women of childbearing age if serum testing was not performed.

C. Stool Tests

Gastrointestinal bleeding is not a common feature of the acute abdomen. Nonetheless, testing for occult fecal blood should be performed on a case-by-case basis. A positive test points to a mucosal lesion that may be responsible for large bowel obstruction or chronic anemia, or it may reflect an unsuspected carcinoma.

Stool samples for culture should be taken in patients with suspected gastroenteritis, dysentery, or cholera. *Clostridium difficile* should be on the differential of anyone with a recent course of antibiotic therapy.

▶ Imaging Studies

Radiographic imaging is now routinely used to aid in the diagnosis and even treatment of the acute abdomen. It is of utmost importance that the surgeon, who is familiar with the clinical scenario of the patient, reviews all images. It should be remembered that patients in distress with concern for abdominal catastrophe may be moved to the operating room without any confirmatory imaging.

A. Plain Chest X-Ray Studies

An upright chest x-ray is essential in all cases of an acute abdomen. Not only is it vital for preoperative assessment, but it may also demonstrate supradiaphragmatic conditions that simulate an acute abdomen (eg, lower lobe pneumonia or ruptured esophagus). An elevated hemidiaphragm or pleural effusion may direct attention to subphrenic inflammatory lesions. Subdiaphragmatic air, if present, suggests perforated viscous and may forego the need for additional imaging. An upright chest radiograph is more sensitive than abdominal plain films for free intraperitoneal air.

B. Plain Abdominal X-Ray Studies

Plain supine films of the abdomen should be obtained only selectively, especially if the facility does not have a computed tomography (CT) scanner. In general, erect (or lateral decubitus) views contribute little additional information except in suspected intestinal obstruction, and they rarely eliminate the need for further imaging. Plain films are indicated in patients with signs and symptoms of intestinal obstruction or in patients with suspected foreign body ingestion. They are inappropriate in pregnant patients, unstable individuals in whom clear physical signs mandating laparotomy already exist, or patients with only mild, resolving, nonspecific pain.

When looking at plain radiographs, one should observe the gas pattern of the hollow viscera; an abnormal bowel gas pattern suggests paralytic ileus, mechanical bowel obstruction, or pseudo-obstruction. Bowel obstructions are usually accompanied by findings of gaseous distention, air-fluid levels, distended cecum, and a paucity of air in the rectum. Colonic dilatation is seen in toxic megacolon or volvulus (see Figures 32–16 and 32-18). "Thumbprint" impressions on the colonic wall are noted in about half of patients with ischemic colitis. Radiopaque densities may be seen with biliary, renal, or ureteral calculi, as well as in the case of foreign bodies.

Free air under the hemidiaphragm suggests a perforated viscous, although it does not identify the source. Its presence in approximately 80% of perforated ulcers corroborates the clinical diagnosis. Massive pneumoperitoneum is observed in free colonic perforations. Biliary tree air designates a biliary-enteric communication, such as a gallstone ileus. Air delineating the portal venous system characterizes pylephlebitis.

C. Ultrasonography

The role of ultrasonography is becoming increasingly important in the early evaluation of abdominal pain because it is often used bedside by a trained physician. It is one of the first exams for right upper quadrant pain that is biliary in nature. Ultrasonography has a diagnostic sensitivity of about 80% for acute appendicitis and is most useful in pregnant patients due its safe modality and lower cost. It becomes technically difficult in the third trimester due to the large gravid uterus and is also difficult in obese patients. Ultrasound also plays a role in evaluating a variety of gynecologic causes of abdominal pain. Color Doppler studies can distinguish avascular cysts and twisted masses from inflammatory and infectious processes.

Ultrasound with Doppler may also be useful in evaluating for flow through the mesenteric vessels. The bedside test can also be helpful in quickly assessing unstable patients where transfer for CT might not be possible. The focused assessment with sonography for trauma (FAST) is a limited ultrasound examination directed at identifying presence of free intraperitoneal fluid, especially in the trauma setting.

D. Computed Tomography Scan

CT scan of the abdomen has proved extremely useful in the evaluation of abdominal complaints for patients who do not already have clear indications for laparotomy or laparoscopy. CT provides excellent diagnostic accuracy and is often readily available. Whether contrast is used should be carefully weighed on an individual basis. Intravenous (IV) contrast administration may be limited by creatinine impairment. Oral contrast is useful to distinguish bowel from remaining abdominal contents and also to diagnose bowel perforations or anastomotic leaks. It can be administered orally or rectally, but oral administration adds significant time to obtaining imaging and may not be appropriate in severely ill patients. CT scans should be used sparingly in pregnancy because of the risk radiation poses to the fetus, especially in the first trimester. Ultrasound and magnetic resonance imaging (MRI) are preferred imaging techniques in pregnancy.

CT can identify small amounts of free intraperitoneal gas and sites of inflammatory diseases that may prompt (appendicitis, tubo-ovarian abscess) or postpone (noncomplicated diverticulitis, pancreatitis, hepatic abscess) operation. It should not replace or delay operation in a patient for whom the findings will not change the decision to operate. CT has proven helpful in the diagnosis of appendicitis, especially where exam and laboratory data may not be clear, and is recommended in females, in whom other pelvic pathology may explain the presence of right lower quadrant pain.

E. Angiography

CT angiography (CTA), percutaneous invasive angiographic studies, or magnetic resonance angiography (MRA) is indicated if intestinal ischemia or ongoing hemorrhage is suspected. They should precede any gastrointestinal contrast study that might obscure film interpretation. Selective visceral angiography is a reliable method of diagnosing mesenteric infarction. Emergency angiography may be diagnostic (eg, confirm a ruptured liver adenoma or carcinoma or an aneurysm of the splenic artery or other visceral artery) as well as therapeutic (eg, for coiling or embolizing aneurysmal disease). In patients with massive lower gastrointestinal bleeding, angiography may identify the bleeding site, suggest the likely diagnosis (eg, vascular ectasia, polyarteritis nodosa), and be therapeutic if embolization can be performed. Angiography is of little value in ruptured aortic aneurysm or if frank peritoneal findings (peritonitis) are present. It is contraindicated in unstable patients with severe shock or sepsis and seldom warranted if other findings or tests already dictate the need for laparotomy or laparoscopy. A patient's renal function should be considered before contrast is administered. MRA is useful when a patient is unable to undergo IV contrast administration (due to either renal impairment or contrast dye allergy). It is additionally used as an alternative imaging modality in pregnancy.

F. Gastrointestinal Contrast X-Ray Studies

Gastrointestinal contrast studies should not be requested routinely or be regarded as screening studies. They are helpful only if a specific condition being considered can be verified or treated by a contrast x-ray examination. For suspected perforations of the esophagus or gastroduodenal area without pneumoperitoneum, a water-soluble contrast medium (eg, meglumine diatrizoate [Gastrografin]) is preferred. If there is no clinical evidence of bowel perforation, a barium enema may identify the level of a large bowel obstruction or even reduce a sigmoid volvulus or intussusception. Upper gastrointestinal contrast studies can also be helpful in the bariatric patient population to evaluate for leak or gastric pouch emptying.

G. Radionuclide Scans

The utility of radionuclide scans has been greatly decreased by the routine availability of urgent CT scans. Liver-spleen scans, hepatobiliary iminodiacetic acid (HIDA) scans, and gallium scans may be useful for localizing intra-abdominal abscesses in rare cases. Radionuclide blood pool or Tc-sulfur colloid scans may identify sources of slow or intermittent intestinal bleeding. Technetium pertechnetate scans may reveal ectopic gastric mucosa in Meckel diverticulum.

▶ Endoscopy

Proctosigmoidoscopy is indicated in any patient with suspected large bowel obstruction, grossly bloody stools, or a rectal mass. Minimal air should be used for bowel insufflation to minimize iatrogenic bowel perforation. Besides reducing a sigmoid volvulus, colonoscopy may also locate the source of bleeding in cases of lower gastrointestinal hemorrhage that has subsided. Gastroduodenoscopy and endoscopic retrograde cholangiopancreatography (ERCP) are usually done electively to evaluate less urgent inflammatory conditions (eg, gastritis, peptic disease) in patients without alarming abdominal signs. However, urgent ERCP may be indicated in cases of suspected cholangitis.

▶ Paracentesis

Although performing paracentesis is becoming increasingly rare, it is important to understand that in patients with free peritoneal fluid, aspiration of blood, bile, or bowel contents is a strong indication for laparotomy. On the other hand, infected ascitic fluid may establish a diagnosis in spontaneous bacterial peritonitis, tuberculous peritonitis, or chylous ascites, which rarely require surgery.

Laparoscopy

Laparoscopy is a therapeutic as well as diagnostic modality. The role of laparoscopy has broadened to be a useful modality in the treatment of abdominal emergencies. In certain cases, it has been associated with decreased pain and faster recovery times. Its use is dependent on surgeon experience and hospital and operating room equipment and staffing.

In cases of unclear diagnosis, laparoscopy helps guide surgical planning and avoid unneeded laparotomies. In young women, it may distinguish a nonsurgical problem (ruptured graafian follicle, pelvic inflammatory disease, tubo-ovarian disease) from appendicitis. In obese patients, it may allow for a smaller, less morbid incision. In obtunded, elderly, or critically ill patients, who often have deceptive manifestations of an acute abdomen, it may facilitate earlier treatment in those with positive findings while eliminating the added morbidity of a laparotomy in negative cases. Any patient undergoing laparoscopy must be suited to tolerate conversion to an open procedure when necessary. This aspect must be communicated with the patient and discussed prior to proceeding to the operating room.

DIAGNOSTIC UNCERTAINTY

As the surgeon gathers data, the differential diagnosis is narrowed and associated with a clear direction of plan. The plan of action should focus on whether the patient will need to:

- Go directly to the operating room
- Be admitted for surgical observation and expected operative intervention
- Be admitted for surgical observation or further diagnostics
- Be admitted to medical service for nonoperative abdominal pain

Several patient populations may fall out of the expected presentation of the patient with an acute abdomen. The clinical picture in early cases is often unclear. The following observations should be borne in mind:

1. Acute abdominal pain persisting for over 6 hours should be regarded as indicating a surgical problem requiring in-hospital evaluation. Well-localized pain and tenderness usually indicate a surgical condition. Systemic hypoperfusion with generalized abdominal pain is seldom nonsurgical.

2. Acute appendicitis and intestinal obstruction (usually small bowel) are the most frequent final diagnoses in cases erroneously believed at first to be nonsurgical. Appendicitis

should remain a foremost concern if sepsis or an inflammatory lesion is suspected. It is the most common cause of bizarre peritoneal findings producing ileus or intestinal obstruction. Pelvic appendicitis, with mild abdominal pain, vomiting, and frequent loose stools, simulates gastroenteritis. Atypical presentations of appendicitis are encountered during pregnancy.

3. Salpingitis, dysmenorrhea, ovarian lesions, and urinary tract infections complicate the evaluation of the acute abdomen in young women. Diagnostic errors can be avoided by taking a careful gynecologic history and performing a pelvic examination and urinalysis. Always consider a pregnancy test. CT scan can help confirm the diagnosis.

4. Unusual types or atypical manifestations of intestinal obstruction are easily missed. Emesis, abdominal distention, and air-fluid levels on x-ray may be negligible in Richter hernia, proximal or closed-loop small bowel obstructions, and early cecal volvulus. Intestinal obstruction in an elderly woman who has not had a previous operation suggests an incarcerated femoral hernia or, rarely, an obturator hernia or gallstone ileus.

5. Elderly or cardiac patients with severe unrelenting diffuse abdominal pain but no peritoneal signs may have intestinal ischemia. Arterial blood pH and lactate should be measured and visceral angiography or CTA performed expediently.

6. Medical causes of the acute abdomen should be considered and excluded if possible before exploratory laparotomy is planned (Table 23–5). Upper abdominal pain may

Table 23–5. Medical causes of an acute abdomen for which surgery is not indicated.

Endocrine and metabolic disorders	Infections and inflammatory disorders
Uremia	Tabes dorsalis
Diabetic crisis	Herpes zoster
Addisonian crisis	Acute rheumatic fever
Acute intermittent porphyria	Henoch-Schönlein purpura
Acute hyperlipoproteinemia	Systemic lupus erythematosus
Hereditary Mediterranean fever	Polyarteritis nodosa
Hematologic disorders	**Referred pain**
Sickle cell crisis	Thoracic region
Acute leukemia	Myocardial infarction
Other dyscrasias	Acute pericarditis
Toxins and drugs	Pneumonia
Lead and other heavy metal poisoning	Pleurisy
	Pulmonary embolus
Narcotic withdrawal	Pneumothorax
Black widow spider poisoning	Empyema
	Hip and back

be encountered in myocardial infarction, acute pulmonary conditions, pancreatitis, and acute hepatitis. Generalized or migratory abdominal discomfort may be felt in acute rheumatic fever, polyarteritis nodosa, and other vasculitides. Acute bursitis and hip joint disorders can produce pain radiating into the lower quadrants.

7. Beware of acute cholecystitis, acute appendicitis, and perforated peptic ulcer in patients already hospitalized for an illness affecting another organ system. Always perform a systematic evaluation as previously emphasized.

SPECIAL POPULATIONS

▶ Elderly

Physicians are increasingly exposed to elderly patients given the rising population of older patients. Most often, elderly patients presenting with an acute abdomen are more likely to require surgical intervention. However, the presence of comorbidities adds complexity to their presentation and overall risk of surgical intervention. For example, patients with cardiovascular disease, whether known or unknown, will be more likely to present with acute mesenteric ischemia as a cause of abdominal pain. One of the most frequent causes of acute abdominal pain in the elderly is bowel obstruction. The etiology of these bowel obstructions will differ from younger populations, with malignancy and hernias higher on the differential. Elderly patients tend to present later in their course of illness. Many will have past surgical history, which can make operative intervention technically challenging.

▶ Bariatrics

Obesity is increasingly prevalent in the United States, and weight-loss surgery (either gastric bypass surgery or sleeve gastrectomy) has become relatively common. This patient population presents both its own differential for the acute abdomen and its own anatomic challenge to the surgeon. Physical exam findings may be vague due to the patient's body habitus. Tachycardia is an ominous sign that should not be dismissed. Common causes of acute abdomen in the bariatric population include marginal ulcers, obstruction due to internal hernias or adhesions, and gastric band complications. Due to the common formation of gallstones following rapid weight loss, cholecystitis is another frequent cause of the acute abdomen in post-bypass patients. These patients almost always need a CT scan for further evaluation.

▶ Pregnancy

Prompt diagnosis and management of acute abdomen in pregnant women can be particularly challenging, as they often present with confounding symptoms. Normal pregnancy may be associated with nausea and vomiting or mild leukocytosis.

Physical exam may also be misleading due to the shift in organs secondary to their enlarged uterus. Thus, importantly, abdominal pain problems must be dealt with immediately because delay may be detrimental to both the mother and the fetus. The most common cause of the acute abdomen in pregnancy is appendicitis. Appendicitis in pregnancy may present with pain in atypical locations due to displacement by the uterus. As the gravid uterus pushes the appendix cephalad and often posteriorly, right lower quadrant pain remains the most consistent symptom in any trimester. Pain may also be present in the right upper quadrant, or if the appendix is pushed posteriorly, patients may not demonstrate peritoneal pain. One way to differentiate pain due to appendicitis from uterine pain is with the help of the **Adler sign**: if the point of maximal tenderness shifts medially with repositioning on the left lateral side, then the etiology is usually (not always) due to adnexa or uterine. It should be noted that guarding and rebound tenderness may not manifest in the third trimester given the relative laxity of the abdominal wall muscles.

Once diagnosed, early operative intervention is indicated because ruptured appendicitis leads to increased risk of fetal loss. However, it should be noted that the risk of spontaneous abortion at operation tends to be highest in the first trimester. If the patient is hemodynamically stable and the appendix is not ruptured, treatment with IV antibiotics may be appropriate in certain scenarios, although nonoperative management of acute appendicitis is associated with higher rate of recurrence. These risks should be weighed against the benefits of the procedure itself at the time of evaluation.

▶ Immunocompromised

Immunosuppressed patients present a unique challenge, because their immune response will not mount the same presentation as an otherwise healthy patient. This population includes patients with HIV/AIDS, diabetics, patients on chemotherapy, transplant patients, and patients on steroid therapy. Immunosuppressed patients have a wider differential including many obscure medical etiologies, such as various opportunistic infections. Due to the lack of inflammatory response, physical exam may present as not concerning. The examiner should be wary of a "benign exam" in light of an otherwise concerning clinical picture. These patients often do not mount an expected leukocytosis. Delayed diagnosis may be devastating because patients often present with advanced disease, shock, or peritonitis, with limited reserve.

INDICATIONS FOR SURGICAL EXPLORATION

The need for operation is apparent when the diagnosis is certain, but surgery sometimes must be undertaken before a precise diagnosis is reached. Table 23–6 lists some indications for urgent laparotomy or laparoscopy. Among patients with acute abdominal pain, those over age 65 more often require operation (33%) than do younger patients (15%).

Table 23–6. Indications for urgent operation in patients with an acute abdomen.

Physical findings
Involuntary guarding or rigidity, especially if spreading
Increasing or severe localized tenderness
Tense or progressive distention
Tender abdominal or rectal mass with high fever or hypotension
Rectal bleeding with shock or acidosis
Equivocal abdominal findings along with septicemia (high fever, marked or rising leukocytosis, mental changes, or increasing glucose intolerance in a diabetic patient)
Bleeding (unexplained shock or acidosis, falling hematocrit)
Suspected ischemia (acidosis, fever, tachycardia)
Deterioration on conservative treatment
Radiologic findings
Pneumoperitoneum
Gross or progressive bowel distention
Free extravasation of contrast material
Space-occupying lesion on scan, with fever
Mesenteric occlusion on angiography
Endoscopic findings
Perforated or uncontrollably bleeding lesion

A liberal policy of exploration is advisable in patients with inconclusive but persistent right lower quadrant tenderness. Pain in the left upper quadrant infrequently requires urgent laparotomy, and its cause can usually await elective confirmatory studies.

PREOPERATIVE MANAGEMENT

After initial assessment, parenteral analgesics for pain relief should not be withheld. In moderate doses, analgesics neither obscure useful physical findings nor mask their subsequent development. Indeed, abdominal masses may become obvious once rectus spasm is relieved. Pain that persists despite adequate doses of narcotics suggests a serious condition often requiring operative correction.

Resuscitation of acutely ill patients should proceed based on their intravascular fluid deficits and systemic diseases. Medications should be restricted to essential requirements. Particular care should be given to use of cardiac drugs and corticosteroids and to control of diabetes. Antibiotics are indicated for some infectious conditions or as prophylaxis in the perioperative period. They should be immediately initiated if sepsis due to perforated viscous is suspected.

A nasogastric tube should be inserted in patients with hematemesis or copious vomiting, suspected bowel obstruction, or severe paralytic ileus. This precaution may prevent aspiration in patients suffering from drug overdose or alcohol intoxication, patients who are comatose or debilitated, or elderly patients with impaired cough reflexes. A urinary catheter should be placed in patients with systemic hypoperfusion. In some elderly patients, it eliminates the cause of pain (acute bladder distention) or unmasks relevant abdominal signs.

Informed consent for surgery may be difficult to obtain when the diagnosis is uncertain. It is prudent to discuss with the patient and family the possibility of multiple staged operations, temporary or permanent stomal openings, impotence or sterility, and postoperative mechanical ventilation. Whenever the exact diagnosis is uncertain—especially in young, frail, or severely ill patients—a frank preoperative discussion of the diagnostic dilemma and reasons for laparotomy or laparoscopy will reduce postoperative anxieties and misunderstanding. Discussing goals of care, especially in frail and elderly patients, is also key.

References

Flum D: Acute appendicitis: appendectomy or the "antibiotics first" strategy. *N Engl J Med.* 2015;372:1937-1943.
Gans S, Pols M, Stoker J, et al: Guideline for the diagnostic pathway in patients with acute abdominal pain. *Dig Surg.* 2015;32(1):23-31.
Lewis K, Takenaka K, Luber S: Acute abdominal pain in the bariatric surgery patient. *Emerg Med Clin.* 2016;34:387-407.
Spangler R, Van Pham T, Khoujah D, et al: Abdominal emergencies in the geriatric patient. *Int J Emerg Med.* 2014;7:43.
Strasberg S: Acute calculous cholecystitis. *N Engl J Med.* 2008;358:2804-2811.

MULTIPLE CHOICE QUESTIONS

1. A 50-year-old white woman presents to the emergency department with a 24-hour history of right upper quadrant abdominal pain, fever, and a white blood cell count of 14,000/μL. What is the initial imaging study of choice?

   A. 99m-Tc hepatobiliary scintigraphy (hepatic iminodiacetic acid [HIDA]) scan
   B. Computed tomography (CT) scan of the abdomen
   C. Kidney, ureter, and bladder radiograph
   D. Abdominal ultrasound
   E. Magnetic resonance cholangiopancreatography

2. A 75-year-old man has a right hemicolectomy performed for cecal polyps. The patient has return of bowel function. On postoperative day 10, the patient complains of worsening abdominal pain and a low-grade fever. A CT scan is performed that shows evidence of a high-grade small bowel obstruction. A nasogastric (NG) tube is placed. The patient is observed over the next 2 days, and he has no return of bowel function. The next step in management is to

   A. Start Reglan and encourage ambulation
   B. Diagnostic laparoscopy
   C. Exploratory laparotomy
   D. NG tube decompression and continued observation
   E. Repeat CT scan

3. Which of the following is true regarding small bowel obstruction (SBO)?

   A. The most common worldwide etiology is adhesions from prior surgery.
   B. It is more frequent with upper intestinal than lower intestinal surgeries.
   C. In a complete closed-loop obstruction, serum lactate can be normal.
   D. Partial SBO symptoms typically improve within 24 hours of nonoperative management.
   E. Abdominal pain disproportionate to exam findings occurs early in the setting of obstruction.

4. An 89-year-old man who is currently a resident in a senior assisted living facility comes to the emergency department with an 8-day history of nausea, vomiting, abdominal pain, and profound abdominal distention. The patient states that his last bowel movement was 9 days ago. He is afebrile with stable vital signs. His physical examination is consistent with a distended and tender abdomen without evidence of peritoneal signs. A CT of the abdomen and pelvis with intravenous contrast only shows a diffusely dilated colon, without evidence of perforation. Which one of the following steps is the most appropriate next step in the management of this patient?

   A. Colonoscopy
   B. Barium enema
   C. Watchful waiting
   D. Docusate
   E. Cholinesterase inhibitor

5. A 90-year-old man, currently living in a skilled nursing facility, presents to the emergency department with a 2-day history of progressively worse nausea, vomiting, abdominal distention, and pain. His nurse indicates that his last bowel movement was 5 days ago. His past medical history is significant for hypertension, hyperlipidemia, senile dementia, and chronic constipation. Upon physical examination, he is afebrile with stable vital signs and is in visible discomfort due to the abdominal pain. His abdomen is distended, with lower quadrant tenderness and no peritoneal signs. His rectal examination shows a hypotonic sphincter with no feces on the rectal vault. His white blood cell (WBC) count is 10,000/µL. A plain film of the abdomen is done and shows a dilated sigmoid with a coffee bean shape. Which one of the following steps is the most appropriate next step in the management of this patient?

   A. Admission to hospital, bowel rest, intravenous (IV) fluids, barium enema
   B. Observation in the emergency department
   C. Admission to hospital, bowel rest, IV fluids, colonoscopy
   D. Admission to hospital, bowel rest, IV fluids, IV antibiotics
   E. Admission to hospital, bowel rest, IV fluids, exploratory laparotomy

Peritoneal Cavity

Anupamaa Seshadri, MD

Erika Rangel, MD, MS, FACS

THE PERITONEUM AND ITS FUNCTIONS

The peritoneum is a thin serous membrane that lines the peritoneal cavity. It is the largest serous surface layer in the human body, and its surface area is comparable to the skin. The structure is made up of a single flat layer of mesothelial cells, rich in microvilli. Beneath the mesothelium are a basement membrane and a loose collagen network containing vascularized connective tissue with scattered fibroblasts and macrophages. Normally there is between 5 and 20 mL of free peritoneal fluid. This can vary in women, peaking after ovulation. Normal peritoneal fluid has a specific gravity of less than 1.016, protein concentration of less than 3 g/dL, pH between 7.5 and 8, and white blood cell count (WBC) of less than 3000/μL.

Once thought to be a passive barrier, the peritoneum is now understood to have numerous functions.

- The mesothelial cells provide a near-frictionless environment within the peritoneum and allow intraperitoneal organs to glide over one another during peristalsis and movement.

- The peritoneum participates in transport of fluid and cells across serosal cavities, which is facilitated by its large surface area and semipermeable nature. Fluid exchange with the extracellular fluid space occurs at rates of over 500 mL/h. The circulation of peritoneal fluid is directed toward lymphatics on the undersurface of the diaphragm. Particulate matter up to 20 μm in size is cleared via stomas in the diaphragmatic mesothelium and emptied into the right thoracic duct.

- The peritoneum, usually sterile, participates in recognizing and eliminating bacteria. Mesothelial cells secrete opsonins that promote bacterial destruction, aid in antigen presentation, and express intercellular adhesion molecule 1 (ICAM-1) and vascular cell adhesion molecule 1 (VCAM-1). These are involved in attachment and activation of lymphocytes, granulocytes, and monocytes in response to infectious pathogens.

- The mesothelial cells participate in intraperitoneal adhesiolysis by secreting tissue plasminogen activator under normal conditions. Impaired healing and cell transformation lead to formation of serosal adhesions.

- The peritoneum has significant wound healing functions and secretes inflammatory mediators in response to trauma and injury, including vascular endothelial growth factor, plasminogen activator inhibitor, nitrogen monoxide, transforming growth factor-β, and tumor necrosis factor-α. The proinflammatory response causes fibrin deposition and activation of coagulation pathways. There is uniform re-creation of the mesothelial monolayer within 5-10 days after injury.

Arung W, Meurisse M, Detry O: Pathophysiology and prevention of postoperative peritoneal adhesions. *World J Gastroenterol.* 2011;17(41):4545-4553.

Beyene RT, Kavalukas SL, Barbul A: Intra-abdominal adhesions: anatomy, pathophysiology, and treatment. *Curr Probl Surg.* 2015;52(7):271-319.

Hellebrekers BW et al: Pathogenesis of postoperative adhesion formation. *Br J Surg.* 2011;98:1503-1516.

ANATOMY OF THE PERITONEUM

BOUNDARIES OF THE PERITONEAL CAVITY

The peritoneum is divided anatomically into parietal and visceral components. The parietal peritoneum underlies the anterior, lateral, and posterior abdominal walls as well as the undersurface of the diaphragm and pelvic basin. The visceral peritoneum is reflected over the viscera within the abdominal cavity. Because organs are not densely packed into the abdomen, the peritoneal lining of the abdominal wall and the viscera creates spaces or basins that are physiologically important.

▲ Figure 24–1. Supracolic compartment, subdiaphragmatic spaces. **A:** Anterior view. **B:** Right lateral view. **C:** Left lateral view.

- *Supracolic compartment*: Located above the transverse mesocolon, the supracolic compartment broadly defines the subphrenic spaces (Figure 24–1A), which are divided as follows:
  - Subdiaphragmatic suprahepatic space: Located between the domes of the hepatic lobes and the diaphragm. The falciform ligament separates the right and left subdiaphragmatic divisions. The inferior limits of the subdiaphragmatic spaces are the attachments of the coronary and triangular ligaments on the diaphragm.
  - Subhepatic spaces
    - Right subhepatic space (Figure 24–1B): Located between the undersurface of the liver and gallbladder superiorly and the right kidney and mesocolon inferiorly. The anterior bulge of the kidney partitions this space into an anterior (gallbladder fossa) and posterior (Morrison pouch) section.
    - Left subhepatic space (Figure 24–1C): The smaller anterior subhepatic space lies between the undersurface of the left lobe and the anterior surface of the stomach, and left subdiaphragmatic collections often extend into this area. The posterior subhepatic space is the lesser sac, which is located behind the lesser omentum and stomach and lies anterior to the pancreas, duodenum, transverse mesocolon, and left kidney. It extends posteriorly to the attachment of the left triangular ligament superiorly onto the hemidiaphragm. The lesser sac communicates with both the right subhepatic and right paracolic spaces through the narrow foramen of Winslow.

- *Infracolic compartment*: Located below the transverse mesocolon and includes the pericolic and pelvic areas (Figure 24–2). The diagonally aligned root of the small bowel mesentery divides the midabdominal area between the fixed right and left colons into right and left infracolic spaces. Each lateral paracolic gutter and lower quadrant area communicates freely with the pelvic cavity.

THE OMENTUM

The omentum is an organ consisting of highly vascularized tissue containing mostly adipose and some lymphoid tissue within folds of peritoneum. It is pliable and mobile and concentrates itself in areas of inflammation within the peritoneal cavity.

Right paracolic space

Phrenicocolic ligament

Left paracolic space

Pelvic cavity

▲ **Figure 24–2.** Infracolic peritoneal compartment.

Anatomically, it consists of both greater and lesser components. The greater omentum is a double-layered fibroadipose tissue that drapes from the greater curvature of the stomach anteriorly, descends to cover the small intestines, and turns back on itself, inserting onto the transverse colon posteriorly. Therefore, it comprises four layers of peritoneum when fused. Its blood supply is from the right and left gastroepiploic arteries, which arise from the gastroduodenal and splenic arteries, respectively, and its venous drainage exits to the portal system. The lesser omentum is a much thinner structure and extends from the porta hepatis to the inferior curvature of the stomach.

The omentum has active roles in immune function, inflammation, and infection control within the peritoneal cavity. Described as "the abdominal policeman" by Rutherford Morrison in the early 20th century, the omentum enlarges in size and mass with expansion of stromal cells in response to foreign bodies in the peritoneal cavity. This response is essential to the omentum's ability to fight infections and to assist with tissue repair.

THE RETROPERITONEUM

The retroperitoneal space includes the space posterior to the posterior peritoneum and extends from the diaphragm to the pelvis. It is divided into anterior and posterior compartments by the perinephric fascia (Figure 24–3).

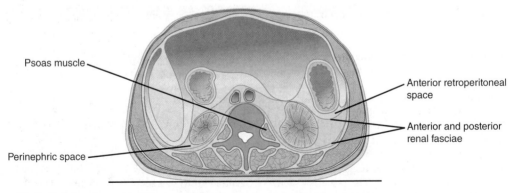

Psoas muscle

Perinephric space

Anterior retroperitoneal space

Anterior and posterior renal fasciae

▲ **Figure 24–3.** Retroperitoneal space.

- Anterior portion: Includes the pancreas, parts of the duodenum, and the ascending and descending colon.
- Posterior portion: Contains the adrenals, kidneys, and perinephric spaces.

▼ DISEASES OF THE PERITONEUM

The etiologies of peritonitis are divided into primary and secondary causes and are summarized in Table 24–1.

PRIMARY PERITONITIS

▶ Epidemiology & Pathogenesis

Primary ("spontaneous") bacterial peritonitis (SBP) is defined as an ascitic fluid infection occurring in the absence of a surgically treatable gastrointestinal source. It is typically associated with advanced liver disease, with other cirrhosis-related complications, and with poor prognosis, with a mortality rate of approximately 20%. It occurs in 8%-30% of hospitalized patients with ascites. Cirrhosis may predispose to small bowel dysmotility and intestinal bacterial overgrowth, with portal hypertension increasing risk of bacterial translocation. In addition, portosystemic shunting leads to decreased clearance of gut-derived bacteria and their products from the peripheral blood. Recurrence of bacterial peritonitis in these patients is common and is often fatal. Other patients may acquire primary peritonitis through hematogenous spread from sites outside the gut, such as urinary tract infections, pneumococcal sepsis, cellulitis, pharyngitis, and dental infections.

▶ Clinical Findings

Clinical presentation of SBP is very heterogenous, but the diagnosis should be suspected in patients with abrupt onset

Table 24–1. Common causes of peritonitis.

Primary
  Spontaneous bacterial peritonitis
Secondary
  Catheter-associated peritonitis
  Acute bacterial peritonitis
    Proximal gastrointestinal tract perforation
    Small bowel perforation
    Colonic perforation
    Mesenteric ischemia
    Cholecystitis
    Appendicitis
  Trauma
  Intra-abdominal abscess
  Pancreatitis
  Salpingitis

of fever over 37.8°C (100.0°F), abdominal pain, distention, rebound tenderness, and altered mental status, although 25% of patients have minimal or no peritoneal symptoms. Most have clinical and biochemical manifestations of advanced cirrhosis or nephrosis. Leukocytosis, hypoalbuminemia, and a prolonged prothrombin time are common.

The diagnosis of SBP requires abdominal paracentesis for examination of the ascitic fluid, with fluid polymorphonuclear cell (PMN) count ≥ 250 cells/μL, fluid culture positivity, and exclusion of secondary causes of peritonitis. A blood-ascitic fluid albumin gradient (serum albumin–ascites albumin) > 1.1 g/dL supports a diagnosis of portal hypertension, which is an useful information because SBP rarely occurs in the absence of portal hypertension. Fluid lactate and pH are nonspecific and tend to be of limited utility. Gram stains must be interpreted with caution, because they are notoriously insensitive for detecting SBP and carry a high rate of false positives. However, the Gram stain may be able to help differentiate between SBP and secondary bacterial peritonitis (see later section), in which bowel perforation may show multiple bacterial forms on Gram stain. Fluid cultures are performed by inoculating ≥ 10 μL of ascites immediately into blood culture media at the bedside. This usually reveals a single enteric organism, most commonly *Escherichia coli*, *Klebsiella*, or streptococci. *Listeria monocytogenes* has been reported in immunocompromised hosts.

▶ Treatment

The use of primary prophylaxis against spontaneous peritonitis remains controversial, with opponents citing concerns for antibiotic resistance and increasing rates of *Clostridium difficile* infections. However, some studies have demonstrated a benefit in high-risk patients with advanced cirrhosis and ascitic fluid protein of < 1.5 g/dL. Typical antibiotics used for primary prophylaxis include norfloxacin and rifampin.

Empiric treatment for SBP is initiated with systemic antibiotics using a third-generation cephalosporin (eg, cefotaxime) or a fluoroquinolone (eg, levofloxacin) for all patients with an ascitic PMN count ≥ 250 cells/μL. Antibiotics are subsequently tailored to cultures obtained from paracentesis. Nonselective beta-blockers, which are associated with increased risk of hepatorenal syndrome and mortality in patients with SBP, should be discontinued. It is important to perform the paracentesis before receiving any antibiotics because a single dose of a broad-spectrum antibiotic can lead to no culture growth in up to 86% of patients. This underscores the importance of timely paracentesis in patients with suspected SBP, with significantly higher mortality (27% vs 13%, $P = 0.007$) in patients who undergo paracentesis more than 12 hours after hospitalization. A 5-day course of antibiotic treatment is recommended because it has an equivalent cure and recurrence rate compared to a 10-day regimen.

Kim JJ et al: Delayed paracentesis is associated with increased in-hospital mortality in patients with spontaneous bacterial peritonitis. *Am J Gastroenterol.* 2014;109(9):1436-1442.

Mandorfer M et al: Nonselective β blockers increase risk for hepatorenal syndrome and death in patients with cirrhosis and spontaneous bacterial peritonitis. *Gastroenterology.* 2014;146(7):1680-1690.

Pericleous M et al: The clinical management of abdominal ascites, spontaneous bacterial peritonitis, and hepatorenal syndrome: a review of current guidelines and recommendations. *Eur J Gastroenterol Hepatol.* 2016;28(3):e10-18.

Solà E et al: Management of uninfected and infected ascites in cirrhosis. *Liver Int.* 2016;36(cuppl 1):109-115.

Strauss E et al: Spontaneous bacterial peritonitis: a therapeutic update. *Expert Rev Anti Infect Ther.* 2006;4(2):249-260.

SECONDARY PERITONITIS

CATHETER-ASSOCIATED PERITONITIS

▶ Epidemiology

In patients undergoing peritoneal dialysis (PD), peritonitis is a source of significant morbidity and mortality, with up to 20% of affected patients needing to transfer to hemodialysis and up to a 6% risk of death after infection. Prolonged peritonitis can lead to structural changes in the peritoneum that eventually lead to membrane failure and inability to continue with this mode of dialysis. Catheter-associated peritonitis is usually caused by introduction of microbes to the sterile peritoneum due to suboptimal sterile technique while connecting or disconnecting the catheter to perform exchanges. Rarely, such infections can also be caused by hematogenous spread or translocation of bacteria from bowel or genitourinary tracts. Biofilms on the dialysis catheter may contribute to relapsing or recurrent infections. PD patients have compromised peritoneal defense mechanisms, impaired by the continuous presence and exchange of large amounts of fluid in the peritoneal cavity. Risk factors include recent invasive procedures, nasal *Staphylococcus aureus* colonization, exit site or tunnel infections, smoking, constipation, and chronic obstructive pulmonary disease. Coagulase-negative *Staphylococcus* is the most common cause of peritonitis in this population, but *Streptococcus* species, *Enterococcus* species, and gram-negative organisms can be seen as well. Fungal peritonitis occurs in up to 13% of infections and is usually due to *Candida* species.

▶ Prevention

Given the morbidity and mortality of catheter-associated infections, the International Society for Peritoneal Dialysis (ISPD) provides guidelines for the prevention and management of peritonitis.

Preoperative systemic prophylactic antibiotics should be administered immediately prior to surgical catheter insertion. Although intravenous (IV) vancomycin has been found to be more effective than cefazolin in prevention of infection, cefazolin is more commonly used because of concern for antibiotic resistance. Therefore, institutional antibiograms should be used to determine which antibiotics are ideal for prophylaxis. Patients then undergo extensive training to ensure they are familiar with sterile technique.

Because exit site or catheter tunnel infections are typically the prelude to peritonitis, daily topical application of antibiotic cream or ointment to the catheter exit site and prompt treatment of superficial infection are recommended.

A lower-grade recommendation includes administration of prophylactic antibiotics for PD patients undergoing procedures that involve instrumentation of intraperitoneal organs, including colonoscopy, cystoscopy, and hysteroscopy. This is still a topic under debate, and the ideal antibiotic regimen has not yet been determined.

Finally, PD patients on antibiotics for other indications are at risk for fungal peritonitis, and antifungal prophylaxis is recommended.

▶ Clinical Findings

Clinical findings of peritonitis are similar to SBP, with abdominal pain and cloudy effluent when the dialysate is removed from the abdomen. The patient should also be examined for superficial infection of the catheter exit site and tunnel because this is a common source of peritonitis. The major laboratory finding is a peritoneal fluid WBC count > 100/μL (normal WBC < 8/μL). However, approximately 10% of PD patients with bacterial peritonitis have dialysate WBC counts < 100/μL, such as those with poor host immune response and those on automatic PD. In the latter patient population, rapid exchanges and brief dwell times may lower the WBC in the dialysate, and a presumptive diagnosis should be made if there are > 50% neutrophils in the effluent.

▶ Treatment

Empiric antibiotics should be started as soon as there is a suspicion for peritonitis in PD catheter patients, including those with cloudy effluent, following culture and sensitivity and cell count. The recommended route is intraperitoneal, as opposed to IV, and treatment should include empiric coverage of both gram-positive and gram-negative organisms. Although institution-specific antibiograms should inform antibiotic choice, the ISPD suggests that gram-positive organisms should be covered by vancomycin or a first-generation cephalosporin and gram-negative organisms should be covered by a third-generation cephalosporin or aminoglycoside.

Indications for catheter removal include lack of clinical improvement in response to appropriate antibiotics within 5 days of treatment, clinical deterioration, or confirmed fungal infections.

Szeto CC et al: ISPD catheter-related infection recommendations: 2017 update. *Perit Dial Int.* 2017;37(2):141-154.

ACUTE BACTERIAL PERITONITIS

▶ Epidemiology & Pathogenesis

Secondary peritonitis occurs as a result of perforating, inflammatory, infectious, or ischemic injuries of the gastrointestinal or genitourinary system, in which breach of the intrinsic mucosal defense barrier allows bowel flora to inoculate the abdominal cavity. These cases typically follow disruption of a hollow viscus, and presentation varies by the viscus involved.

The immune response against bacterial infection is limited by dilution of opsonic proteins in intraperitoneal fluid, which impairs phagocytosis. When hemoglobin is present in the peritoneal cavity, *E coli* can elaborate leukotoxins that reduce bactericidal activity. Limited, localized infection can be eradicated by host defenses, but continued contamination leads to generalized peritonitis and eventually to sepsis and organ failure.

Factors that influence the severity of peritonitis include the type of bacterial or fungal contamination, the nature and duration of the injury, and the host's nutritional and immune status. Cleaner (eg, proximal gut perforations) or well-localized (eg,, ruptured appendix) contaminations progress to fulminant peritonitis relatively slowly (approximately 12-24 hours). In contrast, bacteria associated with distal gut or infected biliary tract perforations quickly overwhelm host peritoneal defenses. The degree of toxicity seen in the latter type of perforations is also characteristic of postoperative peritonitis due to anastomotic leakage or contamination. Of note, conditions that ordinarily cause mild peritonitis may produce life-threatening sepsis in an immunocompromised host.

Secondary peritonitis is almost always polymicrobial; cultures usually contain more than one aerobic and more than two anaerobic species. The microbial picture reflects the bacterial flora of the involved organ. If gastric acid secretion and gastric emptying are normal, perforations of the proximal bowel (stomach or duodenum) are generally sterile or associated with relatively small numbers of gram-positive organisms. Perforations of the distal small bowel lead to infection with aerobic bacteria in about 30% of cases and anaerobic organisms in about 10% of cases. Fecal spillage, with a bacterial load of 10^{12} or more organisms per gram, is extremely toxic.

Aerobic infections include both gram-negative and gram-positive species. The most frequent gram-negative organisms encountered include coliforms (*E coli, Klebsiella, Enterobacter, Proteus mirabilis*) and, infrequently, *Pseudomonas aeruginosa*. The more common gram-positive organisms include *Enterococcus, Streptococcus,* and less commonly

Table 24–2. Mortality related to acute bacterial peritonitis.

Cause	Mortality With Treatment
Appendicitis	0.2%-0.8%
Cholecystitis	1%
Proximal gastrointestinal tract perforation	7%
Small bowel perforation	4%-10%
Colonic perforation	17%
Acute bacterial peritonitis	22%-55%
Mesenteric ischemia	20%-70%

S aureus and coagulase-negative *Staphylococcus*. Anaerobic pathogens include *Bacteroides,* including *Bacteroides fragilis,* and *Clostridium*. Fungi are rarely encountered, although they may be present in immunocompromised patients. When present, *Candida* are the predominant species.

The mortality of generalized peritonitis varies widely (Table 24–2). Many factors contribute to determining the risk of death, including the etiology of peritonitis, the duration of contamination, presence of organ failure before treatment, and the age and general health of the patient. Mortality rates are consistently below 10% in patients with perforated ulcers or appendicitis, in young patients, in those having less extensive bacterial contamination, and in those promptly diagnosed and operated upon. Patients with distal small bowel or colonic perforations, bowel ischemia, or postoperative sepsis tend to be older, to have concurrent medical illnesses and greater bacterial contamination, and to have a greater propensity for renal and respiratory failure. Mortality rates in these patients are as high as 50%. Poor preoperative physiologic indices (eg, APACHE II or Mannheim Peritonitis Index), reduced cardiac status, and low preoperative albumin levels identify high-risk patients who require intensive treatment to reduce a daunting mortality rate.

Recent studies have increased understanding of risk factors for poor outcome in patients with peritonitis. Emergency surgery is an independent risk factor for increased morbidity and mortality. Frailty, or reduced physiologic reserve to compensate for stress, and sarcopenia, or the loss of lean muscle mass, confer significant risk for poor outcomes. The publicly available National Surgical Quality Improvement Project (NSQIP) risk calculator can be used for prognostication in these settings to provide patients and families with general estimates of the risk of death or serious complications. However, although the NSQIP risk calculator accounts for several comorbidities and for emergency cases, it is not yet clear that it adequately risk stratifies the emergency general surgery patient.

A. Proximal Gastrointestinal Tract Perforation

Proximal gastrointestinal tract (gastroduodenal) perforation is usually caused by peptic ulcer disease, although the epidemiology and management of this entity have been revolutionized by the development of medical therapies for acid hypersecretion. Currently, the worldwide incidence of peptic ulcer disease is 1.5%-3%, with < 10% lifetime prevalence of perforation in these patients. Peptic ulcer disease may be caused by uncontrolled or inadequately controlled acid hypersecretion, use of nonsteroidal antiinflammatory drugs (NSAIDs) or steroid medications, or *Helicobacter pylori* infection. Marginal ulceration leading to perforation may be seen in patients who have undergone gastrojejunostomies in the past (eg, bariatric surgery or partial gastric resection). Less commonly, gastroduodenal perforation may be caused by perforating or obstructing tumors, iatrogenic perforation (eg, during endoscopy), gastric volvulus and subsequent necrosis, and violent retching.

B. Small Bowel Perforation

The leading causes of small bowel perforation are trauma (see later in chapter) and small bowel obstruction. In the latter, obstruction leads to proximal small bowel dilation, bowel wall ischemia and necrosis, and perforation. Malignancy is a rare cause of perforation in this location, with small bowel cancers only representing < 5% of all gastrointestinal cancers. Neoplasms cause perforation through obstruction and ischemia or by direct penetration and necrosis. Some medications (including chemotherapeutic agents such as bevacizumab and anti–tumor necrosis factor agents used to manage Crohn disease) can lead to small bowel perforation. Infectious etiologies, including typhoid, tuberculosis, and cytomegalovirus in the immunosuppressed patient, occasionally cause small bowel perforation.

C. Colonic Perforation

Like small bowel perforation, colonic perforation can be caused by both blunt and penetrating trauma. Other common causes include diverticulitis, obstructive or perforating tumors, and diseases that cause marked colonic dilation such as Ogilvie syndrome and *C difficile* infection.

D. Ischemic Causes

Acute mesenteric ischemia is a surgical emergency if it leads to bowel necrosis and peritonitis. It occurs secondary to embolic or thrombotic events and rarely from dissection. Patients at higher risk for embolic causes include those with cardiac arrhythmias such as atrial fibrillation. Those with atherosclerotic disease or diabetes are at increased risk of thrombotic causes. Nonocclusive mesenteric ischemia (NOMI) can be distinguished from acute mesenteric ischemia by the etiology of ischemia and management; NOMI

occurs in patients who suffer from low-flow hypotensive states, such as those undergoing cardiac surgery or dialysis or in septic shock. Care of these patients should be focused on reversing the underlying etiology of the low-flow state because there is no specific anatomic target for revascularization in these patients.

▶ Clinical Findings

The clinical manifestations of peritonitis reflect the severity and duration of infection and the age and general health of the patient. Physical findings can be divided into (1) local or abdominal signs arising from the initial injury and (2) manifestations of systemic infection.

Local findings include those of an acute abdomen, with pain, tenderness, guarding or rigidity, distention, and diminished bowel sounds. These reflect parietal peritoneal irritation and resulting ileus. **Systemic findings** include fever, chills or rigors, tachycardia, sweating, tachypnea, dehydration, oliguria, and disorientation. Shock may occur due to the combined effects of hypovolemia and sepsis with organ dysfunction. Physical signs of peritonitis are subtle or difficult to interpret in very young or elderly patients, postoperative patients, and those who are chronically debilitated, immunosuppressed, or receiving corticosteroids.

Laboratory studies reveal leukocytosis or leukopenia and may show elevated amylase and C-reactive protein. Paracentesis or diagnostic peritoneal lavage may be occasionally useful in equivocal cases. A WBC count of > 200 cells/μL is indicative of peritonitis, with virtually no false-positive and minimal false-negative errors.

Although gastrointestinal perforation may be suspected based on history and exam findings, imaging that shows air outside the gastrointestinal tract in the abdomen (pneumoperitoneum) or mediastinum (pneumomediastinum) is diagnostic with rare exception. Upright plain chest films detect extraluminal air with 50%-70% sensitivity, but cannot rule out perforation if negative. Computed tomography (CT) is highly sensitive and specific for extraluminal air and is the most useful imaging modality for diagnosis. It can be completed expeditiously and has the advantage of helping to localize the site and cause of perforation. If imaging is equivocal but the diagnosis is strongly suspected, abdominal exploration may be necessary. Delayed recognition is a major cause of high mortality.

▶ Treatment

Prompt initiation of treatment is necessary to reduce patient morbidity and mortality. Initial management consists of IV fluid therapy, cessation of oral intake, and broad-spectrum antibiotics. These supportive measures should be initiated while workup continues to determine underlying pathology.

Antibiotics should cover aerobic and anaerobic organisms commonly encountered in gut perforation. IV antibiotics should be used to ensure therapeutic serum levels in the early course of treatment, given ileus and impaired oral absorption. Precise selection of antibiotics depends on patient risk factors for resistant bacteria and local antibiograms.

The primary principle in the management of peritonitis is source control. Selected cases with contained leakage and infection may be managed with percutaneous drainage. However, for many of the etiologies listed earlier, the underlying source of the peritoneal inflammation is either an ongoing leak from a perforation or the presence of ischemic bowel, both of which require an operation to obtain source control. Unstable patients may require a staged approach to management, with an initial damage control operation to address immediately life-threatening conditions. These cases focus on controlling ongoing contamination by resecting or oversewing perforated viscera and maintaining optimal blood flow to vital organs. Operative time during this first-stage procedure is limited to minimize hypothermia, coagulopathy, and acidemia, which can significantly increase morbidity and mortality. Bowel is often left in discontinuity, and the abdominal fascia is left open with a temporary abdominal closure placed to facilitate subsequent exploration. Definitive operations to restore bowel continuity and close the abdomen take place after the patient has been stabilized in the intensive care unit.

Intraoperative cultures were obtained frequently in the past if purulence was encountered in the surgical field. Although there is controversy regarding whether intraperitoneal purulent collections should be cultured routinely, these cultures are still commonly performed to help guide antibiotic therapy if the need for a prolonged antibiotic course is expected, particularly in high-risk or immunosuppressed patients.

Observational studies show that antibiotic therapy is often administered for 10-14 days, but infectious complications occur in approximately 20% of patients after treatment regardless of antibiotic regimens. The 2015 Study to Optimize Peritoneal Infection Therapy (STOP-IT) was a randomized controlled trial performed to determine the optimal antibiotic course after adequate source control in patients with peritonitis. This trial showed similar mortality and infectious outcomes in those who received a short fixed-duration course of antibiotics (4 days following source control) and those who received a longer course of antibiotics that extended to resolution of physiologic abnormalities (approximately 8 days). Therefore, we recommend nonimmunosuppressed patients with peritonitis receive 4 days of antibiotics after source control.

In diffuse peritoneal contamination, irrigation with warm isotonic crystalloid solution removes gross particulate matter as well as blood and fibrin clots. There is no clear evidence supporting the addition of antiseptics or antibiotics to the irrigating solution. All fluid in the peritoneal cavity should be aspirated because it may hamper local defense mechanisms by diluting opsonins and removing surfaces upon which phagocytes destroy bacteria.

Postoperative complications are common and may be divided into local and systemic problems. Deep wound infections, residual abscesses and intraperitoneal sepsis, anastomotic breakdown, and fistula formation usually manifest toward the end of the first postoperative week. Persistent high fevers, inability to wean off pressors, unexplained continued high fluid requirements, increased abdominal distention, prolonged delirium and weakness, or general failure to improve despite intensive treatment may be the sole indicators of residual intra-abdominal infection. This should prompt an abdominal CT scan. Percutaneous catheter drainage of localized abscesses or open reexploration is undertaken as needed.

Clair DG et al: Mesenteric ischemia. *N Engl J Med.* 2016;374:959-968.

Columbus AB et al: Critical differences between elective and emergency surgery: identifying domains for quality improvement in emergency general surgery. *Surgery.* 2018;163(4):832-838.

Lubitz AL et al: American College of Surgeon NSQIP Risk Calculator accuracy for emergent and elective colorectal operations. *J Am Coll Surg.* 2017;22(5):601-611.

Sawyer RG et al: Trial of short-course antimicrobial therapy for intraabdominal infection. *N Engl J Med.* 2015;372(21):1996-2005.

Weber DG, Bendinelli C, Balogh ZJ. Damage control surgery for abdominal emergencies. *Br J Surg.* 2014;101(1):e109-118.

TRAUMA

▶ Epidemiology

After both blunt and penetrating injury, peritonitis can be an ominous but nonspecific sign of intra-abdominal injury. Peritonitis can be caused by bleeding from solid organ injury, by hollow viscus injury leading to leakage of enteric contents, and by devascularization of organs leading to ischemia. Furthermore, biliary or pancreatic injury can also lead to peritonitis. The clinical finding of peritonitis should lead to immediate operative intervention for the unstable patient or expeditious workup with a CT scan for hemodynamically stable patients.

▶ Clinical Findings

Solid organ injury, specifically liver or splenic injury, is typically associated with abdominal pain and potential hemodynamic changes depending on the amount of hemoperitoneum associated. CT scan evaluation is very sensitive for this injury, and IV contrast can be helpful to evaluate for an active extravasation.

Findings on CT scan that suggest hollow viscus injury include pneumoperitoneum, mesenteric air, mesenteric vessel extravasation or beading, extraluminal enteric contrast, free fluid in the abdomen in the absence of a solid organ injury, bowel wall thickening or edema, or a mesenteric hematoma. Hollow viscus injury can be missed on CT scan if there is no significant free air or fluid. Therefore, patients with a history of a substantial mechanism or concomitant injuries associated with gastrointestinal injury should be monitored for 24 hours with serial abdominal exams. For example, flexion-distraction injuries of the spine (Chance fractures), solid organ injuries, and injuries of the genitourinary tract are commonly associated with hollow viscus injuries.

▶ Treatment

Blunt solid organ injury can often be managed nonoperatively. Those with more extensive injuries should be monitored in the intensive care setting with serial hemoglobin levels to ensure there is no active bleeding and that intervention can occur expeditiously for those who decompensate. Patients who are hemodynamically stable but have active extravasation on CT or an ongoing transfusion requirement should be evaluated for angiography and selective embolization by interventional radiology. Operative intervention and vascular control are required for hemodynamically unstable patients.

Patients with suspected hollow viscus injuries should undergo immediate operative intervention and repair. Absolute indications for surgical exploration include hemodynamic instability, peritonitis or diffuse abdominal pain, or findings on initial CT scan suspicious for gastrointestinal perforation (pneumoperitoneum, bowel infarction, extraluminal enteric contrast). Mesenteric hematomas may resorb spontaneously without further sequelae, but patients warrant close observation as they may develop delayed bowel ischemia secondary to devascularization of the mesenteric vessels. Vigilance and early intervention are required in the management because a missed hollow viscus injury can lead to death.

Atri M et al: Surgically important bowel and/or mesenteric injury in blunt trauma: accuracy of multidetector CT for evaluation. *Radiology.* 2008;249(2):524-533.

INTRA-ABDOMINAL ABSCESSES

▶ Epidemiology

An intra-abdominal abscess is a collection of infected fluid within the abdominal cavity, typically caused by gastrointestinal perforations, postoperative complications, and penetrating injuries. Abscesses can form adjacent to a diseased viscus (eg, with perforated appendix, Crohn enterocolitis, or diverticulitis) or secondary to external contamination (eg, postoperative subphrenic abscesses). Interloop and pelvic abscesses form if infected fluid settles into a dependent or localized area.

The organisms involved in intra-abdominal abscesses are similar to those responsible for peritonitis, with coliforms (*E coli, Klebsiella* species, *Proteus* species, *Enterobacter* species, *B fragilis*) seen in colonic perforations and flora of the upper gastrointestinal tract (aerobic and anaerobic gram-positive bacteria and *Candida* species) seen in perforations of the proximal bowel.

▶ Clinical Findings

Patients with intraperitoneal abscesses may present with fever, tachycardia, leukocytosis, hyperglycemia, metabolic acidosis, or bacteremia. Although these are nonspecific findings, the diagnosis should be suspected in any patient with a predisposing condition, such as recent abdominal surgery or gastrointestinal inflammation. Those receiving antibiotics may have milder presentations, and deep-seated or retroperitoneal abscesses have few physical exam changes. The initial symptoms in postoperative patients may be as subtle as prolonged ileus or increasing leukocytosis. A mass is seldom felt except late in patients with lower quadrant or pelvic lesions. Irritation of contiguous structures may produce secondary symptoms. For example, subphrenic abscesses may present with referred shoulder pain, hiccups, basilar atelectasis, or effusion. Pelvic abscesses may present with diarrhea or urinary frequency. The diagnosis is more difficult in postoperative, frail, immunosuppressed, or diabetic patients, who are particularly susceptible to septic complications. Multiple organ dysfunction can occur rapidly in patients who are not treated promptly, with respiratory, renal, cardiac, or hepatic dysfunction contributing to mortality as high as 50%.

CT scan of the abdomen is rapid, efficient, accurate, and suitable for ill patients. Abscesses appear as fluid collections with density measurements between 0 and 50 Hounsfield units. Resolution is increased by contrast media, with IV contrast demonstrating rim enhancement of abscesses and oral contrast providing the ability to delineate bowel from the mesentery and other peritoneal content. Iodinated IV contrast improves diagnostic accuracy for many intra-abdominal pathologies but increases the risk for contrast-induced nephropathy in patients with severely impaired renal function (estimated glomerular filtration rate < 30 mL/min/1.73 m^2) or acute kidney injury. Other diagnostic tests such as noncontrast CT, magnetic resonance imaging (MRI), or ultrasound should be considered in these patients. Although data are limited, IV volume expansion with isotonic fluids may be helpful to avoid contrast-induced nephropathy, but sodium bicarbonate and *N*-acetyl cysteine have not been proven to be protective. Patients who are at risk for bowel perforation or leak should not receive barium-based oral contrast, which increases the risk for mediastinitis or peritonitis. Water-soluble contrast agents should be used in these patients, but judgment should be used in those at risk for aspiration because aspirated oral contrast can cause pneumonitis. Rectal contrast is used to help detect rectal or distal colonic leaks but is unnecessary for other indications.

Treatment

Treatment consists of prompt and complete drainage of the abscess, control of the primary cause, and appropriate antibiotics. Depending on the abscess site and the condition of the patient, drainage may be achieved by operative or nonoperative methods.

Percutaneous drainage is preferred for single, well-localized abscesses without solid debris that are > 3 cm and anatomically accessible. Certain collections not accessible by anterior abdominal wall drain placement may be amenable to transgluteal or transpleural approaches. However, other locations, including interloop abscesses, are not amenable to drainage because of the high likelihood of injury to adjacent bowel. The technique of drainage is similar to the Seldinger technique employed for numerous procedures. Under CT scan or ultrasound guidance, a needle is guided into the abscess cavity, infected material is aspirated for culture, and a suitably large drainage catheter is inserted. Complications include sepsis, fistula formation, bleeding, contamination of adjacent sterile body cavities (eg, during transpleural drainage), and potential damage to nearby structures during the procedure.

Open drainage is reserved for abscesses for which percutaneous drainage is inappropriate or unsuccessful. These include many cases where there is a persistent focus of infection (eg, diverticulitis, fistula, or anastomotic dehiscence) that needs to be controlled. This can be performed laparoscopically or via laparotomy.

Pelvic abscesses can often be detected on pelvic or rectal examination as a fluctuant mass distorting the contour of the vagina or rectum. If needle aspiration directly through the vaginal or rectal wall returns pus, the abscess is best drained by making an incision in that area. In all cases, digital or direct exploration must ensure that all loculations are broken down. Penrose and sump drains are used to allow continued drainage postoperatively until the infection has resolved.

Satisfactory drainage is usually evidenced by improving clinical findings within 3 days after starting treatment. Failure to improve may indicate inadequate drainage, inappropriate antibiotic selection, or another source of sepsis and must be addressed to avoid higher mortality. Additional imaging studies should be undertaken urgently, and repeated percutaneous or operative drainage performed as appropriate. As in cases of secondary bacterial peritonitis, antibiotics should be continued for 4 days after appropriate source control.

Merten GJ et al: Prevention of contrast-induced nephropathy with sodium bicarbonate: a randomized controlled trial. *JAMA.* 2004;291(19):2328-2334.

Trivedi HS et al: A randomized prospective trial to assess the role of saline hydration on the development of contrast nephrotoxicity. *Nephron Clin Pract.* 2003;93(1):C29-34.

Vaitkus PT et al: N-acetylcysteine in the prevention of contrast-induced nephropathy: publication bias perpetuated by meta-analyses. *Am Heart J.* 2007;153(2):275–80.

ADHESIVE DISEASE

Epidemiology

Peritoneal adhesions are fibrous connections that develop in response to trauma or surgical interventions in the abdomen or pelvis. They occur in > 90% of open abdominal or pelvic operations and are a source of major morbidity and healthcare spending. Adhesions are the leading cause of mechanical small bowel obstruction (SBO), with over 300,000 laparotomies performed yearly for this indication, and are an important cause of infertility in women. The risk of SBO varies by surgery type, with an estimated risk of 1%-10% after appendectomy and 10%-25% after open intestinal surgery. The impact that laparoscopy and other surgical advances have had on rates of SBO and need for adhesiolysis remains controversial.

Current strategies to minimize adhesions include careful operative technique and barrier methods. Gentle tissue handling minimizes peritoneal and serosal damage and limits the inflammatory response responsible for adhesion formation. Commercially available agents to reduce postoperative adhesion formation include a bioresorbable membrane made of hyaluronic acid and carboxymethycellulose, such as Seprafilm® (Genzyme, Cambridge, MA). These function as a mechanical barrier between two damaged surfaces during the most active early stages of adhesiogenesis and exist in solid, liquid, and sprayable forms. However, they are only effective at the site it is placed and can be difficult to handle, particularly during laparoscopy. Additionally, they are associated with an increased risk of anastomotic leak if placed around fresh bowel anastomoses and a small increased risk of fistula formation. Despite documented local antiadhesive effects, the long-term benefit of Seprafilm is controversial, with several studies failing to show reduction in overall long-term SBO rates.

Clinical Findings

Intra-abdominal adhesions do not usually cause discomfort in the absence of obstruction, and elective adhesiolysis in the absence of SBO symptoms is not recommended. Bowel obstructions typically present with abdominal pain, distention, nausea, emesis, and obstipation. Hemodynamic changes, peritoneal signs, and elevated lactate may indicate bowel compromise.

Abdominal x-ray can be used to identify air-fluid levels in distended small bowel loops. However, CT scan is typically the modality of choice in evaluation of SBO, as it allows for identification of the site of adhesion (known as a "transition point"), evaluation for a closed-loop obstruction, and assessment for bowel ischemia and integrity. CT should be obtained with IV contrast, and findings suggestive of small bowel strangulation and compromise include high-density bowel wall on precontrast scans, diminished or absent contrast enhancement of the bowel wall, mesenteric congestion, or pneumatosis. "Whirling" of the mesentery with an adjacent U-shaped, distended, fluid-filled loop of bowel and two adjacent collapsed loops of bowel are suggestive of a closed-loop intestinal obstruction.

Treatment

Most stable SBO patients with no evidence of bowel compromise can be managed with nonoperative strategies, with up to 80% of adhesive SBOs resolving without surgery. Nonoperative management includes admission to the hospital, IV fluid resuscitation, bowel decompression with a nasogastric tube, and symptomatic management of pain and nausea. Water-soluble contrast can be administered through a nasogastric tube and serial abdominal radiographs obtained. The appearance of contrast in the colon on an abdominal x-ray within 24 hours predicts patients who are likely to respond with nonoperative therapy with fairly high sensitivity and specificity and reduces hospital stay by permitting early diet advancement. Slow transit or nonopacification of the colon at 24 hours suggests the bowel obstruction is complete and is less likely to respond to nonoperative management and may expedite the decision to operate.

A closed-loop SBO or bowel ischemia is a surgical emergency and warrants immediate operative exploration.

Abbas S et al: Oral water soluble contrast for the management of adhesive small bowel obstruction. *Cochrane Database Syst Rev.* 2007;18(3):CD004651.

Scott FI et al: Secular trends in small-bowel obstruction and adhesiolysis in the United States: 1988-2007. *Am J Surg.* 2012; 204(3):315-320.

Taylor GW et al: Adhesions and incisional hernias following laparoscopic versus open surgery for colorectal cancer in the CLASICC trial. *Br J Surg.* 2010;97(1):70-78.

Van der Wal JB et al: Adhesion prevention during laparotomy: long-term follow-up of a randomized clinical trial. *Ann Surg.* 2011; 253(6):1118-1121.

Zeng Q et al: Efficacy and safety of Seprafilm for preventing postoperative abdominal adhesion: systematic review and meta-analysis. *World J Surg.* 2007;31(11):2125-2131.

▼ TUMORS OF THE PERITONEUM

PERITONEAL MESOTHELIOMA

Epidemiology

Malignant peritoneal mesothelioma (MPM) is one of few primary peritoneal neoplasms. It accounts for only about 10%-15% of all cases of mesothelioma diagnosed annually in the United States (approximately 400 cases per year), the majority being pleural mesothelioma. Although asbestos is a shared risk factor, gene expression profiles and molecular pathogenesis of MPM are quite different from pleural mesothelioma, suggesting they are clinically very different entities.

The lifetime risk for mesothelioma in any location is as high as 10% in asbestos workers, with a latency of 20-40 years between exposure and development of disease. The mean age of presentation is in the fifth decade of life.

Four subtypes exist: epithelioid, sarcomatoid, mixed, and well-differentiated papillary. Well-differentiated papillary is usually found in women of reproductive age and is distinguished by a high cure rate following resection. The epithelioid subtype has a more favorable prognosis compared to the more aggressive and rare sarcomatoid subtype.

Clinical Findings

Clinical manifestations of MPM develop secondary to ascites or tumor progression within the abdominal cavity. Common complaints include abdominal pain, increased abdominal girth, nausea, and weight loss. These vague and nonspecific symptoms frequently delay diagnosis, with many patients presenting at an advanced stage.

Lab tests are often unrevealing. CA125, carcinoembryonic antigen (CEA), and soluble mesothelin-related protein (SMRP) are commonly elevated, although they have a low specificity. CT with IV contrast typically demonstrates sheet-like thickening of the peritoneum, with peritoneal nodules in diffuse cases, and distinct masses with peritoneal studding in localized subtypes. Ascites is present in 60%-100% of cases. In patients who cannot receive iodinated contrast for CT imaging, MRI can be used.

Although MPM may be suspected based on clinical and radiographic evaluation, diagnosis requires tissue sampling via core needle or laparoscopic biopsy, with immunohistochemical staining for calretinin, cytokeratins 5 and 6, mesothelin, and Wilms tumor 1 antigen. Cytology of ascitic fluid is often inconclusive because it does not establish stromal invasion into the peritoneum or viscera, which is the defining factor in malignancy. If peritoneal mesothelioma is suspected, laparoscopic tracts should be excised at the time of operation given its propensity to seed port sites.

Treatment

Peritoneal mesothelioma is highly malignant. Mean time from diagnosis to death is less than 1 year without treatment. Current advances in the past decade with debulking surgery and intraperitoneal chemotherapy have extended median survival up to 5 years in many patients with epithelioid tumors, although these treatments are not yet standardized. The goal of surgery is complete or near-complete cytoreduction of affected surfaces, which may require multiple visceral resections. The extent of peritonectomy is somewhat controversial, with some centers advocating complete parietal peritonectomy and others recommending removal of only peritoneal surfaces visibly infiltrated by disease. Completeness of cytoreduction is the most important factor influencing survival.

Hyperthermic (40-42°C) intraperitoneal chemotherapy (HIPEC) is performed at the time of debulking. Common regimens include intraperitoneal doxorubicin and cisplatin, but mitomycin-based regimens are also used in some centers. Contraindications to surgery include sarcomatoid or mixed subtypes, inability to perform adequate cytoreduction, advanced age, poor functional status, extra-abdominal metastases, hepatic parenchymal metastases, and bulky retroperitoneal disease.

PSEUDOMYXOMA PERITONEI

▶ Epidemiology

This unusual disease is caused by a low-grade mucinous cystadenocarcinoma of the appendix or ovary that secretes large amounts of mucus-containing epithelial cells. It should be distinguished from benign appendiceal mucocele, which may also have local mucinous deposits but carries a favorable outlook. The mucin-producing neoplastic cells spread freely to two main areas: the upper abdominal sites of peritoneal fluid resorption (undersurface of diaphragm and omentum) and the dependent peritoneal areas (pelvis and paracolic gutters), causing accumulation of copious amounts of mucinous fluid in the abdomen, termed "jelly belly." Distant metastases and visceral involvement are rare.

▶ Clinical Findings

As with peritoneal mesothelioma, patients seldom complain until they have advanced-stage disease, at which time they have abdominal distention, pain, and intermittent or chronic partial SBO. Weight loss and other features of cancer are uncommon. CT scans show a distinctive peritoneal scalloping of the liver margin, calcified plaques, ascites, and low-density masses.

▶ Treatment

At laparotomy, the surgeon should remove as much of the primary lesion, omentum, and gelatinous material as possible. If there is no apparent primary tumor, the appendix and both ovaries (in women) should be removed. There is controversy on the treatment of pseudomyxoma peritonei, with some recommending periodic surgical debulking for symptomatic disease and others advocating aggressive cytoreductive surgery followed by HIPEC to improve relapse-free survival and potential cure. Larger series have used intraoperative intraperitoneal mitomycin and fluorouracil, although

institutional experiences vary and there is no consensus on the optimal regimen. Recent studies report 10- and 15-year survival rates of 63% and 59%, respectively, when combining cytoreductive surgery with HIPEC. Systemic chemotherapy is generally not beneficial and is reserved for patients with unresectable disease.

Passot G et al: What made hyperthermic intraperitoneal chemotherapy an effective curative treatment for peritoneal surface malignancy: a 25-year experience with 1,125 procedures. *J Surg Oncol.* 2016;113(7):796-803.

Sugarbaker PH et al: Management of malignant peritoneal mesothelioma using cytoreductive surgery and perioperative chemotherapy. *J Oncol Pract.* 2016;12(10):928-935.

Sugarbaker PH et al: Pseudomyxoma peritonei syndrome. *Adv Surg.* 1996;30:233-280.

▼ DISEASES OF THE RETROPERITONEUM

RETROPERITONEAL FIBROSIS

▶ Epidemiology

This rare condition, also known as Ormond disease, is characterized by inflammation and extensive fibrotic encasement of retroperitoneal tissues, often involving the ureters or abdominal organs. Over two-thirds of cases are idiopathic, and the remaining cases are caused by drugs (eg, methysergide, beta-adrenergic blocking agents), retroperitoneal hemorrhage, perianeurysmal inflammation, radiation, urinary extravasation, infection, or malignancy. Idiopathic cases may involve infiltration of immunoglobulin G4–producing plasma cells or autoimmune aortitis with periaortic inflammation from insoluble lipid leaking from atheromatous aortic plaques.

▶ Clinical Findings

Dull and poorly localized pain in the lower back or flank is a common presenting symptom. The urinary tract may be involved in peri-iliac disease, causing hydronephrosis, hydroureter, medial deviation of the ureters, and extrinsic ureteric compression near the L4-5 level. Pyuria and urinary frequency are present in most patients. Compression of mesenteric arteries can cause mesenteric ischemia, and venous compression of the inferior vena cava can cause lower limb edema secondary to lymphatic compression. Because progression is slow, patients have time to develop collateral circulation, and deep venous thrombosis is rare.

The diagnosis is suggested by a CT scan that shows the fibrotic process and any coexisting aneurysmal changes in the aorta. MRI may distinguish fibrosis from lymphoma or metastatic carcinoma.

Treatment

Therapy is aimed at relieving the obstruction caused by fibrosis, ceasing the progression of the fibrotic process, and preventing relapse. If the retroperitoneal fibrosis is due to a secondary cause, treatment is aimed at the underlying condition or stopping the causative drug. Idiopathic cases are targeted with immunosuppressive therapy, including glucocorticoids as first-line therapy. Mycophenolate mofetil, methotrexate, azathioprine, cyclosporine, and cyclophosphamide are added in refractory cases. Few studies have compared the effects or toxicity of steroids alone or steroids plus immunosuppressants. Tamoxifen has resulted in regression of desmoid tumors.

Patients with renal failure due to complete urinary tract obstruction or severe unilateral kidney obstruction require upper urinary tract decompression with ureteric stents or nephrostomy. If surgery becomes necessary, multiple biopsy specimens should be taken to exclude cancer. Ureterolysis should be attempted and can sometimes be performed laparoscopically. There may be some advantage to wrapping omentum around the freed ureters to reduce the risk of subsequent entrapment.

RETROPERITONEAL ABSCESSES

Epidemiology

Abscesses occur less frequently in the retroperitoneum than in the peritoneal cavity. Retroperitoneal abscesses occur from injuries or infections in adjacent structures or by hematogenous spread. Etiologies include appendicitis, pancreatitis, penetrating posterior ulcers, regional enteritis, diverticulitis, pyelonephritis, trauma, and spinal column abscesses secondary to osteomyelitis or disk space infections.

The psoas muscle is a common location for these abscesses. Primary psoas abscesses, which occur without associated disease of other organs, are caused by hematogenous spread of *S aureus* from an occult source and are predominantly seen in children and young adults in underdeveloped countries. Secondary psoas abscesses result from spread of infection from adjacent organs, principally from the intestine, and are therefore most often polymicrobial with enteric organisms. The most common etiology is Crohn disease.

Clinical Findings

Retroperitoneal abscesses manifest with fever, abdominal or flank pain, anorexia, weight loss, nausea, and vomiting. The "psoas sign" may be present, with pain with passive hip extension. These patients often prefer to be in a position of less discomfort with hip flexion and lumbar lordosis. Presentation may be subacute, with symptoms for weeks to months before diagnosis is made.

CT is the optimal imaging modality, although sensitivity is lower early in the disease course. Gas bubbles are diagnostic of an abscess. Awareness of the overall clinical picture is essential for CT scanning to differentiate retroperitoneal abscesses from neoplasms or hematomas. Abscesses are confined to specific compartments, whereas malignant lesions frequently violate peritoneal and fascial barriers and can invade bone.

Treatment

Like intra-abdominal abscesses, antibiotics and drainage are the mainstay of treatment. Catheter-based drainage of retroperitoneal abscesses has a lower rate of success than for intraperitoneal abscesses for the following reasons: (1) they often dissect along planes, giving a stellate instead of globular shape; (2) they often contain necrotic debris that will not pass through catheters; and (3) they often invade adjacent muscle (ie, psoas abscess). Surgical management is indicated if there is no clinical improvement following percutaneous drainage, with resection of necrotic or diseased organs, debridement of the affected compartment, and thorough drainage. An extraperitoneal approach via the flank is preferred for upper retroperitoneal and perinephric abscesses. Transperitoneal exploration may be unavoidable for deep anterior retroperitoneal abscesses.

DISEASES OF THE OMENTUM

OMENTAL INFARCTION AND TORSION

Epidemiology

Torsion of the omentum is a rare condition that develops if a free portion twists around a pivot point or becomes trapped within a hernia. Twisting around the vascular pedicle compromises blood flow, leading to ischemia and necrosis.

Clinical Findings

Clinically, torsion presents as escalating acute abdominal pain, typically in the right lower quadrant. Gastrointestinal symptoms such as nausea and vomiting are absent in over half the patients because intestinal peristalsis is not impacted. A mobile, tender mass is present in one-third of cases. Although some of these features suggest acute appendicitis or cholecystitis, they are not typical of those diseases. CT scans may demonstrate omental edema or swirling of omental vessels.

Treatment

The clinical findings usually warrant surgical exploration. The operation typically reveals serosanguineous fluid, a normal appendix, and the hemorrhagic necrotic segment of omentum. Resection of the affected portion is curative.

OMENTAL TUMORS AND CYSTS

Tumors of the omentum are usually secondary to metastases from gastrointestinal or ovarian malignancies. Although rare, the omentum can be a site of primary cancer. The most common malignant lesions of the omentum are leiomyosarcomas, hemangiopericytomas, and fibrosarcomas. The most common benign lesions of the omentum are gastrointestinal stromal tumors, leiomyomas, lipomas, and fibromas. Primary benign omental cysts are uncommon but can be easily resected if symptomatic.

MULTIPLE CHOICE QUESTIONS

1. Which of the following symptoms should prompt suspicion of spontaneous bacterial peritonitis in a patient with ascites?

   A. Headache
   B. Fever over 37.8°C (100.0°F)
   C. Weakness
   D. Obstipation

2. What route of antibiotics should be given for catheter-associated peritonitis?

   A. Intraperitoneal
   B. Intraperitoneal and intravenous
   C. Intravenous
   D. Intramuscular

3. In a patient with nonocclusive mesenteric ischemia, what is the best management strategy?

   A. Operative revascularization
   B. Systemic heparinization
   C. Reversal of low-flow state
   D. Endovascular revascularization

4. According to the STOP-IT trial, for intra-abdominal infection causing peritonitis, how long should antibiotics be continued after adequate source control?

   A. 2 days
   B. 4 days
   C. 8 days
   D. 14 days

5. What is the best radiologic imaging study for diagnosis of an intra-abdominal abscess?

   A. Computed tomography (CT) scan of the abdomen without contrast
   B. CT scan of the abdomen with intravenous contrast
   C. Abdominal ultrasound
   D. Magnetic resonance imaging (MRI) of the abdomen

25

Stomach & Duodenum

Heather G. Lyu, MD
Douglas Smink, MD, MPH

▼ I. STOMACH

The stomach receives food from the esophagus and has four functions: (1) to act as a reservoir that permits eating boluses of food at intervals of several hours; (2) to mix and deliver food into the duodenum in amounts regulated by its chemical nature and texture; (3) to facilitate the first stages of protein and carbohydrate digestion; and (4) to absorb some small molecules across the gastric mucosa.

ANATOMY

The anatomy of the stomach is illustrated in Figures 25–1, 25–2, and 25–3. Because of its size and varying functions, the stomach is divided into loosely defined areas. The **cardia** is the region of the stomach located at the gastroesophageal junction. The portion of the stomach that lies cephalad to the gastroesophageal junction is known as the **fundus**. The **body** is the capacious central part; division of the body from the pyloric antrum is marked approximately by the **angular incisure**, a crease on the lesser curvature just proximal to the "crow's foot" terminations of the nerves of Latarjet (Figure 25–3). The **pylorus** is the boundary between the stomach and the duodenum.

Different areas of the stomach contain different histologic cell types. The **cardiac gland area** is the small segment located at the gastroesophageal junction. It primarily contains mucus-secreting cells, although a few parietal cells are sometimes present. The **oxyntic gland area** is the portion containing parietal (oxyntic) cells and chief cells (Figure 25–2). The boundary between this region and the adjacent pyloric gland area is reasonably sharp, since the zone of transition spans a segment of only 1-1.5 cm. The **pyloric gland** area constitutes the distal 30% of the stomach and contains the G cells that manufacture gastrin. Mucous cells are common in the oxyntic and pyloric gland areas.

As in the rest of the gastrointestinal tract, the muscular wall of the stomach is composed of an outer longitudinal and an inner circular layer. An additional incomplete inner layer of obliquely situated fibers is most prominent near the lesser curvature but is of less substance than the other two layers.

▶ Blood Supply

The blood supply of the stomach and duodenum is illustrated in Figure 25–3. The blood vessels that supply the stomach originate from the celiac artery, the first major branch off the abdominal aorta. The celiac artery typically gives off the left gastric artery, the common hepatic artery, and the splenic artery. These arteries then branch off to supply various parts of the stomach.

A summary of the gastric and duodenal blood supply is as follows:

Celiac

- Left gastric artery
- Branches of the common hepatic artery
  - Right gastric artery
  - Gastroduodenal artery
    - Right gastroepiploic artery
    - Superior pancreaticoduodenal artery
  - Proper hepatic artery
- Branches of the splenic artery
  - Posterior gastric artery
  - Left gastroepiploic artery
  - Short gastric arteries

Superior mesenteric artery

- Inferior pancreaticoduodenal artery

The left gastric artery supplies the lesser curvature and connects with the right gastric artery. In 60% of people, a

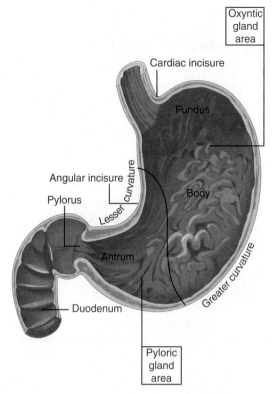

Oxyntic gland area

Cardiac incisure

Fundus

Angular incisure

Pylorus

Lesser curvature

Body

Antrum

Greater curvature

Duodenum

Pyloric gland area

▲ **Figure 25–1.** Names of the parts of the stomach. The line drawn from the lesser to the greater curvature depicts the approximate boundary between the oxyntic gland area and the pyloric gland area. No prominent landmark exists to distinguish between antrum and body (corpus). The fundus is the portion craniad to the esophagogastric junction. The cardiac gland area is adjacent to the gastroesophageal junction, again without a clear anatomic boundary.

posterior gastric artery arises off the middle third of the splenic artery, which runs posterior to the stomach and terminates in branches on the posterior surface of the body and the fundus. The greater curvature is supplied by the right gastroepiploic artery and the left gastroepiploic artery. The mid-portion of the greater curvature corresponds to a point at which the gastric branches of this vascular arcade change direction. The fundus of the stomach along the greater curvature is supplied by the short gastric arteries or the vasa brevia.

The blood supply to the duodenum is from the superior and inferior pancreaticoduodenal arteries. The stomach contains a rich submucosal vascular plexus. Venous blood from the stomach drains into the coronary, gastroepiploic, and splenic veins before entering the portal vein. The lymphatic drainage of the stomach, which largely parallels the arteries, partially determines the direction of metastasis of gastric neoplasms.

Nerve Supply

The parasympathetic nerves to the stomach are shown in Figure 25–3. As a rule, two major vagal trunks pass through the esophageal hiatus in close approximation to the esophageal muscle. The nerves are originally located to the right and left of the esophagus and stomach during embryonic development. When the foregut rotates, the lesser curvature turns to the right and the greater curvature to the left, and corresponding shifts in location of the vagal trunks follow. Hence, the right vagus supplies the posterior and the left vagus supplies the anterior gastric surface. About 90% of the vagal fibers are sensory afferent; the remaining 10% are efferent.

In the region of the gastroesophageal junction, each trunk of the vagus nerve bifurcates. The hepatic branch of the anterior trunk travels to the liver through the lesser omentum. The bifurcation of the posterior trunk gives rise to fibers that enter the celiac plexus and supply the parasympathetic innervation to the remainder of the gastrointestinal tract as far as the mid-transverse colon. Both trunks, after giving rise to their extragastric divisions, send some fibers directly onto the surface of the stomach and others along the lesser curvature (anterior and posterior nerves of Latarjet) to supply the distal part of the organ. As shown in Figure 25–3, a variable number of vagal fibers ascend with the left gastric artery after having passed through the celiac plexus.

The preganglionic motor fibers of the vagal trunks synapse with ganglion cells in the Auerbach plexus (plexus myentericus) between the longitudinal and circular muscle layers. Postganglionic cholinergic fibers are distributed to the cells of the smooth muscle layers and the mucosa.

The adrenergic innervation to the stomach consists of postganglionic fibers that pass along the arterial vessels from the celiac plexus.

PHYSIOLOGY

Motility

Storage, mixing, trituration, and regulated emptying are accomplished by the muscular apparatus of the stomach. Peristaltic waves originate in the body and pass toward the pylorus. The thickness of the smooth muscle increases in the antrum and corresponds to the stronger contractions that can be measured in the distal stomach. The pylorus behaves as a sphincter, although it normally allows a little to-and-fro movement of chyme across the junction.

Peristalsis begins with regular (3/min) electrical impulses from an electrical pacemaker in the fundal musculature that pass toward the pylorus in the outer longitudinal layer. Not all impulses are followed by a peristaltic muscular contraction, but they determine the maximal peristaltic rate. Peristaltic contractions are more forceful in the antrum than the body and travel faster as they progress distally. Gastric chyme is forced into the funnel-shaped antral chamber by

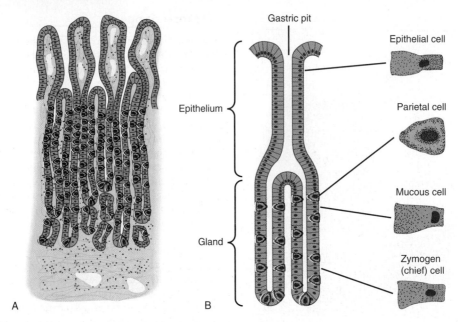

▲ **Figure 25–2.** Histologic features of the mucosa in the oxyntic gland area. Each gastric pit drains three to seven tubular gastric glands. **A:** The neck of the gland contains many mucous cells. Oxyntic (parietal) cells are most numerous in the mid-portion of the glands; peptic (chief) cells predominate in the basal portion. **B:** Drawing from photomicrograph of the gastric mucosa.

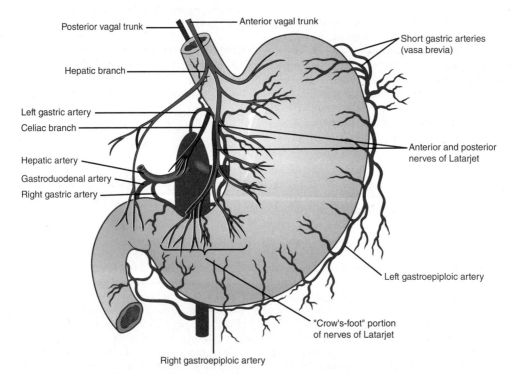

▲ **Figure 25–3.** Blood supply and parasympathetic innervation of the stomach and duodenum.

peristalsis; the volume of contents delivered into the duodenum by each peristaltic wave depends on the strength of the advancing wave and the extent to which the pylorus closes. Most of the gastric contents that are pushed into the antral funnel are propelled backward as the pylorus closes and pressure within the antral lumen rises. Five to 15 mL enter the duodenum with each gastric peristaltic wave.

The frequency of peristalsis is governed by a variety of stimuli. Peristalsis is initiated by the stimulus of distention after eating. Vagal reflexes from the stomach have a facilitating influence on peristalsis. The texture and volume of the meal both play a role in the regulation of emptying; small particles are emptied more rapidly than large ones, which the organ attempts to reduce in size (trituration). The osmolality of gastric chyme and its chemical makeup are monitored by duodenal receptors. If osmolality is greater than 200 mosm/L, a long vagal reflex (the enterogastric reflex) is activated, delaying emptying. Gastrin causes delay in emptying. Gastrin is the only circulating gastrointestinal hormone to have a physiologic effect on emptying.

The storage capacity of the stomach is variable. The volume of the empty gastric lumen is only 50 mL. By a process called receptive relaxation, the stomach can accommodate about 1000 mL before intraluminal pressure begins to rise. Receptive relaxation is an active process mediated by vagal reflexes; hence, it is abolished by vagotomy.

Gastric Juice

The output of gastric juice in a fasting subject varies between 500 and 1500 mL/d. After each meal, about 1000 mL are secreted by the stomach.

The components of gastric juice are mucus, pepsinogen, intrinsic factor, and electrolytes.

A. Mucus

Mucus is a heterogeneous mixture of glycoproteins manufactured in the mucous cells of the oxyntic and pyloric gland areas. Mucus provides a weak barrier to the diffusion of H^+ and probably protects the mucosa. It also acts as a lubricant and impedes diffusion of pepsin.

B. Pepsinogen

Pepsinogens are synthesized in the chief cells of the oxyntic gland area (and to a lesser extent in the pyloric area) and are stored as visible granules. Cholinergic stimuli, either vagal or intramural, are the most potent pepsigogues, followed by gastrin and secretin. Pepsinogen is activated to pepsin when the pH falls below 5.00 by a process that entails severance of a polypeptide fragment. Pepsin cleaves peptide bonds, especially those containing phenylalanine, tyrosine, or leucine. Its optimal pH is approximately 2.00. Pepsin activity stops at pH greater than 5.00, and the molecule is irreversibly denatured at pH greater than 8.00.

C. Intrinsic Factor

Intrinsic factor, a mucoprotein secreted by the parietal cells, binds with vitamin B_{12} of dietary origin and greatly enhances absorption of the vitamin. Absorption occurs by an active process in the terminal ileum.

Intrinsic factor secretion is enhanced by stimuli that evoke H^+ output from parietal cells. Pernicious anemia is characterized by atrophy of the parietal cell mucosa, deficiency in intrinsic factor, and anemia. Subclinical deficiencies in vitamin B_{12} have been described after operations that reduce gastric acid secretion, and abnormal Schilling tests in these patients can be corrected by the administration of intrinsic factor. Total gastrectomy creates a dependence on parenteral administration of vitamin B_{12}.

D. Electrolytes

The unique characteristic of gastric secretion is its high concentration of HCl (hydrochloric acid), a product of the parietal cells. As the concentration of H^+ rises during secretion, that of Na^+ drops in a reciprocal fashion. K^+ remains relatively constant at 5-10 mEq/L. Chloride concentration remains near 150 mEq/L, and gastric juice maintains its isotonicity at varying secretory rates.

The Parietal Cell & Acid Secretion

Many of the key events in acid secretion by gastric parietal cells are illustrated in Figure 25–4. The onset of secretion is accompanied by striking morphologic changes in the apical membranes. Resting parietal cells are characterized by an infolding of the apical membrane, called the secretory canaliculus, which is lined by short microvilli. Multiple membrane-bound tubulovesicles and mitochondria are present in the cytoplasm. With stimulation, the secretory canaliculus expands, the microvilli become long and narrow and filled with microfilaments, and the cytoplasmic tubulovesicles disappear. The proton pump mechanism for acid secretion is located in the tubulovesicles in the resting state and in the secretory canaliculus in the stimulated state.

The basal lateral membrane contains the receptors for secretory stimulants and transfers HCO_3^- out of the cell to balance the H^+ output at the apical membrane. Active uptake of Cl^- and K^+ conduction also occur at the basal lateral membrane. Separate membrane-bound receptors exist for histamine (H_2 receptor), gastrin, and acetylcholine. The intracellular second messengers are cyclic adenosine monophosphate (cAMP) for histamine and Ca^{2+} for gastrin and acetylcholine.

Acid secretion at the apical membrane is accomplished by a membrane-bound H^+/K^+-ATPase (the proton pump); H^+ is secreted into the lumen in exchange for K^+.

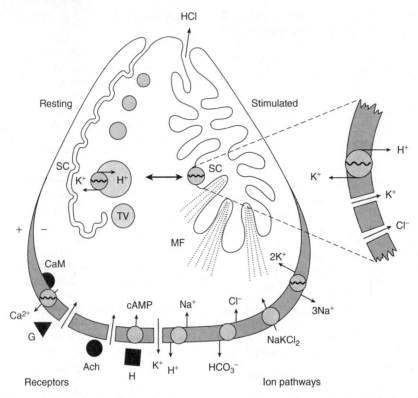

▲ **Figure 25–4.** Diagram of a parietal cell showing the receptor systems and ion pathways in the basal lateral membrane and the apical membrane transition from a resting to a stimulated state. Ach, acetylcholine; CaM, calmodulin; G, gastrin; H, histamine; MF, microfilaments; SC, secretory canaliculus; TV, tubulovesicles. (Reproduced with permission from Malinowska DH, Sachs G: Cellular mechanisms of acid secretion, *Clin Gastroenterol.* 1984 May;13(2):309-326.)

▶ Mucosal Resistance in the Stomach & Duodenum

The healthy mucosa of the stomach and duodenum is provided with mechanisms that allow it to withstand the potentially injurious effects of high concentrations of luminal acid. Disruption of these mechanisms may contribute to acute or chronic ulceration.

The surface of the gastric mucosa is coated with mucus and secretes HCO_3^- in addition to H^+. Protected by the blanket of mucus, the surface pH is much higher than the luminal pH. HCO_3^- secretion is stimulated by cAMP, prostaglandins, cholinomimetics, glucagon, cholecystokinin (CCK), and as yet unidentified paracrine hormones. Inhibitors of HCO_3^- secretion include nonsteroidal anti-inflammatory agents, alpha-adrenergic agonists, bile acids, ethanol, and acetazolamide. Increases in luminal H^+ result in increased HCO_3^- secretion, probably mediated by tissue prostaglandins.

Gastric mucus is a gel composed of high-molecular-weight glycoproteins and 95% water. Because it forms an unstirred layer, it helps the underlying mucosa to maintain a higher pH than that of gastric juice, and it also acts as a barrier to the diffusion of pepsin. At the surface of the layer of mucus, peptic digestion continuously degrades mucus, while below it is continuously being replenished by mucous cells. Gastric acid is thought to enter the lumen through thin spots in the mucus overlying the gastric glands. Secretion of mucus is stimulated by luminal acid and perhaps by cholinergic stimuli. The layer of mucus is damaged by exposure to nonsteroidal anti-inflammatory agents and is enhanced by topical prostaglandin E_2.

Mucosal defects produced by mechanical or chemical trauma are rapidly repaired by adjacent normal cells that spread to cover the defect, a process that can be enhanced experimentally by adding HCO_3^- to the nutrient side of the mucosa.

Similarly, the duodenal mucosa also possesses the ability to secrete HCO_3^- and mucus and rapidly repair mucosal injuries.

▶ Regulation of Acid Secretion

The regulation of acid secretion can best be described by considering separately those factors that enhance gastric acid production and those that depress it. The interaction of these forces is what determines the levels of secretion observed during fasting and after meals.

A. Stimulation of Acid Secretion

Acid production is usually described as the result of three phases that are stimulated simultaneously after a meal. The separation into phases is of value principally for descriptive purposes.

1. Cephalic phase—Stimuli that act upon the brain lead to increased vagal efferent activity and acid secretion. The sight, smell, taste, or even thought of appetizing food may elicit this response. The vagal stimuli directly affect the parietal cells to increase acid output. This process is vagally mediated and is abolished by vagotomy.

2. Gastric phase—Food in the stomach (principally protein hydrolysates and hydrophobic amino acids) stimulates gastrin release from the antrum. Gastric distention has a similar but less intense effect.

The presence of food in the stomach excites long vagal reflexes, impulses that pass to the central nervous system via vagal afferents and return to stimulate the parietal cells. A third aspect of the gastric phase involves the sensitizing effect of distention of the parietal cell area to gastrin that is likely mediated through local intramural cholinergic reflexes.

3. Intestinal phase—The role of the intestinal phase in the stimulation of gastric secretion has been incompletely investigated. Various experiments have shown that the presence of food in the small bowel releases a humoral factor, named entero-oxyntin, that evokes acid secretion from the stomach.

B. Inhibition of Acid Secretion

Without systems to limit secretion, unchecked acid production could become a serious clinical problem. Examples can be found (eg, Billroth II gastrectomy with retained antrum) where acid production rises after surgical procedures that interfere with these inhibitory mechanisms.

1. Antral inhibition—A pH below 2.50 in the antrum inhibits the release of gastrin regardless of the stimulus. When the pH reaches 1.20, gastrin release is almost completely blocked. If the gastric anatomy is changed so that acid does not flow past the site of gastrin production, serum gastrin may never be inhibited. In those situations, gastrin increases to high levels, with marked acid stimulation. Somatostatin in gastric antral cells serves a physiologic role as an inhibitor of gastrin release (a paracrine function).

2. Intestinal inhibition—The intestine participates in controlling acid secretion by liberating hormones that inhibit both the release of gastrin and its effects on the parietal cells. Secretin blocks acid secretion under experimental conditions but not as a physiologic action. Fat in the intestine is the most potent method of inhibition, affecting gastrin release and acid secretion.

▶ Integration of Gastric Physiologic Function

Ingested food is mixed with salivary amylase before it reaches the stomach. The mechanisms stimulating gastric secretion are activated. Serum gastrin levels increase from a mean fasting concentration of about 50 pg/mL to 200 pg/mL, with the peak occurring about 30 minutes after the meal. Food in the lumen of the stomach is exposed to high concentrations of acid and pepsin at the mucosal surface. Food settles in layers determined by sequence of arrival, but fat tends to float to the top. Mixing of gastric contents mostly occurs in the antrum. Antral contents therefore become more uniformly acidic than those in the body of the organ, where the central portion of the meal tends to remain alkaline for a considerable time, allowing continued activity of the amylase.

Peptic digestion of protein in the stomach is only about 5%-10% complete. Carbohydrate digestion may reach 30%-40%. A lipase originating from the tongue initiates the first stages of lipolysis in the stomach.

The gastric contents are delivered to the duodenum at a rate determined by the volume and texture of the meal, its osmolality and acidity, and its content of fat. A meal of lean meat, potatoes, and vegetables leaves the stomach within 3 hours. A meal with a very high fat content may remain in the stomach for 6-12 hours.

PEPTIC ULCER

Peptic ulcers result from the corrosive action of acidic gastric juice on a vulnerable epithelium. Depending on circumstances, ulcers may occur in the esophagus, the duodenum, the stomach itself, the jejunum after surgical construction of a gastrojejunostomy, or the ileum secondary to ectopic gastric mucosa in Meckel diverticulum. When the term *peptic ulcer* was first used, it was thought that the most important factor was the peptic activity in gastric juice. Since then, evidence has implicated acid as the chief injurious agent; in fact, it is axiomatic that if gastric juice contains no acid, a benign peptic ulcer cannot be present. Appreciation of the role of acid has led to the emphasis on therapy with antacids and H_2 blocking agents for the medical therapy of ulcers. In the case of duodenal and gastric ulcers, *Helicobacter pylori* colonize and weaken the mucosa before acid is able to do the damage, and therapy directed against this organism has a more definitive effect on the disease. Antisecretory medications and *H pylori* eradication have led to a significant reduction in the surgical management of peptic ulcer disease.

It has been estimated that about 2% of the adult population in the United States suffers from active peptic ulcer disease, and about 10% of the population will have the disease during their lifetime. Men are affected three times as often as women. Duodenal ulcers are 10 times more common than gastric ulcers in young patients, but in older age groups, the frequency is about equal. Likely due to a declining prevalence of *H pylori* infection, the incidence has declined to less than half what it was 30 years ago.

In general terms, the ulcerative process can lead to four types of disability: (1) **Pain** is the most common. (2) **Bleeding** may occur as a result of erosion of submucosal or extraintestinal vessels as the ulcer becomes deeper. (3) Penetration of the ulcer through all layers of the affected gut results in **perforation** if other viscera do not seal the ulcer. (4) **Obstruction** may result from inflammatory swelling and scarring and is most likely to occur with ulcers located at the pylorus or gastroesophageal junction, where the lumen is the most narrowed.

The clinical features and prognosis of duodenal and gastric ulcers are sufficiently different, so they are dealt with separately later in this chapter.

DUODENAL ULCER

ESSENTIALS OF DIAGNOSIS

▸ Epigastric pain often relieved by food or antacids.

▸ Epigastric tenderness.

▸ Normal or increased gastric acid secretion.

▸ Signs of ulcer disease on endoscopy.

▸ Evidence of *H pylori* infection.

▶ General Considerations

Duodenal ulcers may occur in any age group but are most common in the young and middle-aged (20-45 years) populations. They appear in men more often than women. About 95% of duodenal ulcers are within 2 cm of the pylorus, in the duodenal bulb. Ulcers identified in more distal portions of the duodenum, while rare, may be a result of a gastrinoma and warrant appropriate investigation.

Considerable evidence implicates *H pylori* as the principal cause of duodenal ulcer disease. This microaerophilic gram-negative curved bacillus can be found colonizing patches of gastric metaplasia within the duodenum in 90% of patients with this disease. The bacilli remain on the surface of the mucosa rather than invading it. They act by rendering the duodenum more vulnerable to the injurious effects of acid and pepsin by releasing urease or other toxins and increasing acid secretion through the excretion of histamine N-methyltransferase.

The epidemiology of peptic ulcer disease reflects the prevalence of *H pylori* infection in different populations. In areas of the world where peptic ulcer is uncommon (eg, rural Africa), human infection is rare. Duodenal ulcer disease has emerged

as a major clinical entity in Western society only since the latter part of the 19th century. The incidence reached a peak about 35 years ago and then declined to reach a lower plateau in the early 2000s. These changes are thought to be explained by variations in *H pylori* infection resulting from public health factors. Within countries like the United States, the distribution of *H pylori* is explainable by fecal–oral transmission. The prevalence of infection is higher among lower socioeconomic groups. Interestingly, only a minority of infected persons develop ulcers. *H pylori* also has an important role in the etiology of gastric ulcers, gastric cancer, and gastritis. The 10% of duodenal ulcers that are not associated with *Helicobacter* infection are caused by nonsteroidal anti-inflammatory drugs and other agents. Very rarely, duodenal ulcers are caused by gastrinomas or Zollinger-Ellison syndrome.

Gastric acid secretion is characteristically higher than normal in patients with duodenal ulcers compared with normal subjects, but only one-sixth of the duodenal ulcer population have secretory levels that exceed the normal range (ie, acid secretion in normal subjects and those with duodenal ulcer overlaps considerably), so the disease cannot be explained simply as a manifestation of increased acid production. Whether acid secretion increases in response to *Helicobacter* infection is questionable; however, recent studies have proposed that gastric acid secretion may increase in response to increased gastrin production stimulated by the transformation of urea to ammonia. One possibility is that the colonized patches of metaplastic gastric epithelium in the duodenum, on which *Helicobacter* is present, result from the action of acid. The colonized patches then undergo ulceration.

Chronic liver disease, lung disease, and pancreatitis have all been implicated as increasing the possibility of duodenal ulceration.

▶ Clinical Findings

A. Symptoms and Signs

Epigastric pain is the most common presenting symptom in patients and is variably described as aching, burning, or gnawing. The daily cycle of the pain is often characteristic. The patient usually has no pain in the morning until an hour or more after breakfast. The pain is relieved by lunch, only to recur later in the afternoon. Pain may appear again in the evening, and in about half of cases, it arouses the patient during the night. Food, milk, or antacid preparations give temporary relief.

When the ulcer penetrates the head of the pancreas posteriorly, back pain is noted. Concomitantly, the cyclic pattern of pain may change to a steadier discomfort, with decreased relief from food and antacids. Varying degrees of nausea and vomiting are common. Vomiting may be a major feature even in the absence of obstruction.

Abdominal examination may reveal localized epigastric tenderness to the right of the midline, but in many instances, no tenderness can be elicited.

B. Endoscopy

Gastroduodenoscopy is useful in evaluating patients with an uncertain diagnosis, those with bleeding from the upper intestine, and those who have obstruction of the gastroduodenal segment and for assessing response to therapy. Gastric mucosal biopsies should be taken to test for *H pylori*.

C. Diagnostic Tests

1. Gastric analysis—A gastric analysis may be indicated in certain cases. The standard gastric analysis consists of the following: (1) Measurement of acid production by the unstimulated stomach under basal fasting conditions; the result is expressed as H^+ secretion in mEq/h and is termed the **basal acid output (BAO)**. (2) Measurement of acid production during stimulation by histamine or pentagastrin given in a dose maximal for this effect. The result is expressed as H^+ secretion in mEq/h and is termed the **maximal acid output (MAO)**.

Interpretation of the results is outlined in Table 25–1.

2. Serum gastrin—Depending on the laboratory, normal basal gastrin levels average 50-100 pg/mL, and levels over 200 pg/mL are typically considered elevated.

Gastrin concentrations may rise in hyposecretory and hypersecretory states. In the former conditions (eg, atrophic gastritis, pernicious anemia, acid-suppressant medications), the cause is higher antral pH with loss of antral inhibition for gastrin release. More important clinically is elevated gastrin levels with concomitant hypersecretion, where the high gastrin level is responsible for the increased acid and resulting peptic ulceration. The best-defined clinical condition in this category is Zollinger-Ellison syndrome (gastrinoma). Antrum out of continuity with the gastric alimentary flow after gastrectomy ("retained antrum") is another cause of elevated gastrin driving excess gastric acid secretion due to the bypass of inhibitory cells in the antrum.

Table 25–1. Mean values for acid output during gastric analysis for normals and patients with duodenal ulcer. The upper limits of normal are basal, 5 mEq/h; maximal, 30 mEq/h.

	Sex	Mean Acid Output (mEq/h)	
		Normal	Duodenal Ulcer
Basal	Male	2.5	5.5
	Female	1.5	3
Maximal (pentagastrin)	Male	30	40
	Female	20	30

A fasting serum gastrin determination should be obtained in patients with peptic ulcer disease that is unusually severe or refractory to therapy.

3. *H pylori* testing—Patients with a new diagnosis or a past history of peptic ulcer disease should be tested for *H pylori* with a urea breath test or fecal antigen test. Patients who undergo gastroduodenoscopy should have gastric biopsies, which are diagnostic.

D. Radiographic Studies

On an upper gastrointestinal series or computed tomography (CT) scan with gastrointestinal contrast, the changes induced by duodenal ulcer consist of duodenal deformities and an ulcer niche. Inflammatory swelling and scarring may lead to distortion of the duodenal bulb, eccentricity of the pyloric channel, or pseudodiverticulum formation. The ulcer itself may be seen either in profile or, more commonly, *en face*.

▶ Differential Diagnosis

The most common diseases simulating peptic ulcer are (1) chronic cholecystitis, in which cholecystograms show either nonfunctioning of the gallbladder or stones in a functioning gallbladder; (2) acute pancreatitis, in which the serum amylase and/or lipase is elevated; (3) chronic pancreatitis, in which endoscopic retrograde cholangiopancreatography (ERCP) shows an abnormal pancreatic duct; (4) functional indigestion, in which x-rays are normal; and (5) reflux esophagitis.

▶ Complications

The common complications of duodenal ulcer are hemorrhage, perforation, and duodenal obstruction. Each of these is discussed in a separate section. Less common complications are pancreatitis and biliary obstruction.

▶ Prevention

Prevention of duodenal ulcer disease entails avoidance of *H pylori* infection.

▶ Treatment

Acute duodenal ulcers can be controlled by suppressing acid secretion in most patients. For patients with an *H pylori* infection, symptoms will continue without combination therapy. Surgical therapy is recommended principally for the treatment of complications: bleeding, perforation, or obstruction.

A. Medical Treatment

The goals of medical therapy are (1) to heal the ulcer and (2) to cure the disease. Treatment in the first category is aimed at decreasing acid secretion or neutralizing acid. The principal drugs consist of H_2 receptor antagonists (eg, cimetidine, ranitidine) and proton pump blockers (eg, omeprazole, pantoprazole).

After the ulcer has healed, discontinuation of therapy results in an 80% recurrence rate within 1 year, which may be avoided by chronic nighttime administration of a single dose of an acid-suppressive agent. A better approach is to treat the *H pylori* infection along with the ulcer, because eradication of *H pylori* diminishes recurrent ulceration unless the infection recurs—an uncommon event. All patients who test positive for an active infection with *H pylori* should be treated with either of the following: (1) triple therapy consisting of a proton pump inhibitor (PPI) such as omeprazole 20 mg or lansoprazole 30 mg twice daily; amoxicillin 1000 mg twice daily; and clarithromycin 500 mg or metronidazole 500 mg twice daily for 14 days; or (2) quadruple therapy consisting of a PPI such as omeprazole 20 mg or lansoprazole 30 mg twice daily, bismuth 525 mg four times daily, tetracycline 500 mg four times daily, and a metronidazole 500 mg three times daily.

Patients with complicated peptic ulcer disease will need to continue PPI therapy indefinitely.

B. Surgical Treatment

Surgical management is now uncommon due to appropriate medical management of duodenal ulcers. Typically, an operation is reserved for complications of ulcer disease and focuses on damage control followed by subsequent medical management of an *H pylori* infection. However, if ulcers persist despite medical treatment, surgical treatment is indicated.

The surgical procedures that can cure peptic ulcer are aimed at reduction of gastric acid secretion. Excision of the ulcer itself is not sufficient for either duodenal or gastric ulcers; recurrence is nearly inevitable with such procedures.

The surgical methods of treating duodenal ulcer are vagotomy with or without a drainage procedure and antrectomy plus vagotomy. All of these procedures can be performed laparoscopically. With rare exceptions, any one of the vagotomy operations is sufficient (Figure 25–5).

1. Vagotomy—Truncal vagotomy consists of resection of a 1- or 2-cm segment of each vagal trunk as it enters the abdomen on the distal esophagus. The resulting vagal denervation of the gastric musculature produces delayed emptying of the stomach in many patients unless a drainage procedure is performed. The method of drainage most often selected is **pyloroplasty (Heineke-Mikulicz procedure; Figure 25–6); gastrojejunostomy** is used less often. Neither procedure gives a superior functional result, and pyloroplasty is less time consuming.

Preservation of certain branches of the vagal nerves can reduce the morbidity of vagotomy. Selective vagotomy consists of the resection of the vagal nerves distal to the take-off of the celiac branches posteriorly and hepatic branches

anteriorly. Even more conservative is a **parietal cell vagotomy** or **highly selective vagotomy.** The technique spares the main nerves of Latarjet (Figures 25–3 and 25–5) but divides all vagal branches that terminate on the proximal two-thirds of the stomach. Because antral innervation is preserved, gastric emptying is relatively normal, and a drainage procedure is unnecessary. Nevertheless, parietal cell vagotomy plus pyloroplasty gives better results (ie, fewer recurrent ulcers) than parietal cell vagotomy alone. Parietal cell vagotomy appears to have about the same effectiveness as truncal or selective vagotomy for curing the ulcer disease, but dumping and diarrhea are much less frequent.

The vagotomy procedures have the advantages of technical simplicity and preservation of the entire gastric reservoir capacity. The principal disadvantage is recurrent ulceration in about 10% of patients. The recurrence rate after parietal cell vagotomy is about twice as high in patients with prepyloric ulcer, and most surgeons use a different operation for an ulcer in this location.

2. Antrectomy and vagotomy—This operation entails a distal gastrectomy of 50% of the stomach, with the line of gastric transection carried high on the lesser curvature to conform with the boundary of the gastrin-producing mucosa. The incisura is typically used as the proximal margin. The distal transection margin is located on the duodenum, just distal to the pylorus.

The terms antrectomy and hemigastrectomy are loosely synonymous. The proximal remnant may be reanastomosed to the duodenum (**Billroth I reconstruction**) or to the side of the proximal jejunum (**Billroth II reconstruction**). The Billroth I technique is used most frequently, but there is no conclusive evidence that the results are superior. When creating a Billroth II (gastrojejunostomy) reconstruction, the surgeon may bring the jejunal loop up to the gastric remnant either anterior to the transverse colon or posteriorly through a hole in the transverse mesocolon. Because either method is satisfactory, an antecolic anastomosis is elected in most cases because it is simpler. Truncal vagotomy is performed as described in the preceding section; antrectomy by itself will not prevent a high recurrence rate. In most instances, the surgeon will be able to remove the ulcerated portion of duodenum in the course of resection.

Vagotomy and antrectomy are associated with a low incidence of marginal ulceration (2%) and a generally good overall outcome, but the risk of complications is higher than after vagotomy without resection.

3. Subtotal gastrectomy—This operation consists of resection of two-thirds to three-fourths of the distal stomach. After subtotal gastrectomy for duodenal ulcer, a Billroth II reconstruction is preferable. Subtotal gastrectomy is considered the last line of definitive surgical treatment reserved for patients who have undergone multiple failed procedures for refractory ulcer disease.

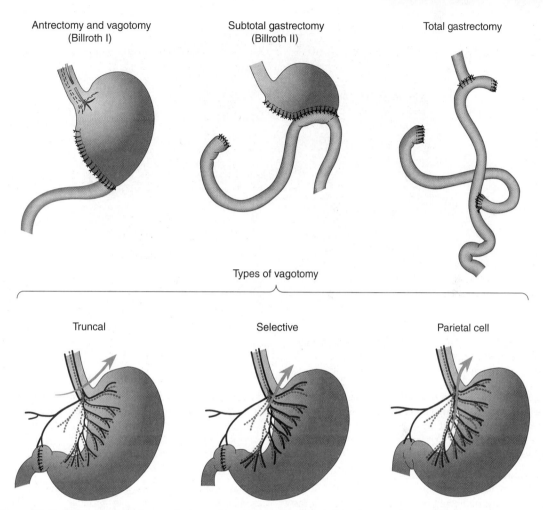

▲ **Figure 25–5.** Various types of operations used to manage duodenal ulcer disease. The choice among the other procedures should be individualized according to principles discussed in the text.

▶ Complications of Surgery for Peptic Ulcer

A. Early Complications

Postgastrectomy patients can develop early complications associated with their anastomoses including postoperative hemorrhage, anastomotic leaks, duodenal stump leaks, and strictures. Any anastomoses created to achieve continuity can lead to a leak, most commonly within the first 7-10 days after surgery. Patients typically present with fever, abdominal pain, and unexplained tachycardia or hypotension.

Similarly, duodenal stump leaks following a Billroth II or Roux-en-Y bypass can cause similar symptoms. These typically present between 5 and 7 days after surgery. Duodenal stump leaks can be managed several ways. In stable patients,

patients can undergo percutaneous or endoscopic drainage of fluid collections. Conservative management heals duodenal stump leaks in most patients. For patients who have persistent leaks up to 6 weeks, the duodenal defect should be closed. Small defects can be closed primarily. Large defects can be patched with a loop or jejunum, or a duodenojejunostomy can be created. Unstable patients must undergo surgical exploration immediately for drainage and biliary diversion.

Anastomoses can also be complicated by postoperative edema and/or scarring, leading to gastric outlet obstruction. Patients typically present with bloating and vomiting. These patients sometimes require endoscopic dilation, but patients who develop recurrent strictures can be offered stricturoplasty.

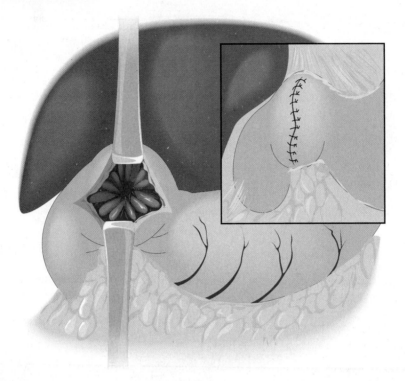

▲ **Figure 25–6.** Heineke-Mikulicz pyloroplasty. A longitudinal incision has been made across the pylorus, revealing an active ulcer in the duodenal bulb. The insert shows the transverse closure of the incision that widens the gastric outlet. The accompanying vagotomy is not shown.

B. Late Complications

1. Recurrent ulcer (marginal ulcer, stomal ulcer, anastomotic ulcer)—Recurrent ulcers form in about 10% of duodenal ulcer patients treated by vagotomy and pyloroplasty or parietal cell vagotomy and in 2%-3% of patients after vagotomy and antrectomy or subtotal gastrectomy without chronic acid suppression. Recurrent ulcers nearly always develop immediately adjacent to the anastomosis on the intestinal side.

The usual complaint is upper abdominal pain, which is often aggravated by eating and improved by antacids. In some patients, the pain is felt more to the left in the epigastrium, and left axillary or shoulder pain is occasionally reported. About a third of patients with marginal ulcer have major gastrointestinal hemorrhage. Free perforation is less common (5%).

For patients who have undergone antrectomy, retained gastric antrum should be ruled out with a fasting serum gastrin level. If the patient has hypergastrinemia, a secretin test should also be performed to rule out Zollinger-Ellison syndrome; serum gastrin levels rise with a secretin test in patients with Zollinger-Ellison syndrome, whereas they decrease in cases with retained antrum. In patients with low serum gastrin, recurrent ulcers can be due to incomplete vagotomy and can be treated with PPIs.

2. Gastrojejunocolic and gastrocolic fistula—A deeply eroding ulcer may occasionally produce a fistula between the stomach and colon. Most examples have resulted from recurrent peptic ulcer after an operation that included a gastrojejunal anastomosis.

Severe diarrhea and weight loss are the presenting symptoms in over 90% of cases. Abdominal pain typical of a recurrent peptic ulcer often precedes the onset of the diarrhea. Bowel movements number 8-12 or more a day; they are watery and often contain particles of undigested food.

The degree of malnutrition ranges from mild to very severe. Laboratory studies reveal low serum proteins and manifestations of fluid and electrolyte depletion. Appropriate tests may reflect deficiencies in both water-soluble and fat-soluble vitamins.

An upper gastrointestinal series reveals the marginal ulcer in only 50% of patients and the fistula in only 15%. Barium enema has 95% sensitivity in diagnosing gastrojejunocolic and gastrocolic fistulas.

Initial treatment should include replenishing fluid and electrolyte deficits. The involved colon and ulcerated gastrojejunal segment should be excised and colonic continuity reestablished. Vagotomy, partial gastrectomy, or both are required to treat the ulcer diathesis and prevent another recurrent ulcer. Results are excellent in benign disease. In general, the outlook for patients with a malignant fistula is poor.

3. Dumping syndrome—Symptoms of the dumping syndrome are noted to some extent by most patients who have an operation that impairs the ability of the stomach to regulate its rate of emptying. For most patients, these symptoms resolve; within several months, however, dumping is a clinical problem in only 1%-2% of patients. Symptoms fall into two categories: cardiovascular and gastrointestinal. Shortly after eating, the patient may experience palpitations, sweating, weakness, dyspnea, flushing, nausea, abdominal cramps, belching, vomiting, diarrhea, and, rarely, syncope. The degree of severity varies widely, and not all symptoms are reported by all patients. In severe cases, the patient must lie down for 30-40 minutes until the discomfort passes.

Diet therapy to reduce jejunal osmolality is successful in all but a few cases. The diet should be low in carbohydrate and high in fat and protein content. Sugars and carbohydrates are least tolerated; some patients are especially sensitive to milk. Meals should be taken dry, with fluids restricted to between meals. This dietary regimen ordinarily suffices, but anticholinergic drugs may be of help in some patients. Others have reported improvement with supplemental pectin in the diet or the use of somatostatin analogues.

4. Alkaline gastritis—Reflux of duodenal juices into the stomach is an invariable and usually innocuous situation after operations that interfere with pyloric function, but in some patients, it may cause marked gastritis. The principal symptom is postprandial pain, and the diagnosis rests on endoscopic and biopsy demonstration of an edematous inflamed gastric mucosa. Because a minor degree of gastritis is found in most patients after Billroth II gastrectomy, the endoscopic findings are to some degree nonspecific. Persistent severe pain is an indication for surgical reconstruction. Roux-en-Y gastrojejunostomy with a 40-cm efferent jejunal limb is the treatment of choice.

5. Anemia—Iron deficiency anemia develops in about 30% of patients within 5 years after partial gastrectomy. It is caused by failure to absorb ingested iron bound in an organic molecule. Before this diagnosis is accepted, the patient should be checked for blood loss, marginal ulcer, or an unsuspected tumor. Inorganic iron—ferrous sulfate or ferrous gluconate—is indicated for treatment and is absorbed normally after gastrectomy.

Vitamin B_{12} deficiency and megaloblastic anemia appear in a few cases after gastrectomy and may require indefinite supplementation.

6. Postvagotomy diarrhea—About 5%-10% of patients who have had truncal vagotomy require treatment with antidiarrheal agents at some time, and approximately 1% are seriously troubled by this complication. The diarrhea may be episodic, in which case the onset is unpredictable after symptom-free intervals of weeks to months. An attack may consist of only one or two watery movements or, in severe cases, may last for a few days. Other patients may continually produce three to five loose stools per day.

Most cases of postvagotomy diarrhea can be treated satisfactorily with constipating agents.

7. Chronic gastroparesis—Chronic delayed gastric emptying is seen occasionally after gastric surgery. An upper gastrointestinal series and endoscopy can rule out a mechanical obstruction. Delayed gastric emptying can be definitively diagnosed with a nuclear medicine food emptying test. These patients can have symptom improvement with small, frequent feedings. Prokinetic agents (eg, metoclopramide) are often helpful, but some cases are refractory to any therapy except a completion gastrectomy and Roux-en-Y esophagojejunostomy (ie, total gastrectomy).

8. Late duodenal stump leak—Some patients who have undergone a Billroth II reconstruction can present with a duodenal stump leak at any time after their operation. Duodenal stump leaks can be managed with drain placement or, in some cases, exploratory laparotomy, washout, and closure.

Chey WD, Leontiadis GI, Howden CW: Treatment of *Helicobacter pylori* infection. *Am J Gastroenterol.* 2017;112:212-238.

Costa F, D'Elios MM: Management of *Helicobacter pylori* infection. *Expert Rev Anti Infect Ther.* 2010;8(8):887-892.

Schubert ML, Peura DA: Control of gastric acid secretion in health and disease. *Gastroenterology.* 2008;134:1842.

Waldum HL, Kleveland PM, Sordal OF: *Helicobacter pylori* and gastric acid: an intimate and reciprocal relationship. *Ther Adv Gastroenterol.* 2016;9(6):836-844.

ZOLLINGER-ELLISON SYNDROME (GASTRINOMA)

 ESSENTIALS OF DIAGNOSIS

▸ Peptic ulcer disease (often severe) in 95%.

▸ Gastric hypersecretion.

▸ Elevated serum gastrin.

▸ Non-B islet cell tumor of the pancreas or duodenum.

▸ General Considerations

Zollinger-Ellison syndrome is manifested by gastric acid hypersecretion caused by a gastrin-producing tumor (gastrinoma). Most gastrinomas occur in the submucosa of the duodenum; others are found in the pancreas and rarely as primary tumors of the liver or ovary. About one-third of patients have the multiple endocrine neoplasia type 1 syndrome (MEN 1), which is characterized by a family history of endocrinopathy and the presence of tumors in other glands, especially the parathyroid glands and pituitary. Patients with MEN 1 usually have multiple gastrinomas. Those without MEN 1 usually have solitary gastrinomas that are often malignant. The tumors may be as small as 2-3 mm and are often difficult to find.

The diagnosis of cancer can be made only with findings of metastases or blood vessel invasion, because the histologic pattern is similar for benign and malignant tumors.

▶ Clinical Findings

A. Symptoms and Signs

Symptoms associated with gastrinoma are principally a result of acid hypersecretion, usually from peptic ulcer disease. Some patients with gastrinoma have severe diarrhea from the large amounts of acid entering the duodenum, which can destroy pancreatic lipase and produce steatorrhea, damage the small bowel mucosa, and overload the intestine with gastric and pancreatic secretions. About 5% of patients present with diarrhea only. Other less common symptoms include nausea and vomiting, gastrointestinal bleeds secondary to erosive ulcers, and weight loss.

Ulcer symptoms are often refractory to large doses of antacids or standard doses of H_2 blocking agents. Hemorrhage, perforation, and obstruction are common complications. Marginal ulcers appear after surgical procedures that would cure the ordinary ulcer diathesis.

B. Laboratory Findings

Hypergastrinemia in the presence of acid hypersecretion is necessary for the diagnosis of gastrinoma. In normal patients, gastrin levels are inversely proportionate to gastric acid output; therefore, diseases that result in increased gastric pH may cause a rise in serum gastrin concentration (eg, pernicious anemia, atrophic gastritis, postvagotomy state, acid-suppressing medications). Serum gastrin levels should be measured in any patient with suspected gastrinoma or ulcer disease severe enough to warrant consideration of surgical treatment. H_2 receptor blocking agents, omeprazole, or antacids frequently increase serum gastrin concentrations and should be avoided for several days before gastrin measurements are made. It is often helpful to measure concurrently gastric acid secretion to rule out H^+ hyposecretion as a cause of hypergastrinemia. Patients should also be fasting prior to testing gastrin levels.

The normal gastrin value is less than 200 pg/mL. Patients with gastrinoma usually have levels exceeding 500 pg/mL and sometimes 10,000 pg/mL or higher. Patients with borderline gastrin values (eg, 200-500 pg/mL) and acid secretion in the range associated with ordinary duodenal ulcer disease should have a secretin provocative test. Following intravenous administration of secretin (2 units/kg as a bolus), a rise in the gastrin level of > 150 pg/mL within 15 minutes or > 200 pg/ml above baseline is diagnostic.

Marked basal acid hypersecretion (> 15 mEq H^+ per hour) occurs in most Zollinger-Ellison patients who have an intact stomach. In a patient who has previously undergone an acid-reducing operation, a basal acid output of 5 mEq/h or more is suggestive. Because the parietal cells are already under near-maximal stimulation from hypergastrinemia, there is little increase in acid secretion following an injection of pentagastrin, and the ratio of basal to maximal acid output (BAO/MAO) characteristically exceeds 0.6.

Hypergastrinemia and gastric acid hypersecretion may occur in patients with gastric outlet obstruction, retained antrum after a Billroth II gastrojejunostomy, and antral gastrin cell hyperactivity (hyperplasia). These conditions are differentiated from gastrinoma by use of the secretin test. Because of the possibility of MEN 1, serum calcium, PTH, prolactin, and insulin levels should be measured in all patients with gastrinoma. Genetic testing should also be considered in patients with relevant family history.

Serum levels of neuron-specific enolase, β-human chorionic gonadotropin, and chromogranin-A are often elevated in patients with functioning neuroendocrine tumors. Although they are probably of no physiologic importance, the high levels of these peptides may be useful in following the results of therapy.

C. Imaging Studies

A CT or magnetic resonance imaging (MRI) scan often demonstrates a gastrinoma if it is in the pancreas. However, gastrinomas located within the submucosa of the duodenum are difficult to identify with these modalities. Somatostatin-receptor scintigraphy can be extremely sensitive for detection of gastrinoma primary and metastatic sites. Transhepatic portal vein blood sampling to find gradients of gastrin production has been supplanted by the intra-arterial secretin test. Infusion of secretin into the artery supplying a functional gastrinoma causes an increase in hepatic vein gastrin levels. This invasive test is usually reserved for difficult situations and is often completed intraoperatively.

Although used less frequently now with the availability of endoscopy, an upper gastrointestinal series can show ulceration in the duodenal bulb, although ulcers sometimes appear in the distal duodenum or proximal jejunum. The presence of ulcers in these distal ("ectopic") locations is nearly diagnostic of gastrinoma. The stomach contains prominent rugal folds, and secretions are present in the lumen despite overnight fasting. The duodenum may be dilated and exhibit hyperactive peristalsis. Edema may be detected in the small bowel mucosa. The barium flocculates in the intestine, and transit time is accelerated.

Treatment

A. Medical Treatment

Initial treatment should consist of PPI (eg, omeprazole, 20-40 mg, once or twice daily) or H_2 blocking agents (eg, cimetidine, 300-600 mg, four times daily; ranitidine, 300–450 mg, four times daily). The dose should be adjusted to keep gastric H^+ output below 5 mEq in the hour preceding the next dose. Somatostatin receptor analogues can be used to reduce gastrin secretion.

B. Surgical Treatment

Resection is the ideal treatment for gastrinoma and is appropriate in all patients with apparently localized disease and no other significant limitations to their survival. Surgical cure may be possible when there are resectable metastases in peripancreatic lymph nodes or the liver. Overall, about 70% of patients have immediate biochemical cure, and about 30% of patients remain disease free after 5 years.

Every patient with sporadic Zollinger-Ellison syndrome should be considered a candidate for tumor resection. The preoperative workup should include a CT or MRI scan of the pancreas and somatostatin-receptor scintigraphy. Regardless of other findings, exploratory laparotomy is then recommended in the absence of evidence of unresectable metastatic disease. If the tumor is found in the pancreas, it is enucleated if possible. Most lesions will be found in the gastrinoma triangle, an area confined within the following three points: the cystic and common bile duct, the second and third portions of the duodenum, and the neck of the pancreas. All patients should have longitudinal duodenotomy and palpation of the duodenal mucosa to identify the frequent primary tumors in this site. Intraoperative ultrasound may help in further examination of the pancreas and duodenum for lesions that are difficult to find.

Prognosis

Because H_2 blocking agents become less effective with time, omeprazole is eventually required in medically treated patients. Because it is usually multifocal, the disease can rarely be cured surgically in patients with MEN 1. Malignant gastrinomas can cause death from growth of metastases.

Ito T, Igarashi H, Jensen RT: Zollinger-Ellison syndrome: recent advances and controversies. *Curr Opin Gastroenterol.* 2013;29(6):650-661.

Norton JA, Fraker DL, Alexander HR, et al: Value of surgery in patients with negative imaging and sporadic Zollinger-Ellison syndrome. *Ann Surg.* 2012;256(3):509-517.

GASTRIC ULCER

ESSENTIALS OF DIAGNOSIS

▶ Epigastric pain.

▶ Ulcer demonstrated on endoscopy.

▶ Acid present on gastric analysis.

General Considerations

The peak incidence of gastric ulcer is in patients aged 40-60 years, or about 10 years older than the average for those with duodenal ulcer. Ninety-five percent of gastric ulcers are located on the lesser curvature, and 60% of these are within 6 cm of the pylorus. The symptoms and complications of gastric ulcer closely resemble those of duodenal ulcer.

Gastric ulcers may be separated into five types with different causes and different treatments. **Type I ulcers,** the most common variety, are found in patients who on the average are 10 years older than patients with duodenal ulcers and who have no clinical or radiographic evidence of previous duodenal ulcer disease; gastric acid output is normal or low. The ulcers are usually located within 2 cm of the boundary between parietal cell and pyloric mucosa, but always in the latter. As noted earlier, 95% are on the lesser curvature, usually near the incisura angularis.

Antral gastritis is universally present, being most severe near the pylorus and gradually diminishing. This is associated in most cases with the presence of *H pylori* beneath the mucus layer, on the luminal surface of epithelial cells, and gastric ulcer disease is probably the result of infection with this organism.

Type II ulcers are found along the lesser curvature, close to the pylorus (prepyloric ulcers) and occur in association with (and most often following) duodenal ulcers. The risk of cancer is very low in these gastric ulcers. Acid secretion measured by gastric analysis is in the range associated with duodenal ulcer.

Type III ulcers are also prepyloric ulcers also associated with high acid secretion. For both type II and III ulcers, vagotomy is recommended due to high acid levels.

Type IV ulcers are found proximally on the lesser curvature near the gastroesophageal junction and often require a much larger gastric resection due to their location.

Type V ulcers are diffuse ulcerations throughout the stomach secondary to the use of nonsteroidal anti-inflammatory agents or steroids. Type V ulcers typically do not require surgery and resolve with cessation of the nonsteroidal anti-inflammatory drugs or steroids along with the addition of PPIs and H_2 blockers.

The ulcers described earlier are typically benign, but any ulcers with malignant features should be biopsied. Malignant features include an ulcerated, protruding mass; nodular, fused folds surrounding the ulcer crater; or irregular and thickened ulcer margins. Efforts must be expended during the *initial* stage of the workup to establish this distinction. Despite the generally discouraging results of surgery for gastric adenocarcinoma, those whose tumors are difficult to distinguish from benign ulcer have a 50%-75% chance of cure after gastrectomy.

Clinical Findings

A. Symptoms and Signs

The principal symptom is epigastric pain relieved by food or antacids, as in duodenal ulcer. Epigastric tenderness is a variable finding. Compared with duodenal ulcer, the pain in gastric ulcer tends to appear earlier after eating, often within 30 minutes. Vomiting, anorexia, and aggravation of pain by eating are also more common with gastric ulcer.

Achlorhydria is defined as no acid (pH > 6.00) after pentagastrin stimulation. Achlorhydria is incompatible with the diagnosis of benign peptic ulcer and suggests a malignant gastric ulcer. About 5% of malignant gastric ulcers will be associated with this finding.

B. Upper Endoscopy and Biopsy

Upper endoscopy should be performed as part of the initial workup to attempt to identify malignant lesions. The rolled-up margins of the ulcer that produce the meniscus sign on x-ray can often be distinguished from the flat edges characteristic of a benign ulcer. Multiple (preferably six) biopsy specimens and brush biopsy should be obtained from the edge of the lesion. False positives are rare; false negatives occur in 5%-10% of malignant ulcers.

C. Imaging Studies

Upper gastrointestinal x-rays can show an ulcer, usually on the lesser curvature in the pyloric area. In the absence of a tumor mass, the following suggest that the ulcer is malignant: (1) the deepest penetration of the ulcer is not beyond the expected border of the gastric wall; (2) the meniscus sign is present (ie, a prominent rim of radiolucency surrounding the ulcer), caused by heaped-up edges of tumor; and (3) cancer is more common (10%) in ulcers greater than 2 cm in diameter. Coexistence of duodenal deformity or ulcer favors a diagnosis of benign ulcer in the stomach.

Differential Diagnosis

The characteristic symptoms of gastric ulcer are often clouded by nonspecific complaints. Uncomplicated hiatal hernia, atrophic gastritis, chronic cholecystitis, irritable bowel syndrome, and undifferentiated functional problems are distinguishable from peptic ulcer only after appropriate radiologic studies and sometimes not even then.

Gastroscopy and biopsy of the ulcer should be performed to rule out malignant gastric ulcers.

Complications

Bleeding, obstruction, and perforation are the principal complications of gastric ulcer. They are discussed separately elsewhere in this chapter.

Treatment

A. Medical Treatment

Medical management of gastric ulcer is the same as for duodenal ulcer. *H pylori* treatment should only be initiated in patients with evidence of active infection. The patient should be questioned regarding the use of ulcerogenic agents, which should be eliminated as far as possible.

Repeat endoscopy should be obtained to document the rate of healing. After 4-16 weeks (depending on the initial size of the lesion and other factors), healing usually has reached a plateau. To cure the disease and avoid recurrent ulcers, *H pylori* must be eradicated. The success of therapy in this regard can be checked by serologic testing for *H pylori* antibodies.

B. Surgical Treatment

Before the significance of *H pylori* in the etiology of gastric ulcer was appreciated, the most effective surgical treatment was distal hemigastrectomy (including the ulcer); somewhat less effective but still useful in high-risk patients was vagotomy and pyloroplasty. Parietal cell vagotomy for prepyloric ulcers was followed by a high (eg, 30%) recurrence rate, but vagotomy followed by a gastric drainage procedure such as a Heineke-Mikulicz pyloroplasty to avoid gastric stasis typically leads to improved outcomes.

Intractability to medical therapy has now become a rare indication for surgery in gastric ulcer disease, because H_2 receptor antagonists or omeprazole can bring the condition under control, and treatment of *H pylori* infection can almost eliminate recurrence. Consequently, surgery is indicated principally for complications of the disease: bleeding, perforation, or obstruction.

Lee CW, Sarosi GA Jr: Emergency ulcer surgery. *Surg Clin North Am.* 2011;91(5):1001-13.

UPPER GASTROINTESTINAL HEMORRHAGE

Upper gastrointestinal hemorrhage may be mild or severe but should always be considered an ominous manifestation that deserves thorough evaluation. Bleeding is the most common serious complication of peptic ulcer, portal hypertension, and gastritis, and these conditions taken together account for most episodes of upper gastrointestinal bleeding in the average hospital population.

The major factors that determine the diagnostic and therapeutic approach are the amount and rate of bleeding. Estimates of both should be made promptly and monitored and revised continuously until the episode has been resolved. It is important to know at the outset that bleeding stops spontaneously in 75% of cases; the remainder includes those who will require surgery, experience complications, or die.

Hematemesis or melena is present except when the rate of blood loss is minimal. **Hematemesis** of either bright red or dark blood indicates that the source is proximal to the ligament of Treitz. It is more common from bleeding that originates in the stomach or esophagus. In general, hematemesis denotes a more rapidly bleeding lesion, and a high percentage of patients who vomit blood require surgery. Coffee-ground vomitus is due to vomiting of blood that has been in the stomach long enough for gastric acid to convert hemoglobin to methemoglobin.

Most patients with **melena** (passage of black or tarry stools) are bleeding from the upper gastrointestinal tract, but melena can be produced by blood entering the bowel at any point from mouth to cecum. The conversion of red blood to dark depends more on the time it resides in the intestine than on the site of origin. The black color of melenic stools is probably caused by hematin, the product of oxidation of heme by intestinal and bacterial enzymes. Melena can be produced by as little as 50-100 mL of blood in the stomach. When 1 L of blood was instilled into the upper intestine of experimental subjects, melena persisted for 3-5 days, which shows that the rate of change in character of the stool is a poor guide to the time bleeding stops after an episode of hemorrhage.

Hematochezia is defined as the passage of bright red blood from the rectum. Bright red rectal blood can be produced by bleeding from the colon, rectum, or anus. However, if intestinal transit is rapid during brisk bleeding in the upper intestine, bright red blood may be passed unchanged in the stool.

▶ Tests for Occult Blood

Normal subjects lose about 2.5 mL of blood per day in their stools, presumably from minor mechanical abrasions of the intestinal epithelium. Between 50 and 100 mL of blood per day will produce melena. Tests for occult blood in the stool should be able to detect amounts between 10 and 50 mL/d. False-positive results may be due to dietary hemoglobin, myoglobin, or peroxidases of plant origin. Iron ingestion does not give positive reactions. The sensitivity of the guaiac slide test (Hemoccult) is in the desired range, and this is the best test available at present.

▶ Initial Management

In an apparently healthy patient, melena of a week or more suggests that the bleeding is slow. In this type of patient, admission to the hospital should be followed by a deliberate but nonemergent workup. However, patients who present with hematemesis or melena of less than 12 hours in duration should be handled emergently. The approach entails a simultaneous series of diagnostic and therapeutic steps with the following initial goals: (1) assess the status of the circulatory system and replace blood loss as necessary; (2) determine the amount and rate of bleeding; and (3) discover the lesion responsible for the episode. The last step may lead to more specific treatment appropriate to the underlying condition.

The patient should be admitted to the hospital and a history and physical examination performed. Experienced clinicians are able to make a correct diagnosis of the cause of bleeding from clinical findings in only 60% of patients. Peptic ulcer, acute gastritis, esophageal varices, esophagitis, and Mallory-Weiss tear account for over 90% of cases (Table 25–2). Questions concerning the symptoms and predisposing factors should be asked. The patient should be questioned about anticoagulation medications, salicylate intake, and any history of bleeding.

Of the diseases commonly responsible for acute upper gastrointestinal bleeding, only portal hypertension is associated with diagnostic clues on physical examination. However,

Table 25–2. Causes of massive upper gastrointestinal hemorrhage. Note that cancer is rarely the cause.

	Relative Incidence	
Common causes		
Peptic ulcer		45%
Duodenal ulcer	25%	
Gastric ulcer	20%	
Esophageal varices		20%
Gastritis		20%
Mallory-Weiss syndrome		10%
Uncommon causes		5%
Gastric carcinoma		
Esophagitis		
Pancreatitis		
Hemobilia		
Duodenal diverticulum		

gastrointestinal bleeding should not be automatically attributed to esophageal varices in a patient with jaundice, ascites, splenomegaly, spider angiomas, or hepatomegaly; over half of cirrhotic patients who present with acute hemorrhage are bleeding from gastritis or peptic ulcer.

Blood should be drawn for cross-matching, hematocrit, hemoglobin, creatinine, and tests of liver function. An intravenous infusion should be started and, in the presence of massive bleeding, a large-bore nasogastric tube inserted. In cases of melena, the gastric aspirate should be examined to verify the gastroduodenal source of the hemorrhage, but about 25% of patients with bleeding duodenal ulcers have gastric aspirates that test negatively for blood. A large nasogastric tube (16F or larger) can be used to lavage the stomach and remove liquid blood and clots prior to endoscopy. For patients with acute, rapid hematemesis, a Sengstaken-Blakemore tube may be used to temporarily tamponade the hemorrhage.

Patients should be started on intravenous PPI therapy on admission. Randomized controlled trials have shown that patients on intravenous PPI therapy are less likely to have recurrent bleeding within 72 hours than those receiving placebo. Use of H_2 blockers is not recommended for patients with gastrointestinal bleeding. If bleeding continues or if tachycardia or hypotension is present, the patient should be monitored and treated as for hemorrhagic shock.

In acute rapid hemorrhage, the initial hematocrit may be normal or only slightly low. A very low hematocrit without obvious signs of shock may indicate more gradual blood loss.

All of the previously described tests and procedures can be performed within 1 or 2 hours after admission. By this time, in most instances, the patient has been adequately resuscitated and is being adequately monitored so that recurrent bleeding can be detected promptly. When this stage is reached, additional diagnostic tests should be performed to identify and control the source of bleeding.

Diagnosis of Cause of Bleeding

Once the patient is stabilized, flexible endoscopy should be performed. In general, endoscopy should be performed within 24 hours after admission, and under these circumstances, the source of bleeding can be demonstrated in about 80% of cases. Longer delays have a lower diagnostic yield. An upper gastrointestinal series should be performed if endoscopy is equivocal or unavailable. Endoscopic sclerosis of varices or injection of a bleeding ulcer can result in decreased blood loss and improved outcomes. Patients who have nontherapeutic endoscopic studies still have diagnostic benefit, particularly for surgical planning if an operation becomes necessary.

Rarely, selective angiography will have diagnostic or therapeutic usefulness. For diagnosis, it is most helpful when other studies fail to demonstrate the cause of bleeding. Infusion through the angiographic catheter of vasoconstrictors (eg, vasopressin) and embolization of the bleeding vessel with Gelfoam may be able to halt the bleeding in special cases.

Later Management

Although a precise diagnosis of the cause of the bleeding may be valuable in later management, the patient must not be allowed to slip out of clinical control during the search for definitive diagnostic information. *The decision for emergency surgery depends more on the rate and duration of bleeding than on its specific cause.*

The need for transfusion should be determined on a continuing basis, and blood volume must be maintained. Blood pressure, pulse, central venous pressure, hematocrit, hourly urinary output, and amount of blood obtained from the gastric tube or from the rectum all enter into this assessment. Many studies have shown the tendency to underestimate blood loss and inadequately transfuse massively bleeding patients who truly need aggressive therapy. Continued slow bleeding is best monitored by serial determinations of the hematocrit.

Several factors are associated with a worse prognosis with continued medical management of a bleeding episode. These are not absolute indications for laparotomy, but they should alert the clinician that emergency surgery may be required.

High rates of bleeding or amounts of initial blood loss predict high failure rates with medical treatment. Hematemesis is usually associated with more rapid bleeding and a greater blood volume deficit than melena. The presence of hypotension on admission or the need for more than four units of blood to achieve circulatory stability implies a worse prognosis; if bleeding continues and subsequent transfusion requirements exceed 1 unit every 8 hours, surgical management should be considered.

Total transfusion requirements also correlate with death rates. Mortality is uncommon when fewer than 7 units of blood have been used, and the death rate rises progressively thereafter.

In general, bleeding from a gastric ulcer is more dangerous than bleeding from gastritis or a duodenal ulcer, and patients with gastric ulcers should always be considered for early surgery. Regardless of the cause, if bleeding recurs after it has once stopped, the chances of success without operation are lower. Patients who rebleed in the hospital should be considered for surgical intervention.

Patients over age 60 are unable to tolerate continued blood loss as well as younger patients, and their hemorrhage should be controlled before secondary cardiovascular, pulmonary, or renal complications arise.

In 85% of patients, bleeding stops within a few hours of admission. About 25% of patients rebleed once bleeding has stopped. Rebleeding episodes are concentrated within the first 2 days of hospitalization, and if the patient has had no further bleeding for a period of 5 days, the chance of rebleeding is low. Rebleeding is most common in patients with varices, peptic ulcers, anemia, or shock. About 10% of patients require surgery to control bleeding, and most of these patients have bleeding ulcers or, less commonly, esophageal varices. Mortality from gastrointestinal bleeds is 30% among patients who rebled and 3% among those who do not. The mortality rate is also high in the elderly and in patients who are already hospitalized at the onset of bleeding.

Barkun AN, Bardou M, Kuipers EJ, et al: International Consensus Upper Gastrointestinal Bleeding Conference Group. International consensus recommendations on the management of patients with nonvariceal upper gastrointestinal bleeding. *Ann Intern Med.* 2010;152(2):101-113.

Cheung FK, Lau JY: Management of massive peptic ulcer bleeding. *Gastroenterol Clin North Am.* 2009;38(2):231-243.

Greenspoon J, Barkun A: The pharmacological therapy of nonvariceal upper gastrointestinal bleeding. *Gastroenterol Clin North Am.* 2010;39(3):419-432.

Sung JJ, Barkun A, Kuipers EJ, et al: Peptic Ulcer Bleed Study Group. Intravenous esomeprazole for prevention of recurrent peptic ulcer bleeding: a randomized trial. *Ann Intern Med.* 2009;150(7):455=464.

HEMORRHAGE FROM PEPTIC ULCER

Approximately 20% of patients with peptic ulcer experience a bleeding episode, and this complication is responsible for about 40% of the deaths from peptic ulcer. Peptic ulcer is the most common cause of massive upper gastrointestinal hemorrhage, accounting for over half of all cases. Chronic gastric and duodenal ulcers have about the same tendency to bleed, but the former produce more severe episodes.

Bleeding ulcers in the duodenum are usually located on the posterior surface of the duodenal bulb. As the ulcer penetrates, the gastroduodenal artery is exposed and may become eroded. Since no major blood vessels lie on the anterior surface of the duodenal bulb, ulcerations at this point are not as prone to bleed. Patients with concomitant bleeding and perforation usually have two ulcers, a bleeding posterior ulcer and a perforated anterior one. Postbulbar ulcers (those in the second portion of the duodenum) bleed frequently, although ulcers are much less common in this site than near the pylorus.

In some patients, the bleeding is sudden and massive, manifested by hematemesis and shock. In others, chronic anemia and weakness due to slow blood loss are the only findings. The diagnosis is unreliable when based on clinical findings, so endoscopy should be performed early (ie, within 24 hours).

In the preceding section, the management of acute upper gastrointestinal hemorrhage, the selection of diagnostic tests, and the factors suggesting the need for operation were discussed. Although most patients (75%) with bleeding peptic ulcer can be successfully managed by medical means alone,

early upper endoscopy is recommended because it can confirm the diagnosis of peptic ulcer disease and allow for targeted treatment including epinephrine injection, thermocoagulation, clip application, and banding. This can reduce the risk of recurrent bleeding and result in overall reduced morbidity. The indications for treatment are (1) active bleeding at the time of endoscopy and (2) the presence of a visible vessel in the base of the ulcer. When treatment fails the first time, it may often be repeated with a good chance of success.

Rebleeding in the hospital has been associated with a death rate of about 30%. Patients with rebleeding can undergo a second endoscopy followed by arteriography with embolization prior to surgery. Considering early surgery for those who rebled, however, is recommended. Patients who are over age 60, present with hematemesis, are actively bleeding at the time of endoscopy, have fresh clots and/or visible vessel on endoscopy, have large ulcers of 2 cm or greater, or whose admission hemoglobin is below 8 g/dL have a higher risk of rebleeding. About three times as many patients with gastric ulcer (30%) rebled compared with those with duodenal ulcer. Most instances of rebleeding occur within 2 days from the time the first episode has stopped. In one study, only 3% of patients who stopped bleeding for this long bled again.

▶ Endoscopic Therapy

Treatments administered through the endoscope may stop active bleeding or prevent rebleeding. Effective methods include injection into the ulcer of epinephrine, epinephrine plus 1% polidocanol (a sclerosing agent), or ethanol; application of clips to bleeding areas; or cautery using the heater probe, monopolar electrocautery, or cautery using the Nd:YAG laser. At least two modalities should be available to the endoscopist in the event one is unsuitable for a specific case or fails to work. Except for the laser, all are inexpensive. It is important, however, not to allow the patient to deteriorate during nonoperative attempts at halting the bleeding.

▶ Emergency Surgery

Less than 10% of patients bleeding from a peptic ulcer require emergency surgery. Selection of those most likely to survive with surgical compared with medical treatment rests on the rate of blood loss and the other factors associated with a poor prognosis. Patients who fail multiple endoscopic efforts and interventional angiography with embolization as well as hemodynamically unstable patients and patients with evidence of perforation should undergo emergent surgery.

In patients with hemodynamic instability, bleeding ulcers should be oversewn with no other intervention. Definitive ulcer management with vagotomy should only be considered in patients who are hemodynamically stable. The overall death rate is significantly less after vagotomy and pyloroplasty than after gastrectomy for bleeding ulcer, and rebleeding occurs with about equal frequency after either procedure.

During laparotomy, if the endoscopic diagnosis is a bleeding duodenal ulcer, the first step is to make a pyloroplasty incision longitudinally across the pylorus from the distal stomach to the proximal duodenum. If a duodenal ulcer is found, the bleeding vessel should be suture-ligated and the duodenum and antrum inspected for additional ulcers. Suture ligation typically requires three stitches—above and below the ulcer to ligate the gastroduodenal artery as well as medial to the ulcer to control the transverse pancreatic artery. The pyloroplasty incision should then be closed and a truncal vagotomy performed. If the posterior wall of the duodenal bulb has been destroyed by a giant duodenal ulcer, a gastrectomy and Billroth II gastrojejunostomy may be preferable, since this somewhat uncommon ulcer is especially prone to bleed again if left in continuity with the stomach. Gastric ulcers can be handled by either gastrectomy or vagotomy and pyloroplasty. A thorough search should always be made for second ulcers or other causes of bleeding.

Prognosis

The death rate for an acute massive hemorrhage is about 15%. Careful study of the causes of death suggests that this figure could be improved by (1) appropriate blood replacement, because undertransfusion is the cause of some complications and deaths; and (2) earlier surgery in selected patients who fall into high-risk categories.

Cappell MS, Friedel D: Initial management of acute upper gastrointestinal bleeding: from initial evaluation up to gastrointestinal endoscopy. *Med Clin North Am.* 2008;92:491.

Cheung FK, Lau JY: Management of massive peptic ulcer bleeding. *Gastroenterol Clin North Am.* 2009;38(2):231-243.

Wilkin T, Khan N, Nabh A, et al: Diagnosis and management of upper gastrointestinal bleeding. *Am Fam Physician.* 2012;85(5):469-476.

MALLORY-WEISS SYNDROME

Mallory-Weiss syndrome is responsible for about 10% of cases of acute upper gastrointestinal hemorrhage. The lesion consists of a 1- to 4-cm longitudinal tear in the gastric mucosa near the gastroesophageal junction usually following a bout of forceful retching. The disruption extends through the mucosa and submucosa but not usually into the muscularis mucosae. About 75% of these lesions are confined to the stomach, 20% straddle the gastroesophageal junction, and 5% are entirely within the distal esophagus. Two-thirds of patients have a hiatal hernia.

The majority of patients are alcoholics, but the tear may appear after severe retching for any reason. Several cases have been reported following closed-chest cardiac compression.

Clinical Findings

Typically, the patient first vomits food and gastric contents. This is followed by forceful retching and then bloody vomitus. Rapid increases in gastric pressure, sometimes aggravated by a hiatal hernia, cause the linear mucosal tears that cause upper gastrointestinal bleeding. Actual rupture of the distal esophagus can also be produced by vomiting (Boerhaave syndrome).

Esophagogastroscopy is the most practical means of making the diagnosis.

Treatment & Prognosis

Initially, the patient is handled according to the general measures prescribed for upper gastrointestinal hemorrhage. Bleeding from Mallory-Weiss tears typically stops on its own without intervention. However, endoscopy is still performed to determine the cause of the bleed. Patients who are still bleeding vigorously by the time endoscopy is performed are more likely to require surgery. The bleeding can usually be controlled by endoscopic therapy (eg, electrocautery, clipping, banding). If bleeding persists, angiography and intra-arterial embolization should be considered. If bleeding continues despite endoscopic therapy and angiography, surgical repair of the tear will be required.

If the diagnosis has been made before laparotomy, the surgeon should make a long, high gastrotomy after the abdomen is opened. The tear may be difficult to expose adequately. The search must be thorough because in about 25% of patients there are two tears. A running absorbable acid suture should be used to oversew the lesion. Postoperative recurrence is rare.

PYLORIC OBSTRUCTION DUE TO PEPTIC ULCER

The cycles of inflammation and repair in peptic ulcer disease may cause obstruction of the gastroduodenal junction as a result of edema, muscular spasm, and scarring. To the extent that the first two factors are involved, the obstruction may be reversible with medical treatment. Obstruction is usually due to a duodenal ulcer and is less common than either bleeding or perforation. Gastric ulcers that obstruct are close to the pylorus. Obstruction due to peptic ulcer must be differentiated from that caused by a malignant tumor of the antrum or of the pancreas.

Clinical Findings

A. Symptoms and Signs

Most patients with obstruction have a long history of symptomatic peptic ulcer, and as many as 30% have been treated for perforation or obstruction in the past. The patient often notes gradually increasing ulcer pains over weeks or months, with the eventual development of anorexia, vomiting, and failure to gain relief from antacids. The vomitus often contains food ingested several hours previously, and absence of bile staining reflects the site of blockage. Weight loss may be marked if the patient has delayed seeking medical care.

Dehydration and malnutrition may be obvious on physical examination but are not always present. A succussion splash or a splashing sound heard with a stethoscope can often be elicited on exam from the retained gastric contents. Peristalsis of the distended stomach may be visible on gross inspection of the abdomen, but this sign is relatively rare. Most patients have upper abdominal tenderness. Tetany may appear with advanced alkalosis.

B. Laboratory Findings

Anemia is present in about 25% of patients. Prolonged vomiting leads to metabolic alkalosis with dehydration. Measurement of serum electrolytes shows hypochloremia, hypokalemia, hyponatremia, and increased bicarbonate. Vomiting depletes the patient of Na^+, K^+, and Cl^-; the latter is lost in excess of Na^+ and K^+ as HCl. Gastric HCl loss causes extracellular HCO_3^- to rise, and renal excretion of HCO_3^- increases in an attempt to maintain pH. Large amounts of Na^+ are excreted in the urine with the HCO_3^-. Increasing Na^+ deficit evokes aldosterone secretion, which in turn brings about renal Na^+ conservation at the expense of more renal loss of K^+ and H^+. Glomerular filtration rate (GFR) may drop and produce a prerenal azotemia. The eventual result of the process is a marked deficit of Na^+, Cl^-, K^+, and H_2O. Treatment involves replacement of isotonic saline until a satisfactory urine flow has been established. KCl replacement should then be started.

C. Saline Load Test

This is a simple means of assessing the degree of pyloric obstruction and is useful in following the patient's progress during the first few days of nasogastric suction.

Through the nasogastric tube, 700 mL of normal saline (at room temperature) is infused over 3-5 minutes, and the tube is clamped. Thirty minutes later, the stomach is aspirated and the residual volume of saline recorded. Recovery of more than 350 mL indicates obstruction. It must be recognized that the results of a saline load test do not predict how well the stomach will handle solid food. Solid emptying can be measured with a gastric emptying study using technetium-99m–labeled food.

D. Imaging Studies

Plain abdominal x-rays may show a large gastric fluid level. An upper gastrointestinal series should not be performed until the stomach has been emptied, because dilution of the barium in the retained secretions makes a worthwhile study impossible.

E. Endoscopy

Upper endoscopy is usually indicated to rule out the presence of an obstructing neoplasm.

▶ Treatment

A. Medical Treatment

Treatment chosen is dependent on the duration of the obstruction. Acute obstruction is often managed conservatively with nasogastric decompression, fluid resuscitation, and intravenous PPIs. A saline load test after 48-72 hours of decompression should be performed. If this indicates sufficient improvement, the tube should be withdrawn and a liquid diet may be started. Gradual resumption of solid foods is permitted as tolerated.

No improvement after 48-72 hours may indicate chronic obstruction. If chronic obstruction has produced severe malnutrition, total parenteral nutrition should be instituted and surgical intervention should be considered.

B. Surgical Treatment

If 5-7 days of gastric aspiration do not result in relief of the obstruction, the patient should be treated surgically. Persistence of nonoperative effort beyond this point in the absence of progress rarely achieves resolution of the obstruction. Failure of the obstruction to resolve completely (eg, if the patient can take only liquids) and recurrent obstruction of any degree are indications for surgery.

Surgical treatment may consist of a truncal or parietal cell vagotomy and drainage procedure (Figure 25–5). Truncal vagotomy and gastrojejunostomy are the easiest procedures to perform laparoscopically.

▶ Prognosis

About two-thirds of patients with acute obstruction fail to improve sufficiently on medical therapy and require operation to relieve the blockage. Patients who respond to medical treatment should be treated as outlined in the section on duodenal ulcer.

PERFORATED PEPTIC ULCER

Perforation complicates peptic ulcer approximately half as often as hemorrhage. Most perforated ulcers are located anteriorly, although occasionally, gastric ulcers perforate into the lesser sac. The 15% death rate correlates with increased age, female gender, and gastric perforations.

Anterior ulcers tend to perforate instead of bleed because of the absence of protective viscera and major blood vessels on this surface. In less than 10% of cases, acute bleeding from a posterior "kissing" ulcer complicates the anterior perforation, an association that carries a high death rate. Immediately after perforation, the peritoneal cavity is flooded with gastroduodenal secretions that elicit a chemical peritonitis. Early cultures show either no growth or a light growth of streptococci or enteric bacilli. Gradually, over 12-24 hours, the process evolves into bacterial peritonitis. Severity of illness and occurrence of death are directly related to the interval between perforation and surgical closure.

In an unknown percentage of cases, the perforation becomes sealed by adherence to the undersurface of the liver. In such patients, the process may be self-limited, but patients may develop an intraperitoneal abscess.

Clinical Findings

A. Symptoms and Signs

Perforation usually elicits a sudden, severe upper abdominal pain whose onset can be recalled precisely. The patient may or may not have had preceding chronic symptoms of peptic ulcer disease. Perforation rarely is heralded by nausea or vomiting, and it typically occurs several hours after the last meal. Shoulder pain, if present, reflects diaphragmatic irritation. Back pain is uncommon.

The initial reaction consists of a chemical peritonitis caused by gastric acid or bile and pancreatic enzymes. The peritoneal reaction dilutes these irritants with a thin exudate, and as a result, the patient's symptoms may temporarily improve before bacterial peritonitis occurs. The physician who sees the patient for the first time during this symptomatic lull must not be misled into interpreting it as representing bona fide improvement.

On examination, the patient appears severely distressed, lying quietly with the knees drawn up and breathing shallowly to minimize abdominal motion. Fever may or may not be present. The abdominal muscles are rigid owing to severe involuntary spasm. Epigastric tenderness may not be as marked as expected because the boardlike rigidity protects the abdominal viscera from the palpating hand. Escaped air from the stomach may enter the space between the liver and abdominal wall, and upon percussion, the normal dullness over the liver will be tympanitic. Peristaltic sounds are reduced or absent due to reactive ileus. If delay in treatment allows continued escape of air into the peritoneal cavity, abdominal distention and diffuse tympany may result.

The above description applies to the typical case of perforation with classic findings. In as many as one-third of patients, the presentation is not as dramatic, diagnosis is less obvious, and serious delays in treatment may result from failure to consider this condition and to obtain the appropriate abdominal imaging. Many of these atypical perforations occur in patients already hospitalized for an unrelated illness, and the significance of the new symptom of abdominal pain may not be appreciated.

Lesser degrees of shock with minimal abdominal findings occur if the leak is small or rapidly sealed. A small duodenal perforation may slowly leak fluid that runs down the lateral peritoneal gutter, producing pain and muscular rigidity in the right lower quadrant, thus raising concerns for acute appendicitis.

B. Laboratory Findings

A mild leukocytosis in the range of 12,000/μL is common in the early stages. After 12-24 hours, this may increase to 20,000/μL or more if treatment has been inadequate. The mild increase in the serum amylase value that occurs in many patients is probably caused by absorption of the enzyme from duodenal secretions within the peritoneal cavity. Direct measurement of fluid obtained by paracentesis may show very high levels of amylase.

C. Imaging Studies

Plain x-ray or CT scan of the abdomen reveals free subdiaphragmatic air in 85% of patients.

If no free air is demonstrated and the clinical picture suggests perforated ulcer, an emergency CT scan with gastrointestinal contrast or upper gastrointestinal series should be performed. If the perforation has not sealed, the diagnosis is established by the extravasation of contrast material from the lumen.

Differential Diagnosis

The differential diagnosis includes acute pancreatitis and acute cholecystitis. The former is typically more subtle in presentation and is usually accompanied by high serum levels of lipase and amylase. Acute cholecystitis with a perforated gallbladder could mimic perforated ulcer closely, but free air would not be present with ruptured gallbladder. Intestinal obstruction has a more gradual onset and is characterized by less severe pain that is crampy and accompanied by nausea and vomiting.

The simultaneous onset of pain and free air in the abdomen in the absence of trauma commonly indicates a perforated peptic ulcer. Other potential causes include perforation of colonic diverticulitis and acute appendicitis.

Treatment

The diagnosis is often suspected before the patient is sent for confirmatory imaging. Whenever a perforated ulcer is considered, the first step should be to pass a nasogastric tube and empty the stomach to limit further contamination of the peritoneal cavity. Blood should be drawn for laboratory studies, and broad-spectrum intravenous antibiotics and a PPI should be started. If the patient is hemodynamically unstable, the patient should be adequately resuscitated prior to any diagnostic measures. Imaging should be obtained as soon as the patient is stable.

The simplest surgical treatment, laparoscopy (or laparotomy) and suture closure of the perforation, solves the immediate problem. The closure most often consists of securely plugging the hole with omentum (Graham-Steele closure) sutured over the defect. Gastric ulcers should be biopsied prior to closure. All fluid should be aspirated from the peritoneal cavity, and copious irrigation of the abdomen should be performed. A drainage catheter can be left in the hepatorenal space to monitor for leakage; however, reperforation is rare in the immediate postoperative period.

About three-fourths of patients whose perforation is the culmination of a history of chronic symptoms continue to have clinically severe ulcer disease after simple closure. In the past, patients underwent more aggressive treatment involving a definitive ulcer operation for most patients with acute perforation (eg, parietal cell vagotomy plus closure of the perforation or truncal vagotomy and pyloroplasty). Now, patients with perforated ulcers are treated with PPI and antibiotic therapy to eradicate *H pylori*. However, patients who must continue nonsteroidal anti-inflammatory drugs postoperatively or who have previously failed medical management should be considered for vagotomy and drainage procedures. More extensive surgeries should only be considered in hemodynamically stable patients.

Concomitant hemorrhage and perforation are most often due to two ulcers, a perforated anterior ulcer and a bleeding posterior ulcer. Obstructing perforated ulcers cannot be treated by suture closure of the perforation alone. Vagotomy plus gastroenterostomy or pyloroplasty should be performed. Perforated anastomotic ulcers require a vagotomy or gastrectomy, since in the long run, closure alone is nearly always inadequate.

Nonoperative treatment of perforated ulcer consists of continuous gastric suction and the administration of antibiotics in high doses. Although this has been shown to be effective, with a low death rate, it is occasionally accompanied by a peritoneal and subphrenic abscess.

▶ **Prognosis**

About 15% of patients with perforated ulcer die, and about a third of these ulcers are undiagnosed before surgery. The death rate of patients with early perforated ulcers is low. Delay in treatment, advanced age, and associated systemic diseases account for most deaths.

STRESS GASTRODUODENITIS, STRESS ULCER, & ACUTE HEMORRHAGIC GASTRITIS

The term *stress ulcer* has been used to refer to a heterogeneous group of acute gastric or duodenal ulcers that develop following physiologically stressful illnesses. There are four major etiologic factors associated with such lesions: (1) shock, (2) sepsis, (3) burns, and (4) central nervous system tumors or trauma.

▶ **Etiology**

A. Stress Ulcer

Acute ulcers following major surgery, mechanical ventilation, shock, sepsis, and burns (Curling ulcers) have enough common features to suggest they evolve by a similar pathogenetic mechanism.

Hemorrhage is the major clinical problem, although perforation occurs in about 10% of cases. Despite the predilection of stress ulcers to develop in the parietal cell mucosa, in about 30% of patients, the duodenum is affected, and sometimes both stomach and duodenum are involved. Morphologically, the ulcers are shallow, discrete lesions with congestion and edema but little inflammatory reaction at their margins. Gastroduodenal endoscopy performed early in traumatized or burned patients has shown acute gastric erosions in the majority of patients within 72 hours after the injury. Such studies illustrate how frequently the disease process remains subclinical; clinically apparent ulcers develop in about 20% of susceptible patients. Clinically evident bleeding is usually seen 3-5 days after the injury, and massive bleeding generally does not appear until 4-5 days after that.

Decreased mucosal resistance is the first step, which may involve the effects of ischemia (with production of toxic superoxide and hydroxyl radicals) and circulating toxins, followed by decreased mucosal renewal, decreased production of endogenous prostanoids, and thinning of the surface mucus layer. Decreased gastric mucosal blood flow also plays a role by decreasing the supply of blood buffers available to neutralize hydrogen ions that are diffusing into the weakened mucosa. Experimental evidence has implicated platelet-activating factor, released by endotoxin, as a possible mediator of gut ulceration in sepsis. The mucosa is thus rendered more vulnerable to acid-pepsin ulceration and lysosomal enzymes. Acid hypersecretion may be involved to some extent, because burn-patients who manifest serious bleeding have higher gastric acid output than patients with a more benign course. Disruption of the gastric mucosal barrier to back diffusion of acid has been found in less than half of patients and is now thought to be a manifestation of the disease rather than a cause.

B. Cushing Ulcers

Acute ulcers associated with central nervous system tumors or injuries differ from stress ulcers because they are associated with elevated levels of serum gastrin and increased gastric acid secretion. Morphologically, they are similar to ordinary gastroduodenal peptic ulcers. Cushing ulcers are more prone to perforate than other kinds of stress ulcers.

C. Acute Hemorrhagic Gastritis

This disorder may share some causative factors with the conditions described earlier, but the natural history is different and the response to treatment considerably better. Most of these patients can be controlled medically. When surgery is required for alcoholic gastritis, a high proportion of patients are cured by pyloroplasty and vagotomy.

▶ Clinical Findings

Hemorrhage is nearly always the first manifestation. Pain rarely occurs. Physical examination is not contributory except to reveal gross or occult fecal blood or signs of shock.

▶ Prevention

Acid-suppressing medications including H_2 antagonists and PPIs are given prophylactically to critically ill patients to decrease the incidence of stress erosions and overt bleeding. Sucralfate is also effective by creating a cytoprotective barrier. Patients receiving total parenteral nutrition appear to be protected by this therapy and experience no increased benefit from H_2 antagonists. Early enteral nutrition has also been found to contribute to reducing stress ulcer–related complications for critically ill patients.

▶ Treatment

Initial management should consist of gastric lavage with chilled solutions and measures to combat sepsis if present. H_2 receptor blockers are of no value in the actively bleeding patient, but they probably decrease the rate of rebleeding once bleeding has stopped. PPIs have been found to be more effective than H_2 blockers in resolving gastric bleeding, although these data are largely collected from patients with bleeding peptic ulcers.

If nonoperative treatment, including endoscopy, fails to halt the bleeding, a laparotomy should be considered. Surgical treatment should consist of vagotomy and pyloroplasty, with suture of the bleeding points, or vagotomy and subtotal gastrectomy. There is a trend toward the first of these options, particularly in unstable patients. When it occurs, rebleeding is nearly always from an ulcer left behind at the initial procedure. Rarely, total gastrectomy has had to be used because of the extent of ulceration and severity of bleeding or because of rebleeding after a lesser operation.

Ali T, Harty RF: Stress-induced ulcer bleeding in critically ill patients. *Gastroenterol Clin North Am.* 2009;38(2):245-265.

Plummer MP, Balser AR, Deane AM: Stress ulceration: prevalence, pathology, and association with adverse outcomes. *Crit Care.* 2014;18(2):213.

GASTRIC CARCINOMA

There are about 26,000 new cases of carcinoma of the stomach in the United States annually. The incidence has dropped to one-third of what it was 40 years ago. This may reflect changes in the prevalence of *H pylori* infection, which has a role in the etiology of this disease. *H pylori* is known to be a cause of chronic atrophic gastritis, which in turn is a recognized precursor of gastric adenocarcinoma. Epidemiologic studies have linked gastric *H pylori* infection with a 3.6-fold to 18-fold (all patients versus women) increase in the risk of developing carcinoma of the body or antrum (not the cardia), and the risk is proportionate to serum levels of *H pylori* antibodies.

The present incidence in American men and women is 7.2 new cases per 100,000 population per year. The highest rate, 41.8 per 100,000 men and women, is observed in South Korea. Epidemiologic studies suggest that the incidence of gastric carcinoma is related to low dietary intake of vegetables and fruits and high intake of salt and starches, as well as smoking. Carcinoma of the stomach is rare under age 40, from which point the risk gradually climbs. The mean age at discovery is 63 years. It is about twice as common in men as in women.

Gastric epithelial cancers are nearly always adenocarcinomas. Squamous cell tumors of the proximal stomach involve the stomach secondarily from the esophagus. Five morphologic subdivisions correlate loosely with the natural history and outcome.

1. Ulcerating carcinoma (25%)—This consists of a deep, penetrating ulcer-tumor that extends through all layers of the stomach. It may involve adjacent organs in the process. The edges are shallow by contrast with overhanging edges noted in benign ulcers.

2. Polypoid carcinomas (25%)—These are large, bulky intraluminal growths that tend to metastasize late.

3. Superficial spreading carcinoma (15%)—Also known as early gastric cancer, superficial spreading carcinoma is confined to the mucosa and submucosa. Metastases are present in only 30% of cases. Even when metastases are present, the prognosis after gastrectomy is much better than for the more deeply invading lesions of advanced gastric cancer. In Japan, screening programs have been so successful that early gastric cancer now constitutes 30% of surgical cases, and survival rates have improved accordingly.

4. Linitis plastica (10%)—This variety of spreading tumor involves all layers with a marked desmoplastic reaction in which it may be difficult to identify the malignant cells. The stomach loses its pliability. Cure is rare because of early spread.

5. Advanced carcinoma (35%)—This largest category contains big tumors that are found partly within and partly outside the stomach. They may originally have qualified for inclusion in the preceding groups but have outgrown that early stage.

Gastric adenocarcinomas can also be classified by degree of differentiation of their cells. In general, rate and extent of spread correlate with lack of differentiation. Some tumors are found histologically to excite an inflammatory cell reaction at their borders, and this feature indicates a relatively good prognosis. Tumors whose cells form glandular structures (intestinal type) have a somewhat better prognosis than tumors whose cells do not (diffuse type); the diffuse type is often associated with a substantial stromal component. The intestinal type of tumor accounts for a much larger proportion of cases in countries such as Japan and Finland where gastric cancer is especially common. The gradual decline in incidence in these areas is due principally to decreased occurrence of the intestinal type of tumor. Signet ring carcinomas, which contain more than 50% signet ring cells, have become increasingly more common and now constitute one-third of all cases. They behave as the diffuse type of cancer and occur more frequently in women, in younger patients, and in the distal part of the stomach. Previous *H pylori* infection is not associated with the development of any specific histologic type of gastric cancer.

Extension occurs by intramural spread, direct extraluminal growth, and lymphatic metastases. Pathologic staging, which correlates closely with survival, is demonstrated in Table 25–3. Three-fourths of patients have metastases when diagnosed. Within the stomach, proximal spread exceeds distal spread. The pylorus acts as a partial barrier, but in 25% of cases, tumor is found in the first few centimeters of the duodenal bulb.

Table 25–3. American Joint Committee on Cancer (AJCC) gastric cancer staging.

DEFINITIONS OF AJCC TNM	
Definition of Primary Tumor (T)	
N Category	**T Criteria**
TX	Primary tumor cannot be assessed
T0	No evidence of primary tumor
Tis	Carcinoma *in situ*: intraepithelial tumor without invasion of the lamina propria, high-grade dysplasia
T1	Tumor invades the lamina propria, muscularis mucosae, or submucosa
T1a	Tumor invades the lamina propria or muscularis mucosae
T1b	Tumor invades the submucosa
T2	Tumor invades the muscularis propria*
T3	Tumor penetrates the subserosal connective tissue without invasion of the visceral peritoneum or adjacent structures**,***
T4	Tumor invades the serosa (visceral peritoneum) or adjacent structures**,***
T4a	Tumor invades the serosa (visceral peritoneum)
T4b	Tumor invades adjacent structures/organs

*A tumor may penetrate the muscularis propria with extension into the gastrocolic or gastrohepatic ligaments, or into the greater or lesser omentum, without perforation of the visceral peritoneum covering these structures. In this case, the tumor is classified as T3. If there is perforation of the visceral peritoneum covering the gastric ligaments or the omentum, the tumor should be classified as T4.

**The adjacent structures of the stomach include the spleen, transverse colon, liver, diaphragm, pancreas, abdominal wall, adrenal gland, kidney, small intestine, and retroperitoneum.

*** Intramural extension to the duodenum or esophagus is not considered invasion of an adjacent structure, but is classified using the depth of the greatest invasion in any of these sites.

Definition of Regional Lymph Node (N)	
N Category	**N Criteria**
NX	Regional lymph node(s) cannot be assessed
N0	No regional lymph node metastasis
N1	Metastasis in one or two regional lymph nodes
N2	Metastasis in three to six regional lymph nodes
N3	Metastasis in seven or more regional lymph nodes
N3a	Metastasis in seven to 15 regional lymph nodes
N3b	Metastasis in 16 or more regional lymph nodes

(Continued)

Table 25–3. American Joint Committee on Cancer (AJCC) gastric cancer staging. (*Continued*)

Definition of Distant Metastasis (M)

M Category	M Criteria
M0	No distant metastasis
M1	Distant metastasis

AJCC PROGNOSTIC STAGE GROUPS

Clinical (cTNM)

When T is...	And N is...	And M is...	Then the stage group is...
Tis	N0	M0	0
T1	N0	M0	I
T2	N0	M0	I
T1	N1, N2, or N3	M0	IIA
T2	N1, N2, or N3	M0	IIA
T3	N0	M0	IIB
T4a	N0	M0	IIB
T3	N1, N2, or N3	M0	III
T4a	N1, N2, or N3	M0	III
T4b	Any N	M0	IVA
Any T	Any N	M1	IVB

Pathological (pTNM)

When T is...	And N is...	And M is...	Then the stage group is...
Tis	N0	M0	0
T1	N0	M0	IA
T1	N1	M0	IB
T2	N0	M0	IB
T1	N2	M0	IIA
T2	N1	M0	IIA
T3	N0	M0	IIA
T1	N3a	M0	IIB
T2	N2	M0	IIB
T3	N1	M0	IIB
T4a	N0	M0	IIB
T2	N3a	M0	IIIA
T3	N2	M0	IIIA
T4a	N1	M0	IIIA
T4a	N2	M0	IIIA
T4b	N0	M0	IIIA
T1	N3b	M0	IIIB
T2	N3b	M0	IIIB

(*Continued*)

Table 25–3. American Joint Committee on Cancer (AJCC) gastric cancer staging. (*Continued*)

When T is...	And N is...	And M is...	Then the stage group is...
T3	N3a	M0	IIIB
T4a	N3a	M0	IIIB
T4b	N1	M0	IIIB
T4b	N2	M0	IIIB
T3	N3b	M0	IIIC
T4a	N3b	M0	IIIC
T4b	N3a	M0	IIIC
T4b	N3b	M0	IIIC
Any T	Any N	M1	IV

Post-Neoadjuvant Therapy (ypTNM)

When T is...	And N is...	And M is...	Then the stage group is...
T1	N0	M0	I
T2	N0	M0	I
T1	N1	M0	I
T3	N0	M0	II
T2	N1	M0	II
T1	N2	M0	II
T4a	N0	M0	II
T3	N1	M0	II
T2	N2	M0	II
T1	N3	M0	II
T4a	N1	M0	III
T3	N2	M0	III
T2	N3	M0	III
T4b	N0	M0	III
T4b	N1	M0	III
T4a	N2	M0	III
T3	N3	M0	III
T4b	N2	M0	III
T4b	N3	M0	III
T4a	N3	M0	III
Any T	Any N	M1	IV

HISTOLOGIC GRADE (G)

G	G Definition
GX	Grade cannot be assessed
G1	Well differentiated
G2	Moderately differentiated
G3	Poorly differentiated, undifferentiated

Used with the permission of the American College of Surgeons. Amin MB, Edge SB, Greene FL, et al. (Eds.) *AJCC Cancer Staging Manual*, 8th Ed. Springer New York, 2017.

Early gastric cancer, defined as a primary lesion confined to the mucosa and submucosa with or without lymph node metastases, is associated with an excellent prognosis (5-year survival rate of 90%) after resection. In Japan, mass screening programs detect about 30% of patients with this lesion, whereas in the United States, only 10% of patients have early gastric cancer.

Forty percent of tumors are in the antrum, predominantly on the lesser curvature; 30% arise in the body and fundus, 25% arise at the cardia, and 5% involve the entire organ. Frequency of location has gradually changed, so that proximal lesions are more common now than 10-20 years ago. Benign ulcers develop at the greater curvature and cardia less commonly than malignant ones. Ulcers at these points are particularly suspicious for neoplasm.

Clinical Findings

A. Symptoms and Signs

The earliest symptom is usually vague postprandial abdominal fullness. Sometimes the discomfort is no different from other vague dyspeptic symptoms that have been intermittently present for years, but the frequency and persistence are new.

Anorexia develops early and may be most pronounced for meat. Weight loss, the most common symptom, averages about 6 kg. True postprandial pain suggesting a benign gastric ulcer is relatively uncommon, but if it is present, one may be misled if subsequent x-rays show an ulcer. Vomiting may be present and becomes a major feature if pyloric obstruction occurs. It may have a coffee-ground appearance secondary to bleeding from the tumor. Dysphagia may be the presenting symptom of lesions at the cardia.

An epigastric mass can be felt on examination in about one-fourth of cases. Hepatomegaly is present in 10% of cases. Stool will be positive for occult blood in half of patients, and melena is sometimes noted. Otherwise, abnormal physical findings are confined to signs of distant spread of the tumor. Metastases to the neck along the thoracic duct may produce a Virchow node. Rectal examination may reveal a Blumer shelf, a solid peritoneal deposit anterior to the rectum. Enlarged ovaries (Krukenberg tumors) may be caused by intraperitoneal metastases. Further dissemination may involve the liver, lungs, brain, or bone.

B. Laboratory Findings

Anemia is present in 40% of patients. Carcinoembryonic antigen (CEA) levels are elevated in 65% of patients, usually indicating extensive spread of the tumor. Patients with metastatic disease should undergo human epidermal growth factor receptor 2 (HER2) testing; overexpression of HER2 can identify patients who may benefit from the addition of trastuzumab in their chemotherapeutic regimen.

C. Imaging Studies

An upper gastrointestinal series is diagnostic for many tumors, but the overall false-negative rate is about 20%. Major diagnostic problems are posed by ulcerating tumors that may not be distinguishable radiologically from benign peptic ulcers. The differential features are listed in the section on gastric ulcer, but x-rays alone will not establish a diagnosis of benign ulcer. All patients with a newly discovered gastric ulcer should undergo upper endoscopy and gastric biopsy. All confirmed diagnoses should be followed by staging with CT, positron emission tomography, MRIs, and in some cases, laparoscopic staging to rule out widespread metastases. Endoscopic ultrasounds are often indicated to assess the depth of tumor invasion and for lymph node staging.

D. Gastroscopy and Biopsy

Large gastric carcinomas can usually be identified as such by their gross appearance at endoscopy. All gastric lesions, whether polypoid or ulcerating, should be examined by taking multiple biopsy and brush cytology specimens during endoscopy. False-negative results are seen occasionally as a result of sampling error, and a minimum of six biopsies is necessary for greatest accuracy.

Treatment

Surgical resection is the only curative treatment. About 85% of patients are operable, and in 50% of patients, the lesions are amenable to resection; of the resectable lesions, half are potentially curable (ie, no signs of spread beyond the limits of resection). Preoperative chemotherapy with a multidrug regimen is recommended for most patients.

The surgical objective should be to remove the tumor, an adjacent uninvolved margin of stomach and duodenum, the regional lymph nodes, and, if necessary, portions of involved adjacent organs. The proximal margin should be a minimum of 6 cm from the gross tumor. If the tumor is located in the antrum, a curative resection would entail distal gastrectomy with en bloc removal of the omentum, a 3- to 4-cm cuff of duodenum and the subpyloric lymph nodes, and, in some instances, excision of the left gastric artery and nearby lymph nodes. Reconstruction after gastrectomy may be by either a Billroth I or II procedure, but the latter is preferable because postoperative growth of residual tumor near the pylorus may obstruct a gastroduodenal anastomosis early.

Total gastrectomy with splenectomy is required for tumors of the proximal half of the stomach and for extensive tumors (eg, linitis plastica). Whether or not the spleen should be removed in such cases is a subject of debate. Alimentary continuity is most often reestablished by a Roux-en-Y esophagojejunostomy. Construction of an intestinal pouch as a substitute food reservoir (eg, Hunt-Lawrence pouch) is of no nutritional value and increases the risks of immediate complications.

Esophagogastrectomy plus splenectomy with intrathoracic esophagogastrostomy is the operation usually performed for tumors of the cardia. The procedure is usually done through two separate incisions: first, a laparotomy for the gastric part, and then a right posterolateral thoracotomy for the anastomosis.

The propensity for proximal submucosal spread must be appreciated at surgery. It is often advisable to perform a frozen section at the proximal margin before constructing the anastomosis. If tumor is found, the gastrectomy should be extended.

Palliative resection is usually indicated if the stomach is still movable and life expectancy is estimated to be more than 1-2 months. Palliative gastrectomy is usually performed to remove an antral lesion and prevent obstruction, but in selected cases, total gastrectomy is appropriate palliative treatment if the operation can be done safely and the amount of extragastric tumor is minimal. Whenever technically feasible, palliative gastrectomy is preferable to palliative bypass.

Adjuvant chemotherapy after curative surgery is recommended, particularly for patients who have undergone preoperative chemotherapy and had appropriate response.

▶ Prognosis

In the United States, the overall 5-year survival rate for gastric carcinoma is about 31%. The 5-year survival rates are listed in Table 25–3.

Death from tumor may follow dissemination to other organs or may be the result of progressive gastric obstruction and malnutrition.

Ajani JA, D'Amico TA, Almhanna K, et al: Gastric cancer, version 3.2016: NCCN Clinical Practice Guidelines in Oncology. *J Natl Compr Canc Netw*. 2016;14:1286-1312.

American Joint Committee on Cancer. Stomach cancer. In *AJCC Cancer Staging Manual*. 8th ed. New York, NY: Springer; 2017:117-121.

Ferlay J, Soerjomataram I, Ervik M, et al: GLOBOCAN 2012 v1.1, Cancer Incidence and Mortality Worldwide: IARC CancerBase No. 11 [Internet]. Lyon, France: International Agency for Research on Cancer; 2014. http://globocan.iarc.fr

Howlader N, Noone AM, Krapcho M, et al (eds): SEER Cancer Statistics Review, 1975-2014. Bethesda, MD: National Cancer Institute. https://seer.cancer.gov/csr/1975_2014/

GASTRIC POLYPS

Gastric polyps are single or multiple benign tumors that occur predominantly in the elderly. Those located in the distal stomach are more apt to cause symptoms. Whenever gastric polyps are discovered, gastric cancer must be ruled out.

Gastric polyps can be classified histologically as hyperplastic, adenomatous, or inflammatory. Other polypoid lesions, such as leiomyomas and carcinoid tumors, are discussed elsewhere. Hyperplastic polyps, which constitute 80% of cases, consist of an overgrowth of normal epithelium; they are not true neoplasms and have no relationship to gastric cancer. About 30% of adenomatous polyps contain a focus of adenocarcinoma, and adenocarcinoma can be found elsewhere in the stomach in 20% of patients with a benign adenomatous polyp. The incidence of cancer in an adenomatous polyp rises with increasing size. Lesions with a stalk and those less than 2 cm in diameter are usually not malignant. About 10% of benign adenomatous polyps undergo malignant change during prolonged follow-up.

Anemia may develop from chronic blood loss or deficient iron absorption. Over 90% of patients are achlorhydric after maximal stimulation. Vitamin B_{12} absorption is deficient in 25%, although megaloblastic anemia is present in only a few.

Excision with a snare through the endoscope can be performed safely for most polyps. Otherwise, surgical excision is indicated for polyps greater than 1 cm in diameter or when cancer is suspected. Single polyps may be excised through a gastrotomy and a frozen section performed. If the polyp is found to be malignant, an appropriate type of gastrectomy is indicated. Partial gastrectomy should be performed for multiple polyps in the distal stomach. If 10-20 polyps are distributed throughout the stomach, the antrum should be removed and the fundic polyps excised. Total gastrectomy may be required for symptomatic diffuse polyposis.

These patients should be followed because they have an increased risk of pernicious anemia or gastric cancer. Recurrent polyps are uncommon.

GASTRIC LYMPHOMA & PSEUDOLYMPHOMA

Lymphoma is the second most common primary cancer of the stomach but constitutes only 2% of the total number, with 95% being adenocarcinomas. Almost all are non-Hodgkin lymphomas and are generally classified as B-cell mucosa-associated lymphoid tissue (MALT) lymphomas. They are further subclassified as low grade or high grade based on nuclear pattern. About 20% of patients manifest a second primary cancer in another organ.

The principal symptoms are epigastric pain and weight loss, similar to those of carcinoma. Characteristically, the tumor has attained bulky proportions by the time it is discovered; by comparison with adenocarcinoma of the stomach, the symptoms from a gastric lymphoma are usually mild in relation to the size of the lesion. A palpable epigastric mass is present in 50% of patients. Imaging studies will demonstrate the lesion, although it usually is mistaken for adenocarcinoma or benign gastric ulcer. Gastroscopy with biopsy and brush cytology combined with endoscopic ultrasound to detect lymph node involvement approaches 90% accuracy. If a pathologic diagnosis has not been made, the surgeon may incorrectly judge the lesion to be inoperable carcinoma because of its large size. Preoperative staging should include a CT scan and bone marrow biopsy.

Treatment of limited-extent, *H pylori*–positive, low-grade gastric MALT lymphoma consists of antibiotic treatment and PPIs. More extensive disease or *H pylori*–negative lymphoma may require therapy with external beam radiation or rituximab. Surgery is reserved for those with complications such as perforation, hemorrhage, or obstruction.

Gastric pseudolymphoma consists of a mass of lymphoid tissue in the gastric wall, often associated with an overlying mucosal ulcer. It is thought to represent a response to chronic inflammation. The lesion is not malignant, although the presentation, which includes pain, weight loss, and a mass on imaging, cannot be distinguished from that of a malignant lesion.

Treatment of gastric pseudolymphoma consists of resection. The distinction from lymphoma is made on histologic examination of the specimen, which shows mature germinal centers in pseudolymphoma. No additional therapy is indicated postoperatively.

Ghimire P, Wu G, Zhu L: Primary gastrointestinal lymphoma. *World J Gastroenterol.* 2011;17(6):697-707.

Harada N, Wiersema M, Wiersema L: Endosonography guided fine needle aspiration biopsy (EUS FNA) in the evaluation of lymphadenopathy: staging accuracy of EUS FNA versus EUS alone. *Gastrointest Endosc.* 1997;45(abstract).

Zelenetz AD, Wierda WG, Abramson JS, et al: Non-Hodgkin's lymphomas, version 1.2013. *J Natl Compr Canc Netw.* 2013;11(3): 257-272.

GASTRIC LEIOMYOMAS & GASTROINTESTINAL STROMAL TUMOR

Leiomyomas are common submucosal growths that are usually asymptomatic but may cause intestinal bleeding. Gastrointestinal stromal tumors (GISTs; previously called leiomyosarcomas) may grow to a large size and most often present with bleeding. Radiologically, the tumor usually contains a central ulceration caused by necrosis from outgrowth of its blood supply. In most cases, the tumor arises from the proximal stomach. It may grow into the gastric lumen, remain entirely on the serosal surface, or even become pedunculated within the abdominal cavity. GISTs can also be found, although less commonly, in the other parts of the gastrointestinal tract as well as the gallbladder and urinary bladder. Spread is by direct invasion or bloodborne metastases. Common sites of metastasis include the liver, peritoneum, and omentum. CT scans and MRI provide useful information on the amount of extragastric extension. Endoscopic biopsies often have low diagnostic yield; however, endoscopic ultrasound–guided fine-needle aspiration can be helpful to guide treatment because it can provide additional cytology, immunohistochemistry, and mutational analyses.

All gastric GISTs that are 2 cm or larger should be removed by enucleation or wedge resection. GISTs found outside of the stomach are at higher risk for aggressive behavior and should be resected regardless of size. All malignant GISTs require a wedge or segmental resection without the need for the wide margins required for adenocarcinoma; more extensive resections can be performed to remove metastases (eg, peritoneal, hepatic). The prognosis is affected by tumor size, DNA ploidy pattern, and tumor grade. Lesions that exhibit 10 or more mitoses in a high-powered field rarely can be cured. GISTs have a profound expression of the tyrosine kinase KIT as well as mutations in the corresponding *c-KIT* protooncogene. Subsequently, tyrosine kinase inhibitors such as imatinib and sunitinib are used as both neoadjuvant and adjuvant chemotherapeutic agents, although the role of systemic therapy on overall survival in patients with resectable disease remains unclear.

MÉNÉTRIER DISEASE

Ménétrier disease, a form of hypertrophic gastritis, consists of giant hypertrophy of the gastric rugae; high, normal, or low acid secretion; and excessive loss of protein from the thickened mucosa into the gut, with resulting hypoproteinemia. Clinical manifestations include edema, diarrhea, anorexia, weight loss, and skin rash. Chronic blood loss may also be a problem. Indigestion may respond to antacids, but this treatment does not improve the gastric pathologic process or secondary hypoproteinemia. The hypertrophic rugae present as enormous filling defects on upper gastrointestinal imaging and are frequently misinterpreted as carcinoma. The protein leak from the gastric mucosa may respond to atropine (and other anticholinergic drugs), hexamethonium bromide, eradication of *H pylori*, or H_2 blocking agents or omeprazole. Rarely, total gastrectomy is indicated for severe intractable hypoproteinemia, anemia, or inability to exclude cancer. Medical management is best for most patients, although the gastric abnormalities and hypoproteinemia may persist. Some cases gradually evolve into atrophic gastritis. In children, the disease characteristically is self-limited and benign. There is an increased risk of adenocarcinoma of the stomach in adults with Ménétrier disease.

GASTRIC VOLVULUS

The stomach may rotate about its longitudinal axis (organoaxial volvulus) or a line drawn from the mid lesser to the mid greater curvature (mesenteroaxial volvulus). The former is more common and is often associated with a paraesophageal hiatal hernia. In other patients, eventration of the left diaphragm allows the colon to rise and twist the stomach by pulling on the gastrocolic ligament.

Acute gastric volvulus produces severe abdominal pain accompanied by a diagnostic triad (Borchardt triad): (1) vomiting followed by retching and then inability to vomit, (2) epigastric distention, and (3) difficulty passing a nasogastric tube. Nasogastric tube placement should nonetheless be attempted. If decompression is not possible, immediate laparotomy is indicated to prevent death from acute gastric necrosis, perforation, and sepsis. If the patient can be decompressed, adequate resuscitation is recommended prior to urgent operative intervention. Emergency imaging on presentation shows blockage at the point of the volvulus. The associated mortality rate with emergency surgery ranges from 42%-56% and can be attributed to gastric ischemia, necrosis, and perforation.

Chronic volvulus is more common than acute. It may be asymptomatic or may cause crampy intermittent pain secondary to obstruction. Cases associated with a paraesophageal hiatal hernia should be treated by a repair of the hernia and fundoplication, either partial or complete. A gastropexy may also be considered. When cases are due to eventration of the diaphragm, the gastrocolic ligament should be divided the entire length of the greater curvature. The colon rises to fill the space caused by the eventration, and the stomach will resume its normal position, to be fastened by a gastropexy.

GASTRIC DIVERTICULA

Gastric diverticula are uncommon and usually asymptomatic. Most are pulsion diverticula consisting of mucosa and submucosa only, located on the lesser curvature within a few centimeters of the esophagogastric junction. Those in the prepyloric region generally possess all layers and are more likely to be symptomatic. A few patients have symptoms from hemorrhage of inflammation within a gastric diverticulum, but these lesions are usually incidental findings on imaging or endoscopy that do not require treatment. Radiologically, they can be confused with a gastric ulcer.

BEZOAR

Bezoars are concretions formed in the stomach. Trichobezoars are composed of hair and are usually found in young female patients who swallow their own hair. Phytobezoars consist of agglomerated vegetable fibers. Pressure by the mass can create a gastric ulcer that can bleed or perforate.

The postgastrectomy state predisposes to bezoar formation because pepsin and acid secretion are reduced and the triturating function of the antrum is gone. Orange segments or other fruits that contain a large amount of cellulose have been implicated in most cases. Improper mastication of food is a contributing factor that can sometimes be obviated by providing the patient with properly fitted dentures. The fruit may remain in the stomach or pass into the small intestine and cause obstruction.

Large semisolid bezoars of *Candida albicans* have also been found in postgastrectomy patients. Some can be fragmented with the gastroscope. The patient should also be treated with oral nystatin.

Patients with symptomatic gastric bezoars may complain of abdominal pain. Ulceration and bleeding are associated with a mortality rate of 20%.

Nearly all gastric bezoars can be broken up and dispersed by endoscopy. Neglected lesions with complications (ie, bleeding or perforation) require gastrectomy.

▼ II. DUODENUM

DUODENAL DIVERTICULA

Diverticula of the duodenum are found in 20% of autopsies and 5%-10% of upper gastrointestinal imaging. Symptoms are uncommon, and only 1% of those found by imaging warrant surgery.

Duodenal pulsion diverticula are acquired outpouchings of the mucosa and submucosa, 90% of which are on the medial aspect of the duodenum. They are rare before age 40. Most are solitary and are found within 2.5 cm of the ampulla of Vater. There is a high incidence of gallstone disease of the gallbladder in patients with juxtapapillary diverticula. Diverticula do not occur in the first portion of the duodenum, where diverticular configurations are due to scarring by peptic ulceration or cholecystitis.

A few patients have chronic postprandial abdominal pain or dyspepsia caused by a duodenal diverticulum. Treatment is with antacids and anticholinergics.

Serious complications include hemorrhage or perforation from inflammation, pancreatitis, and biliary obstruction. Bile acid-bilirubinate enteroliths are occasionally formed by bile stasis in a diverticulum. Enteroliths can precipitate diverticular inflammation or biliary obstruction and, rarely, cause bowel obstruction after entering the intestinal lumen.

Surgical treatment is required for complications and, rarely, for persistent symptoms. Excision and a two-layer closure are usually possible after mobilization of the duodenum and dissection of the diverticulum from the pancreas. Removal of the diverticulum and closure of the defect are superior to simple drainage in the case of perforation. If biliary obstruction appears in a patient whose bile duct empties into a diverticulum, a side-to-side choledochoduodenostomy may be preferred over a diverticulectomy.

The rare wind sock type of intraluminal diverticulum usually presents with vague epigastric pain and postprandial fullness, although intestinal bleeding or pancreatitis occasionally observed. The diagnosis can be made by imaging studies. The diverticulum can be excised through a nearby duodenotomy. In some cases, the narrow diverticular outlet can be enlarged endoscopically.

DUODENAL TUMORS

Tumors of the duodenum are rare. Carcinoma of the ampulla of Vater is discussed in Chapter 28.

1. Malignant Duodenal Tumors

Most malignant duodenal tumors are adenocarcinomas, leiomyosarcomas, or lymphomas. They appear in the second portion of the duodenum more often than elsewhere. Pain, obstruction, bleeding, obstructive jaundice, and an abdominal mass are the modes of presentation. Patients with periampullary lesions typically present earlier due to biliary obstruction. Duodenal carcinomas, particularly those in the third and fourth portions of the duodenum, are often missed on barium x-ray studies. Endoscopy and biopsy will usually be diagnostic if the examiner can reach the lesion.

If possible, adenocarcinomas and leiomyosarcomas should be resected. Pancreaticoduodenectomy is usually necessary if the tumor is localized. Patients with unresectable or metastatic duodenal adenocarcinoma may require duodenal stent placement, palliative resections, or intestinal bypass to relieve obstruction. For unresectable GISTs in the duodenum, imatinib should be considered for preoperative shrinkage of tumor or to delay tumor progression. Chemoimmunotherapy and radiotherapy are recommended for lymphoma.

After curative resections, the 5-year survival rate is 30%. The overall 5-year survival rate is 18%.

2. Benign Duodenal Tumors

Brunner gland adenomas are small submucosal nodules that have a predilection for the posterior duodenal wall at the junction of the first and second portions. Sessile and pedunculated variants are seen. Common symptoms are bleeding and obstruction. Leiomyomas may also be found in the duodenum and are typically asymptomatic unless they are causing biliary obstruction.

Neuroendocrine tumors of the duodenum are often endocrinologically active, producing gastrin, somatostatin, or serotonin. Simple excision is the treatment of choice.

Heterotopic gastric mucosa, presenting as multiple small mucosal nodules, is an occasional endoscopic finding of no clinical significance.

Villous adenomas of the duodenum may give rise to intestinal bleeding or may obstruct the papilla of Vater and cause jaundice. The risk of malignant transformation is high—about 50%. Small pedunculated villous adenomas may be snared during endoscopy, but sessile tumors must be locally excised via laparotomy. Tumors that contain malignant tissue should be treated with a Whipple procedure.

SUPERIOR MESENTERIC ARTERY OBSTRUCTION OF THE DUODENUM

Rarely, obstruction of the third portion of the duodenum is caused by compression of the bowel between the superior mesenteric vessels and the aorta. It most commonly appears after rapid weight loss following injury, including burns. Patients in body casts are particularly susceptible.

The superior mesenteric artery normally leaves the aorta at an angle of 50 to 60 degrees, and the distance between the two vessels where the duodenum passes between them is 10 to 20 mm. These measurements in patients with superior mesenteric artery syndrome average 18 degrees and 2.5 mm. Acute loss of mesenteric fat is thought to permit the artery to drop posteriorly, trapping the bowel and causing intermittent obstruction.

The patient often complains of epigastric bloating and crampy pain, particularly after eating and relieved by vomiting. The symptoms may remit in the prone position. Anorexia and postprandial pain lead to malnutrition and weight loss.

Upper gastrointestinal x-ray imaging demonstrates a widened duodenum proximal to a sharp obstruction at the point where the artery crosses the third portion of the duodenum. When the patient moves to the knee-chest position, the passage of gastrointestinal contrast is suddenly unimpeded.

Many patients who are found to have a superior mesenteric artery that makes a prominent impression on the duodenum are asymptomatic. In ambulatory patients, other diagnoses should be explored to explain any vague chronic complaints.

Involvement of the duodenum by scleroderma leads to duodenal dilatation and hypomotility. Abdominal imaging and clinical symptoms are highly suggestive of superior mesenteric artery syndrome. In the latter, increased duodenal peristalsis should be demonstrable proximal to the arterial blockage, whereas diminished peristalsis characterizes scleroderma. Patients with duodenal scleroderma usually have dysphagia from concomitant esophageal involvement.

Malrotation with duodenal obstruction by congenital bands can also mimic this syndrome.

Postural therapy may suffice. The patient should be placed prone when symptomatic or in anticipation of postprandial difficulties. Ambulatory patients should be instructed to assume the knee-chest position, which allows the viscera and the artery to rotate forward off the duodenum.

Chronic obstruction may require resection of the suspensory ligament and mobilization of the duodenum or a duodenojejunostomy to bypass the obstruction. Patients with various forms of malrotation should be treated by mobilizing the duodenojejunal flexure, which releases the duodenum from entrapment by congenital bands.

REGIONAL ENTERITIS OF THE STOMACH & DUODENUM

The proximal intestine and stomach are rarely involved in regional enteritis, although this disease has now been reported in every part of the gastrointestinal tract from the lips to the anus. Most patients with Crohn disease in the stomach or duodenum have ileal involvement as well.

Pain can in many instances be relieved by antacids. Intermittent vomiting from duodenal stenosis or pyloric obstruction is a frequent finding. Endoscopic findings are fairly characteristic, and biopsy with the peroral suction device usually gives an adequate specimen for histologic confirmation of the diagnosis.

Medical treatment is nonspecific and consists principally of corticosteroids during exacerbations. Surgery may be indicated for disabling pain or obstruction. If the disease is localized to the stomach, a partial gastrectomy can be performed. Duodenal involvement most often requires a gastrojejunostomy to bypass the obstruction. Vagotomy should also be performed to prevent development of a marginal ulcer. Recurrent Crohn disease involving the anastomosis is an occasional late complication, but it can usually be managed successfully by reoperation.

Internal fistulas involving the stomach or duodenum usually represent extensions from primary disease in the ileum or colon. Surgical treatment consists of resection of the diseased ileum or colon and closure of the fistulous opening in the upper gut.

MULTIPLE CHOICE QUESTIONS

1. The blood supply to the stomach

   A. Typically includes direct branches from the celiac axis and superior mesenteric artery
   B. Includes predominant supply of the greater curve of the stomach by the left gastric artery
   C. Includes the right gastroepiploic artery, which is usually a branch of the splenic artery
   D. May include a posterior gastric artery that is typically a branch of the splenic artery
   E. Is anatomically separate from the blood supply to the spleen

2. Which of the following is *true* about gastric volvulus?

   A. All patients presenting with gastric volvulus must emergently go to the operating room.
   B. Associated mortality rate is as high as 56%.
   C. Acute volvulus is more common than chronic volvulus.
   D. Patients typically present with no symptoms.
   E. Mesenteroaxial volvulus is more common than organoaxial volvulus.

3. The surgical management of gastric cancer

   A. Is better with Billroth I reconstruction
   B. Requires resection of uninvolved margins of stomach, duodenum, and regional lymph nodes
   C. Requires bypass when there is an obstructing tumor at the gastroesophageal junction
   D. Is limited to palliative resection for cancers that are stage III and above
   E. Is often preceded by neoadjuvant chemotherapy

4. Vagotomy

   A. Can impair the appropriate relaxation of the pylorus
   B. Has several variations, but each denervates the pylorus
   C. Has become more widely applied as ulcer therapy since the introduction of acid-suppressing medications (H_2 blockers and proton pump inhibitors)
   D. Impairs gallbladder emptying
   E. Can include division of both the left (posterior) and right (anterior) vagus nerve trunks

5. Management of duodenal ulcers

   A. Is mostly managed surgically in an attempt to reduce gastric acid secretion
   B. Requires surgical resection of duodenal ulcers
   C. Consists of multimodal medical treatment including triple and quadruple therapy
   D. Can be discontinued after 6 months of medical therapy
   E. Requires a combination of medical therapy and surgical vagotomy and drainage procedures

Liver & Portal Venous System

Kevin C. Soares, MD
William R. Jarnagin, MD

SURGICAL ANATOMY

▶ Sections and Segments

The liver develops as an embryologic outpouching from the duodenum. The liver is one of the largest organs in the body, representing up to 2% of the total body weight. The relationship of the liver to the other abdominal organs is shown in Figure 26–1. In classic descriptions, the liver was characterized as having four lobes: right, left, caudate, and quadrate; however, this is an overly simplistic view that fails to consider the more complex segmental anatomy, which is depicted in Figure 26–2.

The anatomical right and left hemilivers are separated by an imaginary line running from the medial aspect of the gallbladder fossa to the inferior vena cava, running parallel with the fissure of the round ligament (Figure 26–3). This division is known as the Cantlie line or the principal plane and marks the course of the middle hepatic vein. The liver is divided into four sections and eight segments based on the branching of the portal triads and hepatic veins. The structures of the portal triad (hepatic artery, portal vein, and biliary duct) are separate in their extrahepatic course but enter the hepatic hilum ensheathed within a thickened layer of the Glisson capsule.

The three main hepatic veins divide the liver into four sections (previously known as sectors), each of which is supplied by a **portal pedicle:** the right posterior section (segments VI and VII), the right anterior section (segments V and VIII), the left medial section (segment IV), and the left lateral section (segments II and III) (Figure 26–2). The caudate lobe (segment I) is an exception because its venous drainage is directly into the vena cava and therefore independent of the major hepatic veins. The four sections delimited by the hepatic veins are called the **portal sections,** and these portions of the parenchyma are supplied by independent

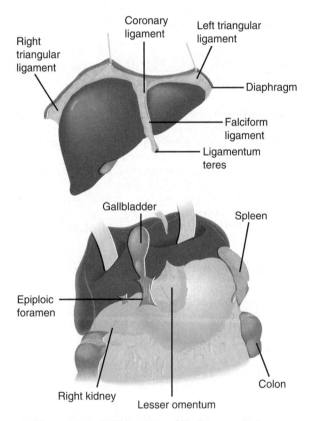

▲ **Figure 26–1.** Relationships of the liver to adjacent abdominal organs. The liver is invested with peritoneum except on the posterior surface, where the peritoneum reflects onto the diaphragm forming the right and left triangular ligaments.

R Extended hepatectomy

R Hepatectomy

M&LHV
RHV
VIII
VII
I
II
VI
V
III
RPV LPV
IV

L Hepatectomy

L Extended hepatectomy

▲ **Figure 26–2.** Segmental anatomy of the liver. Each of the eight segments is numbered. Segment I (caudate) is not shown but is indicated at the back of the liver, posterior to the middle hepatic vein. Segments I-IV compose the anatomical left liver, and segments V-VIII, the right. The most common major hepatic resections performed and the segments removed with each are indicated. LPV, left portal vein; M&LHV, middle and left hepatic veins originating from a common trunk; RHV, right hepatic vein; RPV, right portal vein.

▲ **Figure 26–3.** Anatomy of the veins of the liver. The major lobar fissure, also referred to as the principal plane or Cantlie line, is represented by the dashed line and divides the anatomical right and left liver. Branches of the hepatic artery and biliary ducts follow those of the portal vein. The darker vessels represent the hepatic veins and vena cava; the lighter system represents the portal vein and its branches.

portal pedicles arising from the right or left main pedicles. The divisions separating the sections are called **portal scissurae,** within each of which runs a hepatic vein. Further branching of the pedicles subdivides the sections into segments. The liver is thus subdivided into eight segments, with the caudate lobe designated as segment I. Segments I-IV compose the left liver, and segments V-VIII, the right. Each segment is supplied by an independent portal pedicle, which forms the basis of sublobar segmental resections.

▶ **Portal Circulation**

The portal vein is formed by the confluence of the splenic and superior mesenteric veins at the level of the second lumbar vertebra behind the head of the pancreas (Figure 26–4). It runs for approximately 6-9 cm to the hilum of the liver, where it divides into the main right and left branches. The left gastric vein usually enters the portal vein on its anteromedial aspect just cephalad to the margin of the pancreas, in which case it must be ligated during the surgical construction of a portacaval shunt; in 25% of cases, the left gastric vein joins the splenic vein. Other small venous tributaries from the pancreas and duodenum are less constant but must be anticipated during surgical mobilization of the portal vein.

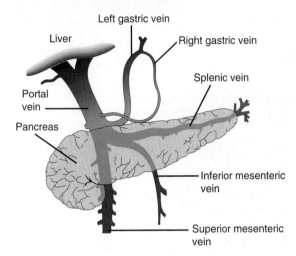

Left gastric vein

Liver

Right gastric vein

Splenic vein

Portal vein

Pancreas

Inferior mesenteric vein

Superior mesenteric vein

▲ **Figure 26–4.** Anatomic relationships of portal vein and branches.

The inferior mesenteric vein often drains into the splenic vein to the left of its junction with the superior mesenteric vein; alternatively, it may empty directly into the superior mesenteric vein.

In the hepatoduodenal ligament, the portal vein lies dorsal and slightly medial to the common bile duct. Portacaval lymph nodes are encountered along the right lateral aspect of the portal vein, running from the level of the duodenum to the base of the liver and extending posteriorly to the common hepatic artery and celiac axis. These lymph nodes are routinely removed during resections for certain malignancies and must be dissected before a portacaval shunt can be created.

▶ Venous Blood Supply

The anatomy of venous blood supply is shown in Figure 26–2. Both the portal and hepatic venous systems lack valves. The main portal vein terminates in the porta hepatis by dividing into right and left branches. The right branch typically has a 1- to 1.5-cm extrahepatic course before subsequently dividing into anterior and posterior sectoral or sectional divisions, often high within the porta hepatis or intrahepatically. A caudate branch is typically seen prior to its division into the anterior and posterior sections. The left branch has a longer extrahepatic course of approximately 3 to 4 cm, running first along the base of segment IV and then entering the umbilical fissure, where it gives rise to branches to segments II, III, and IV; a large branch to the caudate lobe generally arises from the left portal vein prior to its entry into the umbilical fissure. Variations in the normal portal venous anatomy occur but are less common than aberrancies in the arterial supply or the biliary drainage. The most common anomaly of the portal venous system is separate origins of the right anterior and posterior sectional branches. The left portal vein may drain primarily into the right anterior pedicle.

The hepatic veins represent the final common pathway for the central veins of the lobules of the liver. There are three major hepatic veins: left, right, and middle. The right hepatic vein drains into the vena cava independently, whereas the middle and left hepatic veins typically join just outside of the liver, forming a common trunk. The middle hepatic vein runs in the principal plane (Cantlie line) and provides drainage for segment IV and the anterior section of the right liver (segments V and VIII). The left hepatic vein drains segments II and III, whereas the right hepatic vein drains the posterior section (segments VI and VII) and provides additional drainage to the anterior section. The umbilical vein provides additional drainage of segment IV, running along the umbilical fissure and emptying into the left hepatic vein. Several small accessory veins enter the inferior vena cava directly from the posterior aspect of the right lobe and must be carefully ligated during mobilization and resection of the right liver.

▶ Arterial Blood Supply

The common hepatic artery arises from the celiac axis, ascends in the hepatoduodenal ligament, and gives rise to the right gastric, gastroduodenal, and proper hepatic arteries; the proper hepatic artery then divides into the right and left hepatic arterial branches in the liver hilum. The hepatic artery supplies approximately 25% of the 1500 mL of blood that enters the liver each minute; the remaining 75% is supplied by the portal vein.

Variations of the standard arterial anatomy of the liver are relatively common, seen in up to 40% of patients. The most common variants involve different origins of the right or left hepatic artery. A replaced right hepatic artery arises entirely from the superior mesenteric artery and courses posteriorly and to the right of the common bile duct within the porta hepatis, which is in contrast to its normal position to the left of the duct. Recognition of this anatomical variant is critical during operations on the extrahepatic biliary tree. An accessory right hepatic artery also arises from the superior mesenteric artery and is found in the same location within the porta hepatis but supplies only a portion of the right liver; in this situation, a separate right branch arising from its normal position off the proper hepatic artery is typically present. An accessory or replaced left hepatic artery arises from the left gastric artery and enters the liver through the gastrohepatic ligament. Up to 25% of patients have a replaced or accessory right hepatic artery, and a similar proportion have a replaced or accessory left hepatic artery. Another arterial variation includes the common hepatic artery originating from the superior mesenteric artery. Within the liver, the hepatic arterial branches travel with segmental bile ducts and portal vein branches and remain as portal triads in subsegmentations, found at each angle of the hexagon-shaped liver lobules.

▶ Biliary Drainage

The biliary tree arises within the liver from bile canaliculi, formed from specialized segments of the hepatocyte membrane. Bile canaliculi join to form progressively larger channels, resulting in segmental bile ducts that drain each segment. The right anterior and right posterior sectional ducts unite to form the main right hepatic duct, while the union of ducts draining segments II, III, and IV forms the left hepatic duct. The left hepatic duct is typically longer and has a longer extrahepatic course than the right hepatic duct. Drainage of segment I (caudate lobe) is principally into the left hepatic duct, but additional smaller ducts enter the right hepatic duct or drain directly into the hepatic duct confluence, which is formed by the union of the major lobar ducts to form the common hepatic duct. The common hepatic duct descends within the hepatoduodenal ligament for a variable distance to the point of insertion of the cystic duct of the gallbladder to give rise to the common bile duct. The right hepatic artery is usually found posterior to the common bile duct; however, in 20% of patients, it crosses anteriorly. The common bile duct diameter is approximately 6 mm, and it lies to the right of and anterior to the portal vein. It enters behind the pancreas along the pancreatic groove, ultimately entering the second portion of the duodenum along with the duct of Wirsung at the ampulla.

Anatomic variations in the biliary ductal anatomy are seen in approximately 30% of patients and most often involve the right hepatic duct. In approximately 25% of patients, the duct from the right posterior section joins the common hepatic duct or the left hepatic duct independently. Recognition of this variation is crucial for the surgeon performing a left hepatectomy for avoiding injury of the right posterior biliary drainage. Variations are far less common on the left side.

▶ Lymphatics

Lymphatics draining superficial lobules of the liver follow a subcapsular course to the diaphragm, to the suspensory ligaments of the liver, or to the posterior mediastinum, whereas others enter the porta hepatis. Lymphatics arising from lobules deep within the liver travel either with the hepatic veins along the vena cava or with the portal veins into the porta hepatis. Most of the lymphatic drainage of the liver is to the hepatoduodenal ligament.

NERVES

The liver and biliary tree are innervated by sympathetic fibers arising from T7 to T10 and by parasympathetic fibers from the right and left vagus nerves. The postganglionic sympathetic nerves arise from the celiac ganglia. Fibers derived from the celiac ganglia and vagus nerves form a plexus of nerves that run along the anterior and posterior aspects of the hepatic artery.

PHYSIOLOGY

Total hepatic blood flow (about 1500 mL/min; 30 mL/min per kg body weight) constitutes 25% of the cardiac output, although the liver accounts for only 2.5% of body weight. About 30% of the hepatic volume is blood (12% of total blood volume). Two-thirds of the flow enters through the portal vein and one-third through the hepatic artery. Pressure in the portal vein is normally low (10-15 cm H_2O [7-11 mm Hg]). The liver derives half of its oxygen from hepatic arterial blood and half from portal venous blood.

Blood flow within the liver is uniform, as demonstrated by an even distribution of microspheres injected into the hepatic artery or portal vein. Hepatic blood flow to the liver is regulated by a number of factors. Muscular sphincters at the inlet and outlet of sinusoids represent a major control point and respond to a number of different stimuli, including the autonomic nervous system, circulating hormones, bile salts, and metabolites. The cells lining the hepatic sinusoids (endothelial cells, Kupffer cells, and stellate cells) can also regulate flow to some extent.

Portal venous and hepatic arterial blood becomes pooled after entering the periphery of the hepatic sinusoid (Figure 26–5). Hepatic arterial flow increases or decreases reciprocally with changes in portal flow; however, portal venous flow does not increase with reductions in arterial flow. This arterial compensatory response is controlled largely by adenosine, which is released into the space of Mall surrounding the hepatic arterial resistance vessels. High concentrations of adenosine dilate the vessels, which increases flow and washes out the adenosine.

Sudden occlusion of the portal vein results in an immediate 60% rise in hepatic arterial flow. The total flow then gradually returns toward normal. On the other hand, sudden reductions in hepatic arterial supply are not immediately met

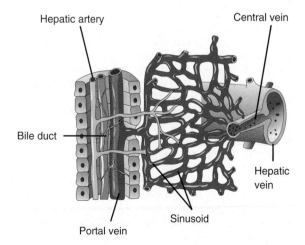

▲ **Figure 26–5.** Vascular anatomy of the liver lobule.

by significant increases in portal vein flow. In both normal subjects and cirrhotics, total hepatic flow and portal pressure drop following hepatic arterial occlusion. Arterial collaterals develop, and arterial perfusion is ultimately restored.

It is for this reason that interruption of hepatic arterial flow to the right or left liver generally has little impact on hepatic function. The one notable exception is in the setting of biliary obstruction. Decreased hepatic arterial flow to portions of the liver with impaired biliary drainage carries a high risk of hepatic necrosis. Clinically, this is an important consideration in patients undergoing hepatic arterial embolization of liver tumors and in patients undergoing resection of periampullary tumors, where jaundice is common and dissection within the porta hepatic could potentially put the hepatic artery at risk for injury. On the other hand, portal venous flow plays a critical role in maintaining normal hepatic architecture and function. This point is underscored by the observation that occlusion of the right or left portal venous branches results in profound ipsilateral hepatic atrophy and contralateral hypertrophy. Portal vein occlusion is clinically relevant in a number of disease processes, particularly carcinoma of the hepatic duct confluence (hilar cholangiocarcinoma), in which portal venous involvement is common and has important therapeutic implications. In addition, intentional occlusion of a major portal vein branch (usually the right side) is used with great frequency prior to major hepatic resection, primarily when the regenerative capacity of the future liver remnant (that portion of the liver that remains behind after the resection) is questionable because of either size concerns (too small) or underlying parenchymal disease (steatohepatitis, cirrhosis). By causing atrophy of the liver to be resected, and therefore hypertrophy of the future liver remnant, the risk of postoperative hepatic failure may be reduced.

HEPATIC RESECTION

Liver resection is most commonly indicated for primary and secondary malignant tumors and symptomatic benign tumors; less common indications include traumatic injury, infection/abscesses, and living donor transplantation. Removal of as much as 75%-80% of the normal liver can be performed with the expectation that the liver remnant will regenerate sufficiently for the patient to survive. It must be emphasized, however, that such extensive resections should be considered only in patients with normal hepatic function; those with cirrhosis or significant fibrosis or steatosis (fatty infiltration of the liver) are less likely to tolerate a major hepatic resection. Liver function may be impaired for several weeks after an extensive resection, but the extraordinary regenerative capacity of the liver rapidly provides new functioning hepatocytes. Within 24 hours after partial hepatectomy, cell replication becomes active and continues until the original volume of hepatic tissue is restored. Considerable

regeneration occurs within 10 days, and the process is largely completed by 8 weeks, although some small amount of regeneration continues well after this time. Excised portions of liver are not re-formed; rather, the remaining liver parenchyma increases in volume and mass. Hepatocyte proliferation begins in the periportal areas of the lobules and then proceeds centrally. The stimuli for hepatic regeneration are thought to include the following: hepatocyte growth factor, transforming growth factor (TGF)-α, heparin-binding growth factor, hepatopoietin B, and disinhibition by TGF-β_1 (ie, decreased levels of this inhibitor of hepatic growth). More specifically, hepatic resection activates Kupffer cells, which release tumor necrosis factor-α and interleukin-6, thereby priming remnant hepatocytes and activating hepatocyte growth factor. This results in hepatocyte cell DNA synthesis and proliferation. TGF-β signaling then blocks further proliferation at the completion of regeneration.

► Preoperative Evaluation

Several different disease-related and patient-related factors must be assessed before deciding to proceed with hepatic resection. Among the most important of these is the preoperative functional status of the liver. Cirrhosis is a relative contraindication for partial hepatectomy because the limited reserve of the residual cirrhotic liver may be insufficient to meet essential metabolic demands and the cirrhotic liver has a reduced capacity for regeneration. Cirrhosis is a particular concern in patients with hepatocellular carcinoma, which frequently arises in the setting of chronic hepatic parenchymal disease. Nonalcoholic steatohepatitis/nonalcoholic fatty liver disease has emerged as a major cause of liver parenchymal disease and an important risk factor for hepatic fibrosis/cirrhosis and primary liver cancer. Patients with severe steatohepatitis are also at significant risk of liver failure after major hepatic resection. An increasingly important concern in patients with hepatic colorectal metastases is chemotherapy-induced liver damage, which may also impair regeneration of the liver remnant.

Several tests are available to assess hepatic function prior to operation, none of which is perfect. The Child-Pugh classification is the oldest and most widely employed and remains the most useful assessment. The Child-Pugh system classifies hepatic function on the basis of the amount of ascites, the degree of encephalopathy, albumin and total bilirubin levels, and the prothrombin time (international normalized ratio [INR]) (Table 26-1). Originally used to assess mortality related to portosystemic shunts, the Child-Pugh score also predicts mortality after hepatic resection in patients with cirrhosis. In general, only Child-Pugh A and highly selected Child-Pugh B cirrhotics would be candidates for resection. To improve allocation of cadaveric liver transplant to cirrhotic patients with the highest risk of death, the Model for End-Stage Liver Disease (MELD) score has been

Table 26–1. Child-Pugh classification of functional status in liver diseases.

	Points		
	1	2	3
Ascites	Absent	Slight to moderate	Tense, refractory
Encephalopathy[1]	None	Grades I-II	Grades III-IV
Serum albumin (g/dL)	> 3.5	3.0-3.5	< 3.0
Serum bilirubin (mg/dL)	< 2.0	2.0-3.0	> 3.0
Prothrombin time (seconds above control)/international normalized ratio	< 4.0/< 1.7	4.0-6.0/1.7-2.3	> 6.0/> 2.3
Child-Pugh classification A (low risk) B (moderate) C (high risk)	Scores 5-6 7-9 10-15		

[1]Grade I, altered mood; grade ii, inappropriate behavior, somnolence; grade iii, markedly confused, stuporous but arousable; grade iv, unresponsive.
To convert the values for bilirubin to μmol/L, multiply by 17.1.

validated. Similar to the Child-Pugh classification, the total bilirubin level and the INR are accounted for, combined with the serum creatinine level. The MELD score was originally devised to predict mortality of patients awaiting liver transplantation but is also effective for assessing liver function in patients undergoing resection. The indocyanine green clearance test is commonly used in centers outside of North America but has not been proven superior to the Child-Pugh scoring system.

Extent of Hepatic Resection

Hepatic resections are classified as anatomical (based on the segmental liver anatomy) or nonanatomical. Wedge resections, enucleations, and resectional debridement of devitalized tissue are examples of the latter. In general, anatomical resections are preferred because they are associated with lower blood loss and, when performed for malignancy, a lower incidence of positive resection margins.

Major resections must be performed in accordance with the segmental anatomy (Figure 26–2). Major resections (right or left hepatectomy or extended hepatectomy) are commonly performed; however, the segmental anatomy of the liver allows smaller resections or bilateral resections to be performed when necessary and appropriate. For example, in selected situations, a resection of the anterior (segments V

and VIII) or posterior (segments VI and VII) sections may be performed rather than sacrificing the entire right liver. Such parenchymal-sparing resections on one side would then allow a resection of part of the contralateral lobe, if necessary. Sequential, two-stage hepatectomy has also been proven to benefit patients in the setting of multiple, bilateral liver metastases of colorectal cancer origin, allowing time for the liver remnant to regenerate and compensate for the second resection.

The terminology and extent of the common types of major resections are in Figure 26–2. The operation entails removal of a lobe or segment with its afferent and efferent vessels while avoiding injury to vessels and bile ducts supplying the remnant tissue.

Most elective hepatic resections can be performed through an abdominal incision, although selected situations (very large right lobe tumors) are probably best performed with a thoracoabdominal approach. Laparoscopic resections are being performed with greater frequency, although the open approach is most common and remains the standard. Optimal perioperative results are obtained by minimizing blood loss, which is accomplished by (1) achieving vascular inflow and outflow control prior to parenchymal transaction, (2) performing careful division of the liver with precise control of intrahepatic vascular structures, and (3) using low central venous pressure anesthesia, which reduces hepatic venous blood loss. Clamping of the portal inflow pedicle (Pringle maneuver) for periods of 10-15 minutes is commonly used to minimize blood loss via intrahepatic arterial and portal venous branches, although hepatic venous bleeding is unaffected.

Preoperative Portal Vein Embolization

Preoperative portal vein embolization is a technique that can be used to potentially improve the safety of major hepatic resections. By inducing hypertrophy of the future liver remnant prior to operation, the risk of postoperative liver failure is potentially reduced. The risk of such complications increases significantly with resections that leave behind a liver remnant of less than 25% in patients with normal liver or less than 40% in patients with liver disease.

Future liver remnant is a strong predictor of postoperative liver failure; however, other factors can also be used to independently predict this risk. Degree of hypertrophy is defined as the future liver remnant after portal vein embolization minus the future liver remnant before portal vein embolization. Degree of hypertrophy greater than 5% and a future liver remnant greater than 20% strongly predict good postoperative outcomes. Kinetic growth rate, defined as the degree of hypertrophy divided by the number of weeks since portal vein embolization, also strongly predicts a low risk of postoperative liver failure when this value is greater than 2% per week.

Postoperative Course

Patients submitted to major resections require close monitoring for the first several postoperative days; however, a prolonged stay in the intensive care unit is unnecessary in most cases. The major concern in the immediate postoperative period is hemorrhage, although in practice, reoperation for bleeding is rarely necessary. Patients without cirrhosis usually exhibit some metabolic changes consistent with mild liver insufficiency, but these quickly normalize, and they are often ready for discharge on the seventh or eighth postoperative day. In the presence of significant hepatic parenchymal disease (ie, cirrhosis, fibrosis, steatosis) or septic complications, postoperative liver function may be significantly impaired.

Many of the postoperative abnormalities can be predicted on the basis of the liver's normal function. The serum bilirubin often increases after major resections but returns to normal as regeneration progresses. A persistent or rising serum bilirubin level should raise concern for a perihepatic fluid collection (biloma) or hepatic failure (especially if other measures of hepatic function are also deteriorating). The serum albumin level usually falls, and the prothrombin time (PT) often increases. Abnormalities of the measures of thrombotic cascade (low fibrinogen and elevated PT) generally reflect abnormalities in liver function and do not necessarily imply increased risk of bleeding. Indeed, these patients are usually prothrombotic, and treatment of these laboratory abnormalities with fresh frozen plasma or other blood products is generally needed only when the INR is markedly elevated (> 2) and there is evidence of hemorrhage. Some patients may develop ascites, which can be treated with diuresis. Although the liver's glycogen stores are necessarily reduced after a major partial hepatectomy, hypoglycemia is almost never a problem postoperatively; normoglycemia can be easily maintained with 5% dextrose solutions, and profound hypoglycemia should raise concern for liver failure. Serum levels of phosphate, magnesium, and potassium often decrease during the first several postoperative days and require replacement. The liver enzymes (aspartate aminotransferase [AST], alanine aminotransferase [ALT]) are usually increased in the first few days after operation and then normalize. By contrast, alkaline phosphatase is often initially normal and then increases and can remain elevated for several days to weeks after surgery.

Complications

Complications may occur in up to 40% of patients after major liver resection (three or more segments), but many are relatively minor, and the overwhelming majority resolve without sequelae. Liver-related complications are the most frequent; perihepatic fluid collections requiring drainage occur in approximately 10%-15% of patients. Relative hepatic insufficiency (hyperbilirubinemia, ascites,

coagulopathy) is common but resolves in most patients as the liver regenerates. Hepatic failure is distinctly uncommon in high-volume centers. Pulmonary complications are also seen with some frequency, underscoring the need for aggressive pulmonary toilet postoperatively. The most common pulmonary problems are symptomatic pleural effusions or atelectasis; pneumonia is infrequent. Despite the potential complications associated with major liver resection, mortality rates are low, typically on the order of 1%-3% in high-volume centers. Less extensive liver resections (less than three segments) are associated with even lower morbidity and mortality rates.

Chun YS, et al: Management of chemotherapy-associated hepatotoxicity in colorectal liver metastases. *Lancet Oncol.* 2009;10:278.

Clavien PA, et al: Strategies for safer liver surgery and partial liver transplantation. *N Engl J Med.* 2007;356(15):1545.

Covey AM, et al: Combined portal vein embolization and neoadjuvant chemotherapy as a treatment strategy for resectable hepatic colorectal metastases. *Ann Surg.* 2008;247:451.

Frankel TL, et al: Hepatic resection for colorectal metastases. *J Surg Oncol.* 2014;109(1):2-7.

Kingham TP, et al: Hepatic parenchymal preservation surgery: decreasing morbidity and mortality rates in 4,152 resections for malignancy. *J Am Coll Surg.* 2015;220(4):471-479.

Leung U, et al: Remnant growth rate after portal vein embolization is a good early predictor of post-hepatectomy liver failure. *J Am Coll Surg.* 2014;219(4):520-530.

Rahbari NN, et al: Posthepatectomy liver failure: a definition and grading by the International Study Group of Liver Surgery (ISGLS). *Surgery.* 2011;149(5):713-724.

Riehle KJ et al: New concepts in liver regeneration. *J Gastroenterol Hepatol.* 2011;26-S1:203.

Strasberg SM: Nomenclature of hepatic anatomy and resections: a review of the Brisbane 2000 system. *J Hepatobiliary Pancreat Surg.* 2005;12:351-355.

Wicherts DA, et al: Long-term results of two-stage hepatectomy for irresectable colorectal cancer liver metastases. *Ann Surg.* 2008;248:994.

▼ DISEASES & DISORDERS OF THE LIVER

HEPATIC TRAUMA

The liver is injured in approximately 5% of all trauma admissions. Based on the mechanism of injury, liver trauma is classified as penetrating or blunt. Penetrating wounds, constituting more than half of cases, are typically due to projectiles (eg, bullets or shrapnel) or knives. In civilian practice, most of these tend to be clean wounds that are dangerous because of intra-abdominal bleeding but do not result in much devitalization of liver tissue. In contrast, high-velocity projectiles, commonly associated with military weapons, are associated with greater energy that is transferred to the abdominal viscera and can shatter the parenchyma, even if the projectile does not enter the liver directly.

Blunt trauma can be inflicted by a direct blow to the upper abdomen or lower right rib cage or can follow sudden deceleration, as occurs with a fall from a great height. Most often a consequence of automobile accidents, direct blunt trauma tends to produce explosive bursting wounds or linear lacerations of the hepatic surface, often with considerable parenchymal destruction. The stellate, bursting type of injury tends to affect the posterior and superior aspect of the right liver (segments VI, VII, and VIII) because of its relatively vulnerable location, convex surface, fixed position, and concentration of hepatic mass. Damage to the left liver is much less common than damage to the right. Injuries that involve shearing forces can tear the hepatic veins where they enter the liver substance, producing an exsanguinating retrohepatic injury in an area difficult to surgically expose and repair.

The improvement in image quality and rapidity of execution of computed tomography (CT) scans has transformed the initial management of trauma patients over the past few decades. For patients who can be hemodynamically stabilized with initial resuscitation, CT allows staging of the liver injury, in addition to all other structures from the neck to the pelvis. The staging system described in Table 26–2 is used to categorize liver injuries and provide a common language in order to allow comparisons of results of treatment between institutions. Patients who cannot be stabilized must go directly to the operating room.

There are two main management approaches to traumatic liver injury: nonoperative, which can be combined with angiography and selective embolization, or operative. When angiographic embolization is used as adjuvant to nonoperative management, approximately 85% of patient with blunt hepatic trauma can be successfully managed. A major limitation of arterial embolization is its inability to control bleeding from major venous injuries. Penetrating trauma, however, most often requires surgical intervention. The principal surgical goals are to stop bleeding and debride devitalized liver. Because some degree of liver failure is common postoperatively, efforts should be made during each step to maintain adequate oxygenation and perfusion of the liver. Also, when one is debriding liver tissue, care should be taken to avoid injury to the vascular supply of adjacent viable parenchyma.

▶ **Clinical Findings**

A. Symptoms and Signs

The clinical manifestations of liver injury are those of hypovolemic shock: hypotension, decreased urinary output, low central venous pressure, and, in some cases, abdominal distention. Patients managed nonoperatively are admitted in a monitored setting and closely followed with serial exams and hematocrit assessments. Patients who develop peritoneal signs on physical exam or the onset of hemodynamic instability denote failure of nonoperative management and mandate surgical intervention.

B. Laboratory Findings

With major injuries, particularly those associated with disruption of hepatic veins, the rate of blood loss is usually so rapid that anemia does not develop. Leukocytosis greater than 15,000/μL is common following rupture of the liver from blunt trauma. Polytrauma patients most often develop acidosis and coagulopathy.

C. Imaging Techniques

Focused abdominal sonography for trauma (FAST) in unstable patients has a sensitivity of 97% for detecting hemoperitoneum larger than 1 L, which warrants going directly to surgical management. The exact location of the injury often cannot be reliably identified with FAST. There is no defined role for FAST in stable patients.

High-resolution CT scan with intravenous contrast enhancement should be obtained in all stable patients suspected of having a hepatic injury. The CT provides a detailed

Table 26–2. Liver injury scale.[1]

Grade	Type	Description
I	Hematoma	Subcapsular, nonexpanding, < 10% of liver capsule surface area
	Laceration	Capsular tear, nonbleeding; < 1 cm deep in parenchyma
II	Hematoma	Subcapsular, nonexpanding, 10%-50% surface area; intraparenchymal, nonexpanding, < 10 cm in diameter
	Laceration	Capsular tear, active bleeding; 1-3 cm deep into the parenchyma, < 10 cm long
III	Hematoma	Subcapsular, > 50% surface area or expanding; ruptured subcapsular hematoma with active bleeding; intraparenchymal hematoma > 10 cm or expanding
	Laceration	> 3 cm deep into the parenchyma
IV	Laceration	Parenchymal disruption involving 25%-75% of hepatic lobe or 1-3 Couinaud segments
V	Laceration	Parenchymal disruption involving > 75% of hepatic lobe or > 3 Couinaud segments within a lobe
	Vascular	Juxtahepatic venous injuries; ie, retrohepatic vena cava or major hepatic veins
VI	Vascular	Hepatic avulsion

[1]Increase by one grade when there are two or more injuries to the liver. Grading is applied based on best available evidence, whether from x-rays, operative findings, or autopsy findings.

evaluation of the liver injury and its extent, provides an estimate of the amount of blood loss, and can demonstrate a contrast blush from the liver parenchyma. The findings are useful for triaging, because minor injuries rarely require surgical treatment. One must exercise caution, however, in using CT estimates of injury grade, because they correlate poorly (ie, they both understage and overstage) with what is found at surgery. CT scanning is also useful for identifying injuries to other organs, which are not uncommon, particularly in the setting of high-velocity blunt trauma.

Angiography is generally not helpful in the acute setting for the diagnosis of liver injury but may be used as an interventional adjunct in patients with arterial injuries who are candidates for nonoperative management.

▶ Treatment

Regardless of the grade of blunt liver injury, the hemodynamic stability of patients dictates whether or not a liver trauma should be managed operatively. By contrast, only highly selected patients with penetrating trauma can be managed nonoperatively. In absence of injury to the spleen and the kidneys, CT findings most often associated with successful nonoperative management include small hemoperitoneum, contained subcapsular or intrahepatic hematoma, unilobar fracture, absence of devitalized liver, minimal intraperitoneal blood, and absence of injuries to other intra-abdominal organs. Failure rate of the nonoperative approach increases in patients presenting with clinical signs of shock, a high injury severity score, and associated intra-abdominal injuries. It should be kept in mind that low-grade injuries can bleed significantly. Drop in hematocrit in stable patients should prompt a CT scan to verify that the lesion is stable rather than expanding. A blush of intravenous contrast associated with the liver injury represents bleeding that can often be addressed by angiographic embolization in the stable patient.

Strict contraindications to nonoperative management include hemodynamic instability after initial resuscitation or other indications for abdominal surgery such as peritonitis. Relative contraindications include gunshot injury and the absence of an appropriate clinical setting to monitor the patient (ie, limited embolization resources or inability to provide prompt, urgent exploration should that be necessary). Most patients with CT or clinical evidence of active bleeding or a major injury require prompt exploration. Most minor parenchymal lacerations have stopped bleeding by the time operation is performed. In the absence of active hemorrhage, these wounds should not be sutured. Active bleeding should be managed by clipping or direct suture of identifiable vessels, if possible, rather than by mass ligatures. Subcapsular hematomas often overlie an active bleeding site or parenchyma in need of debridement and should be explored even though the injury appears to be tamponaded and of limited severity. Blunt injuries associated with substantial amounts

of parenchymal destruction may be particularly difficult to manage. Rarely, a very severe pulverizing injury requires formal partial hepatectomy.

Temporary occlusion of the hepatic artery and portal vein can be done quickly by placing a vascular clamp around the entire hepatoduodenal ligament (Pringle maneuver). This can be done for periods of 10-15 minutes and reduces the hemorrhage sufficiently to permit more accurate ligation of bleeding vessels. With major hepatic venous injuries, however, a Pringle maneuver has no effect, and precise repair of the injury may not be possible. Absorbable gauze mesh (ie, polyglycolic acid) can sometimes be wrapped around an injured lobe and sutured in a way that maintains pressure and tamponades the bleeding. This is difficult to accomplish without rendering the involved liver ischemic, however, and such an approach is rarely applicable. In some cases, control of arterial hemorrhage requires ligation of the hepatic artery or one of the accessible major branches (ie, right anterior or right posterior sectional branches) in the hilum.

The most difficult problems involve lacerations of the major hepatic veins behind the liver. With such injuries, temporary clamping of the inflow vessels has little impact on back-bleeding from the inferior vena cava and does not allow adequate inspection and repair of the injured vessels. For persistent bleeding, the abdominal incision can be extended into a median sternotomy or thoracoabdominally to improve exposure. An ancillary technique, which is used only rarely and has been associated with high mortality rates, is to place a tube through the atrial appendage into the inferior vena cava past the origin of the hepatic veins. Appropriately placed ligatures around the suprahepatic and infrahepatic vena cava combined with the Pringle maneuver permit total isolation of the liver circulation. Resection of the right liver improves exposure of the retrohepatic vena cava but is difficult to perform in the face of massive hemorrhage.

In many cases, when bleeding is difficult to control, and especially when other injuries must be addressed, damage control is the best strategy and involves packing the liver to achieve hemostasis. The packs are generally left in place for 24-48 hours, during which time the patient remains sedated and intubated in the intensive care unit. Adequate resuscitative measures are undertaken to correct hypothermia, acidosis, and coagulopathy. The packs are removed in the operating room, and if persistent bleeding is noted, definitive repair of the injury can then be performed in a somewhat more controlled fashion.

The majority of patients who come to operation require little in the way of surgical intervention to control bleeding; drainage of substantial liver lacerations and other injuries is reasonable, since bile leakage can occur. For superficial liver injuries, bleeding can often be controlled with direct compression, topical agents, electrocautery, or argon beam coagulation. Suture ligation of bleeding hepatic vessels and debridement of devitalized tissue are indicated in about 30%

and 10% of cases, respectively. More extensive procedures are indicated even less often.

Penetrating injuries that also involve the small bowel or colon may result in contamination of perihepatic fluid or devitalized liver tissue, leading to a subhepatic abscess. Placement of drains may help prevent this problem, but a high index of suspicion should be maintained during the postoperative period.

Postoperative Complications

The rate of complications correlates with the grade of hepatic injury, reaching up to 50% in patients with grade V injuries. With present techniques, hemorrhage at laparotomy is rarely uncontrollable, except with retrohepatic venous injuries. Patients who rebled early from the liver wound after initial suture ligation should be treated by reexploration and packing; rarely is a major resection required. Angiography and CT scanning may provide useful diagnostic information preoperatively in such patients.

Bile leaks can follow both blunt and penetrating liver injuries when the biliary system is disrupted (1%-21% of cases). Most bilomas can be treated with image-guided percutaneous drainage. Endoscopic retrograde cholangiopancreatography (ERCP) may help identify the site of injury and may be therapeutic in some cases, since stents can be deployed in selected bile ducts and sphincterotomy of the sphincter of Oddi can relieve pressure in the biliary system. It should be noted, however, that such maneuvers have not been shown to expedite the resolution of biliary injuries, provided that adequate drainage of the biloma has been achieved.

Subhepatic sepsis develops in about 20% of cases and is more frequent if a major hepatectomy has been performed. Abscess can occur after blunt trauma, especially with concomitant enteric injuries. Most abscesses can be managed with percutaneous drainage and antibiotic therapy.

Severe hepatic injury and surgery-induced ischemia secondary to arterial inflow ligation increase the risk of hepatic necrosis. Clinically significant hepatic necrosis is managed with broad-spectrum antibiotics and source control generally consisting of a combination of resection/debridement and interventional drainage procedures.

Hemobilia may be responsible for gastrointestinal bleeding in the postoperative period and can be diagnosed by selective angiography. Treatment consists of embolization through the arteriography catheter.

Prognosis

The death rate of 10%-15% following hepatic trauma depends largely on the type of injury and the extent of associated injury to other organs. About one-third of patients admitted to the emergency department in shock cannot be saved. Only 1% of penetrating civilian wounds are lethal, whereas a 20% death rate attends blunt trauma. The death rate in blunt hepatic injury is 10% when only the liver is injured. If three major organs are damaged, the death rate is close to 70%. Bleeding causes more than half of deaths associated with liver trauma.

Boese CK, et al: Nonoperative management of blunt hepatic trauma: a systematic review. *J Trauma Acute Care Surg.* 2015;79(4):654-660.

Kozar RA, et al: Western Trauma Association/critical decisions in trauma: operative management of adult blunt hepatic trauma. *J Trauma.* 2011;71:1.

Navsaria PH, et al: Selective nonoperative management of liver gunshot injuries. *Ann Surg.* 2009;249:653.

Ordonez CA, et al: A comprehensive five-step surgical management approach to penetrating liver injuries that require complex repair. *J Trauma Acute Care Surg.* 2013;75:207.

Saltzherr TP, et al: Improved outcomes in the non-operative management of liver injuries. *HPB.* 2011;13:350.

SPONTANEOUS HEPATIC RUPTURE

Spontaneous rupture of the liver is not common. Most cases of ruptured diseased liver are due to hepatic tumors. Approximately 5% of hepatocellular carcinomas can rupture and manifest as hemoperitoneum. Hepatic adenoma larger than 5 cm carries a risk of spontaneous bleeding of approximately 20%-40%, although the true incidence is difficult to know with certainty.

Many cases of ruptured normal liver occur during or after pregnancy and are related to preeclampsia, eclampsia, and/or HELLP syndrome (hemolysis, elevated liver enzymes, low platelet count). Hepatic rupture should be suspected in any pregnant or postpartum patient (especially if hypertensive) who complains of acute discomfort in the upper abdomen.

Spontaneous rupture has also been reported in association with a number of other conditions, including hepatic hemangioma, typhoid fever, malaria, tuberculosis, syphilis, polyarteritis nodosa, and diabetes mellitus. Rupture of the liver in the newborn is usually related to birth trauma in larger infants after difficult deliveries. The typical progression is intrahepatic hemorrhage expanding to subcapsular hematoma and eventually capsular rupture and free intra-abdominal hemorrhage.

CT scan is the best modality for making the diagnosis. Angiography and hepatic artery embolization can be quite effective for controlling hemorrhage in the setting of spontaneous rupture. Emergency laparotomy and intraoperative management (as one would use for a traumatic liver injury) are reserved for those who fail hepatic artery embolization or are unsuitable for the procedure. Patients who experience hemoperitoneum from spontaneous rupture of hepatocellular carcinoma are at increased risk for peritoneal dissemination of tumor.

Battula N, et al: Spontaneous rupture of hepatocellular carcinoma: a Western experience. *Am J Surg.* 2009;197:164.

Bieze M, et al: Risk factors for bleeding in hepatocellular adenoma. *Br J Surg.* 2014;101(7):847-855.

Deneve JL, et al: Liver cell adenoma: a multicenter analysis of risk factors for rupture and malignancy. *Ann Surg Oncol.* 2009;16:640.

Stoot JH, et al: Life-saving therapy for haemorrhaging liver adenomas using selective arterial embolization. *Br J Surg.* 2007;94:1249.

Zeirideen R, Kadir RA: Spontaneous postpartum hepatic rupture. *J Obstet Gynecol.* 2009;29:155.

PRIMARY LIVER CANCER

Liver malignancy may arise from hepatocytes (hepatocellular carcinoma [HCC], the most common) or biliary epithelial cells (intrahepatic cholangiocarcinoma). Tumors arising from both cell types (mixed HCC/cholangiocarcinoma, also known as biphenotypic tumors) have also been described. Neonates may also develop a variant of HCC called hepatoblastoma because it is morphologically similar to fetal liver and the occasional presence of hematopoietic elements. Primary malignancy arising from other liver cell types (endothelial cells, stellate cells, neuroendocrine cells, or lymphocytes) is exceedingly rare.

Primary liver cancer is relatively uncommon in the United States, with approximately 42,000 new cases diagnosed in the United States in 2018. The incidence of liver cancer has tripled since 1980, largely the result of hepatitis C infection outbreak among individuals born between 1945 and 1965. The median survival time of patients with HCC ranges from 7 to 20 months, with only 17% of patients surviving 5 years. It is the fifth most common cancer worldwide. In Asia and Africa, primary liver cancer is extremely common and, in some areas, represents the single most frequent abdominal tumor and the most common cause of cancer-related death. The etiologic factors in these high-risk areas are environmental or cultural, since persons of similar racial background in the United States are at only slightly greater risk than whites.

▶ Hepatocellular Carcinoma

Chronic hepatitis B and C virus infection is the principal etiologic factor worldwide for HCC. Patients chronically seropositive for hepatitis B surface antigen (HBsAg) constitute a high-risk group for development of HCC. Hepatitis B virus DNA can be integrated into the genome of host hepatocytes and hepatoma cells and has a direct oncogenic effect. Patients with chronic hepatitis B infection may therefore develop HCC in the absence of cirrhosis. By contrast, HCC arising in the setting of chronic hepatitis C infection is typically associated with cirrhotic change. Cirrhosis from almost any cause (eg, alcoholism, hemochromatosis, α_1-antitrypsin deficiency, or primary biliary cirrhosis) is associated with an increased risk of HCC, and the great majority of these tumors arise in the setting of chronic underlying liver disease. With the increase in obesity in the United States, nonalcoholic fatty liver disease has become one of the most common causes of chronic liver disease; a subgroup of these patients with steatohepatitis are at high risk of cirrhosis and malignant transformation. Certain fungal metabolites called aflatoxins have been shown experimentally to be capable of producing liver tumors. These substances are present in staple foods (eg, ground nuts and grain) in some parts of Africa where HCC has a high incidence.

HCC constitutes about 85%-95% of primary hepatic cancers. A number of staging systems for HCC are in current use when considering treatment options for patients with HCC, including the Barcelona Clinic Liver Cancer (BCLC), Cancer of the Liver Italian Program (CLIP), Okuda, Chinese University Prognostic Index (CUPI), and Japan Integrated Staging (JIS). These classifications differ regarding their assessment of tumor burden, related symptoms, and underlying liver dysfunction, and most cannot predict survival in patients with advanced HCC. The eighth edition of the American Joint Commission on Cancer tumor-node-metastasis (TNM) staging system can be used after pathologic examination of the resected liver to determine the prognosis of patients after transplantation. About 50% of resectable tumors are surrounded by a fibrous capsule, which develops as a result of compression of adjacent liver stroma. Encapsulated tumors exhibit a lower incidence of tumor microsatellites and venous permeation compared with non-encapsulated tumors, and the finding is a favorable sign. An uncommon variant, **fibrolamellar HCC,** contains numerous fibrous septa and may resemble focal nodular hyperplasia. Fibrolamellar hepatoma occurs in a younger age group (average age, 25 years), has a female predilection, and is not associated with cirrhosis or hepatitis virus infection.

A large proportion of patients have intrahepatic or extrahepatic metastases at presentation. Multiple intrahepatic tumors can arise as a result of infiltration of the portal venous system with subsequent dissemination of tumor cells. Vascular invasion is more common with larger tumors (> 5 cm). The extrahepatic sites most commonly involved with metastatic disease include the hilar and celiac lymph nodes, adrenals, and the lungs; metastases to bone and brain are less common, and peritoneal disease (ie, carcinomatosis) is distinctly unusual. Major portal or hepatic veins are often invaded by tumor, and venous occlusion may occur as a result.

Microscopically, there is usually little stroma between the malignant cells, and the tumor has a soft consistency. The tumor may be highly vascularized, a feature that can result in massive intraperitoneal hemorrhage following spontaneous rupture.

Intrahepatic Cholangiocarcinoma

Cholangiocarcinoma makes up a small fraction of primary liver cancers, although several reports have documented a marked increase in incidence worldwide. Cirrhosis and chronic liver disease are recognized risk factors. Primary sclerosing cholangitis and choledochal cysts are predisposing conditions in a small minority of patients. Intrahepatic stone disease (recurrent pyogenic cholangitis) has also been associated with an increased incidence of cholangiocarcinoma. Widespread infection with liver flukes (*Clonorchis sinensis*) is at least partly responsible for the higher incidence of these tumors in some parts of Asia. Emerging evidence has implicated chronic hepatitis C infection, obesity, diabetes mellitus, chronic liver disease, and cigarette smoking as risk factors for intrahepatic cholangiocarcinoma. In Western centers, however, the vast majority of intrahepatic cholangiocarcinomas are sporadic. Intrahepatic cholangiocarcinoma generally presents as a large mass within the liver and is therefore clinically distinct from cholangiocarcinoma arising from the extrahepatic biliary tree.

Histologically, these tumors are most often invasive adenocarcinomas, although rare variants have been reported. Intrahepatic or extrahepatic spread of disease is not uncommon by the time the tumor is detected. These tumors infrequently cause symptoms at early stages and therefore often grow to a large size before they become apparent, frequently because of pain. Infrequently, these tumors may contain cells of both cholangiocellular and hepatocellular origin. These mixed tumors are similar to intrahepatic cholangiocarcinoma in that they are infrequently associated with chronic liver disease.

Angiosarcoma of the liver, a rare, aggressive and uniformly fatal tumor, has been seen in workers intensively exposed to vinyl chloride for prolonged periods in polymerization plants. Hepatoblastoma is the most common primary hepatic tumors of childhood and is estimated to affect 1 child younger than 15 years old per 1 million per year, and approximately 50 to 70 new cases are reported in the United States yearly.

Clinical Findings

A. Symptoms and Signs

The diagnosis at early and more treatable stages is often difficult, since symptoms are often absent. Screening and surveillance of high-risk patients (eg, those with cirrhosis, chronic hepatitis) with ultrasonography of the liver has been recommended. Patients with more advanced tumors may have epigastric or right upper quadrant pain, which may be associated with referred pain in the right shoulder. Weight loss may be present. Jaundice is rare in patients with small tumors and good liver function; the presence of jaundice suggests either very advanced cancer or deteriorating liver function or both.

Hepatomegaly or a mass is palpable in many patients. An arterial bruit or a friction rub may be audible over the liver. Intermittent fever may be a presenting feature. Ascites or gastrointestinal bleeding from varices indicates advanced disease, and ascites fluid with blood should always suggest HCC. An acute deterioration in a previously well-compensated cirrhotic patient should also raise the suspicion of HCC.

The patterns of presentation can thus be extremely variable and may include (1) pain with or without hepatomegaly; (2) sudden deterioration of the condition of a cirrhotic patient with the onset of hepatic failure, bleeding varices, or ascites; (3) sudden, massive intraperitoneal hemorrhage; (4) acute illness with fever and abdominal pain; (5) symptoms related to distant metastases; and (6) no clinical findings or symptoms.

B. Laboratory Findings

Depending on the disease extent and underlying hepatic function, laboratory values may range from entirely normal to suggestive of impending liver failure. Serum transaminase levels (AST and ALT) and alkaline phosphatase may be increased, but increased levels are nonspecific and often seen in patients with chronic liver disease without HCC. The presence of a moderate to large liver tumor may bring about an increase in the serum alkaline phosphatase in the absence of underlying liver disease. An elevated serum bilirubin is a more ominous finding and may reflect some degree of liver dysfunction, either from the underlying chronic liver disease or from a large volume of cancer within the liver. Tumor extension within the portal venous system is not uncommon, and involvement of the right and left portal trunks or the main portal vein may result in jaundice due to compromised portal venous inflow. Less often, jaundice is the result of tumor involvement of the biliary confluence by direct compression or by intrabiliary tumor extension. Other signs of compromised hepatic function include hypoalbuminemia, coagulopathy, and thrombocytopenia. A large number of patients are positive for HBsAg or hepatitis C virus antibody; the proportions of each vary somewhat by geography.

C. Liver Imaging

Liver ultrasound, CT scans, and magnetic resonance imaging (MRI) scans demonstrate the principal lesion in nearly all patients. A triple-phase (no contrast, arterial phase, portal venous phase), contrast-enhanced helical CT scan of the chest, abdomen, and pelvis generally provides the best images of disease extent within the liver and also assesses for extrahepatic spread. HCCs are supplied primarily by the hepatic artery, and the vast majority thus enhance on arterial phase more than the adjacent nontumorous liver parenchyma (hypervascular). In some cases, the center of the tumor has become necrotic, and only the peripheral areas are hypervascular. Arterial branches supplying the tumor have an irregular appearance compared to the native hepatic artery, and arteriovenous shunting may be seen. Upon venous phase, the arterial contrast typically has washed out, and the HCC bears similar density to the adjacent parenchyma (isodense).

The Liver Imaging Reporting and Data System (LI-RADS) was developed in 2011 in order to use accepted and consistent terminology and eliminate ambiguity and variability in interpretation of cross-sectional imaging of liver lesions in high-risk patients (Figure 26–6). Lesions are graded from LI-RADS 1 (definitely benign) to LI-RADS 5 (definitely HCC). Arterial phase enhancement, mass diameter (> 1 cm), contrast washout, presence of an enhancing capsule, and threshold growth are all used to determine LI-RADS category. This allows for noninvasive diagnosis of HCC and eliminates the need for biopsy except for LI-RADS 4 lesions (70%-80% likelihood of HCC) or LR-M (probably or definitely malignant but not definitely HCC).

By contrast to HCC, intrahepatic cholangiocarcinomas usually appear less vascular than adjacent liver parenchyma

Untreated observation without pathologic proof in patient at high risk for HCC

- If cannot be categorized due to image degradation or omission → LR-NC
- If definite tumor in vein (TIV) → LR-TIV
- If definitely benign → LR-1
- If probably benign → LR-2
- If probably or definitely malignant but not HCC specific (e.g., if targetoid) → LR-M

Otherwise, use CT/MRI diagnostic table below

- If intermediate probability of malignancy → LR-3
- If probably HCC → LR-4
- If definitely HCC → LR-5

CT/MRI Diagnostic Table

Arterial phase hyperenhancement (APHE)		No APHE		Nonrim APHE		
Observation size (mm)		< 20	≥ 20	< 10	10-19	≥ 20
Count additional major features:	None	LR-3	LR-3	LR-3	LR-3	LR-4
• Enhancing "capsule" • Nonperipheral "washout" • Threshold growth	One	LR-3	LR-4	LR-4	LR-4 / LR-5	LR-5
	≥ Two	LR-4	LR-4	LR-4	LR-5	LR-5

LR-4 / LR-5   Observations in this cell are categorized based on one additional major feature:
- LR-4 – if enhancing "capsule"
- LR-5 – if nonperipheral "washout" **OR** threshold growth

If unsure about the presence of any major feature: characterize that feature as absent

▲ **Figure 26–6.** Liver Imaging Reporting and Data System (LI-RADS) diagnostic algorithm and table. CT, computed tomography; HCC, hepatocellular carcinoma; MRI, magnetic resonance imaging. (Reproduced with permission from Cerny M, Chernyak V, Olivié D, et al: LI-RADS Version 2018 Ancillary Features at MRI, *Radiographics.* 2018 Nov-Dec;38(7):1973-2001.)

on all phase contrast. As an adjunct to CT, MRI scans with magnetic resonance angiography or CT angiography may provide more detail regarding vascular involvement and clarify whether a tumor is surgically removable.

D. Angiography

Diagnostic angiography was previously often used to assess liver tumors but is now rarely needed for this purpose; it is reserved primarily for treatment (ie, transarterial embolization). Angiography may be equivocal in small HCC, which may be demonstrated with greater certainty by a selective injection of iodized oil (Lipiodol) followed 1-2 weeks later by CT scanning. In a normal liver, the contrast medium is cleared quickly, but HCC retains it and remains opacified.

E. Liver Biopsy

The diagnosis can be established by percutaneous core biopsy or aspiration biopsy. Fine-needle aspiration biopsy is associated with an approximately 30% false-negative rate. A negative result, therefore, does not rule out malignant disease, and a core biopsy should be pursued if the index of suspicion is high. Percutaneous biopsy carries some risk of bleeding, although this is rare in experienced hands; tumor dissemination by seeding resulting from a biopsy can occur in 2%-4% of patients. In patients with cirrhosis, the presence of a hypervascular mass larger than 1 cm with typical imaging features on contrast-enhanced CT or MRI has specificity and positive predictive values of nearly 100%, and a biopsy is generally not required in this setting. In other clinical scenarios, a diagnostic biopsy is often requested for nonsurgical candidate to guide appropriate liver-directed or systemic treatment.

F. Tumor Markers

Alpha-fetoprotein (AFP), a glycoprotein normally present only in the fetal circulation, is present in high concentrations in the serum of many patients with HCC, testicular tumors, and hepatoblastomas. Increased levels are rarely seen as a product of other tumor types, such as the lung, stomach, pancreas, and biliary tree.

The upper limit of normal in the serum is 20 ng/mL; values above 200 ng/mL are suggestive of HCC, whereas levels above 400 ng/mL in cirrhotic patients with a hypervascular liver mass larger than 2 cm in diameter are considered diagnostic. Levels in the intermediate range are nonspecific and may occur with benign liver diseases, such as cirrhosis and chronic hepatitis, where they represent a manifestation of liver cell proliferation. As imaging methods have improved, the diagnosis of liver cancer is being made earlier, when AFP levels may be normal or only minimally elevated. Additionally, some patients may have normal AFP levels despite the presence of advanced disease. In general, AFP levels correlate with tumor size and vascular invasion, and a number of studies have shown a correlation between high AFP levels and recurrent cancer after resection. AFP levels can also provide a measure of tumor response in patients treated nonoperatively.

G. Surveillance

In patients with cirrhosis or chronic hepatitis B, surveillance with biannual liver sonography is recommended because early detection and treatment compose the best strategy to achieve long-term survival. The optimal type and timing of imaging studies are the subjects of debate, but imaging typically consists of abdominal ultrasound exams performed by qualified sonographers or physicians every 6 months. AFP level is considered optional and should only be used in conjunction with ultrasound given its high false-positive detection rate as a single surveillance technique. Such programs have proved useful in areas with a high incidence of chronic hepatitis, such as Asia, where a large proportion of patients are now identified with a mass 2 cm in diameter or smaller; other studies in high-risk patients have also proved valuable.

▶ Differential Diagnosis

The clinical picture is often nonspecific, and the presenting symptoms may provide little in the way of diagnostic clues. Primary liver cancer may initially be confused with metastatic cancer arising from other abdominal sites. The presence of cirrhosis and findings consistent with chronic liver disease should make HCC the leading diagnosis, and this is often confirmed with further testing. In patients without cirrhosis or normal AFP levels (or both), a hypervascular mass in the liver should raise other diagnostic considerations, such as hepatic adenoma, which may be difficult to distinguish from HCC on the basis of imaging alone. In addition, certain types of cancer may give rise to hypervascular liver metastases, including melanoma, neuroendocrine carcinoma, and renal cell carcinoma.

When sudden decompensation develops in a cirrhotic patient, the possibility of HCC must always be considered. In rare instances, HCC is associated with metabolic or endocrine abnormalities such as erythrocytosis, hypercalcemia, hypoglycemic attacks, Cushing syndrome, or virilization.

▶ Complications

Sudden intra-abdominal hemorrhage may occur from spontaneous bleeding. Obstruction of the portal vein may produce portal hypertension, and obstruction of the hepatic veins may produce the Budd-Chiari syndrome. Liver failure is a common cause of death in these situations.

▶ Treatment

A. Partial Hepatectomy

Resection is the treatment of choice in selected HCC patients without cirrhosis or in cirrhotics with well-preserved hepatic function (Child-Pugh class A). Initial diagnostic laparoscopy, immediately prior to planned laparotomy, may identify previously undetected spread of tumor within the liver or abdominal cavity that would preclude resection; however, with better imaging, the yield of laparoscopy has decreased. The minimal criteria of resectability that must be met are (1) disease confined to the liver and (2) disease amenable to a complete resection. Multiple tumors in the liver and tumor invasion into major portal or hepatic veins are bad prognostic findings, even if resection is technically feasible, and such patients generally are not good candidates for resection. For small and peripherally placed lesions, particularly in cirrhotics, sublobar, segmental resections are preferred if technically feasible. Anatomical segmentectomies are preferred to nonanatomical resections. Larger or more central tumors require more extensive resections. In Western centers, about 25%-30% of patients with HCC prove to be candidates for resection; this proportion is over 60% in Japan due largely to widespread surveillance programs.

If gross tumor is left behind or if the margins of resection are involved microscopically, progressive disease is the rule. After a complete resection, the prognosis is best for patients with a solitary, small (< 3 cm), and asymptomatic tumor and well-preserved hepatic function. Several adverse predictors of outcome have been identified, which vary somewhat among studies. However, the presence of vascular invasion (even if microscopic) has been identified in nearly all studies to predict recurrent cancer and poor outcome. Large tumor size (> 5 cm), the presence of satellite tumors, and markedly elevated AFP (> 2000 ng/mL) are also associated with a worse outcome, in part because of their correlation with vascular invasion. Additionally, patients with coexistent hepatocellular disease (eg, cirrhosis) do worse, and this is especially true in the face of significant hepatocellular dysfunction or portal hypertension.

In general, cirrhosis constitutes the major obstacle to resection in patients with HCC. Careful patient selection (eg, Child-Pugh class A, no portal hypertension) is critical in order to avoid acute liver failure and provide survival benefit to patients. In addition to this immediate perioperative concern, cirrhotic patients have a late risk of death from progression of the underlying liver disease (bleeding esophageal varices or liver failure) and a high rate (> 75%) of new tumors developing in the residual liver. For these reasons, highly selected HCC patients may be better treated with liver transplantation rather than resection.

Overall, the rate of HCC recurrence is approximately 70% at 5 years (although it is higher, as mentioned earlier, in patients with cirrhosis). Some patients may be candidates for repeat resection or ablative procedures. The 5-year survival rate varies from approximately 40% to 70% but is lower for patients with cirrhosis.

After surgery, patients should be followed by periodic physical examinations and blood work to assess liver function. Imaging studies and AFP measurements (if elevated before resection) at regular intervals may help identify early, localized recurrences that may be amenable to repeat resection or palliative therapy.

For intrahepatic cholangiocarcinoma, complete resection with negative margins is the treatment of choice. Unresectable intrahepatic cholangiocarcinoma includes metastatic disease, locally advanced tumors involving bilateral inflow and/or outflow, and multiple intrahepatic lesions or satellite tumors. Lymph node metastases beyond the porta hepatis and distant metastatic disease contraindicate resection.

Malignant portal lymphadenopathy portends a poor prognosis; however, surgical resection can be performed in highly selected patients. The role of routine portal lymphadenectomy is debated. Although not therapeutic, portal lymph node dissection is certainly prognostic in that an R0 hepatic resection in the absence of lymph node metastases leads to 5-year survival rates of 40% compared to rates of 10%-13% in patients with positive portal nodes. Current National Comprehensive Cancer Network guidelines from 2018 recommend regional lymphadenectomy as a prognostic tool, although the lymph node yield is typically low (one to three nodes).

B. Liver Transplantation

HCC is the only solid neoplasm for which transplantation plays a significant role. Liver transplantation has the advantage of treating not only the malignant disease, but also the underlying cirrhosis. Initially, the selection criteria for transplanting hepatoma patients were broad and included patients with very advanced disease. Consequently, 5-year survival rates were less than 40%—too low to justify use of a scarce resource. The lessons learned from this early experience have allowed identification of patients most likely to benefit, specifically those with a single tumor no larger than 5 cm in diameter or those with up to three tumors with none exceeding 3 cm in diameter and no major vascular invasion. Using these strict criteria (the Milan criteria), 5-year survival rates of 70% can be achieved, a survival benefit similar to transplant patients with advanced cirrhosis but without HCC. Attempts to expand the Milan criteria to include patients with more advanced disease (eg, the University of California San Francisco criteria) have suggested some benefit in highly selected patients, particularly those who respond well to embolic therapy (see later in chapter). In general, however, transplantation outside of the Milan criteria leads to poor results and should be done with caution.

It should be emphasized that the benefit of transplantation is realized only when the waiting time for a new graft is under 6 months. Because waiting times can exceed 12 months in many centers, up to 50% of patients develop cancer progression or otherwise become ineligible. This problem has led a number of centers to adopt living donor transplantation as a means of increasing the donor pool, an approach that remains controversial because of donor-related morbidity and mortality. Another approach to this problem has been to increase the number of MELD points for transplantable liver disease, which effectively places eligible patients higher on the priority list.

A major concern of transplantation in cancer patients has been that the immunosuppressive therapy required to support the graft would remove an important defense mechanism against progression of residual microscopic disease. Indeed, calculated tumor doubling times for lesions in transplanted patients have been shown to be greater compared to patients not on immunosuppressive agents. Despite this possibility and although the logistical problems and expense are enormous, transplantation is a reasonable option in patients with cirrhosis who are not candidates for resection and have limited malignant disease burden, as specified in the selection criteria.

Transplantation for intrahepatic cholangiocarcinoma is rarely indicated and should only be performed in controlled clinical trials. Small case series of unresectable intrahepatic cholangiocarcinoma with no extrahepatic spread treated with orthotopic liver transplant have shown poor outcomes, with a median survival of only 9 months and nearly half of patients experiencing recurrence of disease.

C. Nonoperative Liver-Directed Therapy

Liver directed-therapies have been the subject of multiple investigations for the treatment of HCC. Indications for use of liver-directed therapies include advanced disease (unresectable, large, or multifocal HCC) and HCC in the setting of advanced cirrhosis and no longer suitable for resection (Child-Pugh class B, portal hypertension). In addition, percutaneous ablation is used as a bridge to transplant for eligible patients with expected wait list times greater than 6 months. Radiofrequency ablation and microwave irradiation are the main techniques being used today; however, ethanol injection has also been shown to be effective. Ethanol injection can be particularly useful in the presence of contraindications to radiofrequency or microwave ablation such as tumor proximity to the gallbladder or heart.

The effectiveness of liver-directed approaches for unresectable intrahepatic cholangiocarcinoma is being evaluated.

1. Ethanol injection—Percutaneous ablative techniques are a reasonable option in patients with small, unresectable HCC, of which ethanol injection is the cheapest, easiest, and least morbid. Using ultrasound or CT guidance, 95% ethanol (5-20 mL) is injected through a 22-gauge needle directly into the tumor. This approach can achieve complete necrosis in 90%-100% of tumors smaller than 2 cm, but its efficacy declines rapidly as the tumor size increases. The patient is followed up and retreatment given for residual or new primary tumors. In one multi-institutional series from Italy, survival rates 1, 2, and 3 years after treatment for patients with solitary, small tumors were 90%, 80%, and 63%, respectively.

2. Radiofrequency ablation—Radiofrequency ablation (RFA) is another percutaneous ablative approach that is useful for treating selected patients with small tumors who are not candidates for surgery or liver transplantation. RFA has generally supplanted ethanol injection as the percutaneous treatment of choice. Under ultrasound or CT guidance, a needle is used to access the lesion; the needle is attached to a radiofrequency generator that generates thermal energy to bring about tumor destruction. RFA can be performed percutaneously, laparoscopically, or at laparotomy.

The goal of RFA is the same as that of ethanol injection: to achieve complete tumor necrosis. The efficacy of RFA is limited by tumor size but may be somewhat greater than ethanol injection in this regard. RFA is less effective for tumors adjacent to major vascular structures. A randomized study comparing the two techniques found no differences in survival, although RFA may offer better local tumor control rates. In carefully selected patients, 5-year survival rates of 30%-40% have been reported with RFA. RFA has been compared with resection in early HCC in randomized controlled trials, but results have varied. Generally, RFA appears to be as effective as resection in lesions smaller than 2 cm. Ablation techniques, including RFA, have been studied in the context of controlling disease progression in patients who are candidates for transplantation while on the waiting list, with some suggestion of benefit.

3. Microwave ablation—Microwave ablation uses active and passive heating to destroy tissue. Microwaves emit nonionizing radiation which heats all tissue types equally throughout the entirety of the field. Both microwave ablation and RFA are subject to heat sinking and current sinking in tumors near major blood vessels. Heat sinking is due to the cooling effect of the blood, and current sinking describes diversion of the current by the nearby blood flow. Both processes decrease the amount of energy delivered to the tumor and can lead to incomplete tumor ablation. Microwave ablation for the treatment of HCC has been shown to be safe with acceptable morbidity and reported local recurrence rates of 6% at 5 years.

Irreversible electroporation is an emerging ablative technique that may prove to be an alternative to RFA and microwave ablation.

4. Arterial embolization—Hepatic artery embolization (HAE) is another technique that is more broadly applicable than ablation or ethanol injection. This approach takes advantage of the fact that primary liver cancers derive disproportionately greater blood supply from the hepatic arterial circulation compared to the surrounding liver. The strategy is to combine selective hepatic arterial injection of cancer chemotherapeutic agents with arterial embolization, the latter to produce tumor necrosis and slow the washout of the drugs. Embolization can be used in patients with much larger tumors than can be effectively treated with percutaneous procedures, and the procedure can be staged to treat bilobar disease. Patients must have adequate liver function; those with Child-Pugh class C cirrhosis or thrombosis of the portal vein are not suitable candidates.

A variety of techniques have been used. In the past, HAE has been performed with Gelfoam, which dissolves after a few weeks, and is, therefore, relatively ineffective for providing durable occlusion of arterial flow. Other inert agents (ie, polyvinyl alcohol particles) are also used and are probably more effective for occluding vessels. Some centers use inert particles without chemotherapy (ie, bland embolization), but most employ a chemotherapeutic component (ie, transarterial chemoembolization). Doxorubicin, mitomycin, and cisplatin in various combinations are the drugs most often given. Lipiodol, which lodges in the tumor, has been used as a carrier for the drugs. It remains unclear if the addition of chemotherapeutic agents provides much benefit beyond the necrosis produced by occlusion of the hepatic arterial supply. Many patients require multiple treatments, although the optimal schedule is ill defined. Embolization achieves partial responses in up to 55% of patients. A survival benefit of approximately 10 months has been reported with chemoembolization compared to best supportive care in randomized controlled trials, and 30%-50% of patients are reported to survive at 3 years. Of note, histologic studies of tumors resected shortly after treatment reveal viable neoplastic cells in the tumor capsule, which receives blood from the portal vein as well as the hepatic artery. A randomized prospective trial has shown that the combination of RFA and chemoembolization provided superior disease control rates compared with either technique alone. The advantage of chemoembolization over HAE with bland particles has not been clearly demonstrated, and in a randomized study comparing transarterial chemoembolization with drug-eluting beads to bland embolization, no difference in survival was found.

D. Systemic Therapy

Until recently, no systemic treatment was able to offer improved survival in patients with metastatic HCC. However, the multikinase inhibitor sorafenib, which mainly blocks RAF, VEGF, PDGF, and c-Kit signaling, has been shown to have antitumor efficacy. In two phase III, multicenter, randomized, double-blind, placebo-controlled trials, sorafenib improved overall survival by 2-3 months in patients with advanced HCC and compensated liver function. Combining sorafenib with other biologic and chemotherapeutic agents is being evaluated; however, results up until now have not shown any benefit. More recently, cabozantinib, a small-molecule tyrosine kinase inhibitor, was studied in a phase III, multicenter, randomized, double-blind, placebo-controlled trial of previously treated hepatocellular cancer patients who progressed on sorafenib. Median overall survival was significantly longer in the treatment group (10.2 months) compared to the placebo group (8.0 months).

Gemcitabine based-chemotherapy, in particular in combination with cisplatin, has shown prolongation of survival in patients with metastatic biliary tract cancer. Recently, results of the phase III, randomized controlled BILCAP trial demonstrated a 17-month improvement in median overall survival with adjuvant capecitabine versus placebo after complete resection of cholangiocarcinoma.

Abou-Alfa GK, et al: Cabozantinib in patients with advanced and progressing hepatocellular carcinoma. *N Engl J Med.* 2018;379(1):54-63.

Brown KT, et al: Randomized trial of hepatic artery embolization for hepatocellular carcinoma using doxorubicin-eluting microspheres compared with embolization with microspheres alone. *J Clin Oncol.* 2016;34(17):2046-2053.

Cheng AL, et al: Efficacy and safety of sorafenib in patients in the Asia-Pacific region with advanced hepatocellular carcinoma: a phase III randomized, double-blind, placebo-controlled trial. *Lancet Oncol.* 2009;10:25.

Cheng BQ, et al: Chemoembolization combined with radiofrequency ablation for patients with hepatocellular carcinoma larger than 3 cm: a randomized controlled trial. *JAMA.* 2008; 299:1669.

Clavien PA, et al: Recommendation for liver transplantation for hepatocellular carcinoma: an international consensus conference report. *Lancet Oncol.* 2012;13:e11-22.

De Jong MC, et al: Intrahepatic cholangiocarcinoma: an international multi-institutional analysis of prognostic factors and lymph node assessment. *J Clin Oncol.* 2011;29:3140.

Endo I, et al: Intrahepatic cholangiocarcinoma: rising frequency, improved survival, and determinants of survival after resection. *Ann Surg.* 2008;247:994.

Feng K, et al: A randomized controlled trial of radiofrequency ablation and surgical resection in the treatment of small hepatocellular carcinoma. *J Hepatol.* 2012;57(4):794-802.

Forner A, et al: Hepatocellular carcinoma. *Lancet.* 2012;379:1245.

Hernaez R, et al: How we approach it: treatment options for hepatocellular carcinoma. *Am J Gastroenterol.* 2018;113(6): 791-794.

Kamarajah SK, et al: Critical evaluation of the American Joint Commission on Cancer (AJCC) 8th edition staging system for patients with hepatocellular carcinoma (HCC): a Surveillance, Epidemiology, End Results (SEER) analysis. *J Surg Oncol.* 2018; 117(4):644-650.

Llovet JM, et al: Sorafenib in advanced hepatocellular carcinoma. *N Engl J Med.* 2008;359:378.

Mazzaferro V, et al: Liver transplantation for the treatment of small hepatocellular carcinomas in patients with cirrhosis. *N Engl J Med.* 1996;334:693.

Park SY, et al: Transarterial chemoembolization versus supportive therapy in the palliative treatment of unresectable intrahepatic cholangiocarcinoma. *Clin Radiol.* 2011;66:322.

Primrose JN, et al: Capecitabine compared with observation in resected biliary tract cancer (BILCAP): a randomised, controlled, multicentre, phase 3 study. *Lancet Oncol.* 2019;20(5): 663-673.

Silva MA, et al: Needle track seeding following biopsy of liver lesions in the diagnosis of hepatocellular cancer: a systematic review and meta-analysis. *Gut.* 2008;57:1592.

Takami Y, et al: Evaluation of intraoperative microwave coagulo-necrotic therapy for hepatocellular carcinoma: a single center experience of 719 consecutive cases. *J Hepatobil Pancreat Sci.* 2013;20(3):332-341.

Valle J, et al: Cisplatin plus gemcitabine versus gemcitabine for biliary tract cancer. *N Engl J Med.* 2010;362:1273.

White DL, et al: Association between nonalcoholic fatty liver disease and risk for hepatocellular cancer, based on systemic review. *Clin Gastroenterol Hepatol.* 2012;10:1342-1359.

METASTATIC NEOPLASMS OF THE LIVER

In Western countries, metastatic cancer is much more common than primary liver malignancy. Nearly all solid tumors can potentially give rise to liver metastases; primary cancers of the gastrointestinal tract (colon, pancreas, esophagus, stomach, neuroendocrine), breast, lung, genitourinary system (kidney, adrenal), ovary, and uterus, melanoma, and sarcomas account for the overwhelming majority of cases. Spread to the liver may be via the systemic or portal venous circulation. The cirrhotic liver, which often gives rise to primary hepatic tumors, seems to be less susceptible than normal liver to implantation of metastases.

Individual tumor types have characteristic patterns of spread. For example, colorectal cancer spreads to the liver as the first site of metastatic disease in a very high proportion of patients; the lung is the next most common site, but bone, brain, or adrenal metastases are distinctly unusual. By contrast, metastatic lung cancer to the liver typically occurs concomitantly with spread to other sites, with brain, bone, and adrenal among the most common. In general, the vast majority of patients with metastases to the liver also have disease at other sites. A notable exception is colorectal cancer, which in many cases involves the liver only for a prolonged period.

▶ Clinical Findings

A. Symptoms and Signs

The signs and symptoms vary with the clinical scenario, disease extent within the liver, and the presence or absence of metastatic disease to other sites. Patients with an undiagnosed primary tumor may come to attention because of symptoms caused by the metastatic disease. Weight loss, fatigue, pain, and anorexia are the presenting general complaints in many such patients. Signs of liver failure, such as ascites and jaundice, are uncommon and suggestive of very advanced cancer. Fever without demonstrable infection is present in 15% of cases. By contrast, patients with a known history of cancer undergoing routine surveillance often develop liver metastases that cause no symptoms; in a small proportion of cases, liver metastases are found on studies done for unrelated reasons.

Physical examination is frequently unrevealing. Hepatomegaly or a palpable tumor in the upper abdomen may be present, and either may be tender. Portal hypertension may be manifested by abdominal venous collaterals or splenomegaly. A friction rub is sometimes heard over the liver.

B. Laboratory Findings

Laboratory values may be entirely normal or, at most, reflect only minor nonspecific changes. Patients with advanced cancer can have anemia and hypoalbuminemia. The alkaline phosphatase is increased in most patients. More significant derangements in liver function occurs in patients with a large volume of liver disease, although this is uncommon at initial presentation. Tumor marker levels (carcinoembryonic antigen [CEA], carbohydrate antigen [CA] 19-9, CA-125) are often elevated, depending on the tumor type, and may be helpful for monitoring treatment.

The diagnosis can be established in most cases by CT-guided or ultrasound-guided percutaneous liver biopsy or fine-needle aspiration for malignant cells.

C. Imaging Studies

The detection of liver metastases relies on contrast-enhanced CT and/or MRI scans. Ultrasonography identifies tumors in the liver and distinguishes solid from cystic lesions but cannot provide the same degree of anatomical detail. MRI provides useful additional information and may help distinguish benign from malignant disease. However, a high-quality multiphase CT scan with intravenous and oral contrast provides excellent assessment of disease extent in the liver and elsewhere in the abdomen. In the past, CT portography was superior to ordinary contrast-enhanced CT and was obtained routinely in patients being considered for hepatic resection, but this is no longer the case. Positron emission tomography using ^{18}F-fluorodeoxyglucose (FDG-PET) is a commonly used staging study for many diseases, but the yield is too low to justify its routine use. A recent randomized study of patients with metastatic colorectal cancer showed essentially no benefit of PET beyond good-quality cross-sectional imaging. As such, routine use of FDG-PET in metastatic colorectal cancer is not cost effective, and its utility is limited to patients with an elevated CEA and negative CT. During surgery, intraoperative ultrasound is used to assess the liver for disease not appreciated on imaging studies.

▶ Treatment

For most patients with metastatic liver disease, chemotherapy is the only treatment option, particularly with coexisting metastases outside the liver. Such therapy is usually not curative but rather palliative. A notable exception is metastatic colorectal cancer, for which resection or other treatments aimed at the liver disease are effective and potentially curative; the recent advent of several active chemotherapeutic agents has further improved the results of treatment. Carefully selected patients with metastases from other primary tumors (sarcoma, breast, ovary, lung, neuroendocrine) may also benefit from resection but represent a small minority of cases.

A. Hepatic Resection

Hepatic resection is most commonly indicated in patients with metastatic colorectal cancer. Of the approximately 130,000 patients diagnosed with colorectal cancer annually in the United States, approximately 50% either have liver metastases at diagnosis or develop liver metastases at some point. In 40% of the latter group, the liver is the only demonstrable site of disease. Hepatic metastases from colorectal cancer thus affect approximately 20,000 patients per year.

After a complete resection of colorectal metastatic liver disease, the 5-year survival rate has historically been 25%-40%. Systemic or regional chemotherapy (eg, hepatic arterial chemotherapy) or both are frequently given before or after resection and appear to enhance the results of surgery, with more recent series reporting 5-year survival rates of approximately 50%. The presence of extrahepatic metastases and inability to achieve a complete resection are contraindications to resection in most cases. However, as more effective chemotherapeutic options have emerged, the indications for resection have expanded to include selected patients with multiple bilobar tumors and even some with extrahepatic metastatic disease. Extensive use of chemotherapy prior to surgery can cause changes in the liver, particularly steatosis and steatohepatitis, which can impair the liver's normal regenerative response. Caution is therefore needed when considering such patients for major hepatic resections, since operative morbidity and mortality may be increased. Preoperative portal vein embolization may reduce the incidence of serious postoperative complications, in particular liver failure.

The following variables are associated with a worse prognosis after resection: (1) node-positive primary disease, (2) multiple liver lesions, (3) less than 1-year interval between resection of the primary colorectal tumor and diagnosis of liver disease (disease-free interval), (4) CEA level higher than 200 ng/mL, and (5) tumor size greater than 5 cm. Variables that do not influence the outcome include (1) histologic grade of the tumor, (2) bilateral rather than unilateral disease, and (3) the gender of the patient. In the past, it was believed that location of the primary tumor within the large intestine was not a predictor of outcome. More recently, however, evidence has suggested that tumors arising from the right colon have a more aggressive biology than those arising from the left. The mortality rate for resection of hepatic metastases is 1%-2% in hospitals where this operation is performed frequently.

The liver is the most common site of cancer recurrence after a complete resection. A small proportion of patients with hepatic recurrence may be amenable to a second resection. The use of adjuvant hepatic arterial chemotherapy appears to reduce the risk of intrahepatic recurrence.

The efficacy of liver resection for colorectal cancer has been clearly established and is the most common indication for this procedure. By contrast, for most other tumor types, particularly those arising from the gastrointestinal tract other than the colon or rectum, the benefit of liver resection is much more limited. Rare patients with metastases from renal cell carcinoma, ovarian cancer, adrenocortical carcinoma, or sarcomas appear to derive the most benefit; by contrast, liver resection for metastatic esophageal, gastric, or pancreatic cancer is almost never warranted. In selecting patients with noncolorectal liver metastases for resection, the most important factors are (1) long disease-free interval, (2) solitary resectable liver tumor, and (3) absence of extrahepatic metastases.

Neuroendocrine carcinomas (pancreatic islet cell tumors, carcinoids) represent a unique class of tumors that often give rise to liver metastases. Unlike patients with other metastatic tumor types, those with neuroendocrine tumors often survive for many years. Multiple liver metastases are the rule with this disease, so complete resection is usually not possible. However, debulking liver resections are sometimes indicated to palliate tumor-related pain or hormonal symptoms in patients with functional tumors. Like HCC, metastatic neuroendocrine tumors may also be treated effectively using HAE. Partial hepatectomy is also sometimes worthwhile to extirpate a tumor invading directly from a contiguous organ.

B. Radiofrequency Ablation

RFA has been used to treat metastases to the liver from a variety of tumor types. The indications for this procedure remain ill defined. The best candidates are those with a limited number of small liver lesions with no evidence of extrahepatic cancer. RFA can also be used as part of a combinatorial approach to treat colorectal liver metastases when resection of all lesions is not feasible.

C. Chemotherapy

In a large proportion of patients with metastatic colorectal cancer, the liver is the only evident site of disease. If the lesions cannot be resected, regional intrahepatic chemotherapy can be given by placing a catheter in the gastroduodenal artery (at its origin with the common hepatic artery) connected to an implantable, subcutaneous infusion pump, which allows the delivery of much higher concentrations of drug to the tumor than is possible with systemic administration. This regimen is generally not used for metastases from other tumor types. The pump is primed with floxuridine, which is delivered by continuous infusion (0.1-0.2 mg/kg/d) for 14-day periods alternating with 14-day rests. Systemic chemotherapy is usually given concomitantly. The discovery of extrahepatic lesions at laparotomy for pump placement is a relative contraindication to proceeding with this approach. Treatment is continued until disease progression or excessive toxicity is seen or, less commonly, until the response is complete. Toxicity consists mainly of gastroduodenal erosions (caused by unintentional perfusion of these areas), chemical hepatitis, or chemical sclerosing cholangitis. Survival is related principally to the initial amount of liver involvement by tumor, objective response to treatment (which is seen in about 80% of patients), and extent of prior chemotherapy. The median survival of patients with less than 30% of liver replaced by tumor is 24 months, compared with 10 months if the extent of replacement exceeds 30%. Up to 47% of patients with initially unresectable disease may respond enough to become resectable and potentially benefit from surgery. There is a general perception that hepatic artery infusion therapy improves survival, but the objective evidence is inconclusive.

Hepatic artery infusion chemotherapy may be a useful adjunctive therapy after complete tumor resection. Systemic chemotherapy (eg, with fluorouracil, irinotecan, or oxaliplatin) after complete resection of liver metastases has not been proven to improve survival, although it is often prescribed. Systemic chemotherapy can be given concomitantly with hepatic artery infusion chemotherapy; median overall survival is 67 months with combined pump and modern systemic chemotherapy.

D. Miscellaneous

Hepatic artery ligation or angiographic embolization of the tumor has been of benefit in a few patients with hepatic metastases from specific tumor types, particularly neuroendocrine tumors.

▶ Prognosis

Survival varies with the site of origin of the primary tumor and the extent of metastatic disease. Patients with extensive hepatic replacement by multiple lesions have a dismal outlook, with a survival measured in months, compared to perhaps 2-3 years for patients with small solitary lesions. The range of treatment options and effective chemotherapeutic agents is greatest for metastatic colorectal cancer compared to most other tumor types, and survival is generally better in this group.

Brouquet A, et al: High survival rate after two-stage resection of advanced colorectal liver metastases: response-based selection and complete resection define outcome. J Clin Oncol. 2011; 29:1083.

Cho CS, et al: Histologic grade is correlated with outcome after resection of hepatic neuroendocrine neoplasms. Cancer. 2008; 113:126.

Fong Y, et al: Clinical score for predicting recurrence after hepatic resection for metastatic colorectal cancer: analysis of 1001 consecutive cases. Ann Surg. 1999;230(3):309-318.

Groot Koerkamp B, et al: Perioperative hepatic arterial infusion pump chemotherapy is associated with longer survival after resection of colorectal liver metastases: a propensity score analysis. J Clin Oncol. 2017;35(17):1938-1944.

Kemeny NE, et al: Conversion to resectability using hepatic artery infusion plus systemic chemotherapy for the treatment of unresectable liver metastases from colorectal carcinoma. J Clin Oncol. 2009;27:3465.

Kingham TP, et al: Hepatic parenchymal preservation surgery: decreasing morbidity and mortality rates in 4,152 resections for malignancy. J Am Coll Surg. 2015;220(4):471-479.

Moulton CA, et al: Effect of PET before liver resection on surgical management for colorectal adenocarcinoma metastases: a randomized clinical trial. JAMA. 2014;311(18):1863-1869.

Nordlinger B, et al: Perioperative FOLFOX4 chemotherapy and surgery versus surgery alone for resectable liver metastases from colorectal cancer (EORTC 40983): long-term results of a randomized, controlled, phase 3 trial. Lancet Oncol. 2013;14(12):1208-1215.

Pak LM, et al: Prospective phase II trial of combination hepatic artery infusion and systemic chemotherapy for unresectable colorectal liver metastases: long term results and curative potential. J Surg Oncol. 2018;117(4):634-643.

Tomlinson JS, et al: Actual 10-year survival after resection of colorectal liver metastases defines cure. J Clin Oncol. 2007;25:4575.

Wong SL, et al: American Society of Clinical Oncology 2009 clinical evidence review on radiofrequency ablation of hepatic metastases from colorectal cancer. J Clin Oncol. 2010;28:493.

BENIGN TUMORS & CYSTS OF THE LIVER

▶ Hemangiomas

Hemangioma is the most common benign hepatic tumor, with an incidence of approximately 7%. Except for the skin and mucous membranes, the liver is the most common site of origin. Women are affected more often than men—in some series, up to 75% of patients are female. Histologically, hepatic hemangiomas are of the cavernous type rather than the capillary type. Most are small, solitary, subcapsular asymptomatic growths that are found incidentally during laparotomy or autopsy or on imaging studies. Rarely, hemangiomata grow to very large dimensions (giant hemangiomata) and cause abdominal pain or a palpable mass. Most are small to moderate-sized lesions, however; pain is uncommon in tumors smaller than 8-10 cm in diameter.

Rare complications of liver hemangiomata include hemorrhagic shock resulting from spontaneous rupture and the Kasabach-Merritt syndrome, which is usually seen in children. Kasabach-Merritt syndrome is a rare but devastating complication where a large or rapidly growing hemangioma traps platelets, leading to consumptive thrombocytopenia and eventually consumptive coagulopathy and disseminated intravascular coagulation. This can be triggered by simple dental procedures or other surgeries and is associated with high morbidity and mortality. Large congenital hemangiomas of the liver may be associated with others in the skin. Large hemangiomata may also give rise to large-volume arteriovenous shunting, resulting in cardiac hypertrophy and congestive heart failure.

Large-bore needle biopsy is hazardous due to bleeding risks. Fortunately, biopsy is very rarely indicated because the diagnosis can be made in most cases by contrast-enhanced CT or MRI scans. The hallmark features of hemangiomata are nodular peripheral enhancement on arterial phase with progressive central enhancement on the more delayed images. MRI is a particularly good study for hemangiomata, which appear very bright on the T2-weighted images, and combined with dynamic intravenous contrast, it has a sensitivity and specificity of 98%. Angiography is unnecessary, and nuclear scans lack sufficient sensitivity and specificity.

Deciphering hemangiomata-derived symptoms is critical because this is one of the few indications for surgical intervention. Irrespective of their size, the only reasons to resect hemangiomata are for symptoms, most commonly pain, or diagnostic uncertainty (rare). Symptomatic hemangiomas should be excised by lobectomy or enucleation; however, enucleation is more common. Anatomic resection is typically reserved in cases of diagnostic uncertainty or very large lesions. Hepatic hemangioma blood supply is derived mainly from the hepatic artery; therefore, early control of the hepatic artery during enucleation can minimize blood loss. Even large lesions can be safely enucleated. Radiotherapy or embolization via a catheter in the hepatic artery may be tried in patients who are poor candidates for surgery, but the efficacy of these approaches is limited. The natural history of asymptomatic hemangiomas, whether large or small, is benign. The vast majority of incidentally discovered hemangiomata remain stable in follow-up, do not give rise to symptoms, and therefore do not require resection.

Concejero AM, et al: Giant cavernous hemangioma of the liver with coagulopathy: adult Kasabach-Merritt syndrome. *Surgery.* 2009;145:245.

Duxbury MS, et al: Giant haemangioma of the liver: observation or resection? *Dig Surg.* 2010;27:7.

Liu Y, et al: Enucleation versus anatomic resection for giant hepatic hemangioma: a meta-analysis. *Gastrointest Tumors.* 2017;3(3-4):153.

Van den Bos IC, et al: Magnetic resonance imaging of liver lesions: exceptions and atypical lesions. *Curr Probl Diagn Radiol.* 2008; 37:95.

▶ Cysts

A number of different cystic lesions may affect the liver. Simple hepatic cysts, the most common, are unilocular fluid-filled lesions that generally produce no symptoms. The occasional large cyst may present as an upper abdominal mass or discomfort. Small, simple cysts may be difficult to diagnose on CT and may be confused for metastatic disease; ultrasound and MRI are better modalities to assess the character of cystic lesions. Many patients have multiple simple cysts, which should not be confused with polycystic liver disease,

a progressive condition characterized by cystic replacement of virtually the entire liver. Polycystic liver disease is associated in about half of cases with polycystic renal disease. The possibility of echinococcus (see Chapter 8) should be considered in patients with cystic liver lesions and the appropriate exposure history, although their radiographic appearance is usually quite distinctive.

Most simple cysts have a serous lining and a smooth, thin wall. Intracystic hemorrhage can occur, which can confuse the radiographic appearance. Solitary cysts lined with cuboidal epithelium are classified as cystadenomas and are premalignant. Cystadenomas are characterized radiographically as complex, with internal septae, an irregular lining, and papillary projections. The vast majority of these lesions contain ovarian stroma and are more commonly seen in females. Complex, multilocular (septated) cysts (if not echinococcal) are often neoplastic and should be resected. However, cystadenomas and cystadenocarcinomas are rare, whereas internal hemorrhage into a simple cyst is a more common entity and may have a similar appearance. Nevertheless, complex cysts of the liver must be approached with some caution in order to avoid inappropriate interventions. Unlike simple cysts, fenestration and fulguration of cystadenoma is not recommended. Rather, complete resection is needed given the possibility of neoplastic disease and to limit the likelihood of recurrence. Complete resection of cystadenocarcinoma with negative margins is indicated. There are few indications for aspirating hepatic cysts—simple cysts reaccumulate fluid quickly, neoplastic cysts must be excised, and parasitic cysts might rupture and the parasite thus be allowed to spread. It is possible to eliminate small cysts by aspiration of the contents followed by an injection into the lumen of 20-100 mL of absolute alcohol; however, care must be taken to ensure that there is no communication with the biliary tract prior to ethanol injection, which could lead to biliary sclerosis. Small cysts almost never cause symptoms and generally require no treatment.

Large symptomatic simple cysts are difficult to eradicate with alcohol injections, and serious superinfection of the cyst cavity may occur. The simplest method of treatment consists of laparoscopic cyst fenestration (wide excision of the cyst wall). A tongue of omentum may be fixed so it lies in the residual cyst cavity as an ancillary measure to prevent the edges from coapting. The operation is curative in nearly all patients.

Multiple, small, simple cysts do not usually require treatment, but large polycystic livers that cause discomfort or are associated with obstructive jaundice can be managed by partial resection or surgically unroofing the cysts on the surface of the liver and creating windows between superficial cysts and adjacent deep cysts. The opened cysts are allowed to drain into the abdominal cavity. The results of surgery for polycystic liver disease are often disappointing, with quick return of symptoms in many patients.

Choi HK, et al: Differential diagnosis for intrahepatic biliary cystadenoma and hepatic simple cyst: significance of cystic fluid analysis and radiologic findings. *J Clin Gastroenterol.* 2010;44:289.

Del Poggio P, et al: Cystic tumors of the liver: a practical approach. *World J Gastroenterol.* 2008;14:3616.

Doussot A, et al: The accuracy of pre-operative imaging in the management of hepatic cysts. *HPB (Oxford).* 2015;17(10):889-895.

Kelly K, et al: Cystic diseased of the liber and bile ducts. *J Gastrointest Surg.* 2014;18(3):627-634.

Soares KC, et al: Cystic neoplasms of the liver: biliary cystadenoma and cystadenocarcinoma. *J Am Coll Surg.* 2014;218(1):119-128.

Hepatic Adenoma

Hepatic adenomas occur predominantly in women of child-bearing age and appear to be related to the use of oral contraceptives. The tumors are soft, yellow-tan, well-circumscribed masses that are usually of moderate size (range of 2-15 cm in diameter). Most adenomas that cause symptoms are in the 8- to 15-cm range. Two-thirds of hepatic adenomas are solitary; other benign tumors (eg, focal nodular hyperplasia; see next section) are present in some cases. Transition from benign hepatic adenoma to HCC is estimated to occur in 5% of cases, with liver cell dysplasia as an intermediate step. Histologically, hepatic adenomas consist of an encapsulated homogeneous mass of normal-appearing hepatocytes without bile ducts or central veins. Intratumoral hemorrhage or central necrosis may be present.

Hepatic adenomas can be further divided into four subtypes according to their genetic and pathologic features: hepatocyte nuclear factor-1α mutated, β-catenin mutated, inflammatory hepatic adenomas, and unclassified. B-Catenin–mutated hepatic adenomas represent 10% of all hepatic adenomas and are associated with an increased risk of malignant transformation to HCC. Inflammatory hepatic adenomas are most common (50% of hepatic adenomas), whereas unclassified adenomas represent less than 10% of all hepatic adenomas and have the highest risk of bleeding.

Most patients are asymptomatic. Those with symptoms present with right upper quadrant pain. Spontaneous hemorrhage into the substance of the tumor with subsequent rupture and intraperitoneal bleeding is a well-known potential complication of adenomas. The true risk of spontaneous hemorrhage is difficult to know with certainty, since the overall incidence of adenomas is unknown. This risk increases with size, and there appears to be a strong association of acute bleeding episodes from adenoma with pregnancy. Patients with this life-threatening problem present with acute pain or even hemorrhagic shock.

Liver function tests and AFP levels are usually normal or minimally deranged. Adenomas typically appear hypervascular compared to the surrounding liver parenchyma, a feature that is apparent on contrast-enhanced CT or MRI scans or angiography. Adenomas can be difficult to distinguish from focal nodular hyperplasia, another benign tumor often found in young women. Differences in tumor vascularity may be demonstrated on angiography; however, MRI is probably the best study for differentiating these lesions. Adenomas often cannot be distinguished from well-differentiated HCC on imaging studies and even on biopsy specimens. Needle biopsy is generally safe but often inconclusive and is associated with a small risk of bleeding.

The general recommendation is that adenomas above 5 cm in size should be resected because of the risks of malignant change and spontaneous hemorrhage. Unfortunately, the true likelihood of these events is difficult to estimate, since most series include only treated patients. Lesions measuring less than 5 cm can be observed with serial imaging since the risk of malignant transformation or bleeding at this size appears minimal. Symptomatic and large asymptomatic adenomas clearly should be resected. HAE of the feeding vessel is recommended in hemodynamically stable patients with evidence of hemorrhage. Unstable patients are probably best managed in the operating room, where resuscitation can be carried out along with exploration and achievement of hemostasis; if feasible, the tumor should be resected. Tumor regression after embolization is not uncommon; therefore, lesions are reassessed with cross-sectional imaging. Resection is performed weeks to months after the bleeding event in adenomas remaining greater than 5 cm in size or with concern for malignancy. Small peripheral lesions may be removed with wedge excisions, but larger tumors require more extensive resections. Small adenomas may regress when oral contraceptive agents are discontinued, and close follow-up with imaging studies is not unreasonable in such cases; however, any change in symptoms or imaging characteristics (growth, hemorrhage) should prompt resection. The possibility that a presumed adenoma is actually a well-differentiated HCC or contains a focus of malignancy must always be kept in mind; there is no completely reliable means of making the differentiation other than pathologic analysis of the resected specimen.

Most patients recover without sequelae after surgical removal; recurrence is rare. Oral contraceptives should be avoided permanently in all cases. Radiotherapy and chemotherapy are of no value, but elective HAE may be helpful in patients who are not surgical candidates. Embolization may be particularly helpful in the very rare patient with multiple hepatic adenomas (hepatic adenomatosis), since resection is usually not possible.

Focal Nodular Hyperplasia

Focal nodular hyperplasia (FNH) is the second most common benign liver process after hemangioma. Like hepatic adenoma, FNH is much more common in young women. The average age is about 40 years, but the tumor can occur at any age. Unlike hepatic adenoma, however, the use of oral contraceptive agents does not appear to predispose to the development of FNH, although it has been suggested that these agents may stimulate growth.

Grossly, the tumor is a well-circumscribed, firm, tan, usually subcapsular mass measuring 2-3 cm in diameter. In patients with symptoms, the lesions are much larger, usually around 10 cm. Multiple tumors can occur; however, 80% are solitary. The gross appearance on cut section is quite characteristic, consisting of a central stellate scar (which is actually an aggregation of blood vessels) with radiating fibrous septa that compartmentalize the lesion into lobules. Histologically, there are nodular aggregations of normal-appearing hepatocytes without central veins or portal triads. Bile duct proliferation is present in the nodules.

Most patients with FNH are asymptomatic. The few with symptoms present with right upper quadrant discomfort. Unlike hepatic adenomas, these lesions rarely, if ever, bleed, and the natural history of asymptomatic lesions is benign. Very few patients with diffuse FNH develop portal hypertension.

Hepatic function tests and AFP levels are usually normal. Hepatic scintiscans usually do not show a filling defect but are of little practical value. CT scans demonstrate the tumor and may also show the central stellate scar. The arteriographic pattern is one of hypervascularity. In most cases, the diagnosis of FNH can be made with noninvasive studies, although distinguishing FNH from hepatic adenomas can be difficult, even for experienced radiologists. MRI scanning is the best modality, but the imaging features of both tumors overlap somewhat, and they occur in similar patient populations. Fine-needle aspiration biopsies are generally not helpful.

Symptomatic lesions should be removed, whereas asymptomatic tumors (the majority) should be left undisturbed, provided that the diagnosis has been made confidently. In the latter circumstance, a period of observation with imaging studies is recommended to ensure stability. Inability to distinguish FNH from adenoma or malignant disease is an indication for resection in some patients. Discontinuation of oral contraceptives probably has no impact. FNH can be reliably identified on examination of frozen sections.

Cho SW, et al: Surgical management of hepatocellular adenoma: take it or leave it. *Ann Surg Oncol.* 2008;15:2795.

Dokmak S, et al: A single-center surgical experience of 122 patients with single and multiple hepatocellular adenomas. *Gastroenterology.* 2009;137:1698.

Grazioli L, et al: Hepatocellular adenoma and focal nodular hyperplasia: value of gadoxetic acid-enhanced MR imaging in differential diagnosis. *Radiology.* 2012;262:520.

Torbenson M: Hepatic adenomas: classification, controversies, and consensus. *Surg Pathol Clin.* 2018;11(2):351-366.

Tsillimigras DI, et al: Current approaches in the management of hepatic adenomas. *J Gastrointest Surg.* 2019;23(1):199-209.

CIRRHOSIS

Hepatic cirrhosis remains a major public health problem worldwide, with an annual mortality of approximately 23,000 per year in the United States alone. The incidence of cirrhosis is increasing, due in large measure to hepatitis C, and at present is the third most common cause of death in men in the fifth decade of life. Another contributing factor is the epidemic of obesity, which is associated with nonalcoholic fatty liver disease and progression to cirrhosis in many patients.

Alcohol abuse remains the leading cause of cirrhosis in most Western countries. Alcohol exerts direct toxic effects on the liver that are magnified in the presence of protein and other dietary deficiencies that are often present. Even still, cirrhosis develops in a small minority of patients who abuse alcohol. Alcohol induces a specific cytochrome P450 in the liver (ie, P450 2E1) that participates in its metabolism to acetaldehyde, which has a number of deleterious effects, including antibody formation, decreased DNA repair, enzyme inactivation, and alterations in microtubules, mitochondria, and plasma membranes. Acetaldehyde also promotes glutathione depletion, free radical–mediated toxicity, lipid peroxidation, and hepatic collagen synthesis. Hepatic steatosis and alcoholic hepatitis are stages of alcoholic liver injury that may precede cirrhosis. Alcoholic hyalin, a glycoprotein, accumulates in centrilobular hepatocytes of patients with alcoholic hepatitis. There is some evidence that immunologic responses to alcoholic hyalin may be important in the pathogenesis of cirrhosis.

Regardless of the cause (Table 26–3), collagen deposition in cirrhosis results from increased fibroblastic activity as well as

Table 26–3. Causes of cirrhosis.

I. Drugs and toxins   Alcohol, methotrexate, isoniazid, methyldopa, amiodarone
II. Infections   Viral hepatitis, schistosomiasis
III. Autoimmune disorders   Autoimmune hepatitis, primary biliary cirrhosis, primary sclerosing cholangitis
IV. Inherited metabolic defects   Hemochromatosis, Wilson disease, α_1-antitrypsin deficiency, galactosemia, tyrosinemia, glycogen storage disease, hereditary fructose intolerance, urea cycle disorders, alpha-/beta-lipoproteinemia, progressive familial intrahepatic cholestasis, cystic fibrosis
V. Acquired bile duct disease   Biliary atresia, gallstone obstruction, common bile duct benign stricture
VI. Vascular disorders   Budd-Chiari syndrome, veno-occlusive disease, congestive heart failure, hereditary hemorrhagic telangiectasia
VII. Miscellaneous   Nonalcoholic steatohepatitis (NASH), total parenteral nutrition, Indian childhood cirrhosis, intestinal bypass surgery, hypervitaminosis A, sarcoidosis, cryptogenic

Modified with permission from Jarnagin WR et al: *Blumgart's Surgery of the Liver, Biliary Tract, and Pancreas*, 5th ed. Philadelphia, PA: Elsevier Saunders; 2012.

from repair following hepatocellular injury and necrosis. The ultimate result is a liver containing regenerative nodules and connective tissue septa linking portal fields with central canals. Liver biopsy for cirrhosis has a sensitivity of 80%-100%; however, it is not necessary in the setting of laboratory, radiologic, and clinical data consistent with this diagnosis. However, a liver biopsy can sometimes determine the cause of cirrhosis when the underlying etiology is unknown, such as hemochromatosis, nonalcoholic fatty liver disease, and Wilson disease.

The natural history of cirrhosis is difficult to predict. Once the diagnosis has been established, up to 30% of patients die within a year from hepatic failure or complications of portal hypertension, of which bleeding esophageal varices is the most feared. In newly diagnosed cirrhotics, the chances of dying within the subsequent 2-3 years are influenced by the status of liver function (as reflected by the Child-Pugh classification, Table 26–1), the presence of varices, and the portal pressure. A group of cirrhotics with varices followed by the Boston Interhospital Liver Group experienced a 1-year death rate of 66%. Cirrhotics without varices may benefit substantially by abstaining from alcohol. Bleeding episodes occur in up to 40% of all patients with cirrhosis, and the initial episode of variceal hemorrhage is fatal in 50% or more. At least two-thirds of those who survive their initial hemorrhage bleed again, and the risk of dying from the second hemorrhage is similarly high. It is principally for such patients that portal decompressive procedures are recommended.

Other main complications of cirrhosis include ascites, hepatorenal syndrome with hyponatremia and renal insufficiency, coagulopathy and encephalopathy. Those processes are mainly managed medically to maintain a state of relative physiologic compensation. Liver transplantation for eligible candidates provides the most effective treatment option associated with prolongation of survival.

Bravo AA, et al: Liver biopsy. *N Engl J Med.* 2001;344(7):495-500.

Ginès P, et al: Renal failure in cirrhosis. *N Engl J Med.* 2009;361:1279.

Rahimi RS, et al: Complications of cirrhosis. *Curr Opin Gastroenterol.* 2012;28:223.

Reuben A: Alcohol and the liver. *Curr Opin Gastroenterol.* 2008;24:328.

Schuppan D, et al: Liver cirrhosis. *Lancet.* 2008;371:838.

Tripodi A, Mannucci PM: The coagulopathy of chronic liver disease. *N Engl J Med.* 2011;365:147.

Wong F: Management of ascites in cirrhosis. *J Gastroenterol Hepatol.* 2012;27:11.

Wong RJ, et al: Nonalcoholic steatohepatitis is the second leading etiology of liver disease among adults awaiting liver transplantation in the United States. *Gastroenterology.* 2015;148(3):547-555.

PORTAL HYPERTENSION

▶ Etiology

The major causes of portal hypertension are listed in Table 26–4. In all but a few instances, the basic lesion is associated with increased resistance to portal flow. Those associated with increased resistance can be subclassified according to the site of the block as prehepatic, hepatic, and posthepatic; hepatic causes of portal hypertension are further subclassified as presinusoidal, sinusoidal, and postsinusoidal. Cirrhosis accounts for about 85% of cases of portal hypertension in the United States, most commonly from heavy alcohol use. Postnecrotic cirrhosis is next in frequency, followed by biliary cirrhosis. The other intrahepatic causes of portal hypertension are relatively rare in Western countries, although in some parts of the world, hepatic schistosomiasis constitutes the largest single group. Idiopathic portal hypertension occurs with greater frequency in southern Asia.

After cirrhosis, extrahepatic portal venous thrombosis or occlusion is the most common cause of portal hypertension in the United States. Patients with this condition are

Table 26–4. Causes of portal hypertension.

I. **Increased resistance to flow**
  A. **Prehepatic (portal vein obstruction)**
    1. Congenital atresia or stenosis
    2. Thrombosis of portal vein
    3. Thrombosis of splenic vein
    4. Extrinsic compression (eg, tumors)
  B. **Hepatic**
    1. Cirrhosis
      a. Portal cirrhosis (nutritional, alcoholic, Laënnec)
      b. Postnecrotic cirrhosis
      c. Biliary cirrhosis
      d. Others (Wilson disease, hemochromatosis)
    2. Acute alcoholic liver disease
    3. Chronic active hepatitis
    4. Congenital hepatic fibrosis
    5. Idiopathic portal hypertension (hepatoportal sclerosis)
    6. Schistosomiasis
    7. Sarcoidosis
  C. **Posthepatic**
    1. Budd-Chiari syndrome (hepatic vein thrombosis)
    2. Veno-occlusive disease
    3. Cardiac disease
      a. Constrictive pericarditis
      b. Valvular heart disease
      c. Right heart failure
II. **Increased portal blood flow**
  A. **Arterial-portal venous fistula**
  B. **Increased splenic flow**
    1. Banti syndrome
    2. Splenomegaly (eg, tropical splenomegaly, myeloid metaplasia)

generally younger than cirrhotics, and many are children. Posthepatic obstruction due to Budd-Chiari syndrome or constrictive pericarditis is rare.

Pathophysiology

Portal hypertension is defined as a hepatic venous pressure gradient (the difference between portal vein pressure and hepatic vein pressure) greater than 5 mm Hg, but hypertension usually becomes clinically significant when this gradient reaches 10 mm Hg. Portal venous pressure normally ranges from 7 to 10 mm Hg. In portal hypertension, portal pressure exceeds 10 mm Hg, averaging around 20 mm Hg and occasionally rising as high as 50-60 mm Hg. With those portal pressures, since the venous pressure in the right atrium averages 5 mm Hg, the hepatic venous pressure gradient can easily become greater than 5 mm Hg.

Because pressure in the portal venous system is determined by the relationship Pressure = Flow × Resistance, portal hypertension could result either from increased volume of portal blood flow or increased resistance to flow. Portal hypertension can be classified by pathophysiologic processes, as summarized in Table 26–4. A catheter wedged in a tributary of the hepatic vein permits estimation of the pressure in the afferent veins to the sinusoid. The gradient between the wedged pressure and that in the hepatic vein reflects resistance at any point between the wedged position and the periphery of the sinusoid. The current view holds that the site of principal resistance in normal persons is in reasonably large hepatic veins. In cirrhosis, it is probably in the sinusoids as well as the hepatic veins.

In practice, however, the liver has tremendous reserve capacity to accommodate increased blood flow, and portal hypertension solely due to this mechanism is extremely uncommon. Increased flow may contribute to portal hypertension in patients with arterial-portal venous fistulae (traumatic, congenital). When an arteriovenous fistula occurs, portal hypertension and its clinical manifestations usually do not appear for several months because sinusoidal capacity is so great that the immediate rise in portal pressure is only moderate. With time, however, sinusoidal sclerosis develops, resistance increases, and portal pressure gradually reaches high levels, leading to the formation of varices.

Nearly all clinically relevant cases of portal hypertension result from increased resistance, in itself due to both structural distortion of the liver vascular architecture by fibrosis and dynamic increases in hepatic vascular tone. In addition to increased vascular resistance in the liver, splanchnic vascular bed resistance decreases, a consequence of local production of vasodilators (eg, nitric oxide) and mesenteric angiogenesis, paradoxically worsening the portal hypertension by increasing the splanchnic blood flow to the liver.

The average portal flow in cirrhotic patients with complications of portal hypertension is nonetheless about 30% of normal, ranging from 0 to 700 mL/min. Hepatic arterial flow is usually reduced by a similar proportion. The range of portal flow rates in different patients may vary greatly; in some, blood in the portal vein moves sluggishly or the direction of flow may even be reversed (hepatofugal) so that the portal vein functions as an outflow tract from the liver. These states of low flow predispose to spontaneous thrombosis of the portal vein, a complication of cirrhosis seen in 16% of patients with advanced liver disease per year. Portal thrombosis usually is associated with acute clinical deterioration and renders the portal vein unsuitable for a shunt to decompress the portal venous system.

Fluctuations in the level of portal hypertension may occur in conjunction with changes in blood volume. This is almost never a problem in patients with a normal liver. However, administration of colloid solutions to a patient with underlying liver disease and a normal or expanded blood volume could theoretically aggravate the clinical manifestations of portal hypertension.

Disease-Specific Pathophysiology

In **alcoholic liver disease,** the abnormal resistance is predominantly hepatic and postsinusoidal, as indicated by the results of wedged hepatic vein pressure studies. The causes of increased resistance in this disease are thought to be (1) distortion of the hepatic veins by regenerative nodules and (2) fibrosis of perivascular tissue around the hepatic veins and the sinusoids.

Even in the absence of cirrhosis, acute alcoholic hepatitis can raise portal pressure by producing centrilobular swelling and fibrosis. Sinusoidal resistance to flow is also increased by engorgement of adjacent hepatocytes with fat and resultant distortion and narrowing of vascular channels. Documented cases of normalization or reduction in portal pressure have occurred with resolution of the pathologic changes.

Schistosomiasis can produce a unique form of hepatic presinusoidal obstruction to blood flow from deposition of parasite ova in small portal venules. The subsequent chronic inflammatory reaction leads to fibrosis and cirrhosis. Many patients with schistosomiasis are also at risk for chronic hepatitis, which can exacerbate the liver damage.

Budd-Chiari syndrome (hepatic vein thrombosis) results from obstruction of flow through the hepatic veins. The resulting sinusoidal hypertension produces prominent ascites and hepatomegaly. Conditions (veno-occlusive disease, inferior vena cava obstruction by tumor or congenital webs, right-sided heart failure) that reduce flow through the hepatic veins result in a similar clinical picture.

Banti syndrome was defined as liver disease secondary to primary splenic disease and was incorrectly considered as the cause of portal hypertension now known to result from cirrhosis and other hepatic disorders rather than a consequence of such conditions. Portal hypertension from splenomegaly and increased splenic vein flow has been described in patients with hematologic diseases or tropical splenomegaly and apparently normal liver function. This is extremely uncommon, however, and given the great reserve of the liver to handle increases in portal flow, many such patients probably have some component of liver disease. In cirrhosis, the increased splenic blood flow accompanying "congestive" splenomegaly may occasionally be great enough to warrant splenic artery ligation or splenectomy to decrease portal pressure and improve symptoms, but this situation is rare.

Development of Portosystemic Collaterals and Varices

The obstacle to flow through the liver promotes expansion of collateral channels between the portal and systemic venous systems. As the pathologic process develops, portal pressure increases until a level of about 40 cm H_2O (30 mm Hg) is reached. At this point, increasing hepatic resistance, even to the point of occlusion of the portal vein, diverts a greater fraction of portal flow through collaterals without significant increments in portal pressure.

The type of portosystemic collaterals that develops depends partly on the cause of the portal hypertension. In extrahepatic portal vein thrombosis (without liver disease), collaterals in the diaphragm and in the hepatocolic, hepatoduodenal, and gastrohepatic ligaments transport blood into the liver around the occluded vein (hepatopetal). In cirrhosis, collateral vessels circumvent the liver and deliver portal blood directly into the systemic circulation (hepatofugal); these collaterals give rise to esophageal and gastric varices. Other common spontaneous collaterals are through a recanalized umbilical vein to the abdominal wall, from the superior hemorrhoidal vein into the middle and inferior hemorrhoidal veins, and through numerous small veins (of Retzius) connecting the retroperitoneal viscera with the posterior abdominal wall.

Isolated thrombosis of the splenic vein causes localized splenic venous hypertension and gives rise to large collaterals from spleen to gastric fundus (sinistral, or left-sided, portal hypertension). From there, the blood returns to the main portal system through the coronary vein. In this condition, gastric varices are often present without esophageal varices.

Of the many large collaterals that form as a result of portal hypertension, spontaneous bleeding is relatively uncommon except from those at the gastroesophageal junction. Spontaneous bleeding from gastric varices can sometimes occur and carries a higher rate of death than gastroesophageal varices. Compared with adjacent areas of the esophagus and stomach, the gastroesophageal junction is especially rich in submucosal veins, which expand disproportionately in patients with portal hypertension. The cause of variceal bleeding is most probably rupture due to sudden increases in hydrostatic pressure. Esophagitis is usually mild or absent.

Berzigotti A, et al: Assessing portal hypertension in liver diseases. *Expert Rev Gastroenterol Hepatol.* 2013;7(2):141-155.
Garcia-Pagan JC, et al: Portal vein thrombosis: a predictable milestone in cirrhosis? *J Hepatol.* 2009;51:632.
Hackl C, et al: Liver surgery in cirrhosis and portal hypertension. *World J Gastroenterol.* 2016;22(9):2725-2735.
Merkel C, et al: Hepatic venous pressure gradient measurement in clinical hepatology. *Dig Liver Dis.* 2011;43:762.

ACUTELY BLEEDING VARICES

Varices develop in 5%-15% of cirrhotic patients per year. Most patients with cirrhosis develop varices, but only about one-third experience variceal hemorrhage. Each bleeding episode is associated with a mortality rate of up to 25%, and 70% of untreated patients die within a year of the first episode. This high death rate reflects not only the massive hemorrhage but also the frequent presence of severely compromised liver function and other systemic disease. Malnutrition, pulmonary aspiration, infections, and coronary artery disease are frequent coexisting conditions. Additional complicating factors in this patient population include lack of cooperation with treatment and acute alcohol withdrawal, which in its worst manifestation (delirium tremens) adds greatly to the already high mortality rate.

Clinical Findings

A. Symptoms and Signs

If cirrhosis or varices have been documented on previous examinations, hematemesis would strongly suggest bleeding varices as the cause. Patient with significant hemorrhage present with alteration of mental status, with hypotension and tachycardia, and often in hypovolemic shock. It must be emphasized that bleeding from varices cannot be accurately diagnosed on clinical grounds alone even though the history or the appearance of the patient may strongly suggest the presence of cirrhosis or portal hypertension. Most patients with bleeding varices have alcoholic cirrhosis, and the diagnosis may seem obvious in a patient with hepatomegaly, jaundice, and vascular spiders who admits to recent binge drinking. Splenomegaly, the most constant physical finding, is present in 80% of patients with portal hypertension regardless of the cause. Ascites is frequently present. Massive ascites and hepatosplenomegaly in a nonalcoholic would suggest the much less common Budd-Chiari syndrome.

B. Laboratory Findings

Most patients with alcoholic liver disease and acute upper gastrointestinal bleeding have compromised liver function. The bilirubin is usually elevated, and the serum albumin is often below 3 g/dL. The leukocyte count may be elevated. Anemia may be a reflection of chronic alcoholic liver disease or hypersplenism as well as acute hemorrhage. The development of a hepatoma by a cirrhotic may first manifest by hemorrhage from varices; CT scan and marked elevation of the serum AFP make the diagnosis. Thrombocytopenia and coagulopathy are common.

▶ Treatment of Acute Bleeding

The general goal of treatment is to control the bleeding as quickly and reliably as possible using methods with the fewest possible side effects. The methods in use for acute variceal bleeding are listed in Table 26–5 and presented as a current treatment algorithm in Figure 26–7. Over the past few decades, improvement in medical, endoscopic, and endovascular techniques studied in the setting of randomized controlled trials has lessened the need for surgical interventions to the point that they are rarely used.

The initial management of the patient with massive gastrointestinal hemorrhage is discussed in Chapter 25. Critical initial steps include airway protection, particularly in patients with altered mental status or those with hemodynamic instability, and resuscitation with blood products. In cirrhotic patients, correction of coagulopathy and thrombocytopenia should also be initiated early. Patients admitted with variceal hemorrhage are often bacteremic as a result of a concomitant infectious process (spontaneous bacterial peritonitis, urinary tract infection, or pneumonia). Clinical trials have shown better outcomes when empiric antibiotic

Table 26–5. First-line management of acute bleeding from esophageal varices.

1. **Medical: vasoconstrictor**
   Somatostatin analogues
   Vasopressin, terlipressin
2. **Medical: antibiotic prophylaxis**
   Norfloxacin, ciprofloxacin
   Ceftriaxone (if doubt of quinolone resistance)
3. **Interventional, nonsurgical**
   Endoscopic variceal ligation
   Transjugular intrahepatic portosystemic shunt (TIPSS)
4. **Mechanical**
   Balloon tamponade (Sengstaken-Blakemore)
5. **Surgical**
   Emergency portosystemic shunts
   Esophageal transection and reanastomosis
   Esophagogastric devascularization
   Suture ligation of varices

▲ **Figure 26–7.** Algorithm for the management of acute variceal bleeding. TIPS, transjugular intrahepatic portosystemic shunt.

therapy is initiated during an episode of variceal bleed, and usually a third-generation cephalosporin such as ceftriaxone is favored.

Vasoconstrictive drugs that reduce portal pressure (somatostatin and vasopressin analogues) and endoscopic variceal ablation (ligation and sclerotherapy) are the mainstay of initial management. The combined pharmacologic and endoscopic therapy has been shown in single trials and meta-analyses to be more effective in controlling acute bleeding than endoscopic treatment alone. With this initial strategy, control of bleeding can be achieved in 80%-85% of episodes. Endoscopic intervention requires a skilled endoscopist; banding has been shown to be effective and is considered the treatment of choice, although very profuse bleeding makes ligation a challenge, and sclerotherapy with cyanoacrylate may be useful in this setting if special expertise is available. Balloon tamponade is no longer used routinely but is rather reserved for failure of the pharmacologic/endoscopic therapy for hemodynamically unstable patients and when the next line of treatment cannot readily be implemented.

The failure rate of standard medical therapy for all comers is 10%-20% and is highest in patients with Child-Pugh class C disease. Early rebleeding is reported in up to 30% of patients. Placement of a transjugular intrahepatic portosystemic shunt (TIPSS) is currently considered the salvage therapy of choice in this situation. TIPSS may not be an option in some instances, for example, in the presence of portal thrombosis, in which case surgical shunt or devascularization procedures are indicated.

Death rates rise rapidly in patients requiring more than 10 units of blood, and in general, patients still bleeding after 6 units—or those whose bleeding is still unchecked 24 hours after admission—should be considered for portal decompression procedures. Even when the bleeding is brought under control by the initial intervention, the mortality rate remains high (about 35%) as a result of liver failure and other complications.

Specific Measures

1. Acute endoscopic sclerotherapy or ligation—Emergency esophagogastroscopy is the most useful procedure for the diagnosis and the treatment of bleeding varices and should be performed as soon as the patient's general condition is stabilized by blood transfusion, correction of coagulopathy, and administration of vasoconstrictors and antibiotics. Endotracheal intubation is usually necessary for airway control. Varices appear as three or four large, tortuous submucosal bluish vessels running longitudinally in the distal esophagus. The bleeding site may be identified, but in some cases, the lumen fills with blood so rapidly that the lesion is obscured. Via fiberoptic endoscopy, 1-3 mL of sclerosant solution is injected into the lumen of each varix, causing it to become thrombosed. Variations in the type of endoscope or sclerosant solution or whether or not the varices are physically compressed appear to have little influence on the outcome. Endoscopy is usually repeated within 48 hours and then once or twice again at weekly intervals, at which time any residual varices are injected.

Sclerotherapy controls acute bleeding in 80%-85% of patients, and rebleeding during the same hospitalization is about half (25% versus 50%) the rebleeding rate of patients treated with a combination of vasopressin and balloon tamponade. Even though controlled trials show improvement in the control of bleeding with sclerotherapy, the evidence for increased patient survival is conflicting.

A similar effect is achieved by endoscopic ligation of the varices. The varix is lifted with a suction tip, and a small rubber band is slipped around the base. The varix necroses to leave a superficial ulcer. Several controlled trials have reported rubber band ligation to be more effective in controlling long-term bleeding episodes compared to sclerotherapy, although comparisons in the acute setting are limited. Band ligation is associated with fewer complications, and fewer procedures are needed for complete eradication; thus, band ligation has emerged as the initial endoscopic treatment of choice.

2. Somatostatin and analogue—Octreotide (brand name Sandostatin) is an octapeptide that mimics the hormone somatostatin pharmacologically. Purified somatostatin is not available in the United States. Somatostatin infusion reduces portal pressure without any impact on systemic hemodynamics; this effect may be less pronounced for octreotide. Somatostatin has been shown, in a prospective randomized trial, to effectively control acute bleeding, although other studies have had equivocal results. A meta-analysis of all studies using somatostatin or its analogues did show a significant risk reduction in control of hemorrhage. The efficacy of octreotide remains uncertain, but it appears to reduce the rebleeding rate when used in conjunction with endoscopic therapy. It should be emphasized that no study of somatostatin or octreotide has shown improved survival after an acute bleeding episode. Octreotide is given as an initial bolus of 50 μg followed by a continuous infusion of 50 μg/h for 2 to 5 days.

3. Vasopressin and analogue —Vasopressin and its analogue terlipressin (triglycyl lysine vasopressin) lower portal blood flow and portal pressure by directly constricting splanchnic arterioles, thereby reducing inflow. Vasopressin or terlipressin alone controls acute bleeding in about 80%-85% of patients, and this rate is increased when combined with endoscopic therapy or balloon tamponade. Cardiac output, oxygen delivery to the tissues, hepatic blood flow, and renal blood flow are also decreased—effects that occasionally produce complications such as myocardial infarction, cardiac arrhythmias, and intestinal necrosis. These unwanted side effects may sometimes be prevented without interfering with the decrease in portal pressure by simultaneous administration of nitroglycerin or isoproterenol. Terlipressin has fewer untoward cardiovascular side effects than vasopressin.

Although the results are somewhat contradictory, controlled trials generally indicate that vasopressin plus nitroglycerin is superior to vasopressin alone and that vasopressin alone is superior to placebo in controlling active variceal bleeding. Survival is not increased, however. In fact, although several vasoactive agents effectively stop acute hemorrhage, only terlipressin has been shown to improve survival after an acute event. Vasopressin is given as a peripheral intravenous infusion (at about 0.4 units/min), which is safer than bolus injections. Nitroglycerin can be given intravenously or sublingually. Terlipressin undergoes gradual conversion to vasopressin in the body and is safe to give by intravenous bolus injection (2 mg intravenously every 6 hours); however, this drug is not available in the United States.

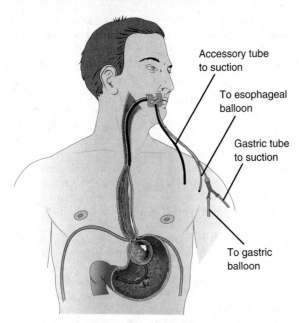

Accessory tube
to suction

To esophageal
balloon

Gastric tube
to suction

To gastric
balloon

▲ **Figure 26–8.** Sengstaken-Blakemore tube with both gastric and esophageal balloons inflated.

4. Balloon tamponade—See Figure 26–8. Tubes designed for tamponade have two balloons that can be inflated in the lumen of the gut to compress bleeding varices. There are three or four lumens in the tube, depending on the type: two are for filling balloons within the stomach and the esophagus, and the third permits aspiration of gastric contents. A fourth lumen in the Minnesota tube is used to aspirate the esophagus through the esophageal balloon. The main effect results from traction applied to the tube, which forces the gastric balloon, generally inflated first and with 200 mL of air, to compress the collateral veins at the cardia of the stomach. Inflating the esophageal balloon probably contributes little, since barium x-rays suggest that it does not actually compress the varices.

The most common serious complication is aspiration of pharyngeal secretions and pneumonitis. Another serious hazard is the occasional instance of esophageal rupture caused by inflation of the esophageal balloon. The esophageal balloon is therefore infrequently used.

About 75% of actively bleeding patients can be controlled by balloon tamponade, usually applied for 6-12 hours. When bleeding has stopped, the balloons are left inflated for another 24 hours. They are then decompressed, leaving the tube in place. If bleeding does not recur, the tube should be withdrawn. The efficacy of other therapies and the potential complications associated with balloon catheters have led to a marked reduction in the use of the latter approach, which is now reserved as a salvage treatment or temporary bridge in patients who fail medical and endoscopic therapy.

5. Transjugular intrahepatic portosystemic shunt (TIPSS)—TIPSS is a minimally invasive means of creating a portosystemic shunt by creating a direct communication between the portal and hepatic venous systems within the liver parenchyma. A catheter is introduced through the jugular vein and, under radiologic control, positioned in the hepatic vein. From this point, the portal vein is accessed through the liver, the tract is dilated, and the channel is kept open by inserting an expandable metal stent, which is left in place. This technique is of great value in controlling portal hypertension and variceal bleeding and is used most commonly as a salvage therapy to stop acute bleeding for the 10%-20% of patients in whom medical and endoscopic therapy fails. TIPSS is also indicated to prevent rebleeding in patients with advanced liver disease at high risk for recurrent variceal bleeding. In this latter category of patients, early use of TIPSS has been shown in randomized controlled trials to improve survival. The shunt remains open in most patients for up to a year, at which point intimal overgrowth leads to thrombosis and occlusion in many cases. The use of polytetrafluoroethylene (PTFE)-covered stents appears to have improved the patency rate.

TIPSS should not be regarded as definitive therapy, however, even though the shunt usually remains patent for many months. Patients with advanced liver disease are the principal candidates for TIPSS, which proved most useful as a bridge to transplantation. Patients with less severe cirrhosis should generally be considered for β-blocker therapy and, in some cases, for surgical devascularization procedure when transplantation is not a suitable option.

6. Surgery—The operative procedures to control active bleeding are emergency portosystemic shunt and variceal ligation or esophageal transection.

A. EMERGENCY PORTACAVAL SHUNT—Although TIPSS, when technically feasible, has largely supplanted more invasive surgical shunts as a salvage procedure for variceal bleed, emergency portacaval shunt has a success rate of 95% in stopping bleeding in this context. The death rate of the operation is not insignificant and is generally related to the status of the patient's liver function (ie, Child-Pugh classification; Table 26–1) as well as the rate and amount of bleeding and its effects on cardiac, renal, and pulmonary function. Some patients with advanced liver disease, especially those with severe encephalopathy and ascites, have an extraordinarily poor survival regardless of the treatment. In such patients, surgery is usually not warranted, even in the face of continued bleeding. On the other hand, patients with good liver function usually recover after an emergency shunt. A controlled trial showed that the death rate in acutely bleeding Child-Pugh C patients was insignificantly lower after endoscopic sclerotherapy (44%) than after emergency portacaval shunt (50%).

All portosystemic shunts reduce varices and decrease the risk of rebleeding. Nonselective portosystemic shunts divert large amounts of portal blood flow to the systemic circulation

▲ **Figure 26–9.** Types of portacaval anastomoses: **A:** Normal. **B:** Side-to-side. **C:** End-to-side. **D:** Mesocaval. **E:** Central splenorenal. **F:** Distal splenorenal (Warren). The H-mesocaval shunt is not illustrated.

without necessarily preserving portal blood flow (ie, end-to-side portacaval shunt). This is associated with an extremely high rate of hepatic encephalopathy. Selective portosystemic shunts preserve portal flow to liver while decompressing gastroesophageal varices; however, they can be more time consuming and technically complicated. For active bleeding, a nonselective end-to-side portacaval shunt is most commonly performed (Figure 26–9). A side-to-side portacaval shunt might be preferable in an acutely bleeding patient with severe ascites (Figure 26–9B), and this approach (or a variant such as an H-mesocaval shunt) would be required for someone with Budd-Chiari syndrome. H-mesocaval shunts are ideal for transplant-eligible patients because they can avoid dissection in the porta hepatis and the shunt can be ligated at the time of transplantation.

The central splenorenal shunt, in which the portal vein is decompressed via the splenic vein into the left renal vein, is more complicated than portacaval shunts and has no specific advantages. Selective shunts, such as the distal splenorenal (Warren) shunt, in which the gastrosplenic collaterals are decompressed via the splenic vein into the left renal vein, leaving the portal vein intact, are usually too time consuming for use in emergency operations.

Although the risk of variceal rebleeding is low, approximately 40% of patients develop encephalopathy after portacaval surgical shunting. Hepatic insufficiency is accelerated, and liver failure is the cause of death in about two-thirds of patients who die after an emergency portacaval shunt. Portacaval shunts can also render liver transplantation more difficult. Renal failure, which is often accompanied by ascites, is another potentially lethal problem. Metabolic alkalosis and delirium tremens are not uncommon postoperatively in alcoholics.

B. Esophageal transection—Varices may be obliterated by firing the end-to-end stapler in the distal esophagus after tucking a full-thickness ring of tissue into the cartridge with a circumferential tie. This procedure has gained popularity over the past decade, and in many surgical units, it is considered a last-resort therapy when nonsurgical methods fail.

If transection is performed, it must be done as soon as it is recognized that a second attempt at sclerotherapy or band ligation has failed. The results (ie, survival) are better in patients with nonalcoholic cirrhosis. Stapled transection has replaced the older technique of direct suture ligation of the varices. Transection must be viewed as an emergency measure to stop persistent bleeding—not as definitive treatment—since the underlying portal hypertension is not corrected and varices recur months later in many patients.

Bosch J, et al: Recombinant factor VIIa for variceal bleeding in patients with advanced cirrhosis: a randomized, controlled trial. *Hepatology.* 2008;47:1604.

Garcia-Pagan JC, et al: Early use of TIPS in patients with cirrhosis and variceal bleeding. *N Engl J Med.* 2010;362:2370-2379.

Gonzalez R, et al: Combination endoscopic and drug therapy to prevent variceal rebleeding in cirrhosis. *Ann Intern Med.* 2008;149:109.

Mercado MA, et al: Comparative study of 2 variants of a modified esophageal transection in the Sugiura-Futagawa operation. *Arch Surg.* 1998;133:1046.

Orloff MJ: Fifty-three years' experience with randomized clinical trials of emergency portacval shunt for bleeding esophageal varices in cirrhosis: 1958-2011. *JAMA Surg.* 2014;149:155-169.

Orloff MJ, et al: Randomized trials of endoscopic therapy and transjugular intrahepatic portosystemic shunt versus portacaval shunt for emergency and elective treatment of bleeding gastric varices in cirrhosis. *Surgery.* 2015;157(6):1028-1045.

Tripathi D, et al: U.K. Guidelines on the management of variceal hemorrhage in cirrhotic patients. *Gut.* 2015;64:1680-1704.

NONBLEEDING VARICES

Gastroesophageal varices are present in almost half of patients with cirrhosis at the time of diagnosis. Development and growth of esophageal varices each occur at a rate of 7% per year. Patients with varices that have never bled have a 30% chance of bleeding at some point; of those who bleed, 50% die. For patients who do not bleed during the first year after diagnosis of varices, the risk of bleeding subsequently decreases by half and continues to drop thereafter. Patients who have bled once from esophageal varices have a 60%-70% chance of bleeding again, and about two-thirds of repeat bleeding episodes are fatal.

▶ Evaluation

A. Portal Flow and Pressure Measurements

Measurements of pressure and flow in the splanchnic vasculature have been used for diagnosis and as a guide to therapy and prognosis in portal hypertension. Portal pressure can be measured directly at surgery or preoperatively by any of the following techniques: (1) Wedged hepatic venous pressure (WHVP) accurately reflects free portal pressure when portal hypertension is caused by a postsinusoidal (or sinusoidal) resistance, as in cirrhosis. The portal pressure can be determined with the catheter in the wedged position, corrected by subtracting the free hepatic venous pressure (FHVP); the hepatic venous pressure gradient (HVPG; the pressure gradient from the portal to the hepatic venous systems) can also be determined. This is the most commonly used technique. (2) Direct measurement of splenic pulp pressure is obtained by a percutaneously placed needle. (3) Percutaneous transhepatic catheterization of the intrahepatic branches of the portal vein is the method of choice in patients thought to have presinusoidal block or Budd-Chiari syndrome. (4) Catheterization of the umbilical vein is accomplished through a small incision, and the catheter is threaded into the portal system. With each of these methods, one may also obtain anatomic information by performing angiography through the catheter.

HVPG predicts decompensation and death. Reduction in the HVPG, either spontaneously or after therapy, may help predict the risk of rebleeding in some patients. It has therefore been suggested that HVPG can be used to guide therapy. However, its value currently has been shown primarily in alcoholic liver disease. Also, it is an invasive study that requires special expertise and is not always readily available. Duplex ultrasonography is an accurate noninvasive means of assessing the amount and direction of flow in the portal vein. Preoperatively, duplex ultrasonography is useful to determine patency of the portal vein and direction of flow. Because of spontaneous thrombosis, about 10% of patients with cirrhosis have a portal vein unsuitable for a portacaval shunt. If flow in the portal vein is reversed (hepatofugal),

a selective shunt (ie, distal splenorenal) is not recommended because it compromises the ability of portal tributaries to serve as an outflow tract for liver blood. Duplex ultrasonography can also be used to follow changes in portal perfusion after shunt operations.

B. Portal Angiography

The portal venous anatomy is often studied preoperatively by angiographic techniques. The objectives are to determine the patency, location, and size of the veins tentatively chosen for a shunt, to demonstrate the presence of varices, and to estimate the degree of prograde portal flow. Some of this information can now be obtained less invasively by duplex ultrasonography. When a splenorenal shunt is contemplated, the left renal vein should be opacified, either by injection of the renal artery or renal vein.

▶ Treatment

The treatment options consist of expectant management, endoscopic sclerotherapy, nonselective β-blocker (eg, propranolol, nadolol), portosystemic shunts, devascularization of the esophagogastric junction, and miscellaneous rarely used operations. The treatment of patients with varices that have never bled is usually referred to as prophylactic therapy (eg, prophylactic endoscopic variceal ligation or prophylactic propranolol). By convention, procedures performed on patients who have bled previously are referred to as therapeutic (eg, therapeutic shunts).

A. Prophylactic Therapy

Prophylactic therapy is of value, since the risk of bleeding and associated mortality are both extremely high, and varices can often be diagnosed before the initial episode of bleeding. In patients who have never had a bleeding episode, the following have been shown to be related to the risk of hemorrhage: Child-Pugh classification, the size of the varices, and the presence of red wale markings (longitudinal dilated venules resembling whip marks) on the varices. This information can be used to identify high-risk patients (up to 65% risk of bleeding within a year) who are most likely to benefit from prophylactic treatment.

In cirrhotic patients without varices, treatment with nonselective β-blockers is not recommended because they do not prevent the development of varices and are associated with side effects. In patients with low-risk varices (small, no red wale marks, no severe liver dysfunction), nonselective β-blockers may delay variceal growth and thereby prevent hemorrhage. The alternative is to schedule periodic endoscopic screening for detection of variceal growth, at which time medical treatment can be initiated.

In patients who have never bled but have a high risk (medium to large varices or small varices with red wale markings and/or decompensated cirrhosis), endoscopic variceal ligation (EVL) and nonselective β-blockers are considered equally adequate, because high-quality randomized controlled trial have shown similar survival of patients with either approach. It has been suggested that β-blocker therapy should be the first-line treatment, with EVL used in patients who cannot tolerate or have contraindications to β-blockade. Endoscopic sclerotherapy is no longer routinely used as primary prophylaxis. Low-dose carvedilol has shown lower rates of first variceal hemorrhage when compared to EVL (10% versus 23%), but those results needs to be validated in other trials.

B. Therapy of Patients Who Have Bled Previously

As noted earlier, patients who recover from an episode of variceal bleeding have an approximately 60%-70% chance of bleeding again. Much effort has been expended to ascertain the best treatment for these patients. The methods of greatest interest include nonselective β-blocker therapy, endoscopic band ligation, and portosystemic shunts.

1. Nonselective β-blocker therapy— As with patients with esophageal varices who have never bled, nonselective β-adrenergic blocking agents (propranolol, nadolol) effectively reduce the risk of recurrent bleeding episodes. These agents work by decreasing cardiac output and splanchnic blood flow and consequently portal blood pressure. Chronic propranolol therapy, 20-160 mg twice daily (a dose that reduces resting pulse rate by 25%), decreases by about 40% the frequency of rebleeding from esophageal or gastric varices, deaths from rebleeding, and overall mortality. The benefits are greater in Child-Pugh class A and B than in Child-Pugh class C cirrhotics. β-Blocker therapy has been compared to endoscopic sclerotherapy, with no difference in rebleeding or mortality seen but with higher complications in the sclerotherapy group. However, randomized controlled trials have shown that the combined use of EVL and nonselective β-blockers could further lower the risk of rebleeding. The addition of nitrate drugs to β-blocker therapy appears to result in a greater reduction of portal pressure compared to β-blockade alone. This approach is often favored in patients who are not candidates for EVL. Abstinence from alcohol should always be emphasized and may help prevent further bleeding but may not necessarily decrease the mortality related specifically to variceal hemorrhage, as was previously thought.

2. Endoscopic band ligation— Endoscopic band ligation, as described earlier, is an effective means of preventing recurrent bleeding episodes and has been shown to be superior to sclerotherapy in this regard. Both band ligation and β-blocker therapy appear to be similarly effective in preventing rebleeding. However, the combination of both therapies has been shown to significantly reduce not only the risk of rebleeding but also the recurrence of varices. Thus, combination therapy appears to be the most effective treatment after an initial bleeding episode.

3. Endoscopic sclerotherapy— The technique of endoscopic sclerotherapy was described earlier in this chapter. Sclerotherapy was previously used routinely to reduce the risk of rebleeding but has been replaced by band ligation.

4. Transjugular intrahepatic portosystemic shunt— The TIPSS technique has been described earlier in this chapter. TIPSS is effective in preventing rebleeding episodes, more so than either endoscopic or pharmacologic therapy alone. However, this advantage is offset by its higher morbidity and mortality rates from the development of hepatic encephalopathy and liver failure. For this reason, as well as the lack of a clear survival or cost-benefit advantage, TIPSS is used mainly to salvage patients who fail endoscopic and/or pharmacologic treatment.

TIPSS has generally replaced shunt surgery in most patients who fail first-line therapy. A recent large, multicenter, randomized trial showed that TIPSS and surgical shunts had similar rates of rebleeding, encephalopathy, and mortality in Child-Pugh class A and B cirrhotic patients. There was a higher incidence of shunt dysfunction in the TIPSS patients, perhaps because of the type of stent used, with the first generation not being covered with PTFE. The use of TIPSS covered with PTFE has a significantly lower occlusion rate. Therefore, the choice between TIPSS and surgical shunts currently depends on expertise, anatomical considerations, and patient's preference.

C. Surgical Approaches

The objective of surgical procedures used to treat portal hypertension is either to obliterate the varices or to reduce blood flow and pressure within the varices (Table 26–6). A third option, liver transplantation, can treat both the underlying liver dysfunction and the portal hypertension.

1. Liver transplantation— Any relatively young patient with cirrhosis who has survived an episode of variceal hemorrhage should be considered a candidate for liver transplantation, since any other form of therapy carries a much higher (about 80%) mortality rate within the subsequent 1-2 years as a result of repeat bleeding or complications of hepatic failure. Obviously, continued alcohol use is a contraindication to transplantation in most patients. The good transplantation candidates, however, should not be subjected to portosystemic shunts or other procedures if it appears that they will come to transplantation in the near future. In general, Child-Pugh class A patients are candidates for portal decompression, whereas Child-Pugh class C patients are candidates for transplantation. A transjugular intrahepatic shunt (see previous section) is an excellent way to control bleeding while the patient is being prepared for a transplant.

Table 26–6. Surgical procedures for esophageal varices.

A. Direct variceal obliteration
  1. Variceal suture ligation
    a. Transthoracic
    b. Transabdominal
  2. Esophageal transection and reanastomosis
    a. Suture technique
    b. Staple technique
  3. Variceal sclerosis
    a. Esophagoscopic
    b. Transhepatic
  4. Variceal resection
    a. Esophagogastrectomy
    b. Subtotal esophagectomy
B. Reduction of variceal blood flow and pressure
  1. Portosystemic shunts
    a. End-to-side
    b. Side-to-side
      1. Side-to-side portacaval
      2. Mesocaval
      3. Central splenorenal
      4. Renosplenic
  2. Selective shunts
    a. Distal splenorenal (Warren)
    b. Left gastric vena caval (Inokuchi)
  3. Reduction of portal blood flow
    a. Splenectomy
    b. Splenic artery ligation
  4. Reduction of proximal gastric blood flow
    a. Esophagogastric devascularization
    b. Gastric transection and reanastomosis (Tanner)
  5. Stimulation of additional portosystemic venous collaterals
    a. Omentopexy
    b. Splenic transposition
C. Measures to preserve hepatic blood flow after portacaval shunt
  1. Arterialization of portal vein stump

2. Portosystemic shunts—The advent of TIPSS has resulted in a marked decline in the number of shunt operations performed. However, surgical shunts are durable, and good-risk patients appear to benefit from these procedures.

Portosystemic shunts can be grouped into those that shunt the entire portal system (total shunts) and those that selectively shunt blood from the gastrosplenic region while preserving the pressure-flow relationships in the rest of the portal bed (selective shunts; see below). All of the shunt operations commonly used today reduce the incidence of rebleeding to less than 10%, compared with about 75% in unshunted patients. Unfortunately, the price of this achievement is an operative mortality rate of 5%-20% (depending on the Child-Pugh classification), further impairment of liver function, and an increase in encephalopathy (greater with total shunts). Therefore, because shunts have these potential drawbacks, clinical trials are needed to pinpoint their place within an overall treatment strategy.

In one well-designed trial, patients who had bled previously were randomized to chronic sclerotherapy or a distal splenorenal shunt (Warren shunt; Figure 26–9F). Patients randomized to chronic sclerotherapy who had recurrent episodes of bleeding during treatment (ie, treatment failures, which amounted to 30% of the sclerotherapy group) were then treated surgically (ie, shunted). The results showed that 2-year survival was better among those originally randomized to sclerotherapy (90%) than among those originally assigned to the shunt group (60%). This trial supports a general treatment plan consisting initially of endoscopic therapy and reserving portosystemic shunts for the patients in whom the former fails to control bleeding adequately (Figure 26–7).

The choice of shunt has been the subject of much debate and several randomized trials. The principal question in recent years has been whether encephalopathy and survival are better with a selective shunt (ie, a distal splenorenal shunt; Figure 26–9F) than with a total shunt (ie, a mesocaval or an end-to-side portacaval shunt; Figure 26–9C and D). The results are conflicting, but in general, they support the contention that there is about half as much severe encephalopathy following selective shunts. None of the trials have shown any particular shunt to be associated with longer survival.

3. Severity of hepatic disease and operative risk—The immediate death rate of an elective shunt procedure can be predicted from the patient's hepatic function as reflected by the Child-Pugh classification (Table 26–1). In addition to operative death rate, the figures also correlate with the death rate in the first postshunt year. Thereafter, survival curves of the different risk classes become reasonably parallel.

The severity of histopathologic changes in liver biopsies correlates with the immediate surgical death rate, the most ominous findings being hepatocellular necrosis, polymorphonuclear leukocyte infiltration, and the presence of Mallory bodies. The extent of histologic change also correlates with the more easily obtained data in the Child-Pugh classification (ie, severe changes occur in class C patients), so results of biopsies have no independent predictive value.

A. TYPES OF PORTOSYSTEMIC SHUNTS—Figure 26–9 depicts the various shunts in use currently. Although they differ technically, physiologically there are only three different types: end-to-side, side-to-side, and selective.

(1) Total shunts—The end-to-side shunt completely disconnects the liver from the portal system. The portal vein is transected near its bifurcation in the liver hilum and anastomosed to the side of the inferior vena cava. The hepatic stump of the vein is oversewn. Postoperatively, the WHVP (sinusoidal pressure) drops slightly, reflecting the inability of the hepatic artery to compensate fully for the loss of portal inflow. The side-to-side portacaval, mesocaval, mesorenal, and central splenorenal shunts are all physiologically similar, since the

shunt preserves continuity between the hepatic limb of the portal vein, the portal system, and the anastomosis. Flow through the hepatic limb of the standard side-to-side shunt is nearly always away from the liver and toward the anastomosis. The extent to which hepatofugal flow is produced by the other types of side-to-side shunts listed previously is not known.

The end-to-side portacaval shunt gives immediate and permanent protection from variceal bleeding and is somewhat easier to perform than a side-to-side portacaval or central splenorenal shunt. Encephalopathy may be slightly more common after end-to-side than side-to-side portacaval shunts. Side-to-side shunts are required in patients with Budd-Chiari syndrome or refractory ascites (when the latter is treated by a portosystemic shunt).

The mesocaval shunt interposes a segment of prosthetic graft or internal jugular vein between the inferior vena cava and the superior mesenteric vein where the latter passes in front of the uncinate process of the pancreas. The mesocaval shunt is particularly useful in the presence of severe scarring in the right upper quadrant or portal vein thrombosis, and in some cases, it may be technically easier than a conventional side-to-side portacaval shunt if a side-to-side type of shunt is necessary. In most cases, portal flow to the liver is lost after this shunt. Evidence has been presented, however, that by limiting the diameter of the prosthetic graft to 8 mm (compared with 12- to 20-mm grafts), antegrade flow is preserved in the portal vein, which decreases the incidence of postoperative encephalopathy while still preventing variceal hemorrhage.

(2) Selective shunts—Selective shunts lower pressure in the gastroesophageal venous plexus while preserving blood flow through the liver via the portal vein.

The distal splenorenal (Warren) shunt involves anastomosing the distal (splenic) end of the transected splenic vein to the side of the left renal vein, plus ligation of the major collaterals between the remaining portal and isolated gastrosplenic venous system. The latter step involves division of the gastric vein, the right gastroepiploic vein, and the vessels in the splenocolic ligament. The operation is more difficult and time consuming than conventional shunts and, except for the experienced operator, is probably too complex for emergency portal decompression. If mobilization of the splenic vein is hazardous, the renal vein may be transected and its caval end joined to the side of the undisturbed splenic vein. The segment of splenic vein between the anastomosis and the portal vein is then ligated. Surprisingly, this seems to have little permanent effect on renal function as long as the remaining tributaries are preserved on the oversewn renal vein stump.

In contrast to total shunts, the Warren shunt does not improve ascites and should not be performed in patients whose ascites has been difficult to control. Preoperative angiography should be performed to determine if the splenic vein and left renal vein are large enough and close enough together for performance of this shunt. Recent pancreatitis may preclude safe dissection of the splenic vein from the undersurface of the pancreas.

Another type of selective shunt (Inokuchi shunt) consists of joining the left gastric vein to the inferior vena cava by a short segment of autogenous saphenous vein. The procedure has not become popular, perhaps because of its technical complexity.

Selective shunts tend to become less selective over several years as new collaterals develop between the high-pressure and low-pressure regions of the portal system. This is accompanied by a gradual decrease in portal pressure (measured by WHVP) and evolution of the procedure into a version of side-to-side total shunt. The enlargement postoperatively of small venous tributaries entering the distal splenic vein from the pancreas suggests that this is the path by which nonselectivity develops. It is possible that this can be avoided by mobilizing the splenic vein all the way to the hilum (dividing these small vessels) before performing the splenorenal anastomosis.

B. Choice of shunt—A reasonable approach to shunt selection is as follows: The distal splenorenal shunt is the first choice for elective portal decompression. If ascites is present or the anatomy is unfavorable, an end-to-side portacaval shunt is preferred. Side-to-side shunts would be done for patients with severe ascites or Budd-Chiari syndrome. The H-mesocaval and central splenorenal shunts are reserved for special anatomic situations in which the above operations are unsuitable. An end-to-side shunt or H-mesocaval shunt is performed for emergency decompression.

Portacaval and distal splenorenal shunts are often followed by a rise in platelet count in patients with secondary hypersplenism. The response is unpredictable, however, and hypersplenism need not necessarily dictate the type of shunt since it rarely produces clinical manifestations. A central splenorenal shunt, in which splenectomy is performed, should not be considered preferable to other kinds of shunt just because the patient has a low platelet count.

C. Results of portosystemic shunts—Over 90% of portosystemic shunts remain patent, and the incidence of recurrent variceal bleeding is less than 10%. The 5-year survival rate after a portacaval shunt for alcoholic liver disease averages 45%. Some degree of encephalopathy develops in 15%-25% of patients. Severe encephalopathy is seen in about 20% of alcoholics following a total shunt; its occurrence is not related to the severity of preshunt encephalopathy.

D. Devascularization Operations

The objective of devascularization is to destroy the venous collaterals that transport blood from the high-pressure portal system into the veins in the submucosa of the esophagus.

The Sugiura-Futugawa procedure initially described in 1973 was done in two stages. The first stage was performed through a thoracotomy and consisted of division of the dilated venous collaterals between esophagus and adjacent structures, transection of the esophagus at the level of the diaphragm, and reanastomosis. The second stage, a laparotomy, was performed immediately after the thoracotomy if the patient was actively bleeding or deferred 4-6 weeks in elective cases. In the second stage of the operation, the upper two-thirds of the stomach was devascularized, and selective vagotomy, pyloroplasty, and splenectomy were performed.

More recently, an analogous one-stage operation has been described in many series and performed through laparotomy that consists of splenectomy, devascularization of 8-10 cm of distal esophagus, devascularization of the lesser and greater curvature with ligation of the left gastric and gastroepiploic vessels, transection and end-to-end anastomosis of the lower esophagus 4-5 cm above the gastroesophageal junction (EEA stapler), pyloroplasty, and insertion of a feeding jejunostomy.

In Eastern and Western series published between 1980 and 1999, the operative mortality ranged from 0%-36% up to 80% in Child-Pugh class C patients, the variceal rebleeding rate ranged from 0% to 37%, encephalopathy ranged from 0% to 22%, and esophageal stenosis ranged from 2% to 37%. For cirrhotic patients with extensive portal thrombosis, for whom portosystemic shunt cannot be performed, devascularization operations offer an alternative, but morbidity can be substantial.

E. Miscellaneous Operations

Attempts have also been made to decrease portal pressure by decreasing splanchnic inflow through splenectomy or splenic artery ligation. Diseases characterized by marked splenomegaly may rarely be associated with portal hypertension as a consequence of increased splenic blood flow, which has been known to reach levels as high as 1000 mL/min. Splenic blood flow may occasionally be increased enough in patients with cirrhosis to contribute significantly to the portal hypertension. However, splenectomy or splenic artery ligation in cirrhosis most often gives only a transient decrease in portal pressure, and over half of patients having these operations bleed again. Some workers have suggested that the absolute size of the splenic artery (a crude index of splenic flow) correlates with the clinical effectiveness of splenic artery ligation, with a good result being predictable if the diameter of the artery is 1 cm or greater.

Bonnel AR, et al: Transjugular intrahepatic portosystemic shunts in liver transplant recipients. *Liver Transpl.* 2013;20:130-139.

Brunner F, et al: Prevention and treatment of variceal haemorrhage in 2017. *Liver Int.* 2017;37:104.

Garcia-Tsao G, et al: Management of varices and variceal hemorrhage in cirrhosis. *N Engl J Med.* 2010;362:823.

Gluud LL, et al: Banding ligation versus beta-blockers as primary prophylaxis in esophageal varices: systematic review of randomized trials. *Am J Gastroenterol.* 2007;102:2842.

Gonzalez R, et al: Combination endoscopic and drug therapy to prevent variceal rebleeding in cirrhosis. *Ann Intern Med.* 2008;149:109.

Henderson JM, et al: Distal splenorenal shunt versus TIPS for refractory variceal bleeding: a prospective randomized controlled trial. *Gastroenterology.* 2006;130:1643.

Tripathi D, et al: Randomized controlled trial of carvedilol versus variceal band ligation for the prevention of the first variceal bleed. *Hepatology.* 2009;50:825.

Villanueva C, et al: A randomized trial to assess whether portal pressure guided therapy to prevent variceal rebleeding improves survival in cirrhosis. *Hepatology.* 2017;65(5):1693-1707.

Voros D, et al: Long-term results with the modified Sugiura procedure for the management of variceal bleeding: standing the test of time in the treatment of bleeding esophageal varices. *Word J Surg.* 2012;36:659.

EXTRAHEPATIC PORTAL VENOUS OCCLUSION

Extrahepatic portal vein obstruction is one of many causes of noncirrhotic portal hypertension, with the other common cause being noncirrhotic portal fibrosis. These disorders are distinct but appear to share several similar etiologic and pathogenetic features, the most notable of which is the clinical manifestation of portal hypertension in the absence of significant hepatic parenchymal dysfunction.

Idiopathic portal vein thrombosis (in the absence of liver disease) is a relatively common cause of portal hypertension in developing countries but is less prevalent in the West. This diagnosis accounts for most cases of portal hypertension in childhood (80%-90%) and for a smaller proportion of cases in adults. Neonatal septicemia, omphalitis, umbilical vein catheterization for exchange transfusion, and dehydration have all been considered as possible causes, but collectively, they can be implicated in less than half of cases. The causes of portal vein thrombosis in adults include hepatic and pancreatic tumors, cirrhosis, trauma, pancreatitis, pancreatic pseudocyst, myelofibrosis, thrombotic states (eg, protein C deficiency), and sepsis; in particular, cirrhosis and/or HCC need to be considered in adult patients. In adults, systemic anticoagulation results in complete portal vein recanalization in approximately 38% of cases and partial recanalization in 15%.

Although clinical manifestations may be delayed until adulthood, 80% of patients with idiopathic portal vein thrombosis present between 1 and 6 years of age with variceal bleeding, although hemorrhage from ectopic varices at other locations in the gastrointestinal tract is not uncommon. About 70% of hemorrhages are preceded by a recent upper respiratory tract infection. Some of these children first come to medical attention because of splenomegaly and pancytopenia. Failure to recognize the underlying problem has occasionally led to splenectomy, with the result that portal decompression using the splenic vein is precluded.

Ascites is uncommon except transiently after bleeding. Liver function is either normal or only slightly impaired, which probably accounts for the low incidence of overt encephalopathy. There is an increased frequency of neuropsychiatric problems, which may represent a subtle form of encephalopathy.

Portal biliopathy refers to abnormalities of the extrahepatic bile ducts, usually the result of bile duct compression from large, dilated venous collaterals within the porta hepatis. These changes result in marked irregularities of the biliary wall that can progress to strictures and even obstructive jaundice and cholangitis in some cases; secondary biliary cirrhosis has been reported. Biliopathy is commonly seen on imaging studies, but most patients remain free of related symptoms.

Because the patient's general condition and liver function are well preserved, the death rate for sudden massive bleeding is below that for other types of portal hypertension. The diagnosis can be confirmed with cross-sectional imaging or direct mesenteric angiography. WHVP is normal to slightly elevated; liver biopsies are normal or may show mild to moderate periportal fibrosis.

Bleeding episodes in children under age 8 are usually self-limited and often do not require endoscopic sclerotherapy, administration of vasopressin, or balloon tamponade. Even if such interventions are necessary, however, the bleeding episodes are self-limited and uncommonly fatal, so emergency operations are rarely necessary.

Thrombosed portal veins are unsuitable for shunt procedures. Cavo-mesenteric shunts are best for young children, whose vessels are small. In older individuals, treatment should be started with sclerotherapy. If that fails to control the bleeding, a distal splenorenal shunt is preferred. Splenectomy alone has no permanent effect and sacrifices the splenic vein, which might be needed later for a shunt operation. Shunts in small children have a high rate of spontaneous thrombosis and should be avoided, if possible, until approximately 8-10 years of age, when the vessels are of larger caliber. Even still, using precise technique, some surgeons have obtained a high rate of anastomotic patency in the very young. Encephalopathy and hepatic dysfunction many years after a total shunt may be improved if converted to a selective shunt.

Splenectomy alone is never indicated in this disease, either for hypersplenism or in an attempt to reduce portal pressure, because the rebleeding rate is 90%. If it is not possible to construct an adequate shunt, expectant management is the best strategy. Repeated severe bleeding episodes should be treated by transendoscopic sclerosis. Esophagogastrectomy with colonic interposition may be effective but should be considered a last resort.

Chattopadhyay S, et al: Portal biliopathy. *World J Gastroenterol.* 2012;18(43):6177-6182.

Hall TC, et al: Management of acute non-cirrhotic and non-malignant portal vein thrombosis: a systematic review. *World J Surg.* 2011;35:2510.

Plessier A, et al: Acute portal vein thrombosis unrelated to cirrhosis: a prospective multicenter follow-up study. *Hepatology.* 2010;51(1):210-218.

SPLENIC VEIN THROMBOSIS

Isolated thrombosis of the splenic vein is a rare cause of variceal bleeding that can be cured by splenectomy. The splenic venous blood, blocked from its normal route, flows through the short gastric vessels to the gastric fundus and then into the left gastric vein, continuing toward the liver. This phenomenon is called left-sided (or sinistral) portal hypertension. As the blood traverses the stomach, large gastric varices are produced that may rupture and bleed. Characteristically, the collateral pattern does not involve the esophagus, so esophageal varices are uncommon.

The principal causes of this syndrome are pancreatitis, pancreatic pseudocyst, pancreatic neoplasm, and trauma. The mean incidence of splenic vein thrombosis associated with chronic and acute pancreatitis is estimated at 12.4% and 22.6%, respectively, with an overall bleeding rate of 12.3%. Splenomegaly is present in two-thirds of patients. Diagnosis can be made by selective splenic arteriography that opacifies the venous phase but now is more commonly made on CT scan with portal phase imaging. Splenectomy is curative. Many cases of splenic vein thrombosis are unaccompanied by bleeding varices, and in such cases, no therapy is required. Treatment of acute bleeding from gastric varices is generally endoscopic, and endoscopic variceal obscuration with tissue glue appears to be superior to band ligation or sclerotherapy.

Butler JR, et al: Natural history of pancreatitis-induced splenic vein thrombosis: a systematic review and meta-analysis of its incidence and rate of gastrointestinal bleeding. *HPB.* 2011;13:1477.

Strasberg SM, et al: Pattern of venous collateral development after splenic vein occlusion in an extended Whipple procedure: comparison with collateral vein pattern in cases of sinistral portal hypertension. *J Gastrointest Surg.* 2011;15:2070.

BUDD-CHIARI SYNDROME

Budd-Chiari syndrome is a rare disorder resulting from obstruction of hepatic venous outflow, which can arise at several different levels, from the small hepatic venous tributaries within the liver parenchyma to the major hepatic venous trunks to the inferior vena cava up to the level of the right atrium. The prevalence of Budd-Chiari syndrome is estimated as 1:100,000, and the largest published series reported on 237 patients treated at four centers in the United States, the Netherlands, and France between 1984 and 2001. Females are more often affected compared to males (3:1), and this is thought to be secondary to the use of estrogen-containing medications in undiagnosed hypercoagulable patients. Most cases are caused by spontaneous thrombosis of the hepatic veins, often associated with myeloproliferative disorders (polycythemia vera, essential thrombocytosis) or the use of birth control pills. Other common associated conditions include factor V Leiden and factor II gene mutations. Other predisposing factors include protein C and S deficiencies, antiphospholipid syndrome, antithrombin III deficiency, paroxysmal nocturnal hemoglobinuria, Behçet syndrome, and trauma. Some patients present with idiopathic membranous stenosis of the inferior vena cava located between the hepatic veins and right atrium, which is usually associated with secondary thrombosis of the hepatic veins; this condition appears to be more common in Asia than in Western countries. Many patients with Budd-Chiari syndrome are HBsAg positive, and others have malignancies (eg, HCC). Vena caval webs were once thought to be congenital, but more recent evidence suggests that they are the consequence of thrombus formation. Primary Budd-Chiari syndrome originates from within the lumen of the hepatic veins or venules, and occlusion results from thrombosis, webs, or endophlebitis. By contrast, secondary Budd-Chiari syndrome results from extrinsic compression of the venous outflow tract, usually related to a neoplasm or abscess.

Veno-occlusive disease and congestive hepatopathy are two conditions that can cause hepatic venous outflow obstruction, and although the clinical picture of both may be indistinguishable from that of Budd-Chiari syndrome, they differ in the level of obstruction and in predisposing conditions. Veno-occlusive disease is primarily a problem affecting the sinusoids and terminal venules, whereas congestive hepatopathy reflects a problem at the level of the heart.

Posthepatic (postsinusoidal) obstruction raises sinusoidal pressure, which is transmitted proximally to cause portal hypertension. Because the parenchyma is relatively free of fibrosis, filtration across the sinusoids and hepatic lymph formation increase greatly, producing marked ascites.

Symptoms usually begin with a mild prodrome consisting of vague right upper quadrant abdominal pain, postprandial bloating, hepatomegaly, and anorexia. After weeks or months, a more florid picture develops consisting of gross ascites, hepatomegaly, hepatic failure, and jaundice. At this stage, the AST is usually markedly increased, the serum bilirubin is elevated, and the alkaline phosphatase is inconsistently abnormal.

Except in patients with membranous obstruction of the vena cava, liver scans (CT or MRI) usually demonstrate a marked perfusion abnormality throughout most of the liver except for a small central area representing the caudate lobe, whose venous outflow is spared (it goes directly to the vena cava through multiple small tributaries). CT scans show pooling of intravenous contrast media in the periphery of the liver; patent hepatic veins cannot be seen on ultrasound scans. An enlarged azygos vein may be seen on chest x-rays of patients with caval obstruction. Liver biopsy reveals grossly dilated central veins and sinusoids, pericentral necrosis, and replacement of hepatocytes by red blood cells. Centrilobular

fibrosis develops late. The clinical diagnosis should be confirmed by venography, which shows the hepatic veins to be obstructed, usually with a beaklike deformity at their orifice. The inferior vena cava should be opacified to verify its patency, which is a requirement for a successful portacaval shunt. Previously, direct venography was used, but the required information may now be obtained using noninvasive methods, such as CT or magnetic resonance angiography. The x-rays may show compression of the intrahepatic cava by the congested liver.

Treatment of Budd-Chiari syndrome relies on expert consensus given the low incidence of this disease. The underlying cause should be investigated and treated immediately. Traditionally, surgical shunts and liver transplantation were considered first-line options; however, improvement in less invasive techniques has changed the treatment algorithm. Anticoagulation is recommended in the presence of recent or long-standing thrombosis to allow recanalization or to avoid propagation of venous thrombosis. Management of ascites and treatment or prevention of portal hypertension and variceal hemorrhage follow the same algorithms as for cirrhotic patients. Surgical or radiologic approaches to relieve sinusoidal pressure have been advocated and are now considered appropriate only for symptomatic patients who do not improve with medical management. In recent years, the development of interventional radiology techniques using thrombolysis and angioplasty has made it possible to insert TIPSS in selected patients with recent thrombosis or with short-length stenosis of the inferior vena cava or hepatic veins with good outcomes. Portosystemic surgical shunts are considered effective for relieving sinusoidal hypertension with the potential to reverse hepatic necrosis and prevent cirrhosis.

Focal membranous obstruction of the suprahepatic cava may be treated by excision of the lesion with or without the addition of a patch angioplasty. Some cases may be managed nonsurgically by percutaneous transluminal balloon dilation of the stenosis. Occlusion of the inferior vena cava by thrombosis or compression from the liver requires a mesoatrial shunt using a prosthetic vascular graft. Because the incidence of graft thrombosis is relatively high, it may be advisable to perform a second-stage side-to-side portacaval shunt a few months after mesoatrial shunt decompression of the liver in patients with hepatic vein thrombosis whose vena cava was originally blocked by a congested liver. Development of HCC is common in patients with membranous obstruction of the vena cava. The postoperative results are excellent in patients without malignant neoplasms.

Liver transplantation is required when medical treatment and portosystemic shunts fail in patients presenting with progressive liver failure either from cirrhosis or as part of the acute syndrome. The 1-, 5-, and 10-year survival rates with transplantation are 76%, 71%, and 68%, respectively, and the risk of later HCC is eliminated.

Bittencourt PL, et al: Portal vein thrombosis and Budd-Chiari syndrome. *Hematol Oncol Clin North Am.* 2011;25:1049.

Das CJ, et al: Role of radiological imaging and interventions in management of Budd-Chiari syndrome. *Clin Radiol.* 2018; 73(7):610-624.

Garcia-Pagan JC, et al: TIPS for Budd-Chiari syndrome: long-term results and prognostic factors in 124 patients. *Gastroenterology.* 2008;135:808.

Qi X, et al: Transjugular intrahepatic portosystemic shunt in the treatment of Budd-Chiari syndrome: a critical review of literatures. *Scand J Gastroenterol.* 2013;48(7):771-784.

Seijo S, et al, European Network for Vascular Disorders of the Liver: Good long-term outcome of Budd-Chiari syndrome with a step-wise management. *Hepatology.* 2013;57(5):1962-1968.

Zhang W, et al: Budd-Chiari syndrome in China: a 30-year retrospective study on survival from a single center. *World J Gastroenterol.* 2018;24(10):1134-1143.

ASCITES

Ascites is a common manifestation of chronic liver disease, resulting from sinusoidal hypertension as the specific pathophysiologic abnormality. Ascites in hepatic disease results from (1) increased formation of hepatic lymph (from sinusoidal hypertension), (2) increased formation of splanchnic lymph (from splanchnic vasodilatation), (3) hypoalbuminemia, and (4) salt and water retention by the kidneys. Before therapy is started, paracentesis should be performed and the following examinations made on a sample of ascitic fluid: (1) Culture and leukocyte count: Spontaneous bacterial peritonitis is common and may be clinically silent. A white count above $250/\mu L$ is highly suggestive of infection. (2) Lactate dehydrogenase (LDH) levels: A ratio of LDH in ascites to serum that exceeds 0.6 suggests the presence of cancer or infection. (3) Serum amylase: A high level suggests pancreatic disease. (4) Albumin: The ratio of serum to ascites albumin concentrations is above 1.1 in liver disease and below 1.1 in malignant ascites. (5) Cytology: This is pertinent only in patients with a cancer diagnosis or a suspicion of cancer.

Nonhepatic ascites can result from congestive heart failure; chylous leak; peritoneal carcinomatosis; infections such as tuberculosis, coccidioidomycosis, and chlamydia; and some autoimmune diseases involving the connective tissues, such as systemic lupus erythematosus. Treatments of ascites in these contexts depend on the underlying cause and are not discussed in this chapter.

Medical Treatment

In general, the intensity of medical therapy required to control ascites can be predicted from the pretreatment 24-hour urine Na^+ output as follows: an Na^+ output below 5 mEq/24 h requires strong diuretics; 5-25 mEq/24 h, mild diuretics; and above 25 mEq/24 h, no diuretics. Initial treatment is usually with spironolactone, 200 mg/d. The objective is to stimulate a weight loss of 0.5-0.75 kg/d except in patients with peripheral edema who can mobilize fluid faster. If spironolactone alone is insufficient, another drug such as furosemide should be added. A loop diuretic (eg, furosemide, ethacrynic acid) should be given only in combination with a distally acting diuretic (eg, spironolactone, triamterene). Alternatively, massive ascites may be treated by one or more large-volume (ie, 5-L) paracenteses; this is often accompanied by an intravenous infusion of albumin, although the benefits of albumin remain controversial. Caution is required in patients with evidence of renal dysfunction, since aggressive fluid removal can result in renal failure. Close monitoring of serum electrolytes should be done. Because the development of ascites in cirrhosis is a result of renal sodium retention, dietary sodium restriction is a mainstay of treatment. A typical American diet contains 4-6 g of sodium per day. Patients are educated to have a dietary maximum of 2 g of sodium per day. Fluid restriction is only indicated in patients with severe hyponatremia, but all patients should avoid excessive fluid intake.

Surgical Treatment

A. Portacaval Shunt

A history of ascites that has been easy to control need not influence the choice of shunt operation intended to treat variceal bleeding. When ascites has been severe, however, a side-to-side shunt (eg,. side-to-side portacaval, H-mesocaval, central splenorenal) may be considered, because it reduces sinusoidal as well as splanchnic venous pressure. A side-to-side portacaval shunt is rarely indicated just to treat ascites (eg, in patients in whom several LeVeen shunts have thrombosed), although the incidence of severe postoperative encephalopathy is high under these circumstances. TIPSS is another effective intervention for refractory ascites and probably a better option than repeated paracentesis in good-risk patients, although there is an associated risk of hepatic encephalopathy.

B. Peritoneal-Jugular Shunt (LeVeen Shunt, Denver Shunt)

Refractory ascites can be treated with a LeVeen shunt—a subcutaneous Silastic catheter that transports ascitic fluid from the peritoneal cavity to the jugular vein. A small unidirectional valve sensitive to a pressure gradient of 3-5 cm H_2O prevents backflow of blood. A modification called the Denver shunt contains a small chamber that can be used as a pump to clear the line by external pressure. In practice, Denver shunts become blocked more often than LeVeen shunts.

In patients with ascites due to cirrhosis, use of a LeVeen shunt should be confined to those who fail to respond to high doses of diuretics (eg, 400 mg of spironolactone and 400 mg of furosemide daily) or who repeatedly develop encephalopathy or azotemia during diuretic therapy.

Peritoneovenous shunts may also be used for ascites associated with cancer. The best results occur in patients whose ascitic fluid contains no malignant cells. A LeVeen shunt is of benefit in Budd-Chiari syndrome but is ineffective for chylous ascites. Because the incidence of complications and early shunt thrombosis is high, a LeVeen shunt is relatively contraindicated if the ascitic fluid is grossly bloody, contains many malignant cells, or has a high protein concentration (> 4.5 g/dL). The incidence of tumor embolization is low (5%).

The ascitic fluid should be cultured a few days before the shunt is inserted. Antibiotic coverage should be given for the procedure. The operation can be done with local anesthesia.

Postoperatively, the patient is outfitted with an abdominal binder and instructed to perform respiratory exercises against mild pressure to increase abdominal pressure and flow through the shunt. Dietary salt should not be restricted. A functioning LeVeen shunt alone is unable to fully eliminate the ascites, but it improves symptoms related to distention and renders the patient much more responsive to diuretics. Therefore, furosemide should be administered postoperatively.

An average of 10 kg of weight is lost during the first 10 days after the operation, and eventually the abdomen assumes a normal configuration. Nutrition and serum albumin levels often improve postoperatively. Urinary sodium excretion increases promptly, and renal function may improve in patients with the hepatorenal syndrome. Serious complications and deaths are most common in patients with advanced hepatorenal syndrome or a serum bilirubin level greater than 4 mg/dL. Although some patients eventually bleed from varices following insertion of a LeVeen shunt, the shunt itself does not increase the risk of bleeding and actually decreases portal pressure. Thus, a previous episode of variceal bleeding is not a contraindication for this procedure. Disseminated intravascular coagulation (eg, manifested by increased fibrin split products, decreased platelet count) occurs in more than half of cases but is clinically relevant in only a few. Lethal septicemia may occur if the ascitic fluid is infected at the time the shunt is inserted. In about 10% of cases, the valve becomes thrombosed and must be replaced.

Hydrothorax, usually on the right side, may develop in patients with cirrhosis and ascites. The fluid reaches the chest through a pinhole opening in the membranous portion of the diaphragm, a pathway that can be demonstrated by aspirating the thoracic fluid, injecting technetium ^{99m}Tc colloid into the ascites fluid, and observing rapid accumulation of the label in the chest. Treatment consists of a peritoneovenous shunt and injection of a sclerosing agent into the pleural cavity after it has been tapped dry. If a leak persists, it may be closed surgically by thoracotomy.

Bernardi M, et al: Does the evidence support a survival benefit of albumin infusion in patients with cirrhosis undergoing large-volume paracentesis? *Expert Rev Gastroenterol Hepatol.* 2017;11(3):191-192.

European Association for the Study of the Liver: EASL clinical practice guidelines for the management of patients with decompensated cirrhosis. *J Hepatol.* 2018;69(2):406-460.

Fede G, et al: Renal failure and cirrhosis: a systematic review of mortality and prognosis. *J Hepatol.* 2012;56:810.

Gordon FD: Ascites. *Clin Liver Dis.* 2012;16:285.

Narahara Y, et al: Transjugular intrahepatic portosystemic shunt versus paracentesis plus albumin in patients with refractory ascites who have good hepatic and renal function: a prospective randomized trial. *J Gastroenterol.* 2011;46:78-85.

White MA, et al: Denver peritoneovenous shunts for the management of malignant ascites: a review of the literature in the post LeVeen era. *Am Surg.* 2011;77:1070.

Wong F: Management of ascites in cirrhosis. *J Gastroenterol Hepatol.* 2012;27:11-20.

HEPATIC ENCEPHALOPATHY

Central nervous system abnormalities may be seen in patients with chronic liver disease and are especially likely after portacaval shunts. Portosystemic encephalopathy, ammonia intoxication, hepatic coma, and meat intoxication are older terms used to refer to this condition. The manifestations range from lethargy to coma—from minor personality changes to psychosis—from asterixis to paraplegia. Hypothermia and hyperventilation may precede coma. The changes may be quite subtle and detectable only with the use of formal neuropsychological or neurophysiologic testing. The differential diagnosis in suspected hepatic encephalopathy is broad and includes diabetic complications, alcohol, drug effects, and infections. The West Haven Criteria for Semiquantitative Grading of Mental State are used to grade hepatic encephalopathy into four grades. Grade 1 is mild and includes trivial lack of awareness and euphoria or anxiety. Grade 2 includes lethargy and inappropriate behavior, which can be treated on an outpatient basis. Grades 3 and 4 are severe and include gross disorientation (grade 3) and coma (grade 4).

Pathogenesis

Hepatic encephalopathy is a reversible metabolic neuropathy that results from the action of chemicals absorbed from the gut on the brain. Increased exposure of the brain to these agents is the result of impaired hepatic metabolism due to cirrhosis or spontaneous or surgically created shunts of portal venous blood around the liver and increased permeability of the blood-brain barrier. The chemical agents responsible for encephalopathy form from the action of colonic bacteria on protein within the gut. Potential aggravating factors include gastrointestinal hemorrhage, constipation, azotemia, hypokalemic alkalosis, infection, excessive dietary protein,

Table 26–7. Factors contributing to encephalopathy.

A. **Increased systemic toxin levels**
1. Extent of portal-systemic venous shunt
2. Depressed liver function
3. Intestinal protein load
4. Intestinal flora
5. Azotemia
6. Constipation

B. **Increased sensitivity of central nervous system**
1. Age of patient
2. Hypokalemia
3. Alkalosis
4. Diuretics
5. Sedatives, narcotics, tranquilizers
6. Infection
7. Hypoxia, hypoglycemia, myxedema

and sedatives (Table 26–7). Four main chemical mediators of this syndrome currently attract the most attention. Low-grade cerebral edema appears to be a major component of the pathophysiologic process.

A. Amino Acid Neurotransmitters

Gamma-aminobutyric acid (GABA), the principal inhibitory neurotransmitter in the brain, produces a state similar to hepatic encephalopathy when given experimentally. It is normally synthesized in the brain and by bacteria within the colon; GABA in the gastrointestinal tract is normally degraded by the liver and is found in increased levels in the serum of patients with hepatic encephalopathy. The passage of GABA across the blood-brain barrier is increased in hepatic encephalopathy. Experiments also indicate the presence of increased numbers of GABA receptors in encephalopathy and increased GABA-ergic tone, perhaps due to a benzodiazepine receptor agonist ligand on the receptor complex (GABA/benzodiazepine receptor). This has raised the possibility of treating encephalopathy with benzodiazepine antagonists, and the drug flumazenil has shown limited promise in preliminary trials.

B. Ammonia

Ammonia is produced in the colon by bacteria and is absorbed and transported in portal venous blood to the liver, where it is extracted and converted to glutamine. Ammonia concentrations are elevated in the arterial blood and cerebrospinal fluid of patients with encephalopathy, and experimental administration of ammonia produces central nervous system symptoms.

C. False Neurotransmitters

According to this theory, cerebral neurons become depleted of normal neurotransmitters (norepinephrine and dopamine), which are partially replaced by false neurotransmitters (octopamine and phenylethanolamine). The result is inhibition of neural function. Serum levels of branched-chain amino acids (leucine, isoleucine, valine) are decreased, and levels of aromatic amino acids (tryptophan, phenylalanine, tyrosine) are elevated in patients with encephalopathy. Because these two classes of amino acids compete for transport across the blood-brain barrier, the aromatic amino acids have increased access to the central nervous system, where they serve as precursors for false neurotransmitters. Trials of therapy with supplements of branched-chain amino acids have given conflicting results.

D. Synergistic Neurotoxins

This theory postulates that ammonia, mercaptans, and fatty acids, none of which accumulate in the brain in amounts capable of producing encephalopathy, have synergistic effects that produce the full-blown syndrome in patients with liver disease.

▶ Prevention

Encephalopathy is a major side effect of portacaval shunt and is to some extent predictable. Elderly patients are considerably more susceptible. Patients with alcoholic liver disease fare better than those with postnecrotic or cryptogenic cirrhosis, apparently owing to the invariable progression of liver dysfunction in the latter. Good liver function partially protects against encephalopathy. If the liver has adapted to complete or nearly complete diversion of portal blood before operation, a surgical shunt is less apt to depress liver function further. For example, patients with thrombosis of the portal vein (complete diversion and normal liver function) rarely experience encephalopathy after portosystemic shunt. Encephalopathy is less common after a distal splenorenal (Warren) shunt than after other kinds of shunts.

Increased intestinal protein, whether of dietary origin or from intestinal bleeding, aggravates encephalopathy by providing more substrate for intestinal bacteria. Constipation allows more time for bacterial action on colonic contents. Azotemia results in higher concentration of blood urea, which diffuses into the intestine, is converted to ammonia, and is then reabsorbed. Hypokalemia and metabolic alkalosis aggravate encephalopathy by shifting ammonia from extracellular to intracellular sites where the toxic action occurs.

▶ Laboratory Findings

Arterial ammonia levels are usually high, although encephalopathy can certainly be present with a normal ammonia level. The presence of high levels of glutamine in the cerebrospinal fluid may help distinguish hepatic encephalopathy from other causes of coma. Electroencephalography is more sensitive than clinical evaluation in detecting minor involvement. The changes are nonspecific and consist of slower mean frequencies. Studies performed at different times can be compared to assess the effects of therapy.

▶ Treatment

Acute encephalopathy is treated by controlling precipitating factors, halting all dietary protein intake, cleansing the bowel with purgatives and enemas, and administering antibiotics (neomycin or ampicillin) or lactulose. Neomycin may be given orally or by gastric tube (two to four times daily) or rectally as an enema (1% solution one or two times daily). At least 1600 kcal of carbohydrate should be provided daily, along with therapeutic amounts of vitamins. Blood volume must be maintained to avoid prerenal azotemia. After the patient responds to initial therapy, dietary protein may be started at 20 g/d and increased by increments of 10-20 g every 2-5 days as tolerated.

Chronic encephalopathy is treated by restriction of dietary protein, avoidance of constipation, and elimination of sedatives, diuretics, and tranquilizers. To avoid protein depletion, protein intake must not be chronically reduced below 50 g/d. Vegetable protein in the diet is better tolerated than animal protein. Lactulose, a disaccharide unaffected by intestinal enzymes, is the drug of choice for long-term control. When given orally (20-30 g three or four times daily), it reaches the colon, where it stimulates bacterial anabolism (which increases ammonia uptake) and inhibits bacterial enzymes (which decreases the generation of nitrogenous toxins). Its effect is independent of colonic pH. A related compound outside the United States, lactitol (β-galactoside sorbitol), is also effective and appears to work faster. As a powder, it is easier to use than liquid lactulose. Intermittent courses of oral neomycin or metronidazole may be given if lactulose therapy and preventive measures are inadequate.

Goh ET, et al: Flumazenil versus placebo or no intervention for people with cirrhosis and hepatic encephalopathy. *Cochrane Database Syst Rev.* 2017;10:8.

Khungar V, Poordad F: Hepatic encephalopathy. *Clin Liver Dis.* 2012;16:301.

Tranah TH, et al: Pathophysiological mechanisms of hepatic encephalopathy. *Clin Liver Dis.* 2015;5:59-63.

Vilstrup H, et al: Hepatic encephalopathy in chronic liver disease: 2014 practice guidelines by the American Association for the Study of the Liver. *Hepatology.* 2014;60:715-735.

HEPATIC ABSCESS

Hepatic abscesses may be bacterial, parasitic, or fungal in origin. In the United States, pyogenic abscesses are the most common, followed by amebic abscesses (see Chapter 8). Unless otherwise indicated, the remarks in this section refer to bacterial abscesses.

Cases are about evenly divided between those with a single abscess and those with multiple abscesses. About 90% of right lobe abscesses are solitary, whereas only 10% of left lobe abscesses are solitary.

In most cases, the development of a hepatic abscess follows a suppurative process elsewhere in the body. Many abscesses are due to direct spread from biliary infections such as empyema of the gallbladder or protracted cholangitis. Abdominal infections such as appendicitis or diverticulitis may spread through the portal vein to involve the liver with abscess formation. Other cases develop after generalized sepsis from bacterial endocarditis, renal infection, or pneumonitis. In 25% of cases, no antecedent infection can be documented ("cryptogenic" abscesses). Rare causes include secondary bacterial infection of an amebic abscess, hydatid cyst, or congenital hepatic cyst. Abscesses may also be caused by trauma or may be secondary to liver-directed therapy. Liver transplant patients are particularly susceptible to pyogenic abscess, especially those with hepatic infarction from vascular complications, or ischemic cholangiopathy.

In most cases, the organism is of enteric origin. *Escherichia coli, Klebsiella pneumoniae, Bacteroides,* enterococci (eg, *Streptococcus faecalis*), anaerobic streptococci (eg, *Peptostreptococcus*), and microaerophilic streptococci are most common. Staphylococci, hemolytic streptococci, or other gram-positive organisms are usually found if the primary infection is bacterial endocarditis or pneumonitis.

▶ Clinical Findings

A. Symptoms and Signs

When liver abscess develops during the course of another intra-abdominal infection such as diverticulitis, it is accompanied by increasing toxicity, higher fever, and a generally deteriorating clinical picture. Right upper quadrant pain, jaundice, and chills may appear.

In other cases, the diagnosis is much less obvious, since the illness develops insidiously in a previously healthy person. In these patients, the first symptoms are usually malaise and fatigue, followed after several weeks by fever. Epigastric or right upper quadrant pain is present in about half of cases. The pain may be aggravated by motion or may be referred to the right shoulder.

The course of fever is often erratic, and spikes to 40-41°C are common. Chills are present in about 25% of cases. The liver is usually enlarged and may be tender to palpation. If tenderness is severe, the condition may be confused with cholecystitis.

Jaundice is unusual in solitary abscesses unless the patient's condition is worsening. Jaundice is often present in patients with multiple abscesses.

B. Laboratory Findings

Leukocytosis is present in most cases and is usually over 15,000/μL. A small group of patients, usually the most seriously ill, may fail to develop leukocytosis. Anemia is frequently seen. The average hematocrit is 33%. Blood cultures are positive in 50% of patients and should be drawn at the time of presentation.

Serum bilirubin is usually normal except in patients with multiple abscesses or biliary obstruction or when hepatic failure has supervened. Alkaline phosphatase is often elevated even in the presence of a normal bilirubin.

C. Imaging Studies

X-ray changes present in the right lung in about one-third of cases and consist of basilar atelectasis or pleural effusion. The right diaphragm may be elevated and less mobile than the left.

Plain films of the abdomen are usually normal or show only hepatomegaly. In a few patients, an air-fluid level in the region of the liver reveals the presence and location of the abscess. Distortion of the contour of the stomach on upper gastrointestinal series may be seen with large abscesses involving the left lobe.

Ultrasound and CT scans are the most useful diagnostic tests, providing accurate information regarding the presence, size, number, and location of abscesses within the liver. CT scans have the added advantage of being able to demonstrate abscesses or neoplasms elsewhere in the abdomen. The radioisotope liver scintiscan is able to demonstrate most liver abscesses but is nonspecific, gives little other useful information, and is therefore not helpful.

▶ Differential Diagnosis

In many cases, early findings may be so vague that hepatic abscess is not even considered. The multiple other causes of malaise, weight loss, and anemia would then enter into the differential diagnosis. With spiking fevers, one must consider all the causes of fever of unknown origin. Failure to entertain the idea of hepatic abscess and to obtain the necessary scans leads to most errors and delays in diagnosis.

Once imaging tests have demonstrated the abscess, the responsible organisms must be identified. Amebiasis should be considered in cases of a solitary abscess. Compared with amebic abscesses, pyogenic liver abscesses are seen more often in patients older than 50 years and are associated with jaundice, pruritus, sepsis, a palpable mass, and elevated bilirubin and alkaline phosphatase levels. Patients with amebic abscesses more often have been to an endemic area and have abdominal pain and tenderness, diarrhea, hepatomegaly, and positive serologic tests for amebiasis.

▶ Complications

Intrahepatic spread of infection may create multiple additional abscesses and is responsible for some failures after treatment of an apparently solitary abscess. As the untreated abscess expands, rupture may occur into the pleural or peritoneal cavity, usually with catastrophic results. Septicemia and septic shock are common terminal complications of diffuse hepatic infection. Hepatic failure may develop in addition to uncontrolled sepsis, or it may predominate over signs of infection.

Hemobilia may follow bleeding from the vascular wall into the abscess cavity. In this case, hepatic artery embolization or ligation may be required to control bleeding.

▶ Treatment

Antibiotics should be started promptly. Most infections are polymicrobial. Initial coverage, before culture results are available, should be adequate for *E coli, K pneumoniae, Bacteroides*, enterococci, and anaerobic streptococci and consequently would usually include an aminoglycoside, clindamycin or metronidazole, and ampicillin. The regimen may be modified later according to the results of cultures. Antibiotics are generally continued for 4-6 weeks total.

About 80% or more of patients with liver abscesses are adequately treated by drainage catheters inserted percutaneously under ultrasound or CT guidance. Whether the patient has a single abscess or multiple abscesses, this is usually the most appropriate initial therapy. Single abscesses less than or equal to 5 cm in size can be drained with needle aspiration or placement of a catheter. Abscesses greater than 5 cm should have a catheter placed. The catheters can be removed in 1-2 weeks after output becomes nonpurulent and scant.

In about 40% of patients, the catheters do not drain well following initial placement and must be repositioned. The principal advantage of percutaneous drainage is lower morbidity compared to open drainage, although not necessarily lower mortality. It is easier to provide thorough drainage surgically, so when difficulties are encountered with percutaneous drainage, laparotomy should be performed promptly. Surgical intervention is more often necessary in cases of multiple, loculated collections or when the abscess cavity contains a large amount of necrotic debris. In such cases, open debridement should be considered early. Likewise, early surgical intervention is indicated for patients who are seriously ill (APACHE II score ≥ 15). Rarely, multiple abscesses are confined to a single lobe and can be cured by lobectomy. Biliary obstruction or other causes of sepsis must also be corrected.

▶ Prognosis

The overall mortality rate of 15% is more closely related to the underlying disease than to any other factor. The mortality rate is about 40% in patients with malignant disease. Pleural effusion, leukocytosis greater than 20,000/μL, hypoalbuminemia, and polymicrobial infection correlate with a poor outcome. In the United States, whether the abscess is solitary or multiple no longer has a major influence on survival, but where benign biliary disease remains a major cause of this disease, multiple hepatic abscesses are associated with a worse prognosis. Death is rare in patients with a cryptogenic liver abscess.

Bächler P, et al: Multimodality imaging of liver infections: differential diagnosis and potential pitfalls. *Radiographics*. 2016; 36(4):1001-1023.
Reid-Lombardo KM, et al: Hepatic cysts and liver abscess. *Surg Clin North Am*. 2010;90:679.
Yu SC, et al: Treatment of pyogenic liver abscess: prospective randomized comparison of catheter drainage and needle operation. *Hepatology*. 2004;39:932-938.

MULTIPLE CHOICE QUESTIONS

1. Which of the following is *not* true about the blood supply to the liver?

   A. The portal vein is formed by the confluence of the splenic and superior mesenteric veins at the level of the second lumbar vertebra behind the head of the pancreas.
   B. The common hepatic artery typically arises from the superior mesenteric artery, ascends in the hepatoduodenal ligament, and gives rise to the right gastric, gastroduodenal, and proper hepatic arteries.
   C. In the hepatoduodenal ligament, the common bile duct lies anteriorly and slightly lateral to the portal vein.
   D. A replaced right hepatic artery typically arises from the superior mesenteric artery and courses posteriorly and to the right of the common bile duct within the porta hepatis.
   E. A replaced left hepatic artery typically arises from the left gastric artery.

2. The Child-Pugh classification of functional status in liver disease does not include

   A. Ascites
   B. Serum bilirubin
   C. Albumin
   D. Serum creatinine
   E. Encephalopathy

3. A grade III liver injury includes

   A. Subcapsular, nonexpanding hematoma occupying 10%-50% of surface area
   B. Laceration greater than 3 cm deep into the parenchyma
   C. Retrohepatic inferior vena cava vascular injury
   D. Parenchymal disruption involving > 75% of hepatic lobe
   E. Hepatic avulsion

4. Which of the following can be a posthepatic cause of portal hypertension?

   A. Wilson disease
   B. Hemochromatosis
   C. Portal vein thrombosis
   D. Budd-Chiari syndrome
   E. Schistosomiasis

5. Which of the following portosystemic shunts is most likely to lead to encephalopathy?

   A. Distal splenorenal shunt (Warren)
   B. End-to-side portocaval shunt
   C. Transjugular intrahepatic portosystemic shunt
   D. Central splenorenal
   E. Left gastric vena caval (Inokuchi)

Biliary Tract

David A. Harris, MD

Eric G. Sheu, MD

EMBRYOLOGY & ANATOMY

The anlage of the biliary ducts and liver is a diverticulum appearing on the ventral foregut in 3 mm embryos. The cranial portion becomes the liver; a caudal bud, the ventral pancreas; and an intermediate bud, the gallbladder. The hepatic diverticulum becomes a solid mass of cells that later recanalizes to form ducts. The smallest, the bile canaliculi, first appear as a basal network between the primitive hepatocytes (Figure 27–1). In most cases, the common hepatic duct is formed by the union of a single right and left duct. In 25% of individuals, the anterior and posterior divisions of the right duct join the left duct separately. The origin of the common hepatic duct is close to the liver but always outside its substance. It runs 4 cm before joining the cystic duct to form the common bile duct. The common duct begins in the hepatoduodenal ligament, passes behind the first portion of the duodenum, and runs in a groove on the posterior surface of the pancreas before entering the duodenum. Its terminal 1 cm is intimately adherent to the duodenal wall. The total length of the common duct is about 9 cm.

In 80%-90% of individuals, the main pancreatic duct joins the common duct to form a common channel about 1 cm long. The intraduodenal segment of the duct is called the hepatopancreatic ampulla, or ampulla of Vater.

The gallbladder is a pear-shaped organ adherent to the undersurface of liver segments 4b and 5 by a veil of peritoneum known as the, cystic plate. The fundus projects 1-2 cm below the hepatic edge. The gallbladder rarely has a complete peritoneal covering. The lumen of the cystic duct contains a thin mucosal septum, the spiral valve of Heister, that offers mild resistance to bile flow. The neck of the gallbladder tapers into the narrow cystic duct, which in 75% of people connects with the common duct. However, biliary anatomy is highly variable. The cystic duct can be short or long and can insert directly into the right hepatic duct, runs parallel to the hepatic duct, or winds around it before joining the common duct. An accessory right hepatic duct is also common (Figure 27–2).

In the hepatoduodenal ligament, the hepatic artery is to the left of the common duct, and the portal vein is posterior and medial. The right hepatic artery usually passes behind the hepatic duct and then gives off the cystic artery before entering the right lobe of the liver, but variations are common. A replaced right hepatic artery is typically found coming off the superior mesenteric artery and will course along the lateral aspect of the common bile duct. The cystic artery can also have varied origins, but its termination is usually found by Calot's node, which sits at the gallbladder infundibular-cystic junction.

PHYSIOLOGY

▶ Bile Flow

Bile is produced from cholesterol at a rate of 500-1500 mL/d, and bile salts are actively secreted into the biliary canaliculus. Na^+ and water follow passively to establish isosmolality and electrical neutrality. Lecithin and cholesterol are secreted at rates that correlate with variations in bile salt output. In addition, bilirubin and a number of other organic anions are actively secreted by the hepatocytes.

The columnar cells of the ducts add a fluid rich in HCO_3^- to that produced in the canaliculus. This involves active secretion stimulated by secretin, vasoactive intestinal peptide (VIP), and cholecystokinin (CCK). K^+ and water are distributed passively across the ducts (Figure 27–3).

Between meals, bile is stored in the gallbladder, where it is concentrated at rates of up to 20% per hour. Na^+ and either HCO_3^- or Cl^- are actively transported from its lumen during absorption. The changes in bile composition brought about by the act of concentration are shown in Figure 27–4.

Three factors regulate bile flow: hepatic secretion, gallbladder contraction, and choledochal sphincteric resistance.

▲ **Figure 27–1.** Scanning electron photomicrograph of a hepatic plate with adjacent sinusoids and sinusoidal microvilli and a bile canaliculus running in the center of the liver cells. Although their boundaries are indistinct, about four hepatocytes constitute the section of the plate in the middle of the photograph. Occasional red cells are present within the sinusoids. (Reduced from ×2000.)

In the fasting state, pressure in the common bile duct is 5-10 cm H_2O, and bile produced in the liver is diverted into the gallbladder. After a meal, the gallbladder contracts, reaching 25 cm H_2O; the sphincter relaxes; and bile is forced into the duodenum as ductal pressure (15-20 cm H_2O) exceeds sphincteric resistance.

CCK is the major physiologic stimulus for postprandial gallbladder contraction and relaxation of the sphincter, but vagal impulses facilitate its action. CCK is released into the bloodstream from the mucosa of the small bowel by fat or lipolytic products in the lumen. Amino acids and small polypeptides are weaker stimuli, and carbohydrates are ineffective. Bile flow during a meal is augmented by turnover of bile salts in the enterohepatic circulation and stimulation of ductal secretion by secretin, VIP, and CCK. Motilin stimulates episodic partial gallbladder emptying in the interdigestive phase.

▶ Bile Salts & the Enterohepatic Circulation

Bile salts, lecithin, and cholesterol compose about 90% of the solids in bile, with the remainder consisting of bilirubin, fatty acids, and inorganic salts. Gallbladder bile contains about 10% solids and has a bile salt concentration between 200 and 300 mmol/L (Figure 27–4).

Bile salts are steroid molecules formed from cholesterol by hepatocytes. The rate of synthesis is under feedback control and can be increased to a maximum of about 20-fold. Two **primary** bile salts—cholate and chenodeoxycholate—are produced by the liver. Before excretion into bile, they are conjugated with either glycine or taurine, which enhances

water solubility. Intestinal bacteria alter these compounds to produce the **secondary** bile salts, deoxycholate and lithocholate. Bile salts function to (1) induce the flow of bile, (2) transport lipids, (3) bind calcium ions in bile, and (4) regulate metabolic functions. The importance of the last of these is unknown, but it is clear that bile acid signaling is capable of affecting global glucose and fat metabolism and likely contributes to the metabolic benefits of bariatric operations such as Roux-en-Y gastric bypass and sleeve gastrectomy.

Bile acid molecules are amphipathic—ie, they have hydrophilic and hydrophobic poles. In bile, they form multimolecular aggregates called micelles in which the hydrophilic poles become aligned to face the aqueous medium. Water-insoluble lipids, such as cholesterol, can be dissolved within the hydrophobic centers of bile salt micelles. Molecules of lecithin, which is water insoluble but polar lipid, aggregate into hydrated bilayers that form vesicles in bile, and they also become incorporated into bile acid micelles to form mixed micelles. Mixed micelles have an increased lipid-carrying capacity compared with pure bile acid micelles. Cholesterol in bile is transported within the phospholipid vesicles and the bile salt micelles.

Bile salts remain in the intestinal lumen throughout the jejunum, where they participate in fat digestion and absorption (Figure 27–5). Upon reaching the distal small bowel, they are reabsorbed by an active transport system located in the terminal 200 cm of ileum. Over 95% of bile salts arriving from the jejunum are transferred by this process into portal vein blood; the remainder enter the colon, where they are converted to secondary bile salts by colonic bacteria. The entire bile salt pool of 2.5-4 g circulates twice through the enterohepatic circulation during each meal, and six to eight cycles are made each day. The normal daily loss of bile salts in the stool amounts to 10%-20% of the pool and is restored by hepatic synthesis.

▶ Bilirubin

About 250-300 mg of bilirubin is excreted each day in the bile, 75% of it from breakdown of red cells in the reticuloendothelial system and 25% from turnover of hepatic heme and hemoproteins. First, heme is liberated from hemoglobin, and the iron and globin are removed for reuse by the organism. Biliverdin, the first pigment formed from heme, is reduced to unconjugated bilirubin, the indirect-reacting bilirubin of the van den Bergh test. Unconjugated bilirubin is insoluble in water and is transported in plasma bound to albumin.

Unconjugated bilirubin is extracted from blood by hepatocytes, where it is conjugated with glucuronic acid to form bilirubin diglucuronide, the water-soluble direct bilirubin. Conjugation is catalyzed by glucuronyl transferase, an enzyme on the endoplasmic reticulum. Bilirubin is transported within the hepatocyte by cytosolic binding proteins, which rapidly deliver the molecule to the canalicular

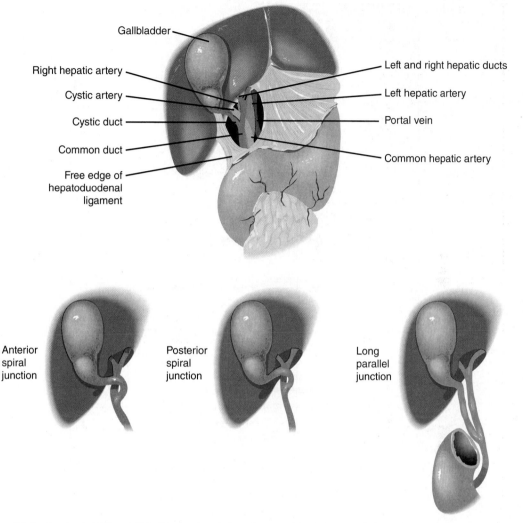

Gallbladder

Right hepatic artery

Cystic artery

Cystic duct

Common duct

Free edge of
hepatoduodenal
ligament

Left and right hepatic ducts

Left hepatic artery

Portal vein

Common hepatic artery

Anterior
spiral
junction

Posterior
spiral
junction

Long
parallel
junction

▲ **Figure 27–2.** Anatomy of the gallbladder and variations in anatomy of the cystic duct.

membrane for active secretion into bile. Within bile, conjugated bilirubin is largely transported in association with mixed lipid micelles.

After entering the intestine, bilirubin is reduced by intestinal bacteria to several compounds known as urobilinogens, which are subsequently oxidized and converted to pigmented urobilins. The term *urobilinogen* is often used to refer to both urobilins and urobilinogens.

PATHOGENESIS OF GALLSTONES

More than 20 million people in the United States have gallstones in their gallbladders; about 300,000-600,000 operations are performed annually for this disease, and at least 6000 deaths result from its complications or treatment. The incidence of gallstones increases with age, so that between 50 and 65 years of age, about 20% of women and 5% of men are affected.

The gallstones in 75% of patients are composed predominantly (70%-95%) of cholesterol and are called cholesterol stones. The remaining 25% are pigment stones. Regardless of composition, all gallstones give rise to similar clinical sequelae.

▶ Cholesterol Gallstones

Cholesterol gallstones result from secretion of bile supersaturated with cholesterol. Influenced by various factors present in bile, the cholesterol precipitates from solution, and the newly formed crystals grow to macroscopic stones. Except

Bile lipids

Bile salts

Bile salts

LIVER

Bile salts

H_2O

Enterohepatic circulation

Mixed micelles

Bile pigments (other organic ions)

Inorganic ions

Vagal tone

Secretin, CCK, gastrin

BILE DUCT

HCO_3^-, Na^+

K^+, Cl^-, H_2O

HCO_3^-, Na^+, H_2O

Bile ⟶ Fat absorption

Jejunum   Ileum

▲ **Figure 27–3.** Bile formation. Solid lines into the ductular lumen indicate active transport; dotted lines represent passive diffusion.

when the common bile duct is dilated or partially obstructed, the stones in this disease form exclusively within the gallbladder. Those found in the ducts usually reach that location after passing through the cystic duct.

The incidence of cholesterol gallstone disease is highest in American Indians, lower in whites, and lowest in blacks, with a twofold gradient from one group to the next. More than 75% of American Indian women over age 40 are affected. Before puberty, the disease is rare but of equal frequency in both sexes. Thereafter, women are more commonly affected than men until after menopause, when the discrepancy lessens. Hormonal effects are also reflected in the increased incidence of gallstones with multiparity and the increased cholesterol saturation of bile and greater incidence of gallstones following ingestion of oral contraceptives. Obesity is the other major risk factor. The relative risk rises proportionately to the extent of overweight due to a progressively increasing output of cholesterol in bile.

▲ **Figure 27–4.** Changes in gallbladder bile composition with time. (Used wth permission from J Dietschy.)

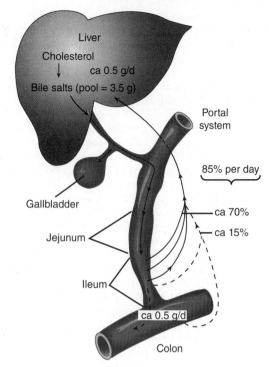

▲ **Figure 27–5.** Enterohepatic circulation of bile salts. (Used with permission from M Tyor.)

As noted previously, cholesterol is insoluble and, in bile, must be transported within bile salt micelles and phospholipid (lecithin) vesicles. When the amount of cholesterol in bile exceeds the cholesterol holding capacity, cholesterol crystals begin to precipitate from the phospholipid vesicles.

The secretion of bile salt and cholesterol into bile is linked. Bile salt elutes cholesterol from the hepatocyte membrane during passage into the bile canaliculus. At higher bile salt output levels, the amount of cholesterol relative to bile salt entering bile decreases. This means that during low bile flow (eg, during fasting), bile holding capacity for cholesterol is more saturated than during high bile flow. In fact, almost half of persons in Western cultures have bile supersaturated with cholesterol in the morning after an overnight fast. The bile salt pool in patients with cholesterol gallstone disease is about half the size of that of normal subjects, but this is a result of the gallstone disease (eg, gallstones displace bile in the gallbladder) and not a cause.

The occurrence of cholesterol gallstone disease requires cholesterol supersaturation of bile, but that in itself is not sufficient. Cholesterol in supersaturated bile from individuals without gallstone disease precipitates spontaneously at a much slower rate than does the cholesterol in similar bile from patients with gallstones. Furthermore, among individuals with supersaturated bile, only those with gallstone disease demonstrate cholesterol crystal formation in vivo. These observations are the result of specific bile proteins that either stabilize or destabilize cholesterol-laden phospholipid vesicles. For gallstone formation, the pronucleating factors (eg, immunoglobulin, mucus glycoprotein, fibronectin, orosomucoid) appear to be more important than the antinucleating factors (eg, glycoprotein, apolipoprotein, cytokeratin). Variations in these proteins may be the critical factor determining which of the many individuals with saturated bile develop gallstones.

The fact that gallstones form almost exclusively in the gallbladder, even though the composition of hepatic bile is abnormal, underscores the important role of the gallbladder in gallstone pathogenesis. This includes concentrating the bile, providing nidi (eg, small grains of pigment) for crystallization of cholesterol, supplying mucoprotein to paste the stones together, and serving as an area of stasis to allow stone formation and growth.

▶ Pigment Stones

Pigment stones account for 25% of gallstones in the United States and 60% of those in Japan. Pigment stones are black to dark brown, 2-5 mm in diameter, and amorphous. They are composed of a mixture of calcium bilirubinate, complex bilirubin polymers, bile acids, and other unidentified substances. About 50% are radiopaque, and in the United States, they constitute two-thirds of all radiopaque gallstones. The incidence is similar in men and women and in blacks and whites. Pigment stones are rare in American Indians.

Predisposing factors are cirrhosis, bile stasis (eg, a strictured or markedly dilated common duct), and chronic hemolysis. Some patients with pigment stones have increased concentrations of unconjugated bilirubin in their bile. Scanning electron microscopy demonstrates that about 90% of pigment stones are composed of dense mixtures of bacteria and bacterial glycocalyx along with pigment solids. This suggests that bacteria have a primary role in pigment gallstone formation, and it also helps to explain why patients with pigment gallstone disease have sepsis more often than do those with cholesterol gallstone disease. It seems likely that bacterial β-glucuronidase is responsible for deconjugating the soluble bilirubin-diglucuronide to insoluble unconjugated bilirubin, which subsequently becomes agglomerated by glycocalyx into macroscopic stones.

JAUNDICE

Jaundice is categorized as prehepatic, hepatic, or posthepatic, depending on the site of the underlying disease. Hemolysis, the most common cause of prehepatic jaundice, involves increased production of bilirubin. Less common causes of prehepatic jaundice are Gilbert disease and the Crigler-Najjar syndrome.

Hepatic parenchymal jaundice is subdivided into hepatocellular and cholestatic types. The former includes acute viral hepatitis and chronic alcoholic cirrhosis. Some cases of intrahepatic cholestasis may be indistinguishable clinically and biochemically from cholestasis due to bile duct obstruction. Primary biliary cirrhosis, toxic drug jaundice, cholestatic jaundice of pregnancy, and postoperative cholestatic jaundice are the most common forms.

Extrahepatic jaundice most often results from biliary obstruction by a malignant tumor, choledocholithiasis, or biliary stricture. Pancreatic pseudocyst, chronic pancreatitis, sclerosing cholangitis, metastatic cancer, and duodenal diverticulitis are less common causes.

The cause of jaundice can be ascertained in the majority of patients from clinical and laboratory findings alone. In the remainder, transhepatic cholangiography (THC) or endoscopic retrograde cholangiopancreatography (ERCP) and ultrasound or computed tomography (CT) scans will be necessary. The indications for these tests are discussed in later sections.

▶ History

The age, gender, and parity of the patient and possible deleterious habits should be noted. Most cases of infectious hepatitis occur in patients under age 30. A history of drug addiction may suggest serum hepatitis transmitted by shared hypodermic equipment. Chronic alcoholism can usually be documented in patients with cirrhosis, and acute jaundice in alcoholics usually follows a recent binge. Obstructing gallstones or tumors are more common in older people.

Patients with jaundice due to choledocholithiasis may have associated biliary colic, fever, and chills and may report previous similar attacks. In contrast, pain is either absent in malignant obstruction or deep-seated and dull. Pain in the region of the liver is frequently experienced in the early stages of viral hepatitis and acute alcoholic liver injury. The patient with extrahepatic obstruction may report that stools have become lighter in color and the urine dark. Cholestatic diseases are often accompanied by pruritus. The cause remains obscure; itching does not correlate with bile salt levels in the skin, as was once believed.

▶ Physical Examination

Hepatomegaly is common in both hepatic and posthepatic jaundice. In some cases, palpation of the liver may suggest cirrhosis or metastatic cancer, but impressions of this kind are unreliable. Secondary stigmata of cirrhosis usually accompany acute alcoholic jaundice; palmar erythema, spider angiomas, ascites, collateral veins on the abdominal walls, and splenomegaly suggest cirrhosis. A nontender, palpable gallbladder in a jaundiced patient suggests malignant obstruction of the common duct (Courvoisier sign), but absence of a palpable gallbladder is of little significance in ruling out cancer.

▶ Laboratory Tests

In hemolytic disease, the increased bilirubin is principally in the unconjugated indirect fraction. Because unconjugated bilirubin is insoluble in water, the jaundice in hemolysis is acholuric. The total bilirubin in hemolysis rarely exceeds 4-5 mg/dL because the rate of excretion increases as the bilirubin concentration rises and a plateau is quickly reached. Greater values suggest concomitant hepatic parenchymal disease.

Jaundice due to hepatic parenchymal disease is characterized by elevations of both conjugated and unconjugated serum bilirubin. An increase in the conjugated fraction always signifies disease within the hepatobiliary system. The direct bilirubin predominates in about half of cases of hepatic parenchymal disease.

Both intrahepatic cholestasis and extrahepatic obstruction raise the direct bilirubin fraction, although the indirect fraction also increases somewhat. Because direct bilirubin is water soluble, bilirubinuria develops. With complete extrahepatic obstruction, the total bilirubin rises to a plateau of 25-30 mg/dL, at which point loss in the urine equals the additional daily production. Higher values suggest concomitant hemolysis or decreased renal function. Obstruction of a single hepatic duct does not usually cause jaundice.

In extrahepatic obstruction caused by neoplasms, the serum bilirubin usually exceeds 10 mg/dL, and the average concentration is about 18 mg/dL. Obstructive jaundice due to common duct stones often produces transient bilirubin increases in the range of 2-4 mg/dL, and the level rarely exceeds 15 mg/dL. Serum bilirubin values in patients with alcoholic cirrhosis and acute viral hepatitis vary widely in relation to the severity of the parenchymal damage.

In extrahepatic obstruction, modest rises of aspartate aminotransferase (AST) levels are common, but levels as high as 1000 units/L are seen (although rarely) in patients with common duct stones and cholangitis. In the latter patients, the high values last for only a few days and are associated with increases in lactate dehydrogenase (LDH) concentrations. In general, AST levels above 1000 units/L suggest viral hepatitis.

Serum alkaline phosphatase comes from three sites: liver, bone, and intestine. In normal subjects, liver and bone contribute about equally, and the intestinal contribution is small. Hepatic alkaline phosphatase is a product of the epithelial cells of the cholangioles, and increased alkaline phosphatase levels associated with liver disease result from increased enzyme production. Alkaline phosphatase levels increase with intrahepatic cholestasis, cholangitis, or extrahepatic obstruction. Because the elevation is from overproduction, it may occur with focal hepatic lesions in the absence of jaundice. For example, a solitary hepatic metastasis or pyogenic abscess in one lobe or a tumor obstructing only one hepatic duct may fail to obstruct enough hepatic parenchyma to cause jaundice but usually is associated with increased alkaline phosphatase. In cholangitis with incomplete extrahepatic obstruction, serum bilirubin levels may be normal or mildly elevated, but serum alkaline phosphatase may be very high.

Bone disease may complicate the interpretation of abnormal alkaline phosphatase levels (Figure 27–6). If one suspects that the increased serum enzyme may be from bone, serum calcium, phosphorus, and 5′-nucleotidase or leucine aminopeptidase levels should be determined. These last two enzymes are also produced by cholangioles and are elevated in cholestasis, but their serum concentrations remain unchanged with bone disease.

Changes in serum protein levels may reflect hepatic parenchymal dysfunction. In cirrhosis, the serum albumin falls and the globulins increase. Serum globulins reach high values in some patients with primary biliary cirrhosis. Biliary obstruction generally produces no changes unless secondary biliary cirrhosis has developed.

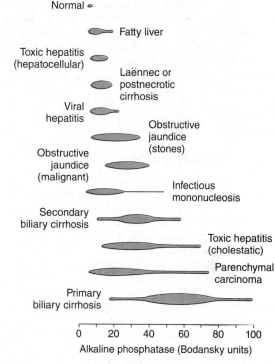

▲ **Figure 27–6.** Range of alkaline phosphatase values in various hepatobiliary disorders.

▶ **Diagnosis**

The principal diagnostic objective is to distinguish surgical (obstructive) from nonsurgical jaundice. The history, physical examination, and basic laboratory data allow an accurate diagnosis to be made in most cases without invasive tests. Most patients with jaundice are not critically ill when first examined; thus, diagnosis and therapy may be conducted in a stepwise fashion. However, severe or worsening cholangitis requires urgent intervention. If the jaundice is mild and recent, it often passes within 24-48 hours, at which time adjunct tests can be ordered to verify gallstone disease.

A comprehensive discussion of available imaging modalities is found in the following sections. In patients with persistent jaundice, the first test is usually an abdominal ultrasound to allow for assessment of ductal dilation and cholelithiasis. Lesions may be further delineated by magnetic resonance cholangiopancreatography (MRCP), ERCP, endoscopic ultrasound (EUS), or THC. ERCP is preferable when the lower end of the duct is believed to be obstructed or if the presence of choledocholithiasis is likely. THC is usually preferred for proximal lesions because it gives better opacification of the ducts proximal to the obstruction and therefore provides more information that can be used in planning surgery. If the clinical presentation suggests neoplastic obstruction, magnetic resonance imaging (MRI) or multiphase, thin-slice CT scan will allow improved definition of the mass, surrounding structures, and general location of bile duct obstruction.

DIAGNOSTIC EXAMINATION OF THE BILIARY TREE

▶ Abdominal Ultrasound

Due to its low risk and high sensitivity and specificity, transabdominal ultrasonography is the primary adjunct test of choice for the detection of cholelithiasis and cholecystitis and evaluation for bile duct dilation. Cholecystitis is suggested by distension of the gallbladder, the presence of stones, pericholecystic edema, and the presence of a sonographic Murphy sign. In the investigation of gallbladder disease, false-positive diagnoses for stones are rare, and false-negative reports due to small stones or a contracted gallbladder occur in only 5% of patients examined by real-time ultrasound. Ultrasound usually misses stones in the common duct, but a dilated common bile duct can hint toward the presence of choledocholithiasis and suggest the need for further intervention or imaging to confirm the presence of choledocholithiasis.

The ultrasonographer occasionally reports that the gallbladder contains "sludge." This material is sonographically opaque, does not cast an acoustic shadow, and forms a dependent layer in the gallbladder. On clinical analysis, it is a fine precipitate of calcium bilirubinate. Sludge may accompany gallstone disease or may be a solitary finding. It is observed in a variety of clinical settings, many of which are characterized by gallbladder stasis. By itself, sludge is not an indication for cholecystectomy.

▶ Abdominal Computed Tomography

Patients presenting with abdominal pain with an unclear history and leukocytosis are often sent for abdominal CT. Although this is not the imaging modality of choice for evaluation of the gallbladder or biliary tree, it does have good specificity and sensitivity for the detection of acute cholecystitis. For the evaluation of the patient with persistent jaundice, it allows for superior detection of pancreatic and distal obstructive pathology.

▶ Radionuclide Scan (Hepatobiliary Iminodiacetic Acid Scan)

Technetium-99m–labeled derivatives of iminodiacetic acid (IDA) are excreted in high concentration in bile and produce excellent gamma camera images. Following intravenous injection of the radionuclide, imaging of the bile ducts and gallbladder normally appears within 15-30 minutes and imaging of the intestine within 60 minutes. In patients with acute right upper quadrant pain and tenderness, a good image of the bile duct accompanied by no image of the gallbladder indicates cystic duct obstruction and strongly supports a diagnosis of acute cholecystitis. The test is easy to perform and is occasionally a useful method of confirming this diagnosis in patients with equivocal history and imaging for acute cholecystitis.

In addition, if biliary dyskinesia is suspected, a hepatobiliary IDA (HIDA) scan can be used to measure the gallbladder ejection fraction after CCK stimulation. Finally, HIDA scanning is useful in the postcholecystectomy patient to diagnose a biliary leak, although the scan usually lacks the fidelity to determine the exact location of the leak.

▶ Magnetic Resonance Cholangiopancreatography

MRCP and ERCP are the two most sensitive (approximately 90% for MRCP and near 100% for ERCP) and specific (approximately 90% for MRCP and 100% for ERCP) modalities for the evaluation of choledocholithiasis. MRCP has resolution to detect stones as small as 2 mm. In patients in whom choledocholithiasis is highly likely, forgoing MRCP for ERCP is prudent because ERCP affords the opportunity for intervention. However, if the diagnosis is in question, MRCP offers the advantage of being noninvasive, without the risk of ERCP-related complications such as pancreatitis, bleeding, or perforation.

▶ Endoscopic Retrograde Cholangiopancreatography

ERCP involves cannulating the sphincter of Oddi under direct vision through a side-viewing duodenoscope. It requires special training involving more than familiarity with the use of fiberoptic endoscopes. Usually it is possible to opacify the pancreatic and bile ducts. It is the preferred method of examining the biliary tree in patients with presumed choledocholithiasis or obstructing lesions in the periampullary region and provides access for therapeutic intervention.

▶ Endoscopic Ultrasound

Using specialized echoendoscopes, EUS allows high-resolution imaging of the biliary tree, pancreas, and stomach. EUS can be used to guide biopsy as well as more advanced interventions. For choledocholithiasis, EUS has a sensitivity of 89%-94% and a specificity of 94%-95%. For small stones in particular, EUS may be more sensitive than MRCP. If choledocholithiasis is detected on EUS, therapeutic ERCP can be immediately performed.

Percutaneous Transhepatic Cholangiography

Percutaneous THC is performed by passing a fine needle through the right lower rib cage and the hepatic parenchyma and into the lumen of a bile duct. Water-soluble contrast material is injected, and fluoroscopy is performed.

The technical success is related to the degree of dilatation of the intrahepatic bile ducts. THC is especially valuable in demonstrating the biliary anatomy in patients with benign biliary strictures, malignant lesions of the proximal bile duct, or when ERCP has been unsuccessful. Patients should be premedicated with antibiotics regardless of whether they have cholangitis—septic shock has been produced by sudden inoculation of organisms from bile into the systemic circulation. Otherwise, the contraindications are the same as for percutaneous liver biopsy.

Intraoperative Imaging

Patients with cholecystitis and equivocal imaging or laboratory testing can undergo intraoperative imaging to assess for common bile duct stones.

Intraoperative cholangiogram (IOC) is performed by direct cannulation of the cystic duct or gallbladder infundibulum during laparoscopic or open cholecystectomy. Contrast material is injected through the cannulation, and fluoroscopy is used to assess for common bile duct stones. Stones present in the duct can sometimes be cleared by flushing and glucagon administration to promote relaxation of the sphincter of Oddi.

Some have recommended routine use of IOC as a means to limit and detect bile duct injuries during cholecystectomy. During routine use of IOC, 2%-10% of patients will have a common bile duct stone, 10% of which will not have been suspected preoperatively, and the majority of incidentally detected common bile duct stones will pass spontaneously without clinical sequelae.

Intraoperative ultrasound is another imaging modality that can be performed to define biliary and vascular anatomy and has a high sensitivity and specificity for the detection of common bile duct stones. However, unlike IOC, ultrasound does not afford the ability to intervene upon any identified pathology. The learning curve for this modality is steep, with upward of 100 cases needed for mastery.

▼ DISEASES OF THE GALLBLADDER & BILE DUCTS

ASYMPTOMATIC GALLSTONES

Data on the prevalence of gallstones in the United States indicate that only about 30% of people with cholelithiasis come to surgery. Symptoms of gallstone disease generally do not change in severity. Each year, about 2% of patients with asymptomatic gallstones develop symptoms, usually biliary colic rather than one of the complications of gallstone disease. Patients with chronic biliary colic tend to have symptoms of the same level of severity and frequency. The present practice of operating only on symptomatic patients, leaving the millions without symptoms alone, seems appropriate. A question is often raised about what to advise the asymptomatic patient found to have gallstones during the course of unrelated studies. The presence of the following portends a more serious course and should probably serve as a reason for consideration of prophylactic cholecystectomy in the asymptomatic patient: (1) large stones (> 1 cm in diameter), because they progress to symptomatic disease more often than small stones; (2) calcified gallbladder, as it may be associated with carcinoma; and (3) enlarging or > 1 cm gallbladder polyps, given the potential risk of malignancy. However, most asymptomatic patients have no special features. If coexistent cardiopulmonary or other problems increase the risk of surgery, operation should not be considered. For the average asymptomatic patient, it is not reasonable to make a strong recommendation for cholecystectomy. The tendency, however, is to operate on younger patients and temporize in the elderly.

BILIARY DYSKINESIA

Patients with histories consistent with biliary colic, but in the absence of stone disease may have a functional gallbladder disorder. Typically, after an overnight fast, a HIDA scan in the presence of CCK is performed over a 45-minute period. A gallbladder ejection fraction less than 40% is considered evidence of gallbladder dyskinesia. Reproduction of symptoms with administration of CCK may also support the diagnosis of biliary dyskinesia. False positives are seen in patients on opioids, with diabetes, and on calcium channel blockers, oral contraceptives, or other medications. In patients with recurring, biliary-type pain and a HIDA-CCK test consistent with dyskinesia, cholecystectomy may be beneficial.

GALLSTONES & CHRONIC CHOLECYSTITIS (BILIARY COLIC)

ESSENTIALS OF DIAGNOSIS

▶ Episodic abdominal pain

▶ Dyspepsia

▶ Gallstones on cholecystography or ultrasound scan

General Considerations

Chronic cholecystitis is the most common form of symptomatic gallbladder disease and is associated with gallstones in nearly every case. In general, the term *cholecystitis* is applied whenever gallstones are present regardless of the histologic appearance of the gallbladder. Repeated minor episodes of obstruction of the cystic duct cause intermittent biliary colic and contribute to inflammation and subsequent scar formation. Gallbladders from symptomatic patients with gallstones who have never had an attack of acute cholecystitis are of two types: (1) In some, the mucosa may be slightly flattened, but the wall is thin and unscarred and, except for the stones, appears normal. (2) Others exhibit obvious signs of chronic inflammation, with thickening, cellular infiltration, loss of elasticity, and fibrosis. The clinical history in these two groups cannot always be distinguished, and inflammatory changes may also be found in patients with asymptomatic gallstones.

Clinical Findings

A. Symptoms and Signs

Biliary colic, the most characteristic symptom, is caused by transient gallstone obstruction of the cystic duct. The pain usually begins abruptly and subsides gradually, lasting for a few minutes to several hours. The pain of biliary colic is usually steady—not intermittent, like that of intestinal colic. In some patients, attacks occur postprandially; in others, there is no relationship to meals. The frequency of attacks is quite variable, ranging from nearly continuous trouble to episodes many years apart. Nausea and vomiting may accompany the pain.

Biliary colic is usually felt in the right upper quadrant, but epigastric and left abdominal pain are common, and some patients experience precordial pain. The pain may radiate around the costal margin into the back or may be referred to the region of the scapula. Pain on top of the shoulder is unusual and suggests direct diaphragmatic irritation. During an attack, there may be tenderness in the right upper quadrant, and rarely, the gallbladder is palpable.

Fatty food intolerance, dyspepsia, indigestion, heartburn, flatulence, and nausea are other symptoms associated with gallstone disease. Because they are also frequent in the general population, their presence in any given patient may only be incidental to the gallstones.

B. Laboratory Findings

An ultrasound of the gallbladder should usually be the first test. Gallstones can be demonstrated in about 95% of cases, and a positive reading for gallstones is rarely in error. About 2% of patients with gallstone disease have normal ultrasound studies.

Differential Diagnosis

Gallbladder colic may be strongly suggested by the history, but the clinical impression should always be verified by an ultrasound study. Biliary colic may simulate the pain of duodenal ulcer, hiatal hernia, pancreatitis, and myocardial infarction. It has been suggested that biliary colic may sometimes aggravate cardiac disease, but angina pectoris or an abnormal electrocardiogram (ECG) should rarely be indications for cholecystectomy.

Right-sided radicular pain in the T6-T10 dermatomes may be confused with biliary colic. Osteoarthritic spurs, vertebral lesions, or tumors may be shown on x-rays of the spine or may be suggested by hyperesthesia of the abdominal skin.

A search for esophageal spasm, hiatal hernia, peptic ulcer, or gastric tumors may be warranted. In some patients, an irritable colon syndrome may be mistaken for gallbladder discomfort. Carcinoma of the cecum or ascending colon may be overlooked on the assumption that postprandial pain in these conditions is due to gallstones.

Complications

Chronic cholecystitis predisposes to acute cholecystitis, common duct stones, and adenocarcinoma of the gallbladder. The longer the stones have been present, the higher is the incidence of all of these complications. Complications are infrequent, however, and the presence of gallstones is not reason enough for prophylactic cholecystectomy in a person with asymptomatic or mildly symptomatic disease.

Treatment

A. Medical Treatment

Avoidance of offending foods may be helpful. Dissolution with ursodiol is generally not recommended due to poor efficacy.

B. Surgical Treatment

Cholecystectomy is indicated in most patients with symptoms. The procedure can be scheduled at the patient's convenience, within weeks or months after diagnosis. Active concurrent disease that increases the risk of surgery should be treated before operation. In some chronically ill patients, surgery should be deferred indefinitely.

Cholecystectomy is most often performed laparoscopically, but when the laparoscopic approach is contraindicated or unsuccessful, it may be performed through a laparotomy. The difference consists of 4 fewer days in the hospital and fewer weeks off work when done laparoscopically. Regardless of how it is done, operative cholangiography may be included to evaluate for common duct stones. If stones are found, common duct exploration may be performed (see section on choledocholithiasis).

Prognosis

Serious complications and deaths related to the operation itself are rare. The operative death rate is about 0.1% in patients under age 50 and about 0.5% in patients over age 50.

Most deaths occur in patients recognized preoperatively to have increased risks. The operation relieves symptoms in 95% of cases.

The historical risk of common bile duct injury is roughly 0.4%. To reduce this catastrophic event, many societies have advocated safe surgical dissection in the form of the "critical view of safety." The goal of this method is to identify the cystic duct and artery prior to division of any tubular structures. The critical view of safety is obtained by dissection of the lower third of the gallbladder free from the liver and identifying two, and only two, tubular structures between the gallbladder and the hepatoduodenal ligament. Studies have shown a reduction in common bile duct injury to 0%-0.03%.

Gurusamy KS, Koti R, Fusai G, et al: Early versus delayed laparoscopic cholecystectomy for uncomplicated biliary colic. *Cochrane Database Syst Rev.* 2013;6:CD007196.

ACUTE CHOLECYSTITIS

 ESSENTIALS OF DIAGNOSIS

- Acute right upper quadrant pain and tenderness
- Fever and leukocytosis
- Palpable gallbladder in one-third of cases
- Sonographic Murphy sign with gallbladder distension, wall thickening, stones, pericholecystic fluid
- Nonopacified gallbladder on radionuclide excretion scan

General Considerations

In 80% of cases, acute cholecystitis results from obstruction of the cystic duct by a gallstone impacted in the Hartmann pouch. The gallbladder becomes inflamed and distended, creating abdominal pain and tenderness. The natural history of acute cholecystitis varies, depending on whether the obstruction becomes relieved, the extent of secondary bacterial invasion, the age of the patient, and the presence of other aggravating factors such as diabetes mellitus. Most attacks resolve spontaneously without surgery or other specific therapy, but some progress to abscess formation or free perforation with generalized peritonitis.

The pathologic changes in the gallbladder evolve in a typical pattern. Subserosal edema and hemorrhage and patchy mucosal necrosis are the first changes. Later, polymorphonuclear leukocytes appear. The final stage involves development of fibrosis. Gangrene and perforation may occur as early as 3 days after onset, but most perforations occur during the second week. In cases that resolve spontaneously, acute inflammation has largely cleared by 4 weeks, but some residual evidence of inflammation may last for several months. About 90% of gallbladders removed during an acute attack show chronic scarring, although many of these patients deny having had any previous symptoms.

The cause of acute cholecystitis is still partially conjectural. Obstruction of the cystic duct is present in most cases, but in experimental animals, cystic duct obstruction does not result in acute cholecystitis unless the gallbladder is filled with concentrated bile or bile saturated with cholesterol. There is also evidence that trauma from gallstones releases phospholipase from the mucosal cells of the gallbladder. This is followed by conversion of lecithin in bile to lysolecithin, which is a toxic compound that may cause more inflammation. Bacteria have a minor role in the early stages of acute cholecystitis, even though most complications of the disease involve suppuration.

Clinical Findings

A. Symptoms and Signs

The first symptom is abdominal pain in the epigastrium or right upper quadrant, sometimes associated with referred pain in the region of the right scapula. In 75% of cases, the patient will have had previous attacks of biliary colic, at first indistinguishable from the present illness. However, in acute cholecystitis, the pain persists and becomes associated with abdominal tenderness. Nausea and vomiting are present in about half of patients, but the vomiting is rarely severe. Mild icterus occurs in 10% of cases. The temperature usually ranges from 38°C to 38.5°C. High fever and chills are uncommon and should suggest the possibility of complications or an incorrect diagnosis.

Right upper quadrant tenderness is present, and in about a third of patients, the gallbladder is palpable (often in a position lateral to its normal one). Voluntary guarding during examination may prevent detection of an enlarged gallbladder. In others, the gallbladder is not enlarged because scarring of the wall restricts distention. If instructed to breathe deeply during palpation in the right subcostal region, the patient experiences accentuated tenderness and sudden inspiratory arrest (Murphy sign).

B. Laboratory Findings

The leukocyte count is usually elevated, but normal counts are common. A mild elevation of the serum bilirubin (in the range of 2-4 mg/dL) is common, presumably due to secondary inflammation of the common duct by the contiguous gallbladder. Bilirubin values above this range would most likely indicate the associated presence of common duct stones. A mild increase in alkaline phosphatase may accompany the attack. Occasionally, the serum amylase concentration transiently reaches 1000 units/dL or more.

C. Imaging Studies

As stated earlier, right upper quadrant ultrasound is the imaging modality of choice. The presence of stones or sludge, thickening of the gallbladder wall, pericholecystic edema, and a sonographic Murphy sign are consistent with acute cholecystitis. Usually, along with a careful history and physical exam, ultrasound is the only test needed to make the diagnosis of acute cholecystitis.

If additional diagnostic information is desirable (eg, if ultrasound is equivocal or negative), a radionuclide excretion scan (eg, HIDA scan) should be performed. This test cannot demonstrate gallstones, but if the gallbladder is imaged, acute cholecystitis is ruled out except in rare cases of acalculous cholecystitis (see later section; the test is positive in most cases of acute acalculous cholecystitis). Imaging of the duct but not the gallbladder supports the diagnosis of acute cholecystitis. A few false positives are seen in advanced gallstone disease without acute inflammation and in acute biliary pancreatitis. The presence of an elevated bilirubin and a dilated common bile duct should suggest the presence of choledocholithiasis (see later in chapter).

▶ Differential Diagnosis

The differential diagnosis includes other common causes of acute upper abdominal pain and tenderness. An acute peptic ulcer with or without perforation might be suggested by a history of epigastric pain relieved by food or antacids. Most cases of perforated ulcer demonstrate free air under the diaphragm on x-ray. An abdominal CT could provide more anatomic detail.

Acute pancreatitis can be confused with acute cholecystitis, especially if cholecystitis is accompanied by an elevated lipase level. Furthermore, HIDA scans fail to outline the gallbladder in most cases of acute biliary pancreatitis. Sometimes the two diseases coexist, but pancreatitis should not be accepted as a second diagnosis without specific findings.

Acute appendicitis in patients with a high cecum may closely simulate acute cholecystitis.

Severe right upper quadrant pain with high fever and local tenderness may develop in acute gonococcal perihepatitis (Fitz-Hugh-Curtis syndrome). Clues to the proper diagnosis may be found in tenderness in the adnexa, vaginal discharge that shows gonococci on a gram-stained smear, and a disparity between the patient's high fever and her general lack of toxicity.

▶ Complications

The major complications of acute cholecystitis are empyema and perforation.

A. Empyema

In empyema (suppurative cholecystitis), the gallbladder contains frank pus, and the patient becomes more toxic, with high spiking fever (39-40°C), chills, and leukocytosis greater than 15,000/μL. Parenteral antibiotics should be given, and percutaneous cholecystostomy or cholecystectomy should be performed.

B. Perforation

Perforation may take any of three forms: (1) localized perforation with pericholecystic abscess; (2) free perforation with generalized peritonitis; and (3) perforation into an adjacent hollow viscus, with the formation of a fistula. Perforation may occur as early as 3 days after the onset of acute cholecystitis or not until late in the second week. The total incidence of perforation is about 10%.

1. Pericholecystic abscess—Pericholecystic abscess, the most common form of perforation, should be suspected when the signs and symptoms progress, especially when accompanied by the appearance of a palpable mass. The patient often becomes toxic, with fever to 39°C and a leukocyte count above 15,000/μL, but sometimes there is no correlation between the clinical signs and the development of local abscess. Cholecystectomy and drainage of the abscess can be performed safely in many of these patients, but if the patient's condition is unstable, percutaneous cholecystostomy is preferable.

2. Free perforation—Free perforation occurs in only 1%-2% of patients, most often early in the disease when gangrene develops before adhesions wall off the gallbladder. The diagnosis is made preoperatively in less than half of cases. In some patients with localized pain, sudden spread of pain and tenderness to other parts of the abdomen suggests the diagnosis. Whenever it is suspected, free perforation must be treated by emergency laparotomy. Abdominal paracentesis may be misleading and has proved to be of little diagnostic usefulness. Cholecystectomy should be performed if the patient's condition will permit; otherwise, cholecystostomy is done. The death rate depends partly on whether the cystic duct remains obstructed or the stone becomes dislodged after perforation. The former leads to a purulent peritonitis that is lethal in 20% of cases. In the latter, a true bile peritonitis ensues and over 50% of patients die. The earlier source control is achieved, the better is the prognosis.

3. Cholecystenteric fistula—If the acutely inflamed gallbladder becomes adherent to adjacent stomach, duodenum, or colon and necrosis develops at the site of one of these adhesions, perforation may occur into the lumen of the gut. The resulting decompression often allows the acute disease to resolve. If the gallbladder stones discharge through the fistula and if they are large enough, they may obstruct the small intestine (gallstone ileus; see later section). Rarely, patients vomit gallstones that have entered the stomach through a cholecystogastric fistula. In most patients, the acute attack subsides and the cholecystenteric fistula is clinically unsuspected. Fistulas arising from gallstones must be differentiated from those caused by perforated peptic ulcers.

Cholecystenteric fistulas do not usually cause symptoms unless the gallbladder is still partially obstructed by stones or scarring. Malabsorption and steatorrhea have been reported in isolated cases of cholecystocolonic fistulas. Steatorrhea in this situation could be due either to absence of bile in the proximal bowel following diversion into the colon or, more rarely, to excess bacteria in the upper intestine. An upper gastrointestinal series or abdominal CT may delineate the fistula, but often, the fistula will be found intraoperatively.

▶ Treatment

The two mainstays of therapy for acute cholecystitis are antibiotics and biliary decompression (Figure 27–7). Intravenous fluids should be given to correct dehydration and electrolyte imbalance. Antibiotics directed against enteric gram-negative rods and anaerobes should be given. Single therapy with piperacillin-tazobactam or imipenem or dual therapy with ceftriaxone plus metronidazole or ciprofloxacin plus metronidazole are appropriate options. Choice of antibiotics should account for known patient- or region-specific bacterial resistance patterns.

The timing and approach to biliary decompression is dependent upon establishment of the diagnosis, the length of disease at presentation, and the patient's preexisting health to undergo surgery. In patients who are reasonable-risk surgical candidates presenting early in their disease course (24-72 hours), the preferred method of treatment is laparoscopic cholecystectomy. Four controlled trials have supported this approach with the following data: (1) the incidence of technical complications is no greater with early surgery; (2) early surgery reduces the total duration of illness by approximately 30 days, length of hospitalization by 5-7 days, and direct medical costs by several thousand dollars; and (3) the death rate is slightly lower with early surgery because of earlier treatment for some patients whose condition would have worsened during expectant management.

In about 30% of cases, the diagnosis of acute cholecystitis is established but the general condition of the patient is unsatisfactory. If possible, surgery should be postponed in these cases until the ancillary disease is controlled. Percutaneous cholecystostomy can be performed in patients whose comorbidities preclude surgery. A catheter is inserted under ultrasound or CT guidance to decompress and drain the gallbladder of bile and/or pus. Along with antibiotics, cholecystostomy controls the acute disease, including any local

▲ **Figure 27–7.** Schema for the management of acute cholecystitis. CBC, complete blood count; ERCP, endoscopic retrograde cholangiopancreatography; HIDA, hepatobiliary iminodiacetic acid; LFTs, liver function tests; MRCP, magnetic resonance cholangiopancreatography; PTC, percutaneous transhepatic cholangiography; RUQ, right upper quadrant; US, ultrasound.

infection, but the gallstones are not removed. Therefore, cholecystectomy should be considered to prevent recurrent disease once the patient recovers and attendant comorbidities are optimized. Alternatively, in nontoxic patients with less severe disease, cholecystitis can be temporized with antibiotics (60% success rate) alone, and an interval cholecystectomy can be performed after medical optimization. However, failure to promptly improve with antibiotics should lead to consideration of cholecystostomy or cholecystectomy.

▶ **Prognosis**

The overall death rate of acute cholecystitis is about 5%. Nearly all of the deaths are in patients over age 60 or those with diabetes mellitus. In the older age group, secondary cardiovascular or pulmonary complications contribute substantially to the death rate. Uncontrolled sepsis with peritonitis and intrahepatic abscesses are the most important local conditions responsible for death.

Common duct stones are present in about 15% of patients with acute cholecystitis, and some of the more seriously ill patients have simultaneous cholangitis from biliary obstruction. Acute pancreatitis may also complicate acute cholecystitis, and the combination carries a greater risk.

Patients who develop the suppurative forms of gallbladder disease such as empyema or perforation are less likely to recover (Figure 27–8). Earlier admission to the hospital and early cholecystectomy reduce the chances of these complications.

Gurusamy KS, Rossi M, Davidson BR: Percutaneous cholecystostomy for high-risk surgical patients with acute calculous cholecystitis. *Cochrane Database Syst Rev.* 2013;8:CD007088.
Okamoto K, Suzuki K, Takada T, et al: Tokyo Guidelines 2018: flowchart for the management of acute cholecystitis. *J Hepatobiliary Pancreat Sci.* 2018;25:55-72.

ACALCULOUS CHOLECYSTITIS

Acute cholecystitis can occur in the absence of cholelithiasis (acalculous cholecystitis). Some of these cases are due to cystic duct obstruction by another process such as a malignant tumor. More cases of acalculous cholecystitis result from primary bacterial infection by *Escherichia coli*, clostridia, or, occasionally, *Salmonella typhi*. Most cases occur in patients hospitalized with some other critical illness. Diagnosis is usually made after fever workup in otherwise critical patients reveals evidence for cholecystitis. Due to the nature of

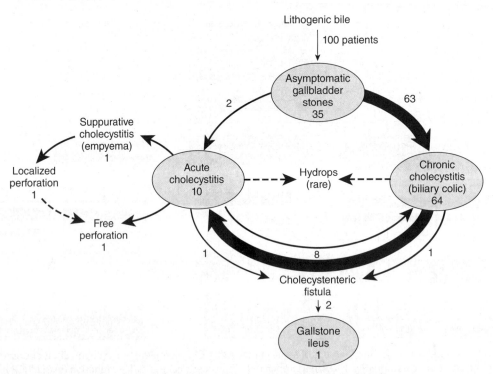

▲ **Figure 27–8.** The natural history of gallbladder stones. The numbers approximate the percentage of patients in each category. Note that most patients with acute cholecystitis have previously had biliary colic.

patients with this diagnosis, antecedent symptoms of disease are rare, save for a new fever and leukocytosis.

Acute acalculous cholecystitis is particularly common in trauma victims, in patients receiving total parenteral nutrition, and in patients with other critical illness. Small-vessel occlusion occurs early, and unless treatment is given promptly, the disease progresses rapidly to gangrenous cholecystitis and septic complications, at which point the death rate is high. Antibiotics and biliary drainage via percutaneous cholecystostomy are the treatment modalities of choice.

EMPHYSEMATOUS CHOLECYSTITIS

Emphysematous cholecystitis is a rare condition in which bubbles of gas from anaerobic infection appear in the lumen of the gallbladder, its wall, the pericholecystic space, and, on occasion, the bile ducts. Clostridia species are the most commonly implicated organisms, but other gas-forming anaerobes such as *E coli* or anaerobic streptococci may be found. Three times as many men as women are affected, and 20% of patients have diabetes mellitus. In contrast to the usual form of acute cholecystitis, the disease probably is a bacterial infection from the earliest moment. In many cases, the gallbladder contains no stones.

The disease begins with sudden and rapidly progressive right upper quadrant pain. Fever and leukocytosis reach high levels quickly, and the patient is considerably more toxic than is usually the case in acute cholecystitis. On examination, a mass can usually be found in the right upper quadrant.

The patient should be treated with antibiotics effective against clostridia and the other species mentioned earlier. Emergency surgical treatment should follow the initial resuscitative measures. Cholecystectomy can be safely performed in most cases, but the most critically ill might fare better with cholecystostomy. The types of complications are the same as in other forms of acute cholecystitis, but illness is more severe and death rates are higher.

GALLSTONE ILEUS

Gallstone ileus is mechanical intestinal obstruction caused by a large gallstone lodged in the ileal lumen. It occurs more often in women, and the average patient age is about 70 years.

▶ Clinical Findings

A. Symptoms

The patient usually presents with obvious small bowel obstruction, either partial or complete. The obstructing gallstone enters the intestine through a cholecystenteric fistula located in the duodenum, colon, or, rarely, the stomach or jejunum. The gallbladder may contain one or several stones, but stones that cause gallstone ileus are almost always 2.5 cm or more in diameter. The lumen in the proximal bowel will allow most of these large calculi to pass caudally until the ileum is reached. Obstruction of the large intestine may follow passage of a gallstone through a fistula at the hepatic flexure or may occur even after the stone has traversed the entire small bowel.

B. Signs

In most patients, the findings on physical examination are typical of distal small bowel obstruction. Obstruction of the duodenum or jejunum may give a perplexing clinical picture because of the lack of distention. Right upper quadrant tenderness and a mass may be present in some cases, but the distended abdomen may be difficult to examine accurately.

C. Imaging Studies

In addition to dilated small intestine, abdominal CT scan with oral and intravenous contrast can show air within the biliary tree and a cholecystenteric fistula.

▶ Treatment

The proper treatment is emergency laparotomy or laparoscopy with removal of the obstructing stone through a small enterotomy. The proximal intestine must be carefully inspected for the presence of a second calculus that might cause a postoperative recurrence. The gallbladder should be left undisturbed at the original operation.

Once the patient has recovered, an elective cholecystectomy should be scheduled if the patient complains of chronic gallbladder symptoms. On this basis, interval cholecystectomy will be required in about 30% of patients. The fistula itself is rarely the source of trouble and closes spontaneously in most patients.

▶ Prognosis

The death rate from gallstone ileus remains about 20%, largely because of the poor general condition of elderly patients at the time of laparotomy. In many cases, the patient has developed cardiac or pulmonary complications during a preoperative delay when the diagnosis was unclear.

CHOLEDOCHOLITHIASIS

ESSENTIALS OF DIAGNOSIS

▶ Biliary pain

▶ Jaundice

▶ Episodic cholangitis

▶ Gallstones in gallbladder or previous cholecystectomy

General Considerations

Approximately 15% of patients with stones in the gallbladder harbor calculi within the bile ducts. Common duct stones are usually accompanied by others in the gallbladder, but in 5% of cases, the gallbladder is empty. The number of duct stones may vary from 1 to more than 100.

There are two possible origins for common duct stones. The evidence suggests that most cholesterol stones develop within the gallbladder and reach the duct after traversing the cystic duct. These are called secondary stones. Pigment stones may have a similar pedigree or, more often, develop de novo within the common duct. These are called primary common duct stones. About 60% of common duct stones are cholesterol stones and 40% are pigment stones. The latter are, on average, associated with more severe clinical manifestations.

Patients may have one or more of the following principal clinical findings, all of which are caused by obstruction to the flow of bile or pancreatic juice: biliary colic, cholangitis, jaundice, and pancreatitis (Figure 27–9). It seems, however,

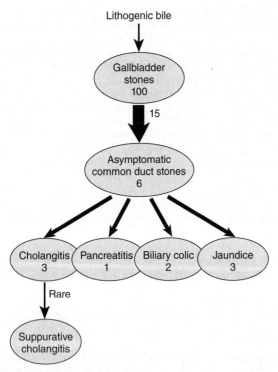

▲ **Figure 27–9.** The natural history of common duct stones. Of every 100 patients with gallbladder stones, 15 will have common duct stones, which will produce the spectrum of syndromes illustrated. Note that the individual syndromes overlap, indicating that they may appear together in various combinations.

that as many as 50% of patients with choledocholithiasis remain asymptomatic.

The common duct may dilate to 2-3 cm proximal to an obstructing lesion, and truly huge ducts develop in patients with biliary tumors. In choledocholithiasis or biliary stricture, the inflammatory reaction restricts dilation, so the dilatation is less marked. Dilation of the ductal system within the liver can also be limited by cirrhosis.

Biliary colic is the result of rapid rises in biliary pressure whether the block is in the common duct or neck of the gallbladder. Gradual occlusion of the duct—as in cancer—rarely produces the same kind of pain as gallstone disease.

Clinical Findings

A. Symptoms

Choledocholithiasis may be asymptomatic or may produce sudden toxic cholangitis, leading to a rapid demise. The seriousness of the disease parallels the degree of obstruction, the length of time it has been present, and the extent of secondary bacterial infection (see later section on cholangitis). Biliary colic, jaundice, and pancreatitis may be isolated findings or may occur in any combination along with signs of cholangitis.

Biliary colic from common duct obstruction cannot be distinguished from that caused by stones in the gallbladder. The pain is felt in the right subcostal region, epigastrium, or even the substernal area. Referred pain to the region of the right scapula is common.

Choledocholithiasis should be strongly suspected if intermittent chills, fever, or jaundice accompanies biliary colic. Some patients notice transient darkening of their urine during an attack even though jaundice is not evident.

Pruritus is usually the result of persistent long-standing obstruction. The itching is more intense in warm weather when the patient perspires and is usually worse on the extremities than on the trunk. It is much more common with neoplastic obstruction than with gallstone obstruction.

B. Signs

The patient may be icteric and toxic, with high fever and chills, or may appear to be perfectly healthy. A palpable gallbladder is unusual in patients with obstructive jaundice from common duct stone because the obstruction is transient and partial, and scarring of the gallbladder renders it inelastic and nondistensible. Tenderness may be present in the right upper quadrant but is not often as marked as in acute cholecystitis, perforated peptic ulcer, or acute pancreatitis. Tender hepatic enlargement may occur.

C. Laboratory Findings

In cholangitis, leukocytosis of 15,000/μL is usual, and values above 20,000/μL are common. A rise in serum bilirubin often appears within 24 hours after the onset of symptoms.

The absolute level usually remains under 10 mg/dL, and most levels are in the range of 2-4 mg/dL. The direct fraction exceeds the indirect, but the latter becomes elevated in most cases. Bilirubin levels do not ordinarily reach the high values seen in malignant tumors because the obstruction is usually incomplete and transient.

The serum alkaline phosphatase level usually rises and may be the only chemical abnormality in patients without jaundice. When the obstruction is relieved, the alkaline phosphatase and bilirubin levels should return to normal within 1-2 weeks, with the exception that the former may remain elevated longer if the obstruction was prolonged.

Mild increases in AST and alanine aminotransferase (ALT) are often seen with extrahepatic obstruction of the ducts.

D. Imaging Studies

Ultrasound will usually show gallbladder stones and, depending on the degree of obstruction, dilatation of the bile duct. Ultrasound and CT scans are insensitive in the search for stones in the common duct. Strong predictors of choledocholithiasis are cholangitis, bilirubin > 4 mg/dL, and a dilated common bile duct on ultrasound and are indications for ERCP. Intermediate evidence of choledocholithiasis warrants evaluation with intraoperative cholangiogram or ultrasound or preoperative MRCP. EUS is another sensitive technique for detection of choledocholithiasis and a cost-effective technique to guide subsequent ERCP.

▶ Differential Diagnosis

The workup should consider the same possibilities in the differential diagnosis as for cholecystitis.

Elevated serum lipase levels are diagnostic of pancreatitis, which may be the result of choledocholithiasis in the appropriate clinical setting.

Alcoholic cirrhosis or acute alcoholic hepatitis may present with jaundice, right upper quadrant tenderness, and leukocytosis. The differentiation from cholangitis may be impossible from clinical data. A history of a recent binge suggests acute liver disease. A percutaneous liver biopsy may be specific.

Intrahepatic cholestasis from drugs, pregnancy, chronic active hepatitis, or primary biliary cirrhosis may be difficult to distinguish from extrahepatic obstruction. MRCP/ERCP would be appropriate to make the distinction, particularly if other studies (eg, ultrasound scan) failed to provide evidence of gallstone disease. If jaundice has persisted for 4-6 weeks, a mechanical cause is probable. Because most patients improve during this interval, persistent jaundice should never be assumed to be the result of parenchymal disease unless imaging rules out obstruction of the major ducts.

Intermittent jaundice and cholangitis after cholecystectomy are compatible with biliary stricture or a retained common bile duct stone, and the distinction requires MRCP/ERCP.

Biliary tumors usually produce intense jaundice without biliary colic or fever, and once it begins, the jaundice rarely remits.

▶ Complications

Long-standing ductal infection can produce intrahepatic abscesses. Hepatic failure or secondary biliary cirrhosis may develop in unrelieved obstruction of long duration. Because the obstruction is usually incomplete and intermittent, cirrhosis develops only after several years in untreated disease. Acute pancreatitis, a fairly common complication of calculous biliary disease, is discussed in Chapter 28. In brief, patients should undergo supportive care for pancreatitis and undergo cholecystectomy with symptomatic improvement on the indexed operation. There is a nearly 25% recurrence of gallstone pancreatitis treated without cholecystectomy within the following 3 months.

Rarely, a stone in the common duct may erode through the ampulla, resulting in gallstone ileus. Hemorrhage (hemobilia) is also a rare complication.

▶ Treatment

Patients with acute cholangitis should be treated with systemic antibiotics and other measures, as described in the following section, followed by urgent or emergent, depending on the patient's condition, decompression of the bile duct through either endoscopic sphincterotomy or surgical common bile duct exploration.

The typical patient presents with mild cholangitis and evidence on ultrasound scans of gallbladder stones. Laparoscopic cholecystectomy is indicated along with, depending on the experience of the surgeon, laparoscopic exploration of the common duct if an operative cholangiogram or laparoscopic ultrasound demonstrates the expected common duct stones. Laparoscopic common duct exploration is usually accomplished through the cystic duct (which may have to be dilated), but when the common duct is enlarged (> 1.5 cm), it may be accomplished through a choledochotomy incision, just as in open surgery. If the surgeon thinks the common duct stones cannot be removed laparoscopically, it is probably best to remove the gallbladder laparoscopically and the common duct stones by endoscopic sphincterotomy. If the stones cannot be removed by sphincterotomy, a second (open) operation may be necessary. To avoid the need for a second operation, ERCP to remove common duct stones may be considered prior to proceeding to the operating room for cholecystectomy.

There is also a lack of consensus regarding the importance of operative cholangiography or ultrasound during cholecystectomy when there are no clues suggesting stones in the duct. In such cases, the chances of finding a stone are only 3%-5%, and because many of these stones will pass spontaneously without clinical sequelae, some consider the effort unwarranted. However, operative cholangiograms also provide confirmation of the biliary anatomy, which contributes to avoidance of bile duct injuries and allows prompt treatment of those stones that would go on to cause symptoms.

When the common duct is explored through the cystic duct and gallstones are removed, the cystic duct must be ligated, but a drainage catheter is not usually left within the common duct. When the common duct is explored through a choledochotomy (either during a laparoscopic or open operation), a T tube is usually left in the duct, and cholangiograms are taken a week or so postoperatively. Any residual stones discovered on these postoperative x-rays can be extracted 4-6 weeks later through the T tube tract.

Patients with common duct stones who have had a previous cholecystectomy are best treated by endoscopic sphincterotomy. Using a side-viewing duodenoscope, the ampulla is cannulated, and a 1-cm incision is made in the sphincter with an electrocautery wire. The opening created in the sphincter permits stones to pass from the duct into the duodenum. Endoscopic sphincterotomy is less likely to be successful in patients with large stones (eg, > 2 cm), and it is contraindicated in the presence of stenosis of the bile duct proximal to the sphincter. In these cases, common duct exploration is required.

Stones in the intrahepatic branches of the bile duct can usually be removed without difficulty during common duct exploration. In some cases, however, one or more of the intrahepatic ducts have become packed with stones, and the associated chronic inflammation has produced stenosis of the duct near its junction with the common hepatic duct. It is often impossible in these cases to clear the duct of stones, and if the disease involves only one lobe (usually the left lobe), hepatic lobectomy is indicated.

ASGE Standards of Practice Committee: The role of endoscopy in the evaluation of suspected choledocholithiasis. *Gastrointest Endosc.* 2010;71:1-9.

CHOLANGITIS (BACTERIAL CHOLANGITIS)

Bacterial infection of the biliary ducts always signifies biliary obstruction because, in the absence of obstruction, even heavy bacterial contamination of the ducts fails to produce symptoms or pathologic changes. The block to flow may be partial or, less commonly, complete. The principal causes are choledocholithiasis, biliary stricture, and neoplasm. Less common causes are chronic pancreatitis, ampullary stenosis, pancreatic pseudocyst, duodenal diverticulum, congenital cyst, and parasitic invasion. Iatrogenic cholangitis may complicate transhepatic or T tube cholangiography. Not all obstructing lesions are followed by cholangitis, however. For example, biliary

infection develops in only 15% of patients with neoplastic obstruction. The likelihood of cholangitis is greatest when the obstruction occurs after the duct has acquired a resident bacterial population.

With obstruction, ductal pressure rises, and bacteria proliferate and escape into the systemic circulation via the hepatic sinusoids. Experimentally, the incidence of positive blood cultures with ductal infection is directly proportionate to the absolute height of the pressure in the duct.

The symptoms of cholangitis (sometimes referred to as the Charcot triad) are biliary colic, jaundice, and chills and fever, although a complete triad is present in only 70% of cases. Laboratory findings include leukocytosis and elevated serum bilirubin and alkaline phosphatase levels. The predominant organisms in bile (in approximately decreasing frequency) are *E coli, Klebsiella, Pseudomonas,* enterococci, and *Proteus. Bacteroides fragilis* and other anaerobes (eg, *Clostridium perfringens*) can be detected in about 25% of cases, and their presence correlates with multiple previous biliary operations (often including a biliary enteric anastomosis), severe symptoms, and a high incidence of postoperative suppurative complications. Anaerobes are nearly always seen in the company of aerobes. Two species of bacteria can be cultured in about 50% of cases. Bacteremia probably occurs in most cases, and blood cultures obtained at the appropriate time contain the same organisms as the bile. An ultrasound will often give useful diagnostic information suggestive of biliary obstruction.

The term *suppurative cholangitis* has been used for the most severe form of this disease, when manifestations of sepsis overshadow those of hepatobiliary disease. The diagnostic pentad of suppurative cholangitis consists of abdominal pain, jaundice, fever and chills, mental confusion or lethargy, and shock. The diagnosis is often missed because the signs of biliary disease are overlooked.

Most cases of cholangitis can be controlled with intravenous antibiotics, as stated earlier, followed by prompt ERCP with sphincterotomy and bile duct decompression. In the uncommon case where this is unsuccessful, laparotomy is indicated in order to decompress the bile duct through a formal common bile duct exploration or, in the most extreme instances, direct common bile duct decompression. Cholangitis accompanying neoplastic obstruction may be managed by insertion of a transhepatic drainage catheter into the bile duct.

Miura F, Okamoto K, Takada T, et al: Tokyo Guidelines 2018: initial management of acute biliary infection and flowchart for acute cholangitis. *J Hepatobiliary Pancreat Sci.* 2018;25:31-40.

POSTCHOLECYSTECTOMY SYNDROME

The term *postcholecystectomy syndrome* has been used to signify the heterogeneous group of disorders affecting patients who continue to complain of symptoms after cholecystectomy. It is not really a syndrome, and the term is confusing.

The usual reason for incomplete relief after cholecystectomy is that the preoperative diagnosis of chronic cholecystitis was incorrect. The only symptom entirely characteristic of chronic cholecystitis is biliary colic. When a calculous gallbladder is removed in the hope that the patient will gain relief from dyspepsia, fatty food intolerance, belching, and other symptoms, the operation may leave the symptoms unchanged.

The presenting symptom may be dyspepsia or pain. An organic cause for the symptoms is more likely to be discovered in patients with severe episodic pain than in those with other complaints. Abnormal liver function studies, jaundice, and cholangitis are other manifestations that indicate residual biliary disease. Patients with suspicious findings should be studied by MRCP, ERCP, or THC. Choledocholithiasis, biliary stricture, and chronic pancreatitis are the most common causes of symptoms. Occasionally, there is sufficient evidence to implicate sphincter of Oddi dysmotility as a cause of pain. Relief of pain may follow endoscopic sphincterotomy. Stenosis of the hepatobiliary ampulla, a long cystic duct remnant, and neuromas have been blamed for continued symptoms.

CARCINOMA OF THE GALLBLADDER

Carcinoma of the gallbladder is an uncommon neoplasm that occurs in elderly patients. It is associated with gallstones in 70% of cases, and the risk of malignant degeneration correlates with the length of time gallstones have been present. The tumor is twice as common in women as in men, as one would expect from the association with gallstones.

Most primary tumors of the gallbladder are adenocarcinomas that appear histologically to be scirrhous (60%), papillary (25%), or mucoid (15%). Dissemination of the tumor occurs early by direct invasion of the liver and hilar structures and by metastases to the common duct lymph nodes, liver, and lungs. In an occasional case, where carcinoma is an incidental finding after cholecystectomy for gallstone disease, the tumor is confined to the gallbladder as a carcinoma in situ or an early invasive lesion. Most invasive carcinomas, however, have spread by the time of surgery, and spread is virtually certain if the tumor has progressed to the point where it causes symptoms.

Clinical Findings

A. Symptoms and Signs

The most common presenting complaint is of right upper quadrant pain similar to previous episodes of biliary colic but more persistent. Obstruction of the cystic duct by tumor sometimes initiates an attack of acute cholecystitis. Other cases present with obstructive jaundice and, occasionally, cholangitis due to secondary involvement of the common duct.

Examination usually reveals a mass in the region of the gallbladder, which may not be recognized as a neoplasm if the patient has acute cholecystitis. If cholangitis is the principal symptom, a palpable gallbladder would be an unusual finding with choledocholithiasis alone and should suggest gallbladder carcinoma.

B. Imaging Studies

CT and ultrasound scans may demonstrate the extent of disease, but more often, they show only gallstones. The correct diagnosis is made preoperatively in only 10% of cases.

Complications

Obstruction of the common duct may produce multiple intrahepatic abscesses. Abscesses in or next to the tumor-laden gallbladder are frequent.

Prevention

The incidence of gallbladder cancer has decreased in recent years as the frequency of cholecystectomy has increased. It has been estimated that one case of gallbladder cancer is prevented for every 100 cholecystectomies performed for gallstone disease.

Treatment

If a localized carcinoma of the gallbladder is recognized at laparotomy, cholecystectomy should be performed along with en bloc wedge resection of an adjacent 3-5 cm of normal liver and dissection of the lymph nodes in the hepatoduodenal ligament. If a small invasive carcinoma overlooked during cholecystectomy for gallstone disease is later discovered by the pathologist, reoperation is indicated to perform a wedge resection of the liver bed plus regional lymphadenectomy. Some surgeons also recommend that the common duct be included routinely (ie, even in the absence of gross invasion) in the lymph node dissection for any lesion that involves the full thickness of the gallbladder wall. In the few cases when cancer has not penetrated the muscularis mucosae, cholecystectomy alone should suffice. More extensive hepatectomies (eg, right lobectomy) are not worthwhile. Lesions that invade the bile duct and produce jaundice should be resected if possible. When not possible, a stent should be inserted endoscopically or percutaneously. There is little that surgery can offer in cases with hepatic metastases or more distant spread.

Prognosis

Radiotherapy and chemotherapy are not effective palliative measures. About 85% of patients are dead within a year after diagnosis.

The 10% of patients who presently survive more than 5 years consist of those whose carcinoma was an incidental finding during cholecystectomy for symptomatic gallstone disease and those in whom an aggressive resection has removed all gross tumor.

Mayo SC, Shore AD, Nathan H, et al: National trends in the management and survival of surgically managed gallbladder adenocarcinoma over 15 years: a population-based analysis. *J Gastrointest Surg.* 2010;14(10):1578-1591.

Wu LM, Jiang XX, Gu HY, et al: Endoscopic ultrasound-guided fine-needle aspiration biopsy in the evaluation of bile duct strictures and gallbladder masses: a systematic review and meta-analysis. *Eur J Gastroenterol Hepatol.* 2011;23(2):113-120.

MALIGNANT TUMORS OF THE BILE DUCT

 ESSENTIALS OF DIAGNOSIS

▸ Intense cholestatic jaundice and pruritus

▸ Anorexia and dull right upper quadrant pain

▸ Dilated intrahepatic bile ducts on ultrasound or CT scan

▸ Focal stricture on transhepatic or retrograde endoscopic cholangiogram

▸ General Considerations

Primary bile duct tumors are not more common in patients with cholelithiasis, and men and women are affected with equal frequency. Tumors appear at an average age of 60 years. Ulcerative colitis is a common associated condition, and in occasional cases, bile duct cancer develops in a patient with ulcerative colitis who has been known to have sclerosing cholangitis for several years. Chronic parasitic infestation of the bile ducts may be responsible for the greater incidence of bile duct tumors in Asia.

Most malignant biliary tumors are adenocarcinomas located in the hepatic or common bile duct. The histologic pattern varies from typical adenocarcinoma to tumors composed principally of fibrous stroma and few cells. The acellular tumors may be mistaken for benign strictures or sclerosing cholangitis if adequate biopsies are not obtained. About 10% are bulky papillary tumors, which tend to be less invasive and less apt to metastasize.

At presentation, metastases are uncommon, but the tumor has often grown into the portal vein or hepatic artery.

▸ Clinical Findings

A. Symptoms and Signs

The illness presents with gradual onset of jaundice or pruritus. Chills, fever, and biliary colic are usually absent, and except for a deep discomfort in the right upper quadrant, the patient feels well. Bilirubinuria is present from the start,

and light-colored stools are usual. Anorexia and weight loss develop insidiously with time.

Icterus is the most obvious physical finding. If the tumor is located in the common duct, the gallbladder may distend and become palpable in the right upper quadrant. The tumor itself is never palpable. Patients with tumors of the hepatic duct do not develop palpable gallbladders. Hepatomegaly is common. If obstruction is unrelieved, the liver may eventually become cirrhotic, and splenomegaly, ascites, or bleeding varices become secondary manifestations.

B. Laboratory Findings

Because the duct is often completely obstructed, the serum bilirubin is usually over 15 mg/dL. Serum alkaline phosphatase is also increased. Fever and leukocytosis are not common, because the bile is sterile in most cases. The stool may contain occult blood, but this is more common with tumors of the pancreas or hepatopancreatic ampulla than those of the bile ducts.

C. Imaging Studies

Ultrasound or CT scans usually detect dilated intrahepatic bile ducts. MRCP, ERCP with EUS, or THC clearly depicts the lesion. THC better demonstrates the ductal anatomy on the hepatic side of the lesion. With tumors involving the bifurcation of the common hepatic duct (Klatskin tumors), it is important to determine the proximal extent of the lesion (ie, whether the first branches of the lobar ducts are also involved). ERCP is of value with proximal tumors because if it shows concomitant obstruction of the cystic duct, the diagnosis will most often prove to be gallbladder cancer invading the common duct (not a primary common duct neoplasm). The typical pattern with distal bile duct cancers consists of stenosis of the bile duct with sparing of the pancreatic duct. Adjacent stenoses of both ducts (the double-duct sign) indicate primary cancer of the pancreas. MRCP may be useful if high-quality studies are available.

Occasionally, bile samples obtained at the time of THC will show malignant cells on cytologic study, but this is not a particularly useful test since the diagnosis of cancer must be presumed from the cholangiographic findings and a negative cytologic study is unreliable. Angiography may suggest invasion of the portal vein or encasement of the hepatic artery. False positives may occur, however.

▸ Differential Diagnosis

The differential diagnosis must consider other causes of extrahepatic and intrahepatic cholestatic jaundice. Choledocholithiasis is characterized by episodes of partial obstruction, pain, and cholangitis, which contrast with the unremitting jaundice of malignant obstruction. Bilirubin concentrations rarely surpass 15 mg/dL and are usually below 10 mg/dL in gallstone obstruction, whereas bilirubin levels almost always exceed 10 mg/dL and are usually above 15 mg/dL in neoplastic obstruction. A rapid rise of the bilirubin level to above 15 mg/dL in a patient with sclerosing cholangitis should suggest superimposed neoplasm. Dilatation of the gallbladder may occur with tumors of the distal common duct but is rare with calculous obstruction.

The combination of an enlarged gallbladder with painless, obstructive jaundice is usually recognized as being due to tumor. If the gallbladder cannot be felt, primary biliary cirrhosis, drug-induced jaundice, chronic active hepatitis, metastatic hepatic cancer, and common duct stone must be ruled out. In general, any patient with cholestatic jaundice of more than 2 weeks in duration whose diagnosis is uncertain should be studied by THC or ERCP. The finding of focal bile duct stenosis in the absence of previous biliary surgery is almost pathognomonic of neoplasm.

Treatment

Patients without evidence of metastases or other signs of advanced cancer (eg, ascites) are candidates for laparotomy. The 30% of patients who do not qualify may be treated by insertion of a stent into the bile duct transhepatically under radiologic control or from the duodenum under endoscopic control. The tube is positioned so that holes above and below the tumor reestablish flow of bile into the duodenum. If both lobar ducts are blocked by a tumor at the bifurcation of the common hepatic duct, it is usually necessary to place a transhepatic tube into only one lobar duct. If the lesion blocks the takeoff of the segmental ducts, stents are rarely beneficial.

Laparotomy is indicated in most cases, however, with the objective of removing the tumor. Preoperative decompression of the bile duct with a percutaneous catheter to relieve jaundice does not lower the incidence of postoperative complications. At operation, which may be immediately preceded by diagnostic laparoscopy, the extent of the tumor should be determined by external examination of the bile duct and the adjacent portal vein and hepatic artery.

Tumors of the distal common duct should be treated by radical pancreaticoduodenectomy if it appears that all tumor would be removed. Secondary involvement of the portal vein is the usual reason for unresectability of tumors in this location. Mid common duct or low hepatic duct tumors should also be removed if possible. If the tumor cannot be excised, bile flow should be reestablished into the intestine by a cholecystojejunostomy or Roux-en-Y choledochojejunostomy. The choice is based on technical considerations.

Tumors at the hilum of the liver should be resected if possible and a Roux-en-Y hepaticojejunostomy performed. The anastomosis is usually between hilum and bowel rather than between individual bile ducts and bowel. A curative operation nearly always requires resection of either the right or the left lobe of the liver and, in all cases, the caudate lobe.

Extension into the lobar and segmental ducts and secondary involvement of the hepatic artery and portal vein are the most common reasons for inability to resect the tumor. Subtotal resections offer little in the way of palliation.

Postoperative radiotherapy is commonly recommended.

Prognosis

The average patient with adenocarcinoma of the bile duct survives less than a year. The overall 5-year survival rate is 15%. Following a thorough radical operation, 5-year survival is about 40%. Biliary cirrhosis, intrahepatic infection, and general debility with terminal pneumonitis are the usual causes of death. Palliative resections and stents may improve the length and quality of survival in this disease even though surgical cure is uncommon. Limited experience with liver transplantation for this disease has been discouraging: tumor has recurred postoperatively in most patients.

American Society for Gastrointestinal Endoscopy (ASGE) Standards of Practice Committee: The role of endoscopy in the evaluation and treatment of patients with biliary neoplasia. *Gastrointest Endosc.* 2013;77(2):167-174.

National Comprehensive Cancer Network: NCCN guidelines Version 3.2018 Hepatobiliary Cancers. https://www.nccn.org/professionals/physician_gls/default.aspx

BENIGN TUMORS & PSEUDOTUMORS OF THE GALLBLADDER

Various unrelated lesions appear on ultrasound as projections from the gallbladder wall. The differentiation from gallstones is based on observing whether a shift in position of the projections follows changes in posture of the patient, since stones are not fixed. Cancer should be suspected in any polypoid lesion that exceeds 1 cm in diameter.

Polyps

Most of these are not true neoplasms but cholesterol polyps, a local form of cholesterolosis. Histologically, they consist of a cluster of lipid-filled macrophages in the submucosa. They easily become detached from the wall when the gallbladder is handled at surgery. It is not known whether cholesterol polyps are important in the genesis of gallstones. Some patients experience gallbladder pain, but whether this is related to the presence of the polyps per se or is a manifestation of functional gallbladder disease has not been established.

Inflammatory polyps have also been reported, but they are quite rare.

Adenomyomatosis

On cholecystography, this entity presents as a slight intraluminal convexity that is often marked by central umbilication. It is usually found in the fundus but may occur elsewhere.

It is unclear whether adenomyomatosis is an acquired degenerative lesion or a developmental abnormality (ie, hamartoma). The following synonyms for this lesion appear in the literature: adenomatous hyperplasia, cholecystitis glandularis proliferans, and diverticulosis of the gallbladder. Although the condition is probably asymptomatic in many cases, adenomyomatosis can cause abdominal pain. Cholecystectomy should be performed in such patients.

▶ Adenomas

These appear as pedunculated adenomatous polyps, true neoplasms that may be papillary or nonpapillary histologically. In a few cases, they have been found in association with carcinoma in situ of the gallbladder.

▶ Treatment of Polyps

In patients with polyps with coincident gallstones or symptoms of biliary colic, cholecystectomy is recommended. Not uncommonly, pathology will reveal gallstones rather than polyps. In those with polyps that are asymptomatic, cholecystectomy is recommended for polyps > 1 cm in size or with concerning radiologic features, given the possible association with gallbladder cancer. Serial ultrasounds are recommended for smaller polyps; enlargement and development of concerning radiologic features are indications for cholecystectomy.

BENIGN TUMORS OF THE BILE DUCTS

Benign papillomas and adenomas may arise from the ductal epithelium. Only 90 cases have been reported to date. The neoplastic propensity of the ductal epithelium is widespread, so the tumors are often multiple, and recurrence is common after excision. The affected duct must be radically excised for permanent cure to result.

BILE DUCT INJURIES, BILE LEAK, STRICTURES, & RETAINED STONES

ESSENTIALS OF DIAGNOSIS

▸ Episodic cholangitis

▸ Previous biliary surgery

▸ HIDA scans, ERCP, MRCP, and THC can aid in the diagnosis

▶ General Considerations

Benign biliary injuries and strictures are caused by surgical trauma in about 95% of cases. The remainder result from external abdominal trauma or, rarely, from erosion of the duct by a gallstone. Prevention of injury to the duct depends on a combination of technical skill, experience, and a thorough knowledge of the normal anatomy and its variations in the hilum of the liver. The number of bile duct injuries rose sharply with the advent of laparoscopy; however, with the increased experience with this technique, bile duct injury rates have improved

The most common lesion consists of excision of a segment of the common duct as a result of mistaking it for the cystic duct. Partial transection, occlusion with metal clips, injury to the right hepatic duct, and leakage from the cystic duct are other examples. A full discussion of how these injuries occur and how they can be prevented is beyond the scope of this text. However, as described earlier, identification of the critical view of safety has been advocated as a method to reduce the incidence of bile duct injury in laparoscopic cholecystectomy.

▶ Clinical Findings

A. Symptoms

Manifestations of postoperative complications are variable. Patients with a retained stone, bile duct injury, or leak often present within days to weeks of their index operation with recurrent right upper quadrant pain. In the case of biliary leak, biliary ascites leads to abdominal distention, bloating, pain, and mild jaundice. Retained common bile duct stones typically result in biliary colic–type pain. Jaundice may accompany both retained bile duct stones and bile duct stricture.

B. Signs

Findings are not distinctive. Bile ascites produces abdominal distention and ileus and, rarely, true bile peritonitis with toxicity. The right upper quadrant may be tender but usually is not. Jaundice is usually present during an attack of choledocholithiasis or cholangitis.

C. Laboratory Findings

The serum alkaline phosphatase and bilirubin concentration are often elevated in cases of stricture or retained bile duct stones. Leukocytosis is often present in patients with biliary ascites.

D. Imaging Studies

Bile ascites can be suspected on ultrasound or CT scan. The fluid should be aspirated, and if it is bile, the diagnosis is clear. Alternatively, a HIDA scan can be used to identify a biliary leak. ERCP can identify the leak and its location and also allow treatment of leaks from the cystic duct or ducts of Luschka by placement of a common bile duct stent.

After laparoscopic cholecystectomy, the most common pattern of iatrogenic stricture is from focal narrowing of the common hepatic duct within 2 cm of the bifurcation and mild to moderate dilatation of the intrahepatic ducts.

Differential Diagnosis

Choledocholithiasis is the condition that most often must be differentiated from biliary stricture because the clinical and laboratory findings can be identical. A history of trauma to the duct would point toward stricture as the more likely diagnosis. Other causes of cholestatic jaundice may have to be ruled out in some cases.

Complications

Complications develop quickly if the leak is not controlled. Bile peritonitis and abscesses may form. With stricture, persistent cholangitis may progress to multiple intrahepatic abscesses and a septic death.

Treatment

Bile leak from a cystic duct stump, liver edge, or duct of Luschka can often be managed via ERCP with biliary stenting. Surgical exploration with direct ligation of the leak and drainage is also an option.

Bile duct strictures should be surgically repaired in all but a few patients who are likely to improve with a nonoperative approach. Depending on the injury pattern, ERCP with stenting may be a therapeutic option, but excision of the damaged duct and Roux-en-Y hepaticojejunostomy are ultimately indicated for most acute and chronic injuries. The entire biliary tree must be outlined by cholangiograms preoperatively. The key to success is the thoroughness of the dissection and the ability ultimately to suture healthy duct to healthy bowel. This, in turn, depends on the experience of the surgeon with this particular operation.

When a definitive repair is technically impossible, the stricture may be dilated with a transhepatic balloon-tipped catheter. This is particularly applicable to patients with portal hypertension, whose hepatic hilum contains numerous venous collaterals that make operation hazardous.

Prognosis

The death rate from biliary injuries is about 5%, and severe illness is frequent. If the stricture is not repaired, episodic cholangitis and secondary liver disease are inevitable.

Surgical correction of the stricture should be successful in about 90% of cases. Experience at centers with a special interest in this problem indicates that good results can be obtained even if several previous attempts did not relieve the obstruction. There is essentially no place for liver transplantation in this disease.

Strasberg SM: A teaching program for the "culture of safety in cholecystectomy" and avoidance of bile duct injury. *J Am Coll Surg.* 2013;217(4):751.

UNCOMMON CAUSES OF BILE DUCT OBSTRUCTION

Congenital Choledochal Cysts

About 30% of congenital choledochal cysts produce their first symptoms in adults, usually presenting with jaundice, cholangitis, and a right upper quadrant mass. Diagnosis can be made by THC or ERCP. The optimal surgical procedure is excision of the cyst and construction of a Roux-en-Y hepaticojejunostomy. If this is not technically possible or if the patient's condition will not permit a prolonged operation, the cyst should be emptied of precipitated biliary sludge and a cystenteric anastomosis constructed. Congenital cysts of the biliary tree have a high incidence of malignant degeneration, which is another argument for excision rather than drainage.

Caroli Disease

Caroli disease, another form of congenital cystic disease, consists of saccular intrahepatic dilatation of the ducts. In some cases, the biliary abnormality is an isolated finding, but more often, it is associated with congenital hepatic fibrosis and medullary sponge kidney. The latter patients often present in childhood or as young adults with complications of portal hypertension. Others have cholangitis and obstructive jaundice as initial manifestations. There is no definitive surgical solution to the problem except in rare cases with isolated involvement of one hepatic lobe, where lobectomy is curative. Intermittent antibiotic therapy for cholangitis is the usual regimen.

Hemobilia

Hemobilia presents with the triad of biliary colic, obstructive jaundice, and occult or gross intestinal bleeding. Most cases in Western cultures follow several weeks after hepatic trauma with bleeding from an intrahepatic branch of the hepatic artery into a duct. It is seen with less frequency now because the general principles of management of hepatic trauma are better understood. Hemobilia can also follow ductal parasitism (*Ascaris lumbricoides*) or cholangiohepatitis. Other causes are hepatic neoplasms, rupture of a hepatic artery aneurysm, hepatic abscess, and choledocholithiasis. The diagnosis may be suspected from a CT angiogram or technetium-99m–labeled red blood cell scan. Sometimes the bleeding can be stopped by embolizing the lesion with stainless steel coils, Gelfoam, or autologous blood clot infused through a catheter selectively positioned in the hepatic artery. If this is unsuccessful, either direct ligation of the bleeding point in the liver or proximal ligation of an upstream branch of the hepatic artery in the hilum is required.

Pancreatitis

Pancreatitis can cause obstruction of the intrapancreatic portion of the bile duct by inflammatory swelling, encasement with scar, or compression by a pseudocyst. The patient may present with painless jaundice or cholangitis. Occasionally, a distended gallbladder can be felt on abdominal examination. Differentiation from choledocholithiasis and secondary acute pancreatitis depends on biliary imaging and evaluation. Jaundice due to inflammation alone rarely lasts more than 2 weeks; persistent jaundice following an attack of acute pancreatitis suggests the development of a pseudocyst, underlying chronic pancreatitis with obstruction by fibrosis, or even an obstructing neoplasm.

Biliary obstruction from chronic pancreatitis may have few or no clinical manifestations. Jaundice is usually present, but the average peak bilirubin level is only 4-5 mg/dL. Some patients with functionally significant stenosis have persistently elevated alkaline phosphatase levels as the only abnormality; when surgical decompression of the bile duct is not performed, these patients often develop secondary biliary cirrhosis within a year or so. Diagnosis of stricture is made by MRCP or ERCP, which shows a long stenosis of the intrapancreatic portion of the duct, proximal dilatation, and either a gradual or abrupt tapering of the lumen at the pancreatic border, occasionally accompanied by ductal angulation. If cholangiograms show stenosis and if alkaline phosphatase or bilirubin levels remain more than twice normal for longer than 2 months, the stenosis is functionally significant and unlikely to resolve and requires surgical correction. Choledochoduodenostomy is done in most cases. Cholecystoduodenostomy is unreliable because the cystic duct is often too narrow to provide continued biliary decompression.

Patients with obstructive jaundice and pseudocyst usually respond to endoscopic or surgical drainage of the pseudocyst. However, occasionally they do not respond, because chronic scarring—not the cyst—is the cause of obstruction. Procedures to drain both the bile duct and the pseudocyst are indicated if there is persistent bile duct obstruction after the cyst has been decompressed.

Ampullary Dysfunction & Stenosis

Stenosis of the hepatopancreatic ampulla (ampullary stenosis) has been implicated as a cause of pain and other manifestations of ampullary obstruction and is often considered as a cause of postcholecystectomy complaints. Some cases are idiopathic, whereas others may be the result of trauma from gallstones. If the patient has secondary manifestations of biliary obstruction (eg, jaundice, increased alkaline phosphatase

concentration, cholangitis) in the absence of gallstones or some other obstructing lesion and cholangiography shows dilatation of the common duct, ampullary stenosis is a plausible explanation. However, the diagnosis is more often proposed as a reason for upper abdominal pain without these more objective findings. Ampullary dysfunction is postulated in these cases.

Sphincter of Oddi dysfunction may be the cause of biliary-like pain and is often considered in patients who remain uncomfortable after cholecystectomy. The pathogenesis of the symptoms is thought to be similar to that of esophageal dysmotility and irritable bowel syndrome. Patients typically experience severe, intermittent upper abdominal pain that lasts for 1-3 hours, sometimes following a meal.

Residual gallstone and pancreatic disease must first be ruled out. Ampullary dysfunction can then be diagnosed by sphincter of Oddi manometry. Patients are placed in one of three groups depending on the presence of three objective manifestations of biliary obstruction: abnormal liver function tests, prolonged (> 45 minutes) common bile duct emptying of contrast media after ERCP, and a common duct greater than 12 mm in diameter. Patients in group I have all three findings; patients in group II have one or two findings; and patients in group III have none of the findings. Group I patients are thought to have enough evidence of disease that sphincterotomy should be performed without manometry. Group I patients have abnormal motility so rarely that they should not be considered further for sphincterotomy. Thus, motility studies are most often of value in determining which of the group II patients will improve after sphincterotomy.

The abnormalities sought on the motility studies include an elevated (> 40 mm Hg) basal sphincter pressure and a paradoxic rise in sphincter pressure in response to CCK. The former is most reliable. About 50% of group II patients have elevated sphincter pressures, and these are the patients who benefit from sphincterotomy.

A scintigraphic test may be just as accurate. The patient is given a bolus of CCK followed by technetium-99m–diisopropyl iminodiacetic acid (DISIDA). Gamma camera images of the liver and bile duct are obtained for 60 minutes. A scoring system (score: 0-12) is based on the rate of passage of the imaging agent past various relevant points (eg, appearance and clearance through the liver, bile duct, and bowel). The normal range is 0-5; abnormal is 6-12.

Sphincter of Oddi dysfunction is an uncommon explanation for abdominal pain, and it is appropriate to remain skeptical unless the objective findings of biliary obstruction are clear-cut. In well-selected cases, however, endoscopic sphincterotomy is beneficial.

Heetun ZS, Zeb F, Cullen G, et al: Biliary sphincter of Oddi dysfunction: response rates after ERCP and sphincterotomy in a 5-year ERCP series and proposal for new practical guidelines. *Eur J Gastroenterol Hepatol.* 2011;23(4):327-333.

Duodenal Diverticula

Duodenal diverticula usually arise on the medial aspect of the duodenum within 2 cm of the orifice of the bile duct, and in some individuals, the duct empties directly into a diverticulum. Even in the latter circumstance, duodenal diverticula are usually innocuous. Occasionally, distortion of the duct entrance or obstruction by enterolith formation in the diverticulum produces symptoms. Either choledochoduodenostomy or Roux-en-Y choledochojejunostomy is usually a safer method of reestablishing biliary drainage than attempts to excise the diverticulum and reimplant the duct.

Ascariasis

When the worms invade the duct from the duodenum, ascariasis can produce symptoms of ductal obstruction. Air may sometimes be seen within the ducts. Antibiotics should be used until cholangitis is controlled, and anthelmintic therapy (mebendazole, albendazole, or pyrantel pamoate) should then be given. The acute symptoms usually subside with antibiotics, but if they do not, endoscopic sphincterotomy should be performed and attempts made to extricate the worms. If this is unsuccessful and the patient remains acutely ill, the duct should be emptied surgically.

Recurrent Pyogenic Cholangitis

Cholangiohepatitis is a type of chronic recurrent cholangitis prevalent in coastal areas from Japan to Southeast Asia. In Hong Kong, it is the third most common indication for emergency laparotomy and the most frequent type of biliary disease. The disease is currently thought to result from chronic portal bacteremia, with portal phlebitis antedating the biliary disease. *E coli* causes secondary infection of the bile ducts, which initiates pigment stone formation within the ducts.

Biliary obstruction from the stones gives rise to recurrent cholangitis, which, unlike gallstone disease in Western countries, may be unaccompanied by gallbladder stones. The gallbladder is usually distended during an attack and may contain pus.

Chronic recurrent infection often leads to biliary strictures and hepatic abscess formation. The strictures are usually located in the intrahepatic bile ducts, and for some unknown reason, the left lobe of the liver is more severely involved. Intrahepatic gallstones are common, and their surgical removal may be difficult or impossible. Acute abdominal pain, chills, and high fever are usually present, and jaundice develops in about half of cases. Right upper quadrant tenderness is usually marked, and in about 80% of cases, the gallbladder is palpable. ERCP, MRCP, or THC is the best way to study the biliary tree and can help in determining the need for surgery and the type of procedure.

Systemic antibiotics should be given for acute cholangitis. Surgical treatment consists of cholecystectomy, common duct exploration, and removal of stones. Sphincteroplasty should also be performed to allow any residual or recurrent stones to escape from the duct. A Roux-en-Y choledochojejunostomy is indicated for patients with strictures, markedly dilated ducts (eg, > 3 cm), or recurrent disease after a previous sphincteroplasty. The results of surgery are good in 80% of patients. Chronic intrahepatic stones and infection, which often involve only one lobe, may require hepatic lobectomy.

Although many patients are cured, prolonged illness from repeated infection is almost unavoidable once strictures have appeared or the intrahepatic ducts have become packed with stones.

Sclerosing Cholangitis

Sclerosing cholangitis is a rare chronic disease of unknown cause characterized by nonbacterial inflammatory narrowing of the bile ducts. About 60% of cases occur in patients with ulcerative colitis, and sclerosing cholangitis develops in about 5% of patients with that disorder. Other less commonly associated conditions are thyroiditis, retroperitoneal fibrosis, and mediastinal fibrosis. The disease chiefly affects men 20-50 years of age. In most cases, the entire biliary tree is affected by the inflammatory process, which causes irregular partial obliteration of the lumen of the ducts. The narrowing may be confined, however, to the intrahepatic or extrahepatic ducts, although it is almost never so short as to resemble a posttraumatic or focal malignant stricture. The woody-hard duct walls contain increased collagen and lymphoid elements and are thickened at the expense of the lumen.

The clinical onset usually consists of the gradual appearance of mild jaundice and pruritus. Symptoms of bacterial cholangitis (eg, fever and chills) are uncommon in the absence of previous biliary surgery. Laboratory findings are typical of cholestasis. The total serum bilirubin averages about 4 mg/dL and rarely exceeds 10 mg/dL. MRCP/ERCP is usually diagnostic, demonstrating ductal stenoses and irregularity, which often gives a beaded appearance. Liver biopsy may show pericholangitis and bile stasis, but the changes are nonspecific.

The complications of sclerosing cholangitis include gallstone disease and adenocarcinoma of the bile duct. The latter is most common in patients with ulcerative colitis. Furthermore, patients with ulcerative colitis and sclerosing cholangitis appear to be at greater risk for colonic mucosal dysplasia and colon cancer than those with ulcerative colitis not associated with sclerosing cholangitis.

Ursodiol (ursodeoxycholic acid), 10 mg/kg/d, improves liver function tests and symptoms. Cholestyramine will give relief from pruritus. Percutaneous transhepatic balloon dilatation can be of value to treat dominant strictures. In cases where the disease is largely confined to the distal extrahepatic duct and the proximal ducts are dilated, a Roux-en-Y hepaticojejunostomy may be indicated. For patients with severe intrahepatic involvement, hepatic transplantation should be considered.

The natural history of sclerosing cholangitis is one of chronicity and unpredictable severity. Some patients seem to obtain nearly complete remission after treatment, but this is not common. Bacterial cholangitis may develop after operation if adequate drainage has not been established. In these cases, antibiotics will be required at intervals. Most patients experience the gradual evolution of secondary biliary cirrhosis after many years of mild to moderate jaundice and pruritus. Liver transplantation is indicated when the disease becomes advanced. The results are good.

MULTIPLE CHOICE QUESTIONS

1. All of the following are current useful imaging modalities for the biliary tree and gallbladder, except

   A. Abdominal ultrasound
   B. Endoscopic retrograde cholangiopancreatography
   C. Abdominal computed tomography scan
   D. Oral cholecystography
   E. Transhepatic cholangiography

2. Serum alkaline phosphatase can come from

   A. Lung
   B. Muscle
   C. Skin
   D. Intestin
   E. Red blood cells

3. Gallstones

   A. Are symptomatic in > 50% of people
   B. Are nearly always present in people with chronic cholecystitis
   C. Are not detected in the gallbladder by ultrasound in about 50% of cases (false negative)
   D. Are usually detectable by ultrasound if present in the common bile duct
   E. Are composed of bile pigment in the majority of cases in the United States

4. Acute cholecystitis can be commonly confused with each of the following, except

   A. Diverticulitis
   B. Pancreatitis
   C. Peptic ulcer disease
   D. Acute appendicitis
   E. Fitz-Hugh-Curtis syndrome

5. Management of acute cholangitis

   A. Typically requires emergent operation
   B. Should not include antibiotics until bile cultures are pending
   C. Should usually include draining the biliary tree
   D. Is commonly required in the management of chronic pancreatitis
   E. Should reserve invasive procedures for patients who have required more than 3 days of antibiotics

Pancreas

Heather G. Lyu, MD
Thomas E. Clancy, MD

EMBRYOLOGY

The pancreas appears in the fourth week of fetal life from the caudal part of the foregut as dorsal and ventral pancreatic buds. Both buds rotate to the right and fuse near the point of origin of the ventral pancreas. Later, as the duodenum rotates, the pancreas shifts to the left. In the adult, only the caudal portion of the head and the uncinate process are derived from the ventral pancreas. The cranial part of the head and all of the body and tail are derived from the dorsal pancreas. Most of the dorsal pancreatic duct joins with the duct of the ventral pancreas to form the main pancreatic duct **(duct of Wirsung)**; a small part persists as the accessory duct **(duct of Santorini)**. In 5%-10% of people, the ventral and dorsal pancreatic ducts do not fuse, a condition known as pancreatic divisum, and most regions of the pancreas drain through the duct of Santorini and the orifice of the minor papilla. In this case, only the small ventral pancreas drains with the common bile duct through the papilla of Vater.

ANATOMY

The pancreas is a thin elliptic organ that lies within the retroperitoneum in the upper abdomen (Figures 28–1 and 28–2). In the adult, it is 12-15 cm long and weighs 70-100 g. The gland can be divided into three portions—head, body, and tail. The head of the pancreas is intimately adherent to the medial portion of the duodenum and lies in front of the inferior vena cava and superior mesenteric vessels. A small tongue of tissue called the uncinate process lies behind the superior mesenteric vessels as they emerge from the retroperitoneum. Anteriorly, the stomach and the first portion of the duodenum lie partly in front of the pancreas. The common bile duct passes through a posterior groove in the head of the pancreas adjacent to the duodenum. The body of the pancreas is in contact posteriorly with the aorta, the left crus of the diaphragm, the left adrenal gland, and the left kidney.

The tail of the pancreas lies in the hilum of the spleen. The main pancreatic duct (the duct of Wirsung) courses along the gland from the tail to the head and joins the common bile duct just before entering the duodenum at the ampulla of Vater. The accessory pancreatic duct (the duct of Santorini) enters the duodenum 2-2.5 cm proximal to the ampulla of Vater (Figure 28–1).

The blood supply of the pancreas is derived from branches of the celiac and superior mesenteric arteries (Figure 28–2). The superior pancreaticoduodenal artery arises from the gastroduodenal artery, runs parallel to the duodenum, and eventually meets the inferior pancreaticoduodenal artery, a branch of the superior mesenteric artery, to form an arcade. The splenic artery provides tributaries that supply the body and tail of the pancreas. The main branches are termed the dorsal pancreatic, pancreatica magna, and caudal pancreatic arteries. The venous supply of the gland parallels the arterial supply. Lymphatic drainage is into the peripancreatic nodes located along the veins.

The innervation of the pancreas is derived from the vagal and splanchnic nerves. The efferent fibers pass through the celiac plexus from the celiac branch of the right vagal nerve to terminate in ganglia located in the interlobular septa of the pancreas. Postganglionic fibers from these synapses innervate the acini, the islets, and the ducts. The visceral afferent fibers from the pancreas also travel in the vagal and splanchnic nerves, but those that mediate pain are confined to the latter. Sympathetic fibers to the pancreas pass from the splanchnic nerves through the celiac plexus and innervate the pancreatic vasculature.

PHYSIOLOGY

▶ Exocrine Function

The external secretion of the pancreas consists of a clear, alkaline (pH 7.0-8.3) solution of 1-2 L/d containing digestive

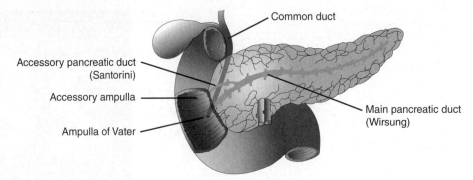

▲ **Figure 28–1.** Anatomic configuration of pancreatic ductal system. (Used with permission from W Silen.)

enzymes. Exocrine functions are stimulated by the hormones secretin and cholecystokinin and by parasympathetic vagal discharge. Secretin and cholecystokinin are synthesized, stored, and released from duodenal mucosal cells in response to specific stimuli. Acid in the lumen of the duodenum causes the release of secretin, and luminal digestion products of fat and protein cause the release of cholecystokinin.

The water and electrolyte secretion is formed by the centroacinar and intercalated duct cells principally in response to secretin stimulation. The secretion is modified by exchange processes and active secretion in the ductal collecting system. The cations sodium and potassium are present in the same concentrations as in plasma. The anions bicarbonate and chloride vary in concentration according to the rate of secretion: with increasing rate of secretion, the bicarbonate concentration increases and chloride concentration

falls, so that the sum of the two is the same throughout the secretory range. Pancreatic juice helps neutralize gastric acid in the duodenum and adjusts luminal pH to the level that allows optimal activity of pancreatic enzymes.

Pancreatic enzymes are synthesized, stored (as zymogen granules), and released by the acinar cells of the gland, principally in response to cholecystokinin and vagal stimulation. Pancreatic enzymes are proteolytic, lipolytic, and amylolytic. Lipase and amylase are stored and secreted in active forms. The proteolytic enzymes are secreted as inactive precursors and are activated by the duodenal enzyme enterokinase. Other enzymes secreted by the pancreas include ribonucleases and phospholipase A. Phospholipase A is secreted as an inactive proenzyme activated in the duodenum by trypsin. It catalyzes the conversion of biliary lecithin to lysolecithin.

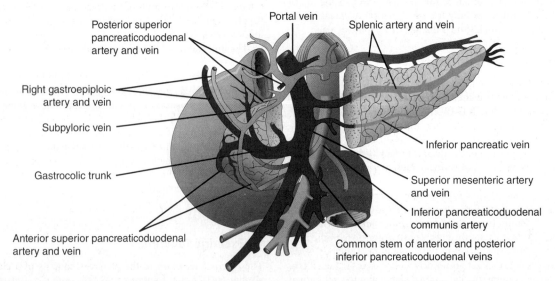

▲ **Figure 28–2.** Arterial supply and venous drainage of the pancreas. (Used with permission from W Silen.)

Turnover of protein in the pancreas exceeds that of any other organ in the body. Intravenously injected amino acids are incorporated into enzyme protein and may appear in the pancreatic juice within 1 hour. Three mechanisms prevent autodigestion of the pancreas by its proteolytic enzymes: (1) The enzymes are stored in acinar cells as zymogen granules, where they are separated from other cell proteins. (2) The enzymes are secreted in an inactive form. (3) Inhibitors of proteolytic enzymes are present in pancreatic juice and pancreatic tissue.

Endocrine Function

The function of the endocrine pancreas is to facilitate storage of foodstuffs by release of insulin after a meal and to provide a mechanism for their mobilization by release of glucagon during periods of fasting. Insulin and glucagon, as well as pancreatic polypeptide and somatostatin, are produced by the islets of Langerhans.

Insulin, a polypeptide (molecular weight [MW] 5734) consisting of 51 amino acid residues, is formed in the beta cells of the pancreas via the precursor proinsulin. Insulin secretion is stimulated by rising or high serum concentrations of metabolic substrates such as glucose, amino acids, and short-chain fatty acids. The major normal stimulus for insulin release appears to be glucose. The release and synthesis of insulin are stimulated by activation of specific glucoreceptors located on the surface membrane of the beta cell. Insulin release is also stimulated by calcium, glucagon, secretin, cholecystokinin, vasoactive intestinal polypeptide, and gastrin, all of which sensitize the receptors on the beta cell to glucose. Epinephrine, tolbutamide, and chlorpropamide release insulin by acting on the adenylyl cyclase system.

Glucagon, a polypeptide (MW 3485) consisting of 29 amino acid residues, is formed in the alpha cells of the pancreas. The release of glucagon is stimulated by a low blood glucose concentration, amino acids, catecholamines, sympathetic nervous discharge, and cholecystokinin. It is suppressed by hyperglycemia and insulin.

The principal functions of insulin are to stimulate anabolic reactions involving carbohydrates, fats, proteins, and nucleic acids. Insulin decreases glycogenolysis, lipolysis, proteolysis, gluconeogenesis, ureagenesis, and ketogenesis. Glucagon stimulates glycogenolysis from the liver and proteolysis and lipolysis in adipose tissue as well as in the liver. With the increase in lipolysis, there is an increase in ketogenesis and gluconeogenesis. Glucagon increases cyclic adenosine monophosphate (cAMP) in the liver, heart, skeletal muscle, and adipose tissue. The short-term regulation of gluconeogenesis depends on the balance between insulin and glucagon. Studies on insulin and glucagon suggest that the hormones exert their effects via receptors on the cell membrane. Before entering the systemic circulation, blood draining from the islets of Langerhans perfuses the pancreatic acini, and this exposure to high levels of hormones is thought to influence acinar function.

ANNULAR PANCREAS

Annular pancreas is a rare congenital condition in which a ring of pancreatic tissue from the head of the pancreas surrounds the descending duodenum. The abnormality usually presents in infancy as duodenal obstruction with postprandial vomiting. Patients will present with bilious emesis if the constriction is distal to the entrance of the common bile duct. X-rays show a dilated stomach and proximal duodenum (double bubble sign) and little or no air in the rest of the small bowel.

After correction of fluid and electrolyte imbalance, the obstructed segment should be bypassed by a duodenojejunostomy or other similar procedure. No attempt should be made to resect the obstructing pancreas because a pancreatic fistula or acute pancreatitis often develops postoperatively.

Occasionally, annular pancreas will present in adult life with similar symptoms.

PANCREATITIS

Pancreatitis is a common nonbacterial inflammatory disease caused by activation, interstitial liberation, and autodigestion of the pancreas by its own enzymes. The process may or may not be accompanied by permanent morphologic and functional changes in the gland. Much is known about the causes of pancreatitis, but despite the accumulation of much experimental data, understanding of the pathogenesis of this disorder is still incomplete.

In **acute pancreatitis,** there is sudden upper abdominal pain, nausea and vomiting, and elevated serum amylase. **Chronic pancreatitis** is characterized by chronic pain, pancreatic calcification on x-ray, and exocrine (steatorrhea) or endocrine (diabetes mellitus) insufficiency. Attacks of acute pancreatitis often occur in patients with chronic pancreatitis. **Acute relapsing pancreatitis** is defined as multiple attacks of pancreatitis without permanent pancreatic scarring, a picture most often associated with biliary pancreatitis. The unsatisfactory term **chronic relapsing pancreatitis,** denoting recurrent acute attacks superimposed on chronic pancreatitis, will not be used in this chapter. Alcoholic pancreatitis often behaves in this way. The term **subacute pancreatitis** has also been used by some to denote the minor acute attacks that typically appear late in alcoholic pancreatitis.

Etiology

Etiologies of pancreatitis can be grouped into four major categories: **metabolic** (eg, alcohol, hyperlipidemia, hypercalcemia, drugs, genetic, scorpion venom), **mechanical** (eg, cholelithiasis, postoperative, pancreas divisum, posttraumatic, endoscopic retrograde cholangiopancreatography [ERCP], pancreatic duct obstruction, pancreatic ductal bleeding, duodenal obstruction), **vascular** (eg, postoperative after cardiopulmonary bypass, periarteritis nodosa, atheroembolism), and **infectious** (eg, mumps, coxsackie B, cytomegalovirus, *Cryptococcus*). The most common etiologies are described in the following sections.

A. Biliary Pancreatitis

Up to 50% of cases of pancreatitis are associated with gallstone disease, which, if untreated, usually gives rise to additional acute attacks. For unknown reasons, even repeated attacks of acute biliary pancreatitis seldom produce chronic pancreatitis. Eradication of the biliary disease nearly always prevents recurrent pancreatitis. The etiologic mechanism most likely consists of transient obstruction of the ampulla of Vater and pancreatic duct by a gallstone. Choledocholithiasis is found in only 25% of cases, but because over 90% of patients excrete a gallstone in feces passed within 10 days after an acute attack, it is assumed that most attacks are caused by a gallstone or biliary sludge traversing the common duct and ampulla of Vater.

B. Alcoholic Pancreatitis

In the United States, excessive alcohol use accounts for about 40% of cases of pancreatitis. Most commonly, 6 years or more of alcoholic excess precede the initial attack of pancreatitis. Microscopic signs of chronic pancreatitis can be detected on initial presentation.

Acute administration of alcohol stimulates pancreatic secretion and induces spasm in the sphincter of Oddi. This has been compared to experiments that produce acute pancreatitis by combining partial ductal obstruction and secretory stimulation. If the patient can be persuaded to stop drinking, acute attacks may be prevented, but parenchymal damage continues to occur due to persistent ductal obstruction and fibrosis.

C. Hypercalcemia

Hyperparathyroidism and other disorders accompanied by hypercalcemia are occasionally complicated by acute pancreatitis. With time, chronic pancreatitis and ductal calculi appear. The resulting increased calcium concentrations in pancreatic juice may prematurely activate proteases, which can facilitate precipitation of calculi in the ducts.

D. Hyperlipidemia

In patients with primary hyperlipidemia (especially that associated with elevated chylomicrons and very-low-density lipoproteins), pancreatitis seems to be a direct consequence of the metabolic abnormality. Hyperlipidemia during an acute attack of pancreatitis is usually associated with normal serum amylase levels, because the lipid interferes with the chemical determination for amylase; urinary output of amylase may still be high. If a primary lipid abnormality is present, dietary control reduces the chances of additional attacks of pancreatitis and associated complications.

E. Familial Pancreatitis

In this condition, attacks of abdominal pain usually begin in childhood. Some affected families also have aminoaciduria, but this is not a universal finding. Chronic calcific pancreatitis develops eventually in most patients, and many patients become candidates for operation for chronic pain. Pancreatic carcinoma is more frequent in patients with familial pancreatitis.

F. Protein Deficiency

In certain populations where dietary protein intake is markedly deficient, the incidence of chronic pancreatitis is high. The reason for this association is obscure, especially in view of the observation that pancreatitis afflicts alcoholics with higher dietary protein and fat intake than those who consume less protein and fat.

G. Iatrogenic Pancreatitis

Pancreatitis can be a complication following endoscopic retrograde pancreatography or endoscopic sphincterotomy. Approximately 75% of patients undergoing ERCP have an elevation in serum amylase concentration; however, only 3%-15% of patients fully develop pancreatitis. Both patient factors (female sex, age < 55 years, history of pancreatitis, history of post-ERCP pancreatitis, normal bilirubin, nondilated bile ducts, suspicion of sphincter of Oddi dysfunction, and presence of intraductal papillary mucinous neoplasm) and procedure-related factors (difficult cannulation of the bile duct, sphincterotomy, balloon dilation of sphincter, wire cannulation of the pancreatic duct, contrast injection in the pancreatic duct, placement of a self-expanding metal stent, and ampullectomy) play a role in post-ERCP pancreatitis.

Most cases of postoperative pancreatitis follow common bile duct exploration, especially if sphincterotomy was performed. Two practices, now largely abandoned, were often responsible: (1) use of a common duct T tube with a long arm passing through the sphincter of Oddi, and (2) dilation of the sphincter to 5-7 mm during common duct exploration. Operations on the pancreas, including pancreatic biopsy, are another cause. A few cases follow gastric surgery or even operations remote from the pancreas. Pancreatitis is particularly common after cardiac surgery with cardiopulmonary bypass, where the risk factors are preoperative renal failure, valve surgery, postoperative hypotension, and (particularly) the perioperative administration of calcium chloride (> 800 mg calcium chloride per square meter of body surface area).

H. Drug-Induced Pancreatitis

Drugs are probably responsible for more cases of acute pancreatitis than is generally suspected. The most common inciting drugs are corticosteroids, estrogen-containing contraceptives, azathioprine, thiazide diuretics, and tetracyclines. Pancreatitis associated with use of estrogens is usually the result of drug-induced hypertriglyceridemia. The mechanisms involved in the case of other drugs are unknown.

I. Obstructive Pancreatitis

Chronic partial obstruction of the pancreatic duct may be congenital or may follow healing after injury or inflammation. Over time, the parenchyma drained by the obstructed duct is replaced by fibrous tissue, and chronic pancreatitis develops.

Pancreas divisum may predispose patients to obstructive pancreatitis. If this anomaly is present and further narrowing of the opening of the minor papilla occurs (eg, by an inflammatory process), the orifice may be inadequate to handle the flow of pancreatic juice. The diagnosis of pancreas divisum is made by ERCP or magnetic resonance cholangiopancreatography (MRCP). If a patient with the anomaly is found to have documented episodes of acute pancreatitis and no other cause is found, it is reasonable to assume that the anomaly is the cause.

Surgical sphincteroplasty of the minor papilla or the insertion of a stent has been proposed as treatment, but results have been suboptimal. This may be due to the presence of irreversible parenchymal changes and the persistence of chronic inflammation. Endoscopic sphincteroplasty is a more commonly employed intervention. In patients with obvious changes of chronic pancreatitis, surgical treatment should consist of pancreatic resection or drainage.

J. Idiopathic Pancreatitis and Miscellaneous Causes

In about 15% of patients, representing the third largest group after biliary and alcoholic pancreatitis, there is no identifiable cause of the condition. If investigated in greater than usual detail (eg, duodenal drainage examination for cholesterol crystals), many of these patients are found to have gallstones or biliary sludge undetectable by ultrasound scans. Recent data have linked mutations of the cystic fibrosis gene to idiopathic pancreatitis.

▶ Pathogenesis

The concept that pancreatitis is due to enzymatic digestion of the gland is supported by the finding of proteolytic enzymes in ascitic fluid and increased amounts of phospholipase A and lysolecithins in pancreatic tissue from patients with acute pancreatitis. Although the available evidence is inconclusive, the autodigestion theory is almost universally accepted. Other proposed factors are vascular insufficiency, lymphatic congestion, and activation of the kallikrein-kinin system. Experimentally, pancreatitis can be re-created if activated enzymes are injected into the pancreatic ducts under pressure.

Recent evidence has emphasized phospholipase A, lipase, and elastase as the principal injurious agents. Phospholipase A, in the presence of small amounts of bile salts, attacks free phospholipids (eg, lecithin) and those bound in cellular membranes to produce extremely potent lyso-compounds. Lysolecithin, which would result from the action of phospholipase A on biliary lecithin, or phospholipase A itself, plus bile salts, is capable of producing severe necrotizing pancreatitis.

If autodigestion is the final common pathway in pancreatitis, earlier steps must account for the presence of active enzymes and their reaction products in the ducts and their escape into the interstitium.

A. Common Channel Theory

Flow between the biliary and pancreatic ducts requires a common channel connecting these two systems with the duodenum. Although these ducts converge in 90% of humans, only 10% have a common channel long enough to permit biliary-pancreatic reflux if the ampulla contained a gallstone. Experimentally, pancreatitis produced by pancreatic duct obstruction alone is similar in severity to pancreatitis following obstruction of a common channel, so biliary reflux is discounted as an etiologic factor in this disease.

Some studies have shown that a very early event in several forms of experimental pancreatitis, including that due to pancreatic duct obstruction, consists of zymogen activation within acinar cells by lysosomal hydrolases (eg, cathepsin B). Additionally, the activation of the inflammatory response and irregular elevation of intracellular calcium have been found to play a key role in alcoholic pancreatitis. Other factors must be postulated, however, to account for the variations in severity of the disease. In biliary pancreatitis, transient obstruction of the ampulla of Vater by a gallstone is most likely the first event.

B. Systemic Manifestations

Severe acute pancreatitis may be complicated by multiple organ failure, principally respiratory insufficiency (acute respiratory distress syndrome [ARDS]), myocardial depression, renal insufficiency, and gastric stress ulceration. The pathogenesis of these complications is similar in many respects to that of multiple organ failure in sepsis, and in fact, sepsis due to pancreatic abscess formation is a contributing factor in some of the most severe cases of acute pancreatitis. During acute pancreatitis, pancreatic proteases, bacterial endotoxins, and other active agents are liberated into the systemic circulation. The endotoxin probably originates from bacteria that translocate through the intestinal mucosa.

Within the circulation, the proteases and the endotoxin activate the complement system (especially C5) and kinins. Complement activation leads to granulocyte aggregation and accumulation of aggregates in the pulmonary capillaries. The granulocytes release neutrophil elastase, superoxide anion, hydrogen peroxide, and hydroxide radicals, which in concert with bradykinin exert local toxic effects on the pulmonary epithelium that result in increased permeability. Arachidonate metabolites (eg, prostaglandin E_2, prostaglandin I_2, leukotriene B_4) may also be involved. Analogous events are thought to occur in other organs.

Ceppa EP, et al: Hereditary pancreatitis: endoscopic and surgical management. *J Gastrointest Surg.* 2013;17(5):847-856.

Clemens DL, et al: Alcoholic pancreatitis: new insights in to the pathogenesis and treatment. *World J Gastrointest Pathophysiol.* 2016;7(1):48-59.

Morales SJ, et al: A review of prevention of post-ERCP pancreatitis. *Gastroenterol Hepatol.* 2018;14(5):286-292.

Spanier BW, et al: Epidemiology, aetiology and outcome of acute and chronic pancreatitis: an update. *Best Pract Res Clin Gastroenterol.* 2008;22(1):45-63.

Working Group IAP/APA Acute Pancreatitis Guidelines: IAP/APA evidence-based guidelines for the management of acute pancreatitis. *Pancreatology.* 2013;13(4 Suppl 2):e1-1.

1. Acute Pancreatitis

ESSENTIALS OF DIAGNOSIS

- ▸ Abrupt onset of epigastric pain, frequently with back pain
- ▸ Nausea and vomiting
- ▸ Elevated serum lipase
- ▸ Cholelithiasis or alcoholism (many patients)

▶ General Considerations

Early diagnosis and appropriate disease staging for acute pancreatitis are important to guide therapy and prevent highly morbid or fatal complications. The Atlanta classification requires patients to have two or more of the following criteria: (1) abdominal pain consistent with acute pancreatitis, (2) amylase or lipase elevation to more than three times the upper limit of normal; and (3) evidence of pancreatic inflammation revealed by abdominal imaging. After initial diagnosis, patients present with one of two distinct subtypes: necrotizing pancreatitis or interstitial edematous pancreatitis (IEP) based on the presence or absence of necrosis. IEP is more common, and although there is evidence of pancreatic edema and small amounts of fluid, there is no necrosis. Necrotizing pancreatitis accounts for 5%-10% of cases. Patients often develop areas of pancreatic and peripancreatic necrosis later in the course of their disease.

▶ Clinical Findings

A. Symptoms and Signs

Patients often present with nonspecific severe epigastric pain that radiates to the back. Depending on the severity of the disease, there may be profound dehydration, fever, tachycardia, and postural hypotension. Myocardial function is depressed in severe pancreatitis, presumably because of circulating factors that affect cardiac performance. Examination of the abdomen reveals decreased or absent bowel sounds and tenderness that may be generalized but more often is localized to the epigastrium. Clinical evidence of pleural effusion, left greater than right, may be present. In 1%-2% of patients, bluish discoloration is present in the flank (**Grey Turner sign)** or periumbilical area (**Cullen sign),** indicating dissection of blood retroperitoneally into these areas.

B. Laboratory Findings

The hematocrit may be elevated as a consequence of dehydration. There is usually a moderate leukocytosis, but total white blood cell counts over $12,000/\mu L$ are unusual in the absence of suppurative complications.

Serum amylase and lipase levels can peak within the first 24 hours after the onset of an acute episode. Lipase has a longer half-life and is more sensitive when labs are drawn after the initial 24 hours after onset of symptoms. Amylase is not sensitive (low levels can be identified in patients with severe pancreatitis) or specific for pancreatitis (high levels may occur in other acute abdominal conditions, such as gangrenous cholecystitis, small bowel obstruction, mesenteric infarction, and perforated ulcer). Episodes of acute pancreatitis may occur without rises in serum amylase; this is the rule if hyperlipidemia is present. Furthermore, amylase has a shorter half-life than lipase, and levels may return to normal before blood is drawn. Elevated serum lipase is detectable early and for several days after the acute attack; therefore, lipase may have greater sensitivity in predicting pancreatitis.

In severe pancreatitis, the serum calcium concentration may fall as a result of calcium being complexed with fatty acids (liberated from retroperitoneal fat by lipase) and impaired reabsorption from bone due to the action of calcitonin (liberated by high levels of glucagon). Relative hypoparathyroidism and hypoalbuminemia have also been found.

C. Classification and Scoring of Acute Pancreatitis

The revised Atlanta classification stratifies patients into three categories: mild, moderately severe, and severe pancreatitis. Mild pancreatitis is not associated with organ failure or local complications, and patients are often discharged within the first week with low rates of mortality. Moderately severe

Table 28–1. Ranson criteria for severity of acute pancreatitis.[1]

Criteria present initially
Age > 55 years
White blood cell count > 16,000/μL
Blood glucose > 200 mg/dL
Serum lactate dehydrogenase > 350 IU/L
Aspartate aminotransferase (serum glutamic oxaloacetic transaminase) > 250 IU/dL
Criteria developing during first 24 hours
Hematocrit decrease > 10%
Blood urea nitrogen increase > 8 mg/dL
Serum Ca^{2+} < 8 mg/dL
Arterial Po_2 < 60 mm Hg
Base deficit > 4 mEq/L
Estimated fluid sequestration > 600 mL

[1]Morbidity and mortality rates correlate with the number of criteria present. Mortality rates correlate as follows: 0-2 criteria present = 2%; 3 or 4 = 15%; 5 or 6 = 40%; 7 or 8 = 100%.

pancreatitis patients have transient organ failure and local complications but experience little mortality. Patients with severe pancreatitis have organ failure longer than 48 hours and have the highest rates of mortality.

Clinical scoring systems to predict the prognosis for patients presenting with pancreatitis include the Ranson and Glasgow scores. In both scoring systems, patients are evaluated at admission and again in 48 hours. Ranson criteria scores are listed in Table 28–1. Just the single finding of fluid sequestration (ie, fluid administered minus urine output) exceeding 2 L/d for more than 2 days is a reasonably accurate dividing line between severe (life-threatening) disease and mild to moderate disease. The Acute Physiology and Chronic Health Evaluation II (APACHE II) score is also often used to estimate disease severity, although it is not specific to pancreatitis.

D. Imaging Studies

In about two-thirds of cases, a plain abdominal film is abnormal, including dilation of a segment of bowel adjacent to the pancreas. These findings, however, are nonspecific. Glandular calcification can be indicative of chronic pancreatitis. Chest films may reveal pleural effusion on the left side. Occasionally, radiopaque gallstones will be apparent on plain x-rays. An ultrasound study may demonstrate gallstones early in the attack.

A computed tomography (CT) scan of the pancreas using intravenous contrast media may be obtained to determine the severity of acute pancreatitis. CT findings often include enlargement and stranding of the pancreas with loss of peripancreatic fat planes, areas of decreased density, and the occasional presence of fluid collections. CT scans can also

be used in the setting of clinical deterioration or failure to respond to therapy to identify pancreatic necrosis, emphysematous pancreatitis indicating infection, or the formation of pancreatic pseudocysts. Necrotic pancreas is diagnosed with nonenhancement of more than 30% of the pancreatic parenchyma. Magnetic resonance imaging (MRI) can also be used for diagnostic imaging.

▶ Differential Diagnosis

To some extent, acute pancreatitis is a diagnosis of exclusion, because other acute upper abdominal conditions such as acute cholecystitis, penetrating or perforated duodenal ulcer, high small bowel obstruction, acute appendicitis, and mesenteric infarction must always be seriously considered. In most cases, the distinction is possible based on the clinical picture, laboratory findings, and CT scans. The critical point is that the diseases with which acute pancreatitis is most likely to be confused are often lethal if not treated surgically.

▶ Complications

Gastrointestinal bleeding may occur from adjacent inflamed stomach or duodenum, ruptured pseudocyst, or peptic ulcer. Intraperitoneal bleeding may occur spontaneously from the celiac or splenic artery or from the spleen following acute splenic vein thrombosis. Involvement of the transverse colon or duodenum by the inflammatory process may result in partial obstruction, hemorrhage, necrosis, or fistula formation.

Local complications of acute pancreatitis are best described using the Atlanta classification, which was developed in 1992 and revised in 2012 to standardize the terminology used to describe pancreatitis and its associated complications. For patients with IEP, complications include acute peripancreatic fluid collections (APFCs) and pseudocysts. In cases of necrotizing pancreatitis, patients can develop acute necrotic collections (ANCs) and walled-off necrosis (WON).

A. Acute Peripancreatic Fluid Collections

APFCs develop in patients with IEP. Extravasation of pancreatic juices form a sterile pocket of fluid that is not reabsorbed as inflammation subsides. APFCs have no evidence of necrotic debris and are not contained within true epithelial walls. These simple pancreatic and peripancreatic fluid collections typically resolve without drainage. In fact, drainage is typically not recommended due to risk of infection of a sterile space.

B. Pseudocysts

Unresolved APFCs can develop into more organized and larger collections contained within an epithelialized wall. At this point, this is called a pseudocyst. They are usually located either within or adjacent to the pancreas in the lesser sac.

▲ **Figure 28–3.** CT scan of a large pancreatic pseudocyst impinging on the posterior wall of the stomach. The large arrow indicates the pseudocyst; the smaller arrow indicates the stomach. **A:** More cephalad in the abdomen, the pseudocyst abuts the stomach and liver. **B:** More caudad in the abdomen, the pseudocyst is immediately posterior to the gastric antrum. The stomach is compressed against the anterior wall of the abdomen, and the duodenum is stretched over the pseudocyst, causing early satiety. A cyst in this location is usually best drained into the stomach.

The walls of a pseudocyst are formed by inflammatory fibrosis of the peritoneal, mesenteric, and serosal membranes.

In some instances, pseudocysts can appear without preceding acute pancreatitis. The mechanism in these cases consists of ductal obstruction and formation of a retention cyst that loses its epithelial lining as it grows beyond the confines of the gland. In posttraumatic pseudocyst, symptoms usually do not appear until several weeks after the injury. Some are iatrogenic (eg, occurring during splenectomy); others follow an external blow to the abdomen.

Pseudocysts are best diagnosed by CT scan (Figure 28–3). A dilated common bile duct would suggest biliary obstruction, either from the cyst or from underlying chronic pancreatitis. MRIs can be used to help differentiate pseudocysts from walled-off pancreatic necrosis. MRCP should be performed if there is concern about significant abnormalities of the bile or pancreatic duct as suggested by CT scans.

In the absence of symptoms or radiographic evidence of enlargement (and irrespective of cyst size), expectant management is reasonable. Expectant management is especially important in the first 6-12 weeks of pseudocyst formation secondary to acute pancreatitis. For symptomatic cysts or pseudocysts greater than 5 cm, percutaneous catheter drainage or endoscopic or surgical drainage into the stomach or intestine can be offered. External drainage is often complicated by a pancreatic fistula or recurrent pseudocysts. For mature and large pseudocysts with thick walls in stable patients, endoscopic drainage of pancreatic pseudocysts is the preferred method of drainage. Stents can be placed between the cyst and the gastric or duodenal wall or in the pancreatic duct for cysts that communicate with the main duct. For patients who fail external or endoscopic drainage, surgical drainage can be offered. Operative management of pseudocysts is composed of three operations: the cyst is anastomosed to a Roux-en-Y

limb of jejunum (**cystojejunostomy**), to the posterior wall of the stomach (**cystogastrostomy**), or to the duodenum (**cystoduodenostomy**). The interior wall of the cyst should be inspected for evidence of a tumor, and biopsy of the wall should be performed.

C. Acute Necrotic Collections and Walled-Off Necrosis

ANCs are found in patients with necrotizing pancreatitis. They are distinguishable from APFCs by the presence of liquefied debris along with fluid. ANCs will typically form a thick wall and develop into WON.

D. Infected Peripancreatic Fluid Collection

All of these collections can become infected, and infection is diagnosed by the presence of gas within the collections on imaging. Infected fluid collections, which complicate about 5% of cases of acute pancreatitis, are invariably fatal if it is not treated surgically. This complication tends to develop in severe cases accompanied by hypovolemic shock and pancreatic necrosis and is an especially frequent complication of postoperative pancreatitis. Gas formation follows secondary bacterial contamination of necrotic pancreatic debris and hemorrhagic exudate. The organisms may spread to the pancreas hematogenously as well as directly through the wall of the transverse colon.

Gas in the collection on plain films or CT scans is virtually diagnostic. Percutaneous CT scan–guided aspiration may be used to aid in diagnosis and obtain a specimen for Gram stain and culture. Infected collections must be drained. Drainage procedures are described later in this chapter.

Treatment

A. Medical Treatment

The goals of medical therapy are reduction of pancreatic secretory stimuli and correction of fluid and electrolyte derangements.

1. Nutritional support—Historically, oral intake was withheld and parenteral nutrition was used for nutritional support for patients in prolonged starvation. Recent studies have shown that enteral nutrition is safe and allows avoidance of total parenteral nutrition (TPN), which is associated with significant catheter-related complications. There have been significant cost savings cited with enteral feeding as well as documented evidence of improved mucosal permeability and inflammatory markers. Although TPN should still be considered for nutrition, particularly for patients with a prolonged ileus, early enteral nutrition via a nasogastric or nasojejunal tube should be considered.

2. Fluid replacement—Patients with acute pancreatitis sequester fluid in the retroperitoneum and bowel, and large volumes of intravenous fluids up to 200 mL/h are necessary to maintain circulating blood volume and renal function. Most recent guidelines suggest the use of goal-directed fluid resuscitation to serially reduce serum blood urea nitrogen. However, there are no firm guidelines for how much and what specific type of fluid to use. The adequacy of fluid replacement is the single most important aspect of medical therapy. In fact, undertreatment with fluids may contribute to the progression of pancreatitis. Fluid replacement may be judged most accurately by monitoring the volume and concentration of the urine.

3. Antibiotics—Antibiotics are not useful in mild cases of acute pancreatitis. Some studies have shown the benefit of antibiotics that penetrate pancreatic tissue for patients with severe pancreatitis. Imipenem is the most commonly used antibiotic, although its use is not universally supported even in patients with severe disease. However, recent randomized controlled trials as well as a meta-analysis have shown that antibiotic prophylaxis does not reduce mortality or protect against infected necrosis or frequency of surgical interventions. Given recent evidence, antibiotics should be not be used in the absence of a documented infection.

4. Calcium and magnesium—In severe attacks of acute pancreatitis, hypocalcemia may require calcium replacement in amounts determined by serial calcium measurements. Recognition of hypocalcemia is important because it may produce cardiac dysrhythmias. Hypomagnesemia is also common, especially in alcoholics, and magnesium should also be replaced as indicated by serum levels.

5. Oxygen—Hypoxemia severe enough to require therapy develops in about 30% of patients with acute pancreatitis. It is often insidious, without clinical or x-ray signs, and out of proportion to the severity of the pancreatitis. Severe acute pancreatitis may progress to secondary organ compromise, including ARDS.

Oxygen saturation should be monitored periodically or continuously for the first few hospital days. Patients who develop ARDS may require endotracheal intubation and mechanical ventilation. Diuretics may be useful in decreasing lung water and improving arterial oxygen saturation.

6. Other drugs—Octreotide, H_2 receptor blockers, anticholinergic drugs, glucagon, and aprotinin have shown no beneficial effects in controlled trials.

B. Endoscopic Sphincterotomy

Biliary pancreatitis is caused by a gallstone becoming lodged in the ampulla of Vater. In most cases, the stone passes into the intestine, but occasionally it becomes impacted in the ampulla, which results in more severe disease. Less than 10% of cases of biliary pancreatitis are severe (ie, three or more Ranson criteria), but in severe cases in which biliary obstruction or sepsis is evident, endoscopic sphincterotomy performed within 72 hours of the onset of the disease has been shown to decrease the incidence of concomitant biliary sepsis and lower the mortality rate from the pancreatitis. Endoscopic sphincterotomy is not indicated in the absence of biliary obstruction.

C. Surgical Treatment

Surgery is generally contraindicated in uncomplicated acute pancreatitis. However, when the diagnosis is uncertain in a patient with severe abdominal pain, diagnostic laparoscopy or laparotomy is not thought to aggravate pancreatitis.

When operative evaluation has been performed for diagnosis and mild to moderate pancreatitis is found, cholecystectomy should be performed if gallstones are present, but the pancreas should be left undisturbed.

The diagnosis of biliary pancreatitis can usually be suspected based on ultrasound studies of the gallbladder. Cholecystectomy should be performed on these patients during hospitalization (within 48 hours of hospital admission) for the acute attack soon after the attack resolves. Interval cholecystectomy has been shown to be associated with a statistically significantly higher rate of recurrent pancreatitis. However, when the attack is especially severe, elective cholecystectomy should be deferred up to several months to allow complete recovery from pancreatitis.

Surgical interventions are typically reserved for patients with infected pancreatic necrosis or fluid collections who fail less invasive measures. Surgical treatment can be expanded to included cases of complicated pancreatitis including symptomatic WONs and severe sterile necrosis that fail medical management. Sterile pancreatic necrosis can often be managed with percutaneous catheter drainage. Percutaneous catheter drainage has been shown to result in significantly decreased morbidity with equal mortality compared to open necrosectomy. Endoscopic necrosectomy is also available in specialized centers for patients with more organized necrotic collections adjacent to the stomach or duodenum. In many cases, catheter or endoscopic drainage will prove to be definitive, but sometimes the necrotic debris cannot pass through the catheter and surgical debridement is necessary.

At surgery, all peripancreatic spaces are opened and any necrotic tissue is removed by gentle blunt dissection. Drains are usually placed to adequately remove ongoing liquefaction of necrotic parenchyma. For some patients with severe pancreatic sepsis, the abdomen can be left open to allow for multiple explorations and debridements. An alternative to this would be to place large irrigation drains to perform continuous closed postoperative lavage.

▶ **Prognosis**

The mortality rate associated with acute pancreatitis is about 10%, and nearly all deaths occur in a first attack. Respiratory insufficiency and hypocalcemia indicate a poor prognosis. The death rate associated with severe necrotizing pancreatitis is 50% or more, but surgical debridement lowers the rate to about 20%. Persistent fever or hyperamylasemia for 3 weeks or longer after an attack of pancreatitis usually indicates the presence of a fluid collection or pseudocyst.

Binmoeller KF: EUS-guided drainage of pancreatic fluid collections using fully covered self-expandable metal stents. *Gastroenteral Hepatol.* 2013;9(7):442.

Blamey SL, et al: Prognostic factors in acute pancreatitis. *Gut.* 1984;25(12):1340-1346.

Crockett SD, et al: American-Gastroenterological Association institute guideline on initial management of acute pancreatitis. *Gastroenterology.* 2018;154(4):1096-1101.

Foster BR, et al: Revised Atlanta classification for acute pancreatitis: a pictoral essay. *Radiographics.* 2016;36(3):675-687.

Freeman ML, et al: International Multidisciplinary Panel of Speakers and Moderators. Interventions for necrotizing pancreatitis: summary of a multidisciplinary consensus conference. *Pancreas.* 2012;41(8):1176-1194.

Martin RF, Hein AR: Operative management of acute pancreatitis. *Surg Clin North Am.* 2013;93(3):595-610.

Ranson JH, et al: Prognostic signs and the role of operative management in acute pancreatitis. *Surg Gynecol Obstet.* 1974;139(1):69-81.

van Santvoort HC, et al: Dutch Pancreatitis Study Group. A step-up approach or open necrosectomy for necrotizing pancreatitis. *N Engl J Med.* 2010;362(16):1491-1502.

Varadarajulu S, et al: Equal efficacy of endoscopic and surgical cystogastrostomy for pancreatic pseudocyst drainage in a randomized trial. *Gastroenterology.* 2013;145(3):583-590.

Working Group IAP/APA Acute Pancreatitis Guidelines: IAP/APA evidence-based guidelines for the management of acute pancreatitis. *Pancreatology.* 2013;13(4 Suppl 2):e1-15.

2. Pancreatic Ascites & Pancreatic Pleural Effusion

Pancreatic ascites consists of accumulated pancreatic fluid in the abdomen without peritonitis or severe pain. The syndrome is most often due to chronic leakage of a pseudocyst, but a few cases are due to disruption of a pancreatic duct. The principal causative factors are chronic alcoholic pancreatitis in adults and traumatic pancreatitis in children. Marked recent weight loss is a major clinical manifestation, and unresponsiveness of the ascites to diuretics is an additional diagnostic clue. The ascitic fluid, which ranges in appearance from straw colored to blood tinged, contains elevated protein (> 2.9 g/dL) and amylase levels. Once this condition is suspected, definitive diagnosis is based on chemical analysis of the ascitic fluid and endoscopic retrograde pancreatography. The latter procedure frequently identifies the location of the duct disruption, allowing endoscopic therapy or less likely guiding a surgical approach. Endoscopic stenting should be attempted before surgical intervention. Studies have shown that the extent of duct disruption (partial vs complete) is predictive of successful endoscopic bridging of the duct disruption, with up to 98% resolution in partial disruptions versus 62% resolution in patients with complete duct disruptions.

Initial therapy should consist of a period of intravenous hyperalimentation and somatostatin. If considerable improvement has not occurred within 2-3 weeks, endoscopic pancreatic duct catheterization should be attempted in an attempt to bridge the duct disruption. Patients who fail both medical and endoscopic therapy may require surgery. Surgical management is dependent on the site of the leak. The operation involves suturing a Roux-en-Y limb of jejunum to the site of the leak on the surface of the pancreas or a pancreatic pseudocyst. If the abnormality or duct leak is at the tail, a distal pancreatectomy may be warranted.

Chronic pleural effusions of pancreatic origin represent a variant in which the pancreatic fistula drains into the chest. The diagnosis is made by measuring high concentrations of amylase (usually > 3000 IU/dL) in the fluid. A CT scan of the pancreas and ERCP should be obtained. Medical therapy consists of draining the fluid with a chest tube, somatostatin, and TPN. If after several weeks the fistula persists or if it recurs after the tube has been removed, the source of the leak on the pancreas should either be drained into a Roux-en-Y limb of jejunum or excised as part of a distal pancreatectomy.

Martin RF, Hein AR: Operative management of acute pancreatitis. *Surg Clin North Am.* 2013;93(3):595-610.

Nadkarni NA, Kotwal V, Sarr M, et al: Disconnected pancreatic duct syndrome: endoscopic stent or surgeon's knife? *Pancreas.* 2015;44(1):16-22.

Pai CG, Suvarna D, Bhat G: Endoscopic treatment as first-line therapy for pancreatic ascites and pleural effusion. *J Gastroenterol Hepatol.* 2009;24(7):1198.

3. Chronic Pancreatitis

ESSENTIALS OF DIAGNOSIS

▸ Persistent or recurrent abdominal pain

▸ Pancreatic calcification on x-ray in 50%

▸ Pancreatic insufficiency in 30%; malabsorption and diabetes mellitus

▸ Most often due to alcoholism

▸ General Considerations

Repeated inflammation and scarring of the pancreas secondary to recurrent episodes of acute pancreatitis can eventually progress to chronic pancreatitis. Management of chronic pancreatitis is mostly nonoperative and consists of alcohol cessation and pain control.

There are multiple factors contributing to the pathophysiology of chronic pancreatitis. Patients with chronic pancreatitis have increased pancreatic duct pressure (about 40 cm H_2O) compared with normal subjects (about 15 cm H_2O). This is a result of increased viscosity of pancreatic juice, partial obstruction by calculi, and/or impaired distensibility of the gland due to diffuse fibrosis. Pathologic changes in the gland include destruction of parenchyma, fibrosis, dedifferentiation of acini, calculi, and ductal dilation.

▸ Clinical Findings

A. Symptoms and Signs

Patients with chronic pancreatitis can be asymptomatic for a long period of time. Symptomatic patients present with one or more of the following: abdominal pain, steatorrhea secondary to fat malabsorption, and insulin-dependent diabetes mellitus. The pain is typically felt deep in the upper abdomen and radiates through to the back, and it waxes and wanes from day to day. Early in the course of the disease, the pain may be episodic, lasting for days to weeks and then vanishing for several months before returning again. Patients can have superimposed attacks of acute pancreatitis. Patients may develop tolerance to and dependence on narcotics prescribed for pain.

Malabsorption and steatorrhea do not appear until more than 90% of pancreatic exocrine function is lost; with 2%-10% of normal function, steatorrhea is mild to moderate; with less than 2% of normal function, steatorrhea is severe.

B. Laboratory Findings

Abnormal laboratory findings may result from (1) pancreatic inflammation, (2) pancreatic exocrine insufficiency, (3) diabetes mellitus, (4) bile duct obstruction, or (5) other complications such as pseudocyst formation or splenic vein thrombosis.

1. Amylase—Amylase is not diagnostic for patients with chronic pancreatitis, and its measurement should be reserved for patients with acute episodes.

2. Fecal fat balance test—The patient ingests a diet containing 75-100 g of fat each day for 5 days. The amounts of dietary fat should be measured and should be the same each day. Excretion of less than 7% of ingested fat is normal. Clinically significant steatorrhea is present when fat malabsorption exceeds about 25%. Total pancreatectomy results in about 70% fat malabsorption.

Examination of a stool specimen for fat globules (obviously much simpler than the fat balance test) is specific and relatively sensitive for fat malabsorption.

3. Diabetes mellitus—About 75% of patients with calcific pancreatitis and 30% of those with noncalcific pancreatitis have insulin-dependent diabetes. Most of the rest have either abnormal glucose tolerance curves or abnormally low serum insulin levels after a test meal. Consequently, patients with parenchymal fibrosis who undergo a partial pancreatectomy are quite likely to be converted to insulin-dependent diabetics postoperatively.

4. Biliary obstruction—Elevated bilirubin or alkaline phosphatase levels may result from fibrotic entrapment of the lower end of the bile duct. The differential diagnosis of biliary obstruction in these patients must consider acute pancreatic inflammation, pseudocyst, or pancreatic neoplasm.

5. Miscellaneous—Splenic vein thrombosis may produce secondary hypersplenism or gastric varices.

C. Imaging Studies

Calcifications within the duct and parenchyma can often be seen on plain films, CT scans, and MRIs. MRCP or endoscopic retrograde pancreatography is helpful in establishing the diagnosis of chronic pancreatitis, in ruling out pancreatic pseudocyst and neoplasm, and in preoperative planning for patients thought to be candidates for surgery. The typical findings are ductal stones and irregularity, with dilation and stenoses and, occasionally, ductal occlusion. The discovery of small, unsuspected pseudocysts is common. Retrograde cholangiography should be performed simultaneously to determine whether the common bile duct is narrowed by the pancreatitis, to determine whether biliary calculi are present, and to aid the surgeon in avoiding injury to the bile duct during operation.

Endoscopic ultrasound (EUS) is the most sensitive diagnostic tool for chronic pancreatitis. There are two main scoring systems to diagnose chronic pancreatitis using features identified on EUS. The conventional criteria include parenchymal features (hyperechoic foci, hyperechoic strands, lobularity, shadowing calcifications, and cysts) and ductal features (main pancreatic duct dilation, irregular ductal margins, hyperechoic ductal margins, and visible pancreatic duct side branches). Meeting five or more of these criteria precludes the diagnosis of chronic pancreatitis. In 2007, the Rosemont criteria were created for the classification of chronic pancreatitis into the following four separate categories: (1) findings consistent with chronic pancreatitis, (2) findings suggestive of chronic pancreatitis, (3) findings indeterminate for chronic pancreatitis, and (4) normal. Studies comparing the two scoring systems have not found significant differences, but they await further validation studies.

Complications

The principal complications of chronic pancreatitis are pancreatic pseudocyst, biliary obstruction, duodenal obstruction, malnutrition, and diabetes mellitus. Adenocarcinoma of the pancreas occurs with greater frequency in patients with familial chronic pancreatitis than in the general population.

Treatment

A. Medical Treatment

Patients with chronic pancreatitis should be urged to discontinue the use of alcohol. Abstention from alcohol will reduce chronic or episodic pain in more than half of cases even though damage to the pancreas is irreversible.

Patients should limit fat intake to control diarrhea. Patients with diarrhea may be restricted to 50 g of fat and the amount increased until diarrhea appears. Permissible fat intake averages 100 g/d distributed equally among four meals.

Abdominal pain, malabsorption, and steatorrhea are often managed with pancreatic enzyme supplements. Pancrelipase replacement may be accomplished with pancreatic extracts containing 30,000-50,000 units of lipase distributed throughout each of four daily meals.

If enzymes alone do not improve the malabsorption enough, the problem is probably due to destruction of lipase by gastric acid. This can be largely alleviated by adding an H_2 receptor blocking agent to the enzyme regimen. A preparation of enzymes as enteric-coated microspheres (Pancrease) is less vulnerable to low pH and may be more effective in refractory cases.

Medium-chain triglycerides (MCTs), which can be obtained as a powder or an oil, may be used as a caloric supplement. This product is more rapidly hydrolyzed and the fatty acids more readily absorbed than are long-chain triglycerides, which make up 98% of the fat in a normal diet. Unfortunately, MCT oil is relatively unpalatable and is frequently associated with nausea and vomiting, bloating, and diarrhea, which limit patient acceptance.

Analgesics are typically used for pain control; narcotics are often combined with tricyclic antidepressants and nonsteroidal anti-inflammatory drugs.

B. Surgical Treatment

The primary indication for surgical therapy is chronic intractable pain. Celiac plexus block may be used in an attempt to obtain pain relief before proceeding with a major pancreatic drainage procedure or resection.

Surgical treatment in most cases involves drainage of the pancreatic duct and/or resection of diseased pancreas. The choice of operation can usually be made preoperatively based on the findings of a retrograde pancreatogram and CT scans. Patients with a pancreatic duct dilated to 7-8 mm in the body are candidates for drainage procedures such as the longitudinal pancreaticojejunostomy, first described by Puestow. Small duct pancreatitis and the presence of an inflammatory mass are indications for resection to remove the diseased pancreas.

1. Drainage procedures—A dilated ductal system reflects obstruction, and when dilation is present, procedures to improve ductal drainage usually relieve pain. Calcific alcoholic pancreatitis most often falls into this category.

The usual finding is an irregular, widely dilated duct with points of stenosis ("chain of lakes" appearance) and ductal calculi. For such patients, a longitudinal pancreaticojejunostomy (**Puestow procedure**) is appropriate (Figure 28–4). The duct is opened anteriorly from the tail into the head of the gland and anastomosed side-to-side to a Roux-en-Y segment of proximal jejunum. Pain improves postoperatively in about 80% of patients, but improvement of pancreatic insufficiency is uncommon. This procedure, however, has a low rate of success when the pancreatic duct is narrow (ie, < 8 mm). This Roux-en-Y drainage procedure can be combined with removal of the fibrotic pancreatic head tissue (**Frey procedure**).

Sphincteroplasty and distal (caudal) pancreaticojejunostomy (**Du Val procedure**) are other drainage techniques that were used more often in the past. The latter is only of historical interest, but surgical sphincteroplasty plus extraction of pancreatic ductal calculi continues in use, more often now through endoscopic access to the pancreatic duct.

2. Pancreatectomy—In the absence of a dilated duct, pancreatectomy is the best procedure, and the extent of resection can often be determined from a CT scan and pancreatogram. In patients with small ducts, the most severe disease is usually located in the head of the gland, and **pancreaticoduodenectomy** (Whipple procedure) is the operation of choice. A variant of this procedure involves resection of the head of the gland while preserving the duodenum. A Roux-en-Y limb of jejunum is anastomosed to both cut surfaces of the pancreas. If the duct is also dilated in the body and tail, resection of the head can also be combined with longitudinal pancreaticojejunostomy in that part of the gland. Pain relief is satisfactory

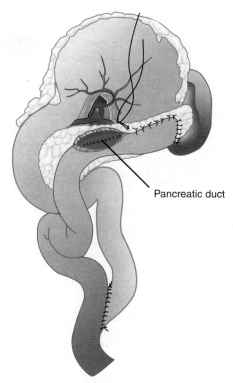

Pancreatic duct

▲ **Figure 28–4.** Longitudinal pancreaticojejunostomy (Puestow procedure) for chronic pancreatitis.

in about 80% of patients treated by these operations. A Beger procedure or a duodenal-preserving pancreatic head resection can be performed to decrease the morbidity of a Whipple procedure. **Total pancreatectomy** is indicated when a previous pancreaticoduodenectomy or distal pancreatectomy has failed to give satisfactory pain relief. Total pancreatectomy may be accompanied by islet cell autotransplantation to preserve endocrine function. Although the procedure has been shown to relieve intractable pain, improve the quality of life for patients with chronic pancreatitis, and decrease costs of long-term medical treatment, up to 30% of patients who undergo total pancreatectomy and islet cell autotransplantation experience brittle diabetes postoperatively. For chronic alcoholic pancreatitis, resections from the left of the gland (eg, **distal subtotal pancreatectomy**) are much less successful than resections of the head and are rarely performed nowadays. The most common indication is chronic focal posttraumatic pancreatitis, in which the head may be normal.

▶ Prognosis

Longitudinal pancreaticojejunostomy relieves pain in about 80% of patients with a dilated duct. Weight gain is common but less predictable. The results of pancreaticoduodenectomy

are good in 80% of patients, but removal of the distal pancreas is less successful. Total pancreatectomy, which is principally reserved for failures of other operations, gives satisfying relief in 30%-90% of patients in various studies. The reasons for these widely differing results are not known. Celiac plexus block is of lasting benefit to no more than 30% of patients. In some patients, pain subsides with advancing pancreatic insufficiency.

Bachmann K, et al: Is the Whipple procedure harmful for long-term outcome in treatment of chronic pancreatitis? 15-years follow-up comparing the outcome after pylorus-preserving pancreatoduodenectomy and Frey procedure in chronic pancreatitis. *Ann Surg.* 2013;258(5):815-820.

D'Souza SL, et al: EUS diagnostic criteria for chronic pancreatitis: a comparison of conventional versus Rosemont criteria. *Dig Dis Sci.* 2015;60(12):3782-3787.

Familiari P, et al: ERCP for biliary strictures associated with chronic pancreatitis. *Gastrointest Endosc Clin N Am.* 2013;23(4): 833-845.

Issa Y, et al: Surgical and endoscopic treatment of pain in chronic pancreatitis: a multidisciplinary update. *Dig Surg.* 2013;30(1): 35-50.

Sutherland DE, et al: Total pancreatectomy and islet autotransplantation for chronic pancreatitis. *J Am Col Surg.* 2012; 214(4):409-424.

ADENOCARCINOMA OF THE PANCREAS

An estimated 55,440 patients will develop pancreatic cancer in the United States in 2018, and 44,330 will die of the disease. These nearly equal numbers illustrate the dismal prognosis generally associated with pancreatic carcinoma. After tumors of the lung and colon, pancreatic carcinoma is the third leading cause of death due to cancer in both men and women. Factors associated with an increased risk of pancreatic cancer are cigarette smoking, dietary consumption of meat (especially fried meat) and fat, previous gastrectomy (> 20 years earlier), and race.

The peak incidence is in the fifth and sixth decades. In two-thirds of cases, the tumor is located in the head of the gland; the remainder occur in the body or tail. Ductal adenocarcinoma, mainly of a poorly differentiated cell pattern, accounts for 80% of the cancers; the remainder are islet cell tumors and cystadenocarcinomas, tumors that are discussed later in this chapter. Pancreatic adenocarcinoma is characterized by early local extension to contiguous structures and metastases to regional lymph nodes and the liver, limiting treatment options. Pulmonary, peritoneal, and distant nodal metastases are present in many patients at initial diagnosis.

▶ Clinical Findings

A. Symptoms and Signs

1. Carcinoma of the head of the pancreas—About 75% of patients with carcinoma of the head of the pancreas present with weight loss, obstructive jaundice, and deep-seated abdominal pain. Back pain occurs in 25% of patients and is associated with a worse prognosis. In general, smaller tumors confined to the pancreas are associated with less pain. Weight loss averages about 20 lb (44 kg). Jaundice may be present in the setting of bile duct obstruction and can occasionally be associated with cholangitis. A palpable nontender gallbladder in a jaundiced patient suggests neoplastic obstruction of the common duct (**Courvoisier sign**), most often due to pancreatic cancer. Jaundice is often accompanied by pruritus, especially of the hands and feet.

2. Carcinoma of the body and tail of the pancreas—Because carcinomas of the body and tail of the pancreas are remote from the bile duct, less than 10% of patients are jaundiced. The presenting complaints are weight loss and pain, which sometimes occurs in excruciating paroxysms. Migratory thrombophlebitis develops in 10% of cases.

The diagnosis of pancreatic carcinoma can be challenging. Patients can present with vague symptoms including weight loss, generalized abdominal pain, and nondiagnostic x-rays. Patients presenting with back pain are often worked up for neurosurgical and orthopedic diagnoses. Sudden onset of diabetes mellitus is an early manifestation in 25% of patients.

B. Laboratory Findings

Elevated alkaline phosphatase and bilirubin levels reflect either common duct obstruction or hepatic metastases. The bilirubin level with neoplastic obstruction averages 18 mg/dL, much higher than that generally seen with benign disease of the bile ducts. Only rarely are serum aminotransferase levels markedly elevated. Repeated examinations of stool specimens for occult blood are usually positive.

Serum levels of the tumor marker CA 19-9 are elevated in most patients with pancreatic cancer, but the sensitivity in resectable (< 4 cm) lesions is too low (50%) for this to serve as a screening tool. Elevated levels also occur with other gastrointestinal cancers. The greatest usefulness of CA 19-9 measurements may be in following the patients after treatment.

C. Imaging Studies

All patients should have a multiphase contrast-enhanced CT or MRI scan to determine resectability.

1. CT scan—CT scans show a pancreatic mass in 95% of cases, usually with a central zone of diminished attenuation, and in over 90% of patients with a mass, there are signs of extension beyond the boundaries of the pancreas. The upstream pancreatic duct is noted to be dilated in 70% of patients, and the bile duct is dilated in 60% (principally in those with jaundice). The presence of both bile duct and pancreatic duct dilation is strong evidence for pancreatic cancer even in the absence of a mass. Locoregional and distant metastases can be assessed on imaging studies. Locoregional involvement

includes superior mesenteric vein/portal vein involvement, superior mesenteric artery involvement, celiac axis involvement, common or proper hepatic artery involvement, regional lymphadenopathy, and invasion of inferior vena cava, left renal vein, and left adrenal vein. Distant metastases are typically seen in the liver or lung. Imaging studies can also be used to look for anatomic variants prior to surgical intervention.

2. ERCP—In patients with a typical clinical history and a pancreatic mass on CT, ERCP is unnecessary. ERCP is helpful in cases where there is biliary duct obstruction.

3. EUS—An EUS is useful in visualizing lesions that are typically not seen on cross-sectional imaging. It can be used to guide and perform fine-needle aspiration biopsies. Biopsy is particularly of value to verify a presumptive diagnosis of adenocarcinoma of the pancreas in patients with radiographic evidence of unresectability when chemotherapy will be indicated. In this case, therapy must be tailored to the tumor's pathology, and it is important to confirm the presence of malignancy prior to initiating therapy.

4. Upper gastrointestinal series—An upper gastrointestinal series is not sensitive in detecting pancreatic cancer, but it provides information about patency of the duodenum that may be useful in deciding whether a gastrojejunostomy will have to be performed. The classic findings consist of widening of the duodenal sweep, narrowing of the lumen, and the "reversed-3 sign," named for the duodenal configuration.

▶ Differential Diagnosis

Other periampullary neoplasms (eg, carcinoma of the ampulla of Vater, distal common bile duct, or duodenum) may also present with pain, weight loss, obstructive jaundice, and a palpable gallbladder. Preoperative cholangiography and gastrointestinal x-rays may suggest the correct diagnosis, but a diagnostic laparoscopy or laparotomy is sometimes required.

▶ Complications

Obstruction of the splenic vein by tumor may cause splenomegaly and segmental portal hypertension with bleeding gastric or esophageal varices.

▶ Treatment

Pancreatic resection for pancreatic cancer is appropriate if all gross tumor can be removed with microscopically negative margins. In general, lesions are considered resectable in the absence of vascular invasion or metastases. Specifically, the following areas must be free of tumor: (1) the superior mesenteric vein; (2) the portal vein; (3) the hepatic artery near the origin of the gastroduodenal artery; (4) the superior mesenteric artery where it courses under the body of the pancreas; and (5) the celiac trunk. Because the pancreas is so close to the portal vein and the superior mesenteric vessels, these structures may be involved early. Tumors abutting the superior mesenteric vein and portal vein are typically considered resectable under most classification systems, although more significant involvement including vascular deformation or circumferential involvement of > 180 degrees suggests a lower probability of margin-negative resection. About 15%-20% of cancers of the head of the pancreas are considered resectable on initial presentation.

Some tumors are considered as borderline resectable based on involvement of adjacent vasculature on cross-sectional imaging. A number of classification systems exist to stratify patients into resectable versus borderline resectable categories. These classification systems differ somewhat in the degree of vascular invasion that is considered sufficient to allow for a given classification. All, however, recognize the designation of borderline resectable as indicating a likelihood of positive surgical margins with attempted resection.

For patients with questionable peritoneal disease not seen on cross-sectional imaging, a histologic diagnosis can be made with a diagnostic laparoscopy. Patients undergoing planned surgical resection should undergo either laparoscopic or open exploration prior to any resections to identify any metastatic disease. For patients with documented metastases, surgical resection is not performed. Surgical bypass to the biliary system may be performed at that time (hepaticojejunostomy) in the absence of preoperative stenting. Enteric

bypass (gastrojejunostomy) is performed only in the presence of symptomatic gastric outlet obstruction. Traditionally, about 15% of patients thought to have localized disease from preoperative studies are found to be unresectable on initial exploration. This number is likely lower in the setting of conventional imaging.

For resectable lesions of the pancreatic head, pancreaticoduodenectomy (**Whipple procedure**) is required (Figure 28–5). This involves resection of the common bile duct, the gallbladder, the duodenum, and the pancreatic head. Resection of the antrum has been performed according to the original description of the procedure, although the operation may also be conducted with preservation of the antrum and pylorus (pylorus-preserving pancreaticoduodenectomy). Data do not support the superiority of either technique. Involvement of the superior mesenteric vein or portal vein is not a contraindication to attempted curative resection, and primary venous repair or venous reconstruction should be performed in these cases. Arterial reconstruction is performed less commonly due to association with poor outcomes.

Pancreaticoduodenectomy outcomes are strongly associated with surgeon volume. When performed by surgeons who do it frequently, the operative mortality rate is less than 5%, although this rate increases to over 20% when performed by less experienced surgeons. Common complications include delayed gastric emptying and non–life-threatening pancreatic fistulas.

Tumors in the body and tail of the pancreas are treated with a distal pancreatectomy, with or without splenectomy.

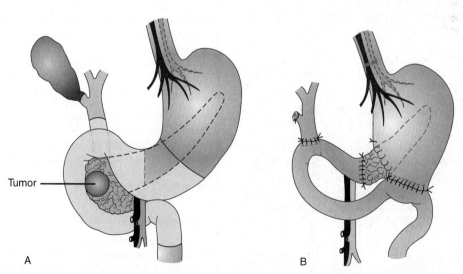

▲ **Figure 28–5.** Pancreaticoduodenectomy (Whipple procedure). **A:** Preoperative anatomic relationships showing a tumor in the head of the pancreas. **B:** Postoperative reconstruction showing pancreatic, biliary, and gastric anastomoses. A cholecystectomy and bilateral truncal vagotomy are also part of the procedure. In many cases, the distal stomach and pylorus can be preserved, and vagotomy is then unnecessary.

Splenectomy is commonly required due to the need to sacrifice the splenic artery and vein, which travel adjacent to the pancreatic body and tail.

Neoadjuvant therapy is increasingly being used for all patients with borderline resectable pancreatic cancer to eventually achieve margin-negative surgical resection. Neoadjuvant therapy has been considered for all patients with pancreatic cancer due to the high likelihood of micrometastatic disease at the time of diagnosis. It can also mitigate delay to chemotherapy for patients who have postoperative complications. However, studies have not definitely shown a benefit to neoadjuvant therapy compared to adjuvant therapy for patients with resectable disease.

Prognosis

The mean survival time following palliative therapy is 7 months. Following a Whipple procedure and adjuvant chemotherapy, median overall survival time has been reported to be as long as 28 months. Factors associated with tumor recurrence and shorter survival include lymph node involvement, tumor size greater than 2.5 cm, blood vessel invasion, and amount of blood transfused. Long-term survival is rare in patients with positive margins at the time of resection. If the margin-negative resection is achieved and adjuvant chemotherapy is completed, 5-year overall survival is approximately 28%.

Clancy TE: Surgery for pancreatic cancer. *Hematol Oncol Clin N Am.* 2015;29:701-716.

Gilbert JW, et al: Borderline resectable pancreatic cancer: conceptual evolution and current approach to image-based classification. *Ann Oncol.* 2017;28(9):2067-2076.

Neoptolemos JP, et al: Comparison of adjuvant gemcitabine and capecitabine with gemcitabine monotherapy in patients with resected pancreatic cancer (ESPAC-4): a multicenter, open-label, randomized, phase-3 trial. *Lancet.* 2017;389(10073): 1011-1024.

Noone AM, et al (eds): SEER Cancer Statistics Review, 1975-2015, National Cancer Institute. Bethesda, MD, https://seer.cancer.gov/csr/1975_2015/, based on November 2017 SEER data submission, posted to the SEER website, April 2018.

Tempero MA, et al: National Comprehensive Cancer Networks: Pancreatic adenocarcinoma, version 2.2012: featured updates to the NCCN guidelines. *J Natl Compr Canc Netw.* 2012;10(6): 703-713.

Visser BC, et al: Failure to comply with NCCN guidelines for the management of pancreatic cancer compromises outcomes. *HPB (Oxford).* 2012;14(8):539-547.

CYSTIC NEOPLASMS

Cystic neoplasms of the pancreas are often diagnosed incidentally on imaging performed for another indication because they are usually asymptomatic. Rarely, symptomatic patients present with abdominal pain, a mass, or jaundice.

Pancreatic cysts increase with age, with up to 10% of patients older than 70 years found to have incidental cysts on cross-sectional imaging.

Most pancreatic cystic lesions may be broadly classified into mucinous and nonmucinous lesions. Nonmucinous lesions predominantly include serous cystadenomas and are not considered premalignant. Mucinous lesions include mucinous cystic neoplasms (MCNs) and intraductal papillary mucinous neoplasms (IPMNs), both with varying premalignant potential.

Serous Cystadenomas

Serous cystadenomas are well-circumscribed lesions consisting of multiple small cysts ranging in size from microscopic to about 2 cm. The multicystic nature of the lesion is often evident on CT scans, which may also show calcifications. Occasionally, serous cystadenoma will present with one or more large cysts (macrocystic serous cystadenoma). The epithelium, which is flat to cuboidal, has no malignant potential. Serous cystadenomas grow slowly, and symptoms are rare until they are large enough to cause fullness and abdominal pain. Nonoperative management is pursued in virtually all cases given the absence of malignant potential. Surgery is only offered for symptomatic patients.

Cystic Pancreatic Endocrine Neoplasms

Cystic pancreatic endocrine neoplasms are a rare variant of neuroendocrine tumors. They are usually nonfunctioning tumors. They are distinguished by prominent septations on imaging, and diagnosis is confirmed with cytology. Immunohistochemical staining is positive for synaptophysin, chromogranin A, pancreatic polypeptide, and glucagon. Given its malignant potential, it is recommended to resect these tumors, but 5-year survival is greater than 87%.

Solid Pseudopapillary Neoplasms

Solid pseudopapillary neoplasms are the rarest cystic neoplasms and often affect young women in their 40s. They are often found incidentally on cross-sectional imaging. Cytology is necessary for diagnosis. Solid pseudopapillary neoplasms have the potential to metastasize, and resection is recommended. Five-year survival is greater than 80%.

Mucinous Cystic Neoplasms

MCNs are much more common in women than in men. They are typically unilocular lesions with a smooth lining with papillary projections. The septate appearance on CT scans is characteristic. The lining consists of tall columnar and goblet cells, which are often arranged in a papillary pattern. MCNs are considered premalignant, so surgical resection is generally indicated for lesions over 3 cm in size.

Rarely, cystadenocarcinomas present as a focus of malignancy within an existing MCN. The tumors are often quite large (eg, 10-20 cm) at the time of diagnosis. Metastases occur in about 25% of cases. Long-term survival rates are excellent unless there is evidence of invasive or malignant disease at time of resection.

Intraductal Papillary Mucinous Neoplasms

IPMNs may involve the main pancreatic or branch ducts. Rarely, IPMNs (mixed IPMNs) involve both pancreatic and branch ducts. Although branch duct IPMNs are more common, main duct and mixed IPMNs compose 60% of all resected IPMNs. In main duct IPMN, the risk of invasive cancer or high-grade dysplasia is over 40%, and therefore, surgical resection is recommended for all main duct and mixed IPMNs. Risk of malignancy in branch duct IPMNs is significantly lower, and surgical intervention must be tailored to the risks in an individual patient. More specific classification and management of IPMNs typically follow the criteria that have come to be known as the Sendai guidelines.

The Sendai guidelines define the classification of IPMNs, diagnostic criteria, and indications for resection. Main duct IPMNs are defined as segmental or diffuse dilation of the main pancreatic duct larger than 5 mm, with no evident etiology for obstruction. Ductal dilation of 5-9 mm is described as a worrisome feature, and dilation greater than 1 cm is a high-risk stigma. Patients with high-risk stigmata, which also include obstructive jaundice secondary to a cystic lesion and an enhancing solid component within a cyst in addition to main pancreatic duct size greater than 1 cm, should undergo resection. Patients with worrisome features, including cyst size greater than 3 cm, thickened or enhancing cyst walls, main duct size of 5-9 mm, a mural nodule, or abrupt change in pancreatic duct size with distal atrophy, should undergo further workup with an EUS. Patients with a definite mural nodule, thickened main duct walls, and positive cytology should also undergo resection.

Patients without high-risk stigmata or worrisome features should undergo close follow-up based on the size of the cyst. Large cysts of 2-3 cm or greater should have imaging and EUS every 3-6 months initially with consideration for surgery in young patients. Patients with smaller cysts up to 2 cm in size can undergo less frequent imaging; small, subcentimeter cysts are followed with imaging every 2-3 years.

Chari ST, et al: Study of recurrence after surgical resection of intraductal papillary mucinous neoplasm of the pancreas. *Gastroenterology.* 2002;123(5):1500.

Farrell JJ, et al: Pancreatic cystic neoplasms: management and unanswered questions. *Gastroenterology.* 2013;144(6):1303-1315.

Greer JB, et al: Spectrum and classification of cystic neoplasms of the pancreas. *Surg Oncol Clin N Am.* 2016;25(2):339-350.

Lee LS, et al: Interdisciplinary management of cystic neoplasms of the pancreas. *Gastroenterol Res Pract.* 2012;2012:513163.

Tanaka M, et al: International consensus guidelines 2012 for the management of IPMN and MCN of the pancreas. *Pancreatology.* 2012;12:183-197.

Vege SS, et al: American gastroenterological association institute guideline on the diagnosis and management of asymptomatic neoplastic pancreatic cysts. *Gastroenterology.* 2015;148(4):819.

ADENOMA & ADENOCARCINOMA OF THE AMPULLA OF VATER

Adenoma and adenocarcinoma of the ampulla of Vater account for about 10% of neoplasms that obstruct the distal bile duct.

CT and ultrasound scans reveal dilation of the biliary tree and pancreatic duct. ERCP can be an important diagnostic study. In 75% of cases, tumor is visible on duodenoscopy as an exophytic papillary lesion, an ulcerated tumor, or an infiltrating mass. An adequate biopsy of these lesions can usually be obtained. In 25% of cases, there is no intraduodenal growth, and endoscopic sphincterotomy is necessary to display the tumor. ERCP also demonstrates dilation of the biliary and pancreatic ducts.

If margin-negative resection is possible, some adenomas may be treated by endoscopic removal. If all tumor cannot be removed endoscopically, surgical resection including local resection or pancreaticoduodenectomy is necessary.

The primary treatment of resectable ampullary adenocarcinoma is surgery via pancreaticoduodenectomy. Endoscopic sphincterotomy alone or with retrograde stent placement (the combination is usually required) is indicated when there is definite evidence of unresectable disease (eg, hepatic metastases). Survival is typically less than a year for these patients.

Tempero MA, et al: National Comprehensive Cancer Networks: Pancreatic Adenocarcinoma, version 2.2012: featured updates to the NCCN Guidelines. *J Natl Compr Canc Netw.* 2012;10(6):703-713.

PANCREATIC NEUROENDOCRINE TUMORS

The incidence of pancreatic neuroendocrine tumors is 1 to 5 per million per year. Pancreatic neuroendocrine tumors may be functioning (ie, hormone-producing) or nonfunctioning, with varying malignant potential. Nonfunctioning tumors are recognized with increasing frequency as incidental findings on cross-sectional imaging. Functioning neuroendocrine neoplasms, or functioning islet cell tumors, are associated with characteristic clinical syndromes. Insulinoma, the most common functioning islet cell neoplasm, arises from beta cells and produces insulin and symptoms of hypoglycemia. Tumors of the delta or alpha$_1$ cells produce gastrin and diffuse gastric ulceration known as the Zollinger-Ellison syndrome. Alpha$_2$ cell neoplasms may produce excess glucagon and hyperglycemia. Non-beta islet cell tumors may secrete serotonin, adrenocorticotropic hormone, melanocyte-stimulating hormone, and kinins. Rare islet cell tumors secrete vasoactive intestinal polypeptide, leading to pancreatic cholera, a severe diarrheal illness.

1. Nonfunctioning Islet Cell Tumors

Most nonfunctioning islet cell tumors are found incidentally because they are usually asymptomatic. For nonfunctioning tumors smaller than 1 cm, conservative management with close monitoring is recommended. Tumors larger than 2 cm or those that grow rapidly within a 3- to 6-month follow-up period should be resected. Surgical intervention is more controversial for tumors between 1 and 2 cm because risk of malignant progression is low. Symptomatic patients may present late in the disease course with abdominal and back pain, weight loss, and, in many cases, a palpable abdominal mass. Jaundice is encountered occasionally. CT scans reveal an enhancing pancreatic mass. The histologic pattern on biopsy specimens is diagnostic of islet cell tumor, but diagnosis of malignancy rests on evidence of invasiveness or metastases, not the histologic appearance of the cells. Immunohistochemical staining of the tissue is positive for chromogranin and neuron-specific enolase (markers of amine precursor uptake and decarboxylation [APUD] tumors). Metastases are present at the time of diagnosis in 80% of symptomatic patients. Resection of all gross tumor (eg, by a Whipple procedure or distal pancreatectomy) is the preferred treatment if possible.

Amin S, et al: Islet cell tumors of the pancreas. *Gastroenterol Clin North Am.* 2016;45(1):83-100.

Anderson CW, et al: Clinical presentation and diagnosis of pancreatic neuroendocrine tumors. *Surg Oncol Clin North Am.* 2016;25(2):363-374.

Kulke MH, et al: National Comprehensive Cancer Networks: Neuroendocrine tumors. *J Natl Compr Canc Netw.* 2012;10(6):724-764.

Oberstein PE, Remotti H, Saif MW, et al: Pancreatic neuroendocrine tumors: entering a new era. *JOP.* 2012;13(2):169-173.

2. Insulinoma

Insulinomas are most frequently solitary and benign. About 10% are malignant, and metastases are usually evident at the time of diagnosis.

Patients may present with neurologic symptoms (related to cerebral glucose deprivation) known as neuroglycopenic symptoms, including memory lapse, vision changes, and unconsciousness. There may be profuse sympathetic discharge, with palpitations, sweating, and tremulousness. Hypoglycemic episodes are usually precipitated by fasting

and are relieved by food, so weight gain is common. The classic diagnostic criteria (**Whipple's triad**) are present in most cases: (1) hypoglycemic symptoms produced by fasting, (2) blood glucose below 50 mg/dL during symptomatic episodes, and (3) relief of symptoms by intravenous administration of glucose.

The most useful diagnostic test and the only one indicated in all but a few patients is demonstration of fasting hypoglycemia in the presence of inappropriately high levels of insulin. The patient is fasted, and blood samples are obtained every 6 hours for glucose and insulin measurements. The fast is continued until hypoglycemia or symptoms appear or for a maximum of 72 hours. Although insulin levels are not always elevated in patients with insulinoma, they will be high relative to the blood glucose concentration. A ratio of plasma insulin to serum glucose greater than 0.3 is diagnostic. Ratios should be calculated before and during the fast. Proinsulin, which constitutes more than 25% of total insulin (the upper limit of normal) in about 85% of patients with insulinomas, should also be measured. Proinsulin levels greater than 40% suggest a malignant islet cell tumor.

Localization of the tumor is important but may be difficult. In about 10% of cases, the tumor is so small or located so deeply that it is difficult or impossible to find at laparotomy. EUS may be successful in locating tumors, and conventional MRI is the most sensitive means of detecting the lesions. Invasive preoperative testing is not routinely indicated but may include transhepatic portal venous sampling and arteriography with selective calcium stimulation. Blood samples from the hepatic veins reveal an increase in insulin level when calcium is infused into an artery supplying the tumor.

▶ **Differential Diagnosis**

Fasting hypoglycemia may be a manifestation of some nonpancreatic, non–islet cell tumors. Clinically, the condition is identical to that resulting from insulinoma, but the cause is rarely secretion of insulin by the tumors, as serum insulin levels are normal. Most non–islet cell tumors associated with hypoglycemia are large and readily detected on physical examination. The majority are of mesenchymal origin (eg, hemangiopericytoma, fibrosarcoma, leiomyosarcoma) and are located in the abdomen or thorax, but hepatoma, adrenocortical carcinoma, and a variety of other lesions may also produce hypoglycemia. The principal means by which these tumors produce hypoglycemia include secretion of insulin-like growth factor II or inhibition of glycogenolysis or gluconeogenesis. Rapid utilization of glucose by the tumor, replacement of liver tissue by metastases, and secretion of insulin are other postulated mechanisms that are probably uncommon.

Surreptitious self-administration of insulin or administration of oral hypoglycemic agents is seen occasionally. Circulating C peptide levels are normal in these patients but elevated in most patients with insulinoma.

▶ Treatment

Surgical procedures for insulinoma include enucleation and resection (distal pancreatectomy, pancreaticoduodenectomy, or total pancreatectomy). Medical treatment is reserved for surgically incurable lesions or patients who cannot undergo surgery.

A. Medical Treatment

Diazoxide is administered to suppress insulin release. Streptozocin is traditionally used with limited success and considerable toxicity. Somatostatin analogs (octreotide) can also be considered for patients who cannot take diazoxide.

B. Surgical Treatment

Intraoperative ultrasound and palpation of the pancreas are routinely utilized. Enucleation is possible for superficial tumors that do not involve the pancreatic duct and is nearly always possible in the pancreatic head.

Tumors that can be localized preoperatively and in favorable anatomic locations can sometimes be resected using a laparoscopic approach. The same principles of local, complete resection should be followed. Laparoscopic ultrasound is often useful to guide this exploration.

In the past, insulinomas could not be detected on preoperative or intraoperative evaluation. Distal or subtotal pancreatectomy with intraoperative blood glucose management was traditionally used in these cases. With current imaging and intraoperative ultrasound, blind distal pancreatectomy is rarely required.

Patients with insulinoma associated with multiple endocrine neoplasia type 1 (MEN 1) usually have multiple (average of three) lesions. Surgery requires resection of all tumors, often including distal pancreatectomy plus enucleation of any lesions found in the head of the gland.

For islet cell hyperplasia, nesidioblastosis, or multiple benign adenomas, distal subtotal pancreatectomy usually decreases insulin levels enough that medical management is simplified. For islet cell carcinomas, resection of both primary and metastatic lesions is warranted if technically feasible.

Patients with sporadic insulinomas lead a normal life after the tumor has been removed. The outcome is less predictable in patients with MEN 1, who may have several insulin-producing tumors.

Kulke MH, et al: National Comprehensive Cancer Networks. Neuroendocrine tumors. *J Natl Compr Canc Netw.* 2012;10(6):724-764.

3. Pancreatic Cholera (WDHA Syndrome: Watery Diarrhea, Hypokalemia, & Achlorhydria)

Most cases of pancreatic cholera are caused by a non-beta islet cell tumor of the pancreas that secretes vasoactive intestinal polypeptide and peptide histidine isoleucine. These tumors are quite uncommon, much less common than other neuroendocrine tumors, and an extremely rare cause of severe diarrhea. The WDHA syndrome is characterized by profuse watery diarrhea, massive fecal loss of potassium, low serum potassium, and extreme weakness. Gastric acid secretion is usually low or absent even after stimulation with betazole or pentagastrin. Stool volume averages about 5 L/d during acute episodes and contains over 300 mEq of potassium (20 times normal). Severe metabolic acidosis frequently results from loss of bicarbonate in the stool. Patients who complain of severe diarrhea must be studied carefully for other causes given the extremely rare nature of the WDHA syndrome.

CT scan is the best initial imaging test; somatostatin receptor scintigraphy is also very useful for localization. Approximately 80% of the tumors are solitary, located in the body or tail, and can be removed easily. About half of the lesions are malignant, and three-fourths of those have metastasized by the time of exploration. Even if all of the tumor cannot be removed, tumor debulking may alleviate symptoms.

Kulke MH, et al: National Comprehensive Cancer Networks: Neuroendocrine tumors. *J Natl Compr Canc Netw.* 2012;10(6):724-764.

4. Glucagonoma

Glucagonoma is another rare functional neuroendocrine tumor. Glucagonoma syndrome is notable for a characteristic rash, necrolytic migratory erythema (usually involving the legs and perineum), weight loss, stomatitis, hypoaminoacidemia, anemia, and mild to moderate diabetes mellitus. Confirmation of the diagnosis depends on measuring elevated serum glucagon levels (> 500 pg/mL). CT scans demonstrate the enhancing tumor and sites of metastases.

Glucagonomas arise from α_2 cells in the pancreatic islets. Most are large at the time of diagnosis. About 25% are benign and confined to the pancreas. The remainder have metastasized by the time of diagnosis, most often to the liver, lymph nodes, adrenal gland, or vertebrae.

Severe malnutrition should be corrected preoperatively with a period of TPN and treatment with somatostatin analogues. Surgical removal of the primary lesion and resectable metastases is indicated if technically feasible. If the tumor is confined to the pancreas, cure is possible. Even if it is not possible to remove all the tumor deposits, considerable palliation may result from subtotal removal. Somatostatin analog therapy normalizes serum glucagon and amino acid levels, clears the rash, and promotes weight gain. The clinical course generally parallels changes in serum levels of glucagon in response to therapy.

Kulke MH, et al: National Comprehensive Cancer Networks: Neuroendocrine tumors. *J Natl Compr Canc Netw.* 2012;10(6):724-764.

5. Somatostatinoma

Somatostatinomas are characterized by diabetes mellitus (usually mild), diarrhea, and malabsorption. Serum calcitonin and IgM concentrations may be elevated. The syndrome results from secretion of somatostatin by an islet cell tumor of the pancreas, half of which are malignant and accompanied by hepatic metastases. The lesion is usually large and readily demonstrated by CT scan or somatostatin receptor scintigraphy. Smaller lesions can be seen on EUS. The diagnosis may be made by recognizing the clinical syndrome and measuring increased concentrations of somatostatin in the serum (>30 pg/mL). Often, however, the somatostatin syndrome is unsuspected until histologic evidence of metastatic islet cell carcinoma has been obtained. When the disease is localized, pancreatic resection is indicated.

Kulke MH, et al; National Comprehensive Cancer Networks: Neuroendocrine tumors. *J Natl Compr Canc Netw.* 2012;10(6): 724-764.

MULTIPLE CHOICE QUESTIONS

1. All of the following are true about the anatomy of the pancreas, except

   A. The head is adherent to the medial duodenum.
   B. The body is in contact posteriorly with the left crus of the diaphragm and the left adrenal gland.
   C. The common bile duct passes through a groove in the posterior aspect of the head.
   D. The uncinate process lies anterior to the superior mesenteric artery.
   E. The main pancreatic duct is also known as the duct of Wirsung.

2. Serum amylase can come from

   A. Lung
   B. Muscle
   C. Skin
   D. Parotid gland
   E. Red blood cells

3. Acute pancreatitis

   A. Is usually caused by acute cholecystitis
   B. Can be complicated by pancreatic necrosis
   C. Causes inflammation of the pancreas that is usually not discernible by computed tomography scan
   D. Is associated with common bile duct stones in > 80% of patients
   E. Progresses to chronic pancreatitis in about 40% of those affected

4. Pancreatic adenocarcinoma

   A. Is unresectable at the time of diagnosis in most people
   B. Is smaller at diagnosis, on average, for tumors in the tail of the pancreas than those in the head
   C. Can be resected by pancreaticoduodenectomy for those tumors limited to the tail
   D. Has a similar prognosis as malignant pancreatic neuroendocrine tumor
   E. Should generally be managed by operative enucleation

5. Management of insulinoma

   A. Typically requires emergent operation
   B. Should not include preoperative imaging
   C. May be treated by enucleation of the pancreatic lesion
   D. Is commonly required in the management of chronic pancreatitis
   E. Is a palliative approach to an incurable problem for most people

Spleen

Matthew A. Nehs, MD

ANATOMY

The spleen is a dark purplish, highly vascular, coffee bean–shaped organ of mesodermal origin situated in the left upper quadrant of the abdomen at the level of the eighth to eleventh ribs between the fundus of the stomach, the diaphragm, the splenic flexure of the colon, and the left kidney (Figure 29–1). The adult spleen weighs 100-150 g, measures about 12 × 7 × 4 cm, and usually cannot be palpated. It is attached to adjacent viscera, the abdominal wall, and the diaphragm by peritoneal folds or "ligaments." The gastrosplenic ligament carries the short gastric vessels. The other ligaments (splenorenal and splenocolic) are avascular except in patients with portal hypertension or myelofibrosis.

The splenic capsule consists of visceral peritoneum overlying a 1- to 2-mm fibroelastic layer that contains a few smooth muscle cells. The fibroelastic layer sends into the pulp numerous fibrous bands (trabeculae) that form the framework of the spleen. The spleen consists of specific segments based on arterial supply numbering between two and six separated by an avascular plane (Figure 29–2).

The splenic artery originates from the celiac artery, it travels posterior to the pancreas, and it enters the hilum of the spleen. It branches into the trabecular arteries and then branches into the central arteries that course through the surrounding white pulp and sends radial branches to the peripheral marginal zone and the more distant red pulp. The white pulp consists of lymphatic tissue including T cells adjacent to the central artery (periarteriolar lymphoid sheets), with a surrounding area containing lymphoid follicles rich in B cells interspersed with dendritic and reticular cells important in antigen presentation. The vascular spaces of the marginal zone between the red and white pulp channel blood into the splenic cords of Billroth and out to the associated venous sinuses. The red pulp vascular structures have a noncontiguous basement membrane that filters cells such as senescent and misshapen erythrocytes into the macrophage-lined sinuses.

Accessory spleens (spleniculi) are seen in 10%-15% of the normal population and are located primarily in the gastrosplenic, gastrocolic, and splenorenal ligaments, but they can also be found throughout the peritoneal cavity in the omentum, bowel mesentery, and pelvis. Accessory spleens probably result from a failure of fusion of the primordial splenic buds during embryogenesis. Ordinarily of no significance, they may play a role in recurrence of certain hematologic disorders for which splenectomy is performed. Removal of accessory spleens may lead to remission of disease in these patients. Accessory spleens can be identified by computed tomography (CT) scan preoperatively and can be resected with a laparoscopic approach in most cases. Patients who

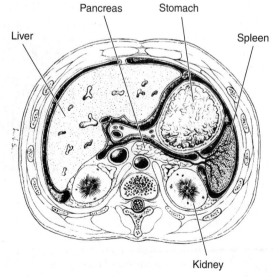

▲ **Figure 29–1.** Normal anatomic relations of the spleen.

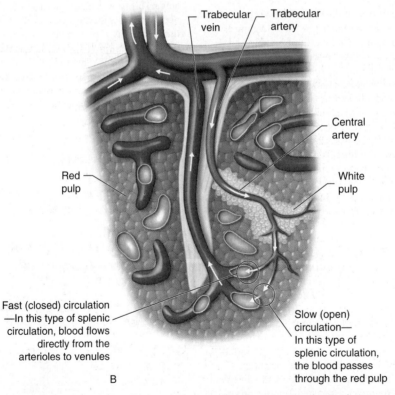

▲ **Figure 29–2.** The internal anatomy of the spleen includes specific segments, numbering between two and six, separated by an avascular plane and based on arterial supply. **A:** Anatomy of a segment. **B:** The internal circulation within the spleen.

fail to respond to initial splenectomy should undergo scanning with technetium-99m–labeled red cells or indium-111–labeled platelets to identify potential sites of missed accessory spleens, which can be identified intraoperatively with a handheld gamma counter.

Ectopic spleen (wandering spleen) is an unusual condition in which a long splenic pedicle allows the spleen to move within the peritoneum. It often resides in the lower abdomen or pelvis, where even a normal-sized spleen can be felt as a mass. The condition is 13 times more common in women than in men. Diagnostic radionuclide scan can diagnose the mass as a spleen. Acute torsion of the pedicle occurs occasionally, necessitating emergency splenectomy, and elective removal of wandering spleens in the pelvis is recommended.

PHYSIOLOGY

The spleen has a dual function as a secondary lymphoid organ important in host immunity and as a large filter for blood, removing senescent erythrocytes. The anatomy of the spleen provides an ideal environment for these two functions with the immune activity in the white pulp and the hematologic/filtration functions in the red pulp.

The spleen receives 5% of the total cardiac output, or approximately 150-300 mL/min, such that each red cell averages 1000 passes through the spleen each day. Normal blood cells pass rapidly through the spleen, whereas abnormal and senescent cells are slowed and entrapped. As they travel through the hypoxic, acidotic, glucose-deprived splenic cords and sinuses of the red pulp, senescent erythrocytes pass into the vascular spaces and are phagocytosed by macrophages in a process called "culling." Part of the membrane of erythrocytes can be removed through the gaps between endothelial cells lining the vascular spaces in a similar process called pitting. In the presence of splenomegaly and other disease states, the flow patterns of the spleen become more circuitous as the red pulp volume expands, so that even normal cells may be trapped.

The spleen is considered to be a secondary organ of the immune system and represents the largest single collection of lymphoid tissue in the body. The white pulp of the spleen contains the various cellular components needed to generate an immune response, with structural and functional relationships similar to those of lymph nodes. Lymphocytes and circulating antigen-presenting cells enter the white pulp via the marginal zone capillaries and traverse the T-cell–rich periarteriolar lymphoid sheets before passing through bridging channels into the red pulp. Primary follicles or germinal centers with secondary follicles at the periphery of the white pulp are sites of B-cell expansion and immunoglobulin (Ig) production. Blood passing through the spleen is exposed to all the key cellular components necessary for both humoral and cellular immune responses. Tissue macrophages in the spleen are key components of generating an immune response particularly against encapsulated organisms. Moreover, the concentration of macrophages in the red pulp vascular spaces facilitates opsonization of particles coated with IgG and plays an important role in the filtration and removal of senescent erythrocytes and in autoimmune hematologic diseases, in addition to explaining the increased risk of sepsis that follows splenectomy in children under 2 years of age. Even in adults, splenectomy leads to a slight but definite reduction in immune function.

Normally, about 30% of the total platelet pool is sequestered in the spleen. Splenomegaly typically involves expansion of the red pulp, which increases this sequestration to between 80% and 95% of the platelet cell mass. Storage of erythrocytes and granulocytes in the spleen is limited in humans, but newly formed reticulocytes released from the bone marrow concentrate in the spleen to undergo a maturational process.

Mebius RE, et al: Structure and function of the spleen. *Nat Rev Immunol.* 2005;5(8):606-616.
Scandella JT, et al: Form follows function: lymphoid tissue microarchitecture in antimicrobial immune defense. *Nat Rev Immunol.* 2008;8:764-775.

OPERATIVE INDICATIONS FOR SPLENECTOMY

To better describe and understand operative indications in surgery of the spleen, one could categorize the indications for splenectomy or procedures of the spleen into eight general areas:

1. **Hypersplenism** is characterized by diffuse enlargement of the spleen by neoplastic disorders, hematopoietic disorders of the bone marrow, and metabolic or storage disorders. These various disease processes result in diffuse enlargement of the spleen and amplify the normal function of elimination of circulating blood cells, resulting in general pancytopenia. Erythrocytes and platelets are most commonly affected. Hypersplenism also may result in symptoms of early satiety due to the mass effect of an enlarged spleen against the stomach.

2. **Autoimmune/erythrocyte disorders.** Specific cytopenias are related to antibodies targeting platelets, erythrocytes, or neutrophils. A second category of diseases relates to intrinsic structural changes within the erythrocyte that lead to a shortened red blood cell half-life with accelerated splenic clearance. In these cases, there is nothing intrinsically wrong with the spleen, and splenic size is typically normal.

3. **Trauma** or injury to the spleen.

4. **Vascular diseases.** Splenic vein thrombosis and splenic artery aneurysm may require splenectomy for treatment.

5. **Cysts, abscesses, and primary splenic tumors** are mass lesions of the spleen. This would include treatment of

simple cysts, echinococcal cysts, splenic abscess, and various benign neoplasms including hamartomas, hemangiomas, lymphangiomas, and rare malignant lesions.

6. **Diagnostic procedures.** This category of splenectomy occurs when the spleen is removed primarily to make a clinical diagnosis when none is available. A subcategory of this would be staging laparotomy for Hodgkin disease, which has all but been eliminated based on alternative imaging techniques and current treatment regimens.

7. **Iatrogenic splenectomy.** Splenectomy that is performed due to an incidental injury to the spleen during surgery within the general abdominal cavity or, specifically, the left upper quadrant can be categorized as iatrogenic splenectomy. This category is likely underreported and may be considered a subcategory of trauma.

8. **Incidental splenectomy.** The spleen may be removed as part of a standard operation to remove the distal pancreas most commonly, and also for gastric cancers, left-sided renal cell carcinomas, adrenal cancers, and retroperitoneal sarcomas in the left upper quadrant. The spleen is removed in these instances due to direct tumor extension, vascular involvement, or the need for excision of splenic hilum lymph nodes.

With the increase in splenic preservation for trauma, many institutional series list medical conditions as the most common indications for splenectomy. Most recent series report 40%-50% performed for hematologic conditions, 35%-40% for trauma, and 20%-30% for neoplastic disease. Within this category, idiopathic thrombocytopenia purpura has the highest incidence of splenectomy, followed by lymphoma and hereditary spherocytosis. Each of these categories of disease will be discussed, including the etiology and pathophysiology of the disorder, the specific indications for splenectomy, alternative treatments, and the results of splenectomy.

Bickenbach KA, et al: Indications for and efficacy of splenectomy for haematological disorders. *Br J Surg.* 2013;100(6):794-800.

Harbrecht BG, et al: Is splenectomy after trauma an endangered species? *Am Surg.* 2008;74:410-412.

Radkowiak D, et al: 20 years' experience with laparoscopic splenectomy. Single center outcomes of a cohort study of 500 cases. *Int J Surg.* 2018;52:285-292.

HYPERSPLENISM

In the past, the term *hypersplenism* or *increased splenic function* has been used to denote the syndrome characterized by splenic enlargement, deficiency of one or more blood cell lines, normal or hyperplastic cellularity of deficient cell lines in the marrow, and increased turnover of affected cells. Increased understanding of the pathophysiology of specific disorders has shown that hypersplenism is not synonymous with splenomegaly. Some disorders in which there is spleen-dependent destruction of blood elements do not manifest all features of hypersplenism. For example, splenomegaly is rarely a feature of immune thrombocytopenic purpura (ITP), and splenectomy is not always curative. Conversely, other conditions that enlarge the spleen may not result in destruction or sequestration of blood elements with resultant cytopenias. In disorders with known pathogenesis, the trend has been to classify them as separate disease entities rather than as hypersplenic conditions.

The defects in hypersplenism are exaggerations of normal splenic functions primarily associated with the red pulp. The principal cause of cytopenias in hypersplenism is increased sequestration and destruction of blood cells in the spleen, which is hypertrophied or increased in volume in a variety of diseases. Etiologic factors include (1) neoplastic infiltration, (2) disease of the bone marrow in which the spleen becomes a site of extramedullary hematopoiesis, or (3) metabolic/genetic disorders such as Gaucher disease. The hyperplastic spleen is not selective in its hyperfunction in most of these disorders. The splenomegaly can lead to an increased turnover in erythrocytes and platelets, with a lesser effect on leukocytes. For example, about 60% of patients with cirrhosis develop splenomegaly, and 15% develop hypersplenism. The hypersplenism of cirrhosis is seldom of clinical significance; the anemia and thrombocytopenia are usually mild and rarely are indications for splenectomy.

▶ Clinical Findings

A. Symptoms and Signs

The clinical findings depend largely on the underlying disorder or are secondary to the depletion of circulating blood elements caused by the hypersplenism (Table 29-1). Manifestations of hypersplenism usually develop gradually, and the diagnosis often follows a routine physical or laboratory examination. Some patients experience left upper quadrant fullness, discomfort (can be severe), or early satiety. Others have hematemesis due to gastroesophageal varices.

Table 29-1. Disorders associated with secondary hypersplenism.

Congestive splenomegaly (cirrhosis, portal or splenic vein obstruction)
Neoplasm (leukemia, metastatic carcinoma)
Inflammatory disease (sarcoid, lupus erythematosus, Felty syndrome)
Acute infections with splenomegaly
Chronic infection (tuberculosis, brucellosis, malaria)
Storage diseases (Gaucher disease, Letterer-Siwe disease, amyloidosis)
Chronic hemolytic diseases (spherocytosis, thalassemia, glucose-6-phosphate dehydrogenase deficiency, elliptocytosis)
Myeloproliferative disorders (myelofibrosis with myeloid metaplasia)

Purpura, bruising, and diffuse mucous membrane bleeding are unusual symptoms despite the presence of thrombocytopenia. Anemia may produce significant fatigue that may be the chief complaint in this patient population. Recurrent infections may be seen in patients with severe leukopenia.

B. Laboratory Findings

Patients with primary hypersplenism usually exhibit pancytopenia of moderate degree and generalized marrow hyperplasia. Anemia is most prominent, reflecting the destruction of erythrocytes in the hypertrophied red pulp of the spleen. Thrombocytopenia occurs due to sequestration of platelets but also possibly due to increased turnover. In most cases, more immature cell types such as reticulocytes are present, reflecting the overactivity of the bone marrow to compensate for the pancytopenias. One exception is myeloid metaplasia, in which dysfunction of the bone marrow is the primary defect.

C. Evaluation of Splenic Size

Before it becomes palpable, an enlarged spleen may cause dullness to percussion above the left costal margin. Splenomegaly is manifested on supine x-rays of the abdomen by medial displacement of the stomach and downward displacement of the transverse colon and splenic flexure. CT scan is useful for differentiating the spleen from other abdominal masses and for demonstrating splenic enlargement or intrasplenic lesions. Some of the largest massive spleens (spleen weight > 1500 g) occur in these types of disease. Finding the edge of the spleen below the iliac crest and crossing the abdominal midline is frequently observed (Figure 29–3).

▶ Differential Diagnosis

Leukemia and lymphoma are diagnosed by marrow aspiration, lymph node biopsy, and examination of the peripheral blood (white count and differential). In hereditary spherocytosis, there are spherocytes, osmotic fragility is increased, and platelets and white cells are normal. The hemoglobinopathies with splenomegaly are differentiated based on hemoglobin electrophoresis or the demonstration of an unstable hemoglobin level. Thalassemia major becomes apparent in early childhood, and the blood smear morphology is characteristic. In myelofibrosis, the bone marrow shows proliferation of fibroblasts and replacement of normal elements. In ITP, the spleen is normal or only slightly enlarged. In aplastic anemia, the spleen is not enlarged and the marrow is fatty.

▶ Treatment & Prognosis

The course, response to treatment, and prognosis of the hypersplenic syndromes differ widely depending on the underlying disease and its response to treatment and will be discussed for each particular disorder below. The indications for splenectomy are given in Table 29–2.

Splenectomy may decrease transfusion requirements, decrease the incidence and number of infections, prevent hemorrhage, and reduce pain. The course of congestive splenomegaly due to portal hypertension depends on the degree of venous obstruction and liver damage. The hypersplenism is rarely a major problem and is almost always overshadowed by variceal bleeding or liver dysfunction.

NEOPLASTIC DISEASES

Neoplastic diseases in which splenectomy may play a role in management of hypersplenism include chronic lymphocytic leukemia (CLL), hairy cell leukemia, and non-Hodgkin

Axial   **Coronal**   **Sagittal**

▲ **Figure 29–3.** Example of a large spleen that has displaced adjacent organs and is palpable and imageable outside of the left upper quadrant.

Table 29–2. Indications for splenectomy.

Splenectomy always indicated
Primary splenic tumor (rare)
Hereditary spherocytosis (congenital hemolytic anemia)
Splenectomy usually indicated
Primary hypersplenism
Chronic immune thrombocytopenic purpura
Splenic vein thrombosis causing gastric varices
Splenic abscess (rare)
Splenectomy sometimes indicated
Splenic injury
Autoimmune hemolytic disease
Elliptocytosis with hemolysis
Nonspherocytic congenital hemolytic anemias
Hodgkin disease (for staging)
Thrombotic thrombocytopenic purpura
Idiopathic myelofibrosis
Splenic artery aneurysm
Wiskott-Aldrich syndrome
Gaucher disease
Mastocytosis–aggressive disease
Splenectomy rarely indicated
Chronic leukemia
Splenic lymphoma
Macroglobulinemia
Thalassemia major
Sickle cell anemia
Congestive splenomegaly and hypersplenism due to portal hypertension
Felty syndrome
Hairy cell leukemia
Chédiak-Higashi syndrome
Sarcoidosis
Splenectomy not indicated
Asymptomatic hypersplenism
Splenomegaly with infection
Splenomegaly associated with elevated IgM
Hereditary hemolytic anemia of moderate degree
Acute leukemia
Agranulocytosis

lymphoma. Lymphoma is discussed in detail in Chapter 46. Related neoplastic disorders of idiopathic myelofibrosis and mastocytosis are also discussed as precursors or variants of neoplastic diseases in which splenectomy is occasionally indicated.

1. Chronic Lymphocytic Leukemia

CLL is a low-grade neoplasm of B-cell lineage characterized by accumulations of populations of lymphocytes that are mature morphologically but functionally incompetent. In the United States, CLL composes 25%-30% of all leukemias, with a mean age at diagnosis of approximately 70 years. The clinical manifestations and natural history are variable, but initially, the disease tends to be indolent. In more advanced stages, splenomegaly, which is frequently massive, is a common characteristic of CLL. Most symptoms related to the

spleen are from thrombocytopenia and anemia due to secondary hypersplenism (80%-90% of splenic symptoms). Ten to 20% of patients may have symptoms primarily related to pressure from the size of the enlarged spleen.

Other causes of cytopenia in CLL relate to decreased cellular production from the bone marrow. Bone marrow failure can be due to replacement with leukemic cells or to depletion of the bone marrow as a toxic effect of prior antitumor chemotherapy.

Splenectomy in patients with CLL corrects thrombocytopenia in 70%-85% of cases, neutropenia in 60%-70%, and anemia in 50%-60% of cases. The median duration of benefit for both platelets and red cell populations is well over 1 year. Patients with smaller spleens preoperatively, lower preoperative platelet counts, and extensive prior chemotherapy are less likely to respond to splenectomy. However, a positive bone marrow aspirate for leukemic cells is not a contraindication to splenectomy in CLL. Patients who do not have a good performance status should not undergo splenectomy because patients in terminal stages have unacceptable operative morbidity.

2. Hairy Cell Leukemia

Hairy cell leukemia (HCL) is a low-grade lymphoproliferative disorder with characteristic "hairy cells" (ie, B lymphocytes with irregular cytoplasmic protrusions positive for tartrate reaction acid phosphatase) that infiltrate the bone marrow and spleen. HCL is a rare malignancy, accounting for just 2% of leukemias. Patients are typically male (~4:1 male-to-female ratio) , and onset of the disease is in the fifth or sixth decade of life. Symptoms relate to pancytopenia, with anemia requiring transfusions; and to neutropenia, characterized by increased susceptibility to infections and increased bleeding tendencies. Some patients may have symptoms from splenomegaly, which is present in 80% of patients at the time of diagnosis of HCL. The cytopenias are due to a combination of bone marrow replacement and secondary hypersplenism.

The standard therapy for HCL between 1960 and 1995 was splenectomy, but recent advances in pharmacotherapy have superseded this surgical approach. First-line therapy is now treatment with purine nucleoside analogues, primarily cladribine and pentostatin, with a complete response rate of 80%-90%. It has never been shown that splenectomy offers survival benefit in this indolent disease. The operation should be reserved for palliation of splenomegaly or in patients with pancytopenia that persists after treatment with purine nucleoside analogues and the second-line agents rituximab and alpha interferon.

3. Myelodysplastic Syndrome

Myelodysplastic syndromes (MDS) are a heterogeneous group of clinical hematopoietic stem cell disorders manifested by pancytopenias and dysplasia of the bone marrow.

Pathologic changes include extensive bone marrow fibrosis, extramedullary hematopoiesis in the spleen and liver, and a leukoerythroblastic blood reaction that may evolve into acute myeloid leukemia over time.

The bone marrow is usually almost completely replaced by fibrous tissue, although in some cases, it is hyperplastic and fibrosis is minimal. Extramedullary hematopoiesis develops mainly in the spleen, liver, and long bones. Symptoms are attributable to anemia (weakness, fatigue, and dyspnea) and to splenomegaly (abdominal fullness and pain, which may be severe). Pain over the spleen from splenic infarcts is common. Spontaneous bleeding, fatigue, secondary infection, bone pain, and a hypermetabolic state are frequent. Portal hypertension develops in some cases as a result of fibrosis of the liver, greatly increased splenic blood flow, or both.

Hepatomegaly is present in 75% of cases, and splenomegaly with a firm and irregular spleen is present in all cases. Striking changes in the peripheral blood (eg, abnormal white blood cell/red blood cell morphology and cytopenias) result from the combination of extramedullary hematopoiesis and hypersplenism. Patients are uniformly anemic, and red cells vary greatly in size and shape, many of them distorted and fragmented. The white blood cell count is usually high (20,000-50,000/µL). The platelet count may be elevated, but values less than 100,000/µL are seen in 30% of cases due to secondary hypersplenism. Bone marrow aspirates frequently result in a dry tap because marrow is replaced with fibrosis. It was once incorrectly thought that the spleen performed a crucial function of extramedullary hematopoiesis in this disease and that splenectomy could be lethal. In fact, many patients with myeloid metaplasia feel better if the massive spleen is removed, and their hypersplenism is often corrected.

About 30% of patients are asymptomatic at the time of initial diagnosis and require no therapy. When cytopenias and splenomegaly produce symptoms, treatment is primarily supportive using transfusions, androgenic steroids, antimetabolites, and hematopoietic growth factors. Newer therapies include treatment with immunomodulatory drugs such as thalidomide or antibodies to vascular endothelial growth factor and tumor necrosis factor. A subset of patients with myeloid metaplasia has a component of autoimmune hemolytic anemia, and in this group of patients, immunosuppressive therapy may be beneficial. Splenectomy is indicated in the following situations: (1) major hemolysis unresponsive to medical management, (2) severe symptoms of massive splenomegaly with mass effect of the spleen, (3) life-threatening thrombocytopenia, and (4) portal hypertension with variceal hemorrhage. This is one of the rare occasions when portal hypertension may be cured by splenectomy.

Splenectomy in myeloid metaplasia is associated with a 7%-10% death rate and frequent complications often related to postsplenectomy hepatic morbidity. Splenectomy best relieves symptoms of splenomegaly and portal hypertension, but only about 75% of patients get relief from anemia and thrombocytopenia. Younger patients with normal platelet counts and symptoms are the best candidates for splenectomy in idiopathic myelofibrosis.

4. Systemic Mast Cell Disease

Systemic mast cell disease, or mastocytosis, is a rare condition characterized by mast cell infiltration of a number of tissues, including the spleen. There are two types: indolent and aggressive. In indolent systemic mass cell disease, there is no need for consideration of splenectomy. The aggressive type is associated with hematologic diseases with characteristics of lymphoma. Splenomegaly may occur, with the predominant symptoms resulting from thrombocytopenia due to hypersplenism. In this subgroup of patients with aggressive disease, splenectomy improves platelet counts and is associated with longer median survival time than for patients with aggressive disease who do not undergo splenectomy, although systemic therapy including alpha interferon has been shown to be effective.

METABOLIC DISORDERS

Metabolic disorders amenable to splenectomy are rare inherited diseases that include as a component splenic enlargement due to the pathologic deposition of material within the spleen. In Gaucher disease, excess sphingolipid is deposited in the spleen. In sarcoidosis, the spleen becomes involved with noncaseating granulomas, as can be seen in lymph nodes. Inherited disorders also include disease in which there is a specific immunologic target with associated destruction in the spleen.

1. Gaucher Disease

Gaucher disease is an autosomal recessive disorder characterized by a deficiency in beta-glucosidase, a lysosomal enzyme that degrades the sphingolipid glucocerebroside. There is an increased incidence of this disorder in Ashkenazi Jews. Three types of this disease exist, and the one amenable to splenectomy is type I, or the adult type. Pathologically, Gaucher disease results in lipid accumulation within the white pulp of the spleen, the liver, or the bone marrow. Predominant symptoms relate to massive splenomegaly from either the direct effects of the size of the spleen or secondary to cytopenias from hypersplenism.

▶ Treatment & Prognosis

Because the metabolic defect in this disease is in production of glucocerebrosidase, the modern first-line treatment is with enzyme replacement therapy. Splenectomy can be reserved for refractory cases with life-threatening thrombocytopenia. In the past, treatment with partial or subtotal splenectomy has been performed in both adults and children with Gaucher disease. However, it was associated with severe complications and incomplete disease treatment. This has largely been abandoned given the success of enzyme replacement therapy.

2. Wiskott-Aldrich Syndrome

Wiskott-Aldrich syndrome is an X-linked disease characterized by thrombocytopenia, combined B- and T-cell immunodeficiency, eczema, and a propensity to develop malignancies (eg, lymphomas, leukemias). Thrombocytopenia is the major feature of this rare disorder, with most patients presenting with bloody diarrhea, epistaxis, and petechiae at a young age. Platelet counts typically range between 20,000/μL and 40,000/μL, and the platelets that are present are between one-fourth and one-half of normal size. The spleen sequesters and destroys platelets in this disease, releasing "microplatelets" back into the circulation. The genetic defect in this disorder may be related to an abnormal adhesion molecule affecting immune as well as platelet cell-to-cell interaction.

▶ Treatment & Prognosis

Typical first-line treatment of Wiskott-Aldrich syndrome includes prophylactic antibiotics to prevent opportunistic infections as well as intravenous (IV) Ig. Additional therapies include interleukin-2 (IL-2) therapy and rituximab, depending on the disease severity. Splenectomy can be considered in patients with severe thrombocytopenia; however, this requires lifelong antibiotic prophylaxis. The optimal treatment for Wiskott-Aldrich syndrome is an human leukocyte antigen–matched bone marrow transplantation, which can be curative in well-matched patients.

3. Chédiak-Higashi Syndrome

Chédiak-Higashi syndrome is a rare autosomal recessive disease characterized by immunodeficiency that increases the susceptibility to bacterial and viral infections and is manifested by recurrent fever, nystagmus, and photophobia. Most patients experience widespread infiltration of tissues with histiocytes similar to a lymphoma. Secondary hepatosplenomegaly with lymphadenopathy, leukopenia, and bleeding complications occur in the accelerated phase of Chédiak-Higashi syndrome. Standard treatment includes chemotherapy, steroids, and ascorbic acid, but these patients have a poor prognosis. Splenectomy has been used in the accelerated phase with beneficial results.

4. Sarcoidosis

Sarcoidosis is a granulomatous disease of unknown origin that can involve virtually any organ or area of the body.

Pulmonary disease is most common, but autopsy studies have shown that the spleen is the second most common site, with enlargement by noncaseating granulomas in 50%-60% of patients. However, most patients do not have massive splenomegaly. When this does occur, patients can have significant cytopenias related to hypersplenism as well as the constitutional symptoms and hypercalcemia of sarcoidosis. In this subgroup of patients, splenectomy is indicated as a potential curative procedure for each of these symptoms.

ERYTHROCYTE DISORDERS

In this category of diseases, there is generally no intrinsic abnormality of the spleen, as opposed to hypersplenism, in which the spleen is primarily infiltrated by neoplasia or storage products and causes cytopenias due to increased volume of splenic tissue. In the autoimmune disorders, there is a humoral antibody response against proteins on circulating blood cells, resulting in depletion primarily within the spleen. Disorders involving platelets, erythrocytes, and neutrophils are listed in decreasing order of incidence. Erythrocyte disorders are genetic defects in structural components or hemoglobin that increase the clearance of red cells in the spleen, causing a significant decrease in erythrocyte half-life.

1. Hereditary Spherocytosis

ESSENTIALS OF DIAGNOSIS

▶ Malaise, abdominal discomfort

▶ Jaundice, anemia, splenomegaly

▶ Spherocytosis, increased osmotic fragility of red cells, negative Coombs test

▶ General Considerations

Hereditary spherocytosis (congenital hemolytic jaundice, familial hemolytic anemia), the most common congenital hemolytic anemia (affecting 1 in 5000 individuals), is transmitted as an autosomal dominant trait. It is caused by a variety of genetic defects related to abnormal cellular structural proteins, primarily ankyrin, band 3, alpha and beta spectrin, and protein 4.2. All of the mutations result in an alteration in binding the cytoskeleton to the cellular membrane, causing a decreased cellular plasticity with membrane loss. The normal shape of the erythrocyte is changed from a biconcave disk into a sphere, and the decreased membrane–to–cell volume ratio causes a lack of deformability that delays passage through the channels of the splenic red pulp. Significant cell destruction occurs only in the presence of the spleen. Hemolysis is largely relieved by splenectomy.

The condition is most common in people of northern European descent because of higher gene frequency in this population. When discovered early in infancy, it may resemble hemolytic disease of the newborn due to ABO incompatibility. Occasionally, the diagnosis is not made until later in adult life, but it is usually discovered in the first three decades.

Clinical Findings

A. Symptoms and Signs

The principal manifestations are splenomegaly, mild to moderate anemia, and jaundice. The patient may complain of easy fatigability. The spleen is almost always enlarged and may cause fullness and discomfort in the left upper quadrant. However, most patients are diagnosed during a family survey at a time when they are asymptomatic.

Periodic exacerbations of hemolysis can occur. The rare hypoplastic crises, which often follow acute viral illnesses, may be associated with profound anemia, headache, nausea, abdominal pain, pancytopenia, and hypoactive marrow.

B. Laboratory Findings

The red cell count and hemoglobin are moderately reduced. Some of the asymptomatic patients detected by family surveys have normal red cell counts when first seen. The red cells are usually normocytic, but microcytosis may occur. Macrocytosis may present during periods of marked reticulocytosis. Spherocytes in varying numbers, sizes, and shapes are seen on a Wright-stained smear. The reticulocyte count is increased to 5%-20%.

The indirect serum bilirubin and stool urobilinogen are usually elevated, and serum haptoglobin is usually decreased to absent. The Coombs test is negative, which rules out autoimmune hemolytic anemia. Infusion of the patient's own blood labeled with chromium-51 (^{51}Cr) shows a greatly shortened red cell life span and sequestration in the spleen. Normal red cells labeled with ^{51}Cr have a normal life span when transfused into a spherocytic patient, indicating that splenic function is normal.

Differential Diagnosis

At present, there is no pathognomonic test for hereditary spherocytosis. Spherocytes in large numbers may occur in autoimmune hemolytic anemias, in which osmotic fragility and autohemolysis may be increased but are usually not improved by incubation with glucose. A positive Coombs test, negative family history, and sharply reduced survival of normal donor red cells are diagnostic of autoimmune hemolysis. Spherocytes are also seen in hemoglobin C disease, in some alcoholics, and in some severe burns.

Complications

Pigment gallstones occur in about 85% of adults with spherocytosis but are uncommon under age 10. However, gallstones in a child should suggest congenital spherocytosis.

Chronic leg ulcers unrelated to varicosities are a rare complication but, when present, will heal only after the spleen is removed.

Treatment

Initial treatments consists of transfusions and erythropoietin for anemic patients. Splenectomy, however, is mainstay of treatment for patients with severe hereditary spherocytosis. At operation, the gallbladder should be inspected for stones, and accessory spleens should be sought. When there is associated cholelithiasis, cholecystectomy should be performed along with the splenectomy. Unless the clinical manifestations are severe, splenectomy should be delayed in children until age 6 to avoid the risk of increased infection due to loss of reticuloendothelial function. For children under age 5 with severe disease and high transfusion requirements, a partial (80%) splenectomy may correct symptoms while maintaining the normal immune functions of the spleen.

Prognosis

Splenectomy cures the anemia and jaundice in all patients. The membrane abnormality, spherocytosis, and increased osmotic fragility persist, but red cell life span becomes almost normal. An overlooked accessory spleen is an occasional cause of failure of splenectomy. The presence of Howell-Jolly bodies in red cells makes an accessory spleen unlikely because an accessory spleen would typically filter out red cells containing these DNA remnants.

Andolfo I, et al: New insights on hereditary erythrocyte membrane defects. *Haematologica*. 2016;101(11):1284-1294.

Gallagher PG: Abnormalities of the erythrocyte membrane. *Pediatr Clin North Am*. 2013;60(6):1349-1362.

Perrotta S: Hereditary spherocytosis. *Lancet*. 2008;372:1411-1426.

2. Hereditary Elliptocytosis

This autosomal dominant genetic disorder, also known as ovalocytosis, is usually of little clinical significance. Normally, up to 15% oval or elliptic red blood cells can be seen on a peripheral blood smear. In elliptocytosis, at least 25% and up to 90% of circulating erythrocytes are elliptic. As with hereditary spherocytosis, this disease is due to a variety of genetic defects in cytoskeletal proteins such as spectrin. The predominant abnormality is that this structural protein exists as a dimer instead of a tetramer, leading to change in the erythrocyte's shape, decreased plasticity, and a shortened life span of the cell.

Most affected individuals are asymptomatic; about 10% have clinical manifestations consisting of moderate anemia, slight jaundice, and a palpable spleen.

Symptomatic patients should have splenectomy and cholecystectomy if gallstones are present. The red cell defect persists after splenectomy, but the hemolysis and anemia are cured.

Gallagher PG: Abnormalities of the erythrocyte membrane. *Pediatr Clin North Am.* 2013;60(6):1349-1362.

3. Hereditary Nonspherocytic Hemolytic Anemia

This is a heterogeneous group of rare hemolytic anemias caused by inherited intrinsic red cell defects that lead to oxidative hemolysis. Included in the group are pyruvate kinase deficiency and glucose 6-phosphate dehydrogenase (G6PD) deficiency. They are usually manifested in early childhood with anemia, jaundice, reticulocytosis, erythroid hyperplasia of the marrow, and normal osmotic fragility. As with other hemolytic anemias, there may be associated cholelithiasis.

Multiple blood transfusions are often required. Splenectomy, although not curative, may ameliorate some of these conditions, especially pyruvate kinase deficiency. In G6PD deficiency, splenectomy is not beneficial, and treatment consists of avoidance of dietary oxidants such as fava beans.

4. Thalassemia Major (Mediterranean Anemia; Cooley Anemia)

In the most common form of this autosomal dominant disorder, a structural defect in the β-globin chain causes excess α chains to precipitate on the inner surface of the membrane of the erythrocyte and produces abnormal red cells (eg, target cells). Heterozygotes usually have mild anemia (thalassemia minor); however, starting early in infancy, homozygotes have severe chronic anemia accompanied by jaundice, hepatosplenomegaly (often massive), retarded body growth, and enlargement of the head. The peripheral blood smear reveals target cells, nucleated red cells, and a hypochromic microcytic anemia. Gallstones are present in about 25% of patients. A characteristic feature is the persistence of fetal hemoglobin.

Because the anemia of thalassemia is due to both increased destruction of red cells and decreased hemoglobin production, splenectomy does not cure the anemia, as in spherocytosis, but it may reduce transfusion requirements by removing an enlarged, uncomfortable spleen. Treatment is by iron chelation and transfusion.

AUTOIMMUNE DISORDERS

The production of IgG autoantibodies specific for cell membrane proteins on erythrocytes causes autoimmune hemolytic anemia; on platelets, it causes ITP and may cause neutropenia in Felty syndrome. Macrophages express Fc receptors for IgG, and antibody-coated cells that pass through the splenic sinuses of the red pulp come into contact with these phagocytic cells. Furthermore, the microenvironment of the red pulp with slow flow of blood with a high cellular content through circuitous spaces facilitates opsonization of cells in the spleen. Production of autoantibodies in the white pulp germinal centers may also enhance cellular destruction, particularly in ITP. Understanding this pathophysiologic mechanism is important because autoimmune hemolytic anemia caused by IgM autoantibodies (ie, cold agglutinin hemolytic anemia) does not respond to splenectomy because macrophages do not have Fc receptors for IgM. This mechanism also explains why treatment with high-dose intravenous immune globulin is beneficial in these diseases because it blocks the macrophage Fc receptor.

1. Acquired Hemolytic Anemia

ESSENTIALS OF DIAGNOSIS

▶ Fatigue, pallor, jaundice

▶ Splenomegaly

▶ Persistent anemia and reticulocytosis

▶ General Considerations

The **autoimmune hemolytic anemias** have also been classified according to the optimal temperature at which autoantibodies react with the red cell surface (warm or cold antibodies). This classification is particularly useful because patients with cold antibodies will not benefit from splenectomy but those with warm antibodies may.

Although hemolysis without demonstrable antibody (Coombs test negative) may occur in uremia, cirrhosis of the liver, cancer, and certain infections, in most cases, the red cell membranes are coated with either Ig or complement (Coombs test positive). The antibody in IgG autoimmune hemolytic anemia is specifically directed against the Rh locus on the erythrocyte. Initiation of this disease is either idiopathic (40%-50%) or secondary to drug exposure, connective tissue disorders, or lymphoproliferative disorders. Hemolytic anemia due to cold antibodies is less common and always a secondary immune response. Cold agglutinin hemolytic anemia is due typically to IgM directed against polysaccharide antigens on the red cell, and hemolysis occurs intravascularly by complement fixation and not within the spleen, making splenectomy not beneficial in the setting of cold antibodies.

About 20% of cases of secondary immune hemolytic anemia are due to drug use, and hemolysis is usually mediated by warm antibodies. Penicillin, quinidine, hydralazine, and

Table 29–3. Disorders associated with immune hemolysis.

Immune drug reaction (penicillin, quinidine, hydralazine, methyldopa, cimetidine)
Collagen vascular disease (lupus erythematosus, rheumatoid arthritis)
Tumors (lymphoma, myeloma, leukemia, dermoid cysts, ovarian teratoma)
Infection (*Mycoplasma*, malaria, syphilis, viremia)

methyldopa have been most commonly implicated drugs in this syndrome (Table 29–3).

Clinical Findings

A. Symptoms and Signs

Autoimmune hemolytic anemia may be encountered at any age but is most common after age 50; it occurs twice as often in women. The onset is usually acute, consisting of anemia, mild jaundice, and sometimes fever. The spleen is palpably enlarged in over 50% of patients, and pigment gallstones are present in about 25%. Rarely, a sudden severe onset produces hemoglobinuria, renal tubular necrosis, and a 40%-50% death rate.

B. Laboratory Findings

Hemolytic anemia is diagnosed by demonstrating a normocytic normochromic anemia, reticulocytosis (> 10%), erythroid hyperplasia of the marrow, and elevation of serum indirect bilirubin. Stool urobilinogen may be greatly increased, but there is no bile in the urine. Serum haptoglobin is usually low or absent. The direct Coombs test is positive because the red cells are coated with Ig or complement (or both).

Treatment

Associated diseases must be carefully sought and appropriately treated. For drug-induced secondary hemolytic anemia, further exposure to the offending agent must be terminated. Corticosteroids produce a remission in about 75% of patients, but only 25% of remissions are permanent. Transfusion should be avoided if possible, because cross-matching may be extremely difficult, requiring washed red cells and saline-active antisera. Rituximab is an effective second-line therapy now producing durable responses in 40% of steroid-resistant cases.

Splenectomy is indicated for patients with warm-antibody hemolysis who fail to respond to 4-6 weeks of high-dose corticosteroid therapy, for patients who relapse after an initial response when steroids are withdrawn, and for patients in whom steroid therapy is contraindicated (eg, those with active pulmonary tuberculosis). Patients who require chronic high-dose steroid therapy should also be considered for splenectomy, because the risks of long-term steroid administration are substantial.

Splenectomy is effective because it removes the principal site of red cell destruction. Occasionally, splenectomy identifies the presence of an underlying disorder such as lymphoma. About half of patients who fail to respond to splenectomy will respond to azathioprine or cyclophosphamide. Plasmapheresis has been employed as salvage therapy in patients with refractory hemolytic anemia.

Prognosis

Relapses may occur after splenectomy but are less frequent if the initial response was good. The ultimate prognosis in the secondary cases depends on the underlying disorder.

Liebman HA, et al: Autoimmune hemolytic anemia. *Med Clin North Am.* 2017;101(2):351-359.

Packman CH, et al: Hemolytic anemia due to warm autoantibodies. *Blood Rev.* 2008;22:17-31.

Valent P, et al: Diagnosis and treatment of autoimmune haemolytic aneaemias in adults: a clinical review. *Wien Klin Wochenschr.* 2008; 120:136-151.

2. Immune Thrombocytopenic Purpura (Idiopathic Thrombocytopenic Purpura)

ESSENTIALS OF DIAGNOSIS

- Petechiae, ecchymoses, epistaxis, easy bruising
- No splenomegaly
- Decreased platelet count, prolonged bleeding time, poor clot retraction, normal coagulation time

General Considerations

ITP is a hemorrhagic syndrome with diverse causes that can occur in an acute or chronic form and is characterized by marked reduction in the number of circulating platelets, abundant megakaryocytes in the bone marrow, and a shortened platelet life span. It may be idiopathic or secondary to a lymphoproliferative disorder, drugs or toxins, bacterial or viral infection (especially in children), systemic lupus erythematosus, or other conditions. Although responses to corticosteroids and to splenectomy in these patients are comparable to the responses observed in other patients with ITP, splenectomy should be reserved for those with signs of blood loss because surgical complications are high and survival may be short. However, due to the incidence of ITP, this disease is typically the most common indication for splenectomy in most institutional series.

The pathogenesis of both primary and secondary disorders involves a circulating antiplatelet IgG autoantibody usually directed against a membrane protein, which is the fibrinogen receptor (glycoprotein IIb/IIIa). In this disorder, the spleen is primarily the site of platelet destruction and may also be a significant source of autoantibody production. Splenomegaly, present in only 2% of cases, is usually a manifestation of another underlying disease such as lymphoma or lupus erythematosus. Five percent to 15% of HIV-positive patients have thrombocytopenia independent of the immunologic state of their disease that is clinically indistinguishable from typical chronic ITP. The precise pathophysiologic mechanism in relation to HIV infection is not known, and some authors advocate for HIV testing in all patients who develop ITP.

► Clinical Findings

A. Symptoms and Signs

The onset may be acute, with ecchymoses or showers of petechiae, and may be accompanied by bleeding gums, vaginal bleeding, gastrointestinal bleeding, and hematuria. Central nervous system bleeding occurs in 3% of patients. The acute form is most common in children, usually occurring before 8 years of age, and often begins 1-3 weeks after a viral upper respiratory illness.

The chronic form, which may start at any age, is more common in women. It characteristically has an insidious onset, often with a long history of easy bruisability and menorrhagia. Showers of petechiae may occur, especially over pressure areas. Cyclic remissions and exacerbations may continue for several years.

B. Laboratory Findings

The platelet count is moderately to severely decreased (always < 100,000/μL), and platelets may be absent from the peripheral blood smear. Although white and red cell counts are usually normal, iron deficiency anemia may be present as a result of bleeding. The bone marrow shows increased numbers of large megakaryocytes without platelet budding.

The bleeding time is prolonged, capillary fragility (Rumpel-Leede test) is greatly increased, and clot retraction becomes poor. Partial thromboplastin time, prothrombin time, and coagulation time are normal. Specific determinations of antiplatelet antibody titers can now be routinely assessed to aid in diagnosis. Reduced red cell or platelet survival can be measured by labeling the patient's cells with ^{51}Cr or the platelets with indium-111 and measuring the rate of disappearance of radioactivity from the blood. The spleen's role in producing the anemia or thrombocytopenia can be determined by measuring the ratio of radioactivity that accumulates in the liver and spleen during destruction of the tagged cells; a spleen-to-liver ratio greater than 2:1 indicates significant splenic pooling and suggests that splenectomy would be beneficial.

► Differential Diagnosis

Other causes of nonimmunologic thrombocytopenia must be ruled out, such as leukemia, aplastic anemia, and macroglobulinemia. Thrombocytopenia and purpura may be caused by ineffective thrombocytopoiesis (eg, pernicious anemia, preleukemic states) or by nonimmune platelet destruction (eg, septicemia, disseminated intravascular coagulation, or other causes of hypersplenism).

► Treatment

Treatment of ITP depends on the age of the patient, the severity of the disease, the duration of the thrombocytopenia, and the clinical variant. Secondary immune thrombocytopenias are best managed by treating the underlying primary disorder (eg, if it is drug induced, the drug should be stopped).

Patients with mild or no symptoms need no specific therapy but should avoid contact sports, elective surgery, and all unessential medications. Corticosteroids are indicated in patients with moderate to severe purpura of short duration. Usually, 60 mg of prednisone (or equivalent) is required daily; this is continued until the platelet count returns to normal and then is gradually tapered after 4-6 weeks. Corticosteroids produce a response in 70%-80% of patients, but sustained remissions occur in only 20% of adults. Second-line therapy with rituximab improves platelet counts in 30%-40% of patients and sustained complete response in 10%-20% of patients. Newer thrombopoietin receptor agonists, such as romiplostim and eltrombopag, are being studied in clinical trials for patients who are refractory to other standard treatments.

Splenectomy is the most effective form of therapy and is indicated for patients who do not respond to corticosteroids, for those who relapse after an initial remission on steroids, and for steroid-dependent patients. Corticosteroid therapy is not necessary in the immediate preoperative period unless bleeding is severe or the patient was receiving steroids before the operation. If indicated, platelet transfusions are given intraoperatively only after ligation of the splenic artery or removal of the spleen, because platelets from earlier transfusion would be rapidly sequestered in the spleen. For temporary treatment of the thrombocytopenia, intravenous Ig is effective.

Splenectomy produces a sustained remission in about 68% of patients. As with corticosteroids, success rates are better with acute than chronic ITP. Two factors associated with better outcomes are shorter duration of disease and younger age. The platelet count usually rises promptly following splenectomy (eg, it may double in 24 hours) and reaches a peak after 1-2 weeks. If the platelet count remains elevated after 2 months, the patient can be considered cured. When corticosteroids and splenectomy have failed, immunosuppressive drugs (azathioprine, vincristine) will achieve a remission in 25% of cases.

The benefit of splenectomy for HIV-associated ITP has been less clear. The risk of infection and the overall shortened survival in this population argue against splenectomy. However, in HIV patients without AIDS, clinically significant thrombocytopenia responds completely in 70%, and there is partial improvement in 20% of patients following splenectomy. Splenectomy does not appear to alter the overall natural history of HIV infection.

▶ Prognosis

Acute ITP in children under age 16 has an excellent prognosis; approximately 80% of patients have a complete and permanent spontaneous remission. This occurs rarely in adults. Splenectomy is successful in about 80% of patients, but more often in idiopathic cases than in those secondary to another disorder. The proportion of patients undergoing splenectomy for ITP has decreased due to medical treatments other than steroids that have efficacy, although the incidence of chronic ITP has increased. Agents that stimulate thrombopoietin may have significant benefit for patients who have no improvement in platelet count after splenectomy.

Auger S, et al: Rituximab before splenectomy in adults with primary idiopathic thrombocytopenic purpura: a meta-analysis. *Br J Haematol.* 2012;158(3):386-398.

Dolan JP, et al: Splenectomy for immune thrombocytopenic purpura. *Am J Hematol.* 2008;83:93-96.

Kuter DJ, et al: Efficacy of romiplostim in patients with chronic immune thrombocytopenic purpura: a double-blind randomized controlled trial. *Lancet.* 2008;371:395-403.

Newland W, et al: Emerging strategies to treat chronic immune thrombocytopenic purpura. *Eur J Haematol.* 2008;69:27-33.

Rodeghiero F, et al: First-line therapies for immune thrombocytopenic purpura: re-evaluating the need to treat. *Eur J Haematol.* 2008;69:19-26.

Shojaiefard A, et al: Prediction of response to splenectomy in patients with idiopathic thrombocytopenic purpura. *World J Surg.* 2008;32:488-493.

Stasi R, et al: Idiopathic thrombocytopenic purpura: current concepts in pathophysiology and management. *Thromb Haemost.* 2008;99:4-13.

Wang L, et al: Efficacy and safety of thrombopoietin receptor agonists in patients with primary immune thrombocytopenia: a systematic review and meta-analysis. *Sci Rep.* 2016;19:6.

3. Felty Syndrome

Approximately 1% of patients with rheumatoid arthritis have splenomegaly and neutropenia, a triad known as Felty syndrome. High levels of IgG have been identified on the surface of neutrophils with evidence of increased granulopoiesis in the bone marrow. Pathologic analysis of the spleen in Felty syndrome patients shows a larger proportionate increase in the white pulp as opposed to most conditions of splenomegaly. There is evidence of excess accumulation of neutrophils in both the T-cell zone of the white pulp as well as the cord and sinuses of the red pulp.

Patients with severe neutropenia have clinical symptoms of recurring infections in Felty syndrome. Symptomatic patients who have evidence of IgG on the surface of neutrophils should be considered for splenectomy. Neutropenia will improve in 60%-70% of these patients, but relapse of neutropenia as well as recurrent infections in the presence of normal neutrophil counts may occur, and these untoward events have dampened enthusiasm for splenectomy in this disease.

4. Thrombotic Thrombocytopenic Purpura

Thrombotic thrombocytopenic purpura (TTP) is a rare disease with a pentad of clinical features: (1) fever, (2) thrombocytopenic purpura, (3) hemolytic anemia, (4) neurologic manifestations, and (5) renal failure. The cause is unknown, but autoimmunity to endothelial cells or a primary platelet defect has been implicated, and its occurrence in patients with AIDS has been reported. It is most common between ages 10 and 40 years.

The thrombocytopenia is probably due to a shortened platelet life span. The microangiopathic hemolytic anemia is produced by passage of red cells over damaged small blood vessels containing fibrin strands. Rigid red cells are trapped and fragmented in the spleen, whereas those that escape the spleen may be more vulnerable to damage and destruction in the abnormal microvasculature. The anemia is often severe, and it may be aggravated by hemorrhage secondary to thrombocytopenia. Hepatomegaly and splenomegaly occur in 35% of cases.

▶ Treatment & Prognosis

Until recently, there was no effective therapy for this disorder, and mortality rates as high as 95% were reported. Most patients died of renal failure or cerebral bleeding. Plasmapheresis with plasma exchange is the first-line therapy, with a complete response rate of 55% to 65%. Rituximab and glucocorticoids are often added to plasma exchange. Plasma exchange failure can be salvaged with splenectomy, with 60% of patients having a substantial response and a 20%-30% relapse rate.

VASCULAR DISORDERS OF THE SPLEEN

Vascular disease of the spleen treated by splenectomy can occur both with the arterial inflow and the venous outflow. The most common disease is splenic vein thrombosis; this can be treated in a straightforward manner by splenectomy. Splenic artery aneurysms are one of the most common sites of visceral aneurysms and may require splenectomy (discussed in Chapter 34).

1. Splenic Vein Thrombosis

▶ Etiology

Thrombosis of the splenic vein can occur as an isolated event not due to any pathologic findings in the spleen but due to diseases that impact on the splenic vein as it travels along the superior border of the pancreas. The most common cause is acute or chronic pancreatitis or a pseudocyst of the body/tail of the pancreas, with the general inflammatory reaction in the pancreas resulting in thrombosis of the splenic vein in 20% of patients. Inflammation from a posterior gastric ulcer is another cause. Direct extension of carcinoma of the pancreas or stomach into the lesser sac may cause splenic vein thrombosis, but the diagnosis is generally not subtle because of other manifestations of these malignancies. Idiopathic retroperitoneal fibrosis may be an alternative cause of splenic vein thrombosis.

Splenic vein thrombosis presents as upper gastrointestinal hemorrhage due to isolated gastric varices. With occlusion of the splenic vein, outflow of blood from the spleen is diverted into the short gastric veins as the remaining collateral vessels. These veins dilate and become varices primarily in the fundus of the stomach, resulting in bleeding in 15%-20% of patients.

▶ Diagnosis

Splenic vein thrombosis is suspected when there are isolated varices of the stomach, particularly in the proximal greater curvature without any esophageal varices. Because there is no portal hypertension, there are no associated signs or symptoms of cirrhosis. Definitive diagnosis is made by confirming that there is no blood flow in the main splenic vein. Invasive venography is no longer needed because this diagnosis can be confirmed by CT scan or magnetic resonance imaging (MRI) scans with contrast material or by high-resolution ultrasound. CT or MRI is preferred because the splenic vein may be hidden from ultrasound by bowel gas and CT or MRI allows characterization of the surrounding structures (pancreas, stomach) to assess for causative pathology.

▶ Treatment & Prognosis

Splenectomy is curative in patients with splenic vein thrombosis. All of the symptoms relate to increased splenic blood flow through collateral vessels; eliminating that blood flow is curative. If a splenic vein thrombosis is diagnosed—even if the patients have not had an episode of upper gastrointestinal hemorrhage—an elective or prophylactic splenectomy is indicated if the patients are otherwise healthy. In patients with portal vein thrombosis, the magnitude of the disease and associated problems is greatly amplified, and splenectomy is almost never indicated because it is not curative.

Agarwal AK, et al: Significance of splenic vein thrombosis in chronic pancreatitis. *Am J Surg.* 2008;196:149-154.

Ruiz-Tovar J, et al: Portal vein thrombosis after splenic and pancreatic surgery. *Adv Exp Med Biol.* 2017;906:241-251.

2. Cysts & Tumors of the Spleen

Parasitic cysts are almost always echinococcal (see Chapter 8). They may be asymptomatic, but usually the patient notices splenomegaly. Calcification of the cyst wall may be seen on x-ray. Eosinophilia may be found, and serologic tests may confirm the diagnosis. The treatment of choice is splenectomy.

Other cysts are dermoid, epidermoid, endothelial, and pseudocysts. The latter are thought to be late results of infarction or trauma. Splenectomy may be indicated to exclude tumor; however, partial splenectomy or observation has been advocated.

The rare primary tumors of the spleen include lymphoma, sarcoma, hemangioma, and hamartoma. Hamartomas may be confused grossly with splenic lymphoma at laparotomy. These lesions are usually asymptomatic until splenomegaly causes abdominal discomfort or a palpable mass. The benign vascular tumors of the spleen (angiomas) can produce hypersplenism. Spontaneous rupture with massive hemorrhage can occur. Splenectomy is indicated if the tumor appears to be limited to the spleen. Inflammatory pseudotumors are benign lesions composed of a mixture of inflammatory cells and a granulomatous reaction that can occur in a variety of organs, including the spleen. Constitutional symptoms of lethargy, weight loss, and fatigue occur and can be alleviated by splenectomy.

The spleen is a common site for metastases in advanced malignancies, especially for lung cancer, breast cancer, and melanoma. Splenic metastases are common autopsy findings but are rarely clinically significant.

INFECTIONS OF THE SPLEEN (SPLENIC ABSCESS)

Splenic abscesses are uncommon but are important because the death rate ranges between 40% and 100%. They may be caused by hematogenous seeding of the spleen with bacteria from remote sepsis such as endocarditis, by direct spread of infection from adjacent structures, or by splenic trauma resulting in a secondarily infected splenic hematoma. Splenic abscess is a complication of intravenous drug abuse. In 80% of cases, one or more abscesses exist in organs other than the spleen, and the splenic abscess develops as a terminal manifestation of uncontrolled sepsis in other organs. Enteric organisms are found in over two-thirds of splenic abscesses, with staphylococci and nonenteric streptococci comprising the majority of the remainder. In some patients, unexplained sepsis, progressive splenic enlargement, and abdominal pain are the presenting manifestations. The spleen may not be palpable, because of left upper quadrant tenderness and guarding. A left pleural effusion combined with unexplained leukocytosis in a septic patient suggests a splenic abscess. The finding of gas in the spleen on plain abdominal x-ray is pathognomonic of splenic abscess, but CT scan is the optimal way to define and diagnose a splenic abscess.

Most splenic abscesses remain localized, periodically seeding the bloodstream with bacteria, but spontaneous rupture and peritonitis may occur. Splenectomy is essential for cure if sepsis is localized to the spleen. Percutaneous drainage of large, solitary juxtacapsular abscesses may occasionally be feasible but is associated with an extremely high mortality rate and should be reserved for patients unable to withstand an operation.

DIAGNOSTIC SPLENECTOMY

One indication for splenectomy is for diagnosis in an otherwise asymptomatic patient. Splenectomy may be needed to make a diagnosis when an asymptomatic mass lesion is seen within the spleen on CT scan, ultrasound, or MRI scan for which a definitive diagnosis cannot be made radiographically. Another example is when a patient has either a palpable spleen on physical examination or an enlarged spleen by scan and otherwise has no clear diagnostic disorder.

▶ Splenic Mass Lesions

In patients who have an isolated splenic mass, 60% turn out to be malignant lesions and 40% turn out to be benign lesions. Most malignant lesions are lymphomas; the next most common lesions are metastatic carcinomas, including some in which the primary diagnosis had not been made previously. In patients with benign lesions, more than half are cysts, and splenic hamartomas and splenic hemangiomas can also be present.

In diagnosing an isolated splenic mass, most of these lesions can be diagnosed by doing a fine-needle aspiration biopsy. Certain lesions, such as the cystic lesions or hemangiomas, have a classic appearance on gadolinium-enhanced MRI scan, and these scans are another imaging modality that can be used to sort out mass lesions without tissue biopsy. Positron emission tomography (PET) scans will reliably identify high-grade lymphoma and metastatic tumors but may miss low-grade or mantle zone lymphoma. The risk of bleeding is significant in patients with hemangiomas. These benign tumors of endothelial cells can be definitively diagnosed with gadolinium-enhanced MRI, and this imaging test is optimal for characterizing an isolated splenic mass.

▶ Splenomegaly Without a Diagnosis

The second diagnostic indication for splenectomy is unexplained splenomegaly. Most of these enlarged spleens will be shown to have lymphoma. The minority will have benign diagnoses including benign lymphoid proliferation, benign vascular lesions, and granulomatous disease, as well as splenic infarction and hemorrhage. The role of the fine-needle aspiration and other percutaneous biopsies for nondiagnosed splenomegaly is quite limited with no distinct mass to biopsy; there would be very low yield in terms of being able to make that diagnosis by that form of biopsy.

▶ Staging Laparotomy for Hodgkin Disease

Historically, Hodgkin disease was staged with laparotomy and splenectomy. Discussion of this procedure is more of a historical note because it has limited use in today's current practice in treating this form of lymphoma.

A standard practice for pathologic staging between 1960 and 1990 was the performance of a staging laparotomy in most patients with Hodgkin disease. The reason for performing this invasive procedure was based on reports that laparotomy altered the clinical stage of disease in approximately 35% of patients. There are several reasons why the incidence of performing staging laparotomy has decreased over the past 10-15 years. The primary reason is that it does not alter treatment of Hodgkin disease based on results of recent clinical series. Because systemic chemotherapy treats the whole patient, accurate pathologic staging has no impact on the treatment outcome or treatment decisions.

▶ Iatrogenic Splenectomy

Procedures in which mobilization of the left upper quadrant is done (eg, reflection of the spleen and pancreas medially to expose retroperitoneal tissue, left adrenalectomy, and left nephrectomy) put the spleen at risk for injury during the dissection. Simple mobilization of the splenic flexure of the colon can lead to bleeding from the inferior pole of the spleen that may be difficult to control. The ligaments that go directly from the omentum to the capsule of the spleen may be the most common location of iatrogenic splenic trauma, because it is a common practice to aggressively retract the omentum as needed for exposure. If there are direct branches that sometimes may be sizable from the omentum to the splenic capsule, this could lead to capsular disruption and troublesome bleeding. A national database on antireflux procedures including 86,411 patients reported an incidence of iatrogenic splenectomy of 2.3%, which translates to 1987 iatrogenic splenectomies for that indication alone over a 6-year period. An outcome study for colon cancer of 42,000 patients reported iatrogenic splenectomy in less than 1% of all patients but 6% of colon cancers at the splenic flexure. Splenectomy resulted in a significant increase in length of stay and a 40% increase in morbidity. Splenectomy has also been reported for splenic trauma following elective colonoscopy, presumably from navigating the colonoscope around the splenic flexure.

Iatrogenic splenectomy is likely an underreported event because the precise reason for splenectomy is not always captured (eg, bleeding, tumor invasion of the spleen or vasculature). There are also probably several-fold more minor or moderate injuries to the spleen during unrelated operations in which the spleen was not removed but was repaired or salvaged. Just as in trauma to the spleen, the techniques of splenorrhaphy can be employed to preserve the spleen. Many techniques of splenorrhaphy have been reported (polyglactin absorbable mesh wrap, suture repair, omental flap, hemostatic glue/foam). For minor capsular disruption, the use of the argon beam coagulator for surface cautery is a helpful technique.

The primary teaching point regarding iatrogenic injuries is that the best way to preserve the spleen is to not damage it in the first place. This requires caution in mobilizing tissue in and around the spleen as well as visual inspection of the attachments of the spleen prior to blunt mobilization. Whenever possible, the spleen should be attempted to be preserved to decrease the risk of postsplenectomy sepsis.

Berg RJ, et al: The contemporary management of penetrating splenic injury. *Injury.* 2014;45(9):1394-1400.

Masoomi H, et al: Predictive factors of splenic injury in colorectal surgery: data from the Nationwide Inpatient Sample, 2006-2008. *Arch Surg.* 2012;147(4):324-329.

INCIDENTAL SPLENECTOMY

In a recent large series evaluating reasons for splenectomy from tertiary institutions, the single most common indication for splenectomy was as an incidental procedure in operations on an adjacent organ. In these situations, the spleen needs to be removed either for completeness of resection or because of division of the splenic vasculature. The actual primary treatments of those various disease entities in adjacent organs are subjects of multiple other chapters within this textbook, but a few comments need to be made regarding the reasons for splenectomy and whether splenic preservation procedures are possible.

One common indication for an incidental splenectomy is to remove tumors located in the distal pancreas. For decades, it was standard practice to remove the spleen when removing the body and tail of the pancreas because the splenic vein is intimately associated with the distal pancreas. Because of the interest in splenic preservation due to the incidence of postsplenectomy infection, operations have been developed to remove the distal pancreas without removing the spleen. The more technically challenging operation is a distal pancreatectomy with preservation of the splenic artery and vein. A second spleen-preserving distal pancreatectomy involves ligation of the splenic artery and vein but preservation of short gastric vessels and utilizing those vessels as collateral inflow and outflow to maintain splenic viability. Removal of the distal

pancreas with splenic preservation has also been reported as a laparoscopic and robotic procedure. For patients with tumors that mandate removal of the lymph nodes of the splenic hilum or with direct association of the tumor with splenic parenchyma, certainly it is more appropriate to do an operation based on neoplastic principles and perform a distal pancreatectomy/splenectomy. In other indications, if the anatomy is appropriate and the completeness of tumor resection is not compromised, splenic preservation is certainly possible.

Additional procedures in which it is common to perform a splenectomy include proximal gastric cancers. The importance of complete nodal dissection in long-term results in gastric resections has been debated for several decades. Level X lymph nodes are located in the splenic hilum, and for 20%-25% of proximal gastric cancers, these nodes will have metastatic cancer mandating removal. A randomized trial showed increased morbidity with a splenectomy and a marginal improvement in survival. Other tumors of the left upper quadrant and retroperitoneum may require splenectomy, including large renal cell carcinomas, left adrenal tumors, and retroperitoneal sarcomas that may infiltrate upward into the spleen. Although the asplenic state does make patients susceptible to infections, the spleen should be viewed as an expendable organ, if necessary, to accomplish complete resection of malignancies, and there should be no hesitation to remove the spleen in these situations to perform an appropriate cancer operation.

SPLENOSIS (SPLENIC AUTOTRANSPLANTATION)

In splenosis, multiple small implants of splenic tissue grow in scattered areas on the peritoneal surfaces throughout the abdomen. They arise from dissemination and autotransplantation of splenic fragments following traumatic rupture of the spleen. Splenic implants or intentional autotransplants are capable of cell culling, and some immunologic function appears to be exhibited in cases of intentional autotransplantation. Aggressive attempts at surgical excision are not warranted. Splenosis is usually an incidental finding discovered much later during laparotomy for an unrelated problem. However, the implants stimulate formation of adhesions and may be a cause of intestinal obstruction. They must be distinguished from peritoneal nodules of metastatic carcinoma and from accessory spleens. Histologically, they differ from accessory spleens by the absence of elastic or smooth muscle fibers in the delicate capsule.

▼ SPLENECTOMY

Preoperative preparation of patients undergoing elective splenectomy should correct coagulation abnormalities and deficits in red cell mass, treat infections, and control immune reactions. Because platelets are removed so rapidly from the circulation, they usually are not given for thrombocytopenia until after the splenic artery has been ligated. Antibodies in the patient's serum may complicate cross-matching of blood. Many patients with autoimmune disorders require corticosteroid coverage in the perioperative period. For emergency splenectomy, hypovolemia should be corrected by whole blood transfusions. For elective cases, prophylactic vaccination with a polyvalent pneumococcal vaccine that protects against a common encapsulated offending organism in postsplenectomy infection is recommended. Elective splenectomy is now most commonly performed as a laparoscopic or robotic procedure. This reduces the recovery period and is significantly better tolerated by most patients.

Details of surgical technique are not within the scope of this text, but it should be noted that there are two approaches to open splenectomy (Figure 29–4). In one, which is of value chiefly in traumatic rupture of the spleen, the organ is immediately mobilized and the splenic artery is secured from behind as it enters the hilum. In the other, which is of vital importance in the removal of massively enlarged spleens, the organ is left in situ. The gastrocolic ligament is opened, and the splenic artery is ligated as it courses along the upper edge of the pancreas. This permits blood to leave the spleen through the splenic vein while all other attachments (ie, the short gastric vessels and splenocolic attachments) are divided before the spleen is delivered. This method permits the removal of massively enlarged vascular spleens with practically no loss of blood.

Splenorrhaphy is operative repair of the spleen following trauma. The principles of splenorrhaphy are to debride the devitalized tissue and to attempt to approximate the normal contour of the spleen with capsular sutures or external wraps of material. Partial splenic resections may be performed for trauma or for disease states in which splenic debulking is indicated but may be unsuccessful with a higher immediate complication rate. Partial splenectomy for Gaucher disease, large cysts, or benign tumors has been reported using automatic stapling devices as well as microwave coagulators. However, for autoimmune disorders, it is absolutely essential for cure to remove the spleen completely, including excision of accessory spleens. There may be some benefit to obtaining a preoperative nuclear scan and intraoperative identification with a handheld gamma counter.

Massive splenomegaly is defined as a spleen with a weight greater than 1500 g or 8 to 10 times the normal size. Disease processes leading to massive splenomegaly include lymphoma, leukemia, and metabolic storage diseases. The morbidity and mortality rates of splenectomy for massive splenomegaly are increased primarily as a result of the risk of severe and rapid intraoperative blood loss. The operative approach in these cases is initial ligation of the splenic artery through the lesser sac at the superior border of the pancreas. Next, ligation of the short gastric vessels along the greater curvature all the way to the gastroesophageal junction is performed, allowing the stomach and left lobe of the liver to be retracted away from the spleen. Only after decreasing the splenic arterial inflow by the above maneuvers should

 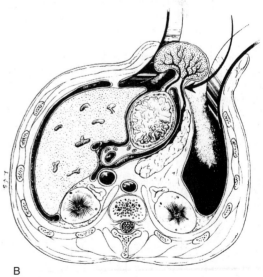

A   B

▲ **Figure 29–4.** **A:** Anterior approach to splenic artery. **B:** Mobilization of spleen with posterior exposure of splenic artery.

mobilization of the lateral and superior attachments be performed, leading to removal of the massive spleen.

Laparoscopic splenectomy is now the standard of care in most major centers with high volumes of splenic surgery. Virtually any indication for elective splenectomy qualifies for a laparoscopic approach, including patients with severe thrombocytopenia, patients with massive splenomegaly, patients needing partial splenectomy, and patients requiring removal of accessory spleens and the wandering spleen. Contraindications to laparoscopic splenectomy include portal hypertension and severe comorbid disease. With improved techniques, laparoscopic partial splenectomy has now been reported for focal mass lesions and hereditary hematologic diseases.

Laparoscopic splenectomy is performed typically using four ports. Midline ports for the cannula as well as for retraction of the stomach away from the splenic hilum are placed. Left subcostal ports are used as operating sites for dissection of the splenic hilum. An angled laparoscope is required for visualization of the superior and lateral attachments of the spleen. Vessels are divided with clips, sutures, or stapling devices. Precise exposure of the hilum with gentle upward traction on the spleen to stretch and expose the vessels is preferred to blind stapling of the hilum. Clinical conditions such as ITP and hereditary spherocytosis are the most common indications for laparoscopic splenectomy as the spleen is of normal size. A thorough search via the laparoscope for accessory spleens is important in these procedures for a successful outcome, and this may be facilitated by reviewing a preoperative CT scan.

HEMATOLOGIC EFFECTS OF SPLENECTOMY

Absence of the spleen in a normal adult usually has few clinical consequences. Red cell count and indices do not change, but red cells with cytoplasmic inclusions may appear (eg, Heinz bodies, Howell-Jolly bodies, and siderocytes). Granulocytosis occurs immediately after splenectomy but is replaced in several weeks by lymphocytosis and monocytosis. Platelets are usually increased, occasionally markedly so, and may stay at levels of 400,000-500,000/μL for over a year. Even more striking thrombocytosis (eg, 2-3 million/μL) may develop after splenectomy for hemolytic anemia. A platelet count of over a million is not an indication for anticoagulants, but antiplatelet agents such as aspirin may help prevent thrombosis.

Davies JM, et al; British Committee for Standards in Haematology: Review of guidelines for the prevention and treatment of infection in patients with an absent or dysfunctional spleen. *Br J Haematol.* 2011;155(3):308-317.

POSTSPLENECTOMY SEPSIS & OTHER POSTSPLENECTOMY PROBLEMS

Complications related to splenectomy per se are relatively few, with atelectasis, pancreatitis, and postoperative hemorrhage being the most common. If splenectomy is done for thrombocytopenia, secondary bleeding may occur even though the platelet count usually rises promptly. Platelet transfusions should be given if primary hemostasis is abnormal (ie, oozing occurs) and the platelet count remains low. Thromboembolic complications may be more common following splenectomy, but this complication does not correlate with the degree of thrombocytosis. The risk of portal vein thrombosis is 3%, and portal vein thrombosis occurs most commonly after splenectomy for massive spleens hemolytic anemia and not after trauma or splenectomy for thrombocytopenia. Symptoms include fever, abdominal pain, diarrhea, and abnormal liver function tests. Treatment consists of anticoagulation plus antibiotics.

Individuals are more susceptible to fulminant bacteremia after splenectomy, and bacteremia has been reported between 1 week and greater than 20 years after splenectomy. This is a result of the following changes that occur after splenectomy: (1) decreased clearance of bacteria from the blood, (2) decreased levels of IgM, and (3) decreased opsonic activity. The risk is greatest in young children, especially in the first 2 years after surgery (80% of cases) and when the disorder for which splenectomy was required was a disease of the reticuloendothelial system. In general, the younger the patient undergoing splenectomy and the more severe the underlying condition, the greater is the risk for developing overwhelming postsplenectomy infection. There is a low but significant risk of infection even in otherwise normal adults following splenectomy. Most of these infections occur after the first year, and nearly half occur more than 5 years after splenectomy. Lethal sepsis is very rare in adults. There is a distinct clinical syndrome: mild, nonspecific symptoms are followed by high fever and shock from sepsis, which may rapidly lead to death. *Streptococcus pneumoniae, Haemophilus influenzae,* and meningococci are the most common pathogens. Disseminated intravascular coagulation is a common complication. Awareness of this fatal complication has led to efforts to avoid splenectomy or to perform partial splenectomy or splenic repair for ruptured spleens (analogous to surgical management of liver trauma) to maintain adequate splenic function. Splenic autotransplantation may also achieve partial restoration of splenic function after splenectomy.

The risk of fatal sepsis is less after splenectomy for trauma than for hematologic disorders, probably due to splenic autotransplantation. Prophylactic vaccination against pneumococcal sepsis should be used in all surgically or functionally asplenic patients. Because splenic function may be important in the immune response to vaccine, early administration of polyvalent pneumococcal vaccine (Pneumovax) is advisable. The vaccine provides protection in adults and older children for 4-5 years, after which revaccination is advisable. Because the vaccine is only effective against about 80% of organisms, some authorities have recommended a 2-year course, treatment until age 16, or lifelong prophylaxis with penicillin following splenectomy. Others have advocated use of ampicillin to provide coverage for *H influenzae* as well as pneumococci. Antibiotic prophylaxis is essential in children under 2 years of age and should be continued until at least age 6. In general, splenectomy should be deferred until age 6 unless the hematologic problem is especially severe.

Davies JM, et al; British Committee for Standards in Haematology: Review of guidelines for the prevention and treatment of infection in patients with an absent or dysfunctional spleen. *Br J Haematol.* 2011;155(3):308-317.

Spelman D, et al: Guidelines for the prevention of sepsis in asplenic and hyposplenic patients. *Int Med J.* 2008;38:349-356.

MULTIPLE CHOICE QUESTIONS

1. Which of the following is true about the spleen?

   A. The red pulp of the spleen is normally a significant contributor to red blood cell hematopoiesis.
   B. The spleen's venous drainage is evenly divided between the splenic vein and direct branches of the left renal vein.
   C. The outer capsule of the spleen is a continuous sheet of smooth muscle.
   D. The gastrosplenic ligament carries the short gastric vessels.
   E. Normally, 80% of the platelet cell mass is sequestered in the spleen.

2. Indications for splenectomy can include

   A. Vascular disease
   B. Splenomegaly associated with infection
   C. Hereditary spherocytosis
   D. Both A and C
   E. A, B, and C

3. Postsplenectomy sepsis

   A. Only occurs within 1 year of operation
   B. Is at greatest risk in young children
   C. Is associated with residual accessory splenules
   D. Is more often lethal in adults than children
   E. Is more common after splenectomy for trauma than for other indications

Appendix

Sabrina E. Sanchez, MD, MPH

Peter A. Burke, MD

ANATOMY & PHYSIOLOGY

In infants, the appendix is a conical diverticulum at the apex of the cecum, but with differential growth and distention of the cecum, the appendix ultimately arises on the left and dorsally approximately 2.5 cm below the ileocecal valve. The taeniae of the colon converge at the base of the appendix, an arrangement that helps in locating this structure at operation. The appendix is freely mobile in the majority of adults and is fixed retrocecally in 16% of adults.

The appendix in children is characterized by a large concentration of lymphoid follicles that appear 2 weeks after birth and number about 200 or more at age 15. Thereafter, progressive atrophy of lymphoid tissue proceeds with fibrosis of the wall and partial or total obliteration of the lumen. If the appendix has a physiologic function, it is probably related to the presence of lymphoid follicles.

ACUTE APPENDICITIS

General Considerations

Approximately 7% of people in Western countries have appendicitis at some time during their lives. With more than 250,000 appendectomies for acute appendicitis performed annually in the United States, it is the most common surgical emergency encountered by the general surgeon and accounts for about 1% of all surgical operations.

Obstruction of the proximal lumen by fibrous bands, lymphoid hyperplasia, fecaliths, calculi, or parasites has long been considered to be the major cause of acute appendicitis. A fecalith or calculus is found in only 10% of acutely inflamed appendices. Although evidence of temporal and geographic clustering of cases has suggested a primary infectious etiology, this remains to be proven.

As appendicitis progresses, the blood supply is impaired by bacterial infection in the wall and distention of the lumen;

gangrene and perforation occur at about 24 hours, although the timing is highly variable. Gangrene implies microscopic perforation, bacterial contamination of the peritoneum, and peritonitis. This process may be effectively localized by adhesions from nearby viscera.

Clinical Findings

Acute appendicitis may simulate almost any other acute abdominal illness and, in turn, may be mimicked by a variety of conditions. Progression of symptoms and signs is the rule—in contrast to the fluctuating course of some other diseases.

A. Signs and Symptoms

Typically, the illness begins with vague midabdominal or periumbilical discomfort followed by nausea, anorexia, and indigestion. The pain is continuous but not severe, with occasional mild cramping. The patient may feel constipated or may vomit. Importantly, within several hours of the onset of symptoms, the pain shifts to the right lower quadrant, becoming localized and causing discomfort upon moving, walking, or coughing.

Physical exam shows localized tenderness to palpation and perhaps slight muscular guarding. Rebound or percussion tenderness (the latter provides the same information more humanely) may be elicited in the right lower quadrant. Rectal and pelvic examinations are likely to be negative; if positive, these more often point to another etiology. The temperature is only slightly elevated in the absence of perforation. Administration of narcotic pain medications does not affect the accuracy of the physical exam.

A common misconception is that inflammation of a retrocecal appendix produces an atypical syndrome. This is incorrect; the clinical findings in this situation are the same as for ordinary (antececal) appendicitis. Acute appendicitis may mimic other surgical diseases if the appendix is located outside the right lower quadrant (ie, sigmoid diverticulitis, acute cholecystitis, or a perforated ulcer). Even when the cecum is normally situated, however, a long appendix may reach to other parts of the abdomen.

Three general points are worth remembering: (1) People with early (nonperforated) appendicitis often do not appear ill. Finding localized tenderness over the McBurney point is the cornerstone of diagnosis. (2) A rule that will help considerably with atypical cases is never to place appendicitis lower than second in the differential diagnosis of acute abdominal pain in a previously healthy person. (3) Patients with appendicitis most commonly have a history of generalized abdominal pain that over time becomes focused in the right lower quadrant.

B. Laboratory Findings

The average leukocyte count is 15,000/μL, and 90% of patients have counts over 10,000/μL. In three-fourths of patients, the differential white count shows more than 75% neutrophils. It must be emphasized, however, that 1 patient in 10 with acute appendicitis has a normal leukocyte count, and many have normal differential cell counts. Appendicitis in HIV-positive patients, although up to three times more common, produces the same syndrome as in healthy adults, but the white blood cell count is usually normal.

Urinalysis is typically normal, but a few leukocytes and erythrocytes, ketones, and occasionally even gross hematuria may be noted, particularly in retrocecal or pelvic appendicitis.

C. Imaging Studies

On plain radiographs, localized air-fluid levels, localized ileus, or increased soft tissue density in the right lower quadrant is present in 50% of patients with early acute appendicitis. Less common findings are a calculus, an altered right psoas shadow, an abnormal right flank stripe, or free peritoneal air (from perforated appendicitis). In general, the findings on plain films rarely aid in diagnosis.

Radiologic evaluation with ultrasound or computed tomography (CT) is often performed to solidify the diagnosis. An enlarged appendix with wall thickening, enhancement, or periappendiceal fat stranding is the most useful CT finding of acute appendicitis. Other findings may be present, including focal cecal thickening, appendicoliths, extraluminal or intramural air, and pericecal phlegmon, with the last finding being concerning for complicated appendicitis. CT scans are also of great value in patients with less than typical clinical and laboratory findings, in whom a positive study would be an indication for appendectomy or indicate a different pathology as the cause of the patient's symptoms. In young adults, low-dose CT with intravenous (IV) contrast is noninferior to standard-dose CT. Oral contrast administration is not necessary. Ultrasound imaging is generally less reliable than CT, although it may become more reliable when

done using a combined transabdominal and transvaginal approach or when performed at a high-volume institution. When appendicitis is accompanied by a right lower quadrant mass, an ultrasound or CT scan should always be obtained to differentiate between a periappendiceal phlegmon and an abscess or tumor.

D. Appendicitis During Pregnancy

Appendicitis is the most common nonobstetric surgical disease of the abdomen during pregnancy, affecting between 1 in 1400 and 1 in 6600 live births, with cases equally distributed through all three trimesters. By far, the most common presentation is right lower quadrant pain, tenderness, and leukocytosis—the classic syndrome—but the enlarged uterus occasionally will have pushed the appendix into the right upper quadrant, which gives rise to pain in this location. Some symptoms, such as nausea and vomiting, occur in normal pregnancy, which may obscure accurate diagnosis. Fever is less common than with appendicitis in the absence of pregnancy. The main problem is to recognize appendicitis and perform appendectomy promptly. Both CT and MRI are highly sensitive and specific for the diagnosis of acute appendicitis during pregnancy. Delay in operation runs a higher than usual risk of perforation and diffuse peritonitis, because the omentum is less available to wall off the infection. Thus, the mother is in greater jeopardy of serious abdominal infection, and the fetus is more vulnerable to premature labor with complications. Laparoscopic appendectomy is well tolerated by the mother and fetus, but the frequency of technical complications is higher than with the open approach. Appendectomy during pregnancy is often followed by preterm labor but rarely by preterm delivery. Early appendectomy in pregnancy has decreased the maternal death rate to less than 0.5% and the fetal death rate to less than 10%. Appendectomy in general does not increase a woman's risk for infertility later in life.

▶ Diagnosis & Differential Diagnosis

The clinical diagnosis of appendicitis rests on a combination of localized pain and tenderness accompanied by signs of inflammation, such as fever, leukocytosis, and elevated C-reactive protein levels. Migration of pain from the periumbilical area to the right lower quadrant is also diagnostically significant. In the absence of signs of inflammation, the diagnosis is less certain.

Imaging with ultrasound, CT, or magnetic resonance imaging (MRI) can significantly improve the certainty of the diagnosis. Over the past 20 years, the overall false-positive rate for the clinical diagnosis of appendicitis has decreased to 5% due to the more common use of confirmatory imaging. Over 90% of patients who proceed to appendectomy for acute appendicitis undergo some sort of imaging, with CT scan being the most common modality.

After equivocal imaging in patients with an atypical presentation, the best strategy is to observe the patient for a period of 6-12 hours or more. During this time, patients with appendicitis without antibiotic treatment often experience increasing pain and signs of inflammation, whereas those without appendicitis generally improve. Some patients experience chronic appendicitis, which involves pain lasting 3 weeks or more and typically includes an acute illness in the recent past compatible with acute appendicitis that was managed nonoperatively.

The diagnosis of acute appendicitis may be difficult in patients at the extremes of age, and it is in these groups that diagnosis is most often delayed. Infants display only lethargy, irritability, and anorexia in the early stages, but may develop vomiting, fever, and pain as the disease progresses. The elderly may not display any classic symptoms.

Clinical scoring systems can be effective in the diagnosis of acute appendicitis. For example, the Alvarado score, which uses both physical exam (anorexia, migration of pain, nausea, right lower quadrant tenderness, rebound pain, and elevated temperature) and laboratory findings (leukocytosis and shift of white blood cell count to the left) has excellent negative predictive value, with a sensitivity of 99%.

▶ Complications

The complications of acute appendicitis include perforation, peritonitis, abscess, and pylephlebitis.

A. Perforation

Perforation follows the natural history of acute appendicitis. It is often accompanied by more severe pain and higher fever (average, 38.3°C) than uncomplicated appendicitis. It is unusual for the acutely inflamed appendix to perforate within the first 12-24 hours. Appendicitis has progressed to perforation by the time of appendectomy in about 50% of patients under age 10 or over age 50. Perforation in young women increases the subsequent risk of tubal infertility about fourfold.

B. Peritonitis

Localized peritonitis often results from microscopic perforation of a gangrenous or necrotic appendix, whereas spreading or generalized peritonitis usually implies gross perforation into the free peritoneal cavity. Increasing tenderness and rigidity, abdominal distention, and adynamic ileus are obvious in these patients. High fever and severe toxicity mark progression of this catastrophic illness.

C. Appendiceal Abscess

Localized perforation occurs when the periappendiceal infection becomes walled off by omentum and adjacent viscera. Clinical presentation consists of the usual findings in appendicitis and may include a right lower quadrant mass. An ultrasound or CT scan should be performed; if an abscess is found, it is best treated by percutaneous image-guided aspiration. Opinion differs about how small abscesses and phlegmons that cannot be drained should be handled. Some surgeons prefer a regimen consisting of antibiotics and expectant management followed by elective appendectomy 6 weeks later. This avoids spreading the localized infection and the need for a more extensive operation and is associated with lower rates of overall complications, abscess formation, bowel obstruction, and reoperation. Other surgeons recommend immediate appendectomy, which some believe shortens the duration of illness.

When an unsuspected abscess is encountered during appendectomy, it is usually best to proceed and remove the appendix. If the abscess is large and further dissection would be hazardous, drainage alone is appropriate. Culturing of intraperitoneal fluid in complicated appendicitis is of little clinical value.

D. Pylephlebitis

Pylephlebitis is suppurative thrombophlebitis of the portal venous system. Chills, high fever, low-grade jaundice, and, later, hepatic abscesses are the hallmarks of this grave but fortunately rare condition, which affects less than 1% of patients. Prompt surgery and antibiotic therapy are indicated.

▶ Prevention

There is no effective prevention strategy for appendicitis. In the past, it was common to perform an incidental appendectomy in young people during the course of an abdominal operation for another illness—as long as the exposure was adequate and there were no specific contraindications. This is no longer practiced. A related question concerns the appropriate course when a laparoscopy is performed for presumptive appendicitis and the appendix looks normal. There is no consensus on these cases, with some surgeons preferring to remove the appendix and some electing to leave it in place. Furthermore, it is not necessary to remove the appendix after an incidentally diagnosed appendicolith.

▶ Treatment

With few exceptions, the treatment of appendicitis is surgical (ie, appendectomy). Patients should receive antibiotics to cover fecal flora as soon as the diagnosis of appendicitis is made and until treatment with appendectomy is completed unless the patient is being managed nonoperatively. The operation can be done open (Figure 30–1) or laparoscopically. A laparoscopic approach is desirable unless comorbidities prevent it. In select patients, outpatient laparoscopic appendectomy may be possible.

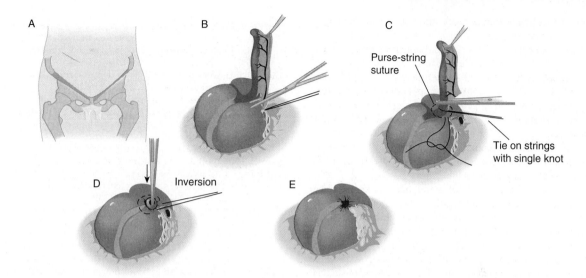

▲ **Figure 30–1.** Technique of open appendectomy. **A:** Incision. **B:** After delivery of the tip of the cecum, the mesoappendix is divided. **C:** The base is clamped and ligated with a simple throw of the knot. The next step—inversion of the stump—is optional. **D:** A clamp is placed to hold the knot during inversion with a purse-string suture of fine silk. **E:** The loosely tied inner knot on the stump assures that there is no closed space for the development of a stump abscess.

Culturing abdominal fluid is not indicated even when the appendix has perforated because the organisms obtained are the typical fecal flora. Abdominal drains are used only to treat established abscesses, and their use is controversial.

If a patient with appendicitis cannot be managed operatively or with drainage, for whatever reason, treatment may consist of antibiotics alone. Appendicitis recurs in only 10% of patients whose initial treatment consists of antibiotics, with or without drainage of an abscess. The complication-free success rate of this approach is greater than 93%. Therefore, when the presence of ancillary conditions increases the risks of surgery, interval appendectomy may be postponed unless symptoms recur.

A. Laparoscopic Versus Open Appendectomy

The laparoscopic approach to appendectomy was first described by Kurt Semm in 1983. There has been much debate over the appropriate role of laparoscopy in the treatment of appendicitis since that initial report, with the large majority of cases in this country performed laparoscopically. In one large study, patients treated laparoscopically had lower overall morbidity (except organ space surgical site infections in patients with complicated appendicitis), but similar serious morbidity, mortality, and length of stay. Generally, patients undergoing laparoscopic appendectomy have less postoperative pain and a shorter length of stay by 1 day. However, laparoscopic appendectomy may be associated with increased overall hospital costs and longer operative times. Conversion rates from laparoscopic to open approach range from

0%-27% and are based on surgeon experience, judgment, and ability to safely perform the procedure. Currently, most patients in the United States undergo laparoscopic treatment, and this approach is safe for both uncomplicated and complicated appendicitis. In select patients, the appendix can be removed using a single-port technique.

B. Outcomes

Although a death rate of zero is theoretically attainable in acute appendicitis, deaths still occur, some of which are avoidable. The mortality rate in simple acute appendicitis is approximately 0.1% and has not changed significantly since 1930. Progress in preoperative and postoperative care has reduced mortality from perforation to about 5%. Nonetheless, postoperative infections still occur in 30% of cases of complicated appendicitis. Although the cases may be more technically challenging, obese patients have similar rates of complication, length of stay, and readmission. The substantial increase in tubal infertility that follows perforation in young women is avoidable using early appendectomy. If the entirety of the appendix is not removed, stump appendicitis can occur in the residual appendix.

C. Controversies

Many controversies exist regarding the treatment of acute appendicitis. Some surgeons routinely irrigate all four quadrants in all appendectomies, whereas others do not. Irrigation has been shown to reduce postoperative abscess rates in perforated appendicitis only. Some surgeons routinely perform interval appendectomies after antibiotic management of perforated appendicitis, with or without drainage, whereas others follow patients clinically and only perform appendectomy in patients with residual or recurrent symptoms.

Although it is clear that postoperative antibiotics are not beneficial for uncomplicated appendicitis after appendectomy, no consensus exists on the drug regimen or duration of antibiotics for complicated disease. Some surgeons advocate treatment for 4 days, as currently recommended for other intra-abdominal infections after source control, whereas others support shorter lengths of treatment or no postoperative antibiotics at all.

The safety and efficacy of antibiotics for the treatment of uncomplicated appendicitis have been well established. However, whether antibiotics could or should be the first-line treatment in patients who are otherwise good surgical candidates is currently under debate. Similarly, it has not been fully established if any specific populations could benefit from initial management with antibiotics instead of surgery. Multiple studies support the possible use of antibiotics for the initial management of uncomplicated appendicitis, but the rates of recurrence are undeniable and postoperative complications in surgical patients are low. Shared decision making could help patients and surgeons decide between surgical and medical management of acute uncomplicated appendicitis.

Akingboye AA, et al: Pus samples in complicated appendicitis: an important investigation or a waste of resources: a prospective cohort study. *Scand J Surg.* 2019;108(1):55-60.

Amoli HA, et al: Morphine analgesia in patients with acute appendicitis: a randomised double-blind clinical trial. *Emerg Med J.* 2008;25(9):586-589.

Basaran A, et al: Diagnosis of acute appendicitis during pregnancy: a systematic review. *Obstet Gynecol Surv.* 2009;64(7):481-488.

Bondi M, et al: Improving the diagnostic accuracy of ultrasonography in suspected acute appendicitis by the combined transabdominal and transvaginal approach. *Am Surg.* 2012;78(1):98-103.

Cardenas-Salomon CM, et al: Hospitalization costs of open vs. laparoscopic appendectomy: 5-year experience. *Cir Cir.* 2011;79(6):534-539.

Cash CL, et al. A prospective treatment protocol for outpatient laparoscopic appendectomy for acute appendicitis. *J Am Coll Surg.* 2012;215(1):101-105.

Coakley BA, et al: Postoperative antibiotics correlate with worse outcomes after appendectomy for nonperforated appendicitis. *J Am Coll Surg.* 2011;213(6):778-783.

Deugarte DA, et al: Obesity does not impact outcomes for appendicitis. *Am Surg.* 2012;78(2):254-257.

Drake FT, et al: Enteral contract in the computer tomography diagnosis of appendicitis: comparative effectiveness in a prospective surgical cohort. *Ann Surg.* 2014;260(2):311-316.

Gilo NB, et al: Appendicitis and cholecystitis in pregnancy. *Clin Obstet Gynecol.* 2009;52(4):586-596.

Hussain A, et al: Prevention of intra-abdominal abscess following laparoscopic appendicectomy for perforated appendicitis: a prospective study. *Int J Surg.* 2008;6(5):374-377.

Ingraham AM, et al: Comparison of outcomes after laparoscopic versus open appendectomy for acute appendicitis at 222 ACS NSQIP hospitals. *Surgery.* 2010;148(4):625-635; discussion 635-627.

Kim K, et al: Low-dose abdominal CT for evaluating suspected appendicitis. *N Engl J Med.* 2012;366(17):1596-1605.

Klein DB, et al: Increased rates of appendicitis in HIV-infected men: 1991-2005. *J Acquir Immune Defic Syndr.* 2009;52(1):139-140.

Korndorffer JR Jr, et al: SAGES guideline for laparoscopic appendectomy. *Surg Endosc.* 2010;24(4):757-761.

Liu K, Fogg L: Use of antibiotics alone for treatment of uncomplicated acute appendicitis: a systematic review and meta-analysis. *Surgery.* 2011;150(4):673-683.

Ohle R, et al: The Alvarado score for predicting acute appendicitis: a systematic review. *BMC Med.* 2011;9:139.

Parks NA, Schroeppel TJ: Update on imaging for acute appendicitis. *Surg Clin North Am.* 2011;91(1):141-154.

Rollins MD, et al: Prophylactic appendectomy: unnecessary in children with incidental appendicoliths detected by computed tomographic scan. *J Pediatr Surg.* 2010;45(12):2377-2380.

Sallinen V, et al: Meta-analysis of antibiotics versus appendicectomy for non-perforated acute appendicitis. *Br J Surg.* 2016;103(6):656-667.

Sauerland S, et al: Laparoscopic versus open surgery for suspected appendicitis. *Cochrane Database Syst Rev.* 2010;10:CD001546.

Sieren LM, et al: The incidence of benign and malignant neoplasia presenting as acute appendicitis. *Am Surg.* 2010;76(8):808-811.

Simillis C, et al: A meta-analysis comparing conservative treatment versus acute appendectomy for complicated appendicitis (abscess or phlegmon). *Surgery.* 2010;147(6):818-829.

St Peter SD, et al: Single incision versus standard 3-port laparoscopic appendectomy: a prospective randomized trial. *Ann Surg.* 2011;254(4):586-590.

Subramanian A, et al: A 60-year literature review of stump appendicitis: the need for a critical view. *Am J Surg.* 2012;203(4):503-507.

Tseng J, et al: Imaging utilization affects negative appendectomy rates in appendicitis: an ACS-NSQIP study. *Am J Surg.* 2019;217(6):1094-1098.

TUMORS OF THE APPENDIX

Benign tumors, including carcinoids, were found in 4.6% of 71,000 human appendix specimens examined microscopically, typically as incidental findings.

▶ Malignant Tumors

Primary malignant tumors of the appendix are present in less than 2% of appendectomies.

Carcinoid and neuroendocrine tumors compose the majority of appendiceal cancers. In addition, the appendix is the most common location of carcinoid tumors of the gastrointestinal tract. Carcinoid tumors of the appendix are most commonly found at the tip and are usually benign, but tumors over 2 cm in diameter may exhibit malignant behavior. About half of these tumors are discovered during appendectomy for acute appendicitis, with the remainder identified incidentally. Lesions less than 2 cm in diameter invade the appendiceal wall in 25% of cases, but only 3% metastasize to lymph nodes. Hepatic metastases and carcinoid syndrome are truly rare. Appendectomy alone is adequate treatment for appendiceal carcinoid unless the lymph nodes are visibly involved, the tumor is more than 2 cm in diameter, mucinous elements are present in the tumor (adenocarcinoid), or the mesoappendix or base of the cecum is invaded; in these cases, right hemicolectomy is recommended. The recurrence rate after surgical treatment is near zero.

Colonic adenocarcinoma can arise in the appendix and spread rapidly to regional lymph nodes or implant on other peritoneal surfaces. Most patients present with advanced disease. Adenocarcinoma is virtually never diagnosed preoperatively, and about half of the cases present as acute appendicitis. Right hemicolectomy should be performed if disease is localized to the appendix and/or regional lymph nodes. The 5-year survival rate is 60% after right hemicolectomy and only 20% after appendectomy alone, but the latter group includes patients with distant metastases at diagnosis.

▶ Mucocele and Pseudomyxoma Peritonei

An appendiceal mucocele is a cystic, dilated appendix filled with mucin. They are very rare. Simple mucoceles are not neoplasms and result from chronic obstruction of the proximal lumen, usually by fibrous tissue. Rarely, mucoceles are associated with mucinous neoplasms of the appendix. Appendectomy is adequate treatment in either case as long as they do not involve the base of the appendix, in which case, a cecal resection should be performed. If a mucinous appendiceal neoplasm ruptures, it can lead to a condition known as pseudomyxoma peritonei (PMP), which is characterized by diffuse mucin production throughout the peritoneal cavity, with variable amounts of tumor cellularity. PMP should be treated with removal of all the mucin deposits from the peritoneum, intraoperative hyperthermic chemotherapy, and postoperative systemic chemotherapy in addition to appendectomy or right hemicolectomy.

Guraya SY, et al: Clinicopathological features and the outcome of surgical management for adenocarcinoma of the appendix. *World J Gastrointest Surg.* 2011;3(1):7-12.

Shapiro R, et al: Appendiceal carcinoid at a large tertiary center: pathologic findings and long-term follow-up evaluation. *Am J Surg.* 2011;201(6):805-808.

Tirumani S, et al: Mucinous neoplasms of the appendix: a current comprehensive clinicopathologic and imaging review. *Cancer Imaging.* 2013;13(1):14-25.

MULTIPLE CHOICE QUESTIONS

1. All of the following are true about the appendix, except

   A. The appendix in children is characterized by a large concentration of lymphoid follicles that appear 2 weeks after birth and number about 200 or more at age 15.
   B. The taeniae of the colon converge at the base of the appendix.
   C. A fecalith or calculus is found in only 10% of acutely inflamed appendices.
   D. The appendix is fixed retrocecally in 65% of adults.
   E. Acute appendicitis may simulate almost any other acute abdominal illness.

2. Helpful tests in the diagnosis of acute appendicitis include

   A. Abdominal computed tomography
   B. Magnetic resonance imaging
   C. Transvaginal ultrasound
   D. A, B, and C
   E. A and C

3. Primary malignant tumors of the appendix

   A. Should prompt right colectomy in nearly all patients
   B. Are most commonly neuroendocrine (carcinoid) tumors
   C. Are the most common etiology of appendicitis
   D. Usually present due to liver metastases
   E. Are usually found at the base of the appendix

Small Intestine

Marco Ettore Allaix, MD, PhD
Alessandro Fichera, MD

ANATOMY

Gross Anatomy

The small intestine is the portion of the alimentary tract extending from the pylorus to the ileocecal valve, and it consists of three segments: the *duodenum*, the *jejunum* (upper two-fifths), and the *ileum* (lower three-fifths). The anatomy, physiology, and pathology of the duodenum are discussed in Chapter 25.

The duodenum is a retroperitoneal structure that is approximately 25 cm long and is divided into four segments: the bulb and the descending, transverse, and ascending segments. Both the celiac trunk, through the gastroduodenal artery, and the superior mesenteric artery (SMA) supply the duodenum.

The jejunum begins at the ligament of Treitz. The jejunum and ileum are suspended on a mobile mesentery covered by a visceral peritoneal lining that extends onto the external surface of the bowel to form the serosa. There is no sharp demarcation between the jejunum and the ileum; as the intestine proceeds distally, the lumen narrows, the mesenteric vascular arcades become more complex, and the circular mucosal folds become shorter and fewer.

The mesentery contains fat, blood vessels, lymphatic channels and nodes, and nerves. The jejunum and ileum are supplied by the SMA. Branches within the mesentery anastomose to form arcades, and small straight arteries from these arcades enter the mesenteric border of the gut. Venous blood is drained through the superior mesenteric vein, which then joins the splenic vein behind the pancreas to form the portal vein.

Lymphatic drainage is abundant, with several levels following the blood vessels. Elliptical, lymphoid aggregates (Peyer's patches) are present in the submucosa on the antimesenteric border along the distal ileum, and smaller follicles are evident throughout the remainder of the small intestine. The lymph is drained into the lymph nodes that follow the mesenteric arcade and then into the lymphatic vessels along the SMA. Eventually, the lymph is drained into the cisterna chyli that is located below the diaphragm.

The innervation for the small intestine is both sympathetic (fibers from the greater and lesser splanchnic nerves) and parasympathetic (from the right vagus nerve). Although both types of autonomic nerves contain efferent and afferent fibers, only the sympathetic afferents appear to mediate intestinal pain.

Microscopic Anatomy

The wall of the small intestine consists of four layers: mucosa (innermost), submucosa, muscularis, and serosa (outermost).

The mucosa is characterized by circular folds about 10 mm high, named *valvulae conniventes*, that are taller and more numerous in the proximal jejunum and project into the lumen (Figure 31–1). These folds, combined with the presence of villi on the surface of the valvulae conniventes, increase the absorptive surface area about eight times. There are approximately 20-40 villi per square millimeter. They are about 0.5-1 mm long, and their walls are made up of epithelial cells with tiny projections named microvilli. The epithelial cells enclose a central axis that contains an arteriole surrounded by blood and lymphatic capillaries, known as a lacteal, and fibers from the muscularis mucosae. The microvilli (1 μm in height) amplify the potential absorptive surface area up to 200-500 m² (Figure 31–2).

The mucosa is microscopically subdivided into three different layers: (1) the muscularis mucosae, the outermost layer, consists of a thin sheet of smooth muscle cells; (2) the lamina propria consists of connective tissue that extends from the base of the crypts up into the intestinal villi; and (3) the epithelium is the innermost layer.

Intestinal epithelium is composed of multiple cell types that rest on a thin basement membrane overlying the lamina

▲ **Figure 31–1.** Blood supply and luminal surface of the small bowel. The arterial arcades of the small intestine increase in number from one or two in the proximal jejunum to four or five in the distal ileum, a finding that helps to distinguish proximal from distal bowel at operation. Plicae circulares are more prominent in the jejunum.

Jejunum

Ileum

▲ **Figure 31–2.** Schematic representation of villi and crypts of Lieberkühn.

propria. There are two major compartments to the intestinal epithelium, the crypt and the villus, each with distinct function and cellular composition. The crypt is populated by cells that are predominantly secretory and that derive from a pluripotent stem cell located above the base of the crypts of Lieberkühn. Paneth cells stay at the base of the crypts; their function is still unknown but may be secretory, as they resemble the zymogen-secreting cells of the pancreas.

Most of the crypt cells are undifferentiated; some mature into mucus-secreting goblet cells and enteroendocrine cells, but the majority become absorptive enterocytes. Enteroendocrine cells include enterochromaffin cells (the most common), N cells that contain neurotensin, L cells (glucagon), and motilin- and cholecystokinin (CCK)-containing cells. Finally, M cells and T lymphocytes play a major role in mucosal cell–mediated immunity.

The villus compartment is nonproliferative. Factors that affect enterocyte differentiation include growth factors, hormones, matrix proteins, and luminal nutrients. The life span of enterocytes is 3-6 days.

The *submucosa* is a dense connective tissue layer populated by different cell types, including fibroblasts, mast cells, lymphocytes, macrophages, eosinophils, and plasma cells. It contains blood vessels, lymphatics, and nerves. Meissner's submucosal neural plexus interconnects with neural elements from Auerbach's plexus. The submucosa is the strongest layer of small bowel wall. The *muscularis* consists of two layers of smooth muscle, a thicker inner circular layer and a thinner outer longitudinal layer. Specialized intercellular junctional structures called gap junctions electrically couple adjacent smooth muscle cells and allow efficient propagation of peristalsis. Ganglion cells and nerve fibers of Auerbach's myenteric plexus interdigitate between layers and communicate with smaller neural elements between cells. The *serosa* consists of a single layer of flattened mesothelial cells that covers the small bowel.

Johansson ME, et al: Composition and functional role of the mucus layers in the intestine. *Cell Mol Life Sci.* 2011;68(22):3635-3641.
Simons BD, et al: Stem cell self-renewal in intestinal crypt. *Exp Cell Res.* 2011;317(19):2719-2724.

PHYSIOLOGY

▶ Motility

Intestinal motility consists of propulsion of luminal contents (peristalsis) combined with mixing action through segmentation. These functions are accomplished by both the outer longitudinal and inner circular muscle layers of the intestinal wall, mainly under the direct control of the myoenteric nervous plexus. The submucosal nervous plexus is primarily involved in the regulation of secretion and absorption. The extrinsic sympathetic input is excitatory and the peptidergic input likely inhibitory. Intestinal motility is also under positive control by local hormones such as motilin and CCK. Smooth muscles of the small intestine undergo spontaneous oscillations of membrane potentials, known as pacesetter potentials, with progressively decreasing frequency from the duodenum to the ileum. The frequency of pacesetter potentials for the entire small intestine is determined by the duodenum, where they originate. A nerve-related cell type known as the interstitial cell of Cajal appears to play a key role in the generation of pacemaker activity. Small bowel motility varies with the fasted and fed state. During the interdigestive or fasting period, a cyclical pattern of motor activity consisting of three phases is observed. Phase I is resting and lasts for about 80% of the cycle. Phase II, about 15%, consists of random contractions of moderate amplitude. Phase III, about 5%, is a series of brief high-pressure waves. This three-phase cycle results in a pattern called the migrating motor complex, which is abolished by ingestion of food. In the fed state, the pattern of contraction is more frequent and consistent over time. Rather than beginning from a proximal site and propagating distally, contractions begin at all levels along the small bowel and spread distally.

Barrier Function

The intestinal epithelium selectively limits the permeation of potentially harmful luminal substances. The anatomic barrier is the intercellular junction complex, a three-level structure that forms a circumferential seal between adjacent cells: the tight junction faces the lumen, the intermediate junction lies deep to the tight junction, and the desmosome is the innermost element of this complex. Several pathologic conditions can alter the barrier function. Certain bacterial toxins, such as *Clostridium difficile*, directly perturb the barrier function through disruption of cytoskeletal-junctional interactions, and various cytokines and proinflammatory mediators can also modulate intestinal permeability.

Digestion and Absorption

Digestion begins in the stomach with the action of gastric acid and pepsin. In the proximal duodenum, ingested food is broken down by pancreatic enzymes such as trypsin, elastase, chymotrypsin, and carboxypeptidases. The activity of intestinal hydrolases and olygopeptidases then accomplishes terminal protein and carbohydrate digestion, and the resulting monosaccharides, amino acids, or di- and tripeptides then serve as substrates for Na^+- or H^+-coupled transporters in the apical membrane of absorptive enterocytes. Fat digestion and absorption occur in the proximal small bowel, where pancreatic lipase partially hydrolyzes triglycerides into two fatty acids and a monoglyceride. These substances are solubilized by bile salts to form micelles that diffuse into enterocytes releasing fatty acid and monoglyceride. Triglycerides are transported intracellularly and incorporated along with cellular protein, phospholipid, and cholesterol to form chylomicrons. They then exit the cell to be absorbed by the lymphatic system. Bile salts are reabsorbed into the enterohepatic circulation in the distal ileum by an ileal Na^+-coupled bile acid transporter.

The small bowel receives about 1-1.5 L/d of ingested fluids and about 8 L of salivary, gastric, and pancreatico-biliary secretions. Most of this fluid is reabsorbed before reaching the colon. Water movement is driven by the active transcellular absorption of Na^+ and Cl^- and by absorption of nutrients such as glucose and amino acids. The energy for many of these processes derives from the activity of an Na^+-K^+ ATPase, which maintains the low Na^+ internal environment that drives uptake via coupled ion exchangers (Na^+/H^+ and Cl^-/HCO_3^-) and Na^+-coupled nutrient transporters.

Secretion

Intestinal crypt cells secrete an isotonic fluid through the active transcellular transport of Cl^-. This process lubricates the mucosal surface and facilitates the luminal extrusion of other secreted substances. Diarrhea results when secretion exceeds intestinal absorptive capacity.

Immune Function

The mucosal immune system is extremely important in defense against toxic and pathogenic threats from the luminal environment. The lamina propria contains numerous immune cells, including plasma cells, mast cells, and lymphocytes, that produce both immunoglobulins and cytokine mediators.

Plasma cells produce immunoglobulin A (IgA) in response to food antigens and microbes. IgA and immunoglobulin M (IgM) are secreted into the lumen by a mechanism that involves transcytosis through epithelial cells after binding to the polymeric immunoglobulin receptor on the basolateral membrane. Secretory IgA prevents microbial pathogens from penetrating the epithelial layer. IgA-antigen interactions also occur within the intraepithelial and subepithelial compartments. Intestinal epithelial cells themselves may also contribute to the immune function of the bowel. These cells express major histocompatibility class I and class II molecules on their surface and may function as weak antigen-presenting cells. The epithelial cell layer may transmit important immunoregulatory signals to the underlying lymphocytic population.

Specialized cells known as M cells are found overlying Peyer's patches and act as the major portal of entry for foreign bodies. Specialized membrane invaginations in these cells create a pocket in which lymphocytes and macrophages gather. Luminal substances are immediately delivered to these antigen-presenting cells, and this information is directly conveyed to the underlying follicles. Intraepithelial lymphocytes (IELs) are specialized T cells that reside in the paracellular space between absorptive enterocytes. The precise role of IELs is still uncertain, but they may mediate cross-talk between epithelial cells and the underlying immune and nonimmune cells of the lamina propria. Within the lamina propria and submucosa, mature T cells, B cells, and macrophages carry out traditional cell-mediated immune response including phagocytosis, cell killing, and cytokine secretion. Mucosal and connective tissue mast cells produce numerous mediators that contribute to overall immune response and modulate the many functions of the epithelial cells.

Neuroendocrine Function

The small bowel is a rich source of regulatory peptides that control various aspects of gut function. These substances, released in response to luminal or neural stimuli, exert their biological actions either at distant sites or locally.

Secretin is a 27-amino-acid peptide released by entero-endocrine cells in the proximal small bowel in response to luminal acidification, bile salts, and fat. Its major function is to stimulate pancreatic ductal alkaline secretion. Secretin inhibits gastric acid secretion and gastrointestinal motility. In addition, it stimulates bile flow by stimulating fluid secretion from cholangiocytes. Other members of the secretin family that share substantial sequence homology and interact with similar receptors include vasoactive intestinal polypeptide (VIP), glucagon, gastric inhibitory polypeptide (GIP), and enteroglucagon. Enteroglucagon and glucagon-like peptides are secreted by neuroendocrine cells in the colon and small bowel and may play an important role in gut adaptation and glucose homeostasis.

CCK is released by specialized enteroendocrine cells in response to luminal amino acids and medium- to long-chain fatty acids. CCK release is inhibited by intraluminal trypsin and bile salts. Two major targets of CCK are the gallbladder and the sphincter of Oddi, where it causes coordinated contraction and relaxation, respectively, to enhance luminal mixing of bile with ingested food. Furthermore, CCK stimulates pancreatic enzyme secretion and cell growth in intestinal mucosa and the pancreas, insulin release, and intestinal motility.

Somatostatin is a 14-amino-acid peptide that exerts a wide variety of inhibitory functions in the gastrointestinal tract. It is released from specialized enteroendocrine cells, and it acts in paracrine fashion to inhibit intestinal, gastric, and pancreatico-biliary secretion and cell growth. Synthetic forms of somatostatin are used in clinical practice in patients with enterocutaneous and pancreatico-biliary fistulae.

Peptide YY is a 36-amino-acid peptide secreted by the distal small bowel, and it inhibits gastric acid and pancreatic secretion, as well as several intestinal hormones, and decreases intestinal motility.

Motilin is secreted by the duodenum and the proximal jejunum, where it acts to enhance contractility and accelerate gastric emptying.

Neurotensin is produced in the ileum and enteric nerves; it appears to affect a variety of enteric functions including gastric acid secretion, gastric emptying, intestinal motility, and secretion.

Other peptides (VIP, calcitonin-related peptide, galanin, bombesin, neuropeptide Y, gastrin-releasing peptides, and substance P) are released from enteric nerves, but their precise role has not been fully clarified.

Crenn P, et al: Citrulline as a biomarker of intestinal failure due to enterocyte mass reduction. *Clin Nutr.* 2008;27:328.
Edholm T, et al: The incretin hormones GIP and GLP-1 in diabetic rats: effects on insulin secretion and small bowel motility. *Neurogastroenterol Motil.* 2009;21(3):313-321.
Jones MP, et al: Small intestinal motility. *Curr Opin Gastroenterol.* 2008;24:164.

SMALL BOWEL OBSTRUCTION

General Considerations

Small bowel obstruction (SBO) is one of the most common disorders affecting the small bowel. It is characterized by impairment in the normal flow of intraluminal contents and can be divided into mechanical obstruction and paralytic ileus. This distinction is critical for the further management of the patient.

Mechanical obstruction implies an extrinsic or intrinsic obstacle that prevents the aboral progression of intestinal contents, and it may be complete or partial. Simple obstruction occludes the lumen only; obstruction with strangulation impairs the blood supply also and leads to necrosis of the intestinal wall. Paralytic (or adynamic) ileus is due to a neurogenic failure of peristalsis to propel intestinal contents with no mechanical obstruction.

A. Etiology

The causes of mechanical obstruction can be divided into three groups according to the relationship to the intestinal wall: (1) intraluminal; (2) intramural; and (3) extrinsic. The three most common etiologies are intra-abdominal adhesions, hernias, and neoplasms.

1. **Adhesions.** Sixty to seventy five percent of cases of mechanical SBO are secondary to adhesions related to prior abdominal surgery. Lower abdominal and pelvic surgery appears to be associated with a higher incidence

of adhesions compared to upper abdominal surgery. Congenital bands are rarely seen in children.

2. **Hernia.** The most common cause of SBO in patients with no history of prior abdominal surgery is a hernia. A careful search for inguinal, femoral, and umbilical hernias must be made during evaluation of every patient presenting with symptoms consistent with obstruction. Internal hernias into the obturator foramen, the foramen of Winslow, or other anatomic defects must also be considered. In patients who have undergone previous surgery, incisional hernias represent another potential cause of SBO, especially after laparotomy in overweight or obese patients, in patients on steroid therapy, or with wound infections.

3. **Neoplasms.** Intrinsic small bowel neoplasms can progressively occlude the lumen or serve as a leading point in intussusception. Symptoms may be intermittent, onset of obstruction is slow, and signs of chronic anemia may be present. Peritoneal carcinomatosis from several tumors is an extrinsic cause of SBO due to adhesions of small bowel loops to neoplastic nodules.

Other causes of SBO include Crohn disease; intussusception, which is most often seen in children without an organic lesion and rarely in adults with a neoplastic intraluminal lesion; volvulus as a consequence of intestinal malrotation in children or of adhesions in adults; and foreign bodies including bezoars, ingested foreign bodies, and gallstones through a cholecystoduodenal fistula. Gallstone ileus is discussed in Chapter 27.

B. Pathophysiology

With onset of obstruction, gas and fluid accumulate and distend the intestinal loops proximal to the site of obstruction. Fluid from the extracellular space also fills the lumen proximal to the obstruction, due to the impaired bidirectional flow of salt and water and fluid secretion enhanced by substances (endotoxins, prostaglandins) released from proliferating bacteria in the intestinal lumen. As a consequence, intraluminal and intramural pressures rise until microvascular perfusion to the intestine is impaired, leading to intestinal wall ischemia and ultimately necrosis.

Activity of the smooth muscle of the small bowel is increased in an attempt to propel its contents past the obstruction consuming all energy sources. At this point, the intestine becomes atonic and enlarges further. Emesis could be feculent due to bacterial overgrowth—particularly with distal obstruction—as the intestinal dilation progresses proximally (Figure 31–3). Bacterial translocation from the lumen to the mesenteric nodes and the bloodstream occurs, and abdominal distention elevates the diaphragm and impairs respiration, resulting in potential pulmonary complications such as pneumonia and atelectasis.

When full-thickness necrosis of the intestinal wall occurs, luminal content with an elevated bacterial load enters the peritoneal cavity and is absorbed by the peritoneum, causing septic shock.

The progression of pathophysiologic events when the bowel is strangulated occurs more rapidly than with simple obstruction and is characterized by an acute impairment of venous return initially followed by arterial flow with subsequent ischemia, necrosis, and perforation of the intestinal wall.

▶ Clinical Findings

Diagnostic evaluation should distinguish mechanical bowel obstruction from ileus, determine the cause of the obstruction, and recognize simple from strangulating obstruction.

Accurate diagnosis requires obtaining a detailed history, paying particular attention to medications known to affect intestinal physiology, previous cancer, inflammatory bowel disease, and abdominal surgery, and performing a meticulous physical examination.

A. Signs and Symptoms

Patients usually present with nausea, vomiting, colicky abdominal pain, and obstipation, although residual gas and stool distal to the obstruction may be expelled. With proximal SBO, emesis is usually profuse, containing undigested food in close temporal association with oral intake; abdominal pain is more often described as upper abdominal discomfort associated with epigastric distension. Distal SBO is characterized by diffuse and poorly localized crampy abdominal pain. Feculent vomiting present in cases of longstanding distal SBO is the consequence of bacterial overgrowth and is pathognomonic for a complete mechanical obstruction. In the presence of strangulation, fever often develops, and previously crampy abdominal pain becomes peritonitis.

Initially, vital signs may be normal, but tachycardia and hypotension usually develop as a result of progressive dehydration. Fever is often present with bowel ischemia or perforation. Inspection of the abdomen usually reveals distension that varies based on the site of obstruction and may be absent in cases of proximal obstruction. Peristalsis is usually tremendously increased in the early phases of mechanical SBO, as a result of intensive intestinal muscular contractions. This so-called "peristaltic rush" progressively decreases until it disappears in the late phase of obstruction. The presence of either surgical scars or hernias should be noted, indicating a possible cause of SBO. Rectal examination is essential to detect rectal lesions and to check for the presence of stool.

B. Laboratory Findings

Laboratory findings reflect intravascular volume depletion and dehydration. An elevated hematocrit is indicative of

High	**Middle**	**Low**
Frequent vomiting. No distention. Intermittent pain but not classic crescendo type.	Moderate vomiting. Moderate distention. Intermittent pain (crescendo, colicky) with free intervals.	Vomiting late, feculent. Marked distention. Variable pain; may not be classic crescendo type.

▲ **Figure 31–3.** Small bowel obstruction. Variable manifestations of obstruction depend on the level of blockage of the small bowel.

hemoconcentration. Leukocytosis is often the result of dehydration and an acute stress response rather than an underlying infection. Blood chemistries may reveal elevated serum creatinine levels, indicating hypovolemia with prerenal failure.

Features of strangulated obstruction or perforation include marked leukocytosis and metabolic acidosis.

C. Imaging Studies

Plain x-rays of the abdomen with the patient in supine and upright positions can confirm the clinical diagnosis of SBO. They reveal dilated small bowel loops with air-fluid levels in a ladder-like appearance and a paucity of air in the colon. These features may be minimal or absent in early or high-grade obstructions.

Computed tomography (CT) scan of the abdomen and pelvis with both intravenous and oral contrast is recommended in patients with suspected SBO. CT scan can visualize the specific location of the obstruction, showing a discrepancy in the caliber between distended proximal bowel loops

and collapsed distal intestine. Moreover, CT scan can also reveal the etiology of SBO and demonstrate signs of strangulation including thickening of the bowel wall, air in the bowel wall or portal venous system, and poor uptake of intravenous contrast by the affected bowel wall. Ascites between dilated bowel loops and in the pelvis is often reported in both simple and strangulated obstruction. Intraperitoneal free air indicates perforation.

In patients who fail to improve after 48 hours of conservative treatment, an abdominal x-ray with water-soluble contrast (Gastrografin) should be obtained for both diagnostic and therapeutic purposes, since it has been demonstrated that the lack of Gastrografin progression into the colon with 24 hours predicts the need for surgery in about 96% of cases.

▶ Differential Diagnosis

Pain in patients with *paralytic ileus* is usually not severe but is constant and diffuse, and the abdomen is often distended and mildly tender. If ileus has resulted from an acute intraperitoneal inflammatory process, there should be symptoms and signs of the primary disease as well as the ileus. abdominal x-rays show the presence of gas in both the colon and the small bowel.

A postoperative ileus may be caused by several factors, including drugs used for anesthesia and analgesia and intraoperative manipulation of intestinal loops and the mesentery. Usually, it is temporary, but if it persists for more than 3-5 days, diagnostic evaluation to rule out mechanical causes of obstruction is mandatory.

Colonic obstruction is usually diagnosed by abdominal x-rays that show colonic dilation proximal to the obstructing lesion. In the presence of a competent ileocecal valve, a closed loop obstruction occurs with an elevated risk of perforation of the colon. If the ileocecal valve is incompetent, the distal small bowel will be dilated, and patients will exhibit abdominal distension, nausea, and vomiting.

Acute gastroenteritis, acute appendicitis, and acute pancreatitis can mimic simple intestinal obstruction, whereas acute mesenteric ischemia must be considered in the differential of small bowel strangulation.

Intestinal pseudo-obstruction comprises a spectrum of specific disorders associated with irreversible intestinal dysmotility, in which there are symptoms and signs of intestinal obstruction without evidence for an obstructing lesion. Acute pseudo-obstruction of the colon carries the risk of cecal perforation and is discussed in Chapter 32. Chronic pseudo-obstruction affecting the small bowel with or without colonic involvement can be idiopathic or secondary to several (sporadic and familial) visceral myopathies and neuropathies that affect intestinal smooth muscle and the intra- and extraintestinal nervous system. Systemic disorders such as scleroderma, myxedema, lupus erythematosus, amyloidosis, drug abuse (phenothiazine ingestion), radiation injury, or progressive systemic sclerosis can be complicated by chronic intestinal pseudo-obstruction. In addition, cytomegalovirus and Epstein-Barr virus infections can cause chronic intestinal pseudo-obstruction.

The clinical manifestations of chronic intestinal pseudo-obstruction include recurrent episodes of vomiting, crampy abdominal pain, and abdominal distention. The diagnosis is suggested by clinical findings and medical history and confirmed by radiologic and manometric studies. Diagnostic laparoscopic full-thickness biopsy of the small bowel may be required to establish the specific cause of the disease. Therapy focuses on palliation of symptoms and nutritional issues.

▶ Treatment

SBO is associated with a marked depletion of liquids caused by decreased oral intake, vomiting, and sequestration of fluid in the bowel lumen. Therefore, vigorous fluid resuscitation and correction of electrolyte disorders (hypochloremic, hypokalemic metabolic alkalosis) are mandatory. A urinary catheter should be placed to monitor urinary output.

Gastrointestinal decompression with a nasogastric tube provides relief of symptoms, prevents further gas and fluid accumulation proximally, and decreases the risk of aspiration. Obstruction that occurs in the early postoperative period is usually partial and only rarely associated with strangulation. Therefore, a period of prolonged total parenteral nutrition and hydration is warranted. Patients who have undergone numerous abdominal operations should initially be conservatively treated with decompression, bowel rest, and serial abdominal exams in hopes of avoiding reentering a hostile abdomen. Patients with Crohn disease rarely present with a complete bowel obstruction, and these patients often benefit from steroids or other immunosuppressive therapy. However, if signs suggestive of ischemia are detected, surgery should be promptly undertaken.

Finally, management of patients with diffuse carcinomatosis is often challenging and, in most of cases, limited to conservative and palliative treatment.

A. Surgery

Major predictors for surgery are persistent abdominal pain, persistent abdominal distention, fever, and high-grade obstruction detected by a CT scan. These findings are associated with failure of conservative management and increased risk of bowel strangulation. The surgical procedure performed varies according to the etiology of the obstruction. However, regardless of the cause of obstruction, all small bowel loops must be examined and nonviable segments resected. Criteria suggesting viability include normal pink color, presence of peristalsis, and arterial pulsation.

Laparoscopic adhesiolysis may be performed in carefully selected patients by surgeons skilled in this procedure. Generally, however, an open procedure is performed through an incision that is partly dictated by the location of scars from previous operations.

If the cause of the obstruction cannot be removed, as in the case of infiltration of vital structures by cancer or in the case of diffuse carcinomatosis, an anastomosis between proximal small bowel and small or large bowel distal to the obstruction (bypass) may be the best procedure in these patients. In some cases, a stoma may be the only choice of treatment.

▶ Prognosis

The vast majority (> 80%) of patients with adhesive SBO do not need an operation because they improve with medical therapy. Among patients who require surgery, the perioperative mortality rate for nonstrangulating obstruction is less than 5%; most of these deaths occur in elderly patients with significant comorbidities. Strangulating obstruction has a mortality rate of approximately 8% if surgery is performed within 36 hours of the onset of symptoms and 25% if operation is delayed beyond 36 hours.

Arung W, et al: Pathophysiology and prevention of postoperative peritoneal adhesions. *World J Gastroenterol.* 2011;17(41):4545-4553.

Branco BC, et al: Systematic review and meta-analysis of the diagnostic and therapeutic role of water-soluble contrast agent in adhesive small bowel obstruction. *Br J Surg.* 2010;97(4):470-478.

Ezer A, et al: Clinical outcomes of manual bowel decompression (milking) in the mechanical small bowel obstruction: a prospective randomized clinical trial. *Am J Surg.* 2012;203(1):95-100.

Maung AA, et al: Evaluation and management of small-bowel obstruction: an Eastern Association for the Surgery of Trauma practice management guideline. *J Trauma Acute Care Surg.* 2012;73(5 suppl 4):S362-S369.

Mullan CP, et al: Small bowel obstruction. *AJR Am J Roentgenol.* 2012;198(2):W105-W117.

O'Connor DB, et al: The role of laparoscopy in the management of acute small-bowel obstruction: a review of over 2,000 cases. *Surg Endosc.* 2012;26(1):12-17.

van der Wal JB, et al: Adhesion prevention during laparotomy: long-term follow-up of a randomized clinical trial. *Ann Surg.* 2011;253(6):1118-1121.

Xin L, et al: Indications, detectability, positive findings, total enteroscopy, and complications of diagnostic double-balloon endoscopy: a systematic review of data over the first decade of use. *Gastrointest Endosc.* 2011;74(3):563-570.

Zielinski MD, et al: Small bowel obstruction-who needs an operation? A multivariate prediction model. *World J Surg.* 2010;34(5):910-919.

CROHN DISEASE

▶ General Considerations

Crohn disease (CD) is a chronic inflammatory disease that commonly affects the small intestine, colon, rectum, and anus, but it can also involve the stomach, esophagus, and mouth. The most commonly affected location is the terminal ileum, and one-fifth of all patients have more than one intestinal segment affected simultaneously.

The United States, Canada, and Europe have the highest incidence of CD. The current estimated incidence of CD in the United States is approximately four new cases per year for every 100,000 persons, whereas the prevalence is much higher, between 80 and 150 cases per 100,000.

It is much less common in Asia, South America, and Japan, whereas accurate data regarding its incidence in Africa are lacking. The peak age for contracting CD is between 15 and 25 years. Familial clusters of disease are not uncommon, with a 6- to 10-fold increase in the risk of CD in first-degree relatives of those affected by CD or its sister ailment, ulcerative colitis. Although familial aggregations are common, the distribution within families does not indicate a pattern of simple Mendelian inheritance.

A. Etiology

The etiology of CD is unknown. CD is an altered immune response that results in inflammation and destruction of intestinal tissues. Whether this altered immune response is the result of a primary dysfunction in the gut-related immune system or whether an unknown pathologic trigger induces an otherwise normal immune system to overreact is still unclear. CD may occur in individuals with a genetic predisposition, whereas environmental triggers may start the pathologic sequence that ultimately manifests as CD.

To date, even though an increase in intestinal permeability in both CD patients and their symptom-free first-degree relatives has been demonstrated, no specific primary defect in the systemic or mucosal immune system has been identified. This may lead to an altered mucosal barrier function with abnormal interactions between the multitude of antigenic substrates normally found in the gut lumen and the immunocompetent tissue of the submucosa.

Concerning genetic predisposition, the *CARD15/NOD2* gene has been linked to susceptibility to CD. *CARD15* is a gene product related to innate immunity, and it is preferentially expressed to Paneth cells of the ileum. Nevertheless, the known mutations of *CARD15* are neither necessary nor sufficient to contract the disease. Hence, it appears that the genetic relationship of *CARD15/NOD2* to CD is complex and still poorly understood.

The hypothesis that infectious agents may play a role, either directly as a primary cause of CD or indirectly as a trigger to stimulate a defective immune system, has always found strength in the identification of noncaseating granulomas as the characteristic histopathologic lesion found in Crohn specimens and in the isolation of *Mycobacterium paratuberculosis* from resected CD specimens. Nevertheless, even sensitive polymerase chain reaction studies have been unable to provide definitive evidence for the presence of *M paratuberculosis*–specific DNA in CD-affected segments of the bowel. Other infectious agents, including measles virus, non-pylori *Helicobacter* species, *Pseudomonas*, and *Listeria monocytogenes* have been studied, but none of them has been consistently associated with CD.

Although diet modification can ameliorate the symptoms of CD, no dietary factor has been identified as a cause of CD. Smoking, however, has been associated with the development of CD. In addition, smoking is known to exacerbate existing CD and can accelerate the recurrence of disease after resection.

B. Pathology

CD has two different phases: the active phase and the remission phase, which is characterized by healing of the inflamed tissue. The histopathologic examination of the active phase of CD typically shows transmural inflammation characterized by multiple lymphoid aggregates in a thickened and edematous submucosa that can be found within the muscularis propria. Another typical microscopic feature of CD is the noncaseating granuloma. However, it is demonstrated in only 50% of resected specimens and is rarely detected on endoscopic biopsies. Additionally, the presence of granulomas does not correlate with disease activity.

Small mucosal ulcerations, called aphthous ulcers, are the earliest gross manifestations of CD. They appear as red spots or focal mucosal depressions, typically directly over submucosal lymphoid aggregates. As the inflammation progresses, the aphthous ulcers enlarge and become stellate. They then coalesce to form longitudinal mucosal ulcerations always along the mesenteric aspect of the bowel lumen. Further progression leads to a serpiginous network of linear ulcerations that surround islands of edematous mucosa producing the classic "cobblestone" appearance. Mucosal ulcerations may penetrate through the submucosa to form intramural channels that can bore deeply into the bowel wall and create sinuses, abscesses, or fistulas.

The inflammation of CD also involves the mesentery and regional lymph nodes such that the mesentery may become massively thickened. With early acute intestinal inflammation, the bowel wall is hyperemic and boggy. As the inflammation becomes chronic, fibrotic scarring develops, and the bowel wall becomes thickened and leathery in texture.

▶ Clinical Findings

A. Symptoms and Signs

The clinical presentation and symptoms of CD depend on the involved segment, the pattern and the severity of disease, and the associated complications. The onset of CD is often insidious, and many patients will experience some symptoms for months or even years before the diagnosis is made. The most common complaints are intermittent abdominal pain, bloating, diarrhea, nausea, vomiting, weight loss, and fever. Abdominal pain occurs in 90% of cases: when related to partial obstruction, it is mostly postprandial and crampy in nature, whereas when it is from septic complications, it is typically steady and associated with fever. Weight loss is usually related to food avoidance, but in severe cases, weight loss may be the result of malabsorption. Symptoms can also be related to complications, including abdominal mass, pneumaturia, perianal pain and swelling, or skin rash. Rarely, some patients can experience a more sudden onset of pain in the right lower quadrant, mimicking an acute appendicitis.

In patients suspected of having CD, a complete physical exam should include a thorough abdominal evaluation. In cases of ileal CD, tenderness is typically present in the right lower quadrant, and occasionally a palpable mass is present. The oral cavity should be examined for aphthous ulcers, whereas the presence of fistulas, abscesses, or enlarged skin tags should be assessed in the perianal area. A digital rectal examination should assess for the presence of anal strictures, fissures, and rectal mucosal ulcerations. The skin in the extremities should be examined for the presence of erythema nodosum and pyoderma gangrenosum.

B. Patterns of Disease

Even though CD can be categorized into three general manifestations, such as stricturing, perforating, and inflammatory disease, these three classes do not represent truly distinct forms of the disease. It is typical that the same patient can present with more than one pattern even in the same segment of bowel. Nevertheless, one pattern tends to be predominant in most cases, determining the clinical presentation and affecting the therapeutic options.

1. Stricturing pattern—Fibrotic scar tissue is the result of chronic inflammation of CD, and it constricts the intestinal lumen, with cicatricial strictures often referred to as "fibrostenotic lesions." Patients with a stricturing pattern of disease generally develop partial or complete intestinal obstruction, and hence their symptoms are primarily obstructive in nature. Being the result of scar tissue, these strictures are not reversible with medical therapy, and surgical intervention is often required.

2. Perforating pattern—Perforating CD is characterized by the development of sinus tracts, fistulae, and abscesses. The sinus tracts penetrate through the muscularis propria and give rise to abscesses or to fistulas if they penetrate into surrounding structures. Inflammatory response around the advancing sinus tract typically results in adhesion to surrounding structures; therefore, free perforation with spillage of intestinal contents into the abdominal cavity is uncommon. Typically, perforating disease is accompanied by a degree of stricture formation, but the fistula or abscess generated by the perforating component of the disease dominates the clinical picture.

3. Inflammatory pattern—The inflammatory pattern of CD is characterized by mucosal ulceration and bowel wall thickening. The edema that results from inflammation can lead to an adynamic segment of intestine and luminal narrowing. This pattern often gives rise to obstructive symptoms. Of the three patterns of disease, the inflammatory pattern is much more likely to respond to medical therapy.

Other common symptoms and findings include anorexia and weight loss. Patients may develop a palpable mass, usually located in the right lower quadrant, related to an abscess or phlegmon in perforating disease or a thickened loop of intestine in obstructive disease. Evidence of fistulization to the skin, urinary bladder, or vagina may also be elicited with an accurate history and physical exam.

C. Laboratory findings

There is no specific laboratory test that is diagnostic for CD. The diagnosis is made by a thorough history and physical examination along with intestinal radiography and endoscopy. Advanced imaging studies such as CT scan or magnetic resonance imaging (MRI) can assess or detect some of the complications and manifestations of CD, but they are generally not useful in making the initial diagnosis of CD.

D. Imaging Studies

Small bowel follow-through or enteroclysis is the best means for assessing the small bowel for CD. The radiographic abnormalities are often distinctive. Mucosal granulations with ulceration and nodularity can be identified in the early stages of the disease. Thickening of the mucosal folds and edema of the bowel wall can be demonstrated as the disease progresses. With more advanced disease, cobblestoning becomes radiographically apparent. Small bowel contrast studies can also provide information regarding enlargement of the mesentery, as well as formation of an inflammatory mass or abscess demonstrated by a general mass effect separating and displacing contrast-filled loops of small intestine. Even though small bowel contrast studies can demonstrate some of the complications of CD, including high-grade strictures and fistulas, they may not identify all such lesions, including ileosigmoid and ileovesical fistulas. In addition, small bowel studies may not demonstrate all the areas of disease with significant strictures. Small bowel radiographs can also help in assessing the extent of the disease by identifying the location and length of involved and uninvolved small bowel and by recognizing whether the disease is continuous or discontinuous, with skip lesions separated by areas of normal intestine. Experienced radiologists can also assess areas of luminal narrowing and determine if they are the result of acute inflammatory swelling or are the result of fibrostenotic scar tissue. Such a distinction provides valuable information regarding the value of medical therapy versus early surgical intervention, as inflammatory stenoses are likely to respond to medical therapy while fibrotic strictures are best treated with surgery.

CT findings of uncomplicated CD are nonspecific, and routine CT is not necessary for the diagnosis of CD. CT, however, is very useful in identifying the complications associated with CD, such as thickened and dilated intestinal loops, inflammatory masses, abscesses and hydronephrosis resulting from retroperitoneal fibrosis, and ureteral narrowing (Figure 31–4). CT is also the most sensitive indicator of an enterovesical fistula, as suggested by the presence of air within the urinary bladder. More recently, cross-sectional imaging techniques have assumed an increasing role in the imaging of patients with CD. CT enterography (CTE) has been shown to have a higher sensitivity than barium small-bowel follow-through. Based on these findings, CTE is often used combined with ileocolonoscopy as a first-line test for the diagnosis and staging of CD. CTE has several potential advantages over barium studies in the identification of

▲ **Figure 31–4.** Computed tomography scan showing a markedly thickened loop of distal ileum (arrow) causing obstruction of the more proximal small bowel in regional enteritis.

fistulizing disease: CTE does not suffer from superimposition of bowel loops, and it displays the mesentery, retroperitoneum, and abdominal wall musculature, typically involved by fistulas. CTE can also readily identify sinus tracts and abscesses. However, recent concerns about radiation-induced cancer arising from medically related CT in young CD patients have encouraged the use of magnetic resonance enterography (MRE). MRE has the same advantages of CTE but does not require ionizing radiation.

E. Endoscopy

Although upper endoscopy is useful in the diagnosis of mucosal lesions of the esophagus, stomach, and duodenum, a colonoscopy often allows the evaluation of the terminal ileum.

1. Capsule endoscopy—Capsule endoscopy can detect subtle mucosal lesions that may not be apparent on small bowel x-rays. The value of capsule endoscopy in the diagnosis of CD has been recently evaluated: the rate of abnormalities detected on capsule endoscopy is higher than that of CTE only for the subgroup of patients with known CD. The need for a preliminary small bowel contrast study to detect asymptomatic partial SBO before the capsule endoscopy and the lack of a clear advantage over other imaging studies limit the utility of capsule endoscopy as a first-line test in CD, and perhaps it is best to reserve this study for patients in whom there is a substantial diagnostic uncertainty.

Differential Diagnosis

The differential diagnosis includes irritable bowel syndrome, acute appendicitis, intestinal ischemia, pelvic inflammatory disease, endometriosis, and gynecologic malignancies. Other disorders include radiation enteritis, *Yersinia* infections, intestinal injury from nonsteroidal anti-inflammatory drugs (NSAIDs), intestinal tuberculosis, and small bowel tumors.

When malignancy is suspected, resection should be undertaken to make the diagnosis certain. The exclusion of intestinal tuberculosis can be difficult, as the inflammation and strictures of the terminal ileum can occur very similarly to CD. A previous exposure to tuberculosis should be evaluated, and a purified protein derivative skin test should be performed, along with chest radiography. Even when the diagnosis of CD is certain, patients who coincidentally are found to also have latent tuberculosis should be treated in accordance with American Thoracic Society guidelines prior to the initiation of immunosuppressive therapy for management of CD.

Intestinal injury from NSAIDs can result in focal enteritis with ulcerations and strictures. These manifestations can be very difficult to distinguish from CD of the small bowel and often require resection or biopsy to confirm the diagnosis.

▶ Treatment

A. Medical

Long-lasting symptomatic relief while avoiding excessive morbidity is the goal of medical treatment of CD. Even though CD cannot be cured by medical treatment, long periods of disease control can be obtained, thus avoiding a surgical intervention. Medical treatment is tailored to the course of the disease, the clinical presentation, and associated complications. Two different CD severity grading systems are used: the Crohn's Disease Activity Index (CDAI) and the Harvey-Bradshaw Index. These two scales identify patients with asymptomatic remission, mild to moderate CD, moderate to severe CD, and severe-fulminant disease.

Two different treatment modalities are used for mild to moderate CD: the step-up approach (starting with the least potent drugs) and the top-down approach (starting with more potent drugs, such as biologics or immunomodulators). The latter approach is more frequently used, aiming at minimizing the risk of dependence to glucocorticoids.

Corticosteroids have been widely used for controlling acute exacerbations of CD in the short term, but their use is limited due to the risk of serious side effects, including diabetes, osteoporosis, cataracts, osteonecrosis, myopathy, psychosis, opportunistic infections, and adrenal suppression, that are related to the dose and duration of steroid therapy. The majority of patients with active small bowel CD will experience clinical remission with a short course of oral prednisone given in a dose between 0.25 and 0.5 mg/kg/d. For patients unable to take oral medications, methylprednisolone can be administered in adults at doses of 40-60 mg given as a daily infusion. Some patients do not respond to corticosteroid therapy (steroid-resistant) or experience disease flares when tapering off the medication (steroid-dependent).

The *aminosalicylates* include sulfasalazine and 5-aminosalicylic acid (5-ASA) derivatives. They inhibit leukotriene production by inhibiting 5-lipooxygenase activity and the production of interleukin-1 and tumor necrosis factor (TNF). Aminosalicylates are effective in the treatment of mild to moderate CD. 5-ASA given in a controlled-release preparation is also effective as maintenance therapy to prevent recurrence after a flare of disease has been effectively managed either medically or surgically.

Aminosalicylates come in a variety of preparations, each designed to deliver the drug in a topical fashion to the affected bowel segments. For instance, Asacol is 5-ASA contained within a pH-dependent resin that releases the drug in the terminal ileum and colon where the pH is > 7.0. Pentasa is 5-ASA contained within ethylcellulose-coated microgranules that slowly releases the active compound throughout the entire small bowel and colon. *Azathioprine* and *6-mercaptopurine (6-MP)* are immunosuppressive agents that inhibit cytotoxic T-cell and natural killer cell function. These agents are effective in treating mild to moderate CD. Azathioprine given at 2.0-2.5 mg/kg/d or 6-MP in doses of 1.0-1.5 mg/kg/d will result in a 50%-60% response rate in patients with active CD. Both 6-MP and azathioprine are also effective in maintaining remission following surgery or successful medical management.

Infliximab is a chimeric mouse-human monoclonal antibody to TNF that is a proinflammatory cytokine that may be important in the pathophysiology of CD. Infliximab binds to both free and membrane-bound TNF and prevents TNF from binding to its cell surface receptors. Clinical trials have demonstrated am 80% response rate with a single dose of infliximab. It is important to note that the doses and dosing intervals of infliximab must be individualized, but a typical regimen would include 5 mg/kg of infliximab given intravenously (IV) at weeks 0, 2, and 6, with a dose of 5 mg/kg every 8 weeks thereafter. Because infliximab is a potent immunosuppressive agent, concerns have been raised about the risk for poor wound healing and postoperative septic complications. Nevertheless, current available data on the perioperative risks associated with infliximab do not seem to support this hypothesis.

Other agents that are used with varying success in the treatment of CD include methotrexate, metronidazole, cyclosporine, tacrolimus, and thalidomide.

B. Surgical Therapy

Similarly to medical treatment, the goal of surgical treatment of CD is to provide long-lasting symptomatic relief while avoiding excessive morbidity. Like medical treatment, surgery should be considered palliative. Therefore, treatment of complications and palliation of symptoms while avoiding excessive resection of small bowel should be the main aims of surgical treatment.

To avoid excessive loss of small bowel, nonresectional techniques such as strictureplasty may be required. In addition, optimal surgical therapy should be the resection of only the areas of severe and symptomatic CD, leaving behind segments of small bowel affected by mild but asymptomatic CD based on the high risks of recurrence and repeated operations.

Adequate preoperative patient preparation is mandatory to reduce the risk of postoperative complications, assessing the nutritional status, the smoking habits, and the entity of small intestine involvement by CD. Recent evidence shows that preoperative immunosuppressive medications have limited impact on the outcomes and can be safely discontinued before surgery. Patients should always be counselled about the possible need for a stoma construction in both elective and emergent settings.

C. Indications for Surgery

1. Failure of medical treatment—The most common indications for surgical treatment of CD are the failure to respond to medical treatment and the inability to tolerate effective therapy, due to the occurrence of complications related to the medical treatment or the progression of disease while on maximal medical treatment. Some patients may respond to the initial medical therapy only to rapidly relapse with tapering of the medical treatment. For example, some patients respond well to steroid therapy but become steroid-dependent as tapering of the steroid dose results in recurrent symptoms. Due to the severe complications that are virtually inevitable with prolonged steroid treatment, surgery is warranted if the patient cannot be weaned from systemic steroids within 3-6 months.

2. Intestinal obstruction—Partial or complete intestinal obstruction is a common indication for operation. The clinical presentation of chronic partial SBO is much more typical than complete obstruction, and postprandial cramps, abdominal distension, borborygmi, and weight loss are common symptoms. To avoid them, many patients restrict the diet to soft foods or even liquids. In case of partial obstruction primarily due to acute inflammation and bowel wall thickening, initial medical therapy is warranted. If, however, the obstructive symptoms are secondary to high-grade fibrostenotic lesions, surgery is indicated because medical treatment will not reverse these lesions.

When complete intestinal obstruction occurs, initial conservative treatment consists of nasogastric decompression and IV hydration along with administration of IV steroids. This treatment leads to decompression of acutely distended and edematous bowel and, in most cases, to resolution of the complete obstruction. However, even patients with complete resolution of the acute obstruction after the initial conservative treatment are at high risk for recurrent episodes of obstruction and are best managed with elective surgery once adequate decompression and resuscitation are achieved. If the obstruction fails to respond to appropriate conservative treatment, then surgery is required. In these situations, a high index of suspicion for small bowel cancer as the cause of the obstruction is mandatory, as obstructions from cancers do not respond to bowel decompression and steroid treatment.

3. Fistulas—Intestinal fistulas occur in one-third of CD patients. However, the presence of an intestinal fistula is not in and of itself an indication for surgery. In general, it is the primary indication for surgery if the fistula is in connection with the genitourinary tract, if its drainage causes personal embarrassment and discomfort (enterocutaneous and enterovaginal fistulas), or if a bypass causing intestinal malabsorption is created.

Fistulas can be classified according to anatomic site, characteristics of the tract (simple vs complex), and volume of output (high vs low). A low-volume output is less than 200 mL/24 h, whereas high-volume output is more than 500 mL/24 h.

4. Ileosigmoid fistulas—Ileosigmoid fistula is a common complication of perforating CD of the terminal ileum. Typically, the inflamed terminal ileum adheres to the sigmoid colon, which is otherwise healthy. Most ileosigmoid fistulas are small and asymptomatic. These ileosigmoid fistulas do not in and of themselves require operative management. However, large ileosigmoid fistulas can result in bypass of the intestinal contents from the terminal ileum to the distal colon and thus give rise to debilitating diarrhea. Such symptomatic fistulas should be managed surgically, because they often fail to respond to medical therapy.

More than half of the ileosigmoid fistulas from CD are recognized intraoperatively. Ileosigmoid fistulas can be managed by simple division of the fistulous adhesion and resection of the ileal disease. The defect in the sigmoid colon is then debrided, and simple closure is undertaken. In about 25% of cases, resection of the sigmoid colon is needed, particularly when primary closure of the fistula is at risk for poor healing. This is the case when the sigmoid is also involved in CD, when the fistulous opening is particularly large, or when there is extensive fibrosis extending along the sigmoid colon. In addition, fistulous tracts that enter the sigmoid colon in proximity to the mesentery can be difficult to close and often require resection and primary anastomosis.

5. Ileovesical fistula—Ileovesical fistulae occur in approximately 5% of CD patients. Although hematuria and fecaluria are virtually diagnostic of ileovesical fistula, these symptoms are absent in almost 30% of cases. Air within the bladder, as noted on CT scan, is often the best indirect evidence for the presence of an enterovesical fistula, whereas small bowel x-rays, cystogram, and cystoscopy often do not detect the fistula. An ileovesical fistula is an indicator of complex fistulizing disease, as most ileovesical fistulas occur along with other enteric fistulae.

The necessity for surgery for ileovesical fistula is controversial. Although it is not mandatory to operate on all cases of enterovesical fistulas, surgery is warranted to avoid deterioration of renal function with recurrent infections or if symptoms persist despite appropriate medical therapy.

Surgical treatment of ileovesical fistulae requires resection of the ileal disease with closure of the bladder defect. Most ileovesical fistulas involve the dome of the bladder, and thus, debridement and primary closure can be accomplished without any risk of injury to the trigone. Decompression of the bladder with an indwelling Foley catheter should be continued postoperatively until the bladder is confidently healed without leaks. A cystogram taken postoperatively is useful to confirm the seal of the bladder repair, before removing the Foley catheter.

6. Enterovaginal and enterocutaneous fistulas—These are rare fistulas caused by perforating small bowel disease draining through the vaginal stump in a female who has previously undergone a hysterectomy or through the abdominal wall, usually at the site of a previous scar. These fistulas often require surgical intervention because they cause physical discomfort and personal embarrassment. Surgical treatment requires resection of the small bowel disease. The vaginal cuff does not need to be closed; the chronic infection along the abdominal wall fistulous tract requires debridement and wide drainage to allow healing by secondary intention.

7. Abscess—Intra-abdominal CD abscesses tend to have an indolent course with modest fever, abdominal pain, and leukocytosis. In up to 30% of cases, preoperative clinical signs of localized infection are absent and the abscesses are discovered only at the time of operation. When an abscess is suspected or an abdominal mass is palpated, a CT scan should be obtained, as 50% of tender intra-abdominal masses will harbor an abscess collection within. The CT scan can detect most chronic abscesses and can also delineate the size and location of the abscess as well as the relationship of the abscess to critical structures such as the ureters, duodenum, and inferior vena cava.

In the majority of cases, abscesses are very small collections contained within the area of diseased small bowel and its mesentery. In the case of small intraloop or intramesenteric abscesses, resection of the involved bowel segment and its mesentery often extirpates the abscess such that drains

are not necessary and primary anastomosis can be performed without risk.

Large abscesses are best managed with CT-guided percutaneous drainage. However, an abscess drained percutaneously is very likely to recur or result in an enterocutaneous fistula, and surgical resection is often advised even after successful drainage. Such a fistula may spontaneously close, or it may persist and the intestine may continue to be a source of sepsis. With successful drainage of the abscess, the sepsis often clears well enough that it can be tempting to try to manage the disease without subsequent surgery. In the absence of symptoms, initial nonoperative management after successful percutaneous drainage can be undertaken in carefully selected patients. If drainage through the fistula continues, surgical resection of the affected segment of intestine becomes necessary.

8. Perforation—Free perforation is a rare complication of CD, occurring in less than 1% of patients, because the chronic progressive inflammation of CD usually leads to adhesions with adjacent structures, and it is an obvious indication for urgent operation with resection of the diseased segment and exteriorization of the proximal bowel as an end ileostomy. The diagnosis of free perforation is made by detecting a sudden change in the patient's symptoms along with the development of the physical findings of peritonitis or the identification of free intraperitoneal air as demonstrated on plain x-rays or CT scan. The use of immunosuppressants and glucocorticosteroids can blunt many of the physical findings of acute perforation; therefore, the index of suspicion for perforation must be higher in immunocompromised patients.

Creation of a primary anastomosis even with a proximal protecting loop ileostomy carries a high risk of anastomotic breakdown and should be avoided. Primary closure of the perforation should never be attempted, as sutures will not be able to approximate the edges of the perforated, edematous, and diseased bowel in a satisfactory and tension-free way and the presence of a distal intestinal stenosis or partial obstruction will cause an increase in the intraluminal pressure at the level of the local repair with subsequent dehiscence.

9. Hemorrhage—Hemorrhage is an uncommon complication from small bowel CD. Angiography in the presence of brisk bleeding leads to localization of the site of bleeding. Bleeding from small bowel tends to be indolent with episodic or chronic bleeding requiring intermittent transfusions, but rarely requires emergent surgery. However, because the risk of recurrent bleeding is high, elective resection of the areas of CD is recommended. Finally, risk for bleeding from peptic ulcer disease is increased in patients, particularly in those receiving corticosteroids.

10. Cancer or suspicion of cancer—The presence of CD increases the risk of adenocarcinoma of the small bowel.

The diagnosis of adenocarcinoma of the small bowel is difficult because symptoms and radiographic findings can be similar to those of the underlying CD. Male patients, patients with long-standing disease, and patients with defunctionalized segments of bowel appear to be at increased risk for small bowel adenocarcinoma. For this reason, bypass surgery should be avoided for CD of the small intestine, and defunctionalized rectal stumps should either be restored to their function or excised.

Adenocarcinoma of the small intestine should be suspected in any patient with long-standing disease whose symptoms of obstruction progress after a lengthy quiescent period.

11. Growth retardation—Growth retardation occurs in a quarter of children affected by CD. Although steroid treatment may delay growth in children, the major cause of growth retardation in CD patients is due to the malnutrition associated with active intestinal disease.

D. Surgical Options

1. Intestinal resection—Intestinal resection with anastomosis is the most common surgical procedure performed for the treatment of small bowel CD. In most cases of CD, only limited resections are required with no risk for short bowel syndrome. Only grossly apparent disease should be resected, as wider resections do not improve the surgical outcomes. Grossly normal resection margins with microscopic evidence for CD activity are not associated with early recurrence or other complications. Therefore, intraoperative frozen section of the resection margins is not necessary.

The extent of mesenteric dissection does not affect the long-term results. Division of the thickened mesentery of small bowel CD can be the most challenging aspect of the procedure, as identification and dissection of individual mesenteric vessels is often not feasible. A common technique consists of the application of overlapping clamps on either side of the intended line of transection. The mesentery is then divided between the clamps, and the tissue contained within the clamps is suture ligated. In severe cases, a vascular clamp may be used at the root of the small bowel mesentery to obtain proximal control: mattress sutures may then need to be applied to the cut edge of the mesentery to control bleeding. Even when tissue-welding devices such as the LigaSure device are used, mattress sutures in the mesentery are commonly needed for complete hemostasis.

2. Anastomosis—There is no consensus regarding the optimal technique for intestinal anastomosis in CD. Recurrent CD after resection of terminal ileum is most likely to occur at the ileocolonic anastomosis or at the preanastomotic ileum. It has been proposed that large-caliber anastomoses require a longer period to stricture down to a critical diameter that becomes symptomatic. The argument is made that a longer side-to-side anastomosis may be beneficial over an end-to-end or end-to-side anastomosis. To date, however, clinical data do not indicate a benefit for one particular intestinal configuration over another. Intestinal anastomosis for CD cases can be fashioned with a stapling device or may be hand sutured. Under selective conditions, small bowel anastomotic dehiscence rates are less than 1%. In the presence of sepsis, severe scarring, malnutrition, or recent treatment with methotrexate or infliximab, it may be wise to protect the anastomosis with a proximal loop stoma or to forego the anastomosis altogether and bring out an end stoma at the point of resection.

3. Bypass procedures—Initially conceived to bypass an area of stricture or obstruction, the use of bypass procedures was eventually extended to CD complicated by septic complications. Increased experience with bypass procedures revealed that patients with persistent disease are at higher risk of persistent sepsis and eventually neoplastic transformation. Therefore, bypass procedures were supplanted by limited intestinal resection as the main surgical option in the late 1960s in all intestinal districts except the duodenum, where a simple side-to-side retrocolic gastrojejunostomy adequately relieves the obstructive symptoms. With increased experience in the performance of strictureplasty, duodenal disease is now more and more commonly handled with strictureplasties.

4. Strictureplasty—Strictureplasties are best performed when resection would otherwise result in loss of a long segment of bowel with an increased risk for short bowel syndrome, including cases of stricturing disease involving long segments of bowel and patients with multiple prior resections. They are also indicated as a simpler alternative to resection in case of short recurrent disease at a previous ileocolic or enteroenteric anastomosis.

There is increased evidence that the acuity of the disease decreases at the site of the strictureplasty and the disease becomes quiescent, maybe in correlation with a simultaneous restoration of absorptive function.

The most commonly performed strictureplasty is the *Heinecke-Mikulicz strictureplasty*, which is appropriate for short segment strictures of 2-5 cm in length. A longitudinal incision is made along the antimesenteric border of the stricture extending for 1-2 cm into the normal elastic bowel on either side of the stricture. Once the enterotomy is made, the area of the stricture should be closely examined to rule out a malignancy. The longitudinal enterotomy of the Heinecke-Mikulicz strictureplasty is then closed in a transverse fashion with either single- or double-layered sutures.

The *Finney strictureplasty* can be used for strictures up to 15 cm in length. The strictured segment is folded onto itself in a U shape, and a row of seromuscular sutures is placed between the two arms of the U. A longitudinal U-shaped enterotomy is then made paralleling the row of sutures.

The mucosal surface is examined, and biopsies are taken as necessary. In essence, the Finney is a short side-to-side functional anastomosis. A very long Finney strictureplasty may result in a functional bypass with a large lateral diverticulum that, in theory, could be at risk for bacterial overgrowth and the blind loop syndrome. However, this theoretical concern has not been observed in clinical practice.

Repeated Heinecke-Mikulicz or Finney strictureplasties to manage multiple strictures should be separated from each other by at least 5 cm, in order to avoid excessive tension on each suture line.

Patients with long-segment stricturing disease and multiple strictures grouped close together are best managed with a side-to-side isoperistaltic strictureplasty, also called *Michelassi strictureplasty*: the segment of stricturing disease is divided at its midpoint. The proximal and distal ends are then drawn onto each other in a side-to-side fashion. Division of some of the mesenteric vascular arcades facilitates the positioning of the two limbs over each other. The proximal and distal loops are then sutured together with a layer of interrupted seromuscular sutures. A longitudinal enterotomy is then made along both of the loops. The intestinal ends are spatulated to provide a smoothly tailored fit to the ultimate closure of the strictureplasty. The outer suture line is reinforced with an interior row of either interrupted or running full-thickness sutures. This inner suture line is continued anteriorly. The anterior closure is then reinforced with an outer layer of interrupted seromuscular sutures to complete the strictureplasty.

Other stricturoplasty techniques are the *Judd stricturoplasty,* the *Moskel-Walske-Neumayer stricturoplasty,* and the *Jaboulay stricturoplasty.*

In appropriately selected patients, perioperative morbidity from strictureplasty appears to be similar to that of resection and primary anastomosis. Specifically, intestinal suture line dehiscence appears to be uncommon with any of the described strictureplasty techniques. The most common postoperative complication directly related to strictureplasty is hemorrhage from the strictureplasty site, in up to 9% of cases. Usually, the gastrointestinal hemorrhage following strictureplasty is minor and can be managed conservatively with transfusions alone. Rarely, a reoperation to control hemorrhage after strictureplasty is necessary. It is by now also well established that strictureplasty techniques provide excellent long-term symptomatic relief, which is comparable to resections with anastomosis.

5. Laparoscopy—Most CD patients are well suited for laparoscopy. They are usually young, otherwise healthy, and interested in undergoing an operation that involves minimal scarring, because they are facing the risk of multiple major abdominal operations in their lifetime.

The indications for laparoscopic surgery for CD should not differ from conventional open surgery, as described earlier. Contraindications to a laparoscopic approach include patients who are critically ill and unable to tolerate the pneumoperitoneum due to hypotension or hypercarbia, patients with extensive intra-abdominal sepsis (abscess, free perforation, or complex fistula), and difficulty in identifying the anatomy (previous surgery, obesity, or adhesions). The same variety of surgical procedures described earlier can be performed laparoscopically.

► Management of Crohn Disease of the Duodenum

Primary CD of the duodenum almost always manifests with stricturing disease that can be managed by strictureplasty or with bypass procedures, whereas resection of the duodenum for CD is almost never required. When CD fistulas involve the duodenum, it is always the result of disease within a distal segment of the small bowel that fistulizes into an otherwise normal duodenum. Heinecke-Mikulicz strictureplasties can be safely performed in the first, second, and proximal third portions of the duodenum, whereas strictures of the last portion of the duodenum are better handled with a Finney strictureplasty constructed by creating an enteroenterostomy between the fourth portion of the duodenum and the first loop of the jejunum.

If the duodenal stricture is lengthy or the tissues around the stricture are too rigid or unyielding, then a strictureplasty should not be performed and an intestinal bypass procedure should be undertaken. The most common bypass procedure performed for duodenal CD is a side-to-side retrocolic gastrojejunostomy. This procedure effectively relieves the symptoms of duodenal obstruction related to CD strictures, but carries a high risk for stomal ulcerations. To lessen the likelihood of ulcerations forming at the anastomosis, it has been recommended that a selective vagotomy be performed along with the gastrojejunostomy in order to reduce the risk of vagotomy-related diarrhea. If only the third or fourth portions of the duodenum are involved by the structuring CD, a Roux-en-Y duodenojejunostomy to the proximal duodenum is preferred over a gastrojejunostomy, with the Roux-en-Y duodenojejunostomy having the advantage of bypassing strictures and eliminating the risk of acid-induced marginal ulceration and the need for vagotomy.

Most of these duodenal fistulas are small in caliber and asymptomatic, but larger fistulas may shunt the duodenal contents to the distal small bowel, resulting in malabsorption and diarrhea. In most cases, duodenoenteric fistulas are identified with preoperative small bowel radiography; however, many are discovered only intraoperatively. Most duodenal fistulas are located away from the pancreaticoduodenal margin, and thus these fistulas can be managed by resection of the primary CD with primary closure of the duodenal defect. In case of larger fistulas or fistulas that are involved with a large degree of inflammation, closure with a Roux-en-Y duodenojejunostomy or with a jejunal serosal patch may be required.

A. Prognosis

The risk for recurrence after surgery is high in CD patients. Most cases of histologic or endoscopically detected recurrences, however, do not produce symptoms of CD. For this reason, histologic or endoscopic evidence of recurrent disease is not typically used as a guide for clinical management.

The development of symptoms related to recurrent CD activity is the most commonly applied definition of disease recurrence, because it is the recurrence of symptoms that has the most relevance to the patient. The onset of symptoms of recurrent CD is often insidious, and the severity of symptoms varies greatly. A CDAI greater than 150 is generally accepted as defining clinical recurrence. Once symptoms suggestive of recurrent disease occur, it is necessary to carry out radiologic and endoscopic tests to confirm that the symptoms are in fact related to CD.

The clearest end point as a definition of recurrence is the need for reoperation. While reoperation is the most precise definition of recurrence, even this standard does not allow for accurate and reproducible comparisons between series, as some centers may submit patients to surgery earlier than other centers.

Reported crude and cumulative recurrence rates vary greatly. Symptomatic recurrence occurs in about 60% of patients at 5 years, and recurrences increase with time such that at 20 years clinical recurrence can occur in between 75% and 95% of cases. Reports of surgical recurrence rates range from 10%-30% at 5 years, 20%-45% at 10 years, and 50%-70% at 20 years. Recurrent CD is most likely to occur in proximity to the location of the previously resected intestinal segment, typically at the anastomosis and preanastomotic bowel, in particular in case of terminal ileal disease. In addition, the length of small bowel involved with recurrent disease parallels the length of disease originally resected. Also, to a lesser degree of concordance, stenotic disease tends to recur as stenotic disease and perforating disease tends to recur as perforating disease.

Although many factors that may influence the risk of recurrence have been studied, the cumulative literature has validated very few as true risk factors. Cigarette smoking has a significant effect on the clinical course of CD. Smoking not only exacerbates existing CD, but also has been identified as a risk factor for the development of CD and for endoscopic, symptomatic, and surgical recurrence. Although the mechanism by which smoking results in exacerbation of CD is not known, the risk from smoking appeared to be dose-related, with heavy smokers being at higher risk, and reversible. There is concern that NSAIDs may exacerbate the activity of both ulcerative colitis and CD, but the data are not conclusive.

The risk for recurrent disease can be reduced with postoperative maintenance therapy. The most common agents are controlled-release 5-ASA and 6-MP. Maintenance with 5-ASA is associated with few side effects, but up to 16 pills have to be taken daily. 6-MP is less expensive and is taken on a once-daily basis. In addition, 6-MP may be more effective in diminishing the risk of recurrence. 6-MP, however, is associated with potential bone marrow suppression, so that patients on 6-MP maintenance must be followed with periodic blood cell counts.

Al-Hawary M, et al: A new look at Crohn's disease: novel imaging techniques. *Curr Opin Gastroenterol*. 2012;28(4):334-340.

Campbell L, et al: Comparison of conventional and nonconventional strictureplasties in Crohn's disease: a systematic review and meta-analysis. *Dis Colon Rectum*. 2012;55(6):714-726.

Choy PY, et al: Stapled versus handsewn methods for ileocolic anastomoses. *Cochrane Database Syst Rev*. 2011;9:CD004320.

Cunningham MF, et al: Postsurgical recurrence of ileal Crohn's disease: an update on risk factors and intervention points to a central role for impaired host-microflora homeostasis. *World J Surg*. 2010;34(7):1615-1626.

Danese S: New therapies for inflammatory bowel disease: from the bench to the bedside. *Gut*. 2012;61(6):918-932.

Fichera A: Crohn's disease: How modern is the management of fistulizing disease? *Nat Rev Gastroenterol Hepatol*. 2009; 6(9):511-512.

Fichera A: Laparoscopic treatment of Crohn's disease. *World J Surg*. 2011;35(7):1500-1504.

Kopylov U, et al: Anti-tumor necrosis factor and postoperative complications in Crohn's disease: systematic review and meta-analysis. *Inflamm Bowel Dis*. 2012;18(12):2404-2413.

Maggiori L, et al: How I do it: side-to-side isoperistaltic strictureplasty for extensive Crohn's disease. *J Gastrointest Surg*. 2012; 16(10):1976-1980.

Turner D, et al: Maintenance of remission in inflammatory bowel disease using omega-3 fatty acids (fish oil): a systematic review and meta-analyses. *Inflamm Bowel Dis*. 2011;17(1):336-345.

SMALL INTESTINAL FISTULAS

General Considerations

Small intestinal fistulas are an abnormal connection between two epithelial lined organs. Enterocutaneous fistulas (ECFs) are the most common small intestinal fistulas, followed by enteroenteric fistulas, enterovesical fistulas, enterovaginal fistulas, and vascular enteric fistulas. Although they may form spontaneously as a result of a disease, about 80% are iatrogenic (anastomotic dehiscence or injury to the bowel during dissection or abdominal wall closure). Fistulas are particularly prone to develop when the surgeon encounters extensive adhesions, inflamed intestine, radiation enteritis, a malnourished patient, or emergency procedures. Ileum is the most common site of ECF. ECF classification is based on the daily output, with an ECF being defined as a low-output (< 200 mL of daily fluid drainage), moderate-output

(200-500 mL of daily drainage), or high-output (> 500 mL of daily drainage) fistula.

Five mechanisms of small intestinal fistulas have been identified: congenital (rare), trauma, infection, perforation/injury, and inflammation/irradiation/tumor.

Clinical Findings

A. Symptoms and Signs

Postoperative fistula formation is heralded by fever, abdominal pain, and distention. Frequently a wound infection is recognized and drained 7-10 days postoperatively with subsequent discharge of enteric contents through the abdominal incision. Spontaneous fistulas from neoplasms or inflammatory disease usually develop in a more indolent manner. ECFs are often associated with abscesses, which often drain incompletely with fistulization, so that persistent sepsis is a common feature. Intestinal fluid escaping through the fistula may severely excoriate the skin and abdominal wall tissues. Persistent sepsis and difficulty in nourishing the patient contribute to rapid weight loss.

B. Laboratory Findings

Routine laboratory tests reflect the severity of deficits in red cell mass, plasma volume, and electrolytes. Hypokalemia is the most common electrolyte abnormality. Ongoing losses may be significant, especially with high-output fistulas necessitating serial measurement of serum electrolytes. Leukocytosis due to sepsis and hemoconcentration is common.

C. Imaging Studies

The goals of imaging are to detect concurrent abdominal pathology and to characterize the fistula. Contrast studies with contrast medium administered orally, per rectum, or through the fistula (fistulogram) delineate the abnormal anatomy, including intrinsic bowel disease, and demonstrate the location and number of fistulae, the length and course of fistula tracts, associated abscess cavities, and the presence of distal obstruction. Radiologists can manipulate catheters into tracts and provide detailed diagnostic information; this procedure may also be therapeutic (see later in chapter). CT scans, endoscopy, and other special studies may be indicated in certain individuals.

Complications

Fluid and electrolyte losses, malnutrition, hemorrhage, and sepsis contribute to multiple-organ failure and death unless effective therapy is instituted promptly.

Treatment

The initial management of an ECF involves recognition of the fistula, control of sepsis, resuscitation, local wound care, and nutritional optimization. A systematic approach combining diagnostic, supportive, and operative procedures is essential in the management of patients with fistulas (Table 31–1). In few other conditions is the proper timing of operative intervention more critical.

Table 31–1. Treatment of fistulas.

First
Restore blood volume and begin correction of fluids and electrolyte imbalance.
Drain accessible abscesses.
Control fistula and measure losses.
Begin nutritional support.
Second
Delineate anatomy of fistulas by radiographic studies.
Third
Maintain caloric intake of 2000–3000 kcal or more per day, depending on status of nutrition and energy expenditure.
Drain abscesses as they appear.
Fourth
Operate if fistula fails to close.

A. Fluid and Electrolyte Resuscitation

Many fistula patients are profoundly depleted of intravascular and interstitial volume, especially if the fistula is large, if it is proximal, or if there is partial or complete intestinal obstruction distal to the fistula, and correction of hypovolemia and electrolyte imbalances is the first priority. Central venous pressure, urine output, and skin turgor are guides to the progress of volume resuscitation. Fluid and electrolyte resuscitation can usually be accomplished within the first day or two. Subsequent maintenance of homeostasis depends on accurately measuring losses and replacing them.

B. Control of Fistula

Fistulous effluent must be collected to avoid excoriation of skin and abdominal wall tissues and to record volume losses. An ostomy appliance or pouch should be placed around the fistula and needs to be tailored based on the characteristics of the fistula. Alternatively, a catheter inserted by a radiologist under x-ray guidance may work best. In selected cases, a vacuum-assisted wound management device can be used to control fistula drainage and accelerate closure of the fistula. The assistance of a skilled and experienced wound care and/or enterostomal nurse is indispensable.

C. Control of Sepsis

Abscesses should be drained as soon as they are diagnosed. While therapy with broad-spectrum antibiotics may be necessary to control infection, they are not a substitute for proper management of abscesses. Most contained abscesses can be drained percutaneously with CT or ultrasound guidance. Drainage catheters should be left in place until the abscess cavity has resolved, which can be confirmed with a drain study once drainage has ceased. A drain study can also demonstrate the presence of persistent communication between the small bowel and the fistula. Free drainage of enteral contents into the abdominal cavity will likely cause peritonitis, necessitating an emergent laparotomy.

D. Delineation of Fistula

Radiographic contrast studies (see earlier in chapter) should be obtained as soon as feasible.

E. Nutrition

Adequate nutrition and control of sepsis make the difference between survival and death for these patients. A useful general rule is to avoid oral intake during the initial stage of treatment. Nasogastric suction may be necessary temporarily. As soon as fluid, electrolyte, and vitamin abnormalities are corrected, parenteral nutrition should be instituted via a central intravenous catheter.

For many patients, total parenteral nutrition is the principal exogenous source of calories and nitrogen until the fistula heals or is closed surgically. For patients with low-output or distal fistulas, the enteral route for nutrition is preferred, and elemental or polymeric diets can be delivered into the distal gut in some patients with proximal fistulas.

F. Other Measures

H_2 receptor antagonists and proton pump inhibitors are useful adjuncts in patients with proximal fistulas. By reducing gastric acid secretion, fistula output is decreased, and fluid and electrolyte management is simplified. Somatostatin analogs decrease fistula output and may accelerate fistula closure.

G. Operation

About 30% of fistulas close spontaneously with proper medical management. CD, irradiated bowel, cancer, foreign body, distal obstruction, extensive disruption of intestinal continuity, and a short (< 2 cm) fistula tract are associated with failure of fistulas to heal. Fibrin glue has been effective in some small bowel fistulas; in particular, it may be considered in complicated patients with a history of a hostile abdomen. Treatment may be successful if the fistula is long and the output is low. If they are going to heal spontaneously, fistulas usually close within 5-6 weeks after eradication of infection and institution of adequate nutritional support. Patients who fail 6 weeks of nonoperative management will often require surgical intervention. Serum levels of short-turnover proteins,

particularly transferrin, might be useful in predicting which patients are unlikely to close their fistulas. The operation should be postponed, however, until one can predict that the phase of dense adhesions associated with ECFs has resolved, and nutrition is optimized typically at least 3 months after the last operation. The fistulous segment should be resected, associated obstruction relieved, and continuity reestablished by a functional end-to-end anastomosis.

▶ Prognosis

The plan of management outlined earlier results in survival rates of 80%-95% in patients with external fistulas. Uncontrolled sepsis is the chief cause of death.

Coughlin S, et al: Somatostatin analogues for the treatment of enterocutaneous fistulas: a systematic review and meta-analysis. *World J Surg.* 2012;36(5):1016-1029.

Lee JK, et al: Radiographic and endoscopic diagnosis and treatment of enterocutaneous fistulas. *Clin Colon Rectal Surg.* 2010; 23(3):149-160.

Martinez JL, et al: Factors predictive of recurrence and mortality after surgical repair of enterocutaneous fistula. *J Gastrointest Surg.* 2012;16(1):156-163.

Visschers RG, et al. Guided treatment improves outcome of patients with enterocutaneous fistulas. *World J Surg.* 2012;36(10): 2341-2348.

BLIND LOOP SYNDROME

The normal concentration of bacteria in the small intestine is about 105/mL. Mechanisms that limit bacterial populations include the continual flow of luminal contents, gastric acidity, local effects of immunoglobulins, and the prevention of reflux of colonic contents by the ileocecal valve. Disturbance of any of these mechanisms can lead to bacterial overgrowth and blind loop syndrome. Strictures, diverticula, fistulas, and defunctionalized segments of bowel allow bacterial proliferation.

This entity is rare, and clinical manifestations include steatorrhea, diarrhea, abdominal pain, vitamin deficiency, neurologic symptoms, anemia, and weight loss. Steatorrhea is the consequence of bacterial deconjugation and dehydroxylation of bile salts in the proximal small bowel. Deconjugated bile salts have a higher critical micellar concentration, and micelle formation is inadequate to solubilize ingested fat in preparation for absorption. The presence of partially digested triglycerides in the distal ileum inhibits jejunal motility; nevertheless, the unabsorbed fatty acids enter the colon, where they increase net secretion of water and electrolytes, and diarrhea results. Hypocalcemia occurs because calcium is bound to unabsorbed fatty acids in the intestinal lumen. Macrocytic anemia is secondary to malabsorption of vitamin B_{12}, largely because it is consumed by anaerobic bacteria. Vitamin B_{12} deficiency also causes neurologic symptoms due to demyelination of the posterior and lateral spinal columns. Malabsorption of carbohydrate and protein is due partly to bacterial catabolism and partly to impaired absorption of these nutrients because of direct damage to the small intestinal mucosa. All of these mechanisms contribute to malnutrition.

Quantitative culture of upper intestinal aspirates is valuable if properly performed; bacterial counts of more than 10^5 per mL are generally abnormal. Endoscopic biopsies of the duodenum can be helpful in patients with suspected small intestinal malabsorption. Laboratory studies reveal impaired absorption of orally administered vitamin B_{12} (Schilling test), D-xylose, and ^{14}C triolein.

Surgical treatment of the underlying disease is carried out whenever possible. If there is no surgical cause of blind loop syndrome, treatment consists of broad-spectrum antibiotics and medications to control diarrhea. It may be necessary to use different antibiotics in sequence, guided by culture results and response to therapy. Damage to enterocytes appears to be reversible with treatment. Octreotide (somatostatin analog) may reduce bacterial overgrowth and improve abdominal symptoms in patients with scleroderma, according to a recent report.

Bures J, et al: Small intestinal bacterial overgrowth syndrome. *World J Gastroenterol.* 2010;16(24):2978-2990.
Rana SV, et al: Small intestinal bacterial overgrowth. *Scand J Gastroenterol.* 2008;43:1030.

ACUTE MESENTERIC ISCHEMIA

▶ General Considerations

Acute mesenteric ischemia (AMI) is a life-threatening clinical condition if not diagnosed promptly and treated adequately. Despite diagnostic and therapeutic advances, morbidity and mortality associated with AMI remain high. A high index of suspicion for this disease is essential since the clinical presentation is often nonspecific. AMI results from four main processes: (1) arterial embolism (50%), most commonly in patients with previous myocardial infarction or atrial fibrillation; (2) acute arterial thrombosis (25%) in patients with diffuse atherosclerosis or, less frequently, with connective tissue disorders; (3) nonocclusive mesenteric ischemia (20%); and (4) venous thrombosis (5%) associated with portal hypertension, abdominal sepsis, hypercoagulable states, or trauma.

The clinical consequences of acute arterial or venous mesenteric ischemia depend on several factors, including the vessel involved, the level of occlusion, the development of collaterals, and reperfusion. Tissue injury caused by the ischemic event compromises the immune and barrier functions of the small bowel, allowing bacterial translocation, cellular degradation, reactive oxygen species formation in case of reperfusion, and intravascular thrombosis. The release of these product into the portal system and the systemic circulation initiates a cascade of events leading to damage of targets organs such as the lungs and kidneys.

A. Symptoms and Signs

The clinical presentation is nonspecific.

Patients with arterial embolism initially present with sudden-onset diffuse abdominal pain that is out of proportion to the clinical exam and often unresponsive to narcotics. The lack of well-developed collaterals causes ischemia, which eventually becomes transmural. As ischemia worsens, patients develop nausea and vomiting, bloody diarrhea, and eventually peritonitis.

Patients with acute thrombotic mesenteric occlusion also present with severe abdominal pain, but it is usually chronic postprandial abdominal pain ("intestinal angina") accompanied by weight loss.

With cardiogenic or hypovolemic shock, blood is shunted away from the mesenteric circulation, and this process is exacerbated by the following local vasoconstriction. Pain in patients with nonocclusive mesenteric ischemia is usually not as sudden as that with embolic or thrombotic occlusion. Moreover, pain is more difficult to assess because many of these patients are hospitalized in intensive care units for life-threatening conditions.

Patients with venous thrombosis commonly complain of nausea, vomiting, diarrhea, and nonlocalized abdominal pain.

B. Laboratory Findings

There are no laboratory tests that are diagnostic for AMI. In most cases, the white blood cell count is elevated, as are lactic acid, amylase (50% of patients), and creatine kinase (BB isoenzyme) levels correlating with intestinal infarction. Significant metabolic acidosis is usually present.

C. Imaging Studies

Abdominal radiographs are not diagnostic but can reveal late signs consistent with bowel ischemia, such as gas in the bowel wall or the portal venous system and free air in the peritoneum.

Duplex ultrasonography plays a limited role in the diagnosis of AMI, given accompanying ileus with air- and gas-filled loops of bowel. Moreover, it cannot assess distal mesenteric blood vessel flow and nonocclusive etiology of ischemia.

Angiography is considered the gold standard for diagnosis for acute embolic and acute thrombotic arterial mesenteric ischemia. Angiography should include both anteroposterior and lateral views of the celiac artery, the SMA, and the inferior mesenteric artery. By selective injection of contrast into the SMA, emboli and thrombi can be identified, whereas patients with nonocclusive mesenteric ischemia typically exhibit evidence of SMA vasospasm. During the same procedure, catheters can be positioned selectively for treatment. Angiography is significantly less useful for the diagnosis of mesenteric venous thrombosis compared to CT scan.

Both CT and magnetic resonance angiography (MRA) have undergone significant advances over the past 10 years. Multislice helical CT scan with three-dimensional spatial resolution of the vascular anatomy allows rapid evaluation of atherosclerosis of the aorta and mesenteric vessels and the status of the small bowel wall and identifies other causes of abdominal pain, such as pancreatitis, bowel perforation, bowel obstruction, and rupture of abdominal aortic aneurism. Nevertheless, it still has some limitations: although the origins of the main abdominal vessels are well visualized, secondary, tertiary, and smaller branches are less well defined compared to angiography. On the contrary, CT is diagnostic for venous thrombosis and is the preferred diagnostic imaging modality in patients with a suspected mesenteric venous thrombosis.

One of the main advantages of MRA is the use of gadolinium, which is significantly less nephrotoxic than the contrast used for CT scan. However, this diagnostic imaging modality is not widely used due to the lack of access in many institutions.

Differential Diagnosis

Acute pancreatitis, intestinal obstruction, aortic dissection, and cholecystitis are the most frequent pathologies that mimic the clinical presentation of AMI.

Treatment

Once the diagnosis is made, fluid resuscitation, antibiotics, and anticoagulants or drugs that inhibit platelet aggregation should be started.

The treatment consists of nonsurgical and surgical options depending on the underlying cause.

The goals of surgery are to restore blood flow when feasible and resect the segments of bowel that are no longer viable. Because the appearance of ischemic bowel may improve dramatically after restoring blood flow, the small bowel should be observed for at least 30 minutes after reperfusion before any decision for resection is undertaken.

For acute SMA embolism, the standard treatment is a laparotomy and embolectomy, with a catheter passed under direct vision into the arterial segment in order to dislodge and retrieve the embolus. Nonsurgical treatments include catheter-directed thrombolytic therapy to treat early acute embolic occlusion in selected patients who present with a partially occluding embolus in the SMA and do not exhibit peritoneal signs on physical examination.

Surgical treatment of acute thrombotic mesenteric occlusion consists of an antegrade or retrograde bypass because a simple thrombectomy usually leads to reocclusion, Revascularization with saphenous vein or prosthetic graft (in the absence of peritonitis) is the most common procedure. Angioplasty can be performed during diagnostic angiography to dilate stenotic lesions; however, clinical findings suspicious for peritonitis frequently make a laparotomy necessary.

In case of nonocclusive mesenteric ischemia, the treatment requires reversal of the underlying causes of the hypoperfusion. Local infusion of vasodilators using selective catheterization of the SMA may also play a role.

Treatment of mesenteric venous thrombosis is nonsurgical and relies on anticoagulation to reverse the hypercoagulable state. Full anticoagulation with heparin is needed with careful monitoring for gastrointestinal bleeding. Long-term oral or subcutaneous anticoagulation therapy is then begun. Exploratory laparotomy is mandatory when clinical conditions worsen and bowel infarction is suspected.

Finally, second-look laparotomy within 24-48 hours is a key point in the management of patients with AMI who require extensive bowel resection during the first operation or have areas of marginally viable bowel after revascularization.

Prognosis

The prognosis of AMI is poor because diagnosis and treatment are often delayed, infarction is extensive, and arterial reconstruction is difficult. Perioperative mortality rates range from 32% to 69%, and 5-year survival ranges from 18% to 50%. Mortality varies substantially according to the cause of AMI, with AMI being lower in cases of venous thrombosis than in cases of arterial origin. The only way to reduce the morbidity and mortality associated with this disease is early diagnosis and treatment, before bowel necrosis develops.

Block TA, et al: Endovascular and open surgery for acute occlusion of the superior mesenteric artery. *J Vasc Surg.* 2010;52(4):959-966.

Meng X, et al: Indications and procedures for second-look surgery in acute mesenteric ischemia. *Surg Today.* 2010;40(8):700-705.

Menke J: Diagnostic accuracy of multidetector CT in acute mesenteric ischemia: systematic review and meta-analysis. *Radiology.* 2010;256(1):93-101.

Renner P, et al: Intestinal ischemia: current treatment concepts. *Langenbecks Arch Surg.* 2011;396(1):3-11.

SHORT BOWEL SYNDROME

General Considerations

Maintenance of adequate nutrition is dependent on the normal digestive and absorptive function of small bowel mucosa. A normal, healthy adult possesses an excess of gut mucosa such that limited resection is well tolerated. However, this depends on the amount of bowel removed and the specific level of resection, the presence or absence of the colon, the absorptive function of the intestinal remnant, adaptation of the remaining bowel, and the nature of the underlying disease process and its complications (Figure 31–5). Symptoms can ensue following surgery, in some cases leading to a condition known as *short bowel syndrome*. This syndrome occurs when there are less than 200 cm of small

NORMAL

Generalized transport of water, electrolytes, sugars, proteins, fats, vitamins; most absorption occurs proximally.

Localized transport of bile salts, cholesterol, vitamin B_{12}; absorption in ileum only.

RESECTION OF JEJUNUM

Generalized transport work load assumed by ileum. Localized transport unaffected. No malabsorption.

RESECTION OF ILEUM

Generalized transport continues. Localized transport lost. Malabsorption of vitamin B_{12}, cholesterol, bile salts, and fats.

▲ **Figure 31–5.** The consequences of complete resection of jejunum or ileum are predictable in part from the loss of regionally localized transport processes.

intestine in place. The patient becomes dependent on parenteral nutrition if there are less than 100 cm of small bowel in the absence of the colon and 60 cm in the presence of well-functioning colon. Because of the important functional capacities of the duodenum in iron and calcium absorption and of the distal ileum in regard to vitamin B_{12} and bile salts,

resections of these specific regions tend to be poorly tolerated. In contrast, up to 40% of the mid-small bowel can be removed with only moderate clinical sequelae. As a general rule, resection of 50% of the small bowel produces significant malabsorption, and if 70% or more of the bowel is resected, survival is threatened. Clinical results in treating short bowel syndrome have improved in recent decades due to recognition of its pathophysiology, improved surgical techniques, and better enteral and parenteral nutritional support.

The most common etiology of short bowel syndrome is a massive resection occurring in the setting of AMI. In children, volvulus of the intestine caused by congenital malrotation can also result in the need for a large resection. Less commonly, patients with neoplasms, trauma, or recurrent CD develop short bowel syndrome.

The minimal amount of small bowel required to sustain life is variable, but in general, survival is threatened in patients with less than 60 cm of intestine beyond the duodenum. Patients with short bowel syndrome have impairment in the absorption of water and electrolytes as well as that of all nutrients (fat, protein, carbohydrates, and vitamins). The colon is vitally important for preventing water loss. In addition, the colon plays an important role in nutrient assimilation by absorbing short-chain fatty acids. The ileocecal valve delays transit of enteric content from the small bowel into the colon, thereby prolonging the contact time between nutrients and the small bowel absorptive mucosa.

Important adaptive changes occur in the remaining intestine following massive resection. In addition to mucosal hyperplasia, there is generally seen to be an increase in the caliber of the remaining small bowel, perhaps adding to the absorptive area. From a functional point of view, the amount of fluid and electrolyte losses following massive resection decrease over time, whereas glucose absorption increases.

Short bowel syndrome is associated with gastric hypersecretion that persists for 1-2 years postoperatively, likely related to loss of the "ileal brake," a mechanism by which luminal fat within the distal small bowel inhibits gastric secretion. The increased acid load delivered to the duodenum inhibits absorption by a variety of mechanisms, including the inhibition of digestive enzymes, most of which function optimally under alkaline conditions. Loss of the terminal ileum also results in impairment in the absorption of conjugated bile salts and fat. With limited ileal resections, an increase in the bile salt load to the colon can cause direct injury to the mucosa and resultant diarrhea. With an ileal resection greater than 100 cm, there is a gradual loss in the total bile salt pool, eventually leading to impairment in fat absorption and the onset of steatorrhea. Ileal resections are also associated with lithogenic bile, such that gallstone formation is seen in approximately 30% of patients who have undergone such surgery. Calcium oxalate urinary tract calculi form in 7%-10% of patients who have extensive ileal resection and an intact colon, due to excessive absorption of oxalate from the colon.

Treatment

Initial therapy involves maintenance of fluid and electrolyte balance. Total parental nutrition is often indicated and, depending on the extent of resection, may be required throughout the lifetime of the patient. It is likely that even small amounts of enteral nutrition are beneficial, however, because the luminal nutrients appear to enhance the adaptive response of the remaining gut. Various antidiarrheal and stool-bulking agents have also been used with some benefits. Gastric hypersecretion should be treated with either H_2-blockers or proton pump inhibitors. Cholestyramine may be beneficial in patients with limited ileal resections, but if the bile salt pool has been depleted, then cholestyramine is contraindicated. The efficacy of intensive medical management, including maintenance of oral hydration, along with a combination of a high-fiber diet, growth hormone, and glutamine, is controversial.

The surgical treatment of patients with short bowel syndrome has been disappointing. Various procedures including intestinal lengthening, reversal of short segments, and placation of excessively dilated bowel have been attempted. Although some improvement has been seen in isolated cases, such operations are not widely performed. The results of small bowel transplantation have also been disappointing because of the high rate of rejection. However, more recent experience with small bowel transplantation suggests that this may become a viable surgical alternative in patients with short bowel syndrome.

Prognosis

Nowadays, mortality in patients with small bowel syndrome is more likely related to complications of the underlying disease rather than parenteral nutrition. It depends on several factors, such as the length of small intestine, the presence of active underlying diseases, the presence of functioning colon, and patient's age.

Thompson JS, et al: Current management of the short bowel syndrome. *Surg Clin North Am*. 2011;91(3):493-510.

Ueno T, et al: Current status of intestinal transplantation. *Surg Today*. 2010;40(12):1112-1122.

Wales PW, et al: Human growth hormone and glutamine for patients with short bowel syndrome. *Cochrane Database Syst Rev*. 2010;6:CD006321.

INTESTINAL DIVERTICULA*

General Considerations

Small bowel diverticular disease is an uncommon clinical entity. However, with progressive aging of the general population, small bowel diverticulosis is encountered more

---

*Meckel diverticulum and other congenital diverticula of the small intestine are discussed in Chapter 43.

often. Overall, the frequency reported in the literature of small bowel diverticula varies with the anatomic location of the disease and the type of investigation used for diagnosis. Clearly, autopsy series report a higher incidence, since small bowel diverticulosis is usually asymptomatic and is found often upon postmortem examination only.

A. Etiology

Diverticular disease of the small bowel is generally classified into two groups: the more common, acquired form and the congenital form, which is somewhat rare, other than Meckel diverticulum in the distal ileum. Primary acquired small bowel diverticula result from the herniation of the mucosa and submucosa through the muscular layer of the bowel wall. These lesions are considered to be false diverticula, with no muscular wall covering. Patients with small bowel diverticula frequently have associated diverticular disease of the colon and diverticula of the esophagus (2%), stomach (2%), or urinary bladder (12%).

In the pathogenesis of small bowel diverticulosis, abnormalities of the myenteric plexus with consequent motor dysfunctions of the small intestine are thought to play a major role. These motility disorders vary in severity and magnitude from localized dysmotility to universal jejunoileal dyskinesia and result in increased intraluminal pressure and ultimately herniation of the mucosa and submucosa through the muscular wall of the small bowel. Usually, diverticula occur where the paired blood vessels penetrate the small bowel wall at the mesenteric site.

In contrast, congenital diverticula are usually considered true diverticula involving the full thickness of the small intestine. Congenital diverticula are often limited to the duodenum (wind-sock diverticulum) and ileum (Meckel diverticulum). Both acquired and congenital diverticula are usually asymptomatic; however, symptoms can originate from small bowel diverticula owing to diverticulitis, perforation, obstruction, or hemorrhage.

B. Duodenal Diverticula

Acquired diverticula are extraluminal and are a fairly common incidental finding usually visualized either upon esophagogastroduodenoscopy (EGD), endoscopic retrograde cholangiopancreatography (ERCP), or barium swallow and small bowel follow-through. Incidences vary significantly in the literature depending on the diagnostic modality used. In the ERCP literature, incidences up to 23% have been reported, usually increasing with advancing age.

In terms of location, these diverticula are generally located within 2 cm of the ampulla. This is an area of weakening of the duodenal wall mucosa, especially around the papilla of Vater, due to the configuration and orientation of the smooth muscle fiber and the sphincter mechanism of Oddi. If the papilla is involved or included in these diverticula, sphincter dysfunction may lead to biliary dyskinesia, formation of biliary stones, cholangitis, and even pancreatitis. Acquired diverticula are also present in the third and fourth portions of the duodenum with decreasing frequency.

Usually, these diverticula are asymptomatic. Symptoms, when present, often are caused by either dysfunction of the sphincter of Oddi or, when the diverticula are significantly large, by obstruction of the biliary and pancreatic ducts due to external compression. Recurrent episodes of pancreatitis potentially evolving into chronic pancreatitis and formation of biliary stones have been reported in patients with large duodenal diverticula. Furthermore, large diverticula can cause bacterial overgrowth, resulting in malabsorption and anemia. Diverticulitis with potential perforation and bleeding from duodenal diverticula has been reported.

Diagnosis is often obtained by EGD or ERCP. An upper gastrointestinal series with a small bowel follow-through is also very helpful in localizing the diverticula and in defining the size of it. When a perforation is suspected, CT scan of the abdomen with oral and IV contrast can accurately define the location of the diverticula and the extent of the inflammatory reaction to the diverticular perforation.

Surgical treatment of duodenal diverticula is complicated by significant morbidity and mortality; therefore, a prophylactic resection of an asymptomatic duodenal diverticulum is not routinely recommended. In presence of perforation or bleeding, a generous Kocher maneuver should be performed in order to identify the posterior aspect of the duodenum. It is very important at this stage of the procedure to have a clear idea of the relationship of the biliary and pancreatic ducts with the ampulla in order to avoid an injury that will be extremely difficult to repair in this setting and location. If the pancreatic and biliary structures are not involved with the diverticulum, in the absence of significant retroperitoneal contamination, a primary excision of the diverticulum is indicated. The resulting defect should be closed in two layers using absorbable suture for the inner layer and nonabsorbable suture for the outer layer. With a large duodenal defect, a serosal patch technique using a defunctionalized loop of jejunum is a useful alternative. However, in presence of significant edema and contamination, primary closure around a T-tube with drainage of the surrounding area may be the only solution. In extreme cases, duodenal diverticulization by gastrojejunostomy with a stapled closure of the pylorus may be necessary. A large diverticulum in the third or fourth portion of the duodenum requires mobilization of the distal duodenum with excision and primary closure. In this area, the relationship with the biliary and pancreatic duct is not obviously as crucial, and therefore, a more aggressive approach can be undertaken.

C. Jejunoileal Diverticula

The acquired forms of jejunoileal diverticula are usually more common in the proximal jejunum, decreasing in frequency throughout the small bowel. Extreme forms of diffuse diverticulosis of the small bowel have been reported. It is a disease of advanced age and is prevalent during the seventh decade of life. These diverticula are located on the antimesenteric border of the small bowel. Due to primary motility disturbances of the small intestine, these patients usually present with chronic abdominal pain, early satiety, and different gastrointestinal conditions, such as diarrhea, malabsorption, steatorrhea, vitamin B_{12} deficiency, and anemia. These patients can present with an acute abdomen in the presence of a free perforation secondary to diverticulitis. Bleeding is also one of the possible complications, and localization of the bleeding diverticulum, in presence of diffuse diverticulosis, may present a significant diagnostic challenge to the clinician.

Jejunoileal diverticula are usually identified by small bowel follow-through or enteroclysis. CT scan can help in the diagnosis of large diverticula or in the presence of acute diverticulitis or perforation. More recently, the use of capsule or wireless endoscopy has helped the clinician in diagnosing patients with unclear gastrointestinal symptoms and especially patients with recurrent significant gastrointestinal bleed secondary to diverticular disease. After the initial experimental papers, several human studies, looking at patients with occult gastrointestinal bleeding, have shown capsule endoscopy to be significantly superior to push enteroscopy and preferred by patients undergoing both procedures. Although small bowel diverticular disease is a rare condition, it may be the cause of a lower gastrointestinal bleed, resulting in a diagnostic dilemma. In the presence of acute significant bleeding, angiography should be attempted for localization of the bleeding diverticulum and possible treatment either by vasopressin injection or, in selected cases, by super-selective embolization. Injection of methylene blue to help identify the bleeding diverticulum at the time of exploration is a helpful technique when the bleeding persists despite medical management.

Asymptomatic jejunoileal diverticula are usually treated conservatively. In the presence of localized segments of multiple diverticula, it has been suggested that a resection, even in the absence of symptomatology, might be indicated because the morbidity from a small bowel resection today is much less than the potential complication from acute diverticulitis. This approach has not been validated by any clinical data thus far. In the presence of diverticulitis and perforation, obviously resection and primary anastomosis are indicated. In the presence of bleeding, if the source is localized by either angiography or capsule endoscopy, the bleeding site should be resected with primary anastomosis. Laparoscopy has been extensively used in the management of this unusual problem.

Woods K, et al: Acquired jejunoileal diverticulosis and its complications: a review of the literature. *Am Surg.* 2008;74:849.

TUMORS OF THE SMALL BOWEL

▶ General Considerations

Although the small bowel accounts for 75% of the gastrointestinal length and 90% of its absorptive surface, neoplasms of this organ, both benign and malignant, are relatively rare. They represent less than 10% of all gastrointestinal tumors, 1%-3% of gastrointestinal malignancies, and 0.4% of all malignancies.

In recent years, the incidence of two small bowel tumors, lymphomas and gastrointestinal stromal tumors (GISTs), has increased substantially. In the case of primary small bowel lymphoma, the incidence in the United States has nearly doubled in the past two decades, due to the increased numbers of immunocompromised patients and immigrants from developing countries. In the case of GIST, the recognition of the KIT protein (CD117) has changed the way spindle cell tumors of the gastrointestinal tract are classified and has led to an increased awareness and recognition.

Several predisposing conditions associated with small bowel malignancies have been identified: CD, familial adenomatous polyposis, hereditary nonpolyposis colorectal cancer, blind loop syndrome, Peutz-Jeghers syndrome, celiac sprue, neurofibromatosis, and IgA deficiency.

The disproportion between the low incidence of malignant tumors of the small bowel and the size of its surface area suggests a significant sparing from or resistance to the development of malignancy. Several hypotheses, based on experimental animal models, have postulated that carcinogens in the enteric content may be in contact with small bowel mucosa over a limited time due to the relatively rapid transit time or may be in a diluted and less carcinogenic form. The preponderance of small bowel adenocarcinomas in the duodenum suggests a role for bile or pancreatic secretions either as primary small bowel carcinogens or even as simple vectors for unknown carcinogens.

Other specific characteristics of the small bowel microscopic and chemical environment might be responsible for the observed cancer resistance. The limited and metabolically inactive bacterial flora of the small bowel is likely unable to transform procarcinogens into their active metabolites, especially in an alkaline milieu. In addition, the proximal small bowel secretes a number of enzymes that detoxify carcinogens.

Finally, the presence of a high concentration of B cells and lymphocytes and high amounts of secretory IgA in the distal small bowel might constitute an effective local immunosurveillance system that prevents carcinogenesis. This theory seems to be supported by the observation that immunocompromised patients have an increased incidence of lymphoma and Kaposi sarcoma of the distal small bowel.

Dietary risk factors, such as high caloric dietary intake in general and more specifically consumption of red meat, fat, and salt-cured smoked foods, have been shown to increase the incidence of small bowel carcinoma in large population-based studies. This similarity in risk factors explains the relatively high risk of synchronous or metachronous colorectal cancer in patients with a known small bowel malignancy.

▶ Pathology

Approximately one-third of primary small bowel neoplasms are benign and two-thirds are malignant. The most common benign tumors are leiomyomas and adenomas; less common lesions include inflammatory polyps, hemangiomas, lipomas, hamartomas (Peutz-Jeghers syndrome), and fibromas. These tumors can occur throughout the small bowel but tend to increase in frequency from proximal to distal, with the exception of adenomas, which occur with the highest frequency in the duodenum.

Adenomas are the most common benign tumors of the small intestine. The duodenum is the most common site of involvement, and the lesion most commonly noted is a villous adenoma. These lesions tend to involve the region of the ampulla of Vater. They may present with obstructive jaundice and are easily diagnosed by upper endoscopy and biopsy. Up to 30% of these tumors may have malignant degeneration. The risk of malignant degeneration in a significant proportion of patients poses challenges to treatment planning.

Leiomyomas arise from smooth muscle and can grow both intra- and extraluminally. They can often become very large before causing symptoms. On gross inspection, it is sometimes difficult to distinguish these lesions from their malignant counterparts. This distinction is made histologically with standard criteria including nuclear pleomorphism, increased mitosis, and the presence of necrosis, although at times, even histologic examination may fail to unequivocally distinguish between benign and malignant histology.

Malignant tumors tend to increase in frequency from proximal to distal, with the exception of adenocarcinomas, which are most frequent in the duodenum. Adenocarcinoma is the most common histologic type (45%), followed by carcinoids (30%), lymphomas (15%), sarcomas, and GISTs (10%). Pathologic staging is performed according to the American Joint Committee on Cancer (AJCC) tumor-node-metastasis (TNM) system.

Most small bowel *adenocarcinomas* are solitary, sessile lesions, often appearing in association with adenomas. They are usually moderately to well differentiated and almost always positive for acid mucin. Most arise in the duodenum: within the duodenum, 15% of these tumors are located in the first portion, 40% in the second portion, and 45% in the distal duodenum. Most of these tumors are sporadic, with the exception of the ones originating in the context of familial adenomatous polyposis. Presenting symptoms include epigastric and abdominal pain or discomfort, and possibly jaundice and gastric outlet obstruction, depending on the location of the tumor. These symptoms and the accessibility of the duodenum and proximal small bowel to endoscopic modalities allow a relatively high rate of diagnosis and resectability.

Carcinoid tumors are the most common endocrine tumors of the gastrointestinal system. In the small bowel itself, carcinoids are the most common distal small bowel neoplasm. These neoplasms arise from enterochromaffin cells and are characterized by the ability to secrete many biologically active substances, including serotonin, bradykinin, dopamine, histamine, and 5-hydroxyindoleacetic acid (5-HIAA). They tend to be small (< 2 cm) and submucosal in location, with a propensity for multicentricity. The most common classification for these tumors is based on embryologic derivation: foregut (stomach and pancreas), midgut (small bowel; 90% or more), and hindgut (colon and rectum). Their presentation depends largely on the hormones elaborated and on the site of origin. Up to 40% of small bowel carcinoids are associated with a second gastrointestinal malignancy, and 30% present as multiple synchronous lesions.

The gastrointestinal tract is the most frequent site of extranodal *lymphoma*: the stomach is the most common site, followed by the small bowel and the colon, respectively. Within the small bowel, lymphomas parallel the distribution of lymphoid follicles, resulting in the ileum being the most common site of involvement. These tumors may be primary or secondary as a manifestation of generalized involvement of systemic lymphoma. For the diagnosis of primary small bowel lymphomas, there must be no peripheral or mediastinal lymphadenopathy, with a normal white cell count and differential, and the tumor must be predominantly in the gastrointestinal tract. When primary, they may be multifocal in as many as 15% of cases. Predisposing conditions include immunodeficiency conditions, CD, and celiac disease.

There are five distinct clinical pathologic subtypes of primary small intestinal lymphoma: the adult Western type, the pediatric type, the immunoproliferative or Mediterranean type, enteropathy-associated (celiac sprue) T-cell lymphoma, and Hodgkin lymphoma. The most common is the adult Western type, occurring in the sixth and seventh decade of life with a male predominance.

Sarcomas make up only 10% of small bowel malignancies. Overall, these tumors are located in the jejunum and ileum, are relatively slow growing, and are locally invasive. Their growth pattern is most commonly extramural, and therefore, they rarely result in obstruction, but sometimes, they present with free intra-abdominal bleeding. Due to their insidious nature and growth pattern, greater than three-fourths of these tumors exceed 5 cm in diameter at the time diagnosis. The most common histologic subtypes are GISTs, leiomyosarcomas, fibrosarcomas, liposarcomas, and malignant schwannomas and angiosarcomas. Similar to sarcomas from other anatomic regions, small bowel sarcomas rarely metastasize to regional lymph nodes. Hematogenous dissemination tends to be the preferred route of distant spread, primarily to the liver, lungs, and bone. Peritoneal sarcomatosis is noted in later stages of the disease.

Malignant *GIST* is now considered the most common sarcoma of the gastrointestinal tract and accounts for about 5% of all small bowel malignancies. Clinical, histopathologic, ultrastructural, and molecular-biological findings have made it clear that GIST is a completely separate entity from leiomyoma and leiomyosarcoma. It is currently thought that GISTs originate from stem cells that differentiate toward the interstitial cells of Cajal (ICCs). ICCs arise from precursor mesenchymal cells and are the pacemaker cells of the gastrointestinal tract. Both ICCs and GISTs express KIT protein, have similar ultrastructural features, and express the embryonic form of the heavy chain of smooth muscle myosin.

KIT immunostaining has become the gold standard for the diagnosis of GIST, and the term *GIST* should apply only to tumors with KIT immunopositivity. In rare situations, a GIST may be immunohistochemically inert, or after therapy with imatinib mesylate, KIT immunostaining may become negative. Furthermore, a minority of GISTs lack demonstrable KIT mutations, but KIT is nonetheless strongly activated. Such GISTs might contain KIT mutations, which are not readily detected by conventional screening methods, or alternately, KIT might be activated by nonmutational mechanisms. To better characterize these tumors, other markers have been studied: about 60%-70% of GISTs show immunopositivity for CD34, 30%-40% for smooth muscle actin, and around 5% for S-100 protein. None of the latter antigens are specific for GIST, but they can help in the differential diagnosis in KIT-negative tumors.

▶ Clinical Findings

A. Symptoms and Signs

The vast majority of patients with benign neoplasms are asymptomatic, whereas most of those with malignancies are symptomatic prior to diagnosis. The most common presentation of benign tumors is intermittent episodes of acute crampy abdominal pain associated with intussusception, followed by chronic bleeding, with iron deficiency anemia in up to 50% of patients.

Malignant lesions are generally associated with weight loss. Symptoms, when they occur, tend to be vague and nonspecific. In general, most symptoms can be attributed to the location of the tumor, its rate of growth, and its size. For example, tumors in the duodenum tend to be symptomatic at an earlier stage, presenting with pain, gastric outlet obstruction, or obstructive jaundice, whereas those in the jejunum or ileum may present at a later stage with obstructive symptoms. Obstruction in this setting tends to be progressive, compared to benign lesions, whose obstructive symptoms tend to be intermittent as they relate to episodes of intussusception. Bleeding and perforation (in up to 10%) may also occur, predominantly in lymphomatous lesions, but this can also be a feature of any malignant tumor because of ulceration or necrosis.

Carcinoid tumors produce symptoms secondary to hormone production, including hot flashes, bronchospasms, and arrhythmias. This constellation of symptoms, called carcinoid syndrome, occurs when the liver is not able to metabolize the active substances produced by the carcinoid tumor. This is usually the case when tumors are either bulky or metastatic or their venous drainage bypasses the liver.

B. Laboratory Findings

A high index of suspicion is required due to the lack of specificity of these tumors' signs and symptoms. A correct preoperative diagnosis is made in up to only 50% of patients. Biochemical and hematologic studies are often not helpful. Iron deficiency anemia may be detected with chronic blood loss; elevated liver enzymes may be noted with periampullary lesions or hepatic metastases; elevated 24-hour urinary 5-HIAA can be detected in more than 50% of patients with carcinoid tumors.

C. Imaging Studies

Radiographic contrast imaging modalities tend to be the most useful in the establishment of the diagnosis. Plain films of the abdomen are generally not helpful and, at best, may demonstrate nonspecific signs of obstruction or a mass effect. Except for the duodenum and the very proximal jejunum, which can often be evaluated by endoscopy, the diagnosis of small intestinal neoplasms depends on contrast studies such as a small bowel follow-through or preferably enteroclysis. Small bowel follow-through is still the most commonly used method in the evaluation of small bowel pathology, although enteroclysis may be a superior imaging modality.

CT, ultrasonography, and MRI are complementary to barium studies in the detection of small bowel neoplasms. Abdominal CT has a sensitivity of 50%-80% in detecting the primary small bowel tumors and occasionally plays an important role in differentiating benign from malignant tumors. Additionally, CT is valuable in staging malignant tumors (presence or absence of hepatic metastases) and in providing important information related to local extent (presence or absence of local invasion, mesenteric implants, and metastatic lymph nodes). More recently, the association of multidetector CT and MRI with small bowel lumen distension (CTE and MRE) has led to a considerable improvement in the diagnosis of small bowel neoplasms. On CTE, small bowel adenocarcinomas may manifest as a discrete tumor mass, a circumferential narrowing with abrupt concentric or irregular edges, or an ulcerative lesion with adjacent enlarged lymph nodes. Mucosal ulceration is a suggestive feature, which is well depicted by CTE. Jejunal lesions have a tendency for being annular. Usually, only a short segment of the small bowel is involved. The mass itself usually shows moderate and heterogeneous enhancement after IV administration of iodinated contrast material. Rarely, adenocarcinoma may present as an aneurismal dilatation of a small bowel segment, similar to that observed in case of lymphoma. On MRI, small bowel adenocarcinomas have morphologic features similar to those observed on CT.

On CTE, small GISTs typically present as regular, round, or lobulated masses with homogeneous and relatively marked enhancement after IV administration of contrast material, whereas larger tumors are heterogeneous with central necrosis and more prone to extraluminal growth. Due to excellent spatial resolution with multidetector CT, the submucosal origin of the tumor may be suspected in case of small tumors. The malignant potential of these lesions cannot be stated with certainty on cross-sectional imaging unless metastases are present. In some instances, GISTs may display an aneurysmal pattern similar to that observed in case of lymphoma, so that differentiation between these two entities is difficult. Mesenteric small bowel tumors are usually hyperintense on T2-weighted MRIs, with variable degrees of enhancement after IV administration of a gadolinium chelate. Because of the lower spatial resolution obtained with MRI by comparison with CT, the submucosal origin of the tumor may be difficult to ascertain.

Angiography is rarely helpful in establishing or refining a diagnosis of small bowel malignancy. In rare cases, angiographic demonstration of tumor neovascularity without contrast agent extravasation may be of diagnostic importance in patients with chronic occult bleeding when other diagnostic studies, such as endoscopy and barium contrast, have been negative. By contrast, this study is rarely beneficial in localizing bleeding tumors since the vast majority bleed at a rate considerably below the limit of detection for this technique. Nuclear medicine scan with technetium-labeled red blood cells may identify bleeding sites with blood loss rates as low as 0.1 mL/min.

Fluorodeoxyglucose (labeled with fluorine-18) positron emission tomography (FDG-PET) has been shown to be highly sensitive to assess disease status in patients with GISTs. FDG-PET is used for preoperative staging but also, more importantly, to assess response to therapy.

D. Endoscopy

Enteroscopy is now available in a fiberoptic form, using conventional endoscopes, or in a wireless form. Push enteroscopy is currently the most frequently used endoscopic method for small bowel examination. The endoscope is introduced orally. After traversing the curve of the second part of the duodenum, the enteroscope is straightened to reduce any loops formed in the stomach. The enteroscope is then pushed to the maximum length of insertion. Dedicated push enteroscopes are 2-2.5 m in length and offer the opportunity to take biopsies when the neoplastic lesion has been identified.

The double balloon (push and pull) enteroscopy system consists of a high-resolution video endoscope with a working length of 200 cm and a flexible overtube 145 cm long. The inflated balloon on the overtube is used to maintain a stable position while the enteroscope is advanced. The overtube balloon is deflated, while the enteroscope balloon is inflated, and the overtube is advanced along the distal end of the enteroscope (push procedure). This is followed by the pull procedure: both the enteroscope and the overtube are pulled back under endoscopic guidance, with both balloons inflated. This procedure is repeated multiple times to visualize the entire small bowel. Few complications have been reported but include the following: postprocedure abdominal pain in up to 20% of patients, pancreatitis, bleeding, and small bowel perforation, which is more common after polypectomy of large polyps (> 3 cm).

The capsule endoscope is a capsule containing a battery-powered imager, a transmitter, antenna, and four light-emitting diodes. The imager takes two images per second through the transparent plastic dome of the capsule. The capsule is swallowed and is propelled through the intestine by peristalsis. Images taken by the capsule are transmitted to a battery-powered data recorder worn on a belt. The equipment is removed after 8 hours, by which time the capsule has reached the cecum in most of cases. The data from the recorder are then downloaded onto a computer workstation, which allows approximately 50,000 images to be viewed as a video. The average reading time of the video images takes between 40 and 60 minutes depending on the experience of the endoscopist. This technique may be affected by two problems: first, the presence of dark intestinal contents in the small bowel may impair visualization of the mucosa, and second, the rate of gastric emptying and small bowel transit could lead to the exhaustion of the capsule batteries before the capsule reaches the ileocecal valve. Incomplete examination occurs in 10%-25% of cases.

The main risk is capsule retention. Therefore, this procedure is contraindicated in patients with known strictures or swallowing disorders.

E. Laparoscopy

Limited information is available regarding the efficacy of diagnostic laparoscopy in the diagnosis and workup of small bowel neoplasms. At present, its usefulness may reside in obtaining staging information and determining resectability prior to formal laparotomy, in the case of tumors of the duodenum, and in obtaining images and potentially tissue diagnoses when other imaging studies have failed to suggest an etiology. It is clear, however, that despite the currently available technology, the diagnosis of these tumors is difficult to establish preoperatively in a significant group of individuals. Laparotomy is often required for definitive diagnosis.

▶ Staging Classification

Radiologic staging is mainly based on the use of CT and MRI. Intraoperative assessment plays a role in clinical staging. Metastatic involvement of the liver may be further evaluated by intraoperative ultrasonography. As far as pathologic staging, the TNM staging system has been recently revised by the AJCC, but no major changes have been implemented for small bowel neoplasms. The primary tumor is staged according to its depth of penetration and the involvement of adjacent structures or distant sites. There is no subdivision within the N category based on the number of nodes involved with tumor. Hematogenous metastases or peritoneal metastases are coded as M1. Cancers of the small intestine can metastasize to most organs, especially the liver, or to the peritoneal surfaces. Involvement of the celiac nodes is considered M1 disease.

For small bowel lymphoma, the most commonly used staging system is the Ann Arbor system based on lymphatic and extralymphatic involvement on either side of the diaphragm.

▶ Treatment

Treatment of *adenocarcinoma* of the small intestine with localized disease is based on oncologic and anatomic principles. For duodenal lesions, the availability of endoscopic ultrasound has allowed better preoperative staging, and the availability of endoscopic resection techniques has offered additional therapeutic options. Ultrasound-proven benign duodenal or ampullary adenomas can be resected endoscopically with excellent results. Invasive lesions of the first and second portion of the duodenum without major vessel involvement and distant spread are best treated by a pancreaticoduodenectomy (Whipple procedure). For tumors in the third or fourth portions of the duodenum, segmental resection with regional lymphadenectomy is indicated. Debate persists about the optimal surgical management of early duodenal cancer. Although early reports suggest that an endoscopic approach could be justified in early favorable lesions, long-term follow-up is still lacking, and surgical resection is to be preferred in good-risk patients. Palliative options for unresectable or metastatic duodenal carcinoma include gastrojejunostomy and/or biliary enteric bypass or endoscopic/interventional placement of stents to relieve the intestinal and/or biliary obstruction.

Adenocarcinoma of the jejunum and ileum is treated by wide excision, including areas of contiguous spread and the associated mesentery, with negative surgical margins.

Although only small series have been published, these tumors do not seem to respond to the conventional flourouracil-based chemotherapy regimens, and there is a radiation dose limitation due to small bowel toxicity. However, for palliation of chronic blood loss in patients with locally advanced unresectable duodenal carcinomas, radiotherapy may provide short-term benefit.

The mainstay of therapy for *carcinoid* tumors is radical surgical excision. In preparation for surgery, a complete assessment of the entire gastrointestinal tract is warranted since up to 40% of midgut carcinoids are associated with a second gastrointestinal malignancy and 30% present with multiple synchronous lesions. In addition, preemptive treatment with octreotide is indicated to prevent carcinoid crisis at the time of surgery. At surgery, wide en block resection including the draining mesentery is the standard approach. This is particularly true for small bowel carcinoids, because these lesions have the propensity to metastasize even when very small. Large lesions near the ampulla may require a pancreaticoduodenectomy for cure, while smaller lesions may be treated with either local excision or endoscopic resection with close endoscopic follow-up. Likewise, lesions of the terminal ileum or carcinoid tumors of the appendix larger than 2 cm require a formal right hemicolectomy for oncologic clearance of disease.

Treatment for advanced locoregional and distant disease includes both medical and surgical modalities. Surgery is indicated in patients with resectable metastatic disease for potential cure or at least meaningful palliation. Orthotopic liver transplantation has been used in the treatment of metastatic neuroendocrine tumors to the liver, with discouraging results.

The role of multimodality therapy, including alpha-2b interferon and octreotide, for metastatic carcinoid remains limited. The addition of liver chemoembolization has not been shown to have a significant effect on survival in patients with metastatic disease to the liver but may have a role in controlling or decreasing the symptoms associated with carcinoid crisis. Octreotide has been effective in the treatment of patients with carcinoid syndrome by improving diarrhea in up to 83% of the patients and abolishing flushing and wheezing, but it has no effect on survival. In consideration of the slow growth rate of many carcinoid tumors, patients with distant metastatic disease can also undergo resection for debulking and palliation of symptoms. For patients with extensive unresectable disease, the indications for surgical intervention are limited to the occurrence of obstruction, perforation, and bleeding. Radiation therapy has not been proven to be effective in either the adjuvant or palliative setting.

Treatment of small bowel *lymphoma* requires conservative resections, with para-aortic and mesenteric lymph node sampling, liver biopsy, and bone marrow biopsy performed for staging. Low-grade localized lesions are treated with resection alone, whereas for intermediate- and high-grade lesions, resection and chemotherapy are recommended. Radiation is used only for palliation in poor-performance patients. This modality is associated with significant side effects, such as bowel necrosis, bleeding, and perforation, and is offered for palliation only to patients unfit for surgery or chemotherapy.

Surgical treatment for small bowel *sarcomas* consists of an en block resection with tumor-free margins. There is no role for extended lymphadenectomy in these tumors. Hematogenous dissemination is the preferred route of metastatic spread to the liver, lungs, and bones. Carcinomatosis is noted in later stages of the disease. In the presence of metastatic disease, local excision or palliative bypass procedure might be indicated to prevent or ameliorate bleeding and obstruction. Furthermore, there is no clear benefit from chemoradiation in the adjuvant setting, because radiation doses are limited due to small bowel toxicity. In the presence of recurrent or metastatic disease, partial response rates after palliative chemoradiation have been reported to be in the 10%-20% range, with minimal improvement in survival at best.

Treatment of localized GISTs is based on surgical resection: the tumor should be removed en block with its pseudocapsule and margins of normal soft tissue or bowel. In the presence of large lesions involving other organs, where an en block resection may be associated with significant morbidity, preoperative neoadjuvant use of imatinib mesylate may be entertained.

A significant breakthrough in the management of small bowel tumors and specifically GISTs has come from the understanding of the molecular and genetic makeshift of these lesions. After the discovery that GISTs characteristically express the KIT protein, a transmembrane tyrosine kinase receptor for a stem cell factor, a specific tyrosine kinase inhibitor, imatinib mesylate (Gleevec, Novartis), has been introduced in clinical practice, with reduced risks of recurrence.

The role of surgery for recurrent or metastatic disease has been questioned since the introduction of imatinib mesylate. Surgery should still be considered in patients with bleeding or obstructive disease and after partial response to imatinib mesylate if the residual disease is deemed to be resectable.

▶ Prognosis

Prognosis for small bowel *adenocarcinoma* is based on similar variables as for colorectal cancer, including stage, perineural and vascular invasion, grade, resectability, and surgical margins. The majority of tumors have regional spread at time of diagnosis, and up to one-fourth of patients have distant organ disease. Overall, the 5-year survival rate is 20%-30%. For resectable disease of the duodenum, the 5-year survival rate approaches 50%.

The prognosis for *carcinoid* tumors with localized disease is excellent, with 5-year survival rates approaching 100% after resection. More than 90% of the symptomatic patients have metastatic disease at the time of surgical exploration. The likelihood of distant disease correlates closely with both the size of the primary lesion and the depth of invasion. For tumors < 1 cm in size, the risk of lymph node metastases is on the order of 2%; for 1- to 2-cm lesions, there is an approximate 50% incidence of lymph node involvement; and 80% of tumors > 2 cm have positive nodes. Survival rates of up to 68% at 5 years have been reported when all gross metastatic disease, including hepatic metastases, is resected. For extensive unresectable disease, debulking has proven to be of some benefit in terms of symptomatic palliation. The 5-years survival for unresectable disease is approximately 35%-40%, reflecting the relatively indolent growth of these tumors.

Prognostic factors for primary small bowel *lymphomas* include higher grade, greater depth of tumor penetration, lymph node involvement, peritoneal disease, and distant metastases. Overall 5-year survival rates range from 20%-40% for all stages. Five-year survivals of up to 60% have been reported for patients with resected localized low-grade tumors.

Sarcomas tend to have an insidious growth pattern, and greater than three-fourths of these tumors are larger than 5 cm at the time of diagnosis and up to 50% of them are not resectable for cure when the diagnosis is established. Prognosis correlates most closely with grade, followed by stage. Five-year survival after curative resection ranges from 60%-80% for low-grade tumors and is no more than 20% for high-grade lesions.

Assessment of the malignant potential of a primary *GIST* lesion is difficult in many cases unless tumor spread can be documented beyond the organ of origin at the time of diagnosis. Historically, size has been used to assess tumor behavior. Although almost all small (< 1 cm) GISTs are clinically benign and tumors larger than 5 cm in diameter are generally malignant, intermediate-size GISTs have uncertain malignant potential, and no cutoff diameter predicts subsequent malignant behavior with certainty.

Other factors that have shown prognostic value include mitotic rate, presence of tumor necrosis, high cellularity, and pronounced pleomorphism; a high S-phase fraction and DNA aneuploidy in flow or image cytometry; a high Ki-67 score; proliferating-cell nuclear antigen expression; and presence of telomerase activity, incomplete surgical resection, tumor rupture at surgery, and invasion of adjacent structures.

Recently, *KIT* mutations have been shown to be an independent prognostic factor for patients with GISTs.

The median disease-specific survival is about 5 years for primary disease, and 10-20 months in recurrent or metastatic disease. Most recurrences take place within 5 years of the primary diagnosis, but in the slowly proliferating subset of GISTs and especially after therapy with imatinib mesylate,

metastases can appear more than 10 years after the primary diagnosis.

The outcome of patients with *metastatic malignancies* to the small intestine (more commonly ovarian, colon, and lung cancers; renal cell carcinoma; and melanoma) is dismal despite palliative therapeutic intervention.

▶ Follow-Up

Routine follow-up for small bowel cancers is accomplished with endoscopy and radiologic imaging. The only exception is GIST. As previously discussed, PET scan is used to follow tumor response to imatinib mesylate; to detect recurrence after either complete response to imatinib mesylate or after curative surgery; and to identify secondary resistance to imatinib mesylate before tumor progression on treatment.

Appelman HD: Morphology of gastrointestinal stromal tumors: historical perspectives. *J Surg Oncol.* 2011;104(8):874-881.

Bilimoria KY, et al: Small bowel cancer in the United States: changes in epidemiology, treatment, and survival over the last 20 years. *Ann Surg.* 2009;249:63-71.

Boudreaux JP, et al: The NANETS consensus guideline for the diagnosis and management of neuroendocrine tumors: well-differentiated neuroendocrine tumors of the jejunum, ileum, appendix, and cecum. *Pancreas.* 2010;39(6):753-766.

Culver EL, et al: Sporadic duodenal polyps: classification, investigation, and management. *Endoscopy.* 2011;43(2):144-155.

Fry LC, et al: Small-bowel endoscopy. *Endoscopy.* 2011;43(11):978-984.

Ghimire P, et al: Primary gastrointestinal lymphoma. *World J Gastroenterol.* 2011;17(6):697-707.

Kamaoui I, et al: Value of CT enteroclysis in suspected small-bowel carcinoid tumors. *AJR Am J Roentgenol.* 2010;194(3):629-633.

Kingham TP, et al: Multidisciplinary treatment of gastrointestinal stromal tumors. *Surg Clin North Am.* 2009;89:217-233.

Learn PA, et al: Randomized clinical trials in gastrointestinal stromal tumors. *Surg Oncol Clin N Am.* 2010;19(1):101-113.

Parc Y, et al: Surgical management of the duodenal manifestations of familial adenomatous polyposis. *Br J Surg.* 2011;98(4):480-484.

Poncet G, et al: Recent trends in the treatment of well-differentiated endocrine carcinoma of the small bowel. *World J Gastroenterol.* 2010;16(14):1696-1706.

Soyer P, et al: Imaging of malignant neoplasms of the mesenteric small bowel: new trends and perspectives. *Crit Rev Oncol Hematol.* 2011;80(1):10-30.

Speranza G, et al: Adenocarcinoma of the small bowel: changes in the landscape? *Curr Opin Oncol.* 2010;22(4):387-393.

MULTIPLE CHOICE QUESTIONS

1. The most common cause of small bowel obstruction is

    A. Intra-abdominal adhesions
    B. Neoplasms
    C. Intussusception
    D. Crohn disease

2. The treatment of small bowel obstruction includes

   A. Nasogastric suction
   B. Fluid and electrolyte resuscitation
   C. Laparoscopic adhesiolysis in highly selected cases
   D. All of above

3. Which of the following statements about acute mesenteric ischemia is incorrect?

   A. The most common cause is the arterial embolism.
   B. Thrombosis of mesenteric veins is often associated with portal hypertension.
   C. Deep venous thrombosis can be a cause.
   D. Abdominal pain is the main clinical finding.

4. Which of the following statements about small bowel tumors is correct?

   A. Adenomas are more common in the distal ileum.
   B. The most common neoplasm is gastrointestinal stromal tumor (GIST).
   C. Peutz-Jeghers syndrome has a very high malignant potential.
   D. Carcinoid syndrome develops in presence of liver metastases.

5. Which of the following is the most common intestinal fistula in patients with Crohn disease (CD)?

   A. Ileosigmoid
   B. Ileovesical
   C. Ileocutaneous
   D. Ileovaginal

Large Intestine

Jessica N. Cohan, MD, MAS
Madhulika G. Varma, MD

ANATOMY

The **colon** begins at the ileocecal valve and ends at the rectum, spanning 140 cm (5 feet) in length. The colon has both intraperitoneal and retroperitoneal components. The cecum and ascending and descending colon are retroperitoneal, whereas the transverse colon and sigmoid are intraperitoneal (Figure 32–1). The diameter of the lumen is greatest at the cecum (approximately 7 cm) and decreases distally. As a result, mass lesions of the cecum are least likely to cause obstruction. However, the wall of the colon is thinnest in the cecum; therefore, it is most vulnerable to ischemic necrosis and perforation from large bowel obstructions.

There are four layers of the wall: mucosa, submucosa, muscularis propria, and serosa (Figure 32–2). The mucosa is composed of three layers: a simple columnar epithelium organized to form crypts, lamina propria, and muscularis mucosa. The submucosa is the strength layer of the colon because it has the highest concentration of collagen. Therefore, this layer is especially important to incorporate during anastomoses. The muscularis propria is composed of an inner circular layer and an outer longitudinal layer that thickens into three bands around the circumference to form the taenia coli. The **appendix** can be found at the point on the cecum where the taenia converge. At the rectosigmoid, these bands fan out to form a uniform layer, marking the end of the colon and the beginning of the rectum. The forces of these muscular components of the wall result in shortening of the colon to form sacculations called haustra (Figure 32–3). These are not fixed structures, but can be observed to move longitudinally. The epiploic appendages are fatty appendages on the serosal surface.

The **rectum** begins at the sacral promontory and ends at the anorectal ring. It lies between the sigmoid colon and the anus and is 12-16 cm in length. There are no tenia as the longitudinal muscle fans out and encompasses the circumference of the rectal wall. The rectum can be further differentiated

from the colon by its lack of appendices epiploicae and haustra. The rectum is both an intra- and extraperitoneal organ. The anterior and lateral walls of the upper rectum are intraperitoneal, and the posterior wall is extraperitoneal. The anterior peritoneal reflection extends low into the pelvis, approximately 5-8 cm above the anal verge, and lies between the rectum and the bladder in men and uterus in women (the pouch of Douglas). Tumors or abscesses in this location can be palpated on digital rectal or vaginal exam. Denonvilliers fascia is the extension of the peritoneum that lies in the plane between the anterior rectum and the seminal vesicles in men and the cervix in women. Luminally, the rectum has three major folds called the valves of Houston. They are variable in location but classically occur every 3-4 cm. The superior and inferior folds are on the left, and the middle fold is on the right. The middle fold marks the anterior peritoneal reflection, where the anterior wall of the rectum is intraperitoneal proximally and extraperitoneal distally.

The pelvic floor is made of three muscles: the pubococcygeus, iliococcygeus, and puborectalis, collectively known as the **levator ani**. The puborectalis forms a sling at the anorectal junction and is an important component of continence and the defecation mechanism.

▶ Blood Supply & Lymphatic Drainage

The arterial supply of the colon is dictated by its embryologic origin. The **superior mesenteric artery** supplies the foregut, which extends to the distal transverse colon, through the ileocolic, right colic, and middle colic arteries. The hindgut, which includes the distal transverse colon to the rectum, is supplied by the **inferior mesenteric artery** (IMA). This gives off the left colic and two to six sigmoid branches, and terminates as the superior rectal (hemorrhoidal) artery. The middle and inferior rectal (hemorrhoidal) arteries originate from the **internal iliac artery**. There is redundancy in the arterial circulation via the meandering mesenteric artery

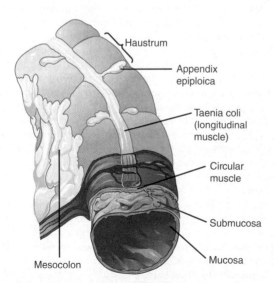

Normal position of colon

▲ **Figure 32–1.** The large intestine: anatomic divisions and blood supply. The veins are shown in black. The insert shows the usual configuration of the colon.

▲ **Figure 32–2.** Cross-section of colon. The muscularis propria consists of the inner circular muscle and the outer longitudinal muscle. The longitudinal muscle encircles the colon but is thickened in the region of the taenia coli. This muscle is responsible for the formation of haustra.

▲ **Figure 32–3.** Barium enema of normal colon. Note the appearance of haustra and the location of the splenic and hepatic flexures.

(arc of Riolan) as well as the **marginal artery of Drummond**, which is a network of arterial branches that runs the length of the colon approximately 2.5 cm from the bowel wall. The vasa recta are the terminal arteries arising from the marginal artery. These penetrate the colon wall, creating focal areas of weakness that have the potential to form false diverticula. The left colic, sigmoid, and superior rectal branches also originate from the IMA in a variable pattern. The venous drainage generally follows the arterial supply with the exception of the inferior mesenteric vein, which runs lateral to the ligament of Treitz to join the splenic vein. The vascular supply is highly variable, and "normal" anatomy is found in only 15% of individuals.

The **lymphatics drain** via continuous plexuses in the submucosal and subserosal layers of the bowel wall. These continue on to the mesenteric lymphatic channels and nodes that accompany the blood vessels, which explains why oncologic resection of the colon and rectum is based on the vascular supply.

▶ Nerve Supply

The nerve supply to the colon and rectum is autonomic and, like the blood supply, is divided according to embryologic development. Sympathetic nerves to the midgut, including the right and proximal transverse colon, originate in T6-12. These synapse in the superior mesenteric plexus and then follow the superior mesenteric artery and its branches to the right colon. The vagus nerve provides parasympathetic fibers to the midgut. Sympathetic innervation to the hindgut (distal transverse colon to the rectum) arises from L1-3. These sympathetic fibers synapse in the preaortic plexus and then follow the IMA to the bowel wall. Nervous impulses to the bowel wall synapse in the myenteric (Auerbach's) plexus and submucosal (Meissner's) plexus. The myenteric plexus is located in between the circular and longitudinal layers of smooth muscle and is responsible for coordinating motility. The submucosal plexus (Meissner's plexus) is located in the submucosa and regulates secretions, blood flow, and absorption.

The distal rectum and anus are innervated by the hypogastric nerves and the nervi erigentes. The hypogastric nerves are sympathetic fibers that originate from L1-3. These fibers course over the sacral promontory to the hypogastric plexus and form the paired **hypogastric nerves** near the root of the IMA. The parasympathetic fibers run in the **nervi erigentes**, which arise from S2-4 and join the hypogastric nerves near the lateral rectal stalks. The fibers continue anterior and laterally to innervate the rectum, pelvic floor muscles, and bladder, as well as the prostate and seminal vesicles in men. The location of these nerves makes them prone to injury during proctectomy. The superior hypogastric plexus is at risk during high ligation of the IMA, the hypogastric nerves are at risk during retrorectal dissection, the inferior hypogastric plexus and nervi erigentes are at risk during mobilization of the lateral stalks, and the periprostatic plexus is at risk during dissection of Denonvillier fascia. Injury to these nerves during proctectomy can cause bladder and sexual dysfunction that is a significant source of postoperative morbidity.

PHYSIOLOGY

The primary functions of the colon are absorption, secretion, motility, and intraluminal digestion. These interrelated processes are responsible for converting ileal effluent into semisolid feces. The rectum functions as a capacitance organ, storing feces produced by the colon and allowing defecation at a convenient time. When surgery or disease results in loss of colonic function, there is a significant increase in intestinal losses of water and electrolytes. If the rectum is overloaded by large-volume watery stool or its capacity to distend is lost or impaired by surgery or disease, fecal urgency and frequency are noted.

▶ Intestinal Gas

Normal volume and composition of intestinal gas have great variation among individuals depending on air swallowing, diet, and the composition of the microbial flora. Small amounts of intestinal gas are absorbed through the bowel wall and excreted through the lungs, but the majority (approximately 400-1200 mL/d) is discharged as flatus.

Intestinal gas is composed of nitrogen, oxygen, carbon dioxide, hydrogen, methane, and trace substances such as methyl sulfide, hydrogen sulfide, indole, and skatole. By far, the largest component is nitrogen, which makes up 30%-90% of intestinal gas. Most nitrogen comes from swallowed air, but some also diffuses from the plasma. Fermentation of nonabsorbed carbohydrates such as fiber is responsible for most of the hydrogen and carbon dioxide in gas. In lactase-deficient individuals, lactose fermentation contributes as well. Methane is produced by specific hydrogen-reducing bacteria (*Methanobrevibacter smithii*) and is only present in 30% of people. Both methane and hydrogen gases are explosive and require caution when using cautery in the bowel lumen.

Patients reporting crampy abdominal pain, bloating, and increased flatus may be suffering from increased gas production. Overproduction may be a result of a malabsorptive state, and eliminating lactose, legumes, and/or wheat in the diet may be of help. More recently, small intestinal bacterial overgrowth (SIBO) has been offered as an explanation. SIBO refers to an excess of bacteria in the upper gastrointestinal tract that causes symptoms such as diarrhea, weight loss, and malabsorption. This can be diagnosed using bacterial culture or breath testing. Treatment consists of nutritional support and antibiotics.

Absorption & Secretion

The colon is primarily an absorptive organ. The absorptive capacity is greatest in the cecum and ascending colon and decreases distally. Most nutrients are absorbed in the small bowel; however, when enteric contents reach the colon, they are still rich in water, electrolytes, and some nutrients. Approximately 1-2 L of ileal effluent containing 250 mEq of sodium reach the cecum every 24 hours. The passive absorption of water and active transportation of sodium allow recovery of more than 90% of the water and sodium content. Every 24 hours, approximately 100-200 mL of water and 2-5 mEq of sodium are excreted in the feces. Table 32–1 gives average values for the composition of ileal effluent and feces. Normal feces are composed of 70% water and 30% solids. Bacteria constitute over half of the solid component. The remaining solids are food waste and desquamated epithelium. Although the absorptive capacity of the colon serves an important role in maintaining homeostasis, it is not essential to life.

Ileal effluent also contains small amounts of nutrients that are absorbed by the colon, including fatty acids, amino acids, and vitamin K. Approximately 10% of undigested starch reaches the colon where colonic bacteria fermentation produces short-chain fatty acids, which are important both systemically and as a nutrient source for colonocytes.

In addition, the colon is part of the enterohepatic circulation. Bile acids not absorbed in the terminal ileum are passively absorbed in the colon. When this capacity is exceeded, the remaining bile acids are metabolized by colonic bacteria into urobilin and stercobilin. Urobilin, stercobilin, and their metabolites are responsible for giving stool its brown color.

The colon also serves an important secretory function. It secretes hydrogen, bicarbonate, chloride, and potassium ions. The colon is in communication with the systemic circulation and is able to adjust over a wide range as needed. Pathologic states such as inflammatory bowel disease, shigellosis, cystic fibrosis, and collagenous colitis cause electrolyte and acid-base disturbances by altering colonic secretion.

Motility

Colonic motility serves to maximize absorption and move feces distally in preparation for excretion. There are numerous types of motility, and these occur with great variation along the length of the colon. Normal movements are slow, variable, and complex and result in nonorganized flow of the fecal stream. In patients with normal bowel function, enteric contents reach the cecum 4 hours after a meal and the rectosigmoid by 24 hours. However, portions of the fecal stream are mixed so that new effluent may bypass old effluent, and residue from a single meal may pass in bowel movements over 3-4 days.

The enteric nervous system coordinates motility. It is increased by physical activity, stress, and diets high in fiber. In addition, the act of eating stimulates colonic transit. The gastrocolic reflex refers to the activation of colonic motor activity in response to a meal. The magnitude is determined by the fat and caloric composition. This increased activity increases ileal and colonic emptying, causing an urge to defecate.

The colon has three distinct patterns of activity that are under control of the enteric nervous system and a postulated pacemaker in the transverse colon. **Retrograde peristalsis** consists of annular contractions occurring most commonly in the right colon. These contractions work to keep the stool in the right colon and therefore facilitate absorption. As ileal effluent continues to empty into the cecum, some of the liquid stool flows to the transverse and descending colon, where **segmentation** predominates. This action consists of random, uncoordinated annular contractions over short segments that propel feces both proximally and distally. Finally, **mass movement** occurs as a strong coordinated contraction that starts proximally and propels colonic contents distally and occurs in concert with the gastrocolic reflex.

Microbiology

The colon of the fetus is sterile, but the process of colonization begins immediately after birth. There is marked variation in

Table 32–1. Mean values for electrolyte and water balance in the normal colon. a plus (+) sign indicates absorption from the colonic lumen; a minus (–) sign indicates secretion into the lumen.

	Ileal Effluent		Feces		Net Colonic Absorption (per 24 h)	
	Concentration (mEq/L)	Quantity (per 24 h)	Concentration (mEq/L)	Quantity (per 24 h)	Normal	Maximal Capacity
Na$^+$	120	180 mEq	30	2 mEq	+178 mEq	+400 mEq
K$^+$	6	10 mEq	67	5 mEq	−5 mEq	±45 mEq
Cl$^-$	67	100 mEq	20	1.5 mEq	+98 mEq	+500 mEq
HCO$_3$	40	60 mEq	50	4 mEq	+56 mEq	
H$_2$O		1500 mL		100 mL	+1400 mL	+5000 mL

the composition of the microbial flora between individuals, likely related to genetic, environmental, and dietary factors. Humans have 10 times more bacterial cells in their bodies than human cells, and in fact, bacteria make up half of the dry weight of feces. Microbes are present throughout the gastrointestinal tract, and their concentration increases from proximal to distal, with the highest concentrations in the colon and rectum. The majority of colonic organisms are anaerobic, but there is a substantial population of facultative anaerobes. *Bacteroides* species account for 60%-70% of the bacterial flora. Other predominant organisms include *Escherichia coli, Lactobacillus bifidus, Klebsiella, Proteus, Clostridium, Enterobacter,* and *Enterococcus. M smithii* is responsible for methane production.

These bacterial populations are instrumental for the health of the colon. They serve a barrier function and maintain epithelial integrity. Fermentation of undigested polysaccharides creates short-chain fatty acids that are an important energy source for colonocytes. In addition, bacteria play an active role in the immune function of the gut. Healthy bacterial populations make it difficult for pathogens to establish infection. In addition, normal microbial flora also serves a role in numerous physiologic processes. They deconjugate unabsorbed bile acids, creating the pigments that give stool its characteristic color; synthesize vitamin K for systemic absorption and use; and recycle colonic nitrogen in the form of urea.

▶ Bowel Habits

There is a broad range of normal bowel habits that varies across cultures. Normal is considered three per day to one every 3 days. A cross-sectional study of 20,000 men and women across all age groups in Britain showed an average of 1-1.5 bowel movements per day, which increased with fiber and fluid intake and physical activity.

▶ Defecation

The urge to defecate is stimulated by rectal stretch in response to feces. This elicits the **rectoanal inhibitory reflex,** which causes temporary relaxation of the internal anal sphincter and allows the rectal contents to be "sampled" by specialized mucosa in the anorectal transition zone. This mucosa contains sensory fibers that can discriminate between flatus and solid and liquid stool. Immediately following this sensory process, the external sphincter contracts and the contents are moved proximally back into the rectum. Flatus and stool can be discharged, if appropriate. If not, the rectum relaxes and the urge to defecate passes. Normal defecation requires regular colonic function, specifically with regard to stool consistency, in addition to coordinated colonic motility, rectal sensation, sphincter function, and pelvic floor relaxation. When the rectum senses presence of feces and the decision is made to defecate, intra-abdominal pressure is increased

and the pelvic floor and anal sphincters relax, allowing the rectum to straighten. After elimination of the stool bolus, the sphincters and pelvic floor resume their tone.

▶ Diarrhea

Diarrhea is defined by the loss of more than 300 mL of fluid per day and chronically affects 5% of the US population. It can result in severe electrolyte disturbances and dehydration. There are four main etiologies of diarrhea: invasive, secretory, osmotic, and malabsorptive. **Invasive diarrhea** results when enterocytes are destroyed by pathogens such as *Shigella, Campylobacter,* and *Entamoeba histolytica,* resulting in low-volume loose bowel movements with blood and leukocytes. **Secretory diarrhea** is the result of excessive secretion by colonocytes or enterocytes. This results in high-volume, isotonic diarrhea with a low osmotic gap. The primary causes are enterotoxins produced by *E coli* and *Vibrio cholerae* and excessive serotonin secretion in the carcinoid syndrome. **Osmotic diarrhea** occurs when an osmotically active substance in the bowel lumen draws hypotonic fluid from the circulation. Osmotic diarrhea is characterized by high-volume output with a high osmotic gap and no leukocytes. Most commonly, this occurs in patients with disaccharidase deficiencies such as lactose intolerance. **Malabsorptive diarrhea** results from the lack of normal digestive or absorptive processes. Pancreatic insufficiency results in loss of proteolytic and lipase activity, causing steatorrhea. Whipple disease (caused by infection with *Tropheryma whipplei*) and celiac sprue (autoantibodies to gluten) are characterized by inflammatory changes with loss of absorptive capacity of the small bowel. Surgery can also cause malabsorption. Extensive small bowel or colonic resections compromise the absorptive capacity and may result in diarrhea. A portion of patients undergoing cholecystectomy will also experience diarrhea with fatty meals due to the loss of the bile reservoir capacity of the gallbladder and subsequent steatorrhea.

CONSTIPATION

▶ Epidemiology

Constipation affects 3%-27% of the general population. The wide variation in reports is likely due to broad definitions of constipation, including infrequent or hard stools, excessive straining, or incomplete evacuation. Incidence is associated with lower socioeconomic and educational status, non-Caucasian ethnicity, female gender, and increasing age. Low fiber intake is especially important, as it normally bulks stool, triggering colonic motility.

▶ Etiology

Although idiopathic constipation occurs, changes in bowel habits should prompt a search for a cause. Numerous medications cause constipation, such as opiates, antiemetics (ondansetron), antipsychotics (chlorpromazine, haloperidol, risperidone, clozapine), antihypertensives (calcium channel blockers, atenolol, furosemide, clonidine), and over-the-counter medications such as ibuprofen, calcium, and iron supplements. The patient should be asked about previous laxative use, as rebound constipation may occur in patients with a history of laxative abuse. Constipation can be a symptom of a systemic disease such as hypothyroidism, hyperparathyroidism, diabetes, electrolyte disturbance, or connective tissue disorders. It may result from a primary colonic disorder such as Hirschsprung disease, endometriosis, and benign or malignant strictures. Neurologic disease or injury, psychiatric illness, and physical or sexual abuse may be contributory.

If none of these factors is present, patients may be suffering from a functional constipation syndrome, such as colonic inertia, irritable bowel syndrome, or pelvic floor dysfunction. Patients with colonic inertia report lifelong constipation with laxative dependence. Irritable bowel syndrome (constipation subtype) causes irregular bowel habits, bloating, and abdominal pain classically relieved with bowel movements. Patients with pelvic floor dysfunction or obstructed defecation syndrome report incomplete evacuation and excessive straining that is often improved with digital manipulation. They may have coexistent urinary dysfunction, pelvic organ prolapse, and sexual dysfunction.

Diagnosis

Evaluation for constipation includes a history and physical examination, including review of medications, and digital rectal and anoscopic evaluation. Metabolic etiologies may be ruled out with laboratory tests including thyroid-stimulating hormone, calcium, electrolytes, and blood sugar in the appropriate patient. Anatomic lesions can be identified by colonoscopy. This should be considered in any patient with alarm symptoms (hematochezia, anemia, or weight loss), patients with refractory constipation, and patients who are due for age-appropriate colon cancer screening. Medical therapy with fiber supplementation and laxatives should be tried first. Patients should be encouraged to keep a written record of their bowel habits. In refractory cases and those in which a functional disorder is suspected, additional testing is indicated.

Pelvic floor testing, such as anorectal manometry and balloon expulsion may be helpful in patients suspected to have pelvic floor dysfunction. Manometry allows evaluation of the rectoanal inhibitory reflex (RAIR), sphincter tone, rectal sensation, and coordination. Patients with Hirschsprung disease will have an absent RAIR. Patients with obstructed defecation will have inappropriate contraction or failure of relaxation of the puborectalis and external anal sphincter. Rectal sensation is determined by placing a balloon in the rectum and filling it until the urge to defecate is perceived.

The patient is then asked to evacuate the balloon. Normal function is indicated by the ability to evacuate a rectal balloon in less than 1 minute. Defecography (barium, scintigraphic, or magnetic resonance) can provide additional functional and anatomic information when the results of manometric testing are not diagnostic.

Colonic transit can be evaluated using radiopaque marker studies. Patients ingest 24 markers and avoid laxatives. An abdominal radiograph is taken on the fifth day, with note made of the distribution and number of retained markers. Normal patients will have fewer than five retained markers. In fact, 80% of normal patients will have passed all markers by the fifth day. Colonic inertia, a primary disorder of colonic motility, is diagnosed when more than five markers are retained and are scattered throughout the colon. Obstructed defecation is suggested if markers have accumulated in the rectum. A more detailed examination involves ingestion of radiopaque markers daily for 3 consecutive days and taking abdominal films on the fourth and seventh days. The number and distribution of retained markers are compared with established normal controls.

Treatment

Initial treatment of constipation should focus on lifestyle and dietary modification. Physical activity, fluid intake, and consumption of fruits, vegetables, and whole grains are increased. A fiber supplement is started in an effort to soften and bulk the stool. A low dose is recommended at first and slowly increased to the desired effect to minimize bloating and flatulence.

Laxatives, stimulants, and enemas should be used only for short periods of time for treatment of acute discomfort. **Osmotic laxatives** include lactulose, magnesium hydroxide, sodium phosphate, and polyethylene glycol. These work by increasing the intraluminal osmolarity, creating a gradient that reduces fluid reabsorption. Magnesium hydroxide should be avoided in patients with renal insufficiency. Polyethylene glycol is one of the most commonly recommended laxatives because it is safe and effective, even for use in the long term. **Colonic irritants** work by increasing motility. Examples include senna, cascara, and bisacodyl. These medications can produce crampy abdominal pain. Long-term use of senna and cascara causes melanosis coli (brown discoloration of the mucosa). **Stool softeners** such as mineral oil and docusate work by increasing stool fluid retention. **Enemas** stimulate bowel movements by causing direct rectal stretch and irrigation (saline, soap suds) or softening of the stool (mineral oil). Colonic irritants and enemas can cause reduced colon and rectal motility and should not be used for prolonged periods of time. Lubiprostone, linaclotide, and plecanatide treat constipation-predominant irritable bowel syndrome by increasing secretion and motility by stimulating the guanylate cyclase-C receptor.

Defecatory disorders, as diagnosed by anorectal manometry, are best managed using biofeedback and pelvic floor retraining. Patients can learn to relax and strengthen the pelvic floor muscles and can develop increased rectal sensation awareness. These techniques have been studied in a randomized fashion and have been shown to be superior to medical management.

Selected patients with constipation may benefit from surgery if all functional aspects of defecation have already been addressed. If there is pelvic floor dysfunction, this should be first addressed using biofeedback. Surgery is considered if patients have obstructed defecation from mechanical reasons such as rectal prolapse, rectocele, enterocele, or sigmoidocele and may benefit from procedures to address the specific condition. Patients with colonic inertia without pelvic floor dysfunction, irritable bowel syndrome, or diffuse stomach or small bowel involvement are treated with **abdominal colectomy with ileorectal anastomosis** with variable results. Multiple other approaches, including segmental colectomy and preservation of the cecum have shown conflicting, but overall worse, outcomes. Complications have been reduced with the use of laparoscopic techniques, which have been shown to be safe and effective. The **antegrade colonic enema** (ACE) procedure is performed successfully in pediatric patients. It involves bringing up a piece of bowel (appendix, ileum, cecum, and left colon have been described) to the abdominal wall to allow intermittent catheterization with antegrade irrigation of the colon. This technique is not generally recommended in adults, where studies have shown only moderate success and relatively high complication rates. Newer therapies such as sacral nerve stimulation show limited efficacy in small studies.

Patel AS, Saratzis A, Arasaradnam R, et al: Use of antegrade continence enema for the treatment of fecal incontinence and functional constipation in adults: a systematic review. *Dis Colon Rectum*. 2015;58(10):999-1013.

Pilkington SA, Emmett C, Knowles CH, et al: Surgery for constipation: systematic review and practice recommendations: Results V: Sacral Nerve Stimulation. *Colorectal Dis*. 2017;19(Suppl 3):92-100.

Rao SS, Rattanakovit K, Patcharatrakul T: Diagnosis and management of chronic constipation in adults. *Nat Rev Gastroenterol Hepatol*. 2016;13(5):295-305.

▼ DISEASES OF THE COLON AND RECTUM

LARGE BOWEL OBSTRUCTION

▶ General Considerations

Fifteen percent of intestinal obstructions in adults occur in the large bowel, and the incidence increases with age. Obstruction can result from pathology of the bowel wall including malignancy and strictures, mechanical problems such as volvulus, incarcerated hernia, and intussusception,

Table 32–2. Causes of colonic obstruction in adults.

Cause	Relative Incidence (%)[1]
Carcinoma of colon	65
Diverticulitis	20
Volvulus	5
Miscellaneous	10

[1]Obstruction due to diverticulitis is usually incomplete; volvulus is second to carcinoma as a cause of complete obstruction.

or intraluminal factors such as fecal or foreign body impaction (Table 32–2). Benign strictures are commonly associated with diverticulitis or inflammatory bowel disease, but may occur as a result of ischemia, radiation, or a surgical anastomosis. Acute colonic pseudo-obstruction (Ogilvie syndrome) can cause the same spectrum of clinical symptoms and is discussed in the following section. It is important to differentiate pseudo-obstruction from mechanical obstruction because the management is different. In contrast to small bowel obstruction, adhesive disease of the colon is a very rare cause of obstruction.

A major factor in the clinical course of large bowel obstruction depends on the competence of the ileocecal valve. Thirty percent of patients have an incompetent ileocecal valve, which allows decompression of the large bowel contents into the ileum. However, in the majority of patients, the ileocecal valve does not allow reflux to occur, resulting in a closed loop obstruction with rapidly increasing intraluminal pressure (Figure 32–4). This results in impaired capillary circulation, mucosal ischemia, and subsequent bacterial translocation with systemic toxicity. This process ultimately progresses to gangrene and perforation. This same process occurs in volvulus, which by definition is a closed loop obstruction. The cecum has the largest diameter and, therefore, by the law of Laplace, is at greatest risk for perforation. The normal diameter is approximately 7 cm. The risk of perforation is high if the diameter increases acutely or to a size greater than 10-12 cm.

▶ Clinical Findings

A. Symptoms and Signs

The history and physical exam can help distinguish a large bowel obstruction from other causes of an acute abdomen and identify patients who require urgent therapy. Obstipation is a universal feature of complete obstruction, although the patient may pass stool and gas located distal to the obstruction after the initial symptoms begin. Classically, the digital rectal exam reveals an empty vault except in cases of distal fecal impaction.

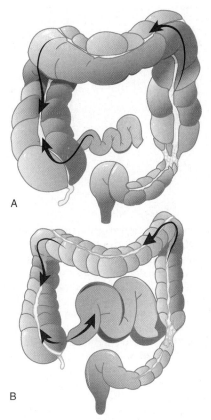

A

B

▲ **Figure 32–4.** The role of the ileocecal valve in obstruction of the colon. The obstruction is in the upper sigmoid. **A:** The ileocecal valve is competent, creating a closed loop between the obstruction and the valve. Tension in the closed loop is increased further by emptying of gas and fluid from the ileum into the colon. **B:** The ileocecal valve is incompetent. Reflux into the ileum is permitted. The colon is relieved of some of its distention, and the small bowel has become distended.

Vomiting is a late finding and may not occur at all if the ileocecal valve prevents reflux. If reflux decompresses the cecal contents into the small intestine, the patient may also present with symptoms of small bowel obstruction.

The onset of symptoms may be acute or gradual, depending on the location and etiology of the obstruction. A patient may report a history of constipation for months preceding any acute obstructive symptoms. Deep, visceral, cramping pain from obstruction of the colon is usually referred to the hypogastrium. Right-sided lesions tend to grow to a large size prior to causing obstruction owing to the larger diameter of the lumen and the liquid stool. Therefore, these lesions may be palpable on abdominal exam. If the patient reports repeated episodes of fever and abdominal pain, a diverticular

stricture is suspected; a history of hematochezia and weight loss suggests colorectal cancer. Alternatively, when symptoms occur acutely, volvulus, incarcerated hernia, or intussusception is more likely. A patient with fever, leukocytosis, and peritonitis has likely progressed to develop intestinal ischemia and/or perforation.

B. Imaging Studies

Abdominal films will frequently reveal dilated colon outlining the abdominal cavity. The colon can be distinguished from the small intestine by its haustral markings, which do not cross the entire lumen of the distended colon. Sigmoid volvulus can be identified by a characteristic "coffee bean" radiographic appearance that represents a dilated loop of colon starting in the left lower quadrant extending medially. Cecal volvulus tends to appear as a dilated loop originating in the right lower quadrant extending medially. In patients with other forms of obstruction, the extent of distention is dependent on the competency of the ileocecal valve and its relation to the location of the obstruction. A transition point with no distal colonic gas indicates complete obstruction. If gas is present in the distal rectum, it can represent residual material present prior to the obstruction or the presence of a partial obstruction. In acute pseudo-obstruction, the colon is diffusely dilated with stool and gas throughout (Figure 32–5).

▲ **Figure 32–5.** Plain radiograph demonstrating acute colonic pseudo-obstruction. (Used with permission from Dr. Santhat Nivatvongs.)

A computed tomography (CT) scan with rectal contrast is the most useful single test for large bowel obstruction because it can yield information regarding the location and etiology of the bowel obstruction. This has largely replaced contrast enema. A water-soluble contrast medium, such as diatrizoate (gastrografin), should be used if strangulation or perforation is suspected.

Treatment

Intervention is almost always required for mechanical large bowel obstructions. The extent of surgery depends on the patient's acuity and the etiology of the obstruction. The primary goals of treatment are resection of all necrotic bowel and decompression of the obstructed segment. Removal of the obstructing lesion is a secondary goal, but a single operation to accomplish both objectives is preferred whenever possible. Options include resection with primary anastomosis, resection with diversion, diversion alone, and endoscopic stent placement.

Endoscopic stents are being used as a bridge to surgery and as palliative therapy. When used in acutely ill patients with a malignancy, there is no clear advantage of endoscopic stent placement as a bridge to surgery in terms of mortality or complications. However, they do allow decompression of the obstruction and time for physiologic optimization. This can increase the chances of resection with primary anastomosis and reduce the chance for diversion. This comes, however, at the risk of stent-related perforation. Stents may be considered also for palliation in high-risk patients whose obstructing cancers are not resectable; however, if the patient can tolerate surgery, a diverting ileostomy or colostomy is a more durable option.

Generally speaking, obstructing lesions of the right colon can be resected in one stage if the patient's condition is stable. If the patient's condition is precarious or if the colon has perforated, other options include diversion alone, resection with anastomosis and diverting ileostomy, or resection with end ileostomy. Intestinal continuity can be restored at a second operation. Intestinal bypass is sometimes used for unresectable lesions, although the relief of the obstruction is not always as effective.

Obstructing lesions of the left colon more commonly require diversion. Ideally, the lesion is resected at the initial operation. After resection, anastomosis may be postponed with creation of a temporary end colostomy and Hartmann pouch (Figure 32–6). If the patient's clinical condition will allow it, a primary anastomosis may be performed with a diverting loop ileostomy if needed to protect the anastomosis. If resection is not possible, the bowel can be decompressed proximally and distally with a colostomy and mucus fistula or loop colostomy, although the latter are much more difficult to manage.

▲ **Figure 32–6.** Primary resection for acute large bowel obstruction or diverticulitis. The affected segment (shaded) has been divided at its distal end. If primary anastomosis is to be done, the proximal margin (dotted line) is transected, and the bowel is anastomosed end to end. If a two-stage procedure will be used, a colostomy is formed at the proximal margin, and the distal stump is oversewn (Hartmann procedure, as shown) or exteriorized as a mucous fistula. The second stage consists of colostomy takedown and anastomosis.

Prognosis

The prognosis depends on the age and general condition of the patient, the extent of vascular impairment of the bowel, the presence or absence of perforation, the cause of obstruction, and the promptness of surgical management.

ACUTE COLONIC PSEUDO-OBSTRUCTION

General Considerations

Acute colonic pseudo-obstruction (Ogilvie syndrome) is characterized by massive colonic distention in the absence of a mechanically obstructing lesion (Figure 32–5). It is a severe form of ileus that occurs most commonly in systemically ill patients of unclear etiology. Electrolyte disturbances and medications are contributing factors. Affected patients are usually recovering from major surgery or are hospitalized for other causes, most commonly cardiac disease, trauma, or infection.

Clinical Findings

Patients usually present with gradual abdominal distention over several days, although some patients will present acutely. Later symptoms include abdominal pain, vomiting, and obstipation and may mimic those of true obstruction. However, 40% of patients will have diarrhea.

The differential diagnosis includes toxic megacolon (in patients with ulcerative colitis and *Clostridium difficile* colitis) and mechanical large bowel obstruction. Plain x-rays of the abdomen show marked distention of the colon, often most severe in the right and transverse colon. A CT scan with rectal contrast is the most useful single test in this situation because it can differentiate true obstruction from pseudo-obstruction. Water-soluble contrast enema can be used to exclude mechanical obstruction, but instillation of contrast should stop as soon as the dilated colon is reached to reduce the chance of colonic perforation.

Treatment

As opposed to a mechanical bowel obstruction, surgical management in acute colonic pseudo-obstruction is reserved for complications including perforation and ischemia. Patients should be fluid resuscitated, and electrolytes should be normalized. Rectal tube placement is unlikely to be helpful for colonic decompression because the colonic distention rarely extends to the distal rectum. Systemic illnesses contribute and should be treated appropriately (respiratory failure, cardiac disease, sepsis). All anticholinergic and narcotic medications should be discontinued. These measures will be effective in 70%-90% of patients. The patient should be followed with serial imaging and abdominal exams to detect signs and symptoms of ischemia or perforation such as fever, tenderness, or leukocytosis. The risk of ischemia and perforation increases with the degree and duration of colon distention. The highest risk patients have a cecal diameter > 12 cm and duration of dilation > 6 days. If there is any sign of clinical deterioration or no improvement in 48 hours, more aggressive treatment is warranted.

The acetylcholinesterase inhibitor neostigmine is an effective treatment for acute colonic pseudo-obstruction in patients without response to conservative measures. This treatment cannot be used until mechanical obstruction has been ruled out. It works by acutely increasing acetylcholine levels in the body, thereby prompting immediate bowel contraction and decompression. Patients require telemetry monitoring during and after administration because symptomatic bradycardia requiring atropine occurs in < 10% of patients. It is also wise to insert a rectal tube prior to administration to aid management of stools. The most common side effects include abdominal cramping, vomiting, and excessive salivation. Neostigmine is successful in approximately 90% of patients with a recurrence rate of 10%-30%. A second dose of neostigmine can be tried (after 80 minutes) if necessary. If neostigmine is contraindicated (renal insufficiency, pregnancy, bronchospasm, bradycardia) or unsuccessful, endoscopic decompression is the next step in management. Endoscopic decompression offers the benefit of visualization of the colonic mucosa for evidence of ischemia but does carry a 2% risk of perforation in experienced centers. Endoscopic decompression is initially successful in 80% of patients, but recurrence is common.

In patients with refractory disease or evidence of ischemia or perforation, surgical intervention is required. Options include percutaneous cecostomy, cecostomy, or loop transverse colostomy for decompression if the cecum is viable. If there is ischemia or colonic perforation, the area of perforation and the surrounding tissue are examined. Depending on the condition of the patient, location of the perforation, and the viability of the surrounding tissue, options include exteriorization of the perforation as a colostomy, resection with end ostomy, and resection with anastomosis with or without diverting stoma.

Prognosis

Acute colonic pseudo-obstruction is associated with an 8% overall risk of mortality, which increases to 40% in patients with ischemia or perforation who require surgery.

COLON CANCER AND POLYPS

Background

In the United States, colorectal cancer ranks third after prostate and lung cancer in men and after breast and lung cancer in women in both incidence and mortality. The American Cancer Society predicts that, in 2018, more than 140,000 patients will be diagnosed and 50,000 will die as a result of their disease. Men have a higher incidence and mortality than women, and black Americans have a higher incidence and mortality than other ethnic groups. The overall incidence and mortality from colorectal cancer has been decreasing since the early 1980s, likely owing to improved screening. The frequency of colorectal cancers by location in the colon is shown in Figure 32-7. The average age at diagnosis is 68 years for men and 72 years for women.

The average lifetime incidence of colorectal cancer in the United States is more than 4%. Multiple risk factors for colorectal cancer have been identified. The most significant are considered nonmodifiable. These include family history of colorectal cancer, or personal history of inflammatory bowel disease (especially pancolitis), adenomatous polyps, diabetes, and truncal obesity. Modifiable risk factors include red and processed meat consumption, smoking, and alcohol.

Genetics

Colorectal cancer develops through a stepwise accumulation of mutations that allow the progression of normal mucosa to adenoma and then to carcinoma. The three well-described pathways for the development of colorectal cancer are chromosomal instability, microsatellite instability, and the methylator phenotype. Although these pathways are distinct, they

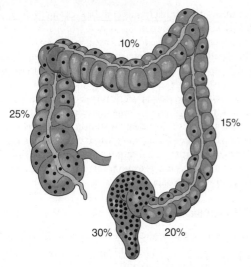

▲ Figure 32–7. Distribution of cancer of the colon and rectum.

can overlap, and some cancers exhibit more than one pathway. Chromosomal instability is the inciting event in 75% of colorectal cancers. In this pathway, the loss of genes or a chromosomal segment results in the accumulation of inactivating mutations in tumor suppressors such as *APC* (adenomatous polyposis coli), *P53*, *DCC* (deleted in colorectal carcinoma) and *SMAD4*, as well as activating mutations in oncogenes such as *KRAS*, *c-myc*, *c-src*, and *BRAF* in a stepwise fashion. Ultimately, this pathway leads to the classically described "adenoma to carcinoma sequence" and is associated with left-sided cancers, older age, and male gender. Microsatellite instability is found in 15% of colorectal cancers, both sporadic and those associated with Lynch syndrome. This pathway involves a loss of normal DNA mismatch repair function that ultimately results in mutations in tumor suppressors and oncogenes such as *TGF-beta2*, *BAX*, and *IGF2R*. The third pathway, the CpG island methylator phenotype (CIMP), is detected in 20% of colorectal cancers. It involves the epigenetic silencing of tumor suppressor genes and oncogenes (most commonly *BRAF*, *p16*, and *MLH1*) through abnormal methylation. These colorectal cancers develop through a serrated polyp pathway (as opposed to adenomatous polyps in the chromosomal instability pathway) and are more common in the right colon, older patients, and women. There is overlap in the microsatellite instability and CIMP pathways because abnormal methylation (CIMP pathway) of *MLH1* is the cause of 85% of microsatellite-unstable cancers (because *MLH1* is a mismatch repair gene).

The familial cancer syndromes are caused by germline (as opposed to sporadic) mutations in genes such as *APC* in familial adenomatous polyposis and mismatch repair genes

in Lynch syndrome. Approximately 5% of colorectal cancers occur in patients with a hereditary syndrome.

LYNCH SYNDROME

The most common genetic colon cancer syndrome is Lynch syndrome, formerly known as hereditary nonpolyposis colorectal cancer. It is an autosomal dominant condition with 80% penetrance in which patients are at increased risk of colorectal cancer as well as extracolonic cancers such as endometrial, ovarian, gastric, urinary tract, biliary, small bowel, and brain (glioblastoma). More recently, there is evidence to suggest an increased risk of breast and prostate cancers as well. The syndrome arises due to a germline mutation in a mismatch repair gene, which results in microsatellite instability. The majority of patients have a mutation in *MLH1*, *MSH2*, *MSH6*, or *PMS2*. The lifetime risk of colorectal cancer is 10%-74%, with mutations in *MLH1* and *MSH2* carrying the highest risk. The average age of colorectal cancer diagnosis is between 44 and 61 years. These cancers tend to occur in the right colon but can occur throughout the colon and rectum, and patients have a tendency to present with synchronous lesions.

The diagnosis can be suspected on clinical grounds using the patient's medical and family history. The Amsterdam criteria (Table 32–3) were initially developed in 1991 to identify individuals and families with Lynch syndrome. These are commonly remembered by trainees using the "3, 2, 1 Rule": 3 relatives with colon cancer in 2 successive generations, 1 must be a first degree relative of another, and 1 must be diagnosed before age 50. In 1999, the Amsterdam II criteria were published, which used the same rules but increased the sensitivity by including extracolonic cancers.

Table 32–3. Amsterdam I and II criteria.

Amsterdam I criteria: At least three relatives must have histologically verified colorectal cancer.	(1) One must be a first-degree relative of the other two. (2) At least two successive generations must be affected. (3) At least one of the relatives with colorectal cancer must have received the diagnosis before age 50.
Amsterdam II criteria: At least three relatives must have a cancer associated with Lynch syndrome (colorectal, endometrial, stomach, ovary, ureter or renal-pelvis, brain, small bowel, hepatobiliary tract, skin (sebaceous tumors)	(1) One must be a first-degree relative of the other two. (2) At least two successive generations must be affected. (3) At least one of the relatives with Lynch syndrome–associated cancer must have received the diagnosis before age 50.

Table 32–4. Revised Bethesda Criteria.

1. Colorectal cancer (CRC) diagnosed in individual under age 50 years.
2. Presence of synchronous, metachronous colorectal or other Lynch syndrome–associated tumors, regardless of age.
3. CRC with the microsatellite instability–high (MSI-H) histology (presence of tumor-infiltrating lymphocytes, Crohn-like lymphocytic reaction, mucinous/signet ring differentiation, or medullary growth pattern) in patient 60 years of age.
4. CRC in one or more first-degree relatives with a Lynch syndrome–related tumor, with one of the cancers being diagnosed under age 50 years.
5. CRC diagnosed in two or more first- or second-degree relatives with Lynch syndrome–related tumors, regardless of age.

When patients present with colorectal cancer, a selective approach to screening uses the Bethesda criteria, published in 1997 and revised in 2004 (Table 32–4). If one criterion is met, the tumor is submitted for microsatellite instability testing or immunohistochemistry for mismatch repair genes. If a tumor is found to have an abnormality in *MLH1* by immunohistochemistry, *BRAF* mutation testing is performed to rule out *MLH* silencing secondary to abnormal promoter methylation. If a *BRAF* mutation is present, this argues against a germline *MLH1* mutation. If absent, a confirmatory genetic test is required. Confirmatory germline testing is similarly required if there are abnormalities in *MSH2*, *MSH6*, and *PMS2* by immunohistochemistry. As molecular testing has become more available and accepted, a universal approach to screening colorectal tumor specimens is being advocated and is included in the National Comprehensive Cancer Network (NCCN) guidelines (v 2.2018). In universal screening, all colorectal cancers are submitted for testing as opposed to only those meeting the Revised Bethesda criteria. In any of the above scenarios, genetic testing should be preceded by genetic counseling.

Once a diagnosis has been made, an aggressive colorectal cancer screening regimen is initiated, including colonoscopy every 1-2 years starting at age 20-25, or 2-5 years prior to the age of onset of colorectal cancer in a family member. There are no widely accepted guidelines for surveillance for extracolonic cancers in patients with Lynch syndrome. The NCCN (v 2.2018) recommends that endometrial and ovarian cancer screening as well as prophylactic hysterectomy and oophorectomy can be considered at the physician's discretion. Further, screening for other extracolonic cancers, including gastric, small bowel, urothelial, central nervous system, pancreatic, breast, and prostate cancers, can be considered in patients with Lynch syndrome, especially in those patients with high-risk mutations or those with a family history. A decision analysis model suggested that prophylactic total abdominal colectomy at age 25 would offer a very small survival benefit (1.8 years) and a decreased quality of life compared with colonoscopic surveillance. Therefore,

surgical intervention is generally reserved for patients who develop a cancer or polyp that is unable to be removed endoscopically.

Surgical planning for patients with Lynch syndrome begins with normal surgical oncologic principles (adequate margins and regional lymphadenectomy). The extent of resection requires careful consideration. If a patient presents with a colon cancer, options include segmental colectomy, total abdominal colectomy, or total proctocolectomy. Segmental colectomy has the benefit of the least impact on bowel and social functioning but the highest risk of metachronous colorectal cancer (40% at 20 years). Total abdominal colectomy with an ileorectal anastomosis results in increased stool frequency, restrictions in diet, and daily medication use with a 6%-20% risk of metachronous cancer. Proctocolectomy with ileal pouch–anal anastomosis (IPAA; J-pouch) can be considered in colon cancer patients who wish to reduce the risk of metachronous cancer as much as possible, but at the cost of the greatest impact on bowel function. In patients presenting with rectal cancer, segmental proctectomy carries a 47% 20-year risk of metachronous colon cancer. Therefore, total proctocolectomy with IPAA or end ileostomy, depending on patient and tumor factors, is often advocated. Decision making for any patient with Lynch syndrome is complex and should consider the patient's age, comorbidities, preoperative continence, compliance with postoperative surveillance, and patient preference.

FAMILIAL ADENOMATOUS POLYPOSIS

The second most common colorectal cancer syndrome is familial adenomatous polyposis (FAP). This syndrome accounts for less than 1% of all colorectal cancers. It is inherited in an autosomal dominant fashion with nearly 100% penetrance. Most cases are a result of a mutation of the DNA mismatch repair gene *APC* located on chromosome 5q21. Depending on the location and type of mutation, the phenotypic presentation can range from mild to severe. Individuals with classic FAP typically have 100-1000 colonic adenomas that develop at an early age and are present in 50% of patients by age 15. Nearly 100% of patients develop colon cancer at a median age of 39 years. Attenuated FAP (aFAP) is a milder form of the condition where patients develop < 100 polyps and can present later in life. The lifetime risk of colorectal cancer in patients with aFAP is 70%, with median age at diagnosis of 58 years.

Management of the colon in patients with FAP involves genetic counseling and testing for family members, aggressive screening, and prophylactic colectomy. Patients at risk for FAP should undergo initial flexible sigmoidoscopy at age 12, followed by a full colonoscopy if polyps are detected. Prophylactic colectomy is warranted in all patients, especially those with severe polyposis, dysplasia, symptoms, or large adenomas. The development of colorectal cancer is rare in patients younger than 20 years, and therefore, surgery can be delayed in asymptomatic teenagers without dysplasia. Surgical options include total proctocolectomy with end ileostomy, restorative proctocolectomy with IPAA, and total abdominal colectomy with ileorectal anastomosis, depending on the burden of disease in the rectum, ability to undergo appropriate surveillance, and patient preference.

All patients require ongoing surveillance after prophylactic colectomy or restorative proctocolectomy with IPAA. Patients undergoing ileorectal anastomosis require surveillance proctoscopy every 6-12 months depending on the polyp burden. Patients undergoing restorative proctocolectomy with IPAA who have a stapled anastomosis will retain about 1 cm of the anal transition zone and are at increased risks of polyps compared with patients undergoing mucosectomy with handsewn anastomosis. For this reason, some surgeons advocate mucosectomy. However, mucosectomy results in a worse functional outcome, and there is no evidence that it decreases the development of cancer or mortality.

A variety of extracolonic manifestations are described in patients with FAP. Duodenal neoplasms are the most common, occurring in > 90% of patients, with 4%-12% going on to develop duodenal cancer. Desmoid disease affects 5% of patients with FAP but is the second most common cause of death. Desmoids generally occur in the small bowel mesentery or in the abdominal wall but can also occur in the subcutaneous tissues. The diagnosis is often made incidentally on imaging or at the time of surgery, but desmoids can have an aggressive course, resulting in their being the second most common cause of death in patients with FAP. Patients are also at increased risk compared with the general population for medulloblastoma, papillary carcinoma of the thyroid, and hepatoblastoma. Other manifestations include gastric fundal gland polyps, retinal pigment epithelium hypertrophy, osteomas, and sebaceous cysts. **Gardner syndrome** is applied to families with the constellation of polyposis, osteoma, dental abnormalities, and soft tissue tumors; **Turcot syndrome** refers to patients affected by polyposis and medulloblastoma.

NCCN recommendations (v 2.2018) for extracolonic surveillance in patients with FAP include annual physical examination, including thyroid and abdominal exams to evaluate for thyroid cancer and abdominal desmoid disease. Routine abdominal imaging is considered in patients with a family history of desmoid disease. Upper endoscopy beginning at age 20-25 years, annual thyroid examination, and consideration for intra-abdominal imaging to detect small bowel polyps if there is advanced duodenal polyposis are recommended.

MUTYH-ASSOCIATED POLYPOSIS

MUTYH-associated polyposis (MAP) is an autosomal recessive condition resulting from a biallelic mutation in the base excision repair gene *MUTYH*. MAP accounts for < 1% of

colorectal cancers and is clinically similar to aFAP. Most patients develop < 100 adenomas, although cases have been documented with 5-750 polyps. Colorectal cancer develops in > 70% of patients, with an average age at diagnosis of 45-55 years. MAP patients are at risk for duodenal adenomas, which occur in 20% of patients, and at an excess risk for duodenal cancer. In addition, there is an association with extracolonic cancers, such as bladder, ovarian, skin, and thyroid cancers. Screening for colon cancer begins at age 25-30 years. Once polyps are detected, surveillance colonoscopy should be performed every 1-2 years. Upper endoscopy is recommended to start at age 30 years and to be repeated every 3-5 years if normal. Consideration for annual thyroid ultrasound is also recommended. Surgery for patients with MAP is indicated when the patient develops colorectal cancer, high-grade dysplasia, or polyp burden that is not manageable endoscopically. Options are similar to those in patients with FAP.

JUVENILE POLYPOSIS

Juvenile polyposis is a rare syndrome characterized by the development of nonadenomatous polyps. It is an autosomal dominant condition, most commonly associated with germline mutations in the *SMAD4* or *BMPR1A* genes. Polyps are typically round, red, and pedunculated, and can be found throughout the gastrointestinal tract. Histologically, juvenile polyps have an overgrowth of lamina propria, mucin, and inflammatory changes. The syndrome is diagnosed by the presence of five or more juvenile polyps in the gastrointestinal tract or the presence of any number of juvenile polyps with a positive family history. There are three associated syndromes: Cronkhite-Canada syndrome (juvenile polyposis and ectodermal lesions), Bannayan-Riley-Ruvalcaba syndrome (juvenile polyposis, macrocephaly, and genital hyperpigmentation), and Cowden disease (juvenile polyposis, facial trichilemmomas, thyroid cancer, goiter, and breast cancer).

Patients with juvenile polyposis are at increased risk of colorectal cancer as well as extracolonic cancer (stomach, duodenum, pancreas, and jejunum). The lifetime risk of colorectal cancer is 39%-68% at an average age of 43 years. Screening colonoscopy is started at age 12-15 years and upper endoscopy at age 15-25 years, or earlier if symptoms develop. Surgery is indicated for patients with high-grade dysplasia or those who fail endoscopic management of their polyps and is considered prophylactically in those unable to adhere to surveillance or with a strong family history of colorectal cancer.

PEUTZ-JEGHERS SYNDROME

Peutz-Jeghers syndrome is a rare autosomal dominant condition (1/200,000 population) caused by a mutation in the *STK11* gene on chromosome 19. The syndrome is characterized by Peutz-Jeghers (hamartomatous) polyps in the gastrointestinal tract (stomach to the rectum) and mucocutaneous pigmentation. Polyps are characterized by an overgrowth of muscularis mucosa and grow to large sizes, becoming symptomatic in 50% of patients by age 20. Symptoms include anemia, abdominal pain secondary to infarction, intussusception, or obstruction. Diagnosis is made in patients with two or more of the following: perioral mucocutaneous pigmentation, family history, or more than one Peutz-Jeghers polyp. The lifetime risk of colorectal cancer is reported to be 39%, and there is an association with gastric, breast, pancreatic, cervical, ovarian, and testicular cancers. Because of the rarity of the condition, management has not been well defined. Screening of the small bowel and testicles is initiated at age 8-10 years; colonoscopy, upper endoscopy, and cervical cancer screening begin in the late teenage years, and pancreatic cancer screening begins at age 30-35. When endoscopic removal of gastrointestinal Peutz-Jeghers polyps is not possible, surgical resection is advised.

COLORECTAL CANCER SCREENING

Colorectal cancer screening is important for two reasons. The first is the early detection of colorectal carcinomas and the second is preventing colorectal cancer through the identification and removal of colorectal adenomas, which are cancer precursors. Trials have shown that the detection of early colorectal cancers by surveillance reduces mortality. Similarly, patients who undergo endoscopic removal of adenomas have a 40%-60% reduction in colorectal cancer–specific mortality at long-term follow-up. The benefit is increased in patients with above average risk for colorectal cancer.

The US Multi-Society Task Force on Colorectal Cancer guidelines on colorectal cancer screening were updated in 2017 (Table 32–5). The updated guidelines include a tier system, with the preferred screening methods in tier 1, and other recommendations in tiers 2 and 3 for patients who decline the preferred tests. For average-risk individuals, the US Multi-Society Task Force recommends initiating screening at age 50. However, the American Cancer Society now recommends that screening is initiated at age 45 for average-risk individuals. It is recommended that consideration is given to stopping screening at age 75 years or when life expectancy is expected to be less than 10 years. All methods have their strengths and weaknesses.

The tier 1 tests include colonoscopy at 10-year intervals or the fecal immunochemical test (FIT) annually. The major drawback to colonoscopy is poor adherence, likely related to the need for bowel preparation, sedation, a chaperone, and time away from work. It is the most expensive screening test and does have a small but real risk of complications, including bleeding, perforation, missed lesions, and incomplete examination. However,

Table 32–5. Colorectal cancer screening.

Risk Factor	Procedure	When to Start
No colorectal cancer or advanced adenoma in any first-degree relative Colorectal cancer or advanced adenoma in first-degree relative ≥ 60 years	**Tier 1[1]:** Colonoscopy every 10 years or fecal immunochemical test (FIT) every year **Tier 2:** CT colonography every 5 years, FIT fecal DNA every 3 years, or flexible sigmoidoscopy every 5 years **Tier 3:** Capsule colonoscopy every 5 years	Age 45-50[2] Age 40
Colorectal cancer or advanced adenoma in first-degree relative age < 60 years, or Colorectal cancer or advanced adenoma in two first-degree relatives of any age	Colonoscopy every 5 years	Age 40, or 10 years before onset in family member, whichever is earlier
Familial adenomatous polyposis: diagnosis or family history and unknown genetic status	Annual flexible sigmoidoscopy until polyps are detected	Age 10-12
Lynch syndrome: genetic or clinical diagnosis	Colonoscopy every 1-2 years	Age 20-25, or 10y before colorectal cancer in family member, whichever is earlier
Ulcerative colitis or Crohn colitis	Colonoscopy with biopsies every 1-2 years	Pancolitis: 8 years after diagnosis Left-sided colitis: 12-15 years after diagnosis

[1]Tiers indicate acceptable screening tests, with the preferred tests in tier 1. If a test in tier 1 is declined, then a test in tier 2 should be offered, etc.
[2]American Cancer Society guidelines recommend starting colorectal cancer screening in all persons with no risk factors at age 45. The US Multi-Society Task Force on Colorectal Cancer recommends starting at age 45 for African Americans and at age 50 for all others.

it is overall a safe and effective screening tool and is the only single-step screening test that allows identification and treatment of polyps or biopsy of colorectal cancer in a single procedure. The FIT stool test is noninvasive, does not require a bowel prep, and has no procedural risk. It is also affordable (approximately US$20 per test). However, there is concern for poor adherence in clinical trials on the part of both the physician and patient, with the exam not being performed at the proper intervals or patients not undergoing colonoscopy for positive tests. It is also important to note that this test is not designed for prevention, but rather for early detection, and although the sensitivity for colorectal cancer is nearly 80%, for advanced adenomas, it is only 30%. In addition, it does not detect sessile serrated polyps.

Tier 2 tests include CT colonography, the FIT-fecal DNA test, and flexible sigmoidoscopy. CT colonography is a radiographic option that has > 80% sensitivity for polyps greater than 1 cm and colorectal cancers. Drawbacks are that the test is expensive, will miss flat polyps, and requires a full bowel preparation. If it appears that there is a polyp 6 mm or greater in size, a colonoscopy with another bowel prep is required. Patients should also be aware that in 5%-15% of cases, there will be an incidental extracolonic finding requiring further evaluation. The FIT-fecal DNA test is performed every 3 years and combines the FIT test with a screen for DNA. The sensitivity for colorectal cancer is > 90%, and there is some sensitivity for adenomas (40% if > 1 cm); however, the specificity is reduced and the cost per test is about 10 times greater than FIT. Flexible sigmoidoscopy is not often used in the United States for screening purposes. Colonoscopic studies have shown that 30% of patients with advanced adenomas have no distal lesions and would therefore have a normal examination to the splenic flexure. This is more common in women and patients over the age of 60 years. This, in combination with the need for bowel preparation and patient discomfort, has made this test infrequently used for screening purposes.

The tier 3 test, capsule colonoscopy, is not been approved by the US Food and Drug Administration for screening in average-risk patients. It is used for patients who have incomplete colonoscopy or are unable to undergo colonoscopy and when CT colonography is not available.

Screening recommendations for high-risk patients are listed in Table 32–5, and colonoscopy surveillance recommendations are listed in Table 32–6. Patients with a family history of colorectal cancer or an advanced adenoma in a first-degree family member initiate screening at age 40 years. Children with a diagnosis of FAP or a family history and no genetic testing should begin screening at age 10-12 years. Patients with a clinical or genetic diagnosis of Lynch syndrome should begin screening at age 20-25 years. Patients with pan-ulcerative colitis or Crohn colitis initiate screening 8 years after diagnosis.

Table 32–6. Colonoscopy surveillance recommendations.

History	Procedure	Interval
Colorectal cancer	Colonoscopy	1, 3, and then every 5 years
1-2 adenomas < 1 cm or sessile serrated polyp < 1 cm	Colonoscopy	5 years
3-10 adenomas < 1 cm, or advanced adenoma (≥ 1 cm, villous, or high-grade dysplasia), or advanced sessile serrated polyp (≥ 1 cm or dysplasia)	Colonoscopy	3 years
≥ 10 adenomas	Colonoscopy	< 3 years
Serrated polyposis syndrome	Colonoscopy	1 year

SPORADIC COLORECTAL POLYPS

The term *polyp* is a morphologic term given to tissue that projects into the lumen of the gastrointestinal tract and therefore is a broad term encompassing many entities, both benign and malignant. Nonneoplastic polyps account for 80% of all colonic polyps. Subtypes include juvenile, hyperplastic, and inflammatory polyps, as well as hamartomas (Table 32–7). There have been rare reports of carcinoma developing within hamartomas, but in general, these polyps do not progress to cancer. Neoplastic polyps, or adenomas, are the precursor lesions to the majority of colorectal adenocarcinomas in a well-studied "polyp to carcinoma" sequence, where colonic mucosa transforms into small tubular adenomas, increases in size, and develops high-risk features prior to frank carcinoma over a period of 10-15 years. The genetic

Table 32–7. Polyps of the large intestine.

Type	Histologic Diagnosis

Neoplastic	Adenoma
	  Tubular adenoma
	  Tubulovillous adenoma
	  Villous adenoma
	  Serrated adenoma
	  Sessile serrated polyp

Hamartomas	Juvenile polyp Peutz-Jeghers polyp
Inflammatory	Inflammatory polyp (pseudopolyp) Benign lymphoid polyp
Unclassified	Hyperplastic polyp
Miscellaneous	Lipoma, leiomyoma, carcinoid

mechanisms behind this process have been well character-ized and are discussed earlier. An exception to this is the more recently recognized CIMP, which involves neoplas-tic transformation via the serrated polyp pathway. Serrated polyps are found more commonly in the right colon and are thought to progress to carcinoma via hypermethylation and epigenetic silencing. This pathway accounts for 20% of colorectal cancers.

Adenomas, although accounting for < 20% of polyps, are common. Screening colonoscopy in asymptomatic patients detects adenomas in 25% of men and 15% of women. In autopsy series, they are detected in up to 60%. They are more common in older age, with a prevalence of 30% at age 50 years and 55% at age 80. About 50% of patients with ade-nomas have more than one lesion, and 15% have more than two. They are predominantly found distal to the transverse colon, and approximately half occur in the rectosigmoid area of the colon.

The presence of an adenoma indicates an increased risk for colorectal cancer. Further, adenomas themselves may harbor malignancy or progress to malignancy. The charac-teristics of the adenoma, including histology, location, shape, and size, significantly influence this risk. Adenomas are sub-divided into tubular, tubulovillous, and villous subtypes, and these exist on a spectrum. If followed over time, only 5% of tubular adenomas will develop into a malignancy; however, 22% of tubulovillous and 40% of villous adenomas will prog-ress. In addition, risk increases with size. Adenomas less than 1 cm harbor carcinoma only 1% of the time; however, this risk increases to 10% in adenomas of 1-2 cm and to 45% in adenomas greater than 2 cm. Other factors include sessile (as opposed to pedunculated) polyps, location in the ascending colon, male sex, age greater than 60 years, and family his-tory. Overall, the greatest risk factors for both the presence of carcinoma within a polyp and the future development of colorectal cancer are size greater than 1 cm and tubulovil-lous or villous histology. These have been termed *advanced adenomas*.

Adenomas, even in the absence of malignancy, are asso-ciated with risk of colorectal cancer. Patients found to have adenomas have a two- to fivefold risk of developing meta-chronous cancers compared with patients without them. The risk is estimated to be 5%-10% per year. For these reasons, the consensus guidelines recommend complete excision of the adenoma plus more frequent colonoscopic surveillance. Colonoscopy is repeated at 5 years for 1-2 low-risk adenomas, at 3 years for 3-10 low-risk or any high-risk adenomas, and at less than 3 years for more than 10 adenomas. Colonoscopy is repeated sooner if there is a question regarding the adequacy of the polypectomy or of visualization of the mucosa.

The majority of polyps are removed using endoscopic instruments such as biopsy forceps and hot or cold snare. However, 10%-15% of polyps cannot be removed with these techniques due to size, location, or sessile morphology.

Table 32–8. Haggitt classification.

Level	Depth
0	Carcinoma in situ or intramucosal carcinoma
1	Carcinoma invading through muscularis mucosa into the submucosa but limited to the head of the polyp
2	Carcinoma invading the neck of the polyp
3	Carcinoma invading any part of the stalk
4	Carcinoma invading into the submucosa of the bowel wall below the stalk of the polyp but above the muscularis propria (T1)
Sessile	By definition, equivalent to level 4

Reproduced with permission from Haggitt RC et al: Prognostic factors in colorectal carcinomas arising in adenomas: implications for lesions removed by endoscopic polypectomy, *Gastroenterology* 1985 Aug;89(2):328-336.

Historically, colectomy was required for these difficult pol-yps; however, there has been increasing use of advanced endoscopic techniques such as endoscopic mucosal resec-tion and endoscopic submucosal dissection in recent years. These are successful in managing difficult colon polyps 90% of the time. Transanal techniques, such as transanal endo-scopic microsurgery (TEM) and transanal minimally inva-sive surgery (TAMIS) can be used for rectal polyps. Surgery is indicated if complete endoscopic resection is not possible using these techniques.

Carcinoma is found in 5% of benign-appearing endo-scopically resected polyps. In 1985, Haggitt reported that depth of invasion was the most important indicator of metastasis and developed a classification system based on depth of invasion (Table 32–8). Levels 1 through 3 with favorable histology have a < 1% risk of nodal metastasis and are adequately treated by endoscopic resection with a margin ≥ 2 mm. However, carcinomas exhibiting evidence of vascular or lymphatic invasion, indeterminate margins, a margin < 2 mm, or level 4 have a 5%-25% chance of lymph node involvement and therefore require formal oncologic resection.

► Clinical Findings

A. Signs and Symptoms

The majority of patients with colorectal cancer are asymp-tomatic. Based on a median doubling time of 130 days, it takes at least 5 years, and often 10-15 years, before a cancer causes symptoms. When symptoms do appear, they are variable, nonspecific, and often indicate an advanced lesion or complications. Colorectal cancers may cause subclinical bleeding, resulting in an asymptomatic iron deficiency anemia. For this reason, any iron deficiency anemia in a man or nonmenstruating woman should prompt a workup to rule out bleeding from the gastrointestinal tract. A minority of patients will present emergently with acute obstruction, perforation, or significant bleeding with symptomatic anemia.

Compared with the left colon, tumors of the right colon may reach a more advanced stage before they cause symptoms. Obstruction is rare because the right colon is larger in diameter and has liquid stool. If these tumors bleed, melena or, more commonly, occult blood will be present in the stool. There may be associated vague abdominal pain. In advanced cases, patients present with a palpable abdominal mass.

In contrast, the left colon and rectum have a smaller diameter and semisolid to solid feces. Tumors here can cause luminal narrowing and obstruction resulting in narrowing of the stool, constipation, and increased frequency of bowel movements. Rectal cancer can produce tenesmus. When bleeding occurs, it tends to be dark to bright red and may streak or be mixed with the stool. Colorectal cancer should be considered as an alternative diagnosis in any patient with ongoing hematochezia, even in the presence of another clinical explanation, such as hemorrhoids.

B. Physical Examination

Physical examination may help localize and determine the extent of disease. The abdomen should be palpated for masses and the liver examined to rule out enlargement. Auscultation of the lungs is poorly sensitive for metastatic disease. A digital rectal examination may detect a distal rectal cancer. Its location, size, and mobility should be noted. Retrorectal nodes or drop metastases in the pouch of Douglas ("Blumer's shelf") may be palpated. In tumors of the rectum, proctoscopy or anoscopy is used to determine the accurate location of the tumor, which is important for treatment planning. Lymph node examination will rarely reveal metastasis in the supraclavicular nodes.

C. Laboratory Findings

Useful laboratory tests include a complete blood count, serum chemistries, and liver function tests as clinically indicated. These will detect anemia and other abnormalities that may need to be addressed prior to initiating treatment. The serum marker for colorectal cancer is carcinoembryonic antigen (CEA). It is a glycoprotein found throughout the gastrointestinal tract as well as other tissues. It is not sensitive or specific for patients with colorectal cancer, specifically for patients without metastatic disease. It is therefore not recommended as a screening test; however, it has been shown to be a useful adjunct to postoperative monitoring for recurrence, specifically in patients with an elevated preoperative CEA that returns to normal after surgery.

D. Colonoscopy

Colonoscopy is the gold standard for the diagnosis of colorectal cancer. Complete colonoscopy is indicated in all patients who have suspected or known colorectal cancer. It allows tissue diagnosis via biopsy, localization of the lesion using tattoo, and evaluation for synchronous neoplasms. Three percent of patients with a known colon or rectal cancer have a synchronous lesion. In patients with obstructing lesions, the remaining colon should be evaluated using contrast enema or CT scan. These patients should undergo postoperative complete colonoscopy 3-6 months after their surgery.

E. Mechanisms of Spread

Invasive colorectal adenocarcinoma is a mucosal-based lesion that by definition has invaded into the submucosa. The tumor grows intraluminally and extends through the wall of the bowel. As the tumor cells infiltrate the bowel wall, they reach the submucosal lymphatic and capillary network and may metastasize through either mechanism. As a colon cancer extends radially, it may penetrate the wall and extend into neighboring structures including the liver, greater curvature of the stomach, duodenum, small bowel, pancreas, spleen, bladder, kidney, ureter, and abdominal wall. Rectal tumors may invade the vaginal wall, bladder, prostate, sacrum, levators, or anal sphincter due to the confined space of the pelvis. The inflammatory response incited by extension of the tumor can be indistinguishable from frank invasion during gross examination at the time of surgery.

Metastatic disease most often occurs through the lymphatics, although it is also known to occur via peritoneal seeding, intraluminal spread, or hematogenously. Rectal cancer metastasizes to the mesorectal, iliac, and inferior mesenteric lymph nodes, as well as radially along the pelvic side walls where obturator nodes can become involved. Very distal rectal cancers can also spread to inguinal lymph nodes. Colon cancer spreads along the superior and inferior mesenteric lymph node basins (Figure 32–8). Approximately half of patients undergoing surgery for colorectal cancer will have lymph node involvement. Hepatic and pulmonary metastases occur via hematogenous invasion. This may occur through the portal system to the liver and, less commonly, the lumbar and vertebral veins to the lungs and other organs. Transperitoneal metastasis or peritoneal "seeding" may occur when a tumor has extended through the serosa, leading to peritoneal implants or generalized carcinomatosis. When found in the pouch of Douglas, these deposits are palpated on digital rectal examination and referred to as Blumer's shelf.

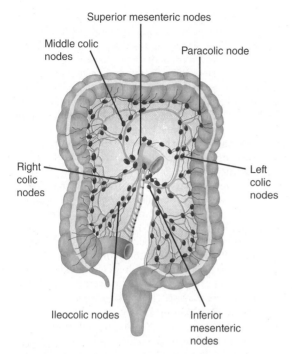

▲ **Figure 32–8.** Lymphatic drainage of the colon. The lymph nodes (black) are distributed along the blood vessels to the bowel.

▲ **Figure 32–9.** Computed tomography scan images. **A:** Primary, circumferential carcinoma of the sigmoid colon (arrow). **B:** Hepatic metastasis (arrow).

F. Staging

Accurately staging patients with colorectal cancer is important as it allows the development of an adequate treatment plan and determination of prognosis. The clinical stage is determined using preoperative imaging. Pathologic staging is based on imaging and information obtained after resection.

The initial step in developing a treatment plan for a patient with colon cancer is to determine if the tumor is resectable and whether or not metastatic disease is present. CT of the chest, abdomen, and pelvis is used routinely for this purpose. Images are examined for extent of tumor and invasion into adjacent structures, signs of obstruction or perforation, presence of lymphadenopathy, and detection of metastatic disease in the liver, lung, or peritoneum. (Figure 32–9). Dedicated magnetic resonance imaging (MRI) of the liver is obtained in patients who are found to have suspicious liver lesions by CT. Positron emission tomography (PET) is not routinely recommended; however, it is indicated in patients with suspicious abnormalities on CT that require evaluation for proper treatment planning.

Treatment planning for rectal cancer requires similar evaluation for metastatic disease with CT scans of the chest, abdomen, and pelvis, as well as staging of the primary tumor with dedicated pelvic imaging. MRI or endorectal ultrasound may be used depending on institutional expertise. Local staging features T stage (depth of invasion through the rectal wall), N stage (nodal involvement), as well as involvement of the mesorectal fascia (circumferential resection margin) and whether the tumor involves nearby pelvic structures, including the levators, sphincter complex, and genitourinary tract. This information is used to make decisions about neoadjuvant therapy and to guide a discussion of surgical options, including the possibility of a sphincter-preserving procedure and the need for en bloc resection of any other pelvic organs.

The standard staging system in the United States is the tumor, node, metastasis (TNM) staging system from the American Joint Committee on Cancer (AJCC). The most recent staging system (8th edition) is shown in Table 32–9. The clinicopathologic stage is the most important determinant of survival. In general terms, stage I includes superficially invasive cancers (T1-2) without lymph node involvement. Stage II includes more deeply invasive lesions (T3-4) without lymph node involvement. Stage III disease is present when there is nodal involvement (T1-4, N+). Stage IV is assigned when any metastatic disease is present regardless of T or N staging. Subclassification within T4 and node-positive disease offers further prognostic information and may be obtained through the AJCC. Stage for stage, patients with colon cancer have a better prognosis than patients with rectal cancer. Similarly, patients with proximal rectal cancers have a better prognosis than those with distal cancers. Poor prognostic factors include complications such as obstruction or perforation, as well as histologic features such as poor differentiation, mucinous histology, tumor budding, and lymphovascular or perineural invasion.

TREATMENT OF COLON CANCER

▶ Segmental Resection

Surgical resection of colon cancer is performed for both treatment and staging. Patients who are stage I-III or stage IV with resectable metastatic disease in the liver and/or lung are candidates for curative surgery. This requires a thorough understanding of the anatomy of the colon vasculature and relationships with the retroperitoneum. Principles include achieving adequate margins, complete mesocolic excision, adequate lymphadenectomy, and high ligation of the vascular supply.

When possible, a minimally invasive approach to colon resection is preferred in most patients. Multiple randomized controlled trials (COST, CLASICC, and COLOR) have compared laparoscopic and open approaches to resection for colon cancer, and none have demonstrated inferior oncologic outcomes. This approach is not always appropriate for patients with obstructive or perforated lesions and prohibitive adhesions.

Upon entering the abdomen, the first step is to explore the abdominal cavity to search for metastatic disease not identified on preoperative imaging. If there are no findings that would preclude colectomy, attention is turned to resection. Although the extent of resection depends on the necessary lymphadenectomy, a margin of 5 cm on each side of the lesion in the bowel wall is generally considered adequate for clearance of any intramural spread. If there is any invasion into adjacent structures, these must be excised en bloc to achieve negative margins.

An important aspect of the surgical management of colon cancer is the removal of the draining lymph node basin. This provides accurate staging and is associated with improved survival. Sentinel lymph node mapping demonstrated poor sensitivity and specificity. Therefore, resection of all draining mesenteric lymph nodes remains the standard of care, often necessitating a larger segmental resection than would otherwise be needed for the purposes of proximal and distal margins. An adequate lymphadenectomy contains 12 or more lymph nodes. The extent of resection of the colon and mesocolon for tumors in various locations is shown in Figure 32–10.

A **right hemicolectomy** is performed for tumors of the cecum and ascending colon. This requires high ligation of the ileocolic, right colic, and right branches of the middle colic artery. If the tumor is at the hepatic flexure or proximal transverse colon, an extended right hemicolectomy is performed with additional ligation of the middle colic artery. During mobilization of the ascending colon and hepatic flexure, the surgeon must identify and protect the right ureter, superior mesenteric vessels, and duodenum.

A **transverse colectomy** with ligation of the middle colic artery is indicated for tumors in the transverse colon. Given the difficulty of mobilizing both the hepatic and splenic flexures for the resection and anastomosis, some surgeons advocate performing an extended right colectomy depending on the precise location of the tumor. If the tumor is in the splenic flexure or descending colon, a **left hemicolectomy** is performed with ligation of the IMA at its origin and resection of the distal transverse, descending, and proximal sigmoid colon. Sigmoid tumors are treated with **sigmoid colectomy** that includes part of the descending colon and proximal rectum. Tumors of the rectosigmoid and upper third of the rectum are removed with an **anterior resection,** requiring distal ligation of the IMA including the sigmoid arteries and superior hemorrhoidal artery, as well as the middle hemorrhoidal arteries. The extraperitoneal rectum is mobilized and the splenic flexure may also be mobilized to ensure a tension-free anastomosis. With all these resections, attention must be paid to the identification and preservation of the ureters, kidney, spleen, and hypogastric nerves. Stapled ileocolic anastomoses are associated with a decreased leak rate compared with handsewn anastomoses. However, there does not appear to be a superior type of anastomosis in colocolonic or colorectal anastomoses. Thus, after resection for non–right-sided colon cancers, the type of anastomosis is best left to the discretion of the surgeon.

▶ Obstructing Colon Cancers

Patients presenting with obstructing colon cancers require special consideration. Stage for stage, patients with clinical signs of obstruction have a worse overall prognosis compared with patients who do not present with obstruction.

Table 32–9. TNM classification of cancer of the colon and rectum.

Primary Tumor (T)	
TX	Primary tumor cannot be assessed
T0	No evidence of primary tumor
Tis	Carcinoma *in situ*, intramucosal carcinoma (involvement of lamina propria with no extension through muscularis mucosae)
T1	Tumor invades the submucosa (through the muscularis mucosa but not into the muscularis propria)
T2	Tumor invades the muscularis propria
T3	Tumor invades through the muscularis propria into pericolorectal tissues
T4	Tumor invades the visceral peritoneum or invades or adheres to adjacent organ or structure
T4a	Tumor invades through the visceral peritoneum (including gross perforation of the bowel through tumor and continuous invasion of tumor through area of inflammation to the surface of the visceral peritoneum)
T4b	Tumor directly invades or adheres to adjacent organs or structures
Regional Lymph Node (N)	
NX	Regional lymph nodes cannot be assessed
N0	No regional lymph node metastasis
N1	One to three regional lymph nodes are positive (tumor in lymph nodes measuring ≥ 0.2 mm), or any number of tumor deposits are present and all identifiable lymph nodes are negative
N1a	One regional lymph node is positive
N1b	Two or three regional lymph nodes are positive
N1c	No regional lymph nodes are positive, but there are tumor deposits in the
	• subserosa
	• mesentery
	• or nonperitonealized pericolic, or perirectal/mesorectal tissues.
N2	Four or more regional nodes are positive
N2a	Four to six regional lymph nodes are positive
N2b	Seven or more regional lymph nodes are positive
Distant Metastasis (M)	
M0	No distant metastasis by imaging, etc.; no evidence of tumor in distant sites or organs (This category is not assigned by pathologists.)
M1	Metastasis to one or more distant sites or organs or peritoneal metastasis is identified
M1a	Metastasis to one site or organ is identified without peritoneal metastasis
M1b	Metastasis to two or more sites or organs is identified without peritoneal metastasis
M1c	Metastasis to the peritoneal surface is identified alone or with other site or organ metastases

AJCC PROGNOSTIC STAGE GROUPS

When T is...	And N is...	And M is...	Then the stage group is...
Tis	N0	M0	0
T1, T2	N0	M0	I
T3	N0	M0	IIA
T4a	N0	M0	IIB
T4b	N0	M0	IIC
T1–T2	N1/N1c	M0	IIIA
T1	N2a	M0	IIIA
T3–T4a	N1/N1c	M0	IIIB
T2–T3	N2a	M0	IIIB
T1–T2	N2b	M0	IIIB
T4a	N2a	M0	IIIC
T3–T4a	N2b	M0	IIIC
T4b	N1–N2	M0	IIIC
Any T	Any N	M1a	IVA
Any T	Any N	M1b	IVB
Any T	Any N	M1c	IVC

Used with the permission of the American College of Surgeons. Amin MB, Edge SB, Greene FL, et al. (Eds.) *AJCC Cancer Staging Manual*, 8th Ed. Springer New York, 2017.

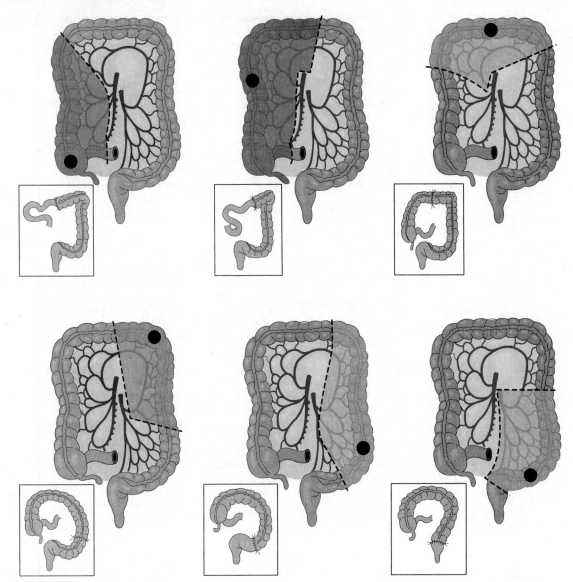

▲ **Figure 32–10.** Extent of surgical resection for cancer of the colon at various sites. The cancer is represented by a black disk. Anastomosis of the bowel remaining after resection is shown in the small insets. The extent of resection is determined by the distribution of the regional lymph nodes along the blood supply. The lymph nodes may contain metastatic cancer.

Surgical options include diversion, urgent resection with or without anastomosis, and endoscopic stenting with or without resection during the same hospitalization. It is important to consider the acuity of the presentation, the degree to which the lumen is obstructed, and whether the cancer is otherwise curable. Simple diversion and endoscopic stenting have the downside of leaving the tumor in place and are therefore reserved for patients who would otherwise not tolerate resection. In centers with experienced endoscopists, colonic stenting as a bridge to surgery can be considered. The data are still mixed, but a meta-analysis comparing endoscopic stenting as a bridge to surgery compared with upfront resection showed a decreased stoma rate in patients undergoing stenting prior to resection. Whether this approach results in improved morbidity or mortality or equivalent oncologic outcomes remains to be seen.

In patients undergoing resection, the physiologic status of the patient, the quality of the tissue, and the location of the tumor are important factors to consider when deciding whether to proceed with an anastomosis. If an anastomosis is feasible, an upstream diverting stoma is an option. If an anastomosis is not feasible, an end stoma can be created and the anastomosis performed after the completion of chemotherapy, when indicated.

▶ Adjuvant Treatment

Adjuvant chemotherapy is the standard of care for patients with stage III (node-positive) disease and has been shown to improve overall survival by 20%-25% and reduce recurrence by 40%. Chemotherapy regimens are based on 5-fluorouracil (5-FU) with levamisole and oxaliplatin (FOLFOX) or capecitabine with oxaliplatin (CapeOx). This should be initiated as soon as the patient has recovered from surgery, generally about a month postoperatively. Each 4-week delay in chemotherapy is associated with a 14% decrease in survival. A delay in chemotherapy beyond 5 months does not improve survival and is usually not offered.

Adjuvant chemotherapy should also be considered in patients with high-risk stage II disease. The idea was initially spurred when it was noted that survival for patients with stage IIB disease (T3-4, N0) was lower than that for patients with stage III (N+) disease. However, there are conflicting data about whether adjuvant chemotherapy improves survival. Analysis of long-term outcomes across multiple trials suggests that there may be a very small (5%) absolute improvement in survival with the addition of chemotherapy in patients with stage II disease. Therefore, the challenge is to identify the patients within the stage II group who could benefit the most. Current NCCN guidelines (v2.2018) advise either adjuvant chemotherapy or no chemotherapy in patients with T3-4, N0 tumors. The benefit of chemotherapy may be greater in patients with high-risk features, which include poor differentiation, lymphovascular or perineural invasion, bowel obstruction or perforation, inadequate lymphadenectomy, and inadequate margins. It is recommended that all tumors are tested for defective mismatch repair to guide treatment planning. Tumors with defective mismatch repair have a lower risk of recurrence and are resistant to treatment with 5-FU–based chemotherapy regimens. Given the uncertain benefit of chemotherapy after resection for stage II disease, it is imperative that patients are referred to an oncologist for a full discussion of the risks and benefits.

Radiation is rarely used in the adjuvant treatment of colon cancer but may be used when there questionable or positive margins are present. Treatment generally includes concomitant 5-FU treatment (chemoradiation) and is guided by preoperative imaging and clips left intraoperatively during surgery.

TREATMENT OF RECTAL CANCER

▶ Chemotherapy & Radiation

Stage I rectal cancers are adequately treated with surgical excision and do not benefit from chemotherapy or radiation. However, patients with locally advanced rectal cancers (ie, stage II and III) have high local recurrence rates and benefit from combined-modality therapy. NCCN guidelines (v2.2018) include three options: (1) neoadjuvant chemoradiation, surgery, and adjuvant chemotherapy; (2) short-course radiation, surgery, and adjuvant chemotherapy; or (3) total neoadjuvant therapy (chemotherapy and chemoradiation or radiation followed by surgery). Chemotherapy for rectal cancer is the same as for colon cancer, as discussed in the previous section.

Developing a multimodal treatment strategy for rectal cancer is complex, and considerations include the size and location of the primary tumor, the extent of nodal disease, patient anatomy, involvement of other organs, and the status of the circumferential margin based on imaging. The addition of radiation and chemotherapy to properly performed mesorectal excision at the time of surgery decreases locoregional recurrence but has not been shown to improve overall survival.

Patients with resectable stage IV disease and asymptomatic primary tumors are commonly treated with neoadjuvant chemotherapy and either chemoradiation or short-course radiation followed by surgery. If a stage II, III, or resectable stage IV rectal cancer is symptomatic, surgery may be required prior to starting neoadjuvant treatment. Bleeding is usually responsive to fulguration or endoscopic coagulation. Patients with impending obstruction or severe tenesmus may benefit from fecal diversion. Following recovery from the diversion procedure, neoadjuvant therapy can be administered, followed by formal oncologic resection.

▶ Surgery

The choice of operation for rectal cancer depends on many factors. These include the location of the lesion; the depth of penetration and invasion into adjacent structures; the patient's individual anatomy, general condition, and preoperative bowel function; and patient preference, if aligned with oncologic goals.

The timing of surgery depends on the need for neoadjuvant treatment and on the patient's symptoms. Patients with stage I disease proceed directly to surgery. Patients with stage II, III, or resectable stage IV disease benefit from neoadjuvant therapy.

A. Local Excision

The surgical management of rectal cancer differs from colon cancer for many reasons, mostly related to its unique anatomy and significant impact on bowel function and quality of life. In patients presenting with what appears to be early-stage disease by clinical staging, local excision can be used to get accurate pathologic staging of the tumor, and in carefully selected patients, it can be used as definitive treatment to avoid the morbidity of proctectomy. This can be performed in one of three ways: transanal excision (TAE), TEM, or TAMIS. TAE is performed for distal lesions that are directly visualized using an anoscope, whereas TEM and TAMIS can be used for more proximal lesions. These techniques utilize a specialized proctoscope (TEM) or a single-port laparoscopic platform (TAMIS) that allow passage of dissecting instruments and insufflation with carbon dioxide.

The goal of local excision is to remove the specimen in a single piece with negative circumferential and deep margins. Benign polyps may be removed in the submucosal plane, but cancers require full-thickness excision. The larger the size of the lesion and the greater the circumferential involvement, the more technically challenging is the procedure. These factors and surgeon experience should be considered in the preoperative plan. A transverse closure of full-thickness defects is performed where possible to avoid a risk of stricture with a longitudinal closure. If there is undue tension on the closure, the defect may be partially closed or left open as long as the defect is extraperitoneal. Morbidity occurs in 5%-25% of patients. Temporary urinary retention is the most common, occurring in about 11% of patients. Bleeding, pelvic sepsis, and temporary fecal seepage are also seen. Suture line dehiscence is fairly common and, in the absence of pelvic sepsis, involves nonoperative management.

Transanal techniques avoid the morbidity of proctectomy but are associated with worse oncologic outcomes. This is in large part due to two factors: the possibility of inadequate excision of the tumor and/or the possibility of nodal involvement that is not detected by imaging. Assuming that the tumor is properly excised, regional recurrence is still a concern. Therefore, patient selection is critical. Appropriate patients include those with benign rectal polyps or very early-stage adenocarcinomas (T1) without high-risk pathologic features or radiographic evidence of nodal metastasis. Lymph node involvement for patients with T1 disease is approximately 10% but is higher in patients with distal rectal cancers and those with high-risk features, such as poor differentiation, lymphovascular or perineural invasion, or mucinous histology. In addition, the depth of invasion into the submucosa is also predictive of risk of lymph node metastasis. Another risk stratification system, the Kikuchi classification, divides the submucosa into thirds during pathologic evaluation. The risk of lymph node metastases in tumors involving the upper third (SM1) is 3%, middle third (SM2) 8%, and lower third (SM3) 24%. In patients with T2 disease, occult lymph node metastases are present in 20%-25% of patients. However, there is a growing body of literature to suggest that the addition of neoadjuvant or adjuvant chemoradiation for high-risk T1 or T2 lesions improves oncologic outcomes. It is likely that a tailored treatment strategy will be needed to optimize oncologic outcomes, and research is ongoing.

Due to the risk of luminal recurrence and the risk of occult metastatic disease in the lymph nodes, patients undergoing local excision have inferior oncologic outcomes compared with patients undergoing upfront proctectomy. Five-year recurrence rates are higher and most studies show a decreased overall survival for patients with T1 and T2 disease undergoing local excision compared with patients undergoing proctectomy. Among patients with locoregional recurrence, curative surgery is not possible in 4%-21%. Current evidence supports consideration of local excision in benign lesions with possible Tis cancer, those with T1 tumors who are highly motivated to avoid proctectomy and understand the risks, or those who are not candidates for proctectomy.

B. Radical Excision

When radical excision of a rectal tumor is considered, planning must include assessment for adequate margins, preoperative bowel function, and patient preference while minimizing morbidity. The options include abdominoperineal resection (APR) with a permanent colostomy or low anterior resection (LAR). For cancers in the distal third of the rectum, an ability to achieve a distal margin of at least 1-2 cm and negative radial margins with complete mesorectal excision is considered the minimum needed to proceed with LAR. Tumors involving the levators or anal sphincter complex require APR. Although avoiding a permanent colostomy is generally considered ideal by patients and surgeons, it is important to recognize that the more distal the anastomosis, the more severe the permanent changes will be in postoperative bowel function. Therefore, a careful evaluation of the patient's preoperative bowel function and a discussion with the patient about postoperative expectations are important aspects of surgical planning.

Historically, recurrence rates were high and survival was low for rectal cancers; however, this has been greatly improved with the technique of total mesorectal excision (TME). According to the *Manual of Total Mesorectal Excision*, principles of proctectomy include (1) sharp, circumferential dissection in the avascular plane between the parietal and visceral layers of the endopelvic fascia that envelop the mesorectum; (2) preservation of the pelvic autonomic nerves; and (3) attaining negative circumferential margins. It is now recognized that formal TME with resection of the entire rectum and mesorectum is not necessary for mid to upper rectal tumors, leading to the concept of tumor-specific TME. This refers to proper mesorectal excision to achieve a distal margin of 5 cm.

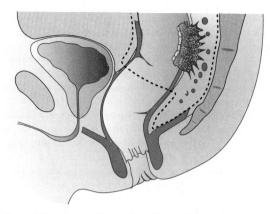

▲ **Figure 32–11.** Total mesorectal excision as depicted in Heald's original publication.

The technique of mesorectal excision is used in both APR and LAR. It requires dissection posteriorly in the avascular plane between the Waldeyer fascia and the presacral fascia, laterally to encompass the peritoneal reflection but medial to the hypogastric plexus, and anteriorly to include Denonvilliers fascia (Figure 32–11). TME is completed by extending the dissection inferiorly to the levators or, in the case of tumor-specific mesorectal excision, to 5 cm distal to the tumor. This allows removal of the mesorectum en bloc with the rectum and ensures adequate lymph node removal. As in colon cancer, a lymph node harvest of at least 12 nodes is standard.

The use of minimally invasive approaches in the treatment of rectal cancer remains controversial. Laparoscopic and robotic techniques are attractive from the standpoint of increasing exposure in the pelvis and minimizing morbidity and length of stay. However, there are concerns about increased cost of care and the ability to achieve adequate margins with laparoscopy. A Cochrane analysis demonstrated no difference in 5-year survival between patients undergoing laparoscopic and open approaches; however, the data were felt to be of only moderate quality. Because randomized controlled trials have demonstrated increased rates of incomplete and near-incomplete TME with laparoscopy, long-term survival data are needed to determine whether this translates into inferior outcomes.

Because LAR and APR are major operations requiring meticulous pelvic dissection in an often radiated field, the morbidity is higher than with colon cancer operations. In addition, LAR includes a technically challenging low anastomosis. Concerns are anastomotic leak, LAR syndrome (bowel dysfunction), urinary and sexual dysfunction, surgical site infection, anastomotic stricture, and injury to the ureters. In cases where identification of the ureters is expected to be difficult (eg, obese patients, those with previous pelvic surgery, and those who have undergone neoadjuvant chemoradiation), preoperative stent placement can assist with intraoperative identification and preservation of the ureters.

1. Low anterior resection—LAR is used when the decision is made to restore intestinal continuity for patients with tumors in the mid to distal rectum who have good preoperative sphincter function and in whom adequate margins can be achieved. It involves resection of the sigmoid colon and the rectum with the distal transection point being determined by the complete mesorectal excision and attainment of an adequate 1- to 2-cm distal margin.

The operation begins with abdominal exploration to assess metastatic disease. The superior hemorrhoidal artery is ligated at its origin, just distal to the takeoff of the left colic artery. A higher ligation at the level of the IMA may be required if there is lymphadenopathy at this level, or to achieve additional length on the colon when a coloanal anastomosis is required. If the IMA is ligated, the left colon (and anastomosis) is dependent on blood supply from the marginal artery, and care must be taken to preserve it. The left colon mesentery is mobilized off the retroperitoneum, and in most cases, the splenic flexure is taken down. Ligation of the inferior mesenteric vein at the ligament of Treitz is a maneuver that will provide additional length to the colonic conduit. The rectum is mobilized using the previously described procedure for TME. The rectum elongates after mobilization, potentially adding length to the distal margin.

The anastomosis is generally performed to the descending colon using a transanal end-to-end stapling device, although a handsewn coloanal anastomosis may be required to achieve an adequate distal margin. Alternatives to the traditional end-to-end anastomosis include the colonic J-pouch and the side-to-end (Baker) anastomosis. Meta-analyses show improvement in bowel function in patients undergoing reconstruction with a colonic J-pouch compared with patients undergoing a straight end-to-end anastomoses for at least for the first year postoperatively. They also show that a Baker anastomosis has equivalent bowel function to a colonic J-pouch. However, these alternative reconstruction options require additional mobilization of the colon and may be too bulky for patients with a narrow pelvis. There is also some concern of a higher anastomotic leak rate given the additional staple lines, particularly in patients undergoing colonic J-pouch reconstruction. Anastomotic technique is therefore at the discretion of the surgeon and dependent on the patient's body habitus.

After the anastomosis is constructed, an anastomotic leak test is performed by filling the pelvis with saline, insufflating the rectum with air, and observing for leakage of bubbles from the rectal lumen into the pelvis. If a leak is identified, the postoperative risk of clinical leak is reduced by either resecting and revising the anastomosis or repairing the leak in addition to performing fecal diversion. Prophylactic pelvic drainage has not been shown to alter leak rates, need for reoperation, or postoperative mortality, and there is evidence to suggest that it results in a higher risk of postoperative bowel obstruction.

Diverting ileostomy or colostomy is commonly performed in patients undergoing proctectomy for rectal cancer. Proximal diversion reduces the incidence and severity of anastomotic leak. However, the protective effect of diversion comes at the price of greater morbidity and the need for an additional operation for stoma reversal. In patients with rectal cancer, the decision to create a diverting stoma takes into consideration technical factors, including the distal location of the anastomosis, concern for leak based on the leak test, and other patient factors.

Anastomotic leak occurs in up to 15% of patients undergoing LAR. Risk factors for anastomotic leak vary by study but generally include male gender, low anastomoses, neoadjuvant radiation, renal disease, smoking, obesity, poor nutrition, emergency surgery, and metastatic disease. Anastomotic leak can be a devastating complication of proctectomy that has both immediate (longer hospitalization, need for additional procedures) and long-term consequences (worse bowel function and oncologic outcomes).

LAR syndrome occurs in 10%-30% of patients after sphincter-preserving operations for rectal cancer and is more pronounced the more distal the anastomosis. Symptoms include clustering (frequent bowel movements in a short period of time), urgency, and incontinence to gas, stool, or both. These symptoms can have a significant impact on quality of life and are the result of a combination of nerve injury, colonic dysmotility, neorectal reservoir dysfunction, sphincter complex damage, and aberrant anal canal sensation. It is worse in patients with a low anastomosis, pelvic radiation, anastomotic leak, and preoperative fecal incontinence. Most patients have improvement of their symptoms with time and, by 6-9 months after surgery, have a decreased, more manageable number of bowel movements per day. Loperamide, fiber supplementation, biofeedback, and sacral nerve stimulation may be useful adjunctive therapies. In patients with intractable symptoms, a permanent stoma may be required.

Other functional complications occur in about 25% of patients as a result of the pelvic dissection in patients undergoing LAR and APR. Urinary dysfunction, specifically urinary retention, is reported in 3%-15% of patients, but this is generally transient. Sexual dysfunction, including impotence, retrograde ejaculation, and dyspareunia, occurs in 10%-15% of patients and tends to become progressively worse with time. Patients undergoing pelvic radiation are at increased risk.

2. Abdominoperineal resection—APR is the operation of choice for tumors in the distal third of the rectum in which achieving negative margins would result in sphincter compromise, as well as in patients who would not tolerate a low anastomosis from a functional standpoint. Resection includes the sigmoid colon, rectum, and anus with creation of an end colostomy. The initial abdominal dissection for APR is similar to that described for LAR. Rectal mobilization is carried down to the levators. The perineal dissection is performed most often with the patient in lithotomy or prone position depending on anatomical factors and surgeon preference. An elliptical incision is made around the anus, and it is circumferentially dissected in the ischiorectal fat to achieve negative margins with care taken anteriorly in the plane between the anus and the vagina or prostate. The dissection is extended through the levators to reach the inferior aspect of the abdominal dissection. The specimen is removed transanally. The perineal wound is washed out and closed in multiple layers. An effort is made to keep intra-abdominal structures out of the pelvis by closure of the pelvic peritoneum and omental interposition. A drain is placed to prevent wound complications.

Postoperative complications occur in up to 50% of patients undergoing APR. Although these patients avoid the risk of anastomotic leak, they are at risk for the functional complications related to pelvic dissection discussed earlier, including urinary and sexual dysfunction. In addition, the perineal wound is at risk in the immediate postoperative period of poor wound healing and wound breakdown. There is limited evidence that myocutaneous flap closure may result in decreased wound complications and is more likely to help in patients requiring pelvic exenteration or wide skin or levator excision and in patients undergoing pelvic radiation. Gracilis, gluteal, or vertical rectus abdominus myocutaneous flaps are commonly used for this purpose. Perineal hernias are a potential long-term complication. These hernias are troublesome and require reoperation, usually with mesh closure of the defect.

Because LAR and APR involve wide dissection in the pelvis, the postoperative complications include those associated with disruption of the pelvic nerves. Urinary dysfunction, specifically urinary retention, is reported in 3%-15% of patients, but this is generally transient. Sexual dysfunction tends to become progressively worse with time. In a recent large survey-based analysis, more than half of men experienced erectile dysfunction and two-thirds experienced problems with ejaculation. One-third of women reported dyspareunia. These factors are also likely related to pelvic irradiation.

▶ Watch and Wait

Typically, in patients with locally advanced rectal cancer, neoadjuvant treatment is administered followed by proctectomy and adjuvant chemotherapy. However, this treatment is associated with substantial morbidity (discussed in detail later in this chapter). In addition, 20%-30% of patients undergoing neoadjuvant treatment have no endoscopically or radiographically detectable disease upon restaging. In patients with this so-called "complete clinical response," there has been a growing interest in utilizing a "watch and wait" approach. Under the watch and wait approach, patients undergo surveillance, and proctectomy is performed only if there is evidence of tumor recurrence.

It is still not clear whether a watch and wait approach will result in equivalent outcomes compared with proctectomy. NCCN guidelines mention watch and wait as an option that may be considered for locally advanced rectal cancers with a clinical complete response, but it is far from the being considered a standard treatment option. Based on meta-analysis, risk of local treatment failure is approximately 30%, and of those cases, salvage surgery is only possible in 80%. Sphincter preservation may also be less likely in a salvage situation. Active research priorities include the need for larger populations followed over longer periods of time and attempts to improve the accuracy of endoscopic and radiologic imaging in detecting a complete clinical response.

METASTATIC DISEASE

Metastatic disease is present in 20% of patients with colorectal cancer at the time of diagnosis. The most common location is the liver. If left untreated, these patients have a 5-year survival of 5%. However, selected patients are candidates for surgical resection with curative intent. Surgery results in an improved 5-year survival of approximately 30%. Unfortunately, after surgery for metastatic disease, recurrence is common, occurring in 50%-70% of patients.

Chemotherapy is the mainstay of treatment for patients with stage IV disease or otherwise unresectable colorectal cancers. These patients are treated with a chemotherapy regimen similar to patients with stage III disease, with the possible addition of irinotecan and/or a vascular endothelial growth factor (VEGF) inhibitor such as bevacizumab. Determination of KRAS mutations may also dictate therapy because research shows that two drugs used for colorectal cancer, cetuximab (Erbitux) and panitumumab (Vectibix), are not effective in tumors that carry a KRAS mutation. In carefully selected patients with metastatic disease, surgery can be performed with curative intent and is associated with increased survival.

Liver and lung metastases are considered resectable if they and all other sites of disease, including the primary tumor, are amenable to a complete oncologic resection (R0). This is based on the anatomic location as well as leaving an adequate quantity of normal liver or lung to maintain normal function. Options for patients with extensive liver disease include preoperative portal vein embolization and staged resection, and in some cases, ablative therapies such as microwave or radiofrequency are used. In the lung, robotic-assisted gamma knife radiotherapy is a promising treatment that minimizes the toxicity historically associated with lung radiation. If a patient presents with borderline resectable metastatic disease, restaging is performed after chemotherapy is administered. This allows an assessment of the biology of the tumor and, in some cases, downstages disease so that an attempt at curative resection is possible.

The peritoneum is the second most common location for colorectal cancer metastases. Peritoneal disease is identified in 10%-15% of patients at the time of diagnosis. This occurs as a result of tumor shedding in T4 or perforated tumors. In women, there is a predilection for ovarian involvement. Median overall survival in patients with peritoneal metastases is 22-24 months and is associated with the burden of disease and the response to chemotherapy. Current guidelines recommend chemotherapy as the primary treatment. Investigational treatments such as cytoreductive surgery and intraperitoneal chemotherapy show promise in improving survival; however, these treatments are associated with significant morbidity and are not currently considered standard of care.

PALLIATIVE PROCEDURES

If a colorectal cancer is unresectable, palliative surgery may be indicated to improve symptoms including obstruction, perforation, bleeding, or tenesmus. Obstructing cancers can be treated with fecal diversion, surgical bypass, or endoluminal stents; however, there is a high risk of stent occlusion and perforation. Perforation can be managed with percutaneous drainage, resection, or fecal diversion. Bleeding and tenesmus may be responsive to fulguration or endoscopic coagulation. It is rare that bleeding will persist and require resection.

POSTOPERATIVE SURVEILLANCE

After appropriate treatment for colorectal cancer, one-third to one-half of patients will experience recurrence. The majority of these (60%-80%) will be in the first 2 years and 95% in the first 5 years after surgery. Postoperative surveillance is therefore conducted in all patients undergoing curative resection of colorectal cancer with the goal of early detection of recurrences, metastases, and metachronous lesions. The exception to this is patients who would not be candidates for surgical management if a lesion were discovered.

After many well-designed randomized trials, there is still no consensus on what constitutes appropriate follow-up for treated colorectal cancer patients. All guidelines recommend some combination of history and physical examination, CEA, imaging, and endoscopy. Current NCCN guidelines (v2.2018) for surveillance of patients with stage II or III colorectal cancer include the following: (1) history, physical exam, and CEA every 3-6 months for 2 years, then every 6 months for a total of 5 years; (2) CT of chest, abdomen, and pelvis every 6-12 months for 5 years; and (3) colonoscopy in 1 year and, if normal, then repeat in 3 years followed by every 5 years. However, there is not strong evidence that any particular surveillance strategy is superior in terms of mortality or cost-effectiveness. It is possible that less intensive surveillance strategies will be shown to be viable alternatives in the future. For example, the COLOFOL trial, which randomized patients to surveillance per guidelines or to a less intensive strategy with CT imaging and CEA at 12 and 36 months, found that the 5-year disease-free and overall survival rates were similar between groups. However, less intensive strategies will need to be tested in larger groups and with longer follow-up before they are adopted into routine practice.

TREATMENT FOR RECURRENT DISEASE

Locoregional recurrence is more common in patients with rectal cancer compared with colon cancer and in patients with locally advanced disease compared with early-stage tumors. When recurrent disease is identified, a thorough search is conducted to rule out metastatic disease. If R0 resection is possible, this can be undertaken in patients who are good surgical candidates, in combination with chemotherapy and possibly radiation depending on the location and any history of radiation. In patients who present with unresectable disease, a combination of palliative chemotherapy and radiation therapy (if appropriate based on location) is administered, although this is unlikely to improve survival. However, the overall prognosis for recurrent colorectal cancer is poor. Survival is 35% at 5 years in patients who are candidates for curative surgical resection.

Kong JC, Guerra GR, Warrier SK, et al: Outcome and salvage surgery following "watch and wait" for rectal cancer after neoadjuvant therapy: a systematic review. *Dis Colon Rectum.* 2017;60(3):335-345.

Menahem B, Vallois A, Alves A, et al: Prophylactic pelvic drainage after rectal resection with extraperitoneal anastomosis: is it worthwhile? A meta-analysis of randomized controlled trials. *Int J Colorectal Dis.* 2017;32(11):1531-1538.

Rex DK, Boland CR, Dominitz JA, et al: Colorectal cancer screening: recommendations for physicians and patients from the U.S. Multi-Society Task Force on Colorectal Cancer. *Gastroenterology.* 2017;153(1):307-323.

Rullier E, Rouanet P, Tuech JJ, et al: Organ preservation for rectal cancer (GRECCAR 2): a prospective, randomised, open-label, multicentre, phase 3 trial. *Lancet.* 2017;390(10093):469-479.

Wille-Jørgensen P, Syk I, Smedh K, et al: Effect of more vs less frequent follow-up testing on overall and colorectal cancer-specific mortality in patients with stage II or III colorectal cancer: the COLOFOL randomized clinical trial. *JAMA.* 2018; 319(20):2095-2103.

Zauber AG, Winawer SJ, O'Brien MJ, et al: Colonoscopic polypectomy and long-term prevention of colorectal-cancer deaths. *N Engl J Med.* 2012;366(8):687-696.

OTHER TUMORS OF THE COLON & RECTUM

▶ Neuroendocrine Tumors

Neuroendocrine tumors (NETs) arise from enterochromaffin cells of the colon and rectum. About 15% of all NETs are located in the colon and rectum. They are rarely symptomatic, but if symptoms arise, rectal bleeding and a change in bowel habits are the most common presenting symptoms. Most are diagnosed incidentally on imaging or during screening colonoscopy. NETs have a characteristic appearance by colonoscopy as a submucosal nodule with normal overlying mucosa. If the mucosa is ulcerated, the lesion is likely to be larger and more deeply invasive into the bowel wall.

Important prognostic factors include tumor size, depth of invasion, location, and pathologic features such as histologic subtype, grade, mitotic index, and lymphovascular invasion. The majority of colon and rectal NETs are low grade (eg, carcinoid tumors). Staging uses the TNM system, similar to that for colorectal cancer. However, unlike in colorectal adenocarcinoma, survival for rectal NETs is better than for colon NETs. Colonic disease tends to be asymptomatic until an advanced stage, and nodal or metastatic disease is present in 60% of patients at the time of diagnosis (compared to 18% of rectal NETs).

Carcinoid syndrome is seen in 8% of localized colorectal NETs and in 35% when distant disease is present. This describes the constellation of symptoms produced by the systemic circulation of bioactive compounds such as serotonin and kallikrein made by the tumor. Symptoms include flushing, diarrhea, and abdominal pain, and in severe cases, right-sided heart failure. Because the liver can deactivate these compounds, the patients at greatest risk are those with liver metastases, because this allows bypass of the portal circulation and secretion of bioactive substances directly into the systemic circulation. However, hindgut tumors rarely produce serotonin, and therefore, even in the presence of liver metastases, rectal carcinoids rarely cause the serotonin syndrome. When present, symptoms may be treated with octreotide, and prophylactic octreotide should be administered preoperatively in patients with a history of carcinoid syndrome or elevated 5-hydroxyindoleacetic acid (5-HIAA) to prevent carcinoid crisis.

Although a NET of the colon or rectum is identified or suspected, the staging workup includes a CT of the chest, abdomen, and pelvis to identify suspicious lymphadenopathy and distant metastatic disease. A full colonoscopy is warranted to rule out synchronous tumors or other colorectal pathology that might influence surgical resection. If a biopsy is not diagnostic, 24-hour urine 5-HIAA and chromogranin A tests may help establish the diagnosis. In patients with advanced disease, somatostatin scintigraphy or PET scan may help identify distant metastases. Rectal lesions undergo additional local staging with endorectal ultrasound or pelvic MRI.

NETs of the colon and rectum should be evaluated for curative resection. Colonic NETs > 2 cm in size should be resected with a formal partial colectomy with lymphadenectomy as would be done for colon adenocarcinoma. Endoscopic resection is an option in tumors < 2 cm with no high-risk features. The management of rectal carcinoids is more controversial. NCCN guidelines (v3.2018) recommend that rectal carcinoids that are T1-2 or less than 1 cm should be treated with local excision (transanal or endoscopic depending on the location) and that all others should be managed with an oncologic resection. In patients with tumors between 1 and 2 cm and no high-risk factors, some authors advocate local excision. However, there is no evidence that a radical resection, even in patients with tumors > 2 cm, results in increased survival. If the patient presents with resectable metastatic disease, an attempt at curative resection is undertaken. If distant disease is not resectable, there may be a role for surgical debulking to palliate symptoms or serotonin syndrome. In all cases with advanced disease, cholecystectomy is recommended at the time of resection to decrease symptomatic gallbladder disease during adjuvant octreotide administration.

▶ Lymphomas

The most common site of extranodal non-Hodgkin lymphoma is the gastrointestinal system; however, the colon and rectum are rarely affected. This disease is more common in middle-aged men and immunosuppressed patients. Symptoms are generally nonspecific, and more than half of patients present with a palpable abdominal mass. On imaging, lymphoma appears as an infiltrating submucosal lesion with associated mesenteric lymphadenopathy, making it difficult to discern from adenocarcinoma. A complete colonoscopy with biopsy establishes the diagnosis. Chemotherapy and/or radiation is the primary treatment. However, surgery may be needed for symptomatic lesions because these tumors may present acutely with intussusception, bleeding, or perforation.

▶ Lipomas

The colon is the most frequent site of gastrointestinal lipomas. They are benign fatty submucosal tumors with an incidence of 1%-4%. They are more common in women and in the right colon. Lipomas are generally asymptomatic; however, they may cause vague abdominal symptoms or intussusception, especially if large in size. Although they can sometimes be difficult to differentiate from other colon polypoid lesions, the diagnosis can be made by characteristic findings on colonoscopy (the pillow sign) or by identification of a hyperechoic submucosal lesion on CT scan or endorectal ultrasound. Resection is indicated for symptomatic lipomas or if the diagnosis is not clear by radiographic or endoscopic findings.

GASTROINTESTINAL STROMAL TUMORS

Gastrointestinal stromal tumors (GISTs) are derived from the pluripotential interstitial cells of Cajal and are associated with activating mutations in a specific tyrosine kinase found in the large intestine called KIT or CD117. They rarely occur in the colon and rectum. Like many of the aforementioned neoplasms, these are submucosal tumors that can grow to a large size before causing symptoms. Workup includes a CT scan of the abdomen and pelvis and colonoscopy with biopsy. MRI is indicated for local staging in rectal tumors. Surgery is the standard treatment for patients with localized tumors > 2 cm, tumors with high-risk features, or symptomatic tumors. Because GISTs spread hematogenously, as opposed to through the lymphatics, local resection with negative margins is adequate. Care must be taken to prevent intraoperative rupture of the tumor pseudocapsule because this is associated with high rates of recurrence. Medical therapy with imatinib mesylate, which selectively inhibits KIT, is used for patients with unresectable or borderline resectable tumors, metastatic disease, or poor prognostic factors. Sunitinib malate has been introduced as salvage therapy for patients with imatinib-resistant disease. Prognostic factors include location in the gastrointestinal tract (stomach most favorable), mitotic index, and size. They are associated with generally good overall survival, but recurrence is common.

ENDOMETRIOMAS

Endometriosis refers to the presence of endometrial tissue that forms implants in the pelvis and abdomen. Deeply infiltrating endometriosis refers to a subtype with locally invasive implants on the bowel wall. Symptoms include abdominal pain, hematochezia, and pain with defecation. Most patients present with palpable, tender nodules on rectal or vaginal exam. The diagnosis is made at the time of surgery for other endometrial disease or occasionally endoscopically during the workup for rectal bleeding. Medical management with nonsteroidal anti-inflammatory drugs (NSAIDs), oral contraceptives, and gonadotropin-releasing hormone agonists is generally limited by side effects and does not appear to prevent progression of the disease. Surgery is indicated for persistent symptoms or if malignancy cannot be excluded. The implants are treated with superficial excision, full-thickness excision with primary defect closure, or resection with anastomosis. Although the majority of patients experience symptomatic improvement, recurrence is greater than 10%, and long-term follow-up is lacking.

OTHER TUMORS

Other rare tumors of the large intestine have been reported, including neurofibromas, teratomas, rectal duplication cysts, lymphangiomas, and cavernous hemangiomas. Rare malignancies include adenosquamous carcinoma, primary squamous cell carcinoma, and melanoma.

Byrne RM, Pommier RF: Small bowel and colorectal carcinoids. *Clin Colon Rectal Surg.* 2018;31(5):301-308.

Ezekian B, Adam MA, Turner MC, et al: Local excision results in comparable survival to radical resection for early-stage rectal carcinoid. *J Surg Res.* 2018;230:28-33.

Roman H, Milles M, Vassilieff M, et al: Long-term functional outcomes following colorectal resection versus shaving for rectal endometriosis. *Am J Obstet Gynecol.* 2016;215(6):762. e1-762.e9.

Wilkinson MJ, Fitzgerald JE, Strauss DC, et al: Surgical treatment of gastrointestinal stromal tumour of the rectum in the era of imatinib. *Br J Surg.* 2015;102(8):965-971.

DIVERTICULAR DISEASE OF THE COLON

Diverticulosis

▶ General Considerations

Diverticula (singular: diverticulum) are more common in the colon than in any other portion of the gastrointestinal tract. Their presence is referred to as diverticulosis. Most colonic diverticula are false, referring to the fact that they consist of mucosa and submucosa that have herniated through the muscular layer of the colon wall. True diverticula, which contain all layers of the bowel wall, are rare in the colon. In the United States, the most common location for diverticula is the sigmoid colon (72%). The descending (33%), ascending (5%), and transverse (3%) portions of the colon may also be involved. One hypothesis is that diverticula form as a result of increased intraluminal pressure, acting at areas of relative weakness on the bowel wall caused by the blood supply. The vasa recta extend onto the colon wall and then penetrate the muscular layer between the tenia to supply the mucosa, creating a region of relative weakness. Therefore, diverticula are most commonly located in the area between the mesenteric tenia and the antimesenteric tenia with a skip area on the antimesenteric border (Figure 32–12).

▶ Epidemiology

In the United States, the prevalence of diverticulosis increases with age, and 60% of people over age 60 are found to have diverticula. Men are affected more than women. In Asian countries, there is a predominance of right-sided diverticula. The geologic differences in the incidence of diverticular disease suggest that cultural and dietary factors may play an etiologic role. There are conflicting data regarding the association of diverticulosis and high-fiber diets, red meat consumption, physical inactivity, constipation, smoking, obesity, alcohol, and NSAID use. Patients with Ehlers-Danlos and Marfan syndrome, both of which involve abnormal connective tissue, are at increased risk.

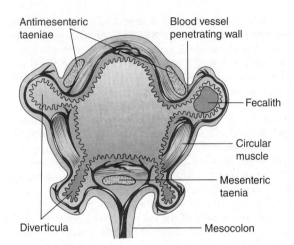

▲ **Figure 32–12.** Cross-section of the colon depicting the sites where diverticula form. Note that the antimesocolic portion is spared.

▶ Symptoms & Signs

Diverticulosis is asymptomatic in more than 80% of people and is usually detected incidentally on colonoscopy or CT scan. When patients develop symptoms, the most common manifestations are diverticulitis (discussed later in this section) and diverticular bleeding (discussed in the acute lower gastrointestinal bleeding section).

▶ Treatment

Asymptomatic patients with diverticulosis do not require any treatment. There is no evidence to suggest that avoiding nuts, seeds, or popcorn has a protective effect. In fact, no dietary change has been conclusively shown to treat diverticulosis or prevent its complications, although weight loss, smoking cessation, and a diet low in red meat have been suggested as possibilities. Surgery is not indicated for uncomplicated diverticulosis.

▶ Prognosis

The natural history of diverticulosis has not been defined. As mentioned previously, complications of diverticulosis occur in approximately 20% of patients with diverticulosis. Because these estimates rely on patients with known diverticulosis, the incidence of complications in the general population (who have undiagnosed, asymptomatic diverticulosis) may be much lower. About 75% of patients who present with complications of diverticular disease report no prior colonic symptoms.

Diverticulitis

▶ General Considerations

The inflammatory response in acute diverticulitis occurs as a result of micro- or macroscopic perforation of a diverticulum; however, the factors that result in perforation of a diverticulum remain unknown. In the United States, the sigmoid colon is the most common location for diverticula and, therefore, is the most common location of diverticulitis. The severity of disease can range from mild inflammation localized to a segment of the bowel wall to colon perforation with feculent peritonitis. The majority of patients (75%) present with uncomplicated diverticulitis. Complicated diverticulitis occurs in 25% of patients. Complications include free perforation, abscess formation, stricture, and fistula (most commonly to the bladder). The presence of extraluminal gas or pericolic phlegmon is not considered complicated disease.

▶ Clinical Findings

A. Symptoms and Signs

Patients with acute diverticulitis classically present with abdominal pain that is progressive over days, usually localized to the left lower quadrant. The severity of abdominal pain ranges from mild to severe and is often described as steady aching or cramping. Occasionally, pain is suprapubic, in the right lower quadrant, or throughout the lower abdomen, depending on the location of the sigmoid and the distribution of disease. Changes in bowel habits, including constipation and diarrhea, are common. Nausea and vomiting may be present depending on the location and severity of the inflammation. Physical findings characteristically include low-grade fever, mild abdominal distention, and left lower quadrant tenderness. There may be a palpable mass. Leukocytosis is common. Hemodynamic instability or diffuse peritonitis is indicative of free perforation and the need for emergency surgery.

Depending on the extent and severity of the disease, patients with diverticulitis can also present with other less typical symptoms. Small bowel obstruction may occur if a loop of small bowel becomes entrapped in inflammatory tissue. Dysuria may be reported in patients with inflammation adjacent to the bladder or as a precursor to development of colovesical fistulae. Colovesical fistulae will typically produce recurrent urinary tract infections, pneumaturia, and fecaluria. Patients with long-standing disease may develop a stricture and present with large bowel obstruction.

B. Imaging Studies

Plain abdominal films are not useful unless they show pneumoperitoneum. Other nonspecific findings include ileus, partial colonic obstruction, or left lower quadrant mass.

CT scan of the abdomen and pelvis with intravenous contrast is the preferred initial imaging study. In most studies, CT has sensitivity, specificity, and accuracy greater than 90%, with other considerations including inflammatory bowel disease, ischemia, and malignancy. Typical findings include wall thickening and pericolic fat stranding or phlegmon in a segment of colon with diverticula. Complications such as

▲ **Figure 32–13.** Computed tomography scan showing sigmoid colon involved with diverticulitis. Note the pericolonic stranding, bowel wall thickening, and intramural abscess.

abscess or fistula may be evident (Figure 32–13). Findings on CT scan may also be predictive of the need for surgical intervention or successful nonoperative expectant management. The Hinchey classification was developed in 1978 to help guide clinical decision making for patients with complicated disease and standardize radiographic reporting. This classification has been updated to reflect improved resolution of CT and currently includes the following stages: 0, mild clinical diverticulitis; 1a, pericolic inflammation or phlegmon; 1b, pericolic or mesocolic abscess; 2, pelvic, intra-abdominal, or retroperitoneal abscess resulting from an extension of a pericolic abscess; 3, purulent peritonitis; and 4, feculent peritonitis.

▶ Differential Diagnosis

Acute diverticulitis presents with such variation that the differential diagnosis is broad and includes most causes of the acute abdomen. The clinical presentation may simulate appendicitis, perforated colonic carcinoma, large bowel obstruction, colonic ischemia, inflammatory bowel disease, cystitis, infectious colitis, and gynecologic disease such as pelvic inflammatory disease, tubal pregnancy, and tubo-ovarian abscess. Differentiation from appendicitis is especially difficult when a redundant sigmoid colon lies in the right lower quadrant. Free perforation with peritonitis is difficult to differentiate from the other causes of perforation. A thorough history and physical exam as well as imaging studies may be helpful in differentiating these conditions.

▶ Complications

The clinical spectrum of diverticulitis includes complications such as free perforation, abscess, fistula, and large bowel obstruction. Fecal and purulent peritonitis require immediate surgery. However, abscesses can often be drained percutaneously and will not require urgent surgical intervention. Fistulae most commonly involve the bladder, but may also extend to involve the ureter, urethra, vagina, uterus, small bowel, ovaries, fallopian tubes, perineum, and abdominal wall. Colonic obstruction is usually slow in onset and incomplete. Small bowel obstruction may rarely result from inflammatory involvement of the small bowel.

▶ Treatment

A. Medical Management

After a patient is diagnosed with acute uncomplicated diverticulitis, a decision is made regarding the need for hospitalization. A meta-analysis demonstrated that in selected patients with uncomplicated diverticulitis, outpatient management is successful in 93% of the time. However, admission should be considered in patients who are pregnant, frail, elderly, or immunosuppressed or in those who have multiple comorbidities or poor social support. To qualify for outpatient management, the patient should have mild symptoms with manageable pain and an ability to keep hydrated. Recommendations include a clear liquid diet and close outpatient follow-up. The use of antibiotics for uncomplicated diverticulitis has been challenged in two trials, which randomized patients to parenteral antibiotics or no antibiotics and found similar rates of recurrence and need for surgery or procedures at up to 2 years of follow-up. However, in both of these trials, patients were hospitalized. Therefore, the safety of outpatient management without antibiotics is not clear.

For patients requiring hospitalization, treatment depends on the severity of presentation. Generally, patients with uncomplicated disease or small abscesses (Hinchey 1b) are managed with bowel rest, intravenous fluids, and systemic broad-spectrum antibiotics. Common regimens cover gram-negative and anaerobic flora and are chosen based on the patient's allergies such as a beta-lactam/beta-lactamase inhibitor, a carbapenem, or the combination of a fluoroquinolone plus metronidazole. As clinical manifestations resolve, oral feeding is resumed gradually. During recovery, a low-residue diet is considered due to the acute inflammatory narrowing of the colon. After recovery, there is no conclusive evidence to support any particular diet to improve recurrence rates, and a normal healthy diet with 25-35 g of fiber per day can be recommended. In patients who do not improve with medical therapy, repeat imaging is considered after the third day to look for the development of complications, such as the development or progression of an abscess that may warrant percutaneous drainage.

B. Interventional Management

Patients who present with Hinchey 1b and 2 diverticulitis with abscesses greater than 3 cm are less likely to respond to medical therapy. These patients should be evaluated for percutaneous drainage. This provides source control and generally results in clinical improvement within days. In patients who go on to require surgery for diverticulitis, percutaneous drainage of an intra-abdominal abscess allows surgery to be performed on an elective basis when there is reduced risk of complications and higher probability of a one-stage operation without a stoma.

The management of the drain is dependent on the quality and quantity of the drainage. In general, if the output is diminished and serous in quality and the patient is doing clinically well, this indicates that the perforation has sealed and the drain can be removed. In patients with ongoing purulent or feculent drainage, a sonogram can be performed to evaluate for a persistent fistula to the colon. If this is demonstrated, the patient can be discharged with the drain and a repeat study performed in 1-2 weeks. Patients with nonhealing fistulae will ultimately require surgery.

C. Surgical Management

1. *Elective surgery*—Patients are often referred for surgical evaluation after recovering from diverticulitis. The American Society of Colon and Rectal Surgeons (ASCRS) guidelines suggest that the decision about elective surgery for diverticulitis should be individualized. Considerations include number of episodes, severity of symptoms, impact on quality of life, comorbidity, anatomic factors, access to medical resources, and patient preference.

One consideration in decision making is the chance of recurrence. Recurrent diverticulitis following nonsurgical management occurs in 15%-36% of patients. In patients who have a recurrence, over 50% will go on to have a third episode. Recurrences tend to occur with severity similar to the previous episode, and patients who require urgent surgery usually do so during the first presentation. In other words, it is rare for a patient with a recurrence after medically managed diverticulitis to require urgent surgery (< 5%). Recurrence is more common in patients with a family history of diverticulitis, retroperitoneal abscess, and more than 5 cm of inflamed colon.

Another consideration is quality of life. Patients are variably bothered by their symptoms depending on the frequency and severity, as well as their lifestyle. The DIRECT trial randomized patients with uncomplicated diverticulitis with either smoldering symptoms or three episodes in 2 years to observation or surgical resection. At 6-month follow-up, quality of life was better in the surgical group. Therefore, patient factors such as symptom severity and the extent to which symptoms interfere with quality of life can be used to help guide surgical decision making.

However, elective sigmoid colectomy, even in the modern age, is not without risks. Anastomotic leak occurs in 5%-10% of patients, which can result in the need for additional procedures or reoperation. Functional results vary widely in studies, but there are reports of sexual dysfunction, alterations in bowel function, and continued chronic abdominal pain after surgery.

When interval colectomy is recommended, it is generally delayed by 6-8 weeks to allow resolution of acute inflammation that may add difficulty to the operation. There is evidence that delaying surgery increases the rate of a successful laparoscopic resection with primary anastomosis, which is possible in > 90% of patients. However, delaying surgery comes with the small but significant risk (2%) of interval development of recurrent severe diverticulitis requiring emergency surgery with high morbidity. Further study is required to determine the optimal timing of surgery.

Surgical planning for patients with a history of diverticulitis begins with a careful review of previous CT imaging. Note is taken of the relationship of the inflamed segment to other abdominal structures, such as the reproductive organs, bladder, ureters, and small bowel. Resection margins for sigmoid diverticulitis should include all radiographically involved areas as well as any abnormal tissue noted intraoperatively. The distal margin should be in soft, healthy upper rectum. Proximal diverticula do not require resection as long as the segment is normal in appearance (Figure 32–6).

Open, robotic, laparoscopic, and hand-assisted approaches to sigmoid colectomy are described. Minimally invasive techniques may provide small improvements in postoperative pain, hospital length of stay, and quality of life. However, the approach to sigmoid resection for diverticulitis should be based on the surgeon's experience and tailored to individual patient factors such as location and severity of inflammation. Prophylactic ureteral stents can be considered in patients in whom the ureter is likely to be difficult to identify intraoperatively.

2. Urgent surgery—Less than 10% of patients will present with complications requiring urgent surgery. Indications include free perforation, uncontrolled sepsis, and failure to improve with nonoperative therapy. There is a lower threshold for surgery for immunocompromised patients given their greater risk of morbidity and mortality with medical management.

At laparotomy for severe acute diverticulitis, exploration may reveal an inflammatory mass involving large bowel, mesocolon, mesentery, omentum, and sometimes small bowel. Except in cases of free perforation with generalized fecal peritonitis, the diseased diverticulum is not often visible. The type of operation performed is dependent on the extent of colonic inflammation; the amount of peritoneal contamination; the patient's general condition, comorbidities, and nutritional status; the extent of blood loss; and the surgeon's experience and preference.

There are three options for surgical management in patients who require urgent surgery for complicated diverticulitis:

Hartmann resection with end colostomy, primary anastomosis with diverting ileostomy, and laparoscopic lavage with drainage. Historically, the two-stage Hartmann resection has been the gold standard. At the initial operation, the diseased bowel is removed, the proximal end of the colon is brought out as a temporary colostomy, and the distal colonic stump is closed (Figure 32–6). Intestinal continuity is restored in a second operation after the inflammation subsides.

If the surgeon determines that the patient can tolerate an anastomosis but remains high risk for leak, resection with primary anastomosis and diverting loop ileostomy is an option. A meta-analysis of randomized controlled trials comparing primary anastomosis with diversion to patients undergoing Hartmann resection for diverticulitis concluded that the risk of mortality, morbidity, and permanent stoma were similar between groups, with a higher risk of intra-abdominal abscess in patients undergoing primary anastomosis.

Another strategy consists of laparoscopic washout and drainage with the hope of performing a one-stage sigmoid colectomy at a later operation. A meta-analysis of randomized controlled trials showed that stoma formation was lower in the laparoscopic washout group, but this came at the cost of increased need for reoperation and percutaneous drainage.

In the absence of strong data to guide surgical management in patients undergoing urgent surgery for diverticulitis, the surgical approach should be chosen after considering the patient's physiology and comorbidities, the contamination of the abdomen, and the condition of the bowel.

▶ Follow-Up

Diverticulitis is often a clinical or radiographic diagnosis made in patients with segmental colonic inflammation in a region of diverticulosis. It is therefore important to rule out other etiologies of segmental colitis in patients with atypical presentations, in patients with nonresolution of symptoms or radiographic findings, and in those who are not up to date on screening colonoscopy. When indicated, colonoscopy is usually deferred for 6-8 weeks after an acute attack in order to allow mucosal healing and minimize complications.

▶ Prognosis

The mortality for diverticulitis can be divided by Hinchey stage. Patients with stage I or II disease have a mortality of < 5%, stage III 13%, and stage IV 43%. The operative mortality rate is about 5% in patients undergoing surgery for diverticulitis.

Diverticulitis recurs in one-third of patients managed conservatively and in 5% of patients after surgical resection. Most postoperative recurrences develop within the first 5 years, and the strongest risk factor is the creation of a colocolic as opposed to a colo-rectal anastomosis.

Abraha I, Binda GA, Montedori A, et al: Laparoscopic versus open resection for sigmoid diverticulitis. *Cochrane Database Syst Rev.* 2017;11:CD009277.

Cirocchi R, Afshar S, Shaban F, et al: Perforated sigmoid diverticulitis: Hartmann's procedure or resection with primary anastomosis-a systematic review and meta-analysis of randomised control trials. *Tech Coloproctol.* 2018;22(10):743-775.

Feingold D, Steele SR, Lee S, et al: Practice parameters for the treatment of sigmoid diverticulitis. *Dis Colon Rectum.* 2014;57(3):284-294.

Galbraith N, Carter JV, Netz U, et al: Laparoscopic lavage in the management of perforated diverticulitis: a contemporary meta-analysis. *J Gastrointest Surg.* 2017;21(9):1491-1499.

Sharma PV, Eglinton T, Hider P, et al: Systematic review and meta-analysis of the role of routine colonic evaluation after radiologically confirmed acute diverticulitis. *Ann Surg.* 2014;259(2):263-272.

Strate LL, Liu YL, Syngal S, et al: Nut, corn, and popcorn consumption and the incidence of diverticular disease. *JAMA.* 2008;300(8):907-914.

van de Wall BJM, Stam MAW, Draaisma WA, et al: Surgery versus conservative management for recurrent and ongoing left-sided diverticulitis (DIRECT trial): an open-label, multicentre, randomised controlled trial. *Lancet Gastroenterol Hepatol.* 2017;2(1):13-22.

van Dijk ST, Daniels L, Unlu C, et al: Long-term effects of omitting antibiotics in uncomplicated acute diverticulitis. *Am J Gastroenterol.* 2018;113(7):1045-1052.

LARGE BOWEL FISTULAE

▶ Colovesical Fistula

Diverticulitis is the etiology of more than half of all colovesical fistulae. This complication occurs in 2%-4% of patients. Other causes include colon cancer, bladder cancer, Crohn colitis, radiation exposure, trauma, and iatrogenic causes. They occur three times more often in men than women. This predilection is likely anatomical: in women, the uterus and adnexa are situated between the colon and the bladder.

The most common presentation is recurrent urinary tract infection. Pneumaturia is reported by up to 70% of patients, and fecaluria is reported in up to 50% depending on the size of the fistula. These symptoms may be intermittent. There are no specific physical exam findings, although some patients may have a palpable pelvic mass. There is usually no leukocytosis. Urinalysis is often indicative of urinary tract infection, and cultures are polymicrobial. The fistula can sometimes be identified by CT imaging with rectal contrast or with CT cystogram. If the fistula itself is not demonstrated, air in the bladder is a common finding. Colonoscopy and cystoscopy may reveal inflammation at the site of the fistula, but the fistula is rarely visualized. These tests are useful for ruling out malignancy prior to surgical intervention. If the diagnosis is still in question, ingestion of charcoal or poppy seeds with elimination in urine is diagnostic.

The treatment for symptomatic colovesical fistula is elective surgery. Although patients may experience bothersome abdominal discomfort or urinary symptoms, the operation should be delayed until any active inflammation has resolved. In most patients, surgery involves resection of the involved colon with a primary anastomosis. Large bladder fistulae are closed in layered repair. If the fistula is small, as is common, the bladder side can be left to heal spontaneously with prolonged Foley catheter drainage. In malignant fistulae, the entire fistula tract should be excised en bloc with the colon and the involved bladder wall, which can usually be repaired primarily. Ideally, healthy omentum is interposed between the anastomosis and the bladder to promote healing. Practice varies in terms of routine prophylactic pelvic drain placement, duration of Foley catheter drainage, and the use of cystograms postoperatively to evaluate for healing of the fistula.

In the majority of patients, surgery can be delayed until medical optimization can be achieved. In minimally symptomatic patients at high risk for surgery, conservative management with intermittent antibiotics may be successful. Fistulae associated with Crohn colitis may also respond to biologic therapy.

The prognosis for colovesical fistula is related to the etiology and the general health of the patient. Recurrence is reported to be 4%-5% overall but is highest in patients with fistulae secondary to radiation therapy and Crohn colitis.

COLOVAGINAL & RECTOVAGINAL FISTULA

Colovaginal fistulae are commonly a complication of diverticulitis, especially in women with a history of hysterectomy. The most common cause of rectovaginal fistula is obstetric injury, followed by Crohn colitis, iatrogenic surgical injury, malignancy, radiation, and trauma. Fistulae between the lower third of the rectum and lower half of the vagina are classified as low rectovaginal fistulae, whereas high fistulae are defined as those between the middle to upper third of the rectum and the posterior vaginal fornix. The most common presentation is feculent vaginal discharge, which may be mistaken for fecal incontinence. Patients may also report vaginal flatus, recurrent genitourinary infections, and dyspareunia. There is a significant negative impact on quality of life. A fistula may be observed on anoscopy, colonoscopy, and/or vaginal speculum examination in 85% of patients. In patients with symptoms but in whom a fistula is unable to be identified on physical exam, imaging can sometime be diagnostic. Useful modalities include CT with rectal contrast, water-soluble enema, or contrast vaginogram.

The treatment for recto- and colovaginal fistula is surgical. Colovaginal fistulae are often successfully managed with resection of the involved colon. The vaginal defect may be closed, but will generally close spontaneously if this is technically challenging. As is done for colovesical fistulae, the interposition of omentum is recommended.

The optimal surgical treatment for rectovaginal fistula, on the other hand, is less clear. The treatment is largely based on etiology, individual patient factors, and surgeon experience. Numerous procedures have been reported, including direct repair, fibrin glue, endorectal advancement flaps, vaginal advancement flaps, biologic mesh, tissue interposition, and rectal resection. Choice of repair depends on the etiology, size, and location of the fistula. However, the recurrence rate is disappointingly high, especially for patients with Crohn disease who have an ongoing source of inflammation. The optimal approach consists of aggressive medical treatment of the colitis and control of pelvic sepsis followed by surgery. However, reported recurrence rates are 25%-50%. Good results have been reported in patients with multiple recurrences using fecal diversion in conjunction with omental, gracilis, and Martius flap reconstruction. In truly refractory cases, proctectomy with permanent stoma can be considered.

ACUTE LOWER GASTROINTESTINAL BLEEDING

▶ Background

Lower gastrointestinal (GI) bleeding refers to bleeding that originates distal to the ligament of Treitz and involves the small bowel, colon, or rectum. Unlike upper GI bleeding, it occurs in predominantly elderly patients. This is because the most common etiologies for lower GI bleeding, such as angiodysplasia and diverticulosis, also increase in prevalence with age. Lower GI bleeding accounts for 20% of all GI bleeds. Patients present with melena (black, tarry stool) or hematochezia (bright red blood, maroon blood, or clots) depending on the rate of bleeding and the time the blood spends in the GI tract. Classically, the more proximal the source, the more likely it is for the patient to present with melena. However, bright red blood may stem from brisk esophageal variceal bleeding, and melena may be the result of slow blood loss from a right-sided colon cancer. The black color of melena is the result of the oxidation of iron in hemoglobin.

▶ Etiology

Lower GI bleeding can originate from numerous sources. In elderly patients, common causes include diverticula, angiodysplasia, malignancy, and ischemia. Younger patients are more commonly affected by inflammatory bowel disease, solitary rectal ulcer, and infection. Anorectal causes include hemorrhoids and fissures. In the appropriate patient, bleeding may be related to coagulopathy, radiation injury, or a recent procedure such as polypectomy or bowel surgery. Chronic, low-volume bleeding is seen in patients with malignancy, polyps, ischemia, hemorrhoids, and fissures. The small intestine can be the source of bleeding in 5% of patients. Other more unusual causes include Meckel

diverticulum (especially with ulceration from ectopic gastric mucosa) and aortoenteric fistula.

Diverticulosis is the most common source of acute lower GI bleeding. Although bleeding occurs in only 5%-15% of patients with diverticulosis, this presentation is common because of the high prevalence of diverticula in the aging population. Diverticula form in areas of weakness where vasa recta penetrate the bowel wall. Structural changes in the bowel wall cause damage to the artery, which can lead to rupture. Diverticular bleeding often presents with painless, massive, and self-limited hemorrhage. NSAID use is a risk factor. About 20% of patients will go on to have another episode of bleeding on long-term follow-up; however, it is often hard to definitively diagnose. Bleeding will spontaneously resolve in 80% of cases, and colonoscopy can definitively diagnose a diverticular bleed less than 25% of the time. If a patient presents with multiple episodes of angiography or colonoscopically confirmed bleeding from a specific location, surgery can be considered to prevent further episodes of bleeding.

Angiodysplasia, also known as vascular ectasia or arteriovenous malformation, consists of dilated submucosal vessels with a central feeding vein that have a propensity to bleed spontaneously. They commonly occur in the jejunum and can also be found in the duodenum, stomach, ascending colon, and ileum in order of decreasing frequency. Two-thirds of patients have more than one lesion, and these are frequently in different anatomic sites. Bleeding is typically intermittent and low volume, and patients often present in the outpatient setting with iron deficiency anemia and heme-positive stool. Angiodysplasia is identified in 2% of asymptomatic patients on screening colonoscopy. Incidentally identified ectasias are not treated prophylactically, as it is estimated that only 15% will cause clinically significant bleeding. If a bleeding lesion is identified, it can be treated with argon plasma coagulation or epinephrine injection. Recurrent bleeding is more common in patients with multiple lesions and need for anticoagulation. Surgery is rarely indicated.

Colitis resulting from inflammatory bowel disease, ischemia, radiation, or infection is a third cause of hematochezia. Colitis tends to cause mild blood loss that rarely requires transfusion. Colitis should be suspected in patients with abdominal pain and diarrhea. Acute ischemia may be caused by an acute decrease in blood supply from embolism, hypotension, or spasm. The watershed areas, including the splenic flexure and rectosigmoid, are most commonly affected. Infectious colitis can be diagnosed by stool culture. The most common organisms causing bloody diarrhea are *E coli* 0157-H7, *Campylobacter*, and *Shigella*. Ulcerative colitis and Crohn colitis can also cause hematochezia during periods of acute inflammation. Ulcerative colitis is more commonly associated with bleeding, although it can sometimes be difficult to distinguish between these two entities during an initial colonoscopy. However, the management in this setting is the same. Treatment with steroids, amino-salicylates, immunomodulators, and biologic agents depends on the severity of the disease. This is discussed further in the section on inflammatory bowel disease.

Neoplastic sources of lower GI bleeding are more common in older adults, paralleling the increase in neoplasia with age. Bleeding will usually be low volume. Right-sided lesions are more likely to result in occult blood loss detected on fecal occult blood tests or by detecting anemia. Left-sided lesions are more likely to cause hematochezia, and patients may describe blood streaked on the outside of the stool.

▶ Management

Chronic rectal bleeding, as seen in patients with colorectal polyps or cancer, and anorectal conditions can be evaluated electively. It is important to include colonoscopy in the evaluation, even if the bleeding can be explained by a benign condition such as hemorrhoids. This is especially true for patients who are not up to date on colorectal cancer screening, have abdominal or constitutional symptoms, or have a family history of colorectal cancer because it ensures that there is not a more proximal lesion that needs to be addressed.

Acute severe hemorrhage is a potentially life-threatening problem, and prompt evaluation and treatment are critical. The first step in the management of these patients is to evaluate and manage the ABCs (airway, breathing, and circulation). A significant portion of these patients have hemorrhagic shock. Resuscitation with intravenous fluids and blood products takes priority over initiation of diagnostic procedures. Large-bore intravenous catheters should be placed, and efforts are made to keep the patient warm. Strong consideration should be given to transferring the patient to the intensive care unit or other closely monitored setting. Patients should be asked about the recent use of NSAIDs, antiplatelet agents, and blood thinners. A focused history includes assessing the onset of bleeding, color and volume of stool, and for symptoms such as abdominal pain and weight loss. Labs are checked for a coagulation profile, platelet count, and hematocrit, and a type and cross should be sent. Any coagulation abnormalities should be corrected. Digital rectal and anoscopic exams are performed first to look for an obvious source of bleeding, and consideration should be given to the possibility of an upper source by examining nasogastric aspirate. Although this is not a perfect test, it can provide quick and useful information in a patient with a life-threatening upper GI bleed. If blood or coffee-ground material is aspirated, there is confirmation of an upper source, and esophagogastroduodenoscopy should be performed. If bile is aspirated, the source is more likely from the lower GI tract, and the diagnostic workup should continue. The next step is determined by patient stability and availability.

A plan of management for acute lower GI hemorrhage is outlined in Figure 32–14. The decision regarding resuscitation and transfusion should be made after evaluating the quality and volume of stool and hemodynamic stability. The hemoglobin value at the time of presentation may not a reliable indicator of blood loss because it can take hours for redistribution of interstitial fluid into the blood and, therefore, for laboratory measurements to accurately reflect the true level of anemia. Bleeding stops spontaneously in 90% of patients before transfusion requirements exceed two units, but there are no reliable methods to predict who will have self-limited bleeding or who will have recurrent bleeding. Therefore, all brisk GI bleeding must be taken seriously.

There is a wide range of procedures that can be used for both diagnostic and treatment purposes in the acute setting. These include endoscopy, CT angiography, mesenteric angiography, and radionuclide scintigraphy. There is no standard algorithm for evaluation, and there is little evidence to support the superiority of any specific test.

Colonoscopy is useful to localize the bleeding in stable patients in whom the colon is the suspected source. It has the advantages of being able to visualize the entire colon and to intervene if the bleeding site is identified. The sensitivity is limited in that active bleeding can obscure visualization, and if the bleeding has stopped, a search for the causative lesion is successful in less than 50% of cases. It can be particularly difficult to identify the source in patients with multiple potential lesions, as in patients with diverticular bleeding or angiodysplasia. Stigmata of recent bleeding, such as an adherent clot or visible vessel, can be used to identify the source of bleeding and are predictive of high recurrence of bleeding if not intervened upon. Depending on the lesion, clips, electrocautery, argon plasma coagulation, epinephrine injection, and/or sclerotherapy may be used. If there is a neoplastic lesion, it can be biopsied or removed. The disadvantages of colonoscopy, including availability of the procedure, need for sedation, and bowel preparation, often preclude its use. It is a generally safe procedure, with complications occurring in less than 2% of cases. When colonoscopy is determined to be necessary, there may be benefit to performing the exam within 12 hours of presentation. Although there are conflicting data, urgent colonoscopy may be associated with increased detection and treatment of bleeding, decreased length of stay, and decreased costs of care. If the patient is stable and esophagogastroduodenoscopy and colonoscopy are both normal, a capsule endoscopy or double-balloon enteroscopy may be performed to evaluate for a small bowel source.

CT angiography is commonly used in the evaluation of active GI bleeding. It has largely replaced radionuclide scanning, as discussed later. It does require active bleeding but can identify the location of bleeding in patients with a rate as low as 0.3 mL/min with a reported sensitivity of 85% and specificity of 92%. Unlike radionuclide scanning, CT angiography can localize bleeding, making for a more accurate and timely intervention by formal angiography. The

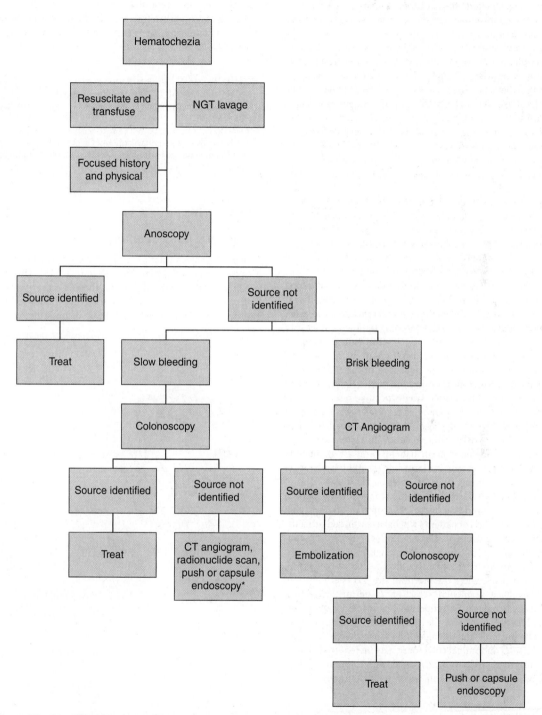

▲ **Figure 32–14.** Algorithm for management of acute lower gastrointestinal hemorrhage. *In patients who undergo a nondiagnostic colonoscopy, the next test should be based on the rate of bleeding and on the suspected source. CT, computed tomography; NGT, nasogastric tube.

disadvantages include the additional radiation and contrast exposure for a diagnostic test that cannot be used to treat any identified lesion.

Selective mesenteric angiography can be used to identify and treat sources of brisk GI hemorrhage and is usually preceded by a positive CT angiogram or radionuclide scan. In order to be detectable by angiography, the rate of hemorrhage must be at least 0.5 mL/min. Benefits of angiography include avoidance of bowel prep, accuracy for localization, and ability to treat active bleeding in sites such as the small bowel that are otherwise not accessible endoscopically. If the site of bleeding is demonstrated, vasopressin or embolization can be used to treat the feeding vessel. Embolism is used if possible because rebleeding is observed in up to 50% of patients treated with vasopressin alone. Embolization is successful in 80%-90% of patients when followed for 30 days. The disadvantage of angiography is that it is resource intensive, requires sedation, and carries a risk of bleeding, bowel ischemia, and renal injury. In addition, after the successful treatment of bleeding, additional evaluation may be required to diagnose the cause.

Radionuclide scanning with 99mTc-labeled red blood cells was historically used to identify patients who would benefit from angiography. Benefits of the test included increased sensitivity (reported to detect bleeding as low as 0.05 mL/min) and the ability to identify intermittent bleeding in patients by repeating scans during symptoms within 24 hours of tracer administration. The downside of the radionuclide scanning, however, is that localization of bleeding is poor and the test is purely diagnostic. After a positive result, another procedure, such as angiography, is required to re-localize the bleeding and then to intervene. This method has been criticized for causing a delay in therapeutic intervention, although it can prevent angiography in patients who are unlikely to benefit. For these reasons, radionuclide scanning is no longer included in algorithms for acute lower GI bleeding.

The majority of lower GI bleeds stop spontaneously or respond to intervention by colonoscopy or angiography. However, 10%-25% of patients will have continued or recurrent bleeding and ongoing shock. Surgery should be considered once the transfusion requirement exceeds six units of blood. However, preoperative localization of bleeding is critical. In cases where the bleeding site has been localized conclusively, a segmental resection is performed. When the source is unclear, intraoperative endoscopy can be performed to try to localize the source. If the patient continues to be unstable and the bleeding is suspected to be in the colon, a total abdominal colectomy may be required. This is a fortunately a rare occurrence today with improvements in imaging, endoscopy, and interventional techniques.

Prognosis

Up to 90% of lower GI bleeds will stop spontaneously; however, 25% of patients will experience recurrent bleeding.

Mortality has been reported in up to 3.6% of patients and is higher in those with refractory bleeding requiring surgery. In patients requiring emergency total abdominal colectomy, mortality is 10%-30%.

García-Blázquez V, Vicente-Bártulos A, Olavarria-Delgado A, et al: Accuracy of CT angiography in the diagnosis of acute GI bleeding: systematic review and meta-analysis. *Eur Radiol.* 2013;23:1181.

Nagata N, Niikura R, Sakurai T, et al: Safety and effectiveness of early colonoscopy in management of acute lower gastrointestinal bleeding on the basis of propensity score matching analysis. *Clin Gastroenterol Hepatol.* 2016;14:558.

VOLVULUS

General Considerations

Volvulus involves rotation of a segment of the intestine on an axis formed by its mesentery (Figure 32–15). This results in a closed-loop obstruction and is therefore a surgical emergency. Luminal obstruction occurs when the bowel rotates 180 degrees. If the bowel rotates 360 degrees, the veins are

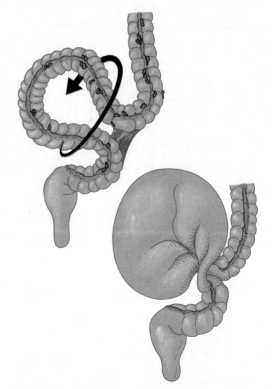

▲ **Figure 32–15.** Volvulus of the sigmoid colon. The twist is counterclockwise in most cases of sigmoid volvulus.

occluded and arterial flow is interrupted. This leads to ischemia, followed by necrosis and perforation if prompt treatment is not instituted. Sigmoid volvulus can be complicated by the additional development of cecal perforation in patients with a competent ileocecal valve. Physiologically, this forms a second closed loop obstruction because the proximal colon is unable to decompress into the small bowel. In this situation, the cecum is at greatest risk of perforation by the law of LaPlace because it has the largest diameter and thinnest wall.

Most cases of volvulus in the United States involve the cecum or sigmoid colon. A minority (2%-3%) of patients present with volvulus of the transverse colon or splenic flexure. Volvulus accounts for 5% of all cases of large bowel obstruction in the United States. Cecal volvulus often occurs in patients with a hypermobile cecum as a result of incomplete embryologic fixation. The average age of presentation is 53 years, and there is a female predilection. This is in contrast to sigmoid volvulus, which tends to occur in elderly or institutionalized patients who experience high rates of constipation and associated motility disorders. It is thought that a long sigmoid colon with an associated narrow-based mesentery are risk factors. In parts of Africa and the Middle East, sigmoid volvulus accounts for about 50% of bowel obstructions and tends to affect younger, healthy, male patients. In South America, it is seen in association with megacolon in patients with Chagas disease.

Cecal bascule accounts for 10% of cecal volvulus. It involves anterior-superior movement of the cecum, causing obstruction at the site of the transverse fold in the ascending colon. Patients may describe intermittent bloating, pain, and obstructive symptoms improved by lying down and massaging the abdomen. Mesenteric blood flow is not compromised because there is no twist in the mesentery.

▷ Clinical Findings

A. Cecal Volvulus

The cecum and terminal ileum are involved in the rotation, so the symptoms generally include those of distal small bowel obstruction. Severe, intermittent, colicky pain begins in the right abdomen. Pain eventually becomes continuous, and the patient will experience the classic symptoms of obstruction: vomiting, distention, and obstipation. Patients may report a history of similar but milder attacks.

Imaging studies are the key to diagnosis. In the early stages, a plain film of the abdomen may show a single fluid level that may be mistaken for gastric dilation. In later stages, there may be a hugely dilated ovoid cecum that favors the epigastrium or left upper quadrant. It is classically described as the "coffee bean" sign and is present in 20% of patients. In cecal volvulus, the apex of the dilated loop points toward the left upper quadrant. If a film is taken later in the course, the x-ray may show classic findings of small bowel obstruction superimposed on the cecal volvulus. The success rate of

diagnosis based on plain abdominal films is extremely variable, ranging from 5% to 90%. CT shows a distended cecum, often with a mesenteric swirl sign, indicating the rotation of the mesentery. Ischemia and necrosis can be identified by a lack of bowel wall enhancement.

B. Sigmoid Volvulus

Sigmoid volvulus presents in a similar fashion to cecal volvulus. Symptoms include intestinal colic, nausea, and obstipation. Distention tends to be more pronounced in sigmoid volvulus. There may be a history of chronic constipation and dysmotility or transient attacks in which spontaneous reduction of the volvulus has occurred. Abdominal x-rays show a markedly distended loop of bowel like a "bent inner tube" that has lost its haustral markings rising up out of the pelvis with the apex pointing toward the right upper quadrant. Contrast enema reveals a pathognomonic "bird's beak" deformity with spiral narrowing of the upper end of the lower segment (Figure 32–16). In the present age, CT

▲ **Figure 32–16.** Volvulus of the sigmoid colon. Barium enema taken with the patient in the supine position. Note the massively dilated sigmoid colon. The distinct vertical crease, which represents juxtaposition of adjacent walls of the dilated loop, points toward the site of torsion. The barium column resembles a "bird's beak" or "ace of spades" because of the way in which the lumen tapers toward the volvulus.

imaging is used with increasing frequency and is especially helpful if the diagnosis is unclear. Findings include a dilated sigmoid loop with a mesenteric swirl sign, indicating the mesenteric twist. As with cecal volvulus, the pattern of bowel wall enhancement may help identify patients with ischemia and necrosis of the bowel wall.

Differential Diagnosis

Volvulus must be differentiated from colonic pseudo-obstruction and from other causes of small and large bowel obstruction, as well as other sources of acute abdominal pain that may mimic the symptoms of volvulus, such as biliary colic, peptic ulcer disease, and nephrolithiasis.

Treatment

Early diagnosis and treatment are imperative because the involved segment of colon is at risk of gangrene and perforation. The first step in the management of these patients is fluid resuscitation and correction of electrolyte imbalances. Vital signs and urine output should be monitored and a nasogastric tube placed. If there is evidence of ischemia, necrosis, or perforation, antibiotics should be administered as the patient is prepared for emergency surgery.

Many techniques have been described for managing patients with cecal volvulus and cecal bascule, but the recommended treatment is ileocecectomy. This can be done via the laparoscopic or open technique depending on the clinical scenario and surgeon preference. If there is necrotic bowel, the blood supply is ideally controlled prior to releasing the volvulus in an attempt to reduce the systemic release of the potentially infected, acidotic, and hyperkalemic fluid that can cause cardiac arrest. Close communication with the anesthesia team is key. In unstable patients, the bowel can be left in discontinuity and anastomosis performed at a second look laparotomy. In patients at high risk for anastomotic leak, an end ileostomy or anastomosis with upstream diverting loop ileostomy can be performed. In otherwise stable patients, a primary ileocolic anastomosis can be performed, although the risk of leak is reported to be 7%-17%, higher than the risk of leak for ileocolic resection performed for other indications. Cecopexy (suture fixation of the bowel to the parietal peritoneum) and tube cecostomy (placement of a decompressive transabdominal drain) have been used to avoid a resection and anastomosis in the acute setting; however, these techniques have generally been abandoned due to high rates of both recurrence (30%) and complications (50%). Colonoscopic decompression is usually unsuccessful and is not recommended.

In contrast, sigmoid volvulus without strangulation is treated initially by urgent endoscopy. A flexible sigmoidoscope or colonoscope is advanced to the obstruction. Under direct visualization, the colon is insufflated, and the tip of the scope is used to apply gentle pressure into the twist of the bowel lumen proximal and distal to the dilated segment. In 70%-90% of patients, decompression is achieved with the immediate release of gas and stool. The mucosa can then be inspected for signs of ischemia. If there is no evidence of ischemia, the patient is scheduled for resection of the affected bowel with primary anastomosis during the same admission. The time between decompression and surgery allows for bowel preparation and for colonic recovery so that a primary anastomosis can be entertained in fit patients. Half of patients managed with decompression alone will have a recurrence within the first year. However, in patients with severe comorbidities, surgery may need to be delayed or may not be an option. Urgent surgery is indicated if strangulation or perforation is suspected or if endoscopic decompression is unsuccessful. In this case, primary anastomosis is not usually possible and a Hartmann procedure is performed.

Prognosis

The outcome for patients with volvulus depends on comorbidities, the urgency of the surgery, and the presence of strangulation or perforation. The mortality rate for patients with cecal and sigmoid volvulus is less than 10%, but this increases to 30%-50% if strangulation or perforation has occurred. Patients who undergo semi-elective resection for sigmoid volvulus after endoscopic decompression have a mortality rate of less than 10%.

Swenson BR, Kwaan MR, Burkart NE, et al: Colonic volvulus: presentation and management in metropolitan Minnesota, United States. *Dis Colon Rectum.* 2012;55:444-449.
Vogel JD, Feingold DL, Stewart DB, et al: Clinical practice guidelines for colon volvulus and acute colonic pseudo-obstruction. *Dis Colon Rectum.* 2016;59(7):589-600.

INFLAMMATORY BOWEL DISEASE

Inflammatory bowel disease (IBD) refers to ulcerative colitis (UC), Crohn disease (CD), and indeterminate colitis. The cause of IBD is not known. The disease is likely the result of a combination of genetic, environmental, and host immune response factors.

There is a positive family history of IBD in 20% of patients. CD seems to have a stronger genetic link than UC. Genome-wide association studies initially identified normal variants of multiple loci associated with the development of IBD. However, these associations are still poorly understood. These genetic associations are heterogeneous and have precluded the development of useful screening and diagnostic tests.

It is postulated that the interplay between the immune system, normal microflora, and colonic epithelium is a factor in the development of IBD, but this is still being investigated.

Patients with UC are known to have an increased concentration of normal bacterial flora compared to healthy controls; however, it is not known if this contributes to the disease process. The mucosal immune system has been implicated by the finding that patients with CD have a predominantly Th1 mucosal population, whereas patients with UC have a Th2 predominance. An autoimmune component is suggested by circulating perinuclear antineutrophil cytoplasmic antibody (pANCA) and abnormally high levels of auto-IgG1 antibodies. These antibodies cross-react with the epithelium of the colon, biliary tract, skin, eye, and cartilage and have been hypothesized to contribute to extraintestinal manifestations.

Environmental factors are also important. The use of NSAIDs has been associated with flares in patients with CD. Smoking has been shown to be a protective factor for UC but is a risk factor for the development and progression of CD. For unclear reasons, UC is also less common in patients who have undergone appendectomy.

ULCERATIVE COLITIS

▶ General Considerations

UC has a bimodal age distribution, with the first peak between ages 15 and 30 years and a second, smaller peak in the sixth to eighth decades. The annual incidence varies from 1 to 20 per 100,000, and the prevalence is 8-246 per 100,000. UC is more common than CD in adults but less common in children. The disease is found worldwide but is more common in Western countries, and the incidence is increasing in Asia. This finding has also contributed to the theory of changes in bacterial flora contributing to the development of the disease.

UC is a diffuse but contiguous mucosal inflammatory disease. Abscesses form in the crypts of Lieberkühn and penetrate the superficial submucosa. In the acute setting, neutrophils predominate, whereas in the chronic setting, the infiltrate is largely composed of lymphocytes and plasma cells. There are no granulomas. The overlying mucosa sloughs as the inflammation spreads. Vascular congestion and hemorrhage are prominent, and there is often diffuse thickening of the muscularis mucosa. The normal tissues surrounding the ulcerated areas appear endoscopically protuberant and thus are called pseudopolyps. Except in the most severe forms, the muscular layers are spared. In fulminant disease, the full thickness of the colon wall can be involved, which leads to dilation and ultimately perforation. In patients with long-standing or severe disease, the colon becomes foreshortened and loses its normal haustral markings.

UC classically starts at the rectum and extends proximally without skip lesions. The disease is confined to the rectum (proctitis) or up to the rectosigmoid region (proctosigmoiditis) in at least half of patients. The disease is classified as left-sided colitis if it involves the descending colon, extensive colitis if it extends proximal to the splenic flexure, and pancolitis if the cecum is involved. In patients with pancolitis, a few centimeters of terminal ileum may be involved by proximity in patients with an incompetent ileocecal valve. This is termed *backwash ileitis* and can make the differentiation of UC from CD challenging. There are no strict diagnostic criteria, but generally, a clinical and histologic appearance of UC without evidence of CD is enough to establish a diagnosis and initiate treatment.

▶ Differential Diagnosis

The differential diagnosis of patients presenting with new-onset IBD is extremely broad. Infectious colitis can mimic IBD but can also be superimposed on patients with underlying IBD. Salmonellosis and other bacillary dysenteries are diagnosed by stool cultures. Shigellosis may be suspected based on a positive methylene blue stain for fecal leukocytes. *Campylobacter jejuni* is a common cause of bloody diarrhea; the organisms can be cultured from the stool, and serum antibody titers rise during the illness. Hemorrhagic colitis—a syndrome of bloody diarrhea and abdominal cramps but no fever—is associated with infection by *E coli* O157:H7. *Legionella* infections can mimic UC. Gonococcal proctitis is detected by culture of rectal swabs. Herpes simplex virus is the most common cause of nongonococcal proctitis in homosexual men. In patients with suspected amoebiasis, corticosteroids should be held until amoebiasis is excluded by microscopic examination of stool, rectal swabs, rectal biopsies, or serologic tests.

Cases of histoplasmosis, tuberculosis, cytomegalovirus disease, schistosomiasis, amyloidosis, or Behçet disease may be very difficult to diagnose. Drug-induced colitis may be suspected based on the patient's history. NSAIDs can cause mucosal inflammation and even strictures in the large intestine. Collagenous colitis may or may not be related to NSAID use. Watery diarrhea is the main symptom of this syndrome, endoscopy is grossly normal, and biopsies show a thickened band of collagen just beneath the mucosa. Ischemic colitis has a segmental pattern of involvement quite unlike the contiguous distribution of UC. Functional diarrhea can mimic colitis, but organic disease must be excluded before it can be concluded that the diarrhea is functional. Diversion colitis refers to inflammation of a previously normal segment of colon or rectum following construction of an intestinal stoma. Deficiency of mucosal nutrients may be responsible, and inflammation may be treated with topical application of short-chain fatty acids or restoration of intestinal continuity.

The most difficult differential diagnosis is between UC and Crohn colitis (Table 32–10). None of the features are

Table 32–10. Comparison of various features of ulcerative colitis with those of Crohn colitis.

	Ulcerative Colitis	Crohn Colitis
Signs and symptoms		
Diarrhea	Marked	Present; less severe
Gross bleeding	Characteristic	Infrequent
Perianal lesions	Not present	When present may be complex
Toxic dilatation	Yes (3%-10%)	Yes (2%-5%)
Perforation	Free (rare)	Localized (in fistulizing disease)
Systemic manifestations (arthritis, uveitis, pyoderma, hepatitis)	Common	Common
X-ray studies	Confluent, diffuse	Skip areas
	Tiny serrations, coarse mucosa, mucosal tags	Longitudinal ulcers, transverse ridges, "cobblestone" appearance
	Concentric involvement	Eccentric involvement
	No fistulae	Fistulae
	Starts in rectum and progresses proximally	Any portion of intestinal tract may be involved
Morphology		
Gross	Confluent involvement	Segmental involvement with or without skip areas
	Rectum usually involved	Rectum often not involved
	Mesocolon not involved; nodes enlarged	Thickened mesocolon; pronounced lymph node enlargement
	Widespread, ragged, superficial ulceration	Large longitudinal ulcers or transverse fissures
	Inflammatory polyps (pseudopolyps) common	Inflammatory polyps not prominent
	No thickening of bowel wall	Thickened bowel wall
Microscopic	Inflammatory reaction usually limited to mucosa and submucosa	Chronic inflammation of all layers of bowel wall; damage to muscle layers usual; submucosal fibrosis
	Crypt abscesses	Granulomas
Natural history	Exacerbations, remissions; may be explosive, lethal	Indolent, recurrent
Treatment		
Response to medical treatment	Good response in majority of cases	Difficult to evaluate; less well controlled over long term
		Repeated episodes of inflammation result in scarring, which is not amenable to medical therapy
Type of surgical treatment and response	Colectomy with ileoanal anastomosis; proctocolectomy with ileostomy	Segmental colectomy; total colectomy with ileorectal anastomosis; proctocolectomy if rectum severely diseased
	No recurrence	Recurrence common

specific for one disease, and often the differentiation can be made only after all the data have been assembled. Luckily, in the acute phase, the medical treatment is similar; however, the differentiation is important because it can dictate appropriate surgical therapy. About 10% of cases cannot be classified (indeterminate colitis). Finally, cancer and diverticulitis should also be considered in the differential as this may affect plans for treatment.

► Clinical Findings

A. Symptoms and Signs

Patients commonly report frequent, small-volume watery stools mixed with blood, pus, and mucus accompanied by tenesmus, urgency, and even fecal incontinence. Many patients will report crampy abdominal pain and variable degrees of fever, vomiting, weight loss, malaise, and dehydration. The symptoms can be episodic with periods of spontaneous improvement, or they can be severe and unrelenting. Mild disease may be manifested by loose or frequent stools or, occasionally, by constipation. In isolated instances, the only symptoms may be from extraintestinal manifestations such as arthropathy or pyoderma.

If the disease is mild, physical examination may be normal, but in severe disease, the abdomen is tender and distended. Severe rectal inflammation may result in considerable tenderness and spasticity of the anus during digital rectal examination. The examining finger may be covered with blood, mucus, or pus. Perianal diseases, such as fissures and hemorrhoids, can occur in UC patients as they do in the general population, but signs of anal disease should prompt a workup for CD.

A simple classification of the severity of an attack was devised by Truelove and Witt in 1955. The assessment of

Table 32–11. Ulcerative colitis disease severity (based on the Truelove and Witt classification).

Symptoms	Mild	Severe	Fulminant
Stools (per day)	< 4	> 6	> 10
Hematochezia	Intermittent	Frequent	Continuous
Temperature	Normal	> 37.5°C	
Pulse (beats/min)	Normal	> 90	
Hemoglobin	Normal	< 75% of normal	Requires transfusion
Erythrocyte sedimentation rate	< 30 mm/h	> 30 mm/h	

disease severity is based on six simple clinical signs including stool frequency, hematochezia, pulse, temperature, hemoglobin, and erythrocyte sedimentation rate (Table 32–11).

B. Laboratory Findings

There is no single diagnostic test for UC, although in unclear cases, serum antibody tests can help differentiate UC from CD. Serum pANCAs are found in 60%-70% of patients with UC but also are found in up to 40% of patients with CD. In patients with IBD for whom the differentiation between UC and CD is unclear, the combination of a positive pANCA and negative anti-*Saccharomyces cerevisiae* antibodies (ASCA) has a specificity of 97%, sensitivity of 48%, and a positive predictive value of 75% for UC. A negative pANCA and positive ASCA has a positive predictive value of 86% for CD. Thus, serologic testing in patients with IBD may be helpful when considered in the context of other clinical factors. However, it is not used as the only basis for differentiating the two entities.

During an acute flare, basic laboratory tests are used to assist in determining the severity of disease. Anemia, leukocytosis, and an elevated sedimentation rate or C reactive protein is usually present. Severe disease leads to hypoalbuminemia, dehydration, and electrolyte abnormalities. There is often evidence of steatorrhea. To look for signs of superinfection, the stool should be sent for ova and parasite examination, culture (*E. coli* 0157:H7 and *Campylobacter*), and *C difficile* toxin assay.

C. Imaging Studies

Abdominal x-rays may show dilation of the colon and can be used to detect free air when perforation is suspected. CT scan has become the most common imaging modality during an acute episode. CT will often show thickened rectum and colon with associated inflammatory changes; however, it does not often lend much to the clinical management of these patients.

▲ **Figure 32–17.** Ulcerative colitis. Barium enema x-ray of colon. Note shortening of colon, loss of haustral markings ("lead pipe" appearance), and fine serrations at the edges of the bowel wall that represent multiple small ulcers.

Barium enema, which is now infrequently used, shows mucosal irregularity that varies from fine serrations to extensive ulceration with pseudopolyps. As the disease progresses, haustra are gradually effaced, and the colon narrows and shortens because of muscular rigidity (Figure 32–17). Widening of the space between the sacrum and rectum is due either to periproctitis or to shortening of the bowel. The presence of a stricture should arouse suspicion of cancer or CD. In cases where the diagnosis is unclear, a small bowel series or CT enterography may be performed to look for involvement suggestive of CD.

D. Colonoscopy

Colonoscopy is an essential part of diagnosis and surveillance. The characteristic mucosal changes in UC include loss of vascular pattern, granularity, friability, hyperemia, and ulceration. Pseudopolyps represent islands of normal mucosa against a background of inflamed, denuded bowel wall. These findings begin in the distal rectum and proceed proximally in a continuous fashion. In more advanced disease, the mucosa is purplish-red, velvety, and extremely friable. Blood mixed with mucus is evident in the lumen. If the mucosa is not grossly diseased, biopsy may be helpful to confirm the diagnosis. In the recovery phase, mucosal hyperemia and edema subside. The healing mucosa is typically dull and granular and has a neovascular pattern of telangiectatic vessels that differs from the normal pink mucosa. These patients are at increased risk for colorectal cancer.

Complications

A. Extraintestinal Manifestations

Extraintestinal manifestations occur in approximately 25% of patients with UC. They are more common in women and patients with pancolitis. The pathogenesis is unknown, but it is thought that they may be a result of a systemic autoimmune process. A genetic component is suggested by the fact that they tend to cluster in families. Nearly 80% of patients who develop extraintestinal manifestations do so after the development of colonic symptoms. The most common extraintestinal manifestations are musculoskeletal (arthralgias, arthritis, and ankylosing spondylitis), anterior ocular chamber inflammation (uveitis, iritis, scleritis, and conjunctivitis), skin (erythema nodosum and pyoderma gangrenosum), and primary sclerosing cholangitis (PSC), in order of decreasing frequency. PSC can lead to cirrhosis requiring liver transplant and puts the patient at increased risk for cholangiocarcinoma. For unclear reasons, patients with PSC also develop colorectal cancer at an increased rate. Most extraintestinal manifestations parallel the course of the colitis and therefore can be expected to improve with medical or surgical treatment. Exceptions to this are PSC and ankylosing spondylitis, which can be persistent despite remission of colonic disease. Most patients will develop only one extraintestinal manifestation, but a subset will develop multiple.

Patients with UC also develop symptoms as a result of the disease process in the colon, including iron deficiency anemia and malnutrition. They are at high risk for thromboembolic disease, especially during flares. Patients are also at risk of developing complications from medical treatment using long-term corticosteroids such as diabetes, osteoporosis, cataracts, and adrenal insufficiency.

B. Hemorrhage

Gross hematochezia is common during acute flares of UC. In the chronic setting, patients frequently develop a chronic iron deficiency anemia. Ten percent of patients will require blood transfusion for bleeding during a flare. Massive hemorrhage is a rare but potentially life-threatening complication. This is an indication for urgent colectomy and accounts for approximately 10% of all urgent colectomies in patients with UC.

C. Fulminant Colitis

Fulminant colitis occurs in less than 10% of all patients with UC, but in up to 50% of these patients, it develops during the initial presentation. This represents the most severe, acute form of the disease. Patients are systemically ill and develop inflammation extending into the muscular layer of the bowel. This is often associated with anorexia, greater than 10 bowel movements per day, bleeding, abdominal pain and distention, and systemic toxicity with fever and tachycardia. Electrolyte disturbances, especially hypokalemia, are common and should be treated aggressively. Opioids and anticholinergics should be avoided. These patients should be fluid resuscitated and treated with broad-spectrum antibiotics. A nasogastric tube is placed for patients with significant signs of distension. A CT scan can detect perforation or ischemia, as well as other causes of abdominal sepsis. Serial abdominal x-rays can be used in conjunction with physical examination to follow colonic distention. However, if there is clinical deterioration or no improvement with maximal medical therapy over the course of 48-72 hours, surgery should be considered. Although barium enema is no longer used to diagnose toxic colitis, one can see the classic findings in Figure 32–18.

D. Perforation

Colonic perforation is the most dreaded complication of severe acute UC and occurs in 3% of hospitalized patients. It is responsible for more deaths than any other complication. The risk of perforation is highest during the initial attack of the disease and correlates well with its extent and severity. It may also occur as a complication of endoscopy or barium enema in acutely ill patients. Patients with toxic colitis are especially vulnerable. Perforation is most common

▲ **Figure 32–18.** Barium enema in a patient with toxic colitis and a history of ulcerative colitis. Note dilation of the transverse colon, the multiple irregular densities in the lumen that represent pseudopolyps, and the loss of haustral markings.

in the sigmoid or splenic flexure and may result in a localized abscess or generalized fecal peritonitis. Systemic therapy (corticosteroids and antibiotics) may mask the development of this complication. Therefore, serial abdominal exams, laboratory tests, and abdominal imaging are important in detecting this complication.

E. Malignancy

Colorectal cancer risk increases above that of the general population 10 years after the onset of UC, although the rates vary widely between studies. The risk increases with the duration and severity of disease and is higher in patients with a family history of colorectal cancer, extensive colitis, and PSC. Decreased risk in recent reports may be associated with improved medical treatment of colitis. Cancers in UC tend to be multicentric and broadly infiltrating. They are difficult to recognize endoscopically because they arise from small, flat areas of dysplasia located in a background of ulceration and inflammation. They do not follow the typical adenoma-carcinoma sequence seen in sporadic colorectal cancers in the general population. Newer techniques, including narrow-band imaging and chromoendoscopy, may improve detection.

Colonoscopic surveillance is recommended beginning 8-12 years after the onset of colitis and continues at 1- to 2-year intervals. Random biopsies are taken in four quadrants every 10 cm throughout the colon and rectum to screen for dysplasia. Synchronous high-grade dysplasia or colorectal cancer is found in 20% of patients undergoing proctocolectomy for low-grade dysplasia, 40% of patients with high-grade dysplasia, and 40%-85% of patients with dysplasia-associated lesion or mass (DALM). Low-grade dysplasia places the patient at a nine-fold increased risk of developing CRC compared to UC patients without dysplasia. In addition, low-grade dysplasia has been reported to progress to carcinoma without progressing to high-grade dysplasia. IBD-associated cancers account for 1%-2% of all colorectal cancers but occur in younger patients and confer a poorer prognosis. High-grade dysplasia and DALM are generally considered indications for proctocolectomy, and there is controversy regarding the need for surgery in patients with low-grade dysplasia. Part of the controversy lies in the interobserver variability in categorizing dysplasia, which is notoriously difficult given the background of chronic inflammation.

▶ Treatment

A. Medical Therapy

The goals of medical therapy are to stop an acute flare as rapidly as possible and to maintain remission of mucosal inflammation. Traditionally, medical management has been approached in a "step-up" fashion, with treatment depending on the severity of disease (classified as mild, moderate, severe, or fulminant), the extent of colonic involvement, and history of previous response to treatment. However, a new paradigm of "top-down" treatment has evolved for patients with severe disease. Both approaches are utilized. The end points of therapy have shifted away from symptomatic improvement to objective mucosal healing and steroid-free remission. Mild to moderate disease usually can be treated on an outpatient basis. If the disease flare is refractory or progressive, hospitalization may be required. Patients with severe or fulminant disease may require inpatient treatment for supportive therapy (intravenous hydration, antibiotics, blood transfusion, and monitoring).

Mild to moderate disease can be treated with sulfasalazine or 5-aminosalicylates, such as mesalamine, olsalazine, or balsalazide. Sulfasalazine is cost effective but associated with more side effects and should not be given to sulfa-allergic patients. These drugs can be administered orally or topically in the form of suppositories or enemas in patients with disease limited to the rectum or sigmoid. A greater response is seen in patients undergoing treatment with both enteral and topical therapy; however, adherence to daily suppositories or enemas is poor. Seventy percent of patients will respond to this regimen within 1 month. In patients who do not exhibit objective evidence of response, steroids are added, and if the disease remains refractory, immunomodulators (azathioprine, 6-mecaptopurine) or biologic agents (infliximab, adalimumab) are additional options to induce and maintain remission.

In patients with severe disease, these initial steps are bypassed, and treatment with intravenous glucocorticoids is initiated. If there is a clinical response, maintenance therapy is initiated. If the disease is refractory, biologic agents or immunomodulators are added. Surgery is considered in patients whose disease remains severe despite a trial of maximal medical therapy.

In the outpatient setting, a similar pathway can be followed beginning with steroids and biologics. If resistance to one biologic agent is discovered, a number of newer drugs may be considered such as the anti–tumor necrosis factor (TNF) agents certolizumab and golimumab, or anti-integrin agent vedolizumab. Surgery may be offered depending on the response to medications and patient preference.

Once remission has been obtained, a maintenance regimen is required to prevent relapse in most patients. These regimens should be individualized based on the response to the induction regimen and revised as clinically indicated. For mild disease, mesalamine is commonly used. Patients unable to wean from steroids require intensified treatment. Azathioprine, 6-mercaptopurine, methotrexate, infliximab, adalimumab, or newer immunomodulators may be needed to successfully wean patients off steroids.

B. Surgical Therapy

1. Indications—Indications for surgery fall under three broad categories: urgent or emergency surgery for patients who are severely ill or develop complications during a flare;

patients who have chronic intractable disease, medication intolerance, or inability to wean from steroids; and as a treatment for dysplasia or carcinoma. Twenty percent of patients who present with fulminant colitis will go on to require surgery. There have been no trials comparing medical therapy to surgery for any of these indications. CD should be ruled out in any patient in whom surgery is being considered, because the surgical approach is different, especially when considering reconstruction with an IPAA.

In the acute setting, emergency surgery is indicated for colonic perforation. Other complications, such as toxic megacolon, fulminant colitis, or uncontrolled hemorrhage, are initially managed medically. However, if there is no improvement with aggressive medical therapy, surgery is warranted. These patients are monitored closely for 48-72 hours. If there is clinical deterioration or no improvement, surgery is indicated.

Another group of patients in whom surgery is considered are those with intractable disease despite maximal medical therapy or those who cannot wean off steroids due to worsening symptoms. In children, this may present with growth retardation. Adults may become physically debilitated and psychosocially limited and experience poor quality of life. There may be medication intolerance, especially in patients who are steroid dependent. Surgery is also considered for patients with severe extraintestinal manifestations that have developed in parallel with the UC flares such as peripheral arthritis, pyoderma gangrenosum, and ocular manifestations. These usually respond to colectomy.

Patients who have biopsy-proven colitis-related carcinoma are offered proctocolectomy as opposed to standard oncologic resection because this treats both the UC and the cancer. In addition, colitis-related colorectal cancer tends to be widely infiltrative, multicentric, and difficult to visualize, making standard oncologic resection dangerous. Patients with dysplasia or DALM are also candidates for surgery due to a high risk of synchronous or metachronous malignancy or dysplasia as discussed previously.

2. Surgical procedures—In the elective setting, there are two surgical options. Proctocolectomy with IPAA is considered by some to be the operation of choice because it provides intestinal continuity (Figure 32–19). However, total proctocolectomy with a permanent end ileostomy is indicated in a subset of patients. Factors include preoperative sphincter function, presence of low rectal cancer, and the patient's age, general health, and preferences. IPAA is contraindicated in patients with poor baseline sphincter tone or in whom a diagnosis of CD cannot be excluded. Both procedures are now increasingly performed with a minimally invasive approach with equivalent functional results and improved short-term outcomes. Because sexual function and fertility may be impaired by the pelvic dissection required for proctectomy in either procedure, consideration is given to subtotal colectomy in patients who have not completed childbearing.

▲ **Figure 32–19.** View of the pelvis after colectomy and ileoanal anastomosis in a male. The J-pouch, shown here, is one of several types of reservoirs and is most commonly utilized.

Patients who have concerns about the postoperative complications or anticipate difficulty managing the changes in bowel function associated with the ileoanal pouch may desire a permanent end ileostomy. Patients frequently experience greater than 10 bowel movements per day during the first 3 months. This eventually decreases to an average of five to seven bowel movements per day. Twenty percent of patients experience nocturnal seepage or incontinence 1 year after surgery. The most common surgical complications include small bowel obstruction, infertility, sexual dysfunction, and pelvic sepsis as a result of anastomotic or pouch leaks. Pelvic sepsis occurs in 25% of patients and is the most common cause of pouch failure. The most common long-term complication is pouchitis, which affects 40% of patients in the first 10 years after surgery. Pouchitis refers to idiopathic inflammation of the ileoanal pouch that causes abdominal pain, increased bowel movements, and bleeding. It is treated with antibiotics.

Proctocolectomy with IPAA can be performed as a one-, two-, or three-stage procedure. In the elective setting, a two-stage procedure is most common, involving procto-colectomy with IPAA and diverting loop ileostomy at the first surgery followed by ileostomy reversal as a second surgery. A single-stage operation (without diverting loop ileostomy) is performed only in the most ideal candidates at specialized centers. This approach eliminates the ileostomy-associated complications and avoids a second surgery at the cost of potentially significant consequences of pelvic sepsis from an undiverted anastomotic leak. The three-stage procedure is reserved for ill patients who would not tolerate the IPAA during the first surgery secondary to malnutrition or severe active disease. It is also useful in patients with indeterminate colitis in whom confirmation of UC may be made after pathologic evaluation of the surgical specimen, allowing the safe formation of the IPAA. The first procedure is a subtotal colectomy with end ileostomy, followed by completion proctectomy and IPAA. Again, at the time of this procedure, an ileostomy may be avoided in selected patients; otherwise, the ileostomy is reversed at a third surgery. In the interval between subtotal colectomy and proctectomy, the residual disease in the rectal remnant improves with fecal diversion, but if symptoms persist, it can be treated locally with suppositories or enemas.

Proctocolectomy involves mobilizing and resecting the entire colon and rectum. If a permanent end ileostomy is planned, an intersphincteric resection of the anus is performed and the perineum is closed primarily. If IPAA is planned, the anal sphincter complex is left in place. The ileum is made into a reservoir, most commonly with a "J" configuration (although multiple configurations have been described), and an anastomosis is created just above the dentate line (Figure 32–19). A diverting loop ileostomy is commonly used to protect the anastomosis, particularly if there is any intraoperative concern about the anastomosis or if the patient has risk factors for impaired healing such as steroid exposure, anemia, diabetes, or malnutrition. Most of these patients will have been treated with immunosuppressants or immunomodulators in the preoperative period. Although these medications theoretically impact healing, there is no clear evidence to suggest that they increase surgical complications in the setting of diversion.

The continent ileostomy, or Kock pouch, was first reported by Kock in 1969. It involves an ileal reservoir and construction of a valve at skin level to allow the patient to catheterize the stoma multiple times per day. This allowed patients not to wear a stoma appliance and to control the timing of stool output. However, this procedure was plagued by a very high complication rate, requiring reoperation in 50% of patients. It has largely been replaced with the IPAA and is mainly mentioned for historical purposes.

► Prognosis

The mortality rate of UC has dropped sharply in the past 2 decades. First attacks are seldom fatal when treated by specialists. In one large series, emergency colectomy was required in 25% of patients with severe first attacks; 60% responded rapidly to medical therapy; and 15% improved slowly on medications alone. Overall, the colitis-related mortality rate during the year after onset is about 1%. Emergency colectomy has a mortality rate of 6%; most of these deaths occur in patients with preoperative perforation, a complication that has a fatal outcome in 40% of cases.

Compared to pancolitis, the long-term prognosis of ulcerative proctitis is excellent; only 10% of patients will develop colonic disease by 10 years, and the mortality rate is very low. In patients with pancolitis, the likelihood of operation during the first year is about 25%, and the mortality rate is 5% over 10 years. Colorectal cancer in UC is more often diagnosed at an advanced stage than is sporadic cancer, but the stage-for-stage prognosis is equivalent. Screening with colonoscopy and biopsies seems to have reduced the cancer mortality rate, but there are still many patients who escape detection until the malignancy has progressed to an advanced stage. The operative mortality rate is less than 1% for elective colectomy.

CROHN COLITIS

► General Considerations

Approximately 45% of patients with CD have diffuse involvement of the GI tract; 30% have disease limited to the small bowel, 20% have disease limited to the colon, and another 5% have isolated anorectal involvement. Symptoms, including diarrhea, abdominal pain, constitutional effects, and extraintestinal manifestations, are approximately the same in colonic and enteric disease. Fistulae, abscesses, and intestinal obstruction are more often complications of small bowel disease. Anorectal complications such as anal fistula, fissure, abscess, rectal stricture, and hemorrhage occur more commonly in patients with disease affecting the large bowel. Smoking is a risk factor for the development of CD as well as severity of disease once it is established.

► Clinical Findings

Patients can develop abdominal pain, diarrhea, and systemic signs of inflammation such as low-grade fevers, weight loss, and malaise. Symptoms are generally dictated by the distribution of disease, but patients with Crohn colitis may report urgency or mucus, blood, or pus per rectum. Patients with perianal disease may present with tenesmus, perianal pain, or discharge from an abscess, fistula, or fissure. If the inflammatory process has caused stricturing, obstructive symptoms may be present.

The differential diagnosis for patients presenting with new-onset Crohn colitis is broad and includes all forms of colitis, including UC, infectious, ischemic, malignancy, and diverticulitis. Features differentiating CD from UC are summarized in Table 32-10.

Clinical Findings

A. Laboratory Findings

Laboratory findings vary based on the severity and extent of disease. In severe or long-standing disease, patients may exhibit anemia or hypoalbuminemia.

B. Imaging Studies

Abdominal x-rays may be useful to exclude the presence of free air in a patient with suspected bowel perforation. CT scan has become the most common imaging modality during an acute episode. CT will often show thickening and inflammation in areas of disease. In CD, there may be pancolitis or patchy involvement of the small bowel, colon, and rectum. CT is also helpful to evaluate for stricture, fistula, and abscess. CT enterography can be particularly helpful in the nonacute phase for staging and detailed evaluation of small and large bowel involvement.

Colonoscopy

Colonoscopy is indicated for diagnosis, evaluation for severity of disease, determining response to treatment, and screening for colorectal cancer. Colonoscopy with biopsy is a mainstay in diagnosis. Patients with Crohn colitis have rectal sparing about 50% of the time. Skip lesions are common, with irregular ulcerations separated by edematous or even normal-appearing mucosa. Patients with pancolitis appear to have similar risk profile for cancer as their UC counterparts. The risk of colorectal cancer in Crohn colitis patients is 4-20 times that of the general population. The 25-year risk of dysplasia in patients with Crohn colitis is 12%-25%. Data to support surveillance and management strategies for patients with Crohn colitis are limited and often extrapolated from UC patients. Routine annual colonoscopy with random biopsies is recommended beginning 8 years after the diagnosis. Surveillance should include high-risk areas, such as segments of intestine excluded from the fecal stream, strictures, and fistulas with focused biopsies performed as needed.

Treatment

A. Medical Therapy

As in UC, medical management for CD can be approached from a top-down or bottom-up strategy. The decision to start a particular therapy takes into account the severity and extent of disease, medication side effects, and patient preference. The medication classes include antibiotics, 5-aminosalicylate compounds, glucocorticoids, immunomodulators, and biologic agents. First, induction therapy is used to achieve remission, and then maintenance therapy is initiated with the goal of sustaining remission. Steroids are effective for acute flares in up to 70% of patients, but they are not used for maintenance therapy because of the associated side effects and complications. Up to 45% of patients who initially improve with steroids will relapse upon tapering or withdrawal. Oral 5-aminosalicylates (sulfasalazine, 4 g/d; or mesalamine, 2-5 g/d) are effective treatment for Crohn colitis. Topical 5-aminosalicylates are beneficial for disease of the rectum and sigmoid and are often used to wean patients off steroids. Anal abscesses and fistulas require surgical drainage and seton placement to treat local sepsis, but healing is improved with biologic agents.

Immunosuppressants (azathioprine, 6-mercaptopurine, methotrexate) are steroid-sparing drugs that can control Crohn colitis well enough so that surgery is delayed or avoided. Biologic agents, including infliximab and other anti-TNF therapies, are effective for inflammatory CD and also specifically indicated for fistulizing or refractory disease. Patients who respond to infliximab induction should receive maintenance therapy. Adalimumab is an effective therapy for patients who are refractory or intolerant to infliximab. Newer human monoclonal antibodies, such as the anti-TNF certolizumab and the integrin-receptor antagonists natalizumab and vedolizumab, are used in patients with moderate to severe disease refractory to other agents.

B. Surgical Therapy

It is estimated that 50%-75% of CD patients will require surgery within 10 years of diagnosis. Because CD cannot be cured with surgery, the primary indications for operation are failure of medical therapy, neoplasia, and complications of CD. Failure of medical therapy is a broad term that refers to symptoms that do not respond to optimal medical management, inability to achieve remission, steroid dependence, intractable weight loss, or unmanageable side effects. The choice of operation depends on the severity and distribution of disease, but the general principle is bowel preservation, with resection of only diseased, actively symptomatic areas. Disease tends to recur, especially at areas of intestinal anastomosis, and short bowel syndrome is a major concern with repeated operations. Resumption of medical therapy after surgery is critical for reducing recurrent disease. Cigarette smoking is an independent risk factor for recurrence of CD after resection.

Strictures are more common in patients with long-standing disease. The use of CT or magnetic resonance enterography is useful to localize the lesion. If the lesion has a significant acute inflammatory component, medical therapy may be successful in treatment. If the stricture is the result of fibrostenotic disease, medical therapy is less likely to be successful. Regardless, if the lesion is symptomatic and unresponsive to medical therapy, surgery is indicated. Asymptomatic strictures do not necessarily require surgery; however, the possibility of an underlying malignancy must be considered. Malignancy is more common in patients with long-standing inflammation. If nonoperative management is chosen, surveillance with biopsies and brushings are critical. If dysplasia is detected or if the lesion prevents colonoscopic surveillance due to obstruction, surgery should be considered.

Surgical options for strictures depend on the degree of obstruction, the length of the stricture, the location of the stricture, and the disease activity in the surrounding bowel. Stricturoplasty is an option for small bowel disease. However, strictures of the terminal ileum and colon require resection. CD patients are at higher risk for anastomotic leak than the general population. The decision about a primary anastomosis versus anastomosis with proximal diversion versus resection with end stoma depends on the overall health of the patient, the location and severity of the stricture, and the condition of the tissues.

Abdominal abscesses may be managed conservatively with percutaneous drainage and antibiotics. Those who do not respond to conservative management may need an operation. Patients with CD are at risk of developing enterocutaneous and enteroenteric fistulas, either spontaneously or after surgical intervention. When they develop, nutritional optimization and control of sepsis are of utmost importance. After sepsis is controlled, medical management is instituted. If disease persists, patients may require resection of the involved segment of bowel and debridement of fistula tracts in the abdominal wall.

Fulminant colitis will occur in less than 5% of patients with CD. These patients should be treated in a similar fashion as patients with UC, including bowel rest, intravenous fluids, broad-spectrum antibiotics, and aggressive CD therapy. They should be closely monitored with serial abdominal exams, laboratory tests, and imaging as indicated. Patients with CD more commonly respond to medical management than patients with UC. When patients require surgery, total abdominal colectomy with end ileostomy is the most common operation performed in the acute setting, although if by operative inspection, the disease is limited to a specific part of the large bowel, this can be resected with creation of an end stoma and Hartmann pouch or mucous fistula.

Perianal complications include perianal abscess, fistula, ulcer, and fissure. The principle of management for infectious complications, such as abscess and fistula, is control of sepsis. Drainage procedures generally need to be done under anesthesia in the operating room to allow thorough evaluation of the perineum and sphincter complex and to assess for fistulas. Fistulas are managed with draining setons. Perianal disease is otherwise optimally managed with medical therapy. For all perianal operations, minimizing trauma, incisions, and damage to the sphincter complex is key. Medical management with biologic agents is the primary treatment. Some patients will require fecal diversion owing to the severity of disease. In refractory cases, patients may require abdominal perineal resection.

Dysplasia or cancer of the colon requires surgical treatment. Depending on the location and extent of disease, proctocolectomy or segmental resection is performed for high-grade dysplasia, dysplasia-associated lesions, or mass lesions. Twenty percent of patients with high-grade dysplasia are found to have carcinoma in the surgical specimen, and half of patients known to have cancer preoperatively are found to have remote dysplasia upon pathologic review. For this reason, total proctocolectomy with end ileostomy should be considered in patients with longstanding pancolitis who develop cancer or high-grade dysplasia on surveillance colonoscopy. IPAA is rarely performed in patients with CD because more than half of patients will develop pouch failure.

Prognosis

Surgical procedures—like medical therapy—should be regarded as palliative, not curative, in patients with CD. Although recurrence rates are high and chronic disease is common, a productive life is usually possible with the aid of combined medical and surgical management. The mortality rate is about 15% over 30 years.

Ng SC, Bernstein CN, Vatn MH, et al, Epidemiology and Natural History Task Force of the International Organization of Inflammatory Bowel Disease (IOIBD): Geographical variability and environmental risk factors in inflammatory bowel disease. *Gut.* 2013;62(4):630-649.

Reinisch, W, Sandborn WJ, Hommes DW, et al: Adalimumab for induction of clinical remission in moderately to severely active ulcerative colitis: results of a randomised controlled trial. *Gut.* 2011;60(6):780-787.

Sandborn WJ, Ghosh S, Panes J, et al: Study A3921063 Investigators: Tofacitinib, an oral Janus kinase inhibitor, in active ulcerative colitis. *N Engl J Med.* 2012;367(7):616-624.

To N, Gracie DJ, Ford AC: Systematic review with meta-analysis: the adverse effects of tobacco smoking on the natural history of Crohn's disease. *Aliment Pharmacol Ther.* 2016;43(5):549-561.

PSEUDOMEMBRANOUS COLITIS

Pseudomembranous colitis is caused by *C difficile*. *C difficile* colitis was first reported in 1978, but the incidence and severity of infection are increasing with time. Of particular concern is the increasing virulence, with reports of antibiotic resistance and mutant strains with uncontrolled toxin production. Infection causes a range of illness from mild diarrhea to fulminant, life-threatening colitis and is particularly dangerous in frail or immunocompromised patients.

Microbiology

C difficile is a spore-forming organism that is ubiquitous in the environment. It is a commensal gut organism that exists in 5%-15% of the general population and up to 57% of patients in long-term care facilities. The spores are dormant and extremely resistant to disinfectants and extreme environments. Spread by health care practitioners is reduced significantly by the use of standard contact precautions including disposable gowns and gloves and hand washing with water and soap. Alcohol-based hand sanitizers are not effective. Once ingested, the spore is reactivated after contact with bile salts in the small intestine.

The bacterium exists in both toxin-producing and non-producing forms. Only the toxin-producing bacterium is capable of causing colitis. Toxins A and B and binary toxin induce apoptosis and provoke inflammation. The epidemic-associated 027 strain is thought to have a mutation causing increased production of toxins A and B, as well as enhanced sporulation, making it particularly virulent and transmittable. These toxins, as well as a variety of nontoxin virulence factors, cause pseudomembranous colitis.

Although *C difficile* is commensal and the spores are easily transmitted, the presence of normal colonic flora is usually enough to prevent infection. Symptoms generally only occur when the normal flora is disrupted. Therefore, pseudomembranous colitis most often occurs in patients taking antibiotics. Clindamycin is historically the most common cause, but all antibiotics that alter the gut flora have the potential to allow symptomatic infection. Pseudomembranous colitis may develop as early as 2 days after exposure to antibiotics but has been reported many weeks after they are discontinued. Other risk factors include advanced age, hospitalization, surgery of the GI tract, immunosuppression, IBD, and use of proton pump inhibitors.

Symptoms and Signs

The most common symptom is diarrhea, which is usually watery, occasionally bloody, and has a characteristic foul odor. Other symptoms include colicky abdominal pain, vomiting, and fever. In severe cases, *C difficile* infection may cause a paralytic ileus and, therefore, can present without diarrhea. Depending on the severity, patients may present with abdominal distention, tenderness, dehydration, and sepsis. The stool is usually positive for leukocytes. Radiographic studies may reveal colonic wall thickening due to submucosal edema. On abdominal films, this may appear as a "target sign." CT scanning is reserved for patients with complicated disease or when the diagnosis is in question. It may show colonic wall thickening and inflammation, most commonly localized to the left colon with or without involvement of the rectum. In more severe cases, patients present with pancolitis. Other findings on CT imaging suggestive of severe disease are ascites and colonic dilation. If left untreated, there may be progression to perforation.

Changes in the colonic mucosa depend on the severity of the infection. Endoscopy performed for mild to moderate cases will show erythema and edema of the mucosa, with occasional hemorrhage. In severe cases, findings include elevated whitish-green or yellow plaque-like "pseudomembranes" overlying inflamed mucosa. The pseudomembrane is made up of leukocytes, necrotic epithelial cells, and fibrin. The rectum is spared in about one-fourth of cases.

Diagnosis

Historically, the gold standard for diagnosis of *C difficile* colitis was a cytotoxin neutralization assay. This has largely been abandoned owing to its technical difficulty and length of time required to obtain a result (24-48 hours). Immunologic assays, such as the enzyme immunoassay (EIA), have greater than 80% sensitivity and 90% specificity. When combined with glutamine dehydrogenase (GDH) assay, the negative predictive value is 98%. To improve the sensitivity, many institutions have adopted the more costly nucleic acid amplification testing (NAAT), which uses polymerase chain reaction to detect toxin A and B sequences. This can be used as a stand-alone test or used as a confirmatory test in patients who screen positive with an EIA test. Retesting stool for cure is not recommended because there is a high rate of positive tests after clinical cure, which may lead to extended and unnecessary treatment.

Treatment

A. Medical

Management is determined by the severity of disease. Any inciting antibiotics are discontinued where possible. Continued antibiotic treatment after diagnosis of *C difficile* infection is associated with lower cure rates. Discontinuation of proton pump inhibitors has not been shown to improve outcomes but is suggested.

Guidelines (2018) from the Infectious Diseases Society of America (IDSA) and the Society for Healthcare Epidemiology of America (SHEA) recommend stratifying patients into nonsevere, severe, and fulminant presentations. Nonsevere disease can be treated with low-dose (125 mg) oral vancomycin or fidaxomicin for 10 days, with oral metronidazole used if vancomycin or fidaxomicin is not available. Severe disease is classified by a white blood cell count of $\geq$ 15,000 cells/μL or a serum creatinine level > 1.5 mg/dL and is treated with low-dose oral vancomycin or fidaxomicin. Fulminant disease is defined by hypotension, shock, ileus, or megacolon and is treated with high-dose vancomycin (500 mg), plus intravenous metronidazole and vancomycin enemas if ileus is present.

Recurrent disease is less well studied. Treatment is tailored based on previous treatments. If the first episode was treated with metronidazole, then a trial of low-dose oral vancomycin is warranted. If the patient previously failed oral vancomycin, then pulsed and tapered vancomycin is initiated. Fidaxomicin is an alternative. For patients with more than two previous episodes, fecal transplant may be effective.

B. Surgical

Although most patients will respond to initial medical management, a subset will develop refractory, progressive, or fulminant disease. In patients at risk, early surgical evaluation is recommended, because retrospective studies have shown that earlier surgical intervention is associated with improved outcomes including mortality. These data must be interpreted with caution, however, because it is not clear if all patients undergoing early surgical intervention would have disease progression in the absence of surgery. For those undergoing surgery, perioperative mortality ranges from 30%-80%. Surgical options include subtotal colectomy with end ileostomy and loop ileostomy with colonic lavage. Subtotal colectomy is required in patients with perforated or nonviable colon at the time of surgery. Loop ileostomy and with intraoperative lavage involves creation of an ileostomy and instilling 8 L of polyethylene glycol into the efferent limb through a catheter. This is left in place and can be used for antegrade vancomycin administration postoperatively. Although there is limited published experience with this technique, small case series report high rates of colon preservation and ileostomy reversal.

Bagdasarian N, Rao K, Malani PN: Diagnosis and treatment of *Clostridium difficile* in adults: a systematic review. *JAMA.* 2015; 313(4):398-408.

Fashandi AZ, Martin AN, Wang PT, et al: An institutional comparison of total abdominal colectomy and diverting loop ileostomy and colonic lavage in the treatment of severe, complicated *Clostridium difficile* infections. *Am J Surg.* 2017;213(3):507-511.

Ferrada P, Velopulos CG, Sultan S, et al: Timing and type of surgical treatment of *Clostridium difficile*-associated disease: a practice management guideline from the Eastern Association for the Surgery of Trauma. *J Trauma Acute Care Surg.* 2014;76(6):1484-1493.

McDonald LC, Gerding DN, Johnson S, et al: Clinical Practice Guidelines for *Clostridium difficile* Infection in Adults and Children: 2017 update by the Infectious Diseases Society of America (IDSA) and Society for Healthcare Epidemiology of America (SHEA). *Clin Infect Dis.* 2018;66(7):987-994.

van Nood E, Vrieze A, Nieuwdorp M, et al: Duodenal infusion of donor feces for recurrent *Clostridium difficile*. *N Engl J Med.* 2013;368(5):407-415.

ISCHEMIC COLITIS

Ischemic colitis refers to colonic inflammation caused by inadequate perfusion. The colon receives blood supply from the superior mesenteric artery and the IMA, and the GI tract has the most variable blood supply of any organ in the body. In times of rest, it receives up to 35% of the cardiac output, and in times of stress, this can drop to as low as 10% under physiologic conditions. There are two "watershed" areas described. The first is at the splenic flexure, where the blood supply transitions from the superior mesenteric artery to the IMA distribution. The second is in the rectosigmoid, where the marginal artery ends.

Ischemic colitis is more common in elderly and frail patients and has a mortality of 13%. It occurs as a result of an occlusive or nonocclusive insult. Examples of occlusive ischemic colitis include embolism, thrombosis (arterial or venous), atherosclerosis, trauma, and postsurgical causes such as patients with loss of inferior mesenteric blood supply after aortic aneurysm repair and those with inadequate perfusion to colonic anastomoses. Nonocclusive injury is the cause of greater than 90% of ischemic colitis cases and occurs as a result of shock, vasopressors, vasospasm, mechanical obstruction of the lumen, or systemic vasculitides.

An important clinical distinction that must be made when evaluating patients is assessing the colon for gangrenous and nongangrenous ischemic colitis. Patients with gangrenous forms have transmural, nonreversible injury that is rapidly fatal without surgery. The nongangrenous type is divided into transient reversible and chronic forms. The chronic form involves the muscularis propria and is prone to stricture development. Transient reversible ischemia involves the submucosa and heals without sequelae. Most cases of ischemic colitis are idiopathic and attributed to a nonocclusive state.

Patients with ischemic colitis have diarrhea (90%), hematochezia (65%), and abdominal pain (58%). A history of atrial fibrillation, thrombophilia, atherosclerotic arterial disease, systemic vasculitis, or recent trauma or surgery should be sought. Recent severe systemic illness with shock is a common suspected cause. There may be localized or diffuse peritonitis. Blood tests may reveal leukocytosis, hyperamylasemia, and acidosis, as well as electrolyte derangements.

The most useful diagnostic tests are colonoscopy and abdominal CT. Colonoscopy is the diagnostic modality of choice (although contraindicated in critically ill patients with peritonitis) as it allows diagnostic confirmation and determination of severity and can exclude other types of colitis. The mucosa of the involved segment is edematous, hemorrhagic, friable, and sometimes ulcerated. A grayish membrane may be present, resembling pseudomembranous colitis, but the presence of hyalinized, hemorrhagic lamina on biopsy will differentiate colonic ischemia from *C difficile* colitis. If full-thickness necrosis is present, surgery is required. Abdominal CT with contrast shows a thickened colonic wall, decreased wall enhancement, pneumatosis, and occasionally a disruption in the arterial circulation. It is also useful to exclude other conditions.

Initial treatment for patients suspected to have reversible ischemic colitis consists of intravenous fluids, bowel rest, broad-spectrum antibiotics, and observation with serial abdominal exams. Less than 20% of patients will have irreversible full-thickness necrosis that requires surgery. The extent of the resection is based on the amount of necrotic or severely diseased colon. Most commonly, a segmental resection is performed, although a subtotal or total colectomy may be required. Depending on the etiology of the ischemia and the appearance of the remaining bowel, a second-look laparotomy may be scheduled 12-24 hours later. Primary anastomosis is rarely performed, and intestinal continuity is restored during a subsequent operation.

NEUTROPENIC COLITIS

Neutropenic colitis, also referred to as neutropenic enterocolitis, necrotizing enteropathy, ileocecal syndrome, and typhlitis, is a syndrome of colonic ischemia occurring in neutropenic patients. The cause is poorly understood but likely involves mucosal injury and unimpeded bacterial translocation as a result of profound immunosuppression. Neutropenic colitis should be on the differential diagnosis for any immunosuppressed patient with abdominal pain; however, it is most common in neutropenic patients undergoing chemotherapy with cytotoxic agents such as the vinca alkaloids and doxorubicin. There are reports in patients with acquired immunodeficiency syndrome (AIDS), aplastic anemia, and cyclic neutropenia and those being treated with a variety of immunosuppressants for other conditions.

The clinical presentation ranges from mild to life threatening, and overall mortality is 30%-50%. Symptoms include fever, nausea, abdominal pain, distention, and watery or bloody diarrhea. These patients often present late and with deceptively benign findings on physical examination owing to the inability to mount a normal inflammatory response. The cecum and right colon are most often affected; however, any part of the small or large bowel, including the appendix, can be involved. Patients are commonly bacteremic and/or fungemic. Causative organisms include gram-negative rods, gram-positive cocci, anaerobes, and *Candida*.

Diagnosis is confirmed using abdominal CT scan, which demonstrates bowel wall thickening and distention and may show pneumatosis or perforation. Initial management consists of bowel rest, intravenous fluids, and broad-spectrum antibiotics. Antifungals are started if there is evidence of fungemia or persistent fevers on antibiotics. Resolution of neutropenia is an important prognostic factor; therefore, discontinuation of immunosuppressants and chemotherapeutics and administration of granulocyte colony-stimulating factor (G-CSF) should be considered. Surgery is recommended for patients with perforation or who do not improve with medical management. Most patients undergo segmental resection with proximal diversion.

MICROSCOPIC COLITIS

Microscopic colitis is a chronic inflammatory disorder of the colon characterized by watery diarrhea but grossly normal colonic mucosa. It is more common in women and in middle age. NSAID use and smoking are risk factors. There are two main subtypes: collagenous colitis and lymphocytic colitis. These are differentiated based on biopsy specimens obtained during colonoscopy. Biopsies in collagenous colitis demonstrate a subepithelial collagen band more than 10 μm in thickness. Lymphocytic colitis is diagnosed by the presence of more than 20 intraepithelial lymphocytes. A diagnosis of incomplete microscopic colitis is assigned if the subepithelial collagen band is less than 10 μm in thickness or if there are less than 20 intraepithelial lymphocytes.

The differential diagnosis for watery diarrhea is extremely broad, and the diagnostic workup should include a thorough search for other causes, including infectious, endocrine, food-related, malabsorption, medication, SIBO, irritable bowel syndrome, and any etiology of colitis. Blood work is generally nonspecific, but patients may have anemia, hypoalbuminemia, and autoantibodies including rheumatoid factor (RF), antinuclear antibody (ANA), antimitochondrial antibody (AMA), antineutrophilic cytoplasmic antibodies (ANCA), and antithyroid peroxidase antibodies (TPO). Evaluation includes upper endoscopy with duodenal biopsies to rule out celiac disease and lower endoscopy with random biopsies from the transverse, ascending colon and rectosigmoid colon because involvement can be patchy and the mucosa generally appears normal.

Treatment begins with the avoidance of inciting agents, such as NSAIDs and tobacco. Antidiarrheal medications, such as loperamide, are used with a goal of preventing dehydration and decreasing stool frequency. If patients remain symptomatic with greater than three bowel movements daily, budesonide and cholestyramine are added. In refractory cases, treatment with bismuth subsalicylate and mesalamine has been successful. Rarely, patients will continue to have severe diarrhea despite maximal therapy. Small studies suggest that anti-TNF agents or immunomodulators may be useful. Surgery is almost never required. However, a total abdominal colectomy with ileorectal anastomosis or ileostomy is an option in patients who have severe and refractory disease.

INTESTINAL STOMAS: ILEOSTOMY AND COLOSTOMY

Creating an intestinal stoma involves exteriorizing a part of the bowel wall onto the surface of the abdomen. This section will focus on the two most common stomas created in colon and rectal surgery: those made from the ileum (ileostomy) and colon (colostomy).

▶ Indications

Stomas are generally created to protect a distal anastomosis temporarily or as a permanent route for enteric contents when the colon and/or rectum is resected. There are two configurations for a stoma. The end ileostomy or colostomy is created by fixing the end of the ileum or colon to the abdominal wall. The loop ileostomy or colostomy involves bringing a segment of ileum or colon to the abdominal wall and opening the side of the bowel, leaving both a proximal and distal opening. In general, very little, if any, stool passes through the distal limb if

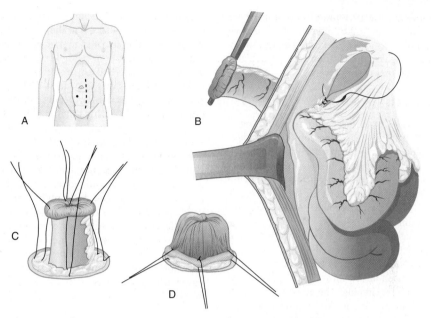

▲ **Figure 32–20.** Ileostomy after colectomy. **A:** A midline incision for colectomy is indicated by the dotted line and the site of the ileostomy by the black dot. **B:** The ileum has been brought through the abdominal wall. **C and D:** The ileostomy stoma has been everted and its margins sutured to the edges of the wound.

the stoma is well constructed. This allows retrograde decompression of the distal bowel and has the benefit of being easier to reverse as both limbs are at the abdominal wall.

In the elective setting, loop ileostomies are commonly used to protect ileoanal anastomoses and low pelvic colorectal or colo-anal anastomoses. These ileostomies are temporary and divert most of the fecal stream away from the anastomosis. End ileostomies (Figure 32–20) are used in the elective setting for patients who require proctocolectomy

and do not desire or are not candidates for IPAA reconstruction. They are also commonly used in patients who require emergency subtotal colectomies and will not tolerate an anastomosis due to severe illness.

Colostomies (Figure 32–21) are used in patients with low rectal cancers requiring either an APR or an LAR who cannot have a low anastomosis for other reasons. In addition, they are useful in patients who require diversion for chronic perianal fistula disease or in the emergency setting for patients

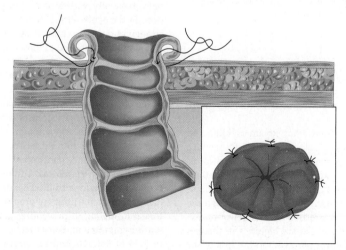

▲ **Figure 32–21.** End colostomy. The margins of the stoma are fixed to the skin with sutures.

with a large bowel obstruction, perforation, or trauma where an anastomosis is unlikely to heal or the patient is too ill to tolerate it. Loop colostomies are created infrequently as they are associated with a higher complication rate, particularly prolapse, although they are easier to reverse.

Technical Aspects

When possible, patients should meet with an enterostomal therapist or surgeon prior to their operation for education, counseling, and stoma marking. Preoperative stoma marking has been shown to reduce complications and improve postoperative quality of life. Ileostomies are typically placed in the right lower quadrant and colostomies in the left lower quadrant. The placement should avoid wrinkles, folds, scars, and hernias on the abdominal wall. It should be at least 2 inches from the surgical incision and have a clear area extending 2-3 inches around it. It must be visible to the patient. Ideally, it is situated below the patient's belt line in the lateral rectus. The patient should be evaluated in the sitting, standing, and lying positions with and without clothing. The mark is made with active patient participation, and it is ideal to provide a stoma appliance for the patient to wear over the mark for several days prior to the operation to ensure it is in the optimal position.

There are several key steps during the operation that, when followed, can reduce the chance of complications. The first step is to ensure adequate mobilization of the bowel so that the stoma will lie without any tension and will not retract into the abdominal wall. The second step is to pay close attention to the blood supply and preserve the mesentery and associated vessels during mobilization to avoid ischemic injury and subsequent stenosis. The third step is to create a defect in the rectus that is as small as possible that will still allow the stoma to pass without ischemia in order to prevent herniation. Lastly, when maturing the stoma, the aim should be to create 2-3 cm of bowel protrusion to ensure good appliance adhesion and improve skin protection.

Management

Having a stoma changes a patient's life in many ways and is associated with an overall complication rate of 20%-70%. For this reason, these patients, especially those with newly created stomas and those experiencing complications, require dedicated management.

An ileostomy has a near-continuous stream of liquid and semi-solid material, whereas a colostomy tends to produce more formed stool. Both generally require an appliance to be worn at all times. Some patients choose to irrigate their colostomies to avoid stool output during the day. Patients cannot control the sound and timing of flatus, although the volume of flatus tends to decrease after the first few months.

After ileostomy creation, there are significant changes in water and electrolyte absorption owing to the loss of the colon (Table 32-1). The small bowel adapts over the first 2 months after surgery. Output increases over the first week up to 1-2 L/d, stabilizes, and then, over the next 2 months, steadily decreases to a steady state of 500-800 mL/d. Output can be higher in patients with diseased small bowel or more proximal stomas. Sodium excretion averages 60 mEq/d, which is 2-3 times that of patients with intact colons. These patients are at risk for developing salt depletion and dehydration, especially during times of illness or exposure to hot weather. They must take care to stay hydrated and to consume enough salt and potassium in their diets to make up for this. Generally, switching to a bland, constipating diet high in breads, cereals, peanut butter, bananas, and rice will help decrease high output and reduce fluid and electrolyte losses. Fiber supplements and antimotility agents such as loperamide or diphenoxylate can be added as needed.

Patients with colostomies are less prone to metabolic disturbances, especially with the more common distal (sigmoid) colostomy configuration. Generally, they will continue to have formed bowel movements similar to their previous bowel habits. Fecal impaction will require irrigation in some patients.

Complications

Stomas are associated with a complication rate of 20%-70%. Ileostomies and colostomies are associated with similar complication rates, although transverse colostomies are harder to manage. The complications seen in ileostomies are different than those seen with colostomies. Ileostomies are more likely to cause high output and peristomal dermatitis, whereas colostomies are more likely to develop parastomal hernia and odor.

A **parastomal hernia** refers to herniation of intraabdominal contents through the defect in the fascia created for the stoma. In the chronic setting, parastomal hernias cause pain, difficulty with stoma appliance fitting, and obstruction. In the acute setting, there is a risk of incarceration and strangulation. Herniation is more common in patients with end stomas as opposed to loop stomas and more common in colostomies than ileostomies. Patient risk factors for hernia development include obesity, chronic obstructive pulmonary disease, poor nutritional status, immunosuppression, and bowel obstruction at the time of colostomy creation. The risk of parastomal hernia increases with time. Creating a fascial defect that is just large enough to accommodate the bowel without ischemia minimizes the risk. Other technical factors that may reduce parastomal hernia include preoperative stoma marking, stoma exit through rectus muscle for support, and fixation with fascial sutures. There are conflicting data regarding the utility of prophylactic mesh and extraperitoneal tunneling in preventing parastomal hernia. If a hernia is symptomatic, conservative management is successful in 70% of patients and includes abdominal binders, stoma belts, and restriction on heavy lifting. Specialized ostomy appliances may decrease leaking. Up to 30% of patients will require surgical revision either for failure of conservative management or for presentation with incarceration or strangulation. Surgical treatments vary depending on individual patient factors. Options include stoma relocation and mesh repair. Mesh repairs can be local or intraperitoneal and open or laparoscopic. Intraperitoneal synthetic mesh repairs using a Sugarbaker technique have the lowest recurrence rates, although this approach involves more surgical risk as well as the risk of mesh erosion or infection.

Stoma prolapse occurs in up to 42% of patients and is associated with similar risk factors as parastomal hernia. In fact, these two complications frequently coexist. It is more common in colostomies and, specifically, in the efferent limb of loop colostomies owing to defunctionalization and atrophy of the distal limb from nonuse. Symptoms include pain and poor fitting of the stoma appliance and may progress to obstruction, incarceration, or strangulation. Indications for repair include intractable symptoms or an acute presentation with bowel compromise. Incarcerated prolapsed stomas can often be reduced using topical sugar, which draws edema fluid out of the bowel wall and allows reduction. Surgical treatment depends on individual patient factors, and options include resection, revision, and relocation. Conservative management can be successful using a stomal belt to keep the prolapse reduced.

High-volume stoma output is defined as effluent greater than 1.5 L or any volume leading to dehydration. It is the most common cause of hospital readmission in patients with ileostomies. Patients with intrinsic small bowel disease (such as CD) or proximal stomas are at particularly high risk. Symptoms include dark urine, fatigue, irritability, muscle cramps, and headache. Patients develop dehydration and hyponatremia, which can result in secondary hyperaldosteronism and urinary potassium and magnesium wasting. Treatment is through rehydration, correction of electrolyte abnormalities, and antimotility medications. In the acute setting, intravenous fluids and electrolyte repletion are used, with some patients requiring total parenteral nutrition for a period of time. For marginally dehydrated patients, an isotonic glucose and sodium oral rehydration solution is effective. Long term, patients can use elemental, high-carbohydrate, low-fat diets to slow output. Helpful foods include breads, cereals, peanut butter, bananas, and rice. Fiber supplementation or medications such as loperamide, diphenoxylate, and tincture of opium can be used as adjunctive therapy. In refractory cases, the addition of proton pump inhibitors and octreotide can be added to decrease GI secretion.

Skin complications are common in patients with ileostomies. This is more common in patients with parastomal hernia, retraction, and prolapse. These factors contribute to poor appliance fitting and high-volume output, which increases leaking. Obese and diabetic patients are more commonly affected. It is most commonly a chemical dermatitis but can result from underlying *Candida* infection or even pyoderma gangrenosum in patients with IBD. Skin irritation can be avoided with dedicated skin care, reducing the number of appliance changes as much as possible (with a goal of one to two times per week), and surgical correction of contributing factors such as hernia or prolapse. *Candida* infections are treated with topical antifungals. Pyoderma gangrenosum is a notoriously difficult condition to treat but may be responsive to local wound care, tacrolimus ointment, and intralesional steroid injections. Occasionally, systemic tacrolimus or steroids are required.

Stoma retraction affects 1%-6% of patients with colostomies and 3%-17% of patients with ileostomies. This generally occurs in the immediate postoperative period as a result of tension on the bowel or poor wound healing and occurs more often in obese patients. It causes poor fitting of the stoma appliance and may lead to severe skin irritation. Some patients will be adequately treated with convex appliances; however, many will require surgery. Local revision may be tried as a first step, but this does not address tension on the bowel. Therefore, some patients will require laparoscopic or open revision.

Stenosis is uncommon, affecting 1%-10% of patients. Patients present with obstructive symptoms or intermittent periods of no stoma output and crampy abdominal pain followed by a sudden large-volume discharge. Most commonly, stenosis is a result of ischemic injury, although in rare cases, it may be due to a technical error (fascia or skin is too tight) or underlying disease of the small bowel such as CD or malignancy. Diagnosis should be made by inspection and digital exploration. Hegar dilation in multiple sessions may be effective, but patients often require stoma revision with resection of the stricture and re-brooking of the distal end. This can be performed through a local or abdominal approach.

Bafford AC, Irani JL: Management and complications of stomas. *Surg Clin North Am.* 2013;93(1):145-166.

Chapman SJ, Wood B, Drake TM, et al: Systematic review and meta-analysis of prophylactic mesh during primary stoma formation to prevent parastomal hernia. *Dis Colon Rectum.* 2017;60(1):107-115.

DeAsis FJ, Lapin B, Gitelis ME, et al: Current state of laparoscopic parastomal hernia repair: A meta-analysis. *World J Gastroenterol.* 2015;21(28):8670-8677.

Hendren S, Hammond K, Glasgow SC, et al: Clinical practice guidelines for ostomy surgery. *Dis Colon Rectum.* 2015;58(4): 375-387.

Rondelli F, Reboldi P, Rulli A, et al: Loop ileostomy versus loop colostomy for fecal diversion after colorectal or coloanal anastomosis: a meta-analysis. *Int J Colorectal Dis.* 2009;24(5): 479-488.

Whitehead A, Cataldo PA: Technical considerations in stoma creation. *Clin Colon Rectal Surg.* 2017;30(3):162-171.

PERIOPERATIVE MANAGEMENT

BOWEL PREPARATION

Because of the high bacterial load of the large intestine, elective colorectal surgery without prophylaxis carries a 40% risk of wound infection. This has also been reported as a cause for anastomotic leakage. It was previously believed that mechanical lavage of the GI tract would prevent these complications by removing fecal waste and the associated bacterial flora. This involves administration of a bowel preparation, commonly polyethylene glycol, sodium phosphate, or magnesium citrate. Bowel preparation can be performed with or without oral antibiotics such as neomycin, erythromycin, and/or metronidazole. Retrograde enemas are used by some groups for patients undergoing distal colon and rectal surgery. Healthy patients usually tolerate bowel preparation; however, the addition of oral antibiotics increases nausea and vomiting. Fragile patients and those with renal failure are at risk for developing dehydration and electrolyte disturbances.

There is active debate about the utility of mechanical bowel preparation for elective colorectal surgery. A 2011 Cochrane analysis of randomized trial data from over 5805 patients concluded that bowel preparation did not result in a significant reduction in anastomotic leak or surgical site infection. Data from subsequent meta-analyses are conflicting about whether there is a benefit to preoperative mechanical bowel preparation in reducing surgical site infection and other perioperative morbidity when used in conjunction with oral and intravenous antibiotics. However, bowel preparation does facilitate laparoscopic manipulation of the colon, and there is limited evidence that bowel preparation may be associated with improved long-term cancer-specific outcomes.

PERIOPERATIVE ANTIBIOTICS

Perioperative parenteral antibiotics significantly reduce surgical wound infections and should be used routinely. There is wide variation in antibiotic choice among surgeons, but considerations include the need for anaerobic and aerobic coverage, cost, side effects, and feasibility of administration. The combination of parenteral antibiotics administered within 1 hour of the incision and preoperative oral antibiotics appears to be most effective and is associated with a decrease in surgical site infection to 6.5%. Oral antibiotics are commonly administered the night before surgery in conjunction with the bowel preparation. There is no evidence to suggest that continuing antibiotics beyond 24 hours postoperatively further reduces infection rates, and this practice is discouraged.

DEEP VENOUS THROMBOSIS PROPHYLAXIS

Colorectal surgery patients are at higher risk than general surgery patients for the development of perioperative thromboembolism. In historical series, deep venous thrombosis was diagnosed in 20% of general surgery patients and 30% of colorectal patients without prophylaxis. The rate of symptomatic pulmonary embolism is four-fold higher in colorectal surgery patients compared with general surgery patients (3.1% vs 0.8%). This is related to a variety of factors, including the prevalence of IBD and malignancy in this patient population. Extended operative times, pelvic dissection, and modified lithotomy position during surgery may also be contributing factors. Subcutaneous heparin and low-molecular-weight heparin are equivalent in reducing both deep venous thrombosis and pulmonary embolism. The American Society of Colon and Rectal Surgeons 2018 Clinical Practice Guidelines recommend early mobilization and intermittent pneumatic compression devices for patients undergoing colorectal surgery. Risk stratification is used to select patients who will benefit from pharmacologic prophylaxis. Extended prophylaxis administered over the first month postoperatively is recommended in high-risk patients with colorectal cancer and can be considered in patients with IBD.

PAIN MANAGEMENT

Postoperative pain management after colorectal surgery has changed dramatically in the past two decades with increased adoption of minimally invasive techniques and enhanced recovery protocols. Although there is debate about which exact techniques or medications are most effective, it is largely accepted that a combination of regional analgesia, such as epidural catheters, rectus sheath catheters, and regional blocks, in addition to the routine use of nonnarcotic pain medications, such as acetaminophen, NSAIDs, and gabapentinoids, is effective in managing pain and in reducing narcotic utilization. This is especially important in an era of a nationwide opioid crisis.

POSTOPERATIVE NUTRITION

Early initiation of nutrition postoperatively has become standard of care for patients undergoing colorectal operations. Although this practice varies widely, evidence suggests that early feeding is not associated with harm. In fact, randomized data and meta-analysis are suggestive that patients receiving early enteral nutrition have decreased length of stay, ileus, and perioperative morbidity compared with patients undergoing delayed feeding.

Fleming F, Gaertner W, Ternent CA, et al: The American Society of Colon and Rectal Surgeons clinical practice guideline for the prevention of venous thromboembolic disease in colorectal surgery. *Dis Colon Rectum.* 2018;61(1):14-20.

Güenaga KF, Matos D, Wille-Jørgensen P: Mechanical bowel preparation for elective colorectal surgery. *Cochrane Database Syst Rev.* 2011;7:9.

Kaslow SR, Gani F, Alshaikh HN, et al: Clinical outcomes following mechanical plus oral antibiotic bowel preparation versus oral antibiotics alone in patients undergoing colorectal surgery. *BJS Open.* 2018;2(4):238-245.

Wick EC, Grant MC, Wu CL: Postoperative multimodal analgesia pain management with nonopioid analgesics and techniques: a review. *JAMA Surg.* 2017;152(7):691-697.

Zhuang CL, Ye XZ, Zhang CJ, et al: Early versus traditional postoperative oral feeding in patients undergoing elective colorectal surgery: a meta-analysis of randomized clinical trials. *Dig Surg.* 2013;30(3):225-232.

MULTIPLE CHOICE QUESTIONS

1. Proctectomy requires pelvic dissection and has the potential to cause injury to the nerves that supply the rectum, pelvic floor muscles, and bladder, as well as the prostate and seminal vesicles in men. Which of the following associations is *incorrect* regarding the nerves at risk at different points in the operation?

   A. Superior hypogastric plexus near root of inferior mesenteric artery
   B. Hypogastric nerves in the retrorectal space
   C. Nervi erigentes near lateral stalks
   D. Inferior hypogastric plexus near Denonvilliers fascia

2. A 60-year-old man presents with abdominal pain, fevers, and nausea. He is febrile, focally tender in the left lower quadrant, and has a white blood cell count of 18,000/μL. Computed tomography (CT) shows sigmoid diverticulitis with a 4-cm pericolonic abscess. What is the optimal management strategy for this patient?

   A. Bowel rest and intravenous fluids
   B. Bowel rest, intravenous fluids, and broad-spectrum antibiotics
   C. Bowel rest, intravenous fluids, broad-spectrum antibiotics, and percutaneous drainage
   D. Urgent exploratory laparotomy

3. An otherwise healthy 60-year-old man presents with abdominal pain. His CT shows an obstructing mass in the sigmoid colon with dilation of the cecum to 13 cm. After fluid resuscitation, what is the next step in management?

   A. Nasogastric decompression and observation
   B. NPO (nothing by mouth), antibiotics, and observation
   C. Flexible sigmoidoscopy with biopsies to further evaluate the mass
   D. Exploratory laparotomy

4. A 65-year-old, asymptomatic woman is found to have a 3-cm sessile polyp in the ascending colon on screening colonoscopy. It was biopsied but could not be resected. Pathology shows tubulovillous adenoma. What is the next step in management?

   A. Colonoscopy in 1 year
   B. Colonoscopy in 3 years
   C. Local excision
   D. Right hemicolectomy

5. What is the most common symptom patients experience after removal of the colon?

   A. Vitamin K deficiency
   B. Renal stones
   C. Dehydration
   D. Hyponatremia
   E. Short-chain fatty acid deficiency

Anorectum

Juliane Y. Cruz, MD
Stephen M. Sentovich, MD, MBA

ANORECTAL ANATOMY

The anatomy of the anus and rectum dictates the clinical evaluation and treatment of patients with anorectal disorders (Figure 33–1).

From external to internal, the surface anatomy of the anorectum is composed of gluteal skin, anoderm, the anal transitional zone, and proximally the rectal mucosa. The gluteal skin includes hair, sebaceous glands, and sweat glands. This area, particularly 3-5 cm of anal margin skin circumferentially around the anus, can commonly become infected with the human papillomavirus, resulting in anal condyloma. Anal condyloma can also affect more proximal tissue in the anoderm and lower rectal mucosa. Perianal hidradenitis is also relatively common and develops in the apocrine sweat glands of the perianal skin. Unlike anal condyloma, perianal hidradenitis can only occur in the gluteal skin because there are no sweat glands in the anoderm.

The anoderm begins at the anal verge and ends at the dentate line. Unlike the gluteal skin, the anoderm is devoid of hair and sweat glands. Anal fissures occur in the anoderm and can be associated with a sentinel tag externally and a hypertrophied anal papilla internally (Figure 33-2). Surgical excision of too much anoderm during hemorrhoidectomy or other anorectal surgery can result in anal stenosis.

The anal transitional zone lies between the squamous anoderm and the rectal mucosa. In this zone, squamous, cuboidal, transitional, and columnar epithelium exist with longitudinal ridges called the columns of Morgagni. Between the columns of Morgagni are anal crypts with associated anal glands that open into their bases. Clinically, the anal transitional zone is important for two main reasons. First, the anal transitional zone is the crossover from somatic to visceral innervation and for lymphatic drainage from the inguinal to the pelvic nodes. Lymphatics from the anal canal above the dentate line drain via the superior rectal lymphatics to the inferior mesenteric lymph nodes and laterally to the

internal iliac nodes. Below the dentate line, drainage occurs to the inguinal lymph nodes but can occur to the inferior or superior rectal lymph nodes. Second, the anal glands in the crypts are the site of anorectal abscesses and anal fistulas. Anatomically the anal glands in the crypts extend to a variable depth, resulting in perianal, intersphincteric, or ischiorectal abscesses when these glands become blocked.

Proximal to the anal transitional zone is the rectal mucosa. Above the dentate line and underlying the rectal mucosa are the vessels that, when abnormally engorged, manifest as internal hemorrhoids. Hemorrhoids are not veins but arteriovenous connections that have pulsatile flow. Patients with bleeding from hemorrhoids can have significant blood loss. Further, internal hemorrhoids are covered by mucosa, and because they are above the dentate line, they are viscerally innervated. This is the reason rubber band ligation of internal hemorrhoids is possible without anesthesia. In contrast, external hemorrhoids are below the dentate line, covered by anoderm and skin. Any surgical intervention on external hemorrhoids requires some type of anesthesia.

Hemorrhoidal vessels are anchored by the Treitz muscle. When the Treitz muscle attachments weaken, internal and external hemorrhoids can prolapse, bleed, and cause perianal irritation and discomfort. Internal hemorrhoids can prolapse and can be confused with rectal prolapse. Generally, internal hemorrhoids prolapse in columns occurring in the right anterior, right posterior, and left lateral quadrants around the anus. When the anus is examined, these prolapsing columns of internal hemorrhoids appear as radial folds. This is distinguished from the circumferential folds of rectal prolapse.

The rectum extends 12-15 cm proximal to the dentate line. The rectum has three curves that create folds called the valves of Houston. The puborectalis and levator muscles provide support of the rectum and are referred to as the pelvic floor. In addition, the rectum is fixed posteriorly by

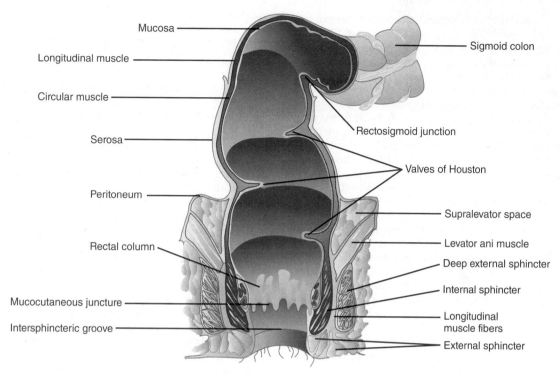

Mucosa
Longitudinal muscle
Circular muscle
Serosa
Peritoneum
Rectal column
Mucocutaneous juncture
Intersphincteric groove

Sigmoid colon
Rectosigmoid junction
Valves of Houston
Supralevator space
Levator ani muscle
Deep external sphincter
Internal sphincter
Longitudinal muscle fibers
External sphincter

▲ **Figure 33-1.** Anatomy of the anorectal canal.

presacral (Waldeyer) fascia, laterally by the lateral ligaments, and anteriorly by Denonvilliers fascia. The arterial supply of the anorectum is via the superior, middle, and inferior rectal arteries. The superior rectal artery is the terminal branch of the inferior mesenteric artery and descends in the mesorectum. It supplies the upper and middle rectum. The middle rectal arteries arise from the internal iliac arteries and enter the rectum anterolaterally at the level of the pelvic floor musculature. They supply the lower two-thirds of the rectum. Collaterals exist between the middle and superior rectal arteries. The inferior rectal arteries—branches of the internal pudendal arteries—enter posterolaterally, do not anastomose with the blood supply to the middle rectum, and supply the anal sphincters and epithelium.

The venous drainage of the anorectum is via the superior, middle, and inferior rectal veins draining into the portal and systemic systems. The superior rectal veins drain the upper and middle thirds of the rectum and empty into the portal system via the inferior mesenteric vein. The middle rectal veins drain the lower rectum and the upper anal canal systemically via the internal iliac veins. The inferior rectal veins drain the lower anal canal, communicating with the pudendal veins and draining into the internal iliac veins. Communication between the venous systems allows low rectal cancers to spread via the portal and systemic systems. Lymphatic drainage of the upper and middle rectum is into the inferior mesenteric nodes. Lymph from the lower rectum may drain into the inferior mesenteric system or into lymphatics around the lower rectum that drain into the inguinal nodes and then into periaortic nodes. Below the dentate line, lymphatic drainage occurs primarily to the inguinal nodes but may drain into the inferior mesenteric lymph nodes.

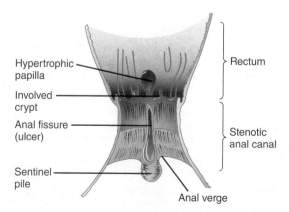

Hypertrophic papilla
Involved crypt
Anal fissure (ulcer)
Sentinel pile
Anal verge
Rectum
Stenotic anal canal

▲ **Figure 33-2.** Diagram of the anorectum showing the fissure or ulcer triad.

The innervation of the rectum is from both the sympathetic and parasympathetic nervous systems. The sympathetic nerves originate from the lumbar segments L1-3, form the inferior mesenteric plexus, travel through the superior hypogastric plexus, and descend as the hypogastric nerves to the pelvic plexus. The parasympathetic nerves arise from the second, third, and fourth sacral roots and join the hypogastric nerves anterior and lateral to the rectum to form the pelvic plexus. Sympathetic and parasympathetic fibers pass from the pelvic plexus to the rectum and internal anal sphincter as well as other pelvic viscera. Injury to these nerves can lead to sexual and bladder dysfunction and loss of normal defecatory mechanisms.

Beneath the surface anatomy of the anus and rectum are the anal sphincter muscles. The internal anal sphincter muscle is involuntary and is responsible for anal canal resting tone. The internal anal sphincter is innervated with sympathetic and parasympathetic fibers. Both are inhibitory and keep the sphincter in a basal state of contraction. The external anal sphincter muscle is voluntary and responsible for anal canal squeezing tone. The external sphincters are skeletal muscles innervated by the pudendal nerve with fibers that originate from S2-4. The external anal sphincter muscle fuses with the pelvic floor muscles to create a bowl-like muscular support of the lower rectum.

Although systemic diseases such as diabetes, scleroderma, and multiple sclerosis can affect the anal sphincter muscles, it is more common to see direct injury to the sphincter muscles from vaginal delivery or surgery. Using transanal ultrasound to evaluate the anal sphincter muscles before and after vaginal delivery, it has been demonstrated that approximately one-third of women injure their anal sphincter at the time of delivery. Fortunately, only one-third of these women with sphincter injury develop fecal incontinence.

Operative intervention for hemorrhoids, anal fissure, and anal fistula can result in anal sphincter injury. Sphincter injury should not occur during hemorrhoid surgery as hemorrhoidal vessels are superficial to the anal sphincter muscles. Division of the anal sphincter is necessary and curative for anal fissure and for anal fistula treated by fistulotomy. While lateral internal sphincterotomy for anal fissure carries a fecal incontinence rate of less than 0.5%, fistulotomy for complex anal fistulas has a rate of over 50%. For this reason, sphincter-sparing approaches to anal fistulas are now the standard of care for patients with anal fistulas involving a significant amount of anal sphincter muscle.

COMMON SYMPTOMS AND THEIR DIFFERENTIAL DIAGNOSIS

▶ Anorectal Pain

Pain is one of the most common presenting symptoms of anorectal disorders. The common causes of anorectal pain are shown in Table 33–1. The vast majority of patients have thrombosed external hemorrhoids, anal fissures, or anorectal

Table 33–1. Causes of anorectal pain.

Thrombosed external hemorrhoids
Anorectal abscess
Anal fissure
Anal mass: anal cancer, anal condyloma
Trauma: direct injury, foreign body
Infections: herpes simplex virus, HIV, cytomegalovirus, and others
Functional: levator spasm, proctalgia fugax

abscesses. The other causes of anorectal pain are relatively unusual. The etiology of anorectal pain can often be determined with a careful history that is then confirmed with the physical examination.

For patients with anorectal pain, the most important aspects of the patient history are the nature and onset of the pain and any associated symptoms. If the pain is acute in onset (< 1-3 days) and associated with a lump at the anus, a diagnosis of a thrombosed external hemorrhoid is highly likely. If the pain is acute in onset and associated with fever and swelling at the anus, then an anorectal abscess should be suspected. Finally, if the pain is described as a "cut," "tear," or "sharp as a knife" and associated with bowel movements, then an anal fissure is the probable cause. Inspection alone will usually confirm the suspected diagnosis, because an external hemorrhoid, abscess or cellulitis, or anal fissure will be present. It is important to efface the anus by pulling the gluteal cheeks apart in order to identify an anterior or posterior anal fissure that occurs just inside the anal canal. Most patients with anorectal pain cannot tolerate a digital examination and anoscopy, but fortunately, these evaluations are often unnecessary. If after obtaining a history and carefully inspecting the anus the diagnosis is still in doubt, an examination under anesthesia may be indicated because a small number of patients may have an intersphincteric or supralevator abscess that usually cannot be diagnosed by inspection alone.

▶ Anorectal Bleeding

Bleeding is the most common presenting symptom in patients with anorectal disorders. Common causes of anorectal bleeding are shown in Table 33–2. Although a careful

Table 33–2. Causes of rectal bleeding.

Hemorrhoids
Anal fissure
Proctitis
Anal fistula
Cancer
Ulceration/infection
Rectal prolapse/solitary rectal ulcer

history may suggest the etiology of bleeding, patients can tolerate and require a thorough physical examination as well as anoscopy and lower endoscopy. Even if anorectal pathology is identified on physical examination or anoscopy, endoscopic evaluation is always necessary in order rule out proximal pathology such as polyps or cancer.

In patients with anorectal bleeding, the history can help to identify the source of the bleeding by fully characterizing the amount, timing, and location of the bleeding. Blood seen just on the toilet paper suggests anal canal pathology, whereas blood seen mixed with the stool suggests a more proximal bleeding source. Inspection of the anus may reveal prolapsing hemorrhoids, an anal fissure, an anal fistula, or an anal ulcer. Anoscopy is necessary to evaluate for possible internal hemorrhoids and distal proctitis. Flexible sigmoidoscopy is typically recommended for younger patients (< 40 years old) who do not have a family history of colon cancer. Colonoscopy is recommended for patients over the age of 40 with anorectal bleeding or patients under 40 who have a family history of colon cancer. Although these general guidelines are appropriate for most patients, the choice between flexible sigmoidoscopy and colonoscopy is individualized to each patient's clinical scenario.

▶ Anorectal Mass

Most anorectal mass lesions are either anal skin tags, a thrombosed external hemorrhoid, or a sentinel pile associated with an anal fissure (Table 33–3). In addition to the history, physical examination, and anoscopy, most patients with mass lesions need either flexible sigmoidoscopy or colonoscopy depending on their age, diagnosis, and whether or not there is a family history of colon cancer. The unusual tumors such as lipoma and gastrointestinal stromal tumor (GIST) that occur deep to the skin, anoderm, and rectal mucosa are difficult to diagnose preoperatively. These tumors often require additional preoperative anatomic evaluation with transanal ultrasonography and/or pelvic magnetic resonance imaging (MRI) to determine their extent and relationship to the anal sphincter muscles.

Table 33–3. Causes of anorectal mass.

Thrombosed external hemorrhoids
Sentinel tag
Anal skin tag
Anal condyloma
Anorectal abscess
Hypertrophied anal papilla
Internal hemorrhoids
Rectal polyp
Anal or rectal cancer
Unusual tumors: gastrointestinal stromal tumor, lipoma, endometriosis

Table 33–4. Causes of anorectal discharge.

Prolapsing internal hemorrhoids
Anal fistula
Proctitis
Rectal polyp (villous adenoma)
Anal or rectal cancer
Anal warts
Mucosal/rectal prolapsed
Fecal incontinence/leakage (multiple etiologies)
Postsurgical: keyhole deformity

▶ Anorectal Discharge

Discharge from the anus is a relatively common complaint and has a wide range of possible etiologies (Table 33–4). The most common causes of anorectal discharge are mucosal prolapse, anal fistula, and fecal leakage. Patients with anal fistula often have a history of perirectal abscess. On examination, the patient should be asked to strain in order to identify mucosal and rectal prolapse. Anal sphincter tone should be assessed during the digital examination. In patients with previous anorectal surgery, careful inspection of the anus is important to identify any anal contour abnormalities (keyhole deformities). In addition to anoscopy, most patients will require lower endoscopy. Patients with fecal leakage or incontinence often require further functional and anatomic studies.

HEMORRHOIDS

Hemorrhoids are blood vessels in the lower rectum and anal canal. They are not veins but rather arteriovenous connections with pulsatile flow. External hemorrhoids are located below the dentate line and anatomically identified by the presence of anoderm or skin overlying the hemorrhoidal vessel. Due to either diarrhea, constipation, or straining, a hemorrhoidal vessel can become thrombosed with a clot, resulting in a painful lump and possibly some bleeding if the clot ruptures through the anoderm. External hemorrhoids typically cause symptoms when they thrombose, prolapse, or cause irritation/hygiene difficulties. Internal hemorrhoids originate from above the dentate line and are covered by mucosa. These blood vessels can become enlarged/engorged (eg, pregnancy) and/or their anchoring muscle, the Treitz muscle, can become weakened (eg, straining, constipation). When either one or both of these circumstances occur, the hemorrhoidal vessels can prolapse into the lumen of the anal canal and can also prolapse externally. This mechanical prolapse of hemorrhoidal vessels can cause bleeding, irritation, and pressure-like pain.

Internal hemorrhoids can be classified as grade I-IV by their symptoms and degree of prolapse. Grade I hemorrhoids are prominent but do not prolapse. Grade II hemorrhoids prolapse but spontaneously reduce. Grade III hemorrhoids prolapse but require manual reduction. Grade IV hemorrhoids prolapse and cannot be manually reduced. The four-level grading system helps guide the choice of treatment of hemorrhoids.

Signs & Symptoms

Patients with thrombosed external hemorrhoids complain of acute pain and swelling or lump at the anus. Patients with external hemorrhoid skin tags will have more chronic symptoms of prolapsed "extra skin," irritation, and difficulty with hygiene after bowel movements. Patients with internal hemorrhoids complain of bleeding, pressure-like pain, and prolapse. Patients with bleeding internal hemorrhoids can have significant blood loss and become anemic acutely or chronically. Other than thrombosed external hemorrhoids, patients with hemorrhoids do not complain of sharp pain but rather bleeding, prolapse, irritation, and sometimes a pressure-like pain due to the prolapse. Both external and internal hemorrhoids can become incarcerated and gangrenous, resulting in necrosis of skin and mucosa as well as bleeding.

Examination of the patient with a thrombosed external hemorrhoid reveals a purple swelling at the anus consistent with a clot in an external hemorrhoid vessel. Patients with external prolapse and tags reveal chronic protrusion and lumps without acute pain and discoloration. Patients with internal hemorrhoids may reveal nothing externally unless the internal hemorrhoids prolapse externally. Digital evaluation of the rectum can rule out any mass lesions or malignancy, but internal hemorrhoids cannot be assessed adequately using digital rectal examination. Anoscopy is necessary to properly evaluate internal hemorrhoids. The examiner asks the patient to push or strain while visualizing each of the three common hemorrhoidal piles in the right anterior, right posterior, and left lateral positions within the anal canal. Internal hemorrhoids are present if prolapse or bleeding occurs in any of the three locations visualized during anoscopy. Physical examination alone establishes a diagnosis of hemorrhoids. Further evaluation with laboratory or imaging studies is unnecessary unless there has been significant hemorrhage. All patients should also undergo evaluation of the more proximal colon with flexible sigmoidoscopy or colonoscopy as indicated.

Differential Diagnosis

Because patients and many primary care providers identify any anorectal symptom as being due to hemorrhoids, nearly all patients complain of "hemorrhoids" or will have been told that they have "hemorrhoids."

Patients with rectal bleeding need to be carefully evaluated not only with anoscopy but also with flexible endoscopy to rule out proximal pathology such as colitis, polyps, or cancer. Patients with rectal bleeding under the age of 40 and without a family history of colon cancer can undergo anoscopy and flexible sigmoidoscopy. Patients with rectal bleeding between 40 and 50 years of age need evaluation with anoscopy and flexible sigmoidoscopy or colonoscopy, with colonoscopy preferred for most patients. Patients over the age of 50 with bleeding need to be evaluated with anoscopy and colonoscopy. Finally, all patients with a significant family history of colon cancer should undergo anoscopy and colonoscopy regardless of age. Thus, it is very important in patients with rectal bleeding to evaluate the whole colon in most circumstances in order to rule out malignancy.

In patients with symptoms of prolapse, the surgeon must differentiate hemorrhoidal prolapse from true rectal prolapse. Patients with hemorrhoidal prolapse have prolapsing hemorrhoids in one or more of the standard hemorrhoid locations: right anterior, right posterior, and/or left lateral position. Because the hemorrhoids prolapse in these specific locations, the examiner sees prolapsing mucosa and underlying hemorrhoidal vessels with radial folds between the various prolapsing hemorrhoids. Patients with true rectal prolapse have circumferential prolapse of mucosa and full-thickness rectal wall that results in concentric folds. Patients with full-thickness rectal prolapse have decreased sphincter tone, whereas patients with prolapsing hemorrhoids typically have normal to increased sphincter tone.

Treatment of External Hemorrhoids

Patients with chronic tags and external hemorrhoids are treated with reassurance, particularly if the tags are small and minimally symptomatic. If they have symptoms of irritation or discomfort, topical hydrocortisone or analgesic creams can be helpful. If the external hemorrhoids are causing recurring symptoms of irritation, discomfort, and difficulty with anal hygiene, then simple surgical excision may resolve them. If a patient with a thrombosed external hemorrhoid is seen within 3 days of the onset of symptoms, then excision of the clot may be beneficial. Excision of the clot in these patients who present early to the surgeon allows for faster resolution of their symptoms. Simple incision of the clot is associated with a higher recurrence rate, so if surgical intervention is undertaken, it should be complete excision of the hemorrhoidal vessel and clot. Most patients with thrombosed external hemorrhoids seek medical attention after 3 days of symptoms. Surgical excision will not hasten resolution of symptoms in these patients, and management is topical and involves oral pain medications, stool softeners, and laxatives. The clot typically resolves in 2 weeks to 2 months. After resolution of their clot, occasionally patients are left with a residual skin tag. Hemorrhoidal disease is common during pregnancy and can be treated postpartum if symptoms persist.

Treatment of Internal Hemorrhoids

Patients with mild to moderate internal hemorrhoids (grades I-II) and constipation are treated with fiber, fluids, and possibly laxatives to improve their bowel habits. In addition, phlebotonics may be used to improve hemorrhoidal symptoms. Phlebotonics are a newer category of medications consisting of plant extracts and synthetic compounds that are thought to increase venous tone, stabilize capillary permeability, and increase lymphatic drainage. They may provide some benefit in regard to discharge, leakage, bleeding, and pruritis. For most of these patients, this medical treatment to improve their bowel function will resolve their hemorrhoidal symptoms. For patients with "hemorrhoids" and hyperactive bowel function, treatment should be directed at the cause of the diarrhea/multiple bowel movements. These patients should not undergo hemorrhoid surgery. Patients with normal bowel habits and persistent hemorrhoidal symptoms are candidates for a surgical approach.

Surgical Treatment of Hemorrhoids in the Office Setting

Internal hemorrhoids can be treated with in-office procedures such as rubber band ligation, sclerotherapy and infrared coagulation. Most patients with grades I-III hemorrhoids can be successfully treated with office-based procedures. Of the office-based procedures, rubber band ligation is typically the most effective option.

A. Rubber Band Ligation of Hemorrhoids

Small to moderate-sized symptomatic internal hemorrhoids (grades I-III) can be treated with rubber band ligation. This in-office treatment involves placement of an anoscope and then grasping the largest hemorrhoidal pile above the dentate line with a clamp and using a rubber band ligator to place a rubber band around the "neck" of the hemorrhoid. Because the rubber band is placed above the dentate line, patients can tolerate this procedure without anesthesia and usually do not have significant postprocedure pain. After banding, patients have either no symptoms or a mild to moderate pressure sensation that resolves in hours to a day or two. The rubber band is a noose around the hemorrhoid's "neck," and the hemorrhoid and rubber band will fall off within 5-10 days, resulting in a scar that reduces the hemorrhoid size and degree of prolapse. When this sloughing of the hemorrhoid and rubber band occurs, the patient may experience bleeding that occasionally is severe enough to require an emergent visit. Patients are banded without antibiotics as sepsis after banding is exceedingly uncommon. Because postbanding sepsis presents with urinary retention, fever, and increasing pain, any rubber band ligation patient with this constellation of symptoms needs to be evaluated urgently. Treatment of postbanding sepsis requires intravenous antibiotics, band removal, debridement of necrotic tissue, and supportive care in an intensive care unit. Banding is usually performed one "pile" at a time, but placement of multiple bands at one setting is possible. Postbanding instructions include keeping the stools soft, using pain medication as needed, and returning for urgent reevaluation if signs and symptoms of sepsis develop. Rubber band ligation is well-tolerated and quite successful for patients with grades I-III internal hemorrhoids but is generally avoided in patients who are taking chronic anticoagulants.

B. Sclerotherapy

Sclerotherapy involves using anoscopy to inject a sclerosing agent into the apex of grades I- II internal hemorrhoids. The agent causes a fibrotic reaction within the submucosa, allowing for fixation of the hemorrhoidal tissue. A variety of sclerosing agents have been used, with a commonly used option being phenol in oil. Typically, 3-5 mL of sclerosing solution is injected. Although the initial success rate approaches that of rubber band ligation, recurrences are common. Complications are unusual, but necrosis, rectal perforation, and sepsis have all been reported.

C. Infrared Coagulation

Infrared coagulation involves application of infrared energy directly to the internal hemorrhoids with an infrared coagulation probe. Using anoscopy, the probe is placed on the hemorrhoid for 1-2 seconds, which results in coagulation of the hemorrhoid with a decrease in size and blood flow through the hemorrhoid. Recent studies have shown that infrared coagulation is as good as rubber band ligation for patients with grades I-II internal hemorrhoids. Complications are unusual but include bleeding, necrosis, and sepsis.

Surgical Treatment of Internal Hemorrhoids in the Operating Room

Patients with persistent symptoms despite in-office treatment of their hemorrhoids are candidates for surgery in the operating room. Surgery is usually performed only for patients with grades III-IV internal hemorrhoids. In the operating room, surgical treatment of internal hemorrhoids can be by surgical excision, stapled hemorrhoidopexy, or Doppler-guided ligation.

A. Excisional Hemorrhoidectomy

Classic excisional hemorrhoidectomy is performed either in the lithotomy or prone position. After the induction of anesthesia, the hemorrhoidal piles are excised with scissors, cautery, bipolar energy device, or vessel sealer. The resulting wounds are closed (Ferguson), partially closed, or left open (Milligan-Morgan), depending on surgeon preference. Care is taken to excise just the mucosa, submucosa, and hemorrhoids and to avoid injury to the underlying anal sphincter muscle. In addition, care is taken not to excise too much mucosa and anoderm because this could result in anal stenosis. The procedure takes less than an hour and is scheduled as outpatient surgery. Given that the incisions start externally and end in the anal canal/lower rectum, patients can have significant discomfort postoperatively. Adequate pain control, keeping the bowel movements soft, and avoiding constipation are all important postoperatively. Early complications after excisional hemorrhoidectomy include bleeding, infection, and urinary retention. The rate of urinary retention can be reduced by limiting the amount of intravenous fluids during surgery. Late complications include anal stenosis and mucosal ectropion and whitehead deformity (circumferential mucosal ectropion). Given its high success rate and low recurrence rate, all other surgical interventions are compared to excisional hemorrhoidectomy to determine their efficacy.

B. Stapled Hemorrhoidopexy

A stapled hemorrhoidopexy is useful for patients with circumferential grade II-III hemorrhoids who fail in-office treatment. The technique involves placement of a purse-string suture 3-4 cm above the dentate line in the submucosal plane. The circular stapler's anvil is then placed proximal to the purse-string suture, and the suture is tied, drawing the internal hemorrhoids into the circular stapler. The stapler is then closed and fired, removing a circumferential strip of internal hemorrhoids. The staple line, 1-2 cm above the dentate line, is inspected and any bleeding oversewn. Thus, the procedure removes a strip of internal hemorrhoids and creates a hemorrhoidopexy at the staple line that reduces hemorrhoidal prolapse. The procedure does not address external hemorrhoids and thus would not be useful for patients with significant external hemorrhoidal disease. Because the procedure's incision (at the staple line) is above the dentate line, stapled hemorrhoidopexy is associated with less pain and discomfort than traditional excisional hemorrhoidectomy. Complications from stapled hemorrhoidopexy are also comparable to excisional hemorrhoidectomy with the exception of including some unique complications such as rectovaginal fistula, rectal obstruction, and staple line bleeding. Long-term follow-up has demonstrated more recurrence of prolapse than initially noted. Appropriate patient selection and meticulous surgical technique are required to achieve the best results with stapled hemorrhoidopexy. Thus, stapled hemorrhoidopexy may be a good option for grade II-III internal hemorrhoids that are not associated with significant external hemorrhoids.

C. Doppler-Guided Hemorrhoidectomy

Doppler-guided hemorrhoidectomy involves the use of a specially designed anoscope with a Doppler probe that allows for precise identification and ligation of the hemorrhoidal vessels. Six to eight hemorrhoidal vessels are identified and suture ligated using the Doppler probe to identify the vessels and then confirm the interruption of blood flow after suture ligation. Early results have demonstrated that this technique is comparable to excisional hemorrhoidectomy for grade II-III internal hemorrhoids. The complication profile is also favorable. More experience with Doppler-guided hemorrhoidectomy is necessary in order to adequately evaluate the long-term effectiveness of the procedure.

▶ Prognosis

The successful treatment of external and internal hemorrhoids is related to changing the patient's bowel habits. Increasing dietary fiber, decreasing constipating foods, introducing exercise, and limiting time spent on the toilet all serve to decrease the amount of time spent straining in the squatting position. These behavioral modifications are the most important steps in preventing recurrence.

Bellio G, Pasquali A, Schiano di Visconte M: Stapled hemorrhoidopexy: results at 10-year follow-up. *Dis Colon Rectum.* 2018;61(4):491-498.

Davis BR, Lee-Kong SA, Migaly J, et al: The American Society of Colon and Rectal Surgeons clinical practice guidelines for the management of hemorrhoids. *Dis Colon Rectum.* 2018;61(3):284-292.

El Nakeeb AM, Fikry AA, Omar WH, et al: Rubber band ligation for 750 cases of symptomatic hemorrhoids out of 2200 cases. *World J Gastroenterol.* 2008;14:6525-6530.

Perera N, Liolitsa D, Iype S, et al: Phlebotonics for haemorrhoids. *Cochrane Database Syst Rev.* 2012;8:CD004322.

Pucher PH, Sodergren MH, Lord AC, et al: Clinical outcome following Doppler-guided haemorrhoidal artery ligation: a systematic review. *Colorectal Dis.* 2013;15(6):e284-94.

Ratto C, Donisi L, Parello A, et al: Evaluation of transanal hemorrhoidal dearterialization as a minimally invasive therapeutic approach to hemorrhoids. *Dis Colon Rectum.* 2010;53:803-811.

Sim HL, Tan KY, Poon PL, et al: Life-threatening perineal sepsis after rubber band ligation of haemorrhoids. *Tech Coloprocotol.* 2009;13:161-164.

ANAL FISSURE

An anal fissure is a tear in the anoderm usually located in the posterior or anterior midline of the anal canal. An anal fissure may be associated with a sentinel tag located at the distal aspect of the anal fissure (anal verge) and/or a hypertrophied anal papilla at the proximal aspect of the fissure. The inciting event causing an anal fissure is thought to be trauma to the anal canal from a hard bowel movement or other cause. This trauma results in a tear that leads to pain and spasm of the internal anal sphincter muscle, particularly during and after bowel movements. The spasm results in elevated anal resting pressures that can unfortunately lead to a vicious cycle of further spasm and pain. With elevated resting pressures, the blood flow to the posterior and anterior midline decreases, inhibiting healing of the fissure. Fissures are usually classified as either acute, with symptoms occurring just over the past month, or chronic, with symptoms present for greater than 2-3 months. Over 90% of fissures are located in the posterior midline, with the rest located in the anterior midline. Given their etiology of spasm and elevated resting pressures resulting in decreased blood flow, chronic anal fissures can be considered "ischemic ulcers" of the anal canal.

Clinical Findings

Patients with an anal fissure complain of sharp pain with or immediately after bowel movements. They may also complain of rectal bleeding and a "hemorrhoid" or sentinel tag. Patients often describe moderate to severe pain, like a "knife" or "razor blade," during defecation. Due to the pain, patients fear going to the bathroom, which can result in delaying defecation, hardened stool, and additional pain. On inspection of the external anus, there may be a sentinel tag in either the posterior or anterior midline. To visualize the fissure, the examiner needs to evert the anus by pulling the right and left anal margin skin laterally. As the anus is everted, the examiner can carefully inspect the anoderm in the posterior and anterior midline for a tear in the anoderm. Patients with significant pain and spasm may not even tolerate this maneuver. In these patients, it is helpful to gently expose the anus and ask the patient to strain to defecate to see if, during straining, self-eversion of the anus occurs. Due to pain, digital rectal examination and anoscopy are not performed immediately but are reserved for when the symptoms resolve or the patient is in the operating room. Laboratory and imaging studies are not necessary, but flexible endoscopy of some type should be scheduled if it has not been performed recently.

Differential Diagnosis

Classic anal fissures occur in either the posterior (90%) or anterior (1%-10%) midline. Not all posterior and anterior anal canal tears are anal fissures. Anal canal ulcers can occur from Crohn disease, leukemia, HIV, cancer, and infections such as herpes, syphilis, cytomegalovirus, and tuberculosis. These anal canal ulcers mimic anal fissures and should be suspected if they are located laterally rather than in the posterior or anterior midline. In addition, typical anal fissures are associated with increased sphincter tone, so any patient with decreased sphincter tone should be suspected of having an anal canal ulcer rather than a fissure. There should be a low threshold to suspect an anal ulcer rather than fissure. A careful history can help identify possible etiologies of an anal ulcer. In these patients, an examination under anesthesia with biopsy of the ulcer is necessary to rule out an infectious or malignant etiology.

Complications

In addition to causing pain and bleeding, anal fissures can become infected and develop a fissure-fistula complex. This relatively unusual complication is easily treated with a posterior intersphincteric fistulotomy.

Medical Treatment

The pathogenesis of an anal fissure is pain and spasm, resulting in increased internal anal sphincter muscle pressures, decreased blood flow, and a nonhealing fissure in the anoderm of the anal canal. Treatment is directed at breaking this pain and spasm cycle to relax the internal sphincter muscle, increase blood flow, and allow the fissure to heal. To do this, patients should keep their stools soft with stool softeners and laxatives to avoid further anal canal trauma. In addition, warm baths are recommended to relax the sphincter muscle and allow the fissure to heal. Stool softeners, bulking agents, and sitz baths will heal 90% of anal fissures. Topical ointments can also be prescribed to decrease the anal sphincter pressure. Nitroglycerin ointment (0.2% or 0.4%) or calcium channel blocker ointment (0.2% diltiazem gel) can be used to chemically relax the internal anal sphincter muscle. Side effects include headache, which occurs more frequently with use of nitroglycerin ointment. Patients who fail this regimen and have a persistent fissure are candidates for surgery or treatment with botulinum toxin. Botulinum toxin injection into the anal sphincter can be successful but is costly and may require more than one treatment. Thus, medical treatment of anal fissures includes stool softeners, bulking agents, warm baths, topical nitroglycerin ointment or diltiazem gel, and possibly botulinum toxin injection. Most patients with acute anal fissures and over 50% of patients with chronic anal fissures are successfully treated without surgery. Patients who fail medical management of their anal fissure should undergo surgical intervention.

Surgical Treatment

Surgical treatment of an anal fissure involves performing a lateral internal sphincterotomy. Although the fissure may be biopsied and a sentinel tag or hypertrophied anal papilla excised, the most important part of an operation for anal fissure is directed via a lateral incision at the internal anal sphincter muscle. In the operating room, a lateral incision is made in the intersphincteric groove between the internal and external anal sphincter muscles, and a submucosal and intersphincteric dissection is performed in order to clearly identify the internal anal sphincter muscle. The internal anal sphincter muscle is then cut the length of the fissure in order to permanently relax the anal canal. After sphincterotomy, relaxation of the anal canal can readily be appreciated by the surgeon. This short, outpatient operation has over a 90% success rate and a recurrence rate of less than 10%. Patients often have less pain *after* surgery. Complications include bleeding, infection, and, rarely, fecal incontinence (< 0.5%).

Patients who have preexisting fecal leakage or lack increased anal sphincter muscle pressures are poor candidates for lateral internal sphincterotomy, as this could result in worsening bowel control. These relatively rare patients are better treated with an anal advancement flap that does not involve dividing any sphincter muscle. For a description of the anal advancement flap, see the later section on anal stenosis.

Barnes TG, Zafrani Z, Abdelrazeq AS: Fissurectomy combined with high-dose botulinum toxin is a safe and effective treatment for chronic anal fissure and a promising alternative to surgical sphincterotomy. *Dis Colon Rectum.* 2015;58(10):967-973.

Lindsey I: To cut or to daub? An algorithmic approach to anal fissure. *Colorectal Dis.* 2012;14(6):657.

Mentes BB, Guner MK, Leventoglu S, et al: Fine-tuning of the extent of lateral internal sphincterotomy: spasm-controlled vs. up to the fissure apex. *Dis Colon Rectum.* 2008;51:128-133.

Nelson RL, Thomas K, Morgan J, et al: Nonsurgical therapy for anal fissure. *Cochrane Database Syst Rev.* 2012;2:CD003431.

Pérez-Legaz J, Arroyo A, Moya P, et al: Perianal versus endoanal application of glyceryl trinitrate 0.4% ointment in the treatment of chronic anal fissure: results of a randomized controlled trial. Is this the solution to the headaches? *Dis Colon Rectum.* 2012;55(8):893-899.

Stewart DB Sr, Gaertner W, Glasgow S, et al: Standards Practice Task Force of the American Society of Colon and Rectal Surgeons clinical practice guideline for the management of anal fissures. *Dis Colon Rectum.* 2017;60(1):7-14.

ANORECTAL ABSCESS AND FISTULA

An anorectal abscess is one of the three common causes of anorectal pain and is the only cause that usually requires urgent surgical treatment. Most anorectal abscesses have a cryptoglandular etiology. When the anal glands in the crypts of the dentate line become blocked, an anorectal abscess can develop. Because these glands extend a variable depth, the developing abscess can track in various anatomic planes. Abscesses are classified by their anatomic location: perianal, ischiorectal, intersphincteric, and supralevator (Figure 33–3). Fortunately, most abscesses are perianal or ischiorectal and can be relatively easily identified on physical examination. Intersphincteric and supralevator abscesses are unusual and often are only identified by MRI or computed tomography (CT) or examination under anesthesia. Most abscesses are cryptoglandular in etiology, but some patients develop abscesses related to another disease process such as Crohn disease, tuberculosis, or cancer. Although many abscesses will heal with simple incision and drainage, some 30%-60% of abscesses will not heal, and patients will complain of persistent drainage and recurrent inflammation related to an anal fistula. In these patients, the cryptoglandular source and external surgical drainage site remain connected, allowing for passage of mucus and stool through

▲ **Figure 33–3.** Composite diagram of acute anorectal abscesses and spaces. (a) Pelvirectal (supralevator) space. (b) Ischiorectal space. (c) Perianal (subcutaneous) space. (d) Marginal (mucocutaneous) space. (e) Submucous space. (f) Intermuscular space.

this tract. The location of the abscess, thus, determines the location and tract of the resulting anal fistula. Anal fistulas are classified by their relationship with the anal sphincter muscle: intersphincteric, transsphincteric, suprasphincteric, and extrasphincteric. Due to the frequency of the abscesses that created them, intersphincteric and transsphincteric fistulas are the most common anal fistulas. Suprasphincteric and extrasphincteric fistulas are exceedingly rare. Due to their relationship with the anal sphincter muscle, anal fistulas should be evaluated and treated by highly specialized surgeons familiar with sphincter-saving techniques in order to avoid complications such as fecal incontinence. Because fistulas occur in 30%-60% of patients after anorectal abscess drainage, patients undergoing abscess drainage should be warned about the possibility of a fistula and should be given appropriate follow-up to ensure healing and absence of a persistent fistula tract.

▶ Clinical Findings

Patients with an anorectal abscess complain of acute pain, swelling, and possibly a fever. An occasional patient may complain of leakage of mucus and pus related to the spontaneous drainage of the abscess. For patients with perianal and ischiorectal abscesses, physical examination often reveals erythema, fluctuance, and asymmetry between the right and left perirectal tissues. An occasional patient will present with a symmetric horseshoe abscess cavity circling half or more of the circumference and may have no left-right asymmetry.

If a patient has an intersphincteric or supralevator anorectal abscess, often none of the above findings are present on physical examination. Thus, patients with a suspicion of an abscess but no obvious physical exam findings should either be imaged with MRI or taken to the operating room for an examination under anesthesia. Laboratory testing is usually not helpful in patients with an anorectal abscess, although frequently these patients will have an elevated white blood cell count. Radiologic studies are also not necessary because the vast majority of anorectal abscesses are obvious based on history and physical examination alone. Some patients with symptoms of an abscess and no physical examination findings may benefit from imaging studies, as may patients with recurrent or complex abscesses such as some patients with Crohn disease. Potential imaging studies include CT, MRI, and anorectal ultrasound (endoanal or transperineal). Anorectal ultrasound is not well tolerated in patients with an acute abscess, and CT will miss some abscesses. Thus, if an imaging study is necessary, MRI is the imaging test of choice because it is able to readily identify complex abscesses and their anatomic extensions.

Patients with an anorectal fistula complain of chronic drainage of mucus and blood and irritation and usually have an antecedent history of an anorectal abscess. If a patient has persistent drainage 6-8 weeks after abscess drainage, then a fistula should be suspected, and evaluation and treatment for an anal fistula should be initiated. Some patients with anal fistulas will have a relatively remote or no history of an abscess. Physical examination reveals the external opening, and often, there is a palpable subcutaneous tract between the external opening and the anus. It is important to remember that any nonhealing wound or opening around the anus should be presumed to be a fistula until proven otherwise. Laboratory testing is not necessary in patients with anal fistulas, but imaging studies may be useful for recurrent and complex anal fistulas. MRI is the imaging procedure of choice to identify anal fistula tracts and side tracts and the relationship of the tracts to the anal sphincter muscle. Transanal ultrasonography can also be useful and can be performed intraoperatively using hydrogen peroxide enhancement to highlight the fistula tract.

Differential Diagnosis

The differential diagnosis for patients with anorectal abscess or fistula includes perianal hidradenitis, pilonidal disease, and rarely Bartholin gland cyst. On physical examination, it may be difficult to differentiate an anorectal abscess/fistula from complex hidradenitis or pilonidal disease. Further, hidradenitis or pilonidal disease can occur concurrently with an anorectal abscess or fistula. Careful evaluation in the operating room is necessary to determine if an abscess is communicating only with the skin (hidradenitis), only with the midline gluteal cleft (pilonidal disease), or with

the anus (fistula). Rare causes of anorectal abscesses and fistulas include tuberculosis, actinomycosis, cancer, and diverticulitis.

Complications

Abscesses can enlarge and spread along various anatomic planes around the anus. Abscesses can form a posteriorly based horseshoe around the anus, usually just sparing the anterior perirectal space. Abscesses can also track around just one side of the anus (1/2 horseshoe). Although it may be unusual for a single abscess to destroy a significant amount of anorectal tissue and diminish anorectal function, multiple recurrent abscesses can result in destruction of anorectal anatomy and muscle function, resulting in a deterioration of anorectal function.

In rare circumstances, an anorectal abscess can result in systemic sepsis. Treatment should include adequate drainage of the abscess, intravenous antibiotics, and supportive intensive care unit care.

Anorectal abscesses can recur after treatment. The reasons for recurrence include inadequate initial drainage (often because deep postanal space was not drained), presence of a fistula, and Crohn disease. Nearly all patients with recurrent or complex abscesses should be evaluated for Crohn disease.

Anal fistulas should be treated when identified because, although they may be minimally symptomatic, they can develop into an acute anorectal abscess. Fistulas, too, may recur after treatment due to undiagnosed side tracts or Crohn disease. Crohn disease should be ruled out in all patients with complicated or recurrent anal fistulas.

Treatment of Anorectal Abscesses

Anorectal abscesses are treated by incision and drainage. For the common perianal and ischiorectal abscesses, a cruciate incision is made over the area of fluctuance as close to the anal verge as possible to decrease the length of a fistula tract if one should develop. Frequently, it is useful to excise the skin tips of the cruciate incision in order to allow for adequate drainage and ensure that the abscess heals from the inside out because premature skin healing could result in a recurrent abscess. When draining an acute abscess, it is very unlikely to be able to identify an internal opening and the course of the fistula tract if one is present. Thus, when draining an abscess either in the office or the operating room, it is important to concentrate effort at ensuring that the abscess is adequately drained and to worry about a fistula later if it should develop. For the relatively rare intersphincteric abscess, transanal drainage is performed. In the operating room, the intersphinteric abscess is palpated within the anal canal, and via an anoscope, a longitudinal incision is made to drain the abscess internally into the rectum. Supralevator abscesses can also be treated in this way. Alternatively, supralevator abscesses can be drained in the interventional radiology suite using CT guidance, but this may result in an extrasphincteric fistula if the etiology of the abscess is cryptoglandular.

Antibiotics have limited use in the treatment of anorectal abscess. Preoperative antibiotics should be given for a patient with a prosthetic valve, history of bacterial endocarditis, congenital heart disease, or a heart transplant. After surgical drainage, only immunocompromised patients or patients with associated sepsis are additionally treated with antibiotics. For large abscesses, placement of a Penrose or mushroom-catheter drain may be necessary to ensure adequate drainage. After draining a horseshoe abscess posteriorly, it is useful to make counter incisions at the anterior extent of the abscess on both sides of the anus and place looped Penrose or vessel-loop drains from the posterior opening to the anterior opening. These drains are left for at least 2-3 weeks and will allow for better drainage of the entire abscess cavity. Finally, follow-up of patients after abscess drainage is important to ensure that the abscess completely heals and does not evolve into a persistently draining fistula tract.

▶ Treatment of Anorectal Fistula

Traditionally, anorectal fistulas have been treated by fistulotomy. Fistulotomy is performed one of three ways. The simplest fistulotomy is a single-stage procedure laying open the fistula tract. This is most commonly used for an intrasphincteric or low transsphincteric fistula. A two-stage approach is used for fistulas that involve a significant amount of sphincter muscle. The two-stage approach uses a seton, which is a suture or vessel loop that is tied to itself after placement in the fistula tract. With the two-stage approach, the first step is a partial fistulotomy and seton placement. After healing from this first step, the second step is a completion fistulotomy. A final method of fistulotomy involves placement of a cutting seton and then gradual division of the fistula tract and involved sphincter muscle by tightening of the cutting seton over time. Although fistulotomy may still be used for subcutaneous, intersphincteric, and low transsphincteric fistulas (all have little or no muscle involvement), fistulotomy has fallen into disfavor because division of the sphincter muscle during fistulotomy and contour deformities associated with fistulotomy can result in fecal incontinence and leakage. Thus, although fistulotomy is a highly successful way to treat subcutaneous and intersphincteric fistulas that involve minimal to no anal sphincter muscle, transsphincteric fistulas are better treated with a sphincter-sparing approach to avoid the complication of fecal incontinence.

Sphincter-sparing treatment approaches for transsphincteric anal fistulas include fibrin glue, anal fistula plug, the LIFT (ligation of the intersphincteric fistula tract) procedure, and the rectal advancement flap. Prior to any of these sphincter-sparing procedures, a vessel loop draining seton is placed into the fistula tract, and the tract is allowed to heal around the seton for 3 months. Although this seton placement procedure step can be omitted, studies have shown that the success rate of the subsequent definitive sphincter-sparing procedure is higher after seton placement. For the fibrin glue procedure, the seton is removed, the internal opening is suture closed, and then fibrin glue is instilled via the external opening to seal the tract. The anal fistula plug procedure is done in a similar fashion, just using the plug rather than the glue. No incisions are made with either of these procedures, which tend to be very well-tolerated by patients. Unfortunately, the success rate is only 60%-70% for fibrin glue and about 50% for the anal fistula plug. Thus, a number of patients will fail glue or plug, at which time further treatment may include repeating the glue or plug or opting for the more invasive LIFT procedure or rectal advancement flap. The main complications for glue/plug are recurrence and abscess (rare).

The LIFT procedure is an outpatient operation that involves ligating the intersphincteric tract and closing the internal opening. The operation starts with removal of any previously placed seton and is followed by making an intersphincteric groove incision that allows for exposure of the fistula tract in the intersphincteric space that can then be circumferentially dissected free. This dissection allows for proximal and distal suture ligation and division of the fistula tract within the intersphincteric space. This procedure is well-tolerated, spares the sphincter muscle, and is successful 80% of the time. Failure may be associated with greater length of fistula tract. Complications include recurrence of a simpler intersphincteric fistula and, rarely, abscess formation.

If the previously mentioned sphincter-sparing techniques are unsuccessful in healing an anal fistula, an anorectal advancement flap can be performed. The LIFT procedure and rectal advancement flap have had comparable results in terms of recurrence and continence. For patients, this is a significantly more involved operation than the previously described options because it involves much larger incisions, longer operative time, and longer healing time. In the operating room, patients are placed prone for an anterior internal opening or placed in lithotomy position for a posterior internal opening. A U-shaped flap of mucosa, submucosa, and some underlying sphincter muscle is dissected proximally, with the base of the "U" just distal to the internal opening. Once the flap is completely mobilized, the internal opening in the underlying sphincter muscle is closed with one or two figure-of-eight sutures. The tip of the flap is then excised, and the flap is advanced distally to cover the suture closure of the internal opening in the sphincter muscle. The flap is then sutured into place, providing a double-layer closure of the internal opening. The external opening is enlarged and left open for drainage. Patients undergoing an anorectal advancement flap are typically observed overnight to control pain and monitor for anorectal bleeding. If the flap remains in place and heals, the internal opening will be closed, and the rest of the fistula tract will heal. The success rate for the rectal advancement flap procedure is about 60%-80%, with the higher success rates associated with preoperative seton drainage.

In patients with Crohn-associated fistulas, the treatment is mainly medical management. Antibiotics can resolve symptoms in the majority of patients. Biologic therapies, most commonly infliximab, remain the best medical therapy for fistulizing Crohn disease. Surgical methods for disease control include long-term seton drainage. Advancement flaps, fistula plug, and the LIFT procedure can also be considered for patients without active proctitis on an individual basis. Finally, in patients with severe uncontrolled disease, fecal diversion or proctectomy may be necessary to control perianal sepsis.

Prognosis

With the exception of Crohn patients, who can develop recurring anal abscesses and fistulas, the prognosis with anorectal abscesses and fistulas is excellent. The new sphincter-sparing techniques for anal fistulas do require multiple operations, but that is a small price to pay in order to minimize the occurrence of fecal incontinence, which can be over 50% in patients after traditional fistulotomy.

Alasari S, Kim NK: Overview of anal fistula and systematic review of ligation of the intersphincteric fistula tract (LIFT). *Tech Coloproctol.* 2014;18:13-22.

Guidi L, Ratto C, Semeraro S, et al: Combined therapy with infliximab and seton drainage for perianal fistulizing Crohn's disease with anal endosonographic monitoring: a single-centre experience. *Tech Coloproctol.* 2008;12:1111-1117.

Liu WY, Aboulian A, Kaji AH, et al: Long-term results of ligation of intersphincteric fistula tract (LIFT) for fistula-in-ano. *Dis Colon Rectum.* 2013;56(3):343-347.

Madbouly KM, El Shazly W, Abbas KS, et al: Ligation of intersphincteric fistula tract versus mucosal advancement flap in patients with high transsphincteric fistula-in-ano: a prospective randomized trial. *Dis Colon Rectum.* 2014;57(10):1202-1208.

Malik AI, Nelson RL, Tou S: Incision and drainage of perianal abscess with or without treatment of anal fistula. *Cochrane Database Syst Rev.* 2010;7:CD006827.

O'Riordan JM, Datta I, Johnston C, et al: A systematic review of the anal fistula plug for patients with Crohn's and non-Crohn's related fistula-in-ano. *Dis Colon Rectum.* 2012;55(3):351-358.

Siddiqui MR, Ashrafian H, Tozer P, et al: A diagnostic accuracy meta-analysis of endoanal ultrasound and MRI for perianal fistula assessment. *Dis Colon Rectum.* 2012;55(5):576-585.

Subhas G, Singh Bhullar J, Al-Omari A, et al: Setons in the treatment of anal fistula: review of variations in materials and techniques. *Dig Surg.* 2012;29(4):292-300.

Vogel JD, Johnson EK, Morris AM, et al: Clinical practice guideline for the management of anorectal abscess, fistula-in-ano, and rectovaginal fistula. *Dis Colon Rectum.* 2016;59(12):1117-1133.

CONDYLOMATA ACUMINATA

Condylomata acuminata are caused by the human papillomavirus (HPV) and are transmitted primarily by sexual contact. In the United States, condylomata acuminatum is the most common sexually transmitted viral disease. It is the most common anorectal infection of men who have sex with men (MSM) and is particularly prevalent in HIV-positive patients. The disease is not limited to men or women who practice anoreceptive intercourse. In women, the virus may track down from the vagina, and in men, it may track from the base of the scrotum. In addition to causing anal warts, HPV infection is the primary cause of anal dysplasia and anal squamous cell cancer. Although HPV strains 6 and 11 can cause benign warts; strains 16 and 18 carry the highest risk of anal cancer. Despite the high prevalence of HPV infection, most HPV-infected individuals will not develop cancer due to the response of the immune system against the virus. Immunocompromised individuals such as patients with HIV or transplant recipients have an increased HPV-related cancer risk.

Clinical Findings

Patients with condylomata acuminata present with wart-like growths around the anus and in the anal canal. Symptoms can include pain, itching, discharge, and bleeding. Due to the high prevalence of HPV in MSM and its risk of causing cancer, screening in high-risk populations can be performed via anal pap smears. Patients with positive anal pap smears are referred for further evaluation. The appearance of condylomata acuminata and HPV disease can be quite variable. Wart-like growths are typical, but flat patches of warty growth can also be seen. Other HPV changes cannot be seen without the assistance of high-resolution anoscopy (HRA). HRA involves applying acetic acid to the anal canal and using a colposcope to look for HPV-related changes in the anoderm and rectal mucosa. These changes are not usually seen proximal to the dentate line. Laboratory and radiographic studies are rarely used in the evaluation of patients with condylomata acuminata. Thus, evaluation of patients with HPV-related condylomata acuminata requires careful external examination, anoscopy, and possibly HRA to determine the extent of disease.

Differential Diagnosis

Because of the variable appearance of condyloma acuminata, hemorrhoids, skin tags, fibroepithelial polyps, and other anal skin conditions can mimic condylomata acuminata. Due to the large differential diagnosis for perianal and anal canal skin changes, it is important that a biopsy is taken of all anal canal lesions in order to make an accurate diagnosis.

Prevention

A quadrivalent HPV vaccine against HPV strains 6, 11, 16, and 18 is available and recommended for both men and women under the age of 26. It has been shown to prevent cancer, precancer, and most types of warts.

▶ Treatment

Condylomata acuminata are treated in the office or the operating room. Significant external disease or any internal anal canal disease is probably best treated in the operating room. Isolated external disease can be safely treated in the office. Condylomata acuminata are treated using a variety of excisional and destructive methods. In the office, anal warts can be excised after injecting local anesthesia or destroyed with bichloroacetic acid, podophyllin, liquid nitrogen, infrared coagulation, or electrocautery. In the operating room, excision and destruction using electrocautery are commonly used. All excised specimens are sent for pathologic analysis. If highly suspicious lesions are excised during an operation, their location should be specified in case the pathology is unfavorable and reexcision is required. Unless a patient has a significant burden of disease, all lesions are either excised or destroyed in the operating room. Some surgeons will use HRA in the office and operating room in order to identify and treat all HPV-related changes. After surgery, pain medication and stool softeners are prescribed, and patients are given appropriate follow-up.

▶ Complications and Prognosis

Bleeding, pain, and rarely infection may occur after excision of condylomata; however, the most common complication is recurrence. Patients should be informed prior to surgery that the recurrence rate is high (30%-80%) but that small areas of recurrence can be treated in the office. Patients should also understand that close follow-up is necessary for early detection of recurrence. This close follow-up is important in order to avoid reoperation and the development of malignancy.

A relatively rare variant of condylomata acuminatum is the giant condylomata acuminatum known as a Buschke-Lowenstein tumor. Some of these tumors have been found to have an in situ or invasive squamous cell cancer component upon pathologic review. Treatment of these lesions is wide local excision with a 1-cm margin. Chemoradiation can be considered when clear margins cannot be obtained or the patient is not a surgical candidate.

After excision of condylomata acuminatum, patients should be informed of their pathology results. If an area of squamous cell cancer has been excised on the anal margin, reexcision of this area may need to be performed if the margins were positive. If squamous cell cancer has been identified in the anal canal or from an unknown location around the anus, then the patient should be treated with chemoradiation (Nigro protocol). However, pathologic analysis may not reveal cancer but rather anal intraepithelial neoplasia (AIN). AIN is a precancerous lesion graded from I (most benign) to III (most ominous and closest to cancer). Further treatment of AIN may consist of topical agents (5-fluorouracil, imiquimod), cryotherapy, excision, or observation. In HIV-positive patients, some grade of AIN is a very common finding. A recent study suggests screening these patients at 3-month intervals due to the high percentage who have progression of disease within 1 year.

Despite the presence of anal warts and HPV, the prognosis of patients with condylomata acuminata is excellent, because anal cancer is still quite rare. Further, the prognosis of anal cancer is favorable if located on the anal margin and completely excised. Chemoradiation is also very successful for most localized anal canal squamous cell cancers. Salvage abdominoperineal resection for recurrence of squamous cell cancer after chemoradiation is unusual.

Fazendin EA, Crean AJ, Fazendin JM, et al: Condyloma acuminatum, anal intraepithelial neoplasia, and anal cancer in the setting of HIV: do we really understand the risk? *Dis Colon Rectum.* 2017;60(10):1078-1082.

Giuliano AR, Palefsky JM, Goldstone S, et al: Efficacy of quadrivalent vaccine against HPV Infection and disease in males. *N Engl J Med.* 2011;364(5):401-411. Erratum in: *N Engl J Med.* 2011;364(15):1481.

Marks DK, Goldstone SE: Electrocautery ablation of high-grade anal squamous intraepithelial lesions in HIV-negative and HIV-positive men who have sex with men. *J Acquir Immune Defic Syndr.* 2012;59(3):259-265.

Salit IE, Lytwyn A, Raboud J, et al: The role of cytology (Pap tests) and human papillomavirus testing in anal cancer screening. *AIDS.* 2010;24(9):1307-1313.

Swedish KA, Factor SH, Goldstone SE: Prevention of recurrent high-grade anal neoplasia with quadrivalent human papillomavirus vaccination of men who have sex with men: a nonconcurrent cohort study. *Clin Infect Dis.* 2012;54:891-898.

Swedish KA, Lee EQ, Goldstone SE: The changing picture of high-grade anal intraepithelial neoplasia in men who have sex with men: the effects of 10 years of experience performing high-resolution anoscopy. *Dis Colon Rectum.* 2011;54(8):1003-1007.

PILONIDAL DISEASE

Pilonidal disease is a chronic gland infection in the depths of the gluteal cleft. Although the glands and resulting pits can occur anywhere along the gluteal cleft, they occur most often in the superior gluteal cleft over the sacrum. The pathogenesis of pilonidal disease is thought to be a process in which the follicles in the midline gluteal cleft get blocked, become infected, and then drain, leaving open midline pits. In the depths of the gluteal cleft, these pits have a vacuum effect on loose hair, and hair is literally sucked into these pits. During surgery, tufts of hair can be found in the pits and chronic abscess cavity. Thus, although the hair does not cause pilonidal disease, the presence of hair in the pits and glands acts as a foreign body and causes the infection and drainage to persist. Pilonidal disease usually occurs in men (3:1 male-to-female ratio) between the ages of 15 and 40, with the peak incidence between 16 and 20 years. Although pilonidal disease is typically chronic with recurrent drainage and inflammation, it often regresses with time and is rare after 40 years of age. The pathogenesis and natural history of pilonidal disease is important to remember when recommending treatment. Given its natural history that involves disease regression with time, conservative treatment and minimal surgery are recommended for most patients.

Clinical Findings

Patients with pilonidal disease present in three main ways: acute abscess, chronic draining pits or complex, or recurrent disease after previous surgery. Patients with an acute pilonidal abscess will have pain and possibly swelling in or along the gluteal cleft. Given the relatively fixed nature of the tissues in this region and how deep a typical pilonidal abscess is located, swelling and cellulitis are often absent, and physical examination often underestimates the size of the abscess. Patients with chronically draining midline pits will have one or more pits in the midline with drainage and recurrent inflammation. Often hair will be seen protruding from the pits. Patients with complex disease after previous surgery may have chronic, nonhealing wounds in the midline of the gluteal cleft. History and physical examination are sufficient to make the diagnosis of pilonidal disease regardless of the type of presentation. Laboratory and imaging studies play no role in the evaluation of patients with pilonidal disease.

Differential Diagnosis

Pilonidal disease occurs in the superior gluteal cleft and is usually relatively easy to diagnose. Pilonidal disease occurring inferior in the gluteal cleft and close to the anus may be difficult to distinguish from an anal fistula. An examination under anesthesia may be required in order to differentiate pilonidal pit and cyst from an anal fistula. Further, pilonidal disease off the midline may mimic hidradenitis. Usually, hidradenitis will occur elsewhere and will not be just limited to the gluteal cleft like pilonidal disease.

Treatment

Patients with an acute abscess related to pilonidal disease should undergo incision and drainage of their abscess. Antibiotics are not necessary unless the patient has significant infection or sepsis or is immunocompromised. The abscess is nearly always located deep to the midline gluteal cleft. Because incisions in the midline heal poorly, an acute abscess should be drained through a lateral incision at least 2 cm off midline. A generous lateral incision allows for adequate drainage of pus and hair from the pilonidal cyst. No packing of the wound is necessary, but shaving a wide area around the gluteal cleft is important to help prevent further accumulation of hair in the cyst. After abscess drainage, patients should be followed to ensure healing, but further operative intervention is usually not necessary.

Patients with chronically draining pilonidal pits should be treated conservatively. The whole gluteal cleft and surrounding gluteal skin should be shaved and all hair in the pits removed. Patients are instructed to bend over in the shower and allow the water to blast the gluteal cleft to help prevent accumulation of hair in the pits. Patients should undergo repeat shaving, and hair should be removed from the pits every week or two until resolution of symptoms. If symptoms recur, conservative treatment with shaving and removal of pit hair should be resumed. Patients with persistent drainage and inflammation despite 2-3 months of conservative treatment are candidates for surgery. Traditionally, surgical treatment of pilonidal disease involved pilonidal cystectomy, which meant complete removal of the midline chronic abscess cavity. This procedure is associated with wound breakdown and possible development of a nonhealing midline wound that may in fact be more debilitating than the disease prior to surgery. Given this possibility, midline incisions are generally avoided. Rather, a minimally invasive operation called a lateral incision and pit closure is performed. After a lateral incision is made, the abscess cavity in the midline is accessed via this lateral incision to remove all pus, hair, and granulation tissue. Next, the pits in the midline are excised, and the minimal 2- to 3-mm wounds are closed with nylon suture. The lateral incision is left open for drainage. If the excised midline pit wounds heal, the pilonidal disease is eliminated, and the lateral incision will heal readily over 2-4 weeks.

Patients with complex, recurrent pilonidal disease with large, nonhealing midline wounds need complex flap surgery to resolve their symptoms. Most of the flaps used today avoid closure at the midline, which has been historically plagued by poor wound healing. The Kardyakis procedure involves making an elliptical incision parallel to the midline followed by excision of the skin and gluteal fat containing the sinus tract down to the sacral fascia. A subcutaneous flap is mobilized across the midline and secured to the sacral fascia, and the skin is then closed off the midline. Another procedure that avoids the midline is the Bascom cleft lift procedure. In this procedure, the skin of the external wound at the gluteal cleft is excised, and this excision is extended laterally off the midline. A flap using the skin and subcutaneous tissues of the gluteal cleft and cheek of the opposite side is then mobilized across the midline to the side with the lateral excision and closed without tension. In addition to avoiding closure at the midline, this flap also eliminates the gluteal cleft. Without a gluteal cleft, further pilonidal disease is unheard of.

Less invasive measures using phenol and thrombin injections have been more recently investigated. Early results appear promising; however, these treatments remain experimental.

Complications and Prognosis

Patients with pilonidal disease are young, active adults and often desire a quick fix for their symptoms. It is important to counsel patients regarding the natural history of the disease. They should understand the chronic nature of the disease, while also being aware that it can naturally regress with time. With this mindset, patients will more readily participate in conservative treatment and understand the goals of minimally invasive surgery, such as lateral incision and pit closure. Overall, the prognosis of patients with pilonidal disease is excellent.

Abdelrazeq AS, Rahman M, Botterill ID, et al: Short-term and long-term outcomes of the cleft lift procedure in the management of nonacute pilonidal disorders. *Dis Colon Rectum.* 2008;51(7):1100-1106.

Al-Khamis A, McCallum I, King PM, et al: Healing by primary versus secondary intention after surgical treatment for pilonidal sinus. *Cochrane Database Syst Rev.* 2010;1:CD006213.

Calikoglu I, Gulpinar K, Oztuna D, et al: Phenol injection versus excision with open healing in pilonidal disease: a prospective randomized trial. *Dis Colon Rectum.* 2017;60(2):161-169.

Humphries AE, Duncan JE: Evaluation and management of pilonidal disease. *Surg Clin North Am.* 2010;90(1):113-124.

Maghsoudi H, Nezami N, Ghamari AA: Ambulatory treatment of chronic pilonidal sinuses with lateral incision and primary suture. *Can J Surg.* 2011;54(2):78-82.

Steele SR, Perry WB, Mills S, et al: Practice parameters for the management of pilonidal disease. *Dis Colon Rectum.* 2013;56(9):1021-1027.

Thompson MR, Senapati A, Kitchen P: Simple day-case surgery for pilonidal sinus disease. *Br J Surg.* 2011;98(2):198-209.

ANAL STENOSIS

Anal stenosis is a relatively unusual condition that is most commonly associated with previous surgery, malignancy, or Crohn disease. Patients often are successful at self-treating their stenosis by keeping their stools soft with stool softeners and laxatives. Complete anal canal obstruction is rare. Identification of the etiology of the anal stenosis is key to successful treatment.

Clinical Findings

Patients with anal stenosis complain of difficult evacuation and possibly rectal bleeding. The history is important to determine the etiology of their symptoms. The most common cause of anal stenosis is previous anorectal surgery, particularly hemorrhoid surgery. Because stenosis often occurs years to decades after hemorrhoid surgery, patients should be specifically questioned regarding prior anorectal surgery. Patients with anal stenosis related to Crohn disease usually have a relatively long history of anorectal Crohn disease that may include treatment of abscesses, fistulas, and anal canal ulcers. Patients with malignancy may have a history of anal condyloma but often will have no antecedent history. Physical examination reveals a narrowed anal canal. Digital examination is still possible in patients with a mild anal stenosis. Moderate to severe anal canal stenosis does not allow digital examination. Due to the severity of stenosis, it may be difficult to determine if the stenosis is due to a mass or tumor. Laboratory and imaging studies play no role in the evaluation of patients with anal stenosis. Flexible endoscopy is important in all patients with anal stenosis. In patients with moderate to severe stenosis, flexible endoscopic evaluation may be impossible prior to treatment and is done after the stenosis is corrected.

Treatment

Mild anal stenosis can be treated with stool softeners and laxatives with good results. Patients with persistent symptoms despite treatment and patients with moderate to severe stenosis require endoscopic or surgical intervention. Because malignancy is always a possibility even after hemorrhoid surgery or in patients with Crohn disease, a biopsy of the anal canal stenosis is mandatory. Of course, any patient diagnosed with malignancy needs appropriate treatment of the malignancy, which may involve chemoradiation (anal cancer) and/or surgery (rectal cancer). For patients without malignancy, the choice of a surgical procedure is dictated by the etiology of the anal stenosis.

Patients with Crohn disease and radiation-induced strictures are at high risk for failure of surgical interventions. Conservative management should be attempted, including manual dilation and medical treatment of Crohn disease. If conservative measures fail, patients can undergo endoscopic balloon dilatation of their anal stricture or operative anal stricturoplasty. During anal stricturoplasty, longitudinal incisions are made through the stricture at one to three locations around the anal canal. Recurrent stricture can be treated with repeat balloon dilatation or operative anal stricturoplasty.

Patients with postsurgical anal stenosis have a deficiency of anoderm related to their previous operation and subsequent scarring. Due to their deficiency of anoderm, these patients are not appropriate candidates for stricturoplasty but rather are better served with a local advancement flap into the anal canal to correct their anoderm deficiency. Many local advancement flaps have been described and used successfully, such as the V-Y, Y-V, diamond, and house flap. During the anal house flap operation, the patient is placed in the prone position, and the anal canal is visualized. Standard operative anoscopes will not fit into the anal canal of patients with moderate to severe stenosis, and thus, use of a nasal speculum is necessary. With the anal canal visualized, the anoderm is divided longitudinally for the length of the strictured anal canal. Transverse incisions are then made at the proximal and distal aspects of this incision, converting the incision wound into a rectangular defect. A house-shaped flap of anal margin skin and subcutaneous tissue is developed and advanced into the anal canal. The flap is then sutured into place, and the donor site is closed. In some cases, two or three separate house flaps around the anus are necessary to adequately correct the anal stenosis. Thus, the advancement of anal margin skin into the anal canal corrects the deficiency of anoderm and relieves the anal stenosis.

The results following anal advancement flap treatment of anal canal stenosis are very good. Potential complications include bleeding, infection, flap necrosis, flap retraction, and recurrence. If an advancement flap fails it can be repeated in another quadrant around the anus.

Brisinda G, Vanella S, Cadeddu F, et al: Surgical treatment of anal stenosis. *World J Gastroenterol.* 2009;15(16):1921-1928.

Brochard C, Siproudhis L, Wallenhorst T, et al: Anorectal stricture in 102 patients with Crohn's disease: natural history in the era of biologics. *Aliment Pharmacol Ther.* 2014;40(7):796-803.

Farid M, Youssef M, El Nakeeb A, et al: Comparative study of the house advancement flap, rhomboid flap, and Y-V anoplasty in treatment of anal stenosis: a prospective randomized study. *Dis Colon Rectum.* 2010;53(5):790-797.

Gülen M, Leventoğlu S, Ege B, et al: Surgical treatment of anal stenosis with diamond flap anoplasty performed in a calibrated fashion. *Dis Colon Rectum.* 2016;59(3):230-235.

Katdare MV, Ricciardi R: Anal stenosis. *Surg Clin North Am.* 2010;90(1):137-145.

PRURITUS ANI

Pruritus ani is a challenging dermatologic disorder characterized by intense itching of the perianal skin. Diagnosis of this problem is typically not straightforward, and subsequently, patients may be evaluated by a variety of specialists including gastroenterologists, dermatologists, and colorectal surgeons. The incidence of pruritus ani ranges from 1%-5% in adults and typically has a male predominance (male-to-female ratio of 4:1).

Pruritus ani is broadly classified either as primary (idiopathic) or secondary. Up to 90% of cases are considered idiopathic, whereas the remaining secondary cases are caused by a variety of local and systemic conditions.

▶ Clinical Findings

Patients typically present with complaints of an unpleasant perianal burning, which usually starts insidiously. As the condition becomes more chronic, this burning is replaced by varying degrees of itching that can become intolerable. Careful history uncovers that symptoms are often more pronounced at night.

Physical findings on examination can be varied. In the early stages, the skin may appear normal; however, as the patient continues to scratch, the local inflammation worsens, resulting in erythematous, excoriated, macerated skin. In the chronic stage, the skin is often lichenified with coarse ridges and ulcerations.

▶ Differential Diagnosis

Identifying the primary etiology of pruritus ani can be very challenging; therefore, a careful history and physical examination is required. Information on diet, medications, synchronous skin conditions, common anorectal disorders, bowel function, and stool consistency, as well as prior anorectal procedures, should be ascertained. A thorough exam of the perianal skin and anoscopy are essential. Skin scrapings, cultures, and biopsy of suspicious lesions are important adjuncts to elucidate the underlying etiology. The routine use of endoscopy and radiologic studies is unnecessary unless there is a high index of suspicion for a colorectal cause. Some of the established causes of secondary pruritus ani are summarized in Table 33–5.

▶ Treatment

The goal of treatment should be directed toward establishing clean and dry perianal skin that is free of ulcerations. If pruritus is found to be secondary to one of the aforementioned causes, then treatment should be directed toward that specific pathology. The management of idiopathic pruritus is more challenging, often requiring intensive patient education and behavior modification.

Meticulous perianal hygiene should be stressed as the first step in management. Patients should focus on keeping the area dry and avoiding soaps and detergents with potential irritants. A high-fiber diet should be encouraged, while eliminating foods that may precipitate pruritus. If symptoms

Table 33–5. Common causes of secondary pruritus ani.

Diet Coffee, tea, caffeinated beverages, alcohol, chocolate, spicy foods, tomatoes (ketchup), dairy products	**Dermatologic Conditions** Psoriasis, contact dermatitis, lichen sclerosus/planus
Local Irritants Topical medications, soaps, detergents, fabric	**Local Malignancies** Bowen disease, Paget disease, squamous cell cancer
Anorectal Diseases Hemorrhoids, fistula, rectal prolapse, fecal incontinence/soiling, skin tags	**Perianal Infections** Bacterial (*Staphylococcus* or *Streptococcus*), fungal, viral (eg, herpes simplex, human papillomavirus), parasitic
Systemic Diseases Diabetes mellitus, liver disease, thyroid disorder, renal disease, leukemia	**Psychological** Anxiety, depression, stress

improve, then these foods may be slowly reintroduced in order to identify the offending product.

In cases of more severe skin excoriation, skin barrier creams may provide symptomatic relief. Topical steroids can be introduced for increased severity of symptoms; however, caution should be applied because they can exacerbate symptoms and thin the perianal skin if used for a prolonged period or at too high a dose. Other topical medications that may provide relief include antibiotics, menthol, and calamine lotion. Additionally, topical capsaicin can be considered. A randomized, placebo-controlled trial comparing topical capsaicin (0.006%) with placebo (1% menthol) in patients with chronic pruritus ani found that of 70% of patients experienced relief of their symptoms.

In patients with refractory symptoms, intradermal injection of methylene blue combined with local anesthetic has been described with limited success. Skin necrosis from inappropriate infiltration has been described.

► Prognosis

The successful identification and treatment of secondary causes of pruritus ani often yield good results. However, relapses can be common with idiopathic pruritus. Every attempt should be made to continue to reinforce patient education.

Ansari P: Pruritus Ani. *Clin Colon Rectal Surg.* 2016;29(1):38-42.

Gooding SM, Canter PH, Coelho HF, et al: Systematic review of topical capsaicin in the treatment of pruritus. *Int J Dermatol.* 2010;4 (8):858-865.

Lacy BE, Weiser K: Common anorectal disorders: diagnosis and treatment. *Curr Gastroenterol Rep.* 2009;11(5):413-419.

Markell KW, Billingham RP: Pruritus ani: etiology and management. *Surg Clin North Am.* 2010;90(1):125-135.

Samalavicius NE, Poskus T, Gupta RK, et al: Long-term results of single intradermal 1% methylene blue injection for intractable idiopathic pruritus ani: a prospective study. *Tech Coloproctol.* 2012;16(4):295-299.

Siddiqi S, Vijay V, Ward M, et al: Pruritus ani. *Ann R Coll Surg Engl.* 2008;90(6):457-463.

Sutherland AD, Faragher IG, Frizelle FA: Intradermal injection of methylene blue for the treatment of refractory pruritus ani. *Colorectal Dis.* 2009;11(3):282-287.

PROCTITIS & ANUSITIS

Proctitis and *anusitis* are general terms referring to inflammation within the anal canal or rectum secondary to infectious pathogens or inflammatory causes. Sexually transmitted infections are an increasingly common cause of proctitis, with an incidence exceeding 15 million new cases annually in the United States. The differential diagnosis can be quite broad, with a variety of bacteria and viruses; therefore, a systematic approach is important. The diagnosis and management of these conditions depend primarily on the underlying etiology.

► Herpes Proctitis

The herpes simplex virus (HSV) is a DNA virus that is the most prevalent sexually transmitted infection in the United States. The majority of anogenital infections are caused by the HSV-2 serotype, accounting for approximately 80%-90% of infections. Anorectal infections typically result from autoinoculation or direct contact with infected partners. The virus travels along peripheral nerves and has a variable incubation period (days to weeks). Prodromal symptoms may consist of burning, tingling, fever, and itching. This typically escalates to more intense, painful proctitis and tenesmus. The characteristic lesions are small vesicles with surrounding erythema, which eventually coalesce and rupture, forming painful ulcerations. In addition, patients may develop tender inguinal adenopathy.

Evaluation of the rectum with a proctoscope will demonstrate erythematous and friable mucosa with ulcerations and mucopurulent discharge. Tzanck smear of the discharge reveals the characteristic multinucleated giant cells with intranuclear inclusion bodies. Viral cultures of the discharge from these vesicles are also highly positive in acute infections.

HSV infections are usually self-limited in the absence of superimposed bacterial infections; therefore, initial treatments, such as sitz baths and oral analgesics, are aimed at controlling symptoms. There is no cure for active infections, but acyclovir, valacyclovir, and famciclovir will shorten the duration of symptoms and may be used for episodic treatment or as chronic suppressive therapy in patients with frequent recurrences.

► Anorectal Syphilis

Syphilis is caused by the spirochete, *Treponema pallidum*, which typically has an incubation period of 2-6 weeks. This disease was once on the verge of elimination, but the incidence has been rising among males.

Acute anorectal infection is characterized by a small papule (chancre) on the anal margin or within the anal canal, which eventually ulcerates and may be mistaken for a routine anal fissure. This eventually regresses spontaneously in 3-4 weeks and is followed by a secondary stage 2-10 weeks later. Secondary syphilis may consist of fever, malaise, arthralgia, a maculopapular rash on the palms and soles of the feet, tenesmus, mucoid discharge, rectal pain, and inguinal adenopathy.

There are several methods for diagnosis. Dark-field microscopy will reveal the spirochetes, which have a corkscrew-shaped appearance. Biopsy shows spirochetes on a Warthin-Starry silver stain. There are also two serologic tests, rapid plasma reagin and VDRL (Venereal Disease Research Laboratory).

Treatment consists of a single dose of penicillin intramuscularly in the early phase. If identified later, three doses are given 2 weeks apart.

Gonococcal Proctitis

Gonococcal proctitis is caused by the organism *Neisseria gonorrhoeae,* which is an intracellular gram-negative diplococcus. It is estimated that there are approximately 3 million people infected yearly worldwide; however, there is a large population of asymptomatic carriers. Anorectal infection results from contiguous spread from the genital area in women and from anal receptive intercourse in men.

The incubation period varies but can last up to 2 weeks. Symptoms then include pruritus, tenesmus, and a thick, purulent discharge that can be expressed from the anal crypts. Proctitis of the mid to distal rectum can be identified on proctoscopy. Standard Gram stains of the discharge are generally unreliable; however, culture on Thayer-Martin medium increases the positive yield.

The first-line treatment of anorectal gonorrhea is an intramuscular dose of ceftriaxone and an oral dose of azithromycin, or oral doxycycline for 7 days. Penicillin is no longer recommended given the high rate of resistance. Infected patients and partners should also be treated for concomitant *Chlamydia* infection, which is very common.

Chlamydial Proctitis & Lymphogranuloma Venereum

Chlamydia trachomatis is the most common sexually transmitted infection worldwide. This intracellular bacterium has several serotypes that have an incubation period up to 2 weeks. Serotypes D-K are responsible for proctitis and genital infections, whereas serotypes L1-L3 are responsible for lymphogranuloma venereum (LGV).

A large portion of patients will be asymptomatic; however, when present, symptoms of an active anorectal infection include rectal pain, tenesmus, and fever. Similar anorectal complaints are present in patients with LGV, but the inguinal adenopathy is often more prominent with large matted nodes with overlying erythema.

Diagnosis of active infections can be challenging with routine culture given the intracellular location of the bacteria. Often patients with suggestive symptoms of proctitis that have a Gram stain demonstrating leukocytes without detectable gonococci are presumed to have a *Chlamydia* infection and are treated accordingly. Cell culture is also possible using a sucrose phosphate media. Treatment consists of a single oral dose of azithromycin or doxycycline twice daily for 7 days. Treatment with doxycycline is extended to 21 days for LGV. Sexual partners should be treated as well to prevent reinfection.

Condyloma Acuminata

Condyloma acuminata, caused by HPV, have a recognizable raised, cauliflower-like appearance and are located on the anal margin, within the anal canal, or surrounding the genitalia. Condyloma acuminatum is one of the most common sexually transmitted infections in the United States for which consultation with a colorectal surgeon is sought. There are more than 60 subtypes of this latent virus, with types 6 and 11 producing benign exophytic lesions. Types 16 and 18 are noted to be more aggressive, often causing lesions with high-grade dysplasia that may progress to cancer if left untreated.

Patients are often asymptomatic but may present with complaints of bleeding, itching, or anal discomfort due to the growths. Once present, there is no way to eradicate the infection surgically. The goal of treatment is to remove the macroscopic burden of disease with excisional biopsies and electrocautery. Recurrences are common; therefore, surveillance of these patients is extremely important. Bichloroacetic acid, trichloroacetic acid, and imiquimod are topical agents that have been used with reasonable success.

Chancroid

Chancroid is a rare sexually transmitted infection in the United States caused by the gram-negative bacteria *Haemophilus ducreyi.* Globally, the incidence is higher in developing countries.

The infection manifests itself days after transmission with painful inguinal adenopathy and erythematous papules around the genitalia that eventually ulcerate. Diagnosis is typically made with routine culture of the fluid from the ulcers. Treatment consists of single doses of azithromycin (orally) or ceftriaxone (intramuscularly).

Inflammatory Proctitis

Inflammatory proctitis refers to a general mild to moderate inflammation of the rectum that is unrelated to an underlying infection or sexually transmitted infection. Symptoms include rectal bleeding, urgency, tenesmus, and often diarrhea. Examination of the rectum is characterized by a continuous erythematous, friable mucosal surface. If applicable, cultures should be taken to elucidate any infectious etiology, and biopsies should be taken to rule out Crohn disease.

This condition can be self-limited, but persistent cases typically respond to short courses of steroid enemas. Additionally, mesalamine enemas are efficacious. If there is no improvement after a few weeks of treatment, the patient should be reevaluated.

Radiation Proctitis

Radiation proctitis is an unfortunate by-product of pelvic irradiation that typically occurs in two phases. Acute injury occurs within 6 weeks of administration of pelvic radiation, while chronic radiation proctitis usually presents 8-12 months after treatment. Acute injury is characterized by direct mucosal damage causing vascular congestion and friable mucosa. Acute symptoms include rectal bleeding, urgency, tenesmus, and diarrhea. The chronic presentation is characterized histologically by fibrosis that can manifest clinically with strictures, fistulas to the urinary tract or vagina, and telangiectasias. Chronic symptoms are similar to those of acute radiation proctitis, with a higher propensity for bleeding. Evaluation should include flexible sigmoidoscopy or colonoscopy and biopsy to make the diagnosis and rule out malignancy.

The initial treatment of acute radiation proctitis incorporates medications that manage symptoms, including bulking agents, antidiarrheals, and antispasmodics. Enemas of steroids, mesalamine, or short-chain fatty acids have been shown to improve proctitis as well. Refractory cases can be treated by topical application of 4% formalin to the rectal mucosa. Radiation proctitis complicated by fistulas is best managed surgically with interposition of normal, healthy tissues.

Assi R, Hashim PW, Reddy VB, et al: Sexually transmitted infections of the anus and rectum. *World J Gastroenterol.* 2014;20(41):15262-15268.

Cernik C, Gallina K, Brodell RT: The treatment of herpes simplex infections: an evidence-based review. *Arch Intern Med.* 2008;168(11):1137-1144.

Davis TW, Goldstone SE: Sexually transmitted infections as a cause of proctitis in men who have sex with men. *Dis Colon Rectum.* 2009;52(3):507-512.

Haas EM, Bailey HR, Faragher I: Application of 10 percent formalin for the treatment of radiation-induced hemorrhagic proctitis. *Dis Colon Rectum.* 2007;50(2):213-217.

RECTOVAGINAL FISTULA

Rectovaginal fistulas can be congenital or acquired and are generally characterized by their abnormal connection between the epithelialized mucosal surfaces of the rectum and the vagina. Distal fistulas arising from the anal canal are appropriately termed *anovaginal fistulas.* Acquired rectovaginal fistulas are generally caused by obstetric injuries, inflammatory bowel disease, trauma, or infection.

▶ Clinical Findings

A. Symptoms and Signs

The diagnosis of a rectovaginal fistula is typically straightforward based on an accurate history; however, in some instances, patients can be asymptomatic. Commonly, patients will present with complaints of the passage of air or feces from the vagina. The degree of distress often depends of the size of the fistulous opening. With smaller fistulas, more subtle complaints of a foul vaginal discharge, recurrent vaginitis, or dyspareunia may be more common, whereas the feculent drainage from larger fistulas may be confused with fecal

incontinence. Patients with obstetric injuries may also have concurrent fecal incontinence. If the etiology of the fistula is due to inflammatory bowel disease, then rectal complaints such as tenesmus or bloody diarrhea may predominate.

On digital rectal examination, the fistula can often be identified as a dimpling or pit in the anterior rectal mucosa, which can be easily be confirmed by anoscopy. Inspection of the vagina will reveal staining of the mucosa with stool, and the hyperemic mucosa of the fistula opening will contrast with the normal pink background of the vaginal mucosa. Occasionally, the identification of the fistula can be more challenging despite very suggestive symptoms. In these instances, a thorough exam under anesthesia may be indicated. With a saline-filled vagina, air can be instilled per rectum via a proctoscope. Air bubbles may help identify fistulas that are not readily apparent. Alternatively, diluted methylene blue can be instilled per rectum with a tampon in place in the vagina. Staining of the tampon with methylene blue will confirm the presence of a fistula.

B. Laboratory Studies and Imaging

Adjunct studies are sometimes necessary to identify the fistula location and to determine the quality of the surrounding tissue. Retrograde contrast enemas and CT scans with rectal contrast may identify contrast extravasation into the vagina. CT scans have the added benefit of identifying any associated inflammatory changes. MRI and endorectal ultrasound have also been used with varying results. Endoanal ultrasound can be used to identify any coexisting sphincter defects. Endoscopy is a valuable diagnostic tool to assess any underlying inflammatory conditions such as Crohn disease and to exclude underlying malignancy. Biopsies should be performed on any abnormal mucosa in the rectum or around the fistula orifice.

▶ Differential Diagnosis

The most common cause of rectovaginal fistulas is obstetrical trauma, accounting for 70%-80% of cases. These fistulas may present immediately, but more frequently, they manifest weeks after delivery, typically after third- and fourth-degree lacerations. In the Western hemisphere, the incidence has been estimated at up to 0.1% of all vaginal deliveries. Other etiologies include inflammatory bowel disease, primarily Crohn disease, postoperative trauma, radiation, malignancy, and infection.

▶ Treatment

The management of rectovaginal fistulas primarily depends on its complexity, as determined by the location, etiology, size, and quality of the surrounding tissue. Simple fistulas are typically small in diameter (< 2.5 cm) and low on the rectovaginal septum and are secondary to either traumatic injury or infection. However, complex fistulas are larger in diameter and higher on the rectovaginal septum and are associated with underlying inflammatory bowel disease, radiation, neoplasm, or previously failed repairs. There are several well-described operative approaches, which can generally be divided into transanal, transvaginal, transperineal, and transabdominal repairs.

Common transanal repairs include fistula excision with layered closure, endorectal advancement flap, and rectal sleeve advancement. The mucosal advancement flap is appropriate for simple, low fistulas. During this procedure, a flap composed of mucosa, submucosa, and a portion of internal sphincter muscle is mobilized proximally and used to cover the fistula defect. The base of the flap should be wider than the apex in order to ensure adequate perfusion of the flap. The muscle is then reapproximated in the midline, closing the fistula. The flap is then advanced into the anal canal and secured with absorbable sutures. Success rates are varied in the literature, ranging from 50%-100%.

Rectal sleeve advancement is a reasonable approach for rectovaginal fistulas with extensive stenosis and anal ulcerations due to Crohn disease. Starting at the dentate line, a circumferential incision is made and extended cephalad. The dissection becomes full thickness above the anorectal ring and is extended until the distal rectum is adequately mobilized. The rectum is then pulled down through the anal canal, and the diseased rectum is transected. The fistula opening in the vagina is closed, and the rectum is sutured to the dentate line. This repair is often done with a protective diverting ostomy.

Perineoproctectomy is a perineal technique that essentially converts a rectovaginal fistula into a fourth-degree laceration. The vaginal mucosa, sphincter muscles, and rectum are divided between the fistula openings and reapproximated in layers, ultimately obliterating the fistula tract.

Tissue interpositions are also typically performed through the perineal approach and include the gracilis muscle flap and the Martius (bulbocavernosus muscle) flap. The fundamental concept in these procedures is that normal, healthy tissue is placed between the fistula openings after dissecting the plane between the rectum and the vagina. Successful closure with these procedures has been reported to be as high as 80%, and they constitute an ideal repair for rectovaginal fistulas that have failed previous repairs or with abnormal surrounding tissues.

Rectovaginal fistulas that are higher in the rectovaginal septum are usually approached through an abdominal approach. There are several potential procedures, ranging from simple fistula division and closure with interposition of pedicled omentum to proctectomy with colorectal or colo-anal anastomosis. The choice of procedure depends on the quality of surrounding tissues, location, and the etiology of the fistula.

Finally, the past decade has seen increasing use of bio-prosthetic plugs and sheets in the management of rectovaginal fistulas. Small series have shown promising results, but there is still a paucity of long-term data.

Prognosis

The prognosis for rectovaginal fistulas is dependent on the overall complexity of the fistula. Crohn-related rectovaginal fistulas and tobacco use have a higher recurrence rate. Simple, low fistulas can be approached with relatively straightforward transanal or perineal techniques with good results. Fistulas that are higher or associated with inflammatory bowel disease, radiation, or neoplasm are understandably more challenging, often requiring multiple repairs.

Champagne BJ, McGee MF: Rectovaginal fistula. *Surg Clin North Am.* 2010;90(1):69-82.

Corte H, Maggiori L, Treton X, et al: Rectovaginal fistula: what is the optimal strategy? An analysis of 79 patients undergoing 286 procedures. *Ann Surg.* 2015;262:855-860.

de Bruijn H, Maeda Y, Murphy J, et al: Combined laparoscopic and perineal approach to omental interposition repair of complex rectovaginal fistula. *Dis Colon Rectum.* 2018;61(1):140-143.

Ellis CN: Outcomes after repair of rectovaginal fistulas using bioprosthetics. *Dis Colon Rectum.* 2008;51(7):1084-1088.

Gosselink MP, Oom DM, Zimmerman DD, et al: Martius flap: an adjunct for repair of complex, low rectovaginal fistula. *Am J Surg.* 2009;197(6):833-834.

Hannaway CD, Hull TL: Current considerations in the management of rectovaginal fistula from Crohn's disease. *Colorectal Dis.* 2008;10(8):747-755; discussion 755-756.

Hotouras A, Ribas Y, Zakeri S, et al: Gracilis muscle interposition for rectovaginal and anovaginal fistula repair: a systematic literature review. *Colorectal Dis.* 2015;17(2):104-110.

Pinto RA, Peterson TV, Shawki S, et al: Are there predictors of outcome following rectovaginal fistula repair? *Dis Colon Rectum.* 2010;53:1240-1247.

Sonoda T, Hull T, Piedmonte MR, et al: Outcomes of primary repair of anorectal and rectovaginal fistulas using the endorectal advancement flap. *Dis Colon Rectum.* 2002;45:1622-1628.

Vogel JD, Johnson EK, Morris AM, et al: Clinical practice guideline for the management of anorectal abscess, fistula-in-ano, and rectovaginal fistula. *Dis Colon Rectum.* 2016;59(12):1117-1133.

ANAL AND PERIANAL NEOPLASMS

▶ General Considerations

Neoplasms of the anus and surrounding skin are uncommon, accounting for only about 3% of all gastrointestinal malignancies. The overall management of these lesions depends primarily on the histology, size, and location of the lesion. While the definitions can be confusing, the anal canal is commonly defined, by surgeons, as the region extending from the anal verge to the anorectal ring at the top of the sphincter complex. The lymphatic drainage in this area is variable but clinically important. Proximal to the dentate line, the lymphatic system drains to the internal iliac and inferior mesenteric nodes, while distal to the dentate line, drainage is typically to the inguinal nodes. It is important to realize that lesions in this area may not be completely visualized on routine inspection of the perineum. The anal margin, or perianal region, is generally defined as the perianal skin extending circumferentially within 5 cm of the anal verge. Lesions in this area are easily visible on exam.

▶ Tumors of the Anal Margin

A. Squamous Cell Carcinoma

The majority of malignant neoplasms of the anal margin are squamous cell cancers (SCCs). They have similar presentation to SCC that occurs elsewhere on the skin and are subsequently staged similarly based on size (< 2 cm, 2-5 cm, > 5 cm, or involving deep structures) and lymph node positivity by the American Joint Committee on Cancer (AJCC) staging system. The overall incidence of anal margin cancers is low, and the prognosis is often more favorable than SCC of the anal canal. These lesions are typically well differentiated and indolent and are rarely associated with distant metastasis.

Lesions in this location may present with pain, bleeding, pruritus, tenesmus, or incontinence if locally advanced. On examination, there are rolled, everted edges often with central ulceration. Palpable lymph nodes may be identified in the inguinal region.

The management of anal margin SCC consists of wide local excision for T1 and early T2 lesions that can be easily resected with a 1-cm margin without compromising sphincter function. For larger tumors, radiation to the inguinal regions and primary tumor can be considered in addition to resection. Poorly differentiated tumors or T3 or T4 cancers should be treated with chemoradiation, including the inguinal and pelvic nodes in the field of treatment. Abdominoperineal resection (APR) should be reserved for recurrent disease, residual disease after radiation, or bulky tumors that are invading the sphincter complex.

B. Basal Cell Carcinoma

Basal cell cancers (BCCs) of the anal margin are exceedingly rare, accounting for 0.2% of anorectal cancers. They typically present in older men, and approximately one-third of patients will have a history of BCC or a synchronous lesion elsewhere. The appearance of these lesions is similar to that of other areas of the body, with irregular, raised, pearly edges with superficial plaques or ulcers. Local invasion and metastatic potential are both typically low, and 5-year survival is 100%.

Wide local excision with an adequate margin is the treatment of choice for small lesions. Local recurrence can occur in up to 30% of patients but can usually be reexcised. Larger, bulky lesions can be treated with APR or radiation.

C. Bowen Disease

Historically, the term *Bowen disease* referred to SCC in situ. This term as well as anal intraepithelial neoplasia (AIN) II and III have largely been replaced by the classification of high-grade squamous intraepithelial lesion (HSIL), which has similar histologic features. HPV infection is common. Patients may complain of itching or pain, and examination reveals scaly, erythematous, and sometimes pigmented lesions.

Traditionally, these lesions have been treated with wide local excision, often with complex reconstructions for larger lesions. This approach has been plagued by high recurrence rates and is generally very morbid. More recent data suggest that HSIL can be adequately treated with targeted biopsy with HRA, ablation, and close surveillance every 3-6 months. The application of topical imiquimod (Aldara) or topical 5-fluorouracil has been proposed to minimize recurrence, but these treatments are generally limited by local skin irritation.

D. Verrucous Carcinoma

Perianal verrucous carcinoma is often referred to as a Buschke-Lowenstein tumor or giant condyloma, given its exophytic, cauliflower-like appearance. They are more common in men and often associated with HPV. These lesions can vary in size but are generally slow growing and locally invasive. Histologically, they are considered benign, but larger lesions may certainly encompass underlying malignancy, usually invasive SCC. Patients frequently present with complaints of an anal mass but may also describe pain, fistulas, or abscesses. Wide local excision is recommended for the majority of these lesions, and if large, the resulting defects may require more complex closure. More advanced cases with invasion into the sphincter complex may require APR.

E. Paget Disease

Paget disease is a rare condition characterized by an intraepithelial adenocarcinoma of the perianal skin. The most common presenting complaint is intolerable pruritus, and examination typically reveals a well-demarcated, erythematous, eczematous rash. Diagnosis is made after a full-thickness biopsy, which shows the pathognomonic Paget cell with pale vacuolated cytoplasm and peripheral nucleus. These lesions often are associated with synchronous gastrointestinal malignancies, so a complete evaluation of the intestinal tract should be performed.

In the absence of invasive disease, wide local excision is the treatment of choice. It is important to obtain intraoperative frozen sections to ensure negative margins. Large defects can be covered with skin grafts or adjacent tissue transfers. Patients with invasive disease have a poor prognosis and should be considered for radical resection with APR. Inguinal lymphadenectomy should be added for clinically positive nodal involvement. The role of chemoradiation is not well defined but has been used as an adjunct in invasive and recurrent disease. Topical imiquimod use has shown promising results in some case reports.

Garrett K, Kalady MF: Anal neoplasms. *Surg Clin North Am.* 2010;90 (1):147-161.

Goldstone SE, Johnstone AA, Moshier EL: Long-term outcome of ablation of anal high-grade squamous intraepithelial lesions: recurrence and incidence of cancer. *Dis Colon Rectum.* 2014;57(3):316-323.

Jiang Y, Ajani JA: Anal margin cancer: current situation and ongoing trials. *Curr Opin Oncol.* 2012;24(4):448-453.

Knight SR, Proby C, Ziyaie D, et al: Extramammary Paget disease of the perianal region: the potential role of imiquimod in achieving disease control. *J Surg Case Rep.* 2016;2016(8):rjw110.

Kyriazanos ID, Stamos NP, Miliadis L, et al: Extra-mammary Paget's disease of the perianal region: a review of the literature emphasizing the operative management technique. *Surg Oncol.* 2011;20(2):e61-71.

Megill C, Wilkin T: Topical therapies for the treatment of anal high-grade squamous intraepithelial lesions. *Semin Colon Rectal Surg.* 2017;28(2):86-90.

Minicozzi A, Borzellino G, Momo R, et al: Perianal Paget's disease: presentation of six cases and literature review. *Int J Colorectal Dis.* 2010;25(1):1-7.

TUMORS OF THE ANAL CANAL

1. Anal Cancer

▶ Clinical Findings

Tumors of the anal canal are rare, accounting for about 2% of all colorectal malignancies. Anal cancer encompasses several histologic subtypes, including squamous cell, basaloid, mucoepidermoid, epidermoid, and cloacogenic cancers. SCC is by far the most common. Risk factors of anal cancer may include HPV infection, HIV or other causes of immunosuppression, anoreceptive intercourse, and tobacco use.

The clinical manifestation of anal canal tumors can be quite variable, and many patients are initially diagnosed with benign anorectal conditions. They are typically slow growing, and symptoms can include pain and bleeding. Digital rectal exam and anoscopy are important tools for an accurate diagnosis, during which the size, location, consistency, and degree of fixation should be noted. A biopsy of the lesion confirms the diagnosis and provides the specific subtype. Additionally, the presence of any palpable inguinal adenopathy should be documented and can be further tested by fine-needle aspiration or core needle biopsy. The staging of anal tumors is based on tumor size (< 2 cm, 2-5 cm, > 5 cm, or involving deep structures) and lymph node positivity by the AJCC staging system. Endoanal ultrasound and MRI can be used in evaluating the primary tumor, and positron emission tomography and CT are important adjuncts that can help identify distant metastases and surrounding adenopathy.

▶ Treatment

Since its introduction in 1974, radiation and chemotherapy with 5-fluorouracil and mitomycin C (Nigro protocol) have largely replaced surgery in the treatment of anal cancer. This treatment has demonstrated good local control, sphincter preservation, and less recurrence. Drawbacks to chemoradiation include toxicity. This can be addressed by considering radiation therapy alone or using intensity-modulated radiation therapy. Approximately 20%-30% of patients have persistent or recurrent disease after chemoradiation for anal SCC. Salvage APR is reserved for recurrent or residual pelvic disease after chemoradiation. After salvage APR, survival rates can vary from 25%-70%. Wound complications are the most common postoperative problem for these patients.

Inguinal node disease is managed by chemoradiation, with response rates up to 90%. Due to the high morbidity rate, prophylactic groin dissection is not recommended; however, selective node dissection may be considered for persistent disease after chemoradiation.

The overall response to chemoradiation should be assessed clinically at about 8 weeks after the completion of treatment. At this point, up to 85% of patients will have a complete clinical response. Those with good partial response may be observed closely to ensure that complete response does occur. Any lesions suspicious for residual disease or progression of disease should be biopsied at that time. For patients with complete clinical response, surveillance entails digital rectal exam, anoscopy, and inguinal node assessment every 3-6 months for the first 2 years and every 6-12 months thereafter up to 5 years. There is no consensus on the routine use of imaging in surveillance, but it is often practiced.

▶ Prognosis

Complete response rates approach 90% for smaller tumors, with 5-year survival that ranges between 70% and 90%. Residual or recurrent disease confers a poorer prognosis, with 5-year survival rates between 24% and 58% after salvage APR.

2. Melanoma of the Anal Canal

The anorectum is the third most common site overall for melanoma, but it is the most common site of primary melanoma of the gastrointestinal tract, making it an exceedingly rare condition. It accounts for up to 2% of all melanomas and 2%-4% of all anorectal tumors.

▶ Clinical Findings

Pain, bleeding, and a palpable mass are the most consistent clinical findings with melanoma of the anal canal. Patients may also present with tenesmus, change in the caliber of stools, inguinal lymphadenopathy, and weight loss. Like its cutaneous counterpart, anal melanomas are raised and pigmented; however, it is important to note that these lesions may be amelanotic, which may mimic more benign disease.

► Treatment

For localized disease, surgery offers the only chance for cure, as there has been no proven benefit for chemotherapy or radiation. Both APR and wide local excision have been advocated. APR does not confer a survival advantage and is associated with high morbidity rates; subsequently, wide local excision is recommended as the initial surgical approach for localized disease. Large, bulky tumors that involve the sphincter complex will require radical resection.

► Prognosis

The prognosis for anorectal melanoma is universally poor because many patients present with metastatic disease. Survival rates generally range from 6% to 28% in the literature. The overall 5-year survival for large, deeply invading, or metastatic disease is less than 10% with a median survival of 12-18 months.

Chen H, Cai Y, Liu Y, et al: Incidence, surgical treatment, and prognosis of anorectal melanoma from 1973 to 2011: a population-based SEER analysis. *Medicine (Baltimore)*. 2016 Feb;95(7):e2770.

Glynne-Jones R, Nilsson PJ, Aschele C, et al: Anal cancer: ESMO-ESSO-ESTRO Clinical practice guidelines for diagnosis, treatment and follow-up. *Ann Oncol*. 2014;25(Suppl 3):iii10-20.

Guerra GR, Kong JC, Bernardi MP, et al: Salvage surgery for locoregional failure in anal squamous cell carcinoma. *Dis Colon Rectum*. 2018;61(2):179-186.

Heeney A, Mulsow J, Hyland JM: Treatment and outcomes of anorectal melanoma. *Surgeon*. 2011;9(1):27-32.

Jiang Y, Mackley H, Cheng H, et al: Anal carcinoma therapy: can we improve on 5 fluorouracil/mitomycin/radiotherapy? *J Natl Compr Canc Netw*. 2010;8:135-144.

Meguerditchian AN, Meterissian SH, Dunn KB: Anorectal melanoma: diagnosis and treatment. *Dis Colon Rectum*. 2011;54(5):638-644.

Steele SR, Varma MG, Melton GB, et al: Practice parameters for anal squamous neoplasms. *Dis Colon Rectum*. 2012;55:735-749.

NORMAL FUNCTION OF THE ANORECTUM

Anorectal physiology is very complex. Coordination between the pelvic nerves, pelvic floor muscles, rectum, and sphincter complex must occur for normal controlled evacuation of intestinal waste.

Like the colon, the rectum is composed of two layers of smooth muscle—an inner circular layer and an outer longitudinal layer. It varies in length from 12-18 cm and is predominantly confined within the bony pelvis. The peritoneum covers the upper two-thirds of the rectum anteriorly and the upper third laterally, and the lower third of the rectum is extraperitoneal. The rectum is very distensible and has the capacity to hold large volumes, which is ideal since its primary function is as a reservoir for stool prior to defecation. Alterations in rectal sensation or compliance due to infection, inflammation, or fibrosis will result in urgency.

The anal canal begins at the anal verge, extending cephalad to the anorectal ring, and is surrounded by the levator ani muscles as well as the internal and external sphincter complex. The internal anal sphincter (IAS) muscle, which accounts for more than 50% of the resting anal pressure, is an involuntary muscle that is the downward continuation of the circular, smooth muscle of the rectum. The IAS is approximately 3 cm in length and supplied by both sympathetic and parasympathetic nerves (S2-4). It is in a constant state of contraction due to intrinsic slow-wave impulses. The IAS muscle is surrounded by the striated muscles of the external anal sphincter (EAS), which is a voluntary muscle but contributes about 30% to the overall resting tone. The EAS is supplied by the pudendal nerves.

The pelvic floor (levator ani muscles) is composed of symmetrical sheets of striated muscles with a central ligamentous attachment—the pubococcygeus, the iliococcygeus, and the puborectalis. These muscles surround and support the rectum, vagina, and urethra as they pass through to the perineum. The puborectalis, which wraps around the anorectal junction posteriorly and inserts on the pubic ramus anteriorly, is particularly important to overall continence by increasing the acute angle between the rectum and anal canal, known as the anorectal angle.

Normal defecation is an intricate sequence of events that relies on proper relaxation of these muscles and a few key anorectal reflexes. The stimulus for initiating defecation is distention of the rectum, which stimulates pressure receptors in the pelvic floor muscles, also known as accommodation. This in turn triggers two key reflexes: (1) relaxation of the internal sphincter, the rectoanal inhibitory reflex (RAIR), and (2) contraction of the external sphincter, the rectoanal excitatory reflex. This process allows sampling of the rectal contents that come into contact with the upper anal canal. This allows us to discriminate between gas, liquid, or solid stools. Once the decision has been made to evacuate the rectum, the puborectalis muscle relaxes and allows straightening of the anorectal angle. Intra-abdominal pressure increases and the EAS relaxes to allow passage of contents through the anus.

In conjunction with a careful history, there are several useful modalities that are employed to investigate evacuation dysfunction. Anal manometry, defecography, endorectal ultrasound, and pudendal nerve terminal motor latency testing can be integral in the diagnosis of fecal incontinence, pelvic dyssynergia, constipation, rectocele, and intussusception, to name a few. A thorough understanding of the anatomy, patient history, and available testing modalities is imperative for diagnosis and treatment.

Bajwa A, Emmanuel A: The physiology of continence and evacuation. *Best Pract Res Clin Gastroenterol.* 2009;23(4):477-485.

Barleben A, Mills S: Anorectal anatomy and physiology. *Surg Clin North Am.* 2010;90(1):1-15.

Cho HM: Anorectal physiology: test and clinical application. *J Korean Soc Coloproctol.* 2010;26(5):311-315.

Stoker J: Anorectal and pelvic floor anatomy. *Best Pract Res Clin Gastroenterol.* 2009;23(4):463-475.

Van Koughnett JA, da Silva G: Anorectal physiology and testing. *Gastroenterol Clin North Am.* 2013;42(4):713-728.

FECAL INCONTINENCE

▶ General Considerations

Complete anal continence results from the complex interactions between stool consistency, rectal capacity and compliance, the sphincter complex, and underlying neurologic function. Impairment in one or all of these components results in varying degrees of fecal incontinence, which is defined as the recurrent, involuntary loss of feces or gas through the anus for a period greater than 1 month.

The true incidence of fecal incontinence is difficult to determine due to lack of standard definitions and underreporting; however, rates up to 20% have been reported in the literature, depending on the study population. Female patients predominate in most series of major incontinence, but men and women are affected equally with minor incontinence. Higher rates have been reported in the elderly and patients with certain neurologic disorders.

There are numerous causes of fecal incontinence; however, the most common is related to obstetric injury. Obstetric tears with vaginal deliveries have been reported in up to 10% of cases. Additionally, occult injuries have been identified by ultrasound in up to 35% of cases; therefore, presentation with symptoms of incontinence or leakage may be delayed. Other causes include congenital anomalies, neurologic disorder (eg, spinal cord injury), pelvic floor denervation (stretch-induced injury of the pudendal nerves), conditions causing poor rectal compliance (eg, Crohn disease, ulcerative colitis, radiation proctitis), functional bowel disorders (diarrhea or fecal impaction with overflow incontinence), and iatrogenic injuries (eg, anorectal surgeries).

▶ Clinical Findings

A. Symptoms and Signs

A detailed history of the presenting symptoms is required to differentiate the patient's ability to control gas, liquid, and solid stools. Frank incontinence must be differentiated from fecal urgency or soiling, which may be associated with other treatable anorectal disorders. Information on diet, activity, medications, and obstetric and anorectal surgical history should also be gathered to provide a more complete picture. This is understandably a potentially devastating disorder, so attempts should also be made to ascertain the overall level of impact of these symptoms on the patient's daily activities and quality of life. To aid in this characterization, there are several validated scoring systems, including the Fecal Incontinence Severity Index (FISI) score, the Cleveland Clinic Florida Incontinence score, and the Fecal Incontinence Quality of Life scale, that can provide a patient's subjective baseline of these symptoms and can be used to track progress throughout treatment.

Physical evaluation should begin with inspection of the anus and perineum, to document any scars from previous obstetric or anorectal procedures. Benign anorectal conditions, such as fistulas, prolapse, and hemorrhoids, may also be readily excluded. Perineal descent during straining is another important finding that indicates an abnormal laxity of the pelvic floor muscles. Digital rectal exam provides useful initial information on the sphincter tone and maximum squeeze pressure. Anoscopy can also be used to rule out other causes of incontinence such as hemorrhoids, a mass, or inflammatory bowel disease.

B. Imaging Studies

Further testing for fecal incontinence often requires an integrated approach. Anal manometry, endoanal ultrasound, MRI, defecography, and pudendal nerve latency studies have all been employed in the evaluation of the patient with fecal incontinence.

Endoanal ultrasound can be used in the evaluation of patients with fecal incontinence who have a history of previous surgery or vaginal delivery. It is an inexpensive office-based procedure that allows visualization of the length and width of the sphincter complex as well as any defects that may be present.

Anal manometry provides an objective assessment of sphincter function, including resting sphincter pressure, maximum squeeze pressure, anal canal pressure, anorectal sensation, and compliance. Resting pressure is in large part a reflection of internal sphincter muscle function, while maximum squeeze pressure reflects external sphincter function. High-resolution anal manometry provides more data than traditional manometry and additionally provides a three-dimensional graphic representation of anal canal anatomy. The advances in high-resolution anal manometry may be as effective as endoanal ultrasound at detecting sphincter defects.

Defecography has a more limited role in the evaluation of incontinence. The study allows visualization of the process of defecation, including the anorectal angle, pelvic floor descent, and internal intussusception.

Pudendal nerve motor latency testing provides information about potential nerve damage to the pelvic floor. It measures the time from nerve stimulation to the onset of response of the pelvic floor muscles. Prolonged times are indicative of neuropathy. The degree of denervation does not influence the severity of incontinence but does seem to provide some prognostic information about the outcomes of surgical repairs. This testing may prove to be more useful in patients who remain incontinent after a repair.

It is important to consider endoscopic workup in patients with fecal incontinence who present with diarrhea, bleeding, or other symptoms concerning for malignancy.

▶ Treatment

The initial management of patients with fecal incontinence should include nonoperative measures that aim to optimize stool consistency and motility. Patients should be educated on keeping a food diary. Diet modification should be tailored to avoid aggravating foods, which may include caffeine, lactose, and sugar substitutes. Several medications may have effects on colonic transit and sphincter relaxation including antidepressants, antidiarrheals, and opioids. Clonidine may also reduce rectal urgency. Fiber supplementation can improve stool consistency. Biofeedback training, or pelvic floor exercises, should be considered in patients who do not respond to the above recommendations alone. If these measures fail, then consideration should be given to surgical repair. Options include sphincteroplasty, sacral nerve stimulation, injectable bulking agents, artificial bowel sphincter, and fecal diversion.

Anterior sphincteroplasty involves direct repair, either in an overlapping or end-to-end fashion, of the external sphincter muscle if a segmental defect is identified on preoperative evaluation. This technique has good short-term results, with up to 85% of patients with obstetrical related injury experiencing improvement in function; however, at 5-10 years of follow-up, function does tend to deteriorate. In the literature, diminished success rates have been associated with age, duration of symptoms, and pudendal neuropathy. Repeat sphincteroplasty has had poor results and is not recommended.

Sacral nerve stimulation treats fecal incontinence through improvement of rectal sensation. It provides the unique advantage of a temporary evaluation phase before permanent implantation. A temporary electrode is placed with the aid of fluoroscopy into the sacral foramen (usually the third), and the patient is subsequently stimulated for 2-3 weeks. If there is at least a 50% reduction in symptoms, then a permanent stimulator is implanted. Success of sacral nerve stimulation does not appear to be affected by different mechanisms of fecal incontinence. A multicenter study reported achieving complete continence in 36% of patients at 5-year follow-up. Complications include infection and need for revision or replacement.

The artificial bowel sphincter is another modality that is approved for treatment of incontinence but is not widely used. The device, which is surgically placed around the sphincter complex, is connected to a tunneled reservoir and pump that inflates and deflates the cuff to allow controlled defecation. This procedure has been limited by infectious complications and device erosion; therefore, it is typically reserved for end-stage incontinence in patients without other alternatives except colostomy.

Passive fecal incontinence caused by internal sphincter dysfunction may respond to injection of bulking agents. Small series have reported the injection of silicone biomaterial into the intersphincteric plane or submucosa with short-term improvement in continence; however, the results remain varied.

Other developing treatments for fecal incontinence include radiofrequency energy delivery and the magnetic sphincter. Radiofrequency energy delivery to the sphincter complex may increase the smooth muscle–to–connective tissue ratio. Early studies suggest some improvement in symptoms. The magnetic sphincter is a string of titanium beads that is implanted into the anus that remains closed until pressure associated with defecation causes the beads to separate.

If conservative and other surgical options have failed, then a diverting colostomy becomes a reasonable solution that can restore a patient's quality of life.

▶ Prognosis

Fecal incontinence is a treatable condition; however, appropriate management requires careful evaluation and proper patient selection. Surgical intervention should be preceded by an initial trial of conservative measures if indicated. Sphincteroplasty has good short-term results with initial success rates of approximately 75%; however, success diminishes over time. Sacral nerve stimulation has been an exciting new surgical development for fecal incontinence with greater than 80% of patients maintaining more than 50% reduction of symptoms after 1-2 years of permanent implantation. Complications requiring explantation of the device are uncommon.

Brown SR, Wadhawan H, Nelson RL: Surgery for faecal incontinence in adults. *Cochrane Database Syst Rev.* 2010;9:CD001757.

Frascio M, Mandolfino F, Imperatore M, et al: The SECCA procedure for faecal incontinence: a review. *Colorectal Dis.* 2014;16(3):167-172.

Glasgow SC, Lowry AC: Long-term outcomes of anal sphincter repair for fecal incontinence: a systematic review. *Dis Colon Rectum.* 2012;55(4):482-490.

Guerra F, La Torre M, Giuliani G, et al: Long-term evaluation of bulking agents for the treatment of fecal incontinence: clinical outcomes and ultrasound evidence. *Tech Coloproctol.* 2015;19(1):23-27.

Hannaway CD, Hull TL: Fecal incontinence. *Obstet Gynecol Clin North Am.* 2008;35(2):249-269.

Norton C, Cody JD: Biofeedback and/or sphincter exercises for the treatment of faecal incontinence in adults. *Cochrane Database Syst Rev.* 2012;7:CD002111.

Rezaie A, Iriana S, Pimentel M, et al: Can three-dimensional high-resolution anorectal manometry detect anal sphincter defects in patients with faecal incontinence? *Colorectal Dis.* 2017;19(5):468-475.

Sugrue J, Lehur PA, Madoff RD, et al: Longterm experience of magnetic anal sphincter augmentation in patients with fecal incontinence. *Dis Colon Rectum.* 2017;60(1):87-95.

Wexner SD, Coller JA, Devroede G, et al: Sacral nerve stimulation for fecal incontinence: results of a 120-patient prospective multicenter study. *Ann Surg.* 2010;251(3):441-449.

PELVIC FLOOR DYSFUNCTION

▶ General Considerations

Pelvic floor dysfunction is a global term that can encapsulate several presentations including dysfunctional urinary and bowel evacuation symptoms, sexual dysfunction, and pain syndromes. Alternative terms, such as *pelvic dyssynergia*, *obstructed defecation*, and *paradoxic puborectalis*, have also been used, further confounding the understanding of the topic. Functional disorders of the pelvic floor are marked by symptoms of obstructed defecation without an anatomic abnormality in the surrounding muscles. As outlined earlier, the process of defecation is intricate. It requires coordination of the pelvic nerves, the rectum, and the surrounding muscles, including the puborectalis and the remaining levator muscles. During normal defecation, these muscles relax, allowing the rectum to empty; however, patients with pelvic floor dysfunction have uncoordinated activity that impairs evacuation of intestinal waste.

Understandably, this is can be a debilitating problem affecting a large number of patients, which are predominantly women. In the United States, approximately 24% of women report at least one pelvic floor disorder, which seems to increase with age, parity, and obesity.

▶ Clinical Findings

A. Symptoms and Signs

Symptoms of pelvic floor dysfunction tend to develop slowly and insidiously; therefore, a careful history is paramount to establishing a working diagnosis and developing a strategy for diagnostic testing. Patients commonly describe constipation, straining with bowel movements, or the sense of incomplete evacuation that may require digital evacuation. The residual soft stool in the rectal vault may cause soiling of the anoderm, triggering the feeling of incontinence. Attention should be paid to diet as well as obstetric, urologic, and surgical histories. Although these symptoms do not impose risk to the patient's health, they do interfere with the overall quality of life. At the time of presentation, patients have often tried a plethora of medications and laxatives.

A focused physical examination should start with inspection of the anus and perineum. Profound perineal descent with straining is an indication of laxity of the pelvic floor, which is common with increasing age and multiparity. Digital rectal examination is important and should be performed to rule out rectal masses, to assess pain with palpation of the puborectalis, and to assess sphincter tone and contraction/relaxation of the levator muscles. Specifically, paradoxic contraction of the puborectalis with simulated straining should be also be assessed.

B. Laboratory and Imaging Studies

A colonoscopy and colon transit study should generally be performed to exclude an underlying malignancy and slow-transit constipation, respectively. Additional adjuncts include anal manometry with balloon expulsion and defecography. Anal manometry should assess resting and maximum squeeze pressure as well as the presence of the RAIR. Patients with pelvic floor dysfunction are typically unable to expel a balloon that is inserted into the rectum.

Fluoroscopic defecography offers a more dynamic view of the rectum, pelvic floor muscles, and anal sphincters. During this exam, the rectum is filled with contrast, and the patient is asked to simulate defecation. Vaginal and oral contrast materials are also usually given to provide additional information about the neighboring structures. Defecography is useful in identifying rectoceles, internal and external rectal prolapse, enteroceles, and a nonrelaxing pelvic floor. Magnetic resonance defecography has been more recently used and can also be helpful for both diagnosis and treatment decisions.

▶ Differential Diagnosis

Symptoms of constipation and defecation problems are quite common and may be due to a myriad of causes. Anatomic disorders, such as anal or rectal cancers, rectoceles, rectal prolapse, internal intussusception, and enteroceles, should be distinguished from functional disorders such as a nonrelaxing puborectalis.

▶ Treatment

A. Medical Treatment

Patients with pelvic floor dysfunction due to a nonrelaxing puborectalis should be referred for pelvic floor retraining, also known as biofeedback, which has become an integral part of treatment. During these sessions with the physical therapist, patients are instructed on how to properly relax the pelvic muscles with the aid of visual feedback. This neuromuscular training program is typically instrument based, employing manometry or electromyography-based biofeedback.

B. Surgical Treatment

Patients with obstructed defecation due to anatomic causes are candidates for surgery if they have failed initial conservative therapy with fiber supplementation and laxatives.

Rectocele repair is indicated for large rectoceles greater than 2 cm that are symptomatic. The two main surgical approaches are transanal and transvaginal. The transanal approach involves plicating the vaginal wall to obliterate the sac, followed by reinforcing the anterior rectal wall. The transvaginal approach involves excising a portion of the vaginal wall from the introitus to the apex, reducing the rectocele, and suturing the vaginal edges closed. The stapled transanal rectal resection (STARR) procedure is another option that uses two circular staplers to produce a circumferential transanal full-thickness resection of the lower rectum.

Internal rectal prolapse (intussusception) can be present in up to 50% of asymptomatic individuals; therefore, the surgical treatment of internal prolapse associated with obstructed defecation symptoms remains controversial. Rectopexy without concomitant resection has been advocated by some, and the STARR procedure has been used by others. Results have been varied in the literature.

Prognosis

Biofeedback has been the mainstay of treatment for nonrelaxing pelvic floor dysfunction. It is minimally invasive and repeatable with good results for those who complete the program. Improvement in symptoms has varied between 40% and 90% in several trials.

Faubion SS, Shuster LT, Bharucha AE. Recognition and management of nonrelaxing pelvic floor dysfunction. *Mayo Clin Proc.* 2012;87(2):187-193.

Liu WC, Wan SL, Yaseen SM, et al: Transanal surgery for obstructed defecation syndrome: Literature review and a single-center experience. *World J Gastroenterol.* 2016;22(35):7983-7998.

McNevin MS: Overview of pelvic floor disorders. *Surg Clin North Am.* 2010;90(1):195-205.

Murad-Regadas SM, Regadas FS, Bezerra CC, et al: Use of biofeedback combined with diet for treatment of obstructed defecation associated with paradoxical puborectalis contraction (anismus): predictive factors and short-term outcome. *Dis Colon Rectum.* 2016;59(2):115-121.

Nygaard I, Barber MD, Burgio KL, et al: Prevalence of symptomatic pelvic floor disorders in US women. *JAMA.* 2008; 300(11):1311-1316.

Piloni V, Tosi P, Vernelli M: MR-defecography in obstructed defecation syndrome (ODS): technique, diagnostic criteria and grading. *Tech Coloproctol.* 2013 Oct;17(5):501-10.

Rao SS: Dyssynergic defecation and biofeedback therapy. *Gastroenterol Clin North Am.* 2008;37(3):569-586, viii.

ABNORMAL RECTAL FIXATION

▶ General Considerations

Abnormal rectal fixation is a general term for a group of diseases in which the attachment of the rectum to its surrounding structures has developed more laxity, allowing the rectum to, completely or incompletely, protrude through the anal canal. The exact pathophysiology is unknown, but in large part, this is related to chronic straining with defecation. Common anatomic variations may include a patulous anus, redundant sigmoid colon, diastasis of the levator ani muscles, and a deep cul-de-sac.

Rectal prolapse is characterized by an intussusception of the rectum. There are three general categories that ultimately influence symptoms and overall management: (1) internal prolapse (intussusception), which does not extend beyond the anal canal; (2) mucosal prolapse; and (3) complete prolapse, which involves full-thickness protrusion of the rectum through the anus.

In adults, older women are six times more likely to develop rectal prolapse, accounting for 80%-90% of the patient populations. The peak incidence is after the fifth decade.

▶ Clinical Findings

A. Symptoms and Signs

Symptoms can vary with the degree of rectal prolapse, but typical complaints include a perianal mass that protrudes with straining, mucoid or bloody discharge, incomplete evacuation, and pain if the rectum becomes incarcerated. Symptoms can also include incontinence or constipation.

On examination, a patulous anus or exaggerated perineal descent may be initial clues to the diagnosis if prolapsing rectal tissue is not evident. Digital rectal examination may reveal diminished or absent tone with complete prolapse but may suggest a mass with straining for internal intussusception. The diagnosis is most easily made with the patient straining in the seated position, which should reproduce the rectal prolapse, identified by the concentric folds of mucosa.

B. Laboratory and Imaging Studies

If the diagnosis remains elusive, defecography should be able to clearly demonstrate either internal prolapse as well as other associated abnormalities such as cystoceles, enteroceles, and rectoceles. In patients who also present with complaints of longstanding constipation, anorectal manometry and colon transit studies are helpful. Patients should also be asked about urinary incontinence and vaginal prolapse because it is not uncommon to have multivisceral prolapse. Prior to any surgical intervention, these patients should also undergo colonoscopy to be sure that a mass is not the cause of prolapse.

Differential Diagnosis

Complete rectal prolapse is often confused with prolapsing internal hemorrhoids; however, the two can easily be separated by close examination of the mucosa. Prolapsing internal hemorrhoids produce radials folds in the visible rectal mucosa, which contrasts with the concentric folds seen with rectal prolapse.

Complications

The most dreaded complication for rectal prolapse is incarceration, which may lead to tissue ischemia and necrosis. Chronic reducible rectal prolapse may also impair fecal continence due to the repeated stretching of the sphincter muscles.

Treatment

A. Medical Treatment

Medical therapy has a limited role in treating rectal prolapse. Associated symptoms of fecal incontinence or constipation can be treated accordingly. A trial of fiber supplementation and diet modification may prove to be beneficial for mild cases of internal intussusception.

B. Surgical Treatment

Surgical treatment is indicated in patients with full-thickness rectal prolapse. Surgical treatment is broadly divided into abdominal and perineal approaches, which are dictated by the patient's age and comorbidities as well as surgeon preference and experience. Perineal approaches generally result in reduced length of hospital stay and less perioperative morbidity and pain; however, they are plagued by higher recurrence rates.

Rectopexy, resection rectopexy, and mesh rectopexy are the three abdominal procedures that are most widely practiced. The principle component of each of these procedures is the posterior mobilization of the rectum down to the level of the levator muscles. The rectum is elevated from the deep pelvis and sutured to the presacral fascia at the level of the sacral promontory. The lateral ligaments are preserved, as this has been shown to decrease postoperative constipation. Sigmoid resection with tension-free anastomosis to the rectum is performed if excessive redundancy is encountered or if there has been a longstanding history of constipation. Mesh has also been used to fix the rectum to the presacral fascia and should be performed without a concomitant resection. Complications include bowel obstruction, erosion of the mesh, and fistulas. All of these abdominal procedures have been approached laparoscopically with similar results, while maintaining the benefits of a minimally invasive technique.

Perineal proctosigmoidectomy, also known as the Altemeier procedure, combines a perineal proctosigmoidectomy with an anterior levatoroplasty. A full-thickness, circumferential incision is made 1 cm proximal to the dentate line. The mesentery of the rectum and sigmoid colon is sequentially divided until no redundant bowel remains. The colon is transected at this level, and an anastomosis is created between the colon and the anal canal with either sutures or a circular stapler. An anterior levatoroplasty is usually added to correct the laxity in the levator muscles commonly associated with this condition

The Delorme procedure is ideal for short segment mucosal prolapse since it entails a mucosal sleeve resection starting at the dentate line. The excess mucosa and submucosa are transected, and the proximal and distal edges are approximated. The muscle is plicated, with interrupted sutures placed circumferentially.

Prognosis

The described abdominal approaches have been shown to be safe and efficacious with approximately a 10% recurrence rate. Perineal approaches are also well tolerated but are associated with higher recurrence rates of 20%-30%.

Blaker K, Amandam JL: Functional disorders: rectoanal intussusception. *Clin Colon Rectal Surg.* 2017;30(1):5-11.

Bordeianou L, Paquette I, Johnson E, et al: Clinical practice guidelines for the treatment of rectal prolapse. *Dis Colon Rectum.* 2017; 60(11):1121-1131.

Cadeddu F, Sileri P, Grande M, et al: Focus on abdominal rectopexy for full-thickness rectal prolapse: meta-analysis of literature. *Tech Coloproctol.* 2012;16 (1):37-53.

Goldstein SD, Maxwell PJ: Rectal prolapse. *Clin Colon Rectal Surg.* 2011;24 (1):39-45.

Sajid MS, Siddiqui MR, Baig MK: Open vs laparoscopic repair of full-thickness rectal prolapse: a re-meta-analysis. *Colorectal Dis.* 2010;12 (6):515-525.

Tou S, Brown SR, Malik AI, et al: Surgery for complete rectal prolapse in adults. *Cochrane Database Syst Rev.* 2008;4:CD001758.

MULTIPLE CHOICE QUESTIONS

1. All of the following are sites of perirectal fistulas, except

    A. Suprasphincteric
    B. Transsphincteric
    C. Intersphincteric
    D. Infralevator
    E. Submucosal

2. Anal bleeding can be commonly caused by

    A. Diverticulitis
    B. Anal condyloma
    C. Anorectal abscess (undrained)
    D. Anal fissure
    E. Thrombosed external hemorrhoids

3. Rectal prolapse

   A. Can be distinguished from prolapsed hemorrhoids based on exam showing concentric folds of the mucosa
   B. Is more common in males
   C. Cannot involve the muscular layers of the rectum due to fixation to the pelvic sidewalls
   D. Is best evaluated by magnetic resonance imaging
   E. Is more common in men than women

4. Squamous cell tumors of the anal canal

   A. Are typically treated with a regimen of chemotherapy and radiation therapy after diagnosis
   B. Are about as common as rectal cancers
   C. Have a 25% response rate to initial therapy regimens
   D. Typically require abdominoperineal resection for complete treatment
   E. Rarely metastasize to regional lymph nodes

5. Condyloma acuminata

   A. Are unlikely to recur after treatment
   B. Are often treated with antiviral therapy as first-line treatment
   C. Can be managed by palliation of macroscopic lesions by operation
   D. Do not carry any risk of dysplasia
   E. Are always asymptomatic

Abdominal Wall Hernias

Sean B. Orenstein, MD
Karen E. Deveney, MD

▼ I. HERNIAS

INTRODUCTION AND DEFINITIONS

Abdominal wall integrity relies on organized anatomic layering of muscle and fascia to contain the intra-abdominal contents. A defect in one or more layers of fasciae can result in a hernia, which represents an abnormal protrusion of intra-abdominal contents through the fascial defect. Groin hernias represent the most common type of abdominal wall hernias (~75%), whereas ventral, umbilical, and other types of hernias compose the rest. Of the various types of ventral hernias, incisional hernias represent the majority of these, stemming from a failure of appropriate healing following a surgical incision. In general, a hernia is composed of covering tissues (eg, skin, subcutaneous tissues), a peritoneal sac (hernia sac), and various contents including preperitoneal fat, omental fat, and/or any visceral organs. In particular, if the neck of the hernia defect is narrow where it emerges from the abdomen, bowel protruding into the hernia may become compromised (obstruction or strangulation). If the hernia is not repaired early, the defect may enlarge, and operative repair may become more complicated. Although some hernias can be observed over time, the definitive treatment of hernias is operative repair.

A **reducible hernia** is one in which the contents of the sac return to the abdomen spontaneously or with manual pressure when the patient is recumbent. An **incarcerated (irreducible) hernia** is one whose contents cannot be returned to the abdomen, usually because they are trapped by a narrow neck. The term *incarceration* does not imply obstruction, inflammation, or ischemia of the herniated organs, although incarceration is typically a requisite for obstruction or strangulation to occur.

Compromise of bowel or other viscera can occur with incarcerated hernias. Bowel **obstruction** results from kinking or twisting of bowel within the hernia, which in turn leads to dilation of the proximal bowel due to blockage of the bowel lumen. However, obstruction does not imply any compromise to the blood supply. Compromise to the blood supply of the hernia contents (eg, omentum or intestine) results in a **strangulated hernia,** in which gangrene of the viscera has occurred. The incidence of strangulation is higher in femoral than in inguinal hernias, but strangulation may occur in any hernia.

An uncommon and dangerous type of hernia, a **Richter hernia**, occurs when only part of the circumference of the bowel becomes incarcerated or strangulated in the fascial defect. Because the bowel is not obstructed, and because only a portion of the bowel wall becomes strangulated, a **Richter hernia** commonly presents late in the clinical course after focal perforation and resultant peritonitis.

HERNIAS OF THE GROIN

▶ Anatomy

All groin hernias protrude through the myopectineal orifice of Fruchaud, a weakness or defect in the **transversalis fascia**, an aponeurosis located just outside the peritoneum. External to the transversalis fascia are found the **transversus abdominis, internal oblique,** and **external oblique muscles,** which are fleshy laterally and aponeurotic medially. Their aponeuroses form investing layers of the strong **rectus abdominis muscles** superior to the arcuate line (linea semicircularis or line of Douglas). Inferior to this line, the aponeurosis lies entirely in front of the muscle, leaving only the transversalis fascia and peritoneum as posterior layers. Between the two vertical rectus muscles, the aponeuroses meet again in the midline to form the **linea alba,** which is well defined above the umbilicus. The subcutaneous fat contains the Scarpa fascia, which is a misnomer, since it is only a condensation of connective tissue with no substantial strength.

In the groin, an **indirect inguinal hernia** results when obliteration of the processus vaginalis, the peritoneal extension accompanying the testis in its descent into the scrotum, fails to occur. The resultant hernia sac passes through the **internal inguinal ring,** a defect in the transversalis fascia halfway between the anterior iliac spine and the pubic tubercle. The sac is located anteromedially within the spermatic cord and may extend partway along the **inguinal canal** or accompany the cord out through the subcutaneous (external) inguinal ring. The sac and the spermatic cord are invested by **cremaster muscles,** an extension of fibers of the internal oblique muscle.

The **Hesselbach triangle** is bounded by the inguinal ligament, the inferior epigastric vessels, and the lateral border of the rectus muscle. A weakness or defect in the transversalis fascia, which forms the floor of this triangle, results in a **direct inguinal hernia.** In most direct hernias, the transversalis fascia is diffusely attenuated, although a discrete defect in the fascia may occasionally occur. Whereas direct inguinal hernias run through the Hesselbach triangle and are located *medial* to the inferior epigastric vessels, indirect inguinal hernias are located *lateral* to the inferior epigastric vessels. The peritoneum may protrude on both sides of the inferior epigastric vessels, giving rise to a combined direct and indirect hernia, called a **pantaloon hernia.**

Other anatomic structures of the groin that are important in understanding the formation of hernias and types of hernia repairs include the **conjoint tendon,** a fusion of the medial aponeurotic transversus abdominis and internal oblique muscles that passes along the inferolateral edge of the rectus abdominis muscle and attaches to the pubic tubercle. Between the pubic tubercle and the anterior iliac spine passes the **inguinal (Poupart) ligament,** formed by the lowermost border of the external oblique aponeurosis as it rolls on itself and thickens into a cord.

Just deep and parallel to the inguinal ligament runs the **iliopubic tract,** a band of connective tissue that extends from the iliopsoas fascia, crosses below the deep inguinal ring, forms the superior border of the femoral sheath, and inserts into the superior pubic ramus to form the **lacunar (Gimbernat) ligament.** The lacunar ligament is about 1.25 cm long and triangular in shape. The sharp, crescentic lateral border of this ligament is the unyielding noose for the strangulation of a femoral hernia.

Cooper ligaments are strong, fibrous bands that extend laterally for about 2.5 cm along the iliopectineal line on the superior aspect of the superior pubic ramus, starting at the lateral base of the lacunar ligament. These ligaments overlie the pubic bone and are useful for securing mesh during inguinal or lower abdominal wall hernias with tacks or sutures.

A **femoral hernia** passes beneath the iliopubic tract and inguinal ligament into the upper thigh. The predisposing anatomic feature for femoral hernias is a small empty space between the lacunar ligament medially and the femoral vein laterally—the **femoral canal.** Because its borders are distinct and unyielding, a femoral hernia carries one of the highest risks of incarceration and strangulation of groin hernias.

Surgeons must be familiar with the pathways of the nerves and blood vessels of the inguinal region to avoid injuring them when repairing groin hernias. The iliohypogastric nerve (T12, L1) emerges from the lateral edge of the psoas muscle and travels inside the external oblique muscle, emerging medial to the external inguinal ring to innervate the suprapubic skin. The ilioinguinal nerve (L1) parallels the iliohypogastric nerve and travels on the surface of the spermatic cord to innervate the base of the penis (or mons pubis), the scrotum (or labia majora), and the medial thigh. This nerve is the most frequently injured in anterior open inguinal hernia repairs. The genitofemoral (L1, L2) and lateral femoral cutaneous nerves (L2, L3) travel on and lateral to the psoas muscle and provide sensation to the scrotum and anteromedial thigh and to the lateral thigh, respectively. These nerves are subject to injury during laparoscopic hernia repairs. The femoral nerve (L2-L4) travels from the lateral edge of the psoas and extends lateral to the femoral vessels. It can be injured during laparoscopic or femoral hernia repairs.

The external iliac artery travels along the medial aspect of the psoas muscle and beneath the inguinal ligament, giving off the inferior epigastric artery, which borders the medial aspect of the internal inguinal ring. The corresponding veins accompany the arteries. These vessels can be injured during hernia repairs of all types.

▶ Etiology

Nearly all inguinal hernias in infants, children, and young adults are **indirect inguinal hernias.** Although these "congenital" hernias are often present during the first year of life, the first clinical evidence of hernia may not appear until middle or old age, when increased intra-abdominal pressure and dilation of the internal inguinal ring allow abdominal contents to enter the previously empty peritoneal diverticulum. An untreated indirect hernia will inevitably dilate the internal ring and displace or attenuate the inguinal floor.

In contrast, **direct inguinal hernias** are acquired as the result of a developed weakness of the transversalis fascia in the Hesselbach area. There is some evidence that direct inguinal hernias may be related to hereditary or acquired defects in collagen synthesis or turnover. **Femoral hernias** involve an acquired protrusion of a peritoneal sac through the femoral ring. In women, the ring may become dilated by physical and biochemical changes during pregnancy.

Any condition that chronically increases intra-abdominal pressure may contribute to the appearance and progression of a hernia. Marked obesity, abdominal strain from heavy exercise or lifting, cough, constipation with straining at stool, and prostatism with straining on micturition are often implicated. Cirrhosis with ascites, pregnancy, chronic ambulatory peritoneal dialysis, and chronically enlarged pelvic organs or pelvic tumors may also contribute. Loss of tissue turgor in the Hesselbach area, associated with a weakening of the transversalis fascia, occurs with advancing age and in chronic debilitating disease.

INDIRECT & DIRECT INGUINAL HERNIAS

▶ Clinical Findings

A. Symptoms

Most hernias produce no symptoms until the patient notices a lump or swelling in the groin, although some patients may describe a sudden pain and bulge that occurred while lifting or straining. Frequently, hernias are detected in the course of routine physical examinations such as preemployment examinations. Some patients complain of a dragging sensation and, particularly with indirect inguinal hernias, radiation of pain into the scrotum. As a hernia enlarges, it is likely to produce a sense of discomfort or aching pain in the groin region, with relief if the patient is able to manually reduce the hernia contents.

B. Signs

Examination of the groin reveals a mass that may or may not be reducible. The patient should be examined both supine and standing and also with Valsalva (coughing and straining), since small hernias may be difficult to demonstrate. The external ring can be identified by invaginating the scrotum and palpating with the index finger just above and lateral to the pubic tubercle (Figure 34–1). If the external ring is very small, the

▲ **Figure 34–1.** Insertion of finger through upper scrotum into the external inguinal ring.

examiner's finger may not enter the inguinal canal, and it may be difficult to be sure that a pulsation felt on coughing is truly a hernia. At the other extreme, a widely patent external ring does not by itself constitute hernia. Tissue must be felt protruding into the inguinal canal during coughing in order for a hernia to be diagnosed.

Differentiating between direct and indirect inguinal hernia on examination is difficult, with identification typically taking place during the operative procedure. Nevertheless, each type of inguinal hernia has specific features more common to it. A hernia that descends into the scrotum is commonly associated with an indirect defect. On inspection with the patient erect and straining, a direct hernia more commonly appears as a symmetric, circular swelling, whereas an indirect hernia appears as an elliptic swelling given its path though the inguinal canal.

On palpation, the posterior wall of the inguinal canal is firm and resistant in an indirect hernia but relaxed or absent in a direct hernia. If the patient is asked to Valsalva while the examining finger is directed laterally and upward into the inguinal canal, an indirect hernia will lead to an impulse felt at the tip of the finger. In a direct hernia, the impulse is felt more medially, on the side of the finger. The fascial edges of a direct hernia defect may also be palpable medially. Many inguinal hernias result in a vague impulse with Valsalva, without knowing the exact type of hernia until time of repair. Compression over the internal ring when the patient strains may also help to differentiate between indirect and direct hernias. A direct hernia bulges forward through the Hesselbach triangle, but the opposite hand can maintain reduction of an indirect hernia at the internal ring.

These distinctions are obscured as a hernia enlarges and distorts the anatomic relationships of the inguinal rings and canal. In many patients, the type of inguinal hernia cannot be established accurately before surgery.

▶ Differential Diagnosis

Groin pain of musculoskeletal or obscure origin that occurs primarily with vigorous physical exertion is called **athletic pubalgia** (ie, "sports hernia") and may be difficult to distinguish from a true hernia, even with thorough physical examination. Magnetic resonance imaging (MRI) may be helpful in identifying the problem, shown as inflammation, edema, or a muscle or tendon tear or strain.

Herniation of preperitoneal fat through the inguinal ring into the spermatic cord ("cord lipoma") is commonly misinterpreted as a hernia. Its true nature may only be confirmed at operation. Cord lipomas are extremely common, and efforts should be made during inguinal hernia repair to find and remove them, since they may cause discomfort if left in place.

Occasionally, a femoral hernia that has extended above the inguinal ligament after passing through the fossa ovalis femoris may be confused with an inguinal hernia. If the examining finger is placed on the pubic tubercle, the neck of the sac of a femoral hernia lies lateral and below, whereas that of an inguinal hernia lies above.

Inguinal hernia must be differentiated from hydrocele of the spermatic cord, lymphadenopathy or abscesses of the groin, varicocele, and residual hematoma following trauma or spontaneous hemorrhage in patients taking anticoagulants. An undescended testis in the inguinal canal must also be considered when the testis cannot be felt in the scrotum.

The presence of an impulse in the mass with coughing, bowel sounds in the mass, and failure to transilluminate are features that indicate that an irreducible mass in the groin is a hernia.

Treatment of Inguinal Hernias

Although inguinal hernias have traditionally been repaired electively to avoid the risks of incarceration, obstruction, and strangulation, asymptomatic or mildly symptomatic hernias may be safely observed in elderly, sedentary patients or those with high morbidity for operation. The annual risk of bowel compromise from an incarcerated hernia is not precisely known but has been estimated at fewer than 2 per 1000 patients per year. However, a high percentage of patients become symptomatic while being observed expectantly. All symptomatic groin hernias should be repaired if the patient can tolerate surgery.

Even elderly patients tolerate elective repair of a groin hernia very well when other medical problems are optimally controlled and local anesthetic is used. Emergency operation carries a much greater risk for the elderly than carefully planned elective operation.

If the patient has significant prostatic hyperplasia, it is prudent to solve this problem first, since the risks of postoperative urinary retention are high following hernia repair in patients with significant prostatic obstruction.

Because of the possibility of strangulation, an acutely incarcerated, severely painful, and tender hernia may require an urgent or emergent operation. Nonoperative reduction of an incarcerated hernia may first be attempted. The patient is placed with hips elevated and given analgesics and sedation sufficient to promote muscle relaxation. Repair of the hernia may be deferred if the hernia mass reduces with gentle manipulation and if there is no clinical evidence of strangulated bowel. Although strangulation is usually clinically evident, gangrenous tissue can occasionally be reduced into the abdomen by manual or spontaneous reduction. It is therefore safest to repair the reduced hernia at the earliest opportunity. At surgery, one must decide whether to explore the abdomen to make certain that the intestine is viable. If the patient has leukocytosis or clinical signs of peritonitis or if the hernia sac contains dark or bloody fluid, the abdomen should be explored, ideally with laparoscopy.

▲ **Figure 34–2.** Indirect inguinal hernia. Inguinal canal opened, showing spermatic cord retracted medially and indirect hernia peritoneal sac dissected free to above the level of the internal inguinal ring.

A. Principles of Operative Treatment of Inguinal Hernia

1. Durable repair requires that any correctable aggravating factors be identified and treated (eg, chronic cough, prostatic obstruction, colonic tumor, ascites) and that the defect be repaired without tension.

2. An indirect hernia sac should be anatomically isolated, dissected to its origin from the peritoneum, and ligated (Figure 34–2). In infants and young adults in whom the inguinal anatomy is normal, repair can usually be limited to high ligation, removal of the sac, and reduction of the internal ring to an appropriate size. For most adult hernias, the inguinal floor should also be reconstructed. The internal ring should be reduced to a size just adequate to allow egress of the cord structures. In women, the internal ring can be totally closed to prevent recurrence through that site.

3. In direct inguinal hernias (Figure 34–3), the inguinal floor is usually so weak that a primary repair using the patient's own tissues would be under tension. Although a vertical relaxing incision in the anterior rectus abdominis sheath was traditionally used, most hernia repairs are now performed using mesh so that a tension-free repair can be accomplished.

▲ **Figure 34–3.** Direct inguinal hernia. Inguinal canal opened and spermatic cord retracted inferiorly and laterally to reveal the hernia bulging through the floor of the Hesselbach triangle.

4. Even though a direct hernia is found, the cord should always be carefully searched for a possible indirect hernia as well. Exploration should include evaluation for cord lipomas.

5. In patients with large hernias, bilateral repair has traditionally been discouraged under the assumption that greater tension on the repair would result and therefore would increase the recurrence rate and surgical complications. If open mesh repair or laparoscopic methods are used, however, bilateral repairs can be done with low risk of recurrence. In children and young adults with small hernias, bilateral hernia repair is usually recommended because it spares the patient a second anesthetic.

6. Hernia recurrence within a few months or a year of operation usually indicates an inadequate repair, such as overlooking a femoral or direct hernia, failing to identify an indirect hernia sac, inadequate mesh fixation, insufficient dissection of the myopectineal orifice, or mesh folding, among other causes. Any repair completed under tension is subject to early recurrence. Recurrences 2 or more years after repair are more likely to be caused by progressive weakening of the patient's fascia. Repeated recurrence after careful repair by an experienced surgeon suggests a defect in collagen synthesis. Because the fascial defect is often small, firm, and unyielding, recurrent hernias are much more likely than unoperated inguinal hernias to develop incarceration or strangulation, and they should nearly always be repaired again.

B. Types of Operations for Inguinal Hernia

The goal of all hernia repairs is to reduce the contents of the hernia into the abdomen and reinforce the fascial defect and/ or inguinal floor. Traditional tissue-only based repairs use native tissues and suture to repair the defect. However, synthetic mesh has supplanted tissue repairs because multiple prospective, randomized studies have shown lower recurrence with tension-free mesh repairs versus traditional primary tissue repair, with the exception of specialty surgery centers that focus on tissue-based repairs.

Over the past 20 years, increased experience has been gained with minimally invasive techniques for hernia repair. Laparoscopic and robotic-assisted approaches offer less pain and more rapid return to work or normal activities. Multiple randomized trials have compared open and laparoscopic hernia repairs. Although details of specific studies vary, long-term recurrence rates of open and laparoscopic repairs are similar. The success of laparoscopic approaches is dependent on the experience of the surgeon, as is also true for open repair.

Although repairs today overwhelmingly employ prosthetic material, the presence of infection or need to resect gangrenous bowel may make use of permanent mesh unwise. In these situations, primary tissue repairs may still be a preferable option. For this reason, surgeons need to know the traditional techniques even though they are rarely used today.

Among the traditional autologous tissue repairs, the **Bassini repair** is one of the most widely used methods. In this repair, the conjoined tendon is approximated to the Poupart ligament, and the spermatic cord remains in its normal anatomic position under the external oblique aponeurosis. The **Halsted repair** places the external oblique beneath the cord but otherwise resembles the Bassini repair. **Cooper ligament (Lotheissen-McVay) repair** brings the conjoined tendon farther posteriorly and inferiorly to the Cooper ligament. Unlike the Bassini and Halsted methods, the McVay repair is also effective for femoral hernias but always requires a relaxing incision to relieve tension. Recurrence rates after these open nonmesh repairs vary widely according to skill and experience of the surgeon, but population studies show them to range from as low as 5%-10% to as high as 33%. Although the **Shouldice repair** has a lower reported recurrence rate, it is not widely used aside from specialty surgery centers, perhaps because of the more extensive dissection required. In the Shouldice repair, the transversalis fascia is first divided and then imbricated to the Poupart ligament.

Finally, the conjoined tendon and internal oblique muscle are also approximated in layers to the inguinal ligament.

A desire to decrease the recurrence rate of hernias prompted the increased use of prosthetic materials in repair of both recurrent and first-time hernias. The most widely used technique is that of **Lichtenstein**, an open mesh tension-free repair that allows an early return to normal activities and a low complication and recurrence rate. In a Lichtenstein repair, a flat piece of mesh is sewn to the inguinal ligament and secured medially to the conjoint tendon, lying in the plane between the external and internal oblique muscle layers. This procedure is sometimes accompanied by a mesh plug that is inserted into the internal ring, the so-called "plug and patch" repair.

The **open preperitoneal approach** exposes the groin from between the transversalis fascia and peritoneum via a lower abdominal incision to effect closure of the fascial defect. Because it requires more initial dissection and is associated with higher morbidity and recurrence rates in less experienced hands, it has not been widely used. For recurrent or large bilateral hernias, a preperitoneal approach using a large piece of mesh to span all areas of potential herniation has been described by Stoppa.

Minimally invasive surgery (MIS) approaches using laparoscopic and robotic-assisted technology have been developed to reduce wound complications and shorten recovery. The vast majority of MIS approaches use mesh in the repair, with the mesh placed in a posterior (preperitoneal) compartment. The visualization and dissection using MIS techniques allow wide overlap of the entire myopectineal orifice and can be used to repair most groin hernias, including indirect and direct defects, femoral hernias, and obturator hernias. Several methods have been explored, with two methods having emerged as most frequently employed: the transabdominal preperitoneal mesh (TAPP) technique and total extraperitoneal (TEP) technique. The high incidence of complications that occurred in early studies prompted revisions in the operative technique to avoid injury to lateral nerves. Several prospective randomized trials have subsequently been conducted comparing open with minimally invasive techniques as well as TAPP versus TEP. These studies have reported decreased pain and faster return to work with the minimally invasive techniques but increased operative time and cost. Laparoscopic procedures also require general anesthesia and therefore are not appropriate for all patients. Long-term hernia recurrence is equivalent with open and laparoscopic mesh repairs, at approximately 4%. TAPP and TEP techniques have demonstrated equivalency with regard to outcomes, with surgeon-specific training as the likely cause of adoption of one technique over another. Specific situations in which laparoscopic procedures often lower recurrence include the repair of recurrent hernias after previous anterior open repairs (eg, previous Lichtenstein repair), repair of bilateral hernias simultaneously, and repair in patients who must return to work particularly quickly. Although the percentage of hernias repaired laparoscopically has increased, the use of this technique varies considerably across different locales and still represents a minority of groin hernia repairs. Even with the widespread adoption of laparoscopic equipment and training, only about a third of inguinal hernias are repaired in an MIS fashion. However, there has been an increase in MIS inguinal hernia repairs being performed with the increased adoption of robotic-assisted repairs. As with many procedures, the success of both open and MIS repairs of groin hernias is highly dependent on the surgeon's skill and experience with the technique.

▶ Preoperative & Postoperative Course

Although groin hernia repair is usually an outpatient procedure, a thorough preoperative evaluation should be completed before the day of surgery. The anesthetic may be general, spinal, or local. Local anesthetic is effective for most patients, and the incidence of urinary retention and pulmonary complications is lowest with local anesthesia. Recurrent hernias are more easily repaired with the patient under spinal or general anesthesia, since local anesthetic does not readily diffuse through scar tissue. A sedentary worker may return to work within a few days; heavy manual labor has traditionally not been performed for up to 4-6 weeks after hernia repair, although recent studies document no increase in recurrence when full activity is resumed as early as 2 weeks after surgery, particularly when mesh has been used in the repair.

▶ Prognosis

In addition to chronic cough, prostatism, and constipation, poor tissue quality and poor operative technique may contribute to recurrence of inguinal hernia. Because tissue is often more attenuated in direct hernias, recurrence rates are slightly higher than for indirect hernias. Placing the repair under tension leads to recurrence. Failure to find an indirect hernia, to dissect the sac high enough, or to adequately cover the internal ring may lead to recurrence of indirect hernia. Postoperative wound infection is associated with increased recurrence. The recurrence rate is considerably increased in patients receiving chronic peritoneal dialysis, cirrhotics with ascites, smokers, and patients on steroids or who are malnourished.

The current recurrence rate after hernia repair in adults is reported at best to be 4%. Reasons for recurrence include failure to identify a femoral or indirect hernia.

An underappreciated sequela of groin hernia repair is chronic groin pain, the incidence of which varies in published series, but is commonly reported at 5%-6%. Causes include recurrent hernia, irritation or inflammation from mesh, or nerve entrapment or neuroma. Laparoscopic repair or prophylactic division of the ilioinguinal nerve in open repairs has been shown to decrease the incidence of chronic groin pain. A discussion of the risk and treatment of chronic groin pain should be a part of the informed consent for repair of groin hernias.

Nonsurgical Management (Use of a Truss)

The surgeon is occasionally called upon to prescribe a truss when a patient declines operative repair or when there are absolute contraindications to operation. A truss should be fitted to provide adequate external compression over the defect in the abdominal wall. It should be taken off at night and put on in the morning before the patient arises. The use of a truss does not preclude later repair of a hernia, although it may cause fibrosis of the anatomic structures, so that subsequent repair may be more difficult.

Alfieri S, et al: International guidelines for prevention and management of post-operative chronic pain following inguinal hernia surgery. *Hernia.* 2011;15:39-49.

Dedemadi G, et al: Laparoscopic versus open mesh repair for recurrent inguinal hernia: a meta-analysis of outcomes. *Am J Surg.* 2010;200:291-297.

Eker H, et al: Randomized clinical trial of total extraperitoneal inguinal hernioplasty vs Lichtenstein repair. *Arch Surg.* 2012;147: 256-260.

Franz M: The biology of hernia formation. *Surg Clin N Am.* 2008;88:1-15.

Gass M, et al: Bilateral total extraperitoneal inguinal hernia repair (TEP) has outcomes similar to those for unilateral TEP: population-based analysis of prospective data of 6,505 patients. *Surg Endosc.* 2012;26:1364-1368.

Hallén M, et al: Laparoscopic extraperitoneal inguinal hernia repair versus open mesh repair: long-term follow-up of a randomized controlled trial. *Surgery.* 2008;143:313-317.

Itani K, et al: Management of recurrent inguinal hernias. *J Am Coll Surg.* 2009;209:653-658.

Mizrahi H, et al: Management of asymptomatic inguinal hernia. *Arch Surg.* 2012;147:277-281.

Nam A, et al: Management and therapy for sports hernia. *J Am Coll Surg.* 2008;206:154-164.

O'Reilly E, et al: A meta-analysis of surgical morbidity and recurrence after laparoscopic and open repair of primary unilateral inguinal hernia. *Ann Surg.* 2012;255:846-853.

Stylianidis G, et al: Management of the hernia sac in inguinal hernia repair. *Br J Surg.* 2010;97:415-419.

Zendejas B, et al: Simulation-based mastery learning improves patient outcomes in laparoscopic inguinal hernia repair. *Ann Surg.* 2011;254:502-511.

Sliding Inguinal Hernia

A sliding inguinal hernia (Figure 34–4) is an indirect inguinal hernia in which the wall of a viscus forms a portion of the wall of the hernia sac. On the right side, the cecum is most commonly involved, and on the left side, the sigmoid colon is most common. The development of a sliding hernia is related to the variable degree of posterior fixation of the large bowel or other sliding components (eg, bladder, ovary) and their proximity to the internal inguinal ring.

▲ **Figure 34–4.** Right-sided sliding hernia seen in sagittal section. At arrow, the wall of the cecum forms a portion of the hernia sac.

Clinical Findings

Although sliding hernias have no special signs that distinguish them from other inguinal hernias, they should be suspected in any large hernia that cannot be completely reduced. Finding a segment of colon in the scrotum on contrast radiograph strongly suggests a sliding hernia. Recognition of this variation is of great importance at operation, since failure to recognize it may result in inadvertent entry into the lumen of the bowel or bladder.

Treatment

Surgical treatment is nearly identical to the aforementioned surgical repair of inguinal hernias; however, it is essential to recognize the entity at an early stage of operation to reduce injury to the viscera. As is true of all indirect inguinal hernias, the sac will lie anteriorly, but the posterior wall of the sac will be formed by colon, bladder, or retroperitoneal ileum.

After the cord has been dissected free from the hernia sac, most sliding hernias can be reduced by a series of inverting sutures (Bevan technique) and one of the standard types of inguinal repair performed. Very large sliding hernias may have to be reduced by entering the peritoneal cavity through a separate incision (La Roque technique), pulling the bowel back into the abdomen, and fixing it to the posterior abdominal wall. The hernia is then repaired in the usual fashion. Sliding hernias can also be repaired successfully by laparoscopic (TAPP or TEP) techniques in experienced hands.

Prognosis

Sliding hernias have a higher recurrence rate than uncomplicated indirect hernias.

The surgical complication most often feared during repair of a sliding hernia is entry into the bowel or bladder, usually due to failure to recognize that the hernia is a sliding hernia.

Adams R, et al: Outcome of sliding inguinal hernia repair. *Hernia.* 2010;14:47-49.

Freundlich R, et al: Laparoscopic repair of an incarcerated right indirect sliding inguinal hernia involving a retroperitoneal ileum. *Hernia.* 2011;15:225-227.

FEMORAL HERNIA

A femoral hernia descends through the femoral canal beneath the inguinal ligament. Because of its narrow neck, it is prone to incarceration and strangulation. Femoral hernias are much more common in women than in men, but in both sexes, femoral hernia is less common than inguinal hernia. Femoral hernias compose about one-third of groin hernias in women and about 2% of groin hernias in men.

Clinical Findings

A. Symptoms

Femoral hernias are notoriously asymptomatic until incarceration or strangulation occurs. Even with obstruction or strangulation, the patient may feel discomfort more in the abdomen than in the femoral area. Thus, colicky abdominal pain and signs of intestinal obstruction frequently are the presenting manifestations of a strangulated femoral hernia, without discomfort, pain, or tenderness in the femoral region. The patient often has a history of previous repair of an inguinal hernia, lending credence to the concept that a femoral hernia may be overlooked if a thorough search for a femoral hernia is not conducted during an operation for an inguinal hernia. One must have high clinical suspicion for an incarcerated obstructed femoral hernia, especially in a clinically obstructed patient without any history of prior abdominal surgeries.

B. Signs

A femoral hernia may present in a variety of ways. If it is small and uncomplicated, it usually appears as a small bulge in the upper medial thigh just below the level of the inguinal ligament. Because it may be deflected anteriorly through the fossa ovalis femoris to present as a visible or palpable mass at or above the inguinal ligament, it can be confused with an inguinal hernia.

Differential Diagnosis

Femoral hernia must be distinguished from an inguinal hernia, a saphenous varix, and femoral adenopathy. A saphenous varix transmits a distinct thrill when a patient coughs, and it appears and disappears instantly when the patient stands or lies down—in contrast to femoral hernias, which are either irreducible or reduce gradually on pressure.

Treatment

A femoral hernia can be repaired through an open or laparoscopic approach, with mesh or primary tissue repair. The traditional primary repair was the McVay (Cooper ligament) repair that employed a relaxing incision in the anterior rectus sheath. More recently, open repair with mesh or laparoscopic preperitoneal repairs with mesh have been used. No matter what the approach, the hernia is often difficult to reduce. Reduction may be facilitated by carefully incising the iliopubic tract, Gimbernat ligament, or even the inguinal ligament. Occasionally, a counterincision in the thigh is required to free attachments below the inguinal ligament. Irrespective of the approach used, successful femoral hernia repair must close the femoral canal.

If the hernia sac and mass reduce when the patient is given opiates or anesthesia and if bloody fluid appears in the hernia sac when it is exposed and opened, one must strongly suspect the possibility of nonviable bowel in the peritoneal cavity. In such cases, it is mandatory to explore the abdomen, an advantage of the laparoscopic approach.

Prognosis

Recurrence rates are equivalent to those of inguinal hernias, at 4%-5%.

Chan G: Longterm results of a prospective study of 225 femoral hernia repairs: indications for tissue and mesh repair. *J Am Coll Surg.* 2008;207:360-367.

Putnis S: Synchronous femoral hernias diagnosed during endoscopic inguinal hernia repair. *Surg Endosc.* 2011;25:3752-3754.

VENTRAL/ABDOMINAL WALL HERNIAS

UMBILICAL HERNIAS

Umbilical hernias occur quite commonly and result from failure of the umbilical fascial ring to properly fuse. This area begins as a natural orifice in utero, through which the umbilical vessels traverse the abdominal wall at the umbilical ring. After the umbilical cord has sloughed off following childbirth, this area of fascial weakness eventually fuses to close the umbilical ring. This process takes place over the first few years of life. Therefore, most umbilical hernias seen in young children are left alone until at least the age of 4 in order to allow time for natural umbilical fascial closure. However, the fascial fusion process can be incomplete or weakened over a patient's lifetime, resulting in herniation at the umbilicus. Predisposing factors include (1) multiple pregnancies with prolonged labor, (2) ascites, (3) obesity, and (4) large intra-abdominal tumors.

Clinical Findings

In adults, umbilical hernia does not usually obliterate spontaneously, as in children, but instead increases steadily in size. The hernia sac is commonly in the form of a single spherical entity, but it may have multiple loculations. Umbilical hernias can contain various tissues, with preperitoneal fat or omentum being the most common incarcerated contents. However, small and large bowel may be present if the defect is large enough. Although most umbilical repairs can take place electively, incarcerated bowel often necessitates emergent repair for obstruction and/or strangulation given the typical narrow neck of the hernia defect compared to the size of the herniated mass.

Umbilical hernias with tight rings are often associated with sharp pain on coughing or straining, even if only fatty tissue (preperitoneal fat or omentum) is present without any bowel. Very large umbilical hernias more commonly produce a dragging or aching sensation.

Treatment

Umbilical hernia in an adult can be repaired electively if only containing fatty tissue contents, or more expeditiously if bowel is involved in order to avoid incarceration and resultant obstruction or strangulation. Although there is debate as to which defect size requires mesh reinforcement, repairs using mesh result in the lowest recurrence rate. Smaller hernias may be amenable to suture-only repairs, whereas patients with larger hernias or patients who are obese, perform manual labor, are bodybuilders, or take steroids should be considered for a mesh-based repair to reduce the risk of hernia recurrence. Minimally invasive approaches are typically associated with less postoperative pain and faster recovery than open techniques.

The presence of cirrhosis and ascites does not contraindicate repair of an umbilical hernia, since incarceration, strangulation, and rupture are particularly dangerous in patients with these disorders. If significant ascites exists, however, it should first be controlled medically or by a transjugular intrahepatic portosystemic shunt, if necessary, because mortality, morbidity, and recurrence are higher after hernia repair in patients with ascites when the procedure must be performed as an emergency. Preoperative correction of fluid and electrolyte imbalance and improvement of nutrition also improve the outcome in these patients.

Prognosis

Factors that lead to a high rate of complications and recurrence after surgical repair include large size of the hernia, old age or debility of the patient, obesity, immunosuppression, and the presence of other intra-abdominal disease. In healthy individuals, surgical repair of the umbilical defects gives good results with a low rate of recurrence.

Aslani N, et al: Does mesh offer an advantage over tissue in the open repair of umbilical hernias? A systematic review and meta-analysis. *Hernia.* 2010;14:455-462.

Farrow B, et al: More than 150 consecutive open umbilical hernia repairs in a major Veterans Administration Medical Center. *Am J Surg.* 2008;196:647-651.

Gray S, et al: Umbilical herniorrhapy in cirrhosis: improved outcomes with elective repair. *J Gastrointest Surg.* 2008;12:675-681.

McKay A, et al: Umbilical hernia repair in the presence of cirrhosis and ascites: results of a survey and review of the literature. *Hernia.* 2009;13:461-468.

EPIGASTRIC HERNIAS

An epigastric hernia (Figure 34–5) protrudes through the linea alba above the level of the umbilicus. The hernia may develop through one of the foramina of egress of the small

▲ **Figure 34–5.** Epigastric hernia. Note closeness to midline and presence in upper abdomen. The herniation is through the linea alba.

paramidline nerves and vessels or through an area of congenital weakness in the linea alba.

About 3%-5% of the population have epigastric hernias. They are more common in men than in women and most common between the ages of 20 and 50. About 20% of epigastric hernias are multiple, and about 80% occur just off the midline. Patients can have both epigastric and umbilical hernias in close proximity.

▶ Clinical Findings

Most epigastric hernias are painless, and many are found on routine abdominal examination. If symptomatic, their presentation ranges from mild epigastric pain and tenderness to deep, burning epigastric pain with radiation to the back or the lower abdominal quadrants. The pain may be accompanied by abdominal bloating, nausea, or vomiting. The symptoms often occur after a large meal and, on occasion, may be relieved by reclining, probably because the supine position causes the herniated mass to reduce back into the abdominal cavity. The smaller masses most frequently contain only preperitoneal fat and are especially prone to incarceration and strangulation. These smaller hernias are often tender. Larger hernias seldom strangulate and may contain, in addition to preperitoneal fat, a portion of the nearby omentum and, occasionally, a loop of small or large bowel.

If a mass is palpable, the diagnosis can often be confirmed by any maneuver that will increase intra-abdominal pressure and thereby cause the mass to bulge anteriorly. While epigastric hernias can be present anywhere along the upper midline, they are most commonly located in the lower epigastrium, just above the umbilicus. The diagnosis is difficult to make when the patient is obese, since a mass is hard to palpate; ultrasound or computed tomography (CT) radiographs may be needed in the very obese patient.

▶ Differential Diagnosis

Differential diagnosis for pain/tenderness in the epigastric region includes peptic ulcer, gallbladder disease, hiatal hernia, pancreatitis, and upper small bowel obstruction. On occasion, it may be impossible to distinguish the hernia mass from a subcutaneous lipoma, fibroma, or neurofibroma.

Another condition that must be distinguished from an epigastric hernia is **diastasis recti**, a diffuse widening and attenuation of the linea alba without a fascial defect. On examination, this condition appears as a fusiform, linear bulge between the two rectus abdominis muscles without a discrete fascial defect with Valsalva. Although this condition may be unsightly, repair is commonly avoided since there is no risk of incarceration, the fascial layer is weak, and the recurrence rate is high. Highly symptomatic diastasis can be repaired with open or laparoscopic plication techniques.

▶ Treatment

Many epigastric hernias are symptomatic and, therefore, should be repaired. Treatment is very similar to that of umbilical hernias. Small defects can usually be closed primarily with sutures alone, with mesh placed for large hernias or for patients with risk factors for recurrence. Herniated fat contents are usually dissected free and removed.

Palanivelu C, et al: Laparoscopic repair of diastasis recti using the "Venetian blinds" technique of plication with prosthetic reinforcement: a retrospective study. *Hernia.* 2009;13:287-292.

VENTRAL & INCISIONAL HERNIAS

Incisional hernias are quite common, with up to 10%-30% of all abdominal operations resulting in an incisional hernia. The incidence of this iatrogenic type of hernia is not diminishing despite an awareness of the many causative factors, especially with the obesity epidemic. There is an increasing need to repair large or complex ventral hernias, and risk factors that impede wound healing such as smoking and diabetes contribute to wound complications as well as hernia recurrence, which makes subsequent repair more difficult.

▶ Etiology

The factors most often responsible for incisional hernia are listed below. When more than one factor coexists in the same patient, the likelihood of postoperative wound failure is greatly increased.

1. Poor surgical technique. Inadequate fascial bites, tension on the fascial edges, and too tight a closure are most often responsible for incisional failure. Additionally, studies have shown that closing fascia with smaller bites (~0.5 cm) instead of traditional large (~1 cm) bites reduces the rate of incisional hernia.

2. Postoperative wound infection. An infection in the wound increases the risk of hernia formation to as high as 80%. Wound infection is one of the single greatest risk factors for hernia formation or hernia recurrence.

3. Age. Wound healing is usually slower and the closure less solid in older patients.

4. General debility. Cirrhosis, carcinoma, and chronic wasting diseases are factors that adversely affect wound healing. Any condition that compromises nutrition increases the likelihood of fascial and wound breakdown.

5. Obesity. Obese patients frequently have increased intra-abdominal pressure. The presence of excessive visceral fat within the abdominal cavity increases intra-abdominal pressure, which puts stress and strain on a closed wound. Additionally, adipose tissue within

the abdominal wound masks tissue layers and increases the incidence of seromas and hematomas in wounds.

6. Diabetes. Uncontrolled diabetes reduces microvasculature. With a diminished blood flow to areas of need (eg, surgical or traumatic wounds), the tissues fail to receive efficient flow of oxygen and nutrients required to support proper wound healing.

7. Smoking. Like diabetes, smoking negatively impacts microvasculature and the tissues that require support. While nicotine is a common culprit cited, it is likely the other components within tobacco that inhibit proper wound healing.

8. Postoperative pulmonary complications that stress the repair as a result of vigorous coughing. Smokers and patients with chronic pulmonary disease are at increased risk of fascial disruption.

9. Intraoperative blood loss greater than 1000 mL.

10. Failure to close the fascia of laparoscopic trocar sites over 10 mm in size.

11. Defects in collagen or matrix metalloprotease.

▶ **Treatment**

There are numerous options for repairing ventral hernias, including primary suture-only repairs, mesh reinforcement, minimally invasive techniques using laparoscopy or robotic technology, open techniques, or a combination of these techniques. Each technique has its own pros and cons, and surgeons should be familiar with multiple techniques in order to tailor the approach to a particular hernia. There are many factors that help determine the proper repair technique, including the size of the hernia(s), location in the abdominal wall, history of previous repairs, patient comorbidities, and the skill set of the surgeon.

Hernias should be addressed if they become symptomatic (eg, pain) or if bowel is involved within the hernia sac. Incarcerated bowel can lead to obstruction and/or strangulation, which can be life threatening if not addressed in a timely fashion. Concerning clinical features for strangulation include a very firm incarcerated hernia, severe tenderness on exam, and redness or other discoloration of the overlying skin. Additionally, obstruction leads to abdominal distention. If the patient does not require urgent or emergent surgery, is unwilling to undergo surgery, or is a poor surgical risk, symptoms may be controlled by an abdominal binder or other type of elastic undergarment for compression.

Small incisional hernias may be amenable to primary suture repair. However, mesh reinforcement greatly reduces the risk of hernia recurrence. Therefore, the vast majority of ventral and incisional hernia repairs are performed with some form of mesh reinforcement. Mesh used in hernia

repairs is manufactured from different materials, such as polypropylene, polyester, or expanded polytetrafluoroethylene (ePTFE), and is produced in varying configurations, including composite meshes with antiadhesion barriers and self-adhering meshes. Biologic and bioresorbable meshes are an alternative to permanent synthetic mesh when there is high concern for infection, because such meshes tend to be more resilient in the setting of contamination. Mesh should not be used when there is active infection or gross contamination present. Biologic meshes are manufactured from various tissues and animal sources, with porcine dermis representing the most commonly used biologically derived collagen-based matrix. Mesh can be placed inside the abdominal cavity directly underneath the abdominal wall as an **underlay**, as long as there is some form of antiadhesion barrier on the mesh to prevent the intestine from adhering to it. Uncoated mesh can be placed within various tissue planes, including the **preperitoneal** space, **retromuscular** space (eg, retrorectus), or on top of the fascia in an **onlay** position after creating skin flaps. Studies have shown that a minimum overlap of 5 cm past the edge of the defect is ideal to reduce the risk of hernia recurrence.

Although surgeons strive to achieve fascial closure with most hernia repairs, some hernia defects are too large for closure of the native fascia. Excessive tension on fascial tissue can lead to fascial dehiscence and subsequent hernia recurrence. Such large hernia defects are commonly repaired using component separation techniques to achieve fascial closure (Figure 34–6). It is important to understand the anatomy of the entire abdominal wall, because these complex hernia repairs use cutting of specific myofascial layers (eg, external oblique release, transversus abdominis release) for medial advancement of the fascial layers and hernia defect closure. Even when the fascia can be closed, these repairs should be reinforced by mesh to support the tissue over the long term.

MIS techniques using laparoscopic and robotic-assisted technology are increasingly being used to repair ventral hernias and perform adhesiolysis and other intra-abdominal procedures. MIS procedures have been shown to greatly reduce the risk of wound complications such as infection, as well as shorten hospitalization and recovery. For many MIS ventral hernia repairs, after closing the hernia defect, a coated sheet of synthetic mesh is secured to the abdominal wall as an underlay mesh; the intraperitoneal placement of the graft greatly enhances the durability of the repair, although it also increases the risk of bowel adhesions or fistula formation.

▶ **Prognosis**

Results of randomized clinical trials show that mesh repair is superior to primary suture repair, even for small incisional hernias. Despite the increasing use of both open and laparoscopic mesh repairs, however, population-based studies show that incisional hernias continue to recur at a high rate

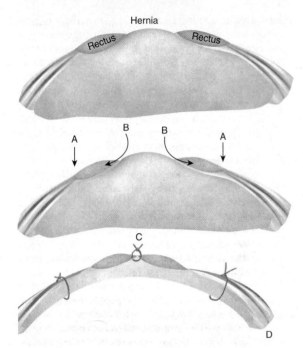

▲ **Figure 34–6.** Component separation technique to allow primary closure in the midline, usually over a mesh underlay. (A) Division of the external oblique aponeurosis. (B) Release of the rectus from the posterior rectus sheath. (C) Closure of the rectus in the midline. (D) Mesh underlay.

after repair, and the recurrence rate increases with each subsequent reoperation for recurrence, reaching almost 40% on average after the third recurrence. Factors shown to increase risk of hernia recurrence include those listed earlier in the "Etiology" section, with obesity, diabetes, and smoking being the three most influential factors. Hernia recurrence and wound complication rates are so high in smokers that many surgeons require patients to stop smoking for a minimum of 1 month prior to the planned hernia repair.

Hernia recurrence rates for commonly used procedures range from approximately 4% up to 30% or more and are highly dependent on the repair technique, type of mesh used, amount of mesh overlap, as well as the patient factors listed earlier. These various factors also determine other patient outcomes related to hernia repair, including surgical site infection, seroma, hematoma, fistula formation, and wound dehiscence. To reduce the risks of hernia recurrence and other complications, effort is devoted in the preoperative setting to optimize the patient (eg, weight loss, diabetes management, smoking cessation). Such preoperative optimization greatly improves outcomes and reduces risks, especially in high-risk patients.

Albright E, et al: The component separation technique for hernia repair: a comparison of open and endoscopic techniques. *Am Surg.* 2011;77:839-843.

Breuing K, et al: Incisional ventral hernias: review of the literature and recommendations regarding the grading and technique of repair. *Surgery.* 2010;148:544-558.

Burger JW, et al: Long-term follow-up of a randomized controlled trial of suture versus mesh repair of incisional hernia. *Ann Surg.* 2004;240:578-585.

Deerenberg EB, et al: Small bites versus large bites for closure of abdominal midline incisions (STITCH): a double-blind, multi-centre, randomised controlled trial. *Lancet.* 2015;386:1254-1260.

den Hartog D, et al: Open surgical procedures for incisional hernias. *Cochrane Database Syst Rev.* 2008;3:CD006438.

Itani KMF, et al: Comparison of laparoscopic and open repair with mesh for the treatment of ventral incisional hernia. *Arch Surg.* 2010;145:322-328.

Jin J, et al: Laparoscopic versus open ventral hernia repair. *Surg Clin N Am.* 2008;88:1083-1100.

Lindström D, et al: Effects of a perioperative smoking cessation intervention on postoperative complications. *Ann Surg.* 2008;248:739-745.

Melvin WS, et al: Laparoscopic ventral hernia repair. *World J Surg.* 2011;35:1496-1499.

Pauli EM, et al: Open ventral hernia repair with component separation. *Surg Clin N Am.* 2013;93:1111-1133.

Poulose BK, et al: Epidemiology and cost of ventral hernia repair: making the case for hernia research. *Hernia.* 2012;16:179-183.

Sauerland S, et al: Laparoscopic versus open surgical techniques for ventral or incisional hernia repair. *Cochrane Database Syst Rev.* 2011;3:CD007781.

PARASTOMAL HERNIAS

A parastomal hernia is a particularly troublesome hernia to repair successfully, since the stoma's course through the abdominal wall is, by its very nature, a hernia. Studies cite an incidence of up to 50% for this type of hernia. Traditional teaching advises that a stoma be placed through the middle of the rectus muscle rather than more laterally to reduce the risk of herniation. However, even perfect stoma placement can result in hernia formation when the fascial opening stretches and allows additional loops of bowel or omentum to herniate adjacent to the stoma. The etiology of parastomal hernias mirrors that of other ventral hernias and includes collagen defects, immunosuppressant therapy, and anything that greatly increases intra-abdominal pressure such as straining, heavy lifting, or obesity.

Parastomal hernias should be repaired if they interfere with stoma function or are difficult to reduce, as they can obstruct and/or strangulate. If the hernia is asymptomatic, repair is not mandatory, although large hernias can diminish the individual's quality of life. Many options for repair of parastomal hernias have been described, with poor results given the need to maintain a fascial defect for the stoma itself. The best way to repair a parastomal hernia is to reverse the ostomy, thus avoiding the need for a fascial defect; however, ostomy takedown might not be possible. Primary suture repair has particularly poor results, with recurrence rates close to 100%. As with other hernia repairs, mesh reinforcement reduces the rate of hernia recurrence. Multiple open and MIS techniques have been described, including the Sugarbaker technique (mesh draped underneath a lateralized bowel, with stoma kept in situ), cruciate technique (mesh is slit and bowel delivered through mesh), keyhole technique (mesh is cut around a stoma kept in situ), and retromuscular techniques.

Due to the significant risk of parastomal hernias, prophylactic mesh can be placed at the time of (permanent) stoma creation to reduce the risk of parastomal hernia formation. Although studies have demonstrated a significant reduction of hernia formation with the placement of prophylactic mesh, this practice has not gained widespread adoption outside of Europe.

Brandsma HT, et al: Prophylactic mesh placement during end colostomy reduces the rate of parastomal hernia. *Ann Surg.* 2017;265(4):663-669.

Hansson BM, et al: Surgical techniques for parastomal hernia repair: a systematic review. *Ann Surg.* 2012;255(4):685-695.

Jones HG, et al: Prosthetic mesh placement for the prevention of parastomal herniation. *Cochrane Database Syst Rev.* 2018;7:CD008905.

Tam KW: Systematic review of the use of a mesh to prevent parastomal hernia. *World J Surg.* 2010;34:2723-2729.

Van Dijk SM, et al: Parastomal hernia: impact on quality of life? *World J Surg.* 2015;39:2595-2601.

VARIOUS RARE HERNIATIONS THROUGH THE ABDOMINAL WALL

▶ Interparietal Hernia

Interparietal hernias are hernias in which the sac insinuates itself between the layers of the abdominal wall. Although interparietal hernias are rare, it is essential to recognize them because obstruction and/or strangulation is common and the mass can easily be mistaken for other pathology (eg, tumor or abscess). The lesion usually can be suspected on the basis of the physical examination provided it is kept in mind. In most cases, extensive studies for intra-abdominal tumors have preceded diagnosis. A lateral film of the abdomen will usually show bowel within the layers of the abdominal wall in cases with intestinal incarceration or strangulation, and an ultrasound or CT scan may be diagnostic. Given the potential threat to bowel, most postoperative interparietal hernias are repaired as soon as the diagnosis is established. For long-standing ventral hernias with an interparietal component, one can plan out the repair and optimize the patient prior to repair.

▶ Spigelian Hernia

A Spigelian hernia is an abdominal wall hernia through the linea semilunaris, which is the lateral border of rectus sheath. Spigelian hernias are nearly always found above the level of the inferior epigastric vessels. They most commonly occur where the semicircular (arcuate) line (fold of Douglas) crosses the linea semilunaris.

The presenting symptom is pain that is usually localized to the hernia site and may be aggravated by any maneuver that increases intra-abdominal pressure. With time, the pain may become more dull, constant, and diffuse, making diagnosis more difficult.

If an incarcerated mass can be demonstrated, the diagnosis presents little difficulty. However, physical exam diagnosis is typically difficult given the occult nature of many Spigelian hernias. Because the hernia defect may lie beneath an intact external oblique layer, representing an interparietal hernia, defects might not be palpable. The hernia often dissects within the layers of the abdominal wall and may not present a distinct mass, or the mass may be located at a distance from the linea semilunaris. Physical exam can be aided with a Valsalva maneuver or by increasing abdominal pressure, such as by coughing or performing a sit-up, to help protrusion of the area of concern. Because of the occult nature of many Spigelian hernias, ultrasound and CT imaging are helpful in confirming.

Spigelian hernias have a high incidence of incarceration and should be repaired. Small hernias may be repaired by primary aponeurotic closure, although fascial defects larger than 2-3 cm should be repaired using mesh, preferable in an underlay, preperitoneal technique. Open or laparoscopic approach may be used according to the surgeon's experience, with laparoscopy affording an advantage in allowing the evaluation and treatment of bilateral hernia.

Bittner J, et al: Mesh-free laparoscopic Spigelian hernia repair. *Am Surg.* 2008;74:713-720.

Saber A, et al: Laparoscopic spigelian hernia repair: the scroll technique. *Am Surg.* 2008;74:108-112.

▶ Littre Hernia

A Littre hernia is a hernia that contains a Meckel diverticulum within the hernia sac. Although Littre first described the condition in relation to a femoral hernia, the relative distribution of Littre hernias is as follows: inguinal, 50%; femoral, 20%; umbilical, 20%; and miscellaneous, 10%. Littre hernias of the groin are more common in men and on the right side. The clinical findings are similar to those of Richter hernia; when strangulation is present, pain, fever, and manifestations of small bowel obstruction occur late.

Treatment consists of repair of the hernia plus, if possible, excision of the diverticulum. If acute Meckel diverticulitis is present, the acute inflammatory mass may have to be treated through a separate abdominal incision.

▶ Amyand Hernia

An Amyand hernia is a groin hernia that contains the appendix. If the appendix is inflamed, it should be removed and the hernia repaired using native tissues or biologic mesh, because the risk of infection to permanent mesh is too great. If the appendix is normal and only an incidental finding in the hernia, it should be returned to the abdomen and a mesh repair employed.

Sharma H, et al: Amyand's hernia: a report of 18 consecutive patients over a 15-year period. *Hernia*. 2007;11:31-35.

Lumbar or Dorsal Hernia

Lumbar or dorsal hernias (Figure 34–7) are hernias through the posterior abdominal wall at some level in the lumbar region. The most common sites (95%) are the superior (Grynfeltt) and inferior (Petit) lumbar triangles. A "lump in the flank" is the common complaint, associated with a dull, heavy, pulling feeling. With the patient erect, the presence of a reducible, often tympanitic mass in the flank usually makes the diagnosis. Incarceration and strangulation occur in about 10% of cases. Hernias in the inferior lumbar triangle are most often small and occur in young, athletic women. They present as tender masses producing backache and usually contain fat. Lumbar hernia must be differentiated from abscesses, hematomas, soft tissue tumors, renal tumors, and muscle strain.

These acquired hernias may be traumatic or nontraumatic. Severe direct trauma, penetrating wounds, abscesses, and poor healing of flank incisions are the usual causes. However, incisional hernias from extended flank procedures can lead to fascial disruption and herniation posterolaterally.

▲ **Figure 34–7.** Anatomic relationships of lumbar or dorsal hernia. On the left, lumbar or dorsal hernia into space of Grynfeltt. On the right, hernia into the Petit triangle (inferior lumbar space).

Congenital hernias occur in infants and are usually isolated unilateral congenital defects.

Lumbar hernias increase in size and should be repaired when found. The approach can be by open or, increasingly, by MIS technique. Repair is by mobilization of the nearby fascia and obliteration of the hernia defect by precise fascia-to-fascia closure for small defects and mesh repair for most defects.

Stamatiou D, et al: Lumbar hernia: surgical anatomy, embryology, and technique of repair. *Am Surg.* 2009;75:202-207.

Obturator Hernia

Herniation through the obturator canal is more frequent in elderly women and is difficult to diagnose preoperatively. Because of the occult nature and difficulty with diagnosis of obturator hernias, the mortality rate (13%-40%) of these hernias makes them one of the most lethal of all abdominal hernias. These hernias most commonly present as small bowel obstruction, with symptoms of abdominal distention, crampy abdominal pain, and vomiting. The hernia is rarely palpable in the groin, although a mass may be felt on pelvic or rectal examination. The most specific finding is a positive Howship-Romberg sign, in which pain extends down the medial aspect of the thigh with abduction, extension, or internal rotation of the knee. Because this sign is present in fewer than half of cases, diagnosis should be suspected in any elderly debilitated woman without previous abdominal operations who presents with a small bowel obstruction. Although diagnosis can be confirmed by CT scan, operation should not be unduly delayed if complete bowel obstruction is present.

Open or laparoscopic transabdominal approach allows the best exposure for repair. Because of the deep inner pelvic location of these hernias, a thigh approach should be avoided. When performed laparoscopically, the repair emulates that of typical MIS inguinal hernia repairs, with wide mesh overlap including deep posterior overlap of the obturator canal. The Cheatle-Henry approach (retropubic) may also be used. Simple repair is most often possible, although bladder wall, pectineal muscle, peritoneum, or mesh has been used when the defect cannot be approximated primarily.

Petrie A, et al: Obturator hernia: anatomy, embryology, diagnosis, and treatment. *Clin Anat.* 2011;24:562-569.
Stamatiou D, et al: Obturator hernia revisited: surgical anatomy, embryology, diagnosis, and technique of repair. *Am Surg.* 2011;77:1147-1157.

Perineal Hernia

A perineal hernia protrudes through the muscles and fascia of the perineal floor. It may be primary but is usually acquired following pelvic procedures such as perineal prostatectomy, abdominoperineal resection of the rectum, or pelvic exenteration. These hernias present as easily reducible perineal bulges and usually are asymptomatic but may present with pain, dysuria, bowel obstruction, or perineal skin breakdown.

Repair is usually done by an abdominal approach, with an adequate fascial and muscular perineal repair. Occasionally, polypropylene mesh or tissue flaps using the gracilis, rectus abdominis, or gluteus may be necessary, when the available tissues are too attenuated for adequate primary repair.

▶ Sciatic Hernia

Sciatic hernias are one of the rarest of abdominal hernias and consist of an outpouching of intra-abdominal contents through the greater sciatic foramen. The diagnosis is typically made after incarceration or strangulation of the bowel occurs, but usually requires CT or MRI for the diagnosis to be made preoperatively. The repair is usually made through the abdominal approach. The hernia sac and contents are reduced, and the weak area is closed by making a fascial flap from the superficial fascia of the piriformis muscle. Reinforcement of the closure with prosthetic mesh provides the most durable repair.

Losanoff JE, et al: Sciatic hernia: a comprehensive review of the world literature (1900-2008). *Am J Surg.* 2010;199:52-59.

TRAUMATIC HERNIAS

Abdominal wall hernias occur rarely as a direct consequence of direct blunt abdominal injury. The patient presents with abdominal pain. On examination, ecchymosis of the abdominal wall and a bulge are usually present. The existence of a hernia may not be obvious, however, and the patient may require CT scan to confirm it. Because of the high incidence of associated intra-abdominal injuries, laparotomy is usually required for further exploration. The defect should be repaired primarily, if possible, at the time of initial exploration, saving more definitive (mesh-based) repair until the patient has fully healed and recovered from the traumatic event.

▼ II. OTHER LESIONS OF THE ABDOMINAL WALL

CONGENITAL DEFECTS

Congenital defects of the abdominal wall other than hernias or lesions of the urachus and umbilicus are rare. The important ones involving the urachus and umbilicus are discussed in Chapter 45.

TRAUMA TO THE ABDOMINAL WALL

▶ Rectus Sheath Hematoma

This is a rare but important entity that may follow mild trauma to the abdominal wall or may occur spontaneously in patients with disorders of coagulation, blood dyscrasia, or degenerative vascular diseases.

Abdominal pain localized to the rectus muscle is the presenting symptom. The pain may be sudden and severe in onset or slowly progressive. The key to diagnosis is the physical examination. Careful palpation will reveal a tender mass within the abdominal wall. When the patient tenses the rectus muscles by raising the head or body, the swelling becomes more tender and distinct on palpation, in contrast to an intra-abdominal mass or tenderness that disappears when the rectus muscles are contracted (Fothergill sign). In addition, there may be detectable discoloration or ecchymosis. If the physical signs are not diagnostic, ultrasound or CT scan will demonstrate the hematoma in the abdominal wall.

The condition does not commonly require an operation. Coagulation abnormalities should be corrected if possible. The acute pain and discomfort usually disappear within 2 or 3 days, although a residual mass and ecchymosis may persist for several weeks. Rarely bleeding persists, requiring embolization by interventional radiology.

PAIN IN THE ABDOMINAL WALL

A number of conditions are characterized by pain in the abdominal wall without a demonstrable organic lesion. Pain from a diaphragmatic, supradiaphragmatic, or spinal cord lesion may be referred to the abdomen. Herpes zoster (shingles) may present as abdominal pain, in which case it will follow a dermatomal distribution.

Scars may be sensitive or painful, particularly in the first 6 months after surgery.

Entrapment of a nerve by a nonabsorbable suture may cause persistent incisional pain, sometimes quite severe. Hyperesthesia of the skin over the involved dermatome may provide a clue to the cause. If local anesthetic nerve block relieves the pain, nerve block with alcohol or nerve excision may be performed.

In all cases of localized pain in the abdominal wall, careful search should be made for a small hernia: MRI or CT scan may be helpful to rule out a hernia.

ABDOMINAL WALL TUMORS

Tumors of the abdominal wall are not unusual, but most are benign, eg, lipomas, hemangiomas, and fibromas. Musculoaponeurotic fibromatoses (desmoid tumors), which often occur in abdominal wall scars or after parturition in women, are discussed in more detail in Chapter 47.

Endometriomas may also occur in the abdominal wall, particularly in the scars from gynecologic procedures and cesarean sections. Most malignant tumors of the abdominal wall are metastatic. Metastases may appear by direct invasion from intra-abdominal lesions or by vascular dissemination. The sudden appearance of a sensitive nodule anywhere in the abdominal wall that is clearly not a hernia should arouse suspicion of an occult cancer, with the lung and pancreas being the more likely primary sites.

MULTIPLE CHOICE QUESTIONS

1. Of the following open repairs, the most effective method of repairing a femoral hernia is a

   A. Lichtenstein repair
   B. Lotheissen-McVay repair
   C. Bassini repair
   D. Shouldice repair
   E. Halsted repair

2. The *least* common reason for recurrence of a groin hernia within the first year after repair is

   A. Overlooking an indirect hernia sac
   B. Tension on the fascial repair
   C. A missed femoral hernia
   D. Failure to close the fascial defect adequately
   E. A defect in collagen synthesis

3. The type of open repair of a groin hernia that is both the most commonly performed and also associated with the lowest rate of recurrence is the

   A. Shouldice repair
   B. Bassini repair
   C. Lichtenstein repair
   D. Halsted repair
   E. Cooper ligament repair

4. Factors associated with a laparoscopic inguinal hernia repair compared to an open repair include all of the following *except*

   A. Less postoperative pain
   B. Faster return to work
   C. Longer operative time
   D. Requires general anesthesia
   E. Lower cost

5. Of the following, the groin hernia that is most likely to incarcerate and strangulate is a

   A. Femoral hernia
   B. Indirect inguinal hernia
   C. Direct inguinal hernia
   D. Pantaloon hernia
   E. Amyand hernia

6. Of the following, the greatest risk for incisional hernia after an abdominal operation is found in patients who

   A. Are greater than 65 years old
   B. Have coronary artery disease
   C. Develop a wound infection
   D. Have diabetes
   E. Have chronic obstructive pulmonary disease

Adrenals

Quan-Yang Duh, MD
Chienying Liu, MD
Carolyn Dacey Seib, MD, MAS

Operations on the adrenal glands are performed for primary hyperaldosteronism, pheochromocytoma, hypercortisolism (Cushing disease or Cushing syndrome), and adrenocortical carcinoma. These conditions are usually characterized by hypersecretion of one or more of the adrenal hormones. Less commonly, surgery may also be performed for nonfunctioning tumors or metastases.

ANATOMY & SURGICAL PRINCIPLES

The normal combined weight of the adrenals is 7-12 g. The right gland lies posterior and lateral to the vena cava and superior to the kidney (Figure 35–1). The left gland lies medial to the superior pole of the kidney, just lateral to the aorta and immediately posterior to the superior border of the pancreas. An important surgical feature is the remarkable constancy of the adrenal veins. The right adrenal vein, 2-5 mm long and several millimeters wide, connects the anteromedial aspect of the adrenal gland with the posterolateral aspect of the vena cava. The left adrenal vein is several centimeters long and travels inferiorly from the lower pole of the gland, joining the left renal vein after receiving the inferior phrenic vein. Variant venous drainage (multiple or anomalous veins) occurs in about 9%-17% of glands and is more common for pheochromocytomas and larger tumors. The adrenal arteries are small, multiple, and inconstant. They usually come from the inferior phrenic artery, the aorta, and the upper pole branch of the renal artery.

With the exception of rare nonsecreting cancers, indications for adrenal surgery result from hypersecretory states. Diagnosis and treatment begin with confirmation of a hypersecretory state (ie, measurement of excess cortisol, aldosterone, or catecholamines in blood or urine). To determine whether the problem originates in the adrenal, levels of the trophic hormone in question (ie, adrenocorticotropic hormone [ACTH] or renin) must be measured. If levels of the trophic hormone are suppressed but hormone secretion is

excessive, autonomous secretion by the adrenal is proved. The next step, except in pheochromocytoma, is to determine the degree of autonomy, a process that usually distinguishes hyperplasias (which respond to most but not all controlling mechanisms) from adenomas and adenomas from cancers. In general, cancers are under little, if any, feedback control. If the primary problem is not in the adrenal, as in Cushing disease, treatment must be directed elsewhere when possible.

The major principles of adrenal surgery are as follows:

1. Whenever possible, the surgeon must be certain of the diagnosis and the location of the lesion before undertaking the operation.

2. The patient must be thoroughly prepared so he or she can withstand any metabolic problems caused by the disease or by the operation.

3. The surgeon and consultants must be able to detect and treat any metabolic crisis that occurs during or after the operation.

SURGICAL APPROACHES

Currently, almost all adrenal tumors are identified preoperatively by localization studies such as computed tomography (CT) and magnetic resonance imaging (MRI), so very few operations require general exploration of the abdomen. This permits the use of minimally invasive surgery. Almost all adrenal tumors can be removed laparoscopically. Traditional open adrenalectomy is necessary only when the tumor is especially large (eg, > 8-10 cm, depending on the surgeon's experience) or for locally invasive adrenocortical cancer where resection of lymph nodes or adjacent organs may be required.

Laparoscopic adrenalectomy can be performed using a transabdominal or retroperitoneal approach. Transabdominal laparoscopic adrenalectomy involves medial rotation of the spleen and pancreas (on the left) or the liver (on the right), using gravity to drop the viscera away from the adrenal.

▲ **Figure 35–1.** Anatomy of the adrenals, showing venous return.

Retroperitoneal adrenalectomy involves the use of high insufflation pressure to maintain the space for dissection and to decrease bleeding during dissection. Although the transabdominal approach is more suitable for larger tumors and the retroperitoneal approach is better for bilateral adrenalectomy and for patients with abdominal adhesions, surgeon preference usually dictates the choice of surgical approach.

The traditional open surgical approach is used when laparoscopic expertise is not available or when required by the size and invasiveness of the tumor. The advantages of laparoscopic operation are so great that it is strongly preferred.

The open anterior approach (midline, subcostal, or "L" incision) allows wide exposure for large tumors but causes more pain and wound complications, and it requires longer hospitalization. The open posterior approach through the bed of the 11th or 12th rib has been superseded by the laparoscopic approach. Thoracoabdominal incision may be used for large or invasive tumors when exposure above the diaphragm is needed.

▼ DISEASES OF THE ADRENALS

PRIMARY ALDOSTERONISM

ESSENTIALS OF DIAGNOSIS

▶ Hypertension with or without hypokalemia.

▶ Elevated aldosterone secretion and suppressed plasma renin activity.

▶ Metabolic alkalosis, relative hypernatremia.

▶ Weakness, polyuria, paresthesia, tetany, cramps due to hypokalemia.

▶ General Considerations

Aldosterone, the most potent mineralocorticoid secreted by the adrenal cortex, regulates the body's electrolyte composition, fluid volume, and blood pressure. Excess aldosterone increases total body sodium, decreases potassium levels, increases extracellular fluid volume (without edema), and increases blood pressure. Under normal conditions, aldosterone secretion is regulated by the renin-angiotensin system in a feedback fashion and is also stimulated transiently by ACTH.

In primary aldosteronism, aldosterone levels are elevated and renin levels are suppressed. In secondary hyperaldosteronism, increased aldosterone is due to increased renin secretion. Examples of secondary hyperaldosteronism include renovascular disease, renin-secreting tumors, and cirrhosis with low intravascular volume or diuretic use. Among the subtypes of primary aldosteronism, aldosterone-producing adenoma (aldosteronoma) and idiopathic hyperaldosteronism with adrenal hyperplasia are the most common types. Unilateral primary adrenal hyperplasia, aldosterone-producing adrenocortical carcinoma, and familial hyperaldosteronism (FH; types I, II, and III) are rare. Surgery is beneficial only in patients with aldosterone-producing adenomas and in patients with unilateral primary adrenal hyperplasia and rarely in FH type III when severe hypertension is refractory to medical therapy.

Primary aldosteronism in its classic form is characterized by hypertension, hypokalemia, increased aldosterone secretion, and suppressed plasma renin activity. However, hypokalemia is not required to make the diagnosis; recent studies have shown that most patients are normokalemic. Primary aldosteronism was once thought to be present in about 1% of patients with mild to moderate hypertension, but more recent studies have demonstrated higher prevalence: 4.3% in primary care setting and 9.5% in specialty setting. Although rare, normotensive primary aldosteronism has been described.

Aldosteronomas are usually solitary and small (0.5-2 cm). They have a characteristic golden-yellow color when sectioned. Tumor cells typically have heterogeneous cytomorphology, resembling those of all three zones of the adrenal cortex, including hybrid cells having cytologic features of the zona glomerulosa and zona fasciculata. Hyperplasia is also often seen in glands harboring adenomas.

▶ Clinical Findings

Aldosterone facilitates the exchange of sodium for potassium and hydrogen ions in the distal nephron. Therefore, when aldosterone secretion is chronically increased, serum potassium and hydrogen ion concentrations fall (hypokalemia and alkalosis), total-body sodium rises, and hypertension results.

A. Symptoms and Signs

Symptoms, if present, are usually those of hypokalemia and depend on the severity of potassium depletion. Patients complain of a sense of malaise, muscle weakness, polyuria, polydipsia, cramps, and paresthesia. Tetany and hypokalemic paralysis occur rarely. Hypertension is usually moderate to severe and may be refractory to medical therapy, but advanced retinopathy is rare. Although extracellular fluid volume is increased, edema is not seen unless renal failure occurs.

B. Laboratory Findings

1. Screening test—Primary aldosteronism should be suspected in patients with hypertension and hypokalemia—either spontaneous or following the administration of diuretics—in patients with resistant hypertension, and in patients with hypertension and adrenal incidentalomas. The diagnostic evaluation should start with screening tests. A simple ambulatory test determines the ratio of plasma aldosterone concentration (PAC), in nanograms per deciliter, to plasma renin activity (PRA), in nanograms per milliliter per hour, performed in the morning in a seated ambulant patient. Although diagnostic protocols are not uniform, a ratio ≥ 20 with an elevated PAC (usually ≥ 15 but may be lower, ie, ≥ 10 ng/dL) and a suppressed PRA (< 1 ng/mL/h) suggests primary aldosteronism and warrants confirmatory biochemical studies. Hypertensive individuals without primary aldosteronism usually have ratios < 20. If the patient is taking an aldosterone receptor antagonist, such as spironolactone or eplerenone, the data can be uninterpretable. These agents should be discontinued for at least 4 weeks before the workup.

Many medications affect PAC and PRA. For example, PAC is decreased by angiotensin-converting enzyme (ACE) inhibitors (inhibitors), angiotensin receptor blockers (ARBs), central α_2 agonists such as clonidine, dihydropyridine (DHP) calcium channel antagonists such as amlodipine, and β-blockers. PRA is increased by ACE inhibitors, ARBs, and DHP-calcium channel antagonists. These medications should be discontinued for 2 weeks if necessary. Peripheral α-adrenergic blockers, such as doxazosin, terazosin, prazosin, hydralazine, and non-DHP calcium channel blockers such as verapamil, are the preferred antihypertensive agents during evaluation. In many patients, it is unwise to withdraw antihypertensive medications, and one must be content with imperfect data.

2. Confirmatory test—If the screening test is positive, failure to suppress aldosterone secretion with sodium loading will confirm the diagnosis of primary aldosteronism in most patients. Normally, aldosterone can be suppressed by oral salt loading or intravenous sodium chloride infusion. The patient should consume a high-sodium diet (6000 mg of sodium for 3 days) or be supplemented with NaCl tablets (2 g with each meal) if necessary. A 24-hour urine sample is collected for both aldosterone and sodium on the third day. Urine sodium should be > 200 mmol/24 h to confirm

adequate salt load. Serum potassium should be monitored because the high-salt diet increases kaliuresis, and potassium chloride should be supplemented to avoid hypokalemia, which interferes with the test results by decreasing aldosterone secretion and may cause cardiac arrhythmias. Urinary aldosterone excretion > 12-14 μg/24 h distinguishes most patients with primary aldosteronism from those with essential hypertension. Alternatively, a PAC higher than 10 ng/mL after an infusion of 2 L of normal saline over 4 hours is also consistent with primary aldosteronism.

▶ Differential Diagnosis

Once the diagnosis is established, the surgically correctable forms—aldosterone-producing adenoma (aldosteronoma), constituting approximately 35% of primary aldosteronism, and the rare unilateral primary adrenal hyperplasia—should be distinguished from idiopathic hyperaldosteronism due to bilateral adrenal hyperplasia, comprising approximately 60%-65% of primary aldosteronism, for which medical therapy is the best management. Aldosteronoma and idiopathic hyperaldosteronism are the most common subtypes. Compared with those with idiopathic hyperaldosteronism, patients with aldosteronoma have more severe hypertension, more severe hypokalemia, and higher aldosterone secretion and are younger. Interestingly, up to two-thirds of aldosteronomas have a somatic *KCNJ5* gene mutation. Somatic mutations have also been described in other genes including *ATP1A1*, *ATP2B3*, and *CACNA1D* genes.

Glucocorticoid-remediable hyperaldosteronism (FH type I) is inherited in an autosomal dominant fashion. The genetic defect results in a chimeric gene. The mutated gene juxtaposes the promoter for expression of the 11-hydroxylase gene, which is ACTH-responsive, with the coding sequence of the aldosterone synthase gene. This leads to aldosterone production under ACTH stimulation in the zona fasciculata. Glucocorticoid therapy reverses this type of hyperaldosteronism. These patients have a family history of onset of hypertension at an early age. The diagnosis can be established by genetic testing. Measurement of 24-hour urine 18-hydroxycortisol and 18-oxocortisol levels is less reliable. The molecular basis for FH type II is not clear, although it is also inherited in an autosomal dominant fashion. Presentation is identical to that of nonfamilial form of primary aldosteronism, and aldosterone-producing adenoma and idiopathic adrenal hyperplasia may coexist in the same family. The cause of FH type III is due to a germline mutation in the *KCNJ5* gene that encodes a potassium channel. Bilateral adrenalectomy has been reported in some patients to control severe resistant hypertension.

Aldosterone-secreting adrenocortical carcinoma is rare and should be suspected if the tumor is larger than 4 cm, especially if it also secrets cortisol and intermediate metabolites.

Tumor Localization

An aldosterone-producing adenoma can frequently be demonstrated by high-resolution CT or MRI scanning. Small aldosteronomas can be missed, and in such cases, a patient with a small aldosteronoma not seen on CT may be misdiagnosed as having adrenal hyperplasia. Aldosteronomas that coexist with nonfunctional adenomas can be mislabeled as adrenal hyperplasia because of multinodularity or bilateral masses on CT. Small abnormalities on CT scans may represent hyperplasia rather than true aldosteronomas. Therefore, unless an unequivocal unilateral tumor, preferably larger than 1 cm, is present on the CT scan and the contralateral gland is normal, the diagnosis and localization of aldosteronoma are not certain. When in doubt, adrenal vein sampling should be done. After venous puncture in the inguinal region, blood is sampled from the adrenal veins and the inferior vena cava to be sent for aldosterone and cortisol levels at baseline and after ACTH infusion. Proper catheter placement is confirmed by finding high cortisol levels in adrenal venous blood compared with the inferior vena cava. Corrected aldosterone levels are calculated from the ratio of aldosterone to cortisol in each venous sample. A lateralization ratio of the corrected aldosterone level higher than 4 indicates unilateral aldosterone secretion, thereby confirming a diagnosis of aldosteronoma in most patients. Adrenal vein sampling is invasive and requires considerable skill and experience. It should only be performed if the patient is a potential candidate for adrenalectomy. The success rate for cannulating both adrenal veins is about 90% (60%-95% depending on the experience of radiologists). Complications of venous sampling, such as adrenal hemorrhage, can occur in 1% of patients. Some recommend adrenal vein sampling to be done routinely regardless of CT findings. However, others advocate using it selectively when CT scan findings are uncertain (no tumor, bilateral tumors, or small tumor < 1 cm in diameter).

Complications

Uncontrolled hypertension can lead to renal failure, stroke, and myocardial infarction. Severe hypokalemia can cause weakness, paralysis, and arrhythmia, especially in patients taking digitalis.

Treatment

The goal of therapy is to prevent the complications of hypertension and hypokalemia. Unilateral adrenalectomy is recommended for patients with aldosteronoma, and medical therapy is recommended for those with idiopathic hyperaldosteronism or those with aldosteronoma who are poor candidates for surgery.

A. Surgical Treatment

1. Preoperative preparation—Blood pressure and hypokalemia should be controlled before surgery. Spironolactone, a competitive aldosterone antagonist, has been the drug of choice. It blocks the mineralocorticoid receptor, promotes potassium retention, restores normal potassium concentrations, and reduces the extracellular fluid volume, thereby controlling blood pressure. Furthermore, it reactivates the suppressed renin-angiotensin-aldosterone system in the contralateral adrenal gland, reducing the risk of postoperative hypoaldosteronism. The medication should be continued to the day of operation. For additional information and medical regimens for preoperative preparation, see the later Medical Treatment section.

2. Surgery—Because aldosteronomas are almost always small and benign, laparoscopic adrenalectomy is the procedure of choice. It can be performed safely and with equally good results by several approaches. The lateral transabdominal approach uses gravity to help medially rotate the viscera (liver on the right and spleen and pancreas on the left) and exposes the adrenal gland. It is the most versatile approach since the anatomy is familiar to most abdominal surgeons. The posterior retroperitoneal approach is best in patients with prior upper abdominal operations, but the working space is more limited. Although some surgeons perform a subtotal resection for aldosteronoma, most excise the whole adrenal gland with the tumor. The surrounding adrenal tissue frequently appears hyperplastic. Small aldosteronomas may not be visible intraoperatively. Bilateral adrenalectomy is not indicated, since hypocortisolism will require steroid replacement treatment. Patients with idiopathic hyperaldosteronism should be treated medically.

3. Postoperative care—Occasional patients may develop transient aldosterone deficiency because of suppression of the contralateral adrenal gland by the hyperfunctioning adenoma. This is uncommon in patients treated with spironolactone preoperatively. Symptoms include postural hypotension and hyperkalemia. Adequate sodium intake is usually sufficient for treatment; rarely, short-term fludrocortisone replacement (0.1 mg/d orally) is required.

B. Medical Treatment

The goal is to control hypertension and hypokalemia. Spironolactone, a competitive aldosterone antagonist, has been the drug of choice. Initial dosages of 200-400 mg/d may be required to control hypokalemia and hypertension. Once blood pressure is normalized and hypokalemia is corrected, the dose can be tapered and maintained at about 100-150 mg/d. Spironolactone may have antiandrogenic side effects, such as impotence, gynecomastia, menstrual irregularity, and gastrointestinal disturbances. These potential side effects may make this medication less desirable for some patients. Unlike spironolactone, which also blocks androgen and progesterone receptors, eplerenone is a selective mineralocorticoid receptor antagonist and has fewer endocrine side effects. It has been approved for treatment of hypertension and for heart failure after myocardial infarction. Eplerenone may become the treatment of choice for primary aldosteronism because of its decreased side effects if it is proven as efficacious as spironolactone, despite its increased cost. Amiloride, 20-40 ng/d, a potassium-sparing diuretic, may be used alternatively or as a supplement to spironolactone. Other medications, such as angiotensin-converting enzyme inhibitors, calcium channel blockers, and diuretics, may be required to control hypertension.

▶ Prognosis

Primary aldosteronism usually follows a prolonged and subtly changing course. Untreated hypertension may cause stroke, myocardial infarction, or renal failure.

Removal of an aldosteronoma normalizes potassium levels in nearly 100% of the patients, but hypertension is cured in about 50% of the patients. Persistent hypertension after operation is more common in overweight men who preoperatively required more than three antihypertensive medications for more than 6 years, but residual hypertension is usually easier to control than before the operation. Essential hypertension and atherosclerosis due to chronic hypertension are contributing factors. Although patients with idiopathic hyperaldosteronism should be treated medically, adrenalectomy is indicated for those with aldosteronoma because side effects of the medications and compliance make long-term medical treatment undesirable. The low morbidity, short hospitalization, and high success rate of laparoscopic adrenalectomy have made surgery preferable to long-term medical therapy.

Åkerström T, et al: Novel somatic mutations and distinct molecular signature in aldosterone-producing adenomas. *Endocr Relat Cancer.* 2015;22:735.

Aronova A, et al: Aldosteronoma resolution score predicts long-term resolution of hypertension. *Surgery.* 2014;156:1387.

Dekkers T, et al, and SPARTACUS Investigators: Adrenal vein sampling versus CT scan to determine treatment in primary aldosteronism: an outcome-based randomized diagnostic trial. *Lancet Diabetes Endocrinol.* 2016;4:739.

Funder JW, et al: Case detection, diagnosis, and treatment of patients with primary aldosteronism: an endocrine society clinical practice guideline. *J Clin Endocrinol Metab.* 2016;101:1889.

Hannemann A, Wallaschofski H: Prevalence of primary aldosteronism in patient's cohorts and in population-based studies: a review of the current literature. *Horm Metab Res.* 2012;44:157.

Rossi GP, et al: The adrenal vein sampling international study (AVIS) for identifying the major subtypes of primary aldosteronism. *J Clin Endocrin Metab.* 2012;97:1606.

Wachtel H, et al: Long-term blood pressure control in patients undergoing adrenalectomy for primary hyperaldosteronism. *Surgery.* 2014:156:1394.

Walz MK, et al: Retroperitoneoscopic adrenalectomy in Conn's syndrome caused by adrenal adenomas or nodular hyperplasia. *World J Surg.* 2008;32:847.

PHEOCHROMOCYTOMA

 ESSENTIALS OF DIAGNOSIS

▸ Hypertension, frequently sustained, with or without paroxysms.

▸ Episodic headache, excessive sweating, palpitation, and visual blurring.

▸ Postural tachycardia and hypotension.

▸ Elevated urinary or plasma catecholamines or their metabolites, hypermetabolism, hyperglycemia.

▶ General Considerations

Pheochromocytomas are tumors of the adrenal medulla and related chromaffin tissues elsewhere in the body (paragangliomas) that secrete epinephrine or norepinephrine, resulting in sustained or episodic hypertension and other symptoms of catecholamine excess.

Pheochromocytoma is found in less than 0.1% of patients with hypertension and accounts for about 5% of adrenal tumors incidentally discovered by CT scanning. Approximately 10% of pheochromocytomas are malignant, compared to 40% of paragangliomas. About one-third of pheochromocytomas are associated with various hereditary syndromes such as multiple endocrine neoplasia (MEN) type 2, neurofibromatosis (NF) type 1, von Hippel–Lindau (VHL) disease, and hereditary pheochromocytoma-paraganglioma (PPGL). Patients with MEN 2A may have medullary thyroid carcinoma, pheochromocytoma, and primary hyperparathyroidism. Those with MEN 2B have medullary thyroid carcinoma, pheochromocytoma, mucosal neuromas, marfanoid habitus, and ganglioneuromatosis. Patients with NF type 1 have café-au-lait spots, neurofibromatosis, and pheochromocytoma. Patients with VHL disease may have retinal hemangioma, hemangioblastoma of the central nervous system, renal cysts and carcinoma, pheochromocytoma, pancreatic cysts or neuroendocrine tumors, and epididymal cystadenoma. Pheochromocytoma can occur in hereditary PPGL syndromes caused by mutations of the succinate dehydrogenase genes (*SDHx*, *SDHB*, *SDHD*, *SDHC*, *SDHA*, and *SDHAF2*). All are associated with extra-adrenal paragangliomas. *SDHB* is particularly associated with malignant pheochromocytomas. These syndromes should be particularly considered in young patients and in patients with multifocal, extra-adrenal, malignant, or recurrent tumors. Pheochromocytoma can also occur in other hereditary PPGL syndromes associated with mutations of the *TMEM127* and *MAX* genes and, much less frequently, mutations of the *FH*, *MDH2*, *PHD1*, *PHD2*, *KIF1Bβ*, and *HIF2α* genes. Because of the higher than previously expected prevalence of hereditary pheochromocytoma, all patients with pheochromocytoma should be considered for genetic counseling and testing. The specific gene tests should depend on clinical and biochemical findings and family history. Family members of patients who have been diagnosed with these syndromes also need screening to determine whether they are gene carriers and are at risk for developing the various tumors, including pheochromocytoma.

On pathologic examination, pheochromocytoma appears reddish-gray and frequently has areas of necrosis, hemorrhage, and sometimes cysts. The usual size is about 100 g, or 5 cm in diameter, but they can be as small as 2-3 cm or as large as 12-16 cm. Cells are pleomorphic, showing prominent nucleoli and frequent mitoses. Cytologic findings cannot be used to determine reliably whether a pheochromocytoma is malignant or benign. The veins and capsules may also be invaded even in clinically benign tumors. Malignancy can only be diagnosed in the presence of metastases in non–chromaffin-cell-bearing tissues (eg, lymph nodes, liver, bone) or invasion into surrounding tissues.

▶ Clinical Findings

A. Symptoms and Signs

The clinical findings of pheochromocytoma are variable, and almost half of them come to attention because of an incidental finding of an adrenal tumor (incidentaloma) on CT or MRI scans performed to evaluate other diseases. Classically, the patient has episodic hypertension associated with the triad of palpitation, headache, and sweating. The patient may also complain of anxiety, tremors, weight loss, dizziness, nausea and vomiting, abdominal discomfort, constipation, and visual blurring. Rarely, pheochromocytomas can secrete vasoactive intestinal peptide (VIP), causing severe diarrhea, or ACTH, causing Cushing syndrome. The physical examination may be unremarkable except during an attack, when pallor and excess sweating may be observed. Tachycardia, postural hypotension, and hypertensive retinopathy are other signs.

Hypertension, the most common feature of pheochromocytoma, occurs in 90% of patients. More than half have sustained hypertension, which may be mild to moderate, with or without other signs and symptoms of catecholamine excess, and the diagnosis may be missed. In some cases, basal blood pressure may not be elevated, and severe hypertension occurs only while the patient is under stress, such as general anesthesia or trauma. Patients with diastolic hypertension and postural hypotension who are not receiving antihypertensive medications may have pheochromocytoma. Hyperglycemia may occur because epinephrine raises blood glucose and norepinephrine decreases insulin secretion.

In children, hypertension is less prominent, and about 50% have multiple or extra-adrenal tumors. Paragangliomas due to *SDHB* mutations are more likely to metastasize. Pheochromocytomas occur in 40%-50% of patients with MEN 2;

they tend to be bilateral and multiple but are rarely extra-adrenal or malignant. Biochemical screening for gene carriers of hereditary pheochromocytoma should be performed routinely. Measurement of plasma free metanephrines (metanephrine and normetanephrine) is the most sensitive test for pheochromocytoma in hereditary syndromes.

B. Laboratory Findings

The diagnosis of pheochromocytoma is best confirmed either by 24-hour urinary fractionated metanephrines or by plasma free metanephrines. Both tests have high sensitivity and specificity (Figure 35–2). Plasma free metanephrines may be more sensitive than the urine test, but has a higher false-positive rate, especially in elderly patients. Assays using liquid chromatography (LC) with electrochemical detection (LC-ECD) or LC with tandem mass spectrometry (LC-MS/MS) perform better than immunoassays and reduce interference by many drugs and diets. However, some drugs can still affect certain LC-ECD methods, including acetaminophen, labetalol, sotalol, alpha-methyldopa, buspirone, and sulfasalazine. The interfering substances vary depending on the specific method used, so a list and protocol for preparing the patient should be obtained from the specific laboratory. LC-MS/MS is a newer assay that has been shown to minimize drug interferences in the measurement of plasma and urinary metanephrines. Some drugs affect secretion and metabolism of catecholamines and will affect all assays, including tricyclic antidepressants; cyclobenzaprine, which is structurally

▲ **Figure 35–2.** Scheme for evaluation of a patient with suspected pheochromocytoma. CT, computed tomography; MRI, magnetic resonance imaging.

related to tricyclic antidepressants; monoamine oxidase inhibitors; most psychotropic drugs (except for selective serotonin reuptake inhibitors) such as buspirone; prochlorperazine; drugs containing catecholamines; amphetamine; withdrawal from clonidine; and alcohol. These agents should be discontinued for 2 weeks, if possible, before biochemical testing. Stress and illnesses can also increase catecholamines, and testing results must be interpreted appropriately. To minimize sympathetic activation, plasma free metanephrines should be measured in the supine position. However, this is frequently not possible. One recent study showed high diagnostic accuracy when the test is measured fasted and seated.

C. Tumor Localization

Localization studies should be performed only after biochemical studies have confirmed the diagnosis of a catecholamine-secreting tumor. Ninety percent of pheochromocytomas are found in the adrenal glands, and most are larger than 3 cm in diameter. Of the extra-adrenal pheochromocytomas (also called paragangliomas), 75% are in the abdomen, 10% in the bladder, 10% in the chest, 2% in the pelvis, and 3% in the head and neck. Both CT and MRI can localize most pheochromocytomas. CT scan is less expensive and gives better anatomic details for the surgeons, but MRI avoids radiation exposure. Pheochromocytoma usually has a characteristic bright appearance on T2-weighted MRI. ^{123}I-MIBG scanning can be considered when searching for extra-adrenal, multiple, malignant, or metastatic pheochromocytomas, especially when they may benefit from ^{131}MIBG-labeled radionuclide therapy for metastatic disease. MIBG is more specific but less sensitive compared with CT or MRI for localization. Positron emission tomography (PET)-CT scans using various PET tracers have been studied. Compared to CT, MRI, and MIBG, ^{18}F-fluoro-2-deoxy-D-glucose (^{18}F-FDG) PET-CT is more sensitive for localizing metastatic paragangliomas in patients with *SDHB* mutations. ^{68}Ga-DOTATATE PET/CT is the most sensitive functional imaging tool in the detection of pheochromocytomas and paragangliomas. Arteriography and fine-needle aspiration biopsy can precipitate a hypertensive crisis. They do not contribute to the diagnosis and should not be performed. Venous sampling for catecholamines is not indicated and can be misleading.

▶ Differential Diagnosis

The differential diagnosis includes all causes of hypertension. Hyperthyroidism and pheochromocytoma have many features in common (weight loss, tremor, and tachycardia). The diagnosis of pheochromocytoma is easier if episodic hypertension is present. Acute anxiety attacks mimic the symptoms and may precipitate hypertensive episodes, but anxiety alone rarely produces severe hypertension. Carcinoid syndrome causing episodes of flushing may also be mistaken

for pheochromocytoma. Urinary 5-hydroxyindoleacetic acid (5-HIAA) level is usually markedly elevated, and CT scan may show liver metastases in patients with carcinoid syndrome. Labile essential hypertension is not associated with elevated catecholamine/metanephrine levels.

Pheochromocytoma in pregnancy, if not recognized, will kill half of the fetuses and nearly half of the mothers. Hypertension in pregnancy is usually ascribed to preeclampsia-eclampsia. The diagnosis of pheochromocytoma requires the same biochemical studies as in nonpregnant patients; MRI is indicated to localize the tumor when a biochemical diagnosis has been established. CT, PET/CT, or MIBG imaging is not used to avoid radiation exposure. α-Adrenergic and β-adrenergic blockers are well tolerated. Timing of the operation is individualized. If recognized early, the tumor is best removed early in the second trimester. Otherwise, α-adrenergic blockade is continued, and a planned cesarean section at term is followed by laparoscopic adrenalectomy a few weeks postpartum.

Pheochromocytoma crisis may develop in patients with pheochromocytoma, usually precipitated by trauma, certain medications, surgery, biopsy, or other procedures. It can also be triggered by glucocorticoids. Crisis usually occurs when α-adrenergic blockade has not been instituted. These patients may develop multisystem failure, especially heart failure and cardiovascular complications. If pheochromocytomas crisis is not recognized, death is the usual result. Once pheochromocytoma is diagnosed, the patient should be started on α-adrenergic blockade. After adequate α blockade (10-14 days), the pheochromocytoma can be resected during the same hospitalization or the patient may be stabilized, discharged, and electively readmitted. Emergency operation is not recommended without stabilization and α blockade.

▶ Complications

Pheochromocytoma causes complications because of hypertension, cardiac arrhythmia, and hypovolemia. The sequelae of hypertension are stroke, renal failure, myocardial infarction, and congestive heart failure. Sudden death can result from ventricular tachycardia or fibrillation. α-Adrenergic stimulation by the catecholamines causes vasoconstriction and a low total blood volume. The patient is therefore unable to compensate for a sudden loss of blood volume (bleeding) or catecholamines (tumor removal) and is at risk of cardiovascular collapse. Preoperative α-adrenergic blockade and restoration of blood volume can prevent these complications.

▶ Treatment

A. Medical Treatment

Treatment with α-adrenergic blocking agents should be started as soon as the biochemical diagnosis is established. The aims of preoperative therapy are (1) to restore the blood volume, which has been depleted by excessive catecholamines; (2) to prevent a severe crisis, with its potential complications; and (3) to allow the patient to recover from cardiomyopathy. Close control of hypertension is necessary in order to keep blood volume normal.

Phenoxybenzamine, a nonselective α-adrenergic antagonist, has a long duration of action and is the preferred drug. It should be started at a dosage of 10 mg/12 h, and the dose should be increased by 10-20 mg every 2-3 days—as postural hypotension allows. Usual doses are 100-160 mg/d; however, dosages as high as 300 mg/d may be necessary. Most patients require 10-14 days of treatment, as judged by stabilization of blood pressure and reduction of symptoms. Nasal stuffiness is usually present when α blockade is well established. Doxazosin, a competitive selective α-adrenergic blocker, may also be effective and less costly. Metyrosine inhibits tyrosine hydroxylase and reduces catecholamine synthesis and can be added to phenoxybenzamine as preoperative therapy.

β-Adrenergic blocking agents are often used to treat arrhythmias and tachycardia but should only be given after α blockade has been achieved. Otherwise, a hypertensive crisis may be precipitated because of the unopposed α-adrenergic effect of the catecholamines. Opioids should be avoided because they may stimulate histamine release and precipitate a crisis.

B. Surgical Treatment

The definitive treatment of pheochromocytoma is excision after preoperative localization and α-adrenergic blockade.

Smaller (< 5-6 cm) adrenal pheochromocytomas can be safely resected by laparoscopic adrenalectomy. Larger (> 8-10 cm), locally invasive, and extra-adrenal tumors are technically more difficult and may require open resection.

During surgery, an arterial line is necessary for continuous blood pressure monitoring. Monitoring of pulmonary artery pressure is usually not necessary in patients who are well blocked.

Nitroprusside should be immediately available to treat sudden hypertension and β-blockers to treat the cardiac dysrhythmias that may occur when the tumor is manipulated. Manipulation of the gland is less with laparoscopic adrenalectomy, which minimizes fluctuations in plasma catecholamine levels.

Very large malignant tumors may require a thoracoabdominal incision. Malignant pheochromocytomas may invade the adrenal vein or vena cava. Extra-adrenal pheochromocytomas (paragangliomas) are usually found along the abdominal aorta and in the organ of Zuckerkandl near the aortic bifurcation around the inferior mesenteric artery. However, tumors have been found in widely scattered sites such as the bladder, the vagina, the mediastinum, the neck, and even the skull base and pericardium. In general, extra-adrenal tumors should be localized preoperatively with MIBG, CT, MRI or PET-CT to avoid a blind exploration.

In patients with MEN 2 or VHL and bilateral pheochromocytomas, cortical-sparing subtotal adrenalectomy on the side of the smaller tumor may avoid postoperative adrenal insufficiency, although it increases the risk for recurrence. In patients with a known hereditary pheochromocytoma syndrome and a unilateral pheochromocytoma, prophylactic resection of the contralateral normal-appearing adrenal gland is not indicated, since bilateral adrenalectomy leads to lifelong hypocortisolism requiring cortisol replacement. These patients should be followed with biochemical evaluations, and the contralateral adrenal gland should be resected only if pheochromocytoma develops.

Patients undergoing resection of pheochromocytoma who are not adequately prepared preoperatively may have hypertensive crises, cardiac arrhythmia, myocardial infarction, or acute pulmonary edema. In addition, these patients may experience intractable hypotension and die in shock after tumor removal. If the patient has been properly prepared with α-blockers, the changes in blood pressure will not be severe. Otherwise, intravenous infusion of large amounts of saline and vasopressors may be necessary to maintain blood pressure after the tumor is removed. Hypoglycemia may develop after tumor removal, so blood glucose level should be checked until the patient is eating.

► Prognosis

Patients with untreated pheochromocytoma are at high risk for complications from hypertensive crisis and cardiovascular disease, whereas the operative mortality rate is 0%-3%. Mild to moderate essential hypertension may persist after surgery. Second tumors in the remaining adrenal or metastatic tumors can occur years after excision of the primary pheochromocytoma; long-term follow-up is mandatory. Patients with pheochromocytoma should be offered genetic counseling and, when appropriate, tested for hereditary causes of pheochromocytoma. Long-term prognosis may depend on the mutation present (eg, risk for malignant pheochromocytoma in SDHB gene mutation carriers). Metastatic or recurrent malignant pheochromocytoma should be resected if possible to reduce the catecholamine load. Treatment with high-dose ^{131}I-MIBG may be helpful in these patients.

Biggar MA, et al: Systematic review of phaeochromocytoma in pregnancy. Br J Surg. 2013;100:182.

Casey R, et al: Screening for phaeochromocytoma and paraganglioma: impact of using supine reference intervals for plasma metanephrines with samples collected from fasted/seated patients. Ann Clin Biochem. 2017;54:170.

Gimenez-Roqueplo AP, et al: An update on the genetics of paraganglioma, pheochromocytoma, and associated hereditary syndromes. Horm Metab Res. 2012;44:328.

Lenders JW, et al: Pheochromocytoma and paraganglioma: an endocrine society clinical practice guideline. J Clin Endocrinol Metab. 2014;99:1915.

Neumann HP, et al: 65 years of the double helix: Genetics informs precision practice in the diagnosis and management of pheochromocytoma. *Endocr Relat Cancer.* 2018;25:T201.

Scholten A, et al: Pheochromocytoma crisis is not a surgical emergency. *J Clin Endocrinol Metab.* 2013; 98:581-91.

Shen WT, et al: One hundred two patients with pheochromocytoma treated at a single institution since the introduction of laparoscopic adrenalectomy. *Arch Surg.* 2010;145:893.

Walz MK, et al. Minimally invasive surgery (MIS) in children and adolescents with pheochromocytomas and retroperitoneal paragangliomas: experiences in 42 patients. *World J Surg.* 2018;42:1024.

HYPERCORTISOLISM (CUSHING DISEASE & CUSHING SYNDROME)

ESSENTIALS OF DIAGNOSIS

▸ Facial plethora, dorsocervical fat pad, supraclavicular fat pad, truncal obesity, easy bruisability, purple striae, acne, hirsutism, impotence or amenorrhea, muscle weakness, and psychosis.

▸ Hypertension, hyperglycemia, and osteopenia or osteoporosis.

▶ General Considerations

Cushing syndrome is due to chronic glucocorticoid excess. It may be caused by excess ACTH stimulation or by adrenocortical tumors that secrete glucocorticoids independently of ACTH stimulation. Excess ACTH may be produced by pituitary adenomas (Cushing disease) or extrapituitary ACTH-producing tumors (ectopic ACTH syndrome). Cushing syndrome not dependent on ACTH is usually caused by primary adrenal diseases such as an adrenocortical adenoma and micronodular or macronodular hyperplasia or carcinoma.

The natural history of Cushing syndrome depends on the underlying disease and varies from a mild, indolent disease to rapid progression and death.

▶ Clinical Findings

A. Symptoms and Signs

See Table 35–1. The classic description of Cushing syndrome includes truncal obesity, hirsutism, moon facies, acne, dorsal fat pad, purple striae, hypertension, and diabetes, but other signs and symptoms are common. Weakness and depression are striking features. Weakness and other features are also seen after prolonged and excessive administration of adrenocortical steroids.

Table 35–1. Frequency of manifestations of hypercortisolism.

	Percentage
Obesity	95%
Hypertension	70%
Glucose tolerance	80%
Centripetal distribution of fat	80%
Weakness	20%
Muscle atrophy in upper and lower extremities	70%
Hirsutism	80%
Menstrual disturbance or impotence	75%
Purple striae	50%
Plethoric facies	85%
Easy bruisability	35%
Acne	40%
Psychological symptoms	40%
Edema	20%
Headache	15%
Back pain	60%

In children, Cushing syndrome is most commonly caused by adrenal cancers, but adenomas and nodular hyperplasia have been described. Cushing syndrome in children also causes growth retardation or arrest.

B. Pathologic Examination

The pathologic features of the adrenal gland depend on the underlying disease. Normal adrenal glands weigh 7-12 g combined. The hyperplastic adrenal glands in patients with Cushing disease weigh less than 25 g combined. In ectopic ACTH syndrome, the combined adrenal weight is greater—from 25 g to 100 g.

Adrenal adenomas in Cushing syndrome range in weight from a few grams to over 100 g, are usually over 3 cm in diameter, and are larger than aldosterone-producing adenomas. The typical cells usually resemble those of the zona fasciculata. Variable degrees of anaplasia are seen, and differentiation of benign from malignant tumors is often difficult on the basis of cytology alone. These adrenal adenomas occur more frequently in women. Adrenal cancers are frequently very large—almost always over 5 cm in diameter. They are undifferentiated, invade the surrounding tissues, and metastasize via the bloodstream.

Rare forms of ACTH-independent Cushing syndrome include ACTH-independent macronodular adrenal hyperplasia, which in some cases is due to aberrant expression of receptors in the adrenals that respond to stimuli other than ACTH. In these cases, the adrenal glands can be massively enlarged. Primary pigmented nodular adrenal disease or micronodular hyperplasia is associated with the syndrome of Carney complex, which also includes cardiac myxoma and lentigines.

Rarely, ectopic adrenal tissue can be the source of excessive cortisol secretion. It has been found in various locations, most commonly near the abdominal aorta.

Cushing disease is caused by ACTH secretion from pituitary adenomas.

Ectopic ACTH syndrome is usually caused by small-cell lung cancer and neuroendocrine tumors (carcinoid tumors) of the pancreas, thymus, thyroid, prostate, esophagus, colon, and ovaries. Pheochromocytoma and malignant melanoma may also secrete ACTH.

C. Laboratory Findings

Because no single test is specific, a combination of tests must be used to diagnosis Cushing syndrome.

Normal subjects have a circadian rhythm of ACTH secretion that is paralleled by cortisol secretion. Levels are highest in the early morning and decline during the day to their lowest levels in the late evening. In Cushing syndrome, the circadian rhythm is abolished, and total secretion of cortisol is increased. In mild cases, the plasma cortisol and ACTH levels may be within the normal range during much of the day but abnormally high in the evening.

When Cushing syndrome is suspected, the first objective is to establish the diagnosis; the second is to establish the cause. An algorithm for the diagnosis is presented in Figure 35–3. When hypercortisolism is suspected, three tests are available as the initial tests to establish the diagnosis: overnight dexamethasone suppression test, measurement of 24-hour urinary free cortisol, and late-night salivary cortisol sampling. Dexamethasone, 1 mg orally, will suppress ACTH secretion and stop cortisol production in most healthy individuals. This low-dose dexamethasone, however, will not suppress excessive cortisol production from autonomous adrenocortical tumors or adrenals that are being stimulated by excess ACTH. Because dexamethasone does not cross-react in the assay for plasma cortisol, suppression of endogenous circulating cortisol is easily demonstrated. The test is done as follows: At 11 PM, the patient is given 1 mg of dexamethasone by mouth. A fasting plasma cortisol is measured the following morning between 8 AM and 9 AM. Suppression of plasma cortisol to 1.8 µg/dL (50 nmol/L) or less excludes Cushing syndrome in most patients. The stringent low cutoff

level of 1.8 µg/dL increases the likelihood of a false-positive result. False-positive results are more common in patients with depression, alcoholism, physiologic stress, marked obesity, obstructive sleep apnea, or renal failure and in those taking estrogens or drugs that accelerate dexamethasone metabolism, such as phenytoin, rifampin, and phenobarbital. Estrogens increase cortisol-binding globulin and elevate total plasma cortisol concentrations. In these situations, measurement of 24-hour urinary free cortisol or salivary cortisol is preferred. The 24-hour urinary cortisol directly measures the physiologically active form of circulating cortisol, integrates the daily variations of cortisol production, and is very sensitive and specific for the diagnosis of Cushing syndrome.

Late-night salivary cortisol sampling can also assist in establishing the diagnosis of Cushing syndrome. The procedure involves chewing a cotton tube for 2-3 minutes between 11 PM and 12 AM. Salivary cortisol levels correlate highly with plasma and serum free cortisol levels. One positive initial screening test result should be confirmed by a second initial screening test to establish the diagnosis. *Once the diagnosis of Cushing syndrome is established,* the next step is to determine the cause. Plasma ACTH measurement by immunoradiometric assay (IRMA) is the most direct method. A normal to elevated ACTH level is diagnostic of hypercortisolism due to pituitary adenoma or ectopic ACTH secretion. Suppressed ACTH levels are diagnostic of hypercortisolism due to a primary adrenal causes such as adenoma, carcinoma, or nodular hyperplasia.

The differential diagnosis of ACTH-dependent Cushing syndrome can be challenging. No test is perfect, and a combination of tests may be necessary. Since 90% of patients have Cushing disease, pituitary MRI is the first test to identify the source of ACTH secretion. However, 10% of normal adults have incidental pituitary lesions 3-6 mm in diameter on MRI, and many patients with Cushing disease have no detectable lesions. Lesions smaller than 3-4 mm are more likely to represent normal variation, artifacts, volume averaging, incidental nonfunctional adenomas, or cysts. An unequivocal pituitary lesion (ie, ≥ 5-6 mm in diameter with decreased signal intensity on gadolinium) strongly suggests Cushing disease.

If the pituitary MRI does not show a definite lesion, the next step is inferior petrosal sinus sampling with corticotropin-releasing hormone (CRH) stimulation. Compared with other biochemical tests, such as high-dose dexamethasone suppression or CRH stimulation, petrosal sinus sampling is the most accurate way to identify an ACTH-secreting pituitary adenoma; the diagnostic accuracy is close to 100%. The test requires simultaneous bilateral venous sampling from the inferior petrosal sinuses. The inferior petrosal sinus connects the cavernous sinus to the jugular bulb and drains the pituitary. A central-to-peripheral ACTH ratio of 2 or greater without CRH stimulation is diagnostic of Cushing disease. CRH, 100 µg given intravenously as a bolus

▲ **Figure 35–3.** Cushing syndrome: diagnosis and differential diagnosis. ACTH, adrenocorticotropic hormone; CRH, corticotropin-releasing hormone; MRI, magnetic resonance imaging.

injection, can increase the diagnostic sensitivity to 100%; a peak central-to-peripheral ACTH ratio of 3 or greater is diagnostic of Cushing disease. The lack of a central-to-peripheral ACTH gradient is diagnostic of an ectopic ACTH-secreting tumor.

In Cushing syndrome caused by primary adrenal diseases, the plasma ACTH level is suppressed. Adenomas are usually 3-5 cm in diameter and secrete only cortisol. Adrenal carcinomas are typically larger than 5 cm in diameter, are usually rapidly progressive, and may co-secrete other hormones, such as adrenal androgens, deoxycorticosterone, aldosterone, and estrogens.

D. Imaging Studies

For Cushing syndrome caused by primary adrenal diseases, thin-section CT or MRI is able to detect virtually all of the adrenal tumors and hyperplasia. MRI of the sella is the imaging study of choice for pituitary adenomas. If a definitive adenoma is not seen, inferior petrosal sinus sampling with CRH stimulation can differentiate Cushing disease from ectopic Cushing syndrome. For ectopic Cushing syndrome, CT or MRI of the chest and abdomen may detect ACTH-secreting tumors. Bronchial carcinoids may be very small and difficult to find; high-resolution thin-cut CT of the chest is indicated. Occasionally, the source of an ectopic ACTH-secreting tumor cannot be determined (occult ectopic ACTH syndrome) by conventional imaging.[68]Ga-DOTATOC-PET/CT is a new imaging technique that may aid in localizing these occult tumors.

▶ Complications

Severe or lethal complications may result from sustained hypercortisolism, including hypertension, cardiovascular disease, stroke, thromboembolism, infection, severe debilitating muscle wasting, and weakness. Psychosis is common. Death may also be caused by the underlying tumors, such as adrenal carcinoma, small-cell lung cancer, and others causing ectopic ACTH syndrome.

The truncal obesity and muscle weakness in patients with Cushing syndrome predispose them to postoperative pulmonary complications. Atrophic skin and easy bruisability also predict poor wound healing.

Nelson syndrome, the progression of an ACTH-secreting pituitary adenoma following bilateral adrenalectomy for Cushing disease, occurred in as many as 30% of patients in the era when bilateral adrenalectomy was used as primary therapy. However, since transsphenoidal resection has become the initial procedure of choice for Cushing disease and because MRI now allows accurate diagnosis of pituitary adenomas larger than 5 mm, Nelson syndrome occurs in less than 5% of patients.

These tumors in patients with Nelson syndrome are among the most aggressive pituitary tumors, causing sellar enlargement and extrasellar extension. Plasma ACTH levels are markedly elevated. Patients are frequently hyperpigmented and hypopituitary, with symptoms of mass effects including headaches, visual field deficits, and even blindness from optic nerve compression. Removal of feedback control from hypercortisolism at the pituitary level probably explains the aggressiveness of these tumors.

▶ Treatment

Resection is the best treatment for cortisol-producing adrenal tumors or ACTH-producing tumors. Other treatment options may be necessary to temporarily control hypercortisolism, for patients not cured by resection, or when complete resection is impossible.

A. Excision of Pituitary Adenoma

Patients with Cushing disease are usually treated by transsphenoidal microsurgical excision of the pituitary adenomas. Relief of symptoms is rapid, and the prognosis for adequate residual pituitary-adrenal function is good. Total or subtotal hypophysectomy may be performed in older patients if a discrete tumor is not found. Pituitary procedures fail in about 15%-25% of patients because of failure to find the adenoma, pituitary hyperplasia, or recurrence of adenoma. When pituitary surgery fails, the disease may respond to pituitary irradiation. In some patients, medical therapy or total adrenalectomy will be necessary. Because of the effectiveness of pituitary microsurgery, radiotherapy is usually not recommended as primary treatment for Cushing disease.

B. Adrenalectomy

Compared with patients with other adrenal tumors, those with severe Cushing syndrome are at a higher risk for postoperative complications such as wound infection, hemorrhage, peptic ulceration, and pulmonary embolism. Adrenalectomy, however, is usually successful in reversing the devastating effects of hypercortisolism.

Laparoscopic adrenalectomy causes less morbidity than open adrenalectomy and is preferred for benign hyperplasia or adenomas. Laparoscopic adrenalectomy for adrenocortical carcinoma is technically challenging. If necessary, the operation should be converted to laparotomy to achieve complete tumor resection without breaching the capsule. Local recurrence may be more common after laparoscopic resection for large and invasive cancers, especially if the capsule is breached during dissection.

Unilateral adrenalectomy is indicated for adrenal adenomas or carcinomas that secrete cortisol. The contralateral adrenal gland and the hypothalamic-pituitary-adrenal axis will usually recover from the suppression 1-2 years after the operation. Subtotal resection is not indicated because adenoma and carcinoma may not be readily distinguishable.

Total bilateral adrenalectomy is indicated for selected patients with Cushing disease or ectopic ACTH syndrome in whom the occult ACTH-secreting tumor cannot be found or resected. It is also indicated for patients with bilateral primary adrenal disease, such as pigmented micronodular hyperplasia or massive macronodular hyperplasia.

Bilateral adrenalectomy can almost always be accomplished by the laparoscopic or posterior retroperitoneoscopic approach.

Subtotal resection is not recommended in patients with Cushing syndrome because it usually leaves inadequate adrenocortical reserve initially, and the disease frequently recurs with continuing ACTH stimulation. Total bilateral adrenalectomy with adrenal gland autotransplantation is rarely successful and offers little advantage over pharmacologic replacement.

C. Medical Treatment

Drugs are mainly used as adjuvant therapy. Hypercortisolism may be controlled with ketoconazole, metyrapone, or aminoglutethimide, all of which inhibit steroid biosynthesis. Ketoconazole is usually the first choice. A combination of drugs may be necessary to control hypercortisolism and to decrease dose-related side effects. Mifepristone (RU 486), a progesterone and glucocorticoid receptor antagonist, is also effective, but it raises cortisol and ACTH levels, making it difficult to monitor the patient. Experience with the medication is still limited.

Mitotane is a dichlorodiphenyltrichloroethane (DDT) derivative that is toxic to the adrenal cortex. It has been used with modest success in the treatment of adrenal hypersecretory states, especially adrenocortical carcinoma. Unfortunately, serious side effects are common at effective doses.

Pasireotide, a somatostatin analog, and cabergoline, a dopamine receptor (type 2) agonist, may be effective in controlling hypercortisolism in small subsets of patients with Cushing disease. Frequently, a combination of drugs is needed.

D. Postoperative Maintenance Therapy

For patients who require total adrenalectomy, lifelong corticosteroid maintenance therapy becomes necessary after total adrenalectomy. The following schedule is commonly used: No cortisol is given until the adrenals are removed during surgery. On the first day, give 50 mg of hydrocortisone intravenously every 8 hours, beginning in the operating room. On the second day, give 25 mg every 6-8 hours. Thereafter, the dose should be tapered as tolerated. The same tapering process is used after excision of a unilateral cortisol-secreting adenoma, because the remaining adrenal may not function normally for months.

As the hydrocortisone dose is reduced below 50 mg/d, it is often necessary to add fludrocortisone (a mineralocorticoid),

0.1 mg daily orally, if patients had bilateral adrenalectomy. The usual maintenance doses are about 15-20 mg of hydrocortisone and 0.1 mg of fludrocortisone daily. More than half the hydrocortisone dose is given in the morning. For patients with Cushing syndrome, rapid taper of hydrocortisone to the usual maintenance dose is not recommended because they will experience withdrawal symptoms including fatigue, weakness, myalgia, arthralgia, nausea, and anorexia.

Patients who have had a total bilateral adrenalectomy and are on maintenance therapy can develop Addisonian crisis when under stress, such as general anesthesia or infection. Adrenal insufficiency causes fever, hyperkalemia, abdominal pain, and hypotension and should be promptly recognized and treated with saline infusion and cortisol.

▶ Prognosis

The prognosis is good after resection of benign adrenal adenomas, pituitary adenomas, or benign ACTH-secreting tumors. Patients with Cushing disease in remission after pituitary surgery have reversal of excess mortality. Symptoms and signs of hypercortisolism resolve, usually over months. Short-term adrenal insufficiency after surgery requires cortisol replacement. Cushing disease can recur after excision of a pituitary adenoma. An occult ACTH-secreting tumor may become apparent later and require removal.

Residual adrenal tissue or embryonic rests are present in up to 10% of patients after total adrenalectomy. Cushing syndrome can then recur if stimulation with ACTH continues.

The prognosis is extremely poor in patients with adrenocortical carcinoma and in those with malignant tumors causing ectopic ACTH syndrome.

Feelders RA, et al: Stepwise medical treatment of Cushing's disease with pasireotide mono- or combination therapy with cabergoline and low-dose ketoconazole. N Engl J Med. 2010;362:1846.

Isidori AM, et al: Conventional and nuclear medicine imaging in ectopic Cushing's syndrome: a systematic review. J Clin Endocrinol Metab. 2015;100:3231.

Nieman LK, et al: The treatment of Cushing's syndrome: an Endocrine Society Clinical Practice Guideline. J Clin Endocrinol Metab. 2015;100:2807.

Sippel RS, et al: Waiting for change: symptom resolution after adrenalectomy for Cushing's syndrome. Surgery. 2008;144:1054.

Toniato A, et al: Surgical versus conservative management for subclinical Cushing's syndrome in adrenal incidentalomas: a prospective randomized study. Ann Surg. 2009;249:388.

Tsinberg M, et al: Subclinical Cushing's syndrome. J Surg Oncol. 2012;106:572.

VIRILIZING ADRENAL TUMORS

In adults, hormonally active benign adrenal adenomas usually secrete aldosterone or cortisol. Virilizing tumors in women are more likely to be caused by ovarian tumors.

Virilizing adrenal tumors are rare, and virilization is usually due to hypersecretion of adrenal androgens, mainly dehydroepiandrosterone (DHEA), its sulfate derivative (DHEAS), and androstenedione, all of which are converted peripherally to testosterone and 5-dihydrotestosterone. Very rarely, virilizing adrenal tumors secrete only testosterone.

The differentiation of benign from malignant adrenocortical tumors may be difficult when based on histologic features; some patients with histologically benign tumors may develop metastases, and others with histologically malignant tumors may never have recurrent disease. Malignancy is only definitely diagnosed from local or distant spread. Seventy percent of virilizing adrenal tumors exhibit malignant behavior. Adrenocortical carcinomas are usually large tumors with local spread or distant metastases. They often secrete multiple steroids, most commonly cortisol and androgens, leading to Cushing syndrome and virilization.

In children, adrenocortical tumors are rare, but virilization with or without hypercortisolism is the most frequent feature. Virilizing adrenal tumors are less likely to be malignant in children than in adults. Histologic features of malignancy do not always predict malignant behavior. Large tumors (> 100 g) have a worse prognosis.

Signs and symptoms of virilization include hirsutism, male-pattern baldness, acne, deep voice, male musculature, irregular menses or amenorrhea, clitoromegaly, and increased libido. Rapid linear growth with advanced bone age is common in children.

CT and MRI are used to image virilizing adrenal tumors. Resection is the only successful treatment.

Virilization can also be caused by congenital adrenal hyperplasia, an autosomal recessive disorder. The mutated genes encode enzymes essential for cortisol and mineralocorticoid synthesis. 21-Hydroxylase deficiency accounts for 90% of cases. The inhibition of cortisol synthesis leads to stimulated ACTH secretion, accumulation of precursors, and overproduction of androgens. Administration of glucocorticoids is the mainstay of treatment in patients with classic congenital adrenal hyperplasia. Mineralocorticoid replacement is also required.

FEMINIZING ADRENAL TUMORS

Estrogens are not normally synthesized by the adrenal cortex. Feminizing adrenal tumors are extremely rare and are almost always carcinomas. They are usually seen in men with feminization or in girls with precocious puberty. Vaginal bleeding may be the presenting symptom in adult women. Feminizing adrenal carcinomas frequently hypersecrete other hormones. The diagnosis is based on a finding of increased plasma estrogens. Ovarian tumors and administration of exogenous estrogen should be ruled out.

Definitive treatment is excision of the tumor. The prognosis is guarded.

Cavlan D, et al: Androgen- and estrogen-secreting adrenal cancers. *Semin Oncol.* 2010;37:638.

Speiser PW, et al: Congenital adrenal hyperplasia due to steroid 21-hydroxylase deficiency: an Endocrine Society Clinical Practice Guideline. *J Clin Endocrinol Metab.* 2018;103:1.

ADRENOCORTICAL CARCINOMA

Adrenocortical carcinomas are rare. More than half of patients have symptoms related to hypersecretion of hormones, most commonly Cushing syndrome and virilization. Feminizing and purely aldosterone-secreting carcinomas are rare. In some cases, hormone hypersecretion is subclinical and only found by biochemical studies. The adrenal mass may be palpable. The mean diameter of adrenal carcinoma is 12 cm (range, 3-30 cm). Adrenocortical carcinoma invades the surrounding tissues, and about half of the patients have metastases (lung, liver, and elsewhere) at the time of diagnosis.

Tumor stage at the initial operation predicts the prognosis. Five-year overall survival was 66%, 58%, 24%, and 0% for stage I, II, III, and IV disease, respectively, from the French Association of Endocrine Surgeons Study Group. Surgery is the only treatment that potentially provides a cure with R0 resection; however, beneficial outcomes are confined to patients with localized disease. When grossly complete resection is possible, the 5-year survival is 55%; recurrence is common despite apparent complete resection due to micrometastases at initial presentation. Laparoscopic adrenalectomy is technically more difficult for adrenocortical carcinomas than for other adrenal tumors because the tumor is fragile and adjacent organs may have to be removed. When the adrenal tumor is small, malignancy is uncertain, and the surgeon is technically capable, starting the operation laparoscopically is acceptable. However, the surgeon should have a low threshold for converting to open or hand-assisted adrenalectomy if a better operation could be accomplished that way. Resection of involved adjacent organs and suspicious lymph nodes should be performed at the time of the initial operation when cancer is suspected. For local recurrent disease, reoperation is indicated and may prolong life. Patients with distant metastases at initial presentation usually die within 1 year. Resecting the adrenal tumor in these patients does not improve survival.

Mitotane, an adrenolytic agent, has been used alone or in addition to surgery in patients with advanced adrenocortical carcinoma. It controls endocrine symptoms in 50% of patients, and the tumor regresses in some in unresectable disease.

Although data on adjuvant mitotane use after complete primary resection are mixed, a recent large retrospective study showed that mitotane improved recurrence-free survival and that the benefit is maintained after an additional 9 years. Dose-related side effects (eg, gastrointestinal symptoms, weakness, dizziness, and somnolence) may limit its use. A variety of other chemotherapeutic agents have been tried with limited success. A recently completed international multicenter prospective randomized study (FIRM-ACT) showed combination chemotherapy of etoposide, doxorubicin, and cisplatin plus mitotane improved the rates of response and progression-free survival over that of mitotane plus streptozocin. However, there was no significant difference in overall survival.

The role of radiation is limited and usually is for palliation, especially for bony metastases. The benefit of adjuvant radiation for local control is limited; survival benefit has not been demonstrated.

Berruti A, et al: Long-term outcomes of adjuvant mitotane therapy in patients with radically resected adrenocortical carcinoma. *J Clin Endocrinol Metab.* 2017;102:1358.

Fassnacht M, et al: Combination chemotherapy in advanced adrenocortical carcinoma. *N Engl J Med.* 2012;366:2189.

Gaujoux S, et al: Recommendation for standardized surgical management of primary adrenocortical carcinoma. *Surgery.* 2012; 152:123.

Icard P, et al: Adrenocortical carcinomas: surgical trends and results of a 253 patient series from the French Association of Endocrine Surgeons study group. *World J Surg.* 2001;25:891.

Margonis GA, et al: Adrenocortical carcinoma: impact of surgical margin status on long-term outcomes. *Ann Surg Oncol.* 2016; 23:134.

Milgrom SA, et al: The role of radiation therapy in the management of adrenal carcinoma and adrenal metastases. *J Surg Oncol.* 2012;106:647.

Miller BS, et al: Resection of adrenocortical carcinoma is less complete and local recurrence occurs sooner and more often after laparoscopic adrenalectomy than after open adrenalectomy. *Surgery.* 2012;152:1150.

Sgourakis G, et al: Laparoscopic versus open adrenalectomy for stage I/II adrenocortical carcinoma: meta-analysis of outcomes. *J Invest Surg.* 2015;28:145.

INCIDENTALOMAS

Adrenal tumors have traditionally been diagnosed after presentation with clinical symptoms of excess hormone secretion. However, the increased use of ultrasonography, CT, and MRI for various diseases in the abdomen has led to the discovery of what are referred to as adrenal incidentalomas. Most are small nonfunctioning adrenal cortical adenomas; some are functioning adenomas or pheochromocytomas with subclinical secretion of hormones; and some are adrenocortical carcinomas or metastases.

Incidentalomas are found in 4% of CT scans and 6% of random autopsies. The incidence increases with age. Based on a review of 10 studies, subclinical Cushing syndrome and Cushing syndrome occur in 6.4% of patients with incidentalomas, 3.1% with pheochromocytoma, 1.8% with adrenocortical carcinoma, 0.7% with metastatic carcinoma, and 0.6% with aldosteronoma (Table 35–2). Thus, 90% of the patients have presumed nonfunctioning cortical adenomas. Simple adrenal cysts, myelolipomas, and adrenal hemorrhages can be identified by the CT characteristics alone.

Table 35–2. Adrenal incidentalomas.[1]

Tumor Types	Percentage
Subclinical Cushing/Cushing	6.4%
Pheochromocytoma	3.1%
Adrenocortical carcinoma	1.9%
Metastatic carcinoma	0.7%
Aldosterone-producing adenoma	0.6%
Presumed nonfunctional adenoma	89.9%
Total	100%

[1]Data from Cawood TJ, Hunt PJ, O'Shea D, et al: Recommended evaluation of adrenal incidentalomas is costly, has high false-positive rates and confers a risk of fatal cancer that is similar to the risk of the adrenal lesion becoming malignant; time for a rethink? *Eur J Endocrinol.* 2009 Oct;161(4):513-527.

Adrenal cysts can be large but are rarely malignant. Adrenal hemorrhage may occur in preexisting adrenal tumors.

The major issues in managing a patient with an incidentaloma is to determine whether the tumor is hormonally active and whether it is a cancer; either would be an indication for resection. All functioning tumors should be excised. Large nonfunctioning tumors also should be excised because of the increased risk of cancer. Small nonfunctioning tumors are almost always benign adenomas; they can be followed with serial CT scans checking for changes in size. Since most incidentalomas are nonfunctioning adenomas, the workup should be selective to avoid unnecessary expense and procedures.

The workup should include a complete history and physical examination with specific reference to a history of previous malignancy and signs and symptoms of Cushing syndrome or pheochromocytoma. Hyperaldosteronism, pheochromocytoma, and virilizing or feminizing adrenocortical carcinoma should be investigated. Further laboratory studies may be indicated depending on the clinical presentation.

All patients—even those who do not have hypertension—should have a 24-hour urine collection for fractionated catecholamines and metanephrines or plasma free metanephrines to search for pheochromocytoma; the risk of unrecognized pheochromocytoma is high, and the hypertension may be absent or episodic. Most pheochromocytomas are over 2 cm in diameter and characteristically bright on T2-weighted MRI. *Almost half of pheochromocytomas are found incidentally because of CT or MRI scans obtained for other indications.*

Subclinical Cushing syndrome refers to autonomous cortisol secretion in patients without typical signs and symptoms of Cushing syndrome. Autonomous cortisol secretion is best assessed by an overnight 1-mg dexamethasone suppression test.

Patients with subclinical Cushing syndrome may experience an Addisonian crisis if the tumor is resected and glucocorticoid replacement is not adequate.

Patients who are hypertensive should also have plasma aldosterone and PRA measured to screen for primary hyperaldosteronism.

If the above studies show that the tumor is nonfunctional, the size and imaging characteristics of the tumor and the patient's overall medical condition should determine the appropriate treatment. Nonfunctioning adrenal tumors larger than 5 cm in diameter should usually be removed because of higher risk of cancer. Nonfunctioning adrenal tumors smaller than 3 cm that are homogeneous and have low density on CT (Hounsfield units < 10) or MRI are unlikely to be cancers and may be safely followed up with one-time serial imaging and biochemical evaluation. The patient's age and overall medical condition and the CT scan findings will usually determine whether a tumor 3-5 cm in size should be resected. High density, delayed wash out of contrast, irregular borders, and heterogeneity make pheochromocytoma, adrenocortical carcinoma, and metastases more likely.

In patients with a previously treated malignancy such as lung or breast cancer, the chance of an adrenal tumor being metastatic is greater than 50%, and even greater if the adrenal mass is larger than 3 cm. CT-guided fine-needle aspiration biopsy is rarely necessary but can be used to diagnose metastatic cancer if it will change management of the patient. Fine-needle aspiration of an adrenocortical cancer may not be diagnostic, and breaching the capsule risks local spread of cancer. Needle biopsy of an unexpected pheochromocytoma can precipitate pheochromocytoma crisis. Biochemical screening for pheochromocytoma should be performed before biopsy of suspected isolated metastasis. Resection of a solitary adrenal metastasis from a primary lung cancer may improve long-term survival (to about 25% at 5 years) if there are no other clinically obvious metastases. Patients with a metachronous solitary adrenal metastasis are more likely to benefit from adrenalectomy than are those with a synchronous metastasis. Patients with adrenal metastases from melanoma or renal cell carcinoma also benefit from resection even when there are other foci of metastases. Adrenal metastasis can be resected laparoscopically with minimal risk of local recurrence.

Chomsky-Higgins K: Less is more: cost-effectiveness analysis of surveillance strategies for small, nonfunctional, radiographically benign adrenal incidentalomas. *Surgery.* 2018;163:197.

Duh QY: Adrenal gland: new guidelines for adrenal incidentalomas. *Nat Rev Endocrinol.* 2016;12:561.

Fassnacht M, et al. Management of adrenal incidentalomas: European Society of Endocrinology Clinical Practice Guideline in collaboration with the European Network for the Study of Adrenal Tumors. *Eur J Endocrinol.* 2016;175:G1.

Iacobone M, et al: Adrenalectomy may improve cardiovascular and metabolic impairment and ameliorate quality of life in patients with adrenal incidentalomas and subclinical Cushing's syndrome. *Surgery.* 2012;152:991.

Pasternak JD, et al: Differences between bilateral adrenal incidentalomas and unilateral lesions. *JAMA Surg.* 2015;150:974.

Taffel M, et al: Adrenal imaging: a comprehensive review. *Radiol Clin North Am.* 2012;50:219.

MULTIPLE CHOICE QUESTIONS

1. The most sensitive and specific test for diagnosis of pheochromocytoma is

    A. Plasma free catecholamines
    B. 24-hour urinary vanillylmandelic acid (VMA)
    C. 24-hour urinary catecholamines
    D. Plasma free metanephrines
    E. Plasma free VMA

2. The workup of an adrenal incidentaloma includes all of the following, *except*

    A. Measurement of 24-hour urinary fractionated metanephrines
    B. Measurement of 24-hour urinary cortisol and creatinine
    C. Fine-needle biopsy of the adrenal tumor
    D. Plasma aldosterone level and renin activity
    E. Obtaining family history of adrenal disease

3. Laparoscopic adrenalectomy is usually *not* indicated for

    A. An aldosteronoma
    B. A feminizing tumor
    C. A pheochromocytoma
    D. A metastasis from melanoma
    E. A symptomatic myelolipoma

4. Adrenal tumor can secrete all of the following, *except*

    A. Normetanephrine
    B. Aldosterone
    C. Cortisol
    D. DHEAS
    E. 5-HIAA

5. All of the following are true about the perioperative care of a patient undergoing unilateral adrenalectomy for pheochromocytoma, *except*

    A. α-Adrenergic blockade is indicated preoperatively to prevent intraoperative hemodynamic instability
    B. An arterial line should be placed for real-time blood pressure monitoring
    C. Nitroprusside should be available to manage severe hypertension
    D. Stress dose steroids and subsequent steroid taper are needed in all patients postoperatively
    E. Glucose should be checked hourly until tolerating a diet to identify hypoglycemia

Arteries

Gaurav Sharma, MD
Samir K. Shah, MD

36

Arterial disease can be broadly classified into two categories: occlusive and aneurysmal. The major sequelae of arterial obstruction are tissue ischemia and necrosis, whereas those of aneurysmal disease are typically rupture and hemorrhage in the aortic position and thrombosis and embolization in the peripheral arteries.

▼ ARTERIAL OCCLUSIVE DISEASE

Although atherosclerosis is the dominant cause of arterial occlusive disease in Western countries, other etiologies such as congenital and anatomical anomalies, autoimmune diseases, and remote thromboembolism can also result in arterial obstruction. Symptoms of occlusive vascular disease primarily are end-organ dysfunction and, in the muscle beds, pain with exercise and tissue necrosis.

ATHEROSCLEROSIS

Atherosclerosis can occur in any artery, with plaques most commonly developing in areas of low shear stress, such as at arterial branch points. Lesions are usually symmetrically distributed, although the rate of progression may vary. Early lesions are confined to the intima. In advanced lesions, both intima and media are involved, but the adventitia is spared. Preservation of the adventitia is essential for the vessel's structural integrity and is the basis for all cardiovascular interventions.

When hemodynamically significant disease affects a major artery, a parallel system of collateral vessels may preserve flow to the peripheral runoff bed. Collateral vessels are smaller, more circuitous, and always have a higher resistance than the original unobstructed artery. The stimuli for collateral development include abnormal pressure gradients across the collateral system and increased flow velocity through intramuscular channels that connect to reentry vessels. Adequate collateral vessels take time to develop but

often maintain tissue viability in patients with chronic major arterial occlusions.

Generally, arterial insufficiency occurs in medium-sized and large arteries with at least a 50% reduction in arterial diameter. This correlates with a 75% narrowing of cross-sectional area and enough resistance to decrease downstream flow and pressure. Early in the process, compensatory dilation of the vessel wall may preserve lumen diameter as the atherosclerotic lesion develops, but with continued growth, lesions overcome this adaptation and result in flow-limiting stenoses. If there is adequate collateral flow, single stenoses or even occlusions are reasonably well-tolerated. Severe ischemia occurs when there are inadequate collaterals or there are multiple levels of disease.

Davì G, Patrono C: Platelet activation and atherothrombosis. *N Engl J Med.* 2008;358:1638.

Libby P, Ridker PM, Hansson GK: Inflammation in atherosclerosis: from pathophysiology to practice. *J Am Coll Cardiol.* 2009; 54:2129.

▼ CHRONIC LOWER EXTREMITY OCCLUSIVE DISEASE

▶ General Considerations

Peripheral arterial insufficiency is predominantly a disease of the lower extremities. Upper extremity arterial lesions are uncommon and confined mostly to the subclavian arteries. Even when present, upper extremity atherosclerosis rarely produces symptoms due to abundant collateral pathways. In the lower extremities, however, obstructive lesions are distributed widely, with lesions of the superficial femoral and iliac arteries the most common (Figure 36–1). Symptoms are related to the location and number of obstructions.

Peripheral arterial disease affects at least 20% of individuals older than 70 years, with the incidence increasing

▲ **Figure 36–1.** Common sites of stenosis and occlusion of the visceral and peripheral arterial systems.

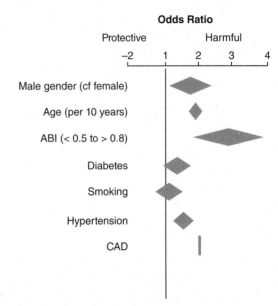

▲ **Figure 36–2.** Odds ratios for risk factors for all-cause mortality. ABI, ankle-brachial index; CAD, coronary artery disease. (Reproduced with permission from Dormandy JA, Rutherford RB: Management of peripheral arterial disease (PAD). TASC Working Group. TransAtlantic Inter-Society Consensus (TASC), *J Vasc Surg* 2000 Jan; 31[1 Pt 2]:S1-S296.)

with the increasing incidence of diabetes. Although most patients with this disorder do not develop gangrene or require amputations, adverse outcomes of systemic atherosclerosis, including myocardial infarction and/or stroke, are common. Even after adjustment for known risk factors, individuals with peripheral arterial disease exhibit a several-fold higher risk of mortality than the nonaffected population. A low ankle-brachial index is one of the strongest risk factors for all-cause mortality. Peripheral arterial disease is more a marker of a more virulent form of atherosclerosis and early death from cardiovascular or cerebrovascular disease than an indicator of imminent limb loss; thus, identifying and treating associated atherosclerotic risk factors is essential (Figure 36–2).

▶ **Clinical Findings**

A. Symptoms

1. Intermittent claudication—Intermittent claudication refers to pain in muscles of the lower extremity associated with walking that is relieved by rest. Tissue perfusion is adequate at rest, and so tissue loss (ie, ulceration or gangrene) does not occur. The risk of major limb amputation is low. The pain is described as a muscle ache, cramp, or fatigue that progresses with exertion and that can be severe enough to force the patient to stop walking. The pain occurs one anatomic level distal to the principal area of disease; thus, disease in the aorta and iliac and common femoral arteries produces buttocks and thigh claudication, and disease in the superficial femoral and popliteal arteries creates calf claudication. Gluteal pain indicates lesions in or proximal to the hypogastric arteries and is often accompanied by impotence. **Leriche syndrome** occurs in men with aortoiliac disease and includes claudication of calf, thigh, and buttock muscles; erectile dysfunction; and diminished or absent femoral pulses. Occasionally, patients describe transient numbness of the extremity accompanying the pain and fatigue of claudication as nerves and muscles become ischemic.

Features of vasculogenic claudication that help in distinguishing it from other diseases include its occurrence only with exertion and the constant relationship between its onset and exertion and lack of relief with positional changes.

The two conditions that most often mimic claudication are osteoarthritis of the hip or knee and neurospinal compression due to congenital or osteophytic narrowing of the lumbar neurospinal canal (spinal stenosis). Osteoarthritis can be differentiated from claudication because pain occurs predominantly in joints, the amount of exercise required to elicit symptoms varies, symptoms are characteristically worse in the morning and upon initiating exercise, rest does not relieve symptoms promptly, the severity of symptoms changes from day to day, and anti-inflammatory agents may relieve the pain. Impingement on the spinal canal or nerve root produces neurospinal compression symptoms; therefore, the pain is typically burning or shooting in nature, and symptoms may occur with sitting or standing. Neurogenic pain may follow a dermatomal distribution, a key factor in differentiating it from vasculogenic claudication.

Uncommon conditions such as coarctation of the aorta, chronic compartment syndrome, popliteal artery entrapment, and vasculitis can mimic symptoms of atherosclerotic arterial insufficiency. Age at presentation and associated findings may aid in diagnosing these conditions.

The correct diagnosis of vascular claudication should be easily established by determining the location of pain with exercise (buttocks, thigh, calf), the quality of the pain (aching or cramping), the length of time required for relief of symptoms after stopping exercise (immediate or nearly immediate), the reproducibility of the distance walked before symptoms begin (initial claudication distance), and most importantly, the reduction or loss of pulses with exercise.

2. Critical limb ischemia—With extensive disease, patients move beyond claudication and develop critical limb ischemia, which includes ischemic rest pain and ulceration. Critical limb ischemia carries a high risk of major limb loss, unlike claudication, and is an indication for revascularization.

Rest pain is severe and burning, usually confined to the forefoot distal to the metatarsals. It may be localized to the vicinity of an ischemic ulcer or pregangrenous toe. It is aggravated by elevation of the extremity. Thus, patients often report a worsening at night while attempting to sleep with improvement with dangling of the limb, which enlists the help of gravity to improve perfusion. In patients who must keep the foot constantly dependent to relieve pain, the leg and foot may be swollen, causing some confusion in diagnosis. The ischemic neuritis of rest pain is severe and resistant to opioids for relief.

Patients with rest pain may give a history of claudication, but rest pain also may occur de novo in diabetics with distal tibial disease or embolic occlusion of the distal tibial arteries and in patients whose walking is limited by other conditions. Differentiating ischemic rest pain from neuropathy in diabetics is critical and may require vascular testing to clarify the diagnosis.

Patients with severe lower extremity arterial insufficiency often develop ulcers or wounds on the feet even from seemingly trivial trauma. These lesions are most commonly located on the distal foot and toes, but on occasion, they can be in the upper foot or ankle. Typically, the wounds are excruciatingly painful, deep, and devoid of any evidence of healing such as contraction or formation of granulation tissue.

3. Erectile dysfunction—Inability to attain or maintain an erection may be produced by lesions that obstruct blood flow through both hypogastric arteries and is commonly found in association with narrowing of the terminal aorta, common iliac, or hypogastric arteries. Vasculogenic erectile dysfunction is less common than that due to other causes.

B. Signs

Physical examination is of paramount importance in assessing the presence and severity of vascular disease. The physical findings of peripheral atherosclerosis are related to changes in the peripheral arteries and to tissue ischemia.

1. Arterial pulse examination—Decreased amplitude of the pulse denotes proximal obstructions to flow, which can help localize disease. For example, an absent femoral pulse usually signifies aortoiliac occlusive disease. It is possible but unusual for collateral flow to be sufficient to produce a pulse distal to an occluded artery.

2. Bruits and thrills—A bruit is the sound produced by dissipation of energy as blood flows through a stenotic arterial segment. With extremely high flows, the energy may vibrate the artery, creating a thrill. The bruit or thrill is transmitted distally along the course of the artery. Thus, when a bruit is heard through a stethoscope placed over a peripheral artery, stenosis is present at or proximal to that level. The pitch of the bruit rises as the stenosis becomes more marked, until a critical stenosis is reached or the vessel becomes occluded, when the bruit may disappear. Thus, absence of a bruit does not indicate insignificant disease.

3. Response to exercise—Exercise in a normal individual increases the pulse rate without producing arterial bruits or reduction in pulse amplitude. In an individual who complains of claudication, there may be minimal findings at rest, but exercise will produce decreased pulse strength, decreased distal arterial pressure, and possibly an audible bruit unmasking a significant stenosis. Exercise is best used in conjunction with noninvasive vascular testing.

4. Integumentary changes—Chronic ischemia commonly produces loss of hair over the dorsum of the toes and foot and may be associated with thickening of the toenails (onychomycosis) due to slowed keratin turnover. With more advanced ischemia, there is atrophy of the skin and subcutaneous tissue so that the foot becomes shiny, scaly, and skeletonized.

5. Pallor—Pallor of the foot on elevation of the extremity with a complete absence of capillary refill indicates advanced ischemia. Pallor on elevation does not occur unless advanced ischemia is present. It is always present with ischemic rest pain.

6. Reactive hyperemia—When pallor is produced with elevation, the ischemia results in maximum cutaneous vasodilation. When the extremity is returned to a dependent position, blood returning to the dilated vascular bed produces an intense color in the foot, called dependent rubor, and denotes advanced disease. The delay in the appearance of color when the extremities return to a dependent position is proportionate to the impairment in circulation. The purple discoloration due to severe chronic *venous* insufficiency does not give way to pallor on elevation.

7. Skin temperature—With chronic ischemia, the temperature of the skin of the foot decreases. Coolness can best be detected by palpation with the back of the examiner's hand with comparison to the contralateral foot.

8. Ulceration—Ischemic ulcers are usually very painful and accompanied by rest pain in the foot. They occur in toes or at a site where minor trauma can initiate the injury. The margin of the ulcer is sharply demarcated or punched out, and the base is devoid of healthy granulation tissue. The surrounding skin is pale and mottled, and signs of chronic ischemia are invariably present. Neuropathic ulcers are surrounded by a callus and occur frequently at areas of repeated trauma, such as plantar surface of the metatarsal heads.

9. Atrophy—Moderate to severe degrees of chronic ischemia produce gradual soft tissue and muscle atrophy and loss of strength. Joint mobility and gait may be altered due to muscle atrophy. Subsequent changes in foot structure and gait increase the possibility of developing foot ulceration.

10. Necrosis—Severe tissue ischemia may progress to necrosis with minor injuries, infection, or swelling. Necrosis halts proximally at a line where the blood supply is sufficient to maintain viability and results in dry gangrene. If the necrotic portion is infected (wet gangrene), necrosis may extend into tissues that would normally remain viable.

C. Noninvasive Vascular Laboratory Tests

Noninvasive assessment is helpful to determine the severity of hypoperfusion and the sites of hemodynamically significant stenoses or occlusions.

The **ankle-brachial index (ABI)** is a quick screening test and the cornerstone of the diagnosis of peripheral vascular disease. The ABI is determined by first determining the systolic pressures obtained by Doppler insonation of the dorsalis pedis and posterior tibial arteries and the bilateral brachial arteries. Next, the highest pedal systolic pressure is divided by the highest brachial pressure to determine the ABI. Normally, the ABI is 0.9 or greater; a lower value indicates occlusive disease proximal to the point of measurement. The ABI correlates roughly with the degree of ischemia: claudication occurs with a value less than 0.7, and rest pain usually appears when the ratio is 0.4 or lower. Patients with diabetic vascular disease may have artificially elevated ABI values due to calcified, noncompressible arteries, and toe-brachial

indices and pulse volume recordings may be used instead to assess arterial perfusion.

Blood pressures can be measured at rest and after exercise in the ankle, and the effect of exercise can be monitored. **Exercise testing** confirms and quantitates the diagnosis of claudication. To perform exercise testing, the patient walks on a treadmill at a standard speed and grade until claudication pain is experienced or a time limit is reached. With significant arterial occlusive disease, there will be a decrease in the ABI with exercise. If the pain is not due to arterial stenosis, no decrease in pressure will occur. This test is particularly useful in differentiating neurogenic pain with walking from claudication.

D. Imaging Studies

Color duplex ultrasound imaging is a mainstay of vascular imaging. It is a painless, relatively inexpensive, and accurate method for acquiring anatomic and functional information (eg, velocity gradients across stenoses). Although the accuracy of this study is operator dependent, it can supply sufficient information to permit intervention in selected cases.

Computed tomography angiography (CTA) is useful for imaging the arterial tree and has the advantage of visualizing cross-sections of the vessel lumen. In many instances, this allows for more accurate determination of vessel diameter and stenosis severity than conventional angiography. It does require the administration of contrast dye and is less useful for tibial disease, and its images may be obscured by the presence of calcification or metallic implants. **Magnetic resonance angiography (MRA)** also can be used to obtain images similar in quality to angiography in most cases. MRA does not show calcifications and gives better visualization of tibial vessels than CTA. MRA also can reveal details of composition of atherosclerotic plaque. Gadolinium-associated nephrogenic systemic fibrosis limits its use in patients with renal insufficiency. The integrated use of computer workstations with computed tomography (CT) and magnetic resonance imaging (MRI) data can provide three-dimensional images that can be useful in visualizing patient anatomy and planning interventional procedures.

Conventional arteriography provides detailed anatomic information about peripheral arterial disease. It is reserved for patients warranting invasive intervention such as percutaneous transluminal angioplasty, stent placement, or planning for open vascular surgery. Complications of angiography are related to technique and contrast media. Technical complications such as puncture site hematomas, arteriovenous fistulas, and false aneurysms are uncommon (1%). Contrast agents may precipitate allergic reactions (0.1%). Patients with renal failure, proteinuria, diabetes, and dehydration are at increased risk for contrast-induced renal failure. Adequate hydration of patients before and after angiography and use of *N*-acetylcysteine may reduce the incidence of this complication. Contrast-sparing techniques and even carbon dioxide–based angiography, which may avoid administration of iodinated contrast altogether, are also in use.

▶ Treatment & Prognosis

The objectives of treatment for lower extremity occlusive disease are relief from symptoms and prevention of limb loss.

A. Nonoperative Treatment

In general, patients with peripheral vascular disease have shortened life expectancies because of their severe atherosclerotic disease. Nondiabetic patients with ischemic disease of the lower extremity have a 5-year survival rate of 70%. The survival rate is 60% in patients with associated ischemic heart disease or cerebrovascular insufficiency. Patients with peripheral vascular disease and renal failure have a 2-year survival rate of less than 50%. Most deaths are due to myocardial infarctions and strokes. Only 20% of deaths are due to nonatherosclerotic causes.

Nonoperative treatment consists of (1) medical management of cardiovascular risk factors, (2) exercise rehabilitation, (3) foot care, and (4) pharmacotherapy.

1. Reduction of cardiovascular risk factors—See Table 36–1. Managing cardiovascular risk in patients with chronic lower extremity ischemia is critical. Although nondiabetics with intermittent claudication carry a less than 5% risk of major amputation at 5 years, in some series, the risk of mortality over that same period exceeds 40%, primarily due to cardiovascular events. Critical limb ischemia (characterized by rest pain and/or tissue loss) patients are at even higher risk of cardiovascular events; mortality in this subset of peripheral arterial disease patients may exceed 25% at 1 year, again primarily due to cardiovascular causes. Cigarette smoking is the single most important risk factor for peripheral vascular disease, and all patients should stop smoking. At high levels of consumption (eg, 2-3 packs per day), claudicants who successfully cease smoking will experience immediate improvement in walking distance.

In the past, elevated lipids were not usually associated with peripheral vascular disease. Hyperlipidemia, however, is often present, especially in patients with early onset of disease. Elevated triglyceride levels and low high-density lipoprotein (HDL) cholesterol levels are more prevalent than elevated levels of low-density lipoprotein (LDL) cholesterol. Reduction of elevated lipid levels is associated with stabilization or regression of arterial plaques. High-intensity, high-dose statin regimens are recommended for all patients with peripheral arterial disease. Statins have other pleiotropic effects that may reduce inflammation, stabilize plaques, and independently increase walking distance in claudicants.

Table 36–1. Summary of risk factor modification in peripheral vascular disease.

Risk Factor	Therapy	Clinical Effect
Tobacco use	Counseling Pharmacotherapy Nicotine replacement Bupropion, varenicline	Reduced overall mortality Reduced cardiovascular events
Antiplatelet	Aspirin Clopidogrel (Plavix)	Antiplatelet therapy gives > 20% reduction in MI, stroke, or vascular death
Hyperlipidemia	Statin Lipid goals in PAD patients: LDL < 100 mg/dL	20%-30% reduction in cardiovascular and all-cause mortality in CAD patients
Hypertension	Target BP < 140/90 in PAD patients Beta-blocker ACE inhibitor	Beta-blocker and ACE inhibitors each associated with > 20% reduction in cardiovascular mortality
Diabetes	Goal hemoglobin A1c < 7%	Benefits in vascular disease unproven
Lifestyle	Daily aerobic exercise Weight loss Healthy, low-fat diet	Reduced lipid levels Reduced cardiovascular events

ACE, angiotensin-converting enzyme; BP, blood pressure; CAD, coronary artery disease; LDL, low-density lipoprotein; MI, myocardial infarction; PAD, peripheral artery disease.

Both type 1 and type 2 diabetes increase the prevalence and severity of cardiovascular disease. Intensive glycemic control reduces the incidence of nephropathy, neuropathy, and retinopathy in diabetes, but it does not correlate with the severity or progression of peripheral arterial disease. In order to reduce all-cause mortality, however, it is recommended that fasting blood sugars should be controlled with hemoglobin A1c levels less than 7%.

2. Exercise rehabilitation—For claudicants, exercise ranging from unsupervised walking to formal supervised exercise on a treadmill significantly improves walking ability. A 21-study meta-analysis of exercise programs showed an average 180% increase in initial claudication distance and a 120% increase in maximal walking distance achieved through exercise. The precise mechanism behind this improvement is not firmly established. Collateral development seems unlikely because ankle pressures and limb flow do not increase substantially. Possible explanations include improved metabolic capacity and conditioning of the muscles.

Because patients with claudication are at a twofold to fourfold greater risk of dying from complications of generalized atherosclerosis than people without claudication, an additional benefit of exercise in these patients is that an improvement in walking distance as part of an aggressive risk factor modification regimen results in an overall decrease in cardiovascular risk.

3. Foot care—The feet of patients with neuropathy or with critical limb ischemia should be inspected and washed daily and kept dry. Mechanical and thermal trauma to the feet should be avoided. Toenails should be trimmed carefully, and corns and calluses should be attended to promptly. Even minor foot infections or injuries should be treated aggressively. Educating the patient to understand neuropathy, peripheral vascular insufficiency, and the importance of foot care is a central aspect of treatment.

4. Pharmacotherapy—The Antiplatelet Trialists Collaboration found an overall 25% decrease in fatal and nonfatal myocardial infarctions, strokes, and vascular deaths in those treated with antiplatelet agents. Aspirin at dosages ranging from 75 to 350 mg/d is the first-line antiplatelet agent recommended, although clopidogrel, which blocks the activation of platelets by adenosine diphosphate (ADP), is a viable alternative. Clopidogrel is also an important adjunctive therapy in reducing thrombogenicity at locations of endovascular arterial treatment. All patients with cardiovascular disease, whether symptomatic or asymptomatic, should be considered for antiplatelet therapy to reduce the risk of cardiovascular morbidity and mortality.

Cilostazol is a phosphodiesterase III inhibitor with vasodilator, antiplatelet, and antilipid activity approved for treatment of intermittent claudication. Randomized, placebo-controlled, blinded trials have shown an increase of about 50% in absolute claudication distance in patients treated with cilostazol. Congestive heart failure is an absolute contraindication, and significant side effects limit its use.

Aboyans V, Criqui MH, Abraham P, et al: Measurement and interpretation of the ankle-brachial index: a scientific statement from the American Heart Association. *Circulation*. 2012;126:2890.

Alonso Coello P, Bellmunt S, McGorrian C, et al: Antithrombotic therapy in peripheral artery disease: Antithrombotic Therapy and Prevention of Thrombosis, 9th ed: American College of Chest Physicians Evidence-Based Clinical Practice Guidelines. *Chest*. 2012;141(2 Suppl):e669S.

Critchley JA, Capewell S: Mortality risk reduction associated with smoking cessation in patients with coronary heart disease: a systematic review. *JAMA*. 2003;290:86.

Dormandy JA, Murray GD: The fate of the claudicant: a prospective study of 1969 claudicants. *Eur J Vasc Surg*. 1991;5:131.

Hamburg NM, Balady GJ: Exercise rehabilitation in peripheral artery disease: functional impact and mechanisms of benefits. *Circulation*. 2011;123:87-97.

McCullough PA: Contrast-induced acute kidney injury. *J Am Coll Cardiol*. 2008;51:1419.

Mills EJ, Wu P, Chong G, et al: Efficacy and safety of statin treatment for cardiovascular disease: a network meta-analysis of 170,255 patients from 76 randomized trials. *QJM*. 2011;104:109.

Momsen AH, Jensen MB, Norager CB, et al: Drug therapy for improving walking distance in intermittent claudication: a systematic review and meta-analysis of robust randomised controlled studies. *Eur J Vasc Endovasc Surg*. 2009;38:463.

Murphy TP, Cutlip DE, Regensteiner JG, et al: Supervised exercise versus primary stenting for claudication resulting from aortoiliac peripheral artery disease: six-month outcomes from the claudication: exercise versus endoluminal revascularization (CLEVER) study. *Circulation*. 2012;125:130.

Rehring TF, Stolcpart RS, Hollis HW Jr: Pharmacologic risk factor management in peripheral arterial disease: a vade mecum for vascular surgeons. Society for Vascular Surgery. *J Vasc Surg*. 2008;47:1108.

B. Operative Treatment

Interventional procedures, open or endovascular, are performed both for limb salvage and for lifestyle-limiting claudication. The choice of operative procedure depends on the location and distribution of arterial lesions and the patient's comorbidities. Recognition of coexistent cardiopulmonary disease is particularly relevant, because many patients with peripheral vascular disease also have ischemic heart disease or chronic lung disease associated with tobacco use. Preoperative cardiac functional assessment is sometimes necessary, but preoperative myocardial revascularization is not beneficial in patients with reasonable cardiac reserve. All patients undergoing vascular surgery should have preoperative risk assessment. Randomized trials have shown that perioperative beta-blocker, angiotensin-converting enzyme (ACE) inhibitor, and statins may reduce cardiac morbidity in patients undergoing vascular surgery.

1. Endovascular therapy—Endovascular therapy consists of image-guided techniques to treat diseased arterial segments from within the lumen of the vessel. Access to the arterial system is established by the insertion of valved sheaths, usually percutaneously, into the access vessel, often the common femoral artery. Steerable wires and catheters are then passed through the vasculature under fluoroscopic guidance to the target lesion (Figure 36–3). Once the target lesion is accessed, therapeutic maneuvers including angioplasty (plain, cutting, or drug-coated balloons), atherectomy (mechanical or laser), and stenting (bare metal or drug-eluting) can be performed. Continued technologic advances have resulted in the ever-expanding application of these interventions to patients with disease characteristics once thought to preclude endovascular interventions, such as high-grade Trans-Atlantic Inter-Society Consensus (TASC) D lesions, chronic total occlusions, infrapopliteal disease, and even common femoral and profunda femoral occlusive disease. In many arterial beds, endovascular therapy is more commonly used than open surgical therapy because of its minimally invasive

▲ **Figure 36–3.** Endovascular gear. **A:** Sheath. Inserted using Seldinger technique into access vessel. Wires, catheters, and devices pass through the sheath. Sheaths provide stable working access points and protect the artery. **B:** Catheter. Variable length, stiffness, coating, and shape (examples: B.1, cobra; B.2, pigtail; B.3, mesenteric selective). Catheters help steer wires through vasculature and also maintain access in vessel. **C:** Guidewire. Variable diameter, length, stiffness, and shape. Used to gain access into vasculature, cross-lesions, and deliver devices. **D:** Balloon catheter. **E:** Peripheral stent graft. **F:** Peripheral nitinol self-expanding stent. **G:** Aortoiliac stainless steel/Dacron stent graft.

nature and reduction of short-term morbidity and mortality. However, many questions remain concerning the long-term durability of endovascular repairs, and open surgery still plays a major role in the treatment of patients with arterial disease.

Percutaneous transluminal angioplasty, with or without placement of an intravascular stent, is often the treatment of choice when stenoses or even occlusions are relatively short and localized. As the angioplasty balloon expands, it stretches the adventitia, fracturing and compressing plaque and expanding the artery to widen the lumen. Energy losses associated with a stenosis are inversely proportionate to the fourth power of the radius; therefore, even small increases in radius can result in substantial increases in blood flow, although durability of the procedure is improved with the reestablishment of a normal lumen. Concomitant stenting is frequently performed to improve luminal expansion. Stent grafts or covered stents (stents lined with an impermeable material) may also be used in selected cases, based on anatomic location of the lesion, or to repair the inadvertent rupture of an artery during angioplasty (Figure 36–4).

Both stents and stent grafts are commonly used from the aortic bifurcation to the distal popliteal artery. Stenting is performed less commonly below the knee, but angioplasty of tibial disease is now increasingly common. Meta-analytic data suggest that infrapopliteal angioplasty in this patient population is associated with less than 50% mid-term primary patency, but 82% limb salvage at 3 years; thus, it may be a viable option in patients who are not candidates for open bypass. Percutaneous mechanical and laser atherectomy are other options in removing obstructing lesions in lower extremity atherosclerotic occlusive disease, although their durability has not been proven.

For short, stenotic segments in larger, more proximal vessels, the results of endovascular therapies are good, with 1-year success rates of 85% in common iliac disease and 70% in external iliac disease. The results with superficial femoral and popliteal lesions are lower (Figure 36–5). The success of endovascular therapy for lower extremity occlusive disease is inversely related to the complexity of the lesion, defined by the number and length of stenoses treated.

Close follow-up of patients after endovascular therapy is required because disease may recur more frequently after angioplasty than after bypass surgery, and the patient should be followed using noninvasive tests. Repeat angioplasty or stenting may be indicated for recurrent disease, but the improvement in morbidity and mortality of endovascular interventions may be offset by the need for multiple repeat procedures. In general, minimally invasive percutaneous treatment of lower extremity occlusive disease is best used in

▲ **Figure 36–4.** Aortoiliac occlusive disease. **A:** Aorta. **B:** Severely stenotic/occluded iliac arteries. **B.1:** Widely patent iliac arteries following balloon angioplasty and stenting (**C**).

patients with high operative risk and severe, limb-threatening ischemia (Figure 36–6).

2. Surgical treatment

A. AORTOILIAC RECONSTRUCTION—Open operations are indicated for aortoiliac occlusive disease in younger patients with low operative risk or patients with severe disease not amenable to endovascular therapy. To completely bypass the aortoiliac segment, an inverted Y-shaped (bifurcated) prosthesis is interposed between the infrarenal abdominal

aorta and the femoral arteries, creating an **aortofemoral bypass.** The goal of operation is restoration of blood flow to the common femoral artery or, when occlusive disease of the superficial femoral artery is present, to the profunda femoris artery. The clinical results of aortofemoral reconstruction are excellent, although the mortality and morbidity clearly are higher than for endovascular therapy. The operative death rate is less than 5%; the early patency rate is 95%; and the late primary patency rate (5-10 years postoperatively) ranges from 72% to 98%. Late complications may be as high as 10%

▲ **Figure 36–5.** Superficial femoral artery occlusion, angioplasty, and stent graft. **A:** Common femoral artery.
B: Occluded superficial femoral artery. **B.1:** Recannalized, stent-grafted superficial femoral artery. **C:** Profunda femoris artery. **D:** Stent graft.

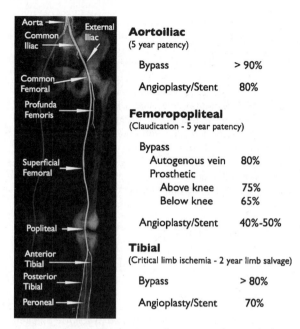

Aortoiliac
(5 year patency)

Bypass	> 90%
Angioplasty/Stent	80%

Femoropopliteal
(Claudication - 5 year patency)

Bypass	
Autogenous vein	80%
Prosthetic	
Above knee	75%
Below knee	65%
Angioplasty/Stent	40%-50%

Tibial
(Critical limb ischemia - 2 year limb salvage)

Bypass	> 80%
Angioplasty/Stent	70%

▲ **Figure 36–6.** Comparison of outcomes for surgical and endovascular intervention in lower extremity occlusive disease.

and include graft-intestinal fistula formation, anastomotic aneurysm formation, renal failure, and erectile dysfunction.

Lower risk procedures may be preferable in high-risk patients. If the clinically important lesions are confined to one side, a femoral-femoral or iliofemoral bypass graft can be used. A graft from the axillary to the femoral artery (ie, axillofemoral graft) can be used for bilateral disease. Unfortunately, these "extra-anatomic" methods of arterial reconstruction are more prone to late occlusion than are direct reconstructions.

B. FEMOROPOPLITEAL RECONSTRUCTION—When disease is confined to the femoropopliteal segment of the superficial femoral artery, **femoropopliteal bypass** is used. The principal indication for these operations is limb salvage. In patients with claudication alone, the indications for femoropopliteal bypass are more difficult to define but must include substantial disability from claudication. For limited lesions of the superficial femoral artery, endovascular therapy is often attempted first, with surgery reserved for extensive disease or angioplasty failure.

The best conduit for femoropopliteal bypass is an autologous greater saphenous vein. The saphenous vein may be left in situ or removed and reversed. Expanded polytetrafluoroethylene (PTFE) may also be used as a conduit, albeit with lower patency. Below the popliteal artery, PTFE conduits produce much lower patency rates than saphenous veins.

Operative death rates are low (2%), and 5-year patency rates range from 60% to 80%. Limb salvage rates are higher than graft patency rates.

The profunda femoris artery perfuses the thigh and acts as an important source of collateral flow to the more distal leg when the superficial femoral artery is diseased. When there is a stenosis of the profunda femoris, **profundoplasty** alone can be performed for limb salvages with success rates of 80% when the suprageniculate popliteal artery is patent and 40%-50% when the popliteal artery is occluded. Isolated profundoplasty is typically inadequate as an isolated procedure for treating claudication.

C. TIBIOPERONEAL ARTERIAL RECONSTRUCTION— Reconstruction of tibial arteries (ie, **distal bypass** to the tibial, peroneal, or pedal vessels) is performed only for limb salvage. Advancing technology allows better endovascular therapy in the tibial vessels, with decreased short-term morbidity and mortality and similar gains in limb salvage when compared to bypass surgery. However, bypass still remains an important mode of therapy for these patients. Autogenous saphenous veins are preferred because prosthetic conduits have high failure rates. Due to smaller vessel size, extensive disease, and probably the length of the bypass conduit, these grafts are not as durable as femoropopliteal bypass, so the limb salvage rate is substantially higher than graft patency. The operative death rate for these procedures is about 5% due to extensive comorbidities.

D. AMPUTATION—Amputation of the limb is necessary within 5-10 years in less than 5% of nondiabetic patients presenting with claudication. Amputation is more common if patients continue to smoke cigarettes. Patients with multiple risk factors for atherosclerosis and short-distance claudication are also at increased risk for eventual limb loss. Of patients who present with ischemic rest pain or ulceration, 5%-10% require amputation as initial therapy, and most eventually will require amputation if not revascularized. Successful revascularization results in lower costs than primary amputation and an improvement in quality of life. Occasionally, primary amputation may be preferable to revascularization if the likelihood of successful bypass is low, extensive foot infection is present, or the patient is nonambulatory. Amputation levels, options, and the special needs of amputees are covered in the section on lower extremity amputation.

Ambler GK, Twine CP: Graft type for femoro-popliteal bypass surgery. *Cochrane Database Syst Rev.* 2018;2:CD001487.

Bradbury AW, Adam DJ, Bell J, et al: Bypass versus Angioplasty in Severe Ischaemia of the Leg (BASIL) trial: an intention-to-treat analysis of amputation-free and overall survival in patients randomized to a bypass surgery-first or a balloon angioplasty-first revascularization strategy. *J Vasc Surg.* 2010;51:5S-17S.

Chung SW, Sharafuddin MJ, Chigurupati R, et al: Midterm patency following atherectomy for infrainguinal occlusive disease: a word of caution. *Ann Vasc Surg.* 2008;22:358-365.

de Vries SO, Hunink MG: Results of aortic bifurcation grafts for aortoiliac occlusive disease: a meta-analysis. *J Vasc Surg.* 1997;26:558-569.

Gerhard-Herman MD, Gornik HL, Barrett C, et al: 2016 AHA/ACC guideline on the management of patients with lower extremity peripheral artery disease: a report of the American College of Cardiology/American Heart Association Task Force on Clinical Practice Guidelines. *Circulation.* 2017;135(12): e791-e792.

Jacobs DL, Motaganahalli RL, Cox DE, et al: True lumen re-entry devices facilitate subintimal angioplasty and stenting of total chronic occlusions: initial report. *J Vasc Surg.* 2006;43:1291-1296.

Nieves JT, Singh G, Laird J, et al: Endovascular versus open bypass surgery for TASC D femoropopliteal lesions in patients with critical limb ischemia. *J Vasc Surg.* 2016;64:545-546.

Norgren L, et al: Inter-Society consensus for the management of peripheral arterial disease (TASC II). TASC II Working Group. *J Vasc Surg.* 2007;45(Suppl S):S5.

Rocha-Singh KJ, Jaff M, Joye J, et al: Major adverse limb events and wound healing following infrapopliteal artery stent implantation in patients with critical limb ischemia: the XCELL trial. *Catheter Cardiovasc Interv.* 2012;80:1042-1051.

Romiti M, Albers M, Brochado-Neto FC, et al: Meta-analysis of infrapopliteal angioplasty for chronic critical limb ischemia. *J Vasc Surg.* 2008;47:975-981.

ACUTE LIMB ISCHEMIA

General Considerations

Sudden occlusion of a previously patent artery is a dramatic event characterized by the abrupt onset of severe pain and absent pulses in the involved extremity. Tissue viability depends on the extent to which flow is maintained by collateral circuits. When ischemia persists, motor and sensory paralysis and muscle infarction become irreversible in a matter of hours.

Acute major arterial occlusion may be caused by an embolus, primary arterial thrombosis, trauma, or dissection. The heart is the embolic source in 80%-90% of episodes, with the remainder from proximal arterial lesions.

Aortic aneurysms often contain thrombus, but this material rarely causes symptomatic emboli. In contrast, femoral and particularly popliteal aneurysms embolize frequently. Ulceration in atherosclerotic plaques also can lead to formation of thrombus, which may fragment. Miscellaneous infrequent sources of emboli include cardiac tumors (including cardiac myxoma) and paradoxical emboli (venous thrombi migrating through a patent foramen ovale). Up to 5%-10% of spontaneous emboli originate from a source that remains unidentified despite thorough diagnostic interrogation.

It may be difficult to differentiate between sudden thrombosis of an atherosclerotic peripheral artery and embolic occlusion. The former patients usually have preexisting atherosclerotic stenosis and low blood flow, which predisposes to stagnation and thrombosis. One should also keep in mind the clinical setting and a history of preexisting symptoms such as atrial fibrillation (embolus) or claudication (primary thrombosis).

Clinical Findings

Acute arterial occlusion is characterized by the *five Ps*: pain, pallor, pulselessness, paresthesias, and paralysis. Severe sudden pain is present in 80% of patients, and its onset usually indicates the time of vessel occlusion. Pain is absent in some patients because of prompt onset of anesthesia and paralysis and portends a poor prognosis.

On examination, the key finding is a lack of palpable pulses in a diffusely painful extremity. Prognosis and management are heavily dependent on physical exam findings, which should include sensorimotor assessment (Table 36–2). Sensory fibers associated with light touch are highly susceptible to ischemia, and their dysfunction heralds the beginning of irreversible ischemic changes. The onset of motor paralysis implies progression to unsalvageable tissue necrosis if not treated immediately. Early intervention is critical. Skin and subcutaneous tissues have greater resistance to hypoxia than nerves and muscles, which may demonstrate irreversible histologic changes after 3 hours or less of ischemia.

Table 36–2. Rutherford classification of acute limb ischemia.

Stage	Limb Description	Prognosis	Sensory Loss	Muscle Weakness	Arterial Doppler	Venous Doppler
I	Viable	Not immediately threatened	None	None	Audible	Audible
IIA	Marginally threatened	Salvageable if promptly treated	Minimal (toes) or none	None	Often inaudible	Audible
IIB	Immediately threatened	Salvageable with immediate revascularization	More than toes, pain at rest	Mild or moderate	Usually inaudible	Audible
III	Irreversibly damaged	Major tissue loss/permanent nerve damage inevitable	Profound, anesthetic	Profound, paralysis (rigor)	Inaudible	Inaudible

Reproduced with permission from Rutherford RB, Baker JD, Ernst C, et al: Recommended standards for reports dealing with lower extremity ischemia: revised version, *J Vasc Surg.* 1997 Sep;26(3):517-538.

▶ Treatment & Prognosis

A. Embolism and Thrombosis

Immediate anticoagulation by intravenous heparin slows the propagation of thrombus and allows time for assessment of adequacy of collateral flow and preparation for operation. Nonoperative management is rarely indicated except in debilitated patients and patients with emboli to major arteries in the upper extremities, which generally have good collateral circulation. If light touch is intact (Rutherford stage I or IIA; Table 36–2), CTA or conventional angiography sometimes may be useful to define the anatomy and assist in planning the operation. Diagnosis of acute embolic occlusion is based on an abrupt cessation of contrast opacification of the artery with little accompanying arterial disease; conversely, acute in situ thrombosis is associated with extensive atherosclerosis and a well-established collateral network. The operative treatment for an embolus, embolectomy, differs from that of preexisting atherosclerosis, which may require bypass. For patients presenting with more advanced ischemia but salvageable limbs (Rutherford stage IIB; Table 36–2), imaging should be deferred in favor of expeditious operative intervention.

Therapeutic options include catheter-directed thrombolysis, percutaneous mechanical thrombectomy, and surgical embolectomy. For patients with severe acute ischemia, operative therapy is preferable because it is usually associated with the least delay in reestablishing perfusion. Surgical embolectomy may be performed through an arteriotomy at the site of the embolic occlusion or, most commonly, by clot extraction with a balloon catheter inserted through a remote arteriotomy. Successful embolectomy requires removal of the embolus and the "tail" of thrombus that extends distally or proximally from it. If operation is not performed within the first few hours, the clot may become adherent, and subsequent revascularization is less successful. Intraoperative infusion of thrombolytic agents is often a useful adjunct to embolectomy.

In patients who will tolerate a delay in revascularization (Rutherford stage I; Table 36–2), particularly in the setting of thromboembolic bypass graft occlusion or extensive tibial artery involvement, intra-arterial thrombolysis should be considered. The usual regimen involves selective intra-arterial infusion of low doses of thrombolytic agent (eg, tissue plasminogen activator) directly into the clot via a remotely placed, indwelling catheter. This activates thrombus plasminogen more efficiently, allows high concentrations in the clot while limiting systemic effect, and has acceptable complication rates. In cases of thrombosis on preexisting atherosclerotic lesions, thrombolysis reveals the underlying lesions that will require treatment to prevent recurrent thrombosis.

If revascularization is successful, a reperfusion injury may develop with significant swelling requiring fasciotomy to treat the compartment syndrome that may accompany the reperfusion injury. Vigilance for compartment syndrome is thus critical, and prophylactic two-incision, four-compartment leg fasciotomies may be undertaken if the period of acute ischemia exceeded 4-6 hours or, even in the presence of lesser durations, if the ischemia was severe. Renal insufficiency from myoglobin release should be anticipated after reperfusion of ischemic muscle. Treatment consists of vigorous hydration and alkalinization of the urine. Administration of free radical scavengers such as mannitol may be helpful in this disorder.

Patients with clearly irreversible limb ischemia (Rutherford stage III; Table 36–2) should undergo amputation without an attempt at revascularization because revascularization may expose the patient to the serious hazards of reperfusion caused by release of acidic and hyperkalemic venous blood from the dying extremity with little benefit given the futility of limb salvage attempts in this setting.

B. Traumatic Arterial Occlusion

An ABI of less than 0.9 in otherwise healthy, peripheral arterial disease–free patients with suspicion of traumatic arterial injury should prompt CTA. Traumatic arterial occlusion must be corrected within a few hours to avoid development of gangrene. Repair of arterial injury is usually performed in conjunction with repair of other injuries. Occasionally, temporary shunts are used to restore flow to the injured extremity while other injuries are addressed and repaired, until definitive vascular reconstruction can be undertaken.

▼ PERIPHERAL MICROEMBOLI

Microemboli are most dramatic when they occlude a digital artery perfusing a toe or finger. This causes sudden pain, cyanosis, and coldness or numbness in the affected digit. These changes characteristically improve over several days. If there are multiple emboli, these symptoms may reappear in a different area of the hand or foot. In the lower extremity, this clinical entity has been called **blue toe syndrome** or trash foot. The sudden onset of pain and purple discoloration of a toe in the presence of palpable pulses is recognized as a potentially limb-threatening arterial problem. With each succeeding episode, recovery is slower and less complete.

The most common source of microembolization is cardiac valvular disease. However, if no cardiac valvular lesions are found, a careful examination of the proximal arterial tree must be done to identify an arterial source shedding atheroemboli.

Sudden onset may differentiate peripheral microembolism from other causes of blue toes, such as vasculitis, thromboangiitis obliterans, trauma, or chronic ischemia. If a single toe is affected, it is more likely to be the result of emboli, whereas multiple cyanotic toes are more likely to be the result of vasculitis or chronic ischemia. It is important to remember that a patent proximal artery is required to serve as a conduit for the embolus, so pulses are intact. Furthermore, a normal blood supply is present in adjacent tissue segments. The appearance of a normally perfused foot with a cyanotic toe is characteristic. However, the waxing and waning symptoms of repeated emboli can make the diagnosis difficult. Unless the syndrome is recognized, alternative diagnoses investigated, and the lesion of origin corrected, survival of the foot or hand may be in peril. Workup may include echocardiography, cross-sectional imaging (eg, CTA), peripheral arterial duplex ultrasonography, and serology if vasculitides are suspected based on history and physical examination.

Dean SM: Atypical ischemic lower extremity ulcerations: a differential diagnosis. *Vasc Med.* 2008;13:47.

DIABETIC VASCULAR DISEASE

Atherosclerotic arterial disease in patients with diabetes mellitus is more diffuse and more severe than in nondiabetics. In diabetic patients, the tibioperoneal vessels frequently contain atherosclerotic changes, and the vessels are often heavily calcified. The degree of ischemia may be severe and extensive, and noninvasive tests (ABIs) may be falsely elevated. Fortunately, in many diabetics, the small arteries in the foot are relatively spared, making distal bypass to these arteries possible and allowing foot salvage in cases of threatened limb loss.

Diabetic patients also have a high incidence of neuropathy and are more apt to ignore minor foot injuries, which can develop into ulcerations. Ulcerations associated with diabetic neuropathy typically occur at pressure points, such as the classic malum perforans ulcer on the plantar surface of the metatarsal heads. In contrast, classic arterial insufficiency ulcers occur at the tips of the toe. Patients often have comorbid arterial insufficiency and neuropathy contributing to complex lesions. Daily foot inspections are essential to avoid progression of minor injuries into limb-threatening lesions. Neuropathy is also responsible for loss of tone of intrinsic foot muscles that leads to subluxation of the metatarsal phalangeal joints, resulting in a "rocker-bottom" foot and ultimately producing complete joint destruction termed *Charcot arthropathy.* These architectural changes also make skin breakdown more likely to occur and require referral to a foot and ankle clinic. In addition to local foot care and glycemic control, assessment for concomitant peripheral arterial disease is essential to ensure that perfusion is optimized for wound healing.

Conte MS: Diabetic revascularization: endovascular versus open bypass—do we have the answer? *Semin Vasc Surg.* 2012;25:108.

Gibbons GW, Shaw PM: Diabetic vascular disease: characteristics of vascular disease unique to the diabetic patient. *Semin Vasc Surg.* 2012;25:89.

Prompers L, et al: Predictors of outcome in individuals with diabetic foot ulcers. *Diabetologia.* 2008;51:747.

NONATHEROSCLEROTIC DISORDERS CAUSING LOWER LIMB ISCHEMIA

Thromboangiitis Obliterans

Thromboangiitis obliterans (Buerger disease) is characterized by multiple segmental occlusions of obliterating tibial and pedal arteries. The most distal arteries are affected, making bypass impossible. Migratory phlebitis may be present. In contrast to atherosclerosis, which involves the intima and media, thromboangiitis obliterans is manifested by infiltration of round cells in all three layers of the arterial wall. The disease occurs principally in young male smokers. Smoking cessation is the cornerstone of therapy. Patients with Buerger disease may have specific cellular immunity against arterial antigens, specific humoral antiarterial antibodies, and elevated circulatory immune complexes, but a precise diagnosis can be made only by tissue histology. Arteriographic findings are distinctive but not pathognomonic. Arterial bypass is not typically feasible because of the lack of distal targets. Amputation is indicated for persistent pain or gangrene and can be performed adjacent to the line of demarcation with satisfactory primary healing.

The disease may become dormant if the patient can stop smoking. Unfortunately, smoking cessation seems particularly difficult in these patients, and many ultimately require multiple amputations.

Popliteal Artery Entrapment Syndrome

This rare cause of popliteal artery stenosis or occlusion occurs as a result of an anomalous course of the popliteal artery. The popliteal artery normally passes between the two heads of the gastrocnemius muscle as it enters the lower leg. In the entrapment syndrome, the artery passes medial to both heads of the gastrocnemius, causing compression of the popliteal artery when the knee is extended. There are five anatomic variants of popliteal artery entrapment, but all produce similar clinical effects. Fibrous thickening of the intima occurs at the site of compression and gradually progresses to total occlusion. Symptoms vary from calf claudication to those of more severe ischemia, depending on lesion severity and embolization. Popliteal artery entrapment should be considered when a young, otherwise healthy patient presents with calf claudication. Until the artery becomes occluded, the only finding is a decrease in strength of the pedal pulses, which is most evident when using provocative maneuvers such as foot passive dorsiflexion or active plantarflexion. Conventional angiography may be useful in demonstrating arterial pathology developing from the repetitive trauma to the vessel and may support the diagnosis by demonstrating stenosis or occlusion with provocative maneuvers but fails to demonstrate the causative extra-arterial, anatomic pathology. MRI and CT studies are most useful in confirmation of

▲ **Figure 36–7.** Popliteal entrapment syndrome. **A:** Gadolinium-enhanced magnetic resonance imaging demonstrating aberrant slip of muscle and fibrous tissue (arrow) overlying the popliteal artery (arrowhead) in a symptomatic patient. **B:** Posterior approach via prone positioning demonstrating fibromuscular abnormality (right angle clamp) with popliteal artery coursing underneath (forceps tip).

the diagnosis (provocative positioning may be performed during image acquisition). Atherosclerotic changes are notably absent. Given the extrinsic pathology responsible for the disorder, open surgery is the mainstay of therapy. Treatment consists of returning the popliteal artery to its normal anatomic course by dividing the aberrant muscle fibers or fibrous band and/or bypass with saphenous vein. Surgery can be performed from a medial or posterior (prone) approach (Figure 36–7).

▶ Cystic Degeneration of the Popliteal Artery

Arterial stenosis is produced by a mucoid cyst in the adventitia, usually located in the middle third of the artery. Calf claudication is the most common symptom, and the only finding is the disappearance of the pedal pulses with knee flexion (Ishikawa sign). Arteriography shows a sharply localized zone of popliteal stenosis with a smooth concentric tapering. Ultrasound or CT scans can be used to demonstrate the cyst within the vessel wall (displacement of the arterial flow lumen, or so-called "scimitar sign" of large lesions). The stenosis may be missed on conventional anteroposterior films and may appear only on lateral exposures. Treatments range from simple cyst aspiration to cyst excision to excision and replacement of the affected arterial segment; more radical treatments appear to reduce the risk of recurrence.

▶ Abdominal Aortic Coarctation

Coarctations of the thoracic or abdominal aorta are rare. They may be congenital or may result from an inflammatory large-vessel arteritis such as Kawasaki or Takayasu disease. These rare disorders may produce symptoms of lower extremity, mesenteric, or renal ischemia depending on the

location of the constriction. The congenital variant of this condition is best managed surgically when it is recognized; autogenous repair may be preferable to the use of prosthetic grafts. Surgical repair in the presence of ongoing inflammation is not recommended because those patients do poorly. However, if the disease is quiescent with a normal sedimentation rate, standard surgical operations appear to produce satisfactory results.

▼ LOWER EXTREMITY AMPUTATION

▶ General Considerations

More than 90% of the 110,000 amputations performed in the United States each year are for ischemic disease or infective gangrene. More than half of lower extremity amputations are performed for complications of diabetes mellitus, and 15%-50% of diabetic amputees will lose a second leg within 5 years. Recent retrospective review has suggested that overall disease-associated amputation rates may actually be increasing. This risk is about two times higher for men than for women. Other indications for amputations are nondiabetic infection with ischemia (15%-25%), ischemia without infection (5%-10%), osteomyelitis (3%-5%), trauma (2%-5%), and frostbite, tumors, neuromas, and other miscellaneous causes (5%-10%).

Many patients facing amputation are near the end of life because of systemic cardiovascular disease. Approximately 20%-30% of patients undergoing major amputation (below-knee or above-knee) will be dead within 2 years. The prevalence of many comorbidities in this population is also reflected in the perioperative mortality rates for major amputation, ranging from 5% to 10% for below-knee amputations to 10% or higher for above-knee amputations.

The level of amputation is determined by assessing the likelihood of healing of the limb in association with the functional potential of the patient. Compared with normal walking, energy expenditure is increased by 10%-40% with a below-knee prosthesis, 50%-70% with an above-knee prosthesis, and 60% with crutches. The clinical conundrum in patients with limb ischemia is twofold: (1) determining which limbs have adequate blood supply to heal at the below-knee level and (2) determining which patients with vascular disease have reasonable rehabilitation potential. The best predictions are based on clinical assessment by an experienced surgeon, assisted by one of the several noninvasive techniques, such as segmental Doppler pressures or transcutaneous measurement of oxygen tension.

► Lower Extremity Amputation Levels

Lower extremity amputations are done most commonly at one of the following levels: toe (called digit amputations, which may be extended to include resection of the metatarsal and called ray amputations), transmetatarsal, below-knee, and above-knee. Amputations at other levels (Syme amputation, Chopart amputation, and hip disarticulation) are infrequently performed for vascular disease.

1. Toe and ray amputations—Toe amputations are the most frequently performed amputation (Figure 36–8). Over two-thirds of amputations in diabetics involve the toes and

▲ **Figure 36–8.** Toe and ray amputations.

forefoot. A guiding principle is midphalangeal or metatarsal resection to assure that all cartilaginous articular surfaces are removed because this material has no blood supply. The indications include gangrene, infection, neuropathic ulceration, frostbite, and osteomyelitis limited to the middle or distal phalanx. Contraindications to digit amputation include indistinct demarcation, infection at the metatarsal level, pallor on elevation, or dependent rubor indicating ischemia of the forefoot.

For dry, uninfected gangrene of one or more toes, autoamputation may be allowed to occur. During this process, epithelialization occurs beneath the eschar, and the toe spontaneously detaches, leaving a clean residual limb at the most distal site. Although preferable in many patients, autoamputation sometimes requires months to complete.

Ray, or wedge, amputation includes removal of the toe and metatarsal head; occasionally, two adjacent toes may be amputated by this method. As with toe amputation, there is modest cosmetic deformity and a prosthesis is not required. Ray amputation of the great toe leads to unstable weight bearing and some difficulty with ambulation resulting from loss of the first metatarsal head.

Complications that may require amputation at higher levels include infection, osteomyelitis of remaining bone, and nonhealing of the incision. These complications have been reported in up to one-third of diabetic patients.

2. Transmetatarsal amputation—Transmetatarsal forefoot amputations preserve normal weight bearing. The principal indication is gangrene of several toes or the great toe, with or without soft tissue infection or osteomyelitis. Good blood supply is needed because the incision creates a generous plantar flap. There is no dorsal flap. On the plantar surface, the incision is continued medially to laterally just proximal to the metatarsophalangeal crease. The metatarsal bones are divided, with the medial and lateral shafts cut shorter than those in the middle to preserve the normal architecture of the foot and assist with orthotic fitting postoperatively, and the tendons are pulled down and transected as high as possible.

Transmetatarsal amputation produces an excellent functional result. Walking requires no increase in energy expenditure, and the gait is usually smooth. A prosthesis is not mandatory, but to achieve optimal gait, the shoes must be modified.

3. Major leg amputations—An attempt at performing a below-knee amputation is warranted in almost any patient who appears to be a potential candidate for rehabilitation.

A. BELOW-KNEE AMPUTATION—The most common procedure for below-knee amputation is the Burgess technique, which uses a long posterior flap (Figure 36–9). The blood supply to a posterior flap is generally better than the supply to an anterior flap or to sagittal flaps, because the sural arteries (which supply the gastrocnemius and soleus muscles)

▲ **Figure 36–9.** Below-knee amputation.

arise high on the popliteal artery, an area not often diseased. The use of rigid dressings and immediate postoperative prostheses has proved advantageous. Application of a rigid cast bandage has several potential advantages: (1) It controls postoperative edema, which may reduce pain; (2) it protects the stump from trauma, particularly when a patient falls during attempts at mobilization; and (3) it allows the patient to be ambulatory with a temporary prosthesis much sooner.

B. ABOVE-KNEE AMPUTATION—Absolute indications for primary above-knee amputation include contracture at the knee joint (observed in debilitated patients with longstanding extremity pain who have been in a prolonged withdrawal posture with the knee flexed) and nonviable calf muscle or skin for creation of the below-knee flap. Patients unlikely to ambulate after below-knee amputation (eg, because of general deconditioning) and those unable to comply with physical therapy and thus at risk for development of a flexion contracture should be considered for above-knee amputation even if able to heal a below-knee amputation.

Above-knee amputation may be performed at several levels, including knee disarticulation. Although it is advantageous to preserve as long a lever arm as possible, knee disarticulation is technically more demanding than transfemoral amputation at a higher level. The technique for standard above-knee amputation is straightforward. Short anterior and posterior flaps, sagittal flaps, or a circular incision may be used. The bone is divided substantially higher than the skin and soft tissue to avoid tension when the wound is closed and later when the muscles of the thigh atrophy. A simple dressing is then applied.

▼ SPECIAL PROBLEMS OF AMPUTEES

▶ Thromboembolism

The amputee is at great risk for deep venous thrombosis (15%) and pulmonary embolism (2%) postoperatively because (1) amputation often follows prolonged immobilization during treatment of the primary disease, and (2) the operation involves ligation of large veins, causing stasis of blood, a situation that predisposes to thrombosis. If immediate-fit prosthetic techniques are not employed, an additional period of inactivity follows the operation, further increasing the risk of thromboembolism.

▶ Rehabilitation After Amputation

The rehabilitation goals following amputation are highly variable. Younger patients universally want to regain ambulatory status and frequently return to work. Elderly patients with significant comorbid conditions may remain wheelchair-bound, and much of their rehabilitation is focused on providing wheelchair access in their living situations and working on independent transfers. It is important to understand that amputation in an elderly patient is frequently an event that occurs near the end of life. For these people, relief of pain and provision for modest function may be the most appropriate outcome in the limited amount of time they have left.

The length of the residual limb correlates well with regaining the ability to walk. Cardiopulmonary disease and physical weakness make walking an overwhelming effort for some patients; this emphasizes the importance of preserving a below-knee amputation if possible, so that walking will require the least possible amount of energy.

▶ Pain & Flexion Contracture

Physical therapy consultation is an important adjunct to prevent contracture. Flexion contractures of the knee or hip occur rapidly in the painful limb because of the relative strength of the flexors over the extensors. Measures to prevent contracture are indicated preoperatively, and application of a rigid dressing postoperatively decreases the incidence of this complication.

▶ Phantom Pain

Persistent sensations in a residual limb are almost universal. Unfortunately, phantom limb pain also is common. Treatment is difficult; improvement has been reported using tricyclic antidepressants and other medications used for neuropathic pain, transcutaneous electrical nerve stimulation, and calcitonin. The incidence and severity of phantom limb pain are increased if there was prolonged ischemia before amputation and decreased if postoperative rehabilitation is rapid.

Brown BJ, Crone CG, Attinger CE: Amputation in the diabetic to maximize function. *Semin Vasc Surg.* 2012;25:115.
Fleury AM, Salih SA, Peel NM: Rehabilitation of the older vascular amputee: a review of the literature. *Geriatr Gerontol Int.* 2013;13:264.

Humphries MD, Brunson A, Li CS, et al: Amputation trends for patients with lower extremity ulcers due to diabetes and peripheral artery disease using statewide data. *J Vasc Surg.* 2016;64:1747-1755.

Landry GJ, Silverman DA, Liem TK, et al: Predictors of healing and functional outcome following transmetatarsal amputations. *Arch Surg.* 2011;146:1005.

CEREBROVASCULAR DISEASE

General Considerations

Unlike in the other vascular beds, symptoms of extracranial carotid disease are most often caused by embolization. Arterial emboli account for approximately one-quarter of strokes in Europe and North America, and 80% of these originate from atherosclerotic lesions in a surgically accessible artery in the neck. The most common lesion is at the bifurcation of the carotid artery. Transcranial Doppler studies have shown that emboli are seen in approximately 20% of patients with moderate (> 50% stenosis) lesions at the carotid bifurcation and even higher rates with more than 70% stenoses. The incidence and frequency of emboli are increased in recently symptomatic patients.

The neurologic dysfunction associated with microemboli may appear as sudden "short-lived," or transient, neurologic symptoms that may include unilateral motor and sensory loss, aphasia (difficulty with understanding and expressing language), or dysarthria (difficulty speaking due to motor dysfunction). These are termed **transient ischemic attacks** (TIAs). Most TIAs are brief, but by convention, a duration of 24 hours is the limit of a TIA. If the symptoms persist, it is a stroke, or **cerebrovascular accident** (CVA). An embolus to the ophthalmic artery, the first branch of the internal carotid artery, produces a temporary monocular loss of vision called amaurosis fugax or permanent blindness. Atherosclerotic emboli may be visible as small bright flecks (Hollenhorst plaques) lodged in arterial bifurcations in the retina.

Characteristically, lesions of atherosclerosis in the internal carotid artery occur along the wall of the carotid bulb opposite to the external carotid artery origin (Figure 36–10). The enlargement of the bulb just distal to this major branch point creates an area of low wall shear stress, flow separation, and loss of unidirectional flow. Presumably, this allows greater interaction of atherogenic particles and the vessel walls at this site and accounts for the localized plaque at the carotid bifurcation.

The accessibility of this localized atheroma allows effective removal of the plaque and a dramatic reduction in stroke risk. Landmark trial data from the 1990s demonstrated that with even the best medical therapy at that time, 26% of patients with TIAs and 70% or greater stenosis of the carotid artery develop permanent neurologic impairment (CVA) from continued embolization at 2 years. The risk of CVA can

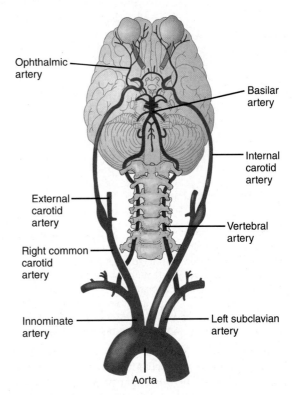

▲ **Figure 36–10.** Cerebrovascular circulation anatomy.

be reduced to 9% with plaque removal. The risk of CVA is lower for patients presenting with amaurosis fugax.

Clinical Findings

A. Symptoms

Patients with cerebrovascular disease can be grouped into three categories based on symptoms at presentation.

1. Asymptomatic disease—An audible bruit heard in the neck may be the only manifestation of cerebrovascular disease. Severe carotid stenosis may also occur in the absence of a bruit with markedly reduced blood flow. Ultrasound screening may identify these patients.

2. Transient ischemic attacks—Sudden onset of a neurologic deficit in the distribution of the anterior or middle cerebral arteries requires investigation of the carotid arteries. Symptoms depend on the ischemic area of the brain, the size of the embolus, and the condition of collaterals to the affected area. Hypoperfusion rarely causes transient neurologic and visual attacks. In symptomatic patients, stroke risk after TIA correlates with the severity of internal carotid artery stenosis.

Patients with multiple TIAs, particularly if these are increasing in frequency or severity, stroke in evolution, or waxing and waning neurologic deficits and high-grade stenoses should be treated urgently, because otherwise they may suffer irreversible deficits.

3. Stroke (CVA)—Intervention is indicated for patients after stroke who have either complete recovery or mild to moderate deficits, because up to one-half will suffer another stroke with further loss of neural function. The timing of intervention is controversial. In select patients, endarterectomy is now recommended within 14 days of the initial neurologic event or earlier. If the infarct is large and the stenosis severe, a healing period prior to revascularization may be advisable to prevent hemorrhage into the necrotic area with restoration of systemic pressure. In stroke patients, the perioperative risk of additional neurologic deficit is higher than in patients after TIA.

4. Distribution—TIAs and strokes attributable to the carotid typically occur in the middle cerebral artery distribution. In the posterior circulation, emboli are less common and hypoperfusion is the dominant pathology. Reduction of flow in the vertebral and basilar arteries may cause drop attacks, clumsiness, and a variety of sensory phenomena. Frequently, the symptoms are bilateral. Vertigo, diplopia, or dysequilibrium occurring individually is rarely due to vertebrobasilar disease, but when these symptoms occur in combination, the diagnosis becomes more likely. It is unusual for dizziness alone to be due to cerebrovascular disease.

B. Signs

A thorough neurologic exam is necessary in all patients both to ensure that the findings are attributable to a carotid stenosis (eg, findings of left arm and leg weakness are not likely to be secondary to high-grade left carotid artery stenosis) and to establish a baseline for comparison on subsequent exam, including after any intervention. Auscultation of the carotid and subclavian arteries is of questionable value because bruits are nonspecific findings.

C. Imaging

1. Doppler ultrasound—The most useful test for the diagnosis of extracranial carotid artery disease is the duplex ultrasound. As the stenosis encroaches on the lumen of the vessel, the velocity of blood increases in the area of the stenosis to maintain distal flow. Doppler spectral velocity analysis determines the flow rate rapidly and with reasonable accuracy. This allows an estimate of the degree of stenosis. Ultrasound can also display plaque morphology but with less reproducibility than stenosis.

2. CTA and MRA—CTA and MRA are often used for confirmation of duplex findings and planning interventional procedures (Figure 36–11). Both types of imaging can assess the degree of stenosis at the carotid bifurcation, providing information on the configuration of the aortic arch and identifying additional disease in the proximal supra-aortic trunk and intracerebral vessels. These studies also delineate regions of ischemic damage in the brain. Diffusion-weighted MRI of the brain is particularly sensitive and will define areas of injury as well as areas of infarction. CTA also displays calcifications, the visualization of which can assist in planning clamp placement and the extent of distal exposure necessary should carotid endarterectomy be undertaken.

▲ **Figure 36–11.** Carotid bifurcation occlusive disease. **A:** Three-dimensional computed tomography (CT) angiogram of neck demonstrating carotid bifurcation stenosis. **B:** Axial CT view demonstrating the lesion.

3. Arteriography—Cerebral arteriography is occasionally performed in patients with symptomatic or asymptomatic cerebrovascular disease. It is most useful for cases in which noninvasive studies are in disagreement or in those patients who are candidates for carotid angioplasty and stenting. Cerebral diagnostic arteriography is invasive and has a low but significant risk of stroke (0.5%-1.0%) due to wire and catheter manipulation within the aortic arch and carotid artery itself.

▶ Treatment

Stroke risk is highest immediately after a TIA, returning to baseline at approximately 6 months. Consequently, in symptomatic patients with carotid stenosis, early intervention is mandatory. Antiplatelet therapy, usually in the form of aspirin or clopidogrel, is particularly important in cerebrovascular patients. Cardiovascular risk factor modification is also imperative in reducing stroke and overall mortality. After a completed stroke, caution must be exercised when planning an intervention.

A. Carotid Endarterectomy

Carotid endarterectomy, the removal of the atherosclerotic lesion at the carotid bifurcation, is the primary operation performed (Figure 36–12). In the North American Symptomatic Carotid Endarterectomy Trial (NASCET), carotid endarterectomy was shown to reduce incidence of ipsilateral stroke from 26% to 9% at 2 years in patients presenting with either TIA or stroke *and* carotid lesions of 70% stenosis or greater. The results also favored surgery in patients with moderate carotid stenosis (50%-69%), but less dramatically. The 5-year risk of ipsilateral stroke was 15.7% among patients treated surgically (n = 1108) and 22.2% among those treated medically (n = 1118; $P = .045$). Patients with stenoses of less than 50% did not significantly benefit from surgery. As such, patients with symptomatic lesions producing a stenosis of 50% or more may be offered surgery provided they are otherwise eligible.

Large clinical trials have also shown a benefit of surgery for asymptomatic carotid stenosis. Both the Asymptomatic Carotid Atherosclerosis Study (ACAS) in North America and the Asymptomatic Carotid Surgery Trial (ACST) in Europe showed that stroke incidence is halved (11%-12% to 5%-6%) by carotid endarterectomy compared to best medical therapy at 5 years of follow-up in patients with at least a 60% stenosis. "Best medical therapy" included antiplatelet agents and statins in the ACST. Although the ACAS did not show a benefit for endarterectomy in women, the larger European study did. Due to the improvement in best medical management

▲ **Figure 36–12.** Technique of carotid endarterectomy.

since the time of these trials, there is no longer a consensus threshold for offering surgery. Many practitioners, including the authors, offer surgery for selected asymptomatic patients with 80% or more stenosis.

Importantly, carotid endarterectomy cannot be performed when the internal carotid artery is completely occluded, because complete thrombectomy is difficult and residual clot may embolize, creating additional lesions. Furthermore, the risk of embolization from a totally occluded carotid is extremely low and generally obviates the need for surgical intervention.

B. Carotid Angioplasty and Stenting

Early studies of carotid angioplasty and stenting (CAS; Figure 36–13) suggested similar morbidity and mortality rates to carotid endarterectomy. Because of the higher rate of emboli with stenting, cerebral protection devices, either filters placed in the distal internal carotid or devices that cause flow cessation or reversal, should always be used. After stenting, clopidogrel is prescribed for at least 30 days to limit late embolization.

Two large randomized studies found more strokes after CAS than after endarterectomy: the International Carotid Stent Study (ICSS) and the Carotid Revascularization Endarterectomy versus Stenting Trial (CREST). Conversely, there were more myocardial infarctions after endarterectomy. All women and men over age 70 did worse with CAS. Younger men did well with CAS. A full discussion of the relative merits of stenting and endarterectomy is beyond the scope of this work, but at present, stenting is reserved for patients with anatomic (hostile neck anatomy due to prior radiation or surgery, prior carotid endarterectomy, or distal lesions not readily accessible via a neck incision) or medical (severe cardiopulmonary disease) contraindications to endarterectomy.

C. Treatment Results

The main complication of cerebrovascular interventions is stroke, which occurs in 2%-7% of patients depending on the operative indications and cerebrovascular anatomy. Higher stroke rates occur in the setting of symptomatic stenosis or contralateral carotid occlusion. Lower stroke rates occur with asymptomatic stenosis. The operative death rate for all extracranial cerebrovascular interventions is less than 1%.

Transient cranial nerve injury occurs in about 10% of cases after endarterectomy and may cause tongue weakness, hoarseness, mouth asymmetry, earlobe numbness, and dysphagia. Less than 2% of peripheral nerve deficits

▲ **Figure 36–13.** Carotid angioplasty and stenting. **A:** Conventional arteriogram demonstrating diffuse occlusive disease of common and internal carotid arteries. **B:** Completion arteriogram following angioplasty and stenting of the lesions.

are permanent, although this number goes up with surgery for recurrent disease, making stenting attractive for this indication.

Restenosis or occlusion is uncommon after carotid endarterectomy (5%-10% at 5 years) and appears to be equally uncommon after carotid stenting. For endarterectomy, randomized controlled trials from the 1980s and 1990s demonstrated that using a prosthetic patch for closure of the arteriotomy reduces stroke and restenosis.

Subclavian Steal Syndrome

The subclavian steal syndrome is characterized by reversal of flow through the vertebral artery due to a more proximal occlusion or stenosis of the subclavian artery (ie, the vertebral artery serves as a collateral to supply blood to the arm). Although this anatomic arrangement is often demonstrated on angiograms, clinical sequelae are rare. Symptoms of effort fatigue in the involved extremity are more common than neurologic complaints. When necessary, treatment consists of stenting or open surgery consisting of bypass grafting from the common carotid to the subclavian artery distal to the lesion or transposition of the subclavian artery beyond the lesion to the side of the nearby common carotid artery.

Concomitant Coronary and Cerebrovascular Disease

When patients have coexistent severe coronary and carotid atherosclerosis requiring treatment, there has been controversy as to which lesion should be addressed first. Most strokes during cardiac procedures are from atheromatous emboli from the aortic arch, not from low flow through a carotid stenosis. Recent trial data failed to demonstrate an advantage to synchronous carotid endarterectomy and coronary artery bypass grafting in the setting of asymptomatic high-grade stenosis and seemed to suggest that such an approach might be associated with poorer outcomes (although underpowered for that treatment effect). In contrast, prior randomized trials with short-term follow-up have suggested equivalent mortality and reduced stroke rates with concomitant carotid endarterectomy and coronary artery bypass graft compared to staged procedures. Thus, the question of optimal timing of extracranial and coronary revascularization remains unanswered.

Other Causes of Cerebrovascular Symptoms

Other than atherosclerosis, primary disease of the extracranial arteries is rare.

A. Takayasu (Giant Cell) Arteritis

Takayasu arteritis is an obliterative arteriopathy principally involving the aortic arch vessels that often affects young women. The pararenal abdominal aorta and pulmonary arteries also may be affected. High-dose corticosteroids and cyclophosphamide have been shown to arrest and, in some cases, reverse the progress of the disease. Operative treatment of nonspecific arteritis should be avoided when the arteritis is active, but it may be successful in quiescent disease.

B. Aortic Dissection with Extension

Aortic dissection may extend into the arch branches, producing obstruction and cerebral symptoms. This is discussed in Chapter 20.

C. Internal Carotid Dissection

Dissection originating in the internal carotid artery and localized to its extracranial segment occurs as an acute event that may narrow or obliterate the internal carotid lumen. The primary lesion is an intimal tear at the distal end of the carotid bulb. It may be associated with other types of neck trauma, severe hypertension, fibrillinopathies, or fibromuscular dysplasia.

Cerebral symptoms are the result of ischemia in the ipsilateral hemisphere. Acute neck pain in association with localized cervical tenderness adjacent to the angle of the mandible is a frequent finding. Patients may also develop unilateral Horner syndrome.

Arteriography shows a characteristic pattern of tapered narrowing at or just beyond the distal portion of the carotid bulb. The lumen beyond this point may be obliterated or may persist as a barely visible narrow shadow. If the lumen persists, it resumes a normal caliber beyond the bony foramen.

Randomized controlled trial data have shown no significant difference in outcomes between antiplatelet and anticoagulation therapy, but event rates were small and the study may have been underpowered. In many patients, the intramural clot will be resorbed, restoring a normal lumen. Intervention is uncommon but may be indicated for patients with recurrent TIAs or pseudoaneurysm formation. Stenting is the procedure of choice and will restore the normal carotid contour.

D. Fibromuscular Dysplasia

Fibromuscular dysplasia is a nonatherosclerotic angiopathy of unknown cause that affects specific arteries chiefly in young women. Symptoms of cerebrovascular disease can occur when the carotid artery is affected. It is usually bilateral and involves primarily the middle third of the extracranial portions of the internal carotid artery. Several pathologic variants of the disease have been described, but in most of them, the primary lesion is overgrowth of the media in a segmental distribution, producing irregular zones of arterial narrowing. The most common result is a series of concentric rings, producing the radiologic appearance of a string of beads in a long internal carotid artery. Approximately one-third of patients are also hypertensive due to renal artery involvement.

The prevalence of fibromuscular dysplasia and the portion of patients who develop symptoms are not known. Once symptoms develop, transient neurologic events are the most common manifestation. However, more than 20% of patients have had a stroke by the time of presentation. Because of the high incidence of neurologic disability, the lesion should be corrected by angioplasty when patients develop symptoms. Fibromuscular dysplasia lesions in the carotid and other arterial beds generally respond well to angioplasty without need for stenting.

Bonati LH, Dobson J, Featherstone RL, et al; International Carotid Stenting Study Investigators: Long-term outcomes after stenting versus endarterectomy for treatment of symptomatic carotid stenosis: the International Carotid Stenting Study (ICSS) randomised trial. *Lancet.* 2015;385(9967):529-538.

Brott TG, Hobson RW, Howard G, et al: Stenting versus endarterectomy for treatment of carotid-artery stenosis. *N Engl J Med.* 2010;363:11.

Endarterectomy for asymptomatic carotid artery stenosis. Executive Committee for the Asymptomatic Carotid Atherosclerosis Study (ACAS). *JAMA.* 1995;273:1421.

Fairman R, Gray WA, Scicli AP, et al: The CAPTURE registry: analysis of strokes resulting from carotid artery stenting in the post approval setting: timing, location, severity, and type. *Ann Surg.* 2007;246:551-556.

Ferguson GG, et al: The North American Symptomatic Carotid Endarterectomy Trial: surgical results in 1415 patients. *Stroke.* 1999;30:1751.

Fusco MR, Harrigan MR: Cerebrovascular dissections—a review part I: spontaneous dissections. *Neurosurgery.* 2011;68(1):242-257.

Halliday A, et al: Prevention of disabling and fatal strokes by successful carotid endarterectomy in patients without recent neurological symptoms: randomized controlled trial. *Lancet.* 2004;363:1491.

Rothwell PM, et al: Prediction and prevention of stroke in patients with carotid stenosis. *Eur J Vasc Endovasc Surg.* 2008;35:255.

Yadav JS, et al: Stenting and angioplasty with protection in patients at high risk for endarterectomy investigators. Protected carotid-artery stenting versus endarterectomy in high-risk patients. *N Engl J Med.* 2004;351:1493.

▼ RENOVASCULAR HYPERTENSION

► General Considerations

More than 23 million people in the United States have hypertension, and renovascular disease is a causative factor in 2%-7% of cases. Atherosclerosis of the aorta and renal artery (two-thirds of cases) and fibromuscular dysplasia are the two primary causes of renovascular hypertension. Less common causes of hypertension include renal artery emboli, renal artery aneurysms, renal artery dissection, hypoplasia of the renal arteries, and stenosis of the suprarenal aorta.

Hypertension due to renal artery stenosis results from the renal response to reduced blood flow. Cells of the juxtaglomerular complex secrete renin, which acts on circulating angiotensinogen to form angiotensin I, which is rapidly converted to angiotensin II by ACE. This octapeptide constricts arterioles, increases aldosterone secretion, and promotes sodium retention. Due to the excess aldosterone, hypertension becomes volume dependent. Over time, pathologic changes occur in the uninvolved kidney, and the hypertension may not be sensitive to ACE inhibition. With sodium restriction and volume reduction (diuretics), the hypertension may once again become sensitive to ACE inhibition. If both kidneys have renal artery stenoses, or if the disease exists in a solitary kidney, renal insufficiency may occur with ACE inhibitor administration with a loss of pressure in the glomerulus due to a reduction of angiotensin II constriction of the efferent arteriole.

Atherosclerosis characteristically produces stenosis at the orifice of the main renal artery. The lesion usually consists of aortic atheroma that protrudes over the renal artery orifice. Less commonly, the atheroma arises in the renal artery itself. Renal artery stenosis is more common in males over age 45 years and is bilateral in about 95% of cases.

Fibromuscular dysplasia usually involves the middle and distal thirds of the main renal artery and may extend into the branches. Medial fibroplasia is the most common variety of fibromuscular dysplasia, accounting for 85% of these lesions. It is bilateral in 50% of cases. Concentric rings of hyperplasia projecting into the arterial lumen cause the arterial stenoses. Renal artery aneurysms frequently coexist. Fibromuscular dysplasia occurs mainly in young women, with onset of hypertension usually occurring before age 45 years. It is the causative disorder in 10% of children with hypertension. Developmental renal artery hypoplasia, coarctation of the aorta, and Takayasu arteritis are other vascular causes of hypertension in childhood.

► Clinical Findings

A. Symptoms and Signs

Most patients are asymptomatic. Persistent elevation of the diastolic pressure is usually the only abnormal physical finding. A bruit is frequently audible on one or both sides of the midline in the flank or upper abdomen. Other signs of atherosclerosis may be present when this is the cause of the renal artery disease.

Other clues to the presence of renovascular hypertension include absence of a family history of hypertension, early onset of hypertension (particularly during childhood or during early adulthood), marked acceleration of the degree of hypertension, resistance to control with antihypertensive drugs, and rapid deterioration of renal function. One should suspect renovascular hypertension if initial diastolic pressure is greater than 115 mm Hg or if renal function deteriorates while a patient is being given ACE inhibitors. Sudden onset of pulmonary edema with severe hypertension also is highly suggestive of renovascular hypertension.

B. Diagnostic Studies

In the past, several diagnostic tests were devised to diagnose renovascular hypertension. Divided urinary excretion studies, selective renin measurement from renal vein sampling, and captopril renal scintigraphy are now rarely used.

Noninvasive or minimally invasive imaging of the renal arteries is justified when the patient has a precipitous drop in blood pressure, decreased renal function with an ACE inhibitor, difficult-to-control hypertension, or an unexplained deterioration in renal function.

C. Imaging Studies

In experienced hands, duplex ultrasound scanning has an overall agreement with angiography of over 90%. Renal artery stenosis is characterized by elevated peak systolic velocities and, in severe cases, elevated renal artery–to–aorta peak systolic velocity ratios. CTA or MRA may provide high-resolution images of diseased renal arteries, although they must be used with caution in patients with renal insufficiency. The contrast required with CTA is nephrotoxic, and gadolinium has been associated with systemic nephrogenic fibrosis in patients with reduced renal clearance. As previously noted, one known disadvantage of MRA is its failure to delineate calcific disease.

Renal arteriography is the gold standard method for delineating the obstructive lesion and also affords the opportunity for simultaneous intervention. Because atherosclerotic disease most often involves the origins of the renal arteries, a midstream aortogram should be obtained in addition to selective renal artery catheterization.

▶ Treatment

A. Medical Management

Patients with renovascular hypertension require aggressive management of modifiable risk factors. If hypertension responds well to medical therapy and the renal function is stable, no intervention on the renal artery stenosis is needed.

B. Percutaneous Transluminal Angioplasty and Stenting

Percutaneous transluminal angioplasty with stenting is the preferred procedure for most patients (Figure 36–14). Although clearly valuable for some patients, the overall results of percutaneous interventions for renal artery stenosis have been mixed, and large randomized clinical trials suggest that medical treatment with angiotensin receptor blockers may be as effective as stenting in most cases. Patients with fibromuscular dysplasia typically respond to angioplasty alone.

C. Surgical Treatment

High-quality, long-term data defining which patients might benefit from open revascularization rather than endovascular intervention are lacking. In the very young with limited comorbidities, surgery may be advisable due to concern regarding the long-term durability of angioplasty and stenting. Patients with anatomically unfavorable lesions (long-segment stenoses over 15-20 mm) or small-caliber (< 6 mm) native renal arteries may be poor candidates for stenting. Surgical repair also is required for failed angioplasty and stenting, renal revascularization during a procedure on the aorta, and lesions that are in branch vessels. As with any operation, the indications for arterial reconstruction are influenced by the extent of disease, the patient's life expectancy, and the anticipated morbidity associated with operation. Nephrectomy may be considered when arterial repair is impossible or especially hazardous and the disease is unilateral.

Options include endarterectomy, which is most easily accomplished through an incision into the adjacent aorta (transaortic), or aortorenal bypass, which can be fashioned in an end-to-side or end-to-end fashion using prosthetic or autogenous (eg, greater saphenous vein) conduits. The sequence of clamping in order to fashion proximal and distal anastomoses should seek to minimize the period of warm ischemia to the affected kidney. An alternative is "nonanatomic" bypass such as an hepato-, spleno-, ilio-, or mesorenal procedure. The celiac and splenic arteries often have coexistent occlusive atherosclerotic disease that mandates preoperative arteriographic assessment of these vessels.

Extracorporeal techniques have been developed for distal branch aneurysms or extensive fibromuscular dysplasia. These require removal of the kidney from the abdomen (ex vivo arterial reconstruction), continuous cold perfusion of its vascular tree, and microvascular techniques for arterial replacement. The kidney is then either returned to a site near its original position or transplanted to the ipsilateral iliac fossa.

▶ Prognosis

Overall, there is no consensus on when to offer percutaneous or open procedures for renovascular hypertension, and results have been mixed. Procedures for revascularization of the renal artery are successful in lowering blood pressure in over 90% of patients with fibromuscular hyperplasia. Open surgery for atherosclerotic stenosis results in improvement or cure of hypertension in about 60%. The results for angioplasty and stenting are not as good, perhaps because of atheroembolization to the kidney during angioplasty.

▲ **Figure 36–14.** Renal artery occlusive disease. **A:** Aortogram demonstrating ostial lesion in left renal artery. **B:** Renal stent constrained on delivery catheter over wire positioned across lesion. **C:** Arteriogram demonstrating widely patent renal artery following balloon angioplasty and stent placement.

The results of intervention for salvage of renal function are better than those for treatment of hypertension. The procedural mortality rate of operative renovascular surgery in children is almost nil, whereas it increases to 2%-8% in adults with diffuse atherosclerosis. Stenting of the renal arteries is also very well tolerated.

Cooper CJ, Murphy TP, Cutlip DE, et al; CORAL Investigators: Stenting and medical therapy for atherosclerotic renal-artery stenosis. *N Engl J Med.* 2014;370(1):13-22.

Mousa AY, Campbell JE, Stone PA, et al: Short- and long-term outcomes of percutaneous transluminal angioplasty/stenting of renal fibromuscular dysplasia over a ten-year period. *J Vasc Surg.* 2012;55:421.

Wheatley K, Ives N, Gray R, et al: Revascularization versus medical therapy for renal-artery stenosis. *N Engl J Med.* 2009;361:1953.

MESENTERIC ISCHEMIA SYNDROMES

General Considerations

The celiac axis and the superior and inferior mesenteric arteries are the principal sources of blood supply to the stomach and intestines, with the inferior mesenteric artery and internal iliac arteries supplying flow to the distal colon (Figure 36–15). The anatomic collateral interconnections between these arteries are numerous. Single or even multiple visceral artery lesions are generally well tolerated, because collateral flow is readily available (Figure 36–16).

Atherosclerosis is the cause of obstructive lesions in the visceral arteries in the vast majority of cases. Vasculitis (eg, Takayasu disease) is much less common. When atherosclerosis is the cause, the usual lesion is a collar of plaque spilling

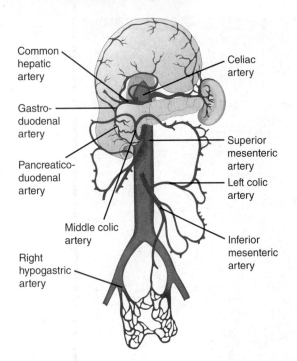

▲ Figure 36–15. Visceral arterial circulation and interconnections.

▲ Figure 36–16. Three-dimensional computed tomography angiogram demonstrating a critical superior mesenteric artery stenosis (arrow) and collateral vessel enlargement originating at the inferior mesenteric artery (arrowhead).

over from the aorta that creates a proximal stenosis or occlusion. Associated atherosclerosis in the aorta and its other branches is common.

CHRONIC MESENTERIC ISCHEMIA

▶ Clinical Findings

The principal complaint is postprandial abdominal pain, which has been labeled abdominal or visceral angina. Pain characteristically appears 15-30 minutes after the beginning of a meal and lasts for an hour or longer. Pain is occasionally so severe and prolonged that opiates are required for relief. Pain occurs as a deep-seated, steady ache in the epigastrium, occasionally radiating to the right or left upper quadrant. Weight loss results from reluctance to eat. Although mild degrees of malabsorption can occur, gastrointestinal absorption studies are not helpful. Diarrhea and vomiting have been described. An upper abdominal bruit may be heard.

Ultrasound can be diagnostic in experienced hands, but CTA or arteriography in the anteroposterior and especially the lateral projections demonstrates both the arterial lesion and the patterns of collateral blood flow.

▶ Treatment

Percutaneous transluminal angioplasty with stenting has gained acceptance as a first line of therapy for mesenteric ischemia (Figure 36–17). Access approaches include transfemoral, transradial/-brachial, and hybrid approach with open exposure of the superior mesenteric artery and retrograde stenting. Results are best for focal, nonorificial stenoses. Embolization to the gut is a rare but potentially fatal complication of instrumentation of these lesions.

Surgical revascularization of the superior mesenteric and celiac axes may be performed by either endarterectomy or graft replacement. During endarterectomy, a sleeve of aortic intima and the orifice lesions in the celiac or superior mesenteric arteries are removed. The operation is performed by a retroperitoneal approach to the aorta through a left thoracoabdominal incision. Alternatively, Dacron grafts may be brought antegrade from the lower thoracic aorta or retrograde from the iliac arteries to the celiac axis or superior mesenteric artery.

Operation should be avoided in patients with acute vasculitis as the underlying cause of mesenteric ischemia; high-dose steroids and immunosuppressive agents are indicated instead, with reassessment once the disease is in a quiescent state.

▶ Prognosis

Opening flow to the mesenteric vascular bed almost always results in relief of symptoms. The endovascular approach

▲ **Figure 36–17.** Lateral projection mesenteric angiogram demonstrating (**A**) celiac artery occlusion (white arrow) and superior mesenteric artery in-stent stenosis (black arrow) and (**B**) resolution of these lesions after placement of a celiac stent and balloon angioplasty of the existing superior mesenteric artery stent.

decreases short-term mortality by up to two-thirds. The limited durability of endovascular therapy necessitates close follow-up and reintervention if symptoms recur.

ACUTE MESENTERIC ISCHEMIA

Acute mesenteric ischemia is a highly morbid disorder. There are four subtypes of acute mesenteric ischemia based on etiology: (1) embolic, (2) thrombotic, (3) venous outflow thrombosis, and (4) nonocclusive ("low-flow"). Patients classically present with excruciating diffuse abdominal pain with a surprising absence of physical findings such as abdominal tenderness or distention ("pain out of proportion to exam")—unless actual bowel perforation produces peritonitis. Symptoms of chronic mesenteric ischemia may precede this catastrophic event, particularly in the case of thrombotic occlusion, or the onset may be sudden and associated with atrial fibrillation or myocardial infarction, if the cause is embolic occlusion of the superior mesenteric artery. The diagnosis can be difficult, and its recognition is often delayed, resulting in irreversible bowel ischemia. The mortality rate from acute mesenteric ischemia remains high, ranging from 50% to 90% in reported series. Patients who require massive bowel resection rarely survive or, if they survive, can develop

incapacitating short-gut syndrome. The prognosis improves dramatically if revascularization can be achieved prior to intestinal infarction. This obviously requires early diagnosis, which will only occur if the practitioner has a high index of suspicion. In addition to clinical suspicion, CTA is often a useful adjunct in evaluating for etiology and for treatment planning. Treatment varies by etiology from embolectomy or bypass for embolic and thrombotic occlusions, to anticoagulation for mesenteric venous thrombosis, to supportive measures to prevent hypotension in nonocclusive mesenteric ischemia.

CELIAC ARTERY COMPRESSION

External compression of the celiac artery, or median arcuate ligament syndrome, is an unusual cause of visceral ischemia. It generally affects young adults, with women more often affected than men, and is commonly associated with rapid weight loss. The precise etiology is controversial, with some arguing that the symptoms represent compression of nerves around the celiac artery rather than true ischemia. CTA or MRA may be helpful in identifying compression; angiography with and without provocative expiration is often the most useful. The difficulty in making the diagnosis is compounded by the presence of celiac artery compression by the arcuate ligament in a fraction of the normal population, in which it is a clinically insignificant incidental finding. As such, surgery should be advised only after an exhaustive search for alternative causes of postprandial pain. The classic sign is a loud epigastric bruit with exhalation as the crus of the diaphragm descends to compress the artery.

Surgery consists of open or laparoscopic division of the median arcuate fibers around the celiac artery. The artery may be fibrotic from chronic compression and may require repair itself as well.

Patients with median arcuate ligament compression respond favorably to operation in many cases; however, some of these patients are not improved even though a technically adequate operation is performed.

Aburahma AF, Campbell JE, Stone PA, et al: Perioperative and late clinical outcomes of percutaneous transluminal stentings of the celiac and superior mesenteric arteries over the past decade. *J Vasc Surg.* 2013;57:1052.

Tallarita T, Oderich GS, Gloviczki P, et al: Patient survival after open and endovascular mesenteric revascularization for chronic mesenteric ischemia. *J Vasc Surg.* 2013;57:747.

Zacharias N, Eghbalieh SD, Chang BB, et al: Chronic mesenteric ischemia outcome analysis and predictors of endovascular failure. *J Vasc Surg.* 2016;63(6):1582-1587.

ARTERIAL ANEURYSMS

▶ General Considerations

An aneurysm is defined as a localized dilation of an artery to at least 1.5 times its normal diameter. The expanding vessel elongates as well as dilates. A true aneurysm involves primary dilation of the artery, including all vessel wall layers (intima, media, and adventitia). A false aneurysm, also called pseudoaneurysm, is characterized by a disruption of the artery wall, does not include all layers of the wall, and may actually be a pulsatile hematoma not contained by the artery wall but by a fibrous capsule. A false aneurysm caused by infection is called a mycotic aneurysm irrespective of the specific pathogen.

Iatrogenic pseudoaneurysms of the femoral artery secondary to catheterization are the most numerous of all aneurysms. Infrarenal abdominal aortic aneurysms are the most common of the true aneurysms. In descending order, other arteries affected are the iliac artery, the popliteal artery, the arch and descending portions of the thoracic aorta (including dilation after aortic dissection), the common femoral artery, the carotid arteries, and other peripheral arteries. Other rare causes of true aneurysms include Marfan syndrome, Ehlers-Danlos syndrome, Behçet disease, and cystic medial necrosis.

ABDOMINAL AORTIC ANEURYSMS

Abdominal aortic aneurysms (AAAs) are found in 2% of the elderly male population, and the incidence may be increasing. In selected groups, the incidence is higher—5% of patients with coronary artery disease and as many as 50% of patients with femoral or popliteal aneurysms have aortic aneurysms. Males are four times as likely to be affected as females. Ruptured aortic aneurysms are a major cause of death of males older than age 65 years in the United States.

Numerous mechanisms have been proposed for the development of AAA. Structural issues may contribute; reductions in the number of elastic lamellae and virtual absence of vasa vasorum in the media of the distal abdominal aorta compared with the thoracic aorta may favor aneurysmal degeneration. Excessive protease activity or local reductions in the concentration of protease inhibitors have been implicated in aneurysm formation, allowing for the enzymatic destruction of the two principle structural elements of the aorta, elastin, and collagen. There may be hemodynamic factors as well, owing to large pulsatile stresses because of tapering geometry, increased stiffness, and reflected pressure waves from branch vessels in the infrarenal aorta. Genetic factors influencing connective tissue metabolism and structure also have been associated with AAA development. Indeed, a positive family history of aortic aneurysms confers a 20% chance that a first-degree family member will have an aneurysm, and some society guidelines suggest screening for family members of appropriate age.

In terms of risk factors, cigarette smoking has a powerful influence on developing an aortic aneurysm. The risk increases in dose-dependent fashion, with those having smoked more than one pack per day for greater than 35 years having an odds ratio of 12 for having an AAA compared to never smokers. The excess prevalence associated with smoking accounted for 78% of all AAAs that were 4 cm or larger in the Veterans Administration ADAM study sample. Hypertension is present in 40% of patients with AAAs but did not correlate with enlargement in the ADAM study. Surprisingly, diabetics appear to have a lower incidence of aortic aneurysm formation.

Ninety percent of aneurysms of the abdominal aorta occur between the takeoff of the renal arteries and the aortic bifurcation but may include variable portions of the common iliac arteries. Rupture with exsanguination is the major complication of AAAs. Unfortunately, neither the expansion rate nor the rupture risk is predictable. Tension on the aneurysm wall is governed by the law of Laplace. Thus, rupture risk is related to diameter. While relating this to an individual risk is not possible, population-wide risks have been established. The Society for Vascular Surgery recommends screening of both men and women who have smoked at least 100 cigarettes at age 65.

Clinical Findings

A. Symptoms and Signs

The vast majority of unruptured aneurysms are asymptomatic. Uncommonly intact AAAs produce back or abdominal pain; such symptoms portend rupture and are an indication or urgent repair.

Eighty percent of AAAs with a diameter of 5 cm are palpable as **pulsatile abdominal masses** in the mid-abdomen just above and to the left side of the umbilicus. Physical examination for an AAA is less reliable in obese patients.

B. Imaging Studies

Plain films of the abdomen reveal calcification in the outer layers of only 20% of abdominal aneurysms.

Ultrasound is the least expensive modality for infrarenal aortic aneurysm surveillance. Repeated ultrasound examinations are cost effective for observing small AAAs and may be used to follow resolution of the aneurysm after endovascular repair. However, ultrasound examinations do not delineate adjacent structures as well as CT or MRI and are less reliable in obese patients.

CT and MRI are both accurate methods for assessing aneurysm diameter (Figure 36–18). An important source of error during interpretation occurs when the course of the aneurysmal aorta is diagonal to the cross-sectional image. This creates an elliptical image of the AAA and a falsely elevated diameter in the larger dimension. Thus, measurement of the short axis is critical to determine true aneurysm diameter. CT scans provide valuable information about aneurysm location and size as well as important adjacent structures that affect AAA repair, such as horseshoe kidneys or other renal abnormalities, and venous anomalies, including retroaortic renal veins, circumaortic renal veins, and left-sided or duplicated vena cavae, which may have important surgical implications. If the patient has a multiplanar CT scan, aortograms, which were once routine studies in planning operative management of AAAs, are not needed.

C. Natural History

Most aneurysms continue to enlarge and will eventually rupture if left untreated. The average expansion rate for an AAA is 2-3 mm per year. The rate of expansion correlates with continued smoking, initial aneurysm diameter, and the degree of obstructive pulmonary disease. An expansion of 0.5 cm in 6 months or 1 cm over 12 months qualifies as rapid enlargement and suggests the aneurysm is unstable and should be repaired.

Aneurysm size is currently the best determinant of rupture risk. About 40% of aneurysms 5.5-6 cm or larger in diameter will rupture within 5 years if untreated, and the average survival of an untreated patient is 17 months. In contrast, the ADAM study found a 0.5% per year rupture rate in AAAs of 4-5.4 cm, an overall rate remarkably similar to a comparable trial in the United Kingdom. Thus, *surgery is recommended for AAAs 5.5 cm or more in size,* but small aortic aneurysms can be safely followed. A threshold of 5 cm is justifiable in women. Regardless of size, repair is mandatory for an aneurysm that is symptomatic or enlarging rapidly.

Treatment

A. Endovascular Repair

Endovascular repair, introduced in 1991, is achieved with a synthetic graft to which metal stents have been attached (Figure 36–19). Endovascular repair requires that the aorta proximal to the aneurysm but inferior to the renal artery ostia ("neck") have a cylindrical configuration of sufficient length to allow for adequate sealing and iliac arteries of sufficient size and limited tortuosity so that the device can be introduced from the femoral arteries. Minimum and maximum parameters for aneurysm neck length and diameter, angulation, length of the distal seal zone proximal to the internal iliac artery ostia, and access vessel diameter are perpetually changing as new devices are introduced. Devices for endovascular repair of AAAs are delivered using a system of guidewires and delivery systems with large-bore sheaths. Several devices are available with unique design features. In series of comparable patients, patients with endovascular repair have less operative blood loss, shorter hospital stays, and reduced operative morbidity compared to those undergoing conventional repair.

The most important intermediate- or long-term adverse outcome of endovascular repair is persistent perfusion of

▲ **Figure 36–18.** Computed tomography showing the typical position of a 5.5-cm abdominal aortic aneurysm and its proximity to the abdominal wall.

▲ **Figure 36–19. A:** Three-dimensional computed tomography (CT) angiogram reconstruction of abdominal aortic aneurysm. White arrow points to aortic flow lumen at same level as that in panel B. **B:** Axial CT view. White arrow points to flow lumen, and black arrow points to thrombus within aneurysm sac. Notice only aortic flow lumen is visualized on CT angiogram, just as in conventional angiography. Total diameter of the aorta, including area containing thrombus, is used in predicting rupture risk and determining need for intervention. **C:** Three-dimensional CT angiogram after aortic stent graft repair.

the aneurysm sac ("endoleak"), which may result in continued aneurysm expansion and rupture. These are divided into types denoting clinical importance. A type 1 endoleak denotes ineffective proximal or distal sealing with pressurization of the aneurysm sac and should be fixed immediately (Figure 36–20). A type 2 endoleak results in persistent flow through the aneurysm from branch vessels, usually the inferior mesenteric artery or a patent lumbar

▲ **Figure 36–20.** Endovascular aneurysm repair (EVAR). **A:** Type 1 endoleak (arrow) after endovascular abdominal aortic aneurysm repair. **B:** Treated with proximal extension via placement of a Palmaz stent with resolution of the endoleak.

artery. These have relatively low pressures and can safely be monitored, with treatment reserved for aneurysm sac enlargement. Aortic stent grafts are typically modular (eg, "main body" and "contralateral limb" grafts), with components overlapped to achieve coverage of the aneurysm while maintaining flow lumens to both lower extremities. Pressurization of the aneurysm through gaps between these components or rents in the graft fabric is a type 3 endoleak. Like type 1 endoleaks, type 3 endoleaks should be treated immediately. Type 4 endoleaks are due to self-limited graft porosity and typically resolve in the first 24 hours following stent graft placement.

Rupture can occur after endovascular aortic aneurysm repair. The rate of late ruptures is low but underscores that patients need extended follow-up to ensure the durability of endovascular aneurysm repair.

B. Open Repair

Conventional open operative AAA repair consists of replacing the aneurysmal segment with a synthetic fabric graft (Figure 36–21). Tubular or bifurcation grafts of Dacron or PTFE are preferred. The proximal anastomosis is made to the aorta above the aneurysm. The site of the distal anastomosis is determined by the extent of aneurysmal involvement of the iliac arteries. Traditionally, a transperitoneal approach via midline laparotomy has been used for AAA repair, but retroperitoneal operations via flank incision

▲ **Figure 36–21.** Replacement of an aortic aneurysm with a synthetic bifurcation graft. The laminated clot within the aneurysm has been removed, and the outer wall is closed over the graft.

may decrease perioperative pulmonary and gastrointestinal complications.

Elective infrarenal abdominal aneurysmectomy has a 2%-4% operative death rate and a 5%-10% rate of complications, such as bleeding, renal failure, myocardial infarction, graft infection, limb loss, bowel ischemia, and erectile dysfunction. Paraplegia is a very rare complication. Malignant tumors are encountered unexpectedly in about 4% of cases, although that rate is now dwindling with the routine use of multiplanar CT scans. If gastrointestinal malignancy is encountered during an aneurysm resection, the aneurysm repair should be done first unless there is impending bowel obstruction, evidence of hemorrhage, or perforation.

Long-term results of open aneurysmectomy are excellent: The graft failure rate is low, and false aneurysm formation at the anastomoses is rare, although approximately 5% of patients develop incisional hernias.

▼ ILIAC ANEURYSMS

Iliac artery aneurysms generally occur in conjunction with AAAs. Isolated iliac aneurysms are unusual, but in some cases, the iliac segment of the aneurysmal artery may enlarge at a greater rate than the aortic segment and is the primary reason for repair. As with aortic aneurysms, most iliac aneurysms are asymptomatic. However, they may present with symptoms related to compression or erosion of surrounding structures, such as obstructive uropathy with ureteral obstruction, neuropathy from compression of local nerves, and unilateral leg swelling from compression of the adjacent iliac vein.

Physical examination can suggest the diagnosis of large (> 4 cm) iliac artery aneurysms if the physician is alert to that possibility. Most symptomatic iliac aneurysms can be palpated as pulsatile masses on abdominal or rectal examinations. However, iliac aneurysms are usually found incidentally on ultrasound or CT.

Similar to aortic aneurysms, iliac aneurysms tend to enlarge and rupture unpredictably, but size is the most important determinant of rupture risk. Iliac aneurysms that are less than 3.5 cm in size should be followed up with serial imaging. Those that enlarge to 3.5 cm or greater should be repaired in patients without serious operative risk factors.

The challenge of iliac aneurysm repair is in preserving flow to the pelvis through at least one internal iliac artery to prevent pelvic ischemia that can present as buttock claudication, impotence, or ischemia of the distal colon. Open repair of isolated iliac arteries is well tolerated and can be done through a transperitoneal or retroperitoneal approach. If the ipsilateral hypogastric artery is also aneurysmal, repair will require opening the sac and ligating the branches from within the aneurysm, taking care not to injure the iliac veins surrounding the aneurysm. New endovascular stent graft technology allows for treatment of extensive common iliac artery aneurysms without sacrificing flow into the hypogastric arteries.

▼ SUPRARENAL AORTIC ANEURYSMS

Aneurysms of the segment of aorta between the diaphragm and the renal arteries account for only 10% of AAAs, with 6% being pararenal and 4% involving the visceral vessels. Resection and graft replacement of the upper abdominal aorta is an operation of far greater magnitude and risk than operations on the infrarenal aorta. Involvement of the renal arteries doubles operative mortality with substantial additional risk for involvement of the visceral vessels. Renal failure and bowel ischemia are much more common after repair of these aneurysms than after repair of infrarenal aortic aneurysms. There is also a risk of paraplegia if flow is interrupted to the artery of Adamkiewicz. An extended incision is usually necessary, and provisions must be made for revascularization of the celiac axis and the superior mesenteric and renal arteries. The use of perfusion catheters for the visceral and renal arteries has improved results, and left heart bypass is used in true thoracoabdominal aneurysms.

Because of the mortality and morbidity of repair of suprarenal aneurysms, there has been considerable interest in endovascular repair of these aneurysms using complex stent grafts with fenestrations or branches for the visceral vessels, allowing seal in the suprarenal aorta. At present, there are multiple viable options including commercially available devices, physician modification of standard commercially available devices, and devices being implanted as parts of trials. A full discussion of these is beyond the scope of this chapter, but results from some of these technologies have been impressive in terms of mortality and early and late morbidity.

RUPTURED AORTIC ANEURYSMS

▶ General Considerations

With increasing aneurysm size, lateral pressure within the aneurysm will eventually lead to spontaneous rupture of the aneurysm wall. Although immediate exsanguination may ensue, there is often an interval of several hours between the first episode of bleeding and death from exsanguination when the initial bleed is contained in the retroperitoneal tissues, a "contained rupture." When the periaortic tissue can no longer contain the expanding hematoma, "free rupture" occurs with exsanguination into the peritoneal cavity.

▶ Clinical Findings

The patient presents with sudden, severe abdominal pain that usually radiates into the back and occasionally into the inguinal region. Lightheadedness or syncope results from blood loss. Pain may lessen and lightheadedness may disappear after the first hemorrhage, only to reappear and progress to shock if bleeding continues. When bleeding remains contained in the periaortic tissue, a discrete, pulsatile abdominal mass may be felt. In contrast with an intact aneurysm, the ruptured aneurysm at this stage is painful to palpation. Signs of an acute abdomen may be present. As bleeding continues, usually into the retroperitoneum, the discrete mass is replaced by a poorly defined midabdominal fullness, often extending toward the left flank.

Shock can be profound, manifested by peripheral vasoconstriction, hypotension, and anuria. Unfortunately, the classic triad of pain, a pulsatile abdominal mass, and hypotension is not always present, and precious time may be lost while confirming the diagnosis. An abdominal ultrasound performed in the emergency room will confirm the presence of an aortic aneurysm but may not disclose hemorrhage. CT scans reliably confirm hemorrhage from an aneurysm, but in a truly unstable patient, the delay in progressing to the operating room precludes their use. It is best to follow the adage that a patient with an AAA, signs of an acute abdomen, and hypotension belongs in the operating room. However, in patients with contained rupture who are not hemodynamically unstable, cross-sectional imaging with CT can provide valuable information such as proximity of the aneurysm to the renal arteries and aberrant arterial, venous, or visceral anatomy that can assist with operative planning. Recent guidelines have been proposed for criteria for transfer should suspected rupture be diagnosed at a facility with limited capabilities in treating the condition.

▶ Treatment & Prognosis

Repair should be performed as soon as intravenous fluids have been started, the airway has been secured, and blood has been sent for cross-matching. Permissive hypotension (systolic blood pressure of 70-90 mm Hg, provided the patient's mentation is preserved) is maintained until the patient is in the operating room. The patient is then prepared and draped prior to induction of general anesthesia so that proximal aortic control can be obtained rapidly should cardiovascular collapse ensue. Surgical control of the aorta proximal and distal to the aneurysm must be obtained immediately; depending on the extent of the aneurysm, prior abdominal surgical history, and surgeon preference, this may performed via a transperitoneal or retroperitoneal approach. Attempts to control the descending thoracic aorta through the chest have been associated with poor outcomes. A successful outcome of the operation is related to the patient's condition on arrival, the promptness of diagnosis, and the speed of operative control of bleeding and blood replacement. The operative death rate is between 30% and 80%, with an average of approximately 50%. Because many patients with ruptured aneurysms die before reaching the hospital, the overall death rate approaches 80%. Without operation, the outcome is uniformly fatal. Many centers are now treating ruptured AAA using endovascular stent grafts; no randomized trial has demonstrated a mortality advantage over open repair as yet.

▼ INFLAMMATORY ANEURYSMS

Inflammatory aneurysms are degenerative aneurysms that elicit a unique inflammatory response adjacent to the external calcified layer of the aneurysm wall. Although similar to retroperitoneal fibrosis, the inflammation is usually confined to the anterior aorta and iliac arteries. The aneurysm may be responsible for chronic abdominal pain and is tender to palpation. One-fourth of patients have some degree of ureteral obstruction. CT scanning reliably demonstrates the characteristic thickened wall and confirms the diagnosis. Characteristic pathologic changes include infiltration of the aortic wall by lymphocytes, plasma cells, occasional multinucleated giant cells, and lymphoid follicles with germinal centers. Inflammation resolves in most cases after successful repair. Inflammatory aneurysms are easily recognized at operation by the dense, shiny, white, fibrotic material that envelops the adjacent viscera, especially the duodenum, left renal vein, and inferior vena cava. Those structures therefore are especially vulnerable to operative injury. Endovascular repair is ideal and is the procedure of choice for inflammatory aneurysms. After repair, the inflammatory tissue often regresses.

▼ INFECTED (MYCOTIC) ANEURYSMS

The confusing term *mycotic aneurysm* is commonly used to denote infected aneurysms in general, which are rarely fungal. The aneurysm is secondary to a microbial aortitis in which virulent bacteria infect the aorta and destroy the aortic wall. Historically, *Salmonella* infection was the most common cause. In the current era, *Staphylococcus* spp. are the more common infection due to intravenous drug use. These organisms may involve every major artery, but aortic involvement predominates.

The typical patient presents with a rapidly enlarging, tender pulsatile mass that may feel warm, if palpable. Fever is present, and half the patients have positive blood cultures. Alternatively, the aneurysm may be discovered late, after successful treatment of the infection. Treatment consists of excision and remote (extra-anatomic) bypass grafting or inline reconstruction with antibiotic-soaked polyester or autogenous conduit. Liberal application of flap coverage techniques facilitates healing. Direct repair has been successful when done after a course of antibiotics. A prolonged course of antibiotics should be given to guard against recurrence.

▼ PERIPHERAL ARTERIAL ANEURYSMS

▶ General Considerations

Popliteal artery aneurysms account for 70% of peripheral arterial aneurysms. Like aortic aneurysms, they are silent until critically symptomatic. However, unlike aortic aneurysms, they rarely rupture. The presenting manifestations are due to peripheral embolization and thrombosis, possibly due to movement of the artery with knee flexion. Popliteal aneurysms may embolize repetitively over time and occlude distal arteries. Due to the redundant parallel arterial supply to the foot, ischemia does not occur until a final embolus occludes flow to the remaining tibial artery. Acute ischemia caused by popliteal aneurysms has a poor prognosis because of the chronicity of the process. The results of both chemical and mechanical thrombolysis may be disappointing because of clot age and adherence to the artery wall. After presentation with acute ischemia, approximately one-third of patients will require an amputation. To prevent embolization and thrombosis, popliteal artery aneurysms should be repaired electively if greater than 2-2.5 cm or symptomatic (eg, distal embolization, deep venous thrombosis, or neurologic symptoms from mass effect).

Primary aneurysms of the femoral artery are much less common than aneurysms of the popliteal artery. However, pseudoaneurysms of the femoral artery following arterial punctures for arteriography and cardiac catheterization occur with an incidence ranging from 0.05% to 6%. The femoral artery is also a common site of puncture for intravenous drug abusers, and mycotic pseudoaneurysms may appear in this setting. Thrombosis and embolization are the main risks of femoral true or false aneurysms and, like popliteal aneurysms, should be repaired when greater than 2-2.5 cm in diameter or if complications such as local compressive symptoms or thromboembolization develop.

▶ Clinical Findings

A. Symptoms and Signs

Until progressive embolization or thrombosis occurs, peripheral artery aneurysms are usually asymptomatic. The patient may be aware of a pulsatile mass when the aneurysm is in the groin, but popliteal aneurysms are often undetected by the patient and physician. Peripheral aneurysms may produce symptoms by compressing a nearby vein or nerve, but this is unusual. In most patients, the first symptom is due to ischemia of acute arterial occlusion. The pathologic findings range from rapidly developing gangrene to moderate ischemia that slowly lessens as collateral circulation develops. Symptoms from recurrent embolization to the leg are often transient if they occur at all. Sudden ischemia may appear in a toe or part of the foot, followed by slow resolution, and the true diagnosis may be elusive. The onset of recurrent

episodes of pain in the foot, particularly if accompanied by cyanosis, suggests embolization and requires investigation of the heart and proximal arterial tree.

Because popliteal pulses are somewhat difficult to palpate even in normal individuals, a particularly prominent or easily felt pulse is suggestive of aneurysmal dilation and should be investigated by ultrasound. Because popliteal aneurysms are bilateral in 60% of cases, the diagnosis of thrombosis of a popliteal aneurysm is often aided by the palpation of a pulsatile aneurysm in the contralateral popliteal space. Approximately 50% of patients with popliteal aneurysms have an aneurysmal abdominal aorta.

B. Imaging Studies

Duplex color ultrasound is the most efficient investigation to confirm the diagnosis of peripheral aneurysm, to measure its size and configuration, and to demonstrate mural thrombus.

Arteriography may not demonstrate aneurysms accurately, because mural thrombus reduces the apparent diameter of the lumen. Three-dimensional imaging by CTA or MRA is required—especially when operation is considered—to define the anatomy and plan intervention.

▶ Treatment

Early operation is indicated for an aneurysm that is greater than 2-2.5 cm in size associated with any peripheral embolization or an aneurysm with mural thrombus. Urgent operation is indicated when acute embolization or thrombosis has caused acute ischemia. Intra-arterial thrombolysis may be done in the setting of acute ischemia if examination suggests that immediate surgery is not imperative to prevent tissue loss (see earlier section, "Acute Limb Ischemia"). Bypass with saphenous vein may include either excision or exclusion, depending on location. If exclusion rather than resection is performed, the geniculate "feeder" arteries within the aneurysm may cause progressive enlargement, mandating surveillance.

Endovascular repair with covered stents can be used but is less durable than open repair and should be reserved for patients at high operative risk and used with caution if the knee joint must be crossed.

Acute pseudoaneurysms of the femoral artery due to arterial punctures can be successfully treated using ultrasound-guided compression and thrombin injections if the aneurysm is not large.

▶ Prognosis

The long-term patency of bypass for femoral and popliteal aneurysms is generally excellent but depends on the adequacy of the outflow tract. Late graft occlusion is less common than in similar operations for occlusive disease.

UPPER EXTREMITY ANEURYSMS

Subclavian Artery Aneurysms

Subclavian artery aneurysms are less common than aneurysms of the lower extremity, and most supraclavicular pulsatile masses represent tortuous vessels, not aneurysms. Pseudoaneurysms due to injections by drug addicts are becoming increasingly frequent. An anomaly, the aberrant right subclavian artery (incidence 0.5%), arises from the aorta distal to the left subclavian and courses behind the esophagus. As found in other aberrant arteries, enlargement is common (eg, a so-called Kommerell diverticulum at the origin of the aberrant right subclavian artery) and may compress the esophagus against the trachea, causing difficulty swallowing (dysphagia lusoria). This anomaly is also commonly associated with a nonrecurrent laryngeal nerve.

A true subclavian artery aneurysm is usually due to poststenotic dilation in a patient with thoracic outlet syndrome or a large callus from a fractured clavicle. As with popliteal aneurysms, the most common manifestation is embolization with episodic distal ischemia. The diagnosis is often missed. A history of waxing and waning digital color changes not otherwise explained is an indication for arterial imaging. Treatment usually consists of resection of the aneurysm and the restricting structures.

Radial Artery False Aneurysms

The incidence of radial artery false aneurysms has increased as a result of increasing use of radial artery catheters. Occasionally, the aneurysm is infected. If the Allen test is normal and adequate collateralization is confirmed with imaging, treatment consists of excision and ligation. If the ulnar collaterals are insufficient to preserve viability of the hand, excision and replacement with vein should be performed.

Small aneurysms of the palmer arch may be due to repetitive trauma. These aneurysms can be responsible for emboli to the digital arteries. Hand ischemia should be investigated with angiography to ensure that all potentially reversible causes of hand ischemia, including these unusual aneurysms, are identified.

Baxter BT, Terrin MC, Dalman RL: Medical management of small abdominal aortic aneurysms. *Circulation.* 2008;117:1883.

Chuter TA, et al: Endovascular treatment of thoracoabdominal aortic aneurysms. *J Vasc Surg.* 2008;47:6.

IMPROVE Trial Investigators, Powell JT, Sweeting MJ, Thompson MM, et al: Endovascular or open repair strategy for ruptured abdominal aortic aneurysm: 30 day outcomes from IMPROVE randomised trial. *BMJ.* 2014;348:f7661.

Lederle FA, Freischlag JA, Kyriakides TC, et al: Long-term comparison of endovascular and open repair of abdominal aortic aneurysm. *N Engl J Med.* 2012;367:1988.

Lindholt JS, Norman P: Screening for abdominal aortic aneurysm reduces overall mortality in men. A meta-analysis of the mid- and long-term effects of screening for abdominal aortic aneurysms. *Eur J Vasc Endovasc Surg.* 2008;36:167.

Mehta M, Byrne J, Darling RC, et al: Endovascular repair of ruptured infrarenal abdominal aortic aneurysm is associated with lower 30-day mortality and better 5-year survival rates than open surgical repair. *J Vasc Surg.* 2013;57:368.

Paravastu SC, Ghosh J, Murray D, et al: A systematic review of open versus endovascular repair of inflammatory abdominal aortic aneurysms. *Eur J Vasc Endovasc Surg.* 2009;38:291.

Tsilimparis N, Dayama A, Ricotta J: Open and endovascular repair of popliteal artery aneurysms: tabular review of the literature. *Ann Vasc Surg.* 2013;27:259.

VISCERAL ARTERY ANEURYSMS

General Considerations

The etiology of this interesting group of aneurysms is generally unknown. Most often, they occur as single lesions in a younger age group than those at risk for aortic aneurysms. Rupture is the primary danger.

Splenic Artery Aneurysms

Aneurysms of the splenic artery account for more than 60% of splanchnic artery aneurysms. Women are affected four times more commonly than men and often during childbearing years. Arterial fibrodysplasia and portal hypertension predispose to formation of splenic artery aneurysms. Rupture, the major complication, has been reported in less than 2% of splenic aneurysms; it rarely occurs with lesions smaller than 2-3 cm in diameter. Rupture during pregnancy tends to occur in the third trimester and is associated with a 75% maternal death rate and 90% fetal death rate. Diagnosis is most often made from plain radiographs of the abdomen, showing concentric calcification in the upper left quadrant.

Intervention is indicated for patients with symptomatic aneurysms, aneurysms in pregnant women, and patients who have a low operative risk profile with aneurysms greater than 2 cm in diameter. Endovascular repair with covered stent grafts is ideal with the use of microcatheters, improving the ability to negotiate the often tortuous splenic artery. Embolization is an alternative. Laparoscopic ligation of the artery is also feasible.

Hepatic Artery Aneurysms

Hepatic artery aneurysms account for 20% of splanchnic artery aneurysms. There is a 2:1 male-to-female ratio, and the frequency of reported rupture is about 20%. Aneurysm rupture is associated with a 35% mortality rate. Rupture into the biliary tree producing hemobilia is as frequent as intraperitoneal rupture. The symptom triad of intermittent abdominal pain, gastrointestinal bleeding, and jaundice strongly suggests the diagnosis and is present in about one-third of patients. Surgery is usually required to control bleeding. If the common hepatic artery is involved, the artery may be safely ligated if collateral flow through the gastroduodenal artery has been demonstrated. Aneurysms in other portions of the artery usually require vascular reconstruction. Endovascular placement with a covered stent is preferred if the anatomy is suitable.

Superior Mesenteric Artery Aneurysms

Aneurysms of the proximal superior mesenteric artery account for 5% of all splanchnic artery aneurysms. Unlike splenic or hepatic aneurysms, 60% of superior mesenteric artery aneurysms are mycotic. The aneurysm may involve the origin or branches of the artery. Symptoms include nonspecific abdominal pain. The diagnosis can be made on CT scan.

Superior mesenteric artery aneurysms should be treated irrespective of size. Operative therapy for mycotic superior mesenteric artery aneurysms includes ligation if there are adequate collaterals or replacement with a segment of autogenous vessel. Endovascular stent graft placement is not advisable in an acute infection. However, it is valuable for true aneurysms as long as critical branches can be avoided. For distal branch aneurysms, bowel resection may be necessary.

RENAL ARTERY ANEURYSMS

This uncommon aneurysm occurs in less than 0.1% of the population and is often associated with hypertension. The aneurysm is usually saccular and located at a primary or secondary bifurcation of the renal arteries. Women are affected slightly more frequently than men. There are three principal categories: (1) idiopathic, (2) aneurysms associated with medial fibrodysplastic disease, and (3) arteritis-related microaneurysms.

Renovascular hypertension may occur because of distortion of the involved or nearby vessels by the aneurysm. Spontaneous rupture of renal artery aneurysms is rare except during pregnancy. CT scans or digital subtraction angiography should be performed to monitor enlargement. Operation is indicated in women of childbearing age or in patients with associated renal artery disease, uncontrolled hypertension, or aneurysms greater than 2 cm in size. Most renal artery aneurysms can be repaired in situ, but ex vivo repair is occasionally required for complex disease. Endovascular options are usually limited due to the involved vessel size and the aneurysm's proximity to artery branch points.

VASOCONSTRICTIVE DISORDERS

General Considerations

Vasoconstrictive disorders are characterized by abnormal activity of the sympathetic nervous system that reduces peripheral blood flow, causing tissue ischemia.

Raynaud Disease/Phenomenon

Raynaud disease/phenomenon consists of sequential pallor, cyanosis, and rubor of fingers or toes after exposure to cold. Excessive vasoconstriction, sluggish flow, and reflex vasodilation produce the characteristic white-blue-red color changes. In Raynaud disease, this response, due to spasm alone without underlying arterial lesions, is quite common and benign.

Sudden onset or progression of symptoms suggests underlying arterial lesions that exaggerate the normal reduction in blood flow caused by vasoconstriction. This is termed Raynaud phenomenon, a more virulent entity associated primarily with immunologic and connective tissue disorders (eg, scleroderma, systemic lupus erythematosus, polymyositis, or drug-induced vasculitis). However, repeated embolization, occupational trauma (vibration injury, cold injury), and other disorders (cold agglutinins, chronic renal failure, and neoplasia) also have been reported.

Hyperreactivity to cold stimuli may be the initial presentation of arterial pathology. In new-onset or severe cases of Raynaud-type symptoms, a search for underlying pathology is required. All patients with Raynaud syndrome should avoid cold exposure, tobacco, oral contraceptives, β-adrenergic blocking agents, and ergotamine preparations. Calcium channel blockers are generally prescribed but may cause hypotension. Transdermal prostaglandins, ketanserin, and cilostazol also have been used, with relief of symptoms in some patients. In rare cases, symptoms progress to tissue loss. Finger amputation is necessary once gangrene has developed.

THORACIC OUTLET SYNDROME

General Considerations

Thoracic outlet syndrome (TOS) refers to the variety of disorders caused by abnormal compression of arterial, venous, or neural structures in the base of the neck. Numerous mechanisms for compression have been described, including cervical rib, anomalous ligaments, hypertrophy of the anterior scalene muscle, and positional changes that alter the normal relation of the first rib to the structures that pass over it. Patients may describe a history of cervical trauma.

Symptoms rarely develop until adulthood. For this reason, it has been assumed that an alteration of normal structural relationships that occurs with advancing years is the primary factor. Even anomalous cervical ribs seem well tolerated during childhood and adolescence.

Symptoms are related to the primary structure that is compressed. Neurogenic TOS is the most common, followed by venous TOS. Arterial TOS is the rarest form. Neurogenic TOS may produce upper extremity pain, paresthesias, and muscle atrophy. Compression of the vein between the anterior scalene, clavicle, and first rib can produce thrombosis, which can result in severe upper extremity pain and swelling. Compression may be exaggerated with exercise precipitating an occlusion. This syndrome is termed effort thrombosis or **Paget-Schroetter syndrome**. Compression of the subclavian artery can produce stenosis and poststenotic dilation of the artery, leading to arterial occlusion or emboli, as discussed earlier.

Clinical Findings

A. Symptoms and Signs

Neural symptoms consist of pain, paresthesias, or numbness in the distribution of one or more trunks of the brachial plexus (usually in the ulnar distribution). Most patients associate their symptoms with certain positions of the shoulder girdle. These may occur from prolonged hyperabduction, as in house painters, hairdressers, and truck drivers. Others may relate their symptoms to the downward traction of the shoulder girdle produced by carrying heavy objects. Numbness of the hands often wakes the patient from sleep. On physical examination, motor deficits are rare and usually indicate severe compression of long duration. Muscular atrophy may be present in the hand. Pulses can be weakened by abduction of the arm with the head rotated to the opposite side (Adson test), although pulse reduction by this maneuver often occurs in completely asymptomatic persons. Light percussion over the brachial plexus in the supraclavicular fossa may reproduce the symptoms in patients with chronic neurologic impingement.

Arterial symptoms are less common and often the result of emboli from an associated subclavian artery aneurysm. A bruit may be heard over the subclavian artery with abduction of the arm, but this is not a specific finding. Venous occlusion results in unilateral arm swelling. There are good collaterals around the shoulder girdle, but symptoms may be debilitating in young active patients, the very patient in whom this is most likely to occur.

B. Diagnosis

Neurogenic thoracic outlet compression must be differentiated from other disorders that mimic this condition (eg, carpal tunnel syndrome and cervical disk disease). Cervical x-rays and peripheral nerve conduction studies are not diagnostic but are valuable to eliminate other possibilities. Unfortunately, there is no recognized objective study to unequivocally confirm the diagnosis of neurogenic TOS. Improvement of symptoms with a scalene nerve block may be both prognostic and therapeutic. Arteriograms may demonstrate subclavian or axillary artery stenosis when the arm is in abduction. This finding is not diagnostic, but poststenotic dilation of the artery is distinctly abnormal and indicates a definite lesion.

Ultrasound, MRI, CT, and angiography can also be used to examine the subclavian artery and vein with and without provocative maneuvers to aid in the diagnosis of venous and arterial TOS.

Treatment

Most patients with neurogenic TOS benefit from postural correction and a physical therapy program directed toward restoring the normal relation and strength of the structures in the shoulder girdle. Surgical techniques for decompression of the thoracic outlet are reserved for patients with neurogenic TOS who have not responded to conservative treatment. Some surgeons prefer transaxillary first rib resection, whereas others prefer a supraclavicular or paraclavicular approach. With either operation, the anterior scalene muscle and any associated fibrous bands should be excised. Up to 90% of patients report cure or significant improvement.

Symptomatic arterial stenoses require decompression of the thoracic outlet in combination sometimes with arterial reconstruction. Effort thrombosis of the subclavian vein is usually best treated by catheter-directed thrombolysis of the venous occlusion followed by thoracic outlet decompression with or without operative venous reconstruction or angioplasty. Outcomes for these patients with vascular TOS symptoms are excellent, with 80%-90% of patients asymptomatic at 6 months.

Hawkins AT, Schaumeier MJ, Smith AD, et al: Concurrent venography during first rib resection and scalenectomy for venous thoracic outlet syndrome is safe and efficient. *J Vasc Surg Venous Lymphat Disord*. 2015;3(3):290-294.

Sanders RJ, Hammond SL, Rao NM: Diagnosis of thoracic outlet syndrome. *J Vasc Surg*. 2007;46:601.

Schneider DB, et al: Combination treatment of venous thoracic outlet syndrome: open surgical decompression and intraoperative angioplasty. *J Vasc Surg*. 2004;40:599.

ARTERIOVENOUS FISTULAS

Arteriovenous fistulas may be congenital, often called "malformations," or acquired. Abnormal communications between arteries and veins occur in many diseases and affect vessels of all sizes and in many locations. In congenital fistulas, the systemic effect is often not great, because although the communications may be multiple, they are small. When a limb is involved, extensive arteriovenous communications may exist with increased flow and increased muscle mass and bone length.

Acquired fistulas are usually the result of trauma, iatrogenic or otherwise. These communications can have considerable flow, and high-output heart failure can occur. The third class of fistulas is surgically created fistulas for hemodialysis access.

Arteriovenous malformations in the gastrointestinal tract may cause hemorrhage. Osler-Weber-Rendu disease or syndrome (also termed hereditary hemorrhagic telangiectasia) is an autosomal dominant disorder characterized by gastrointestinal bleeding and epistaxis due to large arteriovenous anomalies in the gastrointestinal tract and lungs. Pulmonary lesions cause recirculation with lower PO_2, polycythemia, clubbing, and cyanosis.

Penetrating injuries from trauma or iatrogenic ones from arterial punctures are the most common causes of acquired fistulas. Blunt trauma, erosion of an atherosclerotic or mycotic arterial aneurysm into adjacent veins, communication with an arterial prosthetic graft, and neoplastic invasion can all cause arteriovenous fistulas as well. When large vessels are involved, the presentation may be dramatic. For example, if an aortic aneurysm ruptures into the inferior vena cava, the fistula enlarges rapidly and can result in cardiac dilation and failure.

ARTERIOVENOUS FISTULA FOR HEMODIALYSIS

General Considerations

A successful arteriovenous fistula for hemodialysis access may be approximated with the rule of 6s: it requires a large outflow vein (> 6 mm) that lies close to the skin (< 6 mm depth) for a length of a minimum of 6 cm with a flow of at least 600 mL/min. The cephalic vein is ideal for this purpose, but other veins may be used. Veins with diameters of at least 3 mm are ideal. The radial artery to cephalic vein arteriovenous fistula (Brescia-Appel-Cimino fistula) is the classic hemodialysis access fistula. If no suitable vein is available for an autogenous fistula, prosthetic grafts are used, most commonly PTFE, to bridge an artery and vein. In general, upper extremities are preferred over lower extremities, fistulas over grafts, distal upper extremity access over proximal access (eg, radiocephalic fistula is preferred over the brachiocephalic fistula), and the nondominant arm over the dominant. The increased rate of secondary interventions and higher infection risk make grafts generally less desirable, although they typically are ready for use earlier than fistulas. To maximize autogenous vein utilization, current practice includes transposing deep veins such as the basilic vein in the upper arm to the subcutaneous tissue. All veins used for access need to mature—dilate and thicken—prior to use. This process takes at least 6 weeks, but often months.

Patients with a newly created arteriovenous access—particularly with prosthetic graft and/or more proximal arterial inflow—should be watched carefully for arterial steal and distal extremity ischemia. Diabetics is most vulnerable to this complication because of calcified proximal arteries or intrinsic arterial lesions of the arm. High-output cardiac failure occurs infrequently.

Clinical Findings

A. Symptoms and Signs

A typical continuous machinery murmur can be heard over the arteriovenous fistulas and is often associated with a palpable thrill and locally increased skin temperature. Proximally, the arteries and veins dilate, and the pulse distal to the lesion may diminish. There may be signs of venous insufficiency, coolness, and hypertrophy distal to the communication on the involved extremity in the case of fistulas not created for dialysis access. Tachycardia occurs in some patients as a feature of increased cardiac output. The pulse rate slows (Branham sign) when the fistula is occluded by compression.

In contrast, venous malformations rarely produce hemodynamic effects. In this disorder, the presence of a mass, which may or may not be tender, is the principal finding. Because flow rates are low, bruits and thrills are absent.

B. Imaging Studies

MRI has become the imaging study of choice for the evaluation and follow-up of peripheral arteriovenous malformations, but CTA also gives excellent anatomic information. Duplex ultrasonography is also useful, particularly in the extremities. Precise delineation of arteriovenous fistulas can be done with selective angiography.

Treatment

Not all arteriovenous connections require treatment. Most venous malformations should be treated conservatively. In addition, small peripheral fistulas may be observed and will often remain asymptomatic. Some are surgically inaccessible.

The indications for intervention include hemorrhage, local expansion, severe venous or arterial insufficiency, cosmetic deformity, and heart failure. Most fistulas are now managed by embolization under radiographic control. The embolic material used includes blood clot, glass beads, and gelatin powder. Arteriovenous malformations of the head and neck and of the pelvis appear particularly well suited for this form of therapy. Direct injection of sclerosant compounds into venous malformations under fluoroscopic control also has been successful in at least temporarily reducing flow and swelling.

Surgical options are generally reserved for large acquired fistulas. When the fistulous connections involve substantial portions of an extremity, local ligation is invariably followed by recurrence, and only temporary palliation can be expected. Covered stent grafts are now being used for a variety of traumatic fistulas.

Prognosis

The results of therapy vary according to the extent, location, and type of fistula. In general, traumatic fistulas have the most favorable prognosis. Congenital fistulas are more difficult to eradicate because of the numerous arteriovenous connections present.

Sidawy AN, Spergel LM, Besarab A, et al: The Society for Vascular Surgery: clinical practice guidelines for the surgical placement and maintenance of arteriovenous hemodialysis access. *J Vasc Surg.* 2008;48:2S.

MULTIPLE CHOICE QUESTIONS

1. Arterial occlusive disease

   A. Occurs predominantly due to congenital abnormalities or anatomical anomalies
   B. Includes disease caused by atherosclerotic plaques, which typically develop at arterial branch points of high shear stress
   C. Is masked by collateral arterial circulation that typically has a lower resistance than the original unobstructed artery
   D. Typically occurs with at least a 50% reduction in arterial diameter, which correlates with a 75% narrowing of cross-sectional area
   E. Causes symptoms due to high pressure proximal to stenosis

2. Intermittent claudication characteristics include all of the following except

   A. "Cramping" in a muscle
   B. Deep-seated ache in the calf
   C. Can be associated with walking
   D. Pain occurring at rest
   E. Has a low rate of major limb loss

3. Acute lower limb ischemia

   A. Usually is caused by increased muscular demand for blood flow in the distribution of an occluded artery
   B. Can be caused by a major arterial dissection
   C. Causes the five Ps: pain, petechiae, pulselessness, paresthesias, paralysis
   D. Is generally best managed by initial observation to allow recruitment of collaterals
   E. Threatens skin loss before muscle or nerve damage

4. Carotid endarterectomy

   A. Should not be performed when the carotid artery is completely occluded
   B. Has not been shown to be beneficial for any patients in prevention of ipsilateral stroke
   C. Is performed through a catheter placed in the ipsilateral femoral artery
   D. Carries a 30% risk of transient cranial nerve injury
   E. Has a restenosis rate of 35% at 5 years

5. Arterial aneurysm

   A. Management requires operative or catheter-based intervention in nearly all patients
   B. Management should include urgent operation in most patients
   C. Is defined as a localized dilation of an artery to at least 1.5 times its normal diameter
   D. Is caused by a disruption of the artery wall and does not include all layers of the wall
   E. Is most commonly a mycotic aneurysm

Veins & Lymphatics

Ana C. De Roo, MD

Andrea T. Obi, MD

Thomas W. Wakefield, MD

▼ I. THE VEINS

VENOUS ANATOMY

Veins of the lower extremity (Figure 37–1) consist of superficial and deep systems joined by venous perforators. The great and small saphenous veins are superficial veins (the name "saphenous" aptly derived from the Greek word for "manifest, clear," or "visible"). They contain many valves and show considerable variation in their location and branching points. The great saphenous vein may be duplicated in up to 10% of patients. Typically, it originates from the superficial arch of the foot and is found anterior to the medial malleolus at the ankle. As it ascends in the calf just beneath the superficial fascia, it is joined by two major tributaries: an anterior vein, which crosses the tibia; and a posterior arch vein, which arises posterior to the medial malleolus beside the posterior tibial artery. The great saphenous vein then enters the fossa ovalis in the groin to empty into the deep femoral vein.

The saphenofemoral junction is marked by four or five prominent branches of the great saphenous vein: the superficial circumflex iliac vein, the external pudendal vein, the superficial epigastric vein, and the medial and lateral accessory saphenous veins. Another important anatomic landmark is the relationship of the great saphenous vein to the saphenous branch of the femoral nerve; as it emerges from the popliteal space, the nerve follows a course parallel to the vein. Injury during saphenous vein harvest for bypass produces neuropathic pain or numbness along the medial calf and foot. The small saphenous vein arises from the superficial dorsal venous arch behind the lateral malleolus at the ankle and curves toward the midline of the posterior calf, ascending to join the popliteal vein behind the knee.

Deep veins of the leg parallel the courses of the arteries. Two or three venae comitantes accompany each tibial artery. At the knee, these paired high-capacitance veins merge to form the popliteal vein, which continues proximally as the

femoral vein. At the inguinal ligament, the femoral and deep (profunda) femoral veins join medial to the femoral artery to form the common femoral vein. Proximal to the inguinal ligament, the common femoral vein becomes the external iliac vein. In the pelvis, external and internal iliac veins join to form common iliac veins that empty into the inferior vena cava (IVC). The right common iliac vein ascends almost vertically to the IVC, whereas the left common iliac vein takes a more transverse course. For this reason, the left common iliac vein may be compressed between the right common iliac artery and lumbosacral spine, a condition known as May-Thurner syndrome when thrombosis of the left iliac vein occurs.

Muscular sinusoids represent another component of the deep veins of the leg. These thin-walled, nonvalved venous lakes run longitudinally within soleus muscle bellies and then coalesce to join the posterior tibial and peroneal veins. Blood empties from these sinusoids during muscle contraction; inactivity leads to stasis and may contribute to the development of deep venous thrombosis.

Blood flow is directed from superficial to deep veins of the leg via valved perforating (communicating) veins. Perforators are located below the medial malleolus (inframalleolar perforator), in the medial calf (Cockett perforators), at the level of the adductor canal (Hunterian perforator), and just above (Dodd perforator) and below (Boyd perforator) the knee.

Delicate bicuspid venous valves prevent reflux and direct the flow of blood from the foot and leg toward the heart and generally against gravity. Valves are more numerous in the distal part of the extremity, decrease in number proximally, and are virtually absent in the IVC itself.

The IVC ascends in the abdomen and ends at the right atrium. It lies to the right of the midline, lateral to the aorta, and receives a number of lumbar veins that connect with the vertebral and paravertebral venous plexuses. The IVC and its tributaries are derived in the 6th to 10th week of life

Superf. epigastric a. & v.

Femoral v.

Superf. circumflex iliac a. & v.

Superf. ext. pudendal a. & v.

Lateral accessory saphenous v.

Medical accessory saphenous v.

Ant. cut. branches of femoral n.

Greater saphenous v.

Hunter's perforator

Dodd's perforator

Saphenous n.

Ant. tributary of greater saphenous v.

Boyd's perforator

Proximal paratibial perforators

Posterior arch v.

"24 cm" perforator

Cockett III perforator

Greater saphenous v.

Cockett II perforator

Superf. peroneal n.

Cockett I perforator

Medial perforators of the foot

▲ **Figure 37–1.** Anatomy of the superficial and perforating veins of the lower extremity.

hepatic veins drain directly into the right atrium in patients with this unusual anomaly.

Veins of the upper extremity are also divided into superficial and deep groups, although direction of flow from superficial to deep is not as distinct as in the lower extremity. Dorsal veins of the hand empty into the cephalic vein ("intern vein") on the radial aspect and into the basilic vein on the ulnar aspect of the forearm. The cephalic vein ascends lateral to the biceps muscle into the deltopectoral groove, where it passes through the clavipectoral fascia to join the axillary vein. The cephalic vein is useful for arteriovenous fistulas, both at the wrist and in the upper arm, because it is superficial and lateral in the arm, allowing easy access for hemodialysis needles. The basilic vein, which runs medially in the arm to become the axillary vein, is deeper and thicker-walled than the cephalic vein. Its many branches make it tedious to harvest, but it can be used for a bypass conduit or for a laterally tunneled upper-arm dialysis fistula (basilic vein transposition). The median cubital vein links the cephalic and basilic veins in the antecubital space.

Paired brachial veins compose the deep system of veins. They accompany the brachial artery and join the basilic vein as it becomes the axillary vein. The axillary vein continues medially as the subclavian vein, which passes through a tight space anterior to the first rib and anterior scalene muscle and posterior to the clavicle. The subclavian vein and the internal jugular vein join behind the clavicular head to form the brachiocephalic vein, which empties into the superior vena cava.

Malaki M, et al: Congenital anomalies of the inferior vena cava. *Clin Radiol* 2012;67(2):165-171.

Reich-Schupke S, et al: Nomenclature of the veins of the lower limbs: current standards. *J Dtsch Dermatol Ges.* 2011;9(3): 189-914.

VENOUS PHYSIOLOGY

Knowledge of lower extremity venous anatomy is essential to understanding the physiology of venous flow. The volume of blood in the lower extremities may increase by one-half liter when an individual changes from a reclining to an erect position (Figure 37–2). Increased blood volume is accommodated by increased venous capacitance, which is regulated by smooth muscle contractility in the vein walls. Erect posture creates a vertical column of blood, exerting a hydrostatic pressure equal to the distance from the foot to the right atrium (about 100–120 mm Hg). This hydrostatic pressure must be overcome to provide venous return to the heart and avoid pooling of blood in the legs. Several aspects of the venous system facilitate venous return against the force of gravity. Because the circulation is a closed system, venous return is affected by arterial inflow and by the negative

from the fusion and obliteration of several paired embryonic veins: the anterior and posterior cardinal veins, the subcardinal veins, the supracardinal veins, and the sacrocardinal veins. Because of this complex embryonic development, anomalies in the venous system are not uncommon. The most common abnormality is a circumaortic left renal vein (1.5%-8.7% incidence), followed by a retroaortic left renal vein (1.2%-3.4% incidence), duplication of the IVC (1%-3% incidence), azygos and hemiazygos continuation of the IVC (0.6%), and left-sided IVC (0.2%-0.5% incidence). An unsuspected retroaortic or circumaortic renal vein can be inadvertently injured during aortic cross-clamping. Most unusual is the congenital absence of the suprarenal IVC, which results from failure of the right subcardinal vein branches to join the veins of the embryologic liver. This ultimately results in the infrarenal segment of the IVC joining the azygoshemiazygos veins to drain into the superior vena cava. The

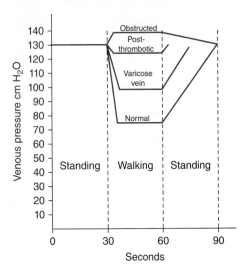

▲ Figure 37–2. Pedal venous pressure measurements with exercise. The normal drop in pressure associated with ambulation is impaired by deep vein incompetence and proximal venous obstruction. (Reproduced with permission from Shives GT, Schwartz S: *Principles of Surgery*, 4th ed. New York, NY: McGraw-Hill Education; 1983.)

intrathoracic pressure created during inspiration. Functional valves ensure unidirectional movement of blood from superficial to deep systems and from the foot back to the heart. Hydrostatic pressure is dissipated by asynchronous opening of the valves. Soleal venous sinusoids are another central component to the system. When the muscle contracts during exercise, blood empties from the sinusoid into the deep veins of the calf and leg. This high-velocity flow siphons blood from deep veins of the foot upward into the calf, analogous to smoke being drawn up a smokestack by wind blowing past the chimney (Venturi effect).

DISEASES OF THE VENOUS SYSTEM

VARICOSE VEINS

▶ General Considerations

Varicose veins are very common, afflicting 10%–20% of the world's population. Abnormally dilated veins occur in several locations in the body: the spermatic cord (varicocele), esophagus (esophageal varices), and anorectum (hemorrhoids). Varicosities of the legs were described as early as 1550 BC and, in the 1600s AD, were correlated with trauma, childbearing, and "standing too much before kings." Modern studies identify female sex, pregnancy, family history, prolonged

standing, and a history of phlebitis as risk factors for varicose veins. The Bonn Vein Study identified higher superficial venous reflux in women, and although the prevalence of superficial venous reflux increased with age for both men and women, men had greater deep venous reflux, but there was no age trend. The Framingham Study found the highest incidence in women between 40 and 49 years of age. The prospective Edinburgh Vein Study followed over half of their initial study population for 13 years and found that greater than 50% of those with baseline venous disease progressed in clinical classification score or development of chronic venous insufficiency. About a third of those with varicose veins progressed to chronic venous insufficiency over the study period. Identified risk factors for progression included family history of varicosities and history of deep venous thrombosis.

Varicose veins are classified as either primary or secondary. Primary varicose veins are thought to be due to genetic or developmental defects in the vein wall that cause diminished elasticity and valvular incompetence. Most cases of isolated superficial venous insufficiency are primary varicose veins. Secondary varicose veins arise from destruction or dysfunction of valves caused by trauma, deep venous thrombosis, arteriovenous fistula, or nontraumatic proximal venous obstruction (pregnancy, pelvic tumor). When valves of the deep and perforating veins are disrupted, chronic venous stasis changes may accompany superficial varicosities. Other causes of varicose veins may include histologic abnormalities, vein wall factors, local hypoxia, hyperplastic and cellular dysfunction, and extracellular matrix abnormalities, in addition to hemodynamic factors. It is important to recognize that untreated, longstanding venous dysfunction from either primary or secondary varicose veins may cause chronic skin changes that lead to infection, nonhealing venous ulceration, and chronic disability. To define the optimal method of treatment, the etiologic factors and distribution of disease must be clearly identified.

▶ Clinical Findings

The clinical presentation of patients with varicose veins can be quite variable. Many varicose veins are asymptomatic and come to medical attention because of aesthetic concerns. If symptomatic, varicose veins may be associated with localized pain, a burning sensation over the vein, a diffuse ache or "heaviness" in the calf (particularly with prolonged standing), or phlebitis. Mild ankle edema may occur. Symptoms generally improve with leg elevation.

The varicosities appear as dilated, tortuous, elongated veins predominantly on the medial aspect of the lower extremity along the course of the great saphenous vein. Overlying skin changes may be absent even in the presence of extensive large varicosities. Smaller, flat, blue-green reticular veins, telangiectasias, and spider veins may accompany varicose veins and are further evidence of venous dysfunction.

A cluster of telangiectasias below the inframalleolar perforator is termed a *corona phlebectatica paraplantaris*. Secondary varicose veins can cause symptoms characteristic of chronic venous insufficiency, including edema, hyperpigmentation, stasis dermatitis, and even venous ulcerations.

Physical examination begins with inspection of the lower extremities to determine the distribution and severity of the varicosities. Bimanual circumferential palpation of the thighs and calves is helpful. Palpation of a thrill or auscultation of a bruit indicates the presence of an arteriovenous fistula as a possible etiologic factor. Today, tourniquet tests have been virtually replaced by venous duplex ultrasound imaging, which is now used as the primary method with which to map the location and extent of reflux. Reflux is determined by valve closure times, which are determined at multiple valve stations (eg, 500 milliseconds for the superficial vein valves and 1000 milliseconds for the deep vein valves). In addition, patients are characterized by the CEAP (Clinical, Etiologic, Anatomic, and Pathophysiologic) system.

▶ Differential Diagnosis

Ulceration, brawny induration, and hyperpigmentation often indicate accompanying chronic deep venous insufficiency. This is important to recognize because the changes generally do not resolve with saphenous vein treatment alone.

Klippel-Trenaunay syndrome (KTS) must be considered if extensive varicose veins are encountered in a young patient, especially if unilateral and in an atypical distribution (lateral leg). The classic triad of KTS is varicose veins, limb hypertrophy, and a cutaneous birthmark (port wine stain or venous malformation). Because the deep veins are often anomalous or absent, saphenous vein ablation or stripping can be hazardous. Standard treatment for patients with KTS is graduated support stockings and a good program of intermittent leg elevation and exercise. Limited ablation or stab avulsion of symptomatic varices after thorough duplex ultrasound vein mapping and occasional surgery for correction of limb length discrepancy may also be indicated.

▶ Treatment

A. Nonsurgical Treatment

Treatment for both primary and secondary varicose veins initially involves a program directed at management of venous insufficiency, including elastic stocking support, periodic leg elevation, and regular exercise. Prolonged sitting and standing are discouraged. For most patients, knee-high or thigh-high gradient compression stockings of 20-30 mm Hg are sufficient, although some patients require 30-40 mm Hg of pressure (especially if associated with significant deep venous insufficiency). The compression stockings are worn all day to diminish venous distention during standing and are removed at night.

B. Surgical Treatment

Today, virtually all open surgical approaches have been replaced with endovenous techniques (see next section). Traditionally, open surgical approaches have been the mainstay of treatment for saphenous vein disease. The preferred surgical option for saphenous veins remains high ligation with stripping or high ligation alone. High ligation and stripping of the saphenous system is performed for patients with an incompetent valve at the saphenofemoral junction and varicosities throughout the length of the great saphenous vein. Ligation of the saphenofemoral junction and the major proximal saphenous vein branches through a small incision in the groin is a historically favored method. A subsequent phlebectomy is performed depending on the size of the saphenous vein. For the small saphenous vein, short-length phlebectomy with local anesthesia is typically performed to minimize risk of sural nerve injury. For larger saphenous veins, a longer phlebectomy is performed to the point of a cluster of varicosities. Epifascial veins may also be treated in an ambulatory setting, with phlebectomy performed under local anesthesia. A new treatment strategy called ASVAL (ambulatory selective varices ablation under local anesthesia) embraces the surgical treatment of epifascial veins while sparing the refluxing saphenous vein, minimizing the need to treat the saphenous vein for many affected patients. Although controversial, the principle of ASVAL is that reflux spreads from epifascial to saphenous veins in an antegrade fashion; thus, the treatment of epifascial veins alone is reported to correct saphenous reflux. Ongoing research has demonstrated that patients with primary varicose veins or less severe disease have done well with this approach.

C. Endovenous Treatment

In recent years, great advances have been made in endovenous techniques for treatment of varicose veins. Ablation techniques include thermal (radiofrequency and laser) and chemical ablation. Thermal ablation causes treated veins to collapse due to vein wall and lumen fibrosis. Both techniques require the use of tumescent solution to surround the vein to protect the surrounding tissues from the heat. The solution usually contains epinephrine for vein contraction and a local anesthetic for pain relief. Vein reabsorption occurs over the course of several months. Both radiofrequency and laser ablation have been found to be safe and effective in the treatment of incompetent greater saphenous veins. A third option is foam sclerotherapy, using either polidocanol or sodium tetradecyl sulfate compounded with carbon dioxide. Compared to liquid sclerotherapy, foam has increased time of endothelial contact as it expands to fill the vein. Foam has the unique advantage to treat both truncal reflux (incompetent saphenous veins) and varicose veins. Emerging technologies for the treatment of saphenous reflux include the use of intravenous glue and mechanicochemical ablation in which mechanical irritation of the endothelium is combined with administration of a sclerosing agent. These techniques do not use heat and, thus, do not need tumescent solution to surround the vein. A recent randomized trial comparing treatments for venous reflux found that the procedural complications were less frequent after laser ablation and that successful ablation of saphenous reflux was less common when foam sclerotherapy was used. The latest Society for Vascular Surgery and American Venous Forum's consensus opinion recommends thermal ablation to surgical or chemical ablation for greater saphenous veins.

Recent guidelines recommend selective treatment of incompetent perforating veins > 3.5 mm in patients with venous ulcers. Options for treatment of these veins include thermal ablation with laser or radiofrequency ablation similar to treatment of axial reflux and ultrasonographically guided sclerotherapy. Alternate options include open ligation and subfascial endoscopic perforating vein surgery.

Brittenden J, et al: A randomized trial comparing treatments for varicose veins. *N Eng J Med.* 2014;371:1218-1227.

Bush RG, et al: histological changes occurring after endoluminal ablation with two diode lasers (940 and 1319 nm) from acute changes to 4 months. *Lasers Surg Med.* 2008;40:676-679.

Gloviczki P, et al: The care of patients with varicose veins and associated chronic venous diseases: clinical practice guidelines of the Society for Vascular Surgery and the American Venous Forum. *J Vasc Surg.* 2011;53:25-485 (suppl).

Jacobs BN, et al: Pathophysiology of varicose veins. *J Vasc Surg Venous Lymphat Disord.* 2017;5:460-467.

Kheirelseid EAH, et al: Systematic review and meta-analysis of randomized controlled trials evaluating long-term outcomes of endovenous management of lower extremity varicose veins. *J Vasc Surg Venous Lymphat Disord.* 2018;6:256-270.

Lee AJ, et al: Progression of varicose veins and chronic venous insufficiency in the general population in the Edinburgh Vein Study. *J Vasc Surg.* 2015;3:18-26.

Maurins U, et al: Distribution and prevalence of reflux in the superficial and deep venous system in the general population–results from the Bonn Vein Study, Germany. *J Vasc Surg.* 2008;48:680-687.

Mowatt-Larssen E, et al: Treatment of primary varicose veins has changed with the introduction of new techniques. *Semin Vasc Surg.* 2012;25(1):18-24.

Pittaluga P, et al: Midterm results of the surgical treatment of varices by phlebectomy with conservation of a refluxing saphenous vein. *J Vasc Surg.* 2009;50:107-118.

DEEP VEIN THROMBOSIS

▶ General Considerations

Deep vein thrombosis (DVT) and pulmonary embolism (PE) affect up to 900,000 people per year in the United States, and incidence increases with age. Acute treatment is estimated to cost billions of dollars per year, not including the cost burden of long-term sequelae.

The Virchow triad (stasis, vascular injury, and hypercoagulability) should be the cornerstone for assessment of risk factors for DVT. In most cases, the cause is multifactorial. In recent years, the role of inflammation has been established in the pathophysiology of DVT.

Acquired risk factors include advanced age, cancer, surgery, trauma, immobilization, hormone replacement therapy, oral contraceptive use, pregnancy, neurologic disease, cardiac disease, and antiphospholipid antibodies. Cancer patients have a several-fold increased risk of venous thrombosis, and approximately 20%-30% of first venous thromboembolic events are cancer associated. Pancreas, brain, lung, and ovarian cancer are reported to induce the highest risks of thrombosis, and lymphomas, myeloma, and kidney, stomach, and bone cancers are also reported to have high risks. Most of these malignancies are associated with increased fibrinogen or thrombocytosis.

Endothelial injury can result from direct trauma (severed vein, venous cannulation, or transvenous pacing) or local irritation secondary to infusion of chemotherapy, previous DVT, or phlebitis. Damaged endothelium leads to platelet aggregation, degranulation, and formation of thrombus as well as vasoconstriction and activation of the coagulation cascade. Thrombin activation from release of tissue factor and diminished fibrinolysis mediated by plasminogen activator inhibitor are intraoperative events that may be related to endothelial disruption.

Hypercoagulable states may also be inherited. Genetic causes include deficiencies of natural coagulation inhibitors (antithrombin III, protein C, and protein S), factor V Leiden, prothrombin 20210A gene variant, blood group non-O, elevated homocysteine levels, plasminogen abnormalities, elevated levels of coagulation factors (eg, factor VIII), and reduced heparin cofactor II activity. Hematologic disorders associated with DVT include disseminated intravascular coagulation, heparin-induced thrombocytopenia, antiphospholipid antibody syndrome, thrombotic thrombocytopenic purpura, hemolytic-uremic syndrome, polycythemia vera, and essential thrombocythemia. Inflammatory bowel disease, systemic lupus erythematosus, and obesity are additionally associated with DVT.

DVT occurs most frequently in the calf veins, although it may arise in the femoral or iliac veins. Thrombi originate in soleal sinusoids or in valve sinuses, where there are flow eddies. Treatment of isolated calf vein thrombosis is controversial, due to its low risk of associated PE. However, a 2011 meta-analysis of studies spanning nearly 25 years demonstrated significant reductions both in progression to PE and in proximal thrombus propagation in patients treated with anticoagulation compared to untreated patients. While the studies were heterogeneous, the pooled data indicated no statistical increased risk of bleeding in patients who received anticoagulation compared to the controls. These observations and the improved safety profile of low-molecular-weight heparin (LMWH) compel practitioners to treat isolated calf DVTs aggressively. In the latest 2016 American College of Chest Physicians (ACCP) guidelines, it is recommended that in patients with acute isolated distal DVT of the leg and without severe symptoms or risk factors for extension, serial imaging of the deep veins for 2 weeks over anticoagulation is recommended, whereas in patients with acute isolated distal DVT of the leg and severe symptoms or risk factors for extension, anticoagulation over serial imaging of the deep veins is recommended. The most recent randomized studies on this topic support the ACCP guidelines. The recommended duration of anticoagulation is 3 months.

▶ **Clinical Findings**

A. Symptoms and Signs

The diagnosis of DVT cannot be made on the basis of presenting symptoms and signs alone. Up to half of patients with acute thromboses have no detectable abnormality in the involved extremity. Homans sign (pain on passive dorsiflexion of the ankle) is nonspecific, positive in only half of cases, and unreliable. Some patients present with acute PE unaccompanied by leg edema or pain.

Symptomatic patients most often complain of a dull ache or pain in the calf or leg associated with mild edema. With extensive proximal DVT, there can be massive edema, cyanosis, and dilated superficial collateral veins. Low-grade fever and tachycardia occasionally occur. Iliofemoral venous thrombosis can result in phlegmasia. In phlegmasia alba dolens, the leg is pulseless, pale, and cool, and the condition may progress to phlegmasia cerulea dolens, which is characterized by cyanosis of the limb and a precursor to gangrene.

B. Imaging Studies

Because DVT is difficult to diagnose on the basis of physical signs or symptoms, an objective diagnostic study is required before treatment is started. Historically, the standard for diagnosis was ascending phlebography, accomplished by fluoroscopic imaging during contrast injection into an intravenous line on the dorsum of the foot. The patient stands but non–weight-bearing on the extremity is studied. An abrupt cutoff of the contrast column indicates DVT. The complications of this procedure included risk of contrast allergy, contrast-induced nephropathy, and phlebitis.

Duplex ultrasound is now the best initial test and the gold standard to detect the presence of DVT. It is a noninvasive examination, does not expose the patient to radiation, is easily reproducible, and has specificity and sensitivity of greater than 95%. In this method, the transducer produces a two-dimensional image of the imaged vein and the surrounding tissue. Normally, veins collapse completely when compressed. Vein incompressibility is the primary ultrasonographic diagnostic criterion for acute lower limb DVT. Secondary diagnostic criteria include vein distention, echogenic thrombus within the vein lumen, absence of spectral or color Doppler signal from the vein lumen, lack of venous collaterals, and loss of venous flow phasicity and/or loss of response to Valsalva maneuver. Additionally, augmentation is expected in normal, compressible veins. When pressure is applied to the lower extremity distal to the area of evaluation, normally there is increased blood through the vein with compression. Lack of augmentation is suggestive of an occlusion in the segment of vein between the site of compression and the transducer. It is worth noting that direct thrombus visualization using B-mode imaging is variable depending on the age of the clot: fresh thrombus is anechoic and therefore not visible. Finally, although duplex ultrasound has a high accuracy for proximal DVT, it is less accurate in distal thrombosis and is highly operator dependent. Magnetic resonance venography shows promise as a diagnostic study for DVT and can be used as an alternative in patients for whom duplex ultrasound is not reliable due to anatomical considerations or to image veins in the pelvis and lower abdomen. The sensitivity and specificity of magnetic resonance venography are 100% and 96%, respectively. The injection of gadolinium may be used and may be helpful for determining the age of the thrombus. Computed tomography (CT) imaging, especially as part of a PE protocol CT image, may also be a good alternative to establish the diagnosis.

Measurement of D-dimer levels is too nonspecific for use alone and, when combined with a negative risk assessment, may be useful to rule out DVT but not to rule in the diagnosis of DVT. Radiolabeled fibrinogen is too sensitive in the pelvis for use in the acute clinical setting and carries with it a risk of transmission of infectious disease. It is no longer used. Older tests such as impedance plethysmography and venous pressure measurements do not achieve the same accuracy as duplex ultrasound and have been largely abandoned. Recent studies have demonstrated the potential for using soluble P-selectin as a marker for diagnosing deep venous thrombosis. P-selectin is a cell adhesion molecule that is the first upregulated glycoprotein on activated endothelial cells and platelets. Because thrombosis and inflammation are interrelated, elevated levels of soluble P-selectin act as an indicator or biomarker of inflammation. Consequently, the combination of soluble P-selectin with a Wells score has been shown to have a positive predictive value of approximately 90% and a negative predictive value of greater than 95% for establishing the diagnosis of DVT. However, this test is not a bedside test and is only available in research protocols at the present time.

Differential Diagnosis

A variety of pathologies may mimic the symptoms of DVT. Lymphatic conditions such as adenopathies or lymphangitis can present with lower extremity pain and edema. Vascular lesions such as hematomas and pseudoaneurysms secondary to catheterization of the common femoral artery may simulate DVTs. These can be differentiated from DVTs under evaluation by gray-scale images showing a delineation of the pseudoaneurysm or hematoma or by color duplex imaging, which will illustrate the typical "yin-yang" sign of bidirectional flow. Muscular lesions of the thigh such as muscle strains, tears, and contusions may result in pain, stiffness, edema, and a mass. Cellulitis may cause edema, localized pain, and erythema. Unilateral leg swelling can also result from lymphedema, obstruction of the popliteal vein by Baker cyst, or obstruction of the iliac vein by retroperitoneal mass or idiopathic fibrosis. Bilateral leg edema suggests heart, liver, or kidney failure or IVC obstruction by tumor or pregnancy.

Prevention

Surgery increases the risk of DVT 21-fold. This disorder is a reported complication for approximately 20%-25% of patients admitted for a general surgical procedure, 20%-30% of those undergoing an elective neurosurgical procedure, and 50%-60% of those undergoing hip or knee arthroplasty. These statistics emphasize the need for routine DVT prophylaxis in the surgical patient. The most commonly used measures are elastic stockings, intermittent pneumatic compression (IPC), low-dose unfractionated heparin (LDUH; 5000 units given by subcutaneous injection), or LMWH given at a prophylactic dose subcutaneously (either once or twice daily).

For general surgical patients, the incidence of DVT is high without prophylaxis, and the risk of PE is 1.6%, with 0.9% being fatal. Patients have been categorized into levels of risk in the current CHEST guidelines based on their risk scoring via the Rogers or Caprini scoring system: very low risk for venous thromboembolism (VTE), < 0.5%; low risk, ~1.5%; moderate risk, ~3%; and high risk, ~6%. In general surgery patients at very low risk for VTE, the recommended prophylaxis is simply early ambulation, with no pharmacologic or mechanical prophylaxis recommended. For patients at low risk, the guidelines suggest mechanical prophylaxis, preferably with IPC. Patients at moderate risk of VTE who are not at high risk for major bleeding complications are suggested to be treated using LMWH, LDUH, or IPC. In those at moderate risk of VTE but at high risk for bleeding, the guidelines suggest IPC. For high risk VTE patients who are not at high risk for major bleeding, the recommendation is pharmacologic prophylaxis with LMWH or LDUH, with the additional suggestion of IPC. In the special case of high VTE risk in patients with cancer who are not at high risk for bleeding complications, the guidelines recommend IPC with LMWH for extended-duration pharmacologic prophylaxis (4 weeks) over a shorter duration.

For orthopedic patients who have undergone major surgery including hip fracture surgery, total hip arthroplasty, or total knee arthroplasty, an evaluation of the extended postoperative VTE risk (postoperative days 0-35) comparing no prophylaxis with LMWH found the total symptomatic VTE rate decreased from 4.3% to 1.8%, a greater than 60% reduction. These values represent a decrease in rates of PE from 1.5% to 0.55% and a decrease in rates of DVT from 2.8% to 1.25%. Therefore, the current guidelines suggest extending thromboprophylaxis for up to 35 days postoperatively (grade 2B). For patients undergoing hip fracture surgery or total knee arthroplasty, the use of LMWH is suggested over fondaparinux, apixaban, dabigatran, rivaroxaban, LDUH, adjusted-dose vitamin K antagonist, or aspirin. In patients undergoing hip fracture surgery, LMWH is also the suggested agent, regardless of concomitant use of mechanical prophylaxis. If started preoperatively, LMWH is suggested to be administered ≥ 12 hours prior to surgery. In patients with increased risk of bleeding or contraindications to both pharmacologic and mechanical thromboprophylaxis, the guidelines suggest against using an IVC filter over no thromboprophylaxis.

For trauma patients, evidence is lacking, and randomized studies are needed. Trauma risk factors include lower extremity or pelvic fractures, surgical procedures, advanced age, femoral vein lines or major venous repairs, prolonged immobility, spinal cord injury, and prolonged duration of hospital stay. In major trauma patients, the guidelines suggest the use of LDUH, LMWH, or IPC. For patients at high risk for VTE, such as those with acute spinal cord injury or traumatic brain injury, IPC is suggested in addition to pharmacologic prophylaxis. Because venous compression ultrasound detection and subsequent treatment of asymptomatic DVT in this population do not reduce the risk of PE or fatal PE, the guidelines do not suggest periodic surveillance with this modality. IVC filters are recommended in patients when anticoagulation is contraindicated but are not suggested for use as primary prevention.

In neurosurgery, DVT and PE occur equivalent to rates in general surgery patients, and risk factors include intracranial surgery, prolonged surgery, malignant tumors, the presence of leg weakness, and increased age. The recommendations differ between craniotomy and spine surgery patients. In craniotomy patients, the suggested prophylaxis is mechanical or pharmacologic or no prophylaxis. However, in craniotomy patients who are at very high risk for VTE, such as those with malignant disease, the guidelines suggest pharmacologic prophylaxis in addition to mechanical prophylaxis when it is safe to do so. For spinal surgery patients, mechanical prophylaxis is suggested over no prophylaxis, unfractionated heparin, or LMWH. Similar to their counterparts, spinal surgery patients at very high risk for VTE are suggested to receive both pharmacologic and mechanical prophylaxis when medically safe.

Treatment

Treatment is aimed at reducing the incidence of complications associated with DVT. Short-term complications include recurrent DVT or pulmonary thromboembolism, whereas long-term complications include the development of varicose veins and chronic venous insufficiency. The primary treatment of DVT is systemic anticoagulation. This reduces the risk of PE and extension of venous thrombosis and also decreases the rate of recurrent DVT by 80%. Systemic anticoagulation does not directly lyse thrombi but stops propagation and allows natural fibrinolysis to occur.

In patients with acute DVT of the leg or acute PE, the most recent 2016 ACCP guidelines suggest direct oral anticoagulants (DOACs; dabigatran, rivaroxaban, apixaban, and edoxaban) over vitamin K antagonist therapy and LMWH, if the patient does not have cancer, for 3 months if provoked or longer if unprovoked. Dabigatran and edoxaban require parenteral anticoagulation prior to initiation, but rivaroxaban and apixaban do not. For patients with cancer and PE or DVT of the leg, LMWH is suggested over vitamin K antagonist therapy and DOACs. Advantages of DOACs include no need for monitoring of levels and decreased risk of intracranial bleeding as compared to vitamin K antagonists. The lack of reversal agents for DOACs was initially an area of concern, with plasma and prothrombin complex concentrates used for reversal, but novel reversal agents have been developed. Regarding LMWH, its advantages over standard heparin include a lower risk of bleeding complications and thrombocytopenia, lower risk of heparin-induced thrombocytopenia, lower recurrence of VTE, decreased mortality, less interference with proteins C and S, less complement activation, and lower risk of osteoporosis. Moreover, recent randomized trials have shown regression of thrombus with LMWH. A disadvantage worth noting is that LMWH accumulates in patients with renal failure. In patients who have renal insufficiency or a contraindication to a DOAC, heparin is dosed to a goal partial thromboplastin time of 1.5 to 2.5 times normal. Heparin cannot be used for outpatient therapy. Warfarin is started after therapeutic heparinization. The two therapies should overlap to diminish the possibility of a hypercoagulable state, which can occur during the first few days of warfarin administration, due to warfarin inhibition of protein C and protein S, which are natural anticoagulants. For both acute lower extremity DVT and acute PE, guidelines recommend starting warfarin on day 1 or 2 of parenteral anticoagulation over delayed initiation, with a continuation of parenteral anticoagulation for a minimum of 5 days until the international normalized ratio is greater than 2.0 for more than 24 hours.

Regarding length of coagulation, in patients with a PE or proximal DVT of the leg provoked by surgery, the recommended treatment is 3 months, compared to a longer or shorter time period. Three months of anticoagulation are similarly recommended in patients with PE/proximal DVT of the leg provoked by a nonsurgical transient risk factor and in patients with PE/isolated distal DVT of the leg provoked by surgery or by a nonsurgical transient risk factor. In patients who have had an unprovoked PE or DVT of the proximal or distal leg, the recommended treatment minimum is 3 months, followed by reevaluation of risk-benefit ratio of extended therapy. Data have now shown that after a course of therapy for unprovoked DVTs and some provoked DVTs, the use of certain DOACs in lower doses may significantly decrease recurrence of DVT by approximately 80% over the next year, compared to low-dose aspirin, which decreases recurrence of DVT by approximately 30%, both compared to placebo. After a second episode of DVT, the usual recommendation is prolonged or lifelong oral anticoagulation in patients with a low or moderate bleeding risk. In patients with a high bleeding risk, the guidelines recommend 3 months of anticoagulation over extended therapy (although in this situation, the patient should be evaluated with the risk-benefit ratio in mind). The risk for recurrent venous thrombosis is increased markedly in the presence of homozygous factor V Leiden mutations, antiphospholipid antibody, antithrombin III, and protein C or protein S deficiencies. Lifelong anticoagulation is usually recommended for these conditions.

An alterative agent for the treatment of acute VTE is fondaparinux. It is a synthetic pentasaccharide that binds to antithrombin and catalyzes the inhibition of factor Xa. It has more specific anti-Xa activity than LMWH and has a longer half-life than LMWH. It is rapidly and almost completely bioavailable after subcutaneous injection and does not require coagulation monitoring. However, due to its dependence on renal clearance, its use is contraindicated in patients with renal insufficiency. For the treatment of VTE, fondaparinux is administered at a fixed dose of 7.5 mg for patients weighing 50-100 kg, with the dose adjusted to 5 mg for patients weighing less than 50 kg and to 10 mg for those weighing more than 100 kg.

The clinical outcome after DVT can be thought of as resulting in valvular reflux, persistent venous obstruction, or their combination. Patients with both obstruction and valvular reflux often have the most severe postthrombotic symptoms. To limit these consequences, thrombus removal has been proposed to alleviate the obstruction. The longer a thrombus is in contact with a vein valve, the more likely the valve will no longer function. Additionally, the thrombus initiates an inflammatory response in the vein wall, which may lead to vein wall and valve dysfunction.

Techniques for early thrombus removal include catheter-directed thrombolytic therapy and open thrombectomy.

In the treatment of acute iliofemoral DVTs, a systematic review and meta-analysis by Casey and colleagues reports that thrombectomy results in significantly decreased risk of developing postthrombotic syndrome and venous reflux and shows a trend for reduced venous obstruction when compared to systemic anticoagulation. A recent randomized controlled trial evaluating patients with acute femoropopliteal or iliofemoral DVT found that there was no difference in development of postthrombotic syndrome, but there was an increase in bleeding in patients undergoing thrombolysis compared to standard treatment with anticoagulation. Analysis of the patient cohorts identified that patients with iliofemoral DVT had decreased development and severity of postthrombotic syndrome, suggesting that this maybe a beneficial therapy in select patients. Following either therapy, it is currently recommended that patients wear knee-high compression stockings (30-40 mm Hg) for at least 2 years following the procedure and be treated with anticoagulation, as indicated earlier. The ability of stockings to prevent postthrombotic syndrome has been recently questioned, but clearly stockings should be used for the pain and swelling related to DVT.

Agnelli G, et al: Apixaban for extended treatment of venous thromboembolism. *N Eng J Med.* 2013;368:699-708.

Bauersachs R, et al: Oral rivaroxaban for symptomatic venous thromboembolism. *N Engl J Med.* 2010;363(26):2499-2510.

Bozzato S, et al: Thromboprophylaxis in surgical and medical patients. *Semin Resp Crit Care Med.* 2012;33(2):163-175.

Casey ET, et al: Treatment of acute iliofemoral deep vein thrombosis. *J Vasc Surg.* 2012;55(5):1463-1473.

De Martino RR, et al: A meta-analysis of anticoagulation for calf deep venous thrombosis. *J Vasc Surg.* 2012;56(1):228-237.e1.

Falck-Ytter Y, et al: Prevention of VTE in orthopedic surgery patients: antithrombotic therapy and prevention of thrombosis, 9th ed: American College of Chest Physicians evidence-based clinical practice guidelines. *Chest.* 2012;141(2 Suppl): e278S-2325S.

Gould MK, et al: Prevention of VTE in nonorthopedic surgical patients: antithrombotic therapy and prevention of thrombosis, 9th ed: American College of Chese Physicians evidence-based clinical practice guidelines. *Chest.* 2012;141 (2 Suppl):e227S-277S.

Guanella R, et al: Serial limited versus single complete compression ultrasonography for the diagnosis of lower extremity deep vein thrombosis. *Semin Respir Crit Care Med.* 2012;33(2): 144-150.

Kahn S, et al: Compression stockings to prevent post-thrombotic syndrome: a randomised placebo-controlled trial. *Lancet.* 2014;383:880-888.

Kearon C, et al: Antithrombotic therapy for VTE disease: antithrombotic therapy and prevention of thrombosis, 9th ed: American College of Chest Physicians evidence-based clinical practice guidelines. *Chest.* 2012;141(2 suppl):e419S-494S.

Meissner MH, et al: Early thrombus removal strategies for acute deep venous thrombosis: clinical practice guidelines of the Society for Vascular Surgery and the American Venous Forum. *J Vasc Surg.* 2012;55(5):1449-1462.

Ramacciotti E, et al: Evaluation of soluble P-selectin as a marker for the diagnosis of deep venous thrombosis. *Clin Appl Thromb Hemost.* 2011;17(4):425-431.

Schulman S, et al: Dabigatran versus warfarin in the treatment of acute venous thromboembolism. *N Engl J Med.* 2009;361(24):2342-2352.

Smith M, et al: New trends in anticoagulation therapy. *Surg Clin J.* 2018;98(2):219-238.

Timp J, et al: Epidemiology of cancer-associated venous thrombosis. *Blood.* 2013;122:1712-1723.

Useche JA, et al: Use of US in the evaluation of patients with symptoms of deep venous thrombosis of the lower extremities. *Radiographics.* 2008;28(6):1785-1797.

van Langevelde K, et al: Magnetic resonance imaging and computed tomography developments in imaging of venous thromboembolism. *J Magn Reson Imaging.* 2010;32(6):1302-1312.

Vedantham S, et al: Pharmacomechanical catheter-directed thrombolysis for deep vein thrombosis. *N Engl J Med.* 2017;377:2240-2252.

Warkentin TE: Aspirin for dual prevention of venous and arterial thrombosis. *N Engl J Med.* 2012;367:2039-2041.

Weitz JI, et al: Rivaroxaban or aspirin for extended treatment of venous thromboembolism. *N Engl J Med.* 2017;376:1211-1222.

AXILLARY-SUBCLAVIAN VENOUS THROMBOSIS

▶ General Considerations

Thrombosis of the axillary or subclavian vein is a relatively uncommon event, accounting for less than 5% of all cases of DVT. Only 12% result in clinically apparent pulmonary thromboembolism, but the incidence is higher if all patients undergo diagnostic testing. Besides PE, the most common consequence of axillary-subclavian vein thrombosis is chronic edema and resultant disability. The effects of postthrombotic syndrome and recurrent thrombosis are not uncommon.

There are two major etiologies. Primary axillary-subclavian thrombosis, also known as Paget-Schroetter syndrome or "effort thrombosis," occurs as a result of intermittent transient obstruction of the vein in the costoclavicular space during repetitive or strenuous activities involving the upper extremity (Figure 37–3). This condition was first described in independent reports by Paget and von Schroetter in the late 19th century. During strenuous repetitive movements of the upper extremity, the subclavian vein is compressed between the first rib and the anterior scalene muscle posteriorly and the clavicle—with underlying subclavius muscle and fibrous costocoracoid ligament—anteriorly. In many cases, the costoclavicular ligament congenitally inserts more laterally than normal, subjecting the anatomically tight space to further compression of the subclavian vein. Primary subclavian vein thrombosis can also occur in patients with hypercoagulable states such as antiphospholipid antibody syndrome or factor V Leiden mutation. Secondary subclavian vein thrombosis,

▲ **Figure 37–3.** **A:** Effort thrombosis in a 13-year-old wrestler. Arrow marks subclavian vein thrombosis refractory to recombinant tissue plasminogen activator thrombolysis. **B:** Arm in abduction. Note disappearance of prominent venous collaterals. **C:** Immediate postoperative venogram following scalenectomy, first rib resection, and thrombectomy.

which is increasing in incidence, results from venous injury by indwelling central venous catheters, external trauma, or pacemaker wires. These patients are less likely to be symptomatic than patients with primary subclavian vein thrombosis.

▶ **Clinical Findings**

A. Symptoms and Signs

Primary axillary-subclavian vein thrombosis usually occurs in healthy young athletes and people who perform repetitive activities that involve hyperabduction of the upper extremities. Most patients present with edema of the affected extremity, diffuse aching pain, and cyanosis of the upper extremity. As venous collaterals develop, dilated veins appear in the chest wall and shoulder region. In less pronounced presentations, patients become symptomatic only when their affected extremity is positioned in a way that predisposes it to vascular occlusion.

Paget-Schroetter syndrome may also be accompanied by symptoms of neurogenic thoracic outlet syndrome, often causing tingling, numbness, and pain in the hand and arm, sometimes in an ulna distribution, indicating compression of the C-8/T-1 roots of the brachial plexus between hypertrophied or anomalous anterior and middle scalene muscles.

B. Imaging Studies

Upper extremity venous duplex ultrasound is a sensitive and reliable modality to diagnose axillary-subclavian vein thrombosis.

Magnetic resonance venography has demonstrated promise with greater than 97% sensitivity and specificity for diagnosis, but its cost and limited availability reduce its widespread use. Although CT venography is widely available, its use exposes the patient to contrast dye. Venography, although invasive, remains the common next step in diagnosis, with a positive venogram indicating subclavian vein compression with the appearance of prominent collateral veins. Obtaining these images allows delivery of catheter-directed thrombolysis and allows for further planning of thoracic outlet decompression surgery.

Chest x-ray should be obtained on all patients to exclude the presence of cervical rib, which can also contribute to compression of the subclavian vein.

▶ **Treatment**

For patients with secondary axillo-subclavian thrombosis, any indwelling central venous lines or pacemaker wires in the thrombosed vein should be removed if possible. If not contraindicated, anticoagulation should be considered, as well as arm elevation and pain control.

Patients who have primary venous thrombosis secondary to thoracic outlet compression should be considered for decompression because, if left untreated, the patients have a 35%-65% risk of postthrombotic syndrome characterized by recurrent episodes of pain, swelling, and chronic venous insufficiency secondary to venous hypertension and valvular damage.

The current standard of care is catheter-directed thrombolysis followed by surgical decompression of the thoracic outlet in the majority of cases. Catheter-directed thrombolysis is beneficial to patients presenting early and offers therapeutic value without the higher rates of bleeding complications seen in systemic fibrinolysis. As the success of thrombolysis decreases as time from onset of symptoms increases, the early initiation of treatment is paramount. Some have advocated a treatment window of 2 weeks, as there is progressive fibrosis of the vein and risk of extension of the thrombus distally into the arm with decreased chance of recovery. In patients who are more than 6 weeks from initial presentation of symptoms, thrombolytic agents are generally ineffective in completely removing the clot. Inflow is typically inadequate by the time patients present with chronic obstruction.

Because the etiology of venous thoracic outlet syndrome is compression of the vein between the first rib–anterior scalene muscle origin and the clavicle, surgery consists of anterior scalenectomy, first rib resection, and venolysis (release of the vein from any externally constricting scar). It is particularly important to resect the entire medial portion of the rib to the sternal junction when an anterior or subclavicular approach is used. Some prefer this to the transaxillary approach because the transaxillary approach prevents full resection of the medial rib and allows for intact subclavius tendons and costoclavicular ligaments, resulting in kinking of the vein on any of these residual structures. However, others find that the transaxillary dissection minimizes the exposure of the neurovascular structures, minimizing their injury. In either case, for patients presenting with acute occlusion, surgical resection of the anterior scalene and first rib with venolysis is preferred to thrombectomy, balloon venoplasty, and stenting.

For patients with chronic obstruction, Molina and colleagues report successful approaches based on length of the obstructed segment. Patients with short-segment chronic obstruction have been successfully treated with saphenous vein patch to the subclavian vein. Patients with a long segment of chronic obstruction have been treated with either a long vein patch with upper thigh saphenous vein or implantation of thoracic aortic homografts with subsequent balloon dilatation and implantation of a stent for reobstruction. Venous bypass has also been successfully used in patients with residual stenosis after thoracic outlet decompression.

The need for and duration of anticoagulation for patients treated with catheter-directed thrombolysis followed by decompression are unclear. Some authors maintain that no anticoagulation is needed when good surgical outcomes are obtained, whereas others have anticoagulated for 2-3 months. All patients who present with primary venous thrombosis should undergo a workup for a hypercoagulable state, the most common of which are mutations in coagulation factor V, protein C and S deficiencies, and antithrombin III. Because of a 40%-60% rate of recurrent thrombosis, these patients are maintained indefinitely on warfarin.

▶ Prognosis

The prognosis after axillary-subclavian vein thrombosis is dependent on the cause of the condition. Most patients experience fairly rapid resolution of their initial presenting symptoms. For patients with secondary forms of this disease, the outcome is dependent on resolution of the underlying condition, such as a malignancy. For patients with Paget-Schroetter syndrome who undergo thoracic outlet decompression, excellent outcomes, characterized by continued venous patency and absence of symptoms of chronic venous insufficiency, occur in 75%-95% of patients. Most patients return to normal activity within 12 weeks of surgical intervention, and up to 20% require long-term anticoagulation. In contrast, chronic axillary-subclavian vein thrombosis with symptoms persisting for over 3 months does not often respond to thrombolysis, mechanical thrombolysis, or prolonged anticoagulation and may cause significant long-term disability.

Alla VM, et al: Paget-Schroetter syndrome: review of pathogenesis and treatment of effort thrombosis. *West J Emerg Med.* 2010;114:358-362.

Molina JE, et al: Protocols for Paget-Schroetter syndrome and late treatment of chronic subclavian vein obstruction. *Ann Thorac Surg.* 2009;87(2):416-422.

Urschel HC Jr, et al: Surgery remains the most effective treatment for Paget-Schroetter syndrome: 50 years' experience. *Ann Thorac Surg.* 2008;86(1):254-260.

Vemuri C, et al: Diagnosis and treatment of effort-induced thrombosis of the axillary subclavian vein due to venous thoracic outlet syndrome. *J Vasc Surg Venous Lymphat Disord.* 2016;4:485-500.

PULMONARY THROMBOEMBOLISM

▶ General Considerations

Pulmonary thromboembolism is responsible for up to 50,000 deaths each year in the United States. It is the third leading cause of death among hospitalized patients, yet only 30%-40% of patients with pulmonary thromboembolism have suspected DVT at the time of diagnosis. Efforts directed at reduction in the mortality rate of pulmonary thromboembolism demand an aggressive approach to the prevention of DVT and diagnosis of pulmonary thromboembolism in patients identified to be at high risk.

Pulmonary thromboemboli arise from a number of sources. Air embolism can occur during the placement or removal of central venous catheters intraoperatively during operation on large venous vessels. Amniotic fluid emboli may occur during active labor. Fat emboli from long bone fractures cause a syndrome characterized by respiratory insufficiency, coagulopathy, encephalopathy, and an upper body petechial rash. Other less common causes of PEs include septic emboli, tumor emboli from atrial myxoma or IVC extension of renal cell carcinoma, and parasitic emboli. However, DVT remains the most common source of pulmonary thromboemboli. Up to 60% of patients with untreated proximal lower extremity DVT may develop pulmonary thromboembolism.

Fewer than 10% of pulmonary thromboemboli will produce pulmonary infarction. The pathophysiology of PE depends on the size and frequency of the emboli as well as the condition of the underlying lung. Obstruction of large pulmonary arteries results in increases in pulmonary artery pressure and acute right ventricular failure, but many of the clinical manifestations of pulmonary thromboembolism result from release of vasoactive amines that cause severe pulmonary vasoconstriction. Vasoconstriction leads to increased physiologic dead space and systemic hypoxia from right-to-left shunt. Reflex bronchial vasoconstriction is also common.

▶ Clinical Findings

A. Symptoms and Signs

Signs and symptoms associated with PE are notoriously vague. Dyspnea and chest pain are present in up to 75% of patients with pulmonary thromboembolism. However, these symptoms are nonspecific, especially in patients who may have underlying cardiopulmonary disease. Tachycardia, tachypnea, and altered mental status are highly suggestive findings in an at-risk population. The classic triad of dyspnea, chest pain, and hemoptysis is present in only 15% of patients with pulmonary thromboembolism. Pleural friction rub and the S1Q3T3 morphology on electrocardiography are even less common findings.

B. Imaging and Other Diagnostic Studies

Chest x-ray is most often normal but may show a pleural cap. Electrocardiography may reveal new-onset atrial fibrillation, evidence of right heart strain, or ischemic changes, but in most cases, only acute sinus tachycardia and nonspecific ST and T-wave changes are identified. Arterial blood gas determination reveals hypoxia and often a respiratory alkalosis or increased arterial-alveolar oxygen gradient. Plasma D-dimer levels are elevated in the presence of both pulmonary thromboembolism and acute DVT, but this test lacks sufficient specificity to be of primary diagnostic value. In acute massive or submassive PE resulting in hemodynamic instability (systolic blood pressure < 90 mm Hg) and right heart strain leading to myocardial ischemia, cardiac troponins may be elevated. Plasma B-type natriuretic peptide may also be elevated in right heart strain, although it is similarly not specific enough to be used alone for diagnosis of PE.

CT angiography is now the preferred imaging modality used for the diagnosis of PE, due to its wide availability, sensitivity and specificity, characterization of vascular and nonvascular structures, and exceptional speed (Figure 37–4).

A

B

▲ **Figure 37–4.** Pulmonary embolism. **A:** Pulmonary angiogram. Arrow marks location of left lower lobe emboli. **B:** Spiral computed tomography. Arrow marks location of large embolus in left main pulmonary artery.

CT angiograms (CTAs) are more accurate than the previously commonly used ventilation-perfusion (VQ) scan, and when compared to pulmonary angiography, CTAs are less invasive, less time consuming, and less expensive. For CTA, the patient presentation must match the results of the CTA for the most accurate determination of the diagnosis of PE. For patients in whom massive PE is suspected but contrast agent administration is undesirable, a bedside echocardiogram may be performed to evaluate for right heart dysfunction as an indication of hemodynamically significant PE. Intravascular ultrasound has also been used for bedside evaluation.

▶ Treatment

A. Anticoagulation and Catheter-Based Techniques

Rapid anticoagulation remains the mainstay of treatment of PE. Heparin, the pentasaccharide fondaparinux, or LMWH anticoagulation is started as soon as the diagnosis is made after initial stabilization with ventilatory support and vasopressor medications. Although these drugs are not thrombolytic, they allow the body's fibrinolytic system to function unopposed. Catheter-directed thrombolysis is considered for large clot burden, severe respiratory compromise, hemodynamic instability, or right heart failure. Catheter techniques involve mechanical thrombolysis or removal of intact PEs using a suction embolectomy device. When compared with heparin alone, thrombolytic therapy speeds the resolution of PE in the first 24 hours. The disadvantages of lytic therapy include its greater cost and higher risk of significant bleeding complications. More efficient care can be provided to patients with symptomatic submassive and massive PE via the use of an organized PE response team (PERT). A PERT team is composed of multiple specialists, including those from pulmonary critical care, radiology, cardiovascular medicine and surgery, emergency medicine, and hematology, who rapidly organize and provide evidence-based care.

B. Inferior Vena Cava Interruption

IVC interruption is considered in patients who have extension of venous thrombus on adequate anticoagulant therapy, patients in whom heparin anticoagulation is contraindicated, patients who have had a complication of anticoagulation, or patients who have had recurrent DVT or PE despite *therapeutic* anticoagulation. Occasionally, temporary or permanent IVC filters have been placed prophylactically in high-risk patients such as those with unresectable cancer or major trauma. Interestingly, because insertion of an IVC filter does not completely eliminate the risk of a PE, may increase the risk of DVT, and does nothing to prevent postthrombotic syndrome, the current guidelines suggest that patients who have an IVC filter should receive the standard course of anticoagulation if the contraindication to anticoagulation resolves.

Historically, IVC interruption was performed as an open surgical procedure, involving ligation or plication of the infrarenal vena cava or placement of a serrated clip to "strain" blood returning to the right atrium. The Greenfield filter, developed in 1973, was initially deployed by venous cutdown. Multiple devices are now available for fluoroscopically guided percutaneous placement through a range of sheath sizes from 6F to 12F and are introduced into the common femoral vein or, in cases of femoral thrombus, into the internal jugular vein. Diagnostic inferior venography is essential prior to placing the filter to exclude the presence of a duplicated IVC because lower extremity DVT might still serve as a source of emboli. The presence of thrombus within the IVC, the diameter of the IVC, and identification of the level of the renal veins are also important to evaluate.

The development and increased use of retrievable IVC filters for both prophylaxis and therapy of VTE are largely driven by the results of the PREPIC study. This study remains only one of two prospective, randomized clinical trials comparing IVC filters to anticoagulation alone. At 8 years, the study suggested a higher incidence of recurrent DVT in patients who were randomized to the IVC filter arm of the study compared to group who received anticoagulation only. This study suggested that patients with IVC filters in place had a significantly higher risk of recurrent DVT than patients treated with anticoagulation alone. There was no difference in the incidence of postthrombotic syndrome between study groups, but patients with IVC filters in place had significantly lower rates of PE over the course of the study compared to the anticoagulation group. These data suggest that the best use of IVC filters may be limited to patients with a high risk of PE. Although there is a multitude of devices available and many small observational studies that suggest that retrievable filters are safe and effective, no other prospective comparison studies have yet to be performed.

Additionally, alternative imaging modalities (other than venography) are successfully being used to place filters. Specifically, devices are being successfully and safely deployed under ultrasound guidance, both intravascular and transabdominal ultrasound. Compared to traditional placement, the use of intravenous ultrasound for IVC filter deployment lacks the risks of prolonged radiation exposure and nephrotoxic contrast agents while diminishing the case duration and overall cost.

C. Surgical Treatment

Hemodynamically unstable patients in whom thrombolytic therapy has failed or cannot be instituted require percutaneous or open surgical extraction of the thrombus. Open surgical pulmonary embolectomy is reserved for patients who develop intractable hypotension, those who fail transcatheter pulmonary embolectomy, and those who have tumor or foreign body emboli.

Prognosis

PE is one of the most frequent causes of preventable hospital death. Prevention by use of DVT prophylaxis and early diagnosis by selective testing of high-risk patients are essential steps to reducing the morbidity of this disease. The placement of IVC filters in selected patients can aid in prevention of pulmonary embolus but does nothing to treat the underlying disease process (venous thromboembolic disease) or prevent the long-term sequelae of DVT-postthrombotic syndrome.

Kabrhel C: Achieving multidisciplinary collaboration for the creation of a pulmonary embolism response team: creating a "team of rivals." *Semin Intervent Radiol.* 2017;34:16-24.

Kassavin DS, et al: The transition to IVUS-guided IVC filter deployment in the nontrauma patient. *Vasc Endovasc Surg.* 2011;45(2):142-145.

Kearon C, et al: Antithrombotic therapy for VTE disease: antithrombotic therapy and prevention of thrombosis, 9th ed: American College of Chest Physicians evidence-based clinical practice guidelines. *Chest.* 2012:141(2 Suppl):e419S-494S.

Kuo WT: Endovascular therapy for acute pulmonary embolism. *J Vasc Interv Radiol.* 2012;23(2):167-179.

PREPIC Study Group: Eight-year follow-up of patients with permanent vena cava filters in the prevention of pulmonary embolism. *Circulation.* 2005;112:416.

Tapson VF: Acute pulmonary embolism. *N Engl J Med.* 2008; 358(10):1037-1052.

SUPERFICIAL THROMBOPHLEBITIS

General Considerations

Superficial thrombophlebitis may appear spontaneously in patients with varicose veins, in pregnant or postpartum women, or in patients with thromboangiitis obliterans or Behçet disease. It may also occur after intravenous therapy or in an area of localized trauma. The presence of superficial phlebitis, particularly if it occurs in a migratory manner, suggests the presence of an abdominal cancer such as carcinoma of the pancreas (Trousseau thrombophlebitis). The most common vein affected is the great saphenous vein and its branches. In up to 40% of cases, a simultaneous DVT exists, and duplex imaging is a must in these situations. PEs are rare unless extension into the deep venous system occurs.

Clinical Findings

The patient usually presents with a complaint of localized extremity pain and redness. Areas of induration, erythema, and tenderness correspond to dilated and often thrombosed superficial veins. Over time, a firm cord may develop. Generalized edema is absent unless the deep veins are involved. The presence of fever and shaking chills suggests septic or suppurative phlebitis, which occurs most commonly as a complication of intravenous cannulation.

Differential Diagnosis

Superficial thrombophlebitis must be distinguished from ascending lymphangitis, cellulitis, erythema nodosum, erythema induratum, and panniculitis. Unlike these other disorders, superficial phlebitis tends to be well localized over a superficial vein.

Treatment

The approach to treating superficial venous thrombophlebitis (SVT) is variable, because there is no general consensus on ideal treatment. Approximately 60%-80% of SVT cases involve the great saphenous vein, and 10%-20% of cases involve the small saphenous veins, followed by upper extremity veins. Reports indicate that < 10% to approximately 40% of patients who present with SVT also present with associated acute DVT. Concurrent PE has been reported in 0.5%-4% of symptomatic patients. The association of SVT with both DVTs and PEs increases as the phlebitis extends toward the saphenofemoral junction. The treatment approach therefore depends on the location, presence of concomitant DVT, and presence of additional risk factors such as hypercoagulable disorders. The primary treatment is the administration of nonsteroidal anti-inflammatory drugs (NSAIDs), local heat, elevation, and support stockings or elastic wraps. Ambulation is encouraged. In most cases, symptoms will resolve within 7-10 days. Both NSAIDS and LMWH reduced extension or recurrence when compared to placebo. When comparing LMWH with surgical intervention (saphenofemoral disconnection), both were comparable in reduction of VTE events, although surgery was associated with a statistically insignificant lower risk of extension or recurrence. Alternatively, venous stripping plus elastic stockings demonstrated a lower, nonsignificant incidence of VTE compared with elastic stockings alone. In general, surgical treatment with ligation of the great saphenous vein at the saphenofemoral junction allows for superior symptomatic relief of pain, whereas medical management with anticoagulants appears superior for minimizing complications and preventing subsequent DVT/PE. In either case, more aggressive treatment is indicated if the thrombus extends toward the saphenofemoral junction (< 3 cm). Regarding thrombi ≥ 3 cm from the saphenofemoral junction, a study treating superficial thrombophlebitis that was at least 5 cm in length demonstrated a benefit to 45 days of fondaparinux therapy compared with less aggressive therapy. Similarly, a Cochrane review involving 26 studies and 5521 participants assessed the current approach to patients with superficial thrombophlebitis of the legs. Fondaparinux at a prophylactic dose given for 45 days was associated with lower rates of recurrence and extension of superficial thrombophlebitis compared to placebo. As a result, the current ACCP guidelines support the use of fondaparinux or LMWH (favoring fondaparinux) in these patients. Of course, if the phlebitis is associated with an underlying DVT, the patient should be treated for the DVT.

Septic thrombophlebitis requires treatment with broad-spectrum intravenous antibiotics. If rapid resolution of the cellulitis occurs, no treatment beyond a short course of antibiotics is required. However, if septic thrombophlebitis progresses to sepsis or demonstrates purulence from the vein, excision of the entire infected vein is required. Catheter removal is required in cases involving central venous catheter infection. In patients refractory to standard medical therapy yet who are poor candidates for invasive surgical therapy, endovascular treatment using thrombectomy devices, balloon angioplasty, and local intraluminal infusion of antibiotics has been reported. Thrombolytic therapy and mechanical thrombectomy remain options for the treatment of the thrombosed vein segment.

▶ Prognosis

Most episodes of uncomplicated superficial thrombophlebitis respond to conservative management. Cases in which extension into the deep venous system occurs can be associated with thromboembolism.

Decousus H, et al: Fondaparinux for the treatment of superficial-vein thrombosis in the legs. *N Engl J Med.* 2010;363:1222-1232.

Di Nisio M, et al: Treatment for superficial thrombophlebitis of the leg. *Cochrane Database Syst Rev.* 2018;2:CD004982.

Enzler MA, et al: Thermal ablation in the management of.superficial thrombophlebitis. *Eur J Vasc Endovasc Surg.* 2012;43(6):726-728.

Kars S, et al: Septic thrombophlebitis: percutaneous mechanical thrombectomy and thrombolytic therapies. *Am J Ther.* 2014;21(2):131-136.

Rathbun SW, et al: A randomized trial of dalteparin compared with ibuprofen for the treatment of superficial thrombophlebitis. *J Thromb Haemost.* 2012:10:833-839.

Smith M, et al: New trends in anticoagulation therapy. *Surg Clin J.* 2018;98:219-238.

CHRONIC VENOUS INSUFFICIENCY

Chronic venous insufficiency can result from congenital venous valvular insufficiency or from previous venous thrombosis. In the former circumstance, it is called chronic venous insufficiency, whereas in the latter circumstance, it is called the postthrombotic syndrome. Varicose veins (also a manifestation of venous insufficiency), chronic venous insufficiency, and postthrombotic syndrome occur in 76/100,000 person-years, and it has been estimated that 6-7 million Americans suffer from stasis pigmentation changes in the legs, with another 400,000-500,000 patients with skin ulceration. Treatment costs are in the billion-dollar range. The basic physiologic abnormality in patients with chronic venous insufficiency is chronically elevated venous pressure.

The normal venous capacitance can accommodate large-volume changes that occur during exercise with only minimal changes in venous pressure. However, with calf muscle pump dysfunction and valvular reflux, blood pools in the lower extremities and leads to venous hypertension. Outflow obstruction from proximal obstruction can also produce venous hypertension, resulting in "venous claudication" as the deep venous system fills with blood during exercise. The severity of chronic venous disease has been associated with older age and higher body mass index.

Valvular incompetence of the deep veins can be congenital or result from damage following phlebitis, varicose veins, or DVT. The best estimate for the incidence of chronic venous insufficiency after DVT is approximately 30% after 8-year follow-up, although it has been seen even more frequently in some studies. Chronic venous stasis changes typically affect the "gaiter areas" around the ankles, a region with sparse soft tissue support to withstand elevated venous pressures and the location of the commonly affected perforator veins. Brawny edema is produced by extravasation of plasma fluid, red blood cells, and plasma proteins. Lysis of red blood cells results in deposition of hemosiderin, which creates a brownish discoloration. Leukocytes become sequestered in the microcirculation, leading to capillary occlusion and release of superoxide radicals, proteolytic enzymes, and growth factors. Macrophages and T lymphocytes are primary mediators of this inflammatory response, which results in fibroblast activation and scarring and fibrosis of the subcutaneous tissues. Ultimately, this fibrosis results in compromised skin perfusion and ulceration.

▶ Clinical Findings

A. Symptoms and Signs

Both isolated saphenous vein incompetence and deep venous insufficiency can lead to venous varicosities and chronic venous stasis changes. The first symptom to develop is usually edema of the ankle and calf. Involvement of the foot and toes suggests lymphedema. Typically, the edema is worse at the end of the day and improves with leg elevation. Additional symptoms may include aching, tingling, burning, muscle cramps, heaviness, sensations of throbbing, and leg fatigue. Longstanding disease is characterized by stasis dermatitis, hyperpigmentation, brawny induration, and ulceration. Venous stasis ulcers are large, painful, and irregular in outline. They have a shallow, moist granulation bed, occur in the "gaiter area" on the medial or lateral aspects of the ankle, and are often accompanied by stasis dermatitis and stasis pigmentation changes.

B. Imaging and Other Diagnostic Studies

Duplex ultrasound can identify the presence and location of incompetent superficial, deep, and perforating veins and has been used to evaluate the function of individual venous valves. Duplex imaging has become the most important test of venous pathophysiology today and should be performed in every patient with chronic venous insufficiency and postthrombotic syndrome. Valve closure times are 500 milliseconds for the superficial vein valves and 1000 milliseconds (1 second) for the deep vein valves. Perforating veins are evaluated with valve closure times of 500 milliseconds. Duplex imaging does not easily assess calf muscle pump function or the presence of proximal obstruction. These concerns are addressed with use of other tests, such as air plethysmography, which gives a quantitative assessment of venous reflux (by the venous filling index), calf muscle pump function (by the ejection fraction), and overall venous function (by residual volume function). These measurements help to stratify patients into treatment groups but are infrequently used compared to duplex imaging.

Determination of outflow obstruction requires venography with or without pressure measurements, although intravascular ultrasound is also very useful to determine the presence or absence of venous obstruction and has become the test of choice in recent years. Descending phlebography involves injection of contrast media into the common femoral vein to test the valves during normal breathing and with a forced Valsalva maneuver. Using this technique, pathologic reflux can be identified in patients with postthrombotic damage. Such testing is reserved in anticipation of surgical correction of the venous pathology if duplex scanning does not provide definite information on pathophysiology. Ascending phlebography, although not used for DVT diagnosis, is used when one is anticipating catheter-directed intervention in the femoropopliteal venous segment for chronic venous changes.

▶ Differential Diagnosis

Congestive heart failure, chronic liver disease, and chronic kidney disease must be considered in the differential diagnosis of bilateral lower extremity edema. Lymphedema is characterized by nonpitting edema of the calf, but also the dorsum of the foot and toes, and generally is not associated with skin pigment changes, dermatitis, or ulceration. Venous edema rarely involves the forefoot out to the toes. Severe arterial insufficiency produces ulcers that are painful, well circumscribed, and located over pressure points on the distal end of the extremity and foot. Ulcers due to autoimmune diseases, erythema nodosum, and fungal infections are distinguished by appearance and distribution.

▶ Treatment

Venous insufficiency is an incurable but manageable problem. Most patients respond well to a conservative treatment program composed of intermittent leg elevation, regular exercise to improve calf muscle pump function, and the use of surgical elastic graduated compression stockings. Although the mechanism by which elastic compression improves the symptoms of chronic venous insufficiency has not been clearly established, recent work suggests that external compression may restore competency of dilated valve cusps and affect venoarterial reflex. Most venous ulceration will improve with leg elevation, external compression, and local wound care. Compression can be achieved with an inelastic bandage such as an Unna boot, an occlusive wound dressing covered by elastic bandage wrapping, or surgical support stockings. Medical management has expanded to include micronized purified flavanoid fraction (MPFF), an orange rind–derived flavonoid that reduces leukocyte adhesion and migration and inhibits endothelial activation and the subsequent increase in capillary permeability. A recent systematic review of 10 studies found beneficial outcomes for patients treated with MPFF, with improved symptoms and ulcer healing and decreased edema, without serious adverse effects.

Surgery is indicated for a small percentage of patients with nonhealing ulcers or disabling symptoms refractory to conservative management. The three main categories of procedures include ablative procedures on the superficial venous system in the face of superficial venous reflux, antireflux procedures, and bypass operations for obstruction. If superficial venous reflux is a significant component of the total venous reflux present, then superficial ablation is appropriate. Such ablation has been found successful in preventing recurrent venous ulceration and has also been found to improve patients' symptoms of both varicose veins and venous reflux. Recently, it has been found that ablation will also heal ulceration in a faster fashion than wound care and compression alone. Ablation may be performed with traditional open surgical ligation and stripping or the more common endovenous procedures such as radiofrequency ablation, endovenous laser therapy, and foam sclerotherapy. The pathology must be accurately characterized so that an appropriate operative strategy can be developed. The most common abnormality in patients with chronic venous insufficiency is incompetence of the popliteal or tibial veins, with or without superficial venous incompetence; 50%-60% of patients have incompetent perforators.

Perforating vein interventions are typically performed in patients with recurrent venous ulcers or demonstrated incompetence of perforating veins under the area of ulceration. Between its inception in the 1980s and the late 2000s, subfascial endoscopic perforator vein surgery (SEPS) was the technique of choice for perforator ablation, as studies revealed that it resulted in a significantly lower rate of wound infections and recurrent ulcers compared to the open Linton procedure. However, continued advancements in perforator ablation techniques in more recent years have led to increased use of percutaneous ablation of perforators, radiofrequency ablation, endovenous laser ablation, and sclerotherapy instead of SEPS. Current guidelines recommend against selective treatment of incompetent perforating veins in patients with simple varicose veins. However, in perforating veins that meet "pathologic" criteria (outward flow ≥ 500 milliseconds in duration, diameter ≥ 3.5 mm, located beneath healed or open venous ulcer), perforating vein interruption is recommended.

Although minimally invasive techniques addressing superficial and perforator reflux have advanced, such treatment of deep reflux disease remains challenging. There are both nonthrombotic and postthrombotic etiologies, either of which contributes to the obstructive component of deep reflux disease. Previous surgical options included venous bypass and reconstruction procedures and patch venoplasty, and specifically in the case of patients for whom iliac-femoral stenosis is confirmed through venography and intravenous ultrasonography, venous stenting has been a successful endovascular treatment option. In the largest series to date, 5-year continued freedom from venous ulcer after iliac stenting was approximately 90%, underscoring both the role of obstruction in the pathophysiology and the effectiveness of relieving such obstruction. Another surgical option is a saphenopopliteal bypass of femorofemoral venous bypass for either iliac vein obstruction or femoropopliteal obstruction without a good profunda vein collateral system. Recently, interventional attempts to open up chronically occluded femoropopliteal venous segments have shown promise. Regarding correction of deep venous reflux, a number of surgical procedures such as valvuloplasty (internal and external), venous transposition, and venous valve transplantation have shown success at very specialized centers. However, these procedures are not in the armamentarium of most venous specialists. Research continues to find a suitable venous valve substitute that is durable and will not thrombose.

Alhalbouni S, et al: Iliac-femoral venous stenting for lower extremity venous stasis symptoms. *Ann Vasc Surg.* 2012;26(2):185-189.

Bush R, et al: Recommendations for the medical management of chronic venous disease: the role of micronized purified flavanoid fraction (MPFF). *Phlebology.* 2017;32:3-19.

Gloviczki P, et al: The care of patients with varicose veins and associated chronic venous diseases: clinical practice guidelines of the Society for Vascular Surgery and the American Venous Forum. *J Vasc Surg.* 2011;53(5 Suppl):2S-48S.

Luebke T, et al: Meta-analysis of subfascial endoscopic perforator vein surgery (SEPS) for chronic venous insufficiency. *Phlebology.* 2008;24(1):8-16.

Musil D, et al: Age, body mass index and severity of primary chronic venous disease. *Biomed Pap Med Fac Univ Palacky Olomouc Czech Repub.* 2011;155(4):367-371.

Raju S, et al: Unexpected major role for venous stenting in deep reflux disease. *J Vasc Surg.* 2010;51(2):401-408.

▼ II. THE LYMPHATICS

LYMPHEDEMA

▶ General Considerations

The lymphatic system fluid dynamics is less understood than those of the venous or arterial system. Most lymph propulsion energy arises from the intrinsic lymphatic smooth muscle contractions that occur rhythmically. Lymphatic luminal pressures are usually 30-50 mm Hg and can exceed arterial pressure under special circumstances. The lymphatic system carries interstitial fluid and macromolecular proteins lost from the capillaries, as well as infectious agents and foreign material, back into the central circulation. Two to 4 L of lymph per day drain into the subclavian vein.

The fundamental mechanism responsible for lymphedema formation is impaired lymph flow out of the extremity. Primary lymphedema causes include abnormal lymphatic development, most often hypoplasia resulting in severe reduction in the number of lymphatics and the lymphatic diameters, and idiopathic lymphedema. Congenital lymphedema develops before 1 year of age, is usually bilateral, and affects males more than females; if familial, it is known as Milroy disease. More often, lymphedema develops during adolescence (lymphedema praecox) and is unilateral; there is a 10:1 female predominance. Lymphedema occurring after age 35 is referred to as lymphedema tarda.

Secondary lymphedema develops from a wide variety of disease processes that cause obstruction to the lymphatic system. The most common of these is surgical excision and radiation to the axillary or inguinal lymph nodes as part of the treatment of breast cancer, cervical cancer, prostate cancer, melanoma, and soft tissue tumors. Many of these neoplasms tend to develop regional lymphatic metastases before progressing to distant metastatic disease, and their treatment commonly involves complete lymph node dissection of the involved territory. Secondary lymphedema may arise at any time postoperatively, including years and decades after the operation. Less common causes of secondary lymphedema are bacterial and fungal infections, trauma, and lymphoproliferative diseases. In many developing countries, lymphatic obstruction due to filariasis is caused by three different parasites: *Wuchereria bancrofti*, *Brugia malayi*, and *Brugia timori*.

▶ Clinical Manifestations

A. Symptoms, Signs, and Assessment

The history of the disease process will usually define the cause of the lymphedema. Development of painless edema in an adolescent girl with a family history of lymphedema would indicate primary lymphedema as a diagnosis. A history of

▲ **Figure 37–5.** Acquired lymphedema. Edema is centered at the ankle and involves the foot and toes.

lymph node dissection or irradiation or the presence of a parasitic infection suggests secondary lymphedema.

Lymphedema development is usually slowly progressive and painless. In the early stages, the edema is pitting, but as the disease progresses, chronic fibrosis occurs and the edema becomes nonpitting. The distribution of edema is also characteristic. It is usually centered on the ankle (Figure 37–5) and is most pronounced on the dorsum of the foot, producing a buffalo hump appearance. Unlike edema of venous stasis disease, lymphedema also often involves the toes. In the early stages, the skin is normal, but skin thickening and hyperkeratosis occur with longstanding disease. A chronic eczematous dermatitis may ensue.

Objective assessment is most commonly performed by measuring the circumference of the extremity, with the difference threshold of > 2 cm to define lymphedema. Additionally, water displacement is used to assess limb volume. The difference between the two arms before and after surgery of over 200 mL has been used to identify secondary lymphedema from lymph node excision.

Rarely, lymphangiosarcoma or angiosarcoma may develop as a complication of chronic lymphedema. This neoplastic transformation of blood vessels and lymphatics is called Stewart-Treves syndrome.

B. Imaging Studies

Venous duplex scans are performed to rule out venous insufficiency and exclude venous obstruction. CT and magnetic resonance imaging (MRI) are useful tests in patients with suspected secondary lymphedema from unknown malignancy. Lymphangiography has largely been replaced by radionuclide lymphoscintigraphy, the gold standard for evaluation of lymphatic function. A subcutaneous injection of 99mTc-labeled substance is injected into the first and second webspace of the toes or fingers, and its movement, transit time, and activity are interpreted. Lymphoscintigraphy carries minimal risk, and its use in conjunction with duplex scans permits the detection of lymphatic dysfunction and lymph nodes and provides information on lymph transport and reflux. Studies show a very high specificity (as high as 100%) and lower but excellent sensitivity (96%).

▶ Differential Diagnosis

A variety of diseases can result in bilateral lower extremity edema. These include congestive heart failure, pulmonary hypertension, chronic renal or hepatic insufficiency, and hypoproteinemia. In patients with unilateral leg edema, differential diagnosis includes congenital vascular malformations, chronic venous insufficiency, and reflex sympathetic dystrophy.

▶ Treatment

Lymphedema is a chronic disease for which there is no complete cure. However, a variety of conservative measures can substantially reduce the risk of further complications and disability.

No drug therapy is effective. Use of benzopyrones (to increase lymphatic transport by macrophages) has shown some benefit. Diuretics can be useful for acute exacerbation of edema secondary to infection, but these agents are not recommended for long-term use in lymphedema.

The mainstay of treatment is external compression and meticulous skin care. Mechanical reduction of lymphedema can best be achieved with a program of frequent leg elevation, manual lymphatic drainage massage, low-stretch wrapping techniques, and IPC. Complete decongestive therapy (CDT) is traditionally the first line of treatment regardless of primary or secondary etiology. CDT is a combination of manual lymphatic drainage, compression therapy with short-stretch bandages and IPC, movement exercises, and skin care. Many different devices are available for use on the leg, and sleeves can be custom fit for patients with postmastectomy arm lymphedema. Graduated compression stockings or short-stretch devices are worn to maintain the results after reduction by IPC or CDT. Good skin care is imperative in order to prevent infection. Moisturizing lotions should be applied regularly, especially after showering or bathing. Drying and cracking of the skin can create portals of entry for bacteria. Infection is difficult to eradicate because of disordered lymphatic drainage and can be limb threatening. Infection can worsen lymphedema, and lymphedema swelling exacerbates infection, so a vicious cycle can occur. This is the reason control of the swelling is so important.

The psychological impact of chronic lymphedema cannot be underestimated. However, with appropriate patient education that results in the prevention of chronic infection or massive edema, this problem can be manageable.

Surgery may be considered in rare cases of severe functional impairment and recurrent lymphangitis. The approaches are either reductive in nature to minimize bulk, or they are reconstructive to rebuild lymphatic channels. Indications for reductive therapies include massive, incapacitating extremities, and the failure of conservative therapy. The Charles procedure involves excision of all skin and subcutaneous tissue from the tibial tuberosity to the lateral head of the fibula and wound coverage by a split-thickness skin graft. Due to unpredictable cosmetic outcomes and associated complications such as cellulitis and sepsis, many variations of this procedure now exist with reported decrease in morbidity. More recently, liposuction-circumferential suction–assisted lipectomy has been successful in treating upper-extremity lymphedema secondary to breast cancer therapy. In this scenario, fat is the primary cause of swelling and not fluid; thus, lymph reconstruction and conservative measurements are ineffective. A recent study describes the outcomes of three patients with lymphoscintigraphy-confirmed lymphedema who underwent circumferential liposuction. With a mean follow-up time of 39 months, distal extremity (hand and foot) edema was improved for all three patients, and lymphoscintigraphy showed improvement in lymphatic flow for two of the patients.

The application of reconstructive techniques is most successful in early disease, when the lymphatics are relatively healthy. Lymphatic channels are rebuilt via microsurgical methods of lymphovenous or lymphovenous-lymphatic bypass anastomosis, lympholymphatic segmental interposition, or free lymph node transplantation. The largest series to date evaluating lymphatic reconstruction, with 1800 patients with primary and secondary lymphedema treated over 30 years with lymphatic-venous anastomoses demonstrates an 87% subject-reported improvement, whereas 83% of patients showed significant volume reduction. Notably, > 90% of these patients were in Campisi stage II and III

lymphedema with persistent edema, but still at a relatively early stage before the onset of fibrosis or severe limb deformation. As the disease progresses and irreversible damage inevitably results, there is little success in restoring flow or reducing fibrosclerotic tissue.

Campisi C, et al: Microsurgery for lymphedema: clinical research and long-term results. *Microsurgery.* 2010;30(4):256-260.

Doscher ME, et al: Surgical management of inoperable lymphedema: the re-emergence of abandoned techniques. *J Am Coll Surg.* 2012;215(2):278-283.

Green AK, et al: Liposuction for swelling in patients with lymphedema. *N Engl J Med.* 2017;377(18):1788-1789.

Hassanein AH, et al: Diagnostic accuracy of Lymphoscintigraphy for lymphedema and analysis of false-negative tests. *Plast Reconstru Surg Glob Open.* 2017;5(7):e1396.

Murdaca G, et al: Current views on diagnostic approach and treatment of lymphedema. *Am J Med.* 2012;125(2):134-140.

LYMPHANGITIS

▶ General Considerations

Lymphangitis is usually caused by a hemolytic streptococcal or staphylococcal infection that arises in an area of cellulitis near an open wound. Multiple long red streaks may be seen coursing toward the regional lymph nodes. Severe systemic manifestations may include tachycardia, fever, chills, and malaise, which left untreated can lead to sepsis and death.

▶ Clinical Findings

A. Symptoms and Signs

Pain at the site of the initial wound is present. High fevers develop rapidly. The streaks may be faint in appearance initially, especially in dark-skinned patients. Regional lymph nodes are often enlarged and tender.

B. Laboratory Findings

An elevated white blood cell count associated with a left shift is almost universally present. Blood and wound cultures should be obtained routinely.

▶ Differential Diagnosis

Lymphangitis should be distinguished from superficial thrombophlebitis, which is usually localized to a single venous segment often with a palpable cord. Patients with thrombophlebitis usually do not appear toxic, although patients with lymphangitis do. Cat-scratch fever should always be considered when lymphadenitis is present. It is also important to differentiate cellulitis and severe soft tissue infections from lymphangitis. In general, lymphangitis is characterized by its superficial location and the linear pattern of erythema.

Treatment

The extremity should be elevated, and warm compresses should be applied. Analgesics and intravenous antibiotics should be instituted immediately. Examination of the wound should be made to determine the need for debridement or incision and drainage of an abscess.

Prognosis

Delayed or inadequate therapy can lead to overwhelming sepsis and death. Aggressive institution of appropriate antibiotic therapy and wound care will usually control the infection within 48-72 hours.

MULTIPLE CHOICE QUESTIONS

1. Which statement regarding the treatment of varicose and perforator veins is true?

   A. Surgical and chemical ablation are preferred compared to thermal ablation of the greater saphenous vein (GSV).
   B. Selective treatment of incompetent perforator veins is recommended in patients with simple varicose veins.
   C. Thermal ablation is an effective approach to the treatment of saphenous veins.
   D. Foam sclerotherapy is associated with improved ablation outcomes compared to all other therapies.

2. A limited duration of 3 months of anticoagulation is recommended for which of the following?

   A. In patients with pulmonary embolism (PE) or isolated distal deep vein thrombosis (DVT) of the leg provoked by surgery
   B. In patients with PE or proximal DVT of the leg provoked by a nonsurgical transient risk factor
   C. All patients with unprovoked DVT
   D. A and B

3. Which imaging study is an appropriate initial evaluation in patients with suspected axillary-subclavian vein thrombosis?

   A. Computed tomography (CT) angiogram
   B. CT venogram
   C. Chest x-ray
   D. Upper extremity venous duplex ultrasound

4. Which of the following regarding superficial thrombophlebitis is true?

   A. Generalized edema is a significant finding in all cases.
   B. Up to 40% of presentations have associated acute DVT.
   C. Ambulation is discouraged due to the painful, inflammatory process.
   D. Most episodes of septic thrombophlebitis require surgical excision.

5. Lymphedema is a chronic condition for which no definitive cure is currently available. Which of the following is true?

   A. The distribution of edema is exactly the same as that of venous stasis disease.
   B. The gold standard for evaluation of lymph function is CT.
   C. Venous duplex scans aid in ruling out venous insufficiency and venous obstruction.
   D. Diuretics are a mainstay of treatment for minimizing the edema.

Neurosurgery

Timothy R. Smith, MD, PhD

Kyle Wu, MD, & Timothy R. Smith, MD, PhD

Consciousness, the complex interplay between wakefulness and awareness, exists on a spectrum from "normal" consciousness to coma, and various states in between. Acute confusional state (delirium) and encephalopathy are among the most common disorders of consciousness encountered in acutely ill patients, especially those recovering from surgery or anesthetic medications or adapting to the hospital environment during the postoperative period. The prevalence of altered mental status in hospitalized patients is high, with reported rates up to 55%, and is associated with increased rates of mortality ranging from 10%-70%. Given the high incidence of altered mental states and their similarity at presentation to various states of primary neurologic disease, an understanding of the pathophysiology, diagnosis, and management of common etiologies is warranted for all medical practitioners.

DEFINITIONS

Consciousness is generally defined as a combination between the experience of the environment and self. It is composed of two components: arousal, a measure of wakefulness, and awareness, a state of perception. This distinction is useful, since the two processes are dissociable. For example, a vegetative state is characterized by a patient who is awake but not necessarily aware of external stimuli or his or her environment (and thus not interactive). On the other hand, the unfortunate patient suffering from locked-in syndrome (due to a structural lesion of the brainstem) is both awake and aware; however, he or she is incapable of movement.

Arousal is generated by activity of the ascending reticular activating system, which is composed of neurons within the central mesencephalic brainstem, the lateral hypothalamus,

and portions of the thalamus. Widespread projections of these nuclei synapse with neurons in the cerebral cortex to generate an arousal response. The arousal response defines the *level* of consciousness (eg, being awake vs asleep vs comatose). **Awareness** is thought to be generated through networks involving the thalamus and association cortices of the frontal, parietal, temporal, and occipital lobes. Processes related to awareness define the *content* of consciousness (eg, seeing a blue circle vs a red triangle). It can be thought of as the way in which one experiences his or her own state of being and relates this to incoming sensory stimuli.

Many terms are used to describe levels of consciousness ranging from alert to comatose. Here we will describe some of the more commonly used terminology. An alert patient is awake and immediately responsive to all stimuli. Stupor is a condition in which the patient is less alert but still responds appropriately to stimulation. An obtunded patient appears to be asleep much of the time but responds, albeit less briskly than expected, to noxious stimuli. A vegetative state is a state of arousal without awareness in which the patient may open his or her eyes, track objects, chew, and swallow, but not respond to auditory stimuli or appear to sense pain (although pain processing is known to occur in the vegetative state). The comatose patient appears to be asleep and does not respond to stimuli. Often, terms used to describe states of consciousness lack consistent definitions, and a clear description of a patient's state of arousal and response to specific stimuli results in more precise communication.

PATHOPHYSIOLOGY OF ALTERED CONSCIOUSNESS

In general, altered states of consciousness occur due to insults to the key anatomic structures or pathways previously mentioned. Owing to the bilateral organization of the brain, typically *both* cerebral hemispheres or thalami, or the reticular activating system within the brainstem itself, must suffer injury to lead to altered states of consciousness. This can arise from causes that may be structural (eg, stroke, hemorrhage, trauma, infection, seizure, tumor) or nonstructural (eg, pharmacologic or altered physiologic states). Structural disease, such as tumor or stroke, will often manifest with a constellation of neurologic symptoms that relate to their anatomic location (alterations in speech, coordination, or movement). Nonstructural disease, such as hypoglycemia, hypoxia, hypercarbia, hyponatremia, and hypothermia, is more likely to manifest with a globally depressed level of consciousness without a clear neurologic motor or sensory localization. Pharmacologic etiologies, such as intoxication or withdrawal, medication overdose, or residual anesthesia after surgery, should be considered and reversed when possible.

Structural Pathology

Structural lesions cause altered consciousness through either insult to the bilateral cerebral hemispheres or thalami or the reticular activating region of the brainstem. Given the anatomic density of brainstem nuclei (ie, a cluster of neurons with similar functions and shared connections), structural lesions affecting the brainstem typically impact multiple functions and manifest with multiple neurologic deficits including cranial neuropathy. Common structural lesions include stroke (both hemorrhagic or ischemic), intracranial hematoma (epidural, subdural, or intraparenchymal), infections (eg, cerebral abscess), or neoplasms.

The reticular activating system is excited by a wide variety of stimuli, particularly somatosensory stimuli. Given that its nuclei are highly concentrated in the midbrain, it may be damaged by central midbrain lesions, resulting in decrease or loss of arousal. Less severe dysfunction of the reticular activating system results in acute confusional state. The cardinal clinical signs of acute confusional state are somnolence, inattention, and disorientation, sometimes with the addition of insomnia and agitation. In addition, perceptions may be distorted, leading to hallucinations and inability to organize and interpret complex stimuli. Disordered perception results in dysfunctional learning, memory, and problem solving. Thought processes can be disorganized and tangential, and the confused patient may develop delusions. In some cases, the acute confusional state presents as delirium, which can, in its hyperactive form, be characterized by heightened arousal, disordered perception, agitation, aggression, delusions, hallucinations, and autonomic hyperactivity (diaphoresis, tachycardia, hypertension, mydriasis). However, it is important to note that hypoactive delirium is the more common variant to manifest in the postoperative setting.

Neurons in the hypothalamus, basal ganglia, midbrain, and pons are thought to be the primary anatomic structures involved in regulation of sleep-wake cycles, as opposed to the midbrain's regulation of arousal. Therefore, lesions involving the pons may preserve a patient's ability to arouse to stimuli but disturb sleep-wake cycles. This contrasts with the typical vegetative state that results from diffuse destruction or injury of the bilateral cerebral cortices (often secondary to global cerebral ischemia) with preservation of the brainstem reticular activating system and sleep centers, leading to a situation of near-normal wakefulness but complete loss of awareness. This leaves the patient with preserved sleep-wake cycles without the ability to interact with the environment.

Nonstructural Pathology

Several nonstructural disorders that diffusely disturb brain function can produce a confusional state or, if severe, may result in coma (Table 38–1). Acute toxic-metabolic encephalopathy (TME), which encompasses delirium and the acute confusional state, is an acute condition of global cerebral dysfunction in the absence of primary structural brain disease. Typically, TME is a reversible consequence of systemic disease, infection, drugs, or metabolic toxins, making prompt recognition and treatment critical.

TME is common among critically ill patients and likely underdiagnosed, especially when occurring in patients who require mechanical ventilation. Risk factors for the development of TME include admission to an intensive care unit (ICU), prolonged hospitalization, advanced age, preexisting primary neurologic disorders, nutritional deficiency, infection, temperature dysregulation, and failure of multiple organ systems.

Table 38–1. Etiology of altered state of consciousness.

Structural	Nonstructural
Trauma: Diffuse axonal injury, contusion, subdural or epidural hematoma	Medication or pharmacologic overdose
Neoplasm (metastatic, primary, or leptomeningeal involvement)	Medication or pharmacologic withdrawal
Infection: meningitis or encephalitis	Alcohol intoxication
Vascular	Hepatic encephalopathy
Ischemic stroke	Infection
Hemorrhagic stroke (intraparenchymal hemorrhage)	Systemic inflammatory response syndrome/sepsis
Ruptured aneurysm, cavernous malformation, or arteriovenous malformation	Global cerebral ischemia
	Myocardial Infarction
Seizures	Pulmonary embolus
Subclinical status epilepticus	Insomnia/iatrogenic sleep prevention
Prolonged postictal state (Todd paresis)	Hypoxia/hypercarbia
Hydrocephalus	Hyperosmolar state
Communicating	Hypo-/hypercalcemia
Noncommunicating	Hypo-/hyperthermia
	Hypo-/hyperglycemia
	Hypo-/hypernatremia
	Hypo-/hyperthyroidism
	Uremia

PATHOPHYSIOLOGY OF ELEVATED INTRACRANIAL PRESSURE

The Monro-Kellie doctrine states that the cranium contains three major components: brain parenchyma, cerebrospinal fluid (CSF), and blood. When healthy, the volumetric sum of these components is maintained at a constant within the rigid and nonexpansile cranial vault. However, in states of pathology, the doctrine states that an increase in one component must be offset by a decrease in another, or else intracranial pressure (ICP) will increase. This offset is normally accomplished by displacement of CSF into the contiguous subarachnoid space of the spinal cord, termed *spatial compensation*. This delicate balance, however, has physiologic limits. Once these compensatory limits are met, an increase in the volume of any component will lead to an exponential increase in ICP, as illustrated by the intracranial elastance curve (Figure 38–1). If pressure in the intracranial compartment increases to nonphysiologic levels, the brain is displaced out of its typical compartment, resulting in "herniation" into another compartment.

Normal ICP in adults is typically cited to be < 10-15 mm Hg. Disease states such as the presence of tumor or blood, the impedance of CSF drainage (hydrocephalus), cerebral edema (commonly due to tumor or stroke), or increased cerebral blood flow (hyperemia as a response to head injury or hypoventilation causing hypercarbia and vasodilation) may raise the ICP to a dangerous level. This creates a positive feedback cycle where increased ICP leads to reduced cerebral perfusion and cytotoxic edema due to neuronal anoxic injury, resulting in worsening edema and further increase in ICP. Furthermore, mass effect from swelling may progress to shifting of the brain parenchyma and devastating herniation.

SIGNS & SYMPTOMS OF INCREASED ICP

Signs and symptoms of increased ICP include altered mental status, headache, vomiting, and papilledema on fundoscopic examination. Cushing triad may be seen in patients with

▲ **Figure 38–1.** Intracranial compliance curve demonstrating the approximate relationship between intracranial pressure (ICP) and an expanding intracranial mass.

severely increased ICP and consists of hypertension, bradycardia, and respiratory irregularity. Obtundation or focal neurologic findings including unilateral pupillary dilation from pressure or traction exerted on the third cranial nerve (ie, the "blown" pupil) are late findings indicative of impending uncal herniation.

▶ Cerebral Herniation Syndromes

Cerebral herniation occurs when increased ICP results in a portion of the brain shifting from one intracranial compartment to another. These shifts may lead to vascular compromise and infarction of portions of the brain or brainstem, disruption of white matter pathways carrying motor and sensory signals, or direct pressure on structures such as cranial nerve III.

Subfalcine Herniation

Subfalcine herniation occurs in patients with a frontal lobe mass causing the cingulate gyrus to herniate beneath the falx into the contralateral frontal lobe. Occasionally, this may result in anterior cerebral artery compression and subsequently ischemic stroke (manifesting as leg weakness).

Uncal Herniation

Uncal herniation occurs in patients with an expanding supratentorial mass. Early symptoms include contralateral hemiparesis, diminished consciousness, and an ipsilateral cranial nerve III palsy. Compression of the Edinger-Westphal nucleus leads to dilation of the pupil due to loss of parasympathetic input. As further herniation and midbrain/reticular activating system compression occur, somnolence ensues. Late-stage herniation may eventually result in brain death and eventual cardiopulmonary collapse.

Cerebellar Tonsillar Herniation

Posterior fossa masses cause symptoms by compressing the brainstem and obstructing the outward flow of CSF (hydrocephalus). As ICP increases in the posterior fossa, the cerebellar tonsils may be pushed into or through the foramen magnum. As the medulla is compressed, apnea results from dysfunction of the medullary respiratory center, ultimately leading to cardiopulmonary arrest.

Upward Transtentorial Herniation

Posterior fossa masses may cause obstructive hydrocephalus, leading to increased pressure in the posterior fossa (ie, infratentorial compartment) that is greater than the pressure of the supratentorial compartment, which in turn leads to upward herniation of the posterior fossa contents, including cerebellum and brainstem. This leads to brainstem dysfunction and eventually brain death.

DIAGNOSTIC EVALUATION OF ALTERED CONSCIOUSNESS

The diagnosis of an altered state of consciousness is provided by general physical examination, neuroradiologic imaging, drug screens, and laboratory studies.

Neurologic Examination

The neurologic exam includes assessment of level of consciousness, brainstem reflexes, and motor activity. Rapid, standardized assessment of the level of consciousness is useful for clinical decision making and communication. The level of alertness reflects the severity of the underlying condition; severely affected patients are comatose. Commonly, the Glasgow Coma Scale (GCS) (Table 38–2) is used to quickly assess and communicate the level of consciousness of a patient. It was initially developed for patients suffering from head trauma, but it is also widely used as assessment of level consciousness regardless of etiology. A patient with a GCS score ≤ 8 is generally considered severe, possibly requiring intubation for ventilation. As opposed to obtundation or somnolence, the cardinal feature of acute confusional state is impaired attention. Simple bedside tasks such as serial subtraction or naming the months of the year in reverse can be used to test attention. Marked fluctuations in mental status over time are characteristic. Other common findings include a disturbed sleep-wake cycle, decreased alertness, hypervigilance, hallucinations, sensory misperceptions, impaired memory, and disorientation. The thought process is often disorganized, manifested by confused or rambling conversation.

Table 38–2. Glasgow Coma Scale.

Eye opening:	
Spontaneous	4
To voice	3
To pain	2
None	1
Verbal response:	
Oriented	5
Confused, disoriented	4
Inappropriate words	3
Incomprehensible sounds	2
None	1
Best motor response:	
Obeys	6
Localizes	5
Withdraws (flexion)	4
Abnormal flexion posturing	3
Extension posturing	2
None	1

The cranial nerves and their corresponding brainstem reflexes, including pupillary response to light, corneal reflexes, oculocephalic reflex (doll's eyes), vestibulo-ocular reflex (cold calorics), breathing patterns, and the cough and gag reflexes, are used to describe accurately the neurologic status and localize the level of brainstem dysfunction. Generally, brainstem reflexes are only affected in severe TME or with structural brainstem lesions. Abnormal patterns of respiration, particularly Cheyne-Stokes respiration, may also occur with significant brainstem dysfunction.

Motor responses may be categorized as either spontaneous or induced by noxious stimuli, purposeful or nonpurposeful, unilateral or bilateral, or involving either the upper or lower extremities. The patient may display withdrawal from a stimulus, abnormal flexion (decorticate posturing), abnormal extension (decerebrate posturing), or absence of motor activity. Both types of posturing are indicative of corticospinal tract damage. A variety of motor abnormalities are also associated with underlying TME; tremor, asterixis, multifocal myoclonus (sudden, nonrhythmic, gross muscle twitching), paratonia (increased tone with variable resistance), diffuse brisk deep tendon reflexes, or bilateral extensor plantar responses may be indicative of a particular underlying pathology.

Laboratory Studies

The laboratory workup for decreased level of consciousness is focused mainly on sorting out toxic-metabolic abnormalities. Basic studies include a complete blood count, coagulation studies, complete metabolic panel, calcium, magnesium, phosphate, glucose, blood urea nitrogen, creatinine, bilirubin, liver enzymes, ammonia, serum osmolality, and arterial blood gases. Toxicology screening should be performed for suspected intoxications. Blood, sputum, urine, or CSF cultures should be considered if there is concern for infection. Further analysis of CSF with white and red blood cell counts, protein, and glucose may suggest an infectious or neoplastic process. Targeted studies may also be performed such as those for encephalitis or meningitis (eg, herpes simplex virus polymerase chain reaction, fungal cultures) or neoplastic processes (eg, cytology, flow cytometry). Thyroid function tests and vitamin B_{12} and serum cortisol concentrations should be assessed if endocrinopathy is suspected.

Neuroradiologic Studies

Emergent computed tomography (CT) imaging to assess for structural lesions (eg, intracerebral hemorrhage, large territory ischemic stroke, hydrocephalus, neoplasm, or diffuse cerebral edema) is strongly recommended for patients presenting with focal neurologic deficits or severe decline in level of consciousness. Acute ischemic stroke within the first 3-4 hours may be clinically occult on CT imaging. Magnetic resonance imaging (MRI) of the head is generally reserved to further assess for acute ischemic stroke as well as further characterization of neoplastic lesions. MRI should not be relied upon for an emergent diagnosis given the time required to obtain the study.

Electroencephalography

The electroencephalogram (EEG) can both confirm global cerebral dysfunction and exclude subclinical status epilepticus with greater sensitivity than clinical examination alone. EEG should be considered in patients with altered consciousness without a clear structural or toxic-metabolic etiology. The degree of diffuse slowing of the normal background plus abnormal mixed rhythms in the EEG correlates with the severity of TME. Slowing can be categorized as follows: mild, with a reduction in the normal alpha frequencies (8-13 Hz); moderate, with theta frequencies (4-8 Hz); and severe, delta frequencies (< 4 Hz).

ICP Monitoring

Quantification of ICP is critical for management of patients with large intracerebral lesions resulting in mass effect and shift of midline structures, diffuse cerebral edema, or hydrocephalus. ICP cannot accurately be estimated based on clinical findings or imaging. There are several methods of direct ICP measurement, but the two most commonly employed in clinical practice are ventricular catheters and intraparenchymal microtransducer "bolt monitor" systems. Other methods such as subarachnoid and epidural devices have much lower accuracy.

The gold standard of ICP monitoring is via an intraventricular catheter connected to a standard pressure transducer. These catheters are usually placed into the lateral ventricle via a small frontal burr hole. The advantages of intraventricular catheters are that they measure global ICP, allow for therapeutic drainage of CSF to lower ICP, and are amenable to external calibration. Disadvantages include risk for infection, catheter-induced hematoma, or misplacement after insertion due to the blind nature of the procedure.

Microtransducer-tipped ICP monitors are most commonly placed in the brain parenchyma through a skull bolt. They are almost as accurate as intraventricular catheters and have the advantages of lower infection and complication rates. The major disadvantages are an inability to drain CSF and inability to recalibrate after placement, with a slight drift of measurements over time. They are generally reserved for situations of trauma or altered consciousness to guide further treatments. Because they are purely diagnostic, in cases where increased ICP is suspected, external ventricular catheter placement is favored.

MANAGEMENT OF ALTERED CONSCIOUSNESS

The initial treatment of a patient with an alteration in consciousness must employ management of the ABCs: airway, breathing, and circulation. Patients who are not responsive enough to protect their own airway require intubation to reduce the risk of aspiration of gastric contents. During intubation, hypoxia and hypotension should be avoided in brain-injured patients and a high suspicion for cervical spine injury should be maintained in cases of trauma. A patient presenting with a GCS score ≤ 8 may require intubation for airway protection and to provide adequate oxygenation and ventilation. Patients presenting with hypotension and shock must be aggressively treated with fluids and vasopressors to maintain adequate perfusion. Sources of shock (septic, cardiogenic, or hypovolemic) should be investigated and treated appropriately.

Regardless of the cause of acute decline in mental status, a number of general measures should be instituted. There should be a discontinuation of all drugs with potential toxicity to the CNS, if possible. Antipsychotic medications such as haloperidol or quetiapine can be used for management of severe agitation. Thiamine should be administered to patients with a history of alcoholism, malnutrition, cancer, hyperemesis gravidarum, or renal failure on hemodialysis in order to prevent the development of Wernicke encephalopathy.

In the event that a patient presents with history or examination findings suggestive of elevated ICP, immediate life-saving measures may be required prior to a detailed laboratory workup. These situations generally rely upon clinical judgment, and expert consultation with a neurologist or neurosurgeon is strongly recommended. An examination consistent with a critically elevated ICP (coma with GCS score < 8, unilateral or bilaterally fixed and dilated pupil[s], decorticate or decerebrate posturing, or Cushing triad of bradycardia, hypertension, and respiratory depression) warrants immediate intervention while delaying additional diagnostic studies. In addition to standard resuscitation measures, other measures include elevation of the head above the heart (usually 30 degrees) to increase cerebral venous outflow, temporary hyperventilation to a goal $PaCO_2$ of 26 to 30 mm Hg, and administration of intravenous hyperosmolar therapy (either mannitol or hypertonic saline infusion). Immediately following these measures, rapid evaluation of the underlying diagnosis by obtaining a thorough history, detailed neurologic examination, and neuroradiologic imaging should be pursued. Neurosurgical consultation should be considered for potential placement of a ventriculostomy as a means to assess ICP and potentially treat with CSF drainage.

If elevated ICP is present, therapy should be directed to maintain ICP < 20 mm Hg. Interventions should be used only when ICP is sustained above 20 mm Hg for more than 5 minutes. Transient physiologic elevations in ICP may be observed in the setting of coughing, movement, suctioning, or ventilator asynchrony and should not be targeted by therapy. During periods of elevated ICP, it is important to maintain adequate mean arterial pressure (MAP) to ensure adequate cerebral perfusion pressure (CPP; which is equal to MAP minus ICP).

GENERAL MANAGEMENT OF ELEVATED ICP

1. Blood pressure control—Therapy with vasopressors should be targeted to maintain an adequate CPP (CPP = MAP – ICP), typically > 60 mm Hg. Hypertension should generally only be treated when CPP > 120 mm Hg. CPP < 50 mm Hg is associated with cerebral ischemia.

2. Head position—Patients with elevated ICP should be positioned with the head elevated 30 degrees above the heart while maintaining the neck in neutral position without excessive flexion or rotation to maximize intracranial venous outflow.

3. Removal of CSF—When hydrocephalus is discovered, a ventriculostomy may be used to reduce intracranial CSF volume and secondarily ICP. Controlled drainage of CSF at a rate of approximately 1-2 mL/min until the goal ICP is reached (ICP < 20 mm Hg) or until CSF is no longer easily obtained is recommended. CSF drainage via an intrathecal lumbar drain is generally contraindicated in the setting of elevated ICP due to the risk of inducing herniation through a pressure differential.

4. Hyperventilation—The use of mechanical ventilation to lower $PaCO_2$ to a goal of 26-30 mm Hg induces cerebral vasoconstriction, decreasing the cerebral blood volume and rapidly reducing ICP. The effect of hyperventilation on ICP typically lasts for a period of hours prior to metabolic compensation. Therapeutic hyperventilation should be used only as an emergent intervention to temporarily control ICP and be replaced by other therapy modalities.

HYPEROSMOTIC THERAPY

1. Mannitol—Osmotic diuretics reduce brain volume by creating an osmotic gradient from the brain parenchyma to the intravascular space, thus drawing free water from the parenchyma. It is also known to decrease blood viscosity by altering red blood cell rheology for more effective oxygen delivery and acts as a free radical scavenger. Mannitol is prepared in a 20% solution and can be given as a bolus of 1-1.5 g/kg. Mannitol can be used in serial doses at intervals of every 6 hours at a reduced dosage of 0.25-0.5 g/kg as needed for continued elevated ICP. The onset of action is within minutes, and the duration of effect varies widely from 4-24 hours. Serial measurements of serum sodium, serum osmolality, and renal function are necessary to prevent overdosage and end-organ failure. Contraindications to the use of mannitol include serum sodium > 150 mEq, serum osmolality > 320 mOsm, or evidence of evolving acute tubular necrosis. In addition, mannitol may induce hypotension and subsequently decrease cerebral perfusion. Mannitol should be used with care in patients with acute or chronic renal disease.

2. Hypertonic saline—Bolus dosing of hypertonic saline (typical tonicity ranging from 1.8%-23.4%) can acutely lower ICP. The typical volume of hypertonic saline varies widely depending on tonicity, ranging from 30 mL of 23.4% to 1 L of 1.8%. Continuous infusion of hypertonic saline (1.8%-3%) to maintain hypernatremia may also be effective in controlling ICP. A meta-analysis of multiple clinical trials comparing the efficacy of mannitol to hypertonic saline for management of elevated ICP from a variety of causes (eg, traumatic brain injury, stroke, tumors) found that hypertonic saline appeared to have greater efficacy in reducing elevated ICP, but clinical outcomes were not examined. Hypertonic saline should generally not be administered through a peripheral intravenous catheter.

3. Fluid management—Typically, patients with elevated ICP should be kept euvolemic and normo- to hyperosmolar. Administration of free water and hypotonic solutions should be strictly avoided, and instead, isotonic fluids should be used in all maintenance fluids and infusions. Serum sodium levels should be closely monitored, and hyponatremia should be appropriately corrected.

4. Sedation—Maintenance of adequate sedation can decrease ICP by reducing cerebral metabolic demand, ventilator asynchrony, and the sympathetic responses of hypertension and tachycardia. Adequate sedation typically requires the establishment of a secure airway. Infusion of propofol is often the drug of choice for sedation because it can be rapidly titrated, thus allowing for frequent neurologic assessments. Adequate pain control, often using fentanyl bolus or infusion, should be maintained while patients are chemically sedated.

5. Fever—Fever increases brain metabolism, which increases cerebral blood flow and thus elevates ICP. Additionally, fever has been demonstrated to worsen brain injury in animal models. Therefore, aggressive treatment of fever, including acetaminophen and cooling, is recommended in patients with increased ICP.

6. Antiepileptic therapy—Seizures, either convulsive or nonconvulsive, increase cerebral metabolism, resulting in ICP elevation. Aggressive treatment of seizures with antiepileptic therapy or infusion of anesthetics and continuous EEG monitoring are warranted. However, prophylactic antiepileptic therapy is not indicated for direct treatment or prophylaxis of elevated ICP, although it may be reasonable to consider in cases of high-risk structural lesions such as tumor or hemorrhage within supratentorial cortical locations or lesions in contact with the cerebral cortex.

7. Glucocorticoids—Glucocorticoids, typically dexamethasone, are reserved for the management of elevated ICP due to vasogenic edema, most often secondary to intracranial neoplasm. Typically, dexamethasone is dosed every 6-24 hours at doses ranging from 2-6 mg. The use of glucocorticoids has been associated with a worse outcome in a large randomized clinical trial in traumatic brain injury and is not recommended. Glucocorticoids are not considered to be useful in the management of cerebral infarction or intracranial hemorrhage.

8. Barbiturates—The use of barbiturates to control ICP is based on the drug's ability to dramatically reduce brain metabolism and secondarily cerebral blood flow. Pentobarbital is most commonly used, with a loading dose of 5-20 mg/kg as a bolus, followed by 1-4 mg/kg/h. The barbiturate infusion is titrated based on assessment of ICP and CPP and tolerance of side effects. Continuous EEG monitoring is generally used, with titration to an EEG burst suppression pattern indicating appropriate suppression of cerebral metabolism. Barbiturate therapy is complicated and fraught with complications, particularly hypotension, adynamic ileus, reduced mucociliary clearance of the airway, and increased risk of infections. In general, the use of barbiturates is reserved for elevated ICP refractory to all other treatment modalities.

9. Therapeutic hypothermia—The use of hypothermia to treat elevated ICP has been controversial for decades, and its use is currently not recommended in cases of trauma. However, out-of-hospital cardiac arrest patients have been shown to have improved neurologic outcomes following targeted therapeutic hypothermia, such that it is now part of the American Heart Association's guidelines. Hypothermia decreases cerebral metabolism and secondarily reduces cerebral blood volume and ICP. When used, hypothermia is achieved by whole-body cooling using surface or intravascular cooling devices to a goal of 32-34°C. Some studies have demonstrated significant adverse effects, including cardiac arrhythmias and severe coagulopathy. Given the uncertainty surrounding appropriate use of therapeutic hypothermia in patients with elevated ICP, this treatment should be limited to post–cardiac arrest patients or those with intracranial hypertension refractory to other therapies.

10. Paralysis—Sustained paralytic use may be employed as an end-of-the-line medical measure to promote ventilator synchrony, prevent brisk bucking and straining, and reduce overall systemic metabolism, allowing for increased oxygen delivery to the cerebrum. The literature generally does not support the use of paralysis, as it has been shown to cause a host of complications and prolong ICU length of stay, without clear benefit.

11. Decompressive craniectomy—Decompressive craniectomy is the surgical removal a large portion of the cranial vault to allow for the edematous intracranial contents to expand into the newly enlarged and soft compartment below the scalp to reduce ICP. At the time of the procedure, any mass lesion (neoplasm or hematoma) is also removed. Decompressive craniectomy is often considered as a last resort for ICP management. There exists evidence that it decreases mortality but increases the number of patients with poor neurologic outcomes in cases of severe traumatic brain injury with refractory ICP. It has also shown potential benefit in healthy younger stroke patients suffering from malignant middle cerebral artery infarction.

Aslaner MA, Boz M, Celik A, et al: Etiologies and delirium rates of elderly ED patients with acutely altered mental status: a multi-center prospective study. *Am J Emerg Med.* 2017;35(1):71-76.

Bhatia A, Gupta AK: Neuromonitoring in the intensive care unit. I. Intracranial pressure and cerebral blood flow monitoring. *Intensive Care Med.* 2007;33:1263-1271.

Diedler J, Sykora M, Blatow M, et al: Decompressive surgery for severe brain edema. *J Intensive Care Med.* 2009;24:168.

Edwards P, Arango M, Balica L, et al: Final results of MRC CRASH, a randomised placebo-controlled trial of intravenous corticosteroid in adults with head injury-outcomes at 6 months. *Lancet.* 2005;365:1957.

Kamel H, Navi BB, Nakagawa K, et al: Hypertonic saline versus mannitol for the treatment of elevated intracranial pressure: a meta-analysis of randomized clinical trials. *Crit Care Med.* 2011;39:554.

The Brain Trauma Foundation; American Association of Neurological Surgeons; Congress of Neurological Surgeons; Joint Section on Neurotrauma and Critical Care. Guidelines for the management of severe traumatic brain injury. VI. Indications for intracranial pressure monitoring. *J Neurotrauma.* 2007;24:S37-S44.

▼ IMAGING OF THE CENTRAL NERVOUS SYSTEM

Kyle Wu, MD, & Timothy R. Smith, MD, PhD

INTRODUCTION

Imaging has become central to medical care over the past 25 years and is one of the fastest-growing components of medical care expenditures in this country. In no field of medicine has imaging made more of an impact than in the neurosciences. The ability to demonstrate anatomy and pathology noninvasively and treat many pathologic central nervous system (CNS) processes using minimally invasive techniques has grown immensely with the recent improvements in imaging technology.

Forty years ago, the only way to image the CNS was to replace CSF with contrast material (dye) or air via a lumbar puncture and take x-rays—a difficult technique called *pneumoencephalography*. Normal and abnormal CNS structures could be crudely outlined in this manner. Pneumoencephalography was abandoned in the late 1970s with the development of CT. Injecting dye directly into major blood vessels of the neck (cerebral angiography) has been available for three-quarters of a century and allows exquisite delineation of intrinsic vascular pathology but still does little to directly visualize the brain or spinal cord. Although angiography is still performed today for both diagnostic and therapeutic purposes, the catheter is now placed via femoral or radial arterial cannulation instead of directly into a neck vessel.

With the advent of CT scanning in the early 1970s, direct visualization of the brain was finally possible, although resolving normal brain parenchymal structures and some pathologic processes remained difficult. MRI first became available for clinical use in the early 1980s and has been the standard for evaluation of most CNS processes since the mid-1980s.

CT and MRI have continued to mature through the 1990s and into the 21st century. In addition to the introduction of lower radiation dose scanner capabilities on the most recent generation (since the late 2000s) of CT scanners, rapid scanning techniques on such scanners (multislice or multidetector CT scanners) now allow for an increasing amount of data collection and resolution in a shorter period of time. Similarly, such state-of-the-art scanners can be used to generate models of the major blood vessels of the brain (CT angiograms), lessening the need for more invasive intravascular catherization in some patients.

MRI advances have been equally as dramatic, particularly with the release of higher field strength magnetic resonance (MR) scanners (3.0 T) for clinical use in 2005. For example, the sensitivity of some of the newer MRI scanning techniques enables identification of physiologic changes in the brain minutes after ischemia occurs, a time frame that can potentially allow for pharmacologic or interventional procedures that might improve clinical outcomes (eg, stroke). Functional MRI can be used to assess eloquent areas of the brain near pathologic lesions (eg, tumors) that should be avoided during surgery. MR spectroscopy (MRS) can identify lesion metabolites that may help discriminate among pathologic processes (eg, tumor, radiation necrosis, ischemia, inflammation, or infection); however, its true clinical utility is still under debate. MRS can also potentially identify metabolites accumulating in the brain in patients with congenital metabolic disorders. MR angiography can be used to image and form three-dimensional reconstructions of blood vessels for evaluation without injection of dye or the use of ionizing radiation.

Endovascular angiography has been available in various forms for over 80 years and has continued to evolve rapidly over past decade. Initially used as a diagnostic tool, the field of interventional neuroradiology now employs a variety of multimodal therapies and continues to experience significant growth, as it exists at the cross-section of multiple disciplines, including radiology, neurology, and neurosurgery. Neuro-interventionalists are now able to visualize and treat vascular abnormalities such as cerebral aneurysms or arteriovenous malformations through a catheter as an adjunct to, or even in lieu of, open surgery. At this time, more than 70% of cerebral aneurysms treated in the United States are currently managed endovascularly, avoiding the need for craniotomy in some patients. Given the less invasive nature yet generally durable outcomes of endovascular treatment, it remains an area of increasing innovation and has been widely adopted across the globe.

BASIC CENTRAL NERVOUS SYSTEM IMAGING TECHNIQUES

1. Plain radiographs (ie, x-rays) are relatively inexpensive, universally available, and sensitive to detecting osseous abnormalities such as fractures or gross destructive lesions (Figure 38–2). The main disadvantage of plain x-rays is that soft tissues (eg, brain and spinal cord) and many pathologic processes (eg, hemorrhage, infarctions, tumors, abscesses, herniated discs) cannot be detected. Even many intrinsic osseous lesions are difficult to delineate. In fact, until 30%-50% of bone marrow trabeculae are replaced by a pathologic process (eg, tumor, infection), no osseous abnormality is seen on a plain radiograph.

Another limitation of plain radiographs is that all structures are superimposed on a single two-dimensional image as the x-ray beam passes through the entire head or spine (as opposed to the multiple "slices" generated on CT and MRI scans).

There is a limited role for plain radiographs during the evaluation of CNS disease as the soft tissue structures within the cranium and spinal canal are not imaged. However, x-rays offer a cost-effective and efficient means to assess spinal column deformity or misalignment and are often used to evaluate for motion between vertebral bodies of the spinal column as they can be performed in

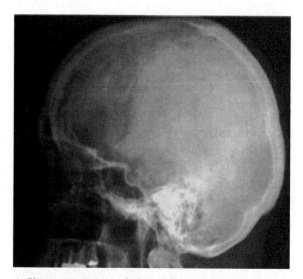

▲ **Figure 38–2.** Lateral plain radiograph (x-ray) of the skull (ionizing radiation). Note the excellent delineation of the osseous structures but poor delineation of soft tissues; specifically, no portion of the brain is imaged. In addition, this study is not tomographic (ie, is not a slice), and therefore, both the left and right sides of the head are superimposed.

a relatively dynamic fashion (ie, lateral flexion/extension/ standing radiographs of the cervical or lumbar spine) compared to CT or MRI imaging. Furthermore, they can be used in the postoperative setting to evaluate placement of internal spinal hardware.

2. Ultrasound of the CNS is predominantly used in the neo-natal period through the anterior fontanelle as a nonin-vasive and radiation-free method by which to screen for intraventricular hemorrhage, abnormal ventricular mor-phology, or gross underlying parenchymal pathology. It is particularly useful for trending ventricular dimensions in infants suffering from hydrocephalus or for viewing the conus medullaris in patients younger than 3 months of age. In addition, prenatal ultrasound as a means of early screening for brain or spinal anomalies is rou-tinely employed. Ultrasound technology also has grow-ing applications in adult patients with neurologic disease, both in and out of the operating room. Intraoperative ultrasound has grown in popularity with neurosurgeons because it offers "live" imaging that can be particularly useful for localizing pathology and evaluating extent of lesion resection and can also be used to help position ven-tricular catheters during surgery.

Adult patients suffering from a ruptured cerebral aneurysm are at increased risk for vasospasm and sub-sequent stroke, and transcranial Doppler examinations to diagnose this disease may be performed by scanning through the thin temporal bone. A specially trained ultrasonographer provides bedside measurements of the velocities of major intracranial arteries (ie, anterior, middle, and posterior cerebral arteries) and compares them to a control, often the internal carotid artery. This provides a noninvasive means to assess for cerebral artery vasospasm in high-risk patients. In addition, the ultraso-nographer may perform a lengthier study to evaluate for "hits" (ie, embolic events) that could be causing symp-toms of transient ischemic attack or stroke.

3. CT scanning with or without intravenous administration of iodinated contrast material is performed using a thin fan-like band of x-rays (ionizing radiation) that are gen-erated by an x-ray–emitting tube that rotates around the patient on the order of seconds. The resultant image, which represents a "slice" of tissue, can be obtained with images as thin as 1 mm. "Reformatted" submillimeter images or three-dimensional models can also be generated in nearly any plane (eg, sagittal, coronal, off-axis) by the CT com-puter software using axial CT scan data in any plane (eg, sagittal, coronal, off-axis,). Three-dimensional images can also be created in this manner. One notable risk of iodin-ated contrast administered during CT angiograms (CTA) is the risk of causing contrast-induced neuropathy, the third most common cause of acute kidney injury in the hospitalized patient.

▲ **Figure 38–3.** Computed tomography scan (ionizing radiation). This image represents a single section ("slice") through the head (ie, it is a tomographic image; the left and right sides of the head can be separately delineated). The brain is directly imaged, although resolving differences in intracranial structures can be difficult (eg, resolving gray and matter structures).

CT demonstrates most osseous abnormalities better than any other imaging test with the possible exception of nondisplaced, nondistracted fractures, which are still often better seen on plain x-rays (Figure 38–3). Soft tissue lesions can also be detected with much better sensitivity than plain x-rays. However, resolving some similar, but not identical, normal soft tissues from one another, delin-eating normal from pathologic soft tissue, and evaluat-ing certain areas of the brain that are limited by scanning artifacts can still be difficult with CT scanning, which is why CT remains inferior to MRI for evaluation of most brain and spinal canal abnormalities.

When discussing CT images, the terms *density* and *attenuation* refer to the same process, namely absorption of the x-ray beam. Areas of increased "density" have greater "attenuation" of the x-ray beam and result in a brighter white appearance on the CT image (eg, bones, iodine-based con-trast material, acute blood, areas of calcification, and some foreign bodies). Areas of lower density have lower attenuation because they absorb less of the x-ray beam as it passes through the patient, resulting in darker areas on the CT scan image (eg, fluid in the ventricles, gas, and fat). CT scans are exceptionally useful for rapid assessment of the intracranial vault, such as in situations of neurologic decline that could be due to a structural cause (eg, hemorrhage, tumor, stroke), with the caveat that acute strokes may be difficult to detect on CT scan and are more readily diagnosed based on clinical assessment and/or MRI. CT scans are also often obtained on an elective basis for patients who will be undergoing certain types of neurologic, sinus, or temporal bone surgery.

The addition of contrast agents to CT scans, CTA, has proven to be exceptionally useful in regard to evaluating extra- and intracerebral vasculature. CTA provides a useful, noninvasive alternative to catheter angiography for assessment of vasculature, although it lacks the dimension of time, which can be useful in assessment of certain pathologies such as dural arteriovenous fistulas or arteriovenous malformations. More recently, advances in technology have allowed for the development of the dynamic CTA (dCTA). This advanced imaging modality allows for the contrast bolus and scan to be timed such that the slices acquired have a temporal component to them much like a traditional catheter angiogram. Although not yet widely available, dCTA is another step toward a noninvasive means to replacing diagnostic cerebral angiograms.

4. Myelography involves performing a lumbar subarachnoid puncture (or a lateral C1-2 subarachnoid puncture) and injecting less than 1 oz of iodinated contrast material to opacify the spinal canal subarachnoid space, which results in contrast filling of the spaces *around* the spinal cord. This is particularly useful for evaluating for areas of cord or nerve root compression from extradural lesions such as epidural tumors, hematomas, bone spurs, abscesses, misplaced spinal hardware, or herniated disks. In addition, some intramedullary lesions, such as spinal cord tumors, may be picked up on myelography.

MRI has replaced myelography as the primary imaging modality for evaluating the contents of the spinal canal. At this time, it is mainly reserved for situations when MRI is not possible to obtain (eg, history of metal foreign body or MR-incompatible cardiac pacemakers) or produces suboptimal images (eg, spinal hardware).

Modern myelography is essentially always followed immediately by CT scanning to better delineate relationships of pathologic processes to the subarachnoid space.

5. MRI is an imaging technique that does not use ionizing radiation.

The physics of creating an MR scan are quite complex. Briefly, a patient is placed in a strong magnetic field (30,000× greater than that of the earth's magnetic field). Radiofrequency pulses are transiently (milliseconds) applied to the patient to briefly perturb the water molecules within the patient by raising them to a slightly higher energy level (quantum mechanical model). After turning off the radiofrequency pulse, these water molecules rapidly return to their respective baseline states and, in the process, release their recently absorbed energy. The rate at which these perturbed water molecules return to their respective baseline states can be measured by using extremely sensitive receiver coils in the MR scanner. As the rates at which these molecules return to their respective baseline states varies by local magnetic environment (eg, the local magnetic environment is different in the ventricular system as opposed to the lentiform nucleus, white matter, the eyeball, muscles, tumors, etc), these detectable differences among tissues can be localized in three-dimensional space and used to generate an image.

MRIs are obtained that highlight different kinds of magnetic field differences between tissues. In general, most MR studies include T1-weighted and T2-weighted scans as part of the overall evaluation of the patient. MRI scans take longer to perform than CT scans in part because T1-weighted and T2-weighted scans and any additional sequences must be obtained separately. T1-weighted images are distinguishable by the black appearance (absence of MR signal) of the CSF over the surface of the brain and in the ventricles. In contrast, on a T2-weighted scan, the CSF over the surface of the brain and in the ventricles appears bright white (Figure 38–4).

In general, T1-weighted scans are best for delineating cerebral anatomy and areas of contrast enhancement, which occur in many tumors. T2-weighted scans are exquisitely sensitive to subtle changes in water concentrations (in both normal and pathologic tissues). This makes them ideal for assessment of many pathologic processes such as stroke, tumor, infection, or edema. These subtle changes manifest as increased signal (brighter) on T2-weighted scans.

Fluid-attenuated inversion recovery (FLAIR) scans are a form of T2-weighted sequence in which normal fluid (eg, in the ventricles and subarachnoid spaces) has no signal (ie, appears black) and, therefore, subtle pathologic process (which still appear bright on FLAIR images, similar to that seen on standard T2-weighted scans) are easier to identify.

Diffusion-weighted imaging (DWI) is obtained by measuring random motion of water molecules within a defined area (voxel) of tissue. In general, highly cellular tissue and tissue with significant cellular swelling (such as seen after stroke) exhibit lower diffusion coefficients, often referred to as *diffusion restriction*. Tissue "restriction" can represent such entities as hypercellular

▲ **Figure 38–4.** Magnetic resonance scan (no ionizing radiation). Similar to computed tomography (CT), this image represents a single section ("slice") through the head. The white matter and gray matter structures are more easily resolved than on a CT scan, and even some gray matter structures can be resolved (eg, putamina and globus pallidae).

neoplasms, ischemic stroke, diffuse axonal injury, cerebral abscesses, or demyelinating disease.

Susceptibility-weighted imaging (SWI) is a sequence that exhibits exquisite sensitivity to compounds that distort the local magnetic field, making them exceptionally useful for detecting blood products or calcium within the brain. In certain vascular pathologies that demonstrate a history of recurrent hemorrhage, the SWI technique offers a sensitive means by which to screen for these lesions. The most notable example of such lesions is cavernous malformation.

Gadolinium-based contrast agents may also be delivered via intravenous injection to enhance the appearance of normal anatomic and vascular structures, as well as pathologic lesions within the brain (primarily neoplasms or infections). Enhancement pattern may differ significantly among various neoplasms, suggesting certain diagnoses. In patients with poor renal function (glomerular filtration rate < 30 mL/min), gadolinium is contraindicated due to the risk of developing nephrogenic systemic fibrosis.

MRI best delineates soft tissues both intrinsic and immediately extrinsic to the brain, can be performed in any plane (including nonorthogonal planes), and has no known adverse effects at the field strengths used for clinical studies. In addition to better demonstrating tissues than CT, MRI is not limited by some of the artifacts that limit evaluation by CT, particularly in the posterior fossa and spinal canal, where CT artifact can be problematic. Although not ideal for directly visualizing dense osseous structures (where fractures, cortical erosions, and degenerative changes often occur), MR excels at detecting intrinsic (ie, bone marrow) osseous abnormalities (eg, primary bone tumors, metastatic neoplasms, lymphoma, vascular anomalies, osteomyelitis).

6. Cerebral angiography is performed by directly placing a catheter into the femoral or radial artery, passing it in a retrograde manner up into either a vertebral or carotid artery, and then directing it further cephalad until it reaches the intracranial vasculature (Figure 38–5). The catheter is moved using intermittent fluoroscopic guidance with small amounts of dye injected at selected intervals to confirm the location of the catheter. When in position, larger amounts of dye are injected, and serial plain digital x-rays are rapidly exposed as the dye passes through the intracranial vessels in the distribution of the injected blood vessel. Hundreds of images might be obtained during a single injection of contrast material. This procedure is associated with a 0.1%-0.5% chance of causing a symptomatic stroke. Embolic events that are clinically silent occur on an even more regular basis.

This technique best delineates intrinsic blood vessel pathology such as arterial stenosis, aneurysms, arteriovenous malformations, fistulas, moyamoya disease, vasculitis, occluded vessels, and other intrinsic vascular disorders. It can be used to inject dye or medications into specific vascular territories for diagnostic or therapeutic purposes. Catheters can be used to deliver a wide variety of therapeutic devices such as prothrombotic coils and intravascular stents for treatment of aneurysms or intravascular glue for embolization of vascular malformations. Balloon angioplasty or stenting can be used to maintain vessel patency in areas of focal stenosis. There are even mechanical or suction-based methods for retrieving intravascular embolic clot for treatment of patients experiencing stroke.

Endovascular (catheter) angiography has come a long way since its inception in the early 1900s; however, it remains expensive and has a non-zero risk of complications. It also requires complex equipment and

▲ **Figure 38–5.** Angiogram (ionizing radiation). A catheter was placed in the right carotid artery in the neck and dye was injected while imaging was performed in a front-to-back projection of the right side of the head. The bones are then digitally "subtracted" from the image. The exquisite delineation of the blood vessels of the right carotid territory are demonstrated but no intra-axial (ie, brain soft tissues) structures.

is performed by highly trained personnel, often at more advanced care centers. In addition, operator skill continues to play an important role in both diagnostic and therapeutic outcomes. Even with advances in x-ray technology, there remains significant exposure to radiation over the lifetime of the operator. There are currently several alternatives to catheter angiography to evaluate for vascular lesions, such as ultrasound (mainly to assess carotid stenosis), CTA, or MR angiography; each is useful for particular situations or pathologies (Figure 38–6). Despite these evolving diagnostic modalities, catheter angiography remains the gold standard for intravascular imaging given its high resolution and temporal component.

▲ **Figure 38–6.** Aneurysm demonstrated by multiple imaging techniques. **A:** Catheter angiogram (ionizing radiation). **B:** Computed tomography (CT) angiogram (ionizing radiation). **C:** Magnetic resonance (MR) angiogram (no ionizing radiation). Note that the catheter angiogram (**A**; an imaging modality that is associated with a risk of causing a stroke) best defines this anterior communicating artery region aneurysm (arrow). However, the aneurysm is still well seen on the CT angiogram (**B**), an imaging technique that is not associated with any risk of causing a stroke, and is also well seen on the MR angiogram (**C**), an imaging technique that is not associated with any risk of causing a stroke and does not employ ionizing radiation.

7. Radionuclide imaging (scintigraphy) includes positron emission tomography (PET) and single-photon emission CT (SPECT) scans, both of which are molecular imaging techniques. Unlike other imaging techniques, these imaging modalities provide information beyond the structural appearance of normal and pathologic tissues. These imaging methods provide physiologic information on the functional state of tissues.

Low doses of radiotracers (positron emitters for PET scanning and single-photon–emitting isotopes for SPECT scanning) are used to label molecules or pharmacologic agents to image molecular interactions of biologic processes in vivo. The nanomolar concentration of the radiotracer allows in vivo assessment of biologic processes without interfering with the process itself.

PET and SPECT cameras are able to detect, localize, and quantify regional distribution of radioactivity within the brain. Reconstruction techniques similar to those used in CT (eg, filtered backprojection and iterative reconstruction) yield two- and three-dimensional images of the brain.

The main advantage of PET over SPECT imaging is that PET uses "coincidence" detection, which is the ability to detect the simultaneous emission of two gamma rays that are generated when positrons annihilate when encountering negative electrons. Practically, this results in the greater spatial resolution of PET compared to SPECT. Both techniques can be used to study the same biologic processes.

The biologic significance of measured radioactivity on PET and SPECT scans depends on the biological function of the molecule that is attached to the radioisotope. For example, radioligands are available to measure cerebral blood flow, blood–brain barrier permeability, neurotransmitter synthesis, enzyme activity, receptor density, glucose metabolic rates, and gene expression, among other physiologic processes. Analysis of regional brain functions can be more specific by performing imaging both before and after specific pharmacologic interventions, specialized motor or mental tasks (so-called "activation" studies), or therapeutic interventions, such as stem cell or gene therapy.

PET or SPECT imaging can also be used in the clinical arena for localization of epileptogenic foci, investigating dementing disorders, distinguishing between tumor recurrence and radionecrosis, and providing a chronologic record of disease progression (or response to therapy).

Finally, the same SPECT radioligands that are used for cerebral blood flow imaging (eg, Tc-99m HMPAO) can also be used to diagnose brain death. Radioligands such as In-111 DTPA can be used intrathecally for radioisotope cisternograms for the clinical evaluation of patients with hydrocephalus or suspected CSF leaks. Radioisotope studies can also be performed to evaluate for leakage of CSF from ventricular shunts.

ADVANCED CENTRAL NERVOUS SYSTEM APPLICATIONS OF MRI, CT, AND ANGIOGRAPHY

▶ Magnetic Resonance Imaging

A. MR Angiography

MR data can be collected using software that images only moving substance. Extravascular stationary soft tissue does not generate any MR signal on such studies, whereas moving blood or CSF will generate signal. Using these techniques, images of blood vessels can be created with a sufficient level of detail that, in some cases, can avoid contrasted scans or formal endovascular catheter angiography (eg, demonstration of significant atherosclerotic disease in the region of the carotid artery bifurcation or surveillance imaging of a known aneurysm). CSF flow evaluation can also be performed (eg, at the craniovertebral junction in Chiari patients).

B. Diffusion MRI and Perfusion MRI

Using rapidly applied magnetic field gradients, random molecular motion of water molecules can be converted to images and can be presented as "diffusion" MRIs. Rapidly applied gradients can also be used with or without contrast agent administration to assess cerebral blood perfusion.

The combination of diffusion and perfusion sequences is used primarily in the field of stroke neurology. Diffusion MRI is sensitive to early cerebral ischemia, often on the order of minutes. In the setting of acute cerebral ischemia, MR diffusion imaging changes (which usually reflect acute irreversible ischemic change) and MR perfusion imaging changes (which reflect cerebral blood flow) can be performed. The MR perfusion and diffusion images are then compared. As diffusion images usually represent permanent injury (infarction) and perfusion (blood flow) deficits are potentially reversible, if an MR perfusion deficit is more extensive than an associated MR diffusion deficit, it is possible that an area of perfusion abnormality without diffusion abnormality represents viable brain that is at risk of developing permanent injury but is not yet irreversibly injured. This so-called "ischemic penumbra" may derive benefit from aggressive medical or interventional therapy. Alternatively, if a diffusion deficit (representing a region of irreversible brain injury) is similar in extent to a perfusion deficit, this suggests that the ischemic changes are permanent and there is no remaining "at-risk" penumbra of tissue that can be saved, and therefore, aggressive therapy may not be warranted.

C. MR Spectroscopy

Using standard MR hardware, MRS can be performed to evaluate brain metabolites. Normal brain tissue includes many metabolites, the most important of which are N-acetyl-aspartate (NAA; which is found in normally functioning neurons and decreases with neuronal injury), choline (Cho; a component of cell membranes that increases in any process that increases cellular turnover, such as tumors, acute infections, etc), and creatine (Cr; a marker of cellular energy). Lactic acid can also be seen in ischemic cells (as a by-product of anaerobic glycolysis) but is not present in detectable amounts on MRS in normal brain tissue. Of note, MRS is commonly used in an attempt to distinguish recurrent tumor from radiation necrosis in postsurgical patients. In cases of recurrent tumor, Cho is elevated, whereas in radiation-induced change, NAA, Cho, and Cr are all low.

▶ Computed Tomography

A. Biopsy

CT can be used for guidance to percutaneously biopsy or drain lesions that previously required an open surgical procedure, such as a spinal epidural abscess or hematoma.

B. Perfusion CT

While rapidly infusing contrast material through a peripheral vein, using a high-speed multidetector CT scanner, data can be collected that reflects how well different portions of the brain are being perfused. In some patients, there are areas of underperfused brain, which may manifest clinically with transient symptoms (eg, transient ischemic attacks [TIAs]); these regions might benefit from revascularization before the patient suffers irreversible injury (ie, stroke). Evaluations similar to brain MRI diffusion/perfusion imaging to assess for penumbra (see earlier) can also be performed.

C. CT Angiography

While rapidly infusing contrast material through a peripheral vein, using a high-speed multidetector CT scanner, data can be collected that can be "reconstructed" with background data removed such that images similar to catheter angiograms can be created without risk of stroke. Although intrinsic vascular detail is not as good as endovascular catheter angiography, in many patients, it is adequate to address the relevant clinical issue. dCTA uses the same principles; however, it adds a temporal component for assessment of flow through vessels.

▶ Angiography

A. Endovascular Coiling of Aneurysms

Small wires can be passed through an endovascular catheter and directly deposited into a saccular aneurysm where they form coils after release from the catheter. An aneurysm can be filled with these wire coils, resulting in the complete obliteration of the patency of the aneurysm lumen, reducing or eliminating the chance that such an aneurysm might rupture in the future and obviating the need for a craniotomy for placement of an aneurysm clip.

B. Stenting

Instead of open surgery to address a narrowed atherosclerotic or dissected blood vessel, affected blood vessels can be treated via an intravascular catheter, which first uses a balloon to dilate the narrowed portion of the blood vessel and then releases a mesh stent to maintain the patency of the newly dilated vessel. Stents can also be placed at the base of wide-necked aneurysms, allowing for the endovascular coiling of aneurysms that otherwise would not be technically possible. This is referred to as stent-assisted coiling.

C. Flow Diversion

In some instances, stent-like flow-diverting devices may be used, offering lower radial opening forces, increased metal coverage, and decreased porosity compared to traditional endovascular stents. These devices are used to provide hemodynamic uncoupling of aneurysms, leading to eventual thrombosis, with endothelialization of the flow-diverting stent to follow. To prevent intraluminal thrombus formation prior to endothelialization, patients require dual antiplatelet agents (eg, aspirin and clopidogrel) to lower the risk of thrombotic complication. In addition, the altered flow and eventual stent endothelialization pose a risk to daughter arteries that take off from the parent artery in a region covered by the flow diverter. However, in practice, this has proven to have a relatively low incidence, occurring in less than 5% of patients. The indications for flow diversion are increasing and often overlap with those of stenting and coiling. At this time, there remains significant provider-dependent variability in regard to the modality chosen; however, as more data are accumulated, a more specific set of indications for each treatment should be reached.

D. Embolization

Although embolization has a significant history in cerebral angiography, its role is somewhat limited in the treatment of intracerebral pathology, and it is mainly used as an adjunct to invasive open surgery. There are many types of embolic materials, such as coils, particles, foam, or microspheres that may be used to occlude blood vessels (eg, those feeding a vascular tumor or the arterial inflow to an arteriovenous malformation) or thrombose aneurysms. Embolization may be employed preoperatively in situations where the surgeon is concerned about a high likelihood of excessive bleeding or to make the surgical procedure simpler and faster. Pure embolization of certain lesions still occurs, although the indications for such treatment seem to become narrower as newer treatments are perfected and developed.

E. Treating Intraluminal Thrombus

An acute (within 6-8 hours of onset of symptoms) intraluminal occluding thrombus or thromboembolus can often be treated with intra-arterial catheter placement within the blood clot and injection of a clot-lysing agent (eg, tissue plasminogen activator) to reestablish blood flow to an affected vascular territory before permanent brain damage occurs. Alternatively, some intravascular clots can be captured and removed from the vascular system using specialized clot retrieval catheters or suction devices.

Brinjikji W, Rabinstein AA, Nasr DM, et al: Better outcomes with treatment by coiling relative to clipping of unruptures intracranial aneurysms in the United States. *AJNR Am J Neuroradiol.* 2011;32:1071-1075.

Fleischmann D, Boas FE: Computed tomography: old ideas and new technology. *Eur Radiol.* 2011;21:510-517.

Hacke W, Kaste M, Bluhmki E, et al: Thrombolysis with alteplase 3 to 4.5 hours after acute ischemic stroke. *N Engl J Med.* 2008;359:1317-1329.

Hopyan J, Ciarallo A, Dowlatshahi D, et al: Certainty of stroke diagnosis: incremental benefit with CT perfusion over non-contrast CT and CT angiography. *Radiology.* 2010;255:142-153.

McKinney AM, Palmer CS, Truwit CL, et al: Detection of aneurysms by 64-section multidetector CT angiography in patients acutely suspected of having an intracranial aneurysm and comparison with digital subtraction and 3D rotational angiography. *AJNR Am J Neuroradiol.* 2008;29:594-602.

Rajah G, Narayanan S, Rangel-Castilla L: Update on flow diverters for the endovascular management of cerebral aneurysms. *Neurosurg Focus.* 2017;42(6):E2.

Schellinger PD, Bryan RN, Caplan LR, et al: Evidence-based guideline: the role of diffusion and perfusion MRI for the diagnosis of acute ischemic stroke: report of the Therapeutics and Technology Assessment Subcommittee of the American Academy of Neurology. *Neurology.* 2010;75:177-185.

▼ CRANIOCEREBRAL TRAUMA

Pui Man Rosalind Lai, MD, & Timothy Smith, MD, PhD, MPH

KEY CONCEPTS

▸ Traumatic brain injury (TBI) is a significant cause of morbidity and mortality in young adults.

▸ Knowledge of the types of primary and secondary brain injury and their sequelae is important in the management of patients with severe TBI.

OVERVIEW

TBI is the leading cause of morbidity and mortality in the United States and is estimated to affect 2.5 million adults every year. Motor vehicle accident is the most frequent cause of TBI in the developed world, accounting for 30%-50% of all serious head injuries. Traumatic falls and recreational injuries account for 10%-15%, and inflicted injury or assaults

account for 10%-20%. Although individuals of all ages can be affected by TBI, peak age is 15-24 years old, with a higher incidence in males. Head injury is frequent in polytrauma patients, and therefore, the basic knowledge of management for these patients by emergency physicians and trauma surgeons is critical.

TBI can range from mild to severe based on clinical presentation. The majority of injuries (80%) are mild, including concussions, and do not require hospitalization. Patients with moderate to severe injuries should be hospitalized and under close observation, as severe injuries can lead to lifelong disability and death.

CLASSIFICATION

The injuries sustained in the setting of TBI can be divided into primary and secondary types. *Primary injury* occurs at the time of trauma and includes deformative or concussive forces applied to the brain. Primary injuries include skull fractures, lacerations, and hemorrhages (which may take time to fully accumulate). Generally, primary injury is considered irreversible and may be minimized with preventive measures, such as the use of a helmet.

Secondary injury is the brain's biologic response to injury, which includes local inflammation, loss of regulation of cerebral blood flow (CBF), brain edema, and global ischemia from increased ICP. At the cellular level, oxidative stresses from free radicals and apoptotic mechanisms are involved, resulting in decreased CBF and tissue ischemia. At the macroscopic level, cerebral edema occurs through both cytotoxic (cell injury and swelling) and vasogenic (incompetent vasculature) mechanisms. Because the skull is a rigid covering that limits space, any increase in amount of material, such as a hematoma or edema, will result in increased ICP. In severe injuries, this increased pressure may result in brain material herniating out from its compartment, causing clinical herniation syndromes, as discussed in the section on concussion in this chapter.

CLINICAL ASSESSMENT

The basic management of patients with severe brain injury can be divided into the following steps: initial resuscitation, primary neurologic survey, immediate surgical management if necessary, and management of cerebral edema and increased ICP. Initial resuscitation (ABCs) is critical because patients with multiple injuries or severe brain injuries may require assistance for critical functions and are unable to protect their airway. Hypoxia is associated with increased mortality in patients with TBI, and therefore, early endotracheal intubation to secure an airway and to maintain ventilation may be critical. Adequate analgesia and sedation are necessary for many trauma patients at intubation and early resuscitation, but the goal should be to use the minimum amount necessary, as the loss of the neurologic examination may delay and impair critical management decisions. Maintenance of blood pressure is also critical because hypotension (systolic blood pressure < 90 mm Hg) has been associated with a twofold increase in mortality in TBI patients. A coagulation profile (complete blood count, prothrombin time, and partial thromboplastin time) is also recommended on admission. Any coagulopathy, including the use of anticoagulant medications, is important to note because patients may develop sudden deterioration if there is an underlying hemorrhage. Aggressive correction of the coagulopathy is prudent for any patients with evidence of bleeding.

The Glasgow Coma Scale

Once initial resuscitation has been established, a primary neurologic survey should be performed to assess the severity of brain injury. The GCS is the most widely used scoring system to evaluate the severity of the injury (see Table 38–2). The three elements of the scoring system are composed of eye opening, verbal communication, and motor function. Patients can be classified as follows:

GCS ≤ 8 = severe

GCS 9-13 = moderate

GCS 14-15 = mild

Intubated patients are given a score of T after the number (eg, a GCS of 3T indicates the patient is intubated). It is critical that the assessment is not clouded by sedatives or other confounding factors.

In addition to the GCS, the primary neurologic survey should also include an assessment of pupils, gross motor function, and brainstem reflexes (Table 38–3). The mass of a hematoma may cause uncal herniation, resulting in contralateral hemiparesis and unilateral pupillary dilation, requiring emergent evacuation, and may be suspected by the examination. Potential presence of concomitant spinal cord injury should also be assessed.

Diagnostic Imaging

Rapid noncontrast head CT is a critical component of all patients with moderate to severe TBI to assess for the extent of brain and skull injury. Importantly, the head CT is reviewed for the presence of intracranial hemorrhage, which may require urgent surgical evacuation. In addition, there are radiographic markers that predict increased ICP (Figure 38–7), which include decrease in basal and convexity subarachnoid spaces (cisternal effacement), compression of adjacent brain structures (local mass effect), and shifting of brain contents from one hemisphere to the other (midline shift). For patients with facial, skull base, or cervical fractures at risk for intracranial vascular injury, dedicated vascular imaging may be additionally acquired. CTA is a convenient and rapid test commonly used as an initial detection for vascular injury, although conventional angiography remains the gold standard. MRI is rarely used on initial neurologic evaluation but may be useful to evaluate brain tissue for more accurate prognostication of injury at a later time.

TYPES AND MANAGEMENT OF PRIMARY TRAUMATIC BRAIN INJURY

Skull Fractures

Skull fractures can be categorized based on their mechanism, extent of injury, and location. Open skull fracture is defined as a fracture that is visible or exposed to air and usually requires surgical management. Closed fracture may be managed surgically or medically depending on its extent of involvement. Depressed fractures can tear the dura or lacerate the cortex of the brain, and those greater than the width of the bone are usually considered for operative repair. Basilar skull fractures, or fractures that involve the base of the brain, are generally managed conservatively, although one should be prudent to look for damages to the vasculature and cranial nerves and CSF leak. Clinically, one may suspect a basilar skull fracture if

Table 38–3. Common brainstem reflexes evaluated in patients with traumatic brain injury.

Reflex	Afferent	Brainstem Level	Efferent	How Tested
Pupillary	Cranial nerve (CN) II	Midbrain	CN III	Light shined in the eye, observed for pupillary constriction.
Corneal	CN V	Pontine	CN VII	Saline dropped into the eye, observe for blink.
Vestibulo-ocular (oculocephalic)	CN VIII		CN III CN IV CN VI	Hold the eyes open and rotate the head side to side or up and down. Reflex present (ie, normal) if eyes move in opposite directions of head movements. Reflex not normally present in awake patients.
Gag	CN IX	Medulla	CN XI	Pharynx stimulated with endotracheal tube or probe; observe for swallow/cough or aversion.

▲ **Figure 38–7. A:** Normal head computed tomography (CT) demonstrating normal basal cisterns (white arrows). **B:** A head CT demonstrating effacement of basal cisterns (black arrow) and global edema after head trauma.

a patient presents with the *Battle sign*, or "racoon eyes," or hemorrhage from the ear.

▶ Penetrating Injury & Gunshot Wounds

A penetrating injury occurs when an object, such as a bullet, causes a focal injury and penetrates the skull and the brain. Multiple factors determine the extent of damage and outcome of the patient, including the velocity of the penetrating injury, the location, and the extent of injury to the brain. An emergent craniotomy for removal of debris and debridement of surrounding tissue may be performed. The presence of contaminated foreign objects increases the risk for local wound infections, meningitis, ventriculitis, and the development of cerebral abscess. The use of broad-spectrum antibiotics is recommended in these cases, although there is variation in practices on the coverage and duration of antibiotic regimens. Head traumas due to gunshot wounds are fatal up to 90% of the time, and for those who survive the initial trauma, half die in the emergency room. Gunshot wounds that cross deep midline structures, the brainstem, or bilateral hemispheres are often fatal.

▶ Intracranial Hematomas

Intracranial hematomas are collections of blood in the brain or between layers of the coverings of the brain usually due to traumatic rupture of blood vessels. The classification of intracranial hematomas depends on the location of the hemorrhage, namely epidural, subdural, intraparenchymal, and subarachnoid.

A. Epidural Hematoma

Epidural hematoma is bleeding that occurs outside of the dura, collecting in the space between the bone and dura. This type of hemorrhage usually occurs from a skull fracture that lacerates a dural artery, classically the middle meningeal artery by the temporal bone, but not infrequently, also involves laceration of a dural venous sinus. The classic presentation of a lucid interval between the initial injury and subsequent neurologic deterioration is only present in 25% of patients with EDH. Some patients suffer no loss of consciousness on initial insult, whereas others decline acutely after injury without a lucid interval. Radiographically, EDH appears as a lens-shaped (lentiform) hyperdense region on CT and is limited by the neighboring dura (Figure 38–8). In general, EDHs larger than 1 cm in depth or rapidly growing hematomas on repeat imaging are considered for emergent surgical removal. The operative approach involves a standard craniotomy over the EDH to allow for hematoma evacuation and to inspect for any active dural vessels that may be coagulated. The outcome for patients with a large EDH can be quite good if managed promptly since the primary injury does not involve the brain.

▲ Figure 38–8. Acute epidural hematoma after head trauma in a 5-year-old patient.

B. Acute Subdural Hematoma

Acute subdural hematoma (SDH) is bleeding that occurs under the inner surface of the dura over the surface of the brain, usually as a result of traumatic rupture of bridging veins. This type of hemorrhage is associated with significant force, usually a diffuse, rotational force, that shears the blood vessels. Compared to an EDH, an SDH has a more crescent shape on head CT and can extend to the entire hemisphere of the brain (Figure 38–9). Associated intraparenchymal hemorrhage, contusion, and edema, may also be found beneath the SDH. Patients usually present with progressively worsening mental status, and emergent operative evacuation of the hemorrhage is critical. Typically, SDHs larger than 1 cm in thickness, causing more than 0.5 cm midline shift, or with any accompanying neurologic deficit are candidates for surgical evacuation. The operative approach involves a large craniotomy to evacuate the hematoma. In large acute SDH, a craniectomy (with the temporary removal of bone) may be needed to allow for underlying brain swelling. In addition, these patients should be watched closely for postoperative elevated ICP due to underlying brain contusion and edema. Outcomes for acute SDH are often poor, with mortality of 50%-90% and with significant neurologic deficits.

SDH is more prevalent in the elderly population due to atrophy of the brain, and as a result, much less force is required to stretch and tear the bridging veins. SDH in the elderly often tends to present more chronically, even several

▲ Figure 38–9. Acute subdural hematoma with an associated intraparenchymal hemorrhage after head trauma in a 25-year-old patient.

months after injury. The timing of the hemorrhage can be discerned on head CT, where the density of the hemorrhage is suggestive of its chronicity (Figure 38–10). The differentiation between an acute and a chronic SDH is important because the management is different in the two scenarios. Due to decreased viscosity of old blood, surgery in chronic SDH generally involves a much smaller craniotomy, such as a mini-craniotomy or a burr hole, to drain the old fluid. Outcomes are better than acute SDH, although recurrence and reoperation are common.

C. Intraparenchymal Hematoma

Intraparenchymal hematoma is bleeding mixed within the brain and is the result of a direct blow to the head or at the region opposite of the point of impact (contrecoup injury). Management for these lesions is generally conservative, although large hemorrhage (> 25 mL) may be considered for evacuation. The relative eloquence of surrounding brain structures is taken into consideration for surgery in these cases. Patients with large intraparenchymal hematoma are at high risk of surrounding brain edema and contusion, and close management of ICP is critical.

▲ **Figure 38–10.** Chronic subdural hematoma with acute blood layering in fluid in a 55-year-old patient.

D. Subarachnoid Hematoma

Trauma is the most common overall cause for a *subarachnoid hematoma* (or *subarachnoid hemorrhage*) (SAH), which is blood collection in the subarachnoid space over the convexity of the brain or in the basal cisterns. Traumatic SAH is typically associated with blood collection in the sulci or near the surface of the brain, but blood in the basal cisterns may also be found. If there is a large density of blood collection in the basal cisterns, one should be suspicious for a ruptured aneurysm and a subsequent angiographic study should be obtained to rule out an alternative cause of the hemorrhage. Traumatic SAH is managed nonoperatively.

▶ Concussion

Concussion is an immediate and transient loss of consciousness after head trauma and is often associated with amnesia. It has been thought that concussion is a result of the disruption of the reticular activating system from the cerebral cortex rotating around the more fixed midbrain and diencephalon.

Concussion is common, and the decision to pursue further workup, such as a CT scan, is important. In general, patients with a GCS < 15 or emesis or who are older than age 60-65 years warrant a head CT. Patients with severe headache, intoxication, persistent anterograde amnesia, seizure, or severe mechanism of injury should also be considered for workup.

Management of concussion includes observation for at least several hours, assuming the individual is neurologically intact. Any patients with abnormal CT findings should be closely monitored. Long-term outcome is generally good for the majority of patients, but it is common for patients to experience transient increased incidence of headache, memory problems, and problems with executive function even after several months.

▶ Diffuse Axonal Injury

Diffuse axonal injury (DAI) results from rotational forces or rapid acceleration or deceleration and the traumatic shearing of axons between gray and white matter. DAI is common and occurs in half of patients with severe TBI. Clinically, DAI can present in varying degrees of severity, from a mild concussive state of confusion to coma. Head CT may demonstrate punctate (< 1 cm) hemorrhages scattered throughout the brain, but this is difficult to visualize with this modality. MRI is more useful for detecting injury resulting from DAI for prognostication. Management of DAI is nonoperative and primarily focused on the prevention of secondary brain injury.

TYPES AND MANAGEMENT OF SECONDARY TRAUMATIC BRAIN INJURY

Maximal medical management is directed at detecting and preventing secondary brain injuries, including increased ICP, cerebral ischemia and hypoxia, and cerebral edema.

▶ Physiology of Increased Intracranial Pressure

The **Monro-Kellie doctrine** states that intracranial volume, which is the sum of the brain, CSF, and blood, is constant. An increase in one compartment would be accommodated by a decrease in the amount of another to maintain a constant ICP. When a mass, such as a hematoma, is introduced into the cranial vault, CSF and venous blood are displaced to make room for the mass with relatively normal ICP. However, if the mass is large enough to overcome these mechanisms, then ICP would rise exponentially. This simplistic model is useful for understanding increased ICP after TBI. As secondary injury evolves with increased cerebral edema, ICP increases and results in brain compression, ischemia from decreased perfusion, and herniation. Increased ICP is a strong predictor for mortality and morbidity after TBI.

The concept of CPP explains how increased ICP leads to decreased tissue perfusion, where CPP is defined as:

$$CPP = MAP - ICP$$

As demonstrated by this equation, an increased ICP results in a decreased CPP, leading to tissue ischemia and damage. Under normal circumstances, MAP is between 60 and 160 mm Hg, and ICP ranges from 5 to 15 mm Hg.

This effect is further worsened by cerebral dysregulation in patients with severe TBI. *Cerebral autoregulation* is the mechanism that maintains CBF by controlling cerebral vascular resistance in response to changing arterial blood pressure. For example, in a normal individual, a lowered blood pressure leads to a decreased CPP, which would result in vasodilation to maintain a constant CBF. However, patients with severe TBI often have disruption to autoregulation. In our example, with a decreased blood pressure and CPP, the patient has no compensatory mechanism for dilation of blood vessels, resulting in decreased perfusion. CPP less than 70 mm Hg and hypotension are associated with increased morbidity and mortality. The intricacies of cerebral pressure autoregulation are beyond the scope of this chapter, but a basic understanding of how increased ICP affects cerebral perfusion is important to understand.

The incidence of raised ICP is found in 50%-60% of patients with severe TBI. Radiographic findings that should raise concerns for increased ICP include the presence of mass effect, midline shift, the loss of sulci and gyri from the displacement of CSF, and the effacement of basal CSF cisterns. However, increased ICP can still occur without any radiographic evidence and should be suspected in patients with severe TBI or with a low GCS score.

ICP can be directly measured by the insertion of a monitoring device into the brain, typically performed by the bedside in the emergency room or the ICU. The device can be placed in the epidural, subdural, intraparenchymal, or intraventricular space. The most common devices currently used are the intraparenchymal ICP monitor and the intraventricular catheter, also more commonly known as the external ventricular drain (EVD). The intraparenchymal monitor is a device that places the sensor directly into brain tissue to monitor ICP. This monitor has a lower rate of intracranial hemorrhage and infection compared with the EVD but is subject to drift in accuracy by 3-4 mm Hg after 4-5 days.

The EVD is a commonly performed procedure that involves the placement of a catheter through the brain parenchyma into the lateral ventricles and serves as both a diagnostic and therapeutic device. The EVD is more invasive but allows for CSF drainage as a therapeutic benefit to decrease ICP.

► Management of Increased Intracranial Hypertension

A. Optimization of Cerebral Venous Outflow

Elevation of the head of the bed to 15-30 degrees is the standard of care to reduce ICP by minimizing venous outflow resistance. In patients with TBI who may also have concurrent or unknown spinal injuries, a tight-fitting cervical collar can increase ICP. Loosening the collar, if deemed safe, may improve ICP.

B. CSF Drainage

Currently, according to the guidelines from the Brain Trauma Foundations, it remains uncertain whether the use of EVD reduces mortality, but a Level III recommendation suggests the use of CSF drainage to lower ICP in patients with GCS < 6 during the first 12 hours after injury. Threshold for treatment after TBI is typically > 20 mm Hg in adult patients.

C. Seizure Prevention

The incidence of seizures after a TBI is estimated to be 5%-15%, with the majority occurring within the first 7 days after trauma. Seizure increases cerebral metabolic rate and ICP and may be subclinical in patients with severe TBI. Prophylactic anticonvulsants, such as phenytoin or levetiracetam, are commonly used to prevent seizures after a moderate to severe TBI during the first week after trauma. Prophylactic use of antiepileptics is not recommended for preventing late seizures or the development of epilepsy.

D. Hyperosmolar Therapy

Mannitol is a commonly used hyperosmolar agent for the reduction of increased ICP. Doses of 0.25-1 g/kg body weight are typically used and usually lower ICP in 1-5 minutes, with peak effects at 20-60 minutes. Arterial hypotension (systolic blood pressure < 90 mm Hg) should be avoided. Mannitol can be redosed every 6 hours for long-term ICP management, although careful attention should be paid to the occurrence of mannitol-induced diuresis and renal impairment. Mannitol has both rheologic and osmotic effects by increasing CBF through the expansion of plasma volume and by acting as a free radical scavenger.

Hypertonic saline, given usually in concentrations of 3% or 23.4%, creates an osmotic force to draw water from interstitial space of the brain parenchyma into the intravascular compartment to reduce ICP. Hypertonic saline is preferred over mannitol in hypovolemic and hypotensive patients because it augments intravascular volume and increases blood pressure. Hyponatremia should be excluded before administering hypertonic saline to reduce the risk of central pontine myelinolysis.

E. Hyperventilation

Hyperventilation decreases $PaCO_2$, leading to vasoconstriction and decreases in cerebral blood volume and ICP. Although hyperventilation was once practiced widely, it has now been regarded to play a limited role in the management of intracranial hypertension, as persistent hyperventilation may lead to ischemia. Hyperventilation is recommended as a temporizing measure for reduction of ICP, but prolonged use is contraindicated.

F. Sedation

Pain and agitation can significantly increase ICP, and therefore, the use of adequate sedation and analgesia is an important element of ICP management. The use of sedation with or without chemical paralysis also aids in reducing excessive brain metabolism that accompanies severe TBI. Shorter-acting agents are preferred to allow for frequent assessment of neurologic examination.

G. Barbiturate Coma

The use of high-dose barbiturates is generally reserved for refractory intracranial hypertension. The exact mechanism by which barbiturates lower ICP is unclear, but it is likely associated with reduction of cerebral metabolism by the coupled reduction in CBF and cerebral metabolic rate of oxygen. However, there are serious complications associated with this treatment, including severe hypotension, metabolic derangements, respiratory complications, infections, and hepatic and renal dysfunction.

H. Fever and Hypothermia

Fever is associated with increased metabolic rate and induces dilation of cerebral vessels, which may increase ICP. Fever has been associated with worse neurologic outcome and should be controlled with antipyretics and cooling blankets.

Hypothermia has been shown to slow edema and injury at a cellular level in experimental settings, and although fever has been shown to be associated with worse outcome, randomized clinical trials of prophylactic hypothermia have failed to show benefit. Current guidelines do not recommend prophylactic hypothermia for the management of elevated intracranial hypertension.

I. Steroids

Large randomized trials of methylprednisolone in severe TBI patients were associated with increased mortality. The use of steroids is not recommended for management of ICP.

J. Surgical Decompressive Craniectomy

Decompressive craniectomy is the maximal aggressive measure for management of increased ICP and involves removal of a portion of the calvarium to allow for increased space. The literature has found surgical decompression to be associated with decreased ICP, but its effect on overall neurologic outcome is debated. In clinical practice, decompressive craniectomy is considered the last resort for when maximal medical treatment has failed to control ICP.

CLINICAL OUTCOMES AFTER TRAUMATIC BRAIN INJURY

The medical literature is mixed on long term clinical outcome after TBI, but it has been reported that up to one-third of patients with severe TBI succumb to death or are severely disabled at 6 months. In those who survive, over 50% have identifiable disability 1 year after injury. Predictors for poor outcome include older age, worse initial GCS score, hypotension, hypoxia, elevated ICP, extent of intracranial injury, and existing comorbidities.

Unfortunately, for some patients with a severe degree of injury, the likelihood of a meaningful recovery may be futile. Once the diagnosis and injury severity are confirmed, with unchanged neurologic condition despite maximal resuscitation, a frank discussion with the family is necessary to make appropriate decisions on the degree of aggressive care as per the patient's and family's wishes.

SUMMARY

TBI is a devastating condition with a high burden on young individuals; it also poses a major societal burden. For patients with severe TBI, initial resuscitation, immediate recognition and diagnosis, emergent surgery if needed, and management of subsequent secondary injuries are critical for optimal outcome. Trauma patients with severe TBI may need to be transferred to an institution well equipped to handle major neurologic injuries after initial assessment and stabilization.

Carney N, et al: Guidelines for the Management of Severe Traumatic Brain Injury, Fourth Edition. *Neurosurgery.* 2017;80(1): 6-15.

Rangel-Castillo L, et al: Management of intracranial hypertension. *Neurol Clin.* 2008;26(2):521-541.

▼ SPINAL CORD INJURY

Ian Tafel, MD, and Timothy R. Smith, MD, PhD

▶ General Considerations

Traumatic spinal cord injury (SCI) primarily affects young people, with a median age at diagnosis of 37.6 years, and often results in significant disability or death. The median age of SCI has increased from 28.7 years in the 1970s largely due to an increase in the incidence of falls causing SCI in patients older than 60 years of age. The main causes in order of incidence are motor vehicle collision, fall, violence, and sports injuries. The prognosis for significant recovery of a complete lesion is poor. Recent research into stem cell technology and other new modalities of therapy is, however, showing promise.

The cost of SCI to the healthcare system and society is significant. A 25-year-old patient with a high cervical cord injury (C1-4) is estimated to incur $741,425 in medical costs in the first year following injury and $132,807 for each year survived thereafter. In addition, the loss of wages and productivity for SCI patients averages $57,000 annually. With 12,000-14,000 Americans suffering SCI per year, the social and economic costs are significant.

Treatment for SCI consists of acute and chronic management. Acutely, the ABCs (airway, breathing, and circulation) must be secured and the spine immobilized to prevent extension of injuries. Compressive lesions must be identified and the need for urgent surgical management determined. Although there is debate as to whether the administration of methylprednisolone after SCI significantly improves motor score, the American Association of Neurological Surgeons/Congress of Neurological Surgeons (AANS/CNS) does not recommend its administration. Other acute nonsurgical treatment options aimed at minimizing secondary injury are modest induced hypothermia and hyperbaric therapy; the former has not been proven to have beneficial effects in humans, whereas the latter increases the speed of neurologic recovery, but does not result in an overall improvement in outcome. Chronic management includes physical and occupational therapy designed to maximize functionality. Specific therapy and improvement depend on the level and completeness of the injury.

Clinical Findings

Clinical findings in SCI depend on the level, mechanism, and severity of injury, with injuries being classified as either complete or incomplete. A complete SCI refers to the lack of motor or sensory function below the level of the lesion, while incomplete lesions have some preserved function. Incomplete lesions often result in recognized SCI syndromes based on the region of the spinal cord affected. The American Spinal Injury Association (ASIA) publishes the International Standards for Neurological Classification of Spinal Cord Injury (ISNCSCI) scale to further classify the severity of SCI (Table 38–4).

Initial clinical findings include motor or sensory deficit and hyporeflexia. Initially, all reflexes below the lesion are lost, including the bulbocavernosus, cremasteric, and abdominal cutaneous reflexes, depending on the level of injury. Over time, these reflexes may return, and the deep tendon reflexes may become hyperreflexive due to the loss of descending tonic inhibition of the reflex arc. Initially, paralysis is flaccid, but eventually, upper motor neuron signs develop, and a spastic paralysis results. If the lesion is in the high cervical region (C1-5), respiratory effort may be compromised due to the loss of innervation to the phrenic nerve. Loss of bowel or bladder function often occurs, and loss of rectal tone and sensation, as well as priapism, may result. The loss of bladder control manifests as urinary retention, and developing urinary incontinence is typically overflow incontinence. Loss of anal sphincter tone and sensation results in leakage of stool and lack of awareness of bowel movements.

Table 38–4. The ASIA classification of spinal cord injury.

A = Complete: No sensory or motor function preserved in the lowest sacral segments (S 4/5).

B = Sensory incomplete: Sensory but no motor function preserved below the neurologic level including the sacral segments S4/5.

C = Motor incomplete: Motor function is preserved below the neurologic level, and more than half of the key muscles below the neurologic level have a muscle grade less than 3. There must be some sparing of sensory and/or motor function in the segments S4/5.

D = Motor incomplete: Motor function is preserved below the neurologic level, and more than half the key muscles below the neurologic level have a muscle grade greater than or equal to 3. There must be some sparing of sensory and/or motor function in the segments S4/5.

E = Normal: Sensory and motor functions are normal. Patient may have abnormalities on reflex examination.

Adapted with permission from American Spinal Injury Association: *Standards for Neurological Classification of Spinal Cord Injury* (rev. 2000). Chicago: ASIA, 2002.

An important early finding that can occur in SCI is "spinal shock." This refers to a drop in the systolic blood pressure with accompanying bradycardia, often to a level of 80 mm Hg systolic, following SCI. This is due to the loss of sympathetic tone to the regions below the lesion and causes venous pooling and decreased venous return to the heart.

Chronic clinical findings in SCI are related to the long-term need for ventilatory support, immobilization, and need for catheterization. Pneumonia, urinary tract infections, and decubitus ulcers are common findings and are often the cause of death in spinal cord–injured patients.

Incomplete SCIs may demonstrate a variable pattern of sensory or motor preservation, although they can often be categorized into recognizable clinical syndromes, depending on the mechanism of injury and the portion of the cord affected.

A. Central Cord Syndrome

Central cord syndrome refers to a pattern of injury that affects the motor strength in the upper extremities more severely than the lower extremities. Sensory function is variable below the level of the lesion, and sphincter control is often affected. This usually occurs in older patients with spinal stenosis following a hyperextension injury. The central cervical cord is a watershed vascular territory that is thought to be disrupted in this syndrome. The spinal cord is somatotopically organized such that cervical fibers are more medial compared to fibers traveling to the lower extremities, resulting in more severely affected upper extremities.

B. Anterior Cord Syndrome

Anterior cord syndrome results from the compression of the anterior portion of the cord by a herniated disk or bone fragment or from occlusion of the anterior spinal artery. The corticospinal tracts and spinothalamic tracts are preferentially affected due to their more anterior location, whereas the posterior columns are relatively spared. This results in loss of motor function and loss of pain and temperature sensation below the level of the lesion, with preserved proprioception, vibration, and pressure sensation. It is important to distinguish surgical from nonsurgical (ie, anterior spinal artery occlusion) etiologies in this condition.

C. Brown-Séquard Syndrome

Brown-Séquard syndrome occurs after spinal cord hemisection. It is usually the result of penetrating trauma and occurs in 2%-4% of SCIs. Motor and posterior column function (proprioception, vibration sense) are disrupted on the side of the lesion. Pain and temperature sensation are diminished on the contralateral side due to the crossing of the spinothalamic tract in the spinal cord at one to two levels above the entrance of the fibers into the cord.

D. Conus Medullaris Syndrome

Conus medullaris syndrome results from injury to the sacral spinal cord. Symptoms include saddle anesthesia, loss of bowel/bladder function, and lower extremity weakness. It includes a combination of both upper and lower motor neuron signs.

E. Cauda-Equina Syndrome

Cauda-equina syndrome refers to compression and dysfunction of the lumbosacral nerve roots. It is not a true SCI because it only affects the nerve roots and not the cord itself. The clinical syndrome is similar to conus medullaris syndrome with saddle anesthesia, loss of bowel/bladder function, and lower extremity weakness, but the findings are all lower motor neuron.

▶ Physical Examination

Initial physical examination in SCI focuses on the ABCs (airway, breathing, and circulation). Special attention must be focused on the airway in high cervical injuries because patients may require endotracheal intubation. Blood pressure must be closely monitored given the possibility of spinal shock. This manifests as a drop in the systolic blood pressure and must be addressed immediately to prevent further cord ischemia.

In the awake patient, a history focusing on the mechanism of injury and detailed neurologic examination is undertaken to determine the level and completeness of the injury. Motor strength should be tested in all muscle groups and sensation should be tested with pinprick, and proprioception. Rectal tone and sensation should be tested with digital examination.

Reflexes should be examined, including the bulbocavernosus, cremasteric, and abdominal cutaneous reflexes. Careful palpation of the spine is important to evaluate for obvious step-offs or tenderness to palpation at all levels. The examination must be carefully documented and a neurologic level and evaluation of completeness of the lesion determined.

In the comatose patient, a complete neurologic examination is often difficult. In this situation, observation of spontaneous movements or movements to painful stimuli is important. Deep tendon reflexes should be examined, and palpation of the spine should be undertaken to observe for obvious step-offs. Radiologic imaging is often required to adequately determine a level of injury and its etiology.

▶ Differential Diagnosis

History, physical examination, and radiographic imaging generally arrive at the diagnosis of SCI. Moreover, radiographic imaging can help determine the mechanism of the injury. Some peripheral nerve lesions may resemble SCI, but these are typically unilateral and affect only lower motor neurons. Malingering and conversion disorders may mimic SCI and should be suspected in the setting of serial examinations showing inconsistencies, as well as imaging findings that do not explain the symptoms.

▶ Radiologic Examination

According to the current recommendations of the AANS/CNS on cervical spine injury, in the awake, asymptomatic patient with no spinal tenderness, distracting injury (eg, long-bone fracture), or evidence of disturbed consciousness or intoxication, no radiographic imaging is necessary and no cervical immobilization is recommended. However, awake patients with spine tenderness, numbness, tingling, or obvious signs of SCI (eg, weakness, loss of bowel/bladder control) require a CT scan, or if one is not available, three-view cervical spine x-rays should be obtained (Figure 38–11). In the awake, symptomatic, patient with a normal CT, an MRI should be obtained within 48 hours of injury to rule out ligamentous injury. If the MRI or flexion/extension x-rays are not concerning for injury, then the cervical immobilization may be removed. Additionally, MRI (particularly T2-weighted sequences) also clearly demonstrates compression of and/or signal change within the spinal cord (Figure 38–12).

Obtunded or unevaluable patients with suspected cervical spine injury require CT or three-view cervical spine x-ray if CT is not available and should have an MRI within 48 hours of injury if no injury is noted on the CT or x-ray. Clearance of the cervical spine in this population is still cause for debate, and recommendations are in flux. Generally, however, a lack of injury noted on CT (or x-ray) and MRI allows for discontinuation of cervical spine immobilization at the discretion of the treating physician.

▲ **Figure 38–11.** Sagittal reconstruction of a cervical computed tomography (CT) scan demonstrating a C6-7 traumatic fracture.

▶ Treatment

Initial treatment of SCI consists of securing the ABCs and immobilizing the spinal column. In the case of high cervical spine injury, the need for endotracheal intubation must be identified, and if it is not immediately necessary, serial arterial blood gas assessments should be monitored to evaluate for hypocapnia and progressive ventilatory failure. Spinal shock and the resultant decrease in blood pressure must be treated aggressively if they occur. Volume expansion should be initiated promptly, and decreased systolic blood pressure refractory to volume expansion should be treated with

vasopressor therapy with a MAP goal of 85-90 mm Hg for 7 days following injury. The choice of pressors has not been conclusively defined, but typically a beta-agonist is followed by an alpha-agonist given the possibility of bradycardia in spinal shock.

Patients should be placed in a hard cervical collar, and cervical immobilization should be ensured until clearance of the cervical spine or definitive treatment has occurred. Patients should be placed on a board for transfers and log-rolled for movement until the thoracic and lumbar spines are cleared as well. Other initial management considerations include placement of an arterial line to monitor blood pressure on a constant basis and placement of a Foley catheter to

▲ **Figure 38–12.** Sagittal T2-weighted magnetic resonance image of a C6-7 traumatic fracture demonstrating spinal cord compression and signal change within the spinal cord (arrow).

decompress the bladder. The AANS/CNS does not recommend administration of methylprednisolone after cervical spine injury, citing inconsistent evidence of its benefit and the risk of adverse events such as wound infection, hyperglycemia, and gastrointestinal hemorrhage.

Following initial stabilization and imaging studies, the need for surgical intervention is assessed. Surgery has two main goals: decompression and stabilization. Surgery is employed on an emergent basis for incomplete lesions in the hopes of preserving or improving neurologic function and on a nonemergent basis for complete lesions, as there is no demonstrated improvement in neurologic function for emergent surgery in these situations. Goals of surgery in this setting are to prevent cranial extension of injury and to prevent progressive deformity. The choice of surgical approach for SCI is not standardized and is dependent on the location of the pathology. Current stabilization procedures typically involve instrumented fusion techniques and may be approached via an anterior, posterior, or combined approach.

Cervical traction may be employed either alone or as an adjunct to surgical therapy to attempt realignment of the spinal column. This is accomplished by fixing a halo ring or specialized devices (eg, Gardner-Wells tongs) to the head, connecting this to a rope and pulley system, and adding weight to adjust the spine in the desired vector.

Chronic treatment of SCI focuses on rehabilitation and adaptation to permanent injury. Rehabilitation can often result in improved neurologic function in incomplete lesions and can help those with complete injuries become as functional as possible. Patients may require ventilatory support, tracheostomy, intermittent catheterization, frequent turning (to prevent decubitus ulcers), and functional accommodations such as wheelchairs and other devices aimed at improving functionality. Attention to long-term care issues can prolong the life and productivity of SCI patients.

Prognosis & Outcome

Death in the acute trauma setting from SCI is 20%. Complete lesions that remain so at 72 hours are unlikely to improve beyond one level above the lesion in the long term. Patients with quadriplegia who have initial ventilator dependency have 5-year survival rates of approximately 33%. Incomplete lesions have a more favorable outcome. Among recognized SCI syndromes, central cord syndrome and Brown-Séquard syndrome have the most favorable outcomes, with up to 90% of patients being able to ambulate independently at 1 year. Anterior cord syndrome patients have a worse prognosis, with 10%-20% recovering functional motor control. Causes of death in long-term SCI patients are usually due to cardiac, respiratory, or infectious causes, often related to the sequelae of SCI.

Current multidisciplinary approaches to SCI involve emergency department, medical, surgical, and rehabilitation staff providing the best possible therapy for patients. Despite this, SCI remains a devastating injury with high rates of mortality and permanent disability. Novel research and innovations will assuredly provide better outcomes for SCI in the future.

Badhiwala JH, Wilson JR, Kwon BK, et al: A review of clinical trials in spinal cord injury including biomarkers. *J Neurotrauma.* 2018;35(16):1906-1917.

Hadley MN, Walters BC: Introduction of the guidelines for the management of acute cervical spine and spinal cord injuries. *Neurosurgery.* 2013;72:5-16.

Ho CH, Wuermser LA, Priebe MM, et al: Spinal cord injury medicine. 1. Epidemiology and classification. *Arch Phys Med Rehabil* 2007;88(Suppl 1):S49-S54.

Hurlbert RJ, Hadley MN, Walters BC, et al: Pharmacological therapy for acute spinal cord injury. *Neurosurgery.* 2013;72:93-105.

Kirshblum S, Waring W 3rd: Updates for the international standards for neurologic classification of spinal cord injury. *Phys Med Rehabil Clin N Am.* 2014;25:505-517.

Kwon BK, Mann C, Sohn HM, et al: Hypothermia for spinal cord injury. *Spine J.* 2008;8(6):859-874.

McKinley W, Santos K, Meade M, et al: Incidence and outcomes of spinal cord injury clinical syndromes. *J Spinal Cord Med.* 2007;30:215-224.

Priebe MM, Chiodo AE, Scelza WM, et al: Spinal cord injury medicine 6. Economic and societal issues in spinal cord injury. *Arch Phys Med Rehabil.* 2007;88(Suppl 1):S84-88.

▼ PERIPHERAL NERVE LESIONS

Ian Tafel, MD, and Timothy R. Smith, MD, PhD

▶ General Considerations

Familiarity with the pertinent aspects of peripheral nerve anatomy and physiology combined with focused history and physical examination aids in the management of peripheral nerve lesions. The history and physical examination may then be complimented by electrodiagnostic and radiographic studies.

▶ Anatomy

Peripheral nerves are composed of varying combinations of sensory and motor axons from more than one spinal nerve root, and each spinal nerve root contributes fibers to more than one peripheral nerve. An axon is a long projection from a nerve cell body that is bounded by a cell membrane as well as a basement membrane. Some axons are surrounded by sheaths of myelin, a fatty substance secreted by Schwann cells. Myelin insulates the axon, thereby increasing the velocity of neurotransmission. The axon is, in turn, surrounded by a layer of connective tissue called endoneurium. Axons travel together in bundles called fascicles, each of which is covered by another layer of connective tissue called perineurium. Fascicles are grouped together to form a peripheral nerve, which is surrounded by a final layer of connective tissue called epineurium.

ACUTE PERIPHERAL NERVE INJURIES

▶ General Considerations

Lesions of spinal nerves manifest as radiculopathies with blurred sensory disturbances, whereas those in peripheral nerves demonstrate sharply demarcated sensory disturbances. Spinal nerve lesions result in mild to moderate weakness in muscles supplied by one spinal nerve but by more than one peripheral nerve. Peripheral nerve lesions manifest more severe muscle atrophy and weakness in muscles supplied solely by the peripheral nerve.

Common etiologies of acute peripheral nerve injury include penetrating or blunt trauma, traction, fractured bones, and compression from hematomas. Minor peripheral nerve injuries arise from blunt trauma that temporarily compresses or stretches a nerve while leaving its axons intact (neurapraxia). In such cases, axonal transport may be temporarily impaired, but Wallerian degeneration, or the death of axons distal to the point of injury, does not occur. These injuries generally recover spontaneously over the course of days to weeks. Slightly more severe injuries may interrupt axons and their myelin sheaths while leaving endoneurium intact (axonotmesis). In these cases, Wallerian degeneration inevitably follows. Axonal regeneration may occur spontaneously, however, guided to areas of previous innervation by intact endoneurial tubes. With this type of injury, there is a good prognosis for spontaneous functional recovery, with axonal regeneration occurring at a rate of about 1 mm/d or 1 inch per month.

If the ends of a completely divided nerve (neurotmesis) remain in proximity, regeneration can occur via axonal sprouting from the proximal stump. These axonal sprouts may bridge the gap to the distal stump, propagating through preserved endoneurial tubes at a rate of 1 mm/d. Severe crush injuries may create internal damage without complete transection, resulting in disruption of axons and their endoneurium and disturbance of the organization of fascicles within the nerve. In these cases, fibrous scar tissue may form within the macerated nerve, which can block the regeneration of axonal sprouts. A tangle of axonal sprouts contained in fibrous scar tissue is called a neuroma, and these act as a barrier to spontaneous peripheral nerve regeneration.

▶ Clinical Findings

A detailed clinical history and neurologic examination help determine which peripheral nerves have been injured and the type of injury present. The type of trauma will generally suggest whether the nerve is in continuity. A penetrating injury with a sharp object, such as a knife, suggests a clean transection that is amenable to immediate surgical repair. Nonpenetrating trauma or a stretch injury is more suggestive of nerve continuity.

Determine the timing of motor and sensory deficits may also aid in the assessment of the nerve injury. For example, in the setting of a penetrating sharp injury, an immediate deficit at the time of the injury would suggest direct involvement of the nerve. However, a delayed deficit would suggest an enlarging adjacent lesion such as a hematoma or pseudoaneurysm.

The physical examination includes inspection, observation, evaluation of the relevant vasculature, range of motion assessment, and neurological examination. A laceration, fracture, or bruising/abrasions may suggest the site of an underlying nerve injury. The Horner sign (ptosis, meiosis, and anhidrosis) is suggestive of a proximal T1/lower trunk brachial plexus lesion. An impaired range of motion can make assessment of strength difficult to evaluate accurately. Furthermore, an elevated hemidiaphragm is suggestive of a phrenic nerve injury.

The sensory and motor findings associated with acute peripheral nerve injury vary widely, depending on which nerve is injured. Pain may also be a symptom, but it usually develops in a delayed fashion. Pain can occur because of neuroma formation, where it is often associated with a tender lump in the area of injury. Neurogenic pain may also develop because of a disturbance in the processing of pain signals. This type of pain, when associated with autonomic hyperfunction, is referred to as complex regional pain syndrome (formally known as causalgia or reflex sympathetic dystrophy), and it is notoriously difficult to treat. When neurogenic pain is associated with nerve root avulsion, it is known as deafferentation pain. Deafferentation pain often responds well to surgical intervention via dorsal root entry zone ablation.

In the diagnosis of acute peripheral nerve injury, electromyography and nerve conduction studies are generally not useful until at least 3 weeks after injury. Nevertheless, it is important to obtain baseline electrodiagnostic studies because they are important for monitoring recovery. In the case of brachial plexus injury, it is useful to obtain an MRI scan or CT myelogram to look for pseudomeningoceles in the vicinity of the nerve roots, which would indicate nerve root avulsion.

Certain peripheral nerve injuries are associated with traumatic fractures of specific bones. For example, traumatic injuries of the radial nerve classically occur with fractures of the shaft of the humerus, at the level of the spiral groove. Such injuries result in weakness of wrist extension, finger extension, and thumb extension, as well as numbness over the radial aspect of the dorsal surface of the hand. In this type of injury, elbow extension is not affected since muscular branches to the triceps are given off proximal to the spiral groove.

Trauma to the brachial plexus can cause a wide array of neurologic signs and symptoms. Clinical manifestations are determined by both the location and severity of the injury. Erb-Duchenne palsy is due to an injury primarily to the upper trunk of the brachial plexus (derived from C5 and C6 nerve roots). It typically results from a stretch injury such as traction on the arm at the time of birth or a fall that forcefully separates the head from the shoulder. The deltoid, biceps, rhomboids, brachioradialis, supraspinatus, and infraspinatus are affected, leaving the arm hanging to the side, internally rotated, and extended at the elbow, which is called the "waiter's tip position."

Differential Diagnosis

In acute trauma, when unilateral limb findings are present, a thorough neurologic exam is critical to differentiate acute radiculopathy from peripheral nerve injury. Several general principles should be considered. Radiculopathy is often accompanied by neck or back pain, which tends to radiate down an arm or a leg. Also the sensory findings of radiculopathy tend to be blurred, reflecting the overlapping nature of dermatomes, while sensory findings in peripheral nerve injuries are sharply demarcated. Weakness from radiculopathy occurs in muscles innervated by one spinal nerve but by more than one peripheral nerve. Thus, it is often only partial weakness, because nearly all muscles are innervated by more than one spinal nerve.

Acute trauma to a peripheral nerve usually results in maximal deficits at the time of injury, but a deficit that progresses should initiate further workup. Immediate surgical exploration should be considered to address compressive lesions such as expanding hematomas or growing traumatic pseudoaneurysms. Sources of ongoing neurologic compression should be removed as soon as possible.

Treatment & Prognosis

Sharp nerve transections with clean ends should be repaired within 3 days. In transections that are less than 5 mm, the repair should be performed in an end-to-end fashion, with no tension across the repair site. However, for larger defects, an autologous nerve graft should be used. Transections from penetrating trauma that do not have clean edges or where significant tissue loss is present should be repaired in a delayed fashion. During exploration of the wound, transected nerve stumps should be identified and tagged. The tagged nerve ends should be attached to fascia to reduce the possibility of retraction. After 3 weeks, the lesion should be reexplored and the injured nerve repaired. At that time, areas of axonal damage and neuroma formation are easier to visualize. Better visualization of damaged axons reduces the possibility of subsequent neuroma formation at the site of repair.

In the case of nonpenetrating injury, recovery often occurs spontaneously without the need for surgery. In these cases, nonoperative management with serial neurologic examinations, including electrophysiologic testing, should be the initial treatment modality. If, after 3 months, there is no sign of clinical recovery, the injured nerve should be explored. Intraoperative electrophysiologic nerve mapping should be performed to determine whether there is conduction across the site of injury. If there is no conduction of evoked potentials, the neuroma should be resected and the stubs should be trimmed and brought together primarily without tension. If intraoperative stimulation reveals conduction across an area of injury, then the nerve should be left intact and allowed to regenerate on its own. A mnemonic for remembering the appropriate timing of operative repair for traumatic nerve injuries is "the rule of threes": 3 days for a sharp transection, 3 weeks for an open ragged transection, and 3 months for a closed stretch injury.

Prognosis for recovery depends on the type of injury as well as the treatment. Axonal regeneration occurs at a rate of 1 inch per month, proximally to distally. Thus, clinical recovery may proceed slowly. Maximal recovery occurs over the course of approximately 1-2 years. Rehabilitation and physical therapy are important for avoiding the development of muscle contractures that may limit mobility when nerve function has returned. Tendon transfers may be of assistance if neural function does not completely recover.

PERIPHERAL ENTRAPMENT NEUROPATHIES

General Considerations

Peripheral nerves are subjected to chronic mechanical forces, such as compression, stretching, and friction. These forces may, over time, lead to peripheral nerve entrapment syndromes, such as carpal tunnel syndrome or ulnar nerve entrapment. Both static and dynamic factors may contribute to chronic peripheral nerve injury. Static factors include musculotendinous anomalies or inflexible anatomic tunnels that compress peripheral nerves. Dynamic factors include mobile joints, muscular contraction, or nerve mobility that leads to stretching of a peripheral nerve or increased friction along its course during movement. Peripheral entrapment neuropathies occur more frequently in upper rather than lower limbs, probably because of the greater mobility of the arms.

Clinical Findings

Entrapment neuropathies are characterized by weakened muscles, as well as sensory disturbances in the distribution of a single peripheral nerve. In general, an individual muscle is supplied by one peripheral nerve, and entrapment of that nerve can lead to severe motor findings as well as muscle atrophy and fasciculations. Marked atrophy is a hallmark of a peripheral nerve lesion. Sensory complaints generally include paresthesias, rather than pain, in the distribution of the involved nerve. Percussion over the nerve may result in an electric sensation radiating along the nerve and its territory, known as the Tinel sign. Electrodiagnostic testing is also useful in the diagnosis of peripheral nerve entrapment, and the finding of a nerve conduction delay at the site of compression is common to all compression neuropathies.

The most common peripheral nerve entrapment syndrome involves the median nerve at the wrist. This condition generally arises from compression of the median nerve by the transverse carpal ligament and is therefore referred to as carpal tunnel syndrome. Carpal tunnel syndrome occurs with higher frequency in patients with conditions leading to connective tissue thickening (eg, rheumatoid arthritis, acromegaly, hypothyroidism, pregnancy) and may be related to repetitive hand or wrist movements. Common presenting symptoms include dysesthetic pain in the hands that is worse at night, often awaking the patient from sleep. This occurs because many people sleep with flexed wrists, a position that exacerbates median nerve compression at the wrist. The pain sometimes radiates upward, into the forearm. Patients also complain of numbness on the palmer side of the hand as well as the first three to three and a half digits. When the ring finger is involved, the sensory disturbance involves only the radial side of the digit. Patients may complain of decreased grip strength or difficulty grasping small objects as well as atrophy of the abductor pollicis brevis, at the lateral base of the thumb, due to involvement of the intrinsic hand muscles innervated by the median nerve (first and second lumbricals, opponens pollicis, abductor pollicis brevis, and flexor pollicis brevis). There is often a positive Tinel sign at the wrist. The Phalen test is a clinical maneuver in which the patient's wrists are held in forced flexion for at least 30 seconds and is considered positive if it produces symptoms of median neuropathy in the hand.

Ulnar nerve entrapment is the second most common peripheral nerve entrapment syndrome and most commonly occurs at the elbow. Patients typically present with upper extremity pain that localizes to the medial aspect of the elbow, as well as paresthesias and numbness of the small finger and the ulnar half of the ring finger. A Tinel sign is often present at the medial aspect of the elbow: tapping over this area sends electric sensations into the fourth and fifth digits. The ulnar nerve innervates most of the intrinsic hand muscles, including the adductor pollicis, the first dorsal interosseous, and the hypothenar muscles, which explains the finding of hand weakness, leading to reduced grip strength and pinch strength. Patients report dropping things or having trouble opening jars, and on exam, atrophy of the hand intrinsic muscles may be marked, particularly the first dorsal interosseous and the muscles of the hypothenar eminence. When nerve dysfunction is severe, the hand may take on a "claw hand" appearance. The patient may also exhibit a Froment sign: when asked to hold a piece of paper between the thumb and index finger, the distal interphalangeal joint will flex because the patient uses the flexor pollicis longus muscle,

innervated by the median nerve, to compensate for lack of abductor pollicis function.

▶ Differential Diagnosis

The differential diagnosis for peripheral nerve dysfunction includes neuropathies of infectious origin (both bacterial and viral), hereditary conditions (eg, Charcot-Marie-Tooth disease), neuropathy associated with nutritional deficiency (eg, vitamin B_{12} deficiency), metabolic or endocrinologic conditions (eg, diabetes), inflammatory or immune-mediated conditions (eg, polyarteritis nodosa), chronic cervical or lumbar radiculopathy, and toxic conditions (eg, lead poisoning). It is important to recognize that sensory changes that "split" the ring finger suggest ulnar nerve dysfunction, rather than C8 radiculopathy. When more than one peripheral nerve is involved, the diagnosis of generalized neuropathy is likely and is typically symmetrical and bilateral. Decreased amplitude on electrodiagnostic studies (which suggests axonal loss) is characteristic of neuropathy of hereditary or metabolic origin. Peripheral nerve entrapment, on the other hand, causes damage to the myelin surrounding an axon, thereby slowing conduction velocity but not affecting amplitude.

▶ Treatment & Prognosis

Surgical management of peripheral nerve entrapment involves decompressing the involved nerve and should be strongly considered when patients present with significant motor weakness or muscle atrophy. Additionally, it should be considered when patients fail to improve with medical treatments. In the case of carpal tunnel syndrome, the transverse carpal ligament is divided, thus relieving compression on the median nerve as it passes from the wrist into the hand. In the case of ulnar neuropathy, simply freeing the nerve from surrounding scar tissue or hypertrophied connective tissue (external neurolysis) is usually sufficient. Carpal tunnel release results in excellent relief of symptoms in 80% of patients and partial relief in another 10%. Similar results are observed for surgical management of ulnar neuropathy.

Nonoperative management strategies include avoidance of repetitive activities that precipitate symptoms or the use of immobilization braces that hold joints in positions that avoid compression or corticosteroid injections.

PERIPHERAL NERVE TUMORS

▶ General Considerations

Peripheral nerve tumors can be divided into nonneoplastic, benign, and malignant masses. The nonneoplastic masses include traumatic neuromas, Morton neuromas, and nerve sheath ganglion cysts. Benign masses include neurofibromas, schwannomas (also known as neurilemmomas), perineuromas, lipofibromatous hamartomas (also known as neural fibrolipomas), nerve sheath myxomas, and granular cell tumors. Malignant masses include the malignant peripheral nerve sheath tumors.

Neurofibromas can be subdivided into solitary, diffuse, and plexiform varieties. The solitary neurofibroma is the most common benign peripheral nerve tumor. Axons are incorporated within the neurofibroma along with Schwann cells, collagen matrix, perineurial cells, and fibroblasts. Because the axons are intermixed within the tumor, the tumor cannot be excised without resecting a portion of the involved nerve. Diffuse neurofibromas and plexiform neurofibromas are less common than the solitary variety. The diffuse neurofibroma typically involves the skin and subcutaneous tissues. Plexiform neurofibromas are large, irregular expansions of nerves ranging from small cutaneous nerves to large trunks. Neurofibromas are commonly found in patients with neurofibromatosis type 1 (von Recklinghausen disease).

Schwannomas are slowly growing lesions made up of Schwann cells in a collagen matrix. Importantly, nerve fascicles run alongside the tumor, rather than through the tumor as in neurofibromas. Schwannomas are the second most common peripheral nerve tumor. Generally, only mild neurologic deficits occur, and operative resection can be considered in the setting of pain, paresthesias, or weakness in the distribution of the nerve.

Malignant peripheral nerve sheath tumors are the most common malignant peripheral nerve tumor. Nearly two-thirds arise from neurofibromas in the setting of neurofibromatosis type 1. The remainder arise either de novo or in patients with a history of prior external-beam radiation.

Clinical Findings

The symptoms of peripheral nerve tumors are generally related to the nerve involved and include weakness, numbness, paresthesias, and pain. MRI with gadolinium contrast can be useful in imaging the tumors.

Differential Diagnosis

The differential diagnosis of peripheral nerve tumors includes entrapment neuropathies, nonneoplastic masses, radiculopathies, and neuropathies associated with infection, malnutrition, and metabolic, endocrinologic, inflammatory, immune-mediated, and toxic conditions. Generally, a symptomatic peripheral nerve tumor will be palpable. Further, the peripheral nerve tumor can occur anywhere along the course of the nerve, whereas entrapment neuropathies typically occur in defined locations, and the various other neuropathies listed are often diffuse processes. Finally, a radiculopathy will be symptomatic in the distribution of the nerve root, likely involving several peripheral nerves.

Treatment & Prognosis

Schwannomas can generally be resected without any neurologic deficit since the nerve fascicles run alongside the tumor and operative resection is curative. Neurofibromas generally cannot be resected without neurologic deficit since the axons run within the substance of the tumor. Indications for surgical resection of solitary neurofibromas are large tumor mass, accelerated growth, neurologic deficit, and pain. Plexiform neurofibromas (excluding superficial ones) can rarely be totally resected and should generally be followed.

Generally, the prognosis for benign peripheral nerve sheath tumors is very good, with improvement in pain, weakness, and paresthesias noted after resection of solitary lesions. Malignant peripheral nerve sheath tumors require aggressive surgical treatment. The expected 5-year survival is 20%-50% and neurofibromatosis type 1–associated tumors do not have a worse prognosis than de novo lesions.

James AW, et al: Malignant peripheral nerve sheath tumor. *Surg Oncol Clin North Am.* 2016;25(4):789-802.

O'Brien M, on behalf of the Guarantors of Brain: *Aids to the Examination of the Peripheral Nervous System.* 5th ed. Edinburgh, United Kingdom: Saunders Elsevier; 2010.

Song JW, et al: An outcome study for ulnar neuropathy at the elbow: a multicenter study by the surgery for ulnar nerve (SUN) study group. *Neurosurgery.* 2013;72(6):971-981.

BRAIN TUMORS

Pablo A. Valdes, MD, PhD, and Timothy R. Smith, MD, PhD

Clinical Presentation

The most common presenting symptoms in patients with intracranial tumors are headaches, seizures, and neurologic deficits. Headaches are the most common presenting symptom in patients with intracranial tumors (50%). The classical presentation is that of headaches that are worse when waking up and that are at times severe enough to wake patients from sleep. Headaches in brain tumor patients can result from a variety of factors, including increased ICP from mass effect in the setting of physiologic elevations in PCO_2 during sleep; maneuvers such as straining, coughing, or bending over; involvement of structures containing pain fibers such as the dura; and visual difficulties through direct or indirect involvement of the optic pathways or oculomotor and abducens nerves. Headaches can be a helpful initial guide in patients who may also show acute and immediately life-threatening conditions such as acute hydrocephalus secondary to tumor obstruction of CSF pathways. Acute hydrocephalus is a neurosurgical emergency requiring prompt intervention (eg, EVD placement). Hemorrhagic tumors with a rapidly expansile mass, patient obtundation, and herniation with compression of brainstem structures can be a neurosurgical emergency requiring craniotomy for evacuation, resection, and decompression.

Seizures are the most common presenting symptom in patients with low-grade gliomas (> 70%) compared to other intracranial tumors such as high-grade gliomas (< 20%) and metastatic lesions (< 10%); greater than 25% of patients with intracranial tumors will experience seizures at some point in their disease course. Seizures can provide useful diagnostic information based on the seizure type and presentation. For example, focal seizures with a motor component can likely be the result of a mass near or at the contralateral primary motor cortex. Seizures with an epigastric or emotional component can be likely secondary to a temporal mass or seizures with a clear language disturbance might point to involvement of the language regions in the left temporoparietal or frontal language regions. Status epilepticus can be a life-threatening condition in the presentation of intracranial tumors requiring emergent management to achieve immediate medical control in collaboration with the neurologists prior to subsequent surgical intervention.

Neurologic deficit is another common presentation of intracranial tumors that can provide a diagnostic clue as to the localization of the lesion. Patients presenting with left-sided arm weakness might have a laterally located lesion of the right primary cortex, whereas patients presenting with left-sided leg weakness might be harboring a right-sided medially located mass affecting the primary motor cortex of the lower extremity homunculus. Patients presenting with cerebellar signs such as ataxia or dysmetria are likely to have a cerebellar mass. Finally, patients presenting with a rapidly deteriorating mental status should elicit prompt medical attention and might require emergent intervention because this could point to a rapidly expansile hemorrhagic mass causing herniation or a metastatic cerebellar hemorrhagic mass causing obstructive hydrocephalus. These are neurosurgical emergencies requiring prompt neurosurgical attention.

Brain tumor patients can also present with a number of additional symptoms including nausea and vomiting due to elevations in ICP or involvement of the area postrema in the fourth ventricle; changes in personality in cases affecting the frontal lobe; changes in hearing or balance due to involvement of the hearing and vestibular systems (cranial nerve VIII); classic bitemporal hemianopsia or homonymous hemianopsia in patients harboring a pituitary tumor impacting the optic pathways; papilledema due to increased ICP; or endocrinologic disturbances in patients with sellar/suprasellar lesions. In summary, a careful history with an accurate neurologic exam can provide the clinician with the necessary tools and knowledge to help guide their subsequent diagnostic workup and urgency of management of the patient with a new intracranial mass.

▶ Diagnostic Workup

A clinical history and exam is the first step to a careful and meticulous workup of the patient with a (tentative) diagnosis of a brain tumor (Table 38–5). Laboratory studies and radiographic imaging are the next steps in helping further hone the diagnosis of the patient with a history concerning for a new intracranial mass. Basic laboratory studies including complete blood count, basic metabolic panel, coagulation markers, and, in cases of a highly suspect pituitary mass, an adequate endocrinologic workup (eg, cortisol, serum sodium, thyroid-stimulating hormone [TSH], luteinizing hormone [LH], follicle-stimulating hormone [FSH], sodium, prolactin).

The next step in the workup of a patient with a newly suspected intracranial process is the use of noncontrast CT given its speed, availability, and affordability to help provide an initial screening test. An initial CT can note any acute process (hemorrhage, hydrocephalus) and also provide information regarding the presence of an intracranial mass that would substantiate further imaging (ie, MRI). Noncontrast CT of the brain provides excellent imaging of hemorrhagic masses, bony structures, and bony infiltration, but poor description regarding soft tissue lesions (eg, gliomas, meningiomas, metastases). If CT imaging notes a likely mass lesion, the next step is MRI imaging of the brain with and without gadolinium contrast (to help highlight tumors that have significant uptake of this contrast agent such as high-grade gliomas, meningiomas, and metastases). The typical MRI sequences provide high-resolution images for the visualization of soft tissue structures and composition of the brain. In brain tumor patients, MRI can provide exquisite details regarding tumor composition including location, size, cellularity, cystic components, hemorrhage, surrounding edema, vascularity, necrosis, and association with surrounding soft tissue structures. MRI sequences, in addition to the standard structural sequences (ie, T1-weighted and T2-weighted), can provide further information to help guide diagnosis and urgency of treatment. Diffusion images can provide clues regarding cellularity and density of tumor or help distinguish between a tumor and abscess, where the latter would require urgent surgical intervention. Perfusion imaging can be used to assess vascularity of tumors as well as help assess tumor recurrence versus treatment-induced changes in the posttreatment period. Spectroscopy can further provide information regarding more subtle molecular changes (eg, lactate contents) to further hone the preoperative presumed diagnosis and assessment of tumor recurrence. All these sequences can help further guide the preoperative diagnosis when distinguishing between a likely brain tumor and an abscess (eg, significant diffusion restriction), in which the latter is a neurosurgical emergency. MRI can provide a good estimate of the preoperative diagnosis (eg, high-grade glioma, meningioma, vestibular schwannoma) of an intracranial lesion, but histology remains the gold standard.

Table 38–5. Brain tumor localizing signs and symptoms.

Location	Sign(s)
Frontal lobe[1]	Impaired intellectual function Language impairment[2], specifically abulia Impaired gait Personality changes Hemiparesis[3]
Dominant temporal lobe	Aphasia Impaired auditory discrimination Memory loss Contralateral superior quadrantanopia
Nondominant temporal lobe	Seizures Visual, auditory, olfactory hallucinations Contralateral superior quadrantanopia
Uncus	CN III palsy
Parietal lobe	Impaired sensory perception Contralateral inferior quadrantanopia Aphasia Anosoagnosia[4]
Occipital lobe	Visual deficits
Posterior fossa	Posterior headache Neck stiffness Opisthotonos
Brainstem	Cranial nerve palsies Long-tract signs
Cerebellopontine angle	Unilateral hearing loss Tinnitus Vertigo Facial palsy Facial anesthesia Cerebellar signs
Sellar region	Endocrime abnormalities Bitemporal hemianopsia CN III palsy
Pineal region	Parinaud syndrome: Upgaze palsy Ptosis Loss of pupillary light reflex Retraction-convergence nystagmus
Meningeal infiltration	Cranial nerve palsies Diffuse headache Meningeal reaction

CN, cranial nerve.
[1]Usually occurs only if both frontal lobes are involved.
[2]Occurs only when dominant hemisphere is involved.
[3]When motor cortex is involved.
[4]When nondominant temporal lobe is involved.

In some special cases, the use of cerebral angiography is warranted for both diagnostic and, more frequently, treatment reasons. In cases of a hemorrhagic mass in which MRI can be equivocal, angiography can be used to help identify a possible vascular nidus to identify a hemorrhagic lesion as an arteriovenous malformation rather than a tumor, which requires a different surgical approach and expertise. In cases of highly vascular tumors such as hemangiopericytomas, some meningiomas, or hemangioblastomas, preoperative angiography can aid in identification of feeding vessels and/or embolization to diminish operative risks and difficulty.

▶ Differential Diagnosis

The differential of possible intracranial lesions is extensive and can include both intra-axial (ie, within the brain parenchyma) and extra-axial (ie, external to the brain parenchyma) lesions. The most common intra-axial tumors are primary brain tumors (eg, high- and low-grade gliomas) and metastases. The most common extra-axial tumors are pituitary tumors, meningiomas, and schwannomas. The differential diagnosis of new intracranial masses is extensive and should be narrowed to ascertain those lesions requiring acute, immediate management (eg, ruptured intracranial aneurysm, hemorrhagic cerebellar tumors with brainstem compression or acute hydrocephalus, brain abscess) and those requiring elective management and workup. The differential diagnosis can be narrowed based on history (patient demographics, chronology of symptoms, past medical history, and specific neurologic deficits), physical exam, and imaging characteristics, including location, size, number, and sequence-specific characteristics. The list is extensive, including neoplastic processes with primary intracranial lesions such as gliomas, meningiomas, schwannomas, pituitary tumors, and lymphoma; metastatic lesions; infectious lesions such as abscesses; vascular masses such as aneurysms, arteriovenous malformations, and cavernous malformations; nonneoplastic processes such as multiple sclerosis, AIDS, dermoid cysts, arachnoid cysts, epidermoid cysts; and hemorrhagic or nonhemorrhagic infarct.

The frequency, types, and presentations of intracranial tumors differ greatly between the adult and pediatric populations. In the adult population, the most common intracranial tumors are metastases, supratentorial gliomas, pituitary tumors, and meningiomas. In the pediatric population, metastases to the brain are rare, and the most common primary brain tumors are infratentorial medulloblastomas, juvenile pilocytic astrocytomas, and ependymomas; more commonly seen in the pediatric population are entities such as embryonal tumors (atypical teratoid/rhabdoid tumor) and pineal tumors (germ cell tumors, such as germinomas, and nongerminomatous germ cell tumors, such as choriocarcinomas, teratomas, and yolk sac tumors). Here, we will focus our discussion on the most common adult pathologies; pituitary tumors are discussed in a separate chapter.

The clinician will a carefully gathered history, physical exam, and imaging workup to help identify the most likely diagnosis(es) to guide management. As such, the use of neurologic expertise working in conjunction with both the neurologist and neurosurgeon can help the general practitioner maximize resource utilization and optimize treatment for these patients.

Tumor Types

A. Intra-axial Tumors

The 2016 World Health Organization (WHO) Classification of Tumors of the CNS provided the community with a conceptual and practical advance in classifying CNS tumors using both novel molecular parameters and traditional histology to define tumor entities. In this new classification, genotype trumps histologic phenotype when providing a diagnosis for tumor entities. Here, will use the newer classification but intermittently refer to the older, more familiar system to help guide the reader.

1. Diffuse gliomas and glioblastoma—Diffuse gliomas encompass the more commonly known WHO grades II to III low- and high-grade gliomas of astrocytic and/or oligodendrocytic lineage. Gliomas account for > 70% of all primary brain tumors (glioblastoma > 60% and diffuse gliomas > 10%). Gliomas are now divided into *IDH* mutant, *IDH* wild-type, and not otherwise specified (NOS; which is usually reserved for cases in which tissue diagnosis is limited due to factors such as limitations in tissue quantity or access to molecular studies). Diffuse WHO grade II and III gliomas are mostly *IDH* mutant. *IDH* mutant diffuse gliomas are further separated into *IDH* mutant with a 1p/19q codeletion, which encompass the majority of the traditional oligodendrogliomas, and *IDH* mutant (without a 1p19q codeletion) with an *ATRX* loss/*TP53* mutation, which are mostly diffuse astrocytomas. Patients harboring *IDH* mutations have a better prognosis (> 5 years) compared to those with an *IDH* wild-type glioma (generally 1-2 years).

Diffuse gliomas constitute the more commonly known low-grade gliomas and are slow-growing lesions within the white matter with modest to low cellularity and no significant endothelial proliferation or necrosis (unlike glioblastoma). WHO grade II *IDH* mutant astrocytomas are usually non–contrast enhancing on T1-weighted imaging but hyperintense on T2-weighted and FLAIR imaging. WHO grade II *IDH* mutant diffuse gliomas with 1p19q codeletion encompass the more commonly known oligodendrogliomas with the classic perinuclear halos or "fried egg" appearance on histologic evaluation. On MRI, these lesions are usually non–contrast enhancing on T1-weighted imaging but hyperintense on T2-weighted and FLAIR imaging. They may demonstrate hypointense regions on MRI that may correspond to hyperdense areas on CT denoting intratumoral calcifications. *IDH* mutant lesions can demonstrate contrast enhancement on T1-weighted imaging usually upon malignant transformation to WHO grade III or IV lesions (eg, secondary glioblastoma). Current treatment varies among institutions but generally includes a combination of watchful waiting, surgery, and/or chemotherapy with procarbazine/lomustine/vincristine or temozolomide with survival rates of approximately 5-20 years. Patients with diffuse low-grade lesions usually do not undergo radiation.

Glioblastomas are generally *IDH* wild-type (90%; de novo or primary glioblastoma) tumors seen in older patients (> 55 years of age), whereas *IDH* mutant glioblastomas are much less common (10%; secondary glioblastoma arising from previously low-grade gliomas) and are seen in younger patients (< 30 years of age). Despite current maximal therapy including surgery, chemotherapy, radiation, and tumor-treating fields, patients have an overall survival of < 2 years. These lesions are highly invasive along white matter tracts and vasculature and demonstrate high cellularity, endothelial proliferation, nuclear atypia, mitotic figures, and necrosis on histologic evaluation. MRI demonstrates a pattern of ring enhancement on T1-weighted imaging with a central area of T1-weighted hypointensity that corresponds to the necrotic core of the tumor with surrounding T2-weighted and FLAIR hyperintensity spanning from the tumor core corresponding to tumor edema and an infiltrative component (Figure 38–13). The mainstay of treatment for glioblastoma involves maximal surgical resection followed by radiation, temozolomide, and more recently, the use of tumor-treating fields, with overall median survival of 21 months.

B. Extra-axial Tumors

1. Meningiomas—Meningiomas are the most common primary intracranial tumors, accounting for one-third of all primary CNS tumors with a pathologically confirmed prevalence of 97.5 in 100,000 in the United States and a peak incidence at 45 years of age. Nevertheless, this is a likely underestimate of the actual prevalence because imaging of asymptomatic meningiomas is 0.9% in adults, and autopsy studies suggest an even higher prevalence of up to 3% in persons over 60 years of age. Meningiomas are generally benign, extra-axial, slow-growing lesions arising from the arachnoid caps cells of the meninges, with lower grade meningiomas more common in women and higher grade more common in men. Ionizing radiation is a known risk factor in patients undergoing prior cranial irradiation (eg, patients with history of irradiated childhood brain tumors). Certain genetic associations have been noted as well. Specifically, neurofibromatosis type 2 greatly increases the risk of meningiomas and schwannomas; other syndromes also increase risk, including neurofibromatosis type 1, Gorlin

▲ **Figure 38–13.** Magnetic resonance imaging of a deep right temporal mass proven to be a high-grade glioma. **A:** Fluid-attenuated inversion recovery imaging demonstrating a mass with significant surrounding white matter edema. **B:** T1-weighted contrast-enhanced image demonstrating smaller enhancing portion of the mass.

syndrome, Li-Fraumeni syndrome, von Hippel-Lindau syndrome, and Cowden disease.

Meningiomas are categorized as WHO grade I (benign, 70%), II (atypical, 30%), or III (anaplastic, ~1%) and include multiple histologic subtypes (eg, meningothelial, fibrous, psammomatous, angiomatous). They are characterized at the histologic level by densely packed sheets of cells (similar to arachnoid cells), psammoma bodies (whorls of calcium and collagen), intranuclear cytoplasmic pseudo-inclusions, and Orphan Annie nuclei (nuclei with central clearing from peripheral migration of chromatin).

Meningiomas can appear slightly hyperdense to normal on brain CT (~60%), contain intratumoral calcification (> 20%), and demonstrate hyperostosis of the skull (5%). MRI is the modality of choice, with meningiomas appearing as extra-axial masses with a dural base or "tail" (secondary to dural thickening rather than invasion of tumor) (Figure 38–14). A vascular cleft sign suggests the extra-axial nature of these lesions. They are typically homogeneous and well circumscribed and have isointense signal on T1-weighted imaging, intense and homogeneous contrast enhancement on T1-weighted postcontrast imaging, and iso- to hyperintense signal on T2-weighted imaging at the tumor core, and in more invasive areas of tumor surrounding brain parenchyma, T2-weighted hyperintense signal suggests edema and possible tumor invasion (60%). Nevertheless, despite all these characteristics, it is virtually

impossible to distinguish between meningioma grades on preoperative imaging.

Most meningiomas are asymptomatic, but symptomatic ones can present with seizures, headaches, or focal

▲ **Figure 38–14.** Sagittal magnetic resonance imaging demonstrating a contrast-enhancing dural-based lesion (arrow) proven to be a meningioma at time of resection.

neurologic deficits (eg, contralateral arms weakness) either directly as space-occupying lesions or indirectly through peritumoral vasogenic edema. As such, treatment with anti-epileptics and steroids should be reserved for patients with seizures or symptomatic patients with imaging evidence of peritumoral edema, respectively. Surgery is the mainstay of treatment for meningiomas, with the goal of surgery entailing complete removal of the lesion, surrounding dura, and any involved bone. The Simpson grading scale provides a clinical risk assessment of recurrence by relating the degree of resection with the risk of recurrence, subsequently helping guide the need for adjuvant treatment. Radiation can serve many roles; for example, it can be used in patients after initial surgery with high risk of recurrence, as primary therapy in patients ineligible for surgery, or for treatment of recurrent disease without a one-size-fits-all approach. At this time, there are no chemotherapy regimens with demonstrated efficacy against meningiomas.

C. Brain Metastases

Brain metastases (BMs) are the most common intracranial tumors, with a yearly incidence of approximately 200,000 cases per year in the United States, affecting up to one-third of adults with cancer and occurring more frequently in adults in their fifth to seventh decades of life. Historically, BM had a dismal prognosis, with median survival of < 6 months, but recent advances with earlier diagnosis, newer treatments, and better understanding of molecular subtypes has led to significant improvements in overall survival. Specifically, in an era of improving systemic therapies, molecular understanding, and personalized medicine, the diagnosis-specific graded prognostic assessment has been used as a means for more accurate patient stratification. This specific stratification reveals the marked heterogeneity in outcomes and important difference in prognostication for the different BM subgroups.

The five most common primary cancers that metastasize to the CNS in adults are lung (20%), melanoma (7%), renal (7%), breast (5%), and colorectal (2%). In the era of immunologic therapies, the natural disease history can be altered, and the risk for BM differs for particular cancers (eg, human epidermal growth factor receptor 2 [HER2]–positive breast cancer, melanoma, and ALK-rearranged non–small-cell lung cancer), with an incidence of BM of up to 40% in HER2-positive breast cancer and overall improved survival. Treatment of melanoma with immune checkpoint inhibitors and targeted treatments can provide survival advantage for systemic disease and CNS control.

Patients will typically present with any combination of symptoms including but not limited to headaches, seizures, changes in mental status, focal neurologic deficits, nausea, and vomiting. Nevertheless, up to 60% of patient are asymptomatic at the time of imaging confirmed BM.

Of note, histologic characteristics are specific to the primary cancer.

CT is the first-line imaging modality to visualize a mass-occupying lesion with varying iso-, hypo-, or hyperdense features and variable associated vasogenic edema. Variable contrast enhancement is noted on CT, including solid, ring, punctuate, or diffuse enhancement. MRI is more sensitive than CT at identifying BM with typical iso- to hypointense T1-weighted signal; uniform, solid, ring, punctuate, and variable patterns of contrast enhancement are noted, with contrast-enhanced sequences used as standard for detection of smaller metastases. Typically, BM demonstrate T2-weighted and FLAIR hyperintense signal with variable degree of peritumoral edema. These lesions are classically found at the gray-white matter interface but can be found anywhere in the brain (Figure 38–15). Specific primary BMs demonstrate a propensity for hemorrhage including melanoma, renal cell carcinoma, and choriocarcinoma. In cases of intratumoral hemorrhage, tumors will show associated CT hyperdense regions and intrinsic hyperintense signal on T1-weighted precontrast imaging.

Treatment of BMs involves a multidisciplinary approach that includes a combination of surgery, stereotactic radiation, whole-brain radiation therapy (WBRT), and/or chemotherapy. Surgery has been typically reserved for patients with a single BM in a favorable location that is large in size (generally > 3 cm) with considerable mass effect and/or edema; patients with a good performance status and limited or absent systemic disease; radioresistant primary cancer (eg, renal cell, melanoma); tissue diagnosis to distinguish necrosis

▲ **Figure 38–15.** Sagittal magnetic resonance image demonstrating multiple contrast-enhancing lesions (arrows) in the infra- and supratentorial spaces. Biopsy demonstrated metastatic adenocarcinoma.

from true recurrence; and cerebellar mass effect causing compression and possible hydrocephalus. More recent data with advances in surgical techniques have shown efficacy in surgical resection of multiple BMs, including resection of a dominant lesion among two to three lesions followed by radiation. As such, data for resection of more than one lesion seem to suggest an advantage in carefully selected patients. Patients can undergo a combination of WBRT and or stereotactic radiation depending on location, number of lesions, and size (generally < 3 cm). With the advent of molecular classification and new targeted therapies, patients with BM undergo specific chemotherapy regimens based on their primary cancer with varied response and highly promising recent results (eg, control of melanoma).

General Surgical Considerations

Every tumor requires an individualized, tailored approach and treatment, but several general principles can help guide and inform management. Surgeons need to decide for each case whether the goal of surgery is biopsy, subtotal resection, or gross total resection, with gross total resection being the gold standard in cases where it is deemed safe, providing the best survival benefit in patients. Tumor resection requires careful consideration of a number of key factors including: (1) tumor size; (2) location; (3) gross, radiographic, and pathologic characteristics; (4) sensitivity to radiation; and importantly, (5) medical and neurologic status of the patient.

Timing is important in preoperative planning, such as in patients with rapid deterioration (eg, elevated ICP may require prompt intervention either by an EVD in cases of acute hydrocephalus or decompression and resection in cases of a rapidly expansile hemorrhagic tumor). Generally, tumor surgery can usually be done on an elective to semi-elective basis depending on neurologic presentation. Some tumors can even be followed long term without any surgical or treatment intervention (eg, small, stable meningiomas).

Modern approaches for tumor resection use a number of intraoperative tools, including head immobilization using a Mayfield head holder; intraoperative imaging including ultrasound, CT, and MRI; intraoperative navigation or frameless stereotaxy, which matches preoperative imaging with the patient's intraoperative location; intraoperative electrophysiologic monitoring to help identify functioning eloquent versus noneloquent brain, which can aid in delineating functional and safe borders during resection; and more recently, the use of intraoperative fluorescent dyes, which help visualize tumors. The approaches have resulted in significant improvement in gross total resection rates. The main goal of brain tumor surgery is maximizing the extent of tumor resection while minimizing damage to surrounding normal brain and vascular structures, and the specific surgical approaches vary based on tumor type (eg, transsphenoidal for a functioning pituitary microadenoma vs retrosigmoid

for a cerebellopontine angle meningioma). Generally, except in rare instances, maximizing the extent of tumor resection provides patients with the greatest survival advantage across tumor pathologies.

Postoperatively patients are observed in an ICU or step-down unit usually overnight with close neurologic monitoring. Steroids are used in some cases depending on associated edema and surgeon preference. Anticonvulsants are used in cases where brain parenchyma has been dissected/contacted and are continued for an extended period only in patients with a history of seizures. Postoperative MRI is done routinely within 48 hours to provide a baseline to evaluate for residual tumor and future evaluation of tumor recurrence.

Arvold ND, Lee EQ, Mehta MP, et al: Updates in the management of brain metastases. *Neuro-Oncology.* 2016;18(8):1043-1065.

Buckner J, Giannini C, Eckel-Passow J, et al: Management of diffuse low-grade gliomas in adults: use of molecular diagnostics. *Nat Rev Neurol.* 2017;13(6):340-351.

Garcia CR, Slone SA, Pittman T, et al: Comprehensive evaluation of treatment and outcomes of low-grade diffuse gliomas. *PloS One.* 2018;13(9):e0203639.

Hervey-Jumper SL, Berger MS: Maximizing safe resection of low- and high-grade glioma. *J Neuro-Oncol.* 2016;130(2):269-282.

Louis DN, Perry A, Reifenberger G, et al: (2016). The 2016 World Health Organization classification of tumors of the central nervous system: a summary. *Acta Neuropathol.* 2016;131(6): 803-820.

Rogers L, Barani I, Chamberlain M, et al: Meningiomas: knowledge base, treatment outcomes, and uncertainties. A RANO review. *J Neurosurg.* 2016;122(1):4-23.

Stupp R, Mason WP, van den Bent MJ, et al: Radiotherapy plus concomitant and adjuvant temozolomide for glioblastoma. *N Engl J Med.* 2005;352(10):987-996.

Wen PY, Chang SM, Van den Bent MJ, et al: Response assessment in neuro-oncology clinical trials. *J Clin Oncol.* 2017;35(21): 2439-2449.

Wiemels J, Wrensch M, Claus EB: Epidemiology and etiology of meningioma. *J Neuro-Oncol.* 2010;99(3):307-314.

TUMORS OF THE SPINE AND SPINAL CORD

Ian Tafel, MD, and Timothy R. Smith, MD, PhD

Introduction

Tumors of the spine and spinal cord are uncommon in the general population but are an important consideration in the evaluation of patients presenting with neck and/or back pain, with or without associated radicular symptoms, sensorimotor deficits, and bowel or bladder dysfunction. An estimated 15% of primary CNS tumors are intraspinal, and most of these are benign. Surgery, radiotherapy, and chemotherapy, alone or in conjunction, remain the best current management of spinal tumors.

In addition to gender and age of presentation, localization of the lesion to the cervical, thoracic, lumbar, or sacrococcygeal spine aids in refining the differential diagnosis because certain tumors demonstrate a predilection for particular regions of the spinal column. Spinal tumors are differentiated based on their location relative to three anatomic compartments: extradural, intradural-extramedullary, and intradural-intramedullary. Extradural tumors are located outside of the thecal sac and arise either from the osseous spine or epidural space. Intradural-extramedullary tumors occur within the thecal sac but are outside of the neural tissues of the spinal cord. These tumors most commonly develop from the leptomeninges or nerve roots. Intramedullary tumors are found within the spinal cord and originate from either the spinal cord parenchyma or pia mater.

Clinical Presentation

Symptoms are more commonly produced by compression than direct invasion of the spinal cord or nerve roots. Classically, the pain associated with neoplasms is unremitting, worse in the supine position, and more noticeable at rest or in bed. Hence, the patient may wake up at night due to pain. Although the progression of symptoms can be insidious, radicular pain, motor weakness, paresthesias, or anesthesia can frequently occur as a result of nerve compression. Long tract myelopathic findings such as ataxia, hyperreflexia, spasticity, fasciculations, sensorimotor loss, or sphincter dysfunction can be caused by spinal cord compression. Recognized unusual findings include muscle wasting or hyporeflexia, referred pain, autonomic changes such as in Horner syndrome, and Brown-Séquard hemi-cord syndrome. Fracture and deformity causing axial pain often occur as well and may be the presenting complaint.

Extradural tumors frequently involve the osseous spine, and so most typically present with axial pain, often increased by motion or Valsalva maneuver. Signs and symptoms of neural compression occur secondarily. Intradural-extramedullary tumors present most commonly with motor deficits and other long tract disturbances. Intramedullary tumors can demonstrate an insidious succession of symptoms including neuralgic pain that can progress to myelopathy.

Diagnosis

A. Radiographic Evaluation

MRI, specifically contrast-enhanced T1-weighted sequences, is the standard imaging modality to assess spinal tumors (Figure 38–16). Nearly all intramedullary lesions demonstrate contrast uptake, and the resolution that MRI provides is typically sufficient for determination of margins and infiltration. The addition of angiography is indicated for the suspicion of a vascular pathology.

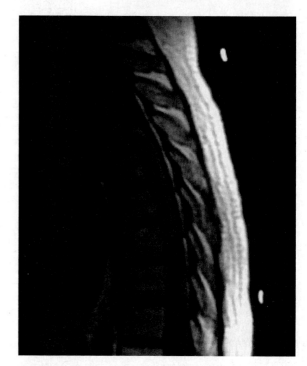

▲ **Figure 38–16.** Sagittal T1-weighted image with contrast of the upper thoracic spinal cord demonstrating an intradural, intramedullary lesion found on biopsy to be a high-grade glioma.

If an MRI is not obtainable, then myelography can still provide excellent structural detail. Fusiform cord widening, a dumbbell-shaped deformity, and complete blockage are classic findings suggesting the presence of a mass lesion. Plain, contrast-enhanced, and postmyelography CT imaging can aid in the assessment of bony spine anatomy. Nuclear scintigraphy is used primarily in the identification of skeletal metastases. Catheter angiography can be employed in the evaluation of suspected vascular lesions. Plain x-rays of the spine have limited utility in the initial assessment of spinal tumors. Findings such as enlarged intervertebral foramina and interpedicular spaces or bone erosion with scalloped edges suggest the presence of an enlarging mass.

B. Laboratory Analysis

Lumbar puncture can provide additional clues to the presence of a spinal cord tumor. Elevated CSF protein is present in approximately 95% of cases, although CSF glucose is normal. Xanthochromia and the presence of fibrinogen causing clotting can also occur. Specific CSF and serum immunocytochemical tests can aid the diagnosis of specific neoplasms.

C. Differential Diagnosis

Extradural lesions compose an estimated 55%-60% of all spinal tumors, and a vast majority of these are metastatic lesions via hematogenous dissemination along Batson venous plexus. The most common primary sources of vertebral metastases are lung, breast, and prostate.

Benign tumors of the osseous spine are very rare and may be incidental findings or may cause pain, radiculopathy, myelopathy, spinal instability, or deformity. Biopsy is used at times, and appropriate management may be observation, as is common in the case of eosinophilic granuloma; ablative, as can be performed for osteoid osteoma; or surgical. Primary benign spine tumors can be classified using the Enneking system.

Approximately 5% of bone malignancies involve the spine, the four most common being osteosarcoma, chondrosarcoma, Ewing sarcoma, and chordoma. Survival varies significantly by pathology. The high rates of recurrence, limited survival duration, and functional morbidity associated with these tumors support the aggressive multimodal strategies typically used in the treatment of these tumors. In some cases, complete resection with negative margins, or en bloc resection, is possible. In other cases, surgical resection may serve to decrease tumor burden, thereby improving the efficacy of adjuvant treatments such as chemotherapy and radiotherapy. At times, surgical intervention is necessary for functional indications, either for neural decompression or spinal stabilization.

Only 0.5% of tumors involving the spinal column are primary neoplasms. Of the intradural tumors, an estimated 70% are extramedullary and consist mainly of schwannoma, neurofibroma, and meningioma. The nerve sheath tumors, schwannoma and neurofibroma, are usually benign and can demonstrate a typical dumbbell-shaped appearance, caused by compression from the neuroforamina through which they sometimes pass. They are an important consideration when deviation of the pleural reflection on x-ray suggests a posterior mediastinal mass. Schwannomas are well-differentiated and typically grossly resectable; however, neurofibromas cannot be resected completely from their parent nerve. In the setting of type 1 neurofibromatosis, suspicion of multiple neurofibromas, meningioma, and ependymoma should be heightened. Schwannoma, neurofibroma, and meningioma multiplicity is associated with type 2 neurofibromatosis. Meningiomas are seen most often in the thoracic spines of middle-aged women and arise from persistent arachnoid cap cells.

Intramedullary tumors compose only approximately 10% of all spinal tumors and arise most commonly in the cervical segment of the spinal cord. Glial tumors are the most common of these, with ependymomas occurring twice as frequently as astrocytomas in adults. In children, the relationship is reversed, with astrocytomas being twice as common as ependymomas. Myxopapillary ependymomas form at the conus medullaris and filum terminale and are a very common tumor to be found at this location.

▶ Treatment

Generally, primary tumors of the spinal column are best treated by complete resection, if possible. In the vertebral column, en bloc resection is frequently the goal of surgery, whereas with any involvement of the spinal cord, gross total resection is the desired treatment. Symptomatic deformity or spinal instability warrants consideration for surgical fixation, as functional deterioration profoundly affects survival.

The role of surgery in epidural disease can include decompressing the spinal cord, obtaining tissue for histologic diagnosis, mechanical stabilization, and decreasing tumor burden to increase the effectiveness of radiotherapy. The role of surgery and its interplay with chemoradiation depends on many factors, including the type of lesion, its location, and the patient's prognosis, and the decision regarding surgery is generally made on an individual basis by a multidisciplinary treatment team.

In 2016, the WHO updated a comprehensive classification of neoplasms affecting the CNS based on molecular parameters and histology that guides therapy and prognosis in most intramedullary tumors. Overall, functional outcome depends heavily on the severity and duration of neurologic symptoms at the time of presentation, whereas survival outcome depends largely on the pathology in question and, less so, on the ability to gain adequate surgical resection.

Intradural-extramedullary tumors are generally best treated by surgical resection; outcomes appear to depend heavily on extent of resection, although preservation of pre-existing neurologic function remains the primary objective in surgery. Radiation and chemotherapy are increasingly important in the management of intradural tumors, especially with recurrence or multiloculated lesions. Determination of a dissection plane between tumor and spinal cord is the initial aim of any resection procedure. Overall, prognosis is excellent in nearly all cases of spinal intradural-extramedullary neoplasms, unless paraplegia is the presenting condition. In contrast, recurrence of infiltrative neoplasms is very common, and progression to paralysis is common. Progressive neurologic deterioration demands particular focus on facilitating appropriate surgical therapy.

Binning M, et al: Spinal tumors in children. *Neurosurg Clin N Am.* 2007;18(4):631-658.

Louis DN, et al: The 2016 World Health Organization classification of tumors of the central nervous system: a summary. *Acta Neuropathol.* 2016;131:803-820.

Mukherjee D, et al: Association of surgical resection and survival in patients with malignant primary osseous spinal neoplasms from the Surveillance, Epidemiology, and End Results (SEER) database. *Eur Spine J.* 2013;22(6):1375-1382.

Ottenhausen M, et al: Intradural spinal tumors in adults—update on management and outcome. *Neurosurg Rev.* 2019;42(2):371-388.

Ozawa H, et al: Spinal dumbbell tumors: an analysis of a series of 118 cases. *J Neurosurg Spine.* 2007;7(6):587-593.

Thakur NA, et al: Benign tumors of the spine. *J Am Acad Orthop Surg.* 2012;20(11):715-724.

Zadnik PL, et al: Spinal cord tumours: advances in genetics and their implications for treatment. *Nat Rev Neurol.* 2013;9(5):257-266.

▼ PITUITARY TUMORS

Pablo A. Valdes, MD, PhD, and Timothy R. Smith, MD, PhD

▶ Clinical Presentation

The pituitary gland is involved in hormonal regulation of the body and is composed of the anterior pituitary (adenohypophysis), posterior pituitary (neurohypophysis), and functionally the pars intermedia separating the two lobes. The anterior pituitary secretes prolactin, adrenocorticotropin hormone (ACTH), TSH, LH, FSH, and growth hormone (GH); meanwhile, the posterior pituitary is a repository of the hypothalamic hormones oxytocin and antidiuretic hormone (ADH; vasopressin).

Pituitary tumors account for 10%-20% of all primary intracranial tumors, making them the third most common after gliomas and meningiomas. The most common are pituitary adenomas. They have a peak incidence at 40-50 years of age, with functioning (ie, secreting) tumors more frequent in young adults and nonfunctioning (ie, nonsecreting) tumors more common in older adults, with a slight female preponderance. They are almost always benign tumors developing from the anterior pituitary (adenohypophysis) and rarely from the posterior pituitary (neurohypophysis).

Pituitary adenomas are classified based on histology, endocrine function, and size. Secreting tumors release supraphysiologic levels of hormones that result in distinct clinical syndromes and account for almost two-thirds of cases (meanwhile, nonsecretory tumors account for the remaining third). The most common adenomas are prolactin secreting (32%-66%), GH secreting (8%-16%), and adrenocorticotropin secreting (2%-6%).

Pituitary tumors can be classified based on size, with approximately 50% of tumors < 10 mm on MRI (known as microadenomas) and approximately 50% of tumors > 10 mm (known as macroadenomas). The new WHO 2017 classification of pituitary adenomas focuses on an adenohypophyseal cell lineage as well as clinical and pathologic prognostic parameters for predicting high risk and aggressive adenomas. The three main adenohypophyseal cell differentiation pathways are corticotrophs, somatotrophs/lactotrophs/mammosomatotrophs/thyrotrophs, and gonadotrophs.

Pituitary tumors can present with a variety of symptoms depending on size, location, and hormonal status (ie, secreting vs nonsecreting). Compression and/or mass effect of an adenoma can lead to a variety of symptoms including headaches, visual field deficits, ophthalmoplegia, and facial pain. The optic chiasm is located superior to the pituitary gland in the majority of cases (80%) such that larger adenomas can grow superiorly, leading to contact, elevation, compression, and/or displacement of the optic chiasm, ultimately leading to the classical bitemporal hemianopsia in patients from compression of the decussating nasal fibers. Visual compromise secondary to optic nerve/chiasm compression is usually an indication for treatment because these can progress to eventual loss of acuity and blindness. Pituitary adenomas also commonly invade the cavernous sinus laterally up to complete 360-degree encasement of the surrounding cavernous internal carotid, which can lead to oculomotor (cranial nerve [CN] III) and abducens (CN VI) palsies, with patients presenting with complaints of diplopia and ophthalmoplegia on neurologic examination. Significant mass effect and encasement of the cavernous sinus can also lead to facial pain due to V1-V2 compression or even proptosis/chemosis due to occlusion of the cavernous sinus. Invasion of the cavernous sinus can be graded and help guide surgical treatment and planning.

Secretory tumors can present with endocrinologic symptoms related to hypersecretion of a specific hormone. Hypersecretion of prolactin may include diminished libido, infertility, and an amenorrhea-galactorrhea syndrome in women and impotence in men. Levels greater than 300 ng/mL are usually associated with a prolactinoma, whereas modestly high levels of 150 ng/mL or less are typically more likely in cases of pituitary stalk interruption (ie, "stalk effect" due to release of tonic inhibition of hypothalamic dopamine on prolactin-producing cells). In cases of extremely elevated prolactin, one should ensure serial dilutions to avoid a false negative by the so-called "hook effect," which results from excess prolactin saturating the laboratory assay causing a false-negative read.

Hypersecretion of GH causes acromegaly in adults and gigantism in children with classical physical changes such as skeletal and soft tissue overgrowth, macroglossia, nerve entrapment syndromes, and associated increased morbidity and mortality due to cardiomyopathy, sleep apnea, and glucose intolerance. Patients can notice changes in shoe sizes as adult or inability to wear a wedding ring, with an overall insidious onset of the disease.

Hypersecretion of ACTH by adenomas accounts for 65% of cases of hypercortisolism, leading to Cushing disease. The signs and symptoms of hypercortisolism are known as Cushing syndrome, with characteristic findings such as moon-shaped face, excess hair growth, easy bruising, menstrual irregularity, hypertension, buffalo hump, obesity, abdominal striae, glucose intolerance, osteoporosis, poor wound healing, amenorrhea, impotence, and hyperpigmentation. Cushing disease patients have up to a two- to fivefold increased morbidity and mortality if left untreated.

Hypersecretion of TSH is rare (< 1%), with classic findings of hyperthyroidism including tachycardia, weight loss, heat intolerance, anxiety, and tremor. Rarely, pituitary adenomas can also hypersecrete gonadotropins (LH and FSH) with a usually silent presentation except in women, in which they can present with amenorrhea and infertility.

Patients can present with excessive thirst and urination as a result of stalk compression and loss of ADH. This is known as diabetes insipidus, in which patients have an inability to concentrate their urine, resulting in dehydration and hypernatremia.

Apoplexy, or acute pituitary failure, is considered a neurosurgical emergency and usually results from hemorrhage and/or necrosis in preexisting adenomas, leading to an acute presentation with severe headache, visual changes, and ophthalmoplegia; changes in mental status; and Addisonian crises. These patients require acute medical management of their endocrinologic and electrolyte status (eg, steroid administration, diabetes insipidus) to avoid cardiovascular collapse. Moreover, surgical decompression is often indicated to prevent blindness from compression of the optic apparatus.

▶ Differential Diagnosis

The differential diagnosis of sellar and suprasellar lesions is broad. It is fundamental to distinguish among the various possibilities by means of a detailed history, physical, MRI, and endocrinologic testing. The differential includes, but is not limited to, pituitary adenoma, craniopharyngioma, Rathke cleft cyst, meningioma, optic pathway glioma, dermoid, epidermoid, lymphoma, carcinoma, pituicytoma, abscess, aneurysm, neurosarcoidosis, Langerhans cell histiocytosis, hypophysitis, and metastases.

▶ Diagnostic Workup

Initial evaluation should include careful note of symptoms related to hyper- or hyposecretion of hormones or compression of surrounding structures. Ideally, a visual field examination with formal visual field testing should be performed. Imaging should be done to help ascertain size, location, and likely preoperative diagnosis. Pituitary tumors are sellar and/or suprasellar masses (specifically with adenomas) that vary in their CT features depending on presence of hemorrhage and cystic and necrotic components. Solid adenomas without cysts or hemorrhage are typically isodense to brain and rarely harbor calcifications (the latter are a more common feature of craniopharyngiomas). MRI should be obtained with and without contrast with thin cuts through the sella in the coronal and sagittal planes to better identify the size, configuration, and extent of invasion of tumor and location of normal gland (Figure 38–17). MRI shows a typically isointense lesion but can vary with a more heterogeneous

A   B

▲ **Figure 38–17.** Magnetic resonance imaging in (**A**) sagittal plain and (**B**) coronal plain of a pituitary macroadenoma.

pattern with hypointense regions (cyst) or hyperintense area (hemorrhage) on T1-weighted imaging; solid components demonstrate contrast enhancement. T2-weighted imaging demonstrates isointense signal but can vary if a more heterogeneous lesion with hyperintense (cyst) or hypointense (hemorrhage) regions is present. Gradient echo/SWI images can provide a more sensitive means of assessing hemorrhagic components.

Laboratory testing should include direct or indirect evaluation of anterior pituitary hormones including prolactin, fasting morning cortisol, free T_4, TSH, insulin-like growth factor-1 (IGF-1), GH, LH, FSH, and testosterone. Studies should also include serum sodium and osmolality as well as urine osmolality or specific gravity to confirm diagnosis. In cases with concern for hypercortisolism, additional studies can be performed including 24-hour urinary free cortisol, low and high dexamethasone suppression tests, and ACTH levels to help confirm location of pathology (eg, pituitary adenoma, adrenal adenoma or carcinoma, or ACTH-producing pulmonary malignancy). IGF-1 is the gold standard for diagnosis of GH-secreting tumors since levels are relatively stable and is a better confirmatory test than the more volatile levels of GH.

▶ Treatment

The mainstay of treatment involves medical and/or surgical approaches that depend on endocrinologic status, location, size, and the patient's health status. Nonsecreting adenomas without compressive symptoms can be managed conservatively and followed with serial imaging. Nonsecreting adenomas causing compressive symptoms and secreting adenomas causing compressive and/or purely endocrinologic disturbance are usually treated surgically. The most common approach is a microscopic or endoscopic transsphenoidal approach (ie, into the nasal cavity, through the sphenoid sinus, and to the sella). This approach provides a more minimally invasive approach to treat these lesions. In some cases with large tumors where a transsphenoidal approach does not provide optimal resection (eg, extensive suprasellar or lateral extension), a craniotomy might be indicated. Prolactinomas are the exception because they can usually respond well to medical treatment alone.

Treatment of hypersecreting adenomas depends on the hormone secreted. Prolactinomas can usually first be treated medically with dopamine agonists such as bromocriptine or cabergoline to decrease size and even result in cure. Most prolactinomas respond well, but 10%-20% of cases do not, in which circumstances surgical treatment is indicated. Other medical options include somatostatin analogs to reduce GH levels and associated symptoms or also control production of TSH. In cases were medical management alone is not indicated or sufficient, patients will undergo surgical treatment. Finally, radiation can be an option, usually in recurrent or aggressive tumors.

Postoperatively patients might require hormonal supplementation, including but not limited to steroids (eg, hydrocortisone), desmopressin (DDAVP), and levothyroxine. Diabetes insipidus following pituitary surgery can occur in up to 30% of cases in the immediate postoperative setting, although a majority will eventually recover function. Some patients maybe undergo a triple-phase response, comprising an early transient diabetes insipidus, followed by antidiuresis and hyponatremia, and finally resolving into a permanent diabetes insipidus.

Inoshita N, Nishioka H. The 2017 WHO classification of pituitary adenoma: overview and comments. *Brain Tumor Pathol.* 2018;35(2):51-56.

Kopczak A, Renner U, Stalla KG: Advances in understanding pituitary tumors. *F1000Prime Rep.* 2014;6:5.

Melmed S: Pathogenesis of pituitary tumors. *Nat Rev Endocrinol.* 2011;7(5):257-266.

Molitch ME: Diagnosis and treatment of pituitary adenomas: a review. *JAMA.* 2017;317(5):516-524.

▼ PEDIATRIC NEUROSURGERY

Kevin T. Huang, MD, and Timothy R. Smith, MD, PhD

CONGENITAL MALFORMATIONS

▶ Craniospinal Dysraphisms

Craniospinal dysraphisms encompass a group of disorders that arise from improper neural tube closure during embryonic development. These may be classified based on whether they are open or closed (with closed defects covered with skin), the location of the lesion, or the embryologic basis for the malformation.

A. Myelomeningocele

Myelomeningocele, also known as spina bifida, occurs in approximately 1 in every 1200-1400 live births. Its incidence has sharply declined in the developed world with prenatal folate supplementation, but cases persist because causative factors include both genetic and environmental factors. The condition arises during primary neurulation from failure of neural tube closure, which occurs between postfertilization days 21 and 28 in humans. The result is a child born with a cutaneous defect in the lumbosacral region, with an exposed sheet of neural tissue known as a neural placode. This is accompanied by several neural dysfunctions and malformations, including congenital dysfunction of the lumbosacral nerves (and associated lower limb paralysis and lack of bowel/bladder function), hydrocephalus, and descended cerebellar tonsils (Chiari II malformation, see below).

The diagnosis of a neural tube defect can be suspected prenatally with an elevated maternal serum alpha-fetoprotein and confirmed by in utero imaging such as a maternal-fetal MRI or ultrasound. Pregnant mothers who have inadequate folate intake or who have other children with neural tube defects are at increased risk for giving birth to a child with a myelomeningocele. Immediately following birth, care of the defect involves placing the baby prone (avoiding pressure on the placode) and keeping the defect moist, followed by prompt closure of the defect. Other considerations include urologic attention for bladder dysfunction and monitoring for any developing hydrocephalus.

B. Closed Neural Tube Defects and Tethered Cord Syndrome

Closed neural tube defects include a wide spectrum of disorders and arise from problems with disjunction, secondary neurulation, or postneurulation events. Types of closed neural tube defects include dermal sinus tracts, spinal lipomas, neurenteric cysts, sacral dysgenesis, and diastematomyelia. They can be suspected in children with certain superficial markers of the lower back, such as a distinct tuft of hair, sacral dimple, visible sinus tract, palpable mass, a prominent port-wine stain, hemangioma, hyper- or hypopigmented macule, or a significantly deviated gluteal cleft. Presence of abnormal cutaneous stigmata should warrant further screening with imaging.

Many of these abnormalities, with some as subtle as a fatty or thickened filum terminale, can tether the spinal cord in an abnormally low position, leading to tethered cord syndrome. It should be noted that the normal spinal cord conus terminates at approximately the level of the L1-2 interspace. Children may initially be asymptomatic, but as the child grows, the tethering can cause traction of the spinal cord. Neuronal dysfunction subsequently ensues with symptoms such as back or leg pain, worsening lower extremity motor and sensory function, decline in bladder and bowel function, worsening lower extremity orthopedic deformities, and progressive scoliosis. Surgical repair is often recommended early in life in order to prevent the onset or halt the progression of neurologic symptoms.

Other specific malformations may require surgical intervention for other reasons as well. Dermal sinus tracts, which can directly communicate the CNS to the outside world, require closure to prevent infection. These can also occur in the cranial region and similarly require repair. Neurenteric cysts, remnants of involuted endodermal material often located intradurally in the ventral thoracic spinal canal, may require resection to prevent enlargement and spinal cord impingement. Lipomyelomeningoceles, involving mesenchymal growth developing into a lipoma involved with the spinal cord itself, may require more complex debulking and detethering procedures. Diastematomyelia, or split-cord malformation, may involve resection of any bony spurs separating the two hemicords and possibly joining of the two thecal sacs.

C. Cranial Dysraphisms

Many cranial dysraphisms are incompatible with life, but when CNS contents are present at birth herniating through a congenital skull defect, they are known as an encephalocele. These herniated tissues include a mixture of neural tissue, meninges, and CSF. Prognosis for the children is dependent on the amount of tissue contained within the encephalocele, and encephaloceles are frequently associated with other congenital anomalies. Surgical repair involves removal of the sac, perseveration of any underlying functional tissue, and closure to prevent egress of CSF.

▶ Arachnoid Cysts

Arachnoid cysts are developmental anomalies that form intradurally, are lined with arachnoid matter, and contain CSF. These cysts most commonly occur in the middle cranial fossa and retrocerebellar region. The brain may be shifted by the arachnoid cyst, but the overall brain volume is usually close to normal. Arachnoid cysts are often asymptomatic, incidental findings that do not require further intervention, and they typically do not expand over time. Occasionally, however, they can present with either symptoms of local compression nearby neural tissue and/or gradual enlargement over time. When clearly symptomatic, they can be surgically treated with cyst fenestration, with cystoperitoneal shunting available for refractory cases.

▶ Chiari Malformations

Chiari malformations encompass a group of congenital malformations of the hindbrain and posterior fossa. Although four different types have been reported, only two are commonly encountered.

▲ **Figure 38–18.** Sagittal T2-weighted magnetic resonance imaging scan of a Chiari I malformation showing typical peg-like appearance of cerebellar tonsils and associated syringomyelia.

Chiari I malformations are most common and are defined as when the cerebellar tonsils are herniated below the level of the foramen magnum (Figure 38–18). It is important to note that many of these are asymptomatic and do not require treatment. Moreover, presenting complains are often nonspecific, such as headaches, which can be difficult to attribute specifically to the Chiari malformation. Symptoms are thought to arise from crowding of the foramen magnum. Symptoms thought to be more specific to a Chiari malformation include occipital headaches that worsen with increased ICP (eg, when coughing or laughing), evidence of syrinx formation in the spinal cord (eg, weakness, numbness, motor regression, or progressive scoliosis), and any evidence of brainstem dysfunction (eg, central sleep apnea). The workup should include imaging of the spine in addition to the brain to assess for the presence of a syrinx. Surgical decision making can be challenging because symptoms can be nonspecific, but patients with symptoms clearly referable to the lesion should be treated. Surgical correction consists of bony decompression of the back of the foramen magnum (suboccipital craniectomy), with the possible addition of a C1 laminectomy and expansile duraplasty for additional decompression.

Chiari II malformations are similarly identified as lowlying cerebellar tonsils herniating through the foramen magnum but arise from the abnormal CNS development secondary to a myelomeningocele. In contrast to Chiari I patients, these patients are more prone to having symptomatic hydrocephalus and are seen as part of a constellation of other CNS developmental abnormalities. Although symptoms can be more complex, surgical treatment similarly involves posterior fossa decompression. Chiari III and IV malformations are very rare. Chiari III malformations include features of Chiari II malformation as well as an occipital encephalocele. Chiari IV malformations are characterized by severe cerebellar hypoplasia without an encephalocele.

▶ Craniosynostosis

Craniosynostosis refers to the premature fusion of one or more cranial sutures. When this occurs, bone growth is restricted in a direction perpendicular to the fused suture, and there is compensatory growth at other sites. The result is a misshapen head, which may worsen as the child grows and possibly restrict brain growth. This can typically be detected on physical examination, where a distinct ridge can be palpated along the abnormally fused suture, one of the classic abnormal head shapes can be observed when viewing the child's head, and the head circumference may be reduced. On careful observation, these findings can often be detected immediately upon birth.

Certain sutures are encountered in synostosis more commonly than others, with sagittal and unilateral coronal synostosis occurring much more commonly than the exceedingly rare lambdoid synostosis. The head shapes they produce are named in Greek for what they resemble, ranging from the elongated head of sagittal synostosis (scaphocephaly or dolichocephaly), to the skewed head shape of unilateral coronal synostosis (plagiocephaly), to the triangle shape of metopic synostosis (trigonocephaly). Notably, craniosynostosis should not be confused with the more common, nonsynostotic condition, positional plagiocephaly, which arises from an infant lying preferentially on one side and will typically resolve with conservative management.

Although most cases of craniosynostosis are sporadic and involve a single suture, multiple-suture craniosynostosis occurs in certain genetic syndromes, such as Crouzon or Apert syndrome. In such cases, treatment is indicated not only for cosmetic reasons, but also because the multiple-suture synostosis is restricting brain growth and causing elevated ICPs.

Operative repair of craniosynostosis is dependent on the age of the child. When performed early enough, endoscopic removal of the fused suture can allow a return to a more normal shape, but cases that are either more severe or present later may require more extensive cranial vault reconstruction.

HYDROCEPHALUS

Disturbances in CSF circulation or absorption result in hydrocephalus. At a basic level, hydrocephalus can be classified into two types: communicating or noncommunicating (sometimes referred to as "obstructive"). In noncommunicating hydrocephalus, there is an identifiable blockage of CSF flow within the ventricular system (eg, by a tumor). In communicating hydrocephalus, no such barrier is clearly identifiable, and CSF absorption is presumed to be blocked at the level of the arachnoid granulations. It is rare for hydrocephalus to be caused by overproduction of CSF (eg, by a choroid plexus tumor). Hydrocephalus can be found in any stage of life but is a particularly salient issue in children because neonatal hemorrhage or meningitis/encephalitis are common causes.

Hydrocephalus can cause elevations in ICP that may manifest in different ways depending on the age of the child. In neonates and infants whose anterior fontanelle is still open, untreated hydrocephalus will present with a tense or bulging fontanelle, apneic and bradycardic episodes, engorgement of the scalp veins, forced downgaze (ie, upward gaze palsy), splayed cranial sutures, rapid increases in head circumference, irritability, poor head control, and poor oral intake. In children with a closed cranial vault whose fontanelle has closed, untreated hydrocephalus will present with symptoms of intracranial hypertension including lethargy or excessive sleepiness, papilledema, headache, nausea, vomiting, gait disturbance, increased fussiness, or upward gaze palsy.

Several surgical options can be considered in the treatment of hydrocephalus. The most common CSF diversionary procedure remains ventriculoperitoneal shunting, which installs tubing that allows the cerebral ventricles to drain into the peritoneal cavity by way of a control valve. Other types of shunts may drain into other locations including the right atrium (ventriculoatrial shunt) or pleural cavity (ventriculopleural shunt). Ventriculosubgaleal shunting may be performed as a temporary measure in infants. Recently, there has also been increased interest in the use of endoscopic third ventriculostomy with choroid plexus cauterization, which involves creating an alternative pathway for CSF flow through fenestration of the floor of the third ventricle. Although traditionally this was applied mostly to cases of noncommunicating hydrocephalus, there is increased interest in its application to cases of communicating hydrocephalus as well.

Shunt failure or infection may manifest with signs and symptoms of acute intracranial hypertension. Importantly, ventricular enlargement may or may not be present in shunt failure. Prompt treatment of acute hydrocephalus and/or shunt failure is indicated to prevent irreversible neurologic injury including herniation, blindness, or death.

PEDIATRIC CENTRAL NERVOUS SYSTEM TUMORS

Brain tumors are the most common solid tumors of childhood. The locations and types of tumors in the pediatric population differ from those in adults, and most tumors in children under the age of 12 occur in the infratentorial space.

In neonates and infants, brain tumors may manifest with nonspecific findings, and mass effect from a tumor may not be clinically evident initially due to a compliant skull and an open fontanelle. In young children, a primary brain tumor may present with symptoms related to intracranial hypertension such as headache, nausea, and vomiting. Papilledema may be evident on funduscopic examination. Older children more often present with focal neurologic signs and symptoms. When a posterior fossa brain tumor is diagnosed, preoperative imaging of the brain and spine should be performed whenever possible to evaluate for drop metastases in the spinal canal.

Medulloblastoma

Medulloblastomas compose approximately 20% of all pediatric brain tumors and 30% of all posterior fossa tumors in children. They are thought to arise from residual embryonic tissue and appear as hyperdense lesions in the region of the fourth ventricle that enhance following contrast administration (Figure 38–19). Although traditionally they have been classified histologically, increasingly it is being viewed as useful to classify them by molecular expression, with consensus of at least four distinct subgroups: WNT, SHH, group 3, and group 4.

When encountered, treatment involves complete or near-complete surgical resection with postoperative craniospinal radiation in children old enough to tolerate it (generally

▲ **Figure 38–19.** Head computed tomography demonstrating large mass (medulloblastoma) within the fourth ventricle causing ventricular dilation.

those age 3 years or older). Patients who are classified as high risk are typically treated with chemotherapy as well. Because of the increased morbidity of radiation in children less than 3 years of age, chemotherapy can be used to delay the radiation dose in such young patients. The 5-year overall survival is reported at between 65% and 75% but is lower in patients with diffuse disease, with postsurgical residuals, or presenting at younger ages.

Cerebellar Astrocytoma/Pilocytic Astrocytomas

Cerebellar astrocytomas (> 75% of which are pilocytic astrocytomas histologically) account for approximately 20% of all pediatric brain tumors. The peak age of presentation is 10 years. The characteristic appearance on imaging studies is an enhancing mural nodule with a surrounding cyst. The goal of treatment is complete surgical resection, as patients with a gross total resection have a 90% long-term survival rate without any need for additional adjuvant therapies.

Ependymoma

Ependymomas arise from the ependymal cells lining the ventricular system and can arise anywhere along the neuraxis with an ependymal surface. In the pediatric population, 90% of ependymomas are intracranial, and of these, two-thirds are located in the posterior fossa. Ependymoma cells are known to migrate through the CSF and can often be found in distal sites within the CNS, underscoring the importance of full neuraxis imaging to properly stage the disease. Treatment usually consists of tumor resection and postoperative focal radiation.

Brainstem Glioma

Brainstem gliomas are a heterogeneous group of tumors of varying histology, biologic behavior, and prognosis. Diffuse brainstem gliomas represent up to 80% of all brainstem gliomas and carry the worst prognosis. Affected children typically present with a relatively short clinical history of unilateral or bilateral cranial neuropathies, progressive ataxia, gait abnormality, and long tract signs. On MRI studies, diffuse brainstem gliomas appear as nonenhancing, T1-hypointense, T2-hyperintense masses that expand the brainstem (typically the pons) (Figure 38–20). Diagnosis of a diffuse brainstem tumor can be made on the basis of imaging alone, and biopsy is usually not recommended. Radiation therapy and steroids may improve symptoms but have not been shown to prolong survival, as these tumors are universally fatal, with a median survival of 8-10 months.

Other types of brainstem gliomas are associated with a better prognosis. Dorsally exophytic brainstem tumors are characterized by slow growth with gradual onset of

▲ **Figure 38–20.** Magnetic resonance imaging appearance of a diffuse pontine glioma.

symptoms and can sometimes be excised with limited morbidity. Moreover, nondiffuse gliomas such as focal intrinsic and dorsally exophytic brainstem gliomas are usually histologically lower grade (WHO grade I or II) lesions.

Tumors of Infancy

Brain tumors that affect infants include medulloblastoma, central neuroblastoma, supratentorial primitive neuroectodermal tumor (PNET), pineoblastoma, and atypical teratoid/rhabdoid tumor. These are all high-grade tumors with a propensity to spread throughout the CSF. Medulloblastoma, central neuroblastoma, supratentorial PNET, and pineoblastomas are all considered PNETs with similar histologies. Atypical teratoid/rhabdoid tumors are usually found in the posterior fossa and are associated with a poor prognosis, as most children die within 1 year of diagnosis.

Pineal Region Tumors

Tumors arising in the region of the pineal gland compose 3%-8% of pediatric brain tumors. Histologically, pineal region tumors are most often germ cell tumors such as germinomas, teratomas (mature and immature), embryonal cell carcinomas, choriocarcinomas, and endodermal sinus tumors. Germinomas are the most common pineal region tumors and demonstrate a gender predilection for males. Pineal parenchymal tumors such as pineocytomas or pineoblastomas occur less frequently. Pineal tumors can compress

the cerebral aqueduct and cause hydrocephalus. Patients may present with Parinaud syndrome consisting of impaired upgaze, convergence-retraction nystagmus, lid retraction, convergence paralysis, pupillary dilatation, and light-near dissociation. Complete neuraxis imaging should be performed because drop metastases can occur via CSF pathways. Serum and CSF should be tested for tumor markers that may be secreted by germ cell tumors including placental alkaline phosphatase, alpha-fetoprotein, and beta-human chorionic gonadotropin. Radiation therapy with or without chemotherapy is the mainstay of treatment for germ cells tumors.

Dysembryoplastic Neuroepithelial Tumors

Dysembryoplastic neuroepithelial tumor is a low-grade cortical based tumor with a median age of presentation of 7 years. They appear as superficial cystic tumors in the temporal or frontal lobes. On MRI, they are hypointense on T1-weighted sequences, hyperintense on T2-weighted sequences, do not enhance, and are often described as having a "bubbly" appearance. Patients with these tumors typically present with a long history of intractable complex partial seizures and have a normal neurologic exam. Gross total resection of the tumor is curative and usually eliminates seizures.

Sellar Tumors

Tumors that arise in the region of the sella turcica and pituitary gland in children include pituitary adenomas and craniopharyngiomas. Pituitary adenomas are relatively rare among children. Craniopharyngiomas, however, represent 6%-9% of all pediatric brain tumors and are the most common nonglial intracranial masses in children. On imaging, craniopharyngiomas appear as cystic tumors that originate from a suprasellar location. Calcification is commonly visible on CT scan and can be helpful in differentiating craniopharyngiomas from other types of tumors. They typically present either with signs of local mass effect (eg, headaches, visual disturbances, and/or noncommunicating hydrocephalus) or symptoms of endocrine dysfunction such as growth failure, diabetes insipidus, hypothyroidism, or menstrual dysfunction. A thorough endocrine workup is warranted in patients with suspected craniopharyngioma. Surgical resection is the mainstay of treatment, but extent of resection is often limited by the tumor's location, and thus radiotherapy is often employed as either primary or adjuvant therapy. Postoperatively, patients should be watched for signs of diabetes insipidus or hypothalamic insufficiency.

Choroid Plexus Tumors

Choroid plexus tumors include choroid plexus papillomas and choroid plexus carcinomas. They represent 2%-4% of all pediatric brain tumors and present as an intraventricular mass that avidly enhances with contrast. For choroid plexus papillomas, prognosis is generally favorable and can typically be treated with gross total resection alone. Choroid plexus carcinomas are malignant tumors for which the average age of diagnosis is 2 years. They are commonly already disseminated at the time of diagnosis, and prognosis is generally poor. Treatment consists of surgical resection, radiation therapy, and possibly chemotherapy.

CEREBROVASCULAR DISEASE IN CHILDREN

▶ Aneurysms and Vascular Malformations

Children may present with a variety of intracranial vascular malformations such as arteriovenous malformations (AVMs), venous angiomas, capillary telangiectasias, and cavernous malformations. AVMs are congenital malformations that often go undetected until they present with an intraparenchymal hemorrhage, which can range in severity from severe headaches to life-threatening increased ICP. AVMs are usually treated with surgery in the pediatric age group but may occasionally be treated with stereotactic radiation or embolization techniques. Cavernous malformations can also present with intracerebral hemorrhage but are more likely to primarily present with seizures. Surgical resection is indicated in symptomatic patients. Although relatively common in the adult population, cerebral aneurysms are rare in the pediatric population. Depending on the size and configuration of the aneurysm, these lesions may be treated by surgical clipping or endovascular coiling or managed conservatively.

▶ Vein of Galen Malformations

Vein of Galen malformations are congenital vascular malformations characterized by extensive arterial feeders draining into an enlarged vein of Galen. Although these malformations are also known as vein of Galen aneurysms, they represent arteriovenous fistulae. Newborns can present with high-output cardiac failure due to the arteriovenous shunting. The extensive arteriovenous shunting can also produce a steal effect and result in cerebral ischemia and infarction. Moreover, hydrocephalus is a common finding due to compression of the cerebral aqueduct by the malformation. The prognosis may be poor for patients diagnosed in early infancy with heart failure but is better for those diagnosed later in life. Treatment usually involves endovascular embolization of feeding arteries.

▶ Moyamoya Disease

Moyamoya disease is an idiopathic vasculopathy that leads to progressive occlusion of one or both internal carotid arteries. Secondary to this phenomenon, there is angiogenesis about the stenotic point, leading to the formation of a capillary network that looks like a "puff of smoke" (translated to "moyamoya" in Japanese) on cerebral angiogram. The disease can also involve the proximal middle and anterior cerebral arteries. Children with moyamoya disease present with ischemic events that may be provoked by straining or hyperventilation. Refractory headaches, seizures, and alternating hemiplegia are also associated with moyamoya disease. Moyamoya is treated with surgical revascularization to improve blood flow via direct or indirect bypass procedures.

SPASTICITY

Spasticity in children is most often due to cerebral palsy, and several surgical interventions exist for treatment. In determining whether a child with hypertonia will benefit from surgical intervention, it is important to assess whether dystonia is present, as well the ambulatory potential of the child, and to what extent the underlying spasticity is useful for the child in terms of providing strength and postural support. In addition to medication, orthopedic procedures, and periodic injections that are used to treat spasticity, the neurosurgical treatments for spasticity include placement of an intrathecal baclofen pump and selective dorsal rhizotomy (SDR).

An intrathecal baclofen pump entails inserting a catheter into the intrathecal space and connecting it to a programmable subcutaneous pump. Depending on at what spinal level the catheter tip is placed, upper and lower extremity spasticity may be treated. Vigilance must be maintained for the possibility of pump malfunction, as symptoms of baclofen withdrawal can be severe and potentially life-threatening. Patients who are ambulatory and whose spasticity primarily affects their lower extremities may be candidates for an SDR. It is thought that inputs entering the spinal cord through the dorsal roots have a net excitatory effect on the ventral motor roots, thus contributing to spasticity. The premise of an SDR is to intraoperatively stimulate lumbosacral dorsal nerve rootlets and record responses from the anterior nerve roots and muscles. This allows for the identification of those nerve rootlets that are relatively more involved in maintaining hypertonia, and such nerve rootlets are sectioned. SDR has been shown to improve ambulation, but the procedure does not confer previously nonambulatory patients with the ability to walk.

PEDIATRIC TRAUMA AND BIRTH INJURIES

▶ General Principles

Head injury and its management are discussed elsewhere, and treatment principles used in the management of adult trauma also apply to the pediatric patient. Certain aspects of trauma that are unique to the pediatric population are highlighted here.

Head injuries are 30 times more common in children than spinal cord injuries, and they represent the most common cause of mortality and morbidity in children. In infants and young children, the brain and head are disproportionately large compared to the trunk and torso, and the neck and paraspinal musculature are incompletely developed. In children younger than 4 years of age, the skull is soft, is more prone to fracture, and provides less protection to the brain. Most skull fractures can be treated conservatively, including some depressed skull fractures. Depressed skull fractures that cause a significant cosmetic defect can be considered for elevation. In children less than 2 years of age, skull fractures associated with a tear in the underlying dura may expand over time. These growing skull fractures are rare but may require operative closure of the dural defect when encountered.

Nonaccidental Trauma

Nonaccidental head trauma is the leading cause of traumatic death and morbidity in children. Diagnosis of nonaccidental head trauma can be challenging, and there may be few signs of external trauma even with significant neurologic injury. The child may present with lethargy, irritability, poor feeding, apneic episodes, or seizures. Multiple skull fractures that are associated with underlying brain injury, bilateral chronic SDHs or SDHs of varying ages, SAH, and retinal hemorrhages should raise the index of suspicion for child abuse. SDHs commonly occur along the bilateral convexities or in the posterior interhemispheric fissure. MRI is best at evaluating SDHs of varying ages, as well as the extent of DAI that occurs with the acceleration-deceleration and rotational forces in shaken baby syndrome. A workup should include imaging of the brain and possibly spine, a skeletal survey to assess for long-bone or rib fractures, a funduscopic examination to check for retinal hemorrhages, and a thorough external exam to assess for bruising. Death from nonaccidental trauma is most often due to refractory intracranial hypertension.

Spine Trauma

SCI is relatively rare in the pediatric population. The pediatric spine continues to develop throughout the first 2 decades of life. Ligamentous injury is more common than bony injury, owing to ligamentous laxity, immature supporting musculature, and the developing bony joints of the spine. The cervical spine is most commonly injured in children, and in children less than 9 years of age, a higher percentage of injuries occur in the upper cervical spine.

Al-Holou WN, Yew AY, Boomsaad ZE, et al: Prevalence and natural history of arachnoid cysts in children. *J Neurosurg Pediatr.* 2010;5(6):578-585.

Klimo P, Rao G, Brockmeyer D: Pediatric arteriovenous malformations: a 15-year experience with an emphasis on residual and recurrent lesions. *Childs Nerv Syst.* 2007;23(1):31-37.

Lew SM, Kothbauer KF: Tethered cord syndrome: an updated review. *Pediatr Neurosurg.* 2007;43:236-248.

Nield LS, Brunner MD, Kamat D: The infant with a misshapen head. *Clin Pediatr.* 2007;46:292-298.

Ramaswamy V, Remke M, Bouffet E, et al: Risk stratification of childhood medulloblastoma in the molecular era: the current consensus. *Acta Neuropathol.* 2016;131(6):821-831.

Shu HG, Sall WF, Maity A, et al: Childhood intracranial ependymomas. Twenty-year experience from a single institution. *Cancer.* 2007;110:432-441.

Tubbs RS, Lyerly MJ, Loukas M, et al: The pediatric Chiari I malformation: a review. *Childs Nerv Syst.* 2007;23(11):1239-1250.

▼ INTRACRANIAL ANEURYSMS AND ARTERIOVENOUS MALFORMATIONS

Pui Man Rosalind Lai, MD, and Timothy Smith, MD, PhD, MPH

INTRACRANIAL ANEURYSMS

KEY CONCEPTS

▸ An intracranial aneurysm is an abnormal dilation or expansion of an artery commonly occurring at branch points in the circle of Willis.

▸ Most aneurysms are asymptomatic, but if they rupture, they carry a significant rate of morbidity and mortality.

▸ Treatment options include surgical clipping or endovascular coiling of the aneurysm to prevent future rupture.

General Consideration

Intracranial aneurysm, or cerebral aneurysm, is an abnormal dilation or expansion of an intracranial artery. Autopsy studies suggest these lesions are relatively common, presenting in 1%-5% of the adult population. Aneurysms are classified into different types based on their morphology: saccular, fusiform, and dissecting. *Saccular aneurysms* are the most common type of aneurysms and are commonly located at the branch points in the circle of Willis. These aneurysms are thought to be sporadically acquired lesions, but rare familial forms have been described in the literature. Intracranial aneurysms are associated with a number of heritable connective tissue disorders, including autosomal dominant polycystic kidney disease, fibromuscular dysplasia, Marfan syndrome, and Ehlers-Danlos syndrome type IV.

The exact pathophysiology of intracranial aneurysms is still to be determined, but it is known that genetics as well as environmental factors, such as hypertension and smoking, play a significant role in the progression of disease. Histologically, the aneurysmal wall has a decreased tunica media, the middle muscular layer of the artery, resulting in structural defects and an outpouching at the arterial branch point.

Diagnosis & Clinical Findings

Most intracranial aneurysms remain asymptomatic and undetected, but if they rupture, they can present as devastating and life-threatening events. The estimated incidence of an aneurysmal rupture in the United States is 1 case per 10,000 persons, with peak incidence in persons 55-60 years old, and they occur more commonly in women. Typically, for less severe bleeds, patients often describe an acute onset of severe headache with nuchal rigidity and lethargy, often known as "the worst headache of life." The Hunt and Hess grading scale is commonly used to convey the severity of symptoms and to risk-stratify patients (Table 38–6). Higher Hunt and Hess grade is associated with worse clinical outcome.

Aneurysms that have hemorrhaged remain at risk for new rebleeding. The estimated rehemorrhage rate of a ruptured aneurysm is approximately 25% within the first 2 weeks and 50% by 6 months. Because mortality of a rebleed approaches 80%, referral to a neurosurgeon for urgent treatment of a ruptured aneurysm is critical for patient outcome.

Anatomically, the intracranial arteries course within the subarachnoid space. An aneurysmal rupture often results in hemorrhage in this space (SAH). Noncontrast head CT has a high sensitivity for the detection of SAH, with a characteristic pattern of blood in the basal cisterns, the CSF spaces surrounding the cortex, and the cerebellum.

An enlarging but unruptured intracranial aneurysm may also present as focal neurologic deficit by its mass effect. The presenting symptom is dependent on the location of the aneurysm. The most common cranial nerve palsy due to mass effect from an aneurysm is a third nerve palsy, through compression of the oculomotor nerve (CN III) by the posterior communicating artery or the posterior cerebral artery. Aneurysms larger than 2.5 cm are called *giant aneurysms* and may lead to more pronounced symptoms including hemiparesis, obstructed hydrocephalus, seizures, and brainstem compression.

▲ **Figure 38–21.** An anterior view of left carotid artery cerebral angiogram demonstrating a large cerebral artery aneurysm (arrow) at the middle cerebral artery bifurcation.

With the increasing availability and advancement of neuroimaging, the detection of unruptured and asymptomatic cerebral aneurysms is increasing (Figure 38–21). Although aneurysms that have ruptured or are causing focal neurologic deficit should be treated as emergencies, the decision for treatment of incidental aneurysms is more complex and is dependent on many factors, including the patient's age and comorbidities and aneurysm location and morphology.

Treatment

A. Initial Management

The determination of a patient's airway, breathing, and circulation (ABCs) should be performed in patients with suspected ruptured intracranial aneurysms. Patients with unstable or unprotected airways should be intubated and placed on mechanical ventilation. The maintenance of PCO_2 values between 28 and 32 mm Hg can help acutely lower ICP. Blood pressure should be maintained with intravenous medications as needed, with close monitoring by placement of an arterial line. Basic laboratory values should be assessed including complete blood count, coagulation levels, sodium level, blood urea nitrogen, and creatinine. An electrocardiogram should be performed to rule out neurogenic stress cardiomyopathy.

The demonstration of SAH on an initial head CT and no traumatic history should raise suspicion for an intracranial vascular lesion and should be immediately followed by an assessment of the cerebral vasculature by

Table 38–6. Hunt-Hess scale.

Grade	Findings
I	Mild headache or nuchal rigidity
II	Severe headache, nuchal rigidity, possible cranial nerve deficit
III	Lethargic, confused, mild focal deficit
IV	Stuporous, moderate to severe hemiparesis, early decerebrate posturing
V	Deep coma, decerebrate posturing, moribund

Reproduced with permission from Hunt WE, Hess RM: Surgical repair as related to time of intervention in the repair of intracranial aneurysms. *J Neurosurg* 1968 Jan;28(1):14-20.

▲ **Figure 38–22.** Classic appearance of a large subarachnoid hemorrhage. Notice the hemorrhage pattern fills the cerebrospinal fluid spaces at the base of the brain and around the brainstem.

CTA or conventional angiography (Figure 38–22). CSF diversion, typically through an EVD, may be required if a patient presents with hydrocephalus or has concerns for elevated ICP.

If an initial head CT did not demonstrate SAH but clinical suspicion is high, a lumbar puncture is often performed to assess for xanthochromia, the yellow discoloration indicating the presence of bilirubin in CSF.

B. Surgical and Endovascular Treatment

The two major modalities for the treatment of an intracranial aneurysm are microsurgical clipping and endovascular coiling. Microsurgical clipping involves an open craniotomy and the application of a surgical clip around the neck of the aneurysm to prevent rupture of the aneurysm. Endovascular treatment uses conventional angiography and navigating a microcatheter to the aneurysmal defect to insert detachable coils into the aneurysm dome. These coils promote thrombus formation to prevent blood entering the aneurysm. More recently, endovascular flow diversion has also been introduced, which involves placing a device in the parent blood vessel to divert blood flow away from the aneurysm. The decision to secure the cerebral aneurysm through microsurgical clipping or endovascular coiling is beyond the scope of this text. Factors for consideration include patient's age, overall medical condition,

aneurysmal characteristics such as size, location, morphology, and rupture status of the aneurysm.

C. Postoperative Management

The management of patients remains particularly challenging, and often, patients require prolonged intensive care hospitalization due to concerns for the development of delayed cerebral ischemia and permanent neurologic deficits, including hemiparesis, aphasia, and visual disturbances. This phenomenon has historically been thought to be due to cerebral vasospasm, the constriction of cerebral blood vessels as a result of the SAH, resulting in ischemia and infarct. The prevalence of vasospasm has been reported in up to 67% of patients presenting with SAH and typically appears between 3 and 14 days after the initial ictus, peaking at 7-10 days. However, only 20%-30% of patients with radiographic findings of vasospasm present with clinical symptoms, and those who develop clinical deficits may not demonstrate radiographic vasospasm, suggesting that the development of neurologic ischemia is not simply due to mechanical constriction of blood vessels. The development of neurologic deficits and infarcts, more recently termed *delayed ischemic neurologic deficits*, is now thought to be more complex, including microthrombosis and the loss of cerebral autoregulation.

The management of cerebral vasospasm often involves a regimen referred to as *triple H therapy*: hypertension (by the use of vasopressors), hemodilution, and hypervolemia (by the use of albumin or hypertonic solution) to increase cerebral perfusion. Patients are typically placed on nimodipine, a calcium channel blocker that has been demonstrated to decrease overall mortality but does not affect vasospasm. For severe cerebral vasospasm, cerebral angioplasty may be performed to inject calcium channel blockers directly into the affected blood vessels.

▶ Outcome/Prognosis

The strongest predictors of outcome after an aneurysmal rupture are patient age, comorbidities, and Hunt and Hess grade. The overall mortality rate of an aneurysmal rupture is 30%-50%, and 10%-20% of patients die before reaching a hospital. For patients who survive the initial insult, mortality rates range from 10%-20%, with morbidity rates of 20%-40% secondary to initial aneurysmal bleed or delayed neurologic ischemia.

▶ Summary

Intracranial aneurysms carry significant morbidity and mortality if they rupture. Because aneurysms have an increased rate of rebleeding after an initial hemorrhage and are often fatal, ruptured aneurysms should be treated urgently by microsurgical clipping or endovascular coiling. Patients remain at risk for delayed neurologic deficits and often require prolonged hospitalization after a ruptured aneurysm.

ARTERIOVENOUS MALFORMATIONS

KEY CONCEPTS

▸ An AVM is a congenital, abnormal collection of arteries and veins that may cause intraparenchymal hemorrhage when ruptured.

▸ Treatment may include surgery and radiosurgery to prevent hemorrhage or observation in some cases.

General Considerations

AVMs are tangles of congenital blood vessels with no intervening capillary bed, forming an abnormal fistula between arteries and veins (Figure 38–23). The majority of AVMs are found in the supratentorial space, but they can also be present in the brainstem and in the spine. Autopsy data suggest that AVMs occur in 1%-4% of the population, estimated to be 10-18 per 100,000 adults. Intracranial AVMs are seen in sporadic cases and rarely in some genetic syndromes, such as Osler-Weber-Rendu syndrome.

▲ **Figure 38–23.** Cerebral angiogram demonstrating a frontal arteriovenous malformation filling from the left anterior cerebral artery.

Diagnosis & Clinical Findings

Hemorrhage is the most common presentation for an AVM, occurring in over 50% of patients. Other common presentations include seizures, headache, and focal neurologic symptoms from mass effect. Initial CT findings most often present as an intraparenchymal hemorrhage, and subsequent angiographic modalities to assess for the cerebral vasculature are critical to confirm the diagnosis of an AVM.

For unruptured AVMs, the estimated rate of hemorrhage is approximately 2%-4% per year. Rebleeding rate in the first year after hemorrhage is 6%.

Treatment

A. Initial Management

The initial evaluation of AVMs depends on the patient's presentation. For patients with hemorrhage from AVM, the fundamentals of emergency care (ABCs) and complete neurologic evaluation are critical. Blood pressure management and the placement of an arterial line may be necessary. Antiepileptics should be administered for seizure prophylaxis.

After the initial confirmation of the diagnosis on CTA, the standard approach often includes a conventional angiography to assess radiographic features of the AVM. The most well-known classification for AVM is the Spetzler-Martin grading scale, which uses AVM size, venous drainage (superficial or deep), and eloquence of surrounding brain tissue, and is used to assess surgical morbidity and mortality (Table 38–7).

B. Treatment for AVM

The treatment modalities for AVM include microsurgical resection, endovascular embolization, stereotactic radiosurgery, or a

Table 38–7. Spetzler-Martin arteriovenous malformation (AVM) grading scale.

Graded Feature	Points Assigned
Size of AVM	
< 3 cm	1
3-6 cm	2
> 6 cm	3
Eloquence[1] of adjacent brain	
Noneloquent	0
Eloquent	1
Venous drainage	
Superficial	0
Deep	1

[1]Eloquent areas include visual, language, and sensorimotor cortex; the thalamus and hypothalamus; the internal capsule; the brainstem; the cerebellar peduncles; and the deep cerebellar nuclei.

combination of the above approaches. The decision on which approach to secure the AVM is beyond the scope of this chapter, but factors considered include AVM location and grade and patient preference.

Microsurgical resection of the AVM is the gold standard, which involves an open craniotomy and complete obliteration of the AVM. Most neurosurgeons agree that Spetzler-Martin grade I-III AVMs that are easily accessible should be surgically resected due to low complication rates. However, grade IV and V lesions carry a much higher risk for morbidity and mortality, up to 30%, and patients should be carefully selected before proceeding with treatment. Endovascular embolization of blood vessels may sometimes assist in reducing the size of AVM prior to surgical resection.

Stereotactic radiosurgery (SRS) may be an alternative for AVMs located in deep locations or patients who are poor surgical candidates. SRS is most ideal for AVMs less than 3 cm. The major disadvantage of this method is the 2-3 years it takes for the AVM to involute, and patients remain at risk of hemorrhage during this time.

Due to the high risk of complications with higher grade AVMs, some surgeons advocate conservative treatment for these AVMS, although opinions on the treatment for AVMs can vary widely among neurosurgeons and neurointerventionalists. AVMs are complex vascular lesions and should be treated by neurosurgeons in high-volume centers with significant experience.

C. Postoperative Management

Patients with hemorrhage from AVMs should be observed in the ICU with close observation of their neurologic status. After the obliteration of a large AVM, a phenomenon known as normal perfusion pressure breakthrough may occur. As the pathologic shunting of blood through the AVM nidus is removed, there is an increase in blood flow to the surrounding blood vessels and brain, which may result in hemorrhage. For these reasons, blood pressure monitoring is critical in postoperative management of AVM.

Spinal Arteriovenous Malformations

Spinal AVMs are rare vascular entities and are commonly classified into four types: (1) dural arteriovenous fistulas; (2) glomus AVMs; (3) juvenile intradural AVMs; and (4) intradural, extramedullary arteriovenous fistulas. Type 1 AVMs are the most common spinal vascular malformations and commonly occur near the thoracolumbar junction, with one arterial feeding vessel that connects to an intradural arterialized vein. Symptoms from spinal AVMs are commonly due to hemorrhage or venous congestion, resulting in acute or subacute lower extremity neurologic deficit, gait difficulties, myelopathy, or loss of bladder or bowel control. Initial diagnostic evaluation should include spinal MRI/MR

angiography, and often, spinal angiography is performed to evaluate the vascular lesion.

Summary

Intracranial aneurysms and AVMs are rare vascular entities that are often asymptomatic but that can be devastating after a hemorrhage. The morbidity and mortality associated with intracranial hemorrhage are high. As such, treatment is often warranted, including open neurovascular or neuroendovascular surgery, and these patients should be referred to and cared for by experienced teams of neurosurgeons, interventionalists, and neurocritical care specialists.

Solomon RA, et al: Arteriovenous malformations of the brain. *N Engl J Med.* 2017;376:1859-1866.

SURGICAL MANAGEMENT OF MEDICALLY INTRACTABLE REFRACTORY EPILEPSY

Pui Man Rosalind Lai, MD, and Timothy Smith, MD, PhD, MPH

KEY CONCEPTS

▸ Epilepsy is a syndrome of recurrent seizures and affects 1% of the population.

▸ Surgery is often reserved for structural lesions causing seizures or patients who have failed maximal medical therapy.

INTRODUCTION

Epilepsy is the second most commonly reported neurologic condition worldwide and affects 1% of the world population. Epilepsy is a syndrome of recurrent seizures, with an onset of seizure due to abnormal neuronal synchronization and propagation to surrounding brain areas. The first-line treatment for epilepsy is medical therapy, which involves pharmacotherapy and lifestyle changes, but those who fail medical treatment may be candidates for surgical intervention.

Seizure Classification

A seizure is an abnormal cerebral neuronal discharge that results in changes in sensation, motor, behavior, or consciousness. Seizures can be classified by their associations with alteration in consciousness and their etiology. Partial seizures involve one hemisphere and can further be categorized as *simple partial*, defined as those that occur with no impairment of consciousness, or *complex partial*, resulting in a loss of awareness. *Generalized seizures* involve synchronous activity in the bilateral hemisphere, and *generalized tonic-clonic seizure* (grand mal seizure) is defined as a specific type of generalized seizure that evolves from tonic to clonic motor activity.

DIAGNOSIS

Several modalities are used in the diagnosis of epilepsy, which include clinical examination, neurophysiology, neuroimaging, and neuropsychologic assessments, and all are critical for consideration for patients who may be candidates for surgery.

▶ Clinical Examination & Laboratory Assessment

The *semiology*, or clinical symptomatology, is a critical component of the diagnosis of epilepsy. The symptoms during the time of seizure may provide localizing clues to the region of onset. For example, seizures starting with motor twitching of the upper extremity likely originate from the vicinity of the primary motor cortex. Serum studies, such as fasting blood glucose, serum electrolyte panel, complete blood count, and toxicology, should also be undertaken to rule out potentially reversible causes of seizures.

▶ Electrophysiology

The standard modality for recording neuronal activity is the scalp EEG. EEG recordings may be obtained between and during seizures to assess for semiology and seizure focus. In patients whose seizure localization cannot be proven by scalp EEG, intracranial EEG electrodes may be placed. These electrodes can either be placed on the surface of the brain for cortical activity (subdural electrodes) or within the brain for deeper structures like the hippocampus (depth electrodes).

▶ Imaging studies

High-resolution MRI of the brain is the gold standard for the evaluation of structural lesions, such as tumors, vascular malformations, dysplastic cortex, and mesial temporal sclerosis (Figure 38–24). For patients who have normal MRIs or those with uncertainty about the site of seizure origin, nuclear medicine may be useful to identify focus area. PET and SPECT may be additionally performed to measure metabolic activity and regional blood flow patterns of the brain. SPECT studies performed at the beginning of a seizure may demonstrate increased blood flow in areas involved in seizure onset. PET studies can be performed during or between seizures and, when performed between seizures, demonstrate hypometabolism with the epileptogenic foci.

▶ Neuropsychological Evaluation

All individuals who are candidate for surgery for the treatment of epilepsy should undergo a neuropsychological evaluation, which is conducted by a neuropsychologist to assess

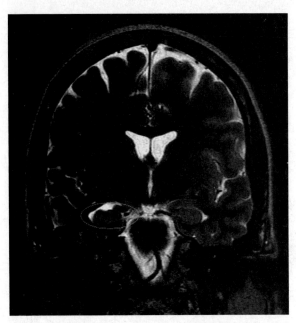

▲ **Figure 38–24.** Coronal magnetic resonance imaging of the brain demonstrating right mesial temporal sclerosis with associated atrophy of the right hippocampus and prominence of the temporal horn of the right lateral ventricle.

a person's cognitive abilities that may have been affected by epilepsy. The testing includes concentration, memory, and a range of verbal and visual abilities.

GOALS OF SURGERY

Surgery is the primary treatment for patients with structural lesions such as tumors and vascular malformations. In these patients, the goal of surgery is curative through complete resection of the affected lesion or cortex, if safe to remove.

Individuals who have failed medical therapy may also be considered for epilepsy surgery. The likelihood of attaining seizure freedom with pharmacotherapies after two drug failures has been shown to be less than 5%, and therefore, a consensus definition of medical failure is currently defined as failure of two or more antiepileptic drugs to reduce seizures to a clinically meaningful level. For these individuals, a palliative surgical approach is often employed for the reduction in seizure frequency and severity.

SURGICAL PROCEDURES FOR EPILEPSY

▶ Surgical Resection or Disconnection

For patients who have identifiable epileptic foci due to a structural lesion, surgical resection is the optimal treatment.

These patients undergo a craniotomy, and the brain tissue containing the epileptic foci is resected, but this operation is limited to noneloquent brain areas. The most common cause of drug-resistant epilepsy is *mesial temporal sclerosis*, and these patients are candidates for *temporal lobectomy*, which involves resection of the amygdala, parahippocampal gyrus, and hippocampus. Observational studies have found long-term seizure-free outcomes to be up to 60%-80%, but potential complications for this procedure include short-term memory problems and minor visual field deficits. An alternative similar technique is the *selective amygdalohippo-campectomy*, which involves the resection of the amygdala and hippocampus only. Comparisons of the standard anterior temporal lobectomy and selective amygdalohippocampectomy have found similar seizure-freedom rates.

In patients without a detectable lesion by MRI or a resectable seizure focus, disconnection procedures may be performed, with the goal of interrupting the synchronous firing of neurons. *Anatomic hemispherectomy* is the complete removal of half of the brain, used in patients with diffuse unilateral hemispheric seizures. More recently, hemispherectomy has been replaced by *functional hemispherectomy*, which involves the disconnection of the corpus callosum and various inter-hemispheric commissures. Functional hemispherectomy is more commonly performed in the pediatric population, such as in patients with Sturge-Weber syndrome, Rasmussen encephalitis, and porencephaly. *Corpus callosotomy* is another palliative disconnective procedure for patients with diffuse epileptic foci involving bilateral hemispheres. This procedure involves resection of the anterior two-thirds of the corpus callosum, with the greatest efficacy for drop attacks, also knowns as sudden atonic seizures (up to 88%).

Ablative Procedures

Ablation of epileptogenic brain tissue using highly focused radiation (SRS) has been used to target a wide variety of brain lesions such as tumors and vascular lesions. The advantage is its less invasive nature and precise targeting of seizure-producing foci, but benefits are delayed (usually starting 12 months after procedure), and there is risk of brain edema in neighboring tissue.

Therapeutic Devices

Electrical stimulation of peripheral nerves, particularly through vagus nerve stimulation, has been used for patients whose disease is not safely amenable to resection. The exact mechanism is unknown but has been postulated to be due to innervation of the nucleus solitarius that sends fibers to hemispheric regions involved in seizure onset. The stimulator electrode is wrapped around the vagus nerve in the neck and connected to a generator implanted on the anterior chest wall. Randomized trials have demonstrated a reduction of seizure frequency to 30%, with greater response rates in the pediatric population.

A more recent advancement includes the placement of an electric stimulator implant into the brain that detects seizure onset and responds by delivering pulsed stimulation to the epileptic focus. The preliminary trials are promising, with up to 50%-70% reduction in seizures. The development of therapeutic devices for refractory epilepsy remains an ongoing research area.

SUMMARY

Epilepsy surgery may be considered for patients with disabling epilepsy who have failed medical therapy. The mapping of epileptogenic origin and careful selection of patients and correct procedures require a multidisciplinary team of epileptologists, neurosurgeons, radiologists, and neuropsychiatrists to best maximize efficacy, with the goal to ultimately improve quality of life for these patients.

Immonen A, Jutila L, Muraja-Murro A, et al: Long-term epilepsy surgery outcomes in patients with MRI-negative temporal lobe epilepsy. *Epilepsia.* 2010;51(11):2260-2269.
Schachter SC, Guttag J, Schiff SJ, et al: Advances in the application of technology to epilepsy: the CIMIT/NIO Epilepsy Innovation Summit. *Epilepsy Behav.* 2009;16:3-46.

▼ SURGICAL MANAGEMENT OF PAIN

Kevin T. Huang, MD, and Timothy R. Smith, MD, PhD

The subjective, emotional, and physical components of pain make its management complex and often require interdisciplinary collaboration. Surgical intervention for pain is uncommon and should be reserved for patients who are refractory to other therapies.

Pain may be classified as *nociceptive* or *neuropathic*. Nociceptive pain results from tissue injury and is often described as a constant aching or throbbing, with responsiveness to opiate medications. Neuropathic pain results from nerve damage and is typically described as electrical, burning, or intense numbness, often with allodynia as well. Neuropathic pain responds poorly to opiate medications. Pain surgeons should be familiar with these concepts to assess medical intractability.

Surgical management of pain typically involves either the interruption or modulation of afferent pain pathways. Ablative surgical techniques involve the destruction of neural tissue, whereas nonablative procedures involve functional modulation of pain transduction pathways.

ABLATIVE PROCEDURES

Neurosurgical procedures to physically interrupt pain signaling have been directed toward the nerves (neurectomy), spinal roots (rhizotomy), dorsal root ganglia (ganglionectomy), dorsal root entry zone (DREZ lesioning), spinal cord (cordotomy, myelotomy), and cerebral cortex (thalamotomy, cingulotomy). Ablative surgery for pain is most often used in the treatment of cancer-related, nociceptive pain, because long-term analgesia is less commonly observed for these procedures.

Neurectomy

Neurectomy involves cutting an injured nerve or the nerve to a specific painful region and can have use in pain following peripheral nerve injury such as from limb amputation and/or neuroma formation. Denervation of joints or distal sensory nerves and neuroma surgery are examples of peripheral neurectomy. The utility of neurectomy is limited, however, because it is rare for the pain to arise from an isolated sensory nerve. More commonly, pain distributions follow a mixed motor-sensory nerve distribution, and the nerve cannot be sectioned without inducing a disabling motor deficit. Moreover, as neurostimulation has gained in popularity, neurectomy has lost ground because it is irreversible and seen as more invasive.

Dorsal Rhizotomy and Ganglionectomy

Dorsal rhizotomy and ganglionectomy target the destruction of the dorsal sensory rootlets or ganglia, respectively, and can produce denervation of a specific dermatome. The procedures are used most commonly for regional cancer-related pain such as thoracic or abdominal wall pain, perineal pain in those with impaired pelvic visceral function, or limb pain in those with preexisting loss of function. Unfortunately, the procedures do not typically have durable results in non–cancer-related pain conditions, although some success in occipital neuralgia, specifically, has been reported. These procedures are rarely used in the treatment of extremity pain because of functional impairment resulting from the loss of proprioception. Ganglionectomy is thought to be slightly more efficacious than rhizotomy due to the ability to catch any afferent fibers that enter through the ventral root, whose bodies nonetheless reside in the dorsal root ganglion.

Dorsal Root Entry Zone Lesioning

Dorsal root entry zone surgery targets the superficial dorsal horn region of the spinal cord, where sensory fibers enter. Levels including and flanking the region of interest, as defined by imaging studies or pain distribution, are typically ablated. A knife or radiofrequency heating is used to make the lesion.

Dorsal root entry zone surgery is most effective in the treatment of regionally specific neuropathic pain following nerve root avulsion and "at-level" or "boundary-level" SCI pain. Risks of surgery include injury to descending motor pathways and decreased sensory function in the territory of the ablated region. In carefully selected patients, rates of successful pain control range from 60% to 80%.

Cordotomy & Myelotomy

Cordotomy is a spinal procedure to interrupt pain transmission along the lateral spinothalamic tract. Cordotomy is most commonly performed in patients with intractable, unilateral, nociceptive cancer pain at the level of the chest or below. The procedure may be performed either with a knife or with radiofrequency heating and can be performed in an open or CT-guided fashion. Risks of surgery include lower extremity weakness, ataxia, and respiratory or urinary dysfunction. These risks are significantly increased when cordotomy is performed bilaterally. As the use of intrathecal analgesics has increased, the popularity of cordotomy has correspondingly declined.

A similar procedure, the midline myelotomy, involves the sectioning of a different spinal cord tract, the mesial dorsal columns, at a single spinal level. It can be useful in treating midline, bilateral, or visceral pain without the associated risks of bilateral cordotomies. The procedure typically preserves dorsal column and spinothalamic signal transmission. Risks include transient lower extremity paresthesias and weakness.

Rates of successful pain control with cordotomy and myelotomy are initially high (60%-90%) but decline over time (40% at 2 years).

Thalamotomy & Cingulotomy

Thalamotomy involves the surgical lesioning of the afferent pain pathway inside the thalamus using stereotactic-guided radiofrequency, radiosurgery, or focused ultrasound ablation. It is used in either cancer- or non–cancer-related pain but is more appropriate for diffuse, widespread, nociceptive pain as opposed to more regionally focused pain. Results are not as favorable as well-selected candidates for other modalities, with 30%-50% of patients achieving acceptable long-term pain relief.

Unlike procedures directed along pathways of pain neurotransmission, cingulotomy is directed toward alteration of the experience of pain. Because the cingulate gyrus is part of the limbic system, radiofrequency ablation of the anterior cingulate gyrus reduces the affective, unpleasant aspects of pain, particularly in patients with obsessive, affective, and/or psychiatric components to their pain. Cingulotomy is performed in relatively few centers and only in carefully selected patients. Following cingulotomy for intractable, cancer-related pain, over 50% of patients have been reported to have moderate to complete pain relief.

PROCEDURES TO MODULATE AFFERENT PAIN PATHWAYS

Intrathecal Analgesic Delivery Pumps

When compared to oral narcotics, intrathecal administration of morphine provides more potent analgesia with reduced side effects, such as nausea, constipation, and sedation.

To benefit from intrathecal delivery, patients should have significant reduction in pain level with oral opiates, limited by intolerable side effects.

Analgesics such as morphine are delivered through a catheter placed into the CSF of the spinal canal. The catheter tubing is then connected to an external or surgically implanted pump. External pumps are used in patients with cancer-related pain and an expected survival of less than 3 months. Principal complications of intrathecal drug delivery include the side effects of the medication, mechanical failure of the system, and infection.

Intrathecal drug delivery may be effective in either nociceptive or neuropathic pain syndromes. However, as with oral opiate administration, long-term tolerance to medications can develop. Hence, these devices are most beneficial for patients with cancer-related pain syndromes and limited life expectancy.

▶ Peripheral Nerve & Spinal Cord Stimulation

Peripheral nerve and spinal cord stimulators deliver regular pulses of electricity to injured nerves or the dorsal columns of the spinal cord, respectively. The mechanism of action by which stimulation works remains unclear but is thought to possibly involve preferential stimulation of large afferent fibers, somehow blocking the pain signals from smaller fibers, as well as possible stimulation of secondary neurohormonal changes.

Although both neurostimulation techniques have been tried in a variety of chronic pain conditions, their use in a few specific indications has met with the most success. Peripheral nerve stimulation is most effective in neuropathic peripheral nerve syndromes that fit well into a known nerve distribution, such as occipital neuralgia. Spinal cord stimulation has been employed successfully in patients with failed back surgery syndrome, ischemic limb pain, and complex regional pain syndrome.

Patient candidates typically undergo an initial trial with a temporary electrode applied to the spinal cord or nerve. After the trial period, permanent placement can be performed if benefit is demonstrated, as evidenced by pain reduction and improvement to go about daily activities. Complications of the therapy include migration or fracture of the simulator leads and infection, and although revisions are common, devastating complications that significantly impact morbidity or mortality are rare.

▶ Deep Brain Stimulation

Deep brain stimulation involves the precise surgical placement of electrodes into the deep nuclei of the brain. Common targets of deep brain stimulation for pain include the thalamus, which is the sensory relay of the brain, and the periaqueductal gray region, which results in the upregulation of endogenous opiates. Once electrodes are implanted, trial stimulation is performed, with success characterized by the experience of pain relief, tolerable off-target sensations, and the absence of an analgesic effect during sham stimulation. Following the trial, a pulse generator is connected to the wires and implanted in the chest. Long-term results in patients with a successful trial are highly variable.

▶ Motor Cortex Stimulation

Electrical stimulation of the region of the motor cortex results in analgesia in neuropathic pain syndromes such as hemibody poststroke pain and trigeminal deafferentation pain. The mechanism of motor cortex stimulation remains unknown.

The surgical procedure involves placement of a stimulating electrode under the skull but over the dura in the region of the motor cortex. Patients undergo a trial of stimulation, and following a successful trial, the electrodes are connected to an implantable pulse generator in the chest. As the neuroanatomic representation of the leg lies further away, in between the two cerebral hemispheres, motor cortex stimulation is typically restricted to those with arm or face pain.

▼ SURGICAL MANAGEMENT OF MOVEMENT DISORDERS

Pablo A. Valdes, MD, PhD, and Timothy R. Smith, MD, PhD

PARKINSON DISEASE

▶ Pathophysiology

Parkinson disease (PD) is the second most common progressive neurodegenerative disease, affecting 2%-3% of patients over 65 years of age. PD is the most common and well-characterized basal ganglia disorder with both motor and non-motor features and is characterized by loss of dopaminergic neurons in the substantia nigra and accumulation of intracellular protein (alpha-synuclein) known as Lewy bodies. The net loss of dopaminergic input in the substantia nigra causes opposing effects in the motor striatum, which leads to increased activity in the indirect pathway through net disinhibition of the subthalamic nucleus (STN) and globus pallidus interna (GPi). As such, surgical approaches generally target either the STN or GPi.

▶ Clinical Features

PD can display both motor and nonmotor symptoms, with the former including tremor, rigidity, akinesia/bradykinesia, postural instability, shuffling gait, masked facies, and micrographia. Non-motor symptoms include cognitive impairment, apathy, fatigue, depression, sleep disorders, and dysautonomia. PD is clinically defined by the presence of bradykinesia and at least one more cardinal feature and supporting/exclusion criteria. A resting tremor characterized as a "pill rolling" tremor is the most common feature and is seen most prominently in the distal extremities. The clinical history and presentation are key to distinguish PD from other parkinsonian syndromes that may be similar but require distinct treatment including multiple system atrophy, corticobasal degeneration, progressive supranuclear palsy, and dementia with Lewy bodies.

▶ Treatment

PD patients first undergo medical treatment for symptomatic control. Mainstay of treatment involves dopaminergic targets given the loss of dopaminergic neurons in the substantia nigra. Levodopa (L-DOPA) is a precursor of dopamine and is the gold standard for PD. It is usually given in combination with carbidopa (an inhibitor of dopamine metabolisms in the bloodstream) to increase its efficiency. Over a period of 5-10 years, patients will naturally develop resistance to L-DOPA with motor response oscillations such as "on-off" fluctuations and drug-induced dyskinesias (involuntary writhing movements of face and extremities at peak dopamine levels). Other medications used in the treatment of PD are monoamine oxidase inhibitors (selegiline) and dopamine agonists (ropinirole).

Once patients start developing medical resistance, they should undergo surgical evaluation. Currently, the preferred surgical treatment options for PD involve pallidotomy or deep brain stimulation (DBS) of the STN or GPi. The ideal DBS patient is generally a healthy patient without psychiatric disorders who is L-DOPA responsive and has disabling idiopathic PD symptoms. In DBS surgery, deep subcortical electrodes are placed into the STN or GPi using stereotactic techniques, with or without intraoperative electrophysiologic monitoring and with or without intraoperative imaging through small burr holes. Stereotactic techniques use known atlas-based distances for each different nuclei (STN, GPi) in relation to the midcommissural point, anterior commissure, and posterior commissure. Electrodes are connected to an implantable pulse generator located in an infraclavicular location. STN and GPi DBS demonstrate comparable efficacy in addressing the cardinal symptoms of PD (bradykinesia, gait, rigidity, tremor) and reducing "on-off" fluctuations. STN is a preferred target based on reduction of medication requirements (> 50% at 12 months) requiring lower stimulation voltage but with more significant cognitive and behavioral side effects. The main complications with DBS include hemorrhage (2%), infection within 6 months (4%), and hardware malfunction (8%). Pallidotomy, or ablation of the GPi, is a surgical option used preferably in patients with asymmetric symptoms and those unable to comply with DBS follow-up and management. Unilateral pallidotomy has similar efficacy as unilateral DBS with the main disadvantage

being that of irreversible damage; otherwise, pallidotomy uses the same localization techniques as DBS, with lesioning performed using radiofrequency ablation.

ESSENTIAL TREMOR

▶ Pathophysiology

Essential tremor (ET) is the most common movement disorder characterized by benign and primary postural or intention tremor with usual age of onset > 70 years of age, a slight female preponderance, and prevalence of 0.4%-6%. There is no consensus regarding the pathophysiologic basis of ET, but the current working understanding suggests a neuronal loop involving the cerebellothalamocortical fibers and the ventral intermediate nucleus (VIM) of the thalamus. The latter contains tremor cells that are posited as tremorigenic pacemakers involved in the tremor circuitry connecting cerebellum and cortical motor pathways.

▶ Clinical Features

ET is characterized by a postural and/or kinetic tremor with frequencies of 4-12 Hz that can be exacerbated by anxiety or improved with alcohol. The intention tremor of ET should be carefully distinguished from physiologic tremor and other disease-associated tremors (eg, resting tremor with a stationary limb seen with PD) or secondary tremors (eg, multiple sclerosis, stroke). Criteria for the diagnosis of ET include bilateral postural tremor with duration greater than 5 years with or without an intentional component of forearms and arms and exclusion of other abnormal signs (eg, causes increasing physiologic tremor, use of drugs inducing withdrawal, trauma, or stepwise deterioration).

▶ Treatment

Similar to PD, ET patients have both medical and surgical options. First-line treatment for ET, especially when the disease impacts the activities of daily living, are β-blockers, (eg, propranolol) and anticonvulsants (eg, primidone), with tremor reduction of up to 60% in 50% of patients. Second-line agents include benzodiazepines, gabapentin, theophylline, calcium channel blockers, and botulinum toxin A. When medical therapy is insufficient, patients should undergo surgical evaluation.

Patients with medically refractory ET notable for distal extremity tremor benefit the most from surgical intervention, with two main surgical options: targeting of the VIM via DBS or thalamotomy using radiofrequency ablation, SRS, or focused ultrasound. DBS of the VIM can be unilateral or bilateral, with success rates of > 70% and studies noting fewer adverse effects than with thalamotomy. Targeting techniques for VIM DBS in ET are similar to those used for PD, with use of different coordinates for the VIM (unlike the GPi or STN for PD). Thalamotomy can be performed by means of the more invasive radiofrequency approach, which, like pallidotomy in PD, is irreversible with reduction of contralateral tremor in > 85% of patients. Thalamotomy is usually reserved for unilateral cases given the high rate (> 50%) of cognitive and bulbar defects with bilateral approaches or for patients who are unable to tolerate or undergo long-term management with DBS. Two noninvasive surgical options for thalamotomy are focused ultrasound and SRS. In focused ultrasound, patients undergo real-time MRI monitoring to target the VIM and undergo highly focused sonication with acoustic energy to ablate tissue to temperatures of 55-60°C. A phase III, randomized controlled trial demonstrated > 50% improvement in tremor scores. SRS has similar clinical outcomes to the aforementioned approaches but with a delayed clinical benefit and inability for intraoperative clinical monitoring.

DYSTONIA

Pathophysiology

Dystonia is a hyperkinetic heterogeneous movement disorder characterized by sustained muscle contractions that generate repetitive movements, abnormal postures, and/or twisting movements. Primary dystonias have no clearly defined etiology (eg, stroke, trauma) and demonstrate a bimodal distribution at age 9 years (with appendicular symptoms) and 45 years (with axial symptoms). A subset of primary dystonias is autosomal dominant with a *DYT1* gene mutation (GAG deletion in chromosome 9 prominently expressed in the substantia nigra) that leads to childhood onset of primary dystonia. Abnormal basal ganglia circuitry leads to imbalance of both the indirect and direct pathways with overactivity of the direct pathway, net decrease in GPi activity, and increase in thalamocortical activation.

Clinical Features

The key characteristics of dystonia include abnormal movements with or without tremor. Abnormal dystonic movements are consistently directional and patterned and involve the same muscle groups, leading to twisting of extremities, trunk, or both, and are usually made worse by voluntary movement. Dystonias are classified based on affected location (generalized, focal, segmental, multifocal, hemidystonia), age of onset (early or late), or etiology (primary/idiopathic or secondary/symptomatic). Secondary dystonias include dystonia-plus syndromes, nondegenerative disorders associated with other movement disorders (eg, DOPA-responsive dystonia), heterodegenerative dystonias (eg, PD, Wilson disease), and those caused by CNS insults (eg, stroke, drugs).

Treatment

Medical treatment seeks to relieve symptoms rather than modify the disease course. Anticholinergics, levodopa, baclofen, and neuroleptics are used for generalized treatment. Botulinum toxin has also shown great results, with focal treatment response rates of 70%-100%. Surgical treatment is reserved for medically refractory patients and requires that patients undergo a trial of levodopa to rule out patients with dopamine-responsive dystonia. The best candidates are those with primary dystonia with a *DYT1* mutation, segmental cervical dystonia, or hemidystonia not responsive to medical treatment, whereas patients with secondary dystonia have much decreased success rates. The preferred surgical treatment is GPi DBS, with improvements of 45%-75% in primary dystonia patients (vs 10%-30% in secondary dystonia). Lesionectomies have been previously performed with both thalamotomy and pallidotomy but are not currently a preferred treatment.

Deuschl G, Raethjen J, Hellriegel H, et al: Treatment of patients with essential tremor. *Lancet Neurol.* 2011;10(2):148-161.

Elias WJ, Lipsman N, Ondo WG, et al: A randomized trial of focused ultrasound thalamotomy for essential tremor. *N Engl J Med.* 2016;375(8):730-739.

Ellis TL: Dystonia and the role of deep brain stimulation. *ISRN Surg.* 2011;2011:193718.

Fukaya C, Yamamoto T: Deep brain stimulation for Parkinson's disease: recent trends and future direction. *Neurol Medico-Chir.* 2015;55(5):422-431.

Odekerken VJJ, Boel JA, Schmand BA, et al: GPi vs STN deep brain stimulation for Parkinson disease: three-year follow-up. *Neurol.* 2016;86(8):755-761.

Poewe W, Seppi K, Tanner CM, et al: Parkinson disease. *Nat Rev Dis Prim.* 2017;3:17013.

Yu H, Neimat JS: The treatment of movement disorders by deep brain stimulation. *Neurotherapeutics.* 2008;5(1):26-36.

INTERVERTEBRAL DISK DISEASE

Kevin T. Huang, MD, and Timothy R. Smith, MD, PhD

General Considerations

The intervertebral disks are fibrocartilaginous joints that connect adjoining vertebral bodies. They consist of an outer annulus fibrosis and an inner nucleus pulposis and serve not only to hold the two vertebral bodies together, but also to help cushion the weight and shock movement of the upper vertebral body on the lower one.

Intervertebral disks degenerate and dehydrate with age. Coupled with degeneration of the facets, this general process is termed *spondylosis*. The process is common and to a certain extent should be expected with age. About 20% of teenagers have signs of mild disk degeneration, whereas by age 70, approximately 60% of disks are severely degenerated. The degenerated and dehydrated disks do not distribute load in the same way and have alterations in their biomechanics. They do not maintain their height under load-bearing conditions, and as a consequence, more stress is placed on the vertebral bodies and adjacent facet joints. This promotes pain, inflammation, ligamentous hypertrophy, and reactionary osteophyte formation. The resulting ligamentous hypertrophy can eventually lead to crowding of the central spinal canal or the exiting neural foramina and neurologic compression. Neural compression can also occur when the degenerated annulus of the disk fissures, allowing the inner nucleus pulposis to herniate out and compress nearby nerves. Disk degeneration can also lead to spondylolisthesis, or subluxation of one vertebral body over another. Degenerative disk disease occurs at all levels of the spine, but the lumbar spine and cervical spine are more commonly impacted as they are more mobile.

CERVICAL SPINE

Degenerative disk disease in the cervical spine is a common finding and frequently features a component of at least some axial neck pain. If there is associated neural compression, symptoms depend on the affected neural structure, with compression of the nerve root leading to radiculopathy and compression of the spinal cord leading to myelopathy.

▶ Symptoms & Signs

Degenerative disease of the cervical spine often presents with a history of neck pain, which may either be abrupt, in the case of disk rupture, or slowly progressive. There is often a loss of cervical lordosis (the normal, backward, C-shaped curvature of the neck), which may be related to muscle spasm or to deformity from chronic degeneration. The characteristic finding in radiculopathy is a sharp, burning pain that radiates down the arm, following a dermatomal distribution. This pain may be exacerbated when the patient tilts the head toward the side of the pain, crowding the neural foramina on the affected side (Spurling maneuver). Indeed, the patient may habitually tilt the head to the opposite side to reduce the pain. Numbness can also often be seen in the same dermatomal pattern, and weakness in the correlating myotome can also sometimes be witnessed. Sensory disturbances (paresthesias, numbness, or allodynia) tend to occur in the terminal distribution of the involved dermatome (ie, in the fingers rather than the proximal arm). Weakness from the radiculopathy can occur in the correlating myotome to the pain. Weakness from radiculopathy is often partial or incomplete, since nearly all muscles are innervated by more than one spinal nerve. Profound weakness, atrophy, and muscle fasciculations are rare in radiculopathy, except in very long-standing cases. The presence of these findings should generate suspicion of a peripheral nerve lesion.

C5 radiculopathy (typically resulting from pathology at the C4-5 level) involves pain radiating into the shoulder (following the distribution of the C5 dermatome). Patients may exhibit weakness of shoulder abduction (deltoids). C6 radiculopathy (as from a C5-6 herniated disk) typically involves pain radiating from the neck into the lateral aspect of the arm and possibly the first two digits. Patients may present with biceps weakness. C7 nerve root compression (from C6-7 pathology) often involves pain radiating from the neck into the back of the shoulder, through the arm, and into the middle finger. Weakness can sometimes be detected in the triceps or in wrist extension. C8 radiculopathy (from C7-T1 pathology) can present with pain and numbness radiating into the medial forearm and fourth and fifth digits. Weakness can occasionally be seen in the hand grip. The lower cervical spine (particularly C5-6 and C6-7) are more commonly affected than the upper cervical spine.

In advanced cases of degenerative disk disease of the cervical spine, signs of myelopathy may develop. These include hyperreflexia, loss of dexterity (eg, difficulty with cooking or buttoning up one's shirt), spasticity, gait disturbance, and sensory disturbances of the upper and lower extremities.

▶ Diagnostic Studies

Not all patients with neck pain require imaging. However, those with prolonged and refractory symptoms, those with increased risk for more serious conditions (eg, tumor or infection), and those with any neurologic deficit should warrant further investigation.

MRI is the primary modality to evaluate potential operative cases (Figure 38–25). Unless infection or tumor is suspected, typically the study need not be performed with gadolinium contrast. MRI allows for the best differentiation between the nerves, CSF, and any potentially compressive structures. Care should be taken in interpretation, as radiographic abnormalities are very common and not always symptomatic. Instead, key to establishing a diagnosis are radiographic findings that correlate with clinical findings (eg, evidence of C5 nerve root compression on MRI in combination with C5 radiculopathy on clinical exam). In cases where an MRI is not able to be obtained, CT myelography can be performed. In CT myelography, a lumbar puncture is performed and contrast dye is injected into the thecal space, allowing for a delineation of the CNS and any compression thereof.

Additional studies that may be of use include plain x-ray films, which can be used to assess for bony alignment of the cervical spine. Similar to their use in the trauma setting, flexion-extension films can also determine any instability as well. CT scans also have a use in perioperative planning, as they provide superior evaluation of the bony anatomy.

Electrodiagnostic studies, particularly electromyography (EMG), may be useful in diagnosing radiculopathy. Nerve conduction studies alone are of little value in identifying radiculopathy and are generally normal, even with severe compression of a nerve root. EMG, on the other hand, is more sensitive

▲ **Figure 38–25.** Sagittal T2-weighted magnetic resonance imaging of cervical spine showing multilevel disk protrusions causing central canal stenosis and cord signal change.

and can help confirm dysfunction isolated to a particular nerve root. Unfortunately, EMG will not reliably detect fibrillations in muscles until at least 3-4 weeks following the onset of radiculopathy and thus may lead to false-negative studies if the test is performed too soon. Even when performed after an appropriate waiting period, EMG findings may be normal in upward of 50% of cases of spinal nerve compression in patients with only complaints of pain without weakness.

▶ **Differential Diagnosis**

In general, severe weakness and muscle atrophy are suggestive of a peripheral nerve lesion, whereas early loss of a reflex (biceps, triceps) suggests radiculopathy. Other conditions that may mimic cervical degenerative disk disease include myocardial infarction, idiopathic brachial plexitis (Parsonage-Turner syndrome), or inflammatory conditions such as ankylosing spondylitis or sarcoidosis. Local conditions affecting the shoulder (eg, rotator cuff tears, acromial bursitis) must also be ruled out. Patients with any atypical features

to their pain, such as fever, night sweats, unexplained weight loss, a history of chronic infections or immunosuppression, or a history of metastatic cancer, should also be evaluated for possible infection or tumor.

▶ **Treatment & Prognosis**

Most conditions that cause pain in the cervical spine (eg, exacerbations of degenerative arthritis, muscle spasm, or minor trauma) are self-limiting and ultimately do not require operation. Acute neck pain may be treated with gentle exercise or a mobilization program, moist heat, or a soft collar to help muscle relaxation. Anti-inflammatory medications are also useful in this regard. For persistent neck pain, intermittent traction is sometimes helpful, either through physical therapy or with a home traction kit. The vast majority of patients improve with medical management alone, although many continue to have mild symptoms they ultimately learn to manage.

Neck pain itself generally responds poorly to operative management, and surgery is typically more targeted at the symptoms of neural compression. Surgical management of cervical degenerative disk disease should be reserved for cases failing medical management and where there is neurologic compression (leading to either myelopathy or radiculopathy). Operative management of the cervical spine involves decompression of the spinal cord or nerve roots, with or without fusion. The cervical spine may be approached either anteriorly or posteriorly, with many pathologies approachable through either route and thus dependent on surgeon preference. Complex cases may require both approaches (combined anterior/posterior).

Options for anterior correction include removal of the disk with either fusion of the adjoining vertebral bodies (anterior cervical discectomy and fusion) or placement of an artificial disk (anterior cervical arthroplasty). It is also possible to drill away the vertebral body itself, with placement of a replacement strut for support (anterior cervical corpectomy). Posterior approaches include removal of the lamina (cervical laminectomy) with or without fusion, removal of lamina with replacement at the end of the surgery (cervical laminoplasty), and opening of the neural foramina (posterior cervical foraminotomy).

Outcomes from surgery are highly dependent on patient selection and the specific scenario. Well-selected patients, with symptoms well-correlated with imaging findings, have a favorable prognosis, with > 80% of patients reporting long-term satisfaction.

THORACIC DISK DISEASE

Thoracic disk herniations are rare, with an incidence between 0.25% and 0.75% of all disk herniations. Often there is a delay in diagnosis because of poorly defined symptoms and the lack of objective findings on physical exam.

Patients can present with symptoms of axial pain, radiculopathy, myelopathy, or some combination of the three. The axial pain may be described as dull, aching, burning, stabbing, or cramping. Load bearing, activity, or Valsalva will often exacerbate the pain. Radicular symptoms generally present in the appropriate dermatomal band. Myelopathy can present as paraparesis, but more often presents with a vague history of lower extremity weakness, gait instability, heaviness, stiffness, or numbness. Bowel and bladder complaints can occur as well.

Treatment for symptomatic lesions is surgical and is directed at alleviating pain or preventing progression of a neurologic deficit. Surgery is more complex than equivalent cervical or lumbar cases as anterior approaches are limited by the thoracic or abdominal viscera and posterior approaches are limited by the spinal cord. Nevertheless, options exist from both anterior and posterior approaches (including transthoracic, lateral extracavitary, costotransversectomy, and transpedicular). In cases of a thoracic disk herniation, a strictly dorsal midline approach (laminectomy) offers poor exposure of the disk and has a high risk of neurologic injury.

LUMBAR SPINE

▶ Symptoms & Signs

As in the cervical spine, degenerative disk disease of the lumbar spine can present as a combination of back pain, radiculopathy, and myelopathy. Similarly, radiculopathy can be identified because symptoms will localize to a particular dermatome and possibly the associated myotome as well. There are a few differences that bear consideration, however.

First, myelopathy is less common in the lumbar spine because the spinal cord itself terminates at the L1-2 level. Instead, any stenosis of the central spinal canal further down may present as neurogenic claudication. Just as in vascular claudication, these patients complain of leg pain upon walking that is alleviated upon sitting down. However, in neurogenic claudication, this is due to nerve compression from the spinal canal narrowing when the back is extended. In addition, severe spinal canal compression below the level of the spinal cord can produce cauda equina syndrome. This is characterized by the presence of saddle anesthesia, bowel and bladder dysfunction, lower extremity weakness (typically severe), and severe pain. Because many patients, especially those with an impaired mental status, can complain of some combination of these symptoms, the diagnosis can sometimes be difficult. Signs that should elevate the suspicion for cauda equina syndrome include a poor rectal tone, an absent bulbocavernosus reflex, and an absent anal wink.

In the lumbar spine, a straight leg raise can be useful in helping diagnose herniated lumbar disks. In such a scenario, the patient presents with radiating leg pain suspicious for a herniated disk. The straight leg raise is positive if raising the affected leg to an angle of 30 degrees reproduces the radiating leg pain. The contralateral leg is then tested in a similar fashion to see if raising it will reproduce the pain in the original leg. These two are then correlated, as a positive *ipsilateral* straight leg raise is sensitive but not specific, while a positive *contralateral* straight leg raise is specific but not sensitive.

As in the cervical spine, determination of dermatomal and/or myotomal pattern of symptoms is key for evaluating radiating pain. Compression of the L4 nerve root (L3/4 herniation) may cause weakness of knee extension (quadriceps) and numbness in the anterior thigh and medial ankle. Compression of the L5 nerve root (L4/5 herniation) may precipitate weakness of the extensor hallucis longus and ankle dorsiflexion (tibialis anterior) and numbness of the dorsal foot and first web space. Finally, compression of the S1 nerve root (L5/S1 herniation) may lead to weakness of ankle plantarflexion (gastrocnemius) and numbness in the lateral ankle and plantar side of the foot.

▶ Imaging Studies

As in the cervical spine, MRI has become the gold standard for diagnosis of degenerative disk disease in the lumbar spine (Figure 38–26). It provides superior evaluation of the soft tissue structures and is used to see if there is a unified clinical and radiographic explanation for the patient's symptoms. CT myelography can be used in its stead when MRI is contraindicated.

CT scans of the lumbar spine are also of significant utility as they identify the nature of previous spine surgery (which patients frequently cannot speak exactly to), the quality of the bones, and the exact bony anatomy. Standing plain-film x-rays are also useful, as increasingly there is an awareness that the balance of the spine in the sagittal plane can have a significant contribution to back pain. These films can help determine any deformities in the spine's overall alignment and may suggest alterations in surgical strategy for certain patients.

As mentioned previously, EMG can be useful when the diagnosis of radiculopathy remains unclear. EMG can help evaluate if pain is radiculopathic in nature and help isolate which myotome is the affected one.

▶ Medical Treatment

The natural history of most acute-onset back pain and radiculopathy associated with disk herniations is that of improvement over time, with significant improvement in the first 4-6 weeks after onset of symptoms. Therefore, conservative measures are recommended initially for patients who present without neurologic deficit. Conservative measures are directed toward initially limiting physical activity, including a brief period of bed rest followed by a gradual exercise program. It is also important for patients to modify their types

▲ **Figure 38–26.** Sagittal T2-weighted magnetic resonance imaging of lumbar spine showing multilevel disk bulges, ligamentum flavum hypertrophy, and retrolisthesis at L2-3.

of movement, for example, to limit heavy lifting, twisting, or bending. Physical therapy can be useful after the acute period for instruction in abdominal and back musculature strengthening exercises. Although of limited utility in radiculopathy, more generalized back pain related to degenerative spine disease can also respond to external bracing.

The core of medical treatment is nonsteroidal anti-inflammatory drugs (NSAIDs). Oral steroids (eg, solumedrol dose pack) also may be useful in the acute setting, and epidural steroid injections and narcotics may be helpful in alleviating pain.

Surgical Treatment

Patients who are refractory to conservative measures or those who present with acute neurologic motor deterioration warrant surgical attention. Surgery is also indicated in patients who fail the conservative measures outlined earlier and continue to suffer from debilitating pain.

For herniated lumbar disks, a microdiscectomy can be performed where the extruded disk material and some of the underlying nucleus pulposus is removed for decompression. Patients primarily presenting with symptoms of stenosis may receive laminectomies, where the lamina and hypertrophied ligamentum flavum in the posterior aspect of the spinal canal are removed.

The use of instrumented spinal fusion has expanded significantly in recent years and remains an area of controversy. It is indicated in patients who present with signs and symptoms of spinal instability or when the spine is deliberately destabilized as part of the surgery (eg, in the process of removing bone to correct a deformity or the complete removal of a facet joint or disk space to facilitate a decompression). Many options exist for fusion, including anterior approaches (eg, anterior lumbar interbody fusion) and posterior approaches (eg, posterolateral fusion with pedicle screws).

Prognosis

Degenerative disk disease in the lumbar spine has varied presentations and sometimes overlapping pathologies. As such, prognosis varies significantly with the condition and presenting symptoms. Generally, acute exacerbations of degenerative spine disease have a favorable prognosis, and most episodes will recover well with conservative management. However, more episodes will likely occur in the future as the patient continues to age.

Outcomes from surgical treatment depend greatly on patient selection and indications for surgery. As a broad generalization, surgery for neural decompression carries a significantly better prognosis than surgery for back pain. Thus, patients undergoing surgery for herniated lumbar disks generally fare well, although approximately 10% may experience reherniations.

Ambrossi GLG, McGirt MJ, Sciubba DM, et al: Recurrent lumbar disc herniation after single-level lumbar discectomy: incidence and healthcare cost analysis. *Neurosurgery.* 2009;65(3):574-578.

Atlas SJ, Keller RB, Wu YA, et al: Long-term outcomes of Surgical and nonsurgical management of sciatica secondary to a lumbar disc herniation: 10 year results from the Maine lumbar spine study. *Spine.* 2005;30(8):927-935.

Boselie TF, Willems PC, van Mameren H, et al: Arthroplasty versus fusion in single-level cervical degenerative disc disease. *Cochrane Database Syst Rev.* 2012;9:CD009173.

Jacobs W, Van der Gaag NA, Tuschel A, et al: Total disc replacement for chronic back pain in the presence of disc degeneration. *Cochrane Database Syst Rev.* 2012;9:CD008326.

Kovacs FM, Urrutia G, Alarcon JD: Surgery versus conservative treatment for symptomatic lumbar spinal stenosis: a systematic review of randomized controlled trials. *Spine.* 2011;36: E1335-E1351.

Matz PG, Anderson PA, Holly LT, et al: The natural history of cervical spondylotic myelopathy. *J Neurosurg Spine.* 2009; 11:104-111.

CHAPTER 38

CSF DIVERSION FOR HYDROCEPHALUS

Kyle Wu, MD, and Timothy R. Smith, MD, PhD

OVERVIEW, EPIDEMIOLOGY, & PATHOPHYSIOLOGY

Hydrocephalus is a common diagnosis in both adult and pediatric patients. Most often, this disease is chronically treated with an implanted catheter system to divert CSF from the ventricles of the brain to an alternative absorptive space such as the pleural or peritoneal space for absorption, known as a CSF shunt. Endoscopic third ventriculostomy is a surgical technique that is commonly used as well that obviates the placement of hardware if successful. The disease is estimated to occur at an incidence of 1 per 1000 live births and has a prevalence of approximately 0.5% within the United States. Shunt failure is common, occurring in up to 30%-35% of individuals within 1 year of initial shunt placement, with about 1% of shunt failures being fatal. Familiarity with the diagnosis and treatment of shunt failure is therefore warranted for providers caring for patients in whom a CSF shunt is present.

In pediatric patients, hydrocephalus is primarily seen in patients with a history of intraventricular hemorrhage, meningitis, congenital cranial malformation, brain tumor, or myelomeningocele. In adults, diseases such as SAH (often from ruptured cerebral aneurysm), brain tumor, or head trauma may lead to development of hydrocephalus. Alternatively, idiopathic intracranial hypertension (IIH; or pseudotumor cerebri) may affect patients, leading to blindness. In older adults, "normal-pressure" hydrocephalus is a potentially treatable cause of dementia.

Hydrocephalus results from an interruption in CSF circulation and drainage. The choroid plexus of the brain's ventricular system makes up about 80% of total adult CSF production, resulting in the generation of about 20 mL/h by an active ion pump–dependent process. The remainder is thought to be generated by general metabolic processes occurring within the brain, as well as via ependymal cells lining the ventricles. Importantly, the production of CSF is minimally affected by the ICP over a wide range of physiologic values. Thus, increases in ICP resulting from increasing CSF volume do not act to significantly slow or stop further production of CSF until relatively high ICP is reached. Once produced, spinal fluid is hypothesized to move in an oscillatory fashion out of the ventricular system and into the subarachnoid space around the brain and spinal cord. From there, it is reabsorbed mainly by passive, pressure-dependent mechanisms into the cerebral venous sinuses via arachnoid granulations, and some is even reabsorbed into the brain parenchyma itself.

The vast majority of hydrocephalus results from interruption in this process of CSF egress. This can occur by either of two mechanisms, often classified as either **noncommunicating/obstructive,** if the blockage to CSF outflow prevents an outlet for CSF drainage from the ventricular system, or **communicating,** if reabsorption is reduced or prevented at the level of the arachnoid granulations. Obstructive etiologies such as tumors, aqueductal stenosis, intraventricular cysts, or even strictures are mainly diagnosed with radiologic imaging. Communicating causes can occur following SAH (after cerebral aneurysm rupture), infection, or tumor spread within the subarachnoid space. This distinction between the mechanism of hydrocephalus is important in determining the expected course of the pathology and appropriate treatment. It is also vital for determining the safety of performing a lumbar puncture. If a patient has obstructive hydrocephalus, a lumbar puncture may be unsafe because of the potential for creating differential pressures between the cranial and spinal spaces after drainage of CSF from the spinal canal. Radiographically, hydrocephalus is sometimes assumed to be communicating when all four ventricles are dilated, as opposed to only the ventricles proximal to the obstruction. However, blockage of CSF outflow from the fourth ventricle to the subarachnoid space at the level of the foramens Luschka or Magendie could produce the same dilated quad-ventricular radiologic picture despite an obstructive physiology. Consultation with a neurosurgeon or neurologist may be helpful if the situation is unclear.

CLINICAL PRESENTATION & ASSESSMENT

The relative difference between the volume of CSF produced and reabsorbed and the relative compressibility of the brain determine the severity and type of clinical symptoms and signs at presentation. Slower buildup of CSF or accumulation within a brain more compliant to compression (such as might occur at the extremes of age or with alcoholism) produces a more protracted course of symptoms. This is in contrast to rapid CSF accumulation within a poorly compressible brain (eg, a young adult's brain) leading to acute neurologic decline. Whether presenting initially or after treatment failure, the symptoms of hydrocephalus can be grouped into two main categories: those related to acute increased ICP, usually seen with rapid accumulation of CSF in a poorly compliant brain, and those related to chronic deformation of the nervous system by slowly accumulating CSF.

Acute, rapidly progressive hydrocephalus presents with headaches, nausea, and vomiting. As it progresses further, patients may experience decreased levels of consciousness and eventually brainstem herniation and coma. Some patients may present with the loss of ability to look upward as part of a constellation of symptoms, known as Parinaud syndrome. This syndrome occurs due to compression of the midbrain tectum resulting in upgaze paralysis, pseudo-Argyll Robertson pupils, convergence-retraction nystagmus, and conjugate downgaze. In some cases, patients may also lose the ability to abduct their eyes due to cranial nerve VI palsy from increased ICP (due to traction on the nerve as it enters the Dorello canal within the skull base). If an open fontanelle is present in the infant, it will be tense and raised. Scalp veins may be distended as well due to decreased blood drainage via the intracranial venous sinuses and subsequent shunting of blood through the valveless scalp veins.

Chronic hydrocephalus presents in a slowly progressive nature that is typically more insidious in nature. In children, an inappropriately large head size that is increasing rapidly over time may suggest hydrocephalus. This may be accompanied by fussiness, frequent vomiting, failure to thrive, and eventually lethargy or coma. In adults, chronic diseases such as IIH may present with a slow but steady visual decline, chronic headaches, nausea, vomiting, dizziness, or tinnitus. This disease often afflicts obese individuals and is associated with certain rheumatologic, endocrinologic, or inflammatory diseases, as well as use of certain medications (eg, birth control, retinoids, lithium, or doxycycline). In the elderly, normal-pressure hydrocephalus presents with the triad of dementia, gait disturbance, and urinary incontinence. The order of symptom onset is important in diagnosis of this disease, with gait issues presenting first, followed by urinary incontinence and finally subacute-onset dementia.

If the patient has already had a CSF shunt placed for such conditions, then additional signs and symptoms to consider include those of hardware infection, such as a stiff neck, fever, confusion, photophobia, nausea, vomiting, abdominal pain, or redness around the device. If the device has broken or malfunctioned, then CSF may accumulate around the disconnected portion of the shunt or shunt valve. If the distal cavity into which a shunt is placed fails to absorb spinal fluid, there may be symptoms related to this, such as abdominal pain from a large sterile intraperitoneal fluid collection (eg, pseudocyst) or intra-abdominal abscess.

The headaches associated with hydrocephalus and/or CSF shunt failure often have morning predominance (occurring after a period of prolonged recumbency) or worsen with Valsalva maneuver (due to transiently increased ICP).

Patients presenting with the clinical features described earlier, especially with a history of a CSF shunt in place for prior treatment of hydrocephalus must be promptly evaluated with imaging studies, usually a CT or MRI scan of the brain. In the setting of a possible shunt failure, it is critical to have prior images available for comparison. Patients with working shunts often have ventricles that are smaller than normal. Radiology reports reading "normal ventricular size" or "no evidence of shunt failure" have been demonstrated to correlate poorly with final diagnosis. Additional studies that can be useful include plain radiographs of the shunt to look for kinks, break, or disconnections. Imaging of the cavity into which the CSF shunt is draining, such as by ultrasound or CT of the abdomen, may be useful in situations where pseudocyst or abscess is suspected. If the diagnosis remains in question, more invasive diagnostic studies may be necessary, usually as directed by a neurosurgical consultant. These can include a CSF shunt tap, in which a portion of the shunt that sits under the scalp is accessed percutaneously similar to a vascular access port. CSF can be removed and sent for analysis and ICP measured during this bedside procedure. In addition, lumbar puncture offers similar benefits; however, there is less of a risk of infecting or damaging the shunt when using this method. It is helpful to know that a high percentage of shunt failures occur within the first 2 years after shunt placement, peaking within the first 6 months and steadily declining thereafter. In children, young age at presentation also appears to be a risk factor for repeated shunt failure. Similarly, most shunt infections occur within 1 year of shunt placement. However, despite these epidemiologic data, a perfectly predictive clinical decision algorithm remains elusive, and a low threshold for obtaining imaging studies and appropriate expert consultations is warranted.

MANAGEMENT

Progressive hydrocephalus must be dealt with in a timely manner to minimize neurologic deterioration. As noted earlier, the rate of pathologic CSF accumulation may vary and produce variable clinical symptoms. However, because of the potential for acute and fatal deterioration from hydrocephalus, the initial presumption should be that rapid intervention is required, subject to reconsideration after all necessary data are available.

Medical management of hydrocephalus may be appropriate in the management of IIH and, in some patients, after SAH. It may also be used in the initial management of hydrocephalus in neonates following intraventricular hemorrhage. The diuretics acetazolamide and furosemide are both used in this context. They act to decrease CSF production by inhibiting carbonic anhydrase, which decreases CSF production at the choroid plexus. Furosemide is also thought to decrease cerebral sodium uptake, thus producing an additive effect when the two medications are used in combination. However, randomized controlled trials of medical therapy in newborns demonstrated no reduction in the need for subsequent shunt placement for patients after medical therapy. If medical management is chosen, patients must be closely monitored for electrolyte imbalances and acetazolamide toxicity (acute gastritis, paresthesias, nephrocalcinosis, and drowsiness). It should be noted that with the exception of IIH, protracted use of diuretics to manage hydrocephalus is rarely successful, and in most cases, surgical therapy is indicated without a trial of diuretics.

Intraventricular administration of fibrinolytic agents (eg, streptokinase) has also been investigated as a treatment for newborns with posthemorrhagic hydrocephalus. However, a systematic review of randomized trials failed to show any benefit in terms of reducing shunt requirement or death.

Furthermore, secondary intraventricular hemorrhage is a potential complication of this treatment.

Temporary drainage techniques include serial lumbar punctures or ventricular taps (either trans-fontanelle or via a surgically created subgaleal fluid collection connected to the ventricle via a shunt). Other techniques include continuous drainage by an external ventriculostomy catheter or via serial taps of an implanted reservoir in communication with the ventricles. These techniques are used when etiology and natural history suggest possible resolution of the hydrocephalus over time, as may occur in intraventricular hemorrhage of the newborn or SAH. In addition, temporary diversion is appropriate when the patient's medical condition precludes definitive treatment.

Endoscopic third ventriculostomy (ETV) is an alternative to CSF shunt placement for the treatment of some forms of hydrocephalus. During the endoscopic procedure, a perforation is made in the floor of the third ventricle (most commonly through the tuber cinereum) communicating the ventricles with the subarachnoid space that exists in the basal cisterns anterior to the brainstem. ETV is currently used as the initial treatment of choice in cases of obstructive hydrocephalus that are not treatable by removal of the obstruction itself and is curative in 80% of properly selected patients, avoiding the need for shunt placement. It is also used frequently in pediatric patients with aqueductal stenosis (narrowing of the CSF drainage pathway) and is combined with choroid plexus cauterization in infants less than 1 year old to achieve superior outcomes. The use of ETV is routinely performed for nonobstructive causes of hydrocephalus as well, such as post-intraventricular hemorrhage, Dandy-Walker malformation, spina bifida, encephalocele, or infection, with varying degrees of success. Given its relatively noninvasive nature and the retained ability to place a shunt in cases of failure, it is sometimes attempted prior to shunt placement as a means of obtaining shunt independence. Similar to shunt epidemiology, ETVs typically will fail within a 1-year time frame (due to closure of the fenestration); however, the incidence of infection is much lower, as would be expected given that no implantable hardware is involved.

CSF shunt treatment is indicated in most cases of progressive hydrocephalus, when conservative management and ETV are not indicated or have previously failed. This procedure involves placement of a mechanical shunt as a means to divert excess CSF from the ventricles or lumbar spinal subarachnoid space (lumbar peritoneal shunts are used infrequently, mainly in IIH) into other body cavities. CSF shunts consist of three major components in continuity: a proximal ventricular catheter, a valve that regulates unidirectional CSF flow, and distal tubing to carry the CSF to its absorption site. Some shunts also have reservoirs at the end of the proximal ventricular catheter that can be percutaneously accessed for diagnostic purposes, to inject intrathecal medications (ie, chemotherapeutic agents), or

as a temporizing measure in case the distal tubing or valve becomes blocked. Most often, the proximal catheter of the shunt system is placed into one of the lateral ventricles, either in the frontal horn via a frontal approach or via the atrium of the lateral ventricle via an occipital (posterior) approach. The technique is mainly provider dependent. Shunt systems may also be used to treat a variety of other conditions such as intracranial cysts or chronic SDHs/hygromas. Shunt valves regulate the amount of fluid drainage from the proximal catheter. Most are differential pressure systems that respond to increasing fluid pressure by allowing more CSF through the valve. Various shunts are designed to open in different pressure ranges (eg, low, medium, or high), and some valves can be externally adjusted to different pressure ranges using a magnet. These adjustable (programmable) valves may be inadvertently reprogrammed by nonmedical external magnets, and although all systems approved for sale in the United States as of this writing are MRI compatible with 1.5-T magnets, the patient must have the valve setting checked (most accurately using a skull x-ray orthogonal to the valve) and reset if necessary following an MRI scan. In certain instances, practitioners may choose to incorporate devices that prevent excessive drainage from the siphoning effect due to a long run of distal tubing running inferiorly when patients assume an upright posture, a phenomenon that may lead to overdrainage of CSF. The distal portion of the shunt system follows the valve and is comprised of a long catheter that terminates within a body cavity, allowing for fluid to be adequately absorbed. A ventriculoperitoneal (VP) shunt, the most commonly used shunt, employs a catheter that terminates in the abdominal cavity so that CSF may be absorbed by the peritoneum. Alternative sites, in order of decreasing usage, include the pleural space (ventriculopleural shunt) or the cardiac atria (ventriculoatrial shunt). These alternative sites are chosen most commonly when there is extensive abdominal scarring or adhesions, recent or active abdominal infection, peritonitis, or morbid obesity that precludes safe peritoneal catheter placement. Major considerations for ventriculopleural shunts include the risk of developing clinically significant pleural effusions. Patients who receive ventriculoatrial shunts are at increased risk of septicemia. Other much less common options for distal placement of a ventricular shunt include the gallbladder or ureter/bladder.

Complications from shunt placement during surgery are infrequent and arise in the context of the surrounding anatomy. Ventricular catheters may be misplaced, resulting in inadequate shunt function or intracranial hemorrhage. Patients undergoing VP shunt may experience bowel perforation or misplacement into the extraperitoneal space, leading to a CSF collection in the nonabsorptive space and subsequent fistulation through the skin. VP shunt patients are also at increased risk of developing hernias and bowel obstruction. Patients with ventriculopleural shunts may develop pleural effusions, leading to shortness of breath and hypoxia. During ventriculoatrial shunt placement, patients may develop cardiac tamponade. Afterward, these patients are at increased risk for septicemia and pulmonary thromboembolism. When evaluating for shunt complications, one must keep in mind the unique anatomy of the particular shunt within that patient and integrate a thorough history, physical exam, laboratory studies, radiologic findings, and possibly invasive diagnostic procedures to make the correct diagnosis.

CSF SHUNT FAILURE

Although the surgical procedure of CSF shunt placement is generally an uncomplicated process, the long-term management of shunted hydrocephalus is more problematic. Multiple clinical studies in both adult and pediatric patients attest to the high rate of device failure, which includes entities such as catheter occlusion, valve malfunction, distal catheter kink or fracture, disconnection of components, infection, or excessive drainage. In young children undergoing first-time shunt placement, roughly one third of shunts will require reoperation in the first year following surgery. Shunt infection rates in children are as high as 10%-12% and are generally higher in patients with shunts placed at a younger age. Adult patients fair somewhat better, but approximately 20% will still require reoperation within the first year after shunt failure. Failure rates for devices drops considerably after the first year or two from surgery, but the threat of failure remains present to some degree as long as the device remains in place.

In evaluating a patient for CSF shunt failure, the above epidemiologic data provide a baseline approximation for the probability of the diagnosis. A history and physical exam, along with images compared to previous findings, as described earlier, help to guide diagnosis. However, several pitfalls deserve mention. First, as has been noted earlier, not all patients with CSF shunt failure will demonstrate significant expansion of the ventricular system. Some patients, particularly those with a long history of shunted hydrocephalus, may present with so-called "slit-ventricle" syndrome, with severely narrowed ventricles on imaging. The clinical slit-ventricle syndrome presents with episodic severe headaches that are thought to occur due to intermittent occlusion of the proximal ventricular catheter within the collapsed ventricles. The diagnosis is often confirmed by direct ICP measurements obtained from a separately placed ICP monitor.

A second group that deserves special attention is children and adults with myelomeningocele. About 70% of patients with this spinal dysraphism will require treatment for hydrocephalus, most with a CSF shunt. Myelomeningocele is associated with a number of abnormalities of the brainstem and foramen magnum. These abnormalities allow CSF shunt failure to produce a much wider array of clinical symptoms. As intracranial CSF and pressure build because of CSF shunt failure, downward pressure on the brainstem may produce lower cranial nerve palsies, including swallowing and breathing irregularities. Mortality rates are higher and rapidity of neurologic decline more precipitous, likely related to the susceptibility of the hindbrain to herniation. In addition, CSF shunt failure may precipitate or exacerbate a preexisting spinal syrinx in these patients, producing symptoms related to spinal cord dysfunction.

Shunt contamination may occur in bacteremic patients, especially in the presence of a ventriculoatrial shunt. It may also arise due to intra-abdominal infections or surgical procedures with nonsterile spillage, as in the case of a VP shunt. Clinically, the presentation of infection can vary greatly. It can range from high-grade fever with overt meningitis and symptoms of acute shunt failure to something more insidious, such as a slight headache, pain along the shunt tract, decreased energy, or subtle recrudescence of the patient's presenting hydrocephalus symptoms. The presence of a large intra-abdominal fluid collection in a patient with a VP shunt should raise suspicion of shunt infection, although sterile fluid collections are not uncommon.

Abdominal surgical procedures in patients with VP shunts raise the issue of how best to manage an intraperitoneal distal shunt catheter during and after the abdominal procedure. While no validated guideline exists, the literature and the author's experience suggest that the infection risk is low during clean and clean-contaminated cases. If an enterotomy or open bladder procedure is to be performed, it is reasonable to relocate the shunt away from this area once the tubing is identified intraperitoneally and protect it with bacitracin-soaked gauze sponges during the procedure. Other than routine preoperative antibiotics, expectant management for shunt infection and failure can be practiced, and the shunt does not require externalization. In situations where there is frank contamination of the shunt catheter in the abdomen, externalization of the shunt would seem prudent. Laparoscopic procedures have been demonstrated to transiently increase ICP due to increased intra-abdominal pressures, but there is no body of literature to suggest that this produces identifiable complications, presumably due to its transient nature. Constipation and ileus, conversely, have been suggested to be a source of at least transient shunt dysfunction due to increased intra-abdominal pressure.

Shunt externalization is most often necessary in cases of distal catheter infection. It involves palpation of the shunt proximal to its entry into the peritoneum, followed by a sterile prep and, if the patient is awake, local anesthesia. If the shunt has been in place for several years, it may be adherent to the surrounding tissues and the procedure is then best performed in the operating room under anesthesia. For recently placed shunts, this is less of an issue and the procedure can be performed at the bedside, assuming a cooperative patient. A cut down is made over the shunt tract, avoiding laceration of the underlying tubing. The catheter is often encased in a thick sheath of scar that must be carefully opened to gain access to the catheter. If a specimen of fluid is required from a peritoneal fluid collection, the tubing is then cut and aspirated distally. In a large pseudocyst, a liter or more of fluid may be withdrawn. The distal catheter is then withdrawn from the patient and the catheter itself sent for culture. The remaining proximal tubing should be observed to confirm CSF drainage and connected to a sterile, enclosed CSF drainage system. Patients with externalized shunts drain isotonic CSF and may suffer hyponatremia if appropriate fluid and electrolyte repletion is not performed. This is of particular concern in young children.

ONGOING CARE

Patients with VP or ventriculopleural shunts do not require prophylactic antibiotics for surgical or dental procedures in which the shunt is outside the operative field. **Prophylactic antibiotics** may be helpful when the shunt is in the operative field, as described earlier, and should be routinely used during a planned CSF shunt revision. For patients with ventriculoatrial CSF shunts in place, an argument can be made for antibiotic prophylaxis prior to procedures likely to result in bacteremia such as dental procedures. Dental practice guidelines suggest this also. American Heart Association guidelines for endocarditis prophylaxis recommend amoxicillin 2 g 30-60 minutes before the procedure for adults and 50 mg/kg for pediatric patients.

Shunt independence has been reported for children with a prior history of shunt placement. In this situation, a child previously dependent on a CSF shunt becomes once again able to drain CSF independently. This most commonly occurs when a shunt has gone without revision for many years or decades. It is discovered most commonly when a shunt is disconnected in the absence of clinical symptoms. One series reported that 3% of children with hydrocephalus became shunt independent later in life. However, in the setting of a shunt found to be fractured on x-ray without ventricular enlargement or clinical symptoms of shunt failure, it has been observed that CSF can drain between the fractured catheter segments through the tunnel of chronic scar tissue that forms around the catheter after shunt placement. Therefore, caution should be exercised in the presumption of shunt independence unless it has been verified by invasive testing. Patients incidentally found to have broken shunt catheters may reasonably be referred to a neurosurgeon for evaluation.

Shunted hydrocephalus during pregnancy frequently raises concerns over management of headaches during pregnancy, mechanism of delivery, and the potential impact of hydrocephalus on the pregnancy outcome. Pregnancy, particularly in the third trimester, increases intra-abdominal pressures. For patients with VP shunts, this can lead to a relative decrease in CSF shunt function. In case series of pregnant patients with hydrocephalus, headaches are not uncommonly reported, particularly during the third trimester. These may herald shunt failure, the evaluation of which may be complicated by a desire to avoid radiation during pregnancy. MRI may be a useful option in these circumstances. In the absence of radiographic manifestations of shunt failure or additional clinical symptoms, safe observation of headaches has been successfully practiced, but treatment decisions must be individualized, and other diagnoses, particularly eclampsia and preeclampsia, must be considered. There is little evidence to suggest that the presence of a CSF shunt is a contraindication to labor and vaginal delivery. It has been argued that patients who are suspected of being symptomatic from increased ICP may benefit from avoiding protracted labor, but no comparative studies exist to provide a clear answer. Hydrocephalus and the presence of a CSF shunt do not, per se, appear to impact pregnancy outcome. However, recalling that hydrocephalus is coincident with other diagnoses, such as epilepsy and myelomeningocele, that do have a significant impact on the potential for birth defects, the importance of prenatal care should be emphasized by providers.

CENTRAL NERVOUS SYSTEM INFECTIONS

Kyle Wu, MD, and Timothy R. Smith, MD, PhD

BRAIN ABSCESS

Brain abscesses are an uncommon entity, with approximately 2000 cases reported in the United States annually. There is a higher incidence in developing countries, and men are affected slightly more often than women. Classically, cerebral abscesses arise locally from otorhinolaryngeal infections or hematogenously from distant infections, although opportunistic infections have become an important consideration upon initial presentation as well. The pathogenic organisms most commonly implicated are of the *Streptococcus* family; *Staphylococcus aureus*, *Klebsiella*, and anaerobes are also frequent. In immunocompromised patients, it is important to include *Toxoplasma*, *Listeria*, and *Nocardia* as possible infectious agents, as well as fungal and mycobacterial pathogens.

A patient with a brain abscess can present with nonspecific symptoms. Headache, nausea, vomiting, and altered mental status can occur due to increased ICP, whereas unilateral headache, seizures, and various focal neurologic deficits may be observed based on location of the mass lesion. Fever and nuchal rigidity are also seen in many cases. Additional findings in the newborn patient may include cranial enlargement, meningeal signs, irritability, and failure to thrive.

Common risk factors for brain abscess include sinus, inner ear, or dental infections. These sources usually lead to formation of frontal or temporal lobe abscesses through contiguous spread. Hematogenous spread from intra-abdominal, pelvic, pulmonary, or cardiac seeding occurs most commonly via the middle cerebral artery. This may lead to septic emboli causing pseudoaneurysm, abscess, or micro-embolic infarction at the gray-white junction. Major risk factors for developing hematogenous infectious processes includes intravenous drug use, access and placement of long-term intravenous hardware, chronic lung infections, pulmonary shunting, osteomyelitis, intracardiac hardware, and congenital cyanotic heart disease. Penetrating head trauma, including neurosurgery, may introduce a nidus for infection with delayed abscess formation. Parasitic infections, such as cysticercosis or toxoplasmosis, should be considered in recent foreign travelers or in immunocompromised patients.

The differential diagnosis for brain abscess is broad, including stroke, TBI, intracranial hemorrhage, subdural empyema, hydrocephalus, dural sinus thrombosis, meningitis, encephalitis, and tumor. Radiographically, abscesses appear most similar to tumor and can often be mistaken. All of these conditions can present with headaches and altered mental status. In the initial evaluation of brain abscess, blood work that should be drawn includes a white blood cell count, pan-cultures, erythrocyte sedimentation rate (ESR), and C-reactive protein (CRP); however, normal test results do not rule out an infectious diagnosis. The key to diagnosing brain abscess is correlating the clinical scenario with an imaging study, such as contrast-enhanced CT or contrasted MRI (the gold standard). The classic finding on CT or MRI is a well-circumscribed circular lesion with a strongly contrast-enhancing rim. CT is typically the first study obtained on presentation, although MRI is the imaging modality of choice as it can provide greater anatomic detail. MRI evaluation for brain abscess should always include DWIs, which can help differentiate between ring-enhancing lesions of infectious and neoplastic origin, as abscesses typically exhibit diffusion restriction, whereas neoplastic lesions generally do not.

Lumbar puncture is not recommended in instances of intracranial abscess because CSF results are often nondiagnostic, and lumbar puncture is associated with a worsened outcome in patients with brain abscesses. Less than one quarter of patients have positive CSF cultures, and with a large enough abscess, there is risk for transtentorial or brainstem herniation. CSF sampling should be considered only if parasitic pathogens are suspected or to guide treatment in clear cases of CSF involvement with an unknown infectious source. A definitive diagnosis is made by biopsy sampling of the abscess through surgical means.

The treatment of brain abscesses can involve medical therapy, surgical intervention, or both. Treatment should incorporate correcting the primary source of infection (eg, treating a cardiac valvular vegetation or repairing a correctable heart defect). Initial surgical treatment may consist of needle aspiration of the abscess, especially if in a deep or difficult-to-access location. The abscess can be monitored serially with imaging, and the procedure repeated as necessary. This reduces the size of the lesion and may provide microbiologic information for tailoring antibiotic treatment. Total excision via a craniotomy may be preferred if the abscess contains multiple loculations or is resistant to antibiotic therapy. Abscesses located near the cerebral ventricles pose a unique problem, as surgical manipulation may introduce infection into the intraventricular space; however, if left uncontrolled, the abscess itself may rupture into the ventricle and seed the CSF. Generally, if the abscess is periventricular, small, and appears stable over serial imaging, it may be managed expectantly with medical therapy. If surgical management for cerebral abscess is chosen, it is advisable to perform surgery before starting antibiotics in medically stable patients to allow for identification of organisms and their antibiotic sensitivities. Antibiotic therapy typically consists of 6-8 weeks of intravenous treatment followed by 4-8 weeks of oral antibiotic medications. Patients should receive routine follow-up imaging and should also be initiated on an antiepileptic medication, which is often continued beyond the initial period of therapy. Glucocorticoids may be considered to mediate symptomatic intracranial hypertension caused by significant vasogenic edema, although there is mixed evidence on the use of steroids, and definitive treatment through mass reduction is favored.

In certain situations, medical therapy may suffice without the need for surgery. These situations include an abscess in its early stages (ie, symptoms for < 2 weeks), a small (< 3 cm) abscess, or definite clinical improvement after 1 week of antibiotic therapy. Medical treatment without surgery should also be considered in poor surgical candidates, patients with multiple abscesses and/or concomitant meningitis, patients with abscesses in eloquent locations, or patients with hydrocephalus and ventricular shunts.

Patients with brain abscess have a reported mortality risk of 0%-30% depending on etiology and presentation. An overall 50% morbidity risk of permanent neurologic deficits is conferred, which depends heavily on the severity of presenting symptoms.

SUBDURAL EMPYEMA

A subdural empyema is a collection of pus that forms in the subdural space. It is less common than brain abscess, but like abscesses, it is more commonly found in males. Subdural empyema is an especially challenging condition because, unlike the brain parenchyma, the subdural space does not pose much of a barrier to prevent the spread of infection. Additionally, antibiotics have poor penetration into the subdural space.

The most common cause of subdural empyema (70%) is contiguous spread from paranasal sinusitis, especially in cases involving the frontal sinus. Chronic otitis media accounts for another 15% of cases. Osteomyelitis of the skull can also result in direct bacterial invasion of the brain and meninges. As such, the organisms typically cultured from a subdural empyema include *Streptococcus* (aerobic and anaerobic) and *Staphylococcus*. Symptoms experienced by patients with subdural empyema include fever, headache, nuchal rigidity, hemiparesis, and altered mental status. Other common symptoms include seizures and sinus tenderness.

CT or MRI imaging will typically diagnose a subdural empyema. Three-fourths of empyemas are located over the convexity, whereas 15% are parafalcine (ie, adjacent to the falx cerebri). Just as with brain abscesses, lumbar puncture should be avoided due to the potential risk of herniation, and generally low culture yield.

The majority of surgical cases of subdural empyema require drainage for removal of mass effect and microbiologic reduction. The two primary surgical options are burr-hole drainage and craniotomy. Although burr-hole drainage is less invasive, it is also less effective in cases of loculated or adherent collections; thus, craniotomy is generally the preferred surgical option. Antibiotics are used for a course of 4-6 weeks, and patients are initiated on therapeutic or prophylactic anti-seizure medication. Medical treatment alone can be effective if the empyema is small, there is minimal neurologic involvement, and early antibiotics demonstrate efficacy.

Subdural empyema carries a 15% mortality rate. Half of patients will have residual neurologic deficits at the time of hospital discharge. Factors known to be associated with poor prognosis include age greater than 60 years, obtunded or comatose state at presentation, and empyema formation secondary to surgery or trauma.

OSTEOMYELITIS

Osteomyelitis can affect the skull or the spinal vertebrae. Osteomyelitis of the skull usually results by contiguous spread from an infected sinus or from penetrating trauma (eg, postoperative). The infectious agents are typically *S aureus* or *Staphylococcus epidermidis*, and treatment consists primarily of prolonged antibiotic therapy (intravenously for the first 1-2 weeks). If resistant to treatment or the patient develops continued spread of the infection, surgical treatment aimed at removing the infected bone may be required. Cranioplasty or other hardware placement is generally avoided until several months later in order to minimize the risk of reestablishing the infection by providing an avascular nidus.

Vertebral osteomyelitis (VO) represents 3% of all cases of osteomyelitis and is more common than cranial osteomyelitis because of the spine's rich vascular supply. Both anterograde arterial seeding as well as retrograde venous plexus spread have been implicated in VO, with *S aureus* being the most common organism. VO caused by *Mycobacterium tuberculosis* is known as Pott disease. Those at higher risk for developing VO include diabetics, intravenous drug users, immunosuppressed patients, patients on hemodialysis, and the elderly.

The most common presentation in patients with VO is that of back pain (> 90%), usually unaffected by activity. Other typical presenting symptoms include fever, weight loss, radicular pain, and myelopathy. Neurologic symptoms are usually a result of spread to the epidural space causing epidural spinal abscess or from destruction of the vertebral body leading to collapse of the neural foramen, which results in nerve root compression. The most commonly affected segment of the spine is the lumbar region followed by the thoracic, cervical, and sacral segments, respectively. Any source of infection can theoretically put one at risk for developing VO, although important sources include infections of the urinary tract, cardiopulmonary system, and mouth. VO also develops at sites of prior spine surgery.

Definitive diagnosis of VO is made with positive cultures, either from biopsy of the tissue itself or via blood cultures in the setting of suggestive radiographic findings. Contrast-enhanced MRI has demonstrated excellent diagnostic sensitivity and is the preferred diagnostic modality. When unable to obtain MRI, bone scintigraphy with SPECT is also highly effective in detection of VO.

The treatment of VO is nonsurgical in the vast majority of cases, with disease resolution being accomplished via antibiotic therapy alone. The goal of therapy should be to minimize neurologic involvement and to maintain structural stability of the spine. Surgical treatment is considered to obtain a tissue diagnosis if both blood cultures and closed-needle biopsy are nondiagnostic. In patients with a worsening neurologic deficit, the onset of structural instability, or a failure of medical management, surgery is warranted for abscess drainage, alleviation of compression, and stabilization.

SPINAL EPIDURAL ABSCESS

Spinal epidural abscesses (SEAs) are often associated with VO, with the microbiologic isolate being *S aureus* in the majority of cases. The *Streptococcus* species are the second most commonly implicated organism (Figure 38–27).

▲ **Figure 38–27.** Sagittal magnetic resonance T1-weighted image with contrast of the lumbar spine demonstrating diskitis/osteomyelitis associated with a spinal epidural abscess.

SEAs are located most often in the thoracic region (50%), followed by the lumbar (35%) and cervical (15%) regions. The vast majority of abscesses (80%) are located posterior to the spinal cord.

The primary infection leading to SEA can be from hematogenous spread or direct extension. Hematogenous spread is more common, with skin infections being the most common originating source. Other sources of hematogenous spread include nonsterile intravenous injections, bacterial endocarditis, urinary tract infections, respiratory infections, and oropharyngeal abscesses. SEAs caused by direct extension can be from decubitus ulcers or penetrating trauma, including after spinal procedures.

Patients with SEA are typically middle-aged. Risk factors for developing SEA include diabetes, peripheral vascular disease, intravenous drug use, chronic renal failure, and alcoholism. Patients often present with back pain, spine tenderness, fever, sweats, and rigors. When motor weakness ensues, there is a very rapid progression to paraplegia and bowel or bladder dysfunction. Thus, the diagnosis and treatment of SEA are emergent for preservation and reversal of neurologic injury.

The workup of spinal epidural abscesses should include a complete blood count, ESR, CRP, and cultures. A lumbar puncture is contraindicated given the potential to spread infection from the epidural to the intradural space. The imaging modality of choice is gadolinium-enhanced MRI, although both contrast CT and myelography (although never used in lumbar SEA for risk of intradural seeding) may also be used to arrive at a diagnosis when the use of MRI is precluded. Standing scoliosis x-rays (ie, 36-inch long cassette stand x-rays) may be used to follow patients at high risk of developing spinal deformity (ie, kyphotic deformity).

The treatment of SEA, as with most infections of the CNS, is a combination of medical therapy plus surgery if needed. In patients who have small spinal epidural abscesses without neurologic deficit, primary management with antibiotics alone is often sufficient. Emergent decompressive surgery via laminectomy and washout is required for patients with new neurologic dysfunction. Surgery may be required on a subacute basis to drain pus and debride granulation tissue if the infection remains treatment resistant. In cases where infection leads to bony instability, most often due to VO, internal fixation with spinal hardware may be necessary, most often following resolution of the acute phase of the infection. Antibiotics are often given intravenously for 4-6 weeks and then orally for another 4 weeks. The overall prognosis for patients with SEA is relatively poor, with a mortality rate of 20%. In patients who survive, restoration of baseline neurologic function is relatively rare.

Arko LT, Quach E, Nguyen V, et al. Medical and surgical management of spinal epidural abscess: a systematic review. *Neurosurg Focus.* 2014;37(2):E4.

Berbari EF, Steckelberg JM, Osmon DR: Osteomyelitis. In: Bennett JE, Dolin R, Blaser MJ, eds. *Mandell, Douglas, and Bennett's Principles and Practice of Infectious Diseases, Updated Edition.* 8th ed. Philadelphia, PA: Elsevier Saunders; 2015: chap 106.

Boody BS, Jenkins TJ, Maslak J, et al: Vertebral osteomyelitis and spinal epidural abscess: an evidence-based review. *J Spinal Disord Tech.* 2015;28(6):E316-E327.

Darouiche RO: Spinal epidural abscess. *N Engl J Med.* 2006;355(19): 2012-2020.

Kusuma S, Klineberg EO: Spinal infections: diagnosis and treatment of discitis, osteomyelitis, and epidural abscess. In: Steinmetz MP, Benzel EC, eds. *Benzel's Spine Surgery.* 4th ed. Philadelphia, PA: Elsevier; 2017:chap 122.

MULTIPLE CHOICE QUESTIONS

1. Intracranial pressure

    A. Is normally between 30 and 40 torr
    B. Is directly (linearly) related to increasing intracranial mass
    C. Cannot be measured directly
    D. Is normally maintained at a stable level by displacement of cerebrospinal fluid (CSF)
    E. Is often affected by changes in the size of the skull after trauma

2. Strategies to reduce intracranial pressure can include all of the following except

    A. Drainage of CSF
    B. Hyperventilation
    C. Treatment with mannitol
    D. Trendelenburg position
    E. Sedation

3. Spinal cord injury

    A. Rarely includes the use of systemic corticosteroid therapy
    B. Is accompanied by initial hyporeflexia
    C. Is termed complete if there is no motor function below the level of injury
    D. Is accompanied by priapism and increased anal sphincter tone
    E. Can cause a Brown-Sequard syndrome, with loss of motor function and loss of pain and temperature sensation below the level of the lesion, with preserved proprioception, vibration, and pressure sensation

4. Peripheral nerve injury recovery
   A. Occurs with axonal regeneration after Wallerian degeneration at a rate of 1 mm/d
   B. Is best treated by delayed (3 months) repair in the case of acute sharp injury
   C. Should be treated by segmental resection and nerve graft in cases of apparent stretch injury
   D. Occurs more quickly with systemic corticosteroid therapy
   E. Is likely to be functionally successful if a neuroma forms

5. Pituitary tumors
   A. Are typically adenocarcinomas
   B. Should be treated by urgent operation in most patients
   C. Can cause symptoms related to the compression of the pituitary stalk causing increased prolactin levels
   D. Can cause Cushing syndrome by overproduction of growth hormone
   E. Cause visual symptoms due to hormonal release

The Eye & Ocular Adnexa

Ian Pitha, MD, PhD

Linda M. Tsai, MD

Ophthalmology is a rapidly progressing specialty that has evolved substantially over the past decade. Innovations in surgical techniques and tissue banking, as well as developments in ophthalmic surgical devices and implants, allow an increasingly sophisticated approach to ophthalmic surgery. Advances in imaging the microanatomy of the eye facilitate diagnosis and guide treatment. Nonetheless, the majority of diagnoses in ophthalmology can be made after a targeted history and careful examination without the need for sophisticated equipment.

EXAMINATION OF THE EYE

Evaluation of the eye and its adnexa requires a good history, assessment of visual function, and physical examination of the eyes. Occasionally, special examinations or tests may be required to identify specific ocular disorders or to establish the presence of associated systemic disease.

The basic equipment required for an eye examination by a nonophthalmologist includes the following: (1) a visual acuity chart, (2) a handheld flashlight, (3) an ophthalmoscope, and (4) a tonometer.

The basic medications required for an eye examination are (1) a local anesthetic such as proparacaine 0.5% or tetracaine 0.5%; (2) fluorescein strips; and (3) dilating drops, such as phenylephrine 2.5% or tropicamide 0.5%-1%.

History

In addition to eliciting a chief complaint, determining whether visual loss is monocular or binocular, central or peripheral, and painful or painless is a key first step in narrowing the differential diagnosis. Prior ophthalmic history (including known ophthalmic conditions, prior eye surgery or trauma, history of contact lens use, and relevant family history) should be obtained. A review of past medical history and all medications should be included as well.

Visual Acuity Testing

Central visual acuity, using the patient's glasses if available, should be determined in all patients. The Snellen chart is most commonly used. The patient faces the test chart at a distance of 6 m (20 ft). Each eye should be tested separately. Visual acuity corresponds to the smallest line the patient can read. The patient who is unable to read the largest letter on the chart (typically a 20/200 letter) should be moved progressively closer until that character can be read and that distance recorded in the chart. If no letters are recognizable, the patient should be tested for the ability to count fingers, see hand motion, or perceive light. If a vision chart is not readily available, the ability to read small print or a name badge can provide useful information. Preschool children or illiterate patients can be tested with the E chart or Allen picture chart.

Visual Field Testing

Confrontation visual fields can be used to detect gross visual field defects such as quadrantanopia, hemianopia, or severe visual field constriction. With one eye occluded, the patient is asked to fixate on the examiner's face and detect finger count or hand motion in each quadrant. Formal visual field testing (perimetry) is used to more carefully examine the central and peripheral visual fields. The technique is performed separately for each eye and measures the function of the retina, the optic nerve, and intracranial visual pathway. Perimetry relies on subjective patient responses, so results will depend on the patient's alertness and cooperation. Several methods are used to assess visual field function, including the tangent screen, Goldmann perimetry, and computerized automated perimetry.

Eye Movements

Ocular motility should be assessed in all positions of gaze. One should also assess the alignment of the eyes when the patient is looking straight ahead. The position of the light reflection from a penlight ("reflex") on the cornea is at the same point in each eye when the eyes are properly aligned. The oculocephalic reflex (doll's head) can be tested. Upward rotation of the eye in response to resistance to forced eyelid closure (Bell phenomenon) should be noted when clinically appropriate. Difficulty with object tracking, random eye movements, and nystagmus (repetitive, uncontrolled movement), may be associated with other medical conditions.

Assessment of Pupillary Function

Examination of the pupils should be performed before any dilating drops are instilled. Both the direct and consensual light reflex should be assessed. The pupils should constrict with accommodation. The size of the pupils should be noted in light and dark conditions, and any difference in size (anisocoria) should be recorded. Irregular pupils may indicate traumatic, postsurgical, neurologic, or congenital defects. In hospitalized patients and those with neurologic disorders requiring monitoring of pupillary reaction to assess clinical status, pupils should be dilated with discretion, using only short-acting mydriatics, and staff should be notified that the patient has been pharmacologically dilated.

Inspection of Anterior Segment & Adnexa

The eyelids, conjunctiva, cornea, sclera, and lacrimal apparatus should be evaluated. Unusual prominence of the globes (proptosis), abnormal eyelid position, and the inability to fully close eyelids are important features that should be documented. Eversion of the upper eyelid to enable inspection of the hidden conjunctival surface should be performed when appropriate. The conjunctiva is inspected for anatomic defects, foreign bodies, lacerations, inflammation, discharge, tearing, dryness, or other abnormalities. In patients who are unconscious, the presence or absence of Bell phenomenon may be an important measure of neurologic function. Corneal sensation should be tested before anesthetic drops are used.

A direct ophthalmoscope focused on the ocular surface can provide magnification for the examination. A magnifying glass and a handheld flashlight can also be used. Shining a light across the eye from the lateral to medial aspects and noting whether or not the nasal iris is shadowed can assess the depth of the anterior chamber. The presence of shadowing may indicate a narrow anterior chamber angle, making the eye prone to an attack of angle closure glaucoma when dilating drops are used. If shadowing is detected, ophthalmologic consultation should be obtained before dilating drops are used.

Ophthalmoscopy

Ophthalmoscopy is important for the diagnosis of both ocular and systemic conditions and can provide critical information in neurologic and neurosurgical contexts. In most instances, the optic nerve head can be clearly seen without dilating the pupils. When describing the optic nerve, it is important to note any nerve head edema and the cup-to-disc ratio. Vessel caliber, tortuosity, arteriovenous nicking, and the presence of retinal hemorrhages are additional findings that can aid in diagnosis. Dilation of the pupils in hospitalized patients with neurologic or neurosurgical conditions should only be done with short-acting agents.

Tonometry

Tonometry measures intraocular pressure. Measurements are taken on the cornea after topical anesthesia has been instilled. Commonly used instruments are the Tono-Pen, iCare rebound tonometer, Perkins tonometer, and Goldmann applanation tonometer. Many of these instruments may only be available in ophthalmology offices. Normal intraocular pressure varies between 10 and 20 mm Hg. Intraocular pressure measurements can vary slightly with corneal thickness.

SYMPTOMS & SIGNS OF OCULAR DISORDERS

Decrease in Visual Acuity

Efforts should be made to determine if the decrease in visual acuity is unilateral or bilateral, painful or painless, persistent or transient, recent or chronic, and isolated or associated with other symptoms. Unilateral acute painful loss of vision may be due to angle-closure glaucoma, endophthalmitis, or uveitis. Painless unilateral loss of vision is often caused by ischemic optic neuropathy, optic neuritis, central retinal artery or vein occlusion, retinal detachment, vitreous hemorrhage, or retinal hemorrhages. Transient painless unilateral loss may be due to retinal migraine or amaurosis fugax. Hemispheric strokes are often responsible for visual field loss with preservation of the central visual acuity.

Disturbances in Vision

A patient's description of visual disturbance can be varied and include image distortion, color change, spots before the eyes, visual field defects, night blindness, momentary loss of vision, or halos around lights. Patients can also note image distortion (metamorphopsia), which is most commonly caused by macular lesions. Abnormally colored vision (chromatopsia) can be caused by cataract formation or systemic medications such as digoxin. Patients with vitreous opacities, intraocular inflammation, or intraocular bleeding may report mobile, floating spots in their vision. Visual field defects may be due to lid edema, retinal and optic nerve lesions, visual pathway lesions, or cortical abnormalities. Night blindness may be genetic (as in patients with retinitis pigmentosa) or acquired. Important causes of acquired night blindness include vitamin A deficiency, glaucoma, optic atrophy, cataract, or retinal degeneration. Transient loss of vision may imply impending cerebrovascular accident or partial occlusion of the internal carotid artery. Colored halos around lights can be caused by elevated intraocular pressure, most commonly due to acute angle-closure glaucoma. Incipient cataract or incorrect refractive error can cause colorless halos around point light sources.

Double Vision (Diplopia)

Diplopia can be constant or intermittent, sudden or gradual, painful or painless, and horizontal, vertical, or torsional. It may occur only in certain gaze positions. The first step should be to determine if the diplopia is monocular or binocular. Binocular diplopia is only present when both eyes are open and disappears when either eye is closed. Binocular diplopia is most often due to misalignment of the eyes from extraocular muscle dysfunction or neurologic abnormalities. Monocular diplopia (multiple images in a single eye) is usually caused by ocular conditions such as refractive error, cataract, and macular lesions but can also be seen in malingering or conversion reactions.

Ocular & Orbital Pain

Ocular pain may result from corneal lesions, inflammation, rapid increase in intraocular pressure, anterior uveitis, cyclitis, scleritis, or optic neuritis. Light sensitivity (photophobia) is a frequent complaint and is most commonly due to corneal inflammation and iritis. However, it can also be associated with rare conditions such as ocular albinism or aniridia. Other causes of pain include inflammation of the orbital contents, tumors in the orbit, and dacryocystitis (lacrimal sac inflammation). Eyelid pain and irritation can also arise from infections of the meibomian glands and the glands of Zeis and Moll.

Redness of the Eye

Acute redness (injection) of the eye not associated with trauma is caused by conjunctivitis, acute anterior uveitis, acute angle-closure glaucoma, corneal infection, or corneal abrasion (Table 39–1). Subconjunctival hemorrhage may also present as a red eye and can be dramatic in appearance but is usually painless and otherwise asymptomatic. Conjunctivitis from bacterial, chlamydial, viral, or allergic causes is a frequent cause of red eye. Nonspecific irritation from exogenous agents or a foreign body can also cause redness. Chemical and thermal injuries cause similar findings. "Dry eye" or ocular surface anomalies can cause redness, a foreign body sensation, and variable degrees of decreased vision.

Discharge

Ocular discharge may be described as watery, mucopurulent, purulent, or crusting of the lid margins. When watery discharge is not associated with redness or pain, it may be due to excessive tear production or obstruction of the lacrimal outflow passages. Watery discharge with photophobia, pain, or irritation indicates possible keratitis or keratoconjunctivitis. Purulent or mucopurulent discharge is a sign of bacterial infection, severe inflammation of the conjunctival surface, or bacterial infection of the lacrimal sac or canaliculus.

Table 39–1. Differential diagnosis of common causes of inflamed eye.

	Acute Conjunctivitis	Acute Iritis[1]	Acute Glaucoma[2]	Corneal Trauma or Infection
Incidence	Extremely common	Common	Uncommon	Common
Discharge	Moderate to copious	None	None	Watery or purulent
Vision	No effect on vision	Slightly blurred	Markedly blurred	Usually blurred
Pain	None	Moderate	Severe	Moderate to severe
Conjunctival injection	Diffuse; more toward fornices	Mainly circumcorneal	Diffuse	Diffuse
Cornea	Clear	Usually clear	Steamy	Change in clarity related to cause
Pupil size	Normal	Small	Moderately dilated and fixed	Normal
Pupillary light response	Normal	Poor	None	Normal
Intraocular pressure	Normal	Normal	Elevated	Normal
Smear	Causative organisms	No organisms	No organisms	Organisms found only in corneal ulcers due to infection

[1] Acute anterior uveitis.
[2] Angle-closure glaucoma.

Pseudomonas or *Haemophilus* species involvement is common in these cases. When the discharge forms mucoid strings, it is characteristic of allergic disorders involving the conjunctiva (vernal conjunctivitis) or dry eye syndrome.

Swelling of the Eyelids

For unilateral swelling, the cause is often a sty or chalazion. Bilateral swelling suggests blepharitis or allergic dermatitis. Systemic diseases associated with water retention, hyperthyroidism, or hypothyroidism can also cause swelling or puffiness of the eyelids.

Displacement of the Eyes

The most common cause of both unilateral and bilateral exophthalmos (proptosis) is hyperthyroidism. Other etiologies include tumors of the orbit.

Strabismus

Strabismus results from misalignment of the eyes due to muscle imbalance. Ocular deviations may be lateral (exotropia), medial (esotropia), upward (hypertropia), or downward (hypotropia). Diplopia is not a frequent complaint in patients with congenital strabismus. Ocular motility is intact in the majority of strabismus cases.

Leukocoria

A white pupil in a child indicates a serious eye disorder. The most frequent cause of leukocoria is congenital cataract, which requires urgent management to prevent amblyopia. Other causes include retinoblastoma, retinopathy of prematurity, toxocariasis, persistent hyperplastic primary vitreous, vitreous hemorrhage, retinal detachment, retinal dysplasia, incontinentia pigmenti, Coats disease, and Norrie disease.

Other Symptoms

Patients may present with other symptoms such as burning, itching, gritty and foreign body sensations, or a "sandy" feeling. These symptoms in elderly patients are suggestive of dry eye syndrome. Itching is also frequently associated with allergic disorders.

DISEASES OF THE EYE & ADNEXA

DISEASES OF THE OCULAR ADNEXA

ACUTE HORDEOLUM

Acute hordeolum (sty) is a common infection of the glands of the eyelids. External hordeolum involve the glands of Zeis or Moll. Internal hordeolum is an infection of the meibomian glands. The usual causative agent is *Staphylococcus aureus*. Acute hordeolum is characterized by pain, localized swelling, and redness of the eyelid. A large hordeolum is rarely associated with a preauricular lymph node.

If there is no abscess formation, treatment with warm compresses three times daily and topical broad-spectrum antibiotic drops such as tobramycin or sulfacetamide three or four times daily for 5-7 days usually suffices. Ophthalmic ointment (erythromycin or bacitracin) twice daily for 5-7 days is also effective but usually not tolerated by adults due to visual blurring. Oral antibiotics, especially tetracycline derivatives, can be useful for patients with acne rosacea. If the infection does not resolve and is localized, treatment consists of making a local horizontal (skin) or vertical (conjunctiva) incision to drain the abscess.

HERPES ZOSTER

Herpes zoster is caused by a reactivation of latent varicella virus (chickenpox) dormant in the dorsal root ganglion. Approximately 15% of herpes zoster cases arise from the ophthalmic division of the trigeminal nerve (herpes zoster ophthalmicus). Hutchinson sign (involvement of the nasociliary nerve, which supplies the tip of the nose) occurs in about one-third of patients with herpes zoster ophthalmicus. If present, it suggests intraocular involvement. Reactivation is associated with decreased cell-mediated immunity, and patients with HIV, blood dyscrasias, neoplasms, or other forms of immunosuppression are at increased risk.

Clinical Findings

Herpes zoster ophthalmicus can involve virtually any ocular and adnexal tissues. Reactivation often starts with headache, malaise, fever, and ocular pain without cutaneous findings. Within 24-48 hours, the classic vesicular lesions develop unilaterally in a dermatomal distribution. Corneal involvement presents with the acute event or may follow it by months or years. A corneal pseudodendritic pattern is common. Conjunctivitis, keratitis, episcleritis/scleritis, and uveitis can also occur. Dry eye and poor corneal sensation are common.

Treatment

Treatments of skin lesions include warm compresses and topical antibiotic ointment. Aggressive lubrication is often needed for maintenance of the ocular surface. Oral antiviral medication is the standard of care. Oral acyclovir (800 mg five times a day) or valacyclovir (1000 mg three times a day) initiated within 72 hours of symptoms has been demonstrated to accelerate the resolution of skin rash and the healing of skin lesions, reduce lesion formation and viral shedding, and reduce the incidence of episcleritis, keratitis, and iritis. Oral antivirals appear to reduce both acute zoster-associated pain and postherpetic neuralgia. Topical antiviral medication and steroids can be used in certain situations to treat corneal lesions or uveitis. The Zostavax vaccine was approved in 2006 for the prevention of herpes zoster in the elderly, although booster shots may be needed to maintain efficacy. An improved recombinant zoster vaccine, Shingrix, was approved in 2017. In patients without known risk factors for herpes zoster ophthalmicus (patients under age 50 without chronic immunosuppression), consider HIV testing.

Baxter R, et al: Long-term effectiveness of the live zoster vaccine in preventing shingles: a cohort study. *Am J Epidemiol.* 2018; 187:161-169.

Dooling KL, et al: Recommendations of the Advisory Committee on Immunization Practices for use of herpes zoster vaccines. *MMWR Morbid Mortal Wkly Rep.* 2018;67:103-108.

Li JY: Herpes zoster ophthalmicus: acute keratitis. *Curr Opin Ophthalmol.* 2018;29:328-333.

Oxman MN, et al: Vaccination against herpes zoster and postherpetic neuralgia. *J Infect Dis.* 2008;197(Suppl 2):S228-S223.

DACRYOCYSTITIS

Dacryocystitis is a common infection of the lacrimal sac. Acute or chronic, it occurs most often in infants and in persons over age 40. It is usually unilateral and always secondary to obstruction of the nasolacrimal duct. In rare instances, the nasolacrimal duct may be obstructed by a tumor.

In children, the nasolacrimal duct opens spontaneously during the first month of life. Failure of canalization leads to obstruction of the sac and secondary dacryocystitis. The cause of acquired nasolacrimal duct obstruction is often unclear, but trauma to the nose or infection may be responsible. In infants, dacryocystitis leading to obstruction may be due to *Haemophilus influenzae*, staphylococci, or streptococci. In patients with trachoma, nasolacrimal and canalicular obstruction is common. The cause of acute dacryocystitis in adults is usually *S aureus* or β-hemolytic streptococci. In chronic dacryocystitis, *Streptococcus pneumoniae* is a common pathogen.

▶ Clinical Findings

A. Symptoms and Signs

Acute dacryocystitis is characterized by pain, swelling, tenderness, and redness in the tear sac area. In chronic dacryocystitis, tearing and discharge are the principal signs. Purulent material can often be expressed through the puncta.

B. Laboratory Findings

Culture and sensitivity of organisms obtained from cotton swab should be performed.

▶ Treatment

A. Adults

Acute dacryocystitis responds well to systemic antibiotic therapy, but recurrences are common if the obstruction is not surgically relieved.

B. Infants

When ductal obstruction is due to failure of canaliculization in the first month of life, daily vigorous massage of the tear sac is indicated. Topical antibiotics should be instilled in the conjunctival sac four or five times daily. If this is not successful, probing of the nasolacrimal duct is indicated. Most ophthalmologists postpone probing until age 6-9 months to allow sufficient time for the passage to open on its own. Both the upper and the lower canaliculi should be probed. In cases of previous failure or in children older than age 2, balloon dacryocystoplasty at the time of probing may increase chances of success. In recalcitrant cases, stenting of the nasolacrimal system or surgical creation of a new tear drain between the eye and nose (dacryocystorhinostomy) is required.

ORBITAL CELLULITIS

Orbital cellulitis is characterized by an abrupt onset of swelling and redness of the lids, accompanied by proptosis, decreased vision, diplopia, and fever. It is usually caused by staphylococci or streptococci. Immediate treatment with intravenous antibiotics is indicated to prevent abscess formation and rapid increase in the orbital pressure with compromise of the blood supply to the eye. The response to antibiotics is usually excellent, but surgical drainage may be required if an abscess forms. Orbital computed tomography (CT) with contrast is indicated to rule out abscess formation. Preseptal cellulitis is limited to the area anterior to the orbital septum and is treated with oral antibiotics while monitoring closely for progression to full-blown orbital infection.

▼ DISEASES OF THE EYE SURFACE

CONJUNCTIVITIS

Acute conjunctivitis is a common cause of red eye. Infectious causes include bacterial, viral, chlamydial, fungal, and parasitic agents. Noninfectious causes include chemical irritation, allergy, hypersensitivity to topical medications, vitamin A deficiency, dry eye syndrome, floppy eyelid syndrome associated with obstructive sleep apnea, and injury.

Clinical Findings

A. Symptoms and Signs

Patients with conjunctivitis complain of redness, irritation, foreign body sensation, and conjunctival discharge. One or both eyes may be affected. The eyelids are often stuck together in the morning. Bacterial conjunctivitis has conjunctival hyperemia with purulent or mucopurulent discharge and variable degrees of lid swelling. Gonococcal conjunctivitis is characterized by hyperacute onset of copious mucopurulent discharge and can be a vision-threatening infection. In viral conjunctivitis, follicles are present in the inferior conjunctival fornix, and preauricular lymph nodes are often involved. The hallmark symptom of allergic conjunctivitis is itching.

B. Laboratory Findings

If bacterial conjunctivitis is suspected, appropriate microbiologic testing should be performed. The AdenoPlus Point-of-Care test for diagnosing adenoviral conjunctivitis is highly specific; however, sensitivity has been reported to be as low as 50%.

Treatment

For patients with suspected bacterial conjunctivitis, topical broad-spectrum antibacterial agents should be prescribed (eg, ciprofloxacin 0.3% eye drops four times a day or tobramycin 0.3% four times a day), with the addition of erythromycin or bacitracin ophthalmic ointment at bedtime if clinical indications warrant.

Viral conjunctivitis is usually self-limited and does not require treatment. If the diagnosis is unclear, topical antibiotics are often used. Contact precautions are necessary in all situations of suspected bacterial and viral conjunctivitis because spread of disease occurs through contact with contaminated tears. Referral to a specialist is indicated if symptoms persist after several weeks or follow a progressive course.

Treatment of patients with allergic conjunctivitis consists of topical decongestants (naphazoline 0.1%) and H_1-receptor blocker (levocabastine) or a mast cell stabilizer (cromolyn). Combination mast cell and antihistamine drops such as olopatadine are also available. In severe cases of allergic conjunctivitis, topical corticosteroids or cyclosporine might be required but should be initiated only with the assistance of an ophthalmologist.

Holtz KK, et al: An Assessment of the AdenoPlus Point-of-Care test for diagnosing adenoviral conjunctivitis and its effect on antibiotic stewardship. *Mayo Clin Proc Innov Qual Outcomes.* 2017;1(2):170-175.

CORNEAL ULCERS

Corneal infections leading to ulceration may be due to bacteria, viruses, fungi, or protozoa.

Clinical Findings

A. Symptoms and Signs

Patients with corneal ulcers complain of pain, photophobia, and blurring of vision. Patients develop conjunctival hyperemia and chemosis with ulceration of the cornea and whitish or yellowish infiltrate. Hypopyon (pus in the anterior chamber) may be present in cases caused by bacterial or fungal infections. Contact lens users and people with diminished corneal sensation or incomplete eyelid closure are at increased risk of developing corneal infections.

B. Laboratory Findings

Laboratory studies include culture and cytologic inspection of corneal scrapings. If contact lenses are involved, the contact lens case should be cultured as well.

Treatment

Corneal ulceration is a serious condition requiring careful management under the direction of an ophthalmologist to avoid permanent visual loss. The most devastating infection of the cornea is caused by *Pseudomonas aeruginosa*. Topical antibiotics should be given on an empirical basis until the results of culture and sensitivity tests are available. Organism-specific antimicrobial treatment should then be started. Patients using topical corticosteroids should stop using them. Central corneal ulcers may leave corneal scars, causing loss of vision. Patients severely affected may require corneal transplantation.

Patients wearing contact lenses (especially extended-wear contacts) are at higher risk of corneal ulcers. Contact lens wear should be stopped if corneal infection is suspected.

HERPES SIMPLEX

Herpes simplex virus (HSV) is a DNA virus that can affect the eye either in a primary ocular reaction or a reactivated state when latent virus travels down the axon of the sensory nerve to its target tissue. HSV is extremely common, with about 90% of the population seropositive for HSV antibodies. HSV-1 usually causes infection above the waist (face, lips, and eyes); HSV-2 infections are usually below. Rarely, HSV-2 is transmitted during birth to the infant eye through infected genital secretions (Table 39–2).

Clinical Findings

A. Symptoms and Signs

Primary infections usually occur in children between ages 6 months and 5 years, accompanied by generalized symptoms of a viral illness. Ocular HSV is usually self-limited, with the most common symptoms being blepharoconjunctivitis and a dendritic keratitis.

Table 39–2. Herpes simplex virus (HSV) versus herpes zoster virus (HZV).

	HSV	HZV
Rash	Clear vesicles on erythematous base; crusting	Vesicular rash along dermatomal distribution, not crossing midline; Hutchinson sign (nasociliary branch of V1) may be present
Epithelial lesion	Dendritic epithelial lesions with heaped edges	Pseudodendrites (mucous plaques without true terminal bulbs)
Staining	Edges stain with rose bengal; central ulceration stains with fluorescein	Minimal fluorescein staining
Patient population	Young	Older or immunocompromised

B. Laboratory Findings

A clinical diagnosis can be made if there is a classic dendritic presentation. However, definitive diagnosis is made using viral culture or Giemsa-stained smears of corneal scrapings that reveal mononuclear cells, polymorphonuclear neutrophil leukocytes, multinucleated giant epithelial cells, and eosinophilic Lipschutz inclusion bodies in the cell nuclei. Enzyme-linked immunosorbent assay (ELISA) can be used to detect live viral particles.

▶ Treatment

The mainstays of treatment are topical and oral antiviral medications. Antibiotic ointment may be used at night to help prevent bacterial superinfection. Topical trifluorothymidine 1% (Viroptic) or ganciclovir ophthalmic gel 0.15% (Zirgan) is used to treat keratitis. Oral acyclovir (400 mg five times a day) or valacyclovir (500 mg three times a day) is usually added. Topical steroids under the direction of an ophthalmologist can be used to treat corneal scarring or uveitis but only with concurrent topical or systemic antiviral therapy. Cost effectiveness of prophylaxis with valacyclovir or acyclovir has been analyzed, but currently, they are rarely used for prolonged periods of time unless significant visual loss has occurred from previous herpetic episodes.

Kalezic T, et al: Herpetic eye disease study: lessons learned. *Curr Opin Ophthalmol.* 2018;29:340-346.

DRY EYE

Dry eye is a disorder of the tear film due to either deficient tear production or excessive tear evaporation. The tear film is composed of mucin, aqueous, and lipid components. Abnormalities of any layer lead to a wide variety of symptoms. Dry eye has become one of the most common reasons for visits to ophthalmologists. Symptoms are often exacerbated by weather, climate, reading, and computer use (decreased blink rate). Women have a much higher incidence of symptomatic dry eye. Primary lacrimal deficiency from diseases such as Riley-Day syndrome and hypoplastic lacrimal glands is rare. Secondary lacrimal deficiency is more common and can be related to prior radiation therapy, lymphoma, sarcoidosis, graft-versus-host disease, HIV, hemochromatosis, and amyloidosis. Systemic medications such as anticholinergics (including antihistamines and antidepressants), antiadrenergics, and diuretics can cause decreased tear production. Dry eye has also been associated with menopause (presumably due to decreased androgens). Evaporative dry eye problems are usually associated with meibomian gland dysfunction. The protective lipid and mucin layers that normally keep the aqueous layer of tears stable are reduced, leading to a poor-quality tear film that breaks up easily. This problem is often associated with acne rosacea and treated conservatively with warm compresses and oral tetracycline if needed. Oral flax or fish oil supplements may help.

▶ Clinical Findings

Symptoms of tear deficiency often include foreign body sensation, redness, decreased vision, and even reflex tearing. Symptoms are usually worse at the end of the day or after prolonged visual tasks.

Symptoms of evaporative tear loss include a chronic "film" over the vision, redness, burning, and itching of the eyelid margin. These symptoms are often worse in the morning. The quick breakup time of the tear film can cause difficulty with reading.

Post–laser in situ keratomileusis (LASIK) patients have decreased corneal sensation, lower tear production, and diminished blink rate, which may cause dry eye symptoms for 6-18 months or more postoperatively.

▶ Treatment

Treatment for aqueous deficiency includes tear supplementation. Over-the-counter lubricant tears (artificial tears) may be used up to four times daily. Preservative-free tear options are available. Punctal occlusion may be used in eyes shown to have decreased tear production.

In meibomian gland disease, eyelid hygiene is extremely important. Hot compresses with eyelid scrubs can improve tear quality and prevent evaporative tear loss. Mild topical corticosteroids or systemic tetracycline may also be used, especially if the patient has associated signs of acne rosacea. Topical cyclosporine A, because of its anti-inflammatory action, has been found to dramatically improve dry eye symptoms, although it may take up to 6 weeks for improvement. More recently, the integrin binding inhibitor lifitegrast (5%) was approved for dry eye treatment in the United States in 2016 and in Canada in 2018.

Sheppard JD, et al; OPUS-1 Study Group: Lifitegrast ophthalmic solution 5.0% for treatment of dry eye disease: results of the OPUS-1 phase 3 study. *Ophthalmology*. 2014;121(2):475-483.

PTERYGIUM

Pterygium is a fleshy, triangular, conjunctival growth that is usually associated with excessive exposure to wind, UV radiation, sand, and dust. Unilateral or bilateral, it is usually on the nasal side of the cornea. There is a likely genetic contribution to the incidence of pterygium; however, the details of inheritance patterns are not presently known.

Treatment is by superficial excision. Excision is indicated if the growth threatens vision by approaching the visual axis. After excising large or recurrent pterygia, autologous conjunctival tissue or amniotic membrane can be used to cover the defect. The conjunctiva is obtained from the upper bulbar conjunctiva and sutured to the denuded area. This leads to rapid restoration of integrity of the epithelial surface and may prevent recurrences. Patients should be advised to wear ultraviolet (UV) protection outdoors. Recurrences can occur in up to 12% of patients.

Zheng K, et al: Comparison of pterygium recurrence rates after limbal conjunctival autograft transplantation and other techniques: meta-analysis. *Cornea*. 2012;31(12):1422-1427.

▼ INTRAOCULAR DISEASES

CATARACT

Cataract is opacity of the lens and is the leading cause of curable blindness in the world. There are three types of cataracts: (1) congenital, (2) those associated with other disorders, and (3) age related. Some cataracts are rapidly progressive, while others may develop more slowly. Surgical removal is indicated when adult patients have difficulty with daily activities or in children if development of amblyopia is a concern. Removal is also indicated for improved visualization of the retina to track diseases such as diabetic retinopathy.

1. Congenital Cataract

Congenital cataract may be genetically determined or may be caused by intrauterine factors that interfere with normal development of the lens. Intrauterine viral infections (most commonly rubella) can cause congenital cataracts. Congenital cataract can be unilateral or bilateral and complete or incomplete. Dense cataract present at birth is an indication for urgent surgical management to ensure proper development of visual function.

Phacoemulsification or simple aspiration with central posterior capsulotomy and limited anterior vitrectomy under general anesthesia is recommended for removal of congenital cataracts. Preservation of the peripheral posterior capsule and zonules is important for future implantation of intraocular lenses. If the cataract is aspirated, leaving the posterior capsule intact, the posterior capsule becomes opaque, requiring capsulotomy at a later stage. Correction with soft contact lenses can be started immediately after surgery. Posterior chamber intraocular lenses can be implanted when the child is older, although children as young as 2 years are being treated with primary intraocular lens implants. Restoration of true binocular vision is seldom achieved after removal of unilateral congenital cataracts.

2. Cataracts Associated with Other Disorders

Many systemic conditions are associated with cataracts, including diabetes mellitus, galactosemia, hypocalcemia, myotonic dystrophy, Down syndrome, and cutaneous disorders such as atopic dermatitis. Certain systemic medications and eye drops containing corticosteroids can also cause cataracts. Other disorders of the eye, such as retinal detachment or chronic uveitis, may also be associated with cataracts. Eyes that have undergone retinal surgical procedures, particularly vitrectomy, have increased risk of cataract development. Physical trauma to the lens as well as injury from thermal and ionizing radiation can cause cataract formation.

3. Age-Related (Senile) Cataract

This is the most common type of cataract. The rate of progression is variable. Diagnosis is by slit-lamp examination. Nuclear changes of the lens produce a brunescent color and often affect distance vision. In advanced cortical cataracts, a white opacity may be seen in the pupillary area upon gross inspection. Monocular diplopia can occur. Posterior subcapsular cataracts are often found in younger patients, causing glare and affecting reading.

▶ Treatment

Once the cataract causes visual impairment, treatment is by surgical removal of the lens. Clinical trials of agents that might delay or prevent the formation of cataracts are under way, but no pharmacologic means of prevention is currently available.

Phacoemulsification of the cataract is the procedure of choice in most developed countries. In developing countries, small incision cataract surgery can produce excellent results. Primary lens implant is preferred unless there is a contraindication to its use. In that situation, optical correction can be achieved with eyeglasses or contact lenses.

A. Extracapsular Extraction

For standard extracapsular cataract extraction, the anterior capsule of the lens is removed, the nucleus of the cataract is expressed, and the residual cortical material is aspirated from the eye through a 9- to 11-mm incision. Smaller incision techniques that involve manual fracturing of the lens nucleus prior to expression are available and have been adopted widely. The posterior capsule is left intact, and an intraocular lens is placed in the capsular bag. The incision is then sutured with 10-0 nylon. In 25%-35% of patients undergoing extracapsular cataract extraction, the posterior capsule will become opacified. This is treated by Nd:YAG laser capsulotomy. If such a laser is not available, surgical incision of the opaque posterior capsule is required.

B. Phacoemulsification

See Figure 39–1. Phacoemulsification is the most common form of extracapsular cataract extraction and involves technology that fragments the nucleus of the lens using a high-frequency ultrasonic probe while simultaneously aspirating these fragments from the eye. The advantage of phacoemulsification is that incision size is reduced, less astigmatism is induced, and the patient can be more quickly rehabilitated. Remaining cortical material is removed by irrigation and aspiration, and an intraocular lens is implanted. Intraocular lenses are folded, which facilitates inserting through a small wound. Local anesthesia (either by injection or topically) is used for most adult patients.

C. Laser Assisted

Femtosecond lasers have been used to perform multiple steps of cataract surgery including wound creation, opening the anterior lens capsule (capsulotomy), and fragmenting the cataractous lens. At the present time, there is no evidence that this technique (which is much more expensive) improves visual outcomes.

Friedman NJ, et al: Femtosecond laser capsulotomy. *J Cataract Refract Surg.* 2011;37(7):1189-1198.

Nagy Z, et al: Initial clinical evaluation of an intraocular femtosecond laser in cataract surgery. *J Refract Surg.* 2009;25(12):1053-1060.

Venkatesh R, et al: Phacoemulsification versus manual smallincision cataract surgery for white cataract. *J Cataract Refract Surg.* 2010;36(11):1849-1854.

A

B

▲ **Figure 39–1.** Phacoemulsification. **A:** Phacoemulsification probe removing lens nucleus through a clear corneal incision. **B:** Implantation of an injectable intraocular lens implant into the capsular bag through a small incision. (Reproduced with permission from Alcon Laboratories, Inc.)

ANGLE-CLOSURE GLAUCOMA

About 1% of people over age 35 have anatomically narrow anterior chamber angles. In such patients, if the pupil dilates spontaneously or is dilated with a mydriatic or cycloplegic agent, there is a small risk that the angle may close and an attack of acute glaucoma precipitated. For this reason, it is a wise to estimate the depth of the anterior chamber angle by slit lamp or penlight before instilling these medications. Acute angle-closure glaucoma is manifested by sudden onset of increased intraocular pressure, which causes pain, headache, blurring of vision, and colored halos around lights. Some patients develop nausea and vomiting. The eye is red, the cornea is hazy, and the pupil is mid-dilated and does not react to light.

The attack can be aborted by use of topical pilocarpine, β-blockers, apraclonidine and latanoprost drops, systemic acetazolamide, and, if necessary, an intravenous hyperosmotic agent such as mannitol. Definitive treatment consists of peripheral iridotomy, which establishes a communication between the posterior and anterior chambers and reopens the angle. This is usually done with an argon or Nd:YAG laser or surgically and should be performed bilaterally. There is now evidence that patients who have had an acute attack of primary angle closure glaucoma should have cataract surgery to improve long-term outcomes.

Azuara-Blanco A, et al: Effectiveness of early lens extraction for the treatment of primary angle-closure glaucoma (EAGLE): a randomised controlled trial. *Lancet.* 2016;388:1389-1397.

OPEN-ANGLE GLAUCOMA

In open-angle glaucoma, the intraocular pressure is elevated, but there are no symptoms. The elevated pressure causes gradual cupping (segmental atrophy) of the optic nerve. The damage to the nerve results in loss of vision ranging in severity from slight constriction of the upper nasal peripheral visual field to complete blindness (absolute glaucoma). The cause of the decreased rate of aqueous outflow that characterizes open-angle glaucoma has not been fully determined. The disease is bilateral but can be asymmetric and is probably genetically influenced. African Americans are at higher risk.

► Clinical Findings

Open-angle glaucoma is painless, so patients are often unaware of damage until late in the course of the disease. On examination, there may be cupping of the optic disc. There is loss of peripheral visual field, but central vision acuity is usually preserved even when peripheral field loss is quite advanced. Tonometry, evaluation of the optic nerve, and visual field testing are the three principal tests used for the diagnosis and continued clinical evaluation of glaucoma. Central corneal thickness should be assessed and included in risk calculations for glaucoma.

The normal intraocular pressure ranges from 10 to 20 mm Hg. Intraocular pressure higher than 21 mm Hg is considered ocular hypertension, although this diagnosis should never be made on the basis of a single tonometric measurement. Fifty percent of glaucoma patients consistently have intraocular pressures less than 21 mm Hg. Transient elevations of intraocular pressure do not constitute glaucoma for the same reason that periodic or intermittent elevations of blood pressure do not constitute hypertensive disease. All persons over age 20 should have tonometric and ophthalmoscopic examinations every 3-5 years. If there is a family history of glaucoma or other risk factors, annual examination is indicated.

► Treatment

See Table 39–3. Most patients can be controlled with topical medications including β-blockers (eg, timolol maleate 0.25%-0.5%, one drop twice daily), α-adrenergic agonists (eg, brimonidine 0.2%, one drop twice daily), carbonic anhydrase inhibitors (eg, dorzolamide 2%, one drop twice daily), or prostaglandins (eg, latanoprost 0.005%, one drop once daily). The recent additions of topical rho-kinase inhibitors and

Table 39–3. Types of glaucoma medications and side effects.

Class	Mechanism	Side Effects	Pregnancy Class
β-Blockers (eg, timolol)	Decrease aqueous production	Hypotension, bradycardia, asthma exacerbation	C
α₂-Adrenergic agonists (eg, brimonidine, Propine)	Decrease aqueous production	Allergy, tachyphylaxis, central nervous system depression	B
Cholinergics (eg, pilocarpine)	Increase outflow	Brow ache, cataract formation, retinal detachment	C
Carbonic anhydrase inhibitors (eg, acetazolamide, dorzolamide)	Decrease aqueous production	Sulfa allergy, systemic metabolic acidosis, tingling, aplastic anemia, metallic taste	C
Prostaglandin analogues (eg, latanoprost)	Increase outflow	Bitter taste, iris color change, red eye	C
Rho-kinase inhibitors (eg, netarsudil)	Increase outflow	Eye redness, subconjunctival hemorrhage, pain	C

nitric oxide–releasing drugs have increased options for topical intraocular pressure reduction. Oral carbonic anhydrase inhibitors (eg, acetazolamide) can be used in patients with persistent elevation of intraocular pressures despite topical treatment. Miotics (eg, pilocarpine 1%-4%, one drop four times daily) and epinephrine eye drops (0.5%-2.0%, one drop twice daily) are less commonly used today.

During laser trabeculoplasty, laser energy is applied to the trabecular meshwork. This technique can lead to significant and sustained decreases in intraocular pressure. Argon laser trabeculoplasty (ALT) and selective laser trabeculoplasty (SLT) may be used in place or along with topical medications. SLT produces similar pressure responses to ALT, but studies suggest it can be repeated multiple times in each eye. In patients with persistent pressure elevation despite maximal medical therapy, surgery is indicated to create an alternate drainage passage for fluid to exit the eye. The most common procedure is trabeculectomy. The success of this procedure has been improved by the use of intraoperative application of mitomycin or fluorouracil to inhibit fibrosis and closure of the newly created filtering channel. Drainage devices are also used to facilitate fluid drainage from the eye to lower intraocular pressure. Recent years have seen an expansion of the options for glaucoma drainage devices, which aim to produce a safer, quicker, and more reproducible result than trabeculectomy. In certain types of glaucoma (eg, neovascular, uveitic, or aphakic glaucoma, or those who have failed previous surgery), insertion of a more complex drainage device is needed, often referred to as a glaucoma valve or tube shunt.

In patients with mild to moderate glaucoma, microinvasive glaucoma surgery, particularly in conjunction with cataract surgery, has become more accepted. An alternative approach that aims to decrease aqueous production through destruction of ciliary body tissue (diode transscleral cyclophotocoagulation or endophotocoagulation) is also employed in some situations.

Gedde SJ, et al: Treatment outcomes in the tube versus trabeculectomy (TVT) study after five years of follow-up. Am J Ophthalmol. 2012;153:789-803 e782.

Pillunat LE, et al: Micro-invasive glaucoma surgery (MIGS): a review of surgical procedures using stents. Clin Ophthalmol. 2017;11:1583-1600.

DIABETIC RETINOPATHY

Diabetes is the leading cause of new blindness in most industrialized countries. Diabetic retinopathy eventually develops in almost half of all diabetics. There are two clinical classifications: (1) **nonproliferative or background diabetic retinopathy** and (2) **proliferative diabetic retinopathy**. The prevalence of retinopathy increases with the duration of diabetes. Patients who have had type 1 diabetes for 5 years or less are at low risk of retinopathy. However, 27% of those with diabetes for 5-10 years and 71%-90% of those with diabetes for longer than 10 years have some form of diabetic

retinopathy. After 20-30 years, the prevalence of retinopathy rises to 95%, with 30%-50% of those patients having proliferative changes. The risk for diabetic retinopathy also increases with duration for type 2 diabetes.

Diabetes can have other effects on the eye. Poor corneal healing and decreased corneal sensation have been noted. Neovascular glaucoma caused by iris neovascularization (which blocks the outflow passage in the anterior chamber angle) is seen in some patients with proliferative disease. Optic neuropathy and cranial neuropathies can also occur.

Clinical Findings

Microaneurysms, intraretinal hemorrhages, cotton wool spots, and lipid deposits due to vascular leakage are the retinal changes seen in early diabetic retinopathy. Later stages include retinal ischemia and neovascularization with subsequent vitreous hemorrhage often associated with retinal detachment. Diabetic retinopathy may be asymptomatic until vision decreases, usually from macular edema or vitreous hemorrhage. The presence of renal microvascular disease correlates well with the presence of diabetic retinopathy.

Treatment

Careful control of blood sugar and blood pressure appears to reduce the incidence and severity of diabetic retinopathy. Recent epidemiologic studies show that many diabetics fail to obtain eye examinations at the recommended intervals. If patients are followed closely and early retinopathy is detected and treated according to the guidelines of the Early Treatment Diabetic Retinopathy Study (ETDRS), the risk of severe visual loss is less than 5%. To meet the screening demands, there is considerable interest in telemedicine in detection of diabetic retinopathy. An artificial intelligence device for detecting diabetic retinopathy was approved by the US Food and Drug Administration in 2017. Treatment consists of photocoagulation, either of the macula to reduce edema or of the retinal periphery to reduce ischemic neovascular changes. Intravitreal injections of agents that neutralize vascular endothelial growth factor (VEGF) now play a central role in treatment of diabetic macular edema. These anti-VEGF agents are be useful for the treatment of proliferative disease. Rare complications from these injections include endophthalmitis and steroid-induced glaucoma.

DeTore J, Rizzolo D: Telemedicine and diabetic retinopathy. JAAPA. 2018;31(9):1-5.

Sivaprasad S, et al: Clinical efficacy of intravitreal aflibercept versus panretinal photocoagulation for best corrected visual acuity in patients with proliferative diabetic retinopathy at 52 weeks (CLARITY): a multicentre, single-blinded, randomised, controlled, phase 2b, non-inferiority trial. Lancet. 2017;389:2193-2203.

van der Heijden AA, et al: Validation of automated screening for referable diabetic retinopathy with the IDx-DR device in the Hoorn Diabetes Care System. Acta Ophthalmol. 2018;96:63-68.

AGE-RELATED MACULAR DEGENERATION

Age-related macular degeneration (AMD) is the leading cause of central visual loss among individuals 65 and older. The pathophysiology is not completely understood, although there is a strong genetic component that interacts with aging and environmental influences such as tobacco use. Regardless of the mechanism, the disease appears to affect the retinal pigment epithelium at the level of Bruch membrane. Drusen (yellowish deposits under the retina caused by the thickening, hyalinization, and calcification of the retinal pigment epithelium) are characteristic of AMD.

1. Atrophic ("Dry") Macular Degeneration

Atrophic ("dry") macular degeneration is the most common form of AMD, occurring in approximately 80% of those with the disease. Drusen, pigment changes, and atrophy are present, but there is no leakage of fluid into the subretinal space. Usually only minimal to moderate visual loss is present, although patients may complain of distorted vision (metamorphopsia).

2. Exudative ("Wet") Macular Degeneration

Exudative ("wet") macular degeneration is characterized by the development of a choroidal neovascular membrane that leaks fluid and blood. This causes a serous detachment of the central fovea that can lead to profound and irreversible vision loss.

▶ Clinical Findings

Visual loss is caused by geographical atrophy, serous detachment of the retinal pigment epithelium, or choroidal neovascularization. Central visual acuity is primarily affected with the peripheral vision remaining intact. Metamorphopsia is a classic patient complaint. Patients can follow their own progression of disease with an Amsler grid.

▶ Treatment

The Age-Related Eye Disease Study (AREDS) is the first large, prospective clinical trial to show the benefit of antioxidant and zinc supplementation on the progression of atrophic AMD and associated visual loss. In evaluating the rate of progression to advanced visual loss, nutritional supplements benefited only patients who had moderate to severe disease. Supplements were not found to prevent the development of AMD or to prevent progression in patients with mild disease. The AREDS2 study started in 2008 and has examined the use of additional alternate micronutrients including omega-3 fatty acids, lutein, and zeaxanthin in preventing the progression of AMD. This study found that lutein and zeaxanthin were safe and effective alternatives to beta-carotene, which was associated with increased risk of lung cancer in smokers. Treatment of exudative AMD was revolutionized through the use of intravitreal injections of anti-VEGF agents. Previously established therapeutic strategies such as standard laser photocoagulation or photodynamic therapy reduced the rate of vision loss when compared to controls but did not improve acuity. These treatments remain beneficial in certain specific situations. Intravitreal injection of anti-VEGF agents such as ranibizumab (Lucentis) and bevacizumab (Avastin) has led to improvements in visual acuity. Intravitreal injection carries a small risk of infection, and treatment resistance can be seen.

Smoking cessation is extremely important in AMD patients and should be stressed. Exercise and control of other systemic diseases such as hypertension and hypercholesterolemia may also help.

Age-Related Eye Disease Study 2 Research Group: Lutein + zeaxanthin and omega-3 fatty acids for age-related macular degeneration: the Age-Related Eye Disease Study 2 (AREDS2) randomized clinical trial. *JAMA*. 2013;309:2005-2015.

Comparison of Age-related Macular Degeneration Treatments Trials (CATT) Research Group: Ranibizumab and bevacizumab for treatment of neovascular age-related macular degeneration: two-year results. *Ophthalmology*. 2012;119(7):1388-1398.

Dhoot DS, et al: Ranibizumab for age-related macular degeneration. *Expert Opin Biol Ther*. 2012;12(3):371-381.

SanGiovanni JP, et al: The relationship of dietary lipid intake and age-related macular degeneration in a case-control study: AREDS Report No. 20. *Arch Ophthalmol*. 2007;125(5):671-679.

Sparrow JR, et al: Complement dysregulation in AMD: RPE-Bruch's membrane-choroid. *Mol Aspects Med*. 2012;33(4):436-445.

RETINAL DETACHMENT

Detachment of the retina is usually spontaneous but may be secondary to trauma. Spontaneous detachment occurs most frequently in persons over 50 years of age. Spontaneous detachments are ultimately bilateral in 20%-25% of cases.

▶ Clinical Findings

Retinal tears or holes are the most important predisposing factor. Increased risk of retinal detachment is also associated with cataract surgery and high myopia. In the presence of a retinal tear or hole, fluid from the vitreous cavity enters the defect, and transudation from choroidal vessels detaches the retina from the pigment epithelium (rhegmatogenous). Small retinal holes may be sealed prophylactically with laser or cryotherapy to prevent detachment.

The superior temporal retina is the most common site of detachment. The size of detachment can rapidly increase, causing progressive visual loss. Central vision remains intact until the macula becomes detached. On ophthalmoscopic examination, the detached retina is seen as an elevated gray membrane.

▶ Treatment

All cases of retinal detachment should be referred immediately to an ophthalmologist. If the patient must be transported a long distance, the head should be positioned to minimize the progression of the detachment. If the upper retina is detached, the head should be kept flat. Patients with an inferior detachment should be kept upright.

Retinal detachment is a true ophthalmic emergency if the macula is threatened. If the macula is detached, permanent loss of central vision may occur even if the retina is successfully reattached by surgery. Treatment consists of drainage of subretinal fluid and closure of retinal tears by cryosurgery, laser, or scleral buckling. This produces an inflammatory reaction that causes the retina to adhere to the choroid. The creation of an inflammatory adhesion between the choroid and the retina helps to prevent future detachment.

In uncomplicated retinal detachment with a superior retinal tear and healthy vitreous, pneumoretinopexy may be performed. The procedure consists of injection of air or certain gases into the vitreous cavity through the pars plana and positioning the patient to allow the gas bubble to seal the retinal hole and permit spontaneous reabsorption of the subretinal fluid.

About 85% of uncomplicated cases can be reattached with one operation. About 10% will need more than one procedure, and the remainder never reattach. The prognosis is worse if the macula is detached or if the detachment is of long duration.

STRABISMUS IN CHILDREN

Any child under age 7 with obvious strabismus should be seen without delay to allow prompt treatment to prevent amblyopia. About 3% of children are born with or develop strabismus. In descending order of frequency, the eyes may deviate inward (esotropia), outward (exotropia), upward (hypertropia), or downward (hypotropia).

▶ Clinical Findings

Children with manifest strabismus suppress the visual image from the deviating eye to avoid diplopia. This causes decreased visual acuity in that eye (amblyopia). Most cases of strabismus are obvious, but if the angle of deviation is small or if the strabismus is intermittent, the diagnosis can be missed.

Fortunately, amblyopia due to strabismus can be detected by routine visual acuity testing of all preschool children. Those who cannot be tested with a standard eye chart can be tested with an illiterate E card or Allen picture chart.

▶ Treatment

The objectives in the surgical treatment of strabismus in children (Figure 39–2) are to achieve good visual acuity in each eye and align the eyes so that normal binocular vision with fusion can occur. Surgery can be performed in infants, and the earlier the problem is detected and corrected, the better the chance of getting a good result. Correcting the strabismus in children above age 7-8 often fails to restore visual acuity to normal.

If the child is under age 6 years and has an amblyopic eye and strabismus, patching of the better eye should be

▲ **Figure 39–2. A:** Exposure of an extraocular muscle in surgery for strabismus. **B:** Recession of the muscle behind its original insertion followed by suturing to the sclera with absorbable suture.

instituted to improve the vision before surgery. At age 1, patching may be successful within 1 week; at age 6, it may take a year to achieve the same result. Surgery to align the eye is usually delayed until maximal visual improvement has been obtained in the amblyopic eye.

Surgery for correction of strabismus consists of weakening or strengthening the extraocular muscles. To weaken the action of a muscle, it is recessed by detaching it from its insertion site and resuturing it to a more posterior location of the sclera. To strengthen a muscle's action, it is separated at the insertion site from the globe a portion resected. It is then resutured to its original insertion site. Muscles should not be recessed more than 8 mm or resected more than 6 mm.

For correction of exotropia, the lateral rectus muscles in both eyes can be recessed. Alternatively, the lateral rectus muscle can be recessed and the medial rectus muscle resected in the same eye. The amount of recession and resection and the number of extraocular muscles chosen are determined by the degree of ocular deviation. The decision to involve one or both eyes is influenced by the visual acuity and potential of each eye. In patients with esotropia, the options are to recess the medial recti of both eyes or to recess the medial rectus in combination with resecting the lateral rectus in the same eye.

For vertical deviation, the vertical muscles are recessed, resected, tucked, or weakened by myectomy.

STRABISMUS IN ADULTS

In adults with mature visual systems, development of strabismus usually produces double vision. Strabismus can arise from head trauma, microvascular infarct as in diabetes, intracranial hemorrhage, elevated intracranial pressure, brain tumor, or orbital disease.

Treatment

Surgical management of strabismus is the same as described for children. Since visual pathways have already been formed, the indications for surgery are for cosmetic reasons or because of diplopia. Care must be taken not to induce diplopia after surgery.

OCULAR MIGRAINE

Migraine is a disorder with multiple clinical presentations. Recurrent headaches are classic, and ocular symptoms are often associated. The pathophysiology of migraine is uncertain, and there may be a genetic component. The differential diagnosis for migraine headaches includes stress-tension headache, cluster headache, sinus congestion/pathology, elevated intracranial pressures, orbital inflammation, orbital neoplasia, and temporal arteritis. A thorough headache history and neurologic examination are important diagnostic tools.

Patients with ocular migraine present with visual symptoms; headache and nausea, if present at all, follow. The ocular symptoms can mimic retinal disease, and a dilated ocular examination is needed to rule out retinal pathology when the symptoms are atypical. The flashing lights from retinal disease are primarily unilateral, while migraine presents with bilateral visual distortion. Asking the patient to cover each eye and see if the symptoms are unilateral or bilateral may clarify the situation. Prophylaxis to prevent migraine with oral β-adrenergic blockers, calcium channel blockers, and tricyclic antidepressants may be used. Triptans such as sumatriptan (Imitrex) are often used to treat the acute episodes. Onabotulinum toxin A (Botox) injections are an effective treatment option for debilitating migraine not controlled by other medications. True acephalgic migraine (migraine with visual symptoms only) typically is not treated with systemic agents because of the self-limited nature of the disease.

Classical Migraines

Classical migraine is characterized by throbbing headaches preceded by visual auras lasting about 20 minutes. The aura may consist of bright or dark spots, zigzag lines (fortification scotoma), heat haze distortions, scintillating scotomas, and tunnel vision. Homonymous or altitudinal hemianopia may rarely occur. The headaches that follow may vary in intensity.

Retinal Migraine

Retinal migraine is characterized by acute, transient unilateral loss of vision that can be identical to that seen in amaurosis fugax. Vascular etiologies must be ruled out with thorough ocular and medical examination before attributing symptoms to a migraine. Amaurosis is often shorter in duration and has a more "curtainlike" quality.

Ophthalmoplegic Migraine

Ophthalmoplegic migraine is very rare and typically starts before the age of 10 years. It is characterized by a recurrent transient third nerve palsy that is associated with a typical migraine headache.

Complicated Migraine

Complicated migraine is associated with neurologic deficits such as tingling in the extremities, hemisensory disturbance, and partial visual loss. Rarely, the deficit persists after the headache has resolved. Antiplatelet therapy with aspirin is often recommended.

Diener HC, et al: OnabotulinumtoxinA for treatment of chronic migraine: results from the double-blind, randomized, placebo-controlled phase of the PREEMPT 2 trial. *Cephalalgia*. 2010; 30(7):804-814.

OCULAR BURNS

CHEMICAL BURNS

Apart from the history, the diagnosis of chemical eye burns is usually based on the presence of swelling of the eyelids and marked conjunctival hyperemia and chemosis. The limbal area may show blanched patchy areas and conjunctival sloughing, especially in the interpalpebral area. There is usually corneal stromal haze and diffuse edema, with wide areas of epithelial cell loss and corneal ulcerations. Defects in the corneal epithelium can be better visualized with the instillation of fluorescein dye.

Alkali burns of the eye are particularly serious because the agents tend to rapidly penetrate intraocularly. Retained particles in the conjunctival fornices may continue to release alkaline material and must be promptly removed. Patients are managed by instilling a topical anesthetic agent and then immediately irrigating copiously (at least several liters) with tap water or any other available solution until a neutral pH is reached. This may require hours of flushing. Double eversion of the upper eyelid should be performed to look for and remove material lodged in the superior fornix. This can be done by using a forceps or moist cotton applicator. Topical dilating drops such as atropine 1% or homatropine 5% are instilled, and a topical antibiotic ointment such as ophthalmic erythromycin and bacitracin should be applied. Severe injuries that result in eyelid destruction require hospitalization and specialized care.

Acid burns cause rapid damage but are in general less serious than alkali burns because of lack of intraocular penetration. Irrigation is carried out as described earlier, the patient is given an analgesic, and the eye is patched for a short time. Close follow-up is needed. Topical antibiotic ointment may also be used.

THERMAL BURNS

The treatment of thermal burns of the eyes is similar to the treatment of burns elsewhere on the body. Adequate systemic analgesia should be provided. A topical anesthetic agent such as proparacaine 0.5% or tetracaine 0.5% is used to minimize pain during manipulation. In cases of burns involving the cornea, topical dilating drops such as atropine 1% or homatropine 5% are instilled. Antibiotic drops are often prescribed for 3-5 days.

BURNS DUE TO ULTRAVIOLET RADIATION

Injuries to the corneal epithelium by UV rays vary in severity. They are described as actinic keratitis, snow blindness, welder's arc burn, or flash burn, depending on the source of UV radiation. Patients present with severe pain, tearing, and photophobia. The examination reveals diffuse punctate staining of the cornea, best seen with fluorescein staining, proper magnification, and a cobalt blue light.

A topical antibiotic such as ophthalmic erythromycin or bacitracin ointment is instilled. Topical nonsteroidal drops such as diclofenac or ketorolac tromethamine can be used for pain.

▼ OCULAR TRAUMA

Eye injuries are common despite the protection afforded by the bony orbit. Blunt trauma is the most common injury, but penetrating injuries of the globe, although less frequent, are often more serious. The use of protective eyewear at work helps prevent most serious occupational injuries.

▶ Clinical Evaluation

A careful history should be obtained from the patient or someone who knows what happened. Visual acuity should be checked. The eyelids, conjunctiva, cornea, anterior chamber, iris, lens, vitreous, and fundus should be evaluated. Corneal damage (eg, abrasions) can be detected by instilling fluorescein dye and using a cobalt blue light to examine the anterior surface. CT scan or x-ray examination is helpful in looking for fractures of the orbital bones or foreign bodies. Patients with severe injuries should have immediate ophthalmic consultation.

PENETRATING OR PERFORATING INJURIES

Penetrating or perforating ocular injuries require immediate treatment and prompt surgical repair to maximize chances for preservation of vision.

Facial injuries—especially those occurring in automobile accidents—can be associated with penetrating ocular trauma. Some injuries may be undetected because of eyelid swelling or because the patient's other injuries have demanded the attention of the emergency room staff. Accurate records and a description of how the injury occurred should be obtained. The eye and ocular adnexa should be examined, including vision testing and testing of ocular motility. *Do not apply pressure on the globe.* X-ray examination and CT scan are performed to rule out fractures of orbital bones or the presence of intraocular foreign bodies. An eye with a penetrating injury should be protected from further injury with a Fox or similar shield and light dressing. Parenteral broad-spectrum antibiotics such as cefazolin or gentamicin should be given. Antiemetics (eg, ondansetron, 4 mg intravenously) should be given to the patient when needed to prevent vomiting, which can lead to extrusion of the intraocular contents.

Careful repair and approximation of corneal and scleral lacerations should be performed in the operating room. Magnetic intraocular foreign bodies can be extracted with a magnet in the operating room. The major objectives in management of ocular penetrating or perforating injuries are to relieve pain, preserve or restore vision, and achieve good cosmetic results. Pain relief may be achieved by the administration of intravenous or subcutaneous morphine or meperidine. Sedatives such as diazepam 5 mg may be given orally as needed.

LACERATIONS OF THE OCULAR ADNEXA

Lacerations of the eyelids and the periorbital skin should be carefully evaluated. Small linear skin lacerations can be easily repaired with 6-0 nylon sutures. The sutures can usually be removed in 3-5 days. In cases of deep eyelid lacerations, intraocular or orbital damage should be ruled out before the repair is performed. The skin of the eyelids has good elasticity and, in adults, is frequently present in surplus quantities. This facilitates the development of flaps and grafts. In deep lacerations of the eyelids, if the wound divides the orbicularis muscle parallel to its fibers, only skin sutures are generally required. When the muscle fibers are transversely divided, they should be approximated with 6-0 absorbable synthetic sutures. The skin can be approximated with nylon sutures. In patients with lacerations resulting in round or oval losses of skin, the skin is undermined and the laceration approximated. For larger defects, reconstruction with flaps may be required. Flaps used in reconstruction of the eyelids are advancement flaps, rotational flaps, transposition flaps, island flaps, and Z-plasty flaps.

When flaps cannot be used, free skin grafts may be obtained from behind the ear or from the skin of the inner upper arm. Special care should be taken with repair of lacerations of the lower lid to be certain that the lid is not closed under tension to prevent eversion and distortion of the lid margin.

Table 39–4. Types of ocular injury associated with blunt trauma.

Eyelids	Ecchymosis, swelling, laceration, abrasions, conjunctival or subconjunctival hemorrhages
Cornea	Edema, lacerations
Anterior chamber	Hyphema, recession of angle, secondary glaucoma
Iris	Iridodialysis, iridoplegia, rupture of iris sphincter
Ciliary body	Hyposecretion of aqueous humor
Lens	Cataract, dislocation
Vitreous	Vitreous hemorrhage
Ciliary muscle	Paralysis
Retina	Commotio retinae, retinal edema, choroidal breaks in Bruch membrane, choroidal hemorrhage

BLUNT TRAUMA TO THE OCULAR ADNEXA & ORBIT

See Table 39–4. Contusions of the eyeball and ocular adnexa may result from blunt trauma. The extent of damage to the vision may not be obvious upon initial examination. A careful dilated eye examination is needed for all patients with this type of injury.

BLOWOUT FRACTURE OF THE FLOOR OF THE ORBIT

Blowout fracture of the floor of the orbit can be associated with enophthalmos, double vision in primary position or upgaze, restriction of ocular movement, hypotropia, and decreased or absent sensation over the maxillary area in the distribution of the infraorbital nerve. CT scan of the orbit will document the extent of the orbital injury that can involve the medial wall as well as the floor. There may be air noted in the sinuses. Evaluation and management of patients with blowout fractures may involve both an ophthalmologist and an otolaryngologist because of potential associated fractures of the maxilla or zygoma. Patients are usually treated with a systemic antibiotic (cephalothin or amoxicillin/potassium clavulanate), told not to blow their nose, and reassessed within 1 week by an ophthalmologist. Many blowout fractures do not require surgical correction. Operative management is recommended if there is significant enophthalmos, continued diplopia in primary gaze, or significant instability of the orbital floor.

CORNEAL & CONJUNCTIVAL FOREIGN BODIES

Patients often give a history of working with high-speed tempered steel tools, drilling, or hammering against a hard object. There may be no history of trauma to the eye, and the patient may have a foreign body. Typically, the patient complains of a foreign body sensation in the eye or under the eyelid with associated pain, tearing, and photophobia.

A corneal foreign body can be seen with the aid of a loupe and diffuse light. Conjunctival foreign bodies often become embedded in the inner surface of the upper lid, which must be everted to facilitate inspection and removal. A topical anesthetic such as proparacaine 0.5% or tetracaine 0.5% is applied. Sterile fluorescein should be instilled to assist in the visualization of small foreign bodies. Some loose foreign bodies can be removed with a moist cotton applicator; others require use of a needle. Topical antibiotic ointment should be instilled (eg, erythromycin or bacitracin) and the eye patched for a few hours if necessary. Patients with continued foreign body sensation, pain, or decreased vision need to be referred to an ophthalmologist to rule out a retained foreign body or corneal ulceration.

Use of topical anesthetic drops for pain control by the patient will slow healing and increase risk of corneal ulceration. Topical anesthetics should be used only for examination purposes, and *never* for treatment. **Note:** If there is any suspicion of penetrating trauma or history consistent with that type of injury, appropriate ultrasound and radiologic tests should be performed.

▼ OCULAR TUMORS

Tumors of the adnexal structures can often be recognized early because they are usually visible and cause local disfigurement, interference with vision, or displacement of the globe. Intraocular tumors are more difficult to diagnose, but in children, ocular tumors such as retinoblastoma that affect visual function may present with strabismus or leukocoria. Tumors of the eye may be primary (affecting only the ocular or adnexal tissues) or secondary to metastatic tumors. In the eye, the highly vascular choroid is the most frequent site of metastasis. The tumors that most frequently metastasize to the eye are carcinoma of the breast and lung.

The history of growth of the lesion is extremely important, as well as recent changes in its size or appearance. Excisional biopsy of lesions of the skin or conjunctiva is indicated if cancer is suspected.

LID TUMORS

▶ Benign Tumors of the Eyelids

The most frequent benign tumors of the eyelids are melanocytic nevi. Excision is indicated primarily for cosmetic reasons (Figure 39–3). Xanthelasma represent lipid deposits in histiocytes in the dermis of the skin of the eyelid. In such patients, a lipid profile is indicated. Treatment is indicated for cosmetic reasons and consists of simple excision. The lesions tend to be larger than the surface size would indicate,

Herlihy EP, et al: Visual acuity and astigmatism in periocular infantile hemangiomas treated with oral beta-blocker versus intralesional corticosteroid injection. *J AAPOS*. 2016;20:30-33.

Missoi TG, et al: Oral propranolol for treatment of periocular infantile hemangiomas. *Arch Ophthalmol*. 2011;129(7):899-903.

Malignant Tumors of the Eyelids

Squamous cell carcinoma tends to grow slowly and painlessly. It begins as a small lesion covered by a layer of keratin. The lesion may erode, causing an ulcer with hyperemic edges. It can enlarge to form a fungating mass and invade the orbit. Early excision is usually curative. If early treatment is not provided, squamous cell carcinoma can spread through the preauricular and submandibular lymph nodes.

Basal cell carcinoma begins as a slowly growing, locally invasive tumor forming the so-called "rodent ulcer" with raised nodular borders. It is the most common malignant eyelid tumor. Inner canthal basal cell carcinoma invades locally and can extend into the orbit. Treatment should include complete excision to prevent recurrence. Mohs surgery is usually performed to assure clean margins prior to eyelid reconstruction. Often, the lesions are more extensive than they appear visually. Systemic metastasis is rare.

Malignant melanomas of the eyelids behave similar to malignant melanomas of the skin.

CONJUNCTIVAL TUMORS

Benign tumors of the conjunctiva include melanocytic nevi (pigmented or nonpigmented), papillomas, granulomas, dermoids, and lymphoid hyperplasia. Malignant tumors of the conjunctiva include carcinoma, malignant melanoma, and lymphoma. Carcinoma of the conjunctiva arises frequently at the limbus or the inner canthus in the exposed area of the bulbar conjunctiva. Early in the course of the disease, the lesion can resemble a pterygium. The tumor is slightly elevated, with a gelatinous surface, and may spread over the corneal surface. These grow slowly. Treatment is by wide excisional biopsy and cryotherapy or topical interferon alpha.

Shah SU, et al: Topical interferon alfa-2b for management of ocular surface squamous neoplasia in 23 cases: outcomes based on American Joint Committee on Cancer classification. *Arch Ophthalmol*. 2012;130(2):159-164.

INTRAOCULAR TUMORS

Benign Intraocular Tumors

Melanocytic nevi of the iris, ciliary body, or choroid are common. No treatment is required. Retinal angioma may be seen in patients with phacomatoses (eg, Bourneville disease). Choroidal hemangioma is another less frequently encountered benign intraocular tumor.

▲ **Figure 39–3.** Tumor of the left lower eyelid involving the lid margin. **A:** Two vertical incisions are made. **B:** The defect after removal of the tumor. **C:** Suturing of the tarsus and orbicularis with absorbable sutures. **D:** Approximation of the eyelid margin. Skin is approximated with 6-0 silk sutures.

and recurrences are common. Care must be taken not to foreshorten the eyelid skin and impair eyelid closure.

Hemangiomas of the eyelids consist of two types: capillary and cavernous. Capillary hemangiomas are composed of dilated capillaries and proliferation of endothelial cells. The lesions appear as bright red spots. They may show rapid growth in early childhood but later often undergo involution and subside spontaneously. Treatment of hemangiomas in infancy and early childhood is not indicated unless they cause interference with vision that may lead to amblyopia. Low-dose oral steroids, local injection of steroids, or systemic use of beta-blockers may cause rapid involution. Cavernous hemangiomas are venous channels in the subcutaneous tissue. They appear bluish in color and are distended. Surgical excision may be required. Radiation is not recommended because it leads to excessive scarring of the eyelid.

Other benign tumors of the eyelids include verrucae and molluscum contagiosum. These lesions are caused by viruses.

Malignant Intraocular Tumors

Malignant intraocular tumors include malignant melanoma of the uvea, retinoblastoma, and a rare tumor of the ciliary body known as diktyoma or medulloepithelioma.

Malignant melanoma of the uvea is the most common primary intraocular tumor in adults. It typically occurs in the fifth or sixth decade and is almost always unilateral. The most frequent site is the choroid, but malignant melanoma can occur also in the ciliary body or iris. Malignant melanomas of the choroid often do not cause decrease in vision. Necrosis of the tumor can lead to intraocular inflammation. Histopathologic examination shows spindle-shaped cells with or without prominent nuclei and large epithelioid tumor cells. Intraocular malignant melanomas may spread directly through the sclera by local invasion or directly into the central nervous system via optic nerve extension.

Malignant melanomas can be detected by ophthalmoscopy after pupillary dilation.

Treatment of malignant melanoma consists of enucleation or radiotherapy with radioactive plaques or charged particles. Extension outside the eye may require exenteration of the orbit. Patients with small melanomas—less than 10 mm in diameter—can be followed with serial fundus photos. Similarly, small melanomas of the iris that have not invaded the iris root can be safely followed and observed until growth is documented. If there is growth of the iris tumor, treatment is by local iridectomy. If the iris malignant melanoma invades the root and ciliary body, it can be removed surgically by iridocyclectomy. Uveal melanoma genotype is predictive of outcome and is part of most melanoma evaluations.

Retinoblastoma is a rare but life-threatening condition in childhood. It is the most frequent intraocular malignant tumor in children. It arises from embryonic cone cells of the photoreceptor layer. Most patients with retinoblastoma present in the first or second year of life. Patients present with leukocoria or strabismus. Retinoblastoma may be unilateral or bilateral and is often multifocal. There are both sporadic and inherited forms of the disease. It may grow slowly to fill the intraocular space and undergo necrosis, leading to calcific deposits. Tumor cells may seed on the iris and in the anterior chamber, causing fluffy whitish exudates.

Spontaneous remission of retinoblastoma has been reported. Treatment options include radiotherapy, cryotherapy, chemotherapy, intra-arterial chemotherapy, and enucleation.

Abramson DH, et al: Chemosurgery for retinoblastoma: what we know after 5 years. *Arch Ophthalmol.* 2011;129(11):1492-1494.
Harbour JW: A prognostic test to predict the risk of metastasis in uveal melanoma based on a 15-gene expression profile. *Methods Mol Biol.* 2014;1102:427-440.

ORBITAL TUMORS

Orbital tumors are of two types: primary and secondary. Benign primary orbital tumors include dermoid cysts, hemangiomas, lipomas, fibromas, osteomas, chondromas, neurofibromas, and lacrimal gland tumors. Malignant tumors include rhabdomyosarcoma, adenocarcinoma of the lacrimal gland, and lymphomas. In children, rhabdomyosarcoma often presents with acute, painless unilateral proptosis and needs to be evaluated immediately. Secondary tumors include extension of malignant melanoma and retinoblastoma from the intraocular structures and malignant melanomas and carcinomas from the skin of the eyelids and conjunctiva. Metastatic lesions commonly are from the lung or breast. Neuroblastoma can also metastasize to the orbit in children. Meningiomas of the cranial nerves may invade the orbit through the optic canal.

Treatment and prognosis in all cases depend on the type of tumor.

LASER TREATMENTS FOR OCULAR DISEASE

The laser has many useful applications in ophthalmology. Using various gases, a single-wavelength beam can be produced that can be absorbed by specific tissues in the eye.

FOCAL DIABETIC TREATMENT

Macular edema occurs in the preproliferative stage of diabetic retinopathy and is characterized by retinal thickening (with or without exudates) within the central macular area. This procedure is performed with a slit-lamp laser delivery system using a contact lens and is aided by fluorescein angiography. Improvement may not occur for several months. Long-term studies by the National Institutes of Health have shown that treatment with an argon laser may improve visual outcome by as much as 50%.

PANRETINAL PHOTOCOAGULATION

Panretinal photocoagulation is indicated for treatment of proliferative diabetic retinopathy. Using a contact lens and a slit-lamp delivery system, extensive destruction of peripheral retina is undertaken to decrease production of vasoproliferative factors and increase retinal oxygenation, causing regression of abnormal blood vessels.

LASER SURGERY FOR CORRECTION OF REFRACTIVE ERROR

LASIK is a lamellar refractive surgical procedure that involves creation of a partial-thickness corneal flap under high suction. The flap is then lifted and an argon-fluoride excimer beam is used to ablate stromal tissue with minimal thermal effect. The flap is then replaced and allowed to heal.

The combination of accurate correction of refractive error, minimal postoperative discomfort, and quick visual recovery make this the most popular refractive technique. A newer technology of flap creation with femtosecond laser instead of microkeratome blades is becoming more popular.

MULTIPLE CHOICE QUESTIONS

1. A 61-year-old Caucasian woman presents with sudden-onset right-sided head pain, right eye redness, and blurred vision. Examination of the right eye is difficult due to the patient's nausea and vomiting but reveals visual acuity of 20/400, a mid-dilated, unreactive pupil, a hazy cornea, and an intraocular pressure of 57. What is the best course of action at this time?

   A. Obtain an immediate head computed tomography (CT) to rule out orbital abscess.
   B. Arrange for follow-up with an ophthalmologist within the next 1-2 weeks.
   C. Medically manage the patient's pain and nausea and arrange an urgent ophthalmology consult.
   D. Start the patient on oral acyclovir as this is likely herpes simplex–induced uveitis

2. A 42-year-old man with a history of chronic sinusitis presents with worsening left eyelid swelling over the preceding 3 days and intermittent double vision for the past 8 hours. Examination reveals swollen, red, and warm left eyelids. Visual acuity is 20/20 in both eyes, and pupillary reactions are normal; however, extraocular motility is limited on lateral gaze in the left eye. What is the best course of action at this time?

   A. Start the patient on a course of oral antibiotics.
   B. Arrange for an outpatient CT scan and endocrine follow-up because this is likely thyroid ophthalmopathy.
   C. Obtain a maxillofacial CT scan and start on intravenous (IV) antibiotics.
   D. Start the patient on a course of valacyclovir 1000 mg three times daily.

3. Which statement regarding herpes simplex virus (HSV) is *true*?

   A. Eye infections are most commonly caused by the HSV-2 virus.
   B. If a vesicular lesion is seen on the tip of the nose, this suggests intraocular involvement of HSV.
   C. Early use of antivirals may help reduce the risk of postherpetic neuralgia.
   D. HSV keratitis classically presents with a dendritic corneal lesion.

4. Which of the following conditions is *not* treated with vascular endothelial growth factor (VEGF)–targeting agents?

   A. Diabetic macular edema
   B. Exudative "wet" macular degeneration
   C. Nonexudative "dry" macular degeneration
   D. Neovascular glaucoma

5. A 25-year-old man reports from his job as a janitor after "ammonia" splashed in his right eye. What is the best course of action at this time?

   A. Send out for special ophthalmic solution, perform a complete dilated exam, and call for an ophthalmology consult.
   B. Use artificial tears to rinse out remaining ammonia.
   C. Instill tetracaine 0.5% and irrigate with approximately 2 L of saline (or any other immediately available fluid) immediately.
   D. Instill topical dilating drops and antibiotic ointment.

40

Urology

Mark H. Katz, MD

Gerard M. Doherty, MD

EMBRYOLOGY OF THE GENITOURINARY TRACT

A basic understanding of genitourinary embryology facilitates learning many aspects of urology. Embryologically, the genital and urinary systems are intimately related. Associated anomalies of the two systems are commonly encountered.

▶ The Kidneys

The kidneys pass through three embryonic phases (Figure 40–1): (1) The **pronephros** is a vestigial structure without function in human embryos that, except for its primary duct, disappears completely by the fourth week. (2) The pronephric duct gains connection to the **mesonephric tubules** and becomes the mesonephric duct. While most of the mesonephric tubules degenerate, the mesonephric duct persists bilaterally; from where it bends to open into the cloaca, the ureteral bud grows cranially to interact with the metanephric blastema. (3) This forms the **metanephros,** which is the final phase. The metanephros develops into the kidney. During cephalad migration and rotation, the metanephric tissue progressively enlarges, with rapid internal differentiation into the nephron and the uriniferous tubules. Simultaneously, the cephalad end of the ureteral bud expands and divides within the metanephros to form the renal pelvis, calices, and collecting tubules.

▶ The Bladder & Urethra

Subdivision of the cloaca (the blind end of the hindgut) into a ventral (urogenital sinus) and a dorsal (rectum) segment is completed during the seventh week and initiates early differentiation of the urinary bladder and urethra. The urogenital sinus receives the mesonephric duct and absorbs its caudal end, so that by the end of the seventh week, the ureteral bud and mesonephric duct have independent openings. The ureteral orifice migrates upward and laterally. The mesonephric

duct orifice moves downward and medially, and the structure in between (the trigone) is formed by the absorbed mesodermal tissue, which maintains direct continuity between the two tubes (Figure 40–2).

The fused müllerian ducts also meet the urogenital sinus at Müller's tubercle. The urogenital sinus above Müller's tubercle differentiates to form the bladder and the part of the prostatic urethra proximal to the seminal colliculus in the male or the bladder and the entire urethra in the female (Figure 40–3). Below Müller's tubercle, the urogenital sinus differentiates into the distal part of the prostatic urethra and the membranous urethra in the male or the distal vagina and vaginal vestibule in the female. The rest of the male urethra is formed by fusion of the urethral folds on the ventral surface of the genital tubercle. In the female, the genital folds remain separate and form the labia minora.

The prostate develops at the end of the 11th week as several groups of outgrowths of urethral epithelium both above and below the entrance of the ejaculatory duct (distal vas deferens). The developing glandular element (seminal colliculus) incorporates the differentiating mesenchymal cells surrounding it to form the muscular stroma and capsule of the prostate. The seminal vesicles form as duplicate buds from the distal end of the mesonephric duct (vas deferens).

▶ The Gonads

The potential to differentiate along male or female lines is present in every embryo initially. The development of one set of sex primordia and the gradual involution of the other are determined by the genetic sex of the embryo and differential secretion of numerous hormones. The *SRY* gene—or testis-determining factor—on the Y chromosome drives the gonad to differentiate into a testicle. Gonadal differentiation begins during the seventh week (Figure 40–3). If the gonad develops into a testis, the germinal epithelium progressively grows into radially arranged, cordlike seminiferous tubules. The production of

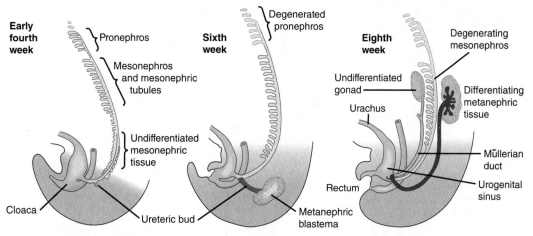

▲ **Figure 40–1.** Schematic of the development of the nephric system. Only a few of the tubules of the pronephros are seen early in the fourth week, while the mesonephric tissue differentiates into mesonephric tubules that progressively join the mesonephric duct. The first sign of the ureteral bud from the mesonephric duct is seen at 4 weeks. At 6 weeks, the pronephros has completely degenerated and the mesonephric tubules start to do so. The ureteral bud grows dorsocranially and has met the metanephric blastema. At the eighth week, there is cranial migration of the differentiating metanephros. The cranial end of the ureteral bud expands and starts to show multiple successive outgrowths (renal calices).

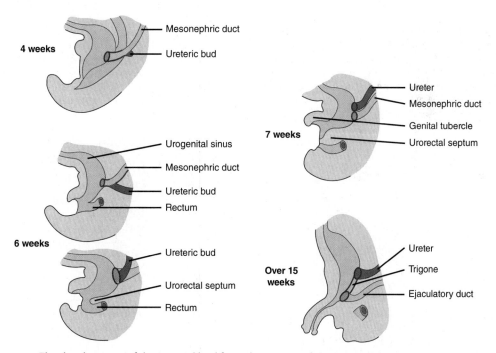

▲ **Figure 40–2.** The development of the ureteral bud from the mesonephric duct and their relationship to the urogenital sinus. The ureteral bud appears at the fourth week. The mesonephric duct distal to this ureteral bud is gradually absorbed into the urogenital sinus, resulting in separate endings for the ureter and the mesonephric duct. The mesonephric tissue that is incorporated into the urogenital sinus expands and forms the trigonal tissue. The mesonephric duct forms the vas deferens in the male and Gartner's duct (if present) in the female.

Undifferentiated (8 weeks)

Mesonephric ducts

Müllerian ducts

Undifferentiated gonads

Primitive testis

Primitive ovary

Fused müllerian duct

Urogenital sinus

Buds to form seminal vesicles

Degenerating mesonephric ducts

Male   (10 weeks)   Female

Müller's tubercle

Sinovaginal node

Vas deferens

Seminal vesicles

Uterine tube

Ejaculatory duct

Ovary

Prostate

Uterus

At birth

Testis

Vagina

Epididymis

Gubernaculum

▲ **Figure 40–3.** Transformation of the undifferentiated genital system into the definitive male and female systems.

müllerian-inhibiting factor (MIF) by the testicle causes regression of the müllerian duct and acts in a local (paracrine) fashion so that only the ipsilateral müllerian duct is affected. The subsequent production of testosterone by the testicle leads to masculinization of the mesonephric (wolffian) duct structures (ie, epididymides, vas deferens, seminal vesicles, and ejaculatory duct). If the gonad develops into an ovary, it becomes differentiated into a cortex and a medulla; the cortex later differentiates into ovarian follicles containing ova. The lack of testosterone leads to the disappearance of the mesonephric duct.

The testes remain in the abdomen until the seventh month and then pass through the inguinal canal to the scrotum, following the path of the gubernaculum. The mechanism of descent remains uncertain. Lack of complete testicular descent is known as cryptorchidism; descent to an abnormal site beyond the external inguinal ring is known as testicular ectopia.

The ovary, which is attached to ligaments, undergoes internal descent to enter the pelvis.

In the female, the genital duct system develops from the müllerian ducts, which fuse at their caudal ends and differentiate into the uterine tubes, the uterus, and the proximal two-thirds of the vagina.

The external genitalia start to differentiate by the eighth week. The genital tubercle and genital swellings develop into the penis and scrotum in the male and the clitoris and labia majora in the female. The external genitalia are masculinized by dihydrotestosterone (DHT), which is created from testosterone under the influence of 5α-reductase.

With the breakdown of the urogenital membrane in the seventh week, the urogenital sinus achieves a separate opening on the undersurface of the genital tubercle. The expansion of the infratubercular part of the urogenital sinus forms the vaginal vestibule and the distal third of the vagina. The two folds on the undersurface of the genital tubercle unite in the male to form the penile urethra; in the female, they remain separate to form the labia minora.

ANATOMY OF THE GENITOURINARY TRACT: GROSS & MICROSCOPIC

The Kidneys

The kidneys lie retroperitoneally in the posterior abdomen and are separated from the surrounding renal fascia (Gerota fascia) by perinephric fat. The renal vascular pedicle enters the renal sinus; the vein is anterior to the artery, and both are anterior to the renal pelvis. The renal artery divides just outside the renal sinus into anterior and posterior branches that undergo further subdivisions with variable extents of distribution. They are end arteries and thus result in segmental infarction when occluded. The venous tributaries anastomose freely and usually drain into one renal vein.

The Renal Parenchyma

The renal parenchyma consists of more than 1 million functioning units (nephrons) and is divided into a peripheral cortex containing secretory elements and a central medulla containing excretory elements. The nephron starts as Bowman's capsule, which surrounds the glomerulus and leads to elongated proximal and distal convoluted tubules with the loop of Henle in between, ending in a collecting duct that opens into a minor calix at the tip of a papilla.

The Renal Pelvis & Calices

The renal pelvis and calices are within the renal sinus and function as the main collecting reservoir. The pelvis, which is partly extrarenal and partly intrarenal (but occasionally is totally extrarenal or intrarenal), branches into three major calices that in turn branch into several minor calices. These calices are directly related to the tips of the medullary pyramids (the papillae) and act as a receiving cup to the collecting tubules. The pelvicaliceal system is a highly muscular structure; the fibers run in many directions and are directly continuous from the calices to the pelvis, allowing synchronization of contractile activity.

The Ureter

The ureter connects the renal pelvis to the urinary bladder. It is a muscularized tube; its muscle fibers lie in an irregular helical arrangement and function primarily in peristaltic activity. Ureteral muscle fibers are directly continuous from the renal pelvis cranially to the vesical trigone distally.

The blood supply to the renal pelvis and ureters is segmental, arising from multiple sources, including the renal, gonadal, and vesical arteries, with rich subadventitial anastomoses.

The Bladder

The bladder is primarily a reservoir with a meshwork of muscle bundles that not only change from one plane to another but also branch and join each other to constitute a synchronized organ. Its musculature is directly continuous with the urethral musculature and thus functions as an internal urethral sphincteric mechanism despite the lack of a true circular sphincter.

The ureters enter the bladder posteroinferiorly through the ureteral hiatus; after a short intravesical submucosal course, they open into the bladder and become continuous with the trigone, which is superimposed on the bladder base though deeply connected to it.

The Urethra

The adult female urethra is about 4 cm long and is muscular in its proximal four-fifths. This musculature is arranged in an inner longitudinal coat that is continuous with the inner longitudinal fibers of the bladder and an outer circular coat that is continuous with the outer longitudinal coat of the bladder. These outer circular fibers compose the sphincteric mechanism. The striated external sphincter surrounds the middle third of the urethra.

In the male, the prostatic urethra is heavily muscular and sphincteric. The membranous urethra is within the urogenital diaphragm and is surrounded by the striated external sphincter. The penile urethra is poorly muscularized and traverses the corpus spongiosum to open at the tip of the glans.

The Prostate

The prostate surrounds the proximal portion of the male urethra; it is a fibromuscular, cone-shaped gland about 2.5 cm long and normally weighing about 20 g in the adult. It is traversed from base to apex by the urethra and is pierced posterolaterally by the ejaculatory ducts from the seminal vesicles and vas deferens that converge to open at the verumontanum (seminal colliculus) on the floor of the urethra.

The prostatic glandular elements drain through about 12 paired excretory ducts that open into the floor of the urethra above the verumontanum. The prostate is surrounded by a thin capsule, derived from its stroma, which is rich in musculature, and part of the urethral musculature and the sphincteric mechanism. A rich venous plexus surrounds the prostate, especially anteriorly and laterally. Its lymphatic drainage is into the hypogastric, sacral, obturator, and external iliac lymph nodes.

The Testis, Epididymis, & Vas

The testis is a paired organ surrounded by the tunica albuginea and subdivided into numerous lobules by fibrous septa. The extremely convoluted seminiferous tubules gather to open into the rete testis, where they join the efferent duct and drain into the epididymis. The epididymis drains into the vas deferens, which courses through the inguinal canal into the pelvis and is joined by the duct from the seminal vesicle to form the ejaculatory duct, which opens before opening into the prostatic urethra on either side of the verumontanum.

Arterial supply is via the spermatic, vas deferential, and external cremasteric arteries. Venous drainage is through the pampiniform plexus, which drains into the internal spermatic veins; the right spermatic vein joins the vena cava, and the left joins the renal vein.

Testicular lymphatics drain into the retroperitoneal lymph nodes; the right primarily into the interaortocaval area, the left into the para-aortic area, both just below the renal vessels.

PHYSIOLOGY OF THE GENITOURINARY TRACT

The Kidneys

The kidneys maintain and regulate homeostasis of body fluids by glomerular filtration, tubular reabsorption, and tubular secretion.

A. Glomerular Filtration

This mechanism is dependent on glomerular capillary arterial pressure minus plasma colloid osmotic pressure plus Bowman's capsular resistance. The resultant glomerular filtration pressure (about 8-12 mm Hg) forces protein-free plasma through the capillary filtering surface into Bowman's capsule. Normally, about 130 mL of plasma is filtered every minute through the renal circulation; the entire volume of plasma recirculates through the kidney and is subjected to the filtration process once every 27 minutes.

B. Tubular Reabsorption

About 99% of the filtered volume is reabsorbed through the tubules, together with all the valuable constituents of the filtrate (chlorides, glucose, sodium, potassium, calcium, and amino acids). Urea, uric acid, phosphates, and sulfates are also reabsorbed to varying degrees. The process of reabsorption is a combination of active and passive transport mechanisms. Reabsorption of water and electrolytes is under the control of adrenal, pituitary, and parathyroid hormones.

C. Tubular Secretion

Tubular secretion helps (1) to eliminate certain substances and thus maintain their plasma levels and (2) to exchange valuable ions from the filtrate for less desirable ions in the plasma (eg, a sodium ion from the urine for a hydrogen ion in the plasma). Failure of adequate secretory function leads to the acidosis commonly encountered in chronic renal disease.

The Ureteropelvicaliceal System

This system is one continuous tubular structure with a syncytial type of smooth musculature that is imperceptibly in motion from one segment to the other. Waves of peristaltic contractions start from the calices and are propagated along the smooth muscle cells to the renal pelvis. At normal urine flow rates, many of these contraction waves are terminated at the ureteropelvic junction; however, some are transmitted to the ureter and down toward the urinary bladder. These peristaltic waves occur at a rate of about 5-8/min, involve a 2- to 3-cm segment at a time, and usually proceed at the velocity of 3 cm/s. Frequency, amplitude, and velocity are influenced by urine output and flow rate. In a state of diuresis, there may be a 1:1 relationship between caliceal contractions and ureteral contractions. Ureteral filling is primarily passive and occurs by reception of a bolus of urine from a renal pelvis contraction. The ureteropelvic junction closes after passing a bolus of urine, preventing back-pressure and back-flow of urine into the renal pelvis secondary to the elevated ureteral contraction pressure. A contraction ring forms in the proximal ureter, and as it migrates down the ureter, it pushes the bolus of urine antegrade. In states of diuresis, the size of the bolus increases and the pressure in the bolus may be greater than the pressure in the contraction ring ahead of it. In this case, the ureteral walls cannot coapt, and urine is transported as an uninterrupted column of fluid.

The Ureterovesical Junction

The ureterovesical junction allows flow of urine from the ureter to the bladder and at the same time prevents retrograde flow. The continuity and the specific muscular arrangement of the intravesical ureter and the trigone provide a muscularly active valvular mechanism that can efficiently adapt itself to the variable phases of bladder activity during filling and voiding.

The normal resting pressure of the ureterovesical junction (10-15 cm H_2O) is greater than the more cephalad ureteral resting pressure (0-5 cm H_2O). Progressive bladder filling leads to firm occlusion of the intravesical ureter against retrograde urine flow and to increased resistance to antegrade flow resulting from trigonal stretching. During voiding, trigonal contraction completely seals the intravesical ureter against any antegrade or retrograde flow of urine.

The Urinary Bladder

The urinary bladder functions primarily as a reservoir that can accommodate variable volumes without increasing its intraluminal pressure. When the bladder reaches full capacity, the detrusor muscle voluntarily contracts following relaxation of the external sphincter and maintains its contraction until the bladder is completely empty. Funneling of the bladder outlet with progressive downward movement of the dome ensures complete emptying.

The vesical sphincteric mechanism is primarily a smooth muscle sphincter in the bladder neck and male prostatic urethra and in the proximal four-fifths of the female urethra. There is no purely circular sphincteric entity, but there are abundant circularly oriented smooth muscle fibers that are directly continuous with the outer coat of the detrusor muscles. The sphincter has an abundance of alpha-receptors that respond to sympathetic neural input from the pelvic nerve to maintain urethral closure. Parasympathetic input from the pelvic nerve facilitates bladder contracture and voiding.

There is a voluntary striated muscle sphincter that is part of the urogenital diaphragm and surrounds the mid urethra in the female and the membranous urethra in the male. It responds to somatic neural input from the pudendal nerve. It is essential for continence when the internal sphincter is nonfunctional. Its pathologic irritability or spasticity can lead to obstructive manifestations.

DEVELOPMENTAL ANOMALIES OF THE GENITOURINARY TRACT

Genitourinary tract anomalies constitute about one-third of all congenital abnormalities and occur in over 10% of the population. The severity varies from lesions incompatible with life to insignificant findings detected during diagnostic studies for unrelated reasons. The anatomic abnormalities are often not intrinsically harmful, yet they may predispose to infection, stone formation, or chronic renal failure.

RENAL ANOMALIES

Bilateral absence of the kidneys is rare and is associated with oligohydramnios, Potter facies, and pulmonary hypoplasia. It occurs more often in males and results in death shortly after birth. Unilateral renal agenesis is seen more often but is not usually associated with illness. **Renal agenesis** is thought to be due to both lack of a ureteral bud and lack of subsequent development of the metanephric blastema. The trigone is absent on the affected side. Because adrenal gland development is unrelated to kidney development, both adrenals are usually present in the normal position. Rarely, more than two kidneys are seen, a condition clearly dissimilar to ureteral duplication, as described later.

Abnormal ascent of the metanephros leads to an **ectopic kidney,** which may be unilateral or bilateral. Lumbar, pelvic, and the less common thoracic and crossed ectopic varieties are seen. Ectopic kidneys are associated with genital anomalies in 10%-20% of cases. Fusion abnormalities are also associated with failure of normal ascent and include fused pelvic kidneys and **horseshoe kidneys** (the most common), which are typically fused at the lower poles. Intravenous urography typically establishes the diagnosis. The relationship of the kidneys to the psoas muscles is abnormal: Instead of an oblique orientation with the medial border of the kidney parallel to the psoas muscle, the kidneys are vertical and the medial border intersects and crosses the psoas muscle. Horseshoe kidneys have an elevated incidence of vesicoureteral reflux and are at increased risk of ureteropelvic junction obstruction. The latter may be related to a high ureteral insertion in the renal pelvis, crossing of the ureter over the isthmus, or compression by one of many anomalous arteries. Failure of rotation during ascent results in "malrotated" kidneys and is rarely significant.

Polycystic Kidneys

Parenchymal anomalies include a variety of cystic and dysplastic lesions. Polycystic kidney disease (PKD) is hereditary and bilateral. Patients with autosomal recessive PKD (ARPKD), previously called infantile PKD, have numerous small cysts that arise only from the collecting ducts and result in bilateral symmetrical enlargement of the kidneys. Patients with autosomal dominant PKD (ADPKD), previously called adult PKD, have cysts arising from all areas of the nephron, which are usually larger and more variable in size than the ARPKD cysts. ARPKD occurs in 1 in 40,000 births and may be detected in utero by the presence of enlarged hyperechogenic kidneys and oligohydramnios. Infants usually die of respiratory failure rather than renal problems; however, the 1-year survival probability after the first month is over 85%. These children have declining renal function as well as severe hypertension and hepatic periportal fibrosis with portal hypertension leading to hypersplenism and esophageal varices.

The genes mutated in ADPKD may include the *PKD1* gene (located on chromosome 16p13.3) in 85% of patients or the *PKD2* gene (on chromosome 4q21-23) in 12%-15% of patients. These genes code for the polycystin-1 and polycystin-2 proteins, respectively. ADPKD occurs in 1 in 1000 individuals and is a major cause of end-stage renal disease in adults. Cysts may also be present in the liver, pancreas, and spleen, and cerebral arterial aneurysms may occur. Renal cystic enlargement exerts pressure on normal parenchyma, leading to its gradual destruction and glomerulosclerosis.

The diagnosis is often made during a workup for hypertension or uremia discovered in the third to sixth decades. Hematuria with or without flank pain is a common finding. An intravenous urogram reveals the enlarged kidneys, with marked elongation of the calices, which are compressed by large cysts. Ultrasonography or computed tomography (CT) scan readily makes the diagnosis.

Surgery is rarely warranted. Therapy is medical and ultimately includes dialysis. The median age for reaching end-stage renal disease is 54 years in PKD1 and 74 years in PKD2. Renal transplantation is often indicated, although potential family donors must be carefully screened to determine whether they have the same disorder. The leading cause of death in ADPKD is cardiovascular disease, which may relate to early untreated hypertension.

▶ Medullary Sponge Kidney

Medullary sponge kidney results from collecting tubular ectasia (see section on polycystic kidneys) and is associated with recurrent urolithiasis and an increased incidence of infection in 50% of patients. The lesion is often bilateral and may involve all of the calices. Intravenous urograms reveal dilated collecting tubules as a "blush" in the renal papilla. Microscopic hematuria is common. Specific antibiotics should be given for documented infections, and prophylactic therapy for renal stones should be recommended on the basis of metabolic stone evaluation.

▶ Simple Renal Cysts

Simple renal cysts are common (approximately 50% after age 50) and are thought to arise from tubular dilation. They may be solitary or bilateral and multiple. They rarely have pathologic significance except in the differentiation from solid renal masses. (See the section on renal adenocarcinoma.)

▶ Multicystic Dysplastic Kidney

Multicystic dysplastic kidney is a congenital abnormality consisting of macroscopic cysts of variable sizes compressing dysplastic renal parenchyma. It is usually associated with an atretic proximal ureter. The disorder occurs in about 1 in 3000 live births and is frequently noted on prenatal ultrasound. Rarely, it may occur bilaterally and is associated with oligohydramnios and renal failure. It may be distinguished from other causes of hydronephrosis by the absence of any renal function on renal scan. There is an increased incidence of contralateral ureteropelvic junction obstruction (5%-10%) and reflux (18%-43%), either of which increases the patient's risk of subsequent chronic renal insufficiency.

The chance of developing a malignancy in multicystic dysplastic kidney appears to be no greater than 1 in 2000. There may also be an increased incidence of hypertension. These two factors constitute a rationale for treatment by nephrectomy. However, conservative management with routine ultrasound examinations at intervals of 6-12 months is a reasonable practice, since about half involute within 5 years.

▶ Renal Vascular Abnormalities

Multiple renal arteries occur in 15%-20% of patients and are significant only when they cause ureteropelvic junction obstruction. Congenital **renal artery aneurysms** are infrequent; they are differentiated from acquired lesions by their location at the bifurcation of the main renal artery or at a distal branch point. The lesions are usually asymptomatic, but they can cause hypertension. They require surgical treatment only if hypertension is uncontrolled, if they are incompletely calcified, or if they have a diameter of more than 2.5 cm. **Congenital arteriovenous fistulas** are rare but may result in hematuria, hypertension, or cardiac failure necessitating operative treatment.

▶ Renal Pelvis Anomalies

Ureteropelvic junction obstruction (UPJO) is the most common cause of antenatal hydronephrosis. The condition may be associated with compression by anomalous renal arteries or intrinsic stenosis of the junction. The diagnosis is not uncommonly made when gross hematuria follows minor trauma. Symptoms include intermittent flank pain, particularly with orally induced diuresis. There is a bimodal age at presentation, with an initial peak in infancy and a secondary presentation in early adulthood. Renal ultrasound provides a safe screening technique in patients suspected of having UPJO. Diuretic renal scan may confirm the diagnosis and suggest functional significance. Intravenous pyelogram or retrograde pyelography may further define the anatomy. Bilaterality is not uncommon, and the condition requires surgical repair if symptomatic or severe. With the advent of laparoscopic and robotic surgery, minimally invasive repair of UPJO with dismemebered pyeloplasty has become standard of care. Success rates with pyeloplasty are superior to endoscopic approaches in the primary setting. Percutaneous or ureteroscopic incision of the obstruction with short-term stenting has been successful in adults, but endoscopic incision is most useful in the setting of recurrent UPJO, when redo pyeloplasty becomes much more difficult, or when patients are poor surgical candidates due to comorbidities.

Light A, Karthikeyan S, Maruthan S, et al: Peri-operative outcomes and complications after laparoscopic vs robot-assisted dismembered pyeloplasty: a systematic review and meta-analysis. *BJU Int.* 2018;122(2):181-194.

URETERAL ANOMALIES

▶ Congenital Obstruction of the Ureter

Congenital obstruction of the ureter may be due to ureterovesical and ureteropelvic junction obstruction or to neurologic deficits such as sacral agenesis or myelomeningocele. Functional ureteral obstruction—also known as **primary obstructive megaureter**—is not uncommon. Symptoms are renal pain during diuresis or resulting from pyelonephritis. Excretory urograms depict dilation above the obstruction. Vesicoureteral reflux is uncommonly associated with megaureter. Milder forms without symptoms or significant hydronephrosis are the rules and do not require treatment if renal function is normal. When treatment is necessary, it consists of division of the ureter proximal to the obstruction and reimplantation of the ureter into the bladder, often involving ureteral tapering or plication.

▶ Duplication of Ureters

Bifurcation of the ureteral bud before it interacts with the metanephric blastema results in incomplete ureteral duplication, commonly in the mid or upper ureter. A second ureteral bud from the metanephric duct leads to complete ureteral duplication (Figure 40–4; right kidney) draining one kidney. This represents the most common ureteral anomaly, occurring in 1 in 125 people. It occurs twice as often in females. The presence of more than two ureters on each side is not common, but bilaterality of ureteral duplication occurs in 40%. Usually, all of the duplicated ureters enter the bladder; the ureter draining the upper pole of the kidney enters closest to the bladder neck (due to its later reabsorption into the bladder). Because of this relationship, the ureter draining the lower pole often has a short intramural tunnel and an inadequate surrounding musculature and is thus prone to vesicoureteral reflux. The ureter draining the upper pole may be ectopic (because of its late absorption) and thus empty into the bladder neck, urethra, or genital structures (vagina or vestibule in the female and seminal vesicle or vas deferens in the male [Figure 40–4; left kidney]). The ureter draining the upper pole is prone to obstruction and may be associated with a ureterocele, which is a common cause of obstruction. Duplication becomes significant when hydronephrosis or pyelonephritis occurs. The diagnosis is made

▲ **Figure 40–4.** Duplication of ureters and ectopic ureteral orifice. Complete duplication with obstruction to one ureter with ectopic orifice on left. The ureter with the ectopic opening always drains the upper pole of the kidney.

by intravenous urography. Ureteral reimplantation to prevent recurrent infection is necessary in some cases. An anastomosis between the upper pole renal pelvis and the lower pole ureter or a low ureteroureterostomy are alternatives in selected cases. The upper pole of the kidney and its ureter may require removal if obstruction is severe and renal function of that segment is poor.

Ectopic Ureteral Orifice

Ureteral ectopia can occur in the absence of duplication and drain into any of the abnormal positions mentioned previously. If the orifice lies proximal to the external urinary sphincter, no incontinence ensues, but vesicoureteral reflux is common. In contradistinction to the female, the ectopic orifice in the male never lies distal to the external sphincter, making incontinence an extremely rare presentation. Should the ectopic orifice in the female drain into the vagina or at the vestibule, there may be continuous leakage of urine apart from voiding. Most ectopic orifices involve the ureter draining the upper pole of a duplicated system, and most are observed in females. Hydroureteronephrosis of the involved segment frequently occurs due to ureteral obstruction as it traverses the muscle of the bladder neck.

An ectopic orifice may be seen beside the urethral orifice or in the roof of the vagina on endoscopy. Renal ultrasound or intravenous urograms often demonstrate hydroureteronephrosis of the upper renal segment. Cystography may show reflux into the ectopic orifice but may require cyclic voiding first to decompress the obstructed segment with bladder neck relaxation and subsequently to permit reflux. In the rare case when there is significant upper pole renal function, the ureter can be divided and reimplanted into the bladder or lower pole ureter. Usually, however, heminephroureterectomy is necessary.

Ureterocele

A ureterocele is a ballooning of the distal submucosal ureter into the bladder. This structure commonly has a pinpoint orifice and therefore leads to hydroureteronephrosis. If large enough, it may obstruct the vesical neck or the contralateral ureter. It is most common in females with ureteral duplication and always involves the ureter draining the upper renal pole.

Most ureteroceles are now detected by prenatal ultrasound. Symptoms are usually those of pyelonephritis or obstruction. Intravenous urograms may show a negative shadow in the bladder cast by the ureterocele. The ureter and renal calices may be normal or may reveal marked dilation or no excretory function at all. A cystogram may show reflux into the ipsilateral lower pole ureter.

Treatment of ureteroceles depends on multiple factors, including the presence or absence of reflux in any or all of the ureters as well as whether or not the ureterocele is completely contained within the bladder (intravesical/orthotopic) or if a portion is at the bladder neck or urethra (extravesical/ectopic). A simple method of establishing drainage involves cystoscopy and puncture of the ureterocele. Associated reflux, if present, can be managed with prophylactic antibiotics until the child has grown larger, at which time a technically easier ureteral reimplant may be performed with a decompressed ureter. In the relatively uncommon situation when there is no associated reflux, an upper pole heminephrectomy is considered. Minimally obstructive ureteroceles within the bladder in adults do not require treatment.

VESICOURETERAL REFLUX

The main function of the ureterovesical junction is to permit free drainage of the ureter and simultaneously prevent urine from refluxing back from the bladder. Anatomically, the ureterovesical junction is well equipped for this function, because the ureteral musculature continues uninterrupted into the base of the bladder to form the superficial trigone. Additionally, the terminal 4-5 cm of ureter are surrounded by a musculofascial sheath (Waldeyer's sheath) that follows the ureter through the ureteral hiatus and continues in the base of the bladder as the deep trigone (Figure 40–5).

Direct continuity between the ureter and the trigone offers an efficient, muscularly active, valvular function. Any

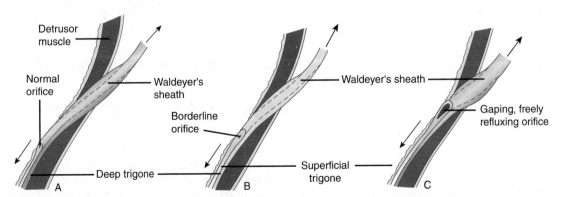

▲ **Figure 40–5.** Vesicoureteral reflux. The length and fixation of the intravesical ureter and the appearance of the ureteral orifice depend on the muscular development and efficiency of the lower ureter and its trigone. **A:** Normal structures. **B:** Moderate muscular deficiency. **C:** Marked deficiency results in a golf hole distortion of the submucosal ureter.

stretch of the trigone (with bladder filling) or any trigonal contraction (with voiding) leads to firm occlusion of the intravesical ureter, thus increasing resistance to flow from above downward and sealing the intravesical ureter against retrograde flow (Figure 40–6).

Etiology & Classification

Vesicoureteral reflux may be classified as primary reflux, due to developmental ureterotrigonal weakness or associated with ureteral anomalies such as ectopic orifice or ureterocele, or secondary reflux, due to bladder outlet or urethral obstruction, neuropathic dysfunction, iatrogenic

causes, and inflammation, especially specific infection (eg, tuberculosis). Primary reflux is associated with some degree of congenital muscular deficiency in the trigone and terminal ureter.

Reflux is associated with an increased incidence of pyelonephritis and renal damage. It also allows bacteria free access from the bladder to the kidney.

Reflux is the most common cause of pyelonephritis and is found in 30%-50% of children presenting with urinary tract infection. It is present in over 75% of patients with radiologic evidence of chronic pyelonephritis and is responsible for end-stage renal disease in a large percentage of patients requiring chronic dialysis or renal transplantation.

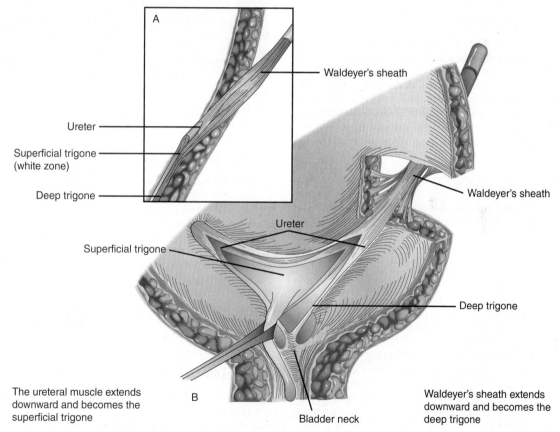

▲ **Figure 40–6.** Normal ureterotrigonal complex. **A:** Side view of ureterovesical junction. The Waldeyer's muscular sheath invests the juxtavesical ureter and continues downward as the deep trigone, which extends to the bladder neck. The ureteral musculature becomes the superficial trigone, which extends to the verumontanum in the male and stops just short of the external meatus in the female. **B:** Waldeyer's sheath is connected by a few fibers to the detrusor muscle in the ureteral hiatus. This muscular sheath, inferior to the ureteral orifices, becomes the deep trigone. The musculature of the ureters continues downward as the superficial trigone. (Adapted with permission from Tanagho EA, Pugh RCB: The anatomy and function of the ureterovesical junction. *Br J Urol.* 1963 June;35(2):151-165.)

In primary reflux, the child (on average, between 2 and 3 years of age) usually presents with symptoms of pyelonephritis or cystitis. Vague abdominal pain is not uncommon. Renal pain and pain with voiding are relatively uncommon. On rare occasions, the patient may present with advanced renal failure with bilateral renal parenchymal damage. Significant reflux and its sequelae are more common in females and are usually detected after a urinary tract infection. About one-third of the siblings of a child with reflux will also have reflux, and one-half of the children of a mother with reflux will also have reflux.

In secondary reflux, manifestations of the primary disease (eg, neuropathic, obstructive) are usually the presenting symptoms.

▶ Clinical Findings

A. Symptoms and Signs

With acute pyelonephritis, fever, chills, and costovertebral angle tenderness may be present. Children usually do not have renal pain but may complain of vague abdominal pain. Occasionally, daytime frequency, incontinence, or enuresis may be caused by infection associated with reflux. In cases of obstruction or neuropathic deficit, a palpable hydronephrotic kidney or a distended bladder may be found. The diagnosis may be elusive in infants who present with ill-defined symptoms.

B. Laboratory Findings

Urinalysis usually reveals evidence of infection (pyuria and bacteriuria). Urine cultures are mandatory when infection is suspected. Renal function tests may be abnormal if reflux and infection have caused renal scarring.

C. Imaging Studies

The most useful study for conclusive diagnosis of reflux continues to be voiding cystourethrography (Figure 40–7). This study demonstrates the grade of reflux as well as the urethral anatomy. Radionuclide voiding studies are extremely sensitive at detecting reflux but do not demonstrate the anatomic detail seen with a voiding cystourethrogram. Radionuclide voiding studies are often performed as follow-up after an initial voiding cystourethrogram because they offer the advantage of decreased radiation exposure.

Radioisotopic renal scanning provides accurate differential renal function data and detection of renal scars. Ultrasound can provide accurate measurement of renal size and may demonstrate the presence of renal scarring and ureteral or caliceal dilation. In many cases, there may be no abnormality visible in the upper urinary tract, or only mild distal ureteral dilatation may be seen.

▲ **Figure 40–7.** Voiding cystourethrogram showing total (grade IV) left vesicoureteral reflux.

D. Urodynamic Considerations

A significant number of children with dysfunctional voiding present with urinary tract infections and are subsequently found to have reflux. These children contract the bladder against a closed external sphincter. Elevated voiding pressures associated with dysfunctional voiding may increase renal damage with an associated urinary tract infection and may also lessen the chance for either spontaneous or surgical resolution of reflux. When the history suggests the possibility of voiding dysfunction (incontinence, frequency, urgency), urodynamic studies are conducted to evaluate the voiding dynamics. Treatment of voiding dysfunction may result in resolution of the reflux.

▶ Treatment

Although some children with lower grades of reflux may not require antibiotics, traditionally any child with reflux was maintained on prophylactic antibiotics to attempt to decrease the incidence of urinary tract infections. Several recent studies suggest that the practice of daily antibiotic prophylaxis in all children with reflux may be of limited benefit in preventing urinary tract infection. Prompt treatment of pyelonephritis prevents renal scar formation. Factors causing secondary reflux—such as dysfunctional voiding or obstruction—should be corrected.

In many children, reflux resolves with time. Reflux is graded as seen on voiding cystourethrography as follows:

Grade I: Contrast enters ureter

Grade II: Contrast enters the renal collecting system

Grade III: Slight dilation of the calices or ureter

Grades IV and V: Progressively increased amounts of caliceal dilation and ureteral dilation or tortuosity

Reflux most likely to resolve is of lower grade or detected at a younger age. Over 70% of children with grades I, II, or unilateral grade III reflux will have resolution within 5 years. Resolution in children with grade V or bilateral grade IV reflux can be anticipated in less than 10% of cases. Other factors that appear to negatively affect the chance for reflux resolution include early reflux during bladder filling, presentation with a febrile urinary tract infection, renal scars, and voiding dysfunction.

In obstructive secondary reflux (eg, posterior urethral valves), release of obstruction may cure reflux. Occasionally, surgical reimplantation is still required. In neuropathic reflux, intermittent catheterization for control of infection may allow return of valvular competence. However, many cases require bladder augmentation for a noncompliant bladder and ureteral reimplantation. In reflux associated with ectopic orifices, duplication with ureterocele, and other congenital malformations, reimplantation is generally required.

The aim of surgery is to correct the reflux. This is accomplished by the creation of a longer submucosal tunnel for the ureter. With bladder filling and increased pressure, the ureter is compressed between the mucosa and underlying detrusor muscle. This flap valve prevents reflux of urine. The necessary length of the tunnel to stop reflux depends on the diameter of the ureter, with a 5:1 length-to-diameter ratio being ideal. One of three methods is used in most cases: (1) In suprahiatal repair (Politano-Leadbetter procedure), a new ureteral hiatus is developed about 2.5 cm above the original one, and the ureter—after passing through a submucosal tunnel—is sutured to the cut edge of the trigone at the level of the original orifice. (2) In the cross-trigonal repair (Cohen procedure), the original hiatus is maintained, and the ureter is advanced through a submucosal tunnel, extending across the trigone to the contralateral bladder wall. (3) A totally extravesical ureteral advancement procedure (extravesical ureteroplasty) achieves results similar to those achieved with the intravesical methods, with a shorter hospital stay and shorter convalescence.

Injections of subureteric bulking agents have also been used to increase submucosal support of the ureter. With proper placement beneath the ureteral orifice under endoscopic vision, these injections act to bolster the deficient antireflux mechanism. Concern regarding late sequelae of Teflon injections (eg, particle migration) has prevented use of this approach in the United States. Currently, hyaluronic acid/dextranomer (NASHA/Dx) gel (Deflux) is the only U.S. Food and Drug Administration (FDA)-approved material for endoscopic injection to manage vesicoureteral reflux in children. Short-term success in stopping reflux with the injection techniques appears to be around 75% overall, with most success with grades I-III reflux. The long-term success rates still need to be evaluated, as many studies only have short-term (ie, 3-month) follow-up.

Prognosis

The long-term prognosis is excellent for patients with mild to moderate reflux successfully treated with antibiotic prophylaxis. There are few instances of recurrent infection or renal insufficiency. Patients with more significant reflux or persistent urinary tract infections may benefit from subureteric injection or surgical reimplantation; the success rate is approximately 95% with the open surgical technique (cessation of reflux, clearance of renal infection, and absence of obstruction). Unfortunately, for patients with advanced disease (irreversible ureteral decompensation and severe bilateral scars), the prognosis is less favorable. These patients account for a significant proportion of patients with end-stage renal disease who ultimately require chronic dialysis, renal transplantation, or both.

BLADDER ANOMALIES

Anomalies of the bladder are infrequent and include the following: (1) **agenesis,** or complete absence, which results in a persistent cloaca; (2) bladder **duplication,** which may be complete, with separate ureteral openings drained by duplicated urethras, or incomplete, with a septum or hourglass deformity; and (3) **urachal anomalies,** which in the most severe forms appear as a patent opening at the umbilicus and are usually associated with some form of bladder outlet obstruction. In less severe forms, a **urachal diverticulum** may be present at the dome of the bladder, or a **urachal cyst** may be present along the course of the partially obliterated urachus. These latter conditions may cause abdominal pain and umbilical or bladder infection requiring surgical treatment. Occasionally, adenocarcinoma develops in a urachal remnant (see section on tumors of the bladder).

Failure of cloacal division results in a persistent cloaca. Incomplete division is more frequent (although still rare) and results in a rectovesical, rectourethral, or rectovestibular fistula (usually with imperforate anus or anal atresia).

Exstrophy of the Bladder

Exstrophy of the bladder is the most severe bladder anomaly—the result of a complete ventral defect of the urogenital sinus and the overlying inferior abdominal wall musculature and integument. The lower central portion is devoid of skin and muscle. The anterior bladder wall is absent, and the posterior wall is contiguous with surrounding skin. Urine drains onto the abdominal wall, the rami of the pubic bones are widely separated, and the open pelvic ring may affect gait. In males, the penis is shortened and the urethra is epispadiac. The exposed bladder mucosa tends to be chronically inflamed.

Currently, the favored treatment is bladder salvage, which includes closure of the bladder in the newborn period. Urethral closure and penile reconstruction have also been advocated at the time of the initial bladder closure. Ureteral obstruction or vesicoureteral reflux may develop and require ureteral reimplantation. The closed bladder may have a small capacity, and incontinence is often a complication. Patients frequently require multiple operations, including bladder augmentation and bladder neck reconstruction. Good results have been observed in more than half of all patients treated, with preservation of renal function and continence.

▶ Prune Belly Syndrome

Prune belly syndrome consists of a triad of abnormalities: deficient abdominal wall musculature, bilateral cryptorchidism, and variable amounts of dilation of the urogenital tract. The cause is not known. Almost all children with prune belly syndrome have reflux. The incidence of eventual renal failure is 25%-30%. Risk factors for renal failure include bilateral abnormal kidneys on ultrasound or renal scan, a serum creatinine that never falls below 0.7 mg/dL, and clinical pyelonephritis. These children are managed with prophylactic antibiotics and frequent urine cultures, followed by prompt treatment of any urinary tract infections. Abdominoplasty may be performed to help correct the abdominal wall defect.

▶ Congenital Neurovesical Dysfunction

Congenital neurovesical dysfunction frequently accompanies a posterior myelomeningocele or sacral agenesis, with associated spinal abnormalities. Both conditions may result in incontinence and recurrent urinary infection with late sequelae (ureteral reflux, pyelonephritis, and renal failure). These children require frequent evaluation of their kidneys and kidney function because high bladder storage pressures may harm the kidneys.

PENILE & URETHRAL ANOMALIES

▶ Hypospadias

Hypospadias results from failure of fusion of the urethral folds on the undersurface of the genital tubercle. The urethral meatus is ventrally displaced on the glans on the shaft of the penis or more proximal at the level of the scrotum or perineum. With more proximal displacement, chordee (ventral curvature of the penile shaft) frequently occurs and requires treatment, or it precludes straight erections and

▲ **Figure 40–8.** Hypospadias, penoscrotal type. Redundant dorsal foreskin that is deficient ventrally; ventral chordee.

normal intercourse (Figure 40–8). The midscrotal hypospadiac penis may resemble female external genitalia with an enlarged clitoris and labia. Sexual assignment in these latter infants requires hormonal and chromosomal analysis.

In hypospadias with the meatus positioned proximal to the corona, the prepuce is abnormal—not forming a complete cylinder due to a ventral defect. Circumcision should not be done in these patients, as the prepuce can be used later in surgical repair.

The degree of hypospadias dictates the need for repair. If the opening is glandular or coronal (85% of patients), the penis is usually functional both for micturition and procreation, and repair is done primarily for cosmetic reasons. Openings that are more proximal on the shaft require correction to allow voiding while standing, normal erection, and proper sperm deposition during intercourse. Surgical plastic repair of hypospadias is currently accomplished by a variety of highly successful one-stage operations and is routinely performed between 6 and 18 months of age. The most common complications of hypospadias surgery include meatal stenosis and fistula formation; however, improved techniques have decreased the incidence of these complications.

Epispadias

Epispadias is a rare congenital anomaly that is commonly associated with bladder exstrophy. When it occurs alone, it is considered a milder degree of the exstrophy complex.

The urethra opens on the dorsum of the penis, with deficient corpus spongiosum and loosely attached corpora cavernosa. If the defect is extensive, it may extend to the bladder neck, causing incontinence because of deficient sphincter muscles. The pubic bones are separated, as in exstrophy. Marked dorsiflexion of the penis is usually present.

Treatment consists of correction of penile curvature, reconstruction of the urethra, and reconstruction of the bladder neck in incontinent patients.

Urethral Strictures

Congenital urethral strictures are rare but, when present, are most common in the fossa navicularis (just proximal to the meatus) and in the bulbomembranous urethra. Commonly, these strictures are thin diaphragms that may respond to simple dilation or to direct vision internal urethrotomy. Rarely is open surgical repair necessary. Congenital urethral strictures in girls and meatal stenosis in boys are uncommon. When the latter does occur, it appears to be acquired, as it is seen only in circumcised boys.

Urethral Diverticulum

In males, urethral diverticula are nearly always in the pendulous or bulbous urethra. They are often associated with an obstructive flap of the urethral mucosa (anterior urethral valve), thought to represent incomplete closure of the urethral folds. Treatment by endoscopic unroofing is usually successful, although most diverticula are small and require no therapy. In females, they occur in adult life and are usually manifested by irritative symptoms and recurrent infection. The cause is unknown, but the disorder is most likely congenital. Treatment is usually by transvaginal excision. Diverticula may occasionally harbor stones or tumors.

Posterior Urethral Valves

Posterior urethral valves are the most common obstructive urethral lesion in newborn and infant males and the most common cause of end-stage renal disease in boys. They consist of obstructive folds of mucosa, which originate at or are attached at some point to the verumontanum in the prostatic urethra. The embryologic derivation is indefinite. They are partially obstructive and thus lead to variable degrees of back-pressure damage to the urinary bladder and upper urinary tract. Dilation and obstruction of the prostatic urethra are always present. Spontaneous urinary ascites from the kidneys is often seen in neonates. This clears when the obstruction is relieved.

About one-third of children with posterior urethral valves are now diagnosed by prenatal ultrasound. Another one-third are diagnosed in the first year of life, with the remaining third presenting later. Clinical manifestations consist of difficult voiding, a weak urinary stream, and a midline lower abdominal mass that represents a distended bladder. In some cases, the kidneys are palpable and the child may have signs and symptoms of uremia and acidosis. Urinary incontinence and urinary tract infection may occur. Laboratory findings include elevated serum urea nitrogen and creatinine and evidence of urinary infection. Ultrasound shows evidence of bladder thickening and trabeculation, hydroureter, and hydronephrosis. Demonstration of urethral valves on a voiding cystourethrogram establishes the diagnosis, as does endoscopic identification of valves. Up to 70% of children with valves may have vesicoureteral reflux.

Treatment consists of destruction of the valves by endoscopic incision. In a premature infant with a small urethra prohibiting transurethral resection, a temporary cutaneous vesicostomy may be required to provide drainage and improve impaired kidney function.

The prognosis depends on the original degree of kidney damage and the success of efforts to prevent or treat infection. Rates of chronic renal failure or end-stage renal disease range from 25% to 67% of boys with valves. Poor prognostic factors include the presence of bilateral reflux or an elevated nadir serum creatinine in the first year of life. Many of these children have delayed development of urinary continence due to bladder changes and impaired urinary concentration.

SCROTAL & TESTICULAR ANOMALIES

Testicular Torsion

Neonatal testicular torsion (extravaginal torsion) is an extremely rare condition. The entire testicle and the tunica vaginalis are twisted. No trigger mechanism associated with the torsion has been identified. Although the vast majority are necrotic and nonsalvageable, several studies have reported salvage of testicular tissue when torsion is detected immediately following birth. Any scrotal swelling in the neonate requires close follow-up. Intravaginal testicular torsion in adolescents is described later in this chapter.

Scrotal Lesions

Congenital scrotal lesions include hypoplasia of the scrotum (unilateral or bilateral) in association with cryptorchidism and bifid scrotum with extensive hypospadias. Midline inclusion cysts may also occur.

CRYPTORCHIDISM

Etiology & Classification

True undescended testicles stop along the normal path of descent into the scrotum. They may remain in the abdominal cavity (least common), in the inguinal canal (canalicular), or just outside the external ring (suprascrotal, most common). Testes may also pass through the external ring and then be located ectopically, most commonly in a superficial inguinal pouch. The incidence of undescended testicles increases from 3% to 5% in full-term infants to 30% in premature infants. Most undescended testicles descend within the first 6 months of life, and by 1 year of age, the prevalence is 1%. The left testicle is affected more often, and 1%-2% of children with cryptorchidism will have both testicles affected. Twenty percent of boys who present with cryptorchidism have one nonpalpable testis. Of nonpalpable testes, 20% are intraabdominal; 40% are canalicular, scrotal, or ectopic testes; and 40% are atrophic or absent.

Clinical Findings

The diagnosis of cryptorchidism relies on physical examination. Absence of an identifiable testicle with ultrasound, CT, or magnetic resonance imaging (MRI) does not prove testicular agenesis and therefore does not alter the need for surgical exploration. Testicular examination in the infant and young child requires two hands, with the first hand being swept from the anterior iliac spine along the inguinal canal to gently express any retained testicular tissue into the scrotum, which is palpated with the other hand. A true undescended or ectopic inguinal testis may slip or "pop" under the examiner's fingers. To distinguish a retractile testicle, the testicle is brought into the scrotal position, holding it in place for a minute to fatigue the cremaster muscle. After this, a retractile testicle remains in the scrotum, whereas an ectopic or undescended testis immediately snaps back out of the scrotum. If a testis cannot be palpated in the inguinal canal or the scrotum, or in the typical ectopic sites, evaluation for a nonpalpable testis must be performed.

A child with bilateral nonpalpable testes should undergo hormonal evaluation for testicular absence. Elevations of luteinizing hormone (LH) and follicle-stimulating hormone (FSH) and absence of detectable müllerian-inhibiting substance suggest testicular absence. Testicular absence is confirmed by a negative human chorionic gonadotropin (hCG) stimulation test. The hCG stimulation test is performed by the administration of intramuscular hCG (2000 IU/d for 3-4 days). Raised gonadotropin levels (FSH and LH) *and* a lack of a testosterone rise from hCG indicate bilateral absent testes, and a formal surgical exploration is unnecessary. When one or both components are lacking or there is detectable müllerian-inhibiting substance, surgical exploration is warranted.

Surgical Therapy

Treatment of the undescended testicle offers the possibility of improved fertility, correction of patent processus vaginalis, prevention of testis torsion, and improvement in body image. There is controversy whether orchidopexy decreases the risk of malignancy, but placement of an undescended testicle in the scrotum assists physical examination of the testis. Histologic changes related to infertility occur in the undescended testicle as young as 1 year of age, and spontaneous descent rarely occurs after 6 months of age, making this the optimal time for surgical correction.

Almost 90% of undescended testes have an associated patent processus vaginalis, which predisposes to formation of a hydrocele or hernia. Occult inguinal hernia in patients with untreated undescended testis can present at any time with the typical symptoms or complications, including incarceration.

Prior to any surgical intervention, the patient is reexamined while under anesthesia because on occasion a retractile testicle descends under anesthesia or a previously nonpalpable testicle becomes palpable. For a palpable testicle, an open inguinal approach is performed. For the nonpalpable testicle in a child, a laparoscopic approach is preferred, but an open inguinal approach may be performed.

Outcomes

Success rates following orchidopexy are 74% for the abdominal testis, 87% for canalicular, and 92% for those distal to the external ring. The most significant complication is testicular atrophy, which occurs in 1%-2% of cases of orchidopexy, whereas complete devascularization of the testis is rare. Paternity rates have been reported at 65%, 90%, and 93% in men with bilateral cryptorchidism, unilateral cryptorchidism, and normally descended testicles, respectively. If only one testis is undescended, the sperm count is subnormal in 25%-33% patients, and serum FSH concentration is slightly elevated. These abnormalities suggest that both testes are abnormal, perhaps congenitally, although only one fails to descend. If both testes are undescended, sperm count usually is severely subnormal, and serum testosterone may be reduced.

Alternative Therapy

Hormonal therapy is an option in the treatment of cryptorchidism because the condition may be related to hypogonadotropic hypogonadism. hCG is the only hormone approved for use in the treatment of cryptorchidism in the United States. Side effects of hCG treatment include enlargement of the penis, growth of pubic hair, increased testicular size, and aggressive behavior during administration. The likelihood of success with hormonal therapy is greatest for the most distal undescended testes or for testes that have been previously descended. Some suggest that hormonal therapy is effective only for retractile and not truly undescended testes. Although hormonal therapy may not be effective in achieving testicular descent, it may improve fertility in cryptorchid boys.

▼ ACQUIRED LESIONS OF THE GENITOURINARY TRACT

OBSTRUCTIVE UROPATHY

Obstruction is one of the most important abnormalities of the urinary tract, since it eventually leads to decompensation of the muscular conduits and reservoirs, back-pressure, and atrophy of renal parenchyma. It also invites infection and stone formation, which cause additional damage and can ultimately end in complete unilateral or bilateral destruction of the kidneys.

Both the level and the degree of obstruction are important to an understanding of the pathologic consequences. Any obstruction at or distal to the bladder neck may lead to back-pressure affecting both kidneys. Obstruction at or proximal to the ureteral orifice leads to unilateral damage unless the lesion involves both ureters simultaneously. Complete obstruction leads to rapid decompensation of the system proximal to the site of obstruction. Partial obstruction leads to gradual progressive muscular hypertrophy followed by dilation, decompensation, and hydronephrotic changes.

► Etiology

Acquired urinary tract obstruction may be due to inflammatory or traumatic urethral strictures, bladder outlet obstruction (benign prostatic hyperplasia or cancer of the prostate), vesical tumors, neuropathic bladder, extrinsic ureteral compression (tumor, retroperitoneal fibrosis, or enlarged lymph nodes), ureteral or pelvic stones, ureteral strictures, or ureteral or pelvic tumors.

► Pathogenesis

Regardless of its cause, acquired obstruction leads to similar changes in the urinary tract, which vary depending on the severity and duration of obstruction.

A. Urethral Changes

Proximal to the obstruction, the urethra dilates and balloons. A urethral diverticulum may develop, and dilation and gaping of the prostatic urethra and ejaculatory ducts may occur.

B. Vesical Changes

Early detrusor and trigonal thickening and hypertrophy compensate for the outlet obstruction, allowing complete bladder emptying. This change leads to progressive development of bladder trabeculation, cellules, saccules, and, finally, diverticula. Subsequently, bladder decompensation occurs and is characterized by the above changes plus incomplete bladder emptying (ie, postvoid residual urine). Trigonal hypertrophy leads to secondary ureteral obstruction owing to increased resistance to flow through the intravesical ureter. With detrusor decompensation and residual urine accumulation, there is stretching of the hypertrophied trigone, which appreciably increases ureteral obstruction. This is the mechanism of back-pressure on the kidney in the presence of vesical outlet obstruction (while the ureterovesical junction maintains its competence). Catheter drainage of the bladder relieves trigonal stretch and improves drainage from the upper tract.

A very late change with persistent obstruction (more frequently encountered with neuropathic dysfunction) is decompensation of the ureterovesical junction, leading to reflux. Reflux aggravates the back-pressure effect on the upper tract by transmitting abnormally high intravesical pressures and favors the onset or persistence of urinary tract infection.

C. Ureteral Changes

The first change noted is a gradual increase in ureteral distention. This increases ureteral caliber and stimulates hyperactive ureteral contraction and ureteral muscular hypertrophy. Because the ureteral musculature runs in an irregular helical pattern, stretching of its muscular elements leads to lengthening as well as widening, causing the dilated ureter to assume a tortuous, serpiginous course, weaving back and forth across the relatively straight course of the ureteral vessels, which are unaffected by the ureteral obstruction. This is the start of ureteral decompensation, where tortuosity and dilation become apparent. These changes progress until the ureter becomes atonic, with infrequent, ineffective, or completely absent peristalsis.

D. Pelvicaliceal Changes

The renal pelvis and calices, subjected to increased volumes of retained urine, distend. The pelvis shows evidence first of hyperactivity and hypertrophy and then of progressive dilation and atony. The calices show similar changes to a variable degree, depending on whether the renal pelvis is intrarenal or extrarenal. In the latter, caliceal dilation may be minimal despite marked pelvic dilation. In the intrarenal pelvis, caliceal dilation and renal parenchymal damage are maximal. The successive phases seen with obstruction are rounding of the fornices, followed by flattening of the papillae and finally clubbing of the minor calices.

E. Renal Parenchymal Changes

With continued pelvicaliceal distention, there is parenchymal compression against the renal capsule, and more importantly, compression of the arcuate vessels results in a marked drop in renal blood flow, leading to parenchymal ischemic atrophy. With increased intrapelvic pressure, there is progressive dilation of the collecting and distal tubules, with compression and atrophy of tubular cells.

Clinical Findings

A. Symptoms and Signs

The findings vary according to the site of obstruction.

1. Infravesical obstruction—Infravesical obstruction (eg, due to urethral stricture, benign prostatic hypertrophy, bladder neck contracture) leads to difficulty in initiation of voiding, a weak stream, and a diminished flow rate with terminal dribbling. Burning and frequency are common associated symptoms. A distended or thickened bladder wall may be palpable. Urethral induration due to stricture, benign prostatic hypertrophy, or cancer of the prostate may be noted on rectal examination. Meatal stenosis and impacted urethral stones are readily diagnosed by physical examination.

2. Supravesical obstruction—Renal pain or renal colic and gastrointestinal symptoms are commonly associated. Supravesical obstruction (eg, due to ureteral stone, UPJO) may be completely asymptomatic when it develops gradually over a period of months. An enlarged kidney may be palpable. Costovertebral angle tenderness may be present.

B. Laboratory Findings

Evidence of urinary tract infection, hematuria, or crystalluria may be seen. Impaired renal function may be noted in cases of bilateral obstruction. Postrenal azotemia (serum changes reflecting impaired renal function due primarily to obstruction) is suggested by elevation of serum urea nitrogen and serum creatinine with a ratio greater than 10:1.

C. Imaging Studies

Radiologic examination is usually diagnostic in cases of stasis, tumors, and strictures. Dilation and anatomic changes occur above the level of obstruction, whereas distal to the obstruction, the configuration is usually normal. This helps in localizing the site of obstruction. Combined antegrade imaging by intravenous urograms and retrograde imaging by ureterograms or urethrograms is sometimes needed to demonstrate the obstructed segment. In supravesical obstruction, demonstration of stasis and delayed drainage is essential to establish and quantitate the severity of obstruction.

1. Ultrasonography—Ultrasonography reveals the degree of dilation of the renal pelvis and calices and allows for diagnosis of hydronephrosis even in the prenatal period. Color Doppler ultrasound can reveal blood flow and restrictive indices to help determine functional impairment.

2. Isotope studies—A technetium-99m DTPA scan or MAG-3 scan portray the degree of hydronephrosis as well as renal function. Use of diuretics during the scan can provide specific data on the significance of the obstruction and the need for treatment. Multiple studies can reveal ongoing functional changes.

3. CT scan—CT scan is of particular value in revealing the degree and site of obstruction as well as the cause in many cases. The use of contrast (CT urogram) agents allows estimation of residual renal function.

4. Magnetic resonance urogram—MRI provides anatomic images and identification of the site of obstruction. With dynamic contrast-enhanced magnetic resonance (MR) urography, functional information is also obtained without the use of ionizing radiation.

5. Antegrade urography—Antegrade urography via percutaneous needle or tube nephrostomy is valuable when the obstructed kidney fails to excrete the radiopaque material on excretory urography. The Whitaker test requires percutaneous catheter access to the collecting system above the site of suspected obstruction. This permits fluid introduction into the renal pelvis and simultaneous measurement of urine flow rate and pressures in the bladder and renal pelvis, thus providing a quantitative assessment of the degree and severity of obstruction. The fluid transport can be measured and the degree of obstruction estimated by the use of a pressure monitor.

Complications

The most important complication of urinary tract obstruction is renal parenchymal atrophy as a result of backpressure. Obstruction also predisposes to infection and stone formation, and infection occurring with obstruction leads to rapid kidney destruction.

Treatment

The first goal of therapy is relief of the obstruction (eg, catheterization for relief of acute urinary retention). Definitive therapy often requires surgery, but minimally invasive techniques are being used more often. Simple urethral stricture may be managed by dilation or internal urethrotomy (incision of the stricture under direct vision through the resectoscope). However, urethroplasty (open surgical graft or flap of skin or buccal mucosa to replace urethral diameter) may be required and have better long-term success. Benign prostatic hyperplasia classically requires excision, but laser techniques are providing satisfactory outcomes with less morbidity. Impacted ureteral stones may either be removed or bypassed by a catheter unless it is thought that they may pass spontaneously.

Ureteral or ureteropelvic junction obstruction requires surgical repair; however, endoscopic approaches within the ureter or by laparoscopy may be equal to open repair. Renal stones may be removed instrumentally via retrograde or antegrade percutaneous approach by direct extraction with baskets or by ultrasonic or laser lithotripsy or by irrigation through a tube placed directly into the kidney.

Preliminary drainage above the obstruction is sometimes needed to improve kidney function. Occasionally, intestinal urinary diversion or permanent nephrostomy is required. If damage is advanced, nephrectomy may be indicated.

▶ Prognosis

The prognosis depends on the cause, site, duration, and degree of kidney damage and renal decompensation. In general, relief of obstruction leads to improvement in kidney function except in seriously damaged kidneys, especially those destroyed by inflammatory scarring.

URETEROPELVIC JUNCTION OBSTRUCTION

Stenosis of the renal pelvis outlet is commonly due to congenital narrowing of the junction or compression by anomalous vessels. However, the lesion may be acquired. Presentation in adults often includes the abrupt onset of flank pain usually following ingestion of large amounts of fluids. Presentation in childhood is now most often made following the diagnosis of hydronephrosis by prenatal ultrasonography.

The diagnosis may be confirmed with a diuretic nuclear renal scan or intravenous urography, which reveals hydronephrosis with a dilated renal pelvis and slow drainage of either radiotracer or contrast medium. Occasionally, patients present with intermittent hydronephrosis and normal urograms, except during attacks of pain, when x-rays show typical obstruction. These patients generally have normal renal parenchyma. Retrograde ureteropyelography is usually needed in patients with chronic moderate to severe obstruction to determine the extent of the lesion and to provide assurance that the distal ureter is normal. Marked obstruction may make it difficult to determine whether kidney function is surgically salvageable. In these cases, it may be necessary to perform either (1) differential radioisotope renography with use of a diuretic during the study or (2) percutaneous nephrostomy and creatinine clearance by 24-hour urine collection.

Severe obstruction with minimal remaining renal function is best treated by unilateral nephrectomy. If renal function is adequate (> 10%-15% of total renal function or > 10 mL/min creatinine clearance), surgical repair of the stenosis, either by creation of a renal pelvis flap or by resection of the stenotic area and reanastomosis (dismembered repair), is warranted. Laparoscopic and/or robotic pyeloplasty has emerged as the standard of care in adults for the repair of UPJO. The use of ureteroscopy or percutaneous nephroscopy with endopyelotomy, incising the strictured ureteropelvic junction, offers an alternative method of therapy and

is most useful in secondary UPJO, after primary repair has failed. Endoscopic approaches are less successful in the presence of a crossing vessel, poor renal function, and significant hydronephrosis. The surgical results of all these methods are excellent in terms of functional preservation, improvement of urine flow, and relief of symptoms, but dilation of the calices may persist.

URETERAL STENOSIS

Ureteral stenosis can be secondary to congenital or acquired lesions. Congenital causes can include compression by an anomalous vessel, such as a lower pole renal artery in UPJO or a retroperitoneal vein, or primary megaureter where the distal ureter is partially obstructed. More commonly, the ureter is secondarily obstructed due to acquired conditions such as inflammation from chronic ureteral stones, trauma secondary to gynecologic or vascular surgery, or external penetrating trauma from a knife or gunshot wound. Enlarged pelvic lymph nodes or an iliac artery aneurysm or retroperitoneal fibrosis may obstruct the ureter, as can intrinsic ureteral cancer or bladder cancer infiltrating the ureter at its insertion into the bladder. Finally, infection such as urinary tuberculosis can cause distal ureteral strictures, and bilateral ureteral obstruction can occur from bladder neck obstruction with urinary retention secondary to benign prostatic hyperplasia.

Chronic conditions with slow development may not cause symptoms, whereas acute obstruction such as that from a stone will cause severe flank pain that may radiate to the groin or testes/labia. Diagnosis is most often made by a CT urogram with contrast that will show delayed function and a dilated renal pelvis and ureter down to the site of the obstruction. This is often an unsuspected finding on a CT done for other reasons in an asymptomatic patient.

Treatment depends entirely on the cause. Severe stenosis may require resection of the lesion and spatulated end-to-end anastomosis of the ureter. Less severe obstruction may be managed by cystoscopy and ureteral or balloon dilation of the narrowed area under direct vision via a ureteroscope. Placement of an indwelling ureteral stent may dilate the stenosis over time and be a useful treatment as well in selected patients.

RETROPERITONEAL FIBROSIS

See also Chapter 24.

One or both ureters may be compressed by a chronic inflammatory process, usually of unknown cause, which involves the retroperitoneal tissues of the lumbosacral area. When the source of fibrosis is unknown, the entity is known as idiopathic retroperitoneal fibrosis. Patients treated for migraine with methysergide may develop this fibrosis. Sclerosing Hodgkin disease and fibrosis from metastatic cancer have also been implicated. Symptoms include flank pain, lower back and abdominal pain (from ureteral obstruction), and those associated with uremia. Some patients present with complete anuria. Urinary infection is unusual. If both ureters are obstructed, the serum creatinine is elevated, but unilateral renal obstruction from fibrosis may present with normal or slightly elevated creatinine levels.

Excretory urograms show hydronephrosis and a dilated ureter down to the point of obstruction. The ureters are displaced medially in the lumbar area. Retrograde ureterograms show a long segment of ureteral stenosis, although a catheter usually passes easily through the ureter. Ultrasound lacks the anatomic specificity to make the diagnosis, but obstruction proximal to the fibrotic mass yields hydronephrosis and hydroureter. Large areas of fibrosis can be identified with ultrasound. CT scans and MRI offer the most diagnostic information about the fibrotic mass and both the degree and level of obstruction. If the patient has significant worsening of renal function, indwelling ureteral stent(s) or percutaneous nephrostomy tube(s) should be placed. When the patient's condition has improved, definitive therapy can be accomplished. If methysergide is suspected to be the causative agent, fibrosis may subside when the drug is discontinued. When malignancy is in the differential diagnosis, a percutaneous or laparoscopic biopsy should be considered prior to treatment. These patients may benefit from administration of corticosteroids and/or other immunosuppressive agents. Chronic indwelling ureteral stents have also been used successfully. If these methods fail, ureterolysis must be performed to free the ureter from the fibrous plaque. The involved ureter should be dissected from the plaque, moved to a lateral position, and wrapped with omentum to prevent recurrent entrapment. This has been accomplished quite successfully with laparoscopic and robotic approaches.

Jadhav KK, Kumar V, Punatar CB, et al: Retroperitoneal fibrosis-clinical presentation and outcome analysis from urological perspective. *Invest Clin Urol.* 2017;58(5):371-377.

BENIGN PROSTATIC HYPERPLASIA

▶ General Considerations

The cause of benign prostatic enlargement is not known but is probably related to hormonal factors. The mechanism for opening and funneling the vesical neck at the time of voiding is altered by hyperplasia of the prostate, which causes increased outflow resistance. Consequently, a higher intravesical pressure is required to accomplish voiding, causing hypertrophy of the vesical and trigonal muscles. This may lead to the development of bladder diverticula—outpocketings of vesical mucosa between the detrusor muscle bundles. Hypertrophy of the trigone causes excessive stress on the intravesical ureter, producing functional obstruction and resulting in hydroureteronephrosis in late cases. Stagnation of urine can lead to infection; the onset of cystitis

exacerbates the obstructive symptoms. The periurethral and subtrigonal prostate enlargement produces the most significant obstruction.

The prostate in young men has an anatomic capsule like an apple peel. In men with prostatic enlargement, there is a thick "surgical" capsule similar to an orange peel, composed of peripherally compressed true prostatic tissue ("peripheral zone"). The hyperplastic benign periurethral glands correspond to the "transition zone" and are the cause of the obstruction (Figure 40–9).

▶ Clinical Findings

A. Symptoms and Signs

Typically, the patient has lower urinary tract symptoms and notices hesitancy and loss of force and caliber of the stream. The urgent need to void when the bladder is nearly full may be an early sign. He may also be awakened by the urge to void several times at night (nocturia). Postvoid dribbling ("terminal dribbling") is particularly disturbing. The complication of infection increases the degree of obstructive symptoms and is often associated with burning on urination. Acute

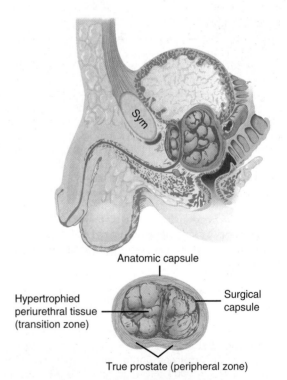

▲ **Figure 40–9.** Benign prostatic hyperplasia. The enlarged periurethral glands are enclosed by the surgical capsule. The true prostate has been compressed.

urinary retention may supervene. This is associated with severe urgency, suprapubic pain, and a distended, palpable bladder.

The size of the prostate rectally is not of primary diagnostic importance, since there is a poor correlation between the size of the gland and the degree of symptoms and amount of residual urine. The American Urological Association (AUA) developed a seven-item, self-administered questionnaire (AUA symptom score) that can assist the patient and physician in evaluating the patient's lower urinary tract symptoms.

B. Laboratory Findings

Urinalysis may reveal evidence of infection. Residual urine is commonly increased (> 50 mL), and a timed urinary flow rate is decreased (< 10-15 mL/s). The serum creatinine may be elevated in cases with prolonged severe obstruction.

C. Imaging Studies

Pelvic ultrasound can easily identify postvoid urine residual as well as estimate prostate size and anatomy, in particular the presence or absence of median lobe tissue. Bladder wall thickness, trabeculation, and diverticula can also be identified with ultrasound. Renal ultrasound can identify hydronephrosis in advanced cases of benign prostatic hyperplasia (BPH). Transrectal ultrasound of the prostate provides better imaging of the prostate than the transabdominal approach but is more invasive and typically not required. CT, MRI, and excretory urography also provide anatomic information for an enlarged prostate but are more time consuming and costly and should only be used in unusual circumstances (eg, ruling out malignancy).

D. Cystoscopic Examination

Cystourethroscopy reveals secondary vesical changes (eg, trabeculation and diverticula) and enlargement of the prostatic urethra. Lateral lobe hypertrophy (so-called "kissing lobes") and median lobe tissue can be easily visualized. Although cystoscopy is not required to make the diagnosis of BPH, it may identify other conditions in the differential diagnosis (eg, urethral stricture, bladder neck contracture, malignancy) as well as complications secondary to BPH (eg, bladder stones).

E. Urodynamic Studies

Simultaneous physiologic monitoring of bladder filling and emptying, urethral sphincter activity, abdominal pressure, and pelvic floor muscle activity (electromyography) can be extremely useful in documenting whether bladder outlet obstruction, poor bladder function, or other causes are responsible for lower urinary tract symptoms. While urodynamic studies are not required for diagnosis in all cases, they are helpful in cases with large postvoid residual volumes or

underlying neurologic disease to help determine appropriate management.

▶ Differential Diagnosis

Neurogenic bladder may produce a similar syndrome. A history suggesting a neuropathic etiology, such as diabetes mellitus, stroke, Parkinson disease, or spinal cord injury or compression, may be obtained. Neurologic deficit involving the spinal nerves S2-4 is particularly significant.

Cancer of the prostate also causes symptoms of vesical neck obstruction. Serum prostate-specific antigen may be elevated in patients with benign prostatic hypertrophy, and the level increases as the volume of the prostate increases. Thus, an absolute value is not diagnostic, but in general, if it is over 10 ng/mL, the possibility of cancer should be evaluated.

Acute prostatitis may cause symptoms of obstruction, but the patient is septic and has infected urine. The prostate is exquisitely tender.

Urethral stricture diminishes the caliber of the urinary stream. There is usually a history of gonorrhea or local trauma. A retrograde urethrogram or cystoscopy shows the stenotic area. A stricture blocks the passage of an instrument or catheter.

▶ Complications

Obstruction and residual urine lead to vesical and prostatic infection and occasionally pyelonephritis; these may be difficult to eradicate. Long-term obstruction can lead to renal failure.

The obstruction may lead to the development of bladder diverticula. Infected residual urine may contribute to the formation of calculi.

Functional obstruction of the intravesical ureter, caused by the hypertrophic trigone, may lead to hydroureteronephrosis.

▶ Treatment

The indications for operative management are impairment of or threat to renal function and bothersome symptoms. Because the degree of obstruction progresses slowly in most patients, conservative treatment may be adequate. Drugs that relax the prostatic capsule and internal sphincter (α-adrenergic blocking agents) or decrease the volume of the prostate (5α-reductase inhibitors or antiandrogens) have been tried with considerable success.

A. Conservative Measures

Treatment of chronic prostatitis may reduce symptoms. The resolution of a complicating cystitis usually affords some relief. In order to protect vesical tone, the patient should be cautioned to void as soon as the urge develops. Forcing fluids over a short time causes rapid vesical filling and decreasing vesical tone; this is a common cause of sudden acute urinary retention and thus should be avoided. Patients with urinary obstructive symptoms should avoid the use of cold remedies, including antihistamines and alpha-agonists, because they are also a common cause of urinary retention. These conservative measures are of only temporary help—if any—in patients with BPH. There has been recent great interest, particularly by patients, in the use of phytotherapy for treatment of lower urinary tract symptoms, including saw palmetto, pumpkin seeds, and other plant extracts. Despite previous claims of efficacy based on small retrospective studies, a recent large, multicenter, randomized trial of 369 men comparing placebo versus saw palmetto showed no improvement in AUA symptom score or secondary outcomes (eg, peak flow and postvoid residual) in the saw palmetto group. Thus, the use of saw palmetto extracts for the treatment of BPH is not recommended.

Barry MJ, et al: Effect of increasing doses of saw palmetto extract on lower urinary tract symptoms: a randomized trial. *JAMA*. 2011;306(12):1344-1351.

Controversy surrounds choices in the treatment of BPH. No treatment (watchful waiting) may be appropriate in patients who complain of mild to moderate symptoms and thus have low AUA symptom scores and residual urine less than 70-100 mL. Interest has also focused on nonoperative medical therapy for those with more significant symptoms. α-Adrenergic blocking agents relax the internal (bladder neck) sphincter and prostatic capsule. Selective agents that are long acting and preferentially work for this purpose include tamsulosin and silodosin. 5α-Reductase inhibitors block conversion of testosterone to dihydrotestosterone (the androgen active in promoting prostate growth) and are useful for large glands, particularly in combination with an alpha-blocker, which has been shown to best prevent urinary retention and other common progressive symptoms of prostatic obstruction. More recently, daily tadalafil, a phosphodiesterase-5 inhibitor commonly used in the treatment of erectile dysfunction, has been shown to have efficacy in treating symptoms related to BPH.

Catheterization is mandatory for acute urinary retention. Spontaneous voiding may return, but a catheter should be left indwelling for at least a few days and preferably 1 week while detrusor tone returns. Several studies have documented improved success of voiding trials after retention if α-blockers are initiated for at least 48 hours prior to catheter removal. If several voiding trials fail, additional treatment is indicated.

B. Surgery

Surgery for BPH is offered to men in whom medical therapy fails to provide adequate symptom relief and/or when objective parameters such as postvoid residual fail to improve. Additionally, men may request surgery because of poor compliance with medical therapy or desire to stop medications. Absolute indications for BPH surgery include recurrent infections, development of bladder stones, renal failure due to BPH, and persistent urinary retention due to obstruction. Men with large amounts of median lobe tissue (intravesical protrusion) tend to have a poor response to medical therapy and benefit most from early surgery.

There are two common approaches used in surgery for BPH: transurethral and transabdominal (open vs minimally invasive). The transurethral route is by far the most common and preferred in patients with glands weighing under 100 g because morbidity rates are lower and the hospital stay is shorter. With new technology, even larger glands can be managed with the transurethral approach. Larger glands, however, may require open surgery (suprapubic or retropubic enucleation), depending on the preference and experience of the urologist. Open surgery for BPH is the exception rather than the rule because of increased morbidity.

Transurethral approaches are the least invasive and require the shortest hospital stay (typically ambulatory or one night). The gold standard is the monopolar transurethral resection of the prostate (TURP), by which a resectoscope with a monopolar loop electrode is used to remove the obstructing BPH tissue. Hypotonic irrigation solution is required, and hyponatremia due to excess systemic absorption (TURP syndrome) is a unique complication of this approach. Additional complications of TURP include hematuria, urinary tract infection, stress incontinence, impotence, retrograde ejaculation, urethral stricture, and bladder neck contracture. Incontinence and impotence are rare complications in the hands of experienced surgeons (< 5%). TURP has reliably demonstrated improvement in AUA symptom score, flow rate, and postvoid residual in randomized controlled trials. The more recent use of bipolar energy has allowed for the use of saline irrigation during TURP, eliminating the risk of hyponatremia.

Transurethral laser vaporization of the prostate with holmium or KTP (potassium titanyl phosphate) laser technology has demonstrated similar efficacy to TURP in well-selected patients with smaller glands. The major advantage of the laser approaches is less risk of bleeding and even the ability to perform the procedure while patients remain on anticoagulation. Holmium-laser enucleation of the prostate (HOLEP) uses laser energy to enucleate the prostate adenoma (rather than vaporize the tissue). The tissue must then be morcellated to be removed via the resectoscope. HOLEP has similar efficacy to TURP and laser vaporization but may be more technically challenging.

An alternative transurethral approach for the treatment of BPH is transurethral incision of the prostate (TUIP). This procedure consists of a linear incision starting at the bladder neck and ending distally at the verumontanum, allowing expansion of the entire prostatic urethra. Typically, two incisions are made with a cutting current at the 5 o'clock and 7 o'clock positions. TUIP is typically reserved for men with a steep/high bladder neck or small, obstructive prostates of 30 g or less in size.

Open and robotic enucleation of the prostate for BPH is reserved for larger glands where transurethral approaches would be unable to remove sufficient tissue to provide long-term relief of the obstruction.

▶ Prognosis

Most patients with marked symptoms receive considerable relief and substantial improvement in urine flow following surgical treatment; however, those with milder forms may benefit from drug therapy. Unless absolute indications for surgery exist (see earlier), most men begin with medical therapy and progress to surgical interventions if substantial symptoms persist.

American Urological Association: American Urological Association guideline: benign prostatic hyperplasia: surgical management of benign prostatic hyperplasia/lower urinary tract symptoms (2018, amended 2019). Available at www.auanet.org. Accessed August 26, 2019.

URETHRAL STRICTURE

Acquired urethral strictures in men may be due to external trauma or to prior instrumentation (most common). Strictures may be inflammatory, due to gonorrhea, tuberculous urethritis, or schistosomiasis, or may rarely be a complication of cancer. The common presenting symptoms are dysuria, weak stream, splaying of the urinary stream, urinary retention, and urinary tract infection. Evidence of scarring due to trauma or induration and perineal fistula may be seen. Urethroscopy reveals the degree of narrowing. A retrograde urethrogram delineates the site and degree of stricture.

Urethral stricture must be differentiated from bladder outlet obstruction due to BPH, impacted urethral stones, urethral foreign bodies, and tumors.

Initial treatment consists of transurethral direct-vision internal urethrotomy (incision of the stricture). Successful results are obtained in 75% of patients. For long, dense strictures or those failing to respond to an initial internal urethrotomy, open surgical repair is indicated. This is probably best achieved by the transpubic or perineal route if the lesion involves the membranous urethra. If the bulbar urethra is involved, the perineal approach is indicated; if the distal/penile urethra is involved, the ventral penile approach is appropriate. End-to-end anastomosis is satisfactory for short segment strictures, usually 2 cm or less, with a > 90% success rate. Longer strictures often require pedicle flaps for distal urethral strictures or onlay grafts (eg, buccal mucosa) for proximal strictures.

HEMATURIA

Hematuria, gross or microscopic, is a common urologic consult because it can be a presenting sign for underlying urologic malignancies. Red-colored urine may not necessarily include blood, and microscopic examination looking for red blood cells is prudent. Microscopic hematuria is defined as three or more red blood cells per high-powered field on urine microscopy in two out of three properly collected specimens. The degree of hematuria bears no relation to the seriousness of the underlying cause. Urine dipstick test is the simplest method to check for blood and has a sensitivity of 91%-100% and a specificity of 65%-99%. Caution should be taken because false positives (menstrual blood, myoglobin, and hemolysis, among others) and false negatives (dipstick exposed to moisture and presence of reducing agents like ascorbic acid) can lead to confusing results. For this reason, further evaluation of microscopic hematuria is performed only when microscopic analysis confirms the diagnosis. Knowledge of the medical history and medications can help rule out other causes of colored urine. Beets, rifampin, and phenazopyridine, among other substances, can cause urine discoloration. Anticoagulation at normal therapeutic levels does not predispose to hematuria, and patients should be evaluated for the hematuria, because 13%-45% of these patients may have significant urologic disease.

Ideally, a clean-catch midstream sample should be collected. If that is not possible, a catheterized specimen is indicated. It is important to note that hematuria can be due to urologic or renal parenchymal disease. The differential diagnosis thus includes benign causes like renal or bladder stones, papillary necrosis, urinary tract infections, prostatitis, or instrumentation, and malignant causes like renal, renal pelvis, bladder, prostate, or urethral cancer. Renal parenchymal causes of hematuria include glomerular and interstitial renal disease. These patients may have proteinuria and casts on the urinalysis, and the red blood cells are typically dysmorphic. Nephrology evaluation is required for hematuria associated with glomerular or interstitial renal disease.

Patients with hematuria referred to urology are classified into low-risk and high-risk groups. High-risk groups include smokers; those age older than 40 years; and those with a history of exposure to pelvic radiation or cyclophosphamide, occupational exposure to chemicals or dyes, or urinary tract infections or other urologic disorders. It is recommended that a complete workup be performed for all patients with symptomatic hematuria, all patients with gross hematuria, and high-risk patients with microscopic hematuria. The workup includes history and physical examination, serum creatinine, upper tract imaging (typically CT urogram), cystoscopy, and urine cytology. Asymptomatic patients younger than 40 years who have microscopic hematuria and have no risk factors can be evaluated with upper tract imaging and either cystoscopy or voided cytology, as the risk of significant pathology in this population is very low. If the workup is negative, it is recommended that the patient be evaluated with urinalysis, voided cytology, and blood pressure check at 6, 12, 24, and 36 months.

URINARY TRACT INFECTIONS

Urinary tract infection is the second most common type of infection in humans and is frequently encountered by primary care physicians as well as urologists.

These infections are caused by a variety of pyogenic bacteria that typically produce a nonspecific tissue response. The most common organisms are gram-negative bacteria, particularly *Escherichia coli*. Less common are *Enterobacter aerogenes, Proteus vulgaris, Proteus mirabilis, Pseudomonas aeruginosa,* and *Enterococcus faecalis.*

Owing to the short length of the female urethra and bacterial colonization of the introitus, ascending infection is a common occurrence in young girls and in sexually active women. In men, ascending infection is often a consequence of urethral instrumentation.

Although relatively uncommon, descending or hematogenous urinary tract infection is usually associated with local urinary tract disorders—most commonly, obstruction and stasis; less commonly, trauma, foreign bodies, or tumors.

Lymphatic spread occasionally occurs from the large bowel or from the cervix and adnexa in the female through the perivesical and periureteral lymphatics.

Direct extension to the urinary bladder of nearby inflammatory processes (eg, appendiceal abscess, enterovesical fistula, or pelvic abscess) may occur.

▶ Predisposing Factors

Infection is usually initiated or sustained by predisposing factors. Predisposing systemic factors include diabetes mellitus, immunosuppression, and malnutrition; these disorders likely interfere with normal bladder and body defense mechanisms. Predisposing local factors include incontinence, constipation, organic or functional obstruction, stasis (residual urine), foreign bodies (especially catheters and stones), tumors, or necrotic tissue. Vesicoureteral reflux facilitates transport of bacteria from the bladder to the kidney, which subsequently predisposes to pyelonephritis.

▶ Classification of Urinary Tract Infection

Urinary tract infection is classified as (1) upper urinary tract infection (most commonly acute or chronic pyelonephritis or infection due to renal abscess), (2) lower urinary tract infection (cystitis or urethritis), or (3) genital infection (prostatitis, epididymitis, seminal vesiculitis, or orchitis).

▶ Urologic Instrumentation or Surgery & Urinary Tract Infection

In the absence of urinary tract infection, surgery of the upper urinary tract should require only short-term prophylactic antibacterial therapy. In the presence of infection, one attempts to sterilize the system before operation. If stenting or tube drainage is required and there are no symptoms of infection, colonization does not call for antibacterial therapy until the stent or tube is to be changed or removed. Broad-spectrum antibacterial prophylaxis is started at that time.

With lower urinary tract surgery, antibacterial therapy is advised before operations involving the urethra and the bladder, especially for women in whom contamination from vaginal organisms is likely. Men undergoing prostatectomy for obstructive prostatism often have urinary tract infection, particularly when catheter drainage is used preoperatively. In these cases, antimicrobial therapy is necessary before and after surgery to prevent bacteremia.

In the presence of urinary tract infection, any urethral instrumentation poses a threat of bacteremia, and possibly sepsis—more apt to occur in men than in women. Appropriate antibacterial coverage should be instituted before manipulation.

A. Principles of Catheterization

After a short-term single catheterization, the rate of infection is 1%-5%. However, in certain patients—pregnant women or elderly or debilitated patients—and in the presence of urologic disease, the risk is much higher. An indwelling catheter often leads to bacterial colonization, especially in women. The incidence is proportionate to the duration of catheterization and reaches approximately 95% after 5 days.

Strict aseptic technique is of critical importance in catheterization. Proper cleansing of the genitalia is essential. Iodophor preparations may be used for cleaning the vaginal introitus or the glans penis. Many common urinary tract pathogens are present in normal colonic flora, and these organisms often gain access to the urinary tract of catheterized patients. Cross-contamination of urinary catheters (passive transmission of bacteria from patient to patient on the hands of hospital personnel) is a frequent mode of transfer of resistant organisms. Measures directed at the prevention of catheter cross-contamination are essential. Closed catheter drainage is probably the best way to reduce cross-contamination.

With sterile technique during catheterization and a closed drainage system, most catheters can be kept sterile for 48-72 hours. In a closed drainage system, an added airlock or one-way valve preventing reflux of urine from the collecting bag to the draining tubes also helps prevent infection. The general principles are as follows: (1) Indwelling catheters should be used only when absolutely necessary. (2) Catheters should be inserted with strict aseptic technique. (3) A closed drainage system, preferably with a one-way valve, is advisable. (4) Nonobstructed dependent drainage is essential. (5) Unnecessary irrigation of the system should be avoided. (6) If the catheter is needed for a prolonged period, it should be changed every 2-4 weeks to minimize encrustation and stone formation. (7) Catheterized patients with asymptomatic catheter colonization should be given antibiotics just before the catheter is changed or removed, not during the period of catheterization, unless symptomatic infection occurs.

B. Evaluation

Imaging of the urinary tract is recommended in every febrile infant or young child following the first urinary tract infection. Imaging includes a renal and bladder ultrasound and a voiding cystourethrogram. The renal ultrasound may detect hydronephrosis, duplication anomalies, stones, or abnormalities of the bladder wall and should be obtained at the earliest convenient time. A cystogram may be obtained by instillation of contrast medium with fluoroscopy or by instillation of a radionuclide. Radionuclide cystography has the advantage of decreased radiation, while the contrast-voiding cystourethrogram has the advantage of providing better anatomic detail, which may help detect bladder or urethral abnormalities. Either method should include a voiding phase because reflux is the most likely abnormality to be detected and may only occur with voiding. The cystogram should be obtained once the child is free of infection.

Imaging recommendations in adults with a urinary tract infection vary depending on the patient's past history and present symptoms. Renal/bladder ultrasound is a good initial study to identify upper (eg, hydronephrosis, stones, or abscess) and lower (eg, urinary retention or bladder calculi) tract sources of infection. CT scan with intravenous contrast can identify stigmata of pyelonephritis (see later in chapter).

C. Antibacterial Therapy

The choice of antibiotics depends on the type of organism and its sensitivity, as determined by urine cultures. For uncomplicated infection, adequate urine concentrations of the antibiotic determine efficacy, but in cases of bacteremia and septic shock, serum concentrations are crucial. Commonly used oral medications are sulfonamides, nitrofurantoin, ampicillin, trimethoprim-sulfamethoxazole, fluoroquinolones, and oxytetracycline. For parenteral therapy, aminoglycosides and cephalosporins are effective against the most common organisms (ie, *P mirabilis, E aerogenes,* and *P aeruginosa*).

ACUTE PYELONEPHRITIS

▶ General Considerations

Except in the presence of stasis, foreign bodies, trauma, or instrumentation, pyelonephritis is an ascending type of infection. Pathogenic organisms usually reach the kidney from the bladder, often via an incompetent ureterovesical junction.

▶ Clinical Findings

A. Symptoms and Signs

In acute attacks, pain is present in one or both flanks. Diagnosis in infants requires a high index of suspicion, since they may present with nonspecific symptoms such as fever and failure to thrive. Young children commonly present with poorly localized abdominal pain; irritative lower urinary tract symptoms may be present. Chills and fever are common. Severe infection may produce hypotension, peripheral vasoconstriction, and acute renal failure. Gross hematuria is not common but can be observed more frequently in women and the elderly.

B. Laboratory Findings

Pyuria and bacteriuria are consistent findings. Leukocytosis with a shift to the left is common. Urine culture identifies the organism.

C. Imaging Studies

In acute attacks, only minimal changes such as delayed visualization and poor concentrating ability are noted on intravenous urography. CT scans may demonstrate zones of decreased enhancement in the renal parenchyma as well as perinephric fat stranding. Renal or ureteral calculi may be seen on plain abdominal x-rays or nonenhanced CT scans. Chest x-ray may show a small ipsilateral pleural effusion.

▶ Differential Diagnosis

Pneumonia, acute cholecystitis, or splenic infarction can be confused with pyelonephritis. Acute appendicitis sometimes causes pyuria and microhematuria. Any acute abdominal illness such as pancreatitis, diverticulitis, or intestinal ischemia can simulate pyelonephritis. Appropriate history, examination, urinalysis, and imaging usually make the distinction.

▶ Complications

If the diagnosis is missed in the acute stage, the infection may become chronic. Both acute and chronic pyelonephritis may lead to progressive renal damage and abscess formation.

▶ Treatment

Specific antibiotic therapy should be given for at least 7 days to eradicate the infecting organism after proper identification and sensitivity determination. Symptomatic treatment is indicated for pain and irritative voiding symptoms.

Adequate fluid intake to assure optimum urinary output is required. Failure to simultaneously identify and treat predisposing factors (eg, obstruction) is the principal cause of failure to respond to therapy, leading to progressive infection, chronic pyelonephritis, and possibly sepsis. Patients not responding to culture-sensitive antibiotics should be imaged, looking for intrinsic (eg, calculi) or extrinsic obstruction or renal abscess.

▶ **Prognosis**

The prognosis is good with adequate treatment of both the infection and its predisposing cause, depending on the degree of preexisting renal parenchymal damage.

EMPHYSEMATOUS PYELONEPHRITIS

Emphysematous pyelonephritis is a form of acute necrotizing pyelonephritis secondary to a gas-producing bacteria (*E coli* in 66% of cases and *Klebsiella* in 26%). It is commonly seen in patients with poorly controlled diabetes (> 90% of cases) or in patients with upper urinary tract obstruction. The diagnosis is made by the usual signs of acute pyelonephritis and by the presence of gas in the renal collecting system and parenchyma seen on plain films, ultrasound, or CT. The condition is life threatening, with a mortality rate of 40%-80% with intravenous antibiotics alone. Obstruction requires drainage either percutaneously or by stent placement. Operative treatment, including nephrectomy and drainage along with antibiotics, decreases the mortality rate to less than 20%.

CHRONIC PYELONEPHRITIS

Chronic pyelonephritis is the result of inadequately treated or recurrent acute pyelonephritis. The diagnosis is primarily made by x-ray, since patients rarely have signs or symptoms until late in the course, when they develop chronic flank pain, hypertension, anemia, or renal failure. Pyuria is not a consistent finding. Because chronic pyelonephritis may be a progressive, localized immune response initiated by bacteria long since eradicated, urine cultures are usually sterile. Early cases may have no findings on intravenous urography, whereas in late cases, it may reveal small kidneys with typical caliceal deformities (clubbing), with evidence of peripheral scarring and a thin cortex. Voiding cystourethrography may document vesicoureteral reflux as the cause. Complications include hypertension, stone formation, and chronic renal failure.

Antibiotic treatment is not helpful in these patients unless ongoing infection can be documented. The prognosis depends on the status of renal function but is generally not good, particularly when the disease is contracted in childhood. Progressive deterioration of renal function usually occurs.

Xanthogranulomatous pyelonephritis is a form of chronic pyelonephritis seen most frequently in middle-aged diabetic women and rarely in children. The disease is usually unilateral and is associated with prolonged obstructing nephrolithiasis. Patients often have nonspecific symptoms similar to those of acute pyelonephritis but have an enlarged kidney with calculi and a mass often indistinguishable from tumor. Proteus species are common causative agents. Nephrectomy is usually the treatment of choice, although a partial nephrectomy may be performed for focal disease. Histologic examination confirms the diagnosis following nephrectomy by the demonstration of foamy lipid-laden macrophages.

PAPILLARY NECROSIS

This disorder consists of ischemic necrosis of the renal papillae or of the entire pyramid. Excessive ingestion of analgesics, sickle cell trait, diabetes, obstruction with infection, and systemic conditions decreasing renal blood flow are common predisposing factors.

The symptoms are usually those of chronic cystitis with recurring exacerbations of pyelonephritis. Renal pain or renal colic may be present. Azotemic manifestations may be the presenting symptoms. In acute attacks, localized flank tenderness and generalized toxemia may occur. Laboratory findings consist of pyuria, hematuria, occasionally glycosuria, and acidosis. Impaired kidney function is shown by elevated serum creatinine and urea nitrogen. Intravenous urography usually shows impaired function and poor visualization in advanced cases. Evidence of ulceration, cavitation, or linear breaks in the base of the papillae and radiolucent defects due to sloughed papillae may be seen; the latter may become calcified. Retrograde urograms may be needed for proper imaging if kidney function is markedly impaired.

Preventive measures consist of proper management of diabetic patients with recurrent infections and avoidance of chronic use of analgesic compounds containing phenacetin and aspirin.

Intensive antibacterial therapy may be needed, although it is commonly unsuccessful in eradicating infection. Little can be done surgically except to remove obstructing papillae and correct predisposing factors (eg, reflux, obstruction) if identified.

In severe cases, the prognosis is poor. Renal transplantation may be required.

RENAL ABSCESS

While renal abscess is occasionally due to hematogenous spread of a distant staphylococcal infection, most abscesses are secondary to chronic nonspecific infection of the kidney, often complicated by stone formation. The onset may be acute, with high fever, but occasionally low-grade fever and general malaise are the presenting symptoms. Localized costovertebral angle tenderness and a palpable flank mass may be present. A mass may be evident on intravenous urograms, DTPA scans, sonograms, CT scans, or renal angiograms.

If the abscess is due to hematogenous spread, the urine does not contain bacteria unless the abscess has broken into the pelvicaliceal system. More frequently, gram-negative organisms are found, as would be expected in light of the preponderance of ascending infection.

If organism sensitivity can be established by appropriate tests (blood and urine cultures and sensitivity tests), treatment with the proper antibiotic is indicated. Many infections have responded to percutaneous drainage and irrigation with antibiotic solutions, especially in cases of unilocular abscess cavity seen on either ultrasound or CT examination. In multilocular abscess or persistent bacteremia despite percutaneous drainage, surgical drainage or even heminephrectomy may be necessary.

When the abscess is found to be secondary to chronic renal infection, nephrectomy is usually indicated because of advanced destruction of the kidney.

PERINEPHRIC ABSCESS

Abscess between the renal capsule and the perirenal fascia most often results from rupture of an intrarenal abscess into the perinephric space. *E coli* is the most common causative organism. The pathogenesis usually begins with severe pyonephrosis secondary to obstruction, as with renal or ureteral calculi. Clinical findings are similar to those of renal abscess. A pleural effusion on the affected side and signs of psoas muscle irritation are common. Abdominal plain films may show obliteration of the psoas muscle shadow, and an intravenous urogram may show poor concentration of contrast medium and hydronephrosis. CT scan is the current study of choice for diagnosis.

Treatment involves prompt drainage of the abscess and use of appropriate systemic antibiotics, including coverage of anaerobes. Percutaneous drainage is often successful; however, open surgical drainage is necessary if percutaneous drainage is incomplete.

CYSTITIS

Cystitis is more common in females and is usually an ascending infection. In males, it usually occurs in association with urethral or prostatic obstruction, prostatitis, foreign bodies, or tumors. The urinary bladder is normally capable of clearing bacterial inoculation unless an underlying pathologic process interferes with its defensive mechanisms.

In the acute phase, the principal symptoms of cystitis are dysuria, frequency, urgency, and hematuria; low-grade fever and suprapubic, perineal, and low back pain may be present. In chronic cystitis, irritative symptoms are usually milder.

Evidence of prostatitis, urethritis, or vaginitis may be present. Laboratory findings, in addition to hematuria, consist of bacteriuria and pyuria. Leukocytosis is not common. Urine culture identifies the organism. Cystoscopy is not advisable in the acute phase. In chronic cystitis, evidence of mucosal irritation may be present.

In any documented recurrent lower urinary tract infection (particularly in males), a complete urologic workup is indicated. Instrumentation is contraindicated in the acute phase, but cystoscopy is essential to identify the predisposing factor in chronic or recurrent bacterial cystitis. Upper tracts should be investigated with renal ultrasound when a lower tract source of infection is not identified.

Specific antibacterial therapy is given according to sensitivity testing of recovered organisms (*E coli* in > 80% of cases). Sterilization of urine should usually be followed by a variable period of continuous antibiotic therapy (depending on the predisposing factor or the chronicity and recurrence of the disease). Prolonged suppressive medication is usually indicated in cases associated with voiding dysfunction.

In females with recurrent postcoital cystitis, premedication (eg, sulfonamides, nitrofurantoin) on the night of intercourse and the following day in addition to immediate postcoital voiding decreases recurrences.

Schneeberger C, Geerlings SE, Middleton P, et al: Interventions for preventing recurrent urinary tract infection during pregnancy. *Cochrane Database Syst Rev*. 2015;7:CD009279.

PROSTATITIS

Acute Bacterial Prostatitis

Acute bacterial prostatitis is a severe acute febrile illness caused by ascending coliform bacteria, which frequently colonize the male urethra. Symptoms include high fever, chills, low back and perineal pain, and urinary frequency and urgency with diminished stream or retention. On examination, the prostate is extremely tender, swollen, and warm to the touch. A fluctuant abscess may be palpable. The prostate must be examined cautiously, because vigorous palpation may cause acute septicemia. Laboratory findings include pyuria, bacteriuria, and leukocytosis.

Transurethral manipulation by catheter or cystoscopy should be avoided if possible; urinary retention should be treated by gently introducing a urethral catheter or introducing a percutaneous suprapubic tube. Treatment with systemic antibiotics (fluoroquinolones or aminoglycosides and ampicillin-cephalosporin) should be started immediately and should be adjusted later when results of urine culture or blood culture (or both) and sensitivity tests are known. *E coli* is found in 80% of cases. Treatment with oral antibiotics for several weeks after the initial phase has subsided is necessary to eradicate the bacteria completely.

Prostate abscess can develop from a smoldering acute prostatitis (typically gram-negative bacteria) or from hematogenous seeding, often from gram-positive *Staphylococcus* species. Pelvic imaging (CT, MRI, or ultrasound) identifies a hypodense fluid collection within the prostate parenchyma. Treatment includes a long course of culture-sensitive antibiotics and drainage of the abscess. Transrectal needle drainage and transurethral unroofing of the abscess are both successful modalities. Ultrasound-guided transrectal needle drainage can be done under local anesthesia, with or without intravenous sedation, whereas transurethral unroofing is performed with a resectoscope in the operating room, typically under general anesthesia. Thus, if feasible, it seems reasonable to attempt transrectal drainage first and, if the abscess recurs or persists, then proceed to transurethral unroofing.

► Chronic Prostatitis

Chronic prostatitis is a common and complex problem. With differential diagnosis including urethritis, bacterial and nonbacterial prostatitis, prostatodynia (chronic pelvic pain syndrome), and seminal vesiculitis, assigning the correct diagnosis may challenge even the expert. The symptoms are varied and include suprapubic pain, low back pain, orchialgia, dysuria at the tip of the penis, and urinary frequency and urgency. The urinalysis may be normal. There may be a clear white urethral discharge. Prostate examination may be normal or reveal a soft, boggy prostate.

Expressed prostatic secretions may contain numerous leukocytes (> 10 per high-power field) in clumps as well as macrophages. Cultures of urine are usually sterile, but cultures of expressed prostatic secretions and urine obtained after prostatic massage are usually positive in bacterial prostatitis. *Chlamydia* or *Ureaplasma* may be an offending organism, particularly in men under age 35. Determination of the site of infection may require differential cultures. The first part of the voided urine stream is collected as VB_1 and the midstream specimen as VB_2. The prostate is then massaged to obtain expressed prostatic secretions, and the postmassage urine is collected as VB_3. The differential leukocyte and bacterial counts from each of these specimens can help localize the site of infection. If VB_1 has high levels of leukocytes and bacteria relative to the other specimens, urethritis is likely; if VB_2 has high levels, a site above the bladder neck is likely; and if the expressed prostatic secretions, VB_3, or both have high counts, prostatitis is likely.

For chronic bacterial prostatitis, at least a 4- to 6-week course of a fluoroquinolone or trimethoprim-sulfamethoxazole is often given. Surgical treatment for prostatitis is rarely indicated or helpful. Some patients improve following discontinuation of caffeine and alcohol, and a few respond to repeated prostatic massage. Patients with no evidence of bacterial infection or obstructive findings and those who have recurrent pelvic pain in association with voiding dysfunction (eg, intermittent or weak urinary stream) may be treated with α-adrenergic blocking agents or biofeedback to decrease the internal and external sphincter tone. 5α-Reductase inhibitors may be helpful.

ACUTE EPIDIDYMITIS

Acute epididymitis is most commonly a disease of young males, caused by bacterial infection ascending from the urethra or prostate. The disease is less common in older males, but when it does occur, it is most often due to infection secondary to urinary tract obstruction or instrumentation.

The symptoms are sudden pain in the scrotum, rapid unilateral scrotal enlargement, and marked tenderness that extends to the spermatic cord in the groin and may be relieved by scrotal elevation (**Prehn sign**). Fever is present. An acute hydrocele may result, and secondary orchitis with a swollen, painful testicle may occur. Laboratory studies reveal pyuria, bacteriuria, and marked leukocytosis.

Epididymitis must be differentiated from torsion of the testis, testicular tumor, and tuberculous epididymitis. A technetium-99m pertechnetate scan reveals increased uptake with epididymitis but decreased uptake with torsion. Scrotal ultrasound distinguishes between the solid mass of a testicular tumor and an enlarged, inflamed epididymis and can also identify epididymal or testicular abscess, which requires operative treatment. Increased blood flow on Doppler ultrasound also helps distinguish epididymitis from torsion, although it is not completely reliable.

Cultured aspirates from inflamed epididymides of males under age 35 tend to show gonococci and chlamydiae; in men older than 35, *E coli* is most common. Epididymal aspiration for culture is not required routinely, however. Pyuria with a negative urine culture suggests the presence of chlamydial infection in both prostate and epididymis. (See also section on tuberculosis.)

Treatment consists of antibiotics, usually ceftriaxone and doxycycline in males under age 35 and fluoroquinolones in those over age 35. In some patients, pain is relieved by scrotal hypothermia, and consideration should be given to infiltration of the spermatic cord by 1% bupivacaine. Nonsteroidal anti-inflammatory drugs are recommended to aid in pain relief. In most instances, prompt treatment results in rapid resolution of pain, fever, and swelling. Patients must refrain from exertion for 1-3 weeks.

Exacerbations can be controlled by treating the predisposing factor. Chronic epididymitis rarely resolves completely; it has no consequences except, occasionally in bilateral cases, sterility due to scarring and obstruction of the delicate epididymal tubules. Rarely, epididymectomy is necessary for severe and refractory pain.

TUBERCULOSIS

Tuberculosis is a commonly missed genitourinary infection that should be considered in any case of pyuria without bacteriuria or in any case of urinary tract infection that does not respond to treatment.

Genitourinary tuberculosis is always secondary to pulmonary infection, though in many cases, the primary focus has healed or is quiescent. Infection occurs via the hematogenous route. The kidneys and (less commonly) the prostate are the principal sites of urinary tract involvement, although any part of the genitourinary system can be affected.

Pathology

Renal tuberculosis usually starts as a tuberculoma that gradually enlarges, caseates, and finally ulcerates, breaking into the pelvicaliceal system. Caseation and scarring are the principal pathologic features of renal tuberculosis. In the ureter, tuberculosis usually leads to distal strictures, periureteritis, and mural fibrosis.

In the bladder, the infection is characterized by areas of hyperemia and a coalescent group of tubercles, followed by ulcerations. Bladder wall fibrosis and contraction are the end results.

Urethral involvement in the male is uncommon but, when present, leads to urethral stricture, usually in the bulbous portion. Periurethral abscess and fistula are possible complications.

Genital tuberculosis may involve the prostate, seminal vesicles, and epididymides, either separately or in association with renal involvement. Tubercle formation with later caseation and fibrosis is the basic pathologic feature. The prostate becomes enlarged, with palpable nodules and an irregular consistency. The affected seminal vesicle is fibrotic and distended. Induration and thickening of the epididymis and beading of the vas deferens are characteristic findings. The testicles are rarely involved.

Clinical Findings

A. Symptoms and Signs

The patient commonly presents with lower urinary tract irritation, usually with pyuria. Less common manifestations are hematuria, renal pain, and renal colic.

B. Laboratory Findings

"Sterile" pyuria is the rule, but 15% of cases have secondary bacterial infection (eg, E coli). Mycobacteria can be identified on an acid-fast stain of the centrifuged sediment of the first morning urine collected on 3 successive days (positive in 90% of cases). Culture of the sediment should yield the mycobacteria, which may then be speciated by niacin and nitrate tests, both of which must be positive for a diagnosis of Mycobacterium tuberculosis.

C. Imaging Studies

Radiologic findings that suggest genitourinary tuberculosis include moth-eaten, caseous renal cavities or bizarre, irregular calices. Strictures in straight, rigid, moderately dilated

ureters and a contracted bladder with vesicoureteral reflux are all suggestive evidence.

Treatment

A. Medical Treatment

Tuberculosis must be treated as a systemic disease. Once the diagnosis is established, medical treatment is indicated regardless of the need for surgery. Whenever possible, medical treatment should be continued for at least 3 months before surgery is considered.

Active medications against tuberculosis include rifampin, isoniazid, pyrazinamide, ethambutol, and streptomycin. Standard initial treatment is with rifampin, isoniazid, and pyrazinamide for 8 weeks. Pyridoxine, 100 mg/d, is given in divided doses to counteract the vitamin B_6 depletion effect of isoniazid. In patients with more severe infections, ethambutol or streptomycin may be added to the initial treatment. Following the initial 8 weeks of therapy, rifampin and isoniazid are continued in combination three times per week for another 8 weeks. Liver function tests must be followed in view of the hepatotoxicity of rifampin, isoniazid, and pyrazinamide.

B. Surgical Measures

If medical therapy fails to cure a unilateral lesion, nephrectomy may be necessary. However, this is rare. In bilateral disease that has seriously damaged one kidney and is in an early stage in the other, unilateral nephrectomy may be considered; in localized polar lesions, partial nephrectomy may be done.

In unilateral epididymal involvement, epididymectomy plus contralateral vasectomy is indicated to prevent descent of the infection to the prostate; bilateral epididymectomy should be done if both sides are involved.

For a severely contracted bladder, augmentation enterocystoplasty increases vesical capacity following eradication of the infection.

Prognosis

In a high percentage of cases, cure is obtained by medical means. Unilateral renal lesions have the best prognosis.

CALCULI

RENAL STONE

General Considerations

Stone disease is common, with the lifetime risk of stone formation in the United States exceeding 12% in males and 6% in females. Prevalence of stone disease varies by racial background and geographic location within the United States, with older white males and southeastern states having the highest prevalence. Seventy-five percent of most stones are composed of calcium salts (oxalate, phosphate), while uric acid and struvite stones (magnesium-ammonium phosphate stones that form secondary to urea-splitting organisms) constitute 10% each. Formation of calcium stones can be due to one or multiple factors that include hypercalciuria, hypocitraturia, hyperoxaluria, and hyperuricosuria. In patients with hyperparathyroidism or those who ingest large amounts of calcium or vitamin D or in patients who are dehydrated or immobilized, hypercalciuria promotes stone formation.

Uric acid stones form in acidic urine. Cystine stones, which make up 1% of all stones, usually form secondary to impaired renal reabsorption of cystine. Owing to the radiodensity of sulfur, cystine stones are radiopaque (albeit less so than calcium stones), whereas uric acid stones are radiolucent. Stones that obstruct the ureteropelvic junction or ureter lead to hydronephrosis and possibly infection.

▶ Clinical Findings

A. Symptoms and Signs

If the stone acutely obstructs the ureteropelvic junction or a calix, moderate to severe renal pain is noted, often accompanied by nausea, vomiting, and ileus. The pain starts in the upper lateral back and may radiate anteriorly and inferiorly toward the groin. Gross or microscopic hematuria is common. Symptoms of infection, if present, are exacerbated. Nonobstructing calculi are usually painless. This includes staghorn calculi, which may form a cast of all calices and the pelvis. In the symptomatic patient, there may be costovertebral angle tenderness and a quiet abdomen. Infection secondary to obstruction may lead to high fever and a rigid abdomen.

B. Laboratory Findings

With acute infection, leukocytosis is to be expected. Urinalysis may reveal red and white blood cells and bacteria. A pH of 7.6 or higher implies the presence of urea-splitting organisms. A pH consistently below 5.5 is compatible with the formation of uric acid or cystine stones. If the pH is fixed between 6.0 and 7.0, renal tubular acidosis should be considered as a cause of nephrocalcinosis. Crystals of uric acid (rhomboid) or cystine (hexagonal) in the urine are suggestive. A 24-hour urine collection can help identify the metabolic effect that predisposes to stone formation (hypercalciuria, hypocitraturia, hyperoxaluria). Hypercalciuria can be resorptive (due to hyperparathyroidism), absorptive (increased gastrointestinal absorption), or renal (increased urine loss of calcium). Citrate is a stone inhibitor, and hypocitraturia predisposes to stone formation.

Increases in urine calcium and phosphate plus hypercalcemia (and hypophosphatemia) suggest the presence of

hyperparathyroidism, and measurement of serum parathyroid hormone is helpful. Excessive urinary uric acid is compatible with uric acid stone formation.

. A qualitative test for urinary cystine should be part of the routine evaluation. If levels are elevated, a 24-hour quantitative measurement should be made. Hyperchloremic acidosis suggests distal renal tubular acidosis with secondary renal calcifications. Total renal function is impaired only if the stones are bilateral and particularly if chronic infection complicates the clinical presentation.

C. Imaging Studies

About 90% of calculi are radiopaque; the majority are calcium stones and can be seen on plain x-ray. However, stones smaller than 5 mm can be difficult to see on plain x-ray, and bowel gas may obscure stone visualization as well.

Renal ultrasound can be an excellent initial and follow-up imaging modality to identify renal calculi, although results depend on the quality of the sonographer. Stones are hyperechoic and cast an acoustic shadow. Small stones can be missed on ultrasound, and sizing estimates can be poor. Hydronephrosis implies a downstream obstruction in the ureter, possibly from obstructing calculus, but ureteral stones are poorly visualized with ultrasound.

Spiral (helical) CT has become the study of choice, because the entire urinary tract can be scanned rapidly and without contrast injection (Figure 40–10). Calculi can be readily

▲ **Figure 40–10.** Computed tomography scan without intravenous contrast demonstrating a left renal calculus (arrow).

identified and distinguished from clot or tumor. Stones are accurately sized and localized with CT, and the anatomic detail is very helpful prior to operative intervention. CT scans deliver significant doses of ionizing radiation, making ultrasound an attractive initial modality to look for stones or obstruction, followed by CT for confirmation and more anatomic detail.

D. Stone Analysis

If a stone has previously been passed or if one is recovered, its chemical composition should be analyzed. Such information may be useful when planning a preventive program.

▶ Differential Diagnosis

Acute pyelonephritis may begin with acute renal pain mimicking that of renal stone. Urinalysis reveals pyuria, and urograms or CT fails to reveal a calculus.

Renal adenocarcinoma may bleed into the tumor, causing acute pain mimicking that of an obstructing stone. Imaging can make the differentiation.

Transitional cell tumors of the renal pelvis or calices mimic uric acid stone; both are radiolucent. CT scan without contrast or ultrasound reveals the stone by virtue of increased density compared with adjacent soft tissues.

Renal tuberculosis is complicated by stone formation in 10% of cases. Pyuria without bacteriuria is suggestive. Urography reveals the moth-eaten calices typical of tuberculosis.

Papillary necrosis may cause renal colic if a sloughed papilla obstructs the ureteropelvic junction. Imaging (particularly CT) settles the issue.

Renal infarction may cause renal pain and hematuria. Evidence of a cardiac lesion, nonfunction of the kidney on urography, and exclusion of a calculus help in differentiation. Infarction is confirmed by angiography, radioisotopic renography, or color Doppler ultrasound.

Other conditions to be considered in the differential diagnosis include UPJO, obstruction due to blood clots, ureteral strictures or fungal bezoars, and renal abscess.

▶ Complications

Acting as a foreign body, a stone increases the probability of infection. However, primary infection may incite stone formation. A stone lodged in the ureteropelvic junction leads to progressive hydronephrosis. A staghorn calculus, as it grows, may destroy renal tissue by pressure, and the infection that is usually present also contributes to renal damage. The presence of an obstructed renal unit with associated infection should be considered a urologic emergency. Drainage of the kidney should be performed promptly with insertion of a ureteral stent or percutaneous nephrostomy tube. Obstruction without infection can be managed without immediate drainage if renal function is preserved and pain is controlled (see later ureteral calculi section). Persistent obstruction for longer than 2-4 weeks requires intervention because permanent renal damage can ensue.

▶ Prevention

An effective preventive regimen depends on stone analysis and chemical studies of the serum and urine.

A. General Measures

Ensure a high fluid intake (3-4 L/d) to keep solutes well diluted. This measure alone may decrease stone-forming potential by 50%. Treat infection, relieve stasis or obstruction, and advise the patient to avoid prolonged immobilization.

B. Specific Measures

1. Calcium stones—Remove the parathyroid tumor, if present. High dietary sodium promotes renal calcium absorption, and restriction to 100 mEq/d may be helpful. Limitation of proteins and carbohydrates may also reduce hypercalciuria. Recent randomized trials have shown that in men with recurrent calcium oxalate stones and hypercalciuria, restricted intake of animal protein and salt, combined with a normal calcium intake, provides greater protection than the traditional low-calcium diet. Potassium citrate can decrease stone formation by increasing urine levels of citrate, which is a stone inhibitor.

Oral orthophosphates are effective in reducing the stone-forming potential of urine by decreasing urine calcium and increasing inhibitor activity. Thiazide diuretics such as hydrochlorothiazide, 50 mg twice daily, decrease the calcium content in urine by 50%. If hyperuricosuria is coincident with calcium urolithiasis, then allopurinol and urinary alkalinization can reduce the formation of urate crystals, which may act as a nidus for calcium crystallization.

For a patient with primary absorptive hypercalciuria, cellulose sodium phosphate can be given. This substance combines with calcium in the gut to prevent absorption.

2. Oxalate stones (calcium oxalate)—Consider a phosphate or a thiazide diuretic (see earlier). Elimination of excessive oxalate in coffee, tea, colas, leafy green vegetables, and chocolate may also be helpful. Excess vitamin C can be metabolized to oxalate and thus should be avoided.

3. Magnesium-ammonium-phosphate stones—These stones are usually secondary to urinary tract infection due to bacteria that produce urease (primarily *Proteus* species). Eradication of the infection prevents further stone formation but is impossible when stones are present. Acetohydroxamic acid, a urease inhibitor, can be used for oral chemolysis and can potentiate antibiotic action. After all calculi have been removed, prevention of stone growth is best accomplished by urinary acidification and suppression antibiotic therapy.

4. Metabolic stones (uric acid, cystine)—These substances are most soluble at a pH of 7.0 or higher. Give potassium citrate, 10-20 mEq by mouth three times a day, and monitor the urine pH with a litmus paper indicator or urine dipstick test. For uric acid stone formers, limit purines in the diet and give allopurinol if they have hyperuricemia. Patients with mild cystinuria may need only urinary alkalinization, as described previously. For severe cystinuria, penicillamine, 30 mg/kg/d orally, reduces urinary cystine to safe levels. Penicillamine should be supplemented with pyridoxine, 50 mg/d orally. Tiopronin, which has fewer side effects than D-penicillamine and captopril, can be used as well.

▶ Treatment

A. Conservative Measures

Intervention is not required for small, nonobstructive, asymptomatic caliceal stones. Hydration and dietary management may be sufficient to prevent growth of existing or new calcium stones in patients without metabolic abnormalities. Those with identifiable metabolic disorders may benefit from the specific measures described previously. Patients with known uric acid stones can be treated with hydration and urinary alkalinization, which can help dissolve the stone. Patients with active infection, obstruction, or intractable nausea or pain may need definitive treatment. In the acute setting, a ureteral stent or percutaneous nephrostomy tube can be inserted.

B. Ureteroscopic Intervention

Patients with small stones can be managed with ureteronephroscopy and laser lithotripsy or basketing of the stones. The presence of a ureteral stent several days prior helps passively dilate the ureter and facilitates the procedure, but new, smaller caliber ureterscopes preclude the need for elective preoperative stenting. As described earlier, stents should be placed emergently in the setting of infection/sepsis with obstructing calculus. After stenting and an appropriate course of antibiotics (typically 10-14 days), the definitive stone surgery is undertaken. Postoperatively, a ureteral stent is often left in place for several days to prevent acute obstruction secondary to edema or small stone fragments.

C. Percutaneous Intervention (Endourology)

In selected patients with symptomatic or large upper tract stones, percutaneous stone removal may be indicated. A percutaneous tract enters the renal collecting system through an appropriate calix (**percutaneous nephrostomy**). The tract is subsequently dilated, and endoscopic extraction of the stones (**percutaneous nephroscopy** and **percutaneous nephrolithotomy**) is done. Pulverization of the fragments is accomplished by means of ultrasonic, electrohydraulic, or laser probes passed through the nephrostomy tract.

For cystine and uric acid stones, alkaline or other irrigants that increase the specific crystal solubility may be used (eg, *N*-acetyl-L-lysine or propionyl glycine for cystine stones). Specific antibiotic treatment for infection must be given before irrigation to prevent sepsis.

Success with these endourologic methods approaches 100%. The advantages over surgical procedures include no incision and rapid recovery and return to full activity. Disadvantages include the occasional need for multiple treatments to completely remove the calculi and the uncommon occurrence of significant hemorrhage, collecting system perforation, or stricture.

C. Extracorporeal Shock Wave Lithotripsy

With this technique, patients are positioned in the path of shock waves focused on the renal calculi with the aid of fluoroscopy or ultrasound. General or regional anesthesia is required in selected patients, but sedation may be sufficient. The shock waves (>1500 are usually given) pulverize the stones, and the small particles pass spontaneously in the postoperative period. With appropriate patient selection, results are excellent. Lower pole renal stones have lower success rates because pulverized fragments are less likely to completely pass. In addition, stones greater than 1.5 cm may produce too many fragments to successfully pass. Percutaneous nephrolithotomy is the treatment of choice for larger stones greater than 1.5-2.0 cm. Calcium stones and magnesium-ammonium-phosphate stones have been treated successfully. Because of the physical properties of the crystal lattice, extracorporeal shock wave lithotripsy (ESWL) is not as effective in fragmenting cystine stones. Radiolucent uric acid stones, which can be visualized using contrast medium are amenable to ESWL treatment. A variety of ESWL devices now effectively pulverize stones using less energy and thus can be used with only intravenous sedation; an increased number of pulses are required to obtain the same results as with previous higher-energy devices. Some instruments use ultrasound instead of x-ray for stone localization. Complications include incomplete fragmentation and need for secondary procedures, ureteral obstruction from stone fragments, and perinephric hematoma.

D. Open and Laparoscopic Surgical Removal of Stones

Endourologic intervention and ESWL have markedly decreased the indications for open surgery. Rarely, both percutaneous nephrolithotomy and ESWL are contraindicated, and open nephrolithotomy is necessary. The goal of any approach is to remove all stone fragments, and the approach chosen must allow for intraoperative localization by radiography or ultrasonography. Incisions into the renal pelvis (pyelolithotomy) or the renal parenchyma (radial nephrotomy or anatrophic nephrolithotomy) may be required for complete stone removal. Instillation of a mixture of thrombin and calcium into the kidney causes the fragments to become trapped in a dense clot, which is removed through a pyelotomy incision (coagulum pyelolithotomy). Operative nephroscopy allows a full view of all the calices and removal of all fragments. "Bench" surgery with autotransplantation of the kidney may be required in very few instances. Rarely, poorly functioning kidneys containing symptomatic stones require nephrectomy, especially in cases of xanthogranulomatous pyelonephritis. Laparoscopic and robotic pyelolithotomy have been used with excellent success and decreased morbidity compared with open surgery. This is especially the case in patients undergoing concomitant robotic pyeloplasty for UPJO.

Prognosis

The recurrence rate of renal stones can be as high as 40% and can be decreased with sufficient attention to measures for prevention of stone formation. The danger of recurrent stones is progressive renal damage due to obstruction and infection.

URETERAL STONE

General Considerations

Ureteral stones originate in the kidney. When symptoms occur, ureteral obstruction is implicit and renal function endangered. Complicating infection may occur. Most ureteral stones pass spontaneously or with the assistance of medical expulsive therapy, especially if they are less than 0.5 cm in greatest dimension.

Clinical Findings

A. Symptoms and Signs

The onset of pain is usually abrupt. Pain is felt in the costovertebral angle and radiates to the ipsilateral lower abdominal quadrant. Nausea, vomiting, abdominal distention, and gross hematuria are common. When the stone approaches the bladder, symptoms mimic cystitis, with frequency and urgency. If the kidney is infected, acute ureteral obstruction exacerbates the infection.

The patient is usually in such agony that only parenteral opioids and nonsteroidal anti-inflammatory drugs will give relief. Costovertebral angle tenderness and guarding may be evident. Absence of bowel sounds and abdominal distention signify ileus. Fever may occur as a result of complicating renal infection.

B. Laboratory Findings

Laboratory findings are similar to those for renal stone. Unilateral obstruction secondary to ureteral stone may cause acute exacerbation of renal function, but not in all cases.

▲ **Figure 40–11.** Computed tomography scan without intravenous contrast demonstrating a left ureteral calculus (arrow).

C. Imaging Studies

CT stone protocol is the gold standard to confirm stone size and location and degree of obstruction (Figure 40–11). Plain films may reveal an opacity in the region of the ureter, and ultrasound will demonstrate ipsilateral hydronephrosis. Excretory urograms and retrograde urography reveal a filling defect (lack of dye) at the location of the stone. Almost all stones are radiopaque on CT scan. The density (hardness) of the stone can be estimated using the Hounsfield units (HU). Calcium-based stones are, on average, greater than 1000 HU. Uric acid and struvite (infection) stones have lower HU.

Differential Diagnosis

A tumor of the kidney or renal pelvis may bleed, and passage of a blood clot may cause ureteral colic. Urograms may reveal a radiolucent area in the ureter surrounded by the radiopaque urine. A CT scan with and without contrast agents reveals no radiopacity in the ureter and helps define the renal parenchymal or renal pelvis tumor.

A primary tumor of the ureter may cause obstructing pain and hematuria. The urogram reveals the ureteral filling defect, often with secondary obstruction. A CT scan can differentiate a stone from tumor. Urinary cytologic study may reveal malignant urothelial cells.

Acute pyelonephritis may cause pain as severe as that seen with stone. Pyuria and bacteriuria are found but do not rule out stone. Stone is absent on noncontrast CT or urography.

A sloughed papilla (consequent to conditions such as diabetes mellitus) traversing the ureter may cause colic and produces a urogram compatible with uric acid stone. Papillary sloughs should be evident, however.

Complications

If obstruction from the ureteral stone is prolonged, progressive renal damage may ensue. Bilateral stones may cause oliguria or anuria, requiring immediate drainage of the proximal collecting system with indwelling ureteral stents or percutaneous nephrostomy. A unilateral obstructing stone in patients with a solitary kidney requires immediate drainage.

Infection may supervene, but many renal infections are iatrogenic (ie, introduced at the time of stone manipulation).

Prevention

See section on renal stones.

Treatment

A. General Measures

Most ureteral stones pass spontaneously—particularly those less than 0.5 cm in diameter. Once the diagnosis has been established, analgesics should be given and the patient hydrated. Recent reports have found alpha-antagonist therapy useful in expulsion of distal ureteral stones by relaxing smooth muscle. Randomized controlled trials have confirmed shorter time to stone passage with the use of alpha-antagonists when compared with placebo. Periodic plain films should be taken to follow the progress of the stone, and interval renal ultrasound studies should be obtained to assess the degree of hydronephrosis. The urine should be strained until the stone passes in order to recover the calculus for analysis. With larger stones, acute obstruction can be temporarily relieved by inserting an indwelling ureteral stent.

B. Specific Measures

If the stone causes intractable pain, progressive hydronephrosis, or acute infection, it should be removed. Obstructing stones in the upper two-thirds of the ureter can often be successfully treated by ureteroscopy or ESWL, with or without ureteral stent insertion to help facilitate stone passage. Ureteroscopy permits laser fragmentation or stone basket retrieval under direct vision. Open and laparoscopic/robotic surgical removal (ureterolithotomy) is only very rarely required for very large ureteral stones. ESWL has been applied to ureteral stones in the proximal ureter but is more problematic in the distal ureter owing to bone interference by surrounding pelvis, which interferes with imaging and attenuates shock wave force. Ureteral stones that have not spontaneously passed with medical expulsive therapy after

4 weeks should be considered for surgical removal with the above techniques.

Prognosis

About 80% of ureteral stones pass spontaneously. Stones larger than 1 cm rarely pass spontaneously. Periodic clinical evaluation, plain films, and renal ultrasound should be performed to document ureteral stone passage and prevent long-term renal damage from obstruction. Patients often do not witness small stones pass if a strainer is not used. If still uncertain about definitive stone passage, repeat CT scan can be obtained with the caveat of additional radiation exposure.

VESICAL STONE

Primary vesical calculi are rare in the United States but are common in Southeast Asia and the Middle East. The cause is probably dietary. Secondary stones usually complicate vesical outlet obstruction with residual urine and infection; 90% of those affected are men. Other causes of bladder stasis such as neurogenic bladder and bladder diverticula also promote vesical stone formation. They are common in vesical schistosomiasis or in association with radiation cystitis. Foreign bodies in the bladder may act as a nidus for the precipitation of urinary salts. Most stones contain uric acid or struvite (in infected urine).

Clinical Findings

A. Symptoms and Signs

Symptoms of bladder neck obstruction are elicited. There may be sudden interruption of the stream and urethral pain if a stone occludes the bladder neck during voiding. Hematuria is common. Vesical distention may be noted; evidence of urethral stricture or an enlarged prostate is usually found.

B. Laboratory Findings

Pyuria and hematuria are almost always present.

C. Imaging Studies

Vesical calculi may be missed on plain x-rays due to the high component of radiolucent uric acid. Excretory urograms reveal a filling defect in the bladder, and ultrasound reveals a large echogenic shadowing focus. CT scan easily identifies the number and size of the stones. Cystoscopy directly visualizes the stone(s) and also evaluates the entire urethra for stricture and/or prostate hypertrophy.

Differential Diagnosis

A pedunculated vesical tumor may suddenly occlude the vesical neck during voiding. Excretory urograms, pelvic ultrasound, CT scan, or cystoscopy leads to definitive diagnosis.

Extravesical opacifications may simulate stones on a plain film.

Complications

Acting as foreign bodies, bladder stones exacerbate urine infection and can cause obstruction at the level of the bladder neck. Antibiotic therapy for concomitant urinary tract infection is often unsuccessful given that the stones harbor persistent bacteria.

Prevention

Prevention requires relief of the primary obstruction, removal of the stones, and sterilization of the urine.

Treatment

A. General Measures

Analgesics should be given for pain and antimicrobials for control of infection until the stones can be removed.

B. Specific Measure

Small stones can be removed or crushed transurethrally (**cystolithalopaxy**). Larger stones are often disintegrated by transurethral electrohydraulic lithotripsy (shock wave–generating probe) or laser destruction, or they may require suprapubic transvesical removal (vesicolithotomy). If the nidus for stone formation is urinary stasis due to BPH, concomitant TURP or suprapubic transvesical prostatectomy should be performed at the time of stone removal.

Prognosis

Recurrent vesical stone is uncommon if the obstruction and infection are treated.

NEPHROCALCINOSIS

Nephrocalcinosis is the precipitation of calcium in the tubules, parenchyma, and, occasionally, the glomeruli. It always causes renal functional impairment, often severe. Stones may be found in the calices and pelvis. The common causes are primary or secondary hyperparathyroidism or excessive milk-alkali or vitamin D intake, or they may be found with severe renal damage associated with renal tubular acidosis or sarcoidosis. Calcifications may also be seen in the skin, lungs, stomach, spleen, and corneas, or around the joints.

Clinical Findings

A. Symptoms and Signs

There are no specific symptoms. In childhood, the patient may merely fail to thrive. Stones or sand may be passed. The complaints are usually those of the primary disease. Physical examination may reveal an enlarged parathyroid gland, corneal calcifications, and pseudorickets.

B. Laboratory Findings

The urine may be infected. In renal tubular acidosis, the pH is fixed between 6.0 and 7.0. Urinary calcium is high in hyperparathyroidism, both primary and secondary. Tests of renal function are depressed; uremia is common. Hypercalcemia and hypophosphatemia are seen with primary hyperparathyroidism; secondary hyperparathyroidism may be associated with a low serum calcium and an elevated serum phosphate. Hyperchloremic acidosis and hypokalemia accompany renal tubular acidosis.

C. Imaging Studies

A plain x-ray reveals punctate calcifications in the papillae of the kidneys. Caliceal or pelvic stones may also be noted. The pattern of calcification may have to be differentiated from renal tuberculosis and medullary sponge kidney.

Complications

Complications include renal damage caused by the calcifications and renal and ureteral calculi. Chronic renal infection may complicate the primary disease.

Treatment & Prognosis

The primary cause should be treated if possible (eg, parathyroidectomy). Hydration with isotonic saline along with furosemide can help enhance calcium excretion. Discontinue vitamin D and milk-alkali producers if the primary cause was due to excessive intake. With hyperchloremic acidosis, alkalinize the urine with potassium citrate. Osteomalacia requires administration of vitamin D and calcium even though nephrocalcinosis is present.

If nephrocalcinosis is secondary to primary renal disease, the outlook is poor. If the cause is correctable and renal function is fairly good, the prognosis is more favorable.

Geraghty RM, Jones P, Herrmann TRW, et al: Ureteroscopy is more cost effective than shock wave lithotripsy for stone treatment: systematic review and meta-analysis. *World J Urol.* 2018;36(11):1783-1793.

Ordonez M, Hwang EC, Borofsky M, et al: Ureteral stent versus no ureteral stent for ureteroscopy in the management of renal and ureteral calculi. *Cochrane Database Syst Rev.* 2019;2:CD012703.

▼ GENITOURINARY TRACT TRAUMA

INJURIES TO THE KIDNEY

▶ General Considerations

Renal injury is uncommon but potentially serious and often accompanied by multisystem trauma. The most common causes are athletic, industrial, or automobile accidents. The degree of injury may range from contusion to laceration of the parenchyma or disruption of the renal pedicle.

▶ Clinical Findings

A. Symptoms and Signs

Gross hematuria following trauma means injury to the urinary tract. Pain and tenderness over the renal area may be significant but could be due to musculoskeletal injury. Hemorrhagic shock may result from renal laceration and lead to oliguria. Nausea, vomiting, and abdominal distention (ileus) are the rule. Physical examination may reveal ecchymosis or penetrating injury in the costovertebral angle or flank. Extravasation of blood or urine may produce a palpable flank mass. Other injuries should be sought.

B. Laboratory Findings

Serial hematocrit determinations will give clues to persistent bleeding. Hematuria is to be expected, but the absence of hematuria does not exclude renal injury (as in renal vascular injury).

C. Imaging Studies

A plain film may reveal obliteration of the psoas shadow; this suggests the presence of a retroperitoneal hematoma or urinary extravasation. Bowel gas may be displaced from the area. Evidence of transverse vertebral process or rib fractures may be noted. In the past, the excretory urogram was used for evaluating renal trauma. Excretory urograms may show a normal kidney if it is mildly contused or may show extravasation of contrast medium if the kidney is lacerated. Nonfunction suggests injury to the vascular pedicle. The excretory urogram should demonstrate that the contralateral kidney is normal. CT scan with intravenous contrast medium is now the method of choice for staging a patient with hemodynamically stable renal trauma. CT scans may miss urinary extravasation if performed too rapidly following intravenous contrast administration—before the contrast is excreted into the collecting system and ureter. Therefore, trauma protocol CT scans should include a delayed phase of imaging, allowing time for contrast to be excreted into the collecting system. If renal vascular damage is suspected and

the patient's condition is stable, preoperative renal angiography may facilitate planning of renovascular reconstruction or permit arterial stenting. In special circumstances, selective renal artery embolization may control segmental arterial bleeding. Renal imaging is indicated in any adult with gross hematuria or microscopic hematuria with shock. Imaging is also required with deceleration injuries and is indicated in children with gross or microscopic hematuria in the setting of trauma.

▶ Differential Diagnosis

Bony fractures or contusion of soft tissues in the region of the kidney may cause confusion. Hematuria might be secondary to ureteral or vesical injury. The absence of a perirenal mass (ie, hematoma or urinoma) or contrast extravasation on urograms or CT scan would rule out significant trauma.

▶ Complications

A. Early

The most serious complication is continued perirenal hemorrhage, which may be fatal. Serial hematocrit, blood pressure, and pulse determinations are essential. Serial CT scans may also be useful. Evidence of an enlarging flank mass implies persistent bleeding. In most cases, bleeding stops spontaneously, probably as a result of tamponade by the perirenal fascia. Delayed bleeding 1-2 weeks later is rare. Infection of the perirenal hematoma may occur.

B. Late

History, examination, and imaging are recommended 1-3 months after management of renal trauma to look for persistent renal damage from prolonged perinephric hematoma, obstruction, and/or urinary extravasation. Ultrasound is a good imaging modality to evaluate the integrity of the kidney and to assess for residual perinephric fluid collections and/or hydronephrosis. The blood pressure should be checked at regular intervals, because hypertension may be a late sequela.

▶ Treatment

Treat shock and hemorrhage with fluids and transfusion. Most patients with blunt renal trauma stop bleeding and heal spontaneously. Bed rest is indicated until hematuria resolves and blood counts stabilize. If bleeding persists, angiography with possible segmental arterial embolization is an option if the patient is hemodynamically stable. Persistent hemodynamic instability requires laparotomy with renorrhaphy or nephrectomy.

Penetrating renal trauma usually requires exploration. Lacerations may be sutured, the collecting system closed, and urinary extravasation drained. Nephrectomy or partial nephrectomy may be necessary to remove devitalized tissue and secure the collecting system.

Late complications may occur. Perinephric abscess/infected hematoma should be drained. Hypertension may be due to renal ischemia and requires medical or surgical correction.

Prognosis

Most injured kidneys heal spontaneously, although the patient must be examined at intervals for the onset of hypertension due to renal ischemia or progressive hydronephrosis due to secondary ureteral stricture. Many patients with genitourinary trauma have associated injuries. In most cases, death is due to associated injury rather than renal injury.

INJURIES TO THE URETER

General Considerations

Most ureteral injuries are iatrogenic in the course of pelvic surgery. Ureteral injury may occur during transurethral bladder or prostate resection or ureteral manipulation for stone or tumor. Ureteral injury is rarely a consequence of penetrating trauma. Unintentional ureteral ligation during operation on adjacent organs may be asymptomatic, although hydronephrosis and loss of renal function results. Ureteral division leads to extravasation and urinoma.

Clinical Findings

A. Symptoms

If the ureteral injury is not recognized at surgery, the patient may complain of flank and lower abdominal pain on the injured side. Ileus and pyelonephritis may develop. Later, urine may drain through the wound (or through the vagina following transvaginal surgery), or there may be increased output through a surgical drain. Wound drainage may be evaluated by comparing creatinine levels found in the drainage fluid with serum levels: Urine exhibits very high creatinine levels when compared with serum. Intravenous administration of 5 mL of indigo carmine causes the urine to appear blue-green; therefore, drainage from a ureterocutaneous fistula becomes blue, compared to serous drainage. Anuria following pelvic surgery not responding to intravenous fluids may rarely signify bilateral ureteral ligation or injury. Peritoneal signs may occur if urine leaks into the peritoneal cavity.

B. Laboratory Findings

Microscopic hematuria is usually found but may be absent. Tests of renal function may be normal unless both ureters are occluded. Drainage fluid will have increased levels of creatinine when compared with serum creatinine.

C. Imaging Studies

Excretory urograms may show evidence of ureteral occlusion. Extravasation of radiopaque fluid may be seen in the region of the ureter. Retrograde ureterography depicts the site and nature (occlusion or division) of the injury.

Ultrasonography may reveal hydroureter and hydronephrosis or a fluid mass representing urinary extravasation. CT urography (including delayed phase imaging) identifies the location of the ureteral injury, surrounding urinary extravasation, and potential urinoma or fistula.

Differential Diagnosis

Ureteral injury may mimic peritonitis if urine leaks into the peritoneal cavity. Excretory urography reveals the ureteral involvement.

Oliguria may be due to dehydration, transfusion reaction, or bilateral incomplete ureteral injury. A survey of fluid and electrolyte intake and output, including serial body weights, should prove helpful in delineating a medical versus surgical etiology for oliguria. Nephrology consultation should be considered. Total anuria may signify bilateral ureteral injury and indicates the need for immediate urologic evaluation.

Vesicovaginal and ureterovaginal fistulas may be confused. Methylene blue solution instilled into the bladder stains the vaginal drainage in the case of vesicovaginal fistula. Cystoscopy may show the vesical defect. Retrograde ureterography should reveal a ureteral fistula. The presence of both injuries occurring simultaneously should also be considered and evaluated.

Complications

These include urinary fistula, ureteral obstruction or stenosis with hydronephrosis, renal infection, peritonitis, and uremia (with bilateral injury).

Prevention

Before operation for large pelvic masses, which may cause displacement of the ureters, catheters should be placed in the ureters to facilitate their identification at surgery. Although the catheters may not prevent injury, they facilitate recognition of a ureteral injury intraoperatively and allow for immediate repair.

Treatment

A. Injury Recognized at Surgery

1. Ureteral division—Repair of a ureter inadvertently cut during surgery consists of anastomosis of the ends over an indwelling stent (**ureteroureterostomy**), reimplanting the ureter into the bladder if the injury is juxtavesical (**neoureterocystostomy**), or anastomosing the proximal segment of divided ureter to the side of the contralateral ureter (**transureteroureterostomy**). The anastomosis must be tension free, and the area of repair must be drained. Injuries resulting from cautery must be adequately debrided prior to reanastomosis.

2. Ureteral resection—Repair of a ureter from which a substantial segment has been removed requires interposition of a ureteral substitute or mobilization of the proximal and distal ureter to provide a tension-free anastomosis. With loss of the distal ureter, the bladder may be hitched cephalad to the psoas muscle, or a bladder flap may be created to facilitate a ureteral implant. In extreme cases, autotransplant of the kidney to the pelvis or bowel interposition may be necessary.

B. Injury Discovered After Surgery

Early intervention is recommended as soon as the ureteral injury is recognized. Depending on the findings, any of the procedures noted earlier may be used. If a long segment of ureter is not viable, an intestinal ureter may be constructed. If hydronephrosis is advanced or if sepsis develops, percutaneous nephrostomy should precede repair. When the patient's condition is stable, definitive repair can be accomplished. If the injury is partial or incomplete, attempted ureteral stent placement for 4-6 weeks followed by repeat evaluation may obviate the need for laparotomy and open repair. Delayed nephrectomy may be indicated if the repair is unsuccessful and the contralateral kidney is normal.

▶ Prognosis

In cases of iatrogenic injury, the results are best if the injury is recognized at the time of surgery. Late repair, if severe periureteral fibrosis has developed, is less likely to afford a good outcome.

INJURIES TO THE BLADDER

▶ General Considerations

The most common cause of vesical injury is an external blow over a full bladder. Rupture of the organ is seen in 15% of patients with pelvic fracture. The bladder may be inadvertently opened during pelvic surgery or injured by cystoscopic maneuvers (eg, transurethral resection of bladder tumor). If the injury is intraperitoneal (40% of all bladder ruptures), blood and urine will extravasate into the peritoneal cavity, producing signs of peritonitis. If it is extraperitoneal (54% of all bladder ruptures), a mass develops in the pelvis. About 6% of all bladder ruptures have a combination of both intraperitoneal and extraperitoneal extravasation.

▶ Clinical Findings

A. Symptoms and Signs

There is usually a history of hypogastric or pelvic trauma. Hematuria and suprapubic pain and possible inability to void are expected. Associated injury may cause hemorrhagic shock. There is suprapubic tenderness and guarding. Intraperitoneal extravasation causes peritoneal signs, whereas extraperitoneal extravasation results in formation of a pelvic urinoma.

B. Laboratory Findings

A falling hematocrit reflects continued bleeding. Hematuria is expected in patients who are able to void. A patient who cannot void should be catheterized unless pelvic fracture (and urethral injury) is suspected or blood is noted at the urethral meatus.

C. Imaging Studies

A plain film may reveal fracture of the pelvis. An extraperitoneal collection of blood and urine may displace the bowel gas laterally or out of the pelvis. If bladder trauma is suspected, cystography should precede excretory urography. Extravasation is most reliably demonstrated by a postdrainage cystogram film showing persistent contrast outside the area of the suspected bladder. If one suspects urethral trauma, a retrograde urethrogram should precede catheter insertion. The excretory urogram may suggest the diagnosis of bladder perforation but by itself is insufficient to exclude bladder injury. A CT cystogram is diagnostic for bladder injury and urinary extravasation. It also reliably distinguishes between intra- and extraperitoneal injury. A catheter is placed, the bladder is filled by gravity with diluted contrast (350-400 mL), and subsequently, the CT scan is performed.

▶ Differential Diagnosis

Renal injury is also associated with bladder trauma and usually presents with hematuria. Imaging shows changes compatible with renal trauma; the cystogram is negative.

Injury to the membranous urethra can mimic extraperitoneal rupture of the bladder. A urethrogram reveals the site of injury. Urethral disruption is a contraindication to urethral catheterization.

▶ Complications

Extraperitoneal extravasation may lead to pelvic abscess. Intraperitoneal extravasation causes delayed peritonitis, oliguria, and azotemia.

▶ Treatment

Treat shock, hemorrhage, and other life-threatening injuries. Marked extraperitoneal extravasation should be drained, the bladder decompressed by either a suprapubic or urethral catheter, and appropriate antibiotics administered. Small extraperitoneal extravasations are treated nonoperatively by urethral catheter.

Intraperitoneal extravasation of bladder urine requires exploratory laparotomy, midline cystotomy, bladder closure, and bladder catheter drainage. Penetrating injuries (ie, gunshot, stabbing) require exploration, with or without debridement, and closure of the bladder. The ureters should also be evaluated in all cases of bladder injury by preoperative imaging or intraoperative assessment, which may be done by injecting indigo carmine and looking for ureteral extravasation or by retrograde passage of 5F feeding tubes through the ureteral orifice. A closed surgical drain is left in place.

Prognosis

Early diagnosis minimizes morbidity and mortality rates. The prognosis depends chiefly on the severity of associated injuries.

INJURIES TO THE URETHRA

Membranous Urethra

Injury to the membranous urethra is usually a consequence of pelvic fracture and thus is associated with hemorrhage and multiorgan injury. The mechanism of injury is blunt trauma and deceleration resulting in shearing forces applied to the prostate and urogenital diaphragm. Penetrating injuries result from external missiles or laceration by bone fragments acting as secondary projectiles.

If the urethral disruption is incomplete, the patient may be able to void, and hematuria would be inevitable. Urethral injury is suspected if blood is expressed from the urethral meatus. In cases of complete avulsion, extravasation causes a suprapubic mass. Rectal examination may reveal a nonpalpable or upwardly displaced prostate.

X-ray reveals a fractured pelvis; urethrography delineates any extravasation, and cystography identifies an associated bladder injury. An immediate excretory urogram or CT scan should be obtained in all cases to assess kidney and ureteral function.

Treatment must be coordinated with care of associated injury. Once a membranous urethral injury with urinary extravasation has been identified, suprapubic cystostomy should be performed either at the time of laparotomy or percutaneously before placement of external pelvic fixation. Definitive urethral repair may be delayed until the patient has recovered from the acute injury and pelvic fractures have healed. Occasionally, when urethral disruption is incomplete, late repair is unnecessary. Primary repair may be indicated in cases of severe prostatomembranous dislocation, major bladder neck laceration, or concomitant pelvic vascular or rectal injury.

Late sequelae are urethral stricture, impotence, and incontinence. Urethral stricture must be identified by retrograde urethrography and may be treated by transurethral incision of the stricture or urethroplasty. Impotence due to injury of nerves to the corpora cavernosa that course adjacent to the membranous urethra may resolve without treatment during the year following injury. Vascular injury of the hypogastric or pudendal arteries may cause impotence following trauma. Cavernosometry and arteriography confirm the diagnosis; appropriate treatment may include vascular reconstruction. Incontinence depends on the neurologic status of the patient. Medical or surgical therapy is used to increase bladder capacity and bladder outlet resistance.

Bulbous Urethra

The bulbous urethra may be injured as a result of instrumentation or, more commonly, falling astride an object (straddle injury). Urethral contusion may cause a perineal hematoma without injury to the urethral wall. Laceration leads to urinary extravasation.

Perineal pain and some urethral bleeding are to be expected. Sudden swelling in the perineum may develop following attempted urination. Examination reveals a perineal mass; swelling due to extravasation of blood and urine involves the penis and scrotum and may spread onto the abdominal wall.

If the patient can void well and the perineal hematoma is small, no treatment is necessary. If urethrography reveals significant extravasation, suprapubic cystostomy should be performed. Minor injury without extravasation (contusion, compression by hematoma) may be managed by careful insertion of a urethral catheter.

The only serious complication is stricture, which requires subsequent internal urethrotomy or surgical repair.

Pendulous Urethra

External injury to this portion of the urethra is not common, since the penis is so mobile. The erect organ, however, is vulnerable, and pendulous urethral injury often occurs in conjunction with penile fracture (see later in chapter). Injury during urethral instrumentation (eg, urethral catheter, urethroscopy) is another common etiology.

Urethral bleeding and penile swelling are to be expected. A urethrogram reveals the site and severity of injury.

If voiding is normal, no treatment is required. A large hematoma may require drainage. If significant injury is present, a suprapubic tube should be inserted and delayed surgical repair performed after swelling and inflammation have resolved.

INJURIES TO THE PENIS

Mechanisms of penile injury include penetration, blunt trauma to the erect penis during sexual activity (eg, fracture of corpora cavernosa), avulsion of skin, and amputation.

Tourniquet injury is also uncommon; the circumferential compression may be due to a rubber band, a steel ring, string, or a hair and may be exacerbated by subsequent erection. The tourniquet may have been applied unintentionally, but child abuse cases have been reported in which the penis has been ligated as punishment for enuresis.

Treatment includes assessment and care of urethral injuries if present. Removal of tourniquet, split-thickness skin grafting of avulsion injuries, and primary closure of corporal lacerations are principles of therapy. Penile fracture is considered a urologic emergency, and immediate repair minimizes the inherent risk of future impotence and penile curvature. The penis may be acutely reimplanted up to 16 hours following amputation using microsurgical techniques.

INJURIES TO THE SCROTUM & TESTIS

Avulsion of the scrotal skin may require a meshed split-thickness skin graft. If the avulsion is severe, involving the skin and dartos muscle, then the testes may be implanted in the subcutaneous tissue of the thigh and dressed outside the wound with 0.25% acetic acid–soaked gauze. Scrotal reconstruction is performed at a later time, frequently by using skin grafts.

Penetrating trauma rarely injures the mobile testes. Lacerations should be explored, debrided, and closed primarily. If hemorrhage into the tunica vaginalis is noted, drainage is indicated.

Blunt trauma to the testes may cause contusion or rupture. Rupture of the tunica albuginea may be demonstrated by ultrasonography as abnormal echotexture of the parenchyma. In cases of rupture, scrotal exploration is imperative and allows debridement and closure of the tunica albuginea. The testes may ultimately undergo atrophy despite these efforts.

▼ TUMORS OF THE GENITOURINARY TRACT

Tumors of the genitourinary tract are among the most common neoplastic diseases found in adults. Prostate cancer, for example, is the most common cancer in men (33%), and renal and bladder cancer account for nearly 10% of all malignant tumors in men, but only about 3% in women. Even though excellent diagnostic methods are available, one-third of all genitourinary tumors are not found until regional or distant spread has occurred. Advances in diagnosis and treatment of genitourinary tract tumors have occurred in recent years, and the prognosis has improved in conditions such as Wilms tumor, testicular cancer, and bladder cancer. The mainstay of diagnosis continues to be physical examination, complete urinalysis, CT urography, and cystoscopy whenever indicated. Curative treatment of these tumors continues to be surgical in most instances.

RENAL ADENOCARCINOMA (RENAL CELL CARCINOMA)

▶ General Considerations

Malignant tumors of the kidney account for approximately 3% of all tumors in adults. Often, the diagnosis is found incidentally on ultrasound, CT scan, or MRI. Microscopic or gross hematuria evaluation can also identify renal cell carcinoma (RCC). Advanced or metastatic disease can present with flank mass, weight loss, or pathologic fracture. Risk factors for RCC include cigarette smoking, obesity, and hypertension. The disease occurs in men three times more commonly than in women. A suppressor gene on chromosome 3p has been shown to be present in von Hippel-Lindau renal cancers as well as in most sporadic RCCs. The most common cell type is clear cell (also called conventional) carcinoma, accounting for 70%-80% of renal carcinomas. The cell of origin is in the proximal convoluted tubule. Other cell types include papillary (10%-15%), chromophobe (3%-5%), and collecting duct renal carcinoma (1%). The tumor metastasizes commonly to the lungs (50%-60%), adjacent renal hilar lymph nodes (25%), ipsilateral adrenal (12%), opposite kidney (2%), and lytic lesions in mainly long bones (30%-40%).

Numerous conditions predispose to RCC, including von Hippel-Lindau syndrome (cerebellar hemangioblastomas, retinal angiomatosis, and bilateral RCC), tuberous sclerosis, and acquired renal cystic disease developing in patients with end-stage renal disease. Paraneoplastic syndromes are common in RCC and are often what suggests the diagnosis, yet they rarely have prognostic significance. These syndromes include hypercalcemia, erythrocytosis, hypertension, fever of unknown origin, anemia, and elevated liver enzymes (**Stauffer syndrome**). RCC has a predilection for producing occlusive tumor thrombi in the renal vein and the inferior vena cava (particularly from the right kidney), manifested by signs of lower extremity edema and acute scrotal varicocele when occluding the left renal vein. This phenomenon of inferior vena cava thrombus occurs in approximately 5%-10% of patients. Occasionally, the tumor thrombus reaches up to the right atrium.

▶ Clinical Findings

A. Symptoms and Signs

Painless gross or microscopic hematuria throughout the urinary stream ("total hematuria") occurs in some patients. The degree of hematuria is not necessarily related to the size or stage of the tumor. Although a triad of hematuria, flank pain, and a palpable flank mass suggests RCC, fewer than 10% of patients will so present. Both pain and a palpable mass are late events occurring only with tumors that are very large or invade surrounding structures or when hemorrhage into the tumor has occurred. Symptoms due to metastases may be the initial complaint (eg, bone pain, respiratory distress). Localized disease is often identified incidentally on imaging.

B. Laboratory Findings

Microscopic urinalysis reveals hematuria in most patients. The erythrocyte sedimentation rate may be elevated but is nonspecific. Elevation of the hematocrit and levels of serum calcium, alkaline phosphatase, and aminotransferases occurs in less than 10% of patients. These findings nearly always resolve with curative nephrectomy and thus are not usually signs of metastases. Anemia unrelated to blood loss occurs in 20%-40% of patients, particularly those with advanced disease.

C. Imaging Studies

The diagnosis of RCC is often made by CT (and, less frequently, by intravenous urography) performed as an initial step in the workup of hematuria, an enigmatic metastatic lesion, or suspicious laboratory findings (Figure 40–12). Ultrasonography and CT scan often reveal incidental renal masses, which now account for 50% of the initial diagnoses of RCC in patients without manifestations of renal disease. Plain abdominal x-rays may reveal a calcified renal mass, but only 20% of renal masses contain demonstrable calcification. (Twenty percent of masses with peripheral calcification are malignant; over 80% with central calcification are malignant.) The initial technique for workup of hematuria is currently CT urography, which can accurately identify an enhancing renal mass, which is diagnostic for RCC. CT scan is also helpful in local staging and can reveal tumor penetration of perinephric fat; enlargement of local hilar lymph nodes, indicating metastases; or tumor thrombi in the renal vein or inferior vena cava. CT angiography can delineate the renal vasculature, which is helpful in surgical planning for partial nephrectomies.

Occasionally, some masses detected on CT require further characterization by ultrasound. Abdominal ultrasonography can define the mass as a benign simple cyst or a solid mass in 90%-95% of cases. Abdominal ultrasound can also identify a vena caval tumor thrombus and its cephalad extent in the cava.

MRI is not more accurate than CT and is much more expensive. It is, however, the most accurate noninvasive means of detecting renal vein or vena caval thrombi. With the further refinement of pulse sequencing and the use of paramagnetic contrast agents, MRI has become one of the primary techniques for staging solid renal masses. Magnetic resonance angiography (MRA) has become particularly useful for mapping the blood supply and the relationship to adjacent structures in candidates for partial nephrectomy.

▲ **Figure 40–12. A:** Adenocarcinoma of the left kidney. Computed tomography (CT) scan of the abdomen shows an exophytic lesion from the midpolar kidney (arrow). **B:** CT scan showing a large left renal mass (arrow) incidentally found on imaging done to evaluate nonspecific abdominal pain. Final pathology revealed clear cell renal carcinoma.

D. Other Diagnostic or Staging Techniques

Isotopic bone scanning is useful in patients with bone pain, elevated alkaline phosphatase, or known metastases. Chest x-ray is sufficient if negative, but if equivocal, then CT scan of the chest can be used to detect metastases. Identification of metastatic disease in the thorax warrants consideration of brain imaging to rule out occult disease. There are currently no tumor markers specific for RCC. Occasionally, biopsy of the mass can be useful when imaging is not definitive or when metastases from another primary malignancy are a possibility. Previously, such procedures were discouraged because of fear of disseminating the tumor along the needle tract, but this has proved to be rare, and the technique is safe. False-negative results and insufficient tissue for diagnosis are limitations of renal mass biopsy. Fortunately, imaging is diagnostic in most cases.

Differential Diagnosis

A variety of lesions in the retroperitoneum and kidney other than renal cysts may simulate renal cancer. These include lesions due to hydronephrosis, adult PKD, tuberculosis, xanthogranulomatous pyelonephritis, metastatic cancer from another primary cancer, angiomyolipoma or other benign renal tumors, or adrenal cancer and retroperitoneal lipomas, sarcomas, or abscesses. In general, one or more of the imaging techniques described earlier should make the differentiation. Percutaneous biopsy is necessary in rare instances when imaging cannot make the diagnosis.

Hematuria may be caused by renal, ureteral, or bladder calculi; renal pelvis, ureteral, or bladder tumors; or many other benign conditions usually delineated by the studies described. Cystoscopy is obligatory in hematuric patients with a normal CT scan or intravenous urogram to rule out disease of the bladder and to determine the source of the hematuria.

Complications

Occasionally, patients may present with acute flank pain secondary to hemorrhage within a tumor or colic secondary to obstructing ureteral clots. Tumor in the renal vein or vena cava may cause an acute left varicocele or lower extremity edema associated with proteinuria. Pathologic fractures are due to osteolytic metastases in long bones. Brain metastases can present with seizure or other neurologic symptoms.

Treatment

Staging is the key to designing the treatment plan (Table 40–1). Patients with disease confined within the renal fascia (Gerota's fascia) or limited to nonadherent renal vein or vena caval tumor thrombi (stages T1, T2, and T3a) are best treated by surgical extirpation with either radical nephrectomy or partial nephrectomy. Radical nephrectomy traditionally includes en bloc removal of the kidney and surrounding Gerota's fascia (including the ipsilateral adrenal), the renal hilar lymph nodes, and the proximal half of the ureter. However, adrenal-sparing radical nephrectomy is routinely performed for mid- and lower-pole renal tumors with equivalent outcomes.

Table 40–1. TNM (tumor, node, metastasis) staging classification and prognosis of renal cell cancer.

Robson Stage	T	N	M	Five-Year Survival (%)
I. Tumor confined by renal capsule	T1 (< 7.0 cm tumor) T2 (> 7.0 cm tumor)	N0 (nodes negative)	M0 (lack of distant metastases)	80-100
II. Tumor extension to perirenal fat or ipsilateral adrenal but confined by Gerota's fascia	T3a	N0	M0	50-60
IIIa. Renal vein or inferior vena caval involvement	T3b (renal vein involvement) T3c (renal vein and caval involvement below the diaphragm) T4b (caval involvement above the diaphragm)	N0	M0	50-60 (renal vein) 25-35 (vena cava)
IIIb. Lymphatic involvement	T1-3	N1 (single regional node involved) N2 (multiple regional, contralateral, or bilateral nodes involved)	M0	15-35
IIIc. Combination of IIIa and IIIb	T3-4	N1-2	M0	15-35
IVa. Spread to contiguous organs except ipsilateral adrenal	T4	N1-2	M0	0-5
IVb. Distant metastases	T1-4	N0-2	M1	0-5

In patients with very large or central tumors and a normal contralateral kidney, radical nephrectomy is recommended. In all other cases, attempts should be made for nephron-sparing surgery. Successful partial nephrectomy with negative surgical margins offers the same survival benefit as radical nephrectomy. Typically, hilar-vessel occlusion with bulldog or Satinsky clamp(s) is performed to allow for resection in a relatively bloodless field.

Laparoscopic radical or partial nephrectomy has been advocated as a method equal to the open approach with the advantages of less blood loss, shorter hospitalization, and earlier return to normal function. It is the gold standard in institutions with appropriate expertise. Laparoscopic or percutaneous cryoablation of RCC has also shown considerable promise. Alternatively, radiofrequency ablation has been used for small renal tumors. These ablative technologies do not provide pathologic diagnosis, so percutaneous biopsy can be performed before the procedure or intraoperatively.

Nephrectomy has not been associated with improved survival rates in patients with multiple distant metastases (stage IV), and the procedure is not recommended unless patients are symptomatic or a promising therapeutic protocol is being studied. Flanigan and others have shown, however, that up to a 6-month improvement in survival can be achieved with nephrectomy—even with soft tissue metastasis—in selected patients who also receive interferon-alfa systemic therapy. Patients with solitary pulmonary metastases have benefited from joint surgical removal of both the primary lesion and the metastatic lesion (30% survival at 5 years). Preoperative arterial embolization in patients with or without metastases does not improve survival rates, although it may be helpful as a single treatment measure in patients with symptomatic but nonresectable primary lesions. Radiation therapy is of little benefit except as treatment for symptomatic bone metastases. Medroxyprogesterone for metastatic RCC has given an equivocal 5%-10% response rate of short duration. Vinblastine has also had a response rate of approximately 20%, again of minimal duration. There are no other cytotoxic chemotherapeutic agents of benefit.

Immunotherapy with interferon-alfa has had a 15%-20% response rate. Other interferons, alone (interferon-beta, interferon-gamma) or in combination with chemotherapeutic agents, have been less effective than interferon-alfa. Adoptive immunotherapy—using lymphocytes (lymphokine-activated killer cells) from exposure of the patient's own peripheral blood lymphocytes to interleukin-2 (IL-2) in vitro followed by reinfusion into the patient along with systemic IL-2 infusion—has shown objective response rates of up to 33%. High-dose intravenous IL-2 causes a profound capillary leak syndrome and substantial toxicity. Subsequent studies have shown only a 16% response rate.

Recent advances in research on the von Hippel-Lindau tumor suppressor gene has led to identification of growth factors including vascular endothelial growth factor (VEGF) and platelet-derived growth factor as molecular targets in treating advanced renal cancer. Initial studies using bevacizumab, an anti–vascular endothelial growth factor antibody, have shown promising results. Sorafenib, a tyrosine kinase inhibitor that blocks the pathway leading to the production of several growth factors, has been studied in patients with metastatic renal cancer and shown longer median progression-free survival than placebo (24 weeks vs 6 weeks). Sunitinib, another tyrosine kinase inhibitor, has shown longer progression-free survival and higher response rates than interferon-alfa in patients with metastatic renal cancer. These oral agents are currently used as first-line therapy in this group of patients.

Temsirolimus is another targeted agent that is a specific inhibitor of the mammalian target of rapamycin kinase (mTOR inhibitor) and has shown promising results. It is now used as first-line therapy in poor-prognosis patients. Many other agents are currently being studied.

▶ Prognosis

Patients with localized RCC (stages T1, T2, and T3a) treated surgically have 5-year survival rates of approximately 70%-80%, whereas rates for those with local nodal extension or distant metastases are 15%-25% and less than 10%, respectively. Most patients who present with multiple distant metastases succumb to disease within 15 months (Table 40–1). The advent of new agents for RCC may improve the outcome in these patients.

RENAL SARCOMA

Renal sarcomas include rhabdomyosarcoma, liposarcoma, fibrosarcoma, and leiomyosarcoma; the latter is the most common, although all are very uncommon. Sarcomas are highly malignant and are usually detected at a late stage and thus have a poor prognosis. The diagnostic approach is similar to that of RCC. The histology of the lesion is rarely suspected preoperatively, although local invasion into surrounding retroperitoneal structures is more common than with RCC. These tumors have a tendency to surround the renal vasculature and do not exhibit neovascularity on MRA.

Treatment is surgical, with wide local excision; however, local recurrence and subsequent distant metastases are the rule. There is no therapy of proved benefit for metastatic disease.

SECONDARY MALIGNANT RENAL TUMORS

Metastatic tumors to the kidney are more common than primary renal tumors and often develop from primary tumors of distant sites, most commonly the lung, stomach, and breast. It is rare for the diagnosis to be made before autopsy; this suggests that renal metastasis is a late event. There are usually no symptoms, although microscopic hematuria occurs in 10%-20% of cases. Imaging reveals a renal mass, often difficult to distinguish from RCC. Contiguous spread of a tumor adjacent to the kidney is not infrequent (eg, tumors of the adrenal, colon, and pancreas and retroperitoneal sarcomas). Tumors such as lymphoma, leukemia, and multiple myeloma may also infiltrate the kidney. Routine radiologic, hematologic, and chemical examinations should demonstrate the primary tumor in most cases. Percutaneous biopsy may be appropriate in certain circumstances.

BENIGN RENAL TUMORS

▶ Renal Oncocytoma

Renal oncocytomas are benign renal neoplasms. The tumors are generally asymptomatic and not associated with the paraneoplastic syndromes. The finding of a central stellate scar on CT or a spoke-wheel pattern of feeding arteries on angiography may suggest the diagnosis, although these findings have been found to be unreliable. Oncocytomas can coexist with renal carcinoma in the same lesion or in other lesions in the same kidney (7%-30%). This finding, along with difficulty differentiating oncocytoma from clear cell or chromophobe renal cancers on fine-needle aspirates, makes it difficult to make a definitive diagnosis preoperatively. Consequently, definitive treatment of these lesions with radical or partial nephrectomy or with ablation (cryoablation or radiofrequency ablation) has been recommended.

▶ Mesoblastic Nephroma

Mesoblastic nephroma is a benign congenital renal tumor seen in early childhood that must be distinguished from the highly malignant nephroblastoma, or Wilms tumor. Unlike Wilms tumor, mesoblastic nephroma is commonly diagnosed within the first few months of life. Histologically, it is distinguished from Wilms tumor by cells resembling fibroblasts or smooth muscle cells and by the lack of epithelial elements. The prognosis is excellent; complete surgical resection is curative, and neither chemotherapy nor radiotherapy is required.

▶ Angiomyolipoma

Angiomyolipoma is a benign hamartoma seen most often bilaterally in adults with tuberous sclerosis (which also includes adenoma sebaceum, epilepsy, and mental retardation). The tumor is also common in middle-aged women but only unilaterally. These tumors can be detected following spontaneous retroperitoneal hemorrhage, although 50% of these lesions are currently diagnosed incidentally. CT scan can be diagnostic, with negative Hounsfield units detected in the fat-containing area of the tumor. Occasionally, an angiomyolipoma eludes diagnosis preoperatively and requires resection (especially the lipid-poor angiomyolipoma). Asymptomatic patients with small (< 4 cm) tumors and typical findings on CT scan of fat within the tumor do not require surgery, as the prognosis is excellent without treatment. These patients can be followed with serial imaging. Those presenting with a retroperitoneal hemorrhage or a size greater than 4 cm should have the tumor removed surgically with partial nephrectomy or embolized via angioinfarction, which has been shown to be effective.

▶ Other Benign Renal Tumors

Other benign renal tumors include (1) **fibroma,** a renal parenchymal capsular or perinephric fibrous mass; (2) **lipoma,** an adipose deposit within or around the kidney, often perihilar or within the renal sinus; (3) **leiomyoma,** a common retroperitoneal tumor that may arise from the renal capsule or renal vascular walls; and (4) **hemangioma,** which is occasionally found to be the elusive cause of hematuria. Hemangiomas are generally quite small, and the diagnosis can be confirmed by direct vision of the lesion in the renal collecting system on ureteroscopy.

TUMORS OF THE RENAL PELVIS & CALICES

▶ General Considerations

In over 90% of cases, tumors involving the collecting system of the kidney are urothelial (or transitional cell) carcinomas. Less than 5% of tumors in this location are squamous carcinomas (often in association with chronic inflammation and stone formation) or adenocarcinomas. The cause of urothelial carcinoma of the upper urinary tract is similar to that of epithelial tumors in the ureter or bladder; there is a strong association with cigarette smoking and exposure to industrial chemicals. Excessive use of phenacetin-containing analgesics and the presence of Balkan nephritis are also predisposing factors.

▶ Clinical Findings

A. Symptoms and Signs

Gross or microscopic painless hematuria occurs in over 70% of patients. The lesions are usually asymptomatic unless bleeding causes acute flank pain secondary to obstructing clots. Presenting symptoms can often be due to metastases to bone, the liver, or the lungs. Physical examination is usually negative for any positive findings.

B. Laboratory Findings

Microscopic hematuria on urinalysis is the rule. Pyuria is not seen. Cytologic examination of voided urine specimens may be diagnostic in high-grade tumors. Urine obtained from the ureter by retrograde catheterization or by brushing with specialized ureteral instruments can improve the diagnostic accuracy of cytologic examinations. Direct biopsy during ureteroscopy is the most accurate. There are no commonly associated paraneoplastic syndromes or diagnostic serum tumor markers in urothelial carcinoma. A large number of urine markers are currently being studied, but only in situ hybridization studies identifying abnormalities in chromosomes 3, 7, 17, and 9p21 can be recommended at present.

C. Imaging Studies

The diagnosis is commonly made on CT urography or intravenous urography and confirmed by retrograde pyelography and ureteroscopy with biopsy. Renal ultrasound or CT scan can be used to rule out calculus. CT scan is also useful in local staging of the tumor. The tumors metastasize to the lungs, liver, and bone, so chest x-ray, CT scan of the lungs and liver, and a bone scan are useful to determine the presence of metastases. Urothelial carcinoma tends to be multifocal in the urinary tract, involving the opposite kidney (1%-2%), ipsilateral ureter, or bladder (38%-50%). Surveillance of these potential sites is important.

D. Endoscopic Findings

Cystoscopy is necessary when gross hematuria is present to determine the location of the bleeding. Lateralizing hematuria can be identified with cystoscopy (bloody efflux from one ureteral orifice). Retrograde pyelography and ureteral cytologic studies or brushing, as described previously, can be useful, although mildly abnormal cytologic findings may occur in patients with upper tract inflammation or calculi. Rigid or flexible ureteroscopes can be used to view the upper ureter and renal pelvis directly. Biopsy of upper tract lesions is possible through these instruments. Although percutaneous approaches to the renal collecting system have been perfected, their use for diagnosis or treatment of suspected urothelial carcinoma in routine cases is not recommended because of the possibility of spreading tumor cells outside the kidney.

Differential Diagnosis

A variety of conditions may mimic transitional cell carcinoma of the renal pelvis, including calculi, sloughed renal papillae, tuberculosis, and RCC with pelvic extension of the tumor. These can usually be ruled out by the diagnostic studies described previously.

Complications

Occasionally, bleeding may be severe enough to require immediate nephrectomy. Infection may develop, particularly when there is obstruction and hydronephrosis, requiring prompt use of systemic antibiotics.

Treatment

Renal urothelial carcinoma is treated by nephroureterectomy (perifascial nephrectomy and removal of the entire ureter, down to and including the ureteral orifice within the bladder). Transureteral or percutaneous endoscopic techniques for resection of selected low-grade lesions have been successful, particularly in patient with significant chronic kidney disease and/or solitary renal units. Upper tract instillation of bacille Calmette-Guérin (BCG) or mitomycin C has been reported with modest results. High recurrence rates and the potential for local tumor spread would argue against this approach in high-grade or extensive lesions. Laparoscopic nephroureterectomy has become common practice, but management of the distal ureter and bladder cuff by this technique has been the subject of controversy. Regional lymph node dissections have not been traditionally performed, although recent reports have shown some benefit for patients with aggressive disease. Because 50% of these patients will develop urothelial carcinoma of the bladder, cystourethroscopy must be performed postoperatively; it is usually done quarterly during the first year, twice the second year, and then annually.

Prognosis

Because most of these tumors are low grade and noninvasive, the 5-year tumor-free survival rate is higher than 90% for lesions treated with complete removal of the ipsilateral upper urinary tract. Survival rates are much lower for lesions that invade the renal parenchyma or are of high histologic grade. A poor prognosis is associated with tumors having histologic features of squamous carcinoma or adenocarcinoma. These tumors are mildly radiosensitive, but preoperative or postoperative radiotherapy has not been particularly helpful. Metastatic lesions are particularly problematic, and survivors are rare. Chemotherapy combinations, which have shown benefit in urothelial carcinoma of the bladder (methotrexate, vinblastine, doxorubicin [Adriamycin], and cisplatin [MVAC] or gemcitabine and cisplatin), are also efficacious in urothelial carcinoma of the upper urinary tract.

TUMORS OF THE URETER

General Considerations

Ureteral tumors are rarely benign, but benign fibroepithelial polyps do occasionally occur within the ureter. More than 90% of ureteral tumors are urothelial carcinomas. The cause is unknown, but tobacco smoking and exposure to industrial chemicals are known to be associated. Ureteral urothelial carcinoma is often found in association with renal pelvis urothelial carcinoma and slightly less often with bladder urothelial carcinoma. The lesions develop in persons aged

60-70 years and are twice as common in men as in women. More than 60% of these tumors occur in the lower ureter.

Clinical Findings

A. Symptoms and Signs

Gross or microscopic hematuria is the rule (80% of cases). Because ureteral tumors grow slowly, they may not cause symptoms even though they completely obstruct the kidney. Occasionally, gross hematuria may cause acute obstruction because of clots. The initial presentation may be due to symptomatic metastases to bone, lungs, or liver.

B. Laboratory Findings

Urinalysis commonly reveals hematuria. There are no biochemical markers specific to the diagnosis, although patients with metastases may have abnormal liver function tests or anemia. Serum creatinine levels may be elevated with complete unilateral obstruction in elderly patients. Cytologic studies of voided urine or ureteral urine or brush biopsy studies may be diagnostic.

C. Imaging Studies

The diagnosis may be made on CT or intravenous urography, although the tumor often obstructs the ureter completely, so that cystoscopy and retrograde pyelography are required for definition of the lesion. These studies often reveal a filling defect in the ureter (classically described as a goblet sign). The ureter is dilated proximal to the lesion. CT scan is useful in ruling out nonopaque calculi and in abdominal tumor staging. Chest x-ray, CT scans, and bone scans are helpful in determining the presence of metastases.

D. Endoscopic Findings

Cystoscopy is necessary when gross hematuria is present to determine the site of bleeding. Retrograde pyelography may then be necessary. Ureteroscopy may provide a direct view of the tumor and access for biopsy.

Differential Diagnosis

Nonopaque calculi, sloughed renal papillae, blood clots, or extrinsic compression by retroperitoneal masses or nodes may all produce signs, symptoms, and x-ray findings similar to those seen with ureteral tumors. The radiographic, cytologic, and endourologic studies listed earlier should make the distinction, but surgical exploration is required occasionally.

Treatment

Most ureteral transitional cell carcinomas are not associated with metastases and can be definitively treated with nephroureterectomy. Selected patients with noninvasive low-grade lesions may be treated by segmental ureteral resection with end-to-end anastomosis (ureteroureterostomy) or ureteral reimplantation for lesions in the distal one-third of the ureter. In some patients who are carefully selected and have low-grade noninvasive tumors, resection or laser ablation can be considered. Regional lymph node dissections have not been traditionally performed, although recent reports have shown some benefit. Preoperative or postoperative radiation therapy appears to be of no benefit. As with renal pelvis and bladder urothelial carcinoma, cystoscopy should be performed periodically postoperatively. Patients with metastases are rarely helped by removal of the primary tumor. These tumors are responsive to chemotherapy. Traditional agents that have been used include cisplatin with gemcitabine or MVAC. These have shown reasonable response rates but poor long-term outcomes.

Prognosis

The 5-year survival rate for patients with low-grade noninvasive lesions treated surgically approaches 100%. Those with high-grade or invasive lesions have a poorer prognosis, and those with metastases have a 5-year survival rate of less than 10%.

TUMORS OF THE BLADDER

General Considerations

Vesical neoplasms account for nearly 6% of all cancers in men and are the second most common cancer of the genitourinary tract in men. In women, these tumors account for 2% of all cancers and are the most common cancer of the genitourinary tract. Men are affected twice as often as women. More than 90% of tumors are urothelial carcinomas, while a few are squamous cell carcinomas (associated with chronic inflammation, as in bilharziasis) or adenocarcinomas (often seen at the dome of the bladder in patients with a urachal remnant).

Most urothelial carcinomas (70%-80%) are non–muscle invasive (not invasive into the bladder detrusor musculature) when recognized. Only 10%-15% of recurrent tumors become invasive.

The cause of urothelial carcinoma is unknown; there is a strong association with chronic cigarette smoking and exposure to chemicals prevalent in dye, rubber, leather, paint, and other chemical industries.

The treatment and prognosis depend entirely on the degree of anaplasia (grade) and the depth of penetration of the bladder wall or beyond (Table 40–2). Most of these tumors develop on the trigone and the adjacent posterolateral wall; thus, ureteral involvement with obstruction is a possibility. Tumors tend to be multifocal within the bladder. Approximately 5% of patients develop upper urinary tract urothelial carcinoma as well.

Table 40–2. Treatment and prognosis of bladder tumors related to stage of disease.

Conventional Stage	TNM Stage	Tumor Involvement	Treatment	Five-Year Survival (%)
0	Ta	Mucosa only	Transurethral resection	85-90
A	T1	Submucosal invasion (lamina propria)	Transurethral resection and intravesical chemoimmunotherapy	60-80
B1	T2a	Superficial muscle invasion	Total cystectomy and pelvic lymphadenectomy	50-55
B2	T2b	Deep muscle invasion		30-50
C	T3	Perivesical fat invasion		30-40
D1	T3-4N+	Regional lymph node invasion	Systemic chemotherapy	6-35
D2	T3-4M1	Distant metastases		0-10

TNM, tumor, node, metastasis.

▶ Clinical Findings

A. Symptoms and Signs

Gross or microscopic hematuria is a common finding that leads to the diagnosis. Patients with diffuse noninvasive tumors, particularly carcinoma in situ, may have urinary frequency and urgency. Occasionally, large necrotic tumors become secondarily infected, and patients exhibit symptoms of cystitis. Pain secondary to clot retention, tumor extension into the bony pelvis, or ureteral obstruction may occur but are not frequent presenting complaints. When both ureters are obstructed, azotemia with attendant secondary symptoms may be the finding that requires diagnostic studies.

External physical examination is not generally revealing, although occasionally a suprapubic mass may be palpable. Rectal examination may reveal large tumors, particularly when they have invaded the pelvic sidewalls. Thus, bimanual examination is a necessary part of staging evaluation.

B. Laboratory Findings

Microscopic hematuria is the only consistent diagnostic finding. Patients with bilateral ureteral obstruction may have azotemia and anemia. Liver metastases may cause elevation of serum transaminases and alkaline phosphatase. There are no paraneoplastic syndromes or tumor markers consistently present in patients with urothelial carcinoma. Urinary markers currently being studied are various tumor-associated antigens, growth factors, and nuclear matrix proteins, but none are proved to be accurate enough to obviate cystoscopy for diagnosis.

C. Imaging Studies

Small bladder tumors are not seen on intravenous urography but may be seen on CT. Larger tumors usually produce filling defects in the bladder on both urography or CT (Figure 40–13). Ureteral obstruction with hydroureteronephrosis may occur as well. Invasion of the bladder wall may be predicted in patients with asymmetry or marked irregularity of the bladder wall. Noninvasive lesions seen on CT or intravenous urography tend to be exophytic within the bladder, without evidence of bladder wall distortion.

Ultrasonography by external, transrectal, or transurethral routes can accurately define moderate-sized bladder tumors and can often depict deep invasion.

CT scan can be useful for staging, but the depth of bladder wall penetration and delineation of tumor deposits in adjacent nonenlarged lymph nodes are not accurately defined. In patients with nodal metastases suspected on CT scans, fine-needle aspiration and cytologic studies may confirm the diagnosis and eliminate the need for surgical exploration.

▲ **Figure 40–13.** Noncontrast computed tomography scan showing space-occupying lesion (transitional cell carcinoma) on the posteroinferior of the bladder (arrow).

MRI is helpful in the pelvis, where motion artifacts are minor and the scant pelvic fat is just enough to provide organ differentiation. However, the information is not superior to that obtained with CT.

D. Urinary Cytologic Studies

Urothelial tumors shed neoplastic cells into the urine in large numbers. Low-grade tumor cells may not appear abnormal on cytologic examination, but higher-grade tumor cells can be detected by cytologic study with high specificity. These studies are most useful in checking for recurrence of urothelial carcinoma. Flow cytometry (differential staining of DNA and RNA within urine cells to measure the amount of nuclear protein and thus the relative number of aneuploid [abnormal] cells) has been used to screen patients with some success. This technique may be useful for early diagnosis of recurrence. The urinary fluorescence in situ hybridization (FISH) assay is more sensitive and comparably specific for bladder cancer cells as compared to cytology.

E. Endoscopic Findings

Cystoscopy is mandatory in any adult patient with unexplained hematuria and a normal upper tract imaging study. Many urothelial carcinomas are not identified on CT or intravenous urography. Cystoscopic examination should detect nearly all tumors in the bladder (Figure 40–14). Only a few patients will have carcinoma in situ (high-grade noninvasive tumor) that is not visible. Any tumor seen should be biopsied and preferably resected to completion if the patient is under anesthesia. The entire bladder, including the bladder neck, should be routinely scrutinized in all patients with microscopic hematuria. In patients without visible tumor and no other causes of hematuria, random biopsies may be

▲ **Figure 40–14.** Transitional cell (papillary) carcinoma of the bladder with minimal invasion of the bladder wall.

diagnostic of carcinoma in situ. A bimanual examination should be done during cystoscopy in all patients with urothelial carcinoma to be certain that the bladder is not fixed, signifying extensive extravesical extension.

F. Staging

Therapy depends on the stage of the tumor as seen on histologic sections and examinations for metastases. Table 40–2 sets forth the stage, treatment, and prognosis of patients with urothelial carcinoma of the bladder. The histologic grade of the tumor is also important in determining treatment and prognosis, but in general, low- and high-grade histologic characteristics tend to occur in low- and high-stage tumors, respectively.

As previously discussed, CT scan, MRI, or both may be helpful in predicting the stage of the tumor. Isotope bone scanning, chest x-ray, and chest CT scan evaluate the possibility of bone or pulmonary metastases and should be done before determining therapy in patients with invasive lesions.

▶ Treatment

A. Transurethral Resection, Fulguration, and Laser Therapy

Endoscopic transurethral resection of superficial and submucosally invasive low-grade tumors can be curative. Nevertheless, because the tumor recurs in more than 50% of patients, cystoscopy should be performed periodically. Quarterly examinations are recommended during the first year following tumor resection, every 6 months during the second year, and annually thereafter. Periodic urinary cytologic examinations can be helpful as well. Upper tract surveillance with CT urography is recommended for high-grade tumors, typically every 2 years. Low-grade tumors do not require upper tract surveillance unless hematuria recurs without evidence for tumor recurrence in the bladder. Recurrent small tumors without obvious invasion may be treated by fulguration only, although biopsy is recommended to document the stage and grade.

Neodymium:YAG lasers have been used for desiccation of low-grade, low-stage tumors. There is as yet no proven advantage to this approach except that patients can be treated under local anesthesia as outpatients and perhaps that tumor cells are rendered nonviable and thus incapable of reimplantation elsewhere in the bladder or urethra. Biopsies for diagnosis and staging are still required.

B. Intravesical Therapy

A variety of chemotherapeutic agents have been used in patients with recurrent low-grade, low-stage tumors. Mitomycin C is instilled into the bladder by catheter (40 mg in 40 mL of water) and left indwelling for 1-2 hours. Patients are treated once a week for 6 weeks and may undergo a less frequent maintenance regimen. Treatment results in decreased frequency of recurrence or no recurrence in nearly 50% of patients. Other agents include thiotepa and doxorubicin.

Immunotherapeutic drugs, which include BCG, are effective in prophylaxis (60%) of recurrent papillary tumors and curative (70%) in carcinoma in situ, a highly malignant lesion less responsive to the cytotoxic agents described earlier. Intravesical BCG is the gold standard first-line therapy for carcinoma in situ of the bladder. Side effects of BCG include vesical irritability (90%), low-grade fever, and systemic BCG-osis (1%). Although the mechanism of action of BCG is not entirely known, it is suspected to induce T-cell recruitment and subsequent cytokine release locally at the tumor site. It is the most effective agent currently used. Interferon-alfa has also been studied and is effective (nearly 50% of cases) for carcinoma in situ, with less toxicity than BCG; however, its durability as a single agent is poor. The combination of BCG and interferon-alfa has shown nearly 50% response rates and is occasionally used in patients who have failed BCG. BCG is contraindicated in immunocompromised patients due to risk of systemic BCG infection and the likely decreased efficacy.

Immediate instillation of mitomycin C after transurethral resection has shown a substantial decrease in recurrence rates and is now standard of care.

C. Radiation Therapy

Definitive radiation therapy should be reserved for patients who have inoperable muscle-invasive bladder cancer localized to the pelvis or who refuse surgical treatment, as the 5-year survival rate is only 30%. In some patients with recurrence after radiation therapy, salvage cystectomy can be curative (in at least 30% of cases), although surgical morbidity rates are high. Radiation, when used, is combined with systemic chemotherapy.

D. Surgical Therapy

Occasional patients are seen with muscle-invasive lesions (T2) localized to an area in the bladder well away from the bladder base or orifices and without tumor in other sites of the bladder (proved by multiple biopsies) or beyond. Partial cystectomy (removal of the tumor with a cuff of normal bladder) may be appropriate in these patients. Such tumors are rare, and patients must be selected carefully for partial cystectomy. All other patients with high-grade or invasive (T2 and T3) lesions without distant spread or a fixed pelvis on bimanual examination are best treated by radical cystectomy and pelvic lymph node dissection. This includes removal of the bladder and the prostate in men. Removal of the entire urethra may be necessary in selected patients with tumors at the bladder neck or in the prostate or in those with diffuse carcinoma in situ in the bladder. In women, the uterus, ovaries, fallopian tubes, urethra, and the anterior vaginal wall are usually removed en bloc with the bladder. Vaginal-sparing cystectomy can be performed as well.

Urinary diversion is required and is accomplished with the use of intestinal conduits, pouches, or neobladders. Ileal conduit urinary diversion creates a urostomy on the skin and requires continuous bag drainage. This is the most common urinary diversion with the lowest complication rates. Continent cutaneous urinary diversions requiring intermittent cutaneous catheterization rather than cutaneous bag drainage became popular in the late 1980s. The basic principles are large-volume reservoirs with detubularization of bowel to maintain low intrapouch pressures and construction of an intussuscepted or plicated ileal segment to provide cutaneous continence. Orthotopic neobladder reservoirs also have been devised using bowel configurations similar to those described earlier to connect directly to the membranous urethra in men and in the distal two-thirds of the female urethra, permitting the patient to void normally. These procedures are appropriate in both men and women and have been shown to be safe, with minimal increase in morbidity over cutaneous diversions.

Robotic cystectomy has been done in large numbers at select centers in the United States and Europe. With short-term follow-up, oncologic outcomes appear equivalent to open surgery with potentially less blood loss and faster convalescence postoperatively. In most cases, the urinary diversion is done via open surgery, but more recently, ileal conduit and neobladder urinary diversions have been performed intracorporeally with robotic assistance.

E. Systemic Chemotherapy

Chemotherapy in the form of CMV (cisplatin, methotrexate, vinblastine) or MVAC (CMV plus doxorubicin [Adriamycin]) has been used before cystectomy (neoadjuvant) or after cystectomy (adjuvant) for muscle-invasive tumors or as treatment of metastatic urothelial cancer. More recently, gemcitabine and cisplatin have become standard of care after a randomized trial showed similar efficacy to MVAC with fewer side effects. A recent randomized trial showed improved survival in patients with locally advanced bladder cancer who received neoadjuvant chemotherapy and cystectomy compared to those who underwent cystectomy alone. Adjuvant chemotherapy has been shown in randomized trials to help patients with locoregional disease but not patients with localized disease (stage T1-T2). Several reports of efficacy with either CMV or MVAC for treatment of metastatic disease have shown a 60% overall objective response rate with a 30% complete response rate. A few long-term survivors with apparent cure have been reported (10%-15%), and thus, either of these regimens appears to be a definite advance in the treatment of urothelial cancer. Other chemotherapeutic agents used in urothelial cancer include paclitaxel and carboplatin in various regimens that appear to have similar efficacy with less toxicity.

Prognosis

Approximately half of the low-grade superficial tumors are controlled by transurethral surgery or intracavitary use of chemotherapeutic agents (Table 40–2). Following radical cystectomy, the 5-year survival rate varies with the extent, stage, and grade of the tumor, but with T2N0M0 tumors, it averages about 50%-70%. The complications of urinary diversion (ureteral obstruction with hydronephrosis, pyelonephritis, and nephrolithiasis) also influence the outcome.

CARCINOMA OF THE PROSTATE

General Considerations

In adult men, prostate cancer is the most common neoplasm (after skin cancer) and the second most common (after lung cancer) cause of death due to cancer. The tumor is more prevalent in black men than in any other group in the United States. The tumor rarely occurs before age 40, and the incidence increases with age such that more than 75% of men older than age 85 have prostate cancer on autopsy. In most of these older men, however, the disease is not clinically apparent; only 10% of men over age 65 develop clinical evidence of the disease. Ninety-five percent of tumors are adenocarcinomas. The tumor arises primarily in the peripheral zone (85%), an area that differs in embryologic derivation from the periurethral (transition) zone, which is the site of formation of BPH. The cause of prostate cancer is unknown, but many factors appear to be involved, including genetic, hormonal, dietary (particular high-fat diets), and perhaps environmental carcinogenic influences.

Screening

Screening with prostate-specific antigen (PSA) monitoring and digital rectal examination (DRE) has been controversial due to conflicting evidence regarding a decrease in mortality. Two very large randomized controlled trials examining the effects of PSA screening on mortality have recently been completed, one in the United States and one in Europe. The US trial did not show a survival benefit in the screening group, although the control group was significantly contaminated with men who had some previous PSA testing. The European study showed a relative survival benefit of 20% in the screening group after 10 years of follow-up, and the data will be reanalyzed with longer follow-up.

Based on all available evidence, the U.S. Preventive Services Task Force released a recommendation against routine screening for prostate cancer in 2011. The AUA recommends a shared decision-making discussion about prostate cancer screening with men between the ages of 55 and 69 and at a younger age for men with a positive family history in a first-degree relative or for African Americans. If screening is agreed upon, serum PSA level and DRE are performed annually or every 2 years based on the clinician's discretion.

Clinical Findings

A. Symptoms and Signs

Nonpalpable (T1) carcinoma of the prostate presents without physical signs and is only diagnosed by the pathologist when prostate tissue is removed as treatment for symptomatic bladder outlet obstruction presumed to be caused by BPH or is found by an elevated PSA (T1c). Patients with T2 or higher disease have a hard nodule on the prostate that can be felt during rectal examination (Table 40–3). T3 disease is palpable (or visible by imaging) beyond the capsule of the prostate or demonstrates seminal vesicle involvement. T4 disease invades adjacent organs including the rectum and pelvic sidewall. Previously, 50% of patients presented with evidence of metastases, including weight loss, anemia, bone pain (commonly in the lumbosacral area), or acute neurologic deficit in the lower limbs. Today, however, fewer than 20% of patients present in this way because of earlier diagnosis due to wide use of PSA screening (stage migration).

B. Laboratory Findings

Patients with extensive metastases may have anemia due to bone marrow replacement by tumor. Those with bilateral ureteral obstruction secondary to trigonal compression by tumor may exhibit azotemia and uremia. Serum alkaline phosphatase is often elevated in patients with bone metastases but not in those with localized disease.

PSA is elevated in the serum of most men with prostate cancer, but high-grade (Gleason score 8-10) cancers and ductal variant adenocarcinomas can present with normal PSA levels. Values above 4 ng/mL are considered abnormal but rise normally with age and significant BPH. PSA can also be falsely elevated due to cystoscopy, prostate biopsy, urethral catheterization, and urinary tract infection. Routine DRE does not usually affect PSA levels.

Methods for enhancing PSA specificity include the following: (1) age-specific PSA (younger men [< age 50 years], normal < 2.5 ng/mL; older men [> age 70 years], normal > 6.5 ng/mL); (2) PSA density (PSA divided by prostate volume), where less than 0.15 ng/mL suggests cancer; and (3) percentage of free PSA (total PSA minus complexed PSA), where lower values signify an increased risk of cancer (useful for total PSA levels between 4 and 10 ng/mL). Although total PSA is useful for staging, it is not absolute. PSA appears to be most helpful in following up on patients after treatment, as levels fall to undetectable after surgery and decrease dramatically after radiation therapy when there is a complete response. There are several new prostate cancer

Table 40–3. Treatment and prognosis of prostate cancer related to tumor stage.

Conventional Stage	TNM Stage Components 2017	Clinical Findings	Treatment	Fifteen-Year Recurrence-Free Survival (%)
A1	T1a	Nonpalpable tumor; incidental finding at transurethral prostatectomy (low-grade cancer seen in < 5% of prostate)	Observation	100
A2	T1b	Same as above, except tumor is high grade, or > 5% of prostate is involved, or both	Radical prostatectomy with pelvic lymphadenectomy	70-80
B1	T2a	Tumor involves one lobe or less	External beam radiation	85
B2	T2b	Tumor involves more than one lobe.	Brachytherapy	60-70
C	T3a	Unilateral extraprostatic extension.	Radiation with or without pelvic lymphadenectomy	20-60
C2	T3b T3c T4a T4b	Bilateral extraprostatic extension Seminal vesicle invasion Invades bladder neck or rectum Invades levator muscle and/or fixed to pelvic sidewall	Hormonal therapy (orchiectomy or LHRH/antiandrogen) when symptomatic. Irradiation for isolated bone pain.	0-10
D	N+ or M+	Pelvic lymph node involvement or distant metastases	Hormonal therapy (orchiectomy or LHRH/antiandrogen) when symptomatic. Irradiation for isolated bone pain.	0-10

LHRH, luteinizing hormone–releasing hormone; TNM, tumor, node, metastasis.

markers currently being investigated, but none have become widely used to date. PCA3 urinary assay shows promise in men with persistently elevated PSA levels and previous negative biopsies.

C. Imaging Studies

Transrectal ultrasound has become very useful for evaluating prostate volume and guiding biopsy needles into the peripheral zone and other specific areas, such as the base, the apex, and the transition zone of the prostate. The study can also reveal typical hypoechoic peripheral zone lesions in 70% of patients with palpable lesions. Because many prostate cancers are not hypoechoic and not all hypoechoic lesions are cancer, transrectal ultrasound alone for screening for prostate cancer is not recommended. CT scan may reveal urinary retention, distal ureteral obstruction with resultant hydronephrosis, and pelvic lymphadenopathy. Locally advanced disease and bony metastases can also be visualized on CT scan. A chest x-ray or CT may help in identifying the uncommon lung metastases but more often shows typical osteoblastic metastases in the thoracic spine or ribs. An abdominal x-ray may reveal metastases in the lumbosacral spine or ilium. Abdominopelvic CT is not usually recommended unless the disease is palpable, Gleason score is ≥ 7, or PSA level is > 20 ng/mL.

Endorectal MRI (eMRI) appears to be more helpful than CT scan in the staging of prostate cancer. This study allows for localization of malignant lesions within the prostate as well as assessment for extracapsular extension, seminal vesical invasion, involvement of adjacent organs, and lymph node involvement. eMRI is useful for clinical staging and preoperative planning but is reliant upon having a radiologist with expertise in this field.

Positron emission tomography is not typically used for prostate cancer staging.

D. Biopsy

The diagnosis is established by transrectal ultrasound–guided biopsies in most instances. Because the great majority of patients have biopsies due to an elevated serum PSA (stage T1c) and no abnormal findings on exam or imaging, biopsies of the base, middle, and apex of the prostate—concentrating on the peripheral zone, with six biopsies per side of the prostate—are required for accurate diagnosis.

Differentiation of the tumor is graded by the pathologist using the Gleason score, which assigns a grade of 1 to 5 (low to high grade) for both the primary and secondary forms of the tumor. The two numbers are added, and the cancer can thus be Gleason sum 2 to 10, with 10 being the most poorly differentiated cancer. Gleason score is an independent predictor of disease recurrence. Typically, pathologists give Gleason scores between 6 and 10.

E. Staging

Rectal examination can provide initial staging in patients with palpable tumors (Table 40–3). Needle biopsy is confirmatory, and histologic grading (Gleason score) can fairly accurately predict the metastatic potential of the tumor. Imaging as described earlier can be useful for staging of the primary tumor (eMRI) and to rule out metastatic disease (eMRI, bone scan).

▶ Differential Diagnosis

Nodules caused by BPH may be difficult to distinguish from cancer; benign nodules are usually rubbery, whereas cancerous nodules have a much harder consistency. Fibrosis following a prior prostatectomy for benign disease or secondary to chronic prostatitis or prior biopsies may be associated with lesions indistinguishable from cancerous nodules and require biopsy for definition. Occasionally, phleboliths or prostatic calculi on the surface of the prostate may be confusing; however, transrectal ultrasound can be helpful in the differentiation and for biopsy guidance.

▶ Treatment

A. Curative Therapy

Curative treatment for localized prostate cancer includes radical prostatectomy and various forms of radiation therapy (external-beam radiation therapy, transperineal radioactive seed placement [brachytherapy with ^{125}I, ^{103}Pd, or ^{192}Ir], and CyberKnife). Complete staging is important so that appropriate candidates will be selected. Patients with localized prostate cancer are stratified into three risk groups (Table 40–4). Low-risk patients have similar 5-year

Table 40–4. Localized prostate cancer risk groups.

Low risk	• PSA ≤ 10 ng/mL • Clinical stage T1c-T2a • Gleason score 2-6
Intermediate risk	• PSA 10-20 ng/mL • Clinical stage T2b • Gleason score 7
High risk	• PSA > 20 ng/mL • Clinical stage ≥ T2c • Gleason 8-10

PSA, prostate-specific antigen.

recurrence survival rates irrespective of the curative treatment modality. Intermediate-risk and high-risk patients have better recurrence-free rates with prostatectomy or external-beam radiation compared to brachytherapy. None of these modalities has been compared in randomized trials. The only reported randomized trial compared watchful waiting to radical prostatectomy and showed improved disease-free as well as overall survival in the prostatectomy group. Studies have shown that compared to external-beam radiotherapy alone, combined androgen deprivation (for 6 months to 3 years) and external-beam radiation improve survival in patients with localized prostate cancer, especially patients in the intermediate- and high-risk groups. Patients with grossly positive pelvic lymph nodes are not candidates for curative therapy. Recent advances in surgical technique have led to a low incidence of incontinence (1%-4%) and preservation of potency in up to 70% of patients. Alternative procedures include external-beam pelvic irradiation plus brachytherapy and transperineal cryoablation of the prostate for primary and recurrent disease after radiation.

Over the past decade, robotic-assisted radical prostatectomy (RARP) has increased in popularity and has been shown to have decreased blood loss and length of hospital stay and more rapid return to normal activity than open surgery. Oncologic and functional (continence and potency) outcomes are equivalent to open surgery. More than 80% of prostatectomies in the United States are now performed with the da Vinci Robot (Intuitive Surgical, Sunnyvale, CA).

B. Palliative Therapy

Patients with metastatic disease cannot be cured, but significant palliation can be offered. Androgen deprivation therapy in the form of luteinizing hormone–releasing hormone (LHRH) agonist or bilateral orchiectomy is effective in 70%-80% of symptomatic patients. Estrogen-based treatments are less commonly used due to the numerous side effects (in about 25% of patients), including congestive heart failure, thrombophlebitis, and myocardial infarction, and thus should not be used except in selected patients. These hormonal treatments are not additive, and use of both treatments simultaneously has no advantages over use of either alone. LHRH agonists have shown efficacy comparable to that of estrogen or orchiectomy, with reduced side effects, and are preferred by patients who find bilateral orchiectomy unacceptable. The drug must be given by injection every 1-6 months (depending on dosage) or via subcutaneous pellet annually. Studies have also shown that if an LHRH agonist is used, concomitant administration of an antiandrogen (flutamide or bicalutamide) may slightly improve survival. Studies to determine if orchiectomy plus an antiandrogen is more effective than orchiectomy alone have not shown an advantage to the combination. Antiandrogens should be administered for at least 1 week prior to inception of LHRH agonists to prevent the short-term flare that occurs with initiation of LHRH monotherapy. LHRH antagonists have more recently become available and have a faster onset to castration and do not require pretreatment with antiandrogens.

Hot flashes, osteoporosis, cardiac disease, and cognitive impairment are all potential long-term side effect of androgen deprivation.

Controversy continues concerning whether to treat asymptomatic patients at the time of diagnosis or to wait until symptoms develop. Because either approach is palliative only and there are no definitive studies showing survival advantages with early treatment, it is recommended that treatment be withheld until PSA is relatively high (> 20 ng/mL) or symptoms occur, except in patients who cannot accept a no-treatment philosophy. Recent studies do show that patients who have had a radical prostatectomy and have node-positive disease do have a slight survival advantage with early hormonal treatment.

Patients whose prostate cancer becomes hormone refractory (median of 18 months after starting treatment) can be treated by ketoconazole (which inhibits adrenal androgen production) with oral corticosteroids for short-term response. Radiation therapy for symptomatic bone lesions can be helpful, as can local irradiation for an obstructing or bleeding prostate tumor. On occasion, transurethral prostatectomy is required to relieve bladder outlet obstruction. Chemotherapy with docetaxel and prednisone has shown a slight survival advantage in phase III trials.

▶ Prostate Cancer Prevention

Because the etiology of prostate cancer is not known, prevention is difficult to determine. However, there is evidence that a low-fat diet and lycopene (found in processed tomatoes) decrease the growth of prostate cancer cells in vitro and in vivo in animals. Further large-scale epidemiologic studies suggest a decrease in prostate cancer in humans who consumed vitamin E and selenium. However, these studies were not planned specifically for this purpose, and thus the results were questionable. A current randomized trial comparing selenium and vitamin E (SELECT) was recently halted due to the lack of evidence of prostate cancer prevention. The largest chemoprevention trial (Prostate Cancer Prevention Trial [PCPT]), with over 18,000 men, compared finasteride (5α-reductase) to placebo and found a 25% reduction in prostate cancer with finasteride but also showed an increased risk of high-grade cancer in the finasteride-treated patients. Although this is thought to be an artifact of the study, these results have limited enthusiasm for recommending prevention therapy with finasteride routinely.

▶ Prognosis

Radical prostatectomy cures 70%-80% of the patients suitable for that operation, but its use should be limited to those with a reasonable life expectancy (Table 40–3). Currently, about 60%-70% of patients with prostatic cancer are amenable to curative therapy when their disease is discovered.

Andriole GL, et al: Mortality results from a randomized prostate-cancer screening trial. *N Engl J Med.* 2009;360:1310.

Bill-Axelson A, et al: Radical prostatectomy or watchful waiting in early prostate cancer. *N Engl J Med.* 2014;370:932-942.

Schroder FH, et al: Screening and prostate-cancer mortality and a randomized European study. *N Engl J Med.* 2009;360:1320.

TUMORS OF THE URETHRA

Malignant tumors of the urethra are rare. The disease is more common in women than in men (4:1). Squamous cell types are seen most often in both sexes.

In women, urethral bleeding is the most common symptom. Distal urethral lesions of low grade and without extension can be treated by radiotherapy or wide local excision. Advanced disease is best treated by combination radiotherapy, chemotherapy, and surgery to achieve good local and distant disease control. Surgery includes anterior exenteration (removal of the bladder, uterus, adnexa, and urethra with the anterior vaginal wall), including pelvic lymphadenectomy and urinary diversion. The prognosis is excellent for distal lesions without extension, but 5-year survival rates are less than 50% for those with proximal lesions.

In men, the lesion is most commonly in the bulbomembranous urethra and is associated with a history of chronic urethral strictures, often secondary to gonorrheal infection. Patients present with urethral bleeding, a weak urinary stream, and a perineal mass. The diagnosis is made by urethroscopy and biopsy. Distal penile urethral lesions can be treated by partial or total penectomy. Lesions in the bulbous urethra or more proximal lesions require extensive surgical resection, including en bloc removal of the penis, urethra, prostate, bladder, pelvic lymph nodes, and urinary diversion. In both men and women with distal lesions, inguinal lymphatics may be involved, but node dissection is required only when gross disease is palpable. Prophylactic node dissection is controversial. Five-year survival rates are 60% for distal urethral tumors but less than 40% for the more common proximal lesions.

Primary irradiation—other than to distal lesions in the female—is rarely helpful. Patients with metastatic disease may respond to methotrexate or cisplatin alone or in combination, but objective remissions are usually of short duration.

TUMORS OF THE TESTIS

▶ General Considerations

Most testicular tumors are malignant germ cell tumors. Non–germ cell tumors such as Sertoli cell tumors and Leydig cell tumors are rare and usually benign. Germ cell tumors are categorized as either seminomatous (35%) or nonseminomatous (embryonal, 20%; teratocarcinoma, 38%; teratoma, 5%; choriocarcinoma, 2%). Cryptorchidism predisposes to testicular cancer, with the incidence increasing inversely with the level of testicular descent (ie, testicles remaining in the abdomen have a much higher incidence of cancer). Metastases first develop in the retroperitoneal nodes; right-sided tumors metastasize primarily to the interaortocaval region just below the renal vessels and left-sided tumors primarily to the left para-aortic area at the same level. Distant spread is to supraclavicular areas (left, primarily) and the lungs. Almost 50% of patients have metastases when first evaluated, and this is more common for nonseminomatous tumors.

▶ Clinical Findings

A. Symptoms and Signs

Testicular tumors present as a painless firm mass within the testicular substance. They often have been present for several months before the patient seeks consultation. Occasionally (10%), a hydrocele is present, obscuring palpation of the mass. A few patients have spontaneous bleeding into the mass, causing pain. Patients with high serum levels of hCG may have gynecomastia. Patients with extensive abdominal metastases may present with abdominal pain, anorexia, and weight loss. Examination may reveal palpable retroperitoneal nodes when spread is extensive or palpable supraclavicular nodes, particularly on the left side.

B. Laboratory Findings

In general, testicular tumors do not alter the usual laboratory parameters, but serum tumor markers are diagnostically helpful. Patients with extensive retroperitoneal metastases may have bilateral ureteral obstruction that causes azotemia and anemia.

Serum lactic dehydrogenase, particularly isoenzyme I, is elevated in approximately 60% of patients. β-hCG, a particularly sensitive marker, is a glycoprotein produced by 65% of nonseminomatous testicular tumors but only 10% of seminomas. The alpha subunit of the molecule is identical to LH, but the beta subunit is unique to testicular tumors in adult men. There is cross-reactivity in some assays between the alpha and beta subunits; treated patients who develop modest elevations should have simultaneous assay of LH to be certain the marker detected is β-hCG.

α-Fetoprotein (AFP) is elevated in 70% of patients with nonseminomatous testicular cancer but is *not* elevated in patients with seminoma. Patients in whom histologic study has shown seminoma but in whom serum AFP is elevated should be suspected of having nonseminomatous elements in the primary specimen or metastatic lesions.

Approximately 85% of patients demonstrate elevation of one of these markers at presentation. Serum levels decrease when the tumor is completely removed or regresses. Markers are used mainly to follow tumor regression or predict recrudescence, as even minute amounts of tumor may cause serum elevations; however, tumor may be present without elevation of serum markers.

C. Imaging Studies

Abdominal CT scan defines enlarged lymph nodes in approximately 90% of cases when they are present. Chest x-ray and CT scan will detect most pulmonary metastases.

Scrotal ultrasound is useful for identifying the typical hypoechoic lesion in the testicle. Regardless of the findings on ultrasound, however, a young man with an intratesticular mass on palpation requires surgical definition of the mass.

▶ Differential Diagnosis

Testicular masses in men aged 18-40 are frequently malignant and should be treated accordingly. Confusion can occur with scrotal hydroceles, cord hydroceles, epididymal masses or cysts, or epididymitis. Most of these can be differentiated from masses within the testicle by palpation, but if not, scrotal ultrasound is usually helpful.

▶ Treatment

See also Table 40–5.

Inguinal orchiectomy with high ligation of the cord at the internal ring is proper initial treatment for all subtypes of testicular cancer. Rarely is incisional biopsy of the testicle advisable. Recommendations for further therapy (retroperitoneal node dissection, chemotherapy, radiation therapy) are then based on the pathologic findings. A staging workup, including postoperative measurement of serum markers, chest x-ray, and chest and abdominal CT scan, is conducted to determine the extent of disease.

A. Nonseminomatous Tumors

Following orchiectomy, three management options are available: (1) active surveillance, (2) retroperitoneal lymph node dissection (RPLND), and (3) systemic chemotherapy. Treatment is based on clinical staging and pathology from the orchiectomy specimen. Patients with no evidence of metastatic disease on imaging and normal serum tumor markers after orchiectomy are candidates for close surveillance with the knowledge that about 20% will relapse and require salvage therapy. This strategy avoids the adverse effects of RPLND and/or systemic chemotherapy. Surveillance, however, is rigorous and should only be offered to motivated and reliable patients.

RPLND is recommended for clinical stage I patients (no evidence of metastatic disease on imaging) or for those with retroperitoneal lymphadenopathy that is not bulky (stage IIA-IIB).

Table 40–5. Treatment and prognosis of testicular cancer related to tumor stage (all patients undergo inguinal orchiectomy).

Conventional Stage	TNM Stage	Clinical Findings	Treatment	Five-Year Survival (%)
I	T1	Confined to testicle	Nonseminoma: RPLND vs surveillance; seminoma: irradiation	> 95
IIA	N1	Regional nodes < 2 cm	Adjuvant chemotherapy Nonseminoma: RPLND or chemotherapy; seminoma: XRT or chemotherapy	> 90
IIB	N2	Nodes 2–5 cm	Adjuvant chemotherapy Nonseminoma; RPLND or adjuvant chemotherapy; seminoma: XRT or chemotherapy	> 85
IIC III	N3 M+	Nodes > 5 cm Distant metastases	Chemotherapy followed by resection of residual disease	~70

RPLND, retroperitoneal lymph node dissection; TNM, tumor, node, metastasis; XRT, radiotherapy.

The extent of lymphadenectomy depends on the testicle involved but, in general, includes para-aortic and paracaval nodes from the renal vessels down to the aortic bifurcation and along the external iliac artery to the internal inguinal ring on the involved side. Adverse effects of RPLND include severe hemorrhage from vascular injury to the vena cava, aorta, or major branches; chylous ascites; loss of seminal emission; and damage to surrounding structures. If necessary, adjacent organs involved are removed en bloc with the lymph node tissue (eg, nephrectomy). Seminal emission can be preserved with modified templates or nerve-sparing techniques that prospectively identify and preserve the sympathetic fibers that coalesce near the bifurcation of the aorta.

Patients with any nonseminomatous cell type who have extensive retroperitoneal or chest metastases are best treated after orchiectomy by multiagent chemotherapy, typically bleomycin, etoposide, and cisplatin. Residual masses after chemotherapy are surgically excised. Combination chemotherapy with bleomycin, etoposide, and cisplatin achieves over a 90% cure rate in stage II patients and a 70% cure rate in stage III patients. Patients who do not respond may be treated with ifosfamide, doxorubicin, or both, with some expectation of success.

B. Seminoma

In the absence of extensive distant spread, patients with pure seminoma should be treated with external-beam radiation therapy (2500 cGy) to the retroperitoneum following orchiectomy. A recent study showed that one cycle of carboplatin is equivalent to radiation therapy for stage I seminoma. In the presence of bulky abdominal disease or more distant metastases, survival rates are better with multiagent chemotherapy (described earlier) given initially in lieu of radiation therapy. Patients with substantial residual retroperitoneal tumor (> 3 cm) after chemotherapy may benefit from surgical removal of the remaining tumor.

 Prognosis

Even in the presence of metastases, many of these patients can be cured, with overall survival rates > 90%. The only exception is patients with pure choriocarcinoma, who still have a poor survival rate (35% at 5 years) despite extensive chemotherapy.

TUMORS OF THE PENIS

Cancer of the penis is a rare disease occurring in the fifth to sixth decades. The cause is uncertain. The disease is rarely seen in circumcised men. The lesion commonly is on the glans penis or foreskin. Early cases may exhibit a painless red, velvety lesion, but most often the lesion is an exophytic nodular or wartlike growth with secondary infection. The initial diagnosis is made by a generous incisional biopsy of the lesion, which reveals squamous cell carcinoma in over 95% of cases. The tumors tend to metastasize to superficial or deep inguinal nodes, although the attendant infection may cause enlarged, tender nodes, which may be difficult to differentiate from metastatic cancer.

The differential diagnosis includes syphilitic chancre, soft chancre due to *Haemophilus ducreyi* infection, and simple or giant condyloma. Biopsy usually differentiates among these conditions.

Small, noninfiltrating lesions (carcinoma in situ) can be treated with fluorouracil cream, external-beam radiation, or laser therapy. However, close follow-up is mandatory in patients so treated. Larger lesions not involving deep structures that are limited to the distal penis are treated by partial penile amputation at least 2 cm proximal to the lesion, leaving enough of the penis for adequate direction of the urinary stream. Deeply infiltrating and proximal lesions require total penectomy, with formation of a perineal urethrostomy.

Patients with high-risk features (high T stage, high grade, or presence of lymphovascular invasion) are at risk of inguinal nodal metastases. Prophylactic node dissection has been associated with improved survival.

Palpable inguinal nodes should be treated with antibiotics for 6 weeks following treatment of the primary lesion to eliminate infection. Persistently palpable nodes require bilateral ilioinguinal lymphadenectomy. An alternative would be fine-needle aspiration of the palpable nodes and node dissection if positive for metastases. Even those who undergo delayed node dissection when the nodes become palpable can be cured, although this is a lower percentage. Radiation therapy for palpable nodes or as prophylaxis for nonpalpable nodes has been occasionally effective but mostly in the palliative setting.

Patients with distant metastases (to the pelvic nodes, lungs, or bone) have a poor prognosis, although cisplatin and methotrexate have shown objective but not durable responses. Five-year survival rates for patients with noninvasive lesions localized to the penis are 80%; for those with inguinal node involvement, 50%; and for those with distant metastases, nil.

NEUROPATHIC (NEUROGENIC) BLADDER

A neuropathic bladder has abnormal activity secondary to a neurologic condition. To understand the variety of neuropathic bladder conditions, a basic understanding of the normal innervation and myoneurophysiology is required.

▶ Myoneural Anatomy

The urinary bladder and its involuntary sphincter develop and differentiate from the tubular urogenital sinus. The differentiation of the encasing mesenchymal cells forms the musculature of the detrusor and urethral sphincter.

▶ Innervation

The innervation of the bladder and its involuntary sphincter is via the autonomic nervous system. The parasympathetic supply to the bladder and the sphincter is via the pelvic nerves, which arise from S2-4. These fibers also carry the stretch sensory receptors to the same spinal cord center (S2-4).

The sensory supply for pain, touch, and temperature is carried via the sympathetic fibers arising from the thoracolumbar segments (T11-L2).

Motor and sensory supply of the trigone is via the thoracolumbar sympathetic fibers.

The striated external sphincter, as well as the entire urogenital diaphragm, receives its motor and sensory innervation from the somatic fibers arising from S2-4 (via the pudendal nerve).

It is clear that the S2-4 segment is the origin of the motor supply to the bladder musculature, to the involuntary sphincter, and to the striated external sphincter. The trigone is the only structure that is partly independent in its innervation. This is why segment S2-4 is called the spinal cord center for micturition. It is located at the level of the T12 and L1 vertebral bodies. There are connections between the spinal reflex center and the midbrain and cerebral cortex. Through these connections, inhibition and control of the spinal cord reflexes can be maintained. The micturition reflex is coordinated in the pontine micturition center.

▶ Myoneurophysiology

The primary functions of the urinary bladder are to store and empty urine at a safe pressure and in a continent fashion. Intact myoneural elements are essential for these functions. The primary reservoir function is possible because of the specialized detrusor muscle arrangement and because of the bladder compliance phenomenon. The normal adult bladder can accommodate volumes up to 400 mL without increasing intravesical pressure. Bladder fullness is perceived through increases in stretching of bladder mechanoreceptors.

Distention and stretch initiate detrusor activity that can be controlled and inhibited by the high cortical centers or can be allowed to progress to active detrusor contraction and voiding. Normally during voiding, detrusor contraction continues until the bladder is completely empty unless voiding is voluntarily interrupted or inhibited.

Before voiding begins, the pelvic floor and the striated external sphincter relax, the bladder base descends, and the bladder outlet assumes a funnel shape. As a result, urethral resistance decreases. This is followed by detrusor muscle contraction and a rise in intravesical pressure to 20-40 cm of water, which results in a urine flow of about 15-30 mL/s. When the bladder is completely empty, the pelvic floor and striated external sphincter contract, elevating the bladder base, increasing urethral pressure, and ending voiding. Intact nerve pathways are essential for these synchronized activities to occur.

▶ Cystometry

Cystometry is a simple method for testing the bladder's storage function and gives the following information: bladder capacity, extent of accommodation or compliance, the ability to sense bladder filling and temperature, and the presence of an appropriate detrusor muscle contraction. In addition, postvoid residual urine can be measured at the same time. A normal cystometrogram is shown in Figure 40-15A.

▶ Uroflowmetry

Uroflowmetry is the measurement of urine flow rate. If detrusor contraction is properly coordinated with sphincter relaxation, then the outlet resistance falls as the bladder pressure

▲ Figure 40–15. Cystometrograms. **A:** Normal cystometrogram. **B:** Cystometrogram in a patient with hyperreflexic bladder caused by transection of the spinal cord above S2. **C:** Cystometrogram in a patient with an areflexic flaccid neuropathic bladder caused by a myelomeningocele.

increases, and the flow rate is adequate. Normally, the flow rate changes with age but is more than 20 mL/s in men under 60 and more than 25 mL/s in women under 50 years of age. Any flow rate below 12 mL/s suggests obstruction or detrusor dysfunction. A flow rate under 10 mL/s strongly suggests underlying pathology.

▶ Urodynamics

Urodynamic studies require measurement of bladder pressure during micturition. The pressure measured within the bladder (intravesical pressure) is a combination of the intra-abdominal pressure and the pressure generated by the detrusor. To determine the detrusor pressure, the intra-abdominal pressure is measured with a rectal catheter, and this pressure is subtracted from the total intravesical pressure (measured by the bladder catheter). The urine flow rates may then be assessed in light of the detrusor pressure. No consensus exists on a critical value for pressure and flow that is diagnostic of obstruction. Nomograms have been developed for evaluating the pressure-flow relationship and

thus to categorize these values as obstructed, equivocal, or unobstructed.

▶ Electromyographic Recording

Needle or patch electrodes may be employed to record the activity of the external sphincter. This information is useful when obtained during micturition. Increased activity in the sphincter after voiding begins suggests detrusor-sphincter dyssynergia.

▶ Classification & Clinical Findings

Several classification systems exist that describe the variety of pathologic bladder conditions that develop secondary to neuropathies. Many bladder conditions are predictable on the basis of the neurologic lesion. A lesion above the brainstem (ie, stroke) affecting micturition frequently results in involuntary bladder contractions (detrusor hyperreflexia) with coordinated (synergistic) sphincter relaxation. These patients have urge incontinence.

A complete lesion of the spinal cord (ie, trauma) above the T12 vertebral body may leave the spinal reflex center intact. This often leads to what has been categorized as an upper motor neuron lesion. These patients have detrusor hyperreflexia and uncoordinated sphincter activity (detrusor-sphincter dyssynergia). Although detrusor contractions can generate abnormally high intravesical pressure, they are not effective in producing adequate urine flow because of the spastic external sphincter. Thus, there is residual urine. Bladder capacity is reduced. Detrusor contraction and mass reflexes can be initiated from certain trigger areas.

Figure 40–15B is a typical cystometrogram of a hyperreflexic bladder.

An injury to the spinal reflex center or below often leads to what has been categorized as a lower motor neuron lesion. These patients often develop detrusor areflexia. Trauma is the most common cause, but tumors, ruptured intervertebral disks, and meningomyelocele may also cause this type of neuropathic bladder. Both motor and sensory fibers are usually affected, and there is loss of sense of fullness (Figure 40–15C). These contractions are usually weak and unsustained, and bladder emptying is incomplete, resulting in large amounts of residual urine.

The bladder dynamics in a person with a neuropathic bladder often change over time. This may occur secondary to changes in innervation (ie, tethering of spinal cord, multiple sclerosis, recovery from spinal shock) or changes in the bladder. For example, a patient with a hyperreflexic bladder and dyssynergic sphincter often develops a trabeculated, noncompliant bladder over time. These changes require periodic reevaluation of all patients with neuropathic bladders regardless of the initial classification.

Differential Diagnosis

Cystitis, interstitial cystitis, and organic obstruction (eg, due to BPH or urethral stricture) are occasionally confused with neuropathic bladder, but associated neurologic lesions usually help make the diagnosis of neuropathic bladder. Psychosomatic disturbances can cause spasm of the external sphincter, incomplete voiding, retention, or incontinence.

Complications

Common complications include urinary tract infection, stone formation, and incontinence. The most serious consequences of these lesions are the hydrodynamic back-pressure on the kidneys, hydronephrosis, infection, decompensation of the ureterovesical junction, and loss of renal function.

Treatment

Immediately following spinal cord injury, there is a shock phase that may last a few weeks up to 2-3 years. The average time is 2-3 months. The bladder is completely dissociated from nervous control and thus has no sensation and is areflexic.

Treatment is aimed at avoiding the aforementioned complications in the hope of partial or complete recovery. During the shock phase, continuous closed drainage or, preferably, clean intermittent (every 4-6 hours) catheterization should be instituted until bladder activity is restored.

A. Hyperreflexic Bladder

In the hyperreflexic bladder, attaining a functional bladder depends on mobilizing residual urine and increasing the bladder capacity. Residual urine volume can be decreased by reducing urethral resistance by several methods: α-antagonists, surgery (eg, TURP), or clean intermittent catheterization.

Functional capacity can be increased by decreasing detrusor instability with anticholinergic drugs (eg, oxybutynin), Botox injection into the bladder with cystoscopic guidance, or operative bladder augmentation. This is often performed with small or large intestine (enterocystoplasty).

Conversion to a flaccid areflexic bladder can be achieved by cord rhizotomy. The storage function of the bladder is preserved, and the patient can be managed by clean intermittent catheterization.

Supravesical urinary diversion may be called for in patients with upper tract deterioration due to elevated storage pressures or female incontinence. Male incontinence may be controlled by a condom catheter.

B. Areflexic Bladder

Function of the flaccid bladder can be improved by measures that facilitate complete emptying; these include voiding by the Credé maneuver (suprapubic pressure), transurethral resection of the bladder neck to reduce outlet resistance, and timed voiding or timed clean intermittent catheterization. An indwelling urethral catheter or suprapubic cystostomy is required in a few cases, but chronic indwelling tubes should be avoided if possible.

Suprapubic urinary diversion (eg, ileal or colon conduit) can circumvent deterioration of upper tracts. Implantable prosthetic sphincters, periurethral bulking agent injections, or urethral slings may also improve urinary control.

A new technique of microanastomosis of a lumbar ventral nerve root to the S3 ventral root has generated promising results in children with spina bifida. This technique is reported to result in improved bladder function in children with an areflexic bladder as well as those with a hyperreflexic bladder.

Prognosis

Renal injury from elevated bladder pressure and infection are the most serious consequences of neuropathic bladder. When diversion or bladder augmentation is required, proper timing of the operation is essential for preservation of kidney function. Patients with a neuropathic bladder require close follow-up of their kidneys with renal ultrasound and serum creatinine determinations.

OTHER DISEASES & DISORDERS OF THE GENITOURINARY TRACT

SIMPLE RENAL CYST

A simple renal cyst is usually unilateral and solitary but may be multiple and bilateral. The cause of this disorder is unclear. The cyst can compress and destroy adjacent parenchyma. Cysts contain fluid that resembles (but is not) urine. Most are diagnosed in patients after the fourth decade. Occasionally, what appears to be a simple cyst may in fact be a papillary cystadenocarcinoma—an uncommon form of renal cancer with both solid and cystic components. In those cases, however, ultrasound usually demonstrates a complex mass with both cystic and solid components.

Flank pain may be a presenting symptom, although most renal cysts are found incidentally on imaging for other purposes. CT scan and ultrasound are the most common imaging modalities. A mass may be felt in the flank or upper quadrant and must be distinguished from tumor. Urinalysis and tests of renal function are normal. If the CT scan or ultrasound reveals an equivocal cystic mass, cyst aspiration may be performed, the fluid submitted for cytologic examination, and the cyst filled with contrast material to delineate its wall. A simple cyst must be distinguished from adenocarcinoma of the kidney; ultrasonography or CT scan usually makes that distinction.

Complications are rare, but bleeding into or infection of a cyst may occur.

If the diagnosis of cyst is established, surgery is not necessary unless the lesion causes pain due to mass effect or endangers renal function. Simple percutaneous aspiration with instillation of 95% ethanol may suffice. If sclerosis fails, laparoscopic or open cyst decortication may be performed.

RENAL ARTERY ANEURYSM

Aneurysm of the renal artery is relatively rare. It results from weakening of the artery wall by arteriosclerosis, poststenotic dilation, intimal or perimedial fibroplasia, or trauma. If the aneurysm causes stenosis of the artery, hypertension may ensue secondary to ischemia and activation of the renin-angiotensin system. A plain abdominal x-ray may reveal a ringlike calcification in the wall. Angiography or CT scan is diagnostic.

Surgery is indicated in the following situations: (1) secondary renal ischemia and hypertension, (2) dissecting aneurysm, (3) aneurysm associated with pain or hematuria, (4) anticipation of pregnancy, (5) aneurysm coincident with significant stenosis, (6) radiographic evidence of incomplete calcification or increase in size on serial films, and (7) aneurysm containing thrombus with evidence of distal embolization. If the aneurysm ruptures, emergency nephrectomy may be necessary.

RENAL INFARCTION

The common causes of renal artery occlusion include emboli due to subacute infective endocarditis, atrial or ventricular thrombi, arteriosclerosis, polyarteritis nodosa, trauma, and, in the neonate, umbilical artery catheterization. Multiple emboli are common and lead to patchy renal ischemia. Occlusion of a main renal artery causes renal total infarction.

The patient may suffer from severe flank pain, or the lesion may be silent. Hematuria is common. Excretory urograms may reveal no excretion of radiopaque material or may only opacify a portion of the kidney. With complete acute occlusion of the main renal artery, a ureteral catheter drains no urine, yet the retrograde urogram reveals normal anatomy. Renal angiography, color Doppler ultrasound, or MR angiography makes the diagnosis by revealing occlusion of the artery or arterioles; a renal scan shows similar findings. CT scan after the intravenous injection of radiopaque medium shows no concentration in the ischemic area. Ureteral stone may mimic renal infarction, but urograms, CT scan, or angiograms distinguish one from the other. Following renal infarction, hypertension may develop secondary to renal ischemia; it may later resolve spontaneously.

If the diagnosis is made promptly (within 5-8 hours), thrombectomy or endarterectomy should be considered. Otherwise, anticoagulation therapy should be instituted (eg, heparin). Thrombolytic therapy (eg, streptokinase) may be used to lyse the clot. If permanent hypertension develops, definitive treatment of the arterial occlusion or nephrectomy (preferably laparoscopic) should be performed.

RENAL VEIN THROMBOSIS

Thrombosis of the renal vein affects both infants and adults and can be either acute or chronic. In children, thrombosis may be caused by severe dehydration (eg, due to ileocolitis and diarrhea or the nephrotic syndrome). In adults, it may be secondary to renal infection, ascending thrombosis of the vena cava, or caval occlusion due to tumor thrombus. There is usually flank pain and a palpable distended kidney. If renal vein thrombosis is secondary to infection, the patient is septic and urinalysis reveals pus cells and bacteria. In noninfectious cases, the urine may reveal microhematuria and mild proteinuria. The patient with bilateral involvement is azotemic. Nephrotic syndrome may develop. Excretory urograms show delayed opacification in an enlarged kidney. The calices are elongated. Later, the kidney may become atrophic. Renal angiography reveals stretching and bowing of arterioles. Selective renal venography demonstrates the thrombus, as does renal ultrasound.

Treatment should attempt to eliminate the underlying cause whenever possible. If the diagnosis of unilateral infected renal vein thrombosis can be established, nephrectomy should be performed. In bilateral disease, anticoagulant or thrombolytic therapy (or both) is required.

VESICAL FISTULAS

Vesical fistulas may be congenital or acquired. Congenital fistulas usually involve the urachus. Acquired fistulas may be iatrogenic or due to trauma, tumor, or inflammation.

The most common types of vesical fistulas are vesicovaginal, vesicointestinal, and vesicocutaneous. Vesicovaginal fistulas are commonly secondary to gynecologic or birth trauma; rarely, they occur as a complication of infiltrating cervical carcinoma. Vesicointestinal fistulas are most often due to inflammatory bowel disease: Crohn disease, diverticulitis, and appendicitis. Cystostomy in the presence of bladder outlet obstruction, bladder cancer, or foreign body may result in vesicocutaneous fistula.

Diagnostic maneuvers include cystoscopy, conventional cystography, barium enema or barium swallow, and CT scan with contrast infusion. Oral charcoal may be useful for detecting a urinary intestinal fistula, as the granules can be seen in spun urine under the microscope.

Therapy for vesicovaginal fistula requires surgical closure, with placement of an omental flap between the bladder and the vagina. For vesicointestinal fistula, the primary intestinal lesion must be resected and the bladder closed. An indwelling urethral catheter is necessary during the healing period.

INTERSTITIAL CYSTITIS

This lesion is most commonly found in middle-aged women. Urinary frequency both day and night is most often accompanied by suprapubic pain with bladder distention. The cause is uncertain, although some suggest an autoimmune collagen disease, while others have documented the presence of mast cells and mast cell mediators (histamine and prostaglandin) in bladder biopsy specimens of affected patients.

The diagnosis is based on the history and the results of cystoscopy under general anesthesia. Cystoscopy reveals a small-capacity bladder and punctate hemorrhage following hydrodistention. (Studies suggest this is a nonspecific finding.) Biopsy may reveal lymphocytic infiltration, mast cell infiltration, and submucosal fibrosis. In patients suspected of having interstitial cystitis, one must rule out carcinoma in situ with cystoscopy, urine cytologic study, and possible bladder biopsies of suspicious areas.

Treatment of established cases of interstitial cystitis often fails. First-line treatment is with dietary modification of foods that can irritate the bladder mucosa (eg, caffeine, spicy foods). If poorly controlled by diet alone, pharmacotherapy with several different agents has shown utility. Pentosan polysulfate sodium is FDA approved for the treatment of interstitial cystitis. Antidepressants, antihistamines, and anticholinergics have also been used with some benefit. Temporary response has been obtained with bladder hydrodistension and intravesical instillations with agents such as dimethylsulfoxide. Systemic corticosteroids have their proponents as well, and BCG has been tried with limited success. Some patients who are refractory to these therapies undergo operative intervention. Neuromodulation with Interstim (Medtronic, Fridley, MN) has demonstrated limited success. Finally, the last resorts of therapy include augmentation of bladder capacity by enterocystoplasty or, rarely, cystectomy and permanent urinary diversion.

URINARY STRESS INCONTINENCE

Involuntary loss of urine during stress (coughing, sneezing, or physical strain) is a common complaint of postmenopausal women. The cause is related to pelvic relaxation with age, resulting in descent of the trigone and proximal urethra. There is obliteration of the urethrovesical angle, which normally provides resistance at the bladder outlet. The diagnosis is made by the history and physical examination and urodynamic evaluation. When the bladder is full, the patient should be asked to cough while in both the supine and upright positions, producing incontinence. Digital pressure applied to the paraurethral tissues in an anterior direction through the vagina reestablishes the urethrovesical angle and prevents stress incontinence (Marshall test).

Treatment in patients with normal bladder function and low residual urine is initiated with behavioral therapy and Kegel exercises; if unsuccessful, pharmacologic methods include anticholinergics to minimize any concomitant urge incontinence. Definitive management is surgical. Currently, the most effective surgical approach is a transvaginal sling procedure with a piece of autologous fascia or synthetic mesh placed at the level of the bladder neck or mid-urethra. Other approaches include the use of bulking agents (eg. calcium hydroxylapatite) injected into the periurethral tissues, resulting in increased urethral outflow resistance.

FEMALE URETHRITIS & PERIURETHRITIS

Urethritis in the female may be acute or chronic. Acute urethritis can be gonorrheal in origin. Chemical urethritis is occasionally acquired from exposure to soap or bath oils. Chronic urethritis is a common problem in women, since the female urethra is exposed to pathogenic bacteria because of its anatomic location. Urethral trauma, instrumentation, and increase in the number of pathogenic organisms lead to infection and overt urethritis. Urethritis usually precedes cystitis.

Hormonal changes associated with menopause cause vaginal and urethral mucosal changes, leading to irritative symptoms and increased susceptibility to inflammation.

Urethritis usually causes irritative voiding symptoms similar to those of cystitis and, occasionally, functional obstructive symptoms. Examination may reveal urethral discharge, marked tenderness, or congested everted mucosa at the external meatus. Induration of the urethra may be associated with vaginitis and cervicitis. Endoscopy may reveal obstruction, mucosal congestion, and inflammatory polyps. Urethral calibration rarely reveals obstruction. Spasm of the external sphincter may be noted.

Treatment is directed to the underlying cause. Estrogen cream is indicated for senile vaginitis. Surgical treatment consists of urethral dilation and opening and draining infected periurethral ducts. Alpha-blockers given orally may also help decrease urethral resistance. Correction of vaginitis, cervicitis, and cervical erosions helps in ameliorating symptoms.

FEMALE URETHRAL CARUNCLE

Urethral caruncle, commonly seen after menopause, represents granulomatous overgrowth of the posterior lip of the external meatus. The caruncle is tender and causes pain with intercourse and urination. The primary concern is exclusion of urethral cancer. Treatment is complete excision.

FEMALE URETHRAL DIVERTICULUM

Urethral diverticulum in the female commonly presents as recurrent lower urinary tract infection. It should be suspected whenever urinary infection fails to resolve with treatment. Symptoms are urinary dribbling and cystic swelling in the anterior vaginal wall during voiding. If diverticulum is suspected, it can usually be identified during panendoscopy and opacified by contrast medium on a voiding cystoure-throgram while occluding the external meatus. Pelvic MRI provides excellent diagnostic detail. These lesions occasionally contain stones or tumors. Treatment consists of transvaginal diverticulectomy.

SPERMATOCELE

Spermatocele is a retention cyst of a tubule of the rete testis or the head of the epididymis. The cyst is distended with a milky fluid that contains sperm. Located at the superior pole of the testis and caput epididymis, the spermatocele is soft and fluctuant and can be transilluminated. No treatment is needed unless the spermatocele is painful, in which case surgical excision may be performed.

VARICOCELE

Varicocele is due to incompetent valves in the testicular vein, permitting transmission of hydrostatic venous pressure; distention and tortuosity of the pampiniform plexus results. Varicocele is found in 15% of male adolescents with left-sided predominance (90%), presumably because of venous drainage of the left testes to the left renal vein, causing increased retrograde venous pressure. Bilateral varicoceles are palpable in less than 2% of male adults.

Mild varicoceles are commonly asymptomatic, but a dragging scrotal sensation may be noted. Varicocele may lead to infertility in some men.

Asymptomatic varicocele is best untreated unless it is a suspected factor in male infertility. Treatment then consists of operative ligation of the spermatic vein at or above the internal inguinal ring. In recurrent varicocele, transfemoral catheterization and occlusion or ablation of the spermatic vein may be performed with a detachable balloon or sclerosing agents. The technical success rate is high.

TORSION OF THE SPERMATIC CORD

Torsion of the spermatic cord (intravaginal torsion or torsion within the space of the tunica vaginalis) is most common in adolescent boys. A twist in the spermatic cord interferes with testicular blood supply. If torsion is complete, testicular infarction may occur within 4-6 hours. The cause is unknown, but an underlying anatomic abnormality (spacious tunica vaginalis, loose epididymotesticular connection, undescended testis) is usually present.

Clinical findings consist of precipitous onset of lower abdominal and scrotal pain and scrotal swelling. There may be a history of previous trauma in young adolescents. The testis is swollen, tender, and retracted. The pain is not relieved by testicular support. The cord above the swelling is normal. The cremasteric reflex is usually absent on the affected side.

Torsion must be differentiated from orchitis, epididymitis, and pain due to testicular trauma. Technetium-99m pertechnetate scan *may* differentiate orchitis-epididymitis from testicular torsion if performed early in the course of symptoms: The former demonstrates increased blood flow, in contrast to the ischemic pattern of torsion. Color Doppler ultrasound is more definitive and less time consuming and can delineate the lack of testicular blood flow. No radiologic study is completely accurate, and imaging should be used to confirm the clinical decision that the cause of the acute scrotum is not torsion. If the diagnosis cannot be established by examination, history, and imaging, exploration is required.

Torsion of the spermatic cord is a surgical emergency! Contralateral orchiopexy is always necessary because of frequent bilateral involvement (ie, the "bell clapper" deformity: lack of fixation of the cord structures by the testicular mediastinum) and the high incidence of recurrent torsion and infertility in bilateral cases.

TORSION OF TESTICULAR APPENDAGES

The epididymis and the testicle often have a vestigial remnant of embryologic ducts known as an appendix testis or appendix epididymis. These structures can undergo spontaneous infarction usually in young boys, causing acute testicular pain and swelling that may be difficult to differentiate from testicular torsion. With torsion of the appendix testis or epididymis, physical examination often demonstrates point tenderness at the site of the torsed appendage. Occasionally, the infarcted appendage can be seen through the scrotal wall as a "blue dot" sign on the scrotum. This sign is only visible early in the course, prior to hydrocele formation and onset of scrotal edema. Scrotal ultrasound occasionally delineates the enlarged appendage and a normal testicle, establishing the diagnosis. In most cases—and certainly in equivocal ones—immediate scrotal exploration and removal of the infarcted appendage is required to rule out testicular torsion. Although the appendages often occur bilaterally, appendiceal torsion does not; thus, removal of the opposite appendage is not indicated.

MALE INFERTILITY

Male infertility accounts for 30%-50% of infertile couples (10%-15% of marriages). Both partners should be evaluated for causes of infertility.

The causes of male infertility include the following: congenital anomalies (genetic, such as Klinefelter syndrome, or developmental, such as absent vas deferens); trauma (both testicular, resulting in atrophy, and neurologic, resulting in erectile or ejaculatory dysfunction); infections (either systemic or reproductive organ specific); endocrine disorders (pituitary insufficiency, androgen deficiency); acquired anatomic abnormalities (varicocele, vasectomy); or drug side effects (nitrofurantoin, estrogens, antineoplastic agents).

▶ Diagnosis

The most important aspect of infertility evaluation is the history, which uncovers the cause in many patients. The physical examination is no less important and may reveal small testicles, a varicocele, or absence of the vas deferens.

A. Semen Analysis

Semen analysis is essential in evaluation of male factor infertility. At least two samples should be analyzed, since values may vary over time and with the method of collection. The specimen is produced by masturbation after 3 days of ejaculatory abstinence and collected in a clean wide-mouth container and examined within 2 hours. Determination of the volume, pH, liquefaction, sperm count, viability, abnormal forms, and motility constitutes a complete analysis. Normal values include volume of more than 2.0 mL, concentration greater than 20 million sperm per mL, more than 50% motile sperm, and 75% or more viable sperm (World Health Organization criteria).

B. Hormone Studies

Patients with no sperm in the ejaculate (azoospermia) or very low counts (oligospermia, < 10 million sperm/mL) should have serum FSH, LH, and testosterone levels measured. Patients with low testosterone should have prolactin levels checked and, if elevated, should be investigated for pituitary tumor. A significant elevation of FSH represents a problem with spermatogenesis.

C. Testicular Biopsy

Testicular biopsies are indicated in azoospermic patients to distinguish obstructive versus parenchymal disease. Testicular biopsy should be performed in patients with unexplained oligospermia to establish a histologic diagnosis, to assess prognosis, and to direct treatment. If the serum FSH is more than two times normal, one may presume the presence of severe and irreversible testicular damage without confirmatory testis biopsy.

Vasography requires injection of contrast material into the vas. The purpose of this study is to delineate obstruction of the vas, epididymis, seminal vesicle, or ejaculatory duct. Vasography is used in patients who are azoospermic and have no evidence of retrograde ejaculation while demonstrating normal spermatogenesis on testicular biopsy. Seminal fructose levels should be obtained before operative exposure of the vas. Absence of fructose would indicate obstruction of the ejaculatory duct, and if this diagnosis is confirmed by vasography, the obstructing tissue may be resected by transurethral methods.

D. Other Diagnostic Studies

The **sperm penetration assay,** performed by incubation of sperm with hamster eggs whose zona pellucida has been enzymatically removed, offers an objective method of determining the ability of sperm to penetrate the ovum. The **cervical mucus penetration test** compares sperm motility in cervical mucus with a known standard. Although these two important parameters of sperm function can be evaluated, neither test alone can establish the cause of male factor infertility.

Antisperm antibodies can be measured in the serum of either the male or female partner or in the seminal fluid. This assessment is indicated when spontaneous sperm agglutination or decreased sperm motility is noted on semen analysis. If antisperm antibodies are found, immunosuppressive therapy in the form of steroids may be effective in reducing agglutination (clumping) and increasing motility. Another method of treating antisperm antibodies is in vitro sperm washing with immunobeads coated by antihuman antibody. The sperm not bound by antibody remain in the supernatant and can be used for intrauterine insemination.

Studies to detect a nonpalpable varicocele are not recommended except in cases in which the physical examination is inadequate. Physical examination is the most effective method of detecting clinically significant varices. Venography is reserved for patients with recurrent varices, since identification of collateral venous channels would direct choice of therapy.

Transrectal ultrasound is used to support the diagnosis of ejaculatory duct obstruction in the azoospermic patient. Absence of the seminal vesicles or distention due to distal obstruction can be identified. This study should be preceded by measurement of fructose in the ejaculate (lack of fructose suggests obstruction of the ejaculatory duct) and examination of postejaculate urine (to determine the presence of sperm, suggesting retrograde ejaculation).

▶ Treatment

A. Nonoperative Treatment

Primary male infertility may be caused by hypogonadotropic hypogonadism, diagnosed by demonstrating low serum levels of FSH, LH, and testosterone. Spermatogenesis may be stimulated by administration of hCG followed by FSH. Isolated absence of either FSH or LH is rare; the LH deficiency is overcome by administration of testosterone, and lack of FSH is treated by administration of menotropins. Hyperprolactinemia may contribute to male infertility and would be treated with bromocriptine.

Infection of the reproductive organs should be treated when found during evaluation of male infertility. Infection may cause infertility immediately by several mechanisms: decreased spermatogenesis due to hyperthermia, immune interaction with sperm causing agglutination and decreased motility, as well as later sequelae such as obstruction of the ejaculatory tract. Pyospermia suggests the diagnosis, and treatment should be designed to eliminate the common pathogens: *Neisseria gonorrhoeae*, *Chlamydia trachomatis,* and *Ureaplasma urealyticum* (all are sensitive to tetracycline).

If antisperm antibodies are found in either partner, steroids may be used to suppress the immune system. One must use steroids with caution and after thorough discussion of possible side effects with the patient; acne, hypertension, gastrointestinal bleeding, and avascular necrosis of the hip have been reported with steroid administration. Response to treatment is assessed by repeat semen analysis and measurement of antisperm antibodies in the patient's serum. Sperm washing in an attempt to remove cytotoxic antibodies may improve motility and decrease clumping; washed semen may then be instilled into the uterus (artificial insemination of the husband's semen) or used in conjunction with in vitro fertilization techniques.

Retrograde ejaculation or lack of seminal emission—usually due to spinal cord injury or sympathetic nerve injury during retroperitoneal surgery leading to bladder neck (ie, internal sphincter) incompetence—can be treated with α-adrenergic drugs or antihistamines to reestablish internal sphincter function and antegrade ejaculation. Alternatively, alkalinized postejaculate urine can be collected and centrifuged and the concentrated sperm instilled into the female partner's uterus.

Clomiphene and tamoxifen are antiestrogens that are currently used in patients with idiopathic oligospermia, although the efficacy of these medications has been doubted.

B. Operative Therapy

Ligation of varicocele yields pregnancy in 30%-50% of patients. Several approaches are available, including inguinal and retroperitoneal. Transvenous occlusion of the spermatic vein by balloon is useful, especially in cases of recurrent varicocele.

Obstruction of the epididymis-vas system may be amenable to vasovasostomy or vasoepididymostomy. Currently, these procedures are performed with the aid of the operating microscope, and patency is established in 50%-90% of cases.

Obstruction of the ejaculatory ducts is rare. When this diagnosis is made, transurethral resection of the ducts may establish patency.

C. Assisted Reproductive Techniques

These include the following: artificial insemination with husband's sperm (AIH), gamete intrafallopian transfer (GIFT), and in vitro fertilization (IVF) using intracytoplasmic sperm injection (ICSI) after retrieving eggs by transvaginal ultrasound guidance and sperm by testicular aspiration in selected partners. In cases of male factor infertility not amenable to treatment, artificial insemination by donor sperm is also available.

PRIAPISM

Priapism is a rare disorder in which prolonged, painful erection occurs, usually not associated with sexual stimulation. The blood in the corpora cavernosa becomes hyperviscous but not clotted. About 25% of cases are associated with leukemia, metastatic carcinoma, sickle cell anemia, or trauma. In most cases, the cause is uncertain.

If the erection does not subside, needle aspiration of the sludged blood of the corpora followed by lavage with α-adrenergic agents such as phenylephrine should be performed. Delayed or unsuccessful treatment may result in impotence. Unsuccessful treatment calls for the Winter procedure, in which a biopsy needle is passed through the glans into one of the corpora, creating a fistula between corpora cavernosa and corpus spongiosum. If this procedure is successful, then potency is usually maintained. Other procedures include excising the tunica albuginea at the tip of the corpora cavernosum, proximal cavernosal-spongiosum shunt, and saphenous vein–cavernous shunt. If priapism persists, impotence results.

In sickle cell anemia, hydration and hypertransfusion often give relief and should constitute initial therapy.

PEYRONIE DISEASE

Fibrosis of the dorsal covering sheaths of the corpora cavernosa occasionally occurs without known cause in men over age 45. Trauma to the penis during intercourse has been implicated in the etiology of Peyronie disease. The fibrosis does not permit the involved surface to lengthen with erection, thus leading to dorsal chordee. The disorder may be due to vasculitis in the connective tissues. Palpation of the penile shaft reveals a raised, firm plaque dorsally. There is an association with Dupuytren contracture.

Controversy exists regarding treatment. Expectant therapy or medical treatment, including vitamin E, para-aminobenzoic acid, colchicine, and intralesional verapamil, may limit progression of disease. Operative therapy is necessary for patients who do not respond or for impotent patients. In the potent patient, either plication of the tunica albuginea on the opposite side of the plaque or a Nesbit procedure—excision of an ellipse of the tunica albuginea from the ventral convex aspect of the shaft and suture closure—or plaque excision and dermal grafting have been used successfully. If the patient is impotent, insertion of a penile prosthesis is the procedure of choice.

Taylor FL, Levine LA: Peyronie's disease. *Urol Clin North Am.* 2007;34:517.

PHIMOSIS & PARAPHIMOSIS

Phimosis—inability to retract the foreskin to expose the glans—may be congenital but is more often acquired. At birth, the foreskin cannot be easily retracted, but by age 3, the prepuce becomes pliant and the glans can be exposed and cleansed. If the foreskin is then retractable, circumcision is not necessary. Acquired phimosis is usually a result of chronic and recurrent bacterial balanitis (infection of the prepuce), common in patients with diabetes or balanitis xerotica obliterans. These patients are best treated by circumcision.

Paraphimosis is the inability to reduce a previously retracted foreskin. The prepuce becomes fixed in the retracted position proximal to the corona. With prolonged retraction, lymphedema of the prepuce exacerbates the condition and increases the circumferential pressure of the shaft proximal to the glans. Manual reduction can usually be accomplished using the index fingers to pull the prepuce distally while pushing the glans into the prepuce. If this measure fails, the preputial cicatrix may be incised (dorsal slit) and the foreskin reduced with relative ease. Circumcision may be performed as an elective procedure once the edema has subsided.

CONDYLOMATA ACUMINATA

Condylomata acuminata are wartlike lesions that occur on the penis, scrotum, urethra, and perineum in men and the vagina, cervix, and perineum in women. They are caused by human papillomavirus and are usually transmitted by sexual contact. Pain and bleeding are common presenting complaints. Warts outside the urethra can be treated with excision, application of podophyllum resin, liquid nitrogen, or CO_2 laser. Urethroscopy is needed to determine the proximal extent of lesions in the urethra. Intraurethral fulguration, CO_2 laser treatment, injection of fluorouracil solution, or interferon-α can be therapeutic.

IMPOTENCE

Impotence is the inability to obtain and sustain an erection satisfactory for sexual intercourse.

▶ Causes of Impotence

Causes can be grouped into the following categories: neurologic, vascular, endocrine, systemic, pharmacologic, and psychological. Treatment is directed accordingly.

A. Neurologic

Reflex erections are mediated by the afferent fibers of the pudendal nerve and efferent fibers of the parasympathetic outflow (S2-4). Psychogenic erections are initiated via cerebral centers. Specific neurologic diseases that may cause impotence may be congenital (spina bifida), acquired (cerebrovascular accident, Alzheimer disease, multiple sclerosis), iatrogenic (electroshock therapy), neoplastic (pituitary or hypothalamic tumors), traumatic (cord compression), infectious (tabes dorsalis), and nutritional (vitamin deficiency).

B. Vascular

Vascular causes of impotence may be cardiac (anginal syndromes, congestive heart failure), aortoiliac disease (Leriche syndrome, atherosclerosis, other embolic phenomena), microangiopathy (diabetes, radiation injury), and abnormal venous drainage.

C. Endocrine

The accepted endocrine causes of impotence are hypogonadism, hyperprolactinemia, pituitary tumors, hypothyroidism, Addison disease, Cushing syndrome, acromegaly, and testicular feminizing syndrome.

D. Pharmacologic

Impotence is a common and often unsuspected complication of many therapeutic and illicit drugs. Major groups that may cause sexual dysfunction are the following: tranquilizers, antidepressants, antianxiety agents, anticholinergic drugs, antihypertensives, and many drugs with abuse potential. One should recognize that virtually all antihypertensives (including diuretics) can be associated with impotence or ejaculatory dysfunction. Drugs with abuse potential include alcohol (both as a direct effect and secondary to cirrhosis) and cocaine.

E. Psychogenic

Up to 50% of cases of impotence are related to psychogenic factors. Establishing an organic cause of impotence is important in choosing appropriate therapy. Factors that indicate a psychogenic cause are the following: selective erectile dysfunction (episodic, normal nocturnal erections, normal erections with masturbation), sudden onset, associated anxiety or external stress, affect disturbances (anger, anxiety, guilt, fear), and patient convinced of an organic cause.

▶ Diagnosis

The history and physical examination suggest the cause in most cases. Confirmatory tests are necessary to ensure an appropriate choice of therapy.

In investigating a possible neurologic cause of impotence, the neurologic examination should include review of systems with respect to bladder and bowel function. More invasive studies include a cystometrogram, electromyography of the external urethral sphincter, and bulbosphincteric reflex latency.

Vascular impotence is suggested by signs of peripheral vascular disease as well as a history of atherosclerotic heart disease. Noninvasive diagnostic testing is performed with penile duplex Doppler studies to assess arterial inflow. Venous leak can be evaluated with cavernosography and cavernosometry. Arteriography is rarely required but may be indicated in patients with a history of pelvic trauma and those considering microvascular arterial revascularization.

Endocrine evaluation mandates measurement of serum testosterone and prolactin; many investigators include assessment of FSH and LH. Routine automated chemical screening may suggest other hormonal abnormalities that require additional testing. These studies should also detect systemic disease capable of causing impotence: cirrhosis, renal failure, scleroderma, and diabetes.

Psychogenic impotence may be established by nocturnal penile tumescence monitoring or outpatient snap-gauge cuffs. Additional testing includes one of the following: Minnesota Multiphasic Personality Inventory, DeRogatis Sexual Function Inventory, and Walker Sex Form.

▶ Treatment

A. Nonoperative Treatment

First-line treatment includes oral phosphodiesterase inhibitors (sildenafil, vardenafil, tadalafil). These medications are contraindicated in men with heart disease who are taking nitroglycerin. These medications work in patients who have normal blood flow and neurologic innervation. In patients without arterial-vascular causes of impotence, intracorporal injections of papaverine, phentolamine, or prostaglandin E_1 (or all three) offer a nonoperative means of restoring sexual function. Intractable psychogenic impotence may also respond to this treatment. Intraurethral pellets of alprostadil (prostaglandin E_1) can also be used; however, they often cause pain and are not favored by most patients. Finally, a vacuum erection device can be used to sustain erection.

Endocrine disturbances responsible for impotence include low testosterone and hyperprolactinemia. Testosterone deficiency is treated by replacement therapy using a once-daily topical testosterone gel or depot testosterone intramuscular injection every 2-3 weeks. Hyperprolactinemia is treated by bromocriptine therapy; the patient should be evaluated to assess the presence of a pituitary tumor.

Pharmacologic causes of impotence require altering medical treatment to ameliorate or eliminate secondary impotence. The ability to change medications depends on the severity of the underlying disease.

Psychogenic impotence is treated by a trained sex therapist, and response may be anticipated in most cases. The importance of eliminating organic causes of impotence before embarking on psychological therapy is obvious: The best psychological methods applied to organic impotence do not resolve the dysfunction but serve to frustrate both the therapist and patient.

B. Operative Treatment

Penile prosthesis insertion is currently the most common operative method for treatment of impotence. Two categories of prosthesis are in use: semirigid and inflatable. The semirigid prostheses are composed of a rigid shaft and a flexible hinge at the penile-pubic junction or a malleable soft metal case within the prosthesis; the erection is constant and is satisfactory to effect vaginal penetration, but the penile circumference is not equal to that of a natural erection.

Inflatable prostheses offer erections more similar in size to those experienced by the patient prior to the onset of impotence when compared to those achieved by semirigid prostheses. Two types of inflatable prostheses are available: The standard inflatable prosthesis consists of two corporal inflatable rods, a reservoir situated in the retropubic space, and a pump placed in the scrotum; the new inflatable rods combine the simplicity of two corporal rods with the sophistication of a self-contained pump and reservoir system (FlexiFlate and Hydroflex), permitting the convenience of inflation and deflation without tubing and multiple components.

Satisfactory results are achieved in 85% of patients. Complications common to both types of prostheses are infection and erosion of skin or urethra. The inflatable prostheses are also at risk for mechanical failure of the pump, tubing or reservoir leak, and aneurysm or rupture of the corporal cylinders.

Arterial revascularization of the penile arteries has met with limited success. Aortoiliac reconstruction improves erectile function in only 30% of cases. Microsurgical revascularization of the penile arteries (dorsal artery of the penis or deep corporal arteries) is successful in about 60% of patients. Although these methods avoid the risks of prosthetic infection and offer the advantage of reestablishing the natural physiologic mechanisms or erection, the mediocre success rate (when compared with the results of prosthetic insertion) would suggest that microsurgical penile revascularization be reserved for carefully selected cases.

MULTIPLE CHOICE QUESTIONS

1. During development, the kidneys pass through three embryonic phases, including all of the following except

   A. Prenephros
   B. Pronephros
   C. Mesonephros
   D. Metanephros

2. The most common site for an undescended testis to reside is

   A. Just outside the external ring
   B. Inside the abdomen
   C. In the inguinal canal
   D. In the wall of a sliding hernia sac
   E. None of the above

3. Patients evaluated for hematuria are considered low risk for malignancy based on all of the following except

   A. Less than 40 years of age
   B. No history of pelvic irradiation or cyclophosphamide exposure
   C. Nonsmokers
   D. Have a history of urinary tract infections
   E. Microscopic hematuria

4. Renal stones composed of calcium salts can be promoted by

   A. Hyperoxaluria
   B. Hypercitraturia
   C. Hypocalciuria
   D. Hypouricosuria
   E. All of the above

5. Palliative therapy for prostate cancer can include

   A. Luteinizing hormone–releasing hormone antagonists
   B. Estrogen blockade
   C. Transurethral prostatectomy
   D. Somatostatin agonists
   E. Depot testosterone therapy

Gynecology

Melissa Brackmann, MD
R. Kevin Reynolds, MD

PERTINENT HISTORY & PHYSICAL EXAM FOR GYNECOLOGIC DISEASES

Accurate diagnosis and treatment of gynecologic disease begins with obtaining a complete history and physical examination. A thorough history should include:

- First day of the most recent menstrual cycle
- Current genital tract symptoms
- Age at first menses (menarche)
- Interval from starting one menses to the next (cycle length)
- Duration and amount of menstrual flow
- Presence or absence of irregular or unexplained bleeding or bleeding between periods
- Symptoms associated with each menstrual cycle such as cramping, nausea, or mood symptoms before or during menses
- Other genital tract symptoms such as urinary or fecal incontinence, vaginal bulge, dyspareunia, discharge, or pruritus
- Sexual history, including assessment of risk factors such as knowledge of safe sex practices, age at first intercourse (coitarche), number and gender of partners, and any history of assault or abuse
- Number of pregnancies and subsequent outcome of each, including term delivery or preterm delivery, (and mode of each delivery), miscarriage, or abortion, and number of living children
- Contraceptive use including type, duration, compliance, and side effects
- History of sexually transmitted diseases such as infection with human papillomavirus (HPV), gonorrhea, chlamydia, herpes, HIV, or syphilis
- Adequacy of cervical cancer screening with Pap tests and HPV testing if appropriate, including date of most recent screen and any prior history of abnormal screens
- History of any gynecologic surgery, including type, date, and indication
- Age of menopause if applicable
- Presence of postmenopausal bleeding, regardless of amount of flow
- Hormone therapy of any type including oral contraceptives, postmenopausal estrogen replacement therapy, or hormone therapy for breast cancer
- Family history of pertinent cancers including ovarian cancer, endometrial cancer, breast cancer, and colorectal cancer, including the age at diagnosis and relationship of the affected individual to the patient
- Ethnicity of the patient regarding potential for hereditary diseases

Perform a complete pelvic examination. Inspect external genitalia including the vulva and urethra for development, symmetry, and visible lesions. Place a vaginal speculum to inspect the vagina and cervix for symmetry and visible lesions, and perform Pap test, cultures, or wet mount as indicated to evaluate symptoms or update screening. Bimanual examination is then performed with careful compression of pelvic viscera between the examiner's hand on the abdominal wall and the finger(s) in the vagina. The process is repeated with the rectovaginal examination, whereby one finger is placed in the vagina and one is inserted into the rectum. The rectovaginal exam allows the examiner to feel higher into the pelvis and improves the ability to feel the cardinal and uterosacral ligaments, cul-de-sac peritoneum, ovaries, rectocele, and sphincter integrity. The rectovaginal exam is particularly important for assessing pelvic masses or malignancies, rectocele, and fecal incontinence.

EMBRYOLOGY & ANATOMY

Development of the reproductive tract in the female fetus results from fusion and differentiation of the Müllerian ducts and the urogenital sinus. Fusion defects may result in duplication, malformation, or absence of genital tract structures. The most common defects are imperforate hymen, presence of longitudinal or transverse septae within the vagina, congenital absence of the vagina, and duplication defects of the uterus (Figure 41–1). The etiology of most of these congenital defects is idiopathic, but some cases arise as a result of teratogens, such as androgen or diethylstilbestrol exposure to the developing fetus during the first and second trimesters.

Careful examination of the female newborn is necessary. Cursory examination of the genital structure of the newborn may result in errors of gender assignment. Ultrasound and/or magnetic resonance imaging (MRI), examination under anesthesia, and possible laparoscopy or hysteroscopy can provide information for accurate diagnosis. One-third or more of children diagnosed with genital tract anomalies will have associated anomalies of the urinary tract, such as absent kidney, horseshoe kidney, and duplication of ureters.

The pelvis is a space constrained by bony architecture and filled with gastrointestinal, urologic, and gynecologic viscera. The blood supply is rich, including the external and internal iliac arteries and veins and their numerous branches within the pelvis. Motor nerves, including the sciatic, obturator, and femoral nerves, transit the pelvis along the pelvic sidewall. Sensory nerves, including the genitofemoral nerve, are superficially located and easily injured.

The ureter courses close to both the ovarian and uterine arteries and is at risk for injury during hysterectomy procedures (Figure 41–2). Thus, a pelvic surgeon must be intimately familiar with the spacing of critical pelvic structures to minimize risk of injury.

THE LOWER GENITAL TRACT: VULVA, VAGINA, & CERVIX

SCREENING & TREATMENT OF PREMALIGNANT LOWER GENITAL TRACT NEOPLASIA

▶ **Screening Guidelines, Colposcopy, Ablative Therapies, Excisional Therapies, & Vaccination**

As recently as 1945, cervical cancer and related lower genital tract cancers were the most common cancers in women. With the advent of the Pap test in the 1940s, cervical cancer incidence began to fall, with more than an 80% reduction of risk of mortality in the ensuing six decades. It is now understood that virtually all cervical cancers and many vaginal and vulvar cancers are caused by persistent infection with oncogenic strains of HPV. There are more than 75 HPV types identified, with types 6 and 11 most commonly associated with condyloma and types 16 and 18 associated with preinvasive and invasive carcinoma. Prevalence of HPV infection is as high as 80% of the population, but most infections are transient in nature. With appropriate screening and treatment to detect

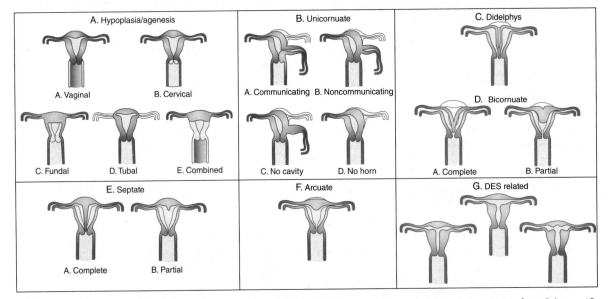

▲ **Figure 41–1.** Classification of Müllerian anomalies. DES, diethylstilbestrol. (Reproduced with permission from Schorge JO, Williams JW: *Williams Gynecology*, New York, NY: McGraw-Hill Education; 2008.)

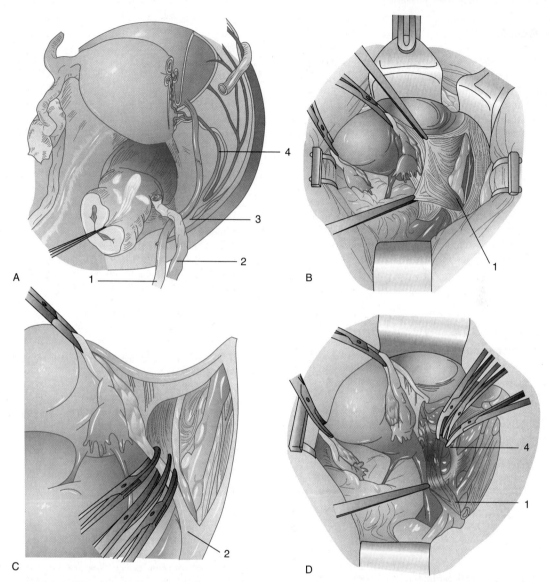

▲ **Figure 41–2.** Pelvic retroperitoneal anatomy. **A:** Dissected right retroperitoneal space illustrating the course of the pelvic ureter. The right uterine adnexa are transected adjacent to the uterus, the ovarian vessels are severed just distal to the pelvic brim, and the peritoneum is removed from the right pelvic sidewall and the right portion of the bladder. The ureter (1) enters the pelvis by crossing over the bifurcation of the common iliac artery just medial to the ovarian vessels (2). It then descends medial to the branches of the internal iliac artery (3). The ureter then courses through the cardinal ligament and passes under the uterine artery (4, "water under the bridge") approximately 1-2 cm lateral to the cervix at the level of the internal cervical os. The origin of the uterine artery from the internal iliac artery (3) is shown. The ureter then courses medially toward the base of the bladder. The distal part of the ureter is associated with the upper portion of the anterior vaginal wall. **B:** The retroperitoneal space is entered, and the peritoneum is retracted medially to show the ureter (1) crossing over the external and internal iliac artery bifurcation. Note that the ureter remains attached to the peritoneum of the pelvic sidewall and the medial leaf of the broad ligament. **C:** The ovarian vessels (2) are clamped and transected after visualization of the ureter. **D:** The uterine artery (4) is being clamped and transected. Note the ureter (1) crossing under this vessel lateral to the cervix.

individuals with persistent high-risk HPV infection, the risk of developing invasive cervical cancer is low. In parts of the world without screening, cervical cancer remains prevalent. A vaccination effective in the prevention of infection with oncogenic HPV strains was first approved by the U.S. Food and Drug Administration (FDA) in 2006. The most recently approved vaccine protects against nine strains of the HPV virus (6, 11, 16, 18, 31, 33, 45, 52, and 58).

A number of professional groups, including the American Cancer Society, American College of Obstetricians and Gynecologists, American Society for Clinical Pathology, American Society for Colposcopy and Cervical Pathology (ASCCP), and the National Comprehensive Cancer Network, have issued consensus guidelines for cervical cancer screening that were updated in 2012. The U.S. Preventive Services Task Force issued nearly identical recommendations in 2012. The guidelines address initiation of screening, screening interval, and discontinuation of screening.

When to Initiate Screening

Begin at age 21

When to Discontinue Screening

1. Age > 65 with adequate negative prior screening

2. Hysterectomy

3. Discontinuation of screening should not occur if the patient has a history of cervical intraepithelial neoplasia (CIN)-2, CIN-3, or adenocarcinoma in situ. In this case, screening should continue for 20 years past the most recent abnormal result.

Screening Interval

1. Women aged 21-29 years
   a. Cytology alone every 3 years
   b. Liquid-based or glass-smear cytology is acceptable

2. Women aged 30-65 years
   a. Cytology with high-risk HPV co-test every 5 years (preferred)
   b. Cytology alone every 3 years (acceptable)

3. Women vaccinated against HPV: Follow age-specific guidelines

The ASCCP has issued an acceptable rating for the use of high-risk HPV testing alone as primary screening for cervical cancer. However, this has not replaced the recommended screening strategy published by ASCCP. If cytology or HPV testing results are abnormal, then further evaluation is warranted. The ASCCP issued guidelines in 2013 that addressed triage and treatment of women with screening test abnormalities. Key points are as follows:

1. Cytologic tests should be reported using standard nomenclature defined by the Bethesda System. Key preinvasive diagnoses with which the clinician should be familiar include:
   a. Atypical squamous cells (ASC). The report will indicate either "uncertain significance" (ASC-US) or "cannot rule out high-grade dysplasia" (ASC-H). ASCUS should be further tested by ordering a reflex hybrid capture assay for high-risk HPV DNA unless the patient is an adolescent. ASC-H has a high risk of high-grade dysplasia and must be evaluated with colposcopy.
   b. Low-grade squamous intraepithelial lesion (LSIL) is virtually always caused by HPV, and HPV testing has been shown not to be cost effective when there is a diagnosis of LSIL. In adolescent patients, a repeat cytology exam in 1 year is recommended. In adults, colposcopy is performed.
   c. High-grade squamous intraepithelial lesion (HSIL) has a high likelihood of high-grade dysplasia on biopsy, and invasive cancer will sometimes be detected. Patients with HSIL, regardless of age, are evaluated with colposcopy.
   d. Glandular abnormalities refer to disease in the endocervical canal. These lesions are difficult to see and may therefore be detected later. Skip lesions occur in 10%-15% of cases, indicating the importance of evaluating the entire canal with curettage or similar sampling methods. All three glandular lesions are reported to have a high likelihood of high-grade dysplasia and a moderate likelihood of associated invasive cancer. Colposcopy and endocervical gland sampling with curettage with possible endometrial sampling are required. Cells in this category will be reported as:

      i. Atypical glands, not otherwise specified (AGC-NOS)

      ii. Atypical glands, favor neoplasia

      iii. Adenocarcinoma in situ (AIS)

2. Adolescents and young adult women, defined as being 24 years of age and younger, have a very high prevalence of HPV infection and a very low likelihood of cervical cancer. Because the disease will often regress in this age range, management guidelines have become progressively more conservative.

3. The colposcope is a binocular microscope (Figure 41–3) that allows close inspection of the squamocolumnar junction on the cervix, where the majority of squamous cervical cancers arise. High-grade lesions have a characteristic appearance, including white light reflection after staining with acetic acid (acetowhite change), abnormal vascular patterns (punctation, mosaic, and atypical vessels), and altered contours. Small biopsies are obtained with colposcopic guidance using cervical biopsy forceps designed

A   B

▲ **Figure 41–3.** Colposcopy. **A:** Zeiss colposcope. (Reproduced with permission from DeCherney AH, Nathan L, Laufer N, et al: CURRENT Diagnosis & Treatment: *Obstetrics & Gynecology,* 12th ed. New York, NY: McGraw-Hill Education; 2019.) **B:** Mosaic vascular pattern with atypical vessels (arrows). (Reproduced with permission from Schorge JO, Williams JW: *Williams Gynecology,* New York, NY: McGraw-Hill Education; 2008.)

for this task. Treatment decisions are based on biopsy results (Figure 41–4).

4. Biopsy proven to be low-grade CIN (CIN-1) has a high likelihood of spontaneous regression with a median time of 2 years and a very low likelihood of progressing to invasive cancer. Management is conservative to minimize treatment morbidity that has been shown to adversely affect fertility. Disease that is persistent for longer than 2 years may be treated, or surveillance may be continued.

5. Biopsy-proven high-grade CIN (CIN-2 or CIN-3) has a much higher risk of progressing to invasive disease if left untreated. Treatment options are discussed in the later section, Surgery for Malignant Cervical Disease.

6. HPV-mediated disease may also affect the vagina and vulva. Colposcopic examination and directed biopsies allow triage of lesions into low-grade and high-grade lesions that are managed either by surveillance or removal, respectively.

7. A new consensus system of nomenclature for squamous neoplasia of the anogenital tract was published in 2012.

In this system, neoplasms of the cervix, vagina, and vulva are now classified as LSIL or HSIL. This two-tiered classification system was designed to reflect the understanding of the biology of these lesions and recognizes that LSIL rarely progresses, whereas HSIL has a significant risk of progression to cancer.

Committee on Practice Bulletins—Gynecology: Screening for cervical cancer. *Obstet Gynecol.* 2012;120:1222-1238.

Darragh TM, Colgan TJ, Cox JT, et al: The lower anogenital squamous terminology standardization project for HPV-associated lesions: background and consensus recommendations from the College of American Pathologists and the American Society for Colposcopy and Cervical Pathology. *J Lower Genital Tract Dis.* 2012;16(3):205-242.

Huh WK, Ault KA, Chelmow D, et al: Use of primary high-risk human papillomavirus testing for cervical cancer screening: interim clinical guidance. *J Lower Gen Tract Dis.* 2015; 19:91-96.

Massad LS, Einstein MH, Huh WK, et al: 2012 updated consensus guidelines for the management of abnormal cervical cancer screening tests and cancer precursors. *J Lower Genital Tract Dis.* 2013;17(5):S1-S27.

Management of the abnormal Pap test in adult women

▲ **Figure 41–4.** Colposcopy triage. Satisfactory colposcopy is defined as complete visualization of the squamocolumnar epithelium, which comprises the cervical region most likely to develop invasive disease. ECC refers to endocervical curettage to obtain tissue from the endocervix above the area that may be inspected with the colposcope. Colposcopically directed biopsies are taken. Low-grade dysplasia usually resolves, and the preferred treatment is observation with periodic retesting for high-risk human papillomavirus (HPV) DNA at 12-month intervals. Any high-grade cervical intraepithelial neoplasia (CIN) in women age 25 years and older must be treated. Persistent low-grade CIN may be treated, or surveillance may be continued. Guidelines treat adolescent and young adult patients differently. See text for details. FIGO, International Federation of Gynecology and Obstetrics; HSIL, high-grade squamous intraepithelial lesion; LSIL, low-grade squamous intraepithelial lesion.

SURGERY FOR BENIGN VULVAR DISEASE

▶ **HPV, Bartholin Abscess, Benign Tumors, Pigmented Lesions, Hidradenitis Suppurativa, Benign Masses, & Tumors of the Vulva**

There are a number of possible masses and benign neoplasms of the vulva. The clinical approach remains to rule out potential malignancies and to treat symptomatic lesions. Biopsy or excision of small masses is usually performed in the office setting under a local anesthetic, either as a punch biopsy or a scalpel excision. Punch biopsy sites are usually left open, whereas elliptical excisions made with a scalpel are closed with fine, interrupted, absorbable sutures. The differential diagnosis for benign lesions is as follows:

1. Solid lesions

    A. Leiomyoma

    Natural History: Uncommon on vulva. Benign smooth muscle tumor that arises from deep connective tissues. Occurs at any age, predominately in fourth and fifth decades. May become very large. Rarely undergoes malignant degeneration.

    Appearance: Slowly growing, firm, usually mobile subcutaneous nodule.

    Diagnosis: Excisional biopsy.

    Treatment: Local complete excision.

    B. Lipoma

    Natural History: Uncommon on vulva. Benign tumor of histologically normal-appearing adipose cells. Large lesions may ulcerate. Usually asymptomatic. Rarely associated with familial lipoma syndrome, an autosomal dominant disease. Rarely undergoes malignant degeneration.

    Appearance: Soft, rounded, slowly growing sessile or pedunculated mass ranging widely in size.

    Diagnosis: Excisional biopsy if symptomatic.

    Treatment: Local excision if symptomatic.

    C. Syringoma

    Natural History: Benign tumor of eccrine ductal origin within fibrous stroma. Occurs mostly after puberty.

    Appearance: Multiple, 1- to 2-mm, flesh-colored or yellow papules on lateral labia major.

    Diagnosis: Biopsy.

    Treatment: Local excision.

    D. Trichoepithelioma

    Natural History: Rare benign tumor on vulva, derived from hair follicle without hair development.

    Appearance: Single or multiple small pink or flesh-colored nodules that can mimic basal cell carcinoma.

    Diagnosis: Biopsy.

    Treatment: Local excision.

    E. Granular cell tumor

    Natural History: Rare benign tumor of nerve sheath. Occurs in adults and children. Usually asymptomatic and solitary in 85%.

    Appearance: Slow-growing subcutaneous nodule, usually on labia majora, clitoris, or mons pubis.

    Diagnosis: Biopsy.

    Treatment: Wide local excision.

    F. Neurofibroma

    Natural History: Rare on vulva. Benign tumor of nerve sheath. Half occur in patients with neurofibromatosis type 1, an autosomal dominant heritable disease affecting skin, nervous system, bone, and endocrine glands. Rare before puberty. Rarely undergoes malignant degeneration.

    Appearance: Solid, cutaneous nodules usually less than 3 cm, but reported as large as 25 cm.

    Diagnosis: Clinical appearance of neurofibromatosis type 1 or biopsy.

    Treatment: In asymptomatic patients with neurofibromatosis type 1, no treatment for a vulvar lesion is needed. For symptomatic patients, local excision.

    G. Schwannoma

    Natural History: Rare on vulva. Benign tumor of neuroectodermal nerve sheath.

    Appearance: Usually solitary.

    Diagnosis: Biopsy.

    Treatment: Local excision.

2. Glandular lesions

    A. Papillary hidradenoma

    Natural History: Benign tumor of apocrine sweat glands. Contains both glandular and myoepithelial elements. Occurs after puberty. Usually asymptomatic. Virtually always in Caucasian women.

    Appearance: Hemispherical in shape, measuring less than 2 cm in diameter. Usually located in labia majora or lateral labia minora.

    Diagnosis: Biopsy.

    Treatment: Local Excision.

    B. Nodular hidradenoma

    Natural History: Benign tumor of eccrine sweat glands. Probably arises from embryonic rests. Clear cells on biopsy. Rare on vulva.

    Diagnosis: Biopsy.

    Treatment: Local excision.

    C. Ectopic breast or nipple tissue

    Natural History: Rare. May occur on the vulva with or without underlying glands, and lactation has been reported. Rarely undergoes malignant degeneration.

    Appearance: Amorphous swelling of the labia most often detected during pregnancy. Pigmented vestigial nipple may or may not be present.

Diagnosis: Biopsy.

Treatment: Local excision if symptomatic.

D. Endometriosis

Natural History: Rare on vulva. Benign ectopic endometrial tissue. May cause cyclic pain, ulceration, or bleeding.

Appearance: Nodule with blue or red-brown appearance. Cyclic tenderness.

Diagnosis: Biopsy.

Treatment: Local Excision.

3. Cysts

A. Bartholin cysts or masses

Natural History: Cysts are common, arising in 1%-2% of women. Cysts often occur after gland abscesses, although the duct may become occluded at any time. Small cysts are usually asymptomatic. Large or infected cysts can be painful.

Appearance: Spherical cyst or nodule in the subcutaneous tissue of posterior labia majora.

Diagnosis:

i. Incise and drain abscesses.

ii. Biopsy recurrent cysts or solid nodules.

Treatment:

i. Incise and drain abscesses using a small balloon-tip catheter (Word catheter) introduced through a stab incision in the medial aspect of the cyst cephalad to the hymen. The catheter should remain in place for 2 weeks to allow tract epithelialization. In the event of surrounding cellulitis, antibiotic therapy should be added.

ii. Marsupialize or resect recurrent cysts.

iii. Resect solid nodules because these may be malignant.

B. Epithelial inclusion cyst (sebaceous cyst)

Natural History: Common. Usually on labia majora. Can occur at any age and may be solitary or multiple. Usually asymptomatic. Caused by trauma to skin or occlusion of a pilosebaceous duct.

Appearance: Single or multiple, round cysts usually ranging from 2-3 mm up to 1-2 cm in diameter. Often have yellow color.

Diagnosis: Clinical appearance.

Treatment: No treatment if asymptomatic. If symptomatic, local excision.

C. Wolffian cyst (mesonephric cyst)

Natural History: Uncommon. Benign, thin-walled cysts on lateral vagina at the introitus.

Appearance: Round cysts with thin smooth walls on lateral vagina at the introitus.

Diagnosis: Clinical appearance or biopsy.

Treatment: No treatment if asymptomatic. If symptomatic, local excision.

D. Cyst of canal of Nuck (mesothelial cyst)

Natural History: Uncommon, Benign cyst

Appearance: Smooth cysts usually located in anterior labia majora or inguinal canal. Thought to be due to peritoneal inclusions. May become large. Differential diagnosis includes inguinal hernia.

Diagnosis: Clinical appearance or excisional biopsy.

Treatment: No treatment if asymptomatic. If symptomatic, local excision.

4. Vascular lesions

A. Angiokeratoma

Natural History: Very common. A clinically insignificant variant of hemangioma that occurs almost exclusively on vulva (and scrotum in men). Occurs during reproductive years. Contains dilated vessels and may have hyperkeratotic overlying epithelium. May resemble Kaposi sarcoma or angiosarcoma. Some forms associated with inborn errors of glycosphingolipid metabolism.

Appearance: Red, purple, or brown-black, 2- to 5-mm papules usually in large numbers anywhere on the vulva.

Diagnosis: Clinical appearance. Occurrence of multifocal lesions in childhood may indicate inborn error of glycosphingolipid metabolism.

Treatment: None, if asymptomatic. Symptomatic lesions treated with laser ablation, electrodessication, or local excision.

B. Capillary hemangioma

Natural History: Capillary hemangioma (strawberry hemangioma) occurs in infants and young children. Usually regresses spontaneously over time. May ulcerate or bleed

Appearance: Well-demarcated, red, slightly raised lesion.

Diagnosis: Clinical appearance.

Treatment: None if asymptomatic.

C. Cavernous hemangioma

Natural History: Rare on vulva. Dilated vessels that may be associated with underlying pelvic hemangioma. Usually regresses spontaneously over time. May ulcerate or bleed.

Appearance: Dilated vessels.

Diagnosis: Clinical appearance.

Treatment: None if asymptomatic.

5. Nevi and pigmented skin lesions

A. Vitiligo

Natural History: Inherited disorder with loss of melanocytes. Asymptomatic.

Appearance: Depigmented skin in well-circumscribed, macular pattern.

Diagnosis: Clinical appearance.

Treatment: Photodynamic therapy. Anti-inflammatory creams.

B. Fibroepithelial polyp (skin tag, acrochordon)

Natural History: Very common. Single or multiple. Hormonal factors are implicated in development, and lesions are more common in obese or diabetic patients (Fisher, Nucci). Also common in axilla.

Appearance: Multiple soft, skin-colored or pigmented lesions. Usually painless unless inflamed or torsed.

Diagnosis: Clinical appearance. Biopsy or excision if symptomatic.

Treatment: Excise, electrodesiccate, or freeze with liquid nitrogen if symptomatic.

C. Seborrheic keratosis

Natural History: Uncommon on vulva. Usually occurs after age 30. Probable autosomal dominant inheritance (Fitzpatrick). Multiple lesions occurring over a short period of time may indicate internal malignancy (Leser-Trélat sign).

Appearance: Lesions appear "stuck on" and are brown to black in color. Most are asymptomatic but can be pruritic. Occur on hair-bearing skin.

Diagnosis: Clinical appearance, biopsy, or excision.

Treatment: If asymptomatic, no treatment. If symptomatic, excise, electrodesiccate, curette, or freeze with liquid nitrogen.

D. Lentigo simplex

Natural History: Most common hyperpigmented lesion on vulva. Occurs on skin and mucous membranes.

Appearance: Usually small, less than 4 mm, macular, uniformly pigmented. Often resemble junctional nevi.

Diagnosis: Clinical appearance. Biopsy only if clinical morphology worrisome. Remember ABCDE signs of melanoma: Asymmetry, Border irregularity, Color variegations, Diameter larger than 6 mm, Evolving.

Treatment: None required.

E. Vulvar melanosis

Natural History: Hyperpigmented macules or freckles are benign and asymptomatic. They are usually acquired, beginning between ages 30 and 40.

Appearance: Asymptomatic brown to black irregular macular patches on vulva.

Diagnosis: Clinical appearance. Biopsy only if clinical morphology worrisome. Remember ABCDE signs of melanoma: Asymmetry, Border irregularity, Color variegations, Diameter larger than 6 mm, Evolving.

Treatment: None required.

F. Acquired melanocytic nevocellular nevus

Natural History: Common, especially in Caucasians. Tends to develop in childhood and early adulthood, followed by gradual involution by age 60. Lesions are usually asymptomatic.

Classification (Fisher)

i. Junctional nevus: Melanocytes at the dermal-epidermal junction above the basement membrane. First stage of nevus evolution. Least common type on vulva.

ii. Compound nevus: Melanocytes in both the dermis and above the basement membrane. Second stage of nevus evolution.

iii. Intradermal nevus: Melanocytes exclusively in the dermis below the basement membrane. Final stage of evolution after which many nevi involute.

iv. Other types include: Halo nevus, blue nevus.

Appearance:

i. Junctional nevus: Macule with smooth border and uniform tan, brown, or dark brown pigmentation.

ii. Compound nevus: Papule with dome shape or macule. Dark brown or black color. May have hairs.

iii. Intradermal nevus: Papule with dome shape or macule. Skin colored, tan, or light brown.

Diagnosis: Clinical appearance. Biopsy if clinical morphology worrisome. Remember ABCDE signs of melanoma: Asymmetry, Border irregularity, Color variegations, Diameter larger than 6 mm, Evolving.

Treatment: None required if asymptomatic and if ABCDE criteria are benign. All others: Local excision.

G. Dysplastic nevus

Natural History:

i. Rare on vulva.

ii. Lesions arise later in childhood than nevi in general and continue to develop throughout life.

iii. Sun exposure contributes to development of these lesions on other areas of the body. Several genetic loci have been implicated for development of melanoma.

iv. Risk of melanoma doubles with one dysplastic nevus and increases 12-fold if 10 or more dysplastic nevi are present.

v. Dysplastic nevi are sometimes associated with a hereditary propensity for melanoma.

Appearance:

i. Tend to be larger in size than nevi (> 10 mm vs < 5 mm, respectively).

ii. Dysplastic nevi are asymmetrical, with variegation of color.

iii. On biopsy, atypical cells are superficial, and the deeper cells are without atypia. Pagetoid spread of cells is noted in lower third of epithelium.

Diagnosis: Excisional biopsy. Wood's lamp accentuates pigmentation, and margins are more easily delineated. Remember ABCDE signs of melanoma: Asymmetry, Border irregularity, Color variegations, Diameter larger than 6 mm, Evolving.

Treatment: Excisional biopsy. Careful longitudinal skin surveillance exams.

SURGERY FOR MALIGNANT VULVAR DISEASE

Vulvar cancer accounts for about 5% of gynecologic malignancies. At least 90% of vulvar cancers are of squamous cell type. Etiology of vulvar carcinoma is grouped into the HPV-associated group and the non–HPV-associated group. The age distribution is bimodal, with younger women more likely to develop HPV-associated disease and older women more likely to develop non–HPV-associated disease. The latter group is often associated with lichen sclerosis of the vulva. Vulvar intraepithelial neoplasia (VIN) is a preinvasive form of HPV-associated neoplasia and is often associated with persistent pruritus. Uncommon histologic types of vulvar cancer include melanoma (6%); Bartholin gland adenocarcinoma (4%); basal cell carcinoma (< 2%); extramammary Paget disease of the vulva (< 1%); rare sarcomas, found arising primarily in the soft tissues; and metastases from other tumor sites.

Lesions arise in the labia majora in about 50% of cases, and about 25% of cases occur on the labia minora. Clitoral lesions and Bartholin gland adenocarcinomas are less common. The natural history of vulvar carcinoma includes local spread and lymphatic spread to inguinal lymph nodes. Lesion depth and diameter are of prognostic value in assessing risk of metastasis and, to a lesser degree, histologic type and presence of lymphatic involvement. Lymph node status is the most significant predictor of survival. Lesions of less than 1 mm depth have a less than 1% risk of nodal metastasis and define the category of microinvasive disease. Microinvasive disease can be treated with radical vulvar resection without inguinal node dissection.

In patients with HPV-mediated disease, multifocal involvement of HPV infection in the vagina and cervix predisposes to a significantly higher risk of cancer at these sites. Smoking is a cofactor for the development of HPV-mediated disease. Smoking cessation may reduce risk of persistent or progressive HPV-mediated disease. Women with extramammary Paget disease, an in situ apocrine adenocarcinoma related to breast tissue development along the milk line in utero, have a significant risk of a second, underlying adenocarcinoma elsewhere. Sites that require evaluation include colon, anus, Bartholin gland, cervix, endometrium, ovary, and breast.

Cancer of the vulva is staged by International Federation of Gynecology and Obstetrics (FIGO) criteria, which is a surgical staging system. Melanoma is staged using American Joint Committee on Cancer (AJCC) staging rules.

▶ Appearance

VIN occurs in women 15-20 years before the average age of invasive disease. Incidence has risen significantly over the past six decades, and the average age at time of diagnosis had decreased from 52.7 years in 1961 to 35 years in 1992. One-third of lesions are solitary, and two-thirds are multifocal. Lesions are widely variable in size and may be slightly raised or papillary. Color variation ranges from white to red or brownish patches on the skin or mucosa. Ulcerated lesions or underlying subcutaneous induration may indicate invasion. Larger lesions have a higher probability of lymph node involvement, but metastatic disease in the lymph nodes may not be palpable. Local spread may involve the urethra, vagina, anus, and rarely the symphysis pubis or other pelvic bones.

▶ Diagnosis

Biopsies are necessary to establish the correct diagnosis. Biopsy of VIN is graded as either LSIL or HSIL, representing low-risk and high-risk lesions, respectively. The differential diagnosis is broad and includes benign lesions discussed earlier as well as infections and vulvar dystrophies. Granulomatous infections, such as lymphogranuloma venereum and granuloma inguinale, of the vulva may be clinically suspicious, and biopsy of the involved areas may need to be supplemented with cultures for documentation of infection. These infections are rare unless a patient has traveled internationally. VIN is best diagnosed by colposcopic examination techniques, including use of magnification and staining the epithelium with 5% acetic acid. Lesions usually appear acetowhite.

▶ Treatment

LSIL, if asymptomatic, does not require treatment. Any HSIL or symptomatic LSIL should be excised or ablated. Focal VIN may be treated by wide local excision or carbon dioxide (CO_2) laser photoablation. Excision is preferred for lesions in the hair-bearing skin, and laser is generally less likely to cause scarring of the mucosal surfaces. Laser ablation is contraindicated if there is any suspicion of invasion.

A skinning vulvectomy with split-thickness skin grafting is effective for widely multifocal disease, but should not be used if there is suspicion for invasion. Extramammary Paget disease requires wide but superficial excision because the tumor cells often spread far wider than the visible lesion. Local recurrences are common in extramammary Paget disease, but invasion is rare.

Vulvar cancer is staged using the international system developed by FIGO. See Table 41–1 for details. Microinvasive lesions with depth of invasion of 1 mm or less are adequately treated by wide and deep local excision with 1 cm margins due to the low likelihood of nodal spread. Stage I lesions are generally treated with radical local excision with a 1- to 2-cm margin. For lesions greater than 1 mm in depth but less than 4 cm in diameter, sentinel lymph node mapping of inguinal lymph nodes is carried out to assess for spread of disease. Larger lesions (> 4 cm in diameter) and those invading local structures require radical local excision and full inguinal lymphadenectomy. Radiation therapy with concurrent chemosensitization is required for inoperable lesions and for patients with positive lymph nodes or resection margins.

▶ Prognosis

Following radical resection with negative lymph nodes and margins, a 5-year survival rate of 90% is anticipated. If lymph nodes are involved, survival is linked to number of nodes involved, unilaterality versus bilaterality, and bulk of disease.

Koh WJ, Greer BE, Abu-Rustum NR, et al: Vulvar cancer, version 1.2017, NCCN Clinical Practice Guidelines in Oncology. *J Natl Compr Canc Netw.* 2017;15(1):92-120.

Levenback CF, Ali S, Coleman RL, et al: Lymphatic mapping and sentinel node biopsy in women with squamous cell carcinoma of the vulva: a Gynecologic Oncology Group study. *J Clin Oncol.* 2012;30:3786-3791.

SURGERY FOR BENIGN VAGINAL DISEASE

▶ Imperforate Hymen

Diagnosis of imperforate hymen is often delayed until puberty, when either a workup for primary amenorrhea has ensued or the patient presents with menstrual symptoms such as cramping, without associated menses. If the patient has obstructed flow of menses, termed *hematocolpos*, examination will reveal a bulging imperforate hymen. Confirmatory rectal exam will detect a bulging, cystic mass. In prepubertal girls, the finding is subtler due to the absence of swelling. Delay of diagnosis may result in backpressure causing an enlarged uterus (hematometra) and possible retrograde menstruation leading to endometriosis. In the presence of a tightly distended hematocolpos, compression of the bladder and ureters may result in urinary obstruction.

Imperforate hymen is treated with a hymenotomy, where the obstructed hymen is incised or resected with either a scalpel or laser.

▶ Longitudinal Vaginal Septum

Duplication of the vagina resulting in a septum may occur with or without similar defects in the uterus based on the exact location of the Müllerian duct fusion defect. The duplication may take the form of a partial longitudinal septum or complete duplication of the vagina. Patients will occasionally report bleeding despite placing a tampon during menses, indicating the possibility of a second passage for menstrual

Table 41–1. International Federation of Gynecology and Obstetrics (FIGO) staging for vulvar cancer.

Stage	Revised 2009
I	Tumor confined to vulva
IA	Lesion ≤ 2 cm in size, and stromal invasion of ≤ 1 mm, nodes negative
IB	Lesion > 2 cm in size, or stromal invasion of > 1 mm, nodes negative
II	Tumor of any size extending to adjacent perineal structures: (anus, lower 1/3 of urethra, lower 1/3 of vagina); nodes negative
III	Tumor of any size with or without extension to adjacent perineal structures: (anus, lower 1/3 of urethra, lower 1/3 of vagina); inguinofemoral nodes positive
IIIA(i)	With 1 lymph node metastasis of ≥ 5 mm
IIIA(ii)	1-2 lymph node metastases of < 5 mm
IIIB(i)	With 2 or more lymph node metastases of ≥ 5 mm
IIIB(ii)	3 or more lymph node metastases of < 5 mm
IIIC	Positive nodes with extracapsular spread
IVA(i)	Invades upper urethra or vagina; bladder or rectal mucosa; or fixed to pelvic bone
IVA(ii)	Fixed or ulcerated inguinofemoral nodes
IVB	Any distant metastases including pelvic nodes

Depth of invasion measured from epithelial-stromal junction of the adjacent most superficial dermal papilla to the deepest point of invasion. This system applies for all tumor types other than melanoma. Melanoma should be staged using the American Joint Committee on Cancer melanoma staging system. Staging assessment may require cystoscopy, sigmoidoscopy, and chest x-ray for locally advanced lesions. (Reproduced with permission from Pecorelli S: Revised FIGO staging for carcinoma of the vulva, cervix, and endometrium. *Int J Gynecol Obstet* 2009; May;105(2):103-4.)

flow. Excision is performed transvaginally for symptomatic patients including those with dyspareunia, obstruction of labor, or similar problems.

Transverse Vaginal Septum

Occasionally, the vagina fails to communicate with the urogenital sinus at the introitus. This may result in formation of a transverse septum, most of which are partial. If the septum is imperforate, hematocolpos will develop following menarche. Marsupialization or excision of the septum restores vaginal patency.

Vaginal Agenesis

Vaginal agenesis, or absence of the vagina, is associated with absence of the uterus in most cases. The lower vagina, derived from the urogenital sinus, may be present, but Müllerian ductal structures comprising the upper two-thirds of the vagina and the uterus are absent or deficient. Diagnosis is usually made at time of evaluation for primary amenorrhea.

Vaginal agenesis is treated by reconstruction of a functional vagina. Treatment is usually deferred until the patient wishes to become sexually active. In a motivated patient, the vagina may be created by nonoperative dilation and elongation of the vulvar vestibule or vaginal introitus. This method, called the Frank nonoperative technique, requires up to 2 hours of dilating per day for 4-6 months. Success has been reported with vaginal dilators, vaginal molds, modified bicycle seat, and intercourse alone. If there is failure to progress or if the patient's anatomy does not favor dilation alone, surgical construction using a skin graft (McIndoe procedure), interposed bowel, or myocutaneous flaps from the perineum can be effective.

SURGERY FOR MALIGNANT AND PREMALIGNANT VAGINAL DISEASE

Vaginal intraepithelial neoplasia (VAIN) is the term used to describe the preinvasive neoplastic changes that arise in the vagina. VAIN is frequently present when HSIL of the cervix or vulva is present, and it may develop in the vagina years after completion of treatment for cancers of these two sites. Vaginal HSIL is most often detected with a Pap test. Subsequent evaluation with colposcopy, staining with 5% acetic acid, and directed biopsies provide an accurate assessment of grade and location of disease.

Treatment

Current terminology for these lesions is low-grade squamous intraepithelial lesion (LSIL) and high-grade squamous intraepithelial lesion (HSIL). LSILs (previously called VAIN-1) have a low probability of progression and may be managed with surveillance using the same principles as for management of low-grade cervical dysplasia. HSILs (previously called VAIN 2-3 and carcinoma in situ) should be treated by local excision of involved areas or with CO_2 laser photoablation. The irregular surface topography of the vagina caused by rugae makes successful visualization of lesions challenging. Recurrence rates for dysplasia are higher for vaginal dysplasia than for similarly treated cervical dysplasia, with a failure rate in the 25% range. Intravaginal placement of topical fluorouracil is an off-label indication that has been reported in the literature, and failure rates are higher than for resection or ablation. Topical fluorouracil has been reported to cause painful vaginal ulcers that heal poorly, limiting the utility of this treatment to carefully selected patients. Extensive involvement of the vagina may require subtotal or complete vaginectomy with skin grafting for maintenance of sexual function. For the elderly, sexually inactive patient, colpocleisis, where the vagina is resected and closed permanently, is an option.

Invasive carcinoma of the vagina is rare, accounting for less than 2% of gynecologic malignancies. Most vaginal cancers involve extension from either cervical or vulvar cancers, both of which are more common than lesions arising in the vagina. By convention, if the cancer involves cervix or vulva in addition to the vagina, the tumor is categorized and staged as either cervical or vulvar cancer, respectively. True vaginal cancer arises only in the vagina. About 85% of vaginal cancers are of squamous type. The next most common type is adenocarcinoma, usually with clear cell type. Rare primary tumors of the vagina include mixed mesodermal tumors, sarcoma botryoides (embryonal rhabdomyosarcoma), sarcoma, adenocarcinoma arising from Gartner duct or Müllerian duct remnants, embryonal carcinoma, and malignant melanoma.

The most common presenting symptoms of vaginal cancer include postmenopausal bleeding in about 65% of patients and persistent vaginal discharge in about 30%. Most tumors arise in the upper third of the vagina along the anterior and posterior surfaces. These sites are usually covered by the vaginal speculum and can easily be missed unless the physician observes all vaginal surfaces upon insertions and withdrawal of the speculum. Diagnosis is confirmed by biopsy.

Staging of carcinoma of the vagina is defined by FIGO and is clinical rather than surgical. See Table 41–2. Squamous cancers are most commonly found in postmenopausal patients, although they may occur even in adolescent patients. Clear cell adenocarcinoma of the vagina is more likely to occur in women below the age of 25, generally arising in vaginal adenosis. Diethylstilbestrol (DES) has been implicated in increasing the incidence of clear cell carcinoma from 1:50,000 in the unexposed population to 1:1000 in women exposed to DES in utero. Although DES is no longer produced or prescribed in this country, DES and similar

Table 41–2. International Federation of Gynecology and Obstetrics (FIGO) staging for vaginal cancer.

FIGO Stage	Description	TNM Class
Stage 0	Carcinoma in situ; intraepithelial neoplasia grade 3	Tis N0 M0
Stage I	The carcinoma is limited to the vaginal wall	T1 N0 M0
Stage II	The carcinoma has involved the subvaginal tissue but has not extended to the pelvic wall	T2 N0 M0
Stage III	The carcinoma has extended to the pelvic wall	T1 N1 M0 T2 N1 M0 T3 N0 M0 T3 N1 M0
Stage IV	The carcinoma has extended beyond the true pelvis or has involved the mucosa of the bladder or rectum. Bullous edema as such does not permit a case to be allotted to stage IV	
IVA	Tumor Invades bladder and/or rectal mucosa and/or direct extension beyond the true pelvis	T4 any N M0
IVB	Spread to distant organs	Any T Any N M1

Reproduced with permission from Benedet JL, Hacker NF, Ngan HYS (editors): FIGO staging classifications and clinical practice guidelines in the management of gynecologic cancers. FIGO Committee on Gynecologic Oncology, *Int J Gynaecol Obstet* 2000 Aug;70(2):209-262.

substances have been detected in the environment and in some food supplies.

Treatment of vaginal cancer is most often a combination of radiation therapy and chemosensitization using treatment plans similar to those for cervical cancer. Radical surgery such as radical hysterectomy with vaginectomy is possible for selected, small, upper vaginal lesions, favoring lesions on the posterior wall due to the improved likelihood of attaining adequate margins. Surgery is preferred for young patients with clear cell carcinoma as long as negative margins can be attained. In over 50% of cases, tumors have penetrated the vaginal wall at the time of the initial examination. Involvement of the bladder and rectum is common. Survival for stage I disease is about 70% but falls to about 40% for stage II and stage III disease.

Darragh TM, Colgan TJ, Cox JT, et al: The lower anogenital squamous terminology standardization project for HPV-associated lesions: background and consensus recommendations from the College of American Pathologists and the American Society for Colposcopy and Cervical Pathology. *J Lower Genital Tract Dis.* 2012;16(3):205-242.

SURGERY FOR MALIGNANT CERVICAL DISEASE

Cervical cancer is the 14th most common cancer of women in the United States but remains the fourth most common cancer of women worldwide. Almost all cervical cancers arise because of persistent infection with high-risk HPV types, most commonly types 16 and 18. Low-risk HPV types such as types 6 and 11 are usually associated with condyloma and are rarely, if ever, associated with cancer. Cervical cancer can be considered a sexually transmitted disease since most HPV infections are transmitted via sexual contact. Early sexual debut (coitarche) and multiple partners increase the risk of exposure to high-risk HPV types. HPV infections are common, and up to 80% of the population will have detectable HPV antibodies indicating prior infection. In most infected individuals, the immune system will mount a successful response, with a median time to regression of infection of about 2 years. Persistent infection with HPV 16 after age 30 increases the relative risk of cervical cancer more than 400-fold. Persistent infections and progression to cancer may be more likely in women who smoke or those with dietary deficiency of folate and β-carotene. Progression to cancer is usually gradual, allowing development of effective screening strategies with Pap tests and testing for high-risk HPV DNA, in addition to effective triage with colposcopy. Low-grade lesions usually regress, making potentially destructive treatments that have an adverse effect on fertility unnecessary. In 2006, the FDA first approved a vaccine for primary prevention of HPV infection. The vaccine is targeted primarily for adolescents prior to sexual debut; however, in 2018, its approval was expanded to include both men and women up to age 45. Widespread vaccination may largely eradicate cervical cancer in the future, although the vaccines are selective only for the most common of high-risk HPV types, raising the possibility of shifting prevalence of HPV types.

Approximately 75% of cervical cancers are squamous type. The remainder consist of adenocarcinomas, mixed carcinomas (adenosquamous), and rare tumors including carcinosarcoma and lymphoma. The relative prevalence of cervical adenocarcinoma has risen in recent years and now accounts for about 25% of cases.

Most cervical cancers arise from a preinvasive dysplastic lesion through a process that generally takes years. HSIL occurs most frequently in the fourth decade of life, whereas invasive carcinoma is encountered most often in perimenopausal women between age 40 and 50 years. Once invasion occurs, there are several routes of potential spread: (1) by direct extension to the vagina and the parametrium or (2) through lymphatic channels to the iliac and obturator lymph nodes, with occasional direct spread to para-aortic nodes. Cervical cancer staging was traditionally clinical because not all stages will require surgery. However, the staging was updated in 2018 to include use of imaging for nodal metastases. See Table 41–3.

Table 41–3. International Federation of Gynecology and Obstetrics (FIGO) staging for cervical cancer.

FIGO Stage	Revised 2018
Stage I	Carcinoma confined to cervix (extension to corpus would be disregarded)
IA	Invasive carcinoma, diagnosed only by microscopy. All macroscopically visible lesions, even with superficial invasion, are stage IB.
IA-1	Measured stromal invasion < 3 mm
IA-2	Measured stromal invasion > 3 mm and < 5 mm
IB	Invasive carcinoma with measured deepest invasion ≥ 5 mm; lesion limited to the cervix
IB-1	Invasive carcinoma ≥ 5 mm depth of stromal invasion and < 2 cm in greatest dimension
IB-2	Invasive carcinoma ≥ 2 cm and < 4 cm in greatest dimension
IB-3	Invasive carcinoma ≥ 4 cm in greatest dimension
Stage II	Tumor invades beyond uterus but not to pelvic wall or to the lower third of vagina
IIA	Tumor without parametrial invasion
IIA-1	Clinically visible lesion < 4 cm in greatest dimension
IIA-2	Clinically visible lesion ≥ 4 cm in greatest dimension
IIB	Tumor with obvious parametrial invasion, but not to pelvic sidewall
Stage III	Tumor extends to the pelvic wall and/or involves lower third of vagina and/or causes hydronephrosis or nonfunctioning kidney and/or involves the pelvic or para-aortic lymph nodes
IIIA	Tumor involves lower third of the vagina, with no extension to pelvic wall
IIIB	Extends to pelvic wall or causes hydronephrosis or nonfunctioning kidney
IIIC	Involves the pelvic or para-aortic lymph nodes, irrespective of tumor size or extent
IIIC1	Pelvic lymph node metastasis only
IIIC2	Para-aortic lymph node metastasis
Stage IV	Carcinoma extends beyond true pelvis or with biopsy-proven spread to bladder or rectal mucosa. Bullous edema does not cause case to be allotted to stage IV
IVA	Spread to adjacent organs
IVB	Spread to distant organs

Reproduced with permission from Bhatla N, Berek JS, Cuello Fredes M, et al: Revised FIGO staging for carcinoma of the cervix uteri, *Int J Gynaecol Obstet.* 2019 Apr;145(1):129-135.

▶ Intraepithelial Lesions (Formerly Dysplasia & Carcinoma In Situ)

Successful screening has greatly reduced the incidence and mortality of cervical cancer and its precursors over the past 50 years. Current screening recommendations for lower genital tract cancers of the vulva, vagina, and cervix have been outlined earlier. When a neoplastic lesion is detected by screening, proper and timely triage is needed. HSILs are typically asymptomatic.

Colposcopic examination of the cervix is the gold standard for assessing intraepithelial lesions and early invasive disease. Application of Lugol's iodine can be a useful adjunct to the colposcopic exam. Normal mature squamous epithelium of the cervix and vagina contains glycogen and stains a dark brown color when Lugol's is applied, whereas dysplastic cells lack glycogen and stain a light yellow color.

Colposcopically directed biopsy is performed for visible abnormalities including acetowhite change, abnormal vessels, ulceration, and papillary lesions. Biopsy-confirmed cervical LSILs (previously called CIN-1) are managed conservatively because most of these lesions regress spontaneously, and there is very little risk of progression to cancer. When a biopsy shows an HSIL (previously called CIN-2, CIN-3, and carcinoma in situ), treatment is either ablative cryotherapy or resection via cold-knife cone biopsy or electrosurgical loop excision. Treatment should include either ablation or removal of the entire transformation zone, defined as the area bounded by the original and current squamocolumnar junction. There are some exceptions when treating adolescents and young adult patients under the age of 25, so the clinician must be familiar with current ASCCP guidelines. Some dysplastic lesions may extend into the endocervical canal, including squamous lesions and most glandular lesions. The preferred treatment for a lesion extending out of colposcopic view into the endocervical canal is excision with a cold-knife cone biopsy in the operating room. Both electrosurgical loop excision and cold-knife cone biopsy increase risk of future preterm delivery, mandating careful triage of only those individuals truly requiring an excisional procedure.

▶ Invasive Carcinoma

Early stromal invasion, defined as microinvasion, is usually asymptomatic. Larger lesions frequently cause postmenopausal bleeding (46%), intermenstrual bleeding (20%), or postcoital bleeding (10%). A watery or malodorous vaginal discharge may be the only symptom. Pain is a manifestation of advanced-stage disease typically extending to the pelvic sidewall with entrapment of the sciatic nerve or femoral nerve. Inspection of the cervix typically reveals an ulcerated or papillary lesion that bleeds on contact. The cytologic examination almost always demonstrates exfoliated malignant cells, although the false-negative rate for an individual Pap test approaches 50% for invasive lesions due to obscuration of malignant cells by inflammation and necrotic debris.

▶ Differential Diagnosis

Chronic cervicitis may appear similar to cancer of the cervix. Polyps of the cervix are often benign, but malignancy can only be ruled out with biopsy. Nabothian cysts are benign, common, and can appear bizarre to the untrained eye but are readily distinguished from cancer by biopsy.

Natural History

Spread of cervical cancer into the parametrium may cause obstruction of the ureter, resulting in hydroureter, hydronephrosis, and uremia. Bilateral obstruction of the ureters leads to kidney failure and death. Involvement of the iliac and obturator lymph nodes may lead to lymphatic obstruction, resulting in lymphedema. Pelvic sidewall nerves, especially the sciatic nerve, may become compressed, causing sciatica or pain in the low back, hip, and leg. Tumor invasion into the bladder or rectum sometimes causes vesicovaginal or rectovaginal fistulae, especially following radiation therapy. Widespread metastases to lung, liver, brain, and bone may occur.

Treatment

Treatment of cervical cancer is stratified by stage. Microinvasive disease, defined as FIGO stage IA-1, has less than a 1% chance of lymphatic metastasis and may be managed conservatively with cone biopsy for preservation of fertility or with simple hysterectomy when preservation of fertility is not desired or relevant. Radical hysterectomy with bilateral pelvic lymph node dissection is the preferred treatment for FIGO stage IA-2 through IIA disease. Radical hysterectomy includes resection of much wider margins than is performed with a simple hysterectomy, including removal of the cardinal and uterosacral ligaments and the upper third of the vagina, in addition to pelvic, obturator, and (optional) para-aortic nodes. Radical hysterectomy procedures have been historically performed either via laparotomy or laparoscopy, although recent randomized trial evidence shows that cancer-related outcomes are greatly improved via the open approach. Procedural details for the most commonly used hysterectomy types (including radical hysterectomy types) are described in Table 41–4.

Complications of radical surgery include hemorrhage, infection, thromboembolism, and a less than 1% risk of uterovaginal, vesicovaginal, or rectovaginal fistula. Early-stage lesions may also be treated with radiation therapy and concurrent chemosensitization with cisplatin with equal likelihood of cure but higher potential morbidity.

The recently developed radical trachelectomy with laparoscopic lymphadenectomy offers a fertility-sparing option for carefully selected individuals with stage IA-2 or stage IB-1 squamous lesions. The cervix, upper vagina, and supporting ligaments are removed as with a radical hysterectomy, but the uterine corpus is preserved. In the posttrachelectomy pregnancies currently reported, there is a 10% likelihood of second-trimester loss, but 72% of patients carry their gestation to 37 weeks or more.

Advanced-stage disease, including FIGO stage IIB and above, requires treatment with external radiation, brachytherapy implants, and concurrent chemosensitization. At least five randomized trials have confirmed a survival advantage for cisplatin-based therapy given weekly during radiation. Uncommon delayed complications of radiation therapy that affect quality of life are cystitis and proctitis. Severe radiation cystitis or proctitis may result in hemorrhage, fistula, or strictures, typically arising several years after treatment in about 1%-3% of patients. Radiation necrosis of the cervix and diffuse radiation pelvic fibrosis are rare complications. Radiating the reproductive tract destroys the function of the uterus, and unless the ovaries have been surgically transposed out of the pelvis, ovarian failure is unavoidable. Recurrent or persistent disease in the central pelvis following radiation therapy may potentially be cured with the ultraradical pelvic exenteration procedure.

Prognosis

Survival is strongly linked to stage at time of diagnosis. Properly treated stage I disease averages 90% survival at 5 years and

Table 41–4. Types of hysterectomy.

	Comparison of Hysterectomy Types		
Anatomic Structure	Extrafascial Type 1	Modified Radical Type 2	Radical Type 3
Uterus	Removed	Removed	Removed
Ovaries	Optional removal	Optional removal	Optional removal
Cervix	Removed	Removed	Removed
Vaginal margin	None	1-2 cm margin	Upper one-third of vagina
Ureters	Not mobilized	Dissected through broad ligament	Dissected through broad ligament
Cardinal ligaments	Divided at uterine border	Divided where ureter transits the broad ligament	Divided at pelvic sidewall
Uterosacral ligaments	Divided at cervical border	Partially resected	Divided near sacral origin
Bladder	Mobilized to base of cervix	Mobilized to upper vagina	Mobilized to middle vagina
Rectum	Not mobilized	Mobilized below cervix	Mobilized below middle vagina

approaches 96% in radical hysterectomy cases with negative margins and negative lymph nodes. For stage II disease, 5-year survival is about 65%, but this rate decreases to about 45% for stage III disease and to less than 10% for stage IV disease.

Koh WJ, Greer BE, Abu-Rustum NR, et al: Cervical Cancer, Version 2.2015. *J Natl Compr Canc Netw.* 2015;13(4):395-404.

Massad LS, Einstein MH, Huh WK, et al: 2012 updated consensus guidelines for the management of abnormal cervical cancer screening tests and cancer precursors. *J Lower Genital Tract Dis.* 2013;17(5):S1-S27.

Schneider A, Erdemoglu E, Chiantera V, et al: Clinical recommendation: radical trachelectomy for fertility preservation in patients with early stage cervical cancer. *Int J Gynecol Cancer.* 2012;22(4):659-666.

US Cancer Statistics Working Group: U.S. Cancer Statistics Data Visualizations Tool, based on November 2017 submission data (1999-2015): U.S. Department of Health and Human Services, Centers for Disease Control and Prevention and National Cancer Institute. www.cdc.gov/cancer/dataviz. Accessed June 2018.

SURGERY FOR PELVIC FLOOR DEFECTS

Cystocele, Rectocele, & Incontinence

An understanding of pelvic support defects requires a thorough knowledge of the anatomic relationships of the pelvic viscera and their supporting tissues. These conditions were originally thought to result from stretching and tearing of the muscles, nerves, and connective tissues of the pelvis during vaginal childbirth. The current understanding is that many pelvic floor defects arise from site-specific tears or breaks of pelvic connective tissue. Causes can include stretching, compression, or tearing during parturition but also include behaviors that increase intra-abdominal pressure such as chronic constipation, heavy lifting, obesity, and chronic cough. Smoking, poor nutrition, and lack of pelvic floor exercise may exacerbate pelvic floor defects. The symptoms of pelvic floor defects may include pelvic pressure or a sensation of "falling out" of the pelvic organs, a mass protruding from the vagina (which may be a cystocele, rectocele, prolapsing cervix, or all of these), stress incontinence, fecal incontinence, and other difficulties with defecation.

Complete examination generally requires evaluating the patient in both the lithotomy and standing positions and by asking her to perform Valsalva or cough. Vaginal support is described with three different levels, illustrated in Figure 41–5. Level I includes the cervix and upper third of the vagina. Level I support is composed superiorly by uterosacral ligaments, endopelvic fascia, and smooth muscle; laterally by support from the cardinal ligaments; and anteriorly from the

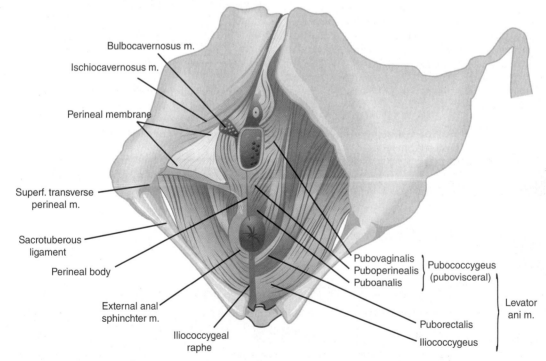

▲ **Figure 41–5.** Anatomy of pelvic support. (Reproduced with permission from Schorge JO, Williams JW: *Williams Gynecology*, New York, NY: McGraw-Hill Education; 2008.)

pubocervical fascia. Level II defines midvaginal support and is composed laterally by attachments to the arcus tendineus fascia pelvis, anteriorly by the pubocervical fascia, and posteriorly by Denonvillier fascia. Level III refers to support of the lower vagina and urethra. Level III support is provided anteriorly by attachment of the urogenital membrane to the symphysis pubis, laterally to the levator ani muscle, and posteriorly to the perineal body. A pelvic organ prolapse quantification profile (POPQ) has been defined by the International Continence Society, the American Urogynecology Society, and the Society of Gynecologic Surgeons (Figure 41–6). Use of the POPQ quantitates the extent and location of defects such that subsequent therapy is directed more specifically. Descent and bulging of the anterior vagina are usually due to a cystocele, a paravaginal defect, or an anterior enterocele. An anatomic defect in the posterior vagina is usually a rectocele or enterocele.

Additional testing that may be necessary for elucidation of the site-specific defect includes assessment of urethral mobility with the Q-tip test, cystourethroscopy, cystometrogram, anoscopy, colonoscopy, anal manometry, and transanal ultrasound. Chronic urinary tract infections must be ruled out prior to deciding upon surgical repair. For fecal incontinence, gastrointestinal disorders such as irritable bowel syndrome, infections such as *Clostridium difficile* or other causes of diarrhea, and malabsorption must be ruled out before proposing surgery.

Repair of pelvic floor defects is based on the principle of identification of the specific site of injury leading to site-specific repair. Pelvic support defects are often treated nonsurgically. For example, postmenopausal women with mild to moderate defects as determined by the POPQ score may experience improvement of symptoms after the administration of a topical estrogen, after initiation of Kegel exercises, or by fitting a pessary to support the pelvic structures. Pessaries are inert material manufactured in many different sizes and shapes that can be fitted to the patient. When inserted in the vagina, a pessary mechanically supports pelvic structures, resulting in temporary correction of the underlying symptoms. A pessary is a good option for patients who choose not to undergo surgery or for those who cannot have surgery.

The Nine–Point POPQ and Staging Definitions		
Point	Description	Range
Aa	Anterior wall 3 cm from hymen	−3 to +3
Ba	Most dependent part of the rest of the anterior wall	−3 to +TVL
C	Cervix or vaginal cuff	+/− TVL
D	Posterior fornix (if no prior total hysterectomy)	+/− TVL
Ap	Posterior wall 3 cm from hymen	−3 to +3
Bp	Most dependent part of the rest of the posterior wall	−3 to +TVL
GH	Genital hiatus (mid-urethra to PB)	No limit

▲ **Figure 41–6.** Pelvic organ prolapse quantification (POPQ) table. Six sites (points Aa, Ba, C, D, Bp, and Ap), genital hiatus (GH), perineal body (PB), and total vaginal length (TVL) are used for quantification of pelvic organ support. Each point is described with respect to position relative to the hymen in centimeters. Positive values represent distance outside the hymen, and negative numbers represent distance superior to the hymen. (Reproduced with permission from Schwartz SI, Brunicardi F: Schwartz's Principles of Surgery: *Self-Assessment and Board Review*, 8th ed. New York, NY: McGraw-Hill Education; 2007.)

Differential Diagnosis

Urethral diverticula may mimic cystocele and produce a bulge of the anterior vaginal wall. A discrete mass is usually palpable. Pressure or massage of the mass may result in turbid or purulent urethral drainage. Vaginal cysts such as Gartner duct or Skene duct cysts are occasionally mistaken for bladder support defects.

Treatment

Categories of pelvic floor defects include anterior compartment, vault prolapse, uterine prolapse, enterocele, posterior compartment, urinary incontinence, and fecal incontinence.

A. Anterior Compartment

Anterior compartment defects, including cystocele and paravaginal defects, are often associated with concurrent urinary incontinence. **Stress incontinence** is involuntary loss of urine caused by increases in intra-abdominal pressure including coughing, heavy lifting, or Valsalva maneuver in the absence of detrusor contraction. Stress incontinence is usually demonstrated during examination by asking the patient to cough. Stress incontinence should be distinguished from other common types of urinary incontinence including urge and overflow incontinence. With **urge incontinence,** the detrussor muscle contracts or spasms, resulting in leakage with associated urgency. **Mixed incontinence** is defined as a combination of stress and urge incontinence. **Overflow incontinence** is often a continual slow leak of urine associated with incomplete emptying and large residual volumes. Stress incontinence is the only type that is amenable to surgical correction. Correction of stress incontinence occasionally produces urge incontinence that may persist in 10%-15% of patients.

Normally, the proximal urethra is supported above the urogenital diaphragm and is subjected to the same intra-abdominal pressure changes as those applied to the bladder. In patients with anterior vaginal compartment defects, the proximal urethra can be hypermobile, and increased intra-abdominal pressure causes the proximal urethra and bladder base to descend into the vagina. Pressure in the bladder thereby exceeds the sphincter pressure, resulting in leakage of urine. Intrinsic sphincter deficiency is a second mechanism of stress incontinence. Risk factors include previous incontinence surgery, prior radiation therapy, and age over 50.

Site-directed repair of anterior compartment defects may include anterior colporrhaphy or repair of paravaginal defects. Repair of stress urinary incontinence can be achieved by retropubic colposuspension using either the Burch or Marshall-Marchetti-Kranz procedure. Success of these two procedures is approximately 85% at 5 years. Recurrent or difficult cases of stress urinary incontinence are often surgically treated with use of slings or grafts to augment support. Grafts may be created from endogenous fascia, usually harvested from the rectus fascia, or exogenous sources including allografts, xenografts, or synthetic mesh. Procedures using the grafts include sling procedures or the tension-free vaginal tape procedure, which has significantly reduced the morbidity of graft procedures compared to historical controls. For patients with intrinsic sphincter deficiency or for patients who are not candidates for more involved surgical procedures, a minimally invasive treatment involves injection of collagen at the urethrovesical junction as a bulking agent to increase outlet resistance.

B. Prolapse

Prolapse, where the level I support involving the upper vagina or uterus is deficient, involves symptomatic descent of the upper vaginal tissues and/or uterus. Prolapse may also be associated with anterior and posterior compartment defects.

Repair of vaginal prolapse is generally performed with a unilateral sacrospinous ligament suspension (SSLS) procedure performed transvaginally or with an abdominal sacrocolpopexy procedure performed via laparotomy or laparoscopy. In the SSLS procedure, the vaginal apex is sutured to the sacrospinous ligament. In the abdominal sacrocolpopexy procedure, a retroperitoneal mesh is sutured from the upper vagina to the anterior longitudinal sacral ligament. Treatment of uterine prolapse sometimes involves hysterectomy combined with SSLS or sacrocolpopexy procedures. Uterine preservation is permissible, combined with plication of uterosacral ligaments or the other procedures described earlier. Surgical correction of prolapse has a 15%-30% failure rate, although patient satisfaction remains high and reoperation low.

C. Enterocele

Enterocele is a hernia that develops between the vagina and the rectum. Diagnosis is confirmed by palpation on pelvic exam and can also be documented on transvaginal ultrasound. Surgical repair requires reapproximation of the fascial defect at the apex of the rectovaginal septum via laparotomy, laparoscopy, or vaginal approach depending on other planned combined procedures.

D. Posterior Compartment

Posterior compartment defects, including rectocele and anal sphincter defects, often are associated with concurrent difficulty with defecation or fecal incontinence (involuntary loss of stool or flatus).

Fecal incontinence alone is not diagnostic of a posterior compartment defect and can also be associated with diarrhea, increased bowel motility, or neurologic disorders such as diabetes, spinal cord injury, or multiple sclerosis. Testing includes careful exam of level II and level III structures, resting anal sphincter tone, and voluntary anal sphincter contraction. Additional tests that may be needed to elucidate the etiology of incontinence include anal manometry, transanal ultrasound, MRI, colonoscopy, defecography, and electromyography. Diarrheal illness and gastrointestinal disorders such as irritable bowel syndrome should be treated prior to consideration of surgery.

Nonsurgical treatment may include use of medications to slow transit time, bulking agents, biofeedback, and electrical stimulation therapy.

Site-directed repair of posterior compartment defects may include posterior colporrhaphy, where posterior fascial defects are repaired primarily or with grafts, sphincteroplasty, or repair of rectal prolapse.

In patients who are no longer planning sexual activity, vaginal closure (colpocleisis) and removal (colpectomy) are also options.

Delancey JO: Why do women have stress urinary incontinence? *Neurourol Urodyn.* 2010;29(suppl 1):S13-S17.

Urinary Tract Fistula

Urinary tract fistulae to the vagina include vesicovaginal, ureterovaginal, and urethrovaginal types. Vesicovaginal fistula is the most common type. In the United States, most urinary tract fistulae occur following pelvic surgery with unrecognized injury or ischemia, particularly ischemia associated with radiation therapy. Worldwide, urinary tract fistulae are more likely to be secondary to prolonged or obstructed labor. Fistulae may also occur as a result of tumor invasion, retained foreign bodies, and chronic inflammation.

Most urologic fistulae arise following gynecologic surgery rather than urologic or colorectal surgery. Total abdominal hysterectomy is the procedure most often complicated by the development of vesicovaginal fistula. A skillful identification of the critical anatomy during surgery can greatly minimize the risk of fistula formation. Injuries recognized at the time of primary surgery should be repaired immediately. Development of postoperative fistulae or delayed recognition of injury may require a waiting period to allow inflammation to subside before undertaking repair.

▶ Symptoms & Signs

Vaginal leakage of urine and constant urinary leakage are symptoms of a urologic fistula. If the fistula involves the distal urethra, the patient may experience vaginal leakage only at the time of voiding. Vesicovaginal and ureterovaginal fistulae almost always develop near the vaginal apex. A urethrovaginal fistula opens into the anterior vaginal wall.

On speculum exam, urine will usually be seen pooling at the vaginal apex. Most fistulae in nonradiated patients are small and may not be readily seen with the naked eye. Confirmation of a suspected vesicovaginal fistula may be demonstrated by instilling dilute methylene blue dye or sterile milk into the bladder with a catheter while inspecting the vaginal vault. A small fistula may leak little and is often better recognized by placing a tampon in the vagina when methylene blue dye is instilled in the bladder and then removing the tampon about 15-20 minutes later to inspect for blue. To detect a ureterovaginal fistula, oral phenazopyridine can be given and will be excreted through the ureters. This is best detected by placement of a tampon for about 30 minutes, followed by inspection for staining. Other useful diagnostic tests include cystoscopy, cystogram, and intravenous pyelogram to assess for the site of injury.

▶ Treatment

In nonradiated, noninfected tissue, many small fistulae will close spontaneously if the bladder is drained with an indwelling catheter to reduce flow through the fistulae. Larger fistulae or small fistulae that fail conservative management must be repaired surgically. One should allow 8-12 weeks for resolution of edema and inflammatory reactions prior to undertaking repair. Premature repair has a high likelihood of being unsuccessful. Urinary tract infections should be treated and skin integrity should be protected with an occlusive barrier cream before surgical correction is attempted.

Repair of vesicovaginal fistulae involves a number of techniques, including layered closure with the Latzko procedure via the vaginal approach or via laparotomy with omental interposition. Principles of repair include meticulous and atraumatic technique using fine suture material; approximation without tension; and bladder decompression postoperatively. Ureterovaginal fistulae are repaired with ureteroneocystotomy if the ureteral injury is in the lower pelvis and with ureteroureterostomy for injury sites higher in the pelvis. These are usually performed via laparotomy, but a laparoscopic approach can be used. Fistulae in radiated tissue cannot be repaired primarily due to chronic tissue ischemia. These fistulae require the introduction of a nonradiated blood supply provided by bulbocavernosus or gracilis myocutaneous flaps for successful repair or, alternatively, permanent urinary diversion.

Rectovaginal Fistula

Rectovaginal fistulae may occur following obstetric injury, pelvic surgery, cervical or rectal cancer, radiation therapy, inflammatory bowel disease, or diverticular disease. The patient will report vaginal passage of flatus or feces, or foul vaginal discharge, sometimes associated with bleeding. The fistula can often be demonstrated upon speculum examination or by palpation on rectovaginal exam. Diagnostic studies such as barium enema x-ray or sigmoidoscopy may be useful for smaller lesions.

To reduce the risk of infection and break down of a planned fistula repair, the bowel should be prepared with a low-residue diet, antibiotics, and a cathartic bowel regimen preoperatively. A rectovaginal fistula in the lower third of the vagina should be repaired after the surrounding inflammation and edema have resolved, usually requiring a delay of approximately 12 weeks. Rectovaginal fistulae in the upper two-thirds of the vagina are best treated with a preliminary diverting colostomy, followed by fistula repair and subsequent colostomy takedown about 2-3 months after the repair.

Fistulae caused by inflammatory bowel disease such as Crohn disease have a high likelihood of recurrence unless the disease is clearly in remission. Ileostomy and abdominoperineal resection are necessary in patients whose symptoms are unacceptable despite medical management. Fistulae associated with radiation therapy can rarely be repaired, and those associated with cancer are not amenable to surgical repair. A diverting colostomy provides considerable relief of symptoms in these situations.

▼ THE UPPER GENITAL TRACT
SURGERY FOR BENIGN UTERINE DISEASE
Congenital Uterine Anomalies

Congenital duplication defects of the uterus are rare, with a reported incidence of 0.4%-1%, and are usually diagnosed during a workup for recurrent spontaneous abortions, premature labor, fetal malpresentation, retained placenta, and postpartum hemorrhage (see Figure 41-1). Anomalies include septate uterus, composed of a simple midline septum; bicornuate uterus, which is a duplication of the uterine horns; and uterus didelphys, consisting of complete duplication of the corpus and cervix. These anomalies can be detected with physical examination, especially during or after pregnancies complicated by malpresentation or preterm labor. Testing with MRI or hysterosalpingogram will usually confirm the diagnosis and is combined with ultrasonography or laparoscopy if the diagnosis remains uncertain. Laparoscopy and hysteroscopy are useful for planning surgical correction.

Surgical correction of uterine anomalies is indicated for prevention of previously experienced or anticipated pregnancy-related complications. A septate uterus is twice as likely to cause a spontaneous abortion than a bicornuate uterus, with an overall pregnancy loss rate of 88% reported

for patients with a complete uterine septum. The septate uterus is treated with a septoplasty, completed in most cases by hysteroscopic division or resection of the septum with up to an 86% success rate for subsequent pregnancies. Alternatively, the abdominal metroplasty is indicated for a large or thick septum or for a bicornuate uterus. A wedge of myometrium is resected, allowing the two horns of the uterus to be joined. This procedure results in measurable loss of uterine volume. Pregnancies occurring after abdominal metroplasty also should be delivered by scheduled, early cesarean section as the risk of uterine rupture with labor is increased.

Abnormal Uterine Bleeding

Abnormal uterine bleeding may occur at any age. It is not unusual for a female infant to have a small amount of self-limited vaginal bleeding attributable to the decline of circulating estrogen from maternal sources after delivery.

Abnormal uterine bleeding during the reproductive years is described according to the chronicity and amount of bleeding because this is often useful in elucidating the etiology. Hypermenorrhea, also referred to as menorrhagia, is defined as excessive or prolonged bleeding at the normal time of menstruation. Polymenorrhea is defined as bleeding that occurs more frequently than every 3 weeks, and metrorrhagia refers to intermenstrual bleeding that occurs in the interval between menses.

Hypermenorrhea may be due to physical/anatomic abnormalities of the uterus including uterine leiomyoma, adenomyosis, and endometrial polyps. Dysfunctional uterine bleeding is abnormal uterine bleeding related to functional response of a normal uterus to extrauterine causes such as abnormal cycling of estrogen and progesterone in patients with anovulation, oligo-ovulation, or persistence of the corpus luteum. Dysfunctional uterine bleeding is seen most often in adolescents and in perimenopausal women. Polymenorrhea is sometimes related to a shortened proliferative phase secondary to hypothyroidism. Causes of metrorrhagia (bleeding between periods) include endometrial polyps, submucosal leiomyoma, coagulopathy, granulomatous infections such as tuberculosis, or cancer of the cervix or uterine corpus. Complications of pregnancy should not be overlooked as a cause of abnormal bleeding in women of reproductive age.

Postmenopausal bleeding is defined as any vaginal bleeding occurring a year or more after menopause and is of concern because it may be a symptom of endometrial cancer. When postmenopausal bleeding is fully evaluated with endometrial biopsy and hormone studies, the majority will be attributed to benign etiologies such as atrophic change, benign polyp, cervicitis, and physiologic withdrawal from exogenous hormones. Endometrial cancer is detected in about 15% of cases of postmenopausal bleeding, but the likelihood increases with increasing age: a 50-year-old woman with postmenopausal bleeding has about a 2% chance of cancer, whereas an 80-year-old woman with the same symptom has about a 60% chance of malignancy. Cervical cancer may also present with postmenopausal bleeding. The exogenous administration of estrogenic substances, including hormone replacement therapy, and use of estrogen analogs such as tamoxifen can cause postmenopausal bleeding as well. Much less likely causes include estrogen-producing tumors of the ovary, coagulopathy, or environmental sources of estrogenic substances. Postmenopausal bleeding in any amount ranging from scant brown vaginal discharge to frank, profuse, bright red bleeding should prompt further workup. Cancer should be considered the likely cause until proven otherwise.

Clinical Findings

Obtain a complete history and perform a careful pelvic examination including a Pap test. The exam will often reveal vaginal, cervical, uterine, or adnexal disease. A complete blood count and measurement of red cell indices will ascertain the degree of chronic blood loss. Additional blood studies, including thyroid function testing and testing for coagulopathy, may be necessary in some cases.

Abnormal bleeding should prompt an endometrial biopsy in any of the following situations: in women over the age of 35, in those with a Pap test result showing atypical glandular cells, or in women with risk factors for gynecologic cancer. The biopsy should be timed at an appropriate time in the menstrual cycle, such as after the 16th day of the cycle if anovulatory bleeding is suspected, but may be performed at any time to evaluate for hyperplasia or carcinoma. Endometrial sampling with a disposable suction device can be accomplished in an office setting in most patients. Obese patients or patients with cervical stenosis may require dilatation and curettage in the operating room. Pregnancy must always be ruled out before performing a biopsy in a woman of reproductive age.

Hysteroscopy, involving insertion of a narrow-diameter videoscope through the cervix while distending the uterine cavity, allows inspection of the endometrium and directed biopsy of suspicious features. Hysteroscopy is very useful for determining the cause of bleeding and offers the opportunity for simultaneous treatment, such as hysteroscopic resection of a polyp. Hysteroscopy can be accomplished in an office or outpatient surgical setting and is recommended when bleeding is recurrent or resistant to therapy or when structural abnormalities of the endometrium, such as polyps or submucous leiomyomata, are suspected.

Transvaginal ultrasound is useful to measure endometrial thickness and structural abnormalities of the uterus, such as a polyp or leiomyoma. In the postmenopausal patient, an endometrial stripe of less than or equal to 4 mm virtually excludes the presence of cancer. However, biopsy is still preferable unless it is unable to be performed for technical reasons. The sonohysterogram, where saline is introduced into the endometrial cavity during ultrasound, increases diagnostic accuracy for defects in the endometrial cavity.

Treatment

Dilation and curettage is both diagnostic and therapeutic for many causes of uterine bleeding. Definitive treatment, however, will be targeted toward the etiology of the abnormal uterine bleeding.

Medical management of most nonneoplastic causes of abnormal uterine bleeding is generally prescribed before considering surgery because many symptoms will resolve or be adequately managed without surgical intervention. Chronic blood loss due to hypermenorrhea produced by leiomyoma or hyperplasia can be reduced by the administration of a progestin. A gonadotropin-releasing hormone agonist will result in amenorrhea and is sometimes prescribed prior to a planned surgery for leiomyomata. The antiprogestin mifepristone may significantly shrink leiomyomata, but a side effect includes increased risk of endometrial hyperplasia. Dysfunctional bleeding due to chronic anovulation is treated with cyclic progestin therapy or oral contraceptives. For women who wish to conceive, ovulation induction with drugs such as clomiphene is prescribed. Control of acute heavy bleeding may be achieved through use of higher doses of combination oral contraceptives prescribed as one pill four times a day for 3 or 4 days, tapered to one pill a day over 1 week. Alternatively, intravenous conjugated estrogen, 25 mg every 4 hours, can also be used to control acute bleeding. Such a regimen must be followed by a progestin to prevent additional subsequent irregular bleeding. Following control of acute bleeding, maintenance therapy with an oral contraceptive is recommended. Another strategy for maintenance includes placement of a progestin-containing intrauterine device (IUD), resulting in amenorrhea in about 25% of women and light menses in the remainder. In the absence of identified intrauterine pathology, pain associated with ovulatory cycles can be ameliorated with nonsteroidal anti-inflammatory drugs.

Persistence of symptoms may require surgical intervention. Surgical treatment of bleeding caused by uterine leiomyoma is discussed later in this chapter. Severe or intractable dysfunctional uterine bleeding may require hysterectomy. Endometrial ablation by hysteroscopically directed electrosurgery or use of proprietary endometrial ablation devices may avoid hysterectomy in the perimenopausal patient with bleeding who cannot be managed medically. Ablation generally requires normal size and shape of the uterine cavity. Up to 55% of women report amenorrhea following endometrial ablation, but about one-third will undergo eventual hysterectomy. Placement of a levonorgestrel-containing IUD is frequently as effective as hysteroscopic endometrial ablation.

Postmenopausal bleeding due to atrophic changes may resolve with estrogen therapy administered with progestin in either a cyclic or continuous fashion. Postmenopausal bleeding attributed to physiologic withdrawal bleeding from prescribed estrogen-based therapy is treated by discontinuing therapy or converting to a continuous regimen. Curettage for removal of benign endometrial polyps is often curative, although polyps may recur. Endometrial carcinoma is a relative contraindication to estrogen therapy and is treated surgically with hysterectomy, with possible postoperative adjuvant radiation or chemotherapy based on stage and grade of the tumor (see later in chapter). Well-differentiated endometrial adenocarcinoma in young women who desire to maintain fertility has been successfully treated using high-dose progestins in about three-fourths of cases. Evidence-based guidelines published by the National Comprehensive Cancer Network (NCCN) provide regularly updated and detailed algorithms for choosing optimal adjuvant therapies.

Adenomyosis

Extension of endometrial glands and stroma into the myometrium is termed *adenomyosis*. Symptomatic adenomyosis is most prevalent between age 35 and menopause. Symptoms include dysmenorrhea, hypermenorrhea, polymenorrhea, metrorrhagia, and dyspareunia. Concurrent endometriosis and adenomyosis is common. Symptoms typically improve after menopause.

Upon pelvic examination, the uterus is slightly to moderately enlarged and is frequently tender to palpation, particularly in the secretory phase of the menstrual cycle. Preoperative confirmation of adenomyosis is challenging. Neither ultrasound nor endometrial biopsy is useful for making the diagnosis. T2-weighted sequences on pelvic MRI are more effective but have a sensitivity of only 70% and specificity of 86%. Definitive diagnosis is confirmed on pathology after hysterectomy.

▶ Differential Diagnosis

Leiomyomata of the uterus are common and cause many symptoms similar to adenomyosis. Low-grade endometrial stromal sarcoma is rare and can be mistaken for adenomyosis. This is an indolent malignancy with a significant likelihood of local recurrence. Distant metastases to the ovary, peritoneal surfaces, and lung are occasionally seen. Tumors of this type should not be morcellated at the time of hysterectomy. Subsequent treatment may include pelvic radiation therapy and hormone therapy based on stage at time of diagnosis and presence of estrogen and progesterone receptors.

▶ Treatment

For adenomyosis, total hysterectomy with or without bilateral salpingo-oophorectomy is the only clearly effective treatment. Hormonal approaches may be successful in treating symptoms, particularly if the patient is nearing menopause, at which time symptoms typically regress.

Leiomyomata

Uterine leiomyomata, or fibroids, are present in 20%-30% of women of reproductive age. The true prevalence is unknown because many fibroids are asymptomatic. Black women have a threefold higher incidence than white, Asian, and Hispanic women. Other risk factors include obesity, nulliparity, early menarche, and infertility. Leiomyomas arise from monoclonal proliferation and are stimulated by estrogen, progesterone, and growth factors. Fibroids increase in growth rate during pregnancy and regress after menopause. Fibroids are usually multifocal and vary greatly in size, ranging from a few millimeters to masses large enough to fill the abdomen. The location of leiomyomata can be nearly anywhere within the uterus. Descriptive terms for location include *intramural* for fibroids arising within the myometrium, *subserosal* for lesions below the exterior surface of the uterus, and *submucosal* for fibroids adjacent to the endometrium. Other types of leiomyomata include pedunculated lesions connected with a narrow vascular stalk to the uterus, intraligamentous lesions within the broad ligament, and parasitic leiomyomata, which are detached from the uterus and derive blood supply from adjacent organs.

▶ Clinical Findings

Symptoms are determined by location, number, and size of the lesions. Common symptoms include hypermenorrhea, prolonged menses, pelvic pressure, increased abdominal girth, urinary frequency, dyspareunia, low back pain, and constipation. Infertility may occur secondary to fibroids, particularly if the uterine cavity is enlarged or distorted by a submucosal lesion. Adverse pregnancy outcomes such as abnormal placentation, fetal malpresentation, placental abruption, and dysfunctional labor are recognized complications associated with fibroids. Degenerative changes may spontaneously occur, potentially causing significant pain that requires treatment. Submucosal leiomyomata are more likely to cause hypermenorrhea, polymenorrhea, and metrorrhagia.

Palpation of the uterus during bimanual examination may reveal a lobular and enlarged structure with a characteristic rubbery consistency. Soft and tender lesions are characteristic of degenerating fibroids. Larger lesions may be felt on abdominal examination.

Anemia may result from acute or chronic abnormal uterine bleeding. Endometrial biopsy should be performed in women with abnormal uterine bleeding to rule out endometrial cancer (see earlier in chapter). Pelvic ultrasound is the most useful study for diagnosis of fibroids. Sonohysterogram and hysteroscopy are also useful for confirmation of submucosal leiomyomata. MRI should be used selectively for evaluation of atypical lesions that could represent sarcoma or for surgical planning prior to myomectomy. Hydronephrosis may be apparent on imaging studies, arising as a result of external compression by an enlarged uterus on the distal ureter.

Differential Diagnosis

Uterine leiomyosarcoma is a rare but aggressive neoplasm. Among women undergoing surgery for fibroids, only 0.23% are found to harbor sarcoma. The rapidly growing leiomyoma, defined as 6 cm of growth in 1 year, will be malignant in less than 0.1% of cases. In a postmenopausal woman with an enlarging uterine mass, sarcoma is more likely. Most sarcomas are not detected prior to surgery, although a high T1/high T2 pattern on MRI has been reported to be predictive of sarcoma. On gross pathologic inspection, leiomyomata are well-circumscribed, solid tumors with a pseudocapsule and an off-white, whorled appearance. If a lesion lacks an apparent capsule, appears necrotic, or is soft or friable, then a frozen section should be submitted because these findings are suggestive of sarcoma.

Other potential diagnoses to consider include solid ovarian tumors. Enlargement of the uterus may arise due to adenomyosis or could represent an undiagnosed pregnancy. A pregnancy test should be considered.

Treatment

Asymptomatic fibroids require no therapy. Women with hypermenorrhea or polymenorrhea often benefit from a trial of cyclic or continuous oral contraceptives or progestins. Gonadotropin-releasing hormone (GnRH) agonists decrease leiomyoma size and stop menstruation prior to surgery. However, long-term use of GnRH agonists causes osteoporosis and is not recommended. Treatment with the antiprogestin mifepristone may result in significant shrinkage of fibroids but may cause endometrial hyperplasia. In premenopausal women, leiomyomata resume growth soon after medication is discontinued.

For women with symptoms unresponsive to medical management, several treatment options are available. Myomectomy is a procedure for removal of leiomyomata with subsequent repair of resultant defects in the uterine wall in order to preserve the uterus. Myomectomy is usually offered to women who desire to retain their fertility. Some women who do not desire pregnancy also choose this option. Myomectomy is performed via laparotomy, laparoscopy, or hysteroscopy depending on the location, number, and size of the leiomyomata. Controversy has arisen over the use of morcellation to reduce a uterine mass to a size amenable to laparoscopic removal because unrecognized malignancy in the specimen can be widely disseminated by this technique. Women who have completed childbearing and desire an alternative to hysterectomy may choose uterine artery embolization or guided focused ultrasound surgery, both of which are designed to decrease the size of lesions. Embolization involves diminishing blood flow to the uterus by occluding vessels to the lesion using angiography, which has been reported to decrease uterine/fibroid size by one-third to one-half. Bleeding and pelvic pressure improve in 80%-90% of women after uterine artery embolization. Hysterectomy is definitive treatment for women with symptomatic uterine fibroids. Alternatives to total abdominal hysterectomy include vaginal hysterectomy, supracervical hysterectomy, and laparoscopic hysterectomy.

Prognosis

Myomectomy results in improvement of symptoms in 80% of women. Fifty percent of women undergoing myomectomy will develop recurrent leiomyomata, and 10% will undergo additional surgery.

SURGERY FOR MALIGNANT UTERINE DISEASE

Endometrial Cancer

Endometrial carcinoma is the most common gynecologic malignancy in the United States. It is primarily a disease of postmenopausal women. Tumors are grouped into type I and II categories based on their underlying etiology. Type I tumors are more common and arise due to prolonged estrogen stimulation of the endometrium. This is most commonly secondary to the conversion of endogenously produced androstenedione to estrone in peripheral adipocytes via the enzyme aromatase. Obese women produce more estrogen and are at much higher risk for developing endometrial cancer. Exogenous estrogens prescribed without accompanying progestins in postmenopausal women also greatly increase the risk of endometrial cancer, as does treatment with other estrogen receptor agonists such as tamoxifen, which is prescribed for treatment or prevention of breast cancer. Other risk factors for the development of endometrial cancer include diabetes (regardless of body mass index), early menarche, late menopause, and low parity. Premenopausal women with chronic anovulation, such as with polycystic ovary syndrome, are also at risk. Oral contraceptives are protective.

Endometrial intraepithelial neoplasia, formerly known as complex atypical hyperplasia, is a precursor lesion for type I endometrial cancer. These tumors usually express estrogen and progesterone receptors. Type II endometrial cancer consists of anaplastic or high-grade endometrioid carcinomas and papillary serous, clear cell, and squamous carcinomas. These tumors rarely express estrogen or progesterone receptors and are not thought to arise as a result of estrogen stimulation. The precursor lesion for type II endometrial cancers is endometrial intraepithelial carcinoma and is distinguished by histologic appearance and loss of native p53 expression on immunohistochemistry. Type II cancers have a significant likelihood of association with *BRCA* gene mutations. Adverse prognostic factors for both types of endometrial cancer include older age, grade, histology, depth of myometrial invasion, cervical extension, tumor size, and extension beyond the uterus.

Endometrial cancer is staged surgically as shown in Table 41–5.

Clinical Findings

Postmenopausal bleeding is the presenting symptom in about 90% of cases of endometrial cancer and should be considered to be cancer until proven otherwise. Common etiologies of postmenopausal bleeding include physiologic bleeding from hormone replacement therapy (27%), benign polyps (7%-23%), cervicitis (6%-14%), endometrial

Table 41–5. International Federation of Gynecology and Obstetrics (FIGO) staging for endometrial cancer.

FIGO Stage	Revised 2009
Stage I	Tumor confined to corpus uteri
IA	No or less than 50% myometrial invasion
IB	Invasion equal to or greater than 50% of myometrium
Stage II	Tumor invades cervical stroma but does not extend beyond uterus
Stage III	Local and/or regional spread. Positive cytology has to be reported separately without changing the stage
IIIA	Tumor invades serosa and/or adnexae.
IIIB	Vaginal and/or parametrial involvement (direct or metastases)
IIIC	Metastases to pelvic and/or para-aortic lymph nodes
IIIC-1	Positive pelvic nodes
IIIC-2	Positive para-aortic nodes with or without positive pelvic nodes
Stage IVA	Tumor invades bladder or bowel mucosa
Stage IVB	Distant metastases, including intra-abdominal and/or inguinal lymph nodes
Grade 1	
Grade 2	
Grade 3	

Grade of tumor is related to the proportion of nonsquamous, solid growth pattern in the tumor. Grade 1 is comprised of ≤ 5% of nonsquamous solid growth pattern; grade 2 is 6%-50% nonsquamous solid growth pattern; and grade 3 is > 50% nonsquamous solid growth pattern. (Reproduced with permission from Pecorelli S: Revised FIGO staging for carcinoma of the vulva, cervix, and endometrium. *Int J Gynecol Obstet* 2009 May;105(2):103-4.)

carcinoma (13%-16%), atrophy (10%), and cervical carcinoma (1%-4%). Despite appropriate workup, up to about one-quarter of cases of postmenopausal bleeding will have no identified etiology. Cervical stenosis with pyometrium or hematometrium is highly suggestive of endometrial carcinoma. Pain is not a common symptom. Vaginal cytology is positive in 40%-80% of cases but is entirely unreliable as a diagnostic tool for endometrial cancer. Endometrial biopsy performed in the office using a disposable biopsy instrument is highly sensitive. If endometrial biopsy fails to provide a definitive diagnosis, dilatation and curettage of the endometrium is definitive.

Type II endometrial carcinoma may disseminate relatively early in the course of the disease. Metastatic spread may occur to the vagina, regional pelvic and para-aortic lymph nodes, ovaries, lungs, brain, and bone. The most frequent site of recurrence following treatment for endometrial carcinoma is the vaginal vault.

Prevention

Oral contraceptives have been shown to reduce the risk of endometrial cancer by up to 50%, depending on duration of treatment. Progestin therapy will reduce the possibility of endometrial carcinoma in the anovulatory patient as well as in postmenopausal women receiving estrogen replacement therapy. Progestins in both oral contraceptive pills and hormone replacement regimens cause downregulation of estrogen receptors and atrophy of endometrium.

Treatment

Endometrial cancer is staged surgically. The route of surgical approach can be either via laparotomy or laparoscopy, with the latter being the preferred approach if feasible. Definitive therapy includes total hysterectomy, bilateral salpingo-oophorectomy, and sentinel lymph node biopsy for type I cancers. For type II lesions, omentectomy is usually added.

If the cervix is grossly involved, patients may receive preoperative radiation followed by surgical staging. Alternatively, a radical hysterectomy (described previously) may be performed without preoperative radiation.

Adjuvant pelvic radiation therapy is administered to patients with cervical extension (stage II); certain patients with deep myometrial invasion and other high-risk characteristics (based on age and grade); or patients with vaginal extension (stage IIIB). Patients with positive lymph nodes (stage IIIC) are treated with postoperative chemotherapy and, in some cases, with radiation as well. Metastatic and type II lesions, such as papillary serous carcinomas, are likely to recur after surgery regardless of stage. These tumors are treated with multimodal therapy using a combination of radiation and chemotherapy.

Metastatic or recurrent disease is treated with multimodal therapy using surgery, tumor-directed radiation, and/or chemotherapy based on the location, size, number, and histology of lesions. Chemotherapy combinations include either a doublet of carboplatin with paclitaxel or cisplatin with doxorubicin. Metastatic type I endometrial cancers may be treated with progestin therapy with good control.

▶ Prognosis

Survival at 5 years is about 70%-90% for stage I disease, depending on grade and myometrial invasion. Survival declines to about 60% in stage II. Higher stage, anaplastic tumors, deep myometrial invasion, and absence of estrogen and progesterone receptors all worsen the prognosis.

Uterine Sarcoma

Uterine sarcomas fall into three histologic groups including leiomyosarcoma, endometrial stromal sarcoma, and carcinosarcoma. These tumors are rare, accounting for about 3% of uterine neoplasms. Sarcomas of the uterus spread via hematogenous and lymphatic pathways in addition to direct extension. Lung and liver are frequent sites of metastases and recurrence.

In patients in whom the tumor is confined to the pelvic organs, treatment consists of total hysterectomy, bilateral salpingo-oophorectomy, pelvic and para-aortic lymphadenectomy, and omentectomy. There are no randomized trials documenting survival benefit for adjuvant therapy with either chemotherapy or radiation. However, individualized postoperative radiation and/or chemotherapy may be offered based on the poor prognosis of these tumors. Radiation reduces pelvic recurrences but does not improve overall survival.

The prognosis for patients with uterine sarcoma is dependent on grade and stage of the tumor. Leiomyosarcomas with more than 10 mitoses per 10 high-power fields carry a poor prognosis, with recurrence within 5 years in about two-thirds of patients. About 40% of patients with early-stage carcinosarcoma survive to 5 years. The clinical course of endometrial stromal sarcomas is highly variable.

The combination of gemcitabine and docetaxel is the chemotherapy regimen with the highest likelihood of response for metastatic or recurrent leiomyosarcoma. Carcinosarcoma was traditionally treated with ifosfamide-based chemotherapy regimens but is increasingly being treated with carboplatin and paclitaxel, similar to other gynecologic malignancies. High-dose progestin therapy is very effective for treatment of metastatic low-grade endometrial sarcoma.

Gestational Trophoblastic Disease

Gestational trophoblastic disease refers to tumors arising from placental tissue. They are unique among all neoplasms in that their genetic complement is provided, at least in part, by the father, thereby resulting in a tumor with genetic material and markers foreign to the patient. Gestational trophoblastic diseases may be divided into preinvasive and invasive types.

The preinvasive types include complete and partial hydatidiform moles. The frequency of hydatidiform mole is about 1:700 to 1:2000 pregnancies in the United States, Canada, and Western Europe and about 1:85 to 1:520 pregnancies in Asia. Hydatidiform mole is more common in women over age 40. A prior history of gestational trophoblastic disease significantly increases the risk of recurrence with a future gestation.

The gross appearance of a hydatidiform mole is related to the hydropic villi in the absence of a fetal circulation. The histologic appearance reveals varying degrees of trophoblastic proliferation. Hydatidiform moles can be classified as either complete or partial, based on cytogenetics and histopathology. These features are compared in Table 41–6. The majority of complete moles carry a 46XX karyotype, with chromosomes exclusively of paternal origin. Partial moles are typically triploid with 69XXX or 69XXY, where two or three sets of chromosomes are paternal in origin. Complete moles are not associated with a developing fetus, and partial moles may include a fetus that is typically small, with multiple anomalies.

Invasive gestational trophoblastic disease types include invasive mole, choriocarcinoma, and placental site trophoblastic tumor (PSTT). Invasive mole is diagnosed after 15% of complete moles and 3.5% of partial moles. Metastases occur following 4% of complete moles and 0.6% of partial moles.

Table 41–6. Features of hydatidiform moles.

Characteristic	Complete Mole	Partial Mole
Karyotype	46XX (90%) 46XY (10%) All paternal chromosomes	Triploid (90%) 69XXX or 69XXY Diploid (10%) 46 paternal chromosomes
Fetus	Absent	Often present
Villous edema	Prominent and diffuse	Focal if at all
Fetal red blood cells	None	Usually present
Proliferation of trophoblast	Prominent	Mild to moderate
Likelihood of local invasion	15%	3.5%
Likelihood of metastasis	4%	0.6%

Choriocarcinoma occurs following 3%-7% of hydatidiform moles and in 1:40,000 term pregnancies. Of all choriocarcinoma cases, 50% are preceded by a mole, 25% by spontaneous abortion, and 25% by term pregnancy. PSTT is a very rare variant with less than 500 cases reported worldwide.

Invasive mole is composed of hyperplastic trophoblasts with villi invading the myometrium. Choriocarcinoma involves sheets of syncitiotrophoblasts with no villi and demonstrates invasion into the myometrium or other tissues. Necrosis and hemorrhage are common. PSTT is composed of intermediate cytotrophoblasts.

β-Human chorionic gonadotropin (β-hCG) is a clinically useful tumor marker for all types of preinvasive and invasive gestational trophoblastic disease except PSTT, where human placental lactogen may be elevated.

Clinical Findings

The most common presenting symptom with hydatidiform mole is vaginal bleeding, occurring in 97% of complete moles and 73% of partial moles. On pelvic exam, about 50% of complete moles and 8% of partial moles will have uterine size greater than expected for a given estimated gestational age. Theca lutein cysts are physiologic ovarian cysts that result from hyperstimulation by very high levels of β-hCG and are apparent in 50% of complete moles. These cysts typically resolve once the β-hCG level regresses following appropriate treatment. Preeclampsia may develop in about one-quarter of women with complete moles and virtually never develops with partial moles. Clinical hyperthyroidism can develop in about 7% of women with complete moles with very high β-hCG levels due to cross-reactivity of this hormone with thyroid-stimulating hormone. A rare but potentially fatal complication is trophoblastic embolization to the lung during or after dilation and evacuation of large complete moles.

Diagnosis is usually confirmed with either ultrasound or β-hCG values. Serum β-hCG levels are above 100,000 mIU/mL in 46% of women with complete moles, and these high values persist beyond the 12th week of gestation, neither of which should be observed in a normal pregnancy. Ultrasound will usually demonstrate multiple small sonolucencies due to the hydropic villi (a "snowstorm" appearance). In a partial mole, the fetus, if present, will usually be small and afflicted with multiple anomalies.

Differential Diagnosis

Threatened abortion or missed abortion will often present with similar symptoms of bleeding, and both are more likely than gestational trophoblastic disease. A multiple gestation must be considered as well because it may produce unusually high levels of β-hCG in addition to uterine size greater than the estimated gestational date.

Complications

Metastasis is most common with choriocarcinoma but may occur with any of the invasive types of gestational trophoblastic disease. The most common sites of spread include lung (80%), vagina (30%), pelvis (20%), brain or liver (10%), and bowel, kidney, or spleen (< 5%). Unlike virtually any other invasive carcinoma, metastatic disease is still potentially curable in most patients with appropriate chemotherapy.

Treatment

Once the diagnosis of a molar pregnancy has been established, the uterus should be evacuated by suction curettage. All specimens are submitted for histology and cytogenetics. Theca lutein cysts regress following treatment of the mole and should not be surgically excised.

Following evacuation of the uterus, weekly serum β-hCG levels should be monitored until normalized for 3 weeks, followed by monthly testing for 6-12 months depending on assessment of pretreatment risk factors. If the β-hCG value plateaus for 3 weeks or rises for 2 weeks, invasive gestational trophoblastic disease should be suspected. Effective contraception during the surveillance phase is important in order not to complicate interpretation of the β-hCG.

Patients with invasive or persistent gestational trophoblastic disease should be evaluated with a metastatic workup including pelvic examination; computed tomography (CT) scan of the chest, abdomen, and pelvis; a complete blood count; and renal and liver function tests. If the chest CT scan shows disease, a scan of the head is indicated.

Staging of gestational trophoblastic tumors is outlined in Table 41-7. Unlike most neoplasms, gestational trophoblastic disease is staged using both an anatomic and a nonanatomic, nonsurgical staging system based on prognostic factors. Current FIGO staging combines anatomic staging with the modified World Health Organization (WHO) prognostic scoring system. For anatomic stage I disease, risk is usually low, and for anatomic stage IV disease, risk is usually high. Stage II and III disease is best stratified with the modified WHO prognostic scoring system. Stage is recorded as anatomic stage and FIGO-modified WHO score.

Single-agent chemotherapy is the preferred treatment for patients with stage I or low-risk disease who wish to maintain reproductive options. If future childbearing is not desired, patients with invasive mole may be treated with a hysterectomy and possible adjuvant chemotherapy. Preferred regimens for single-agent therapy include methotrexate or dactinomycin. Patients with intermediate- and high-risk gestational trophoblastic disease should receive aggressive combination chemotherapy. The most effective regimen reported includes etoposide, methotrexate, dactinomycin, cyclophosphamide, and vincristine. There is occasionally a role for surgery or radiation for selected metastatic disease

Table 41–7. International Federation of Gynecology and Obstetrics (FIGO) anatomic staging for gestational trophoblastic neoplasia (GTN).

FIGO Staging	Description
Stage I	Disease confined to the uterus
Stage II	GTN extends outside of uterus, but is limited to genital structures including adnexa, vagina, broad ligament
Stage III	GTN extends to lungs with or without genital tract involvement
Stage IV	All other metastatic sites

Modified WHO Prognostic Scoring System as adapted by FIGO

Factor	Score			
	0	1	2	4
Age (years)	< 40	> 40		
Antecedent pregnancy type	Mole	Abortion	Term	
Pregnancy to treatment interval (months)	< 4	4–< 7	7–13	> 13
Pretreatment β-human chorionic gonadotropin (mIU/L)	< 10^3	10^3–10^4	10^4–10^5	> 10^5
Tumor size including uterus (cm)	—	3–5	> 5	—
Site of metastases	Lung	Spleen Kidney	Gastrointestinal	Brain Liver
Number of metastases	0	1–4	5–8	> 8
Previous failed chemotherapy regimens			Single	> 2

Total: If score is > 7, then patient is high risk and requires intensive, multiagent chemotherapy Current staging combines anatomic staging with the modified World Health Organization (WHO) prognostic scoring system. Stage is recorded as anatomic stage and FIGO modified WHO score, separated by colon. Example of format: Stage IV: 8. Data from Summary of WHO and FIGO standards.

sites, and intrathecal methotrexate is sometimes needed for treatment of central nervous system disease. The regularly updated evidence-based guidelines published by the NCCN are a source of information for chemotherapy regimens and optimal management.

Prognosis

The potential for cure of gestational trophoblastic tumors is excellent, including cases with pulmonary metastases, which are still considered low risk. Five-year survival of up to 85% is reported in cases with high-risk metastatic disease. The risk of recurrence of gestational trophoblastic disease in a future pregnancy has a relative risk of 20-40, but in absolute terms, this translates to a recurrence risk of less than 5%. During any subsequent pregnancy, early (first-trimester) ultrasound is recommended. The placenta should be examined after delivery, and β-hCG values should be monitored until normalization.

Koh WJ, Greer BE, Abu-Rustum NR, et al. Uterine Neoplasms, version 1.2014. *J Natl Compr Canc Netw.* 2014;12(2):248-280.

Koh WJ, Greer BE, Abu-Rustum NR, et al: Uterine Sarcoma, Version 1.2016: Featured updates to the NCCN guidelines. *J Natl Compr Canc Netw.* 2015;13(11):1321-1331.

SURGERY FOR BENIGN FALLOPIAN TUBE DISEASE

Infertility Attributed to Fallopian Tube Disease

Infertility is defined as failure to conceive after 1 year of normal coital activity without use of contraceptives. Based on this definition, about 15% of couples are infertile. When the etiology of infertility is evaluated, approximately 40% will be attributable to male factor infertility, including low sperm count, impaired motility, or abnormal morphology of the sperm. Anatomic abnormalities of the pelvic organs are the single most common cause of infertility in women, with tubal factor infertility the most common among those.

Common causes for tubal factor infertility include acute and chronic salpingitis, endometriosis, and adhesions from previous appendicitis with rupture or surgery. Chlamydia and gonorrhea infections are the most common causes of direct tubal damage causing infertility. Desire to reverse previous tubal sterilization may also be a reason for tubal surgery. One-third of infertile couples have more than one contributing factor.

History

It is important to elicit any history of sexually transmitted disease, pelvic inflammatory disease, pelvic surgery, cyclic pain, or dyspareunia.

Clinical Findings

The size and mobility of the uterus should be assessed. Adnexae should be palpated for masses, in particular endometrioma or hydrosalpinx. Cul-de-sac or uterosacral ligament nodularity and tenderness suggest endometriosis. Ultrasound may reveal the presence of isoechoic masses suggesting endometriosis or a tubular mass consistent with hydrosalpinx. Hysterosalpingogram, a test that involves fluoroscopic assessment of tubal patency by transcervical injection of the uterus with radiocontrast, may reveal an obstruction, including its location. Use of a water-based dye is indicated for the first attempt, and if occlusion is noted, an oil contrast medium may be used subsequently. The oil-based hysterosalpingogram is reported to have therapeutic benefit.

Laparoscopy is warranted if the evaluation for anatomic abnormalities is inconclusive. Therapeutic interventions including lysis of adhesions or ablation of endometrial implants may be efficacious. If laparoscopy is performed following a normal hysterosalpingogram, 24% of patients will have mild endometriosis, and 6% of patients will have pelvic adhesions.

Treatment

Tuboplasty procedures may be performed to restore tubal patency. However, in vitro fertilization (IVF) has become the standard treatment of infertility attributed to tubal occlusion or when multiple infertility factors affect the couple. Hydrosalpinx is usually treated by salpingectomy in order to optimize subsequent IVF, as a persistent hydrosalpinx has been shown to negatively impact implantation even when IVF is used. Other factors of prognostic significance include age of the couple and presence of other causes of infertility, including ovulatory dysfunction or male factor infertility.

Heterotopic pregnancies and multiple-gestation pregnancies are more likely in patients undergoing IVF than in the general population.

Prognosis

Age and severity of tubal disease are predictors of success. Women with mild adhesive disease and age less than 35 years have the highest success rates, approaching 70%. For severe tubal disease, success is less than 15%. Ectopic pregnancy is 20 times more likely with a history of fallopian tube surgery or preexisting scar, resulting in a 10% incidence. IVF success rates vary by program and have generally been improving steadily in recent years. Decisions regarding planned tubal surgery versus IVF should take into account the relative costs, risks, and success rates.

Ectopic Pregnancy

Ectopic pregnancy is implantation of a viable pregnancy in a location other than within the endometrium lining the uterus. Risk factors for ectopic pregnancy include prior tubal surgery, previous ectopic pregnancy, history of pelvic inflammatory disease or sexually transmitted infection, and pregnancy arising from assisted reproductive technology. Smoking and history of infertility are also associated with increased risk of ectopic pregnancy. Over 95% of ectopic pregnancies occur in the fallopian tube, generally within the ampullary portion. A less common location includes interstitial pregnancy within the tubal lumen where it passes through the myometrium. Rare sites include cervix, ovary, omentum, pelvis, and abdomen. Heterotopic pregnancy refers to the rare occurrence of an intrauterine pregnancy with a synchronous ectopic pregnancy. The incidence of heterotopic pregnancy has increased from a spontaneous rate of 1:30,000 pregnancies to 0.1%-1% for pregnancies arising from assisted reproductive technology.

The incidence of ectopic pregnancy has been reported to occur in approximately 2% of pregnancies, although the true incidence is difficult to ascertain due to the potential for spontaneous resolution of some ectopic pregnancies as well as underreporting of early ectopic pregnancies treated medically rather than surgically. Pregnant women with pain or bleeding have a fourfold higher incidence of ectopic pregnancy than pregnant women without either symptom. The primary potential morbidity of ectopic pregnancy is the potential rupture of the fallopian tube or other implantation site resulting in hemorrhage. Failure to make a timely diagnosis can result in hemorrhagic shock and death.

Symptoms & Signs

Patients will usually present with amenorrhea and a positive pregnancy test. Subsequent irregular bleeding occurs in many but not all cases. In the early course of an ectopic pregnancy, patients may be asymptomatic. Presence of pain is also variable. Classic symptoms of a ruptured ectopic pregnancy include severe abdominal pain, referred pain to the shoulder, and hemodynamic instability. Upon pelvic examination, an adnexal mass may or may not be present. The uterus is usually slightly enlarged and softened secondary to the hormonal influence of the ectopic pregnancy.

Diagnostic Studies

Trophoblastic cells of the blastocyst produce β-hCG that may be detected shortly after implantation. The rise of β-hCG is logarithmic, with a doubling time of about 48 hours. The β-hCG should rise at least 66% every 48 hours in 85% of normal pregnancies and will plateau late in the first trimester. Ectopic pregnancies show a slower rise of β-hCG in all but 15% of cases. An absolute β-hCG does not distinguish between an ectopic and a nonviable intrauterine pregnancy.

Transvaginal ultrasound has almost 100% sensitivity for detection of intrauterine pregnancy as long as care is taken to discriminate between an actual pregnancy and the pseudo-gestational sac, defined as intrauterine fluid that can be mistaken for an intrauterine pregnancy. A true gestational sac is located eccentrically in the uterus and should contained a yolk sac and a fetal pole. The absence of an intrauterine pregnancy in the setting of a positive β-hCG is strongly suggestive of an ectopic pregnancy if the β-hCG value is above the discriminatory threshold of transvaginal ultrasound to detect a gestational sac. The discriminatory threshold has been reported to occur with β-hCG values above 1500 to 3000 mIU/mL, although variables such as body mass index, quality of ultrasound equipment, and experience of the sonographer all impact the threshold value. Diagnosis of ectopic pregnancy by direct ultrasound localization is much less accurate than detection of intrauterine implantation.

Treatment

If the β-hCG shows an abnormal rate of rise, including plateau, slow rise, or declining values, then ultrasound is warranted. However, if the β-hCG value is below the discriminatory threshold, suction curettage is useful to distinguish between a nonviable intrauterine pregnancy and an ectopic gestation. The absence of chorionic villi in the curettage specimen is predictive of an ectopic pregnancy, although in early gestation, the curettage may be falsely negative for villi.

Treatment of ectopic pregnancy is either surgical or medical depending on several variables. The surgical approach is definitive, but invasive and more costly than medical management. Medical management results in successful treatment for 90% of appropriately selected patients. Methotrexate is used for medical management. Appropriate indications for medical management require a hemodynamically stable patient who will be compliant with follow-up and has no medical contraindication to methotrexate. Relative contraindications include a gestational sac greater than 3.5 cm, presence of fetal cardiac motion, or a β-hCG value of greater than 15,000 mIU/mL. Administration of a single dose of methotrexate has a reported efficacy of 84%. Use of multidose regimens increases the rate of success. Failure of the β-hCG value to fall by at least 15% within 4-7 days after treatment indicates that additional methotrexate or surgery is indicated. Patients who are Rh negative are given $Rh_o(D)$ immune globulin whether treated medically or surgically. Other options for medical management include potassium chloride, prostaglandins, and mifepristone, but these have not been studied as well as methotrexate.

Surgical options for treatment of ectopic pregnancy are intended to remove the ectopic gestation and preserve a functional fallopian tube, if possible. If the patient is hemodynamically stable, the laparoscopic approach is usually preferred. If the patient is in shock or if the abdomen is distended with blood, emergent laparotomy is necessary. If the fallopian tube is generally healthy, a salpingostomy is possible whereby the involved section of the fallopian tube is removed through an incision in the antimesenteric portion of the tube, while leaving the remainder of the tube intact. If the tube is more extensively damaged, complete or partial salpingectomy is recommended. If conservative approaches to preserve the fallopian tube are used, β-hCG values should be monitored postoperatively until normalization occurs.

Expectant management of a documented ectopic pregnancy may be an option in stable patients if the β-hCG value is less than 200 mIU/mL and declining. Patients must be counseled regarding the risks of rupture and hemorrhage, and emergency management must be readily available.

Contraception

Contraception to prevent unwanted pregnancy may be attained using either reversible or permanent methods. Reversible methods include hormonal contraceptives via oral, transcutaneous, or subcutaneous routes; injectable long-acting progestins; IUDs; and barrier methods such as condoms. Modern IUD contraceptives contain progestin hormones or copper, delivered in low doses to the uterine cavity where they inhibit sperm motility and block fertilization. They are inserted as an office procedure without requiring local anesthetic or cervical dilation in most cases. Both copper and progestin devices are highly effective and long lasting. Contemporary IUD contraceptives do not increase the risk of pelvic infection. Progestin-releasing IUDs decrease menstrual flow by about 50% and have been shown to be effective for control of abnormal uterine bleeding, prevention of hyperplasia during estrogen replacement therapy, and treatment of hyperplasia. The duration of action of IUDs is from 3-7 years, depending on the formulation.

Subdermal implant contraception uses low serum concentrations of contraceptive progestins found in birth control pills to thicken cervical mucus and inhibit ovulation. These actions result in failure rates comparable to those reported following sterilization and intrauterine contraception. Their duration of action is FDA approved for 3 years. As with intrauterine contraceptives, the principal side effect is change in menstrual bleeding; the majority of users experience a diminution in blood loss but an increase in number of bleeding days, sometimes at unpredictable intervals.

Contraceptive implants require subdermal insertion with a disposable trocar with local anesthetic and are removed under local anesthetic through a small incision. These procedures take only a few minutes and can be performed in an office setting, and pain and infections are rare. Contemporary systems use a single rod and are easier to use, have a shorter life, and are associated with somewhat more acceptable bleeding patterns than the now-discontinued multirod implants.

Unintended pregnancies result in over 1 million therapeutic abortions per year in the United States. Uterine aspiration using either manual or electric vacuum pumps allows safe pregnancy termination in the first trimester, with a mortality rate of less than 1:200,000 procedures. Morbidity and mortality of abortion rise as the gestational age increases.

Permanent sterilization procedures are available for both men and women. Prior to performing any permanent sterilization procedure, the physician must carefully counsel and determine whether a permanent method of contraception is appropriate for the patient. Reversal of permanent sterilization is costly and often ineffective. Permanent male sterilization via vasectomy is safe, minimally invasive, and effective, with reported failure rates of 1.5 per 1000. For women, there are several permanent sterilization options. Most of the procedures for women are designed to occlude or remove the fallopian tube via laparotomy or laparoscopy. These include Pomeroy, Irving, Uchida, and Madelener laparotomy operations in addition to laparoscopic procedures using unipolar or bipolar electrosurgical coagulation of the fallopian tubes or application of silastic bands or proprietary clips (Filshie clips, Hulka clips). Minilaparotomy for Pomeroy-type tubal occlusion is often used for postpartum sterilization. Recent data support the practice of total salpingectomy at the time of permanent sterilization, as there is evidence that this procedure significantly reduces the risk of subsequent ovarian cancer because most high-grade serous ovarian cancers actually originate from the fallopian tube. Total salpingectomy is a safe and effective procedure both postpartum and via an interval laparoscopy. Until recently, there were a limited number of proprietary methods of transcervical tubal occlusion based on intrauterine access to the tubal ostia using a hysteroscope, which have now been taken off the market secondary to postprocedure side effects and complications.

The observed failure rate for tubal ligation procedures ranges from 0.7% to 3.6%, which is comparable to the failure rate of IUDs and subdermal implants.

SURGERY FOR MALIGNANT FALLOPIAN TUBE DISEASE

Benign and malignant tumors isolated to the fallopian tubes are rare. Adenocarcinoma of the fallopian tube was previously thought to account for less than 1% of female reproductive tract cancers. However, recent evidence suggests that a majority of serous ovarian cancers actually start in the fallopian tube.

The most common presenting symptoms for cancer of the fallopian tubes are the same as those for ovarian cancer (see later in chapter). An adnexal mass is sometimes, but not always, palpable. Tumor markers such as CA-125 are usually elevated, although in early-stage disease, elevation of the CA-125 is present in less than half of patients. The diagnosis of fallopian tube carcinoma is usually not made preoperatively.

The differential diagnosis for fallopian tube cancer includes disorders that may result in enlargement or obstruction of the distal fallopian tube. The most common example would be hydrosalpinx whereby obstruction of the fallopian tube results in accumulation of fluid within the lumen and causes distension of the tube. Common causes of hydrosalpinx include prior infection or endometriosis. Another potential confounding diagnosis is the presence of paratubal cysts, which are simple cysts arising in the mesosalpinx or loosely attached to the exterior of the tube. Paratubal cysts are nearly always benign and arise from Müllerian and Wolffian duct remnants. Fallopian tube cancer is staged using the FIGO staging rules for ovarian cancer (see Table 41–10).

Treatment for fallopian tube cancer is identical to treatment for ovarian cancer. Multimodal therapy includes a primary surgery for staging and debulking of disease, followed by adjuvant chemotherapy based on the stage and grade of the disease. A more detailed discussion of the surgery and postoperative adjuvant therapy considerations is provided in the ovarian cancer section of this chapter. If the disease is confined to the tube, the prognosis is good. Like ovarian cancer, most fallopian tube cancers are of advanced stage at the time of diagnosis, and the subsequent survival is much lower than early-stage disease.

SURGERY FOR BENIGN OVARIAN DISEASE

▶ Adnexal Masses

Adnexal masses are abnormal structures arising in the ovary, fallopian tube, or broad ligament. Preoperative assessment can narrow the differential diagnosis, but definitive diagnosis usually requires surgical resection or biopsy.

The differential diagnosis of adnexal masses is broad (Table 41–8). Every structure native to the pelvis can potentially present as a detectable adnexal mass. The majority are benign, but the probability of malignancy increases with age.

Table 41–8. Differential diagnosis of adnexal masses.

Ovarian Etiology	
Functional ovarian cyst	Immature teratoma
Corpus luteum cyst	Endodermal sinus (yolk sac)
Follicular cyst	Embryonal
Theca lutein cyst	Choriocarcinoma
Endometrioma	Epithelial
Polycystic ovaries	Invasive
Benign ovarian neoplasm	Papillary serous
Germ cell	Endometrioid
Mature cystic teratoma	Mucinous
Epithelial	Clear cell
Serous cystadenoma	Transitional cell
Mucinous cystadenoma	Low malignant potential
Stromal	Serous
Adenofibroma	Mucinous
Fibroma	Stromal
Thecoma	Sertoli-Leydig
Malignant ovarian neoplasm	Granulosa cell, adult
Germ cell	Granulosa cell, juvenile
Dysgerminoma	

Fallopian Tube Etiology	
Nonneoplastic fallopian tube conditions	Hydrosalpinx
Ectopic pregnancy	Paraovarian or paratubal cyst
Tubo-ovarian abscess/pelvic inflammatory disease	Malignant fallopian tube neoplasms

Uterine Etiology	
Benign conditions	Malignant neoplasms
Pedunculated leiomyoma	Endometrial carcinoma
Uterine anomalies	Uterine sarcoma
Undiagnosed pregnancy	

Non-Gynecologic Etiology	
Diseases of appendix or colon	Vascular anomalies
Diseases of bladder	Bony deformation

About 10% of persistent ovarian masses are malignant in premenopausal women, but this number rises to nearly 50% in postmenopausal women.

Functional Cysts

Functional cysts are relatively common in reproductive-age women but are also reported in postmenopausal women. These cysts are usually larger than 3 cm in order to be diagnosed and may attain diameters of up to 10 cm or more. Histologic examination reveals no pathologic features such as atypia, necrosis, or invasion. Follicular cysts produce estrogen until resolution of the cyst, and the corpus luteum cyst produces progesterone until resolution. Because of the hormone production by these types of cysts, menses may be delayed or irregular, sometimes leading to an incorrect clinical diagnosis of ectopic pregnancy. The least common type of functional cyst is the theca lutein cyst, which arises as a physiologic response to hyperstimulation by elevated β-hCG values produced by complete hydatidiform moles (see earlier in chapter). Functional cysts usually regress spontaneously within 1-3 months or, in the case of theca lutein cysts, when the β-hCG value normalizes after treatment of the hydatidiform mole.

Correct identification of functional cysts can prevent unnecessary surgical procedures. The functional cyst is typically a smooth, unilateral cyst on pelvic examination. Transvaginal ultrasound will show a simple, sonolucent morphology, and β-hCG is not elevated. Follow-up examination with ultrasound after 4-6 weeks will generally demonstrate resolution without treatment. About 85% of functional cysts smaller than 6 cm regress, but larger masses may be more likely to persist.

The majority of functional cysts remain asymptomatic, but they will occasionally rupture or undergo torsion, resulting in acute colicky abdominal or flank pain. Torsion requires prompt surgical intervention, usually with laparoscopy, in order to restore the blood supply to the ovary by untwisting the vascular pedicle before significant ischemia or necrosis occurs. If the functional cyst ruptures, pain of varying levels may occur. In rare cases, bleeding from the ovary leads to hemodynamic instability requiring surgery. Hospitalization for observation, allowing serial examinations and blood counts, is often appropriate for patients with symptomatic cyst rupture.

Persistent Adnexal Masses

Adnexal masses that persist are likely to be neoplasms. Benign masses can generally be removed effectively by the general gynecologic surgeon, while malignancies should be treated by gynecologic oncologists with expertise in surgical staging, debulking, and administration of adjuvant therapies to optimize outcomes. Triage of adnexal masses provides the best opportunity to serve the patient's interest by having the correct surgical team involved in care of the patient.

The most useful test for assessment of the newly diagnosed adnexal mass is transvaginal ultrasound. Ultrasound is particularly well suited for delineation of the morphologic features of adnexal masses. Medical literature abounds with descriptions of morphology that correlates with benign and malignant neoplasms of the ovary. Figure 41–7 illustrates the morphologic features used to distinguish possible cancers from likely benign lesions. The reported sensitivity of ultrasound for identifying a malignant ovarian neoplasm is 90%-94%, but specificity is only about 60%. Ultrasonographic assessment of Doppler waveforms shows increased flow in neoplasms when compared to functional cysts. Vessels arising in malignant lesions have lower resistance to flow

Benign Pattern

1. Simple cyst without internal echo

2. Simple cyst with scattered echoes

3. Polycystic echo

4. Sessile or polypoid smooth mural echoes

5. Central dense round echoes

6. Thin or thick multiple linear echoes

7. Thin or thick multiple linear echoes with dense part

8. Polycystic echoes with septum

Malignant Pattern

9. Cystic echoes with papillary or indented mural part

10. Polycystic echoes with irregular thick septum and solid part

11. Solid pattern (solid part >50%) heterogeneous component with irregular cystic part

12. Completely solid with homogeneous component

▲ **Figure 41–7.** Differential diagnosis of adnexal masses by ultrasound morphology. (Reproduced with permission from Kawai M, Kano T, Kikkawa F, et al. Transvaginal Doppler ultrasound with color flow imaging in the diagnosis of ovarian cancer, *Obstet Gynecol* 1992 Feb;79(2): 163-167.)

▲ **Figure 41–8.** Doppler waveform and pulsatility index (PI) indicating the objective differences between perfusion in normal versus malignant tissue. If the ratio of 1/PI is greater than 0.8, the likelihood of cancer is 96% (*P* < .01). The waveform on the right has high diastolic flow, and the PI is low, consistent with a cancer diagnosis. PI = (peak systolic flow − peak diastolic flow)/mean flow. S = systolic flow; M = mean flow; D = diastolic flow. (Reproduced with permission from Kawai M, Kano T, Kikkawa F, et al. Transvaginal Doppler ultrasound with color flow imaging in the diagnosis of ovarian cancer, *Obstet Gynecol* 1992 Feb;79(2):163-167.)

Table 41–9. Tumor markers for ovarian cancer.

Tumor Histology	Commonly Used Serum Markers
Epithelial Tumors	CA-125, CA 19-9, CEA, HE-4, OVA1
Papillary serous	CA-125
Endometrioid	CA-125, HE-4
Mucinous	CA 19-9, CEA
Germ Cell Tumors	AFP, β-hCG, LDH
Dysgerminoma	LDH
Endodermal sinus	AFP
Immature teratoma	None
Mixed type	AFP, β-hCG, LDH
Choriocarcinoma	β-hCG
Sex Cord–Stromal Tumors	Testosterone, estradiol, inhibin A and B
Sertoli-Leydig	Testosterone
Granulosa cell	Estradiol, inhibin A and B

AFP, α-fetoprotein; β-hCG, β-human chorionic gonadotropin; CEA, carcinoembryonic antigen; LDH, lactate dehydrogenase.

than in normal tissues: the ratio of diastolic to systolic flow is therefore higher than in normal tissue (Figure 41–8), and this can be quantitated. MRI can frequently predict benign versus malignant morphology but has a limited role in the early workup of adnexal masses due to cost and accessibility.

In addition to ultrasound, tumor markers can be useful for triage of the palpable adnexal mass. The ideal tumor marker is elevated only in the presence of cancer and should correlate with the burden of disease. In reality, no marker is perfect. There are identified markers for ovarian malignancies arising from germ cell, epithelial, and stromal origin. Optimal use of tumor markers involves ordering markers most likely to be clinically useful based on clinical presentation rather than to order all markers for all masses. Commonly used tumor markers are listed in Table 41–9. For example, malignant germ cell neoplasms usually arise in women younger than 35, are almost always unilateral, and typically demonstrate solid morphology on ultrasound evaluation. In this setting, it would be appropriate to order tumor markers including α-fetoprotein, β-hCG, and lactate dehydrogenase. Epithelial tumors are more often complex cystic and solid, bilateral lesions. In this circumstance, CA-125, CA 19-9, HE-4, and carcinoembryonic antigen are better markers. Interpretation of CA-125 is difficult in premenopausal women because benign diseases such as endometriosis, which is much more common than ovarian cancer, will cause false-positive test results. In addition, many tumor markers are normally elevated in pregnancy, thereby complicating evaluation of masses diagnosed during pregnancy.

The American College of Obstetricians and Gynecologists has issued a committee opinion regarding triage of adnexal masses that recommends referral of individuals with high-risk characteristics to gynecologic oncology subspecialists. For postmenopausal women, referral is warranted for patients with a pelvic mass and at least one of the following: CA-125 above 35 U/mL, ascites, a nodular or fixed mass, evidence of abdominal or distant metastasis, or family history of one or more first-degree relatives with ovarian or breast cancer. In premenopausal women, the recommendations are identical, except the threshold for CA-125 is raised to greater than 200 U/mL to account for increased incidence of benign diseases that can elevate the CA-125, such as endometriosis, in this age group. Motivation for referral is based on data showing higher staging accuracy and improved outcome when subspecialists treat ovarian cancer patients.

Low-risk masses thought to be functional cysts are managed expectantly. A mass that persists or demonstrates worrisome features on exam, imaging, or tumor marker measurement should be surgically resected. A basic principle of surgical resection for ovarian neoplasms is not to allow spill or rupture of cyst contents into the abdomen. It is never appropriate to needle aspirate an ovarian mass that may harbor malignancy because of the potential to spread disease intra-abdominally. The surgical procedure to be performed is either oophorectomy or ovarian cystectomy for high-risk and low-risk lesions, respectively. The route of surgical approach may be either with laparoscopy or laparotomy. The laparoscopic approach is better suited for cystic masses that are small enough to be placed in a specimen retrieval bag without spill or rupture. Large or solid masses or those with evidence of metastatic disease, such as ascites or omental caking, require laparotomy for removal. Ovarian conservation is chosen after a balanced assessment of relative risk for cardiac disease versus ovarian cancer. Women with benign-appearing masses under age 60 can expect some cardioprotective benefit from ovarian retention even after menopause.

A simple cystic mass of less than 5 cm with normal CA-125 is considered low risk, even in the postmenopausal woman. Conservative management with serial ultrasounds is reasonable.

SURGERY FOR MALIGNANT OVARIAN DISEASE

Ovarian cancer is stratified into three histologic groups based on the cellular origin of the tumor. Epithelial tumors, germ cell tumors, and sex cord–stromal tumors compose the primary lesions. In addition, cancers arising in other organs such as stomach, breast, and colon frequently metastasize to the ovary. Epithelial carcinoma accounts for about 85% of ovarian cancers, and about 5% arise from each of the remaining categories of germ cell, sex cord–stromal, and metastatic disease from other sites. The peak incidence of epithelial ovarian cancer is in the fifth and sixth decades of life, whereas malignant germ cell tumors are more likely to occur under the age of 30. Stromal tumors have a bimodal distribution, with peaks around ages 25 and 55 years. Malignant ovarian disease spreads by primary extension in the peritoneal cavity, in addition to lymphatic and hematogenous spread.

Epithelial ovarian cancer can be either sporadic or hereditary. The sporadic cases appear to be strongly related to number of lifetime ovulations or chronicity of gonadotropin stimulation. There are also data to suggest an environmental impact with the observation that tubal ligation results in reduction of risk and diets with high lipids relative to omega-3 fatty acids increase risk. About 20% of ovarian cancers are hereditary. Three pedigrees account for most hereditary cases, including ovary site specific, breast-ovary, and Lynch syndrome. Genetic inheritance of a mutation in the *BRCA1* or *BRCA2* gene imparts up to a 40% or a 25% lifetime risk of developing ovarian cancer, respectively. Certain ethnic subgroups, including Ashkenazi Jews and Icelandic peoples, have increased incidence of founder mutations in these genes that increase risk. Other reproductive factors associated with an increased risk include infertility. Recent evidence suggests that most epithelial ovarian cancers actually arise from the fallopian tubes and subsequently spread to the ovaries.

Epithelial tumors are divided into invasive and low malignant potential (borderline) types. The invasive type accounts for 80% of epithelial ovarian cancers and is usually detected in advanced stages. The low malignant potential tumors occur in women at an average age of 10-15 years younger than for invasive disease, and up to 80% are stage I at diagnosis. Destructive stromal invasion is absent in low malignant potential tumors, but these tumors are considered to be malignant and have the potential to metastasize. Epithelial tumors are subcategorized by histology as serous, mucinous, endometrioid, clear cell, transitional cell, or undifferentiated types. Serous tumors are the most common, composing about 50% of epithelial carcinomas. Endometrioid carcinomas are the second most frequent variety, accounting for 24% of ovarian cancers, and are sometimes associated with endometriosis. Clear cell tumors, accounting for less than 5% of epithelial tumors, are also associated with endometriosis and have a more virulent natural history. Mucinous tumors account for 15% of epithelial cancers and may become very large. Epithelial ovarian cancer commonly involves both ovaries.

Germ cell cancer types include dysgerminomas, immature teratoma, endodermal sinus tumor, mixed types, and rare nongestational choriocarcinoma. Germ cell cancers are almost always unilateral and are commonly detected while stage I. Germ cell cancers are three time more common in women of Asian or African descent than in Caucasians. As a separate entity, cancers can also arise in an otherwise benign mature cystic teratoma. This can occur in up to 1% of mature cystic teratomas and is most commonly a squamous cell carcinoma.

The most common sex cord–stromal tumors include Sertoli-Leydig, adult granulosa, and juvenile granulosa cell tumors. These are frequently hormonally active tumors. Sertoli-Leydig cell tumors occur most often in the third decade and arise from Wolffian duct remnants. They are rare and usually produce testosterone, resulting in defeminization (amenorrhea, atrophy of breast tissue) and virilization (deepening of the voice, hirsutism, clitoral hypertrophy). Adult granulosa cell tumors most often arise in the sixth decade and are usually estrogen-producing tumors. Because of the estrogen production, postmenopausal bleeding is common, and endometrial cancer may arise in up to 15% of patients with adult granulosa cell tumors. Juvenile granulosa cell tumors are similar but arise in younger patients. Like germ cell tumors, the sex cord–stromal tumors are unilateral in most cases, and they are usually detected at early stages.

Metastatic carcinoma from other primary sites occurs not infrequently. Common sites include the gastrointestinal tract (Krukenberg tumor), breast, pancreas, lymphoma, colon, and kidney. These tumors are classically solid and bilateral. Prognosis for these tumors is especially poor.

▶ Clinical Findings

Almost 90% of stage I patients have symptoms. The symptoms usually include gastrointestinal complaints that persist for an average of 12 days per month for 3 months. Less often, pelvic pain or metrorrhagia may be present. On examination, any mass should prompt further evaluation. An ovarian mass should be regarded as potentially malignant until proven otherwise. Smooth, mobile masses on exam indicate low risk, and solid, irregular, or fixed pelvic masses are suggestive of malignancy. Triage of the pelvic mass should include transvaginal pelvic ultrasound and selective tumor markers as described earlier. It should be noted that CA-125 may be negative in up to half of early-stage ovarian cancers. If an ovarian malignancy is suspected preoperatively, referral to a gynecologic oncologist is recommended.

Occasionally, ovarian cancer is discovered during an operation for a different indication or when triage of an adnexal mass has not been properly performed. If ascites, peritoneal carcinomatosis, or papillary excrescences are noted, the tumor should be removed intact and submitted for frozen section. If cancer is diagnosed, a gynecologic or surgical oncologist should be consulted intraoperatively for surgical staging and debulking.

▶ Treatment

Ovarian cancer is staged surgically (Table 41–10). When a complex adnexal mass is to be removed, the procedure should begin with obtaining washings for cytology, and

Table 41–10. International Federation of Gynecology and Obstetrics (FIGO) staging for ovarian cancer.

FIGO Staging	Description	TNM class
Stage I	Tumor limited to the ovaries	T1
IA	Limited to one ovary, no tumor on external surface, capsule intact; negative peritoneal cytology	T1a
IB	Limited to both ovaries, no tumor on external surface, capsule intact; negative peritoneal cytology	T1b
IC1	Surgical spill	T1c
IC2	Capsule rupture or surface tumor	
IC3	Positive ascites or peritoneal cytology	
Stage II	Tumor extending to the pelvis	T2
IIA	Metastasis to the uterus or tubes	T2
IIB	Metastasis to other pelvic tissues	T2b
Stage III	Tumor extending outside the pelvis and/or retroperitoneal nodes. Extension to small bowel, omentum, or superficial liver	T3 and/or N1
IIIA1(i)	Retroperitoneal metastases < 10 mm	T3a
IIIA1(ii)	Retroperitoneal metastases > 10 mm	
IIIA2	Microscopic intra-abdominal peritoneal involvement ± positive retroperitoneal nodes	
IIIB	Implants of abdominal or peritoneal surfaces not exceeding 2 cm in diameter	T3b
IIIC	Implants of abdominal or peritoneal surfaces > 2 cm in diameter	T3c and/or N1
Stage IV	Distant metastasis beyond the peritoneal cavity	M1
IVA	Malignant pleural effusion	
IVB	Parenchymal metastases to liver or spleen; metastasis to extra-abdominal organs include inguinal lymph nodes and nodes outside the abdominal cavity	

Modified with permission from Mutch DG, Prat J: 2014 FIGO staging for ovarian, fallopian tube and peritoneal cancer, *Gynecol Oncol.* 2014 Jun;133(3):401-404.

the mass should subsequently be removed intact. Upon removal of the mass, a frozen section should be obtained for diagnosis. If an ovarian malignancy is confirmed, complete staging requires assessment and biopsy of the pelvic and para-aortic nodes, omentum, and peritoneum. All peritoneal surfaces are inspected, and any suspicious lesions are biopsied. If no suspicious lesions are noted, a predetermined pattern of biopsies is taken from the pelvic sidewalls, cul-de-sac, bladder peritoneum, pericolic gutters, and both hemidiaphragms. A decision must be made about possible resection of the uterus and contralateral ovary. If the patient is young and desires to retain her fertility, criteria to identify candidates for conservation of fertility should be applied. Instances that favor preservation of fertility include germ cell and sex cord–stromal tumors because they are usually unilateral, and subsequent chemotherapy, if needed, has curative potential. Low malignant potential tumors affecting one ovary or select cases where extraovarian disease can be completely resected are also candidates. Patients with invasive epithelial tumors are poor candidates for conservative surgery because of the high likelihood of bilateral involvement and the primarily palliative role of chemotherapy for all but early stages of disease. If preservation of fertility is not appropriate, then hysterectomy and removal of the contralateral tube and ovary is completed.

Once the disease spread is documented, debulking of all resectable macroscopic disease is critically important. Numerous randomized clinical trials have demonstrated survival advantage for patients with maximal cytoreduction. Intraoperative decision making for debulking focuses effort on the largest tumor, wherever it may be. If the largest lesion can be resected, attention is directed to the next largest lesion. This process continues until either all measurable disease is removed or a lesion that is unresectable is encountered. To resect the disease at each decision point of this algorithm, the surgeon may need to perform intestinal resection, splenectomy, modified posterior exenteration, culdectomy, diaphragm resection, or other upper abdominal procedures. In two prospective Gynecologic Oncology Group clinical trials, survival for patients with microscopically debulked ovarian cancer (termed R0 disease) was 65% at 4 years and decreased to about 35% if 1 cm or less of macroscopic residual disease remained after surgery. If greater than 2 cm of residual disease remained, the 4-year survival was only 20%. Optimal debulking can be attained in up to 70% of patients who are operated on by subspecialists trained in ovarian cancer surgery.

Patients with stage IA, grade 1 or grade 2 epithelial tumors have a very good prognosis and typically are not treated with additional chemotherapy. For more advanced stages of epithelial cancer, chemotherapy is very effective for inducing clinical remission, but relapses are common, with an average progression-free interval of between 2 and 3 years. The best chemotherapy combination for treating advanced-stage epithelial cancer includes both taxane and platinum agents, administered either intravenously or intraperitoneally for at least six cycles. Intraperitoneal chemotherapy has been demonstrated to induce longer progression-free intervals, but acute toxicity is higher, and only 40% of patients are able to complete all six cycles of planned therapy. The CA-125 tumor marker is useful as a marker for assessing the effectiveness of therapy.

The best current regimen for malignant germ cell tumors is cisplatin, etoposide, and bleomycin, administered as a 3- or 5-day treatment that is continued until at least one cycle after normalization of elevated tumor markers. Sex cord–stromal tumors are treated similarly to germ cell tumors, although clinical trials of combination taxane and platinum agents are currently under way for this tumor type.

The treatment of ovarian cancer is complex and ever changing. The NCCN publishes evidence-based guidelines that are regularly updated to guide decision making.

▶ Prognosis

The prognosis for epithelial ovarian carcinoma is related primarily to stage and histologic grade. Because most ovarian cancers are of advanced stage at the time of initial diagnosis, the long-term survival rate for ovarian cancer is only about 50%. Five-year survival rates for patients with stage III or stage IV disease are around 20%-35%. Prolonged disease-free intervals are best achieved by combining comprehensive surgical staging, aggressive debulking, and adjuvant chemotherapy.

▶ Prevention

Oral contraceptives reduce the risk of ovarian epithelial carcinoma. The magnitude of risk reduction is based on dose and duration of therapy. The protective effects are durable, lasting for a decade or more after discontinuation of the medication.

Any woman with a primary ovarian cancer should be referred for genetic counseling and testing. Patients with a confirmed hereditary risk of ovarian cancer based on careful pedigree analysis or genetic testing benefit from prophylactic removal of ovaries and fallopian tubes. The current recommendation is for removal after completion of childbearing at age 35 or 10 years younger than the earliest incidence of disease in the family. Prophylactic removal of ovaries and tubes reduces the risk of ovarian cancer by at least 95%, but a small number of individuals may still develop a primary peritoneal carcinoma.

To date, no screening test for ovarian cancer has proven to be sufficiently sensitive or specific enough to have earned the recommendation of the U.S. Preventive Services Task Force, American College of Obstetricians and Gynecologists, or American Cancer Society. Prospective ultrasound screening studies and combined CA-125/ultrasound studies show a trend toward earlier stage at time of diagnosis in screened patients, resulting in prolongation of progression-free intervals but no change in overall survival.

Kurman RJ, Chih LM: The origin and pathogenesis of ovarian cancer: a proposed unifying theory. *Am J Surg Pathol.* 2010;34(3):433-443.

Morgan RJ Jr, Armstrong DK, Alvarez RD, et al: Ovarian Cancer, Version 1.2016, NCCN Clinical Practice Guidelines in Oncology. *J Natl Compr Canc Netw.* 2016;14(9):1134-1163.

▼ SURGERY FOR MULTIORGAN DISEASE

Chronic Pelvic Pain

Chronic pelvic pain (CPP) is generally defined as 3-6 months of pain perceived to be in the pelvic area, which is unrelated to pregnancy. Depending on the study, CPP has been reported to affect up to 25% of reproductive-age women. Evaluation and treatment of CPP account for up to 40% of all referrals to gynecologists, leading to up to 40% of all laparoscopies and up to 20% of all hysterectomies.

▶ Diagnosis

The differential diagnosis CPP is complex. Although many patients attribute their pain to a gynecologic cause, the physician must consider nongynecologic diagnoses of the gastrointestinal, urinary, and musculoskeletal systems in addition to psychological and psychosomatic problems. The most common nongynecologic diagnoses include irritable bowel syndrome, inflammatory bowel disease, nephrolithiasis, interstitial cystitis, ventral or inguinal hernia, muscle strain, nerve injury, depression, and somatization. Of note, patients with CPP are more likely to have suffered sexual assault as an adult or child.

The gynecologic causes of CPP are classified as cyclic or continuous in nature. Sources of cyclic pain include primary dysmenorrhea, defined as painful menses without identifiable pelvic pathology, and secondary dysmenorrhea attributable to pathologic conditions such as endometriosis or adenomyosis. Midcycle ovulatory pain may occur that produces unilateral pain at mid-cycle that resolves after a day or two. Continuous pain sources include endometriosis and adenomyosis as well as pelvic organ prolapse, all discussed earlier in this chapter, in addition to chronic salpingitis and pelvic adhesions. Another cause of continuous pain is ovarian remnant syndrome, which occurs when residual ovarian tissue after oophorectomy becomes retroperitoneal in location. Pain may occasionally be caused by degenerating fibroids or by mass effect from large fibroids.

▶ Clinical Findings

The pelvic examination in a patient with CPP requires careful communication of the patient to understand where and when her pain occurs. Identification of palpable abnormalities and localization of focal tenderness are important. If a pelvic mass is detected, it should be triaged as discussed earlier. An abnormal pelvic examination has about an 80% predictive value for pelvic abnormalities noted at laparoscopy.

▶ Treatment

Nongynecologic causes of pain are treated according to the diagnosis. Reproductive-age women with cyclic pain are offered multimodal treatment consisting of nonsteroidal anti-inflammatory drugs and ovulation suppression, usually with continuous oral contraceptives if appropriate for the age and medical risk factors of the patient. Continuous pain attributable to endometriosis or adenomyosis is treated similarly. Other causes of continuous pain include spasm or tension in pelvic floor musculature. Physical therapy and "reverse Kegel" exercises to relax the muscles often result in great improvement. An antibiotic may be prescribed if a chronic infection is suspected, but care should be taken only to treat documented infections and not to overprescribe antibiotics. Concurrent depression is common, usually arising as a secondary effect of the pain rather than as the primary etiology. Treatment with antidepressant medication is often beneficial. The tricyclic antidepressant class is frequently more effective than serotonin reuptake inhibitors for this indication. The physician must use careful judgment regarding initiation of narcotics in a chronic setting due to the potential for dependence and addiction. It is often useful to manage these patients with a narcotic contract between the patient and her physician to regulate drug use. Referral to a multidisciplinary pain service is also often useful for difficult or refractory cases.

If CPP is refractory to medical management or if the physical examination is abnormal, then diagnostic laparoscopy is indicated. During the laparoscopic procedure, upper abdominal structures, pelvic organs and peritoneum, appendix, rectum, and sigmoid colon are carefully inspected. The most commonly identified pathologies are endometriosis (one-third of patients) and adhesions (one-third of patients). Most of the remaining cases will have no identified pathology. The presence of abnormalities may not explain the pain, and treatment of disease such as endometriosis may not resolve the pain.

The evidence for therapeutic benefit of laparoscopy for treatment of pelvic pain is tenuous, at best. Procedures that remove or ablate adhesions or endometriosis may or may not relieve pain. If pain is attributed to the uterus or cervix and cannot be controlled with lesser procedures or medical management, options include hysterectomy or, if fertility preservation is desired, interruption of the autonomic nerve tracts with a presacral neurectomy. Pain attributed to degenerating or large fibroids may be relieved either with uterine artery embolization procedures or surgical removal of the leiomyomata with either hysterectomy or myomectomy. Severe dysmenorrhea that is refractory to medical management may be significantly improved with endometrial ablation or hysterectomy.

Published data indicate that laparoscopic treatment will produce a short-term reduction of pain in about 60%-80% of patients with endometriosis, but long-term benefits are not well documented. In patients who have completed their childbearing or who wish definitive treatment, hysterectomy has reported success rates of up to 95% if identifiable uterine pathology, such as degenerating fibroids, is present. If no pelvic pathology is noted, 50%-91% experience improvement. The success rate of surgical intervention is poor if the patient has concurrent symptoms of depression. Patients with biopsy-proven endometriosis should also be offered bilateral salpingo-oophorectomy to minimize pain from residual implants.

Endometriosis

Endometriosis is defined as extrauterine, functional endometrial tissue. The most common sites include the ovaries, uterosacral ligaments, and cul-de-sac. Less commonly, the fallopian tubes, uterine serosa, sigmoid colon and rectum, peritoneum, and small intestine or small intestine mesentery are involved. Ectopic endometrium is occasionally detected at distant sites including lung, lymph nodes, surgical incision sites, umbilicus, perineum, and breasts.

The etiology of endometriosis is thought to occur via several potential mechanisms: (1) retrograde menstruation with implantation; (2) metaplasia of Müllerian duct remnants or coelomic epithelium; and (3) lymphatic or venous dissemination. Retrograde menstruation through the fallopian tubes is extremely common and yet rarely appears to directly cause endometriosis. It is not known what factors contribute to the implantation and growth of endometriosis. Uterine outflow obstruction from cervical stenosis or congenital anomalies such as imperforate hymen are noted to increase the likelihood of developing endometriosis, lending credence to the theory of retrograde menstruation playing a role.

Endometriosis may develop at any time after onset of menarche and will virtually always regress after menopause. The prevalence of endometriosis is difficult to determine because many women with the disease are asymptomatic, and many women with a reported diagnosis do not have biopsy-proven disease. The estimated prevalence of endometriosis is about 15%-20% of adult women. Endometriosis may cause scar tissue formation that impairs fertility. As a consequence, diagnosis of endometriosis during a workup for infertility is higher, with 20%-47% of patients with infertility being affected. Conversely, in women with proven fertility who elect tubal sterilization, endometriosis is found in only 1%-5% of cases. The incidence of endometriosis is higher in women who choose to delay childbearing and in women with a family history of the disease. There may be environmental factors that predispose to endometriosis, such as dioxin exposure. Pregnancy and hormonal contraceptive hormones are protective.

Carcinoma may arise in endometriosis at any site and is most commonly of endometrioid histology. Clear cell carcinoma can also arise from endometriosis but is rare and more aggressive.

Classification

An anatomic staging system for endometriosis has been developed by the American Society of Reproductive Medicine (Figure 41–9). The Revised American Fertility Society classification system is accepted worldwide. The staging system is broadly predictive of outcome with treatment, but stage does not correlate well with pain symptoms. Alternate systems that recognize the varied presentation of endometriosis in addition to development of serum markers have been proposed.

Symptoms & Signs

Endometriosis frequently causes pain. The pain often begins shortly before menses and continues during menstruation. The presence of pain and its severity are highly variable. Some patients with extensive disease are asymptomatic, while others with small peritoneal implants may be incapacitated. Asymptomatic endometriosis may present as unexplained infertility. Symptoms may occur at any time during reproductive years but are most common in the third and fourth decades of life. Symptoms usually resolve with menopause unless the patient is prescribed a hormone replacement regimen. Patients may also complain of dyspareunia, tenesmus, back pain, or sciatica. Rare manifestations may include ureteral obstruction or bowel obstruction.

Pelvic Examination

Bimanual pelvic examination including the rectovaginal examination should be performed. Common findings include pelvic tenderness, adnexal masses, and soft nodularity in the cul-de-sac or along the uterosacral ligaments. Adnexal masses attributable to endometriosis are often bilateral and are frequently immobile due to adhesions along the posterior broad ligament.

Testing

Ultrasound description of isoechoic masses within the ovaries is highly suggestive of endometrioma. Serum concentrations of CA-125 are elevated above 35 U/mL in about one-third of patients with advanced disease, which complicates triage of adnexal masses. Following surgical and medical treatment, measurement of the CA-125 trend is a useful marker of treatment efficacy and disease recurrence,

similar to how the marker is used for monitoring treatment of ovarian cancer.

Definitive diagnosis requires biopsy, usually obtained with a laparoscopic procedure. The biopsy diagnosis requires the presence of both glands and stroma. Location and extent of disease are noted at the time of surgery to complete disease staging. Characteristic peritoneal implants include the so-called "powder burn" marks of darkly colored endometrium, in addition to red, blue, and white lesions. Peritoneal disease may be flat or raised, including nodular or vesicular appearance. Laparotomy is occasionally necessary for large ovarian masses or bowel and ureteral obstructions that may be present.

Treatment

Treatment should be tailored to severity of symptoms, age of the patient, desire for fertility, and stage of disease. Therapeutic options include a range from observation to medical management, with hormones and analgesics to hysterectomy with bilateral salpingo-oophorectomy. A conservative approach is preferred for patients with minimal symptoms or minimal measurable disease on pelvic exam. Surveillance examinations should be regularly performed, with the interval determined by severity of symptoms, age of the patient, desire for fertility, and stage of disease. If symptoms or physical findings worsen, the management plan may be changed accordingly.

A. Medical Treatment

The goal of medical therapy is to control disease by inducing a remission. There are no known medical therapies that result in a cure for endometriosis. Hormonal therapy is not administered for patients actively attempting to conceive. Upon treatment discontinuation, symptoms commonly recur. Long-term suppression with hormonal contraceptive regimens should be considered as first line.

1. Progestins—Norethynodrel, norethindrone acetate, and medroxyprogesterone acetate are commonly used. Continuous progestins induce amenorrhea, resulting in decreased symptoms in more than three-quarters of patients. Progestin therapy causes downregulation of estrogen receptors in endometrial tissue, resulting in atrophic change in both endometriosis and the endometrium. Breakthrough bleeding may occur. Side effects include weight gain secondary to appetite stimulation, fluid retention, headaches, and mood swings.

2. Oral contraceptives—Oral contraceptives with a low estrogen dose and a high-potency progestin are preferred and may be administered either as cyclic or continuous regimens. Symptoms are relieved in up to 80% of patients. Oral contraceptives may be continued long term as a maintenance therapy in healthy women. Women over 35 who smoke or

American Society for Reproductive Medicine
Revised Classification of Endometriosis

Patient's Name _____ Date _____

Stage I (Minimal) - 1-5	Laparoscopy_____ Laparotomy_____ Photography_____
Stage II (Mild) - 6-15	Recommended Treatment _____
Stage III (Moderate) - 16-40	_____
Stage IV (Severe) - >40	Prognosis _____
Total _____	

	ENDOMETRIOSIS		<1cm	1-3cm	>3cm
PERITONEUM	Superficial		1	2	4
	Deep		2	4	6
OVARY	R	Superficial	1	2	4
		Deep	4	16	20
	L	Superficial	1	2	4
		Deep	4	16	20

POSTERIOR CUL-DE-SAC OBLITERATION	Partial		Complete	
	4		40	

	ADHESIONS		<1/3 Enclosure	1/3-2/3 Enclosure	>2/3 Enclosure
OVARY	R	Filmy	1	2	4
		Dense	4	8	16
	L	Filmy	1	2	4
		Dense	4	8	16
TUBE	R	Filmy	1	2	4
		Dense	4*	8*	16
	L	Filmy	1	2	4
		Dense	4*	8*	16

*If the fimbriated end of the fallopian tube is completely enclosed, change the point assignment to 16.
Denote appearance of superficial implant types as red [(R), red, red-pink, flamelike, vesicular blobs, clear vesicles], white [(W), opacifications, peritoneal defects, yellow-brown], or black [(B) black, hemosiderin deposits, blue]. Denote percent of total described as R ___%, W___% and B ___%. Total should equal 100%

Additional Endometriosis:_____ 　　Associated Pathology: _____
_____ 　　_____
_____ 　　_____
_____ 　　_____

To be used with normal tubes and ovaries	To be used with abnormal tubes and/or ovaries
L ... R	L ... R

▲ **Figure 41–9. Staging of endometriosis.** (Reproduced with permission from American Society for Reproductive Medicine: Revised American Society fro Reproductive Medicine classification of endometriosis, *Fertil Steril* 1997 May;67(5):817-821.)

individuals with hypertension are at increased risk of thromboembolic complications and should not be prescribed estrogen-containing oral contraceptive pills. Side effects include headaches, fluid retention, breast tenderness, breakthrough bleeding, and occasional nausea.

3. GnRH analogs—GnRH analogs act by negative feedback inhibition on the pituitary gland, resulting in prevention of follicle-stimulating hormone and luteinizing hormone secretion. The consequence of low gonadotropin levels is the absence of follicle development and low estrogen production. This treatment strategy induces the medical equivalent of a postmenopausal state. Endometrial implants subsequently become atrophic in the hypoestrogenic environment, and about 80% of patients report clinical improvement. Side effects mimic menopause with vasomotor symptoms, vaginal dryness, and mood swings. Long-term treatment with GnRH analogs can cause osteopenia and osteoporosis. To prevent bone loss, "add-back" therapy with either norethindrone acetate or combined hormone replacement therapy may be prescribed and does not interfere with treatment of the endometriosis.

B. Surgical Treatment

Indications for surgery include treatment of current infertility, treatment to preserve future fertility, or control of symptoms. Medical therapy is unlikely to result in reduction of symptoms for bulky disease, and surgery is recommended for any endometrioma larger than 4 cm. Options for preservation of fertility in symptomatic women who have failed medical therapy include laparoscopic procedures for resection or ablation of implants, lysis of adhesions, or presacral neurectomy. When definitive therapy is necessary and preservation of fertility is not desired, total hysterectomy and bilateral salpingo-oophorectomy is indicated. Endometriosis is dependent on estrogen. Preservation of an ovary in this setting causes symptoms sufficient to prompt additional surgery in 20% of cases. Bowel implants can be locally resected by appropriately trained surgeons.

Postoperative estrogen replacement therapy usually does not lead to exacerbation of endometriosis. The use of estrogen-progestin combinations is generally not required.

Kuznetsov L, Dworzynski K, Davies M, et al; Guideline Committee: Diagnosis and management of endometriosis: summary of NICE guidance. *BMJ*. 2017;358:j3935.

MULTIPLE CHOICE QUESTIONS

1. The differential diagnosis of a vulvar lesion includes all of the following, except

   A. Bartholin abscess
   B. Melanoma
   C. Hidradenitis suppurativa
   D. Luteal cyst
   E. Epithelial inclusion cyst

2. All of the following are true about cervical cancer, except

   A. Most cases are related to high-risk human papillomavirus types.
   B. About 75% are squamous type.
   C. Screening for premalignant lesions is effective because of slow progression through dysplastic precursors.
   D. Carcinoma occurs most frequently in women between the ages of 20 and 30 years.
   E. Vaccination is targeted to both protect individuals and limit prevalence of infection.

3. Treatment of cervical carcinoma

   A. Usually includes hysterectomy for microinvasive disease
   B. Consists of radiation therapy and chemotherapy for advanced disease
   C. Cannot preserve fertility in women with microinvasive disease
   D. Includes systemic therapy only for distant metastases
   E. Often requires radiation therapy for bone metastases

4. Uterine leiomyomata

   A. Are present in 20%-30% of women of reproductive age
   B. Are more common in Caucasian women than in those of African or Asian descent
   C. Often appear after menopause if estrogen supplements are not used
   D. Are usually monofocal, with a single tumor in the uterine wall
   E. Require treatment by hysterectomy

5. The differential diagnosis of adnexal masses includes

   A. Endometrioma
   B. Appendiceal mass
   C. Pedunculated uterine leiomyoma
   D. A, B, and C
   E. A and C only

Orthopedic Surgery

Antonia Chen, MD, MBA

FRACTURES

▶ Definition

A fracture is a break in the continuity of a bone. The severity of fractures ranges from a partial filiform fissure to a complete rupture of the bone in multiple pieces. Most commonly, fractures are the result of high-energy forces, but in the case of a bone weakened by a disease, the bone can break after minimal trauma, or a break can even occur spontaneously.

▶ Classification

Different types of fractures can occur depending on the origin, energy, and direction of the forces applied to the bone and the quality of the bone. It is important to know the etiology and types of forces that can be applied to bones in order to reverse these forces when reducing fractures and understanding the extent of soft tissue disruptions. Several classifications, depending on the bone or joint involved, exist. These will be discussed in their specific sections.

A. Etiology

The different etiologies of fracture (Figure 42–1) are as follows:

Traumatic fracture: Fracture caused by an external high-energy force on a healthy bone.

Pathologic fracture: Fracture caused by a minimal energy (even everyday activities) on a bone weakened by disease. The most common causes of disease that weaken bones are congenital (osteogenesis imperfecta), infectious (osteomyelitis), metabolic (osteomalacia, hyperparathyroidism, osteopenia, osteoporosis), neoplastic (bone cyst, enchondroma), malignant (osteosarcoma, metastasis), and rheumatic (Paget disease).

Periprosthetic fracture: Fracture caused by the application of forces on a point of mechanical weakness in the bone, created by the implantation of a prosthesis.

B. Fracture Patterns

The different fracture patterns (Figure 42–2) are as follows:

Transverse: Fractures induced by a direct impact. The fracture line is at a right angle to the bone's long axis. These fractures are often accompanied by local tissue disruption.

Oblique and spiral: Fractures induced by torsional forces applied distally from the fracture site. The fracture line is diagonal to the bone's long axis. Soft tissue disruptions can be observed in areas other than the fracture site.

Greenstick: Incomplete fracture of the bone, involving only one cortex. The bones of children are more predisposed to this kind of fracture, since they are composed of greater conjunctival tissue and less mineral bone than adult bones.

Compression and wedge: Fractures induced by a direct compression of the cancellous bone that collapses the trabeculae. This type of fracture is usually found in the calcaneus and vertebral bodies in the spine.

Comminuted: Fracture that has more than two fragments. The most severe fractures result from high-energy traumas and are accompanied by significant soft tissue disruption.

Stress: Incomplete or hairline fracture that develops because of repeated or prolonged force against the bone. In fatigue stress fractures, abnormal stresses are applied to a normal bone (eg, overuse injury as in military recruits or marathon runners); in insufficiency stress fractures, normal stresses are applied to an abnormal bone (eg, osteoporotic bone).

A   B

▲ **Figure 42–1.** Images of (**A**) traumatic and (**B**) pathologic fractures. (B, Reproduced with permission from Skinner HB, McMahon PJ: *Current Diagnosis & Treatment in Orthopedics*, 5th ed. New York, NY: McGraw-Hill Education; 2014.)

A   B   C   D   E   F

▲ **Figure 42–2.** Fracture patterns: (**A**) normal, (**B**) transverse, (**C**) oblique, (**D**) spiral, (**E**) segmental, and (**F**) comminuted. (Reproduced with permission from Brunicardi FC, Andersen DK, Billiar TR, et al: *Schwartz's Principles of Surgery*, 11th ed. New York, NY: McGraw-Hill Education; 2019.)

The Arbeitsgemanschaft für Osteosynthesefragen (AO) classification is one of the most widely used comprehensive systems to define fractures. Initially described by Maurice E. Müller, this initial system was further developed by combining the AO and American Orthopaedic Trauma Association (OTA) classifications and now is officially known as the AO/OTA classification. The fracture description is based on a standardized five-element alphanumeric code. First, each fracture is given two localization numbers to describe which bone and what location (proximal, diaphyseal, or distal) of the bone is affected. Then, each fracture is given a letter to describe the type (A = simple, B = wedge, C = complex, if diaphyseal) or joint involvement (A = extra-articular, if proximal or distal). Finally, the fracture is given two further numbers to morphologically describe the fracture pattern and geometry.

C. Displacement

Fractures may be nondisplaced or displaced. Displaced fractures can be translated, angulated, rotated, or shortened depending on the forces applied to the bone and the fracture pattern. Displacement can further be subcategorized into minimally, moderately, or completely displaced.

D. Soft Tissue Involvement

Closed fractures are those in which the overlying skin is intact and the bones are not in contact with the external environment. Soft tissue injury may still occur in a closed fracture and may vary in severity (Table 42–1). On the other hand, open fractures communicate with the external environment, most often via a skin wound overlying the fracture, and may expose the bone to contamination and infection. In skull fractures, the contamination can be through mucosal

Table 42–1. Oestern and Tscherne classification of soft tissue injury in closed fracture.

Grade	Soft Tissue Injury
0	Minimal soft tissue damage Indirect injury to limb (torsion) Simple fracture pattern
1	Superficial abrasion or contusion Mild fracture pattern
2	Deep abrasion Skin or muscle contusion Severe fracture pattern Direct trauma to limb
3	Extensive skin contusion or crush injury Severe damage to underlying muscle Compartment syndrome Subcutaneous avulsion

membranes. Open fractures can be obvious in significant trauma with substantial degloving of the soft tissues, or they can be more subtle, where only a small poke hole in the skin is visible. Open fractures are discussed in more detail in later in section on fracture complications.

Fracture Healing

Most fractures can heal without surgery. However, surgery can assist this natural process by aligning the bones correctly through fracture reduction and immobilization with the help of casts or surgery. The healing process can be divided into three phases that can overlap each other: hematoma formation, callus formation, and consolidation/remodeling. Multiple factors influence bone healing, such as age, bone type, comorbidities, nutritional status, medications, bone malignancy, and smoking.

A. Hematoma Formation and Inflammation

Once a fracture has occurred, vessels of the soft tissues surrounding the bone (periosteum) and bone marrow are injured and result in bleeding into the fracture site. A hematoma forms around the fracture and fills the gap between the fractured bone fragments. This hematoma will act as a template for callus formation. The cells at the edge of the fracture are deprived of blood supply and nutrients, resulting in avascular necrosis. Acute inflammation occurs for 7 days, which induces vasodilatation and the release of platelets, inflammatory cells, and inflammatory mediators. Within 7-14 days, the hematoma organizes into granulation tissue, consisting of a loose aggregate of fibroblasts with conjunctival tissue and interspersed with small blood vessels.

B. Repair and Callus Formation

Seven to nine days after the fracture, mesenchymal stem cells are recruited and come from three different sources: the capillary endothelium, the damaged parts of the periosteum and endosteum, and the systemic circulation. Mesenchymal stem cells near the edge of the fracture develop into chondroblasts, which form hyaline cartilage. Mesenchymal stem cells distal to the fracture edge develop into osteoblasts, which form woven bone. The fibroblasts within the granulation tissue develop into chondroblasts, which also form hyaline cartilage. These two new tissues grow in size until they unite with one other to form an enveloping heterogeneous material called soft callus, which is visible on radiographs 2 weeks after the fracture in children and 3 weeks in adults. This phase mostly requires immobilization, but some micromotion permits healing; rigid internal fixation without micromotion of the fracture fragments prevents soft callus from forming. In the beginning, the soft callus is fragile and flexible. A larger constraint exerted on the fracture at this step generates mobilization of the callus, leading to pain.

At 3 weeks in children and 4 weeks in adults, the hyaline cartilage and woven bone of the callus are progressively replaced by lamellar bone. This new lamellar bone is in the form of trabecular bone. Eventually, all of the cartilage and woven bone of the original soft callus is replaced by trabecular bone and forms a hard callus, restoring most of the bone's original strength. Clinically, a consolidated fracture is not painful to direct pressure, has little or no pain when bending is exerted, and has no mobility.

When the fracture seems to be consolidated, external immobilization should be removed. In general, external immobilization should be maintained 4-8 weeks in cases of cancellous bone fractures and 6-12 weeks in cases of long bone fractures in adults. In children, fracture healing is about twice as fast compared to adults.

C. Consolidation and Remodeling

In the subsequent months, the lamellar bone is substituted by compact bone, and the new bone is remodeled and realigned along the lines where force transmits through the bone. The bone recovers its original strength, and the fracture is finally consolidated. When fracture fragments are fixed through osteosynthesis, consolidation time is considerably increased because of the absence of micromotion.

▶ Patient History

Patient history can clarify the circumstances in which the fracture occurred and underlying causes of fractures. It can also help to target the physical exam, guide a comprehensive diagnostic workup, and implement the right treatment. The keys elements to ask include the following:

- Demographics of the patient (age, gender, and race)
- Comorbidities
- Allergies
- Smoking and alcohol use history
- Hand dominance (in the case of an upper extremity injury)
- Mechanism of injury: magnitude, direction, point of contact, type of force (crushing, compressing, shearing, twisting, pulling, or flexing), and type of trauma (high energy or low energy)
- Snap or crack heard
- Functional impairment
- Pain: progression, frequency, localization, intensity, irradiation, aggravating factors, alleviating factors
- Time since the fracture happened

▶ Clinical Exam

The physical exam should be done in three steps: inspection, palpation, and mobilization.

A. Inspection

Examination should begin with careful inspection of the injured extremity. Look for any signs of shock (pallor, lightheadedness, tachycardia, hypotension), skin cuts, crush to the extremity, abrasions, burns, edema, tenderness, erythema, warmth, ecchymosis, blisters, or angular displacement/rotation.

B. Palpation

Gently palpate the injury to localize any pain, abnormal mobility, or crepitus. Crepitus is a sensation of grinding perceived during the palpation when the bone fragments rub against each other. The vascular examination should be done by checking pulses distal to the injury (palpable, 1+, 2+). Gross sensation, motor function, and reflexes should also be tested to determine if there are any nerve injuries.

C. Mobilization

Ask the patient to try and move the injured limb (passive mobilization) to assess strength, and then carefully manipulate it (active mobilization) to assess the range of motion in all directions (flexion/extension, internal rotation/external rotation, abduction/adduction). Minimize limb mobilization if there is extreme pain or if there is severe soft tissue injury.

▶ Imaging studies

Radiography is the first imaging exam to obtain when evaluating fractures. Images are taken in a minimum of two orthogonal views, usually anteroposterior and lateral, including the full length of the fractured bone and its adjacent joints. For example, in a femur fracture, x-rays of the hip and knee should also be obtained. In certain situations, oblique and tangential views should also be taken to further characterize the fracture. Computed tomography (CT) is helpful to further explore pelvic fractures, and magnetic resonance imaging (MRI) can help characterize vertebrae fractures along with soft tissue disruption and nerve injuries. MRI is also useful for the diagnosis of nondisplaced fractures and stress fractures that are not immediately obvious on radiographs. Scintigraphy allows one to detect zones of increased vascularization, a phenomenon that happens during the inflammatory phase of fracture healing.

▶ Management

A. First Aid

Patients who have sustained a trauma that had the capacity to fracture one of their bones often have associated medical problems that must be investigated because they may be life-threatening. An ABCDE primary survey should be prioritized: airway, breathing, circulation, disability, and exposure. The pain of the patient should also be relieved.

B. Reduction

Reduction refers to the maneuver used to restore proper alignment of the joint or bone. Some fractures do not need to be reduced because they are minimally displaced or nondisplaced or because the displacement has little effect on the final functionality of the limb. Different types of reduction exist:

Closed reduction: This is the preferred method for initially treating fractures. Because the reduction can be as painful as breaking a bone, the maneuver is often done under general anesthesia, under nerve block anesthesia, or after injecting an anesthetic agent into the fracture hematoma. Reduction can be obtained without surgery by exerting longitudinal traction on the injured extremity to disengage all fragments and by applying a force opposite to the one that caused the deformation. After manipulation, the reduction should always be assessed with radiographs.

Mechanical traction: This method can be used to progressively reduce vertebrae or femur fractures. It also allows one to maintain the fragment's position during the fracture healing process.

Open reduction: This is done when closed reduction fails, when the fracture reduction must be perfectly aligned (eg, in intra-articular fracture), or when a fracture has caused vascular or nerve damage. The fracture fragments are surgically exposed, reduced, and usually fixed with internal devices (eg, plates and screws).

C. Immobilization

Immobilization is a process done to maintain a fracture reduction, to reduce pain, to prevent secondary displacement or angulation, and to avoid shearing movements within the fracture hematoma, which can damage the fracture healing process. Occasionally, smaller bones such as ribs, metatarsals, and phalanges do not need immobilization. All immobilization results in immediate muscular atrophy and joint stiffness. This is why immobilization should be terminated as soon as the fracture fragments are consolidated. There are multiple different immobilization methods, including external immobilization (splinting or casting), skeletal traction, and external or internal fixation.

1. External immobilization—Splints and casting are noninvasive ways of stabilizing fractures and maintaining fracture reductions. Splints are typically made of plaster and are not circumferential. Casts are circumferential and can be made of either plaster or fiberglass. Splints are best used for a short period of time (days to up to 1 or 2 weeks) in acute scenarios shortly after injury or operation when swelling is a concern. Because the splint is not circumferential, this avoids compartment syndrome. Cast are sturdier and are used to maintain bones in appropriate alignment for extended periods of time (weeks to months). When casting, the affected limb is first covered with a cloth sleeve or stocking to reduce direct contact of the cast to a patient's skin and hair. For casts, the stocking limb is covered with a generous amount of cotton cast padding interposed between the cloth sleeve and the cast to create an expansion space for the edema during fracture repair and to protect the skin against ulcers. When splinting, cotton cast padding (Webril) is applied directly to the skin, and the plaster is then placed in slabs surrounding the extremity. When immobilizing long bone fractures, the splint or cast should be bent while bone consolidation occurs.

2. Skeletal traction—This method is used when it is difficult to maintain a reduction with external immobilization if the fracture is surrounded by soft tissue or if there are no bony supports above and below the fracture. It is implemented with the use of weights anchored to an adhesive longitudinal bandage or a transosseous wire. Acetabular or femoral shaft fractures can be treated with this method; some centers use this for humeral and tibial shaft fractures. However, attention should be paid to skin disruptions that this method can produce, especially in elderly patients and patients taking corticosteroids. Furthermore, a patient who has skeletal traction is bedridden, which increases the risk of bedsores, pneumonia, osteoporosis, hypercalciuria, and renal lithiasis. This method should be applied for a short period of time and in young patients.

3. External fixation—External fixation is mainly used to treat open or infected fractures, but can be used when there is a comminuted fracture. Long pins are inserted in nonfractured bone at a distance from the injury and fixed to an external fixator, usually metal bars with clamps. This method provides unobstructed access to the fracture and soft tissues for their assessment and healing. A secondary intervention may be performed to restore bone continuity (eg, internal fixation), and soft tissue reconstruction may need to be performed in a staged manner.

4. Internal fixation—This method involves surgical exposure of the fracture and osteosynthesis with sutures, wires, plates, screws, or nails. It secures a reduction of the fracture fragments and accelerates the time to patient mobilization. The advantages of internal fixation are early functional restoration, a shortened length of hospital stay, and faster return to activities of daily living. The disadvantages are increased risk of neurovascular injury, delay in fracture healing because of bone devascularization, and increased risk of infection through an open incision. Internal fixation is indicated in cases of polytrauma, pathologic fractures, associated neurovascular injury, fractures that require a precise reduction, or when a long period of immobilization should be avoided.

D. Observation

During the period that follows reduction and immobilization, attentive, repeated, and close observation should be performed to detect any complications such as neurovascular injuries, fracture malunion, fracture nonunion, and skin disruptions from immobilization. As soon as a complication appears, any bandage, splint, or cast should be removed in order to inspect the fracture site and take necessary steps to correct the complication.

E. Reeducation

Reeducation starts as soon as external or internal immobilization has begun. The patient should mobilize the affected limb as much as the immobilization method allows. Slight movements produce micromotion at the site of the fracture, which stimulates bone union, decreases bone demineralization caused by immobilization, reduces muscular atrophy, and minimizes articular ankylosis if a joint is involved.

▶ Fracture Complications

A. Open Fracture

An open fracture is defined as a bone fracture that communicates with the external environment through a wound of overlying skin. Open fractures have important soft tissue and neurovascular consequences and also carry a serious risk of subsequent osteomyelitis. Open fractures can be characterized using the Gustilo classification (Table 42–2), which also helps in the management of these fractures. The wound must be inspected and then covered with a sterile piece of gauze soaked in normal saline or an antimicrobial of choice. Broad-spectrum antibiotic treatment and tetanus prophylaxis are started as soon as possible, depending on the severity of the injury and the patient's vaccination status. Cephalosporins are used for prophylaxis in grade I and II fractures, whereas cephalosporins and aminoglycosides are used for grade III fracture prophylaxis. Penicillin is administered to patients who sustain farm injuries as prophylaxis against *Clostridium*. A provisional reduction and immobilization should be performed while waiting for surgical management, with a concomitant careful neurovascular examination. Operative intervention should be carried out as soon as possible. Intervention less than 8 hours after injury has been reported to result in a lower incidence of infection and subsequent osteomyelitis. During surgery, the wound should be thoroughly irrigated and debrided in order to excise any devitalized tissues and extract any foreign bodies. Grade I and II

Table 42–2. Gustilo classification of open fractures.

Gustilo	I	II	IIIA	IIIB	IIIC
Description	Clean wound < 1 cm, inside-out perforation, little or no contamination, simple fracture pattern.	Skin laceration > 1 cm, surrounding soft tissue without signs of contusion, vital musculature, moderate to severe fracture instability.	Extensive soft tissue damage, wound contamination, exposed bone, marked fracture instability due to comminution or segmental defects. A: Adequate soft tissue coverage of the fractured bone after surgical debridement. B: Exposed bone with periosteal stripping, requiring flap coverage. C: Any open fracture with associated arterial injury requiring vascular repair.		
Energy	Low	Moderate	High		
Wound size	≤ 1 cm	1-10 cm	> 10 cm		
Soft tissue damage	Minimal	Moderate	Extensive		
Contamination	Clean	Moderate	Extensive		
Comminution	Minimal	Moderate	Severe		
Periosteal stripping	No	No	Yes		
Skin coverage	Local coverage	Local coverage	Local coverage	Requires free tissue flap or rotational flap	Typically requires flap coverage
Neurovascular injury	Normal	Normal	Normal	Normal	Exposed fracture with arterial damage that requires repair
Treatment	First-generation cephalosporin for 24 hours after closure Tetanus booster if not up to date		First-generation cephalosporin + aminoglycoside +/– penicillin (if anaerobic organisms) Tetanus booster if not up to date		
Other antibiotic considerations	Fluoroquinolone for fresh or salt water wounds Doxycycline and third- or fourth-generation cephalosporin for salt water wounds				

open fractures can often be managed with internal fixation, whereas external fixation is often used for grade III open fractures.

B. Compartment Syndrome

In anatomic terms, a compartment is defined as a closed space surrounded by a fascia that contains several muscles. Compartment syndrome may develop wherever a compartment is present. Possible sites include the lower leg, forearm, wrist, hand, and foot. Compartment syndrome primarily occurs in the anterior distal compartment of the lower extremity and in the forearm. This complication can be secondary to trauma (fracture or muscle injury), circumferential thermal injury, surgical procedures, vigorous exercise, and all causes of tissue edema. Compartment syndrome occurs when the pressure within a defined compartmental space increases past a critical threshold, thereby compromising nerve, muscle, and soft tissue perfusion. Tissue ischemia of only 1 hour is associated with reversible neuropraxia, whereas ischemia of 4 hours can induce irreversible axonotmesis. Ischemia of up to 6 hours is associated with irreversible necrosis and is more likely to produce functional impairment.

The classic signs of compartment syndrome include the 6 Ps: pain, poikilothermia, pallor, paralysis, paresthesia, and pulselessness. The initial pain is out of proportion to the injury and is often described as deep, throbbing, and burning in nature. Pain, poikilothermia, and pallor often occur early in compartment syndrome, whereas paralysis, paresthesias, and pulselessness present as late signs of compartment syndrome and often appear after irreversible nerve and muscle damage. Thus, the latter three symptoms should not be a part of the diagnostic criteria for compartment syndrome. When inspecting the extremity in question with compartment syndrome, swelling, pallor, and bullae may be present. A careful neurovascular exam should be performed with an assessment of the peripheral pulses and sensation. A decreased two-point discrimination test is the most consistent early finding. Tenderness may be present to palpation, and if present, the pain could be worsened by passive motion of the involved muscle.

In a patient with classic compartment syndrome symptoms and physical examination findings, no workup is needed. Patients with equivocal clinical findings or those at high risk but without a reliable clinical examination should have compartment pressures measured. A commercially available device, such as the Stryker needle, is often used. After being zeroed, the needle is inserted perpendicular to the skin and then into the muscle compartment in question. A total of 0.3 mL of sterile saline is injected through the needle into the compartment. Equilibrium is reached in a few seconds, and the compartment pressure is then displayed on a digital screen. A difference between the patient's diastolic blood pressure and the compartment pressure under or within 30 mm Hg is considered diagnostic and is an indication for fasciotomy. As soon as the diagnosis of compartment syndrome is obtained, treatment should be performed. This is one of the true orthopedic emergencies. If present, bandages, splints, and casts should be removed immediately. If the tissue pressure remains elevated, adequate decompressive fasciotomies must be performed in the operating room as an emergency procedure.

C. Infection

An infection can happen when a patient sustains an open fracture or a closed fracture treated surgically. Microorganism stimulate local capillary thromboses followed by bone necrosis. The germ isolates itself within the necrotic tissue and is protected from antibiotics. This piece of devascularized and necrotic bone is called the sequestrum. Treatment consists of removal of the necrotic bone, excision of the sequestrum ablation, and local and/or systemic antibiotic treatment.

D. Hemorrhage

Hemorrhage from the bone marrow, periosteum, or surrounding soft tissues may not be obvious initially, but it can be substantial and induce a profound hypovolemia. Generally, blood losses are estimated in adults to be 2-3 L for pelvis fractures, 1-2 L for femoral fractures, and 0.5-1 L for the tibia and humerus. Hemorrhages are more important in open or pathologic fractures. In cases of polytrauma, blood losses can accumulate and can result in hypovolemic shock.

E. Vascular injuries

Vascular injuries can happen in gunshot wounds or following laceration by a bone splinter. Some skeletal injuries are commonly accompanied by arterial or venous injuries. Distal humerus fractures, for example, can cause laceration of the brachial artery, and knee dislocations can be accompanied by an injury of the popliteal artery. Distal ischemia can result in nerve and muscular necrosis or in gangrenous necrosis of the limb, potentially necessitating amputation. If symptoms of ischemia do not resolve within 15 minutes after initial reduction, operative management is necessary.

F. Nerve Injuries

Nerve injuries concomitant with fracture are rare, but if missed, a permanent deficit can result. Certain fractures are more susceptible to nerve injuries than others. For example, shoulder dislocations can result in axillary nerve injury, distal humerus fractures can present with radial nerve injury, and posterior hip dislocations can cause sciatic nerve injury. For any fracture, a careful neurologic examination should be done.

G. Venous Thromboembolism

Venous thromboembolism (VTE), such as deep vein thrombosis (DVT) and pulmonary embolism (PE), can occur after fractures. The following factors increase the risk of DVT after trauma: being bedridden for greater than 3 days, non–weight bearing in the fractured limb, immobilization, fracture or surgery of the pelvis and inferior limb, and age greater than 40 years. VTEs are prevented by elevating extremities, applying compression stockings, mobilizing patients as early as possible, sequential compression devices, extremity exercises, and anticoagulation, such as aspirin, subcutaneous unfractionated heparin, and warfarin.

H. Fat Embolism

Fat emboli mostly occur in polytrauma patients. Fractures of the femur are responsible for 80% of fat emboli. The causes are not well understood; either bone marrow fat from the fracture penetrates the systemic circulation or an unidentified factor provokes chylomicron aggregation in the blood. In either case, large fat globules obstruct the pulmonary circulation, or the cerebral circulation in patients with patent foramen ovale. Patients may develop confusion, tachypnea, and slight hyperthermia within 48 hours of the injury. Cutaneous and mucosal petechiae mostly appear on the neck and conjunctiva, and laboratory studies can reveal reduced Pao_2 and thrombocytopenia. Fat globules can also be detected in the urine. Symptomatic treatment is instituted in these patients by applying oxygen or intubating patients if Pao_2 is less than 60 mm Hg. Antithrombotic medications, such as heparin, should be administered to these patients.

I. Decubitus Ulcers

Decubitus ulcers result from ischemic necrosis following continuous pressure on an area of skin that restricts microcirculation. Ulcers are commonly seen in bedridden patients who lie in the same location for too long. Underlying bony prominences or lack of subcutaneous fat increases the likelihood of ulcer formation. Ulcers are especially seen over the sacrum, ischium, hips, and heels. Prevention of ulcer formation can be performed by routinely moving bedridden patients and by utilizing special beds to more evenly distribute pressure.

J. Malunion

Malunion occurs when a fracture has healed in a suboptimal position, generally after an imperfect reduction or secondary displacement after previous reduction (Figure 42–3). Consolidation at the fracture site still occurs, although the fracture fragments are not anatomically aligned, and there is functional deficiency of the limb.

▲ **Figure 42–3.** Radiograph of malunion. (Reproduced with permission from Moore EE, Feliciano DV, Mattox KL: *Trauma*, 8th ed. New York, NY: McGraw-Hill Education; 2017.)

K. Delayed Union and Nonunion

Delayed union is when a fracture has not consolidated in a normal time frame, although it is correctly aligned (Figure 42–4). A normal delay for a shaft fracture is 3-4 months in adults. Nonunion is diagnosed when the healing fracture process stops before consolidation occurs. Fragments are united only with fibrous tissue (pseudarthrosis). Delayed union and nonunion can be caused by infections, insufficient vascularization, excessive mobility of the fracture site, soft tissue interposition, and loss of contact between the fragments.

L. Complex Regional Pain Syndrome

Complex regional pain syndrome (CRPS) is a complication that can occur within a few months after a fracture. It often presents as pain, dysesthesia, articular ankylosis, and modification of the skin and hair (erythema, cyanosis, alopecia, and abnormal sweating). The cause of CRPS is not well understood, and treatment involves multidisciplinary management to manage the pain.

▲ **Figure 42–4.** Radiograph of scaphoid bone nonunion.

M. Myositis Ossificans

Myositis ossificans is the development of a heterotopic ossification (calcification) in muscles that surround the fracture (Figure 42–5). It occurs most frequently in the elbow.

SUBLUXATIONS AND DISLOCATIONS

Subluxation is a partial loss of contact between two articular surfaces. A dislocation, also called luxation, is a total loss of contact with capsular and ligament tears. Both of these can be associated with fractures. The clinical aspect is the same as fractures in terms of pain, deformation, and functional impairment. Dislocations can be confirmed with orthogonal radiographs, usually anteroposterior and lateral. The integrity of the nerves and vessels surrounding the subluxation or dislocation should be assessed because there is a high incidence of these injuries due to limb elongation or compression. Dislocations are classified by the direction of the distal bone position relative to the proximal bone at the time of dislocation (anterior, posterior, lateral, medial, or other). Treatment is time dependent and closed reduction should be performed as soon as possible given the risk of avascular necrosis. In particular, the risk of necrosis is high in posterior hip dislocations,

▲ **Figure 42–5.** X-ray of the leg with myositis ossificans in adductor muscle. (Reproduced with permission from Skinner HB, McMahon PJ: *Current Diagnosis & Treatment in Orthopedics,* 5th ed. New York, NY: McGraw-Hill Education; 2014.)

unless the femoral head is reduced within the first 6 hours after injury. If reduction is not achieved due to interposition of soft tissue, an open surgical approach should be performed.

SPRAINS

Sprains are traumatic injuries resulting in either ligament elongation or a tear (partial or complete). These injuries affect mainly the ankle, knee, and fingers. Three degrees of injury are classically described, as follows:

First-degree injury: Abnormal elongation of a ligament, producing a minimal disruption of some fibers. Pain and swelling are not pronounced.

Second-degree injury: Stretching of many ligament fibers with a partial tear, but the ligament remains continuous. Symptoms are more pronounced and with associated functional impairment.

Third-degree injury: Complete tear of the ligament with joint instability. Functional impairment is pronounced.

Clinically, the differential diagnosis with a fracture can be difficult, as patients can present with the same amount of functional impairment. Radiography distinguishes complete tear versus bony avulsion. Treatment varies according to the degree of injury, but the first step is RICE (rest, ice, compression, and elevation). Surgery may be required to fix ligament tears in some locations, such as the thumb. In the majority of cases, the joint should be immobilized to allow for healing. In cases of relative immobilization, taping of the joint is performed. In the case where more rigid immobilization is advised, a cast, splint, or boot may be used. It can take up to 6 weeks for ligaments to heal in order to acquire sufficient tensile strength.

TRAUMATIC INJURIES

1. Spine Injuries

▶ **Upper Cervical Spine (C0-2)**

A. Occipital Condyle Fracture

Occipital condyle fractures are rare injuries that involve the craniocervical junction. They can occur following low-energy trauma, such as a blow to the head, or be associated with high-energy trauma, such as a motor vehicle accident. Because of the proximity of the occipital condyles with the medulla oblongata, vertebral arteries, and lower cranial nerves (nerves IX-XII), patients who present with these fractures require careful neurologic exams. CT scans can help with the diagnosis and classification of the fracture. CT should be ordered in cases of high cervicalgia and negative radiographs. These injuries are classified using either the Anderson and Montesano classification, based on mechanism, location, and stability of the fracture, or the Harborview classification, according to MRI findings. Treatment is usually the application of rigid cervical collar immobilization for 8 weeks. In cases of unstable injuries, halo immobilization or surgical stabilization should be performed.

B. Atlas (C1) Fracture

Atlas fractures can involve the anterior arc, posterior arc, or lateral masses. The transverse ligament is the primary stabilizer of the atlantoaxial junction, and its injury can induce instabilities. Atlas fractures occur mostly with head trauma while diving in shallow water or striking the roof of a vehicle during an accident. Fifty percent of these fractures are associated with other cervical spine injuries. However, the risk of neurologic injury is exceptionally rare in these fractures. Vertebral artery injuries may occur concomitantly.

Isolated fractures of the anterior or posterior arc are caused by a trauma in hyperflexion and hyperextension, respectively. Fractures of the lateral masses are usually induced by lateral compression. In these cases, associated fractures of the anterior and posterior arc are named Jefferson fractures. Anteroposterior, lateral, and open-mouth views on radiographs permit diagnosis of these fractures. CT confirms and characterizes the fracture and allows for detection of associated injuries in the cervical spine. The Landells atlas fracture classification, based on fracture location and the transverse ligament involvement, and the Dickman transverse ligament classifications, based on the presence of tear or bony avulsion, can be used to stage these injuries. Stable fractures may be treated with rigid cervical orthosis. Unstable fractures require prolonged halo immobilization. Chronic instability or pain may be treated with C1-2 fusion.

C. Axis (C2) Odontoid Fracture

Axis odontoid fractures (dens fractures) are the most frequent fractures of the upper cervical spine and the axis itself. This type of fracture is caused by an anteroposterior shearing associated with neck hyperflexion or hyperextension, as seen in motor vehicle accidents with posterior or anterior impact. Dens fractures are significantly associated with other cervical spine fractures and a 5%-10% incidence of neurologic injury. The odontoid is vascularized through the base, while the apex has a watershed area, which makes apex fractures highly susceptible to nonunion. Clinical examination of these injuries should include motor, sensory, reflex, and cranial nerve assessments to rule out any neurologic injury. Anteroposterior, lateral, and open-mouth radiographs are adequate to make the diagnosis. However, CT is more accurate for fracture evaluation and displacement. MRI assesses ligamentous, spinal cord, and disk injuries. These fractures can be classified and managed using the Anderson and D'Alonzo classification (Figure 42–6):

- Type I fractures: Oblique avulsion of the tip of odontoid; treated with cervical orthosis

- Type II fractures: Fractures at the junction of the body and neck; treated either with halo or odontoid screw fixation, depending on the risk of nonunion

- Type III fractures: Fractures that extend to the body of the axis; treated with halo immobilization

D. Axis (C2) Hangman's fracture

Hangman's fractures, also known as traumatic spondylolisthesis, are fractures that occur in the thin pars interarticularis of C2 (area between the superior and inferior facets). Originally described in individuals who were hanged, they are generally followed by a sudden hyperextension of the neck after being struck in the face or chin by an object from below. Today, these fractures mainly occur after a fall in elderly patients or a motor vehicle accident in young patients. They are sometimes associated with a fracture of the C3 spinous process or posterior arc of C1. In most cases, these fractures are not associated with narrowing of the spinal canal, and

A

▲ **Figure 42–6.** Anderson and D'Alonzo classification of axis (C2) odontoid fractures. (Reproduced with permission from Skinner HB, McMahon PJ: *Current Diagnosis & Treatment in Orthopedics*, 5th ed. New York, NY: McGraw-Hill Education; 2014.)

patients are usually neurologically intact. Nonetheless, the proximity of the fracture to the vertebral artery and cranial nerves should elicit a thorough neurovascular exam.

These fractures are usually well visualized on a lateral x-ray view of the neck (Figure 42–7). CT demonstrates the exact fracture pattern, whereas MRI can show possible C2-3 disk injuries, which contribute to cervical spine instability. The Levine and Edwards classification, based on mechanism of injury, stages these fractures. Treatment is almost always nonoperative with a cervical orthosis or a halo vest. Surgical treatment with internal fixation should be performed in cases of instability.

E. Axis (C2) Lateral Mass Fracture

C2 lateral mass fractures are usually associated with other C2 or cervical spine injuries, such as occipitocervical or atlantoaxial dislocation. Isolated fractures are extremely rare. The mechanism of these fractures is axial compression and concomitant lateral bending. These injuries are typically diagnosed via CT. Their treatment varies from collar immobilization for uncomplicated, minimally depressed fractures to cervical traction followed by halo immobilization for more complex fractures to fusion for the most extensive fractures.

B

▲ **Figure 42–7.** Lateral x-ray demonstrating an axis hangman's fracture. (Reproduced with permission from Skinner HB, McMahon PJ: *Current Diagnosis & Treatment in Orthopedics*, 5th ed. New York, NY: McGraw-Hill Education; 2014.)

F. Occipitocervical Dislocation

Ligamentous separation of the occiput from the atlas condyles is an extremely serious injury and is often deadly because of the associated damage to the cervical spine or brainstem. Vascular complications are also frequent because of the proximity of the vertebral and carotid arteries to the fracture site and may contribute significantly to mortality. Diagnosis of this type of injury is often made retrospectively in patients with polytrauma following deceleration in a motor vehicle accident. The occipitocervical junction is destabilized by a translation or distraction injury in an accident. Anteroposterior, lateral, and open-mouth radiographs along with CT scans and MRI should be performed. The Traynelis and Harborview classifications, based on the direction of displacement and the degree of instability, respectively, are used to categorize these dislocations. For rare patients who survive, immediate treatment includes halo immobilization with strict avoidance of traction. Definitive surgical treatment with occipitocervical fusion is mandatory in these patients.

Lower Cervical Spine (C3-7)

A. Compression Fracture

A compression fracture is a depression of the superior vertebral endplate with or without anterior cortex involvement, but with preservation of the posterior cortex. This fracture in the cervical spine is rarer than its thoracic counterpart and is mainly caused by an axial load injury. Compression fractures are often associated with posterior longitudinal ligamentous injuries. However, because the posterior cortex stays intact, they are relatively stable injuries and often do not compromise neural element. Patients may present with slight kyphosis. Every lower cervical fracture should be evaluated with anteroposterior, lateral, open-mouth, and left and right oblique radiographs, along with CT or MRI. Usually, these fractures are treated with a cervical brace for 6 weeks.

B. Burst Fracture

A burst fracture is the depression of the superior endplate and anterior and posterior cortex. This fracture is caused by a high-energy axial load following events such as diving accidents or striking a windshield during a motor vehicle accident. The fracture is usually located in C7. Burst fractures are extremely instable because of the concomitant presence of posterior ligamentous injuries. Bony elements are often displaced into the spinal canal, resulting in spinal cord injuries and complications. These fractures are also rarely associated with posterior element fractures. Radiography and MRI should be performed, especially to evaluate ligamentous injuries. Although these fractures can be managed with bed rest and traction in neurologically intact young patients, the treatment of this fracture is mostly surgical, using decompression, reconstruction, and internal fixation for fusion.

C. Cervical Lateral Mass Fracture

A cervical lateral mass fracture is a rare but highly unstable injury that usually follows hyperextension, lateral compression, and rotation trauma of the lower cervical spine during motor vehicle accidents, falls, or a heavy object landing on the head. Neurologic injuries are common in these fractures, necessitating proper clinical evaluation. X-rays and CT and MRI scans should be performed to assess these injuries and their collateral injuries. The Kotani classification, based on the pattern of the fracture and rate of anterior translation, is used to categorize these fractures. Most cases require surgery involving decompression and fusion.

D. Teardrop Fracture

A teardrop fracture is characterized by depression of the anterior cortex with posterior retropulsion of the vertebra due to axial compression and flexion trauma. It is most often caused by diving accidents in shallow water or a motor vehicle accident. If the posterior ligaments are injured, the fracture is unstable; however, if the flexion force from trauma is weak and there is only a bony injury, then the fracture is stable. Unstable injuries are commonly associated with spinal cord injuries. Similar to other injuries, x-rays and CT and MRI scans should be performed. A stable fracture may be managed for 3 months with immobilization, but unstable fractures should undergo surgical treatment with fusion.

E. Clay Shoveler's Fracture

Clay shoveler's fracture is a rare avulsion fracture of the spinous process in the lower cervical and upper thoracic spine due to pulling of the paraspinal muscles. It is most common at the C7 level, but it can also be seen in C6, T1, T2, and T3. These fractures usually occur between the spinous tip and lamina and are often missed. They were originally seen in convicts who would shovel clay and soil. While tossing clay above their heads, the workers would feel a pop and acute pain in their upper back. Now, this fracture is mostly seen in motor vehicle accidents. This is a stable injury and is rarely associated with neural element injuries. Clay shoveler's fractures are difficult to see on radiographs, due to the shadow cast by a patient's shoulders. The method of choice to assess these fractures is CT scan. Treatment is usually only symptomatic with the use of a hard collar for comfort. Surgical treatment is considered in case of persistent pain, nonunion, or failure of conservative treatment.

F. Cervical Facet Dislocation

Cervical facet dislocation can involve one or both of the facet joints. It is usually caused by a trauma in flexion or extension and is associated with distraction and rotation. Cervical facet dislocations can sometimes be associated with facet fractures, but they may also be purely ligamentous sprains. These injuries can be found in whiplash injuries after motor vehicle accidents with restrained passengers. Collateral soft tissue injuries include nerve root impingement and spinal cord injury depending on the severity of the fracture. Anteroposterior x-rays show a spinous process deviated toward the fracture, and the lateral view displays an anterior subluxation depending on the involvement of one or both facets. A CT scan must be performed to demonstrate the anatomy of the injury, evaluate for subtle facet displacement, and determine if there are fractures of other structures. A descriptive classification is usually used as follows: flexion-distraction injuries (only involves disko-ligamentous injury), facet dislocations (unilateral or bilateral), and facet fractures. Treatment should be adapted based on the severity of the injury. Malalignment of the spine and progressive neurologic deterioration are indications that surgical stabilization should be performed.

Thoracolumbar Spine

A. Compression Fracture

Compression fractures of the thoracolumbar spine are common fractures and involve the anterior components of the three columns described by Francis Denis. The anterior column includes the anterior longitudinal ligament, the anterior two-thirds of the vertebral body, and the anterior intervertebral disk. The middle column is composed of the posterior third of the vertebral body, the posterior intervertebral disk, and the posterior ligamentous ligament. The posterior column is made of the pedicles, lamina, facets, ligamentum flavum, spinous process, supraspinous ligament, and interspinous ligament. The posterior vertebral body and posterior longitudinal ligament are spared, making this fracture stable, and it is rarely associated with neurologic injuries. However, these fractures are considered unstable if there is more than a 50% loss of vertebral body height, more than 20-30 degrees of angulation, or multiple adjacent compression fractures present. These fractures can be caused by sudden axial loading following a high-energy trauma during a motor vehicle accident in young patients or low-energy trauma in elderly patients with osteoporosis. In patients over 50 years of age, the diagnosis of pathologic fractures due to metastasis should be excluded. X-rays with anteroposterior and lateral views of the thoracic and lumbar spines are usually sufficient to make the diagnosis. A CT scan is performed to further characterize the fracture. MRIs are performed in cases of neurologic impairment. Treatment is usually conservative with the use of a Jewett brace or thoracolumbar spinal orthosis for comfort, analgesics, and early mobilization. Surgical intervention is required when fractures are unstable or neurologic dysfunction occurs. Pathologic fractures caused by metastasis should undergo a thorough workup to find their origin.

B. Burst Fracture

A burst fracture is caused by more severe axial load forces than those for compression fractures. They are common following a fall or a motor vehicle accident. This type of fracture involves the depression of one of the two endplates and the anterior and posterior cortices and injury to the posterior longitudinal ligament, which causes bony fragments to go into the spinal canal and compress the spinal cord.

With even more severe trauma, lamina fractures and disruption of the posterior ligamentous complex (supraspinous ligament, interspinous ligament, ligamentum flavum, and facet capsule) can occur concomitantly. These two posterior elements can trap dura mater and nerve roots and destabilize the fracture. Similar to compression fractures, radiographs with anteroposterior and lateral views of the thoracic and lumbar spine should be taken. CT scans further characterize the fracture (Figure 42–8), whereas MRI should be performed in cases of neurologic injury. The classification for thoracolumbar injury and the severity score stage the injury, which acts as a guide for management. This score is based on injury morphology, neurologic involvement, and posterior ligamentous complex integrity. Patients with a score of 3 or lower can be treated nonsurgically, a score of 4 is either managed with or without surgery, and a score of 5 or higher is treated surgically. Nonoperative management includes early ambulation and analgesics with or without thoracolumbar spinal orthosis. Surgical decompression and spinal stabilization are indicated in cases of neurologic deficits, unstable fractures (posterior ligamentous complex disruption), and a thoracolumbar injury classification and severity score of 5 or higher.

▲ **Figure 42–8.** Sagittal computed tomography scan of a thoracolumbar burst fracture. (Reproduced with permission from Hall BJ, Schmidt GA, Kress JP: *Principles of Critical Care*, 4th ed. New York, NY: McGraw-Hill Education; 2015.)

C. Chance Fracture

Chance fractures, also known as *seatbelt injuries,* involve vertebrae, disko-ligamentous structures, or both. They are most commonly seen at the thoracolumbar junction (T10-L2) in seatbelt-restrained passengers after a motor vehicle accident. The restraint induced by the lap seatbelt causes a flexion of the spine and then tension in the middle and posterior columns, along with compression of the anterior column. As a result, soft tissue or bony structures can be injured. Soft tissue involvement includes the dorsal fascia, the interspinous ligament, dislocation of the facets, and injury to the disks. Osseous structure involvement includes the vertebral spinous process, lamina, pedicles, and body. The complete involvement of soft tissue elements is called a soft tissue Chance fracture and is more unstable. The involvement of all bony structures is considered a bony Chance fracture and is usually quite stable. Associated abdominal injuries are common. The diagnosis is made with anteroposterior and lateral radiographs of the thoracic and lumbar spines. Chance fractures are usually managed nonoperatively with thoracolumbar spinal orthoses. In cases of neurologic deficiency, unstable spine injuries involving posterior soft tissue elements or polytrauma should be treated with surgical decompression and stabilization.

D. Thoracolumbar Fracture-Dislocation

Thoracolumbar fracture-dislocation is a severe fracture associated with posterior facet dislocation occurring at the thoracolumbar junction (T10-L2). This injury is the result of either translational or rotational deformity after a high-energy injury, such as a motor vehicle accident, fall, or contact sports. It is often associated with neurologic injury and deficit.

The workup should consist of anteroposterior and lateral x-rays, along with CT and MRI scans. These injuries are assessed and managed with the thoracolumbar injury classification and severity score. Patients with a score of 3 or lower can be treated nonoperatively, a score of 4 is managed either nonsurgically or surgically, and a score of 5 or higher is treated surgically. These fracture-dislocations are almost always managed surgically with reduction and fusion.

2. Upper Extremity Injuries

▶ Shoulder

A. Clavicle Fracture

Clavicular fractures are frequent and represent 5%-10% of all fractures. Clavicular fracture is a common fracture in children and young, active patients. It occurs most often in the middle third of the clavicle (approximatively 70%-80%) because this is the thinnest part of the bone (Figure 42–9). Indirect trauma during athletic activities is the most common mechanism of fracture, with a fall on the lateral shoulder or on an outstretched hand. More rarely, direct trauma

▲ **Figure 42–9.** Anteroposterior x-ray of a middle third clavicle fracture. (Reproduced with permission from Ahern G, Brygel M: *Exploring Essential Radiology.* New York, NY: McGraw-Hill Education; 2014.)

may occur due to a motor vehicle accident or a direct blow from an object to the clavicle.

Immediate complications may include disruption of the overlying skin or injury to the subclavian vascular pedicle, brachial plexus injury, or pneumothorax by trauma or a bone fragment. A careful examination of the overlying skin, lungs, pulses, and nerves should be done.

Radiographic imagining should include anteroposterior and 45-degree cephalic views, an x-ray of the shoulder (including axillary view) to rule out additional injury or fractures, and x-ray of the chest to exclude a pneumothorax. Allman, Neer, and AO/OTA classifications categorize these fractures. The Allman classification is based on the localization of the fracture. The Neer classification considers the degree of displacement. The vast majority of clavicle fractures heal with nonoperative management, which includes the use of a simple or figure-of-eight sling for 3-6 weeks. Surgical indications include complete fracture displacement; fractures with greater than 2 cm of shortening; comminuted fracture with a displaced transverse Z-shaped fragment; displaced medial clavicular fracture with mediastinal structures at risk; fracture with interposed muscle, neurovascular compromise, or tenting of the skin with the risk of puncture; open fracture; inability to tolerate closed treatment; polytrauma; concomitant glenoid neck fracture (floating shoulder); and/or symptomatic nonunion.

B. Scapula Fracture

Scapular fractures are rare fractures (< 0.5% of all fractures) that happen mostly in young male adults in a polytraumatic context. They are more frequently caused by high-energy direct trauma with direct blows to the shoulder or from a fall onto an outstretched arm. In about 80% of cases, scapula fractures have associated injuries, such as:

- Thoracic injuries: pneumothorax, pulmonary contusion, rib fractures

- Orthopedic injuries: clavicle fracture, humeral fracture, spine fracture, skull fracture
- Neurovascular injuries: brachial plexus injury, subclavian artery injury, aortic rupture

A careful neurovascular examination must be performed to rule out arterial or brachial plexus injuries. Radiographs with an anteroposterior view of the scapula; lateral, scapular Y, and axillary views of the shoulder; and an x-ray of the chest to exclude a pneumothorax should be obtained. Classification of these fractures can be based on their location (articular fracture or extra-articular fracture) or based on the Ideberg classification of glenoid fractures, the acromial fracture classification, the coracoid fracture classification, or the AO/OTA classifications. These classifications describe the location, displacement, and degree of comminution of the fracture. Most extra-articular fractures can be treated with a sling for 2 weeks. Surgical treatment should be considered for significantly displaced articular fractures, displaced articular fractures involving more than 25% of the articular surface, scapular neck fractures with more than 40 degrees angulation or 1 cm of medial translation, scapula neck fractures with an associated displaced clavicle fracture, acromion fractures that cause subacromial impingement, and coracoid fractures that cause functional acromioclavicular separation.

C. Proximal Humerus Fracture

Proximal humerus fractures are the second most common fractures of the upper extremity after distal radius fractures. These fractures occur primarily in older female patients and are often associated with osteoporosis. The most common mechanism for proximal humerus fractures is an indirect trauma with a fall onto an outstretched hand or elbow. Note that in the elderly, this fracture may be induced by metastases. They can also be the result of violent trauma during motor vehicle accidents or athletic injury in younger patients. Proximal humerus fractures are usually characterized using four anatomic segments, as originally described by Codman: humeral head, greater tuberosity, lesser tuberosity, and metaphysis (Figure 42–10). These fractures are also classified using either the Neer classification, based on the involvement of the four anatomic fragments, or the AO/OTA classification. Complications include injury to the axillary vessels, injury to the circumflex nerve, brachial plexus injury, rotator cuff rupture, skin disruption, and glenohumeral dislocation. A careful neurovascular examination must be performed to rule out arterial or axillary nerve injuries. The assessment of sensation over the deltoid muscle and isometric deltoid motor function is mandatory. Radiographic anteroposterior view of the scapula; lateral, scapular Y, and axillary views of the shoulder; and an x-ray of the chest to exclude a pneumothorax should be obtained. Nondisplaced fractures can be managed with a sling for 3 weeks until consolidation. Premature mobilization elevates the risk

▲ **Figure 42–10.** The four parts of the proximal humerus that can be separated from one another in two-, three-, or four-part proximal humerus fractures.

for secondary displacement. Displaced fractures, including greater tuberosity translation more than 0.5-1 cm or greater than 45 degrees of angulation of fracture fragments relative to others, are usually managed surgically with reduction under general anesthesia and closed reduction with percutaneous pinning, open reduction with internal fixation using either plates or intramedullary nails, or humeral head replacement with hemiarthroplasty or reverse total shoulder arthroplasty.

D. Sternoclavicular Joint Dislocation

The sternoclavicular joint is an extremely powerful and stable joint. That is why this joint is the least dislocated joint in the body. Anterior sternoclavicular joint dislocation occurs more commonly than posterior dislocations and often occurs in patients with an average age of 18 years. Although less common, posterior sternoclavicular joint dislocations are associated with many more complications because of the potential damage to the esophagus, vessels, and trachea. High indirect energy toward the shoulder is the most common cause for anterior and posterior dislocations. An anterior-posterior or a posterior-anterior impact on a lowered shoulder leads to leverage of the clavicle on the first rib, which projects the proximal end forward or backward, respectively. Patients may present with hoarseness, dysphagia, dyspnea, subcutaneous emphysema secondary to tracheal injury, pneumothorax, or vascular/nerve defects.

Radiographic anteroposterior and 45-degree cephalic views of the clavicle, serendipity and Hobbs views, and an x-ray of the chest to exclude a pneumothorax should be obtained. Sternoclavicular joint injuries are graded into three degrees:

- *First-degree injury*: incomplete tear or stretching of the sternoclavicular and costoclavicular ligaments (most common)
- *Second-degree injury*: subluxation with complete tear of the sternoclavicular ligament but incomplete tear of the costoclavicular ligament
- *Third-degree injury*: dislocation with complete tear of both sternoclavicular and costoclavicular ligaments

Treatment usually consists of closed reduction and immobilization in a figure-of-eight sling. Sometimes closed reduction is not possible and the dislocation necessitates an open surgical approach.

E. Acromioclavicular Dislocation

Acromioclavicular sprains or dislocations are mostly seen in active young male adults and athletes. They most commonly occur due to a direct downward blow to the superior or lateral aspect of the acromion or a fall onto the apex of the shoulder with the arm adducted against the body. The context is usually sports trauma (eg, bicycle accident, contact sport) or a motor vehicle accident.

Active mobilization is painful between 120 and 180 degrees of abduction. Passive mobilization is painless and is curative most of the time.

Further maneuvers can be performed to assess the injury:

Piano key sign test (spring test): The examiner applies pressure to the clavicle, resulting in depression of the patient's distal clavicle, and then elevation of the clavicle when the pressure is released. This test demonstrates that the coracoclavicular ligaments are torn.

Anteroposterior drawer sign: The examiner grasps the outer part of the clavicle between two fingers and mobilizes it in all directions. An increase in the mobility of the outer part of the clavicle, with or without pain, demonstrates instability of the joint.

Cross-body adduction test: The patient places the hand of the affected side on the contralateral shoulder with the elbow placed horizontally. The examiner gently pushes against the patient's elbow to bring it closer to the contralateral shoulder. The test is positive if there is pain over the acromioclavicular joint.

Radiographic anteroposterior, lateral, and axillary views of the shoulder and a Zanca view (anteroposterior view with 10-15 degrees of cephalic tilt) should be obtained. The Tossy-Rockwood classification is used to characterize these dislocations and to choose the appropriate treatment. Treatment for an acromioclavicular sprain is usually symptomatic. Significantly displaced injuries sometimes necessitate surgery.

F. Anterior Glenohumeral Joint Dislocation

Anterior glenohumeral joint dislocation is the most common dislocation in the human body and accounts for 90% of shoulder dislocations. It happens mostly in young adults, athletes, and aged females. It most commonly occurs after a fall onto an outstretched hand. Another mechanism is a direct blow to the posterior aspect of an abducted and externally rotated shoulder. In elderly patients or patients with recurrent dislocation episodes, the glenohumeral joint may be extremely unstable and may dislocate during minimal trauma or even during sleep. Associated injuries that can present with shoulder dislocations are Bankart lesions (anterior glenoid labrum tear), fracture of the anteroinferior border of the glenoid rim, Hill-Sachs-Malgaigne lesion at the posterior border of the humeral head secondary to impaction of the humeral head against the anteroinferior border of the glenoid rim, major tubercle fracture, humeral head fracture in the elderly, brachial plexus injury, axillary nerve injury (loss of sensation on the outer surface of the shoulder and loss of isometric deltoid contraction), and rotator cuff tears. Both Bankart and Hill-Sachs-Malgaigne lesions predispose patients to recurrent dislocation. Radiographic anteroposterior and axillary views of the shoulder and a scapular Y view should be obtained (Figure 42–11). Fracture must also be ruled out. The most important treatment of an acute shoulder dislocation is prompt reduction of the glenohumeral joint, after ruling out a fracture. Numerous reduction techniques exist and can be performed after administration of adequate analgesia and relaxation.

Traction-countertraction: The patient is placed in the supine position. Gentle axial traction is applied with progressive abduction with an externally rotated forearm. Countertraction is performed by placing pressure on the thorax with a sheet, while another person pushes on the humeral head. The patient must be anesthetized for this maneuver.

Stimson technique: The patient is placed in the prone position, allowing the affected arm to hang off the bed. Longitudinal traction is applied, and weights can also be added to the patient's wrist to facilitate reduction. The patient can be awake for this maneuver.

Milch technique: The patient is placed in the supine position, with his or her head on a pillow. The dislocated arm is eternally rotated and slowly abducted to 150 degrees. With the patient's elbow flexed, the patient's supine hand is placed under the head. The examiner's hand can help the reduction by applying

▲ Figure 42–11. Scapular Y view of an anterior glenohumeral joint dislocation. (Reproduced with permission from Parks E: *Practical Office Orthopedics*. New York, NY: McGraw-Hill Education; 2018.)

direct pressure to the dislocated humeral head. Once reduced, the arm is internally rotated and placed along the body. The patient can be awake for this maneuver.

Kocher technique: The patient is placed in the supine position. The patient's elbow should be guided with one hand and the ipsilateral wrist with the other hand. The elbow of the affected arm should be flexed 90 degrees at the elbow and brought against the body. The shoulder should be externally rotated until one feels resistance. Subsequently, the arm should be abducted as far as possible. Finally, rotate the shoulder internally until the reduction is obtained. The patient can be awake for this maneuver.

Once the reduction has been accomplished, the arm is placed in a sling for 3-4 weeks for first-time dislocators, and or the arm is placed in a sling for a few days if it is a recurrent dislocation. Neurovascular examination, especially of the axillary nerve, should be performed, and postreduction radiographs are necessary to verify concentric reduction and evaluate for the presence of associated injuries. Surgical treatment should be considered if the reduction is impossible due to interposition of soft tissues or there is

significant bone loss of the anteroinferior border of the glenoid. There is a wide variety of repair procedures with either open or arthroscopic techniques. Surgical reconstruction is indicated for recurrent instability.

G. Posterior Glenohumeral Joint Dislocation

Posterior glenohumeral joint dislocations are much rarer (< 5%) than anterior dislocations and are often underdiagnosed because they are difficult to identify. The most common mechanism of injury is an indirect trauma in a context of epileptic seizure or electrocution. The hypercontraction of the powerful shoulder internal rotator muscles (latissimus dorsi and pectoralis major) is at the origin of the dislocation. Such dislocations often happen bilaterally. They can also occur during a high-energy accident, such as a motor vehicle accident. Associated injuries include reverse Hill-Sachs-Malgaigne lesions (notch on the anterior articular surface of the humerus) and subscapularis injuries. Radiographs with anteroposterior and axillary views of the shoulder and scapular Y (Figure 42–12) or Bloom-Obata views should be obtained. If proper radiographs are not obtained, the diagnosis can be missed. During reduction, the patient should be asleep under general anesthesia and completely relaxed. Reduction is performed either by pulling in line with the axis of the arm with concomitant soft and progressive external rotation of the arm, or by pushing on the humeral head from posterior to anterior. The shoulder should be immobilized in a splint in slight external rotation for 3 weeks.

▲ Figure 42–12. Scapular Y view of a posterior glenohumeral joint dislocation.

H. Rotator Cuff Tear

The shoulder is considered a ball-in-socket joint composed of the humeral head and glenoid fossa. Together, these components provide a great range of mobility, but with limited stability. Shoulder stabilizers can be categorized into two types. *Static stabilizers* include the bony structures, the labrum, the glenohumeral ligaments, the joint capsule, and negative intra-articular pressure. *Dynamic stabilizers* include the rotator and scapular muscles (teres major, rhomboids, serratus anterior, trapezius, and levator scapular). The rotator cuff is composed of the supraspinatus, infraspinatus, subscapularis, and teres minor muscles. The frequency of full-thickness rotator cuff tears ranges from 5%-40%, with an increasing incidence of cuff pathology in older patients. Mechanisms of tear include acute injury, chronic impingement, or a chronic degenerative tear. Tears can occur from violent trauma, such as shoulder dislocations or a fall. Rupture of the supraspinatus muscle occurs most commonly, but these tears can also involve the infraspinatus and subscapularis muscles. The long head of the brachial biceps can also be involved. Anteroposterior and axillary x-ray views of the shoulder should be obtained. An outlet view, which is a lateral radiograph in the scapular plane with the beam tilted 10 degrees caudad, helps identify the acromion shape and slope. Ultrasonography is highly accurate in detecting full-thickness rotator cuff tears. MRI should be used to specify the extent of the cuff rupture and to evaluate tendinous and muscular degeneration (Figure 42–13). Several classifications exist to characterize rotator cuff tears depending on the anatomy, cuff tear size or shape, or cuff atrophy. Nonoperative treatment consists of physical therapy (mobilization, stretching, and strengthening), nonsteroidal anti-inflammatory drugs (NSAIDs), analgesics, and infiltrations of corticosteroids intra-articularly or in the subacromial space. Surgical treatment is considered in the event of failure of conservative treatment, persistence of nocturnal pain, and functional discomfort for performing activities of daily living.

▶ Arm

A. Humeral Shaft Fracture

The humeral shaft is the area extending from the upper border of the pectoralis major tendon to the lower limit of the brachialis tendon muscle. Humeral shaft fractures account for 3%-5% of all fractures. They are more common in young patients with high-energy trauma, but can also be seen in elderly, osteopenic patients with low-energy injuries. They can result from falls or direct trauma. Since the radial nerve and the deep brachial artery cross the posterior border of the humerus, injuries to these two structures can accompany humeral shaft fractures. Radial nerve injuries can be found in 10%-20% of cases and are the result of stretching or contusion. Nerve function usually returns in 3-4 months. Although much rarer, an injury of the deep brachial artery can be present, especially in open fractures. A careful

▲ **Figure 42–13.** Coronal magnetic resonance imaging demonstrating complete rupture of the supraspinous muscle tendon. (Reproduced with permission from Brunicardi FC, Andersen DK, Billiar TR, et al: *Schwartz's Principles of Surgery*, 11th ed. New York, NY: McGraw-Hill Education; 2019.)

neurovascular examination should be performed to evaluate for these potential injuries. Anteroposterior and lateral radiographies of the humerus comprising the shoulder and elbow joints should be taken. These fractures can be classified by descriptive classifications or the AO/OTA classification. More than 90% of these fractures can be treated nonoperatively. Radial paralysis does not contraindicate nonoperative treatment. Treatment consists of a reduction evaluated by anteroposterior and lateral radiographs and immobilization. Immobilization can be achieved by traction, a hanging arm cast, a coaptation splint, a Velpeau dressing, a spica cast, or a functional brace. Surgical treatments are indicated in cases of open fractures, concomitant vascular injury, pathologic fracture, compartment syndrome, floating elbow (concomitant fracture of the forearm bones), segmental fracture, intra-articular extension, and bilateral humeral fracture. Surgery consist of the use of plates and screws, intramedullary wires, intramedullary nails, or external fixators.

▶ Elbow

A. Distal Humerus Fracture

The elbow is a hinged joint that consists of three different articular surfaces: the radiohumeral surface, the ulnohumeral surface, and the proximal radioulnar surface. It has the capacity to flex, extend, and rotate. Fractures of the distal humerus are uncommon. In adults, they do not involve the articular surfaces nearly as often as they do in their pediatric counterparts. They typically occur after high-energy trauma, such as a motor vehicle accident. Fractures that present after low-energy trauma usually occur in osteoporotic females who fall on extended or semi-flexed elbows. The proximity of the brachial artery and median, ulnar, and radial nerves mandates a thorough neurovascular examination to exclude any injuries. Avoid any mobilization of the elbow due to risk of neurovascular damage. Anteroposterior, lateral, and oblique x-rays of the elbow should be obtained. The entire length of the humerus and forearm should also be included in the image. The "fat pad sign," representing displacement of the adipose layer over the joint capsule, may be the only indication of a nondisplaced distal humerus fracture. Distal humeral fractures include intercondylar (most common; Figure 42–14), supracondylar, transcondylar, condylar (Figure 42–15), capitellum (Figure 42–16), trochlear, epicondylar, or supracondylar fractures. These fractures can also be classified using the AO/OTA classification. The patient can be initially managed with a posterior long-arm splint with the elbow flexed at 90 degrees and the forearm in neutral position. Nonoperative treatment is indicated for nondisplaced or minimally displaced fractures. Surgery

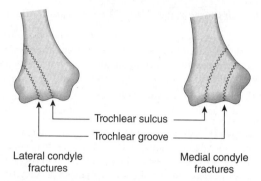

▲ **Figure 42–15.** Distal humerus condyle fracture patterns. The type II fracture involves the lateral lip of the trochlea, thus its inherent instability. (Reproduced with permission from Milch H: Fractures and fracture dislocation of the humeral condyles. *J Trauma.* 1964 Sep;4:592-607.)

is indicated for displaced fractures, open fractures, floating elbow, neurovascular injury, and compartment syndrome. Although a difficult task, emphasis should be put on the precise surgical reconstruction of the articular surface to avoid later complications, such as osteoarthritis.

B. Proximal Ulna Fracture

The proximal ulna (olecranon) is the most important bone that contributes to elbow stability. The subcutaneous position of the olecranon causes it to be especially vulnerable to direct trauma in young adults. Low-energy falls are the cause

▲ **Figure 42–14.** Distal humerus intercondylar fracture patterns. **A:** Type I undisplaced T-condylar fracture of the elbow. **B:** Type II displaced but not rotated T-condylar fracture. **C:** Type III displaced and rotated T-condylar fracture. **D:** Type IV displaced, rotated, and comminuted T-condylar fracture.

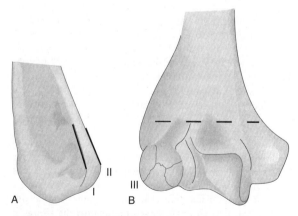

▲ **Figure 42–16.** Distal humerus capitellum fracture patterns. The type I fracture involves a large portion of bone, often the entire structure. **A:** Type II is a shear fracture, often with minimal subchondral bone, and may displace posteriorly. **B:** A type III fracture is a comminuted fracture with varying amounts of displacement of the fracture fragments.

of these fractures in the elderly. The mechanisms of injury include:

- A fall onto an outstretched hand with a semi-flexed elbow accompanied by a strong, sudden triceps contraction resulting in a transverse or oblique fracture of the olecranon
- A direct blow to the olecranon, usually leading to a transverse or comminuted fracture of the olecranon

Isolated fractures of the coronoid process are uncommon and are more frequently associated with posterior elbow dislocations. However, a fracture involving 50% or more of the coronoid process surface alters anteroposterior stability of the elbow. Open fractures can easily occur, which mandates careful examination of the skin. Rarely, arterial injury, neurologic injury (especially the ulnar nerve, despite its proximity), and compartment syndrome can happen. An anteroposterior and lateral radiograph should be done. A true lateral x-ray is essential for determining the fracture pattern and to look for elements that may make treatment difficult, such as articular surface comminution and the involvement of the coronoid process, the radial head, or the capitellum. Several classifications have been suggested to help stage olecranon and coronoid fractures such as the AO/OTA, Schatzker, Colton, Mayo Clinic, and Regan and Morrey classifications. These classifications are all based on the displacement, pattern, and location of the fracture and whether there is an associated dislocation. Among these classifications, none has been proven to be more reliable than the others. Nonoperative management for non- or minimally displaced fractures includes 3 weeks of immobilization in a long-arm splint with the elbow flexed from 45-90 degrees. Splints can also be used for displaced fractures in the elderly for whom the operative management is not ideal due to weak bones. Indications for surgery include any disruption of the extensor mechanism or articular incongruity, fracture with significant displacement (> 1-2 mm), fracture involving more than 50% of the coronoid process, lack of active extension of the elbow, or failure of nonoperative management. Multiple surgical options are available, including intramedullary fixation, tension band wiring, plate and screw constructs, excision, and triceps advancement.

C. Radial Head Fracture

Radial head fractures are among the most common elbow fractures and can be associated with other injuries, such as radial head dislocation, olecranon fracture, coronoid fracture, or elbow dislocation. Most of the time, they result from a fall onto an outstretched hand, with the elbow in extension, causing an indirect axial collision between the radial head and capitellum. The forearm and wrist should be examined for any tenderness, which may indicate the presence of an Essex-Lospreti injury (see later section on this injury). The functional impairment due to radial head fracture is variable, which can lead one to miss the diagnosis.

Radial nerve function is especially important to assess because of its proximity to the radial head. Radiography of the elbow with anteroposterior and lateral x-rays should be ordered. The radial head must be aligned with the capitellum on all views. A nondisplaced fracture should be suspected if a "fat pad sign" is present. If an Essex-Lospreti injury is suspected, additional radiographs of the forearm and wrist are indicated as well. The Mason classification provides staging and management of these fractures (Figure 42–17). Nondisplaced or minimally displaced (< 2 mm) fractures, with no mechanical blockage, can be managed nonoperatively. Any displacement or block should be treated with surgery involving either screws, resection, or radial head prosthesis.

D. Elbow Dislocation

Elbow dislocations are the second most common dislocation after shoulders in adults. They occur more frequently in athletic males, and more than 90% of elbow dislocations are

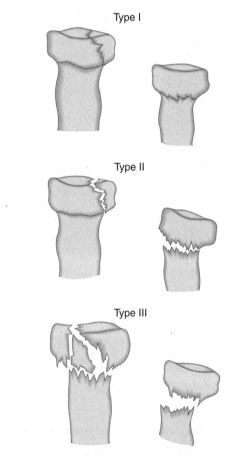

Type I

Type II

Type III

▲ **Figure 42–17.** Mason classification of radial head fractures. (Reproduced with permission from Browner B: *Skeletal Trauma.* Philadelphia, PA: Saunders; 1992.)

posterior dislocations. Other forms of elbow dislocation are anterior, posterolateral, posteromedial, lateral, medial, and divergent. Elbow dislocation most commonly results from a fall on an outstretched hand and a slightly flexed elbow. Extension and valgus deformity of the elbow are almost always present. The anatomic landmark of the medial and lateral epicondyles with the olecranon, which should form an isosceles triangle (Nelaton's triangle), may not be not visible because of edema from the injury. The physical exam should look for an associated fracture. Because of the proximity of the brachial artery and median, ulnar, and radial nerves to the elbow, a careful neurovascular assessment should be performed. Also, edema should be taken as a warning for possible compartment syndrome. Radiographs in the antero-posterior and lateral views confirm the elbow dislocation and its type (ie, anterior vs posterior; Figure 42–18). Oblique views assess the presence of an associated fracture. Acute elbow dislocations should undergo gentle closed reduction with the patient under sedation with adequate relaxation as soon as possible. Hyperextension of the elbow, to open up the coronoid process, should be avoided because of the risk of incarceration of the nerves. The reduction maneuver entails longitudinal traction with a flexed elbow and the forearm in supination. It is essential to have countertraction on the anterior aspect of the humerus performed by another individual in dorsal decubitus or with the table in ventral decubitus. A palpable "clunk" can be appreciated after most reductions. Postreduction range of motion, neurovascular integrity, and radiographic exams should be performed,

▲ **Figure 42–18.** Lateral x-ray view of an elbow dislocation. (Reproduced with permission from Ahern G, Brygel M: *Exploring Essential Radiology*. New York, NY: McGraw-Hill Education; 2014.)

followed by placement of the joint in a posterior splint with 90 degrees of flexion. Surgical treatment is indicated when a closed reduction cannot be performed or if there is persistent instability after reduction, neurovascular compromise, associated fractures, and chronic dislocation.

E. Essex-Lopresti injury

Essex-Lopresti injury is the association of a radial head fracture, proximal radioulnar dislocation, interosseous membrane disruption, and distal radioulnar dislocation. These injuries are often missed, leading to inadequate treatment and definitive destabilization of the forearm. This injury occurs in patients who have fallen from a height on an outstretched hand with a semi-flexed elbow and should be considered in all radial head fractures. The clinical exam should include palpation of the forearm and wrist to exclude these injuries. Radiographic examination is of utmost importance for this diagnosis, with anteroposterior and lateral views containing the elbow, forearm, wrist, and contralateral arm for comparison. The treatment is usually surgical, with fixation of the radial head and reduction and fixation of the distal radioulnar joint.

▶ Forearm

A. Radius and Ulna Shaft Fractures

Fractures of both bones of the forearm (radius and ulna) are common injuries and occur more often in men than women. This is the second most likely location where open fractures occur, only behind tibia fractures. Both-bone forearm fractures are usually the result of direct or indirect high-energy trauma, such as a direct blow on the forearm while protecting one's head, a motor vehicle accident, a fall from a height, or athletic injuries. These fractures are extremely unstable and are most commonly displaced. Compartment syndrome, neurovascular injuries, and open fractures are frequent complications of both-bone forearm fractures. Clinical examination should include a careful evaluation of radial and ulnar pulses, along with documentation of median, radial, and ulnar nerve function. Due to the instability of these fractures, any mobilization should be avoided. Anteroposterior and lateral radiographs of the forearm should be taken to demonstrate the extent of displacement and comminution. Radiographs of the ipsilateral wrist and elbow should be done to assess for associated fractures or dislocation. Fractures of both bones of the forearm are usually classified based on description: whether it is a closed or open fracture, the level of the fracture (proximal, midshaft, or distal), the degree of displacement, angulation and rotational alignment, and the presence or absence of comminution or segmental bone loss. Nonoperative treatment is indicated for pediatric patients but rarely in adults. Nondisplaced fractures require immobilization in a long-arm cast with the elbow bent at 90 degrees for a minimum of 6 weeks. All displaced fractures of both bones of the forearm in adults should be treated with open reduction and internal fixation with plates and screws, intra-medullary nails, or external fixation. The goal is to restore normal ulnar and radial length, rotational alignment, and radial bow, which are essential for rotation of the arm. Open fractures and the presence of a compartment syndrome are other indications for operative management.

B. Ulna Shaft Fracture

An ulna shaft fracture or "nightstick fracture" is common and usually caused by a direct blow to the forearm on the ulnar side while protecting one's head. Evaluation necessitates anteroposterior and lateral radiographs of the elbow, forearm, and wrist to exclude all associated injuries of adjacent joints. Ulna shaft fractures are usually managed nonoperatively with the use of a long-arm splint.

C. Monteggia Fracture

A Monteggia fracture is a fracture of the proximal third ulna with radial head dislocation. These fractures are uncommon and occur after a direct blow on the ulnar diaphysis or after a fall on an outstretched hand. A careful neurovascular exam is necessary due to the potential involvement of the radial and posterior interosseous nerves. Compartment syndrome can complicate the injury. Anteroposterior and lateral x-rays of the forearm with the wrist and elbow joints are needed. Monteggia fractures can be staged using the Bado classification, based on the location of the fracture and the direction of the dislocation. Bado type II Monteggia fractures are further classified using the Jupiter classification, which accounts for the location of the fracture. In almost every case, internal fixation of the ulna is indicated with closed reduction of the radial head. The radial head should be reduced within 6-8 hours of the injury to avoid further articular damage or neurovascular compromise. The interposition of the annular ligament can complicate the reduction, requiring it to be addressed with open surgery. Monteggia fractures can be managed nonoperatively in children.

D. Galeazzi Fracture

A Galeazzi fracture is a fracture of the junction of the middle and distal thirds of the radius within the distal radioulnar joint. It is uncommon, and it is seen most frequently in males. Radioulnar joint injury may be purely ligamentous with subluxation or may present with dislocation or ulnar styloid fracture. These fractures are caused by a direct trauma to the wrist or a fall onto an outstretched hand. Compartment syndrome may occur. The AO/OTA classification categorizes Galeazzi fractures. Anteroposterior and lateral radiographs of the forearm, elbow, and wrist should be performed. Radiographs of the contralateral extremity can be obtained for comparison. In children, these fractures can be managed nonoperatively, but in adults, they must be

addressed surgically to ensure proper anatomic reduction of the distal radioulnar joint.

▶ Wrist

Distal Radius Fracture

A fracture of the distal radius is one of the most common types of fractures and is frequently observed in female over 50 years of age. It is one of three fractures that often result from osteoporosis, along with vertebral compression fractures and femoral neck fractures. They usually occur following a fall onto an outstretched hand from a ground-level fall (Figure 42–19). They are also observed in young patients after a high-energy trauma. Fifty percent of these fractures are intra-articular. Dorsal displacement of the distal segment (Pouteau-Colles fractures) is more common than its volar counterpart (Goyrand-Smith fractures). An avulsion of the ulnar styloid can occur. Other forms of distal radius fractures exist, such as:

- *Volar Barton fracture*: fracture-dislocation of the radiocarpal joint with an intra-articular fracture involving the volar lip

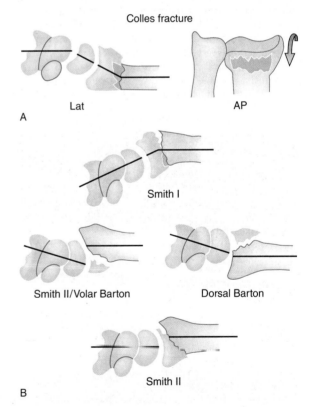

▲ **Figure 42–19.** Schematic drawings of Colles fracture (**A**) and Smith and Barton fractures (**B**). AP, anteroposterior. (Reproduced with permission from Green DP, Hotchkiss RN, Pederson WC: *Green's Operative Hand Surgery*, 4th ed. Philadelpia, PA: WB Saunders; 1999.)

- *Dorsal Barton fracture*: fracture-dislocation of the radio-carpal joint with an intra-articular fracture involving the dorsal lip
- *Backfire, Hutchinson, or chauffeur's fracture*: isolated fracture-avulsion of the radial styloid

A careful evaluation of distal pulses and median nerve function is paramount, since the risk of entrapment is high within the fracture or compression by the fracture hematoma. On physical exam, active extension of the thumb should be assessed due to the risk of extensor pollicis longus tendon incarceration or laceration. Anteroposterior and lateral x-ray views of the wrist should be obtained. CT scans are helpful for detecting intra-articular involvement. The Frykman, Melone, AO/OTA, or Fernandez classifications organize these fractures based on the degree of articular involvement, as well concomitant fractures of the ulna. All displaced distal radius fractures should undergo closed reduction with a hematoma block to limit postinjury swelling, relieve pain, and decompress the median nerve. Nonoperative versus surgical treatment should be guided by the patient's level of activity rather than age alone.

3. Lower Extremity Injuries

▶ Pelvis

A. Pelvic Ring Fracture

Pelvic ring fractures are rare but can potentially be life-threatening injuries. The pelvic ring is composed of the sacrum and the two hip bones (ilium, ischium, and pubis). The weak areas of this ring are the pubic symphysis, the sacroiliac joints, the obturator foramen, the iliac fossa, the acetabular fossa, and the lines of the sacral foramina. These fractures are often caused by high-energy trauma, such as a motor vehicle accident or a fall from height, occurring frequently in a context of polytrauma. They can be stable or unstable fractures. Unstable fractures are further divided into anteroposterior compression, lateral compression, vertical shear, or combined mechanism fractures. Head, chest, vascular, neurologic, genital, rectal, urologic, and perineal skin lesions are frequently associated to these fractures. Hemodynamic instability and shock are other complications encountered with these injuries. Because of the polytrauma context and the risk of complication, a careful physical exam should be conducted using ABCDE (airway, breathing, circulation, disability, exposure) management.

Radiographs with anteroposterior, outlet, inlet, obturator oblique, and iliac oblique views of the pelvis should be done to identify fractures. CT scan is recommended for any suspected pelvis fractures. Fractures of the pelvic ring can be classified and managed according to the Young and Burgess system, based on the mechanism of injury, and the Tile classification, based on the stability of the fracture. The first step of management of these fractures is to wrap a pelvic binder or sheet circumferentially around the pelvis to compress and stabilize it and to control pelvic bone bleeding. The pelvis can then be stabilized with an external fixator until other complications are resolved. Definitive treatment involves either nonoperative treatment for stable fractures or reconstruction of the pelvic ring with open reduction and internal fixation for unstable fractures. Surgical management of pelvic ring fractures are technically challenging, even for experienced trauma surgeons.

B. Pubic Ramus Fracture

Pubic ramus fractures are usually insufficiency fractures caused by normal or physiologic stress upon weakened bone. They are generally stable fractures provoked by a simple fall in elderly patients with osteoporosis. They can be associated with concurrent sacral fractures, which often involve several sacral foramina. Clinical assessment is often vague and nonspecific and does not provide a definitive diagnosis. These injuries must be assessed with anteroposterior radiographs of the pelvis. If there are any doubts or the fracture is not well visualized, a CT scan can help with the diagnosis. Pubic ramus fractures are usually treated nonoperatively with analgesic and full weight-bearing mobilization.

C. Sacral Fracture

Sacral fractures are frequently missed. They can be caused either by high-energy trauma in young patients in the context of motor vehicle accidents or by low-energy trauma in elderly, osteoporotic patients. Complications are lower extremity deficits, along with rectal, urinary, and sexual dysfunction as a result of proximity to the L5-S4 roots. A careful neurologic exam should be performed. Radiographic imaging with anteroposterior, lateral, inlet, and outlet views of the pelvis can be performed but often misses these fractures. CT is the diagnostic study of choice if there is a suspicion for sacral fractures, whereas MRI can reveal nerve injuries caused by the fracture. Fractures of the sacrum can be described using the Denis classification, based on the anatomic location of the fracture. Nonoperative treatment with progressive weight bearing is indicated in osteoporotic nondisplaced fractures. Surgical treatment is indicated in cases of displacement greater than 1 cm, soft tissue compromise, persistent pain, or secondary displacement after nonoperative management.

D. Ilium Fracture

Ilium fractures are typically located between the iliac crest and the greater sciatic notch. They are commonly the result of high-energy trauma and are frequently associated with bowel entrapment and open wounds. Evaluation of these injuries requires anteroposterior, inlet, outlet, obturator oblique, and iliac oblique radiographs of the pelvis. Most of these fractures are unstable and should be treated surgically with open reduction and internal fixation. Nondisplaced stable fractures can be treated nonoperatively.

▶ Hip

A. Acetabular Fracture

An acetabular fracture occurs as a result of forces through the head of the femur to the acetabulum. It can happen through direct lateral trauma on the femoral trochanteric region or indirect axial loading through the lower limb. The position of the femur at the time of impact, the direction of the force, and the quality of the bone all determine the type, pattern, and displacement of the fracture. The fracture can be isolated or associated with a polytrauma. These fractures are seen after high-energy trauma (eg, vehicle accident, fall from height) in young patients or low-energy trauma in elderly, osteoporotic patients. Neurovascular and pelvic organ injuries can complicate these fractures and should be systematically sought and treated. Femoral head dislocation can also present concurrently with these injuries, which can be complicated by avascular necrosis of the femoral head and sciatic nerve injury. Significant bleeding is often present and should be stopped as soon as possible. Anteroposterior, outlet, inlet, obturator oblique, and iliac oblique x-ray views of the pelvis should be obtained, and CT scans can be performed to assess these injuries. These fractures are categorized by the Judet and Letournel classifications, based on the anatomic and radiographic description of fracture patterns, which are correlated with operative findings. Any femoral head dislocation should be treated with closed reduction as soon as possible. Surgical management with open reduction and internal fixation is indicated in cases of displaced roof fractures (> 2 mm), unstable fractures, marginal impaction of the articular surface, intra-articular loose fragments, and failed closed reduction. All other fractures can be treated nonoperatively with either protected weight bearing to reduce forces across the hip or traction for 6-8 weeks.

B. Femoral Head Fracture

Femoral head fractures are rare and are usually associated with hip dislocation. They are often secondary to motor vehicle accidents when the knees strike the car dashboard or after a fall from height. Complications that can consequently occur are sciatic nerve injury and femoral head avascular necrosis. The diagnosis is made with an anteroposterior x-ray view of the pelvis, as well as with anteroposterior and lateral radiographs of the injured hip. A CT scan may be performed to evaluate loose intra-articular fragments and concurrent acetabular or femoral neck fractures. Femoral head fractures can be classified according to the Pipkin classification, based on how much of the femoral head is involved. When there is a concomitant hip dislocation, closed reduction should be performed with a postreduction CT scan to ensure that no fragments are incarcerated in the joint. Nonoperative management with touch-down weight bearing for 4-6 weeks can be pursued if the reduction is adequate, if only the non–weight-bearing surface of the femoral head is involved, and if there are no intra-articular fragments. If these criteria are not met, surgical treatment should be done involving either open reduction and internal fixation or hip arthroplasty, depending if there is preexisting osteoarthritis.

C. Femoral Neck Fracture

Fractures of the femoral neck are common fractures in the elderly. They are intracapsular fractures that can occur from the cartilaginous junction of the femoral head to the base of the neck. They can either be subcapital, transcervical, or basicervical. They are the second most frequent fractures of the hip after trochanteric fractures. Femoral neck fractures are caused either by high-energy trauma in young patients, low-energy trauma in elderly patients following a fall on the trochanteric region, or by a stress fracture in athletes or the elderly because of repeated or prolonged force against the bone. When the fracture is displaced, patients may present with a shortened lower limb that is externally rotated and adducted. Only patients with nondisplaced fractures and/or a stress fracture can ambulate. Radiographically, an anteroposterior view of the pelvis and anteroposterior and lateral views of the hip should be obtained. Internal rotation or traction can help with radiographic evaluation by further delineating the fracture pattern. If no fractures are detected in an elderly patient with persistent hip pain, MRI or a bone scan should be considered to look for nondisplaced or incomplete fractures. The Garden and Pauwels classifications are used to categorize these fractures, based on fracture displacement and orientation patterns. Surgical treatment is the usual choice of treatment for these types of fractures. Nondisplaced stable fractures can be treated by internal fixation using three or four cannulated screws. Care should be taken to place a screw along the inferior femoral neck and to place the remaining screws in a tripod manner to provide the maximum support. Displaced femoral neck fractures are accompanied by disruption of the blood flow to the femoral head. Accordingly, avascular necrosis of the femoral head and nonunion often occur. Therefore, hemiarthroplasty or total hip arthroplasty may be offered to these patients. Basicervical fractures can be fixed with sliding hip screws. Nonoperative management may be considered in some patients who are nonambulatory, have minimal pain, and are at high risk for morbidities if surgical intervention is performed.

D. Trochanteric Fracture

A trochanteric fracture is an extra-articular fracture. This type of fracture is subdivided into either intertrochanteric fractures (between the greater and lesser trochanters) or pertrochanteric fractures (through the trochanters) (Figure 42–20). It

▲ Figure 42–20. Trochanteric fracture patterns: (**A1**) intertrochanteric, (**A2**) pertrochanteric, and (**A3**) reverse obliquity fractures. (Reproduced with permission from Browner BD, Levine A, Jupiter J, et al: *Skeletal Trauma*, 2nd ed. Philadelphia, PA: WB Saunders; 1998.)

is the most frequent hip fracture and occurs most frequently after a fall to the ground in elderly osteoporotic patients, who are usually older than patients with femoral neck fractures. A direct impact or a torsional force transmitted through the leg to the trochanteric area will cause a fracture when such forces are greater than the strength of the bone. These fractures can also be seen after high-energy trauma, mostly in males less than 40 years old. The mortality rate is elevated in the year following these injuries in elderly patients. Unlike displaced femoral neck fractures, these fractures do not often lead to avascular necrosis and nonunion because they occur in cancellous bone, which has an abundant blood supply. Similar to femoral neck fractures, patients with displaced trochanteric fractures often present with a shortened, externally rotated, and adducted lower extremity. The diagnosis is made on anteroposterior radiographs of the femur, and concomitant anteroposterior and lateral x-rays views of the hip should also be obtained. Internal or traction views can help further characterize the fracture line. Typically, trochanteric fractures have an oblique line that extends from the lateral cortex proximally to the medial cortex distally. This standard pattern is considered stable. An oblique

fracture line that extends from the medial cortex proximally to the lateral cortex distally is known as a reverse obliquity fracture and is deemed unstable. Subtrochanteric extension and a large posteromedial fracture (ie, of the lesser trochanter) are also factors of instability. There are several classifications of these fractures, such as the Evans classification, Ender classification, or AO/OTA classification, which define stability and direct treatment. Like femoral neck fractures, treatment is usually operative. Management of these fractures within 48 hours after injury may decrease the 1-year risk of mortality. A dynamic hip screw can be used for stable fractures, while an intramedullary nail is often used for unstable fractures. Nonoperative management includes non–weight bearing of the affected lower extremity with early out of bed to chair mobilization. This may be considered for patients who carry high surgical risk or for demented/nonambulatory patients.

E. Subtrochanteric Fracture

Subtrochanteric fractures occur approximately 5 cm distal to the lesser trochanter. They are usually the result of higher-energy trauma than femoral neck or trochanteric fractures in young patients, either from direct lateral trauma (motor vehicle accident) or from axial loading (fall from height). However, they may also occur in elderly patients with lateral low-energy trauma, especially in patients with a history of long-term bisphosphonate use. Additionally, fractures in this region may be pathologic in nature due to bone metastases. The major muscles that surround the hip create significant forces that contribute to fracture deformity (flexion—iliopsoas; abduction—gluteus medius; and external rotation—external rotators). Subtrochanteric fractures are assessed with anteroposterior radiographs of the femur, along with anteroposterior and lateral views of the injured hip. A full-length image of the femur, including the knee, should also be done. These injuries can be classified with the Russel-Taylor, Seinsheimer, or AO/OTA classifications. These classifications stage the fracture according to the entirety of the piriformis fossa and the number of fracture fragments. These fractures should be treated operatively and may be managed either with fixed-angle plates or intramedullary nailing (Figure 42–21), depending on the fracture pattern. External fixation is indicated in severe open fractures. Secondarily, external fixation is often converted to internal fixation when soft tissue healing has occurred.

F. Hip Dislocation

Hip dislocations are rare and mostly occur after high-energy trauma. They can be posterior (most frequent) or anterior. They are generally seen in young adults after a motor vehicle collision or a fall from height. Causal mechanisms are either direct (trauma on the trochanteric region) or indirect (axial loading through the lower limb or torsion). The femoral head is vascularized by three arteries: the medial circumflex femoral (main supply), the lateral circumflex femoral, and the

▲ **Figure 42–21.** Anteroposterior x-ray of a subtrochanteric fracture treated with an intramedullary nail.

▲ **Figure 42–22.** Anteroposterior x-ray of a posterior hip dislocation.

obturator arteries. The contribution of the medial and lateral circumflex arteries is often disrupted when the hip is dislocated and avascular necrosis of the femoral head is then a major concern. The sciatic nerve can be injured with posterior hip dislocations, and these patients should receive a thorough neurologic examination. Clinically, the patient presents with a limb that is shortened and adopts a classic position that is flexed, adducted, and internally rotated (posterior dislocation) or flexed, abducted, and externally rotated (anterior dislocation). Radiographic studies with anteroposterior views of the pelvis, along with anteroposterior, lateral, external oblique, and internal oblique views of the injured hip should be performed (Figure 42–22). CT scans can further be done to evaluate the direction of dislocation, presence of intra-articular fragments, and associated fractures. Hip dislocations are classified as either simple (isolated) or complex (accompanied by a femoral head fracture, acetabular fracture, or proximal femur fracture).

The dislocated hip should be treated with closed reduction within 6 hours from the injury to limit the risk of avascular necrosis. The only contraindication to emergent closed reduction is the presence of a concomitant femoral head

fracture. For reduction, the patient should be placed in the dorsal decubitus position, be sedated, and have adequate muscular relaxion. An assistant should bilaterally maintain the pelvis with hands on the anterosuperior iliac spines. Anterior dislocations are reduced with in-line longitudinal traction and internal rotation. Posterior dislocations are first reduced with in-line longitudinal traction and then flexion, slight internal rotation, and adduction of the hip to open up the femoral head. Next, the hip is externally rotated and abducted until the head is rearticulated with the acetabulum. Indications of a good reduction include experiencing an audible pop, the disappearance of the classical injured position, and restoration of limb lengths. Following reduction, the hip should be evaluated for stability, and postreduction CT scan can be performed to rule out any intra-articular fragments. Open reduction is indicated in case of irreducible dislocation or incarcerated fragments or tissue. Associated fractures should be stabilized surgically.

▶ Thigh

A. Femoral Shaft Fracture

The femoral diaphysis is the area 5 cm distal to the lesser trochanter to an area 5 cm proximal to the adductor tubercle. Femoral shaft fractures are common fractures and usually occur after a high-energy trauma in young patients or, less commonly, after a low-energy trauma in elderly patients. Pathologic fractures induced by metastatic disease can also occur in this location. Immediate complications that may occur are open wounds and associated fracture of the acetabulum, hip, or knee. Due to the large volume of the three fascial compartments of the thigh, significant blood loss and hemodynamic instability can occur. The appearance of sudden confusion, tachypnea, cutaneous and mucosal petechia, and a slight hyperthermia within 48 hours after the injury should make the diagnosis of fat embolism. Radiographs with anteroposterior and lateral views of the entire femur, including the hip and the knee, should be performed. Fractures of the femoral shaft can be classified descriptively (open vs closed, location, pattern, degree of comminution, angulation, rotational deformity, displacement, and amount of shortening) or using the Winquist and Hansen classification, which is based on the pattern, stability, and amount of comminution of the fracture, or the AO/OTA classification. Ideally, surgical stabilization with plate or intramedullary nailing should occur within 24 hours of injury. External fixators may be used in cases of open fracture, vascular injury, or unstable polytrauma victims.

▶ Knee

A. Distal Femur Fracture

A distal femur fracture can be either supracondylar (between the femoral condyles and 5 cm above the adductor tubercle), intercondylar (between the two condyles), or condylar. It is mostly caused by high-energy trauma with significant displacement in young patients, but can also be seen after a low-energy trauma with less displacement in older, osteoporotic patients. The popliteal artery may be injured in cases of significant posterior displacement of the distal fragment, and the sciatic nerve can also be stretched. Therefore, a careful neurovascular exam should be performed. Open wounds and knee dislocation may complicate these fractures. Additionally, meniscal and ligament injury of the knee can occur. The analysis of the fracture is done with anteroposterior, lateral, and oblique radiographic views of the entire femur. Adjacent joints should also be assessed. Traction views and CT scan may be useful to delineate the fracture and establish intra-articular involvement. MRI is done to assess soft tissue injury. The proximal fracture fragment is typically pulled superiorly by the quadriceps and hamstrings, whereas the distal fragment is typically displaced and angulated posteriorly due to the pull of the gastrocnemius muscle. These injuries can be classified descriptively (open vs closed, intra-articular vs extra-articular, location, pattern, degree of comminution, angulation, rotational deformity, displacement, and amount of shortening) or using the AO/OTA classification. Immediate closed reduction is indicated to avoid impingement of the popliteal artery. If reduction fails to restore pulses, an immediate arteriogram and vascular operative intervention are indicated. Nonoperative management with a hinged brace, immediate range of motion, and non–weight bearing should be considered in nondisplaced fractures, non-ambulatory patients, or patients with high surgical risk. Displaced distal femur fractures are best treated with plates and transfixing screws. Great effort should be made to anatomically reduce the fracture and precisely reconstruct and realign the joint surfaces in order to delay osteoarthritis.

External fixation may be used as temporary treatment in cases of open fractures.

B. Patella Fracture

The patella is an important part of the extensor mechanism of the knee. The subcutaneous location of the patella makes it prone to injury. Patella fractures are commonly the result of a direct trauma on the patella with a flexed knee, such as toward the dashboard in an unrestrained vehicle passenger. Fracture displacement depends on the degree of flexion of the knee and contraction of the quadriceps during impact. Rarely, the mechanism is indirect by rapid knee hyperflexion against a contracted quadriceps, provoking an avulsion of the tip of the patella. Skin injuries are a common complication of this fracture. Cartilaginous and ligamentous injuries of the knee should be ruled out. Patients may be unable to actively extend the knee in case of complete disruption of the extensor mechanism. Anteroposterior, lateral, and axial (sunrise or Merchant) radiographs of the knee should be taken. These fractures can be classified descriptively (displacement, location, and degree of comminution). Nonoperative treatment with the knee immobilized in extension using a cylinder cast for 4-6 weeks and full weight bearing may be performed if there is an intact extensor mechanism, the fracture is nondisplaced, and there is a vertical fracture pattern. Open reduction and internal fixation with a tension band, cerclage wiring, screws, or a combination of these is indicated in cases of extensor mechanism disruption, displaced fractures greater than 3 mm, and articular incongruity with greater than 2 mm of step-off. Partial patellectomy may be performed in the setting of large salvageable fragments with a smaller, comminuted polar fragment not amenable to stable fixation. Total patellectomy is rarely indicated and is only reserved for extensive patella fractures with severe comminution.

C. Tibial Plateau Fracture

The tibial plateau is composed of the medial condyle (large, concave, strong) and lateral condyle (small, convex, weak). It supports 85% of the transmitted load. Tibial plateau fractures can involve the lateral condyle (mostly), the medial condyle, or both condyles and are accompanied by significant angular deformities. They are usually the result of axial loading coupled with varus or valgus forces. Medial condyle fractures typically result from high-energy trauma (motor vehicle accident, a fall from height). Lateral condyle fractures often result from low-energy trauma (fall from ground). The pattern of the fracture can be split, depressed, or both. Meniscal, ligamentous, popliteal artery, or fibular nerve injuries and compartment syndrome can complicate these fractures. A thorough physical exam with vascular and neurologic assessment should be done. Anteroposterior, lateral, and oblique radiographic views of the knee should be taken. CT scans are

A   B   C   D   E   F

▲ **Figure 42–23.** Schatzker classification of tibia plateau fractures. **A**, type I: lateral split; **B**, type II: lateral split depression; **C**, type III: lateral depression; **D**, type IV: medial plateau; **E**, type V: bicondylar; **F**, type VI: bicondylar with separation of metaphysis from diaphysis. (Reproduced with permission from Rockwood CA, Green DP, Bucholz RW, et al: *Fractures in Adults*, 4th ed. Philadelphia, PA: Lippincott; 1996.)

often obtained to evaluate articular surface depression and comminution. The Schatzker classification stages these injuries according to the anatomic location of the fracture and the pattern presented (Figure 42–23). Nonoperative treatment with a hinged brace for 4-6 weeks, non–weight bearing, and early knee range of motion can be performed in minimally or nondisplaced fractures, nonambulatory patients, or elderly osteoporotic patients. Surgical management using external fixation or open reduction and internal fixation is indicated in case of open fractures, displacement of articular surfaces, compartment syndrome, or associated vascular injury. The surgical reconstruction of these fractures is particularly challenging and involves anatomic restitution of the articular surface and limb alignment.

D. Knee Dislocation

The knee is a very stable joint, and knee dislocations are rare injuries. However, when they occur, these dislocations may be limb threatening due to disruption of the popliteal artery. These dislocations result from the disruption of three of four major ligaments (anterior cruciate, posterior cruciate, medial collateral, and lateral collateral). High-energy trauma, such as a motor vehicle accidents, a fall from height, or athletic injuries, is the most common cause of knee dislocations. These injuries may also occur in patients with connective tissue disorders, such as Ehlers-Danlos or Marfan syndrome. Many knee dislocations also have associated fractures of the femur and tibia, common fibular nerve injury, skin disruption, and risk of compartment syndrome. A careful neurovascular exam is required. Radiographs with anteroposterior, lateral, notch, and axial (sunrise or Merchant) views should be performed to assess these injuries and their associated fractures. An MRI should be obtained to evaluate other soft tissue damage that

may need to be repaired in a simultaneous or staged manner. Knee dislocations can be classified according to the Schenck classifications system, which describes the injury according to ligamentous and periarticular structures involvement. They can also be categorized according to the displacement of the proximal tibia in relation to the distal femur (anterior, posterior, lateral, medial, and rotational) in the Kennedy classification. Half of these dislocations spontaneously reduce. If the knee remains dislocated at presentation, closed reduction should be performed in a sedated patient with longitudinal traction to restore limb vascularization. If pulses are absent after reduction, immediate surgical exploration should be performed. If pulses are diminished, arteriography is indicated to assess the blood flow. Once reduced and adequate vascular status is confirmed, the knee should be splinted at 20-30 degrees of flexion. Postreduction radiographs should always be obtained. Open reduction is indicated for unsuccessful closed reduction and soft tissue interposition. If the joint does not stay reduced, if there is an open injury, or if vascular repair is needed, external fixation may be initially performed to stabilize the joint. Repair of the ligamentous structure with special attention to the posterior capsule and posterolateral corner should be performed to definitively stabilize the knee.

E. Patella Dislocation

Dislocation of the patella is a relatively common injury in adolescent females and athletes in general (soccer, gymnastics, and ice hockey). It may also occur in patients with connective tissue disorders (Ehlers-Danlos and Marfan syndromes) due to increased soft tissue laxity. These injuries may be due to direct trauma to the patella or due to a valgus stress combined with flexion and external rotation. Dislocation of the patella can be acute (traumatic) or chronic (recurrent). Radiographic evaluation includes anteroposterior, lateral, and axial (sunrise or Merchant) views. These injuries are typically treated with closed reduction performed by pushing the patella toward the midline with the knee in full extension. Immobilization with casting and bracing in extension for 6 weeks is indicated. Surgical management is usually reserved for recurrent dislocations.

F. Quadriceps Tendon Rupture

The quadriceps tendon is part of the extensor mechanism of the knee joint. Ruptures are uncommon and usually occur within the 2 cm of the quadriceps tendon before it inserts into the patella. It can result from a direct blow on the tendon or an indirect eccentric contraction of the quadriceps muscle, with the foot planted and the knee partially flexed. The rupture may be partial or complete. Risk factors for quadriceps tendon rupture include age greater than 40 years, diabetes mellitus, inflammatory arthropathy, chronic renal failure, hyperparathyroidism, connective tissue disorder, and systemic and intra-articular steroid use. Patients are unable to actively extend the knee or perform a straight leg raise due to a complete disruption of the extensor mechanism. Radiographs should include anteroposterior and lateral views of the knee. In cases of complete rupture, the patella migrates inferiorly (patella baja). Ultrasonography or MRI may help differentiate between partial and complete disruption to make a definitive diagnosis. Nonoperative treatment with knee immobilization in a brace is indicated in case of partial ruptures or patients who cannot tolerate surgery. Complete ruptures of the quadriceps tendon are managed operatively.

G. Patella Tendon Rupture

Patella tendon ruptures are less frequent than quadriceps tendon ruptures and occur mostly in patients under 40 years of age. They are the third most common injury to the extensor mechanism of the knee, following patellar fractures and quadriceps tendon ruptures. They usually occur after a sudden eccentric contraction of the quadriceps with a flexed knee. Ruptures can involve either avulsion from the inferior pole of the patella or midsubstance of the patellar tendon or avulsion from the tibial tubercle. They can be partial or complete. Risk factors for patellar tendon ruptures include diabetes mellitus, inflammatory arthropathy, chronic renal failure, patellar tendinopathy, and systemic and local corticosteroid treatment. Patients may present with an inability to actively extend the knee. If only the tendon is ruptured and the retinaculum is intact, active extension may remain possible. Radiographs in the anteroposterior, lateral, and axial (sunrise or Merchant) views should be performed. In cases of complete rupture, the patella often migrates superiorly (patella alta). Ultrasonography can be used to assess the tendon, whereas MRI is the most sensitive imaging study that can differentiate between partial and complete patella tendon disruption. Partial ruptures are usually treated

nonoperatively with cast or brace immobilization in full extension for 6 weeks, whereas complete tendon ruptures are managed operatively.

H. Meniscal Injuries

Menisci are C-shaped wedges of fibrocartilage located between the tibial plateau and femoral condyles that directly influence the transmission of forces, distribution of load, amount of contact force, and pressure distribution pattern. Menisci are important stabilizing structures of the knee. The blood supply to menisci is limited to the outer third portion. Meniscal injuries can be acute or degenerative. Acute meniscal injuries usually occur after rotational trauma and commonly occur during athletic activities. Medial meniscus tears are more frequent than lateral meniscus tears. However, when associated with anterior cruciate ligament tears, lateral meniscus tears are more common. Chronic or repetitive stress may cause degenerative tears of the menisci. Tear patterns include longitudinal, flap, radial, horizontal, bucket handle, and complex tears (Figure 42–24). Patients may complain of locking and catching while mobilizing their knee, which are highly

▲ **Figure 42–24.** Patterns of meniscal tears: bucket handle, flap, horizontal cleavage, radial, degenerative, and double radial tear of a discoid meniscus.

suggestive physical symptoms of meniscal tear. Radiographic evaluation should include anteroposterior, lateral, and axial (sunrise or Merchant) views of the knee. MRI can help confirm the diagnosis and can provide additional information concerning the status of ligaments and cartilage. Conservative treatment is indicated as the first-line treatment for degenerative tears. Patients should undergo physical therapy and intra-articular corticosteroid injections. If physical symptoms persist that affect activities of daily living, surgery may be indicated. Meniscal arthroscopic surgery is the most commonly performed surgery of the knee for this type of injury. Options for treatment include partial meniscectomy for small and central meniscal tears. Meniscal repair may be an option for large tears located in the outer third of the menisci in young patients. Meniscal transplantation is occasionally used in young patients with complete destruction of the meniscus, but an exact cadaver match must be obtained. Total meniscectomies are no longer performed because they accelerate osteoarthritis. Physical rehabilitation should be performed immediately after meniscal surgery. Rehabilitation starts with isometric quadriceps exercises and range-of-motion exercises. Once the arthroscopic incisions are healed after meniscal debridement, patients can begin strengthening activities such as swimming, biking, and muscular strengthening. As soon as the patient is able to perform these exercises comfortably, weight-bearing exercises can be resumed until the motion and strength are equal to the other healthy knee. For meniscal repair and transplantation, the rehabilitation process is gradually increased until full weight bearing is obtained.

I. Anterior Cruciate Ligament Injuries

The anterior cruciate ligament (ACL) is a sagittal stabilizer of the knee that prevents anterior displacement of the tibia relative to the femur. The greatest restraint is in full extension. ACL injuries mostly result from sports-related trauma, such injuries seen in soccer, basketball, football, and skiing. Female athletes are more susceptible to these injuries, especially when there is eccentric loading of the lower extremity. ACL injuries can occur after sudden contraction of the quadriceps with internal rotation of the extremity with a planted foot or after noncontact active hyperextension of the knee. The injury stretches the ligament, leading to a partial tear or complete tear; the most common injury is a complete tear. ACL tears are often associated with meniscal tears, often involving the lateral meniscus. ACL tears can also be associated with medial collateral ligament injury and chondral injury. The ACL may also be avulsed with part of the tibial tubercle. The diagnosis for ACL tears is made by physical examination of the patient using a Lachman test (Figure 42–25). This is performed by placing the patient in a supine position with the knee flexed to 30 degrees. The examiner uses the nondominant hand to stabilize the patient's thigh, while the other hand holds the patient's proximal tibia and pulls the tibia forward. The amount of anterior displacement and the quality of the end point (firm, marginal, soft) determine the diagnosis and should be compared with the noninjured knee. This test is more sensitive than the anterior drawer test, where the patient is placed supine, the knee is flexed to 90 degrees, and the examiner pulls the proximal tibia forward. Radiographs with anteroposterior and lateral views of the knee may reveal bony injuries. MRI confirms the diagnosis of ACL tear and associated injuries. These injuries can be classified and managed according to the American Academy of Orthopaedic Surgeon classification. Management of ACL tears can be either nonoperative or operative. Nonoperative treatment includes physical therapy and the use of a hinged knee brace; this is indicated in low-demand patients and athletes who may not participate in any pivoting sports. Surgical arthroscopic reconstruction with either autograft or allograft is usually required in younger, active patients. Any bony avulsion should be surgically fixed.

▲ **Figure 42–25.** The Lachman test.

J. Posterior Cruciate Ligament Injuries

The posterior cruciate ligament (PCL) is both a sagittal stabilizer of the knee that prevents posterior displacement of the tibia relative to the femur and an important rotational stabilizer. This ligament is less frequently injured than the ACL, and injury to the PCL is often missed. PCL tears occur after a direct blow to the proximal tibia on a flexed knee; an anteriorly directed force to the anterior tibia in a hyperextended knee with the foot planted; a fall onto a hyperflexed knee; or noncontact hyperextension. PCL tears can also be associated with bony avulsion, as well as chondral, meniscal, or other ligamentous injuries similar to ACL tears. These injuries are clinically diagnosed when performing the posterior drawer sign (Figure 42–26). To perform this maneuver, the patient is placed supine, the knee is flexed to 90 degrees, and the examiner pushes the proximal tibia backward. The amount of displacement should be compared to the contralateral knee. Anteroposterior and lateral radiographs of the knee should be done to assess for bone injuries. MRI confirms the diagnosis of a PCL tear. There are three grades of posterior cruciate ligament injury: partial tear, complete isolated tear, and complete tear with combined capsuloligamentous injuries. Isolated posterior cruciate ligament tears are usually treated nonoperatively with bracing and physical therapy. If a bony avulsion or other associated ligamentous injuries are present, surgical treatment is indicated.

K. Medial Collateral Ligament Injuries

The medial collateral ligament (MCL) is a valgus stabilizer of the knee, and it is the most commonly torn ligament due to sport-related injuries. Contact sports are responsible for most MCL injuries. These injuries are frequently associated with ACL tears and medial meniscus injuries. They are the result of a valgus and external rotation force to the lateral knee that can occur with direct or indirect trauma. Injuries vary from strain to complete rupture. Physical examination of MCL tears demonstrates laxity with valgus stress test of the knee at 0 and 30 degrees of flexion. Anteroposterior and lateral radiographs of the knee should be performed, and the

▲ **Figure 42–26.** Posterior drawer sign.

diagnosis of MCL tear is confirmed by MRI. Isolated tears are usually treated nonoperatively with analgesics, rest, ice, bracing, and physical therapy. The presence of associated injuries should prompt surgical management.

L. Lateral Collateral Ligament Injuries

The lateral collateral ligament (LCL) is a varus stabilizer of the knee. Injuries to the LCL most frequently result from motor vehicle accidents and athletic injuries. LCL tears can be caused by a direct blow to the ligament, excessive varus stress, external rotation, or hyperextension. Tears can be described as a strain, partial, or complete. These injuries may occur concomitantly with other ligamentous injuries, such as injury to the popliteus muscle tendon or iliotibial band in the setting of a multiple ligamentous knee injury. Avulsion of the apex of the fibular head may occur, and the fibular nerve may be injured. Instability of these injuries is clinically assessed while placing a varus stress to the knee at 0 degrees and flexed to 30 degrees. Anteroposterior and lateral radiographs of the knee should be done, while MRI confirms the tear. Isolated partial tears are treated nonoperatively with analgesia, ice, rest, bracing, and physical therapy. Complete tears or tears with associated injuries should be managed operatively.

▶ Leg

A. Tibial Shaft Fracture

Tibial shaft fractures are the most common long bone fractures in the body. They are mostly caused by direct high-energy trauma from a motor vehicle accident. This mechanism of injury is often associated with transversal, oblique, or comminuted fractures and is complicated by open wounds. Fractures of the tibial shaft can also result from indirect torsional injury during a fall or sport-related injuries (eg, skiing) that often result in spiral fractures. These fractures frequently lead to associated fractures of the femur or fibula. Concomitant vascular and nerve injuries may also occur. It is imperative to carefully check pulses and perform a thorough neurologic examination. Compartment syndrome is another frequent complication of this type of injury, and the compartments of the lower leg should be monitored. Full-length radiographs of the tibia with anteroposterior and lateral views should be performed, along with imaging of the knee and ankle. These fractures can be classified using a descriptive classification (open vs closed, location, pattern, degree of comminution, angulation, rotational deformity, displacement, and amount of shortening) or the AO/OTA classification. Nonoperative treatment with closed reduction and immobilization in a long-leg cast is indicated in cases of minimally or nondisplaced, closed, and stable fractures. Surgical treatment with external fixation, intramedullary nailing, or plate and screws is indicated for high-energy, displaced, or comminuted fractures.

B. Fibula Shaft Fracture

Isolated fractures of the fibula are uncommon but can occur after a direct blow to the lateral side of the leg. Anteroposterior and lateral radiographs of the leg, including the knee and ankle joint, should be performed. If no other injury is present, immobilization is for comfort only. Three to four weeks of treatment in a walking cast or removable cast boot are usually sufficient, and complete healing can be expected.

C. Achilles Tendon Rupture

The Achilles tendon is the largest tendon in the body. Achilles tendon ruptures are common athletic injuries that are often seen in jumping sports or sports that require rapid change of direction while running. They may occur after a sudden forced plantarflexion or violent dorsiflexion in a plantarflexed foot. Other mechanisms involve sudden direct trauma to the tendon or sudden activation of the Achilles tendon after atrophy from prolonged periods of inactivity. Risk factors for Achilles tendon ruptures are being a recreational athlete, diabetes mellitus, inflammatory arthropathy, chronic renal failure, hyperparathyroidism, connective tissue disorder, fluoroquinolone antibiotic use, and systemic or local corticosteroid treatment. Ruptures can be either partial or complete. Patients usually report a sudden snap or an audible "pop" that feels like someone shot them in the back of the leg. The provocative Thompson test helps make the diagnosis of complete rupture. This test is positive when there is a lack of plantarflexion after the examiner squeezes the calf of the injured limb while the patient lies prone, with the foot hanging over the edge of the examination table. Ultrasound may be useful to confirm the diagnosis and distinguishes between partial and complete rupture. MRI can provide a definitive diagnosis of a disrupted tendon. Achilles tendon rupture can be managed either nonoperatively or surgically. Nonoperative treatment is usually recommended in older patients with moderate athletic ambitions. Nonoperative treatment involves a cast or boot in resting equinus for 2 weeks, followed by 6-8 weeks of casting or booting with progressive dorsiflexion to neutral and slow advancement of weight bearing. Surgery is often reserved for active patients, and surgical treatment involves suture of the ruptured tendon, sometimes reinforced by the gastrocsoleus aponeurosis or plantaris tendon.

D. Peroneal Tendon Subluxation and Dislocation

Peroneal tendon subluxations and dislocations are often misdiagnosed as ankle sprains and may go unrecognized. They can be the result of a sports-related injury with forced dorsiflexion of the foot on contracted peroneal muscles. Consequently, injury to the superior peroneal retinaculum can occur, and both peroneal tendons (brevis and longus) can be injured. Evaluation of these injuries starts with anteroposterior, lateral, and mortise radiographic views of the ankle, as well as anteroposterior, lateral, and oblique view of the foot. Although the tendon cannot be imaged on radiograph, a cortical avulsion of the distal malleolus is suggestive of tendon subluxation/dislocation. MRI and dynamic ultrasound are the imaging studies of choice to diagnose these injuries. Treatment involves reduction of the tendon and short-leg cast or tall boot immobilization, with the foot in slight plantarflexion and mild eversion. Patients are made non–weight bearing for acute injuries for 6 weeks, followed by progressive weight bearing. If dislocation of the tendon continues, operative intervention with repair of the superior peroneal retinaculum may be considered.

▶ Ankle

A. Tibial Plafond Fracture

A tibial plafond fracture, also called a pilon fracture, is a fracture of the distal portion of the tibia, involving the articular surface at the ankle joint. It is caused by high-energy rotational or axial loads from motor vehicle accidents or a fall from height, which drives the talus into the tibial plafond. Associated fibula or talus fractures, open wounds, and compartment syndrome may complicate these injuries. Radiographic images with anteroposterior, lateral, and mortise views of the ankle should be obtained. Additionally, full-length leg and foot radiographs should be done to asses fracture extension. A CT scan may be necessary in some cases where there is significant comminution and can assist with preoperative planning. These fractures can be classified with the AO/OTA and Ruedi and Allgower classifications. The latter is based on the degree of displacement and comminution of the fracture. Tibial plafond fractures represent one of the most difficult challenges for surgical fixation. Treatment depends on bone and soft tissue involvement, the fracture pattern, and patient characteristics. In most cases, an external fixator is placed to primarily stabilize the fractures and allow for soft tissues to heal. Subsequently, definitive reconstruction using internal fixation can be performed with the goals of restoring fibula length and stability along with the tibial articular surface.

B. Ankle Fracture

Fracture of the ankle are extremely common. They can involve the lateral malleolus, the medial malleolus, and the posterior portion of the tibia (often referred as the posterior malleolus). They are usually described according to the number of fractures (unimalleolar, bimalleolar, or trimalleolar). Indirect mechanisms include torsion, inversion, and eversion injuries. Excessive inversion stress is the most common cause of ankle fractures, making the lateral malleolus the most injured portion of the ankle. Ankle fractures can be complicated by ligamentous injuries, syndesmosis injuries, skin wounds, ankle dislocation, pilon fracture, talar fracture, and Maisonneuve-type fracture (associated spiral fracture of the proximal third of the fibula seen in medial malleolus fractures). Clinical evaluation of ankle injuries is done using the Ottawa ankle rules, which help select patients who require radiographic imaging. If one criterion is positive, radiographic anteroposterior, lateral, and mortise views should be performed. A proximal tibia radiograph should be obtained to rule out Maisonneuve-type fracture (Figure 42–27). Ankle fractures can be categorized using the Lauge-Hansen (rotational mechanism of injury), Danis-Weber (the position of distal fibular fracture in relation to

▲ **Figure 42–27.** Schematic of a Maisonneuve-type fracture showing proximal fibular fracture and associated ankle injury with disruption of syndesmosis.

the syndesmosis), or the AO/OTA classifications. Nonoperative management with reduction and immobilization in a splint and then a cast or brace may be performed for nondisplaced and stable unimalleolar fractures. Surgical treatment with open reduction and internal fixation is indicated for displaced and unstable unimalleolar fractures, bimalleolar fractures, and trimalleolar fractures.

C. Talus Fracture

Talus fractures are the second most common tarsal fracture after calcaneal fractures. The tarsal neck is the most vulnerable to fracture. A talus fracture is frequently the result of a high-energy forced dorsal flexion of the foot and ankle with an axial load. These injuries most commonly occur from high-energy trauma, such as motor vehicle accidents or falls from a height. Associated fractures of the foot and ankle are common. Because the talus is mostly covered in cartilage and most of the blood supply of the talus comes from its neck, talus fractures are subject to avascular necrosis. Radiographic imaging should include anteroposterior, lateral, and mortise views of the ankle, as well as anteroposterior and oblique views of the foot. A canal view provides optimal visualization of the talar neck. A CT scan is indicated when radiographs are negative and there is high suspicion for this injury, and better characterization of these fractures is needed. These injuries are classified based on of their anatomic location: neck, body, head, lateral process, and posterior process. Fractures of the talar neck are classified using the Hawkins classification, based on the degree of displacement of the fracture and dislocation of the subtalar, tibiotalar, or talonavicular joints. Nondisplaced fractures can be treated with short-leg casts and non–weight bearing for at least 6 weeks. Displaced and comminuted fractures should be treated surgically with open reduction and internal fixation as soon as possible.

D. Ankle Syndesmosis Injuries

The ankle syndesmosis is a robust membrane between the distal fibula and tibia that helps to stabilize the ankle joint. Ankle syndesmosis injuries, also known as a *high ankle sprains*, generally occur with external rotation injuries. They often present with concomitant injuries such as fractures, sprains, or dislocations around the ankle. Clinically, the diagnosis can be determined by performing the squeeze test (compression of the leg at midcalf level that causes pain at the syndesmosis) or the external rotation stress test (external rotation of the foot that causes pain at the syndesmosis). Radiographic anteroposterior, lateral, mortise, and external rotation stress views should be obtained. These injuries are staged using the Edwards and DeLee classification, according to the degree of diastasis (latent or frank). Disruption of the ankle syndesmosis is usually managed surgically with a syndesmotic screw or braided suture that fixes the fibula and tibia together at the lower joint. The screw is left in place for

a minimum of 4 months and can be removed to avoid screw breakage, while the braided suture remains in place.

E. Ankle Dislocation

Ankle dislocations are common injuries and are frequently associated with fractures of the ankle. They are seen after high-energy trauma that causes plantarflexion of the ankle with either inversion or eversion of the foot. Four types of dislocation can occur: anterior, posterior, lateral, and superior. Neurovascular injuries are the main concern of these injuries, and a careful neurovascular evaluation should be performed in these patients. The diagnosis is often made clinically: the distal tibia protrudes anteriorly under the skin, and the foot is posteriorly displaced. Ankle dislocations are confirmed with anteroposterior, lateral, and mortise radiographs. Closed reduction should be performed in a sedated patient as soon as possible to limit neurovascular injuries and to avoid the risk of compartment syndrome. The knee can be flexed to 90 degrees to reduce tension on the Achilles tendon. The examiner places one hand on the heel and another on the dorsum of the foot. In-line traction is then applied while another individual applies countertraction at the knee. Postreduction radiographs should be obtained to confirm proper joint alignment. Open reduction is indicated in cases of irreducible dislocation or an incarcerated fragment or tissue. The joint is then stabilized nonoperatively or surgically, depending on concomitant injuries and stability of the ankle joint.

F. Ankle Sprains

Ankle sprains are the most common injuries of the ankle. They are usually the result of forced rotation, inversion, or rotation of the foot. The most commonly injured site is the lateral ligamentous complex composed of the anterior talofibular (most commonly involved ligament), calcaneofibular (second most commonly involved ligament), and posterior talofibular ligaments. The deltoid ligament on the medial side can also be injured. Ankle sprains can be associated with fractures of the fifth metatarsal, Achilles tendon rupture, and fibular tendon subluxation. The need for radiographic studies should be dictated by the Ottawa ankle rules (Figure 42–28). Ankle and foot radiographic series should be done if the patient has pain in the malleolar zone along with any of the following five findings: bone tenderness along the lower 6 cm of the posterior edge of the fibula or the tip of the lateral malleolus; bone tenderness along the lower 6 cm of the posterior edge of the tibia or the tip of the medial malleolus; bone tenderness at the base of the fifth metatarsal; bone tenderness on the navicular bone; or inability to bear weight immediately after the injury and in the emergency department. Ankle sprains are diagnoses of exclusion. If no fractures, dislocation, or widening (> 4 mm) is appreciated between either malleolus or the talus, then an ankle sprain is

The Ottawa rules

- History of trauma and malleolar ankle pain

and any *one* of:

- Age greater than 55
- Inability to bear weight
- Tender over posterior 6 cm of medial *or* lateral malleolus

6 cm

Lateral view

6 cm

Medial view

▲ **Figure 42–28.** The Ottawa ankle rules regarding which ankle injuries should be screened with an x-ray to look for fractures.

a reasonable diagnosis. These injuries are usually treated with RICE (rest, ice, compression with elastic bandage wrap, and elevation), analgesics, NSAIDs, and non–weight bearing or protected weight bearing with crutches for 3-5 days. Splinting or use of an immobilization ankle device is optional. Ankle braces can also be applied. Surgical treatment is reserved for chronic instability of the ankle after failure of conservative treatments.

Foot

A. Calcaneus Fracture

Calcaneus fractures are the most common fractures of the tarsal bones. They can be intra-articular or extra-articular according to the involvement of the subtalar, calcaneal cuboid, or calcaneal navicular joint. Most of these fractures are intra-articular and are frequently comminuted and impacted. The most frequent causal mechanism for intra-articular fractures is a high-energy axial load, which drives the talus bone downward onto the calcaneus. These fractures are seen after motor vehicle accidents or falls from height. Extra-articular calcaneus fractures may be the result of twisting injuries. Calcaneus fractures are often associated with lumbar spine fractures, and a careful physical exam of the back should be performed. Stress fractures can also appear in the lumbar spine. Radiographic anteroposterior, lateral, and oblique views of the foot are necessary, along with

anteroposterior and lateral views of the lumbar spine. CT is the imaging study of choice and should be performed to fully assess these injuries and to plan for surgery. Extra-articular fractures include fractures of the anterior process, calcaneal tuberosity, medial process, sustentaculum tali, and body. The Sanders classification is used to classify intra-articular fractures based on the fracture pattern using a CT. Non-operative treatment with cast immobilization is indicated for small extra-articular fractures (< 1 cm), nondisplaced intra-articular fractures, and stress fractures. Operative treatment with open reduction and internal fixation is indicated for large extra-articular fractures (> 1 cm) and displaced intra-articular fractures. However, surgery should not be performed until the swelling of the operative extremity has decreased and will allow for appropriate skin closure. Patients with calcaneus fractures can be placed in a bulky splint with extra thick cotton padding. The goals of surgery are to restore the heel length and height, restore the mechanical axis of the hindfoot, and realign the posterior facet of the subtalar joint.

B. Metatarsal Fractures

Metatarsal fractures are common injuries of the foot. The fifth metatarsal is the most commonly fractured metatarsal in adults (see next section), followed by fractures of the second, third, and fourth metatarsals. The first metatarsal is the least commonly fractured metatarsal. These injuries may occur after a direct blow from a heavy object or rotation of the hindfoot on a fixed forefoot. Stress fractures are common, especially in the second metatarsal. Anteroposterior, lateral, and oblique x-ray views of the foot should be obtained. MRI can be performed to detect stress fractures of the metatarsals. Classification of metatarsal fractures is descriptive (open vs closed, location, pattern, degree of comminution, angulation, rotational deformity, displacement, and amount of shortening). Nonoperative treatment with a stiff-soled shoe or a short walking boot with weight bearing as tolerated is indicated if the fractures are isolated, are minimally displaced or nondisplaced, or are stress fractures. Displaced and multiple metatarsal fractures are usually managed surgically with open reduction and internal fixation. The treatment should restore the transverse and longitudinal arch of the foot and restore metatarsal alignment to allow for normal force transmission across the metatarsal heads.

C. Fifth Metatarsal Base Fracture

Fifth metatarsal base fractures are the most common metatarsal fractures. These often occur when performing athletic activities. Anteroposterior, lateral, and oblique radiographs of the foot should be obtained. This type of fracture is classified in zones: zone 1, pseudo-Jones fracture (proximal tubercle avulsion, which is the insertion of the peroneal brevis); zone 2, Jones fracture (metaphyseal-diaphyseal junction fracture in which the fracture line extends into the joint between the fourth and fifth metatarsals); and zone 3, proximal diaphyseal fracture, generally a stress fracture. Zone 1 fractures are treated nonoperatively with a stiff-soled shoe. Zone 2 and 3 fractures may be managed either nonoperatively or surgically, depending on the level of a patient's activity. Nonoperative treatment involves non–weight bearing in a short-leg cast or boot for 6-8 weeks. Surgical treatment is performed with percutaneous screw fixation or open reduction and internal fixation.

D. Lisfranc Injuries

The Lisfranc joint consists of the tarsometatarsal, intermetatarsal, and intertarsal joints. Lisfranc injuries, also known as tarsometatarsal fracture-dislocation injuries, encompasses sprains, fractures, and dislocations through the tarsometatarsal joints. Lisfranc injuries usually occur after high-energy trauma (eg, motor vehicle accidents, athletic injuries, a fall from height) caused by a direct blow to the joint or by indirect rotational and axial load. The diagnosis is not always obvious, particularly in a polytrauma context, and these injuries are often undiagnosed, which results in progressive foot deformity, pain, and loss of function. Open wounds and associated fractures of the tarsals or metatarsals may complicate Lisfranc injuries. The proximity of the dorsalis pedis artery mandates a careful vascular exam. Anteroposterior, lateral, oblique, stress (to assess joint stability), and weight-bearing radiographic views should be obtained if possible. CT scan is useful to confirm the diagnosis and can be used for preoperative planning. MRI can be performed to identify ligamentous injuries. Stable injuries are treated nonoperatively with a short-leg cast or boot, and patients are initially made non–weight bearing. Operative management with open reduction and internal fixation is indicated for any displacement of the tarsometatarsal joints greater than 2 mm.

JOINT ASPIRATION/INJECTION

▶ **Definitions**

A. Synovial Fluid

Normal synovial joint fluid is yellow, clear, and highly viscous because of its high content of hyaluronic acid. Synovial fluid provides joint lubrication and nutrient transport to the cartilage.

B. Joint Effusion

Joint effusion is a pathologic accumulation of synovial fluid in the joint and may be a sign of joint pathology. If the synovial fluid is a sufficient quantity, a joint effusion can be diagnosed with physical examination. For smaller volumes or in a deep joint such as the hip, imaging is necessary to diagnose a joint effusion. Although radiography can show widening of the joint space or modification of the surrounding soft tissues, ultrasound and MRI are best for visualizing joint effusions.

C. Aspiration

Joint aspiration (arthrocentesis) involves sampling synovial fluid through the placement of a needle into the joint cavity for diagnostic or therapeutic purposes. Synovial fluid analysis can distinguish between inflammatory and noninflammatory conditions and can provide direct proof of crystal arthropathy, infection, and hemarthrosis (Table 42–3). It also helps evacuate the joint effusion, relieves pain by decreasing joint pressure, and prevents joint damage. Aspiration may be considered in cases of hemarthrosis to prevent adhesions and relieve pressure. Aspiration may also be performed immediately prior to injecting intra-articular medications, such as corticosteroids, to improve efficacy.

Periarticular aspiration is a puncture of a periarticular structure, such as a bursa in the olecranon or prepatellar bursitis in the knee, and is done for diagnostic and therapeutic purposes. Aspiration carries minimal risk when properly indicated and performed. However, caution is advised in certain situations:

- Infection risk or bacteremia if there is dermatitis/cellulitis on the skin overlying the aspiration location

Table 42–3. Parameters of synovial fluid analysis.

Parameter	Normal	Osteoarthritis	Hemorrhagic	Gout	Pseudogout	Inflammatory Arthritis	Septic Arthritis
Gross appearance	Clear	Clear	Bloody	Opaque	Opaque	Opaque	Opaque
Volume (mL)	0-1	1-10	5-50	5-50	5-50	5-50	5-50
Viscosity	High	High	Low	Low	Low	Low	Low
Total white blood cells count (cells/µL)	< 200	200-10,000	> 2,000	500-75,000	500-75,000	500-75,000	> 50,000
Polymorphonuclear cells (%)	< 25	< 50	0.3	> 50	> 50	> 50	> 75
Crystal analysis	None	None	None	Negatively birefringent	Positively birefringent	None	None
Glucose concentration (mg/dL)	Serum glucose	Serum glucose	Serum glucose	Serum glucose	Serum glucose	< 25	< 25

- Intra-articular bleeding risk in patients with coagulopathy or bleeding diathesis
- Adjacent osteomyelitis
- The presence of orthopedic implants or intra-articular fracture; an orthopedic consult is recommended in these cases

D. Infiltration

Joint infiltration is the injection of medical products, such as corticosteroids, anesthetics, antibiotics, contrast fluid, or hyaluronic acid, into a joint cavity for therapeutic and diagnostic purposes.

Periarticular infiltration is the injection into a periarticular structure (bursa, enthesis) in order to control periarticular pathology through corticosteroids, with or without anesthetics. Some examples of locations for injections include subacromial, olecranon, trochanteric, or prepatellar infiltration for ailments such as bursitis, rotator cuff tendinitis, or epicondylitis.

The greatest contraindication for infiltration is hypersensitivity to one of the constituents (active ingredients or excipient) of the medical product.

Equipment

Equipment usually needed includes the following:

- Sterile gloves, drape, and gauze; surgical mask; adhesive bandage; collecting tubes
- Alcohol, povidone-iodine solution, or chlorhexidine for sterilization (allow the skin to dry for 3-5 minutes prior to introduction of the needle)

- Needles: 1.5-inch, 21- to 18-gauge for large joints (eg, knee, ankle, or shoulder); 1-inch, 21-gauge for medium joints; 1-inch, 25-gauge for small joints
- 5-, 10-, 20-, or 60-mL syringes, as appropriate for the joint and the size of the effusion

Procedure

Any joint can be blindly aspirated or infiltrated by using anatomic landmarks. However, some deep joints, such as the hip, require the use of ultrasound or fluoroscopic guidance. Informed consent should be obtained before starting the procedure in order to explain the risks and benefits of the procedure. Once the aspiration/infiltration site is determined, sterilize the surrounding skin with alcohol, povidone-iodine solution, or chlorhexidine using a circular motion, progressively moving away from the puncture site. Drape the approach site in a sterile manner. Depending on the practitioners' preferences, anesthesia of the overlying skin by injecting lidocaine may be performed for the patient's comfort before approaching the joint. Insert and advance the needle slowly until synovial fluid is obtained. If bone is encountered, slowly withdraw the needle without exiting the skin, and then redirect it. The aspiration/injection should be performed without resistance. Once the aspiration/infiltration is performed, remove the needle, apply pressure, and then apply a bandage.

Common Joint Approaches

A. Shoulder Joint

1. Glenohumeral joint—The patient should be seated in a comfortable position, arms along the body, with the palms

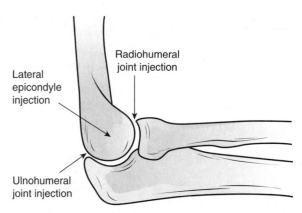

▲ **Figure 42–29.** Anterior approach to the glenohumeral joint for aspirations and injections.

▲ **Figure 42–30.** Approach to the elbow joint for aspirations and injections.

of the hand on the lap, and head turned away from the aspiration/infiltration site for aseptic reasons. Palpate the coracoid process and the joint space, which can be felt as a groove lateral to the coracoid process. Mark the needle insertion site located approximately 0.4 inches inferiorly and 0.4 inches laterally from the coracoid process. Sterilize the skin surrounding the insertion site. Insert an 18- or 21-gauge needle. Direct the needle posteriorly and slightly inferiorly into the glenohumeral joint (Figure 42–29).

2. Subacromial space—The patient should be seated in the same position as the glenohumeral joint approach. Palpate the posterolateral angle of the acromion. Mark the needle insertion site located in the groove below the acromion angle. Insert an 18- or 21-gauge needle. Direct the needle horizontally toward the contralateral sternoclavicular joint.

B. Elbow Joint

The patient should be comfortably seated upright, with the elbow flexed at 90 degrees and resting on a table with the palm on the table. Palpate and identify the triangle formed by the olecranon process, the radial head, and the lateral epicondyle. Mark the needle entry site in the depression located in the middle of the triangle, just proximal to the radial head. Insert an 18- or 21-gauge needle perpendicular to the skin and direct it toward the joint space (Figure 42–30).

C. Wrist Joint

The patient should be comfortably seated upright or in a supine position. The patient's wrist is pronated, with slight palmar flexion, and held in a straight line with the forearm

while resting on a side table. Palpate and identify the extensor pollicis longus muscle tendon and the common extensor muscle tendon of the index finger. Mark the needle site that is located between these two tendons, ulnar to the anatomic snuff box, and at the distal end of the radius. Insert a 21-gauge needle and direct it perpendicularly to the skin (Figure 42–31).

D. Metacarpophalangeal and Interphalangeal Joints

The patient should be comfortably seated upright or in a supine position. The patient's hand should be resting on a

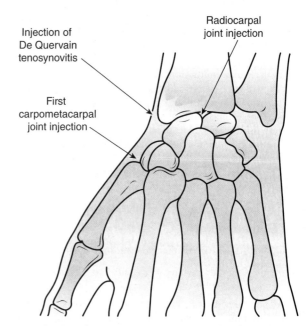

▲ **Figure 42–31.** Approach to the wrist joint for aspirations and injections.

table with the palm facing down. Palpate and identify the joint line. Apply gentle traction, and mark the needle site dorsally and on either the medial or lateral side to the extensor tendon. Insert a 25-gauge needle into the joint space directed toward the center of the joint.

E. Knee Joint (Suprapatellar Approach)

The patient should be lying supine. The knee should be fully extended, and the quadriceps relaxed. Palpate and identify the lateral border of the patella. Mark the midpoint of the lateral border, where the needle should be inserted. The nondominant hand can push on the medial border of the patella in order to open the femoropatellar joint and facilitate needle entry. Insert an 18- or 21-gauge needle perpendicularly to the limb axis and direct it toward the center of joint (Figure 42–32).

F. Ankle Joint

The patient should be lying supine. The ankle is held at a 90-degree angle. Identify the joint line and palpate the sulcus between the lateral malleolus and the extensor digitorum longus muscle tendon. Mark the insertion site located in the middle of the sulcus and insert an 18- or 21-gauge needle. Insert the needle perpendicular to the fibula shaft and direct it medially toward the joint space (Figure 42–33).

G. Metatarsophalangeal and Interphalangeal Joints

The patient should be lying supine. Apply gentle traction, and mark the needle site dorsally on either the medial or

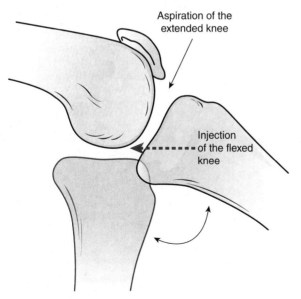

▲ **Figure 42–32.** Approach to the knee joint for aspirations and injections.

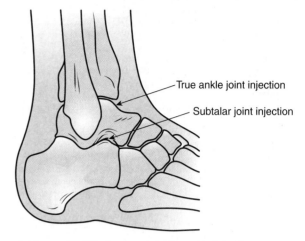

▲ **Figure 42–33.** Approach to the ankle joint for aspirations and injections.

lateral side to the extensor tendon. Insert a 25-gauge into the joint space directed toward the center of the joint.

AO Foundation. Homepage. https://www.aofoundation.org/Structure/Pages/default.aspx

Bartonícek J: Pauwels' classification of femoral neck fractures: correct interpretation of the original. *J Orthop Trauma.* 2001;15(5):358-360.

Bellabarba C, Mirza SK, West GA, et al: Diagnosis and treatment of craniocervical dislocation in a series of 17 consecutive survivors during an 8-year period. *J Neurosurg Spine.* 2006;4(6):429-440.

Brunicardi FC (ed): *Schwartz's Principle of Surgery.* 11th ed. New York, NY: McGraw-Hill; 2019.

Dwyer AJ, John B, Singh SA, et al: Complications after posterior dislocation of the hip. *Int Orthop.* 2006;30(4):224-227.

Joglekar SB, Lindvall EM, Martirosian A: Contemporary management of subtrochanteric fractures. *Orthop Clin North Am.* 2015;46(1):21-35.

Kellam JF, Meinberg EG, Agel J, et al: Introduction: fracture and dislocation classification compendium-2018: International Comprehensive Classification of Fractures and Dislocations Committee. *J Orthop Trauma.* 2018;32(Suppl 1):S1-S10.

Kotani Y, Abumi K, Ito M, et al: Cervical spine injuries associated with lateral mass and facet joint fractures: new classification and surgical treatment with pedicle screw fixation. *Eur Spine J.* 2005;14(1):69-77.

Lee JY, Vaccaro AR, Lim MR, et al: Thoracolumbar injury classification and severity score: a new paradigm for the treatment of thoracolumbar spine trauma. *J Orthop Sci.* 2005;10(6):671-675.

Marsh JL, Slongo TF, Agel J, et al: Fracture and dislocation classification compendium - 2007: Orthopaedic Trauma Association classification, database and outcomes committee. *J Orthop Trauma.* 2007;21(10 Suppl):S1-133.

Meyer N, Pennington WT, Dewitt D, et al: Isolated cerebral fat emboli syndrome in multiply injured patients: a review of three cases and the literature. *J Trauma.* 2007;63(6):1395-1402.

Sanders RJM, Swierstra BA, Goosen JHM: The use of a dual-mobility concept in total hip arthroplasty patients with spastic disorders: no dislocations in a series of ten cases at midterm follow-up. *Arch Orthop Trauma Surg.* 2013;133(7):1011-1016.

Shea KG, Carey JL: Management of anterior cruciate ligament injuries: evidence-based guideline. *J Am Acad Orthop Surg.* 2015;23(5):e1-5.

Skinner HB (ed): *Current Diagnosis and Treatment in Orthopedics.* 5th ed. New York, NY: McGraw-Hill; 2014.

Tartaglione JP, Rosenbaum AJ, Abousayed M, et al: Classifications in brief: Lauge-Hansen classification of ankle fractures. *Clin Orthop Relat Res.* 2015;473(10):3323-3328.

Teefey SA, Hasan SA, Middleton WD, et al: Ultrasonography of the rotator cuff. A comparison of ultrasonographic and arthroscopic findings in one hundred consecutive cases. *J Bone Joint Surg Am.* 2000;82(4):498-504.

Wiegand L, Bernstein J, Ahn J: Fractures in brief: olecranon fractures. *Clin Orthop Relat Res.* 2012;470(12):3637-3641.

MULTIPLE CHOICE QUESTIONS

1. Open fractures, defined as a break in the bone with violation of the skin and soft tissues requires the following management

   A. Splinting
   B. Bedside irrigation and splinting
   C. Formal irrigation and debridement in the operating room with stabilization of fracture and antibiotics
   D. VAC dressing
   E. Plastic surgery consultation

2. A 57-year-old woman is involved in a motor vehicle collision. She is transferred to the Emergency Department where radiographs confirm a closed pelvic fracture with symphyseal widening. She becomes acutely hypotensive in the resuscitation bay. The next important step in her treatment is

   A. Immediate transfusion
   B. Exploratory laparotomy
   C. Move blood pressure cuff to the leg
   D. Apply sheet or pelvic binder around the patient
   E. Obtain more x-rays

3. A 23-year-old man presents to the Emergency Room with an acute injury to his left knee sustained playing football. He is unable to weight bear and on exam demonstrates anterior dislocation of the tibia. The next steps in management include

   A. Emergent reduction, splinting, vascular studies, and neurologic exam
   B. Knee immobilizer and outpatient follow-up
   C. Urgent MRI
   D. Transport to operating room for open reduction of the knee
   E. Reduction and casting

4. A 3-year-old child fell from the monkey bars sustaining an acute injury to her left elbow. She demonstrates good strength with the exception of the anterior interosseous nerve. Radiographs confirm a displaced supracondylar humerus fracture. Parents are informed

   A. Splint will be applied and patient can return for outpatient follow-up.
   B. Patient will require closed reduction and pinning of the elbow in the operating room. The AIN will require exploration and repair.
   C. Patient will require closed reduction and pinning of the elbow in the operating room. The AIN will recover in most cases with observation over the next 3-6 months.
   D. Patient can be observed for recovery of nerve overnight in the emergency room.
   E. AIN is rarely injured with this type of fracture.

Plastic & Reconstructive Surgery

Erin M. Taylor, MD
Yoon S. Chun, MD

43

INTRODUCTION

Plastic surgery is a diverse, comprehensive surgical field that involves treatment of almost all aspects of the human body from the newborn to elderly. The field includes reconstructive surgery, aesthetic surgery, microsurgery, craniofacial surgery, and hand surgery. Plastic surgery tackles a variety of surgical problems through problem solving and use of a comprehensive surgical toolbox that continually expands.

Plastic surgeons routinely collaborate with other subspecialties given the broad range of plastic surgery reconstructive techniques. Reconstruction of wounds after oncologic resection, radiation, trauma, wound breakdown, or infectious processes often requires assistance with plastic surgery reconstruction. For example, neurosurgery collaborates with plastic surgery in cranioplasty, craniosynostosis, spinal surgery requiring flap coverage, and oncologic resection of brain tumors in radiated fields requiring complex reconstruction. Orthopedic surgery frequently collaborates with plastic surgery in the setting of traumatic injuries with soft tissue damage, prosthetic joint complications requiring soft tissue and bone reconstruction, and oncologic excision of sarcoma, chordoma, or bone tumors requiring reconstruction. General surgery collaborates with plastic surgery for abdominal wall reconstruction, ventral hernia repair, reconstruction after abdominoperineal resection, oncologic reconstruction such as breast reconstruction after mastectomy, necrotizing soft tissue infections requiring subsequent soft tissue coverage, or traumatic degloving injuries requiring coverage of vital structures. Cardiac surgery collaborates with plastic surgery for sternal nonunion requiring sternal fixation and sternal wounds requiring flap coverage. Thoracic surgery collaborates with plastic surgery in chest wall reconstruction after oncologic resection, reconstruction after lobectomy or pneumonectomy with filling of pleural cavity with flaps, and soft tissue coverage after infection with empyema or sternum or rib osteomyelitis. Pediatric surgery

collaborates with plastic surgery for esophageal reconstruction in tracheoesophageal fistula with supercharged jejunal flaps, hypospadias repair, and myelomeningocele repair. Urology collaborates with plastic surgery in phalloplasty, urethroplasty, and penile transplant. Gynecology collaborates with plastic surgery in perineal reconstruction after oncologic resection of the vagina, vulva, uterus, and pelvic floor.

Given the field encompasses most of the human body, knowledge of anatomy is essential in plastic surgery. Detailed knowledge of anatomy of vessels, nerves, muscles, tendons, bone, and perforator zones of soft tissue allows for the complex reconstruction, aesthetic procedures, craniofacial surgery, and hand surgery. The hand is one of the most anatomically intricate areas of the body, with complex relationships that allow for the unique and precise mechanics of hand function. Microsurgery requires comprehensive knowledge of vascular and microvascular anatomy. Angiosomes, a concept first described by Dr. Ian Taylor in 1987, are vascular regions perfused by a single artery. The more recently described perforator zones are regions perfused by small branches, or perforators, of larger vessels. Both angiosomes and perforator zones are critical to consider when designing a flap for reconstruction to ensure flap perfusion and survival.

Innovation has long been an essential component of plastic surgery. Dr. Joseph Murray, a plastic surgeon, was instrumental to the field of transplant surgery, for both his clinical work in transplantation and basic science research in immunology. In 1954, Dr. Murray performed the first successful renal transplant between identical twins, for which he was awarded the Nobel Prize in Physiology or Medicine in 1990. The field of microsurgery was developed in the 1960s, first with the use of a modified microscope to perform the first vascular anastomosis on dogs and rabbits. In 1962, Drs. Malt and McKhann performed the first forearm replantation. In 1964, Dr. Nakayama and his team performed the first free flap with intestinal segments for cervical esophageal reconstruction. The first large-volume microvascular tissue transfer was performed by Drs. Bunke and Mclean who transferred an omental free flap for reconstruction of a cranial defect in 1971, followed soon after by Drs. Daniel and Taylor, who performed the first free groin flap for lower extremity reconstruction. Microsurgical replantation of the upper extremity, lower extremity, scalp, lip, penis, and soft tissue has been made possible with these techniques. Microsurgery has further advanced with transfer of perforator flaps, perforator-to-perforator microvascular transfer, and supermicrosurgery, which involves anastomosis of vessels < 0.3 mm in diameter. Lymphatic surgery is an emerging field in microsurgery and supermicrosurgery with the goal to prevent or treat lymphedema with lymphatic to venous transfer or free tissue transfer of lymph nodes to a region of lymphedema.

Transplantation of vascular composite allografts (VCAs) has been made possible by improvements in not only microvascular instruments and techniques but also immunologic therapy. VCAs include partial or full face transplantation, scalp and cranium transplantation, abdominal wall with rib transplantation, hand and upper extremity transplantation, and more recently, penile transplantation. Any VCA that includes skin is extremely immunoreactive and would not have been possible without modern immunologic therapy.

Tissue bioengineering research has been closely tied to the field of plastic surgery, as it provides options for reconstruction of skin, soft tissue, vasculature, nerve, cartilage, and bone. Burn reconstruction often requires skin substitutes, such as cultured epithelial autografts, when limited donor skin is available for autograft. Scaffolds have been developed for reconstruction of cartilaginous structures, such as trachea or ear cartilage. More recent research has focused on the creation of composite grafts and flaps for use in complex reconstruction.

Plastic surgery is an exciting field that involves a broad range of surgical procedures, treatment of diverse clinical problems, collaboration with surgeons from many other subspecialties, detailed knowledge of anatomy, high technical skill, and constant advancement through innovation.

Elliott RM, Tintle SM, Levin LS: Upper extremity transplantation: current concepts and challenges in an emerging field. *Curr Rev Musculoskelet Med.* 2014;7(1):83-88.

Koshima I, Yamamoto T, Narushima M, et al: Perforator flaps and supermicrosurgery. *Clin Plast Surg.* 2010;37(4):683-689, vii-iii.

Pomahac B, Pribaz JJ, Bueno EM, et al: Novel surgical technique for full face transplantation. *Plast Reconstr Surg.* 2012;130(3):549-555.

I. WOUND HEALING AND CLOSURE

Multiple factors must be considered when evaluating a wound and determining the best treatment approach to achieve wound healing. Patient comorbidities, smoking status, nutritional status, wound bed tissue quality, bacterial or fungal colonization of wound, presence of vital structures within wound bed, and size and location of the wound are all essential to consider.

Wounds may heal by primary, secondary, or tertiary or delayed primary closure. Primary closure includes closure of the wound by reapproximation of the wound edges; secondary closure includes allowing a wound to heal by contraction and epithelialization over time; and tertiary, or delayed primary, closure includes sharp debridement and reapproximation of the wound edges as performed in primary closure.

WOUND HEALING

▶ Phases of Wound Healing

Wound healing occurs in four phases: hemostasis, inflammatory, proliferative, and remodeling. Tissue insult leads to vascular endothelial injury with exposure of the basal lamina and release of blood into surrounding soft tissue. This leads to initiation of hemostasis with platelet activation and vasoconstriction of the damaged vessel. Clot forms with platelet activation and fibrin through the coagulation cascade. Growth factors assist in extracellular matrix deposition (transforming growth factor beta [TGF-β]), chemotaxis (platelet-derived growth factor), epithelialization (fibroblast growth factor [FGF]; epidermal growth factor [EGF]), and angiogenesis (vascular endothelial growth factor [VEGF]).

The inflammatory phase occurs within the first 1-2 days and continues through day 6. Neutrophils are the first inflammatory cells to arrive to the wound in the first 24-48 hours, which are closely followed by monocytes after the first 48 hours. The monocytes are activated into macrophages, which are essential in the inflammatory phase of wound healing due to their ability to debride tissue and contribute cytokines and growth factors essential in fibroblast proliferation and angiogenesis. Furthermore, macrophages are believed to induce apoptosis of neutrophils, which is important in prevention of prolongation of inflammation and chronic wounds. Lymphocytes, which arrive in wounds on days 5-7, affect collagenase activity and assist in tissue remodeling.

The proliferative phase, which begins during week 1 and lasts through week 3, includes epithelialization, angiogenesis, collagen formation, and granulation tissue development. Epithelialization occurs through keratinocyte activity along wound edges and in dermal appendages. The growth factors EGF, FGF, and TGF-β cause mobilization, migration, mitotic division, and differentiation of epithelial cells. Angiogenesis, stimulated by VEGF, leads to development of endothelial vessel walls. Fibroblasts produce collagen through a high metabolic process requiring sufficient oxygen for hydroxylation of the amino acids to form mature collagen. Fibroblasts also organize the extracellular matrix and form elastin, which helps create granulation tissue.

The final phase of wound healing, maturation and remodeling, occurs at 3-4 weeks, when the rates of collagen breakdown and formation are equivalent. Stronger cross-linking in the tissue lattice structure leads to more organized collagen. Type III collagen, which is composed of approximately 30% of granulation tissue, is replaced by type I collagen, resulting in a more normal 4:1 ratio of type I to type III collagen composition. The tensile strength of a healing wound is greatest at 60 days and achieves 80% of the original pre–tissue injury strength.

Janis JE, Harrison B: Wound Healing: Part I. Basic Science. *Plast Reconstr Surg.* 2016;138(3 Suppl):9S-17S.

RECONSTRUCTION AND CLOSURE OF WOUNDS

There are many types of wounds and factors to consider when deciding on the optimal reconstruction procedure to achieve definitive coverage and closure. Skin type and color, glandular association, and hair-bearing characteristics must be considered. Avascular wound beds, such as exposed bone, cartilage, or tendon, will not accept skin grafts unless viable periosteum, perichondrium, or paratenon is present. Other areas with poor vascularity are joint capsules, radiation-damaged tissue, and heavily scarred tissue. Exposed or implanted alloplastic material cannot be used as a graft bed. Such areas must be covered with tissue that is attached to its own blood supply. Skin flaps can be considered but are sometimes inadequate because their blood supply is tenuous. Furthermore, the subcutaneous fat layer has even less reliable vascularity and may not adhere to the underlying avascular surface. Muscle or musculocutaneous flaps are generally required for successful reconstruction coverage of avascular areas.

The pros and cons of all reconstructive options must be carefully weighed prior to finalizing the reconstructive decision. The concept of the "reconstructive ladder" describes the treatment steps to consider in order of complexity: wound closure by secondary intention, primary intention, skin graft, local tissue rearrangement, local or regional flap, and free flap reconstruction. The ladder has transitioned to a "reconstructive elevator" in recent years of reconstructive surgery, with more complex reconstructive options higher on the ladder chosen over those lower on the ladder due to superior functional and aesthetic outcomes in some clinical settings. Additional treatment modalities, such as negative-pressure wound therapy, do not fit in any one particular location on the reconstructive ladder but can be used as a useful adjunct to other reconstructive options.

Tissue coverage may require more bulk in areas with significant dead space or vulnerable to significant pressure, such as bony surfaces and prominences, weight-bearing surfaces, densely scarred areas, and areas of potential future breakdown secondary to pressure. Skin grafts may not be of adequate thickness for successful long-term coverage even though they initially may survive and cover the wound. Musculocutaneous flaps provide adequate bulk in these cases but may also atrophy over time. Bulkiness may be undesirable in areas such as the scalp, face, neck, or hand, which may require secondary debulking. Fasciocutaneous flaps may provide thin or thick soft tissue coverage depending on the type of flap, donor site, and patient body habitus. Additionally, fasciocutaneous flaps can be innervated to provide sensory feedback of the skin resurfacing the wound.

Contraction begins during the proliferative phase of healing and continues to a large degree in wounds covered only by split-thickness skin grafts. The grafted area may shrink by up to 50% of its original size, and both the graft and surrounding tissue may become distorted. Splinting of the area for 10 days or longer may favorably alter contraction. Full-thickness skin grafts rich in dermis, attached to a fresh wound bed, will considerably reduce contraction, and skin flaps will eliminate it altogether. In an orifice or tubular passageway, such as the nasal airway, pharynx, esophagus, or vagina, absence of contraction is critical.

The effects of atrophy and gravity should also be considered when the technique of coverage is chosen. A denervated muscle will atrophy up to 60% of its regular size. The muscle tissue in a musculocutaneous flap will atrophy even when the nerve to the muscle is preserved in the pedicle, because the muscle's functional tension is generally not restored. Gravity will cause sagging of any tissue that does not have enough plasticity or muscle dynamics to counteract gravitational pull.

▶ Primary Closure

The ideal wound closure is primary approximation of the skin and subcutaneous tissues immediately adjacent to the wound defect, producing a fine-line scar and the optimal aesthetic result in skin texture, thickness, and color match.

All excisions and wound closures should be planned with this goal in mind. However, primary closure is limited by the size of the defect, and large lesions may not be excised and closed primarily. With invasive cancers, such as sarcomas, the primary treatment goal is achieving adequate en bloc resection, with the type of wound closure being of secondary importance.

In most cases, minimal scars can be achieved only if the line or lines of incision are placed in, or parallel to, the relaxed skin tension lines. These lines lie perpendicular to the underlying muscles. On the face, they are commonly seen as wrinkles or lines of facial expression that become more pronounced with age as a result of repeated muscle contraction over time. On the neck, trunk, and extremities, the lines of minimal tension are most noticeable as horizontal lines of skin relaxation on the anterior and posterior aspects of areas of flexion and extension. Langer lines, which were originally determined by cadaver study, probably show the direction of fibrous tissue bundles in the skin and are no longer considered accurate landmarks for placing skin incisions.

If the lines of expression cannot be followed, the line of incision should attempt to be placed at the junction of unlike tissues such as the hairline of the scalp and the forehead, the eyebrow and the forehead, the mucosal and skin junction of the lips, or the areolar and skin margins of the breast. Scars will be partially hidden if incisions are placed in inconspicuous areas such as the crease of the nasal ala and cheek, the auricular-mastoid sulcus, or the submandibular-neck junction. Lines of incision should never purposely cross flexor surfaces such as the neck, axilla, antecubital fossa, or popliteal space or the palmar skin creases of the fingers and hand, because of the risk of contracture formation. A transverse oblique or S incision should be incorporated when crossing these sites.

If a lesion is to be excised, an elliptic incision placed parallel to the relaxed skin tension lines will provide the best cosmetic result if the amount of tissue to be excised does not preclude primary closure (Figure 43–1). If the ellipse is too broad or short, a protrusion of skin, commonly called a "dog-ear," will occur at each pole of the wound closure. This is most easily corrected by excising the dog-ear as a small ellipse. A dog-ear may also be present if one side of the ellipse is longer than the other. In this case, it may be easier to excise a small triangle of skin and subcutaneous tissue from the longer side (Figure 43–2).

Secondary Closure

Closure by secondary intention occurs when a wound heals by contraction and epithelialization over time, generally in conjunction with local wound care. Wound contraction occurs due to myofibroblasts, which express alpha-smooth muscle actin that allows the myofibroblast cells to contract.

▲ **Figure 43–1.** Sites of elliptic incisions corresponding to wrinkle lines on the face.

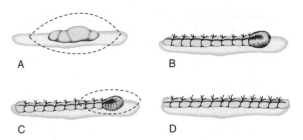

▲ **Figure 43–2.** Correction of a dog-ear.

Epithelialization occurs from wound edges and dermal appendages, such as sweat glands, sebaceous glands, and hair follicles.

Tertiary (Delayed Primary) Closure

Closure by tertiary intention, or delayed primary intention, occurs when a chronic wound is transformed into an acute wound and closed through surgical approximation. For example, a wound is left open due to high bacterial contamination and treated with wet-to-dry dressings for a period of time. Once the wound has been cleared of its high bacterial load and the wound has a clean granulating base, it can be left to heal by secondary intention through contraction, or it can be treated through conversion to an acute wound and primary closure (ie, healing by tertiary intention), which can accelerate the time to a closed wound. Importantly, wounds should not be converted to acute wounds with primary closure if they are infected, heavily colonized with bacteria, perpetuated by a chronic deeper draining sinus, or will be under significant tension with a risk of dehiscence. If significant tension is anticipated following excision and primary closure, other reconstructive options from the reconstructive ladder should be considered, including skin graft or flap coverage.

Vacuum-Assisted Closure

Negative-pressure wound therapy, or vacuum-assisted closure (VAC) therapy, assists wound healing through application of differential suction to wound beds. This technique entails the application of a sealed sponge-like dressing connected to a vacuum pump device that removes excess fluid and exudates. The controlled application of negative pressure to the local wound environment has a positive effect on healing and increased revascularization. It has become a popular method of preparing a wound for definitive closure and can be used until the wound is small enough to heal by secondary intention. VAC therapy has been shown to increase wound bed vascularity and cell proliferation, both of which are essential in wound healing. Newer VAC therapy models include an option for infusion and soaking of wounds with normal saline between negative-pressure therapy cycles, which allows for periodic irrigation of wounds in an effort to provide a moist environment and decrease bacterial colonization.

Contraindications to wound VAC therapy include untreated soft tissue infection or osteomyelitis, exposure of critical structures (blood vessels, anastomoses, organs, nerves), and malignancy.

Liu DS, Sofiadellis F, Ashton M, et al: Early soft tissue coverage and negative pressure wound therapy optimises patient outcomes in lower limb trauma. *Injury.* 2012;43(6):772-778.
Scherer SS, Pietramaggiori G, Mathews JC, et al: The mechanism of action of the vacuum-assisted closure device. *Plast Reconstr Surg.* 2008;122(3):786-797.

CHALLENGING WOUNDS

Risk factors for poor wound healing include infection, pressure, smoking, poor nutrition, steroids, immune compromise, diabetes, peripheral vascular disease, and radiation.

Infected Wounds

Bacteria thwart wound healing at almost every stage: bacteria affect platelets, thus impairing coagulation during hemostasis; bacterial virulence factors decrease the functioning of leukocytes, which leads to prolongation of the inflammatory phase; and bacteria can both increase the amount of granulation tissue formed and decrease the ability of a wound to mature with organized collagen. A wound is classified as infected if it has greater than 10^5 colony-forming bacteria per gram of tissue.

Smoking

Tobacco products and resulting smoke have multiple ingredients and by-products that affect wound healing, including nicotine, carbon monoxide, and hydrogen cyanide. Nicotine causes vasoconstriction and thrombosis, both of which lead to decreased oxygen and nutrient delivery to wounds, as well as decreased activation of macrophages and fibroblasts. Carbon monoxide decreases oxygen transport to the wound through binding to hemoglobin as its binding affinity is 200-fold greater than oxygen. Smoking and nicotine cessation is essential to heal wounds and prevent wound breakdown with surgical procedures. Recommendations regarding the duration of smoking cessation pre- and postoperatively vary, but typically, patients should be free of smoking and nicotine replacement products for at least 4 weeks preoperatively and as long as possible postoperatively for both wound healing and systemic health benefits.

Poor Nutrition

Poor nutrition, which can be caused by poor nutrient intake or malabsorption, leads to decreased ability to heal wounds. Amino acids, and thus protein, are essential components to wound healing. Protein deficiency leads to delayed wound healing and increased risk of dehiscence after wound closure. Carbohydrates and glucose are essential in wound healing as metabolic requirement significantly increases, with an approximate 900 kcal required for every 3 cm² by 1 mm deep wound to heal.

Vitamins are also essential in the formation of collagen. Vitamin C helps to catalyze collagen formation by acting as a cosubstrate for hydroxylase. Deficiency in vitamin C leads to delayed wound healing and, in severe cases, scurvy. In the setting of steroid use, vitamin A increases epithelialization and collagen synthesis.

Immune Compromise

Immune compromise, which may be caused by comorbidities such as diabetes, systemic infectious such as HIV, and medical therapies such as steroids or chemotherapy, leads to decreased ability to mount the inflammatory phase of wound healing and subsequent formation of a strong collagen matrix. Immunocompromised patients are also at greater risk for developing wound infections from inability to clear bacteria from a contaminated wound, which also prevents wound healing.

Steroids in particular have negative impact on multiple areas of the wound-healing process, including inhibition of inflammation, epithelialization, and collagen production. Vitamin A is often supplemented in patients on steroids to help promote wound healing because vitamin A increases epithelialization and formation of collagen.

Chemotherapy has damaging effects on the wound-healing process depending on the mechanism of action of the drug, such as targeting cell division or DNA, RNA, or protein synthesis.

Diabetic Wounds

Wounds that develop in the diabetic patient are often due to a combination of microvascular disease, hyperglycemia, neuropathy, and immune compromise. Diabetics develop microvascular disease that impairs local oxygen transport to the wound, as well as macrovascular disease, which further contributes to a hypoxic environment. Poor glucose control leads to dysfunction of proteins and enzymes, thus affecting wound healing.

Peripheral Vascular Disease Wounds

Wounds that develop from peripheral vascular disease are from macrovascular disease, leading to ischemia and subsequent hypoxia of the wound. The increased metabolic activity of the wound bed requires appropriate oxygen delivery, which is impaired in patients with macrovascular disease. Revascularization, performed by endovascular or open bypass procedures, may reestablish appropriate blood flow and thus oxygen and nutrient delivery to the wound. If feasible, revascularization procedures should be performed in conjunction with local wound care and prior to any reconstructive procedures for limb salvage to ensure wounds have the greatest chance of healing.

Radiated Wounds

Radiation leads to damage to DNA through electron excitement, leading to breaks in the double helix crosslinking, DNA double-strand, or DNA single-strand structures. Resulting free radicals further cause harm to protein and cell membranes. In the acute setting, radiation causes thrombosis, edema, and impairment in fibroblast activity, leading to delayed wound healing, decreased strength of wound repair, and increased risk of infection. Tissue in radiated beds develops chronic long-term fibrosis, poor tissue quality, and microvascular disease.

Pressure Sores

Pressure sores, also less precisely called bedsores or decubitus ulcers, generally occur in patients who are bedridden and unable or unwilling to change position; patients who cannot change position because of a cast or appliance; and patients who have no sensation in an area that is not moved even though they may be ambulatory. The underlying cause of sores in these patients is ischemic necrosis resulting from prolonged pressure against the soft tissue overlying bone. There is also some evidence that local factors in denervated skin predispose to pressure breakdown because there is atrophy of the skin and subcutaneous tissue.

Absence of normal protective reflexes must be compensated for. Prevention is clearly the best treatment for pressure sores. Casts and appliances must be well padded, and points of pressure or pain should be relieved. Bedridden patients must be turned to a new position at least every 2 hours. Water and air mattresses, sheepskin pads, and foam cushions may help relieve pressure but are not substitutes for frequent turning. The introduction of the flotation bed system, which distributes pressure uniformly over a large surface area, has greatly aided in the management of these patients. The pressure on the skin at any time is less than the capillary filling pressure, avoiding many ischemic problems. Paraplegics should not sit in one position for more than 2 hours. Careful daily examination should be made for erythema, the earliest sign of ischemic injury. Erythematous areas should be freed from all pressure. Electrical stimulations, biomaterials, and growth factors are additional modalities available to expedite wound repair, but the results are variable.

Once pressure necrosis is established, it is important to determine whether underlying tissues such as fat and muscle are affected, since they are much more likely than skin to become necrotic. A small skin ulcer may be the manifestation of a much larger area of destruction below. If the area is not too extensive and if infection and abscess due to external or hematogenous bacteria are not present, necrotic tissue may be replaced by scar tissue. Continued pressure

will not only prevent scar tissue from forming, but will also extend the injury. A surface eschar or skin may cover a significant abscess and must be debrided to treat the underlying infection.

If the pressure sore is small and noninfected, application of drying agents to the wound and removal of all pressure to the area may permit slow healing by secondary intention. Wounds extending down to bone rarely heal without surgery. Infected wounds must be debrided down to clean tissue. The surgical objectives are to debride devitalized tissue, including bone, and to provide healthy, well-vascularized padded tissue as coverage. All of the original tissue that formed the bed of the ulcer must be excised.

Only when the patient's nutritional status and general condition of health are optimal, definitive coverage can be performed. Coverage is usually accomplished with a muscle, musculocutaneous, or, sometimes, an axial flap. Well-vascularized muscle appears to help control established low-grade bacterial contamination. The muscle flaps used for the more common bedsores are as follows: greater trochanter: tensor fasciae lata; ischium: gracilis, gluteus maximus, or hamstrings; and sacrum: gluteus maximus. Occasionally, it is possible to provide sensibility to the area of a pressure sore with an innervated flap from above the level of paraplegia. The most common example is the tensor fasciae latae flap with the contained lateral femoral cutaneous nerve from L4 and L5, which is used to cover an ischial sore. Rarely, an innervated intercostal flap from the abdominal wall may be used to cover an insensible sacrum. Unfortunately, attempts to provide protective sensibility with sensory flaps have not demonstrated good results. The tissue expansion techniques should not be the primary surgery treatment of decubitus ulcers but can be used in difficult cases where available tissue is insufficient to close the wound.

Postoperatively, the donor and recipient areas must be kept free of pressure for 2-3 weeks to allow for complete healing. This puts significant demands on other areas of the body that may be equally at risk or may already have areas of breakdown. The use of the air-fluidized bed has greatly aided in such situations.

Unfortunately, recurrence of pressure sores is the most common long-term problem despite surgical reconstruction if the underlying etiology is not treatable. Prevention of sores is even more important for these patients.

HYPERTROPHIC SCARS AND KELOIDS

In response to any injury severe enough to break the continuity of the skin or produce necrosis, the skin heals with scar formation. Under ideal circumstances, a fine, flat hairline scar will result. However, hypertrophy may occur, causing the scar to become raised and thickened, or a keloid may form. A keloid is a true tumor arising from the connective tissue elements of the dermis. By definition, keloids grow

▲ **Figure 43–3.** Keloid scar.

beyond the margins of the original injury or scar; in some instances, they may grow to enormous size (Figure 43–3).

Hypertrophic scars and keloids are distinct entities, and the clinical course and prognosis are quite different in each case. The overreactive process that results in thickening of the hypertrophic scar ceases within a few weeks, and in most cases, some degree of maturation occurs and gradual improvement takes place.

In the case of keloids, the overreactive proliferation of fibroblasts continues for weeks or months. By the time it ceases, an actual tumor is present that typically extends well beyond the limits of the original scar, involves the surrounding skin, and may become quite large. Maturation with spontaneous improvement does not usually occur.

More recent research has shown differences on a biochemical level that can be quite complex. Fibroblasts in both disorders display an increase in procollagen. This is compensated for in hypertrophic scars but not in keloids. This results in an increased ratio of type I to type III collagen in keloids.

▶ **Treatment**

The most frustrating aspect of hypertrophic and keloid treatment for both patient and care provider alike is the high incidence of recurrence. Much work has gone into developing techniques to avoid and treat these scar problems, with mixed results. As this has become more evident, providers have become more specialized and aggressive with treatment options. More recent studies looking at treatments such as interferon, 5-flurouracil injections, and bleomycin injections have shown some promise. But no therapy has been shown to conclusively treat these problems.

Because nearly all hypertrophic scars undergo some degree of spontaneous improvement, they do not require treatment in the early phases. If the scar is still hypertrophic after 6 months, surgical excision and primary closure of the wound may be indicated, but recurrence is between 45% and 100% if no other treatments are provided. Improvement may be expected when the hypertrophic scar was originally produced by excessive endothelial and fibroblastic cell proliferation, as is present in open wounds, burns, and infected wounds. However, little or no improvement can be anticipated if the hypertrophic scar followed uncomplicated healing of a simple surgical incision. Improvement of hypertrophic scars across flexion surfaces such as the antecubital fossa or the fingers requires a procedure such as a Z-plasty to change the direction of the scar.

Pressure may help flatten a potentially hypertrophic scar. It is particularly useful for burn scars. A measured elastic garment or face mask is applied to the scarred area and provides continued pressure that causes realignment and remodeling of the collagen bundles. Pressure should be applied early, continuously, and for 6-12 months. Use of intermittent pressure, such as pressure only at night, or pressure applied after the hypertrophic scar is established (6-12 months) is of little value.

Additional methods of decreasing the thickness of hypertrophied scars include silicone sheeting applied early and continuously for weeks or months. Laser therapy, such as carbon dioxide (CO_2), pulse dye, and flash lamps, has been examined with no definitive long-term success noted when used alone. Radiotherapy has a place in scar management, although it is somewhat controversial due to potential carcinogenesis following the procedure.

The first-line treatment for keloids and second-line therapy for intractable hypertrophic scars is still injection of triamcinolone acetonide, 10 mg/mL (Kenalog-10), directly into the lesion. Corticosteroid injection decreases fibroblast proliferation and collagen synthesis and suppresses proinflammatory markers. There is some evidence that keloids may respond better to early treatment rather than to late treatment. Lesions are injected every 3-4 weeks, and treatment should not be carried out longer than 6 months. A general rule of thumb is to inject 10 mg of triamcinolone for each centimeter in length of the scar. The following dosage schedule is used:

Size of Lesion	Dose
1-2 cm^2	20-40 mg
2-6 cm^2	40-80 mg
6-10 cm^2	80-110 mg

For larger lesions, the maximum dose should be 120 mg. The maximum doses for each treatment for children are as follows:

Age	Dose
1-2 years	20 mg
3-5 years	40 mg
6-10 years	80 mg

There is a tendency to inject the drug into the scar too often or in too high a dosage. An additional common mistake is to inject into the subjacent tissue, which may result in excessive atrophy of the skin and subcutaneous tissues surrounding the lesion. Cushing symptoms have also been reported with the overuse of corticosteroids for scar management. Topical corticosteroid therapy is of little or no value for substantial scarring but may have a role with more superficial scarring, such as in the case of dermabrasion.

At present, surgical excision is used only in conjunction with intralesional corticosteroid therapy. Excision is usually confined to the larger lesions in which steroid therapy would exceed safe dosages. The wound is injected at the time of surgery and then postoperatively. Care should be taken so that surgical incisions are not extended into the normal skin around the keloid, since the growth of a new keloid may occur in these scars.

Hayashi T, Furukawa H, Oyama A, et al: A new uniform protocol of combined corticosteroid injections and ointment application reduces recurrence rates after surgical keloid/hypertrophic scar excision. *Dermatol Surg.* 2012;38(6):893-897.

CONTRACTURES

Contraction is a normal process of wound healing. Contracture, on the other hand, is a pathologic end stage related to the process of contraction. Generally, contractures develop when wounds heal with too much scarring and contraction of the scar tissue results in distortion of surrounding tissues. Although scar contractures can occur in any flexible tissue, such as the eyelids or lips, contractures usually occur across areas of flexion, such as the neck, axilla, or antecubital fossa.

The contracted scar brings together the structures on either side of the joint space and prevents active or even passive extension. Exceptions to this pattern of flexion contractures are extension contractures of the toes and metacarpophalangeal joints of the digits. Contraction is thought to occur via smooth muscle elements in myofibroblasts. In one vertical abdominal scar, there may be an area of normal scar formation and an area of hypertrophic scar formation with visible contracture. Contracture can occur in response to the presence of foreign material such as breast implants. Myofibroblasts are thought to play an important role, but the actual cause is not known. Furthermore, subacute infections with bacteria, such as *Staphylococcus epidermidis*, create a biofilm and may contribute to implant contracture and complications.

The best treatment of contractures is prevention. Incisions should not be made at right angles to flexion creases or should be reoriented with Z-plasty. Wounds in areas of flexion can be covered with flaps or grafted early with thick split-thickness or full-thickness grafts to stop the process of contraction. Such wounds should also be splinted in a position of extension during healing and for 2-3 weeks after

healing is complete. Physical therapy and occupational therapy can also be helpful.

Once a contracture is established, stretching and massage are rarely beneficial. Narrow bands of contracture may be excised and released with one or more Z-plasties. Larger areas must be incised from the medial to the lateral axis across the flexion surface and completely opened up to full extension. The resulting defect can be extensive and must be resurfaced with a skin flap or skin graft. In recurrent contractures, a local or free flap may be helpful. If a skin graft is used, the area must be splinted in extension for approximately 2 weeks after the graft has healed. Less aggressive surgery is likely to result in recurrence.

SUTURE PRINCIPLES

Suture technique in primary closure is important but will not compensate for poorly planned flaps, excessive tension across the incision, traumatized skin edges, bleeding, or other problems due to poor reconstructive design. Sometimes even a skillfully executed closure may result in an unsightly scar because of healing problems beyond the control of the surgeon.

The goal of closure is level apposition of dermal and epithelial edges with minimal or no tension across the incision and no strangulation of tissue between sutures. This is usually accomplished by placement of a layer of interrupted or running absorbable sutures in the superficial fascia and subdermal level at the base of the dermis (Figure 43–4). This suture prevents tension from forming in the upper dermis and epithelium and also causes the surface planes to be level. The epithelial edges can then be opposed with interrupted or running monofilament sutures of absorbable or permanent material. The absorbable suture is placed in the subcuticular or intradermal plane and is left in place. The permanent sutures are removed quickly according to the region of the body, for instance within 5 days in the face, so the suture tracks can be avoided. Sterile adhesive tape (Steri-Strips) placed across the incision will also prevent surface marks and can be used either primarily or after surface sutures have been removed. Taping will not correct errors in suturing that have resulted in uneven edges or tension across the incision. Tape burns may occur if there is excessive tension or swelling around the incision.

The size and even the type of suture material are less important than careful suture placement and observance of previously mentioned factors. Almost any suture properly placed and removed early enough will provide closure without leaving suture marks. The use of monofilament nylon or polypropylene suture material is advised because they create less reaction than gut sutures. Running subcuticular, pullout-type monofilament sutures may be left in for up to 3 weeks without causing reactions. Even buried nylon sutures are well tolerated and generally cause fewer problems than braided or absorbable sutures.

Epidermis
Dermis
Subcutaneous fat
Fascia

A. The strength of the closure lies in the dermis. Occasionally, the subcutaneous fat is incorporated to obliterate dead space.

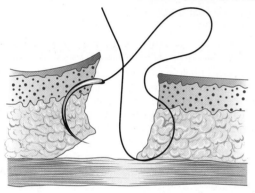

B. The suture is placed so that the knot will lie in the deepest part of the wound. Take care to avoid incorporating the epidermis with this suture, since epithelial cysts will form and result in suture extrusion.

C. The dermal suture is tied just tightly enough to approximate the wound margins. Synthetic absorbable sutures are most commonly used for closure of the dermis.

D. After the dermis is approximated, a fine "epidermal" suture is placed to align the wound edges. This suture adds little to the tensile strength of the wound closure.

E. The epidermal suture is tied just tightly enough to approximate the epidermal edges of the wound. Since the strength of this closure lies in the dermis, the epidermal suture can be removed after 2-3 days. Skin tapes are often used to support the wound for an additional 7-10 days.

▲ **Figure 43–4.** Layered cutaneous closure. (Reproduced with permission from Saunders CE, Ho MT: *Current Emergency Diagnosis & Treatment*, 4th ed. New York, NY: McGraw-Hill Education; 1992.)

An alternative to sutures is the use of skin adhesives such as 2-octylcyanoacrylate (Dermabond). These adhesive glues work well in small areas without much tension or shearing. Some advocate for use in children with superficial lacerations after thorough washout because it avoids the need for sutures, sedation, and suture removal. Further studies are needed to evaluate its wider applicability.

Closure technique is as important as elevation and transposition technique. Flaps should not be allowed to dry out. The wound bed should be irrigated. Closed-system, nonreactive suction drains are routinely used in both the wound bed and the donor defect for most flaps of any significant size. Suction evacuates blood or serum that may accumulate and keeps the flap firmly pressed against the wound bed. External pressure is both ineffective and detrimental for these purposes. Sutures should accurately and completely appose skin edges without strangulating the epithelium, particularly on the flap side, to prevent strangulation and necrosis. Dressings should not cause pressure or constriction. Emollient dressings, such as petrolatum gauze, antibiotic ointment, or silver sulfadiazine cream, have been shown to aid in preventing desiccation and subsequent necrosis of areas of marginal vascularity.

▶ Z-Plasty

One of the most useful and commonly used techniques in primary wound closure is the Z-plasty (Figure 43–5). The angles formed by the Z-shaped incision are transposed as shown in order (1) to gain length in the direction of the central limb of the Z or (2) to change the line of direction of the central limb of the Z. Ninety-degree angles would provide the greatest gain in length of the central limb, but smaller angles, such as 60-degree angles, are usually used, because the incision is easier to close and significant gain in length is still achieved (Table 43–1). The Z-plasty is used for scar revision and reorientation of small wound incisions so that the main incision will be in a more ideal location. The lengthening function is used for the release or breakup of scar contractures across flexion creases. Frequently, many small Z-plasties are created in series rather than one large one.

Table 43–1. Z-plasty angle affects length of central limb increase.

Z-Plasty Angle (degrees)	Central Limb Length Increase (%)
45	50
60	75
75	100
90	120

Occasionally, incisions will be placed under excessive vertical tension after the release of an underlying contracture, such as Dupuytren contracture in the hand.

▼ II. GRAFTS AND FLAPS

Flaps bring their own blood supply versus grafts that require reestablishment of a blood supply within the wound bed. Examples of grafts include skin grafts, fat grafts, bone grafts, cartilage grafts, and composite grafts that are composed of multiple tissue types. Graft vessels are too small to anastomose to recipient bed vessels and must first undergo diffusion of oxygen and nutrients by the recipient wound bed and then undergo subsequent revascularization from the wound bed.

Conversely, flaps receive blood supply through a dominant artery and vein(s). Flaps are either pedicled, where the vessels are never disconnected, or free, where the donor vessels are cut and reanastamosed to new donor vessels. Examples of flaps include muscle flaps, fasciocutaneous flaps, and osteocutaneous flaps.

GRAFTS

▶ Skin Grafts

A graft of skin detaches epidermis and varying amounts of dermis from its blood supply in the donor area and is placed in a new bed of blood supply from the base of the wound or

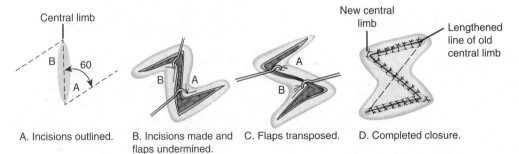

A. Incisions outlined.   B. Incisions made and   C. Flaps transposed.   D. Completed closure.
                             flaps undermined.

▲ **Figure 43–5.** Z-plasty.

recipient area. The way a skin graft survives or "takes" is first by diffusion of nutrient elements from the graft bed, known as **imbibition**. After 48 hours, **inosculation** occurs where the graft vessels make contact with the recipient bed vessels, opening channels for blood flow. The final step of skin graft take is **revascularization**, at which point new vessels form from the recipient bed into the transplanted graft.

Although the technique is relatively simple to perform and generally reliable, definite considerations about the donor area and adequacy of the recipient area are important. Skin grafting is a quick, effective way to cover a wound if vascularity is adequate, infection is not present, and hemostasis is assured. Color match, contour, durability of the graft, and donor morbidity must be considered.

Skin grafts can be either split-thickness or full-thickness grafts. Each type has advantages and disadvantages and is indicated or contraindicated for different kinds of wounds (Figure 43–6).

Split-Thickness Skin Grafts

Thinner split-thickness grafts (10-15/1000th inch) become vascularized more rapidly and survive transplantation more reliably. This is important in grafting on less than ideal recipient sites, such as contaminated wounds, burn surfaces, and poorly vascularized surfaces, such as after radiation. A second advantage is that donor sites heal more rapidly and can be reused within a relatively short time (7-10 days) in critical cases such as major burns.

In general, the disadvantages of thin split-thickness grafts outweigh the advantages. Thin grafts exhibit the highest degree of postgraft contraction, offer the least amount of resistance to surface trauma, and are least like normal skin in texture, suppleness, pore pattern, hair growth, and other characteristics. Thicker split-thickness skin grafts

▲ **Figure 43–6.** Depths of full-thickness and split-thickness grafts.

(> 15/1000th inch) contract less, are more resistant to surface trauma, and are more similar to normal skin than are thin split-thickness grafts. They are also aesthetically more acceptable but not as acceptable as full-thickness grafts.

The disadvantages of thick split-thickness grafts are relatively few but can be significant. They are less easily vascularized than thin grafts and thus result in fewer successful takes when used on less than ideal surfaces. Their donor sites are slower to heal (requiring 10-18 days) and heal with more scarring than donor sites for thin split-thickness grafts.

Meshed grafts are usually thin or intermediate split-thickness grafts that have been rolled under a special cutting machine to create a mesh pattern. Although grafts with these perforations can be expanded from 1.5 to 9 times their original size, expansion to 1.5 times the unmeshed size is the most useful. Meshed grafts are advantageous because they can be placed on an irregular, possibly contaminated wound bed and will usually take. Complications of hemostasis are fewer because blood and serum exude through the mesh pattern. The disadvantage is poor cosmetic appearance following healing, with a meshed appearance. Some advocate for pie crusting of the split-thickness skin graft, which can result in less noticeable pattern and better appearance.

Donor sites for split-thickness grafts heal spontaneously by epithelialization. During this process, epithelial cells from the sweat glands, sebaceous glands, or hair follicles proliferate upward and spread across the wound surface. If these three structures are not present, epithelialization will not occur.

Obtaining Skin Grafts

Instruments used for obtaining skin grafts include razor blades, skin grafting knives (Blair, Ferris Smith, Humby, Goulian), manual drum dermatomes (Padgett, Reese), and electric or air-powered dermatomes (Brown, Padgett, Hall, Zimmer). The electric and air-powered dermatomes are the most widely used because of their reliability and ease of operation. A surgeon, even with only limited experience, can successfully obtain sheets of split-thickness skin grafts using the electric dermatomes.

The Skin Graft Recipient Area

To ensure survival of the graft, there must be (1) adequate vascularity of the recipient bed, (2) complete contact between the graft and the bed, (3) adequate immobilization of the graft-bed unit, and (4) relatively few bacteria in the recipient area.

Because survival of the graft is dependent upon growth of capillary buds into the raw undersurface of the graft, vascularity of the recipient area is of prime importance. Avascular surfaces that will not generally accept free grafts are tissues with severe radiation damage, chronically scarred ulcer beds, bone or cartilage denuded of periosteum or perichondrium, and tendon or nerve without their paratenon or perineurium, respectively. For these surfaces, a bed capable of producing capillary buds must be provided; in some cases, debridement of the recipient site must be debrided. All unhealthy granulation tissue must be removed, because bacterial counts in granulation tissue are often very high. If bone is exposed, it can be decorticated down to healthy cancellous bone with the use of a chisel or power-driven burr, and a meshed split-thickness skin graft can be applied. If an adequate vascular bed cannot be provided or if the presence of essential structures such as tendons or nerves precludes further debridement, skin or muscle flaps are generally indicated for coverage.

Inadequate contact between the graft and the recipient bed can be caused by hematoma, seroma, shearing, or infection. The use of fibrin sealants has more recently been developed to assist with skin graft take. This is sprayed over the wound bed prior to placement of any skin graft. After 60-90 seconds, a fibrin clot develops that better holds the skin graft in place and diminishes potential spaces between the wound bed and the skin graft, which can negatively affect skin graft survival.

After the graft has been applied directly to the prepared recipient surface, it may or may not be sutured in place and may or may not be dressed. Whenever the maximum aesthetic result is desired, the graft should be cut exactly to fit the recipient area and precisely sutured into position without any overlapping of edges. Very large or thick split-thickness grafts and full-thickness grafts will usually not survive without a pressure dressing. In areas such as the forehead, scalp, and extremities, adequate immobilization and pressure can be provided by circular dressings. Tie-over pressure stent dressings are advisable for areas of the face, where constant pressure cannot be provided by simple wraparound dressings; areas where movement cannot be avoided, such as the anterior neck, where swallowing causes constant motion; and areas of irregular contour, such as the axilla. The ends of the fixation sutures are left long and tied over a bolster of gauze fluffs, cotton, a sponge, or other suitable material (Figure 43–7).

Grafts applied to freshly prepared or relatively clean surfaces are generally sutured or stapled into place and dressed with pressure. The use of fibrin sealants has helped minimize the need for these usually uncomfortable bolster techniques. A single layer of damp or other nonadherent fine-mesh gauze is applied directly over the graft. Immediately over this are placed several thicknesses of flat gauze cut in the exact pattern of the graft. On top of these is placed a bulky dry dressing of gauze fluffs, cotton, a sponge, or other material. Pressure is then applied by wraparound dressings, adhesive tape, or a tie-over pressure stent dressing. An alternative dressing is to place a nonadherent fine-mesh gauze atop the graft followed by a negative-pressure dressing. The vacuum-assisted dressings may be useful for irregular contours, such as around digits and webspaces or joint surfaces,

▲ **Figure 43–7.** Tie-over stent dressing.

by maintaining wound-to-graft interface, immobilizing the grafted area, suctioning serosanguineous fluid, and possibly promoting neovascularization. In some cases, it is preferable to leave a skin graft site open with no dressing, such as with skin grafts over free flap reconstruction to allow for monitoring of the underlying muscle flap.

In severely ill patients, such as those with major burns, where time under anesthesia must be kept to a minimum, large sheets of meshed split-thickness skin grafts are rapidly applied but not sutured. Skin staples may be used to fix the graft rapidly. Grafts need not be dressed if the area is small, but if the area is large or circumferential, a dressing should be applied. Meshed grafts should generally be covered for 24-48 hours to prevent dryness, because their dermal barrier has been partly disrupted.

Skin graft dressings may be left undisturbed for 5-7 days after grafting if the grafted wound was free of infection, complete hemostasis was obtained, fluid collection is not expected, and immobilization is adequate. If any one of these conditions is not met, the dressing should be changed within 24-48 hours and the graft inspected. If blood, serum, or purulent fluid collection is present, the collection should be evacuated, usually by making a small incision through the graft with a scalpel blade and applying pressure with cotton-tipped applicators. The pressure dressing is then reapplied and changed daily so that the graft can be examined and fluid expressed as it collects.

▶ The Skin Graft Donor Site

The ideal donor site would provide a graft identical to the skin surrounding the area to be grafted to avoid patch-like appearance. Because skin varies greatly from one area to another as far as color, thickness, hair-bearing qualities, and texture are concerned, the ideal donor site, such as upper eyelid skin to replace skin loss from the opposite upper eyelid, is usually not found. However, there are definite principles that should be followed in choosing the donor area.

Color Match

In general, the best possible color match is obtained when the donor area is located close to the recipient area. Color and texture match in facial grafts will be much better if the grafts are obtained from the preauricular region or above the region of the clavicles. However, the amount of skin obtainable from the preauricular and supraclavicular areas is limited. If larger grafts for the face are required, the immediate subclavicular regions of the thorax will provide a better color match than areas on the lower trunk or the buttocks and thighs. When these more distant regions are used, the grafts will usually be lighter in color than the facial skin in Caucasians. In people with dark skin, hyperpigmentation occurs, producing a graft that is much darker than the surrounding facial skin.

Thickness of the Graft & Donor Site Healing

Donor sites of split-thickness grafts heal by epithelialization from the epithelial elements remaining in the donor bed. The ability of the donor area to heal and the speed with which it does depends on the number of these elements present. Donor areas for very thin grafts will heal in 7-10 days, whereas donor areas for intermediate-thickness grafts may require 10-18 days and those for thick grafts 18-21 days or longer.

Because there is a normal anatomic variation in the thickness of skin, donor sites for thicker grafts must be chosen with the potential for healing in mind and should be limited to regions on the body where the skin is thick. Infants, debilitated adults, and elderly people have thinner skin than healthy younger adults. Grafts that would be split-thickness in the normal adult may be full-thickness in these patients, resulting in a donor site that has been deprived of the epithelial elements necessary for healing.

Management of the Donor Site

The donor site itself can be considered a clean open wound that will heal spontaneously. After initial hemostasis, the wound will continue to ooze serum for 1-4 days, depending on the thickness of the skin taken. The serum should be collected and the wound kept clean so that healing can proceed at a maximal rate. The wound should be cared for as described earlier for clean open wounds in either of two ways.

One technique of donor site management is an open, dry technique. The donor site is dressed with porous, sterile, fine-mesh or nonadherent gauze. After 24 hours, the dry gauze is changed, but the nonadherent gauze is left on the wound and exposed to the air. A scab will form on the gauze and will peel off from the edges as epithelialization is completed underneath. This method has the advantage of simple maintenance once the wound is dry.

The second method that has become more popular is the closed, moist technique. Studies have demonstrated that the rate of epithelialization is enhanced in a moist environment. In contrast to the dry technique, pain can be reduced or virtually eliminated. Moist-to-moist gauze dressings that require frequent wetting have been replaced by newer synthetic materials. A gas-permeable membrane, such as Tegaderm, that sticks to the surrounding skin provides an artificial blister over the wound. Occasionally, there is a break in the protective seal covering leakage of serum collected under the membrane. This increases the risk of infection, especially in a contaminated zone. Newer hygroscopic dressings actually absorb and retain many times their weight in water. They are permeable to oxygen yet impervious to bacteria. Infection is still a concern, however, because of occasional exposure of the wound during healing. Dressings such as Mepilex contain silver-impregnated ions that control bacterial contamination and may hasten healing and reepithelialization while keeping the patient more comfortable. Silver ion is exquisitely antimicrobial and is used for burn dressing care as well as skin graft sites.

Full-Thickness Skin Grafts

Full-thickness skin grafts include the epidermis and all the dermis. They are the most aesthetically desirable of the free grafts because they include the highest number of skin appendage elements, undergo the least amount of contracture, and have a greater ability to withstand trauma. There are several limiting factors in the use of full-thickness grafts. Since no epidermal elements remain to produce epithelialization in the donor site, it must be closed primarily, and a scar will result. The size and number of available donor sites is therefore limited. Furthermore, conditions at the recipient site must be optimal in order for transplantation to be successful.

Areas of thin skin are the best donor sites for full-thickness grafts, such as the eyelids and the skin of the postauricular, supraclavicular, antecubital, inguinal, and genital areas. Submammary and subgluteal skin is thicker but allows camouflage of donor area scars. In grafts thicker than approximately 15/1000th inch, the results of transplantation are less reliable, except on the face or hand, where vascularity is usually superior.

Cultured Epithelial Grafts

Epithelial cells, grown or cultured in a special medium in vitro, will coalesce into thin sheets that can be used to cover full-thickness wounds. Although these cultured epithelial sheets were first used in the treatment of burns, the result was somewhat unsatisfactory because the coverage was very fragile and disfiguring. More recently, success has been obtained with artificial dermis, which when placed in an appropriate bed will revascularize and can then be covered by a very thin split-thickness skin graft, cultured or otherwise. This artificial dermis is increasingly being used in the treatment of burns. Modifications of this concept have also been applied to the care of chronic ulcers, particularly in the leg. The artificial dermis is made out of a collagen matrix and has very low or no antigenicity.

▶ Biologic Skin Substitutes

Research continues to develop bioengineered products that are becoming more common in plastic surgery and general wound management. The source of these products varies (eg, human, porcine, or bovine) and can alter the products' indications and overall ability to assist with wound management. Some of the more common products used are Integra and acellular dermal matrices (ADMs). Integra is a bilayer material consisting of interwoven bovine collagen and shark glycosaminoglycan that mimics the dermal layer of skin. This has made it ideal for reconstruction cases where more than simple skin grafts will suffice, such as over a tendon. ADM is acellular cadaver skin that is chemically prepared. Although initially designed for burn reconstruction, it has been used in wound care and general reconstruction cases from head to toe.

Haddad AG, Giatsidis G, Orgill DP, et al: Skin substitutes and bioscaffolds: temporary and permanent coverage. *Clin Plast Surg.* 2017;44(3):627-634.

▶ Fat Grafts

With the continued interest in lipectomy and the desire for contouring of other body regions, the use of fat grafting has continued to gain popularity. In essence, fat is removed from one part of a patient, prepared via several different techniques, and then placed where further soft tissue enhancement is required. It can be used in the face, the breast, and soft tissue defects in almost all areas of the body. With the discovery of adipose-derived stem cells, this technique will continue to gain popularity. Risks with fat grafting include fat necrosis, oil cysts, and lack of improvement of contour as well as contour defects on the donor site.

▶ Bone Grafts

Bone grafts are often used for bone nonunion, bone malunion, and bone defects of < 6 cm. When defects are greater than 6 cm, free osseous flaps with an established blood supply are required to ensure donor bone survival. Common donor sites for bone grafts include the iliac crest, radius, split calvarium, femur, fibula, and rib.

▶ Cartilage Grafts

Cartilage grafts are used commonly in facial reconstruction, particularly in cosmetic and functional rhinoplasty and ear reconstruction for microtia or anotia. Donor sites include nasal cartilaginous septum, auricular cartilage, and rib cartilage. Cartilage from different donor sites has varying characteristics, pliability, and size. Scoring of the cartilage can cause the cartilage to curl toward the contralateral side. The most common complications of cartilage graft placement are malposition and warping.

▶ Composite Grafts

A composite graft is a free graft that must reestablish its blood supply in the recipient area. It consists of a unit with several tissue planes that may include skin, subcutaneous tissue, cartilage, or other tissue. Dermal fat grafts, hair transplant grafts, and skin and cartilage grafts from the ear fall into this category. Composite grafts must be small or at least relatively thin and will require recipient sites with excellent vascularity to take successfully. These grafts are generally used in the face, such as a conchal bowl auricular composite graft for repair of full-thickness nasal ala or soft triangle defect.

FLAPS

Flap refers to any tissue used for reconstruction or wound closure that retains part or all of its original blood supply after the tissue has been raised and moved to a new location. That part still connected through which the blood supply enters and exits is referred to as the flap base, or pedicle. With local skin flaps, a section of skin and subcutaneous tissue is raised from one site and moved to a nearby area, with the base remaining attached at its original location.

Flaps can be classified according to the pattern of blood supply to the skin into random or axial pattern. Flaps can further be classified according to their tissue content into muscle, musculocutaneous, fasciocutaneous, osteocutaneous, and others.

▶ Random Pattern Flaps

Random pattern flaps consist of skin and subcutaneous tissue cut from any area of the body in any orientation, with no distinct pattern or particular relation to the blood supply of the skin of the flap. Such flaps receive their blood supply from vessels in the subdermal tissue. Although commonly used, this is the least reliable type of flap, and its use should be minimized. With the exception of those designed from facial and scalp skin, the flap ratio of length to width cannot safely exceed 1.5:1. In any reconstructive effort, one should use a flap with known reliability and a predictable blood supply.

Axial Pattern Flaps

The axial pattern flap has a well-defined arteriovenous system running along its long axis. Because of good vascular supply, it can be safely designed comparatively long in relation to width. Foremost among the axial flaps are the deltopectoral flap, based on perforating branches of the internal mammary artery, and forehead flaps, which depending on location can be based on the supraorbital, supratrochlear, or superficial temporal vessels. Additional axial flaps include the groin flap, based on the superficial circumflex iliac artery; dorsalis pedis flap, based on the dorsalis pedis artery; radial forearm flap, based on the radial artery; scapular flap, based on the transverse branch of the circumflex scapular artery; and the lateral upper arm flap, based on the posterior radial collateral artery flap.

Pedicled Flaps

Pedicled flaps remain attached to their original blood supply, whereas free flaps are detached from an artery and vein(s) and reanastamosed to a new blood supply. Pedicled flaps are within the local or regional area of the recipient site, whereas free flaps can be harvested from one region of the body and used for reconstruction in a separate region of the body.

Free Flaps

Free flaps involve tissue transplantation using microvascular surgery. The blood supply from the main axial pedicle of the flap is completely detached and then reattached at a distance to recipient vessels near the recipient site or wound. An operating microscope with two viewing binocular lenses, specialized instruments, and swaged-on needles of 60-80 μm are required for microsurgery; 8-0, 9-0, or 10-0 suture is used to anastamose vessels as small as 0.5 mm in diameter. Supermicrosurgery, an emerging field of anastomosis of vessels even smaller than 0.5 mm, allows for perforator-to-perforator anastomosis and reconstruction of very fine defects, such as the pulp of digits.

Examples of free flaps in current use include axial pattern skin and fasciocutaneous flaps, such as scapular, groin, radial forearm, and anterolateral thigh, which are used when only skin and subcutaneous tissue are needed. Free muscle and musculocutaneous flaps, such as latissimus dorsi, gracilis, and rectus abdominis flaps, are commonly used when the bulk and vascularity of muscle are needed.

The vascular pedicle areas of some flaps contain functional nerves, which can also be reattached using microscopic guidance. Examples are inferior gluteal, thigh, and tensor fascia lata flaps, which contain sensory nerves. Attempts using sensory flaps to provide protective sensation in critical areas such as the feet or the ischium in paraplegic patients have so far been clinically unsuccessful. More encouraging is the work being done to provide sensibility to the floor of the mouth with a sensory innervated radial forearm flap. Motor flaps can restore functions such as forearm flexion or facial expression.

Muscle Flaps

Muscle flaps can include muscle alone or can be combined with a cutaneous component, or "skin paddle," which is perfused by the perforators from the muscle, also known as a musculocutaneous flap (Figure 43–8). The use of the musculocutaneous unit has developed as surgeons have gained more knowledge of the way in which blood is supplied to the skin. The subdermal plexus of vessels from which skin flaps derive their blood supply is augmented or directly supplied in many areas by sizable perforating vessels arising from underlying muscles. Many muscles receive their blood

Epidermis
Dermis
Subdermal plexus
Subcutaneous fat
Fascia
Muscle
Musculocutaneous perforating vessels
Dominant muscular vascular pedicle

▲ Figure 43–8. Musculocutaneous flaps perforating vessels.

supply from a single axial vessel, with only minor contributions from other sources. The skin over these muscles can be completely circumscribed and elevated in continuity with the underlying muscle up to its major vascular pedicle. If the vessels in the pedicle are preserved, the unit can be moved in wide arcs to distant areas of the body while maintaining normal or near-normal blood flow to the muscle as well as the skin island. The donor sites of such flaps can often be closed primarily.

Knowledge of the anatomy of muscles and their nerve and blood supply is necessary for the successful design of musculocutaneous flaps. Although almost any skeletal muscle can be used, muscles with a dominant arterial pedicle and reliable perforating vessels to the skin are most useful.

The most commonly used muscles and musculocutaneous flaps are the latissimus dorsi, pectoralis major, tensor fasciae latae, rectus femoris, rectus abdominis, trapezius, temporalis, serratus anterior, gluteus maximus, gracilis, and gastrocnemius muscles.

▶ Mathes & Nahai Flap Classification

Mathes and Nahai (1981) created a classification system of muscle flaps based on the pattern of vascular anatomy to the flap. Type I has one vascular pedicle; type II has a dominant pedicle and minor pedicle(s); type III has two dominant pedicles; type IV has segmental vascular pedicles; and type V has both a dominant and a segmental blood supply. Muscle flaps have the ability to survive off of one dominant pedicle or the majority of its segmental blood supply (Table 43–2).

Type I includes muscle flaps with one vascular pedicle, such as the tensor fascia lata, gastrocnemius, vastus lateralis, and first dorsal interosseous muscles. The muscle flap survives based on its one vascular pedicle and must not be divided in the case of pedicled flap reconstruction.

Table 43–2. Mathes and Nahai muscle flap classification.

Mathes and Nahai Type	Pedicle Type	Flaps
I	One dominant	Tensor fascia lata, gastrocnemius, vastus lateralis, first dorsal interosseous
II	One dominant and minor	Gracilis, rectus femoris, soleus, trapezius
III	Two dominant	Rectus abdominis, gluteus maximus, serratus, temporalis
IV	Segmental	Sartorius, external oblique, tibialis anterior
V	One dominant and segmental	Latissimus dorsi, pectoralis major, internal oblique

Type II includes muscle flaps with one dominant and minor pedicle(s), such as the gracilis, rectus femoris, soleus, and trapezius. Minor pedicles can be divided in type II muscle flaps, as long as a dominant blood supply remains to perfuse the flap. For example, the gracilis flap, which is a type II muscle, survives off of its dominant pedicle from the medial femoral circumflex system when the more distal minor pedicles are divided. This allows the flap to be rotated proximally into the groin or perineal area for local pedicled flap reconstruction or free flap reconstruction based on a single vascular pedicle.

Type III includes muscle flaps with two dominant vascular pedicles, such as the rectus abdominis, gluteus maximus, serratus, and temporalis muscles. Muscles with two dominant pedicles have the ability to live off of one of the dominant pedicles with the other divided; for example, the rectus abdominis muscle can be perfused by the deep inferior epigastric pedicle once the superior epigastric pedicle is ligated and vice versa, which allows the muscle to be used in reconstruction for both the pelvis, when based on the inferior epigastric vessels, or the chest/breast, when based on the superior epigastric vessels.

Type IV includes muscle flaps with a segmental blood supply, including the sartorius, external oblique, and tibialis anterior muscles. The segmental blood supply includes multiple vessels of near equivalent size, and each supplies a portion of the muscle. Care must be taken not to divide too many of the vessels for transposition to ensure muscle viability.

Type V includes muscle flaps with a dominant vascular pedicle as well as a segmental blood supply, such as the latissimus dorsi, pectoralis major, and internal oblique muscles. The muscle can survive based solely on the dominant blood supply with the segmental blood supply divided; conversely, the muscle also can be perfused by the secondary segmental blood supply if the dominant blood supply is divided. This versatility allows the muscle to be used as a transposition flap with one of two different origins.

Mathes SJ, Nahai F: Classification of the vascular anatomy of muscles: experimental and clinical correlation. *Plast Reconstr Surg.* 1981;67(2):177-187.

▶ Latissimus Dorsi

The latissimus dorsi muscle flap is supplied by the thoracodorsal vessels. This flap has been widely utilized in both one- or two-stage reconstruction of the breast following radical or modified radical mastectomy. The entire latissimus dorsi muscle can be detached from its origin and transposed to the anterior chest. An island of skin can also be included in the center of the muscle to restore the skin lost on the anterior chest wall. The thoracodorsal artery is typically accompanied by a single venae commitans. Pedicle length is typically around 12 cm but can range from 8 to 14 cm. Flap size is typically 20 × 40 cm. Innervation to the flap is from the thoracodorsal nerve. The latissimus flap is useful for regional coverage of defects on the anterior chest, shoulder, head and neck, and axilla as well as restoration of flexion of the elbow. Additionally, it is a popular muscle for free tissue transfer because of its long and relatively large and reliable vascular pedicle.

A partial superior latissimus flap can be harvested, based on the transverse branch of the thoracodorsal artery, where only a superior portion of the muscle is harvested. This leaves the longitudinal branch to the remaining latissimus intact with the longitudinal nerve, preserving an innervated component of the muscle, thus preserving a portion of a functional latissimus muscle on the back.

Pectoralis Major

The pectoralis major musculocutaneous unit obtains its vascular supply from the thoracoacromial axis of the subclavian artery just medial to the medial border of the pectoralis minor. The pectoralis flap derives a dual blood supply from the thoracoacromial artery and the medial intercostal perforators branching from the internal mammary artery. The entire unit may be transposed medially, especially after disinsertion from the humerus, to cover defects of the sternum, neck, and lower face. The flap can be muscle only or include a skin paddle. These flaps are often used for sternal reconstruction or head and neck oncologic reconstruction. A skin island can be outlined low on the chest and made to reach intraoral defects following cancer excision. Although primarily used as a local/regional pedicled flap, the pectoralis flap can also be used as a free flap based on the thoracoacromial artery and venae commitans. Innervation to the flap is provided by the anterior cutaneous branches of intercostal nerves (sensory) and lateral and medial pectoral nerves (motor). The disadvantage of this flap as a free flap is the short pedicle length, at 4.5 cm.

Temporalis

The temporalis muscle extends from the temporal fossa to the coronoid process of the mandible. It is supplied by the deep and superficial temporal systems. It is commonly used to fill orbital defects. However, it can also provide coverage for the neighboring cranial, maxillary, palatal, and pharyngeal regions.

Tensor Fascia Lata

The tensor fascia lata musculofascial unit is supplied by the lateral femoral circumflex artery, a branch of the profunda femoris. It has a wide arc of rotation anteriorly and posteriorly. The flap is elevated with the fascia lata and thus can be used to reconstruct the lower abdominal wall. The flap can be been used to cover defects following excision of osteoradionecrotic ulcers of the pubis or groin. The tensor fascia lata flap is the reconstruction of choice for coverage of greater trochanteric pressure ulcers.

Rectus Femoris

The rectus femoris, a more robust flap than the tensor fascia lata with a shorter arc of rotation, has supplanted the latter for reconstruction of the lower abdominal wall and for coverage to postradiation ulcers in the pubis and groin. It has a dual blood supply: a muscular branch from the profunda femoris and an axial branch from the superficial femoral artery to the overlying skin and fascia.

Rectus Abdominis

The rectus abdominis is supplied by the deep superior epigastric vessels and inferior epigastric vessels that run in the deep surface of the muscle and anastomose with the segmentally arranged intercostal vessels. These vessels send perforating branches throughout the length of the muscle, perforating the anterior rectus sheath and supplying the overlying skin and soft tissue.

The transverse rectus abdominis myocutaneous (TRAM) flap, when based on the superior epigastric vessel and including the infraumbilical skin, has become a workhorse for autologous tissue breast reconstruction. In situations of marked deformity with significant skin deficit, such as a radical mastectomy associated with radiation therapy, reconstruction of the breast can be accomplished reliably with infraumbilical skin and adipose tissue based on both rectus muscles. One of the benefits of the TRAM is improvement in abdominal contour by removing excess tissue while creating a very natural breast reconstruction. Using the inferior epigastric vessels to transport the skin and adipose tissue by means of microvascular surgery has become another popular method of breast reconstruction. This includes free TRAM flap where the rectus abdominis muscle is harvested along with the overlying skin paddle. The deep inferior epigastric perforator (DIEP) flap spares the muscle and transfers only the overlying fat and skin perfused by a main perforator vessel (see section on perforator flaps). In addition, a vertical rectus abdominis myocutaneous (VRAM) flap is a pedicled rectus abdominis muscle flap with a vertically based overlying skin paddle that can be used to cover defects of the abdominal wall, flank, groin, and thigh.

Gluteus Maximus

The gluteus maximus is useful as a muscle or musculocutaneous unit for covering pressure sores or traumatic defects over the sacrum and ischium. The muscle has a double blood supply from the superior and inferior gluteal arteries to the respective halves of the muscle. In ambulatory patients, it is advisable to perform a function-preserving operation by advancing the muscle medially and preserving its insertion laterally.

▶ Gracilis

The gracilis muscle receives its dominant blood supply proximally from the medial femoral circumflex artery. Its arc of rotation makes it an excellent source of coverage for ischial pressure sores and vaginal reconstruction. Other recent uses have included transportation of the muscle alone for repair of a persistent perineal sinus following abdominal-perineal resection. The gracilis muscle can also be used as a free flap by microsurgery for distant reconstruction.

▶ Gastrocnemius

The gastrocnemius musculocutaneous unit is based on either the medial or lateral head of the muscle. Each head is supplied by a sural artery, a branch of the popliteal artery that enters the muscle at its most proximal third near its origin. The flap is most useful to cover defects of the knee and proximal one-third of the anterior tibia. The medial gastrocnemius is preferred for coverage as the medial head of the gastrocnemius provides more bulk than the lateral head of the gastrocnemius. Wound coverage of the middle one-third of the anterior tibia, where the gastrocnemius flap cannot reach, can be accomplished by use of the soleus. Complex bone and soft tissue injuries of the lower one-third of the leg may require reconstruction with free flaps.

▶ Perforator Flaps

A sophisticated variation on the use of the musculocutaneous principle has been the development of perforator flaps. This usually entails taking a branch from the major vascular pedicle that may perforate the muscle to arborize and form a subcutaneous vascular plexus that will supply a considerable amount of overlying skin. Perhaps the greatest benefit from a perforator flap is decreased donor site morbidity. Structures such as the fascia, muscle, and associated nerves may be preserved while allowing the skin to be used for reconstruction. The perforator concept has been applied to further territories of skin over the perforator segments of the gluteal, thoracodorsal, and medial plantar arteries, among others.

The deep inferior epigastric perforator flap, or DIEP flap, is an excellent perforator flap option for autologous tissue breast reconstruction through free tissue transfer. The flap takes skin and fat from the abdomen based on perforating vessels through the rectus muscle, but it spares the rectus abdominus muscle. The DIEP flap uses the same skin territory as the TRAM flap, but the perforating vessels are carefully dissected away from the rectus abdominis muscle, thus sparing the muscle with the goal to prevent excessive abdominal wall weakness at the donor site.

The deep inferior epigastric artery is accompanied by typically paired venae, which join just distal to the external iliac. The pedicle length is very long, as the deep inferior epigastric vessels can be traced to the point of origin from the external iliac. The artery is sizable with a diameter ranging from 2-4 mm. If chosen to be innervated, the flap can have sensory innervation from the intercostal T11 and T12 nerves.

The superficial inferior epigastric artery flap (SIEA flap) can also be used for autologous breast reconstruction when there is a dominant superficial inferior epigastric artery and vein system (SIEA and SIEV), Although the SIEA flap avoids any abdominal wall morbidity, most abdominal flaps are perfused more robustly by the deep system and the SIEA and SIEV typically have short length.

When used for breast reconstruction, the perforator flap vessels are typically anastomosed to the internal mammary artery and vein as recipient vessels, which requires exposure at the third rib space. If the recipient vessels are not large enough, the internal mammary vessels can be traced more proximally to the second rib space.

▶ Fasciocutaneous Flaps

A plexus of vessels is located on top of the muscular fascia and is supplied from vessels that run within the intermuscular septa. These vessels tend to run axially along the fascia, sending perforators to the skin. These flaps spare muscle and are safer than random-patterned flaps given their axial blood supply and more predictable perforator zones. Furthermore, it is possible to make fasciocutaneous or septocutaneous flaps that safely exceed the traditional limits of a 1.5:1 ratio between length and width. Examples of fasciocutaneous flaps are those overlying the gastrocnemius, quadriceps, and rectus abdominis muscles. Other commonly used flaps are the radial forearm, lateral arm, scapular, and deltopectoral flaps.

▶ Anterolateral Thigh Flap

The anterolateral thigh (ALT) flap, harvested from the anterior lateral thigh and composed of skin, adipose tissue, and fascia, is based on the descending branch of the lateral femoral circumflex vessels. The ALT flap perforators are typically musculocutaneous perforators through the vastus lateralis muscle or less commonly septocutaneous perforators through the septum between the rectus femoris and vastus lateralis muscles. The pedicle can be harvested up to 7 cm in length or longer depending on the anatomy of branching vessels. The artery has a diameter of 1.5-2.5 mm with venae slightly larger in size.

The thin facial flap can have an area of 8 × 25 cm with the donor site still closed primarily. If greater than 8 cm width needs to be taken from the thigh, the donor site can be skin grafted. Depending on the thickness of subcutaneous tissue of the patient's thigh, the flap can be relatively thin. The flap can be harvested "super-thin" when dissected suprafacially as long as the perforators to the soft tissue are captured. Variations of the flap can include vastus lateralis muscle if increased tissue bulk is required for reconstruction. The ALT flap can be used as a pedicled flap to the groin, perineum, or lower abdomen or as a free flap.

Radial Forearm Flap

The radial forearm flap is a fasciocutaneous flap based on the radial artery and its perforators. The pedicle length is very long as it can be dissected to the radial artery origin from the brachial artery at the level of the antecubital fossa. The radial artery venae are small, but there are multiple venous options from the subdermal system as well as the cephalic vein. The Allen test is important to perform preoperatively to ensure appropriate blood flow to the hand if the radial artery is harvested. This includes blood flow through the palmar arch when the radial artery is occluded, signifying that the ulnar artery has the ability to perfuse the hand if the radial artery were taken.

The flap provides thin, pliable skin and fascia for resurfacing of wounds. The flap can be harvested with bone by including a segment of the distal radius, as well as tendon by including a segment of palmaris longus. Complex flap designs are possible given the perforator pattern to the skin flap, allowing for multiple skin paddles to be designed. The radial forearm flap is frequently used in head and neck reconstruction.

Scapular & Parascapular Flaps

The scapular flap, based on the transverse branch of the circumflex scapular artery, provides a fasciocutaneous flap. The scapular flap can be incorporated into many flap variations based on the subscapular artery, including an osseous component of scapular bone, a muscular component of latissimus muscle based on the thoracodorsal branch, and a muscular/osseous component of serratus muscle with or without rib. The fascial component is the dorsal thoracic fascia, which can also be harvested without a skin paddle. The pedicle length of the scapular flap is up to 7 cm and has accompanying venae.

The parascapular flap is a fasciocutaneous flap based on the descending branch of the circumflex scapular artery, which can also be included in the subscapular artery tree for combination of multiple components to a chimeric flap. The pedicle is up to 7 cm in length and has accompanying venae. The fasciocutaneous flap size can be up to 15 × 25 cm, providing a large area of tissue to be used for resurfacing.

Lateral Arm & Reverse Lateral Arm Flaps

The lateral arm flap is based on the posterior radial collateral artery, which originates from the brachial artery. The posterior radial collateral artery perfuses the skin, subcutaneous tissue, and fascia of the lateral arm. The pedicle length is short, so this flap is often preferentially used as a pedicled flap for more proximal arm coverage. The innervation is the cutaneous nerve of the forearm. The flap can be taken as an osteocutaneous flap with a portion of humerus.

The same area of skin, adipose tissue, and fascia of the lateral arm can be taken as a reverse lateral arm flap, which is based on the radial recurrent artery. The lateral arm tissue has perfusion from both the posterior radial collateral artery as well as collateral flow from the radial recurrent artery, which makes this variation possible. With distal collateral perfusion present, the flap can be raised to cover defects of the distal arm, antecubital fossa, and proximal forearm.

Groin Flap

The groin flap, also known as the superficial circumflex iliac artery perforator (SCIP) flap, provides a thin adipocutaneous flap based on a perforator from the superficial circumflex iliac artery (SCIA). The SCIA originates from the superficial femoral artery at the level of the inguinal ligament with a cutaneous vein that drains into the saphenous system. The pedicle length is very short at 2-5 cm, which can be a limiting factor for use of the flap.

Osteocutaneous Flaps

Bone and functional joints can be transplanted as free flaps. Flaps from the fibula, femur, iliac crest, and ribs have been successfully transferred for reconstruction of bone defects. The medial femoral trochlea (MFT) flap, uses the concavity and surface of the trochlea to reconstruct defects of the wrist carpus in cases of scaphoid and lunate nonunion and avascular necrosis. Composite free flaps such as the fibular flap with its bone and overlying skin are the most helpful free flaps for reconstruction of the mandible as well as the floor of the mouth following head and neck tumor resections. The toe-to-thumb transfer is an example of a complex transplantation, which includes bone with a functional joint, tendons, and nerves, as well as skin.

Flap Prefabrication & Prelamination

Flap prefabrication and prelamination are two similar yet distinct two-staged techniques to further enhance flap reconstruction in complex defects where traditional techniques are not feasible. Flap prefabrication involves first bringing an axial blood supply to a desired donor tissue that does not have an axial blood supply. Neovascularization of the tissue requires approximately 8 weeks, and then transfer of the prefabricated donor tissue with the newly created axial blood supply is performed as a second-stage procedure to complete the reconstruction. In contrast, flap prelamination involves first construction of a three-dimensional composite or multilayered flap on tissue with native blood supply as the preparation stage. Following approximately 2 weeks of maturation, the prelaminated flap can be transferred to the recipient site for reconstruction. For example, a prelaminated radial forearm free flap with cartilage or bone can be used for complex nasal reconstruction.

Guo L, Pribaz JJ: Clinical flap prefabrication. *Plast Reconstr Surg.* 2009;124(6 Suppl):e340-350.

Hong JP, Choi DH, Suh H, et al: A new plane of elevation: the superficial fascial plane for perforator flap elevation. *J Reconstr Microsurg.* 2014;30(7):491-496.

Wei F-C, Mardini S: *Flaps and Reconstructive Surgery.* New York, NY: Elsevier; 2009.

▶ Reconstruction of Soft Tissue Injury

The plastic surgeon is often involved in emergency department assessment and treatment of soft tissue injuries. Many aspects of wound management must be considered. Careful analysis of the soft tissue injury should include (1) the type of wound or wounds; (2) the cause of injury; (3) the age of the injury; (4) the location of injured tissues; (5) the degree of contamination of the injured area; (6) the nature and extent of associated injuries; and (7) the general health of the patient, including chronic or acute illnesses.

The location of the wound must be noted during evaluation given variable healing characteristics based on anatomic location and the types of skin. The face and scalp are highly vascular and therefore resist infection and heal faster than other areas. However, there are many important structures in and around the face, and scars and defects are cosmetically more noticeable. Skin of the trunk, upper arms, and thighs is fairly thick and heals more slowly than facial or scalp skin and is more susceptible to infection. The hands are a critical anatomic area because there are important structures near the surface, and the destruction caused by infection can be devastating and potentially cause significant functional compromise. The lower legs are particularly challenging given their relatively poor blood supply and have much lower threshold for delayed healing and infectious complications.

▶ Treatment

The type of wound must be determined so that proper treatment can be given. Contusions and swelling require ice packs for 24 hours, rest, and elevation. Abrasions should be cleaned and dressed in a sterile manner similar to a skin graft donor site or must be washed daily until a dry scab forms or healing takes place. Ground-in dirt or gravel must be entirely scrubbed out or picked out with a small blade within 24 hours after injury, or foreign material will be sealed in and traumatic tattooing will result. Extensive local anesthesia may be required to accomplish this. Imbedded particulate matter from an explosion must be removed in a similar manner. Antibiotic coverage is generally not necessary unless heavy contamination is a concern, which may require both gram-positive and gram-negative coverage.

Hematomas may require evacuation if there is concern for soft tissue compromise, such as in the location of the forehead or near ear or nasal septal cartilage, which can sustain permanent damage and alteration in structure with hematomas.

Puncture wounds and bites are notoriously innocuous in appearance but may result in severe destruction or tetanus or gas gangrene. Antibiotic coverage, irrigation, open treatment, and observation are indicated. Most bites on the face, however, can be cleaned and safely closed. Wounds that create flaps of skin or avulsions are difficult to manage. Careful debridement and judicious use of full-thickness or split-thickness grafts from the avulsed tissue are recommended.

Timing is the first factor to consider. Wound contamination can be caused by bacteria on the surface of the wounding agent, such as rust on a nail or saliva on a tooth, or bacteria that enter the wound when the skin is broken. Bacteria driven into tissue become more established as time passes, and it is therefore important to know the age of the wound at the time of the presentation for treatment. Other injuries associated with cuts almost always take precedence in treatment. In general, wounds other than those on the face or scalp should not be closed primarily if they occurred 8-12 hours or longer before presentation unless they were caused by a very clean agent and have been covered by a sterile bandage in the interim. Delayed primary closure, as described previously, is an excellent and safe alternative. Nearly any facial wound up to 24 hours old can be safely closed with careful debridement, irrigation, and antibiotic coverage.

The surgeon must decide whether or not antibiotic treatment is indicated. In general, wounds treated appropriately and early do not call for antibiotic therapy. Antibiotics should be given for wounds with delayed presentation or those for which treatment is delayed by choice: wounds with known contamination; wounds in compromised patients, such as very young or old persons, debilitated persons, or persons with general ill health; wounds in areas where infection may have serious consequences, such as the lower legs and the hands; and wounds in persons in whom bacteremia might have serious sequelae, such as those with prosthetic heart valves or orthopedic appliances. Antibiotics should be started before debridement and closure. Only a few days of coverage are necessary, usually until the wound is examined at 2-3 days and found free of infection. Wounds are usually contaminated by *Staphylococcus aureus,* so an antibiotic effective for penicillin-resistant *S aureus* is typically appropriate. Methicillin-resistant *S aureus* (MRSA) must also be considered in higher risk populations and patients with repeat exposure to hospitals. If gram-negative or anaerobic contamination is suspected, wound closure is risky, and hospitalization of the patient for treatment with parenteral antibiotics should be considered. Tetanus prophylaxis should be given to all patients who have not received current immunizations or who have wounds likely to lead to tetanus.

Anesthesia is an important part of adequate soft tissue wound care and closure. Local anesthesia with either 0.5% or 1% lidocaine with epinephrine 1:200,000 or 1:100,000 is recommended. Lidocaine without epinephrine or smaller amounts of epinephrine may be used in areas of appendages, such as earlobes, toes, and the penis. The injection may be given through the wound edge before debridement and irrigation for maximum patient comfort. Epinephrine vasoconstrictor effect occurs within 7 minutes. Overdose of epinephrine and lidocaine injection into vessels or use of the drugs in patients sensitive to these agents should be avoided.

The importance of irrigation cannot be overstated. Over 90% of bacteria in a recently sustained and superficially contaminated wound can be eliminated by adequate irrigation. Ideally, a physiologic solution such as lactated Ringer solution or normal saline should be forcefully ejected from a large syringe with a 19-gauge needle or from other equipment designed for this purpose such as a water-jet apparatus. The wound is irrigated once to remove surface clots, foreign material, and bacteria and is then debrided and irrigated again. Detergents and antiseptic solutions are toxic to exposed tissue and should not be used.

Debridement must include removal of all obviously devitalized tissues. In special areas such as the eyelids, ears, nose, lips, and eyebrows, debridement must be done cautiously, since the tissue lost by debridement may be difficult to replace. Where tissues are more abundant, such as in the cheek, chin, and forehead areas, debridement may be more extensive. Small irregular or ragged wounds in these areas can be excised completely to produce clean, sharply cut wound edges, which, when approximated, will produce the finest possible scar. Because the blood supply in the face is plentiful, damaged tissues of questionable viability should be retained rather than debrided away. The chances for survival are good.

Following adequate anesthesia, debridement, and irrigation, the wound is ready for final assessment and closure. Lighting must be adequate, and appropriate instruments should be available. The patient and the surgeon must be positioned comfortably. The skin surrounding the wound is prepared with an antiseptic solution, and the area is draped. A final check of the depth and extent of the wound is made, and vital structures are inspected for injury. Hemostasis must be achieved by use of epinephrine, pressure, cautery, or suture ligature. Important structures in facial wounds include the parotid duct, lacrimal duct, and branches of the facial nerve. These should be repaired in the operating room by microsurgical techniques.

Layers of tissue should be closed to achieve strong wound closure. Dead space should be closed with advancement of local tissue or triple-point stitches. If dead space cannot be closed, external pressure or small drains are sometimes effective. Skin closure should begin at the most important points of the laceration, such as the borders of the ears and nose, the vermilion border or margins of the lip, the margins of the eyebrow, or the scalp hairline. Subcuticular sutures are very helpful. Skin edges can be approximated without tension or strangulation with 5-0 or 6-0 monofilament suture material, as outlined earlier under wound closure.

Complicated lacerations, such as complex stellate wounds or avulsion flaps, often heal with excessive scarring. Because of the associated subcutaneous tissue injury, U-shaped or trap-door avulsion lacerations almost always become unsightly as a result of wound contracture. Small lacerations of this type are best excised and closed in a straight line initially; larger flaps that must be replaced usually require secondary revision. Extensive loss of skin is generally best treated by initial split-thickness skin grafting followed later by secondary reconstruction. Primary attempts to reconstruct with local flaps may fail because of unsuspected injury to these adjacent tissues. The decision to convert avulsed tissues to free grafts that may not survive and thus delay healing requires sound surgical judgment.

Small or moderate-sized closures on the face may be dressed with antibiotic ointment alone. The patient may cleanse the suture lines with hydrogen peroxide to clear away crusts and dirt and then reapply the ointment. Elsewhere, closures benefit from the protection of a sterile bandage. Pressure dressings are useful in preventing hematoma formation and severe edema that may result in poor wound healing. Dressings should be changed early and the wound inspected for hematoma or signs of infection. Hematoma evacuation, appropriate drainage, and antibiotic therapy based on culture and sensitivity studies may be required. Removal of sutures within 5 days, followed by splinting of the incision with sterile tape, will minimize scarring from the sutures themselves.

The final result of facial wound repair depends on the nature and location of the wounds, individual propensity to scar formation, and the passage of time. A year or more must often pass before resolution of scar contracture and erythema results in maximum improvement. Only after this time can a decision be made regarding the desirability of secondary scar revision. In wounds involving the major joints, the extracapsular soft tissue and the intracapsular structures should be considered individually to assess accurately the magnitude of the injury and to provide a prognosis. Open joint injuries that are single penetrating and without extensive soft tissue damage permit uncomplicated joint and wound closure. Injuries that are single or multiple penetrations with extensive soft tissue disruption, such as flaps, avulsions, or degloving, often require secondary operations to attain closure. In injuries that show open periarticular fractures with extension through the adjacent intra-articular surface and with associated nerve or vascular injury requiring repair, the cornerstone for successful management is debridement, antibiotic therapy properly timed and performed, joint closure, and aggressive treatment of the bony injury. Newer techniques such as free-tissue transfer can expedite wound care, decrease morbidity, and spare some limbs from amputation.

▼ III. SKIN LESIONS AND TUMORS

Tumors of the skin are by far the most common of all tumors in humans. They arise from each of the histologic structures that make up the skin: epidermis, connective tissue, gland, muscle, and nerve elements. Skin tumors are classified as benign, premalignant, and malignant.

BENIGN

The many benign tumors that arise from the skin rarely interfere with function. Since most are removed for aesthetic reasons or to rule out malignancy, they are quite commonly treated by the plastic surgeon. The majority are small and can be simply excised under local anesthesia following the principles of elliptical excision and wound closure discussed earlier. General anesthesia may be necessary for larger lesions requiring excision and repair by skin grafts or flaps or those occurring in young children.

When the diagnosis is not in doubt, most superficial lesions, including seborrheic keratoses, verrucae, and squamous cell papillomas, can be treated by simple techniques such as electrodesiccation, curettage and electrodesiccation, cryotherapy, and topical cytotoxic agents.

▶ Seborrheic Keratosis

Seborrheic keratoses are superficial noninvasive tumors that originate in the epidermis. They appear in older people as multiple slightly elevated yellowish, brown, or brownish-black irregularly rounded plaques with waxy or oily surfaces. They are most commonly found on the trunk and shoulders but are frequently seen on the scalp and face.

Because the lesion is raised above the epidermis, treatment usually consists of shave excision. Care should be exercised to avoid shaving a melanoma because if that is done it will interfere with the determination of the depth of invasion by the Breslow or Clark classifications. If there is any question about a pigmented lesion, it is preferable to do an excisional biopsy rather than to shave.

▶ Verrucae

Verrucae, or common warts, are usually seen in children and young adults, typically on the fingers and hands. They appear as round or oval elevated lesions with rough surfaces composed of multiple rounded or filiform keratinized projections. They may be skin colored or gray to brown. Verrucae are caused by a virus and are autoinoculable, which

can result in multiple lesions around the original growth or frequent recurrences following treatment if the virus is not completely eradicated. They may disappear spontaneously.

Treatment by electrodesiccation is effective but is frequently followed by slow healing. Repeated applications of bichloroacetic acid, liquid nitrogen, or liquid CO_2 are also effective. Surgical excision alone is not recommended, because the wound may become inoculated with the virus, leading to recurrences in and around the scar. However, surgical excision in conjunction with electrodesiccation can be an effective form of treatment. Recurrence remains a common problem; therefore, it is reasonable to delay treatment of asymptomatic lesions for several months to determine if they will disappear spontaneously.

▶ Epidermal Inclusion Cyst

Although sebaceous cyst is the commonly used term, these lesions more properly should be called epidermal inclusion cysts because they are composed of thin layers of epidermal cells filled with epithelial debris. True cysts arising from sebaceous epithelial cells are uncommon.

Epidermal inclusion cysts are soft to firm, usually elevated, and filled with an odorous cheesy material. Their most common sites of occurrence are the scalp, face, ears, neck, and back. They are usually covered by normal skin, which may show dimpling at the site of skin attachment. They frequently present as infected cysts. Treatment consists of surgical excision.

▶ Dermoid Cyst

Dermoid cysts are deeper than epidermal cysts. They are not attached to the skin but frequently are attached to or extend through underlying bony structures. They may appear in many sites but are most common around the nose or the orbit, where they may extend to meningeal structures, necessitating computed tomography (CT) scans to determine their extent. Treatment is by surgical excision, which may necessitate sectioning of adjacent bony structures.

▶ Pigmented Nevi

Nevocellular nevi are groups of cells of probable neural crest origin that contain melanocytes that form melanin more rapidly upon stimulation than surrounding tissue. These cells migrate to different parts of the skin to give different types of nevi. They may also be distinguished by their clinical presentation.

A. Junctional Nevi

Junctional nevi are well-defined pigmented lesions appearing in infancy. They are usually flat or slightly elevated and light brown to dark brown. They may appear on any part of the body, but most nevi seen on the palms, soles, and genitalia are of the junctional type. Histologically, a proliferation of melanocytes is present in the epidermis at the epidermal-dermal junction. It was formerly thought that these nevi give rise to malignant melanoma and that all junctional nevi should be excised for prophylactic reasons. However, most investigators now feel that the risk is very slight. If there is no change in their appearance, treatment is unnecessary. Any change such as itching, inflammation, darkening in color, halo formation, increase in size, bleeding, or ulceration calls for immediate treatment. Surgical excision is the only safe method of treatment.

B. Intradermal Nevi

Intradermal nevi are the typical dome-shaped, sometimes pedunculated, fleshy to brownish pigmented moles that are characteristically seen in adults. They frequently contain hairs and may occur anywhere on the body. Microscopically, melanocytes are present entirely within the dermis and, in contrast to junctional nevi, show little activity. They are rarely malignant and require no treatment except for aesthetic reasons. Surgical excision is nearly always the treatment of choice. Pigmented nevi should never be treated without obtaining tissue for histologic examination.

C. Compound Nevi

Compound nevi exhibit the histologic features of both junctional and intradermal nevi in that melanocytes lie both at the epidermal-dermal junction and within the dermis. They are usually elevated, dome shaped, and light brown to dark brown in color. Because of the presence of nevus cells at the epidermal-dermal junction, the indications for treatment are the same as for junctional nevi. If treatment is indicated, surgical excision is the method of choice.

D. Spindle Cell–Epithelioma Cell Nevi

These nevi, formerly called benign juvenile melanomas, appear in children or adults. They vary markedly in vascularity, degree of pigmentation, and accompanying hyperkeratosis. Clinically, they simulate warts or hemangiomas rather than moles. They may increase in size rapidly, but the average lesion reaches only 6-8 mm in diameter, remaining entirely benign without invasion or metastases. Microscopically, the lesion can be confused with malignant melanoma by the inexperienced pathologist. The usual treatment is excisional biopsy.

E. Blue Nevi

Blue nevi are small, sharply defined, round, dark blue or grayish-blue lesions that may occur anywhere on the body but are most commonly seen on the face, neck, hands, and arms. They usually appear in childhood as slowly growing,

well-defined nodules covered by a smooth, intact epidermis. Microscopically, the melanocytes that make up this lesion are limited to, but may be found in all layers of, the dermis. An intimate association with the fibroblasts of the dermis is seen, giving the lesion a fibrotic appearance not seen in other nevi. This, together with extension of melanocytes deep into the dermis, may account for the blue rather than brown color. Treatment is not mandatory unless the patient desires removal for aesthetic reasons or fear of cancer. Surgical excision is the treatment of choice.

F. Giant Hairy Nevi

Unlike most nevi arising from melanocytes, giant hairy nevi are congenital. They may occur anywhere on the body and may cover large areas. They may be large enough to cover the entire trunk. They are of special significance for several reasons: (1) their large size is especially deforming from an aesthetic standpoint; (2) they show a predisposition for developing malignant melanoma; and (3) they may be associated with neurofibromas or melanocytic involvement of the leptomeninges and other neurologic abnormalities. Microscopically, a varied picture is present. All of the characteristics of intradermal and compound nevi may be seen. Neurofibromas may also be present within the lesion. Malignant melanoma may arise anywhere within the large lesion; the reported rate of occurrence ranges from 1% to as high as 13.7% in one study. Malignant melanoma with metastases rarely arises in childhood or infancy.

The only full treatment is complete excision, which may require local advancement flaps or skin grafting for coverage of the resulting defect. Large lesions may require excision and grafting in stages. Some lesions are so large that excision is not possible and the most effective approach is using tissue expansion in combination with flaps. Split-thickness excision or dermabrasion has been successful when done in infancy. Some have reported the use of laser photothermolysis of pigmented lesions that cannot be excised with favorable reconstructive outcomes. However, there is still concern over malignant transformation of remaining melanocytes, and close long-term follow-up is recommended when laser ablation is used.

Samarasinghe V, Madan V: Nonmelanoma skin cancer. *J Cutan Aesthet Surg.* 2012;5(1):3-10.

▶ Vascular Tumors & Vascular Malformations

Our understanding of vascular tumors and vascular malformations has evolved a great deal since the description by Mulliken and Glowacki in 1982 of the biologic classification of vascular anomalies based on their endothelial properties. In this way, infant hemangiomas appear within the first 3 weeks of life and have a proliferative endothelium that grows rapidly at first and commonly involutes usually in the first few years of life. Vascular malformations, on the other hand, have stable endothelium, grow proportionally with the child, and persist into adulthood. They can be associated with various complications, such as skeletal abnormalities, ischemia, coagulopathy, heart failure, and death.

Glucose transporter isoform 1 (GLUT1) is a distinguishing feature among various forms of vascular anomalies. It is an immunohistochemical marker that is normally restricted to endothelial cells with blood–tissue barrier function as in the brain and placenta. North and colleagues retrospectively studied specimens from vascular tumors for GLUT1. Specimens from infantile hemangiomas were universally positive. In contrast, biopsies of other vascular anomalies, including rapidly involuting congenital hemangioma, noninvoluting congenital hemangioma, pyogenic granuloma, granulation tissue, vascular malformations, and tufted angioma and kaposiform hemangioendothelioma, were all negative. In addition to providing an early diagnostic assay for hemangiomas, GLUT1 can be useful in research and in trying to explain the pathophysiology.

▶ Vascular Tumors

A. Congenital Hemangiomas

Congenital hemangiomas are present at birth, fully grown, which is in contrast to infantile hemangiomas, which undergo rapid growth during the first 4-6 months of life. Because of their natural history, they are divided into two subtypes: rapidly involuting congenital hemangiomas (RICHs) and noninvoluting congenital hemangiomas (NICHs). RICHs are more common than NICHs, although both are rare. The diagnosis of RICH is confirmed when they rapidly involute by 6-10 months of age. The NICH anomalies, on the other hand, persist into adulthood and may require surgical excision or other ablative measures. Imaging may be helpful, such as ultrasound or magnetic resonance imaging (MRI), in order to evaluate location and extent of the tumor. Both congenital hemangiomas, RICH and NICH, are GLUT1 negative, in contrast to infantile hemangiomas.

B. Infantile Hemangiomas

Infantile hemangiomas are the most common tumors that occur in childhood and constitute at least 95% of all the hemangiomas that are seen in infancy and childhood. They are true neoplasms of endothelial cells but are unique among neoplasms in that they undergo complete, spontaneous involution. GLUT1 is the mutation associated with infantile hemangiomas, which can be identified on pathologic analysis.

Typically, they are present shortly after birth or appear during the first 2-3 weeks of life. They grow at a rather rapid rate for 4-6 months; then growth ceases and spontaneous involution begins. Involution typically starts at age 3-4 years and progresses slowly. However, approximately 50% are involuted by age 5, 70% by age 7, and 90% by age 9. Involuting hemangiomas appear on all body surfaces but are seen more often on the head and neck. They have a 3:1 female-to-male ratio and present 60% in the head and neck region.

Three forms of infantile hemangiomas are seen: (1) superficial, (2) combined superficial and deep (mixed), and (3) deep. Superficial involuting hemangiomas appear as sharply demarcated, bright red, slightly raised lesions with an irregular surface that has been described as resembling a strawberry. Combined superficial and deep involuting hemangiomas have the same surface characteristics, but beneath the skin surface, a firm bluish tumor is present that may extend deeply into the subcutaneous tissues. Deep involuting hemangiomas present as deep blue tumors covered by normal-appearing skin.

Hemangiomas are the result of angiogenic dysfunction. Multiple markers of angiogenesis are increased during the proliferative flow, including fibroblast growth factor, vascular endothelial growth factor, and matrix metalloproteinases. These all decrease with the exception of basic fibroblast growth factor during the involution phase. As the phase of involution progresses, the histologic picture changes, with the solid fields of endothelial cells breaking up into closely packed, capillary-sized, vessel-like structures composed of several layers of soft endothelial cells supported by a sparse fibrous stroma. These vascular structures gradually become fewer and spaced more widely apart in a loose, edematous fibrous stroma. The endothelial cells continue to disappear, so that by the time involution is complete the histologic picture is entirely normal, with no trace of endothelial cells.

Treatment is not usually indicated, since the appearance following spontaneous regression is nearly always superior to the scars that follow surgical excision. Surgical excision of lesions that involve important structures such as the eyelids, nose, or lips may sometimes be necessary in order to avoid serious functional disturbances of vision and airway. Complete excision is usually not necessary.

When treatment is indicated, multiple options have been described. The use of the beta-blocker propranolol has been promising, with slowing of hemangioma progression and dramatically shortened involution time. Usual doses are from 1-3 mg/kg/d for up to 12 months. Side effects include bradycardia, hypotension, and bronchoconstriction. Infants are usually admitted for 24 hours upon starting this therapy for cardiac monitoring. Although the actual mechanism of action remains unknown, it most likely has to do with downregulation of angiogenic growth factors. It has shown such good results that some institutions are using this as a first-line treatment for complicated infantile hemangiomas. If hemangiomas are causing visual or airway compromise, other therapies such as surgery, corticosteroids, laser, and injectable bleomycin or corticosteroids have been used.

Ulceration is a painful and dangerous complication with hemangiomas that can develop in approximately 8% of patients. This may be accompanied by infection, which is treated by the use of compresses of warm saline or potassium permanganate and by the application of antimicrobial powders and creams. Bleeding from the ulcer can occur if there is constant irritation and inflammation. When it occurs, gentle pressure should be applied. In some situations, such as the perianal region, specific measures may be needed to keep the area clean and dry including a diverting colostomy combined with judicious serial excision. In rare cases, the platelet trapping of these lesions leads to the clinical picture of disseminated intravascular coagulopathy called Kasabach-Merritt syndrome.

▶ Vascular Malformations

Vascular malformations are present at birth and typically grow with the patient. They do not involute spontaneously. Types of vascular malformations include capillary, venous, lymphatic, and arteriovenous (AV) malformations. Diagnosis of the lesion is helpful with history, physical exam, imaging, including MRI to better characterize, and Doppler exam. AV malformations are high flow and can be suspected on Doppler exam.

A. Capillary Malformations

Capillary malformations, often referred to as "port wine stains," are the most commonly encountered vascular malformations. They may involve any portion of the body but most commonly appear on the face as flat patchy lesions that are reddish to purple in color. When on the face, they are located in areas supplied by the sensory branches of the trigeminal cranial nerve (cranial nerve V). Capillary malformations are initially light red in color yet have a propensity to deepen in color. Presentation and growth of capillary malformations are variable. If not treated, they commonly will persist into adulthood, and subsequently, 70% will develop into cobblestone ectasia (Figure 43–9).

Microscopically, port wine stains are made up of thin-walled capillaries arranged throughout the dermis. The capillaries are lined with mature, flat endothelial cells. In lesions with surface growth, groups of round proliferating endothelial cells and large venous sinuses are seen. The *RASA1* gene has been identified in association with capillary malformations.

Treatment of capillary malformations has significantly improved with the use of pulsed dye or Nd:YAG lasers. The pulsed dye laser, most often used in treatment of capillary malformations, produces a light with a specific wavelength of 585 nm, which is selectively absorbed by red-pigmented material such as hemoglobin in the blood vessels of the lesion, causing selective photothermolysis. This produces selective heat destruction of these structures, and the treated area becomes whiter. When started early, these treatments can be very effective. Multiple treatments are necessary to obtain a satisfactory result. In darker and more advanced nodular

A

B

▲ **Figure 43–9.** Untreated capillary malformation or "port wine stain" of the left face.

lesions, the laser is less effective because of the thickness of the lesion and the hyperpigmentation that may develop.

In the case of longstanding untreated lesions, surgical excision may be necessary. Certain fast-growing capillary or primarily arterialized hemangiomas have been managed successfully with superselective embolization, either alone or in conjunction with surgery; however, there have been reports of slough of large portions of the face as a result of misdirected embolization. Superficial methods of treatment such as dry ice, liquid nitrogen, electrocoagulation, and dermabrasion have been tried but are ineffective unless they destroy the upper layers of the skin, which can produce severe scarring.

B. Venous Malformations

Venous malformations are typically raised, bluish or purplish lesions. They are composed of mature, fully formed venous structures that are present in tortuous masses, or a "bag of worms." Although they occur anywhere on the body, like other vascular lesions, they are more common on the head and neck. Microscopically, venous malformations are made up of large, dilated, closely packed vascular sinuses that are engorged with blood. They are lined by flat endothelial cells and may have muscular walls like normal veins. Venous malformations are usually present at birth but do not usually grow except to keep pace with normal body growth. In many cases, growth occurs later in life and may interfere with normal function. Puberty and pregnancy can increase the size of the lesions. Many lesions improve when elevated and swell when in a dependent position.

Sclerotherapy is the preferred treatment for venous malformations. The injection of sclerosing agents directly into the venous channels leads to involution or may make surgical excision more amenable. Great care must be used so that areas of overlying skin do not slough. Some lesions can be approached with surgical excision alone; however, many lesions involve deeper structures, such as muscle and bone, so complete excision would be harmful. Laser therapy can be performed with Nd:YAG with some improvement.

C. Lymphatic Malformations

Lymphatic malformations are lesions composed of lymphatic channels, which often appear as clear vesicles within and below the dermis. Lymphatic and venous malformations often appear together. Infections of lymphatic lesions are common, requiring antibiotic therapy and subsequent treatment of the lymphatic lesion after clearance of the infection to prevent recurrence.

MRI should be obtained to determine if the lymphatic lesion is macrocystic or microcystic. If macrocystic, the lesion should be treated with intralesional sclerotherapy. If microcystic, the lesion should be more amenable to resection. Intralesional bleomycin has also been reported as treatment for lymphatic lesions.

D. Arteriovenous Malformations

AV malformations are high-flow lesions having a direct connection between an artery and a vein, bypassing the capillary bed. AV malformations are typically recognized at birth but are misdiagnosed as capillary malformations or involuting hemangiomas. Periods of rapid growth are found after trauma and during periods when the body is under the influence of hormonal changes.

Clinical diagnosis can be confirmed with color Doppler examination, but this does not give information concerning extent of the lesion or relation to surrounding structures. This information can be obtained via MRI or angiography, which has the additional benefit of therapeutic embolization.

Treatment for AV malformations is based on clinical stage of the lesion. Smaller AV malformations can be primarily resected. Larger, more diffuse AV malformations are best managed with superselective arterial embolization followed by surgical resection 24-48 hours after embolization in order to minimize intraoperative blood loss. Surgery must be approached carefully because resection can lead to massive blood loss, consumptive coagulopathy, and heart failure. Strong consideration must be made for correction of coagulopathy preoperatively, blood pressure control, cell-saver use, and even cardiopulmonary bypass.

Couto RA, Maclellan RA, Zurakowski D, et al: Infantile hemangioma: clinical assessment of the involuting phase and implications for management. *Plast Reconstr Surg.* 2012;130(3):619-624.

Mulliken JB, Glowacki J: Hemangiomas and vascular malformations in infants and children: a classification based on endothelial characteristics. *Plast Reconstr Surg.* 1982;69(3):412-422.

PREMALIGNANT SKIN LESIONS

▶ Actinic Keratoses

Actinic keratoses are the most common of the precancerous skin lesions. They usually appear as small, single or multiple, slightly elevated, scaly or warty lesions ranging in color from red to yellow, brown, or black. Because they are related to sun exposure, they occur most frequently on the face and the backs of the hands in fair-skinned Caucasians whose skin shows evidence of actinic elastosis. Microscopically, actinic keratoses consist of well-defined areas of abnormal epithelial cells limited to the epidermis. Approximately 15%-20% of these lesions become malignant, in which case invasion of the dermis as squamous cell carcinoma occurs.

Since the lesions are limited to the epidermis, superficial treatment in the form of curette and electrodesiccation or the application of chemical agents such as liquid nitrogen, phenol, bi- or trichloroacetic acid, or fluorouracil is curative. The application of fluorouracil cream is of particular benefit in preventive treatment in that it destroys lesions of microscopic size, before they can be detected clinically, without causing damage to uninvolved skin.

▶ Chronic Radiation Dermatitis & Ulceration

There are two distinct types of radiation dermatitis. The first and most common follows the acute administration of relatively high dosages of ionizing orthovoltage radiation over relatively short periods, which is almost always performed for the treatment of cancer. Dermatitis is characterized by an acute reaction that begins near the third week of therapy, when erythema, blistering, and sloughing of the epidermis start to occur. Burning and hyperesthesia are commonly present. This initial reaction is followed by scarring characterized by atrophy of the epidermis and dermis along with loss of skin appendages, including sweat glands, sebaceous glands, and hair follicles. Marked fibrosis of the dermis occurs, with gradual endarteritis and occlusion of the dermal and subdermal vessels. Telangiectasia of the surface vessels is seen, and areas of both hypopigmentation and hyperpigmentation occur.

The second type of radiation dermatitis follows chronic exposure to low doses of ionizing radiation over prolonged periods. It is usually seen in professional personnel who handle radioactive materials or administer x-rays or in patients who have been treated for dermatologic conditions such as acne or excessive facial hair. Therefore, the face and hands are most commonly involved. The acute reaction described earlier does not usually occur, but the same process of atrophy, scarring, and loss of dermal elements occurs. Drying of the skin becomes more pronounced, and deepening of the skin furrows is typically present. Fortunately, this second type of radiation dermatitis is rarely seen today.

In both types of radiation dermatitis, late changes such as the following may occur: (1) the appearance of hyperkeratotic growths on the skin surface, (2) chronic ulceration, and (3) the development of either basal cell or squamous cell carcinoma. Ulceration and cancer, however, are seen much less commonly in the first type of radiation dermatitis than in the second. When malignant growths appear, basal cell carcinomas are seen more frequently on the face and neck and squamous cell carcinomas more frequently on the hands and body.

Surgical excision is the treatment of choice. Excision should include all of the irradiated tissue including the area of telangiectasia, whenever possible, and the defect should be covered with an appropriate axial or musculocutaneous flap to provide a new blood supply. Primary wound closure is feasible for only the smallest lesions, and even so, at some risk. Free-skin grafting is usually unsuccessful because of the damage to the vascular supply of the subcutaneous structures. Adjacent random flaps are unreliable because they depend on blood supply from the surrounding irradiated area.

MALIGNANT SKIN LESIONS

1. Intraepidermal Carcinoma

Intraepidermal carcinoma includes Bowen disease and erythroplasia of Queyrat.

▶ Bowen Disease

Bowen disease is characterized by single or multiple, brownish or reddish plaques that may appear anywhere on the skin surface but often on covered surfaces. The typical plaque is sharply defined, slightly raised, scaly, and slightly thickened. The surface is often keratotic, and crusting and fissuring may be present. Ulceration is not common but when present suggests malignant degeneration with dermal invasion.

Histologically, hyperplasia of the epidermis is seen, with pleomorphic malpighian cells, giant cells, and atypical epithelial cells that are limited to the epidermis.

Treatment of small or superficial lesions consists of total destruction by curette and electrodesiccation or by any of the other superficially destructive methods, including cryotherapy and cytotoxic agents. Excision and skin grafting are preferred for larger lesions and for those that have undergone early malignant degeneration and invasion of the dermis.

▶ Erythroplasia of Queyrat

Erythroplasia of Queyrat is almost identical to Bowen disease both clinically and histologically but is confined to the glans penis and the vulva, where the lesions appear as red, irregular, and with slightly raised plaques. Treatment is as described for Bowen disease.

2. Basal Cell Carcinoma

Basal cell carcinoma is the most common skin cancer. The lesions usually appear on the face and are more common in men than in women. Since exposure to ultraviolet rays of the sun is a causative factor, basal cell carcinoma is most commonly seen in geographic areas where there is significant sun exposure and in people whose skin is most susceptible to actinic damage from exposure.

The growth rate of basal cell carcinoma is usually slow but nearly always steady and insidious. Several months or years may pass before the patient becomes concerned. Without treatment, widespread invasion and destruction of adjacent tissues may occur, producing massive ulceration. Penetration of the bones of the facial skeleton and the skull may occur late in the course. Basal cell carcinomas rarely metastasize, but death can occur because of direct intracranial extension or erosion of major blood vessels.

Typical individual lesions appear as small, translucent or shiny ("pearly") elevated nodules with central ulceration and rolled, pearly edges. Telangiectatic vessels are commonly present over the surface, and pigmentation is sometimes present. Superficial ulceration occurs early.

A less common type of basal cell carcinoma is the sclerosing or morphea carcinoma, consisting of elongated strands of basal cell cancer that infiltrate the dermis, with the intervening corium being unusually compact. These lesions are usually flat and whitish or waxy in appearance and firm to palpation—similar in appearance to localized scleroderma. They are particularly difficult to treat because it is difficult to clinically predict the extent of the margins of growth.

The superficial erythematous basal cell cancer occurs most frequently on the trunk as reddish plaques with atrophic centers and smooth, slightly raised borders. These lesions are capable of peripheral growth and wide extension but do not become invasive until late.

Pigmented basal cell carcinomas may be mistaken for melanomas because of the large number of melanocytes present within the tumor. They may also be confused with seborrheic keratoses.

▶ Treatment

There are several methods of treating basal cell carcinoma. All may be curative in some lesions, but no one method is applicable to all. The special features of each basal cell cancer must be considered individually before proper treatment can be selected.

Because most lesions occur on the face, aesthetic and functional results of treatment are important. However, the most important consideration is whether or not therapy is curative. If the basal cell carcinoma is not eradicated by the initial treatment, continued growth and invasion of adjacent tissues will occur, resulting not only in additional tissue destruction but also in invasion of the tumor into deeper structures, making cure more difficult. Adequate treatment of basal cell carcinoma by different modalities achieves a cure rate of approximately 95%.

The principal methods of treatment are curettage and electrodesiccation, surgical excision, and radiation therapy. Chemosurgery, topical chemotherapy, and cryosurgery are not often used but may have value in selected cases.

A. Curettage and Electrodesiccation

Curettage plus electrodesiccation is the usual method of treatment for small lesions. After infiltration with suitable local anesthetic, the lesion and a 2- to 3-mm margin of normal-appearing skin around it are thoroughly curetted with a small skin curette. The resultant wound is then completely desiccated with an electrosurgical unit to destroy any tumor cells that may not have been removed by the curette. The process is then repeated once or twice if necessary. The wound is left open and allowed to heal secondarily.

B. Surgical Excision

Surgical excision, following the principles outlined earlier in this chapter, offers many advantages in the treatment of basal cell carcinoma: (1) Most lesions can be quickly excised in one procedure. (2) Following excision, the entire lesion can be examined by the pathologist, who can determine if the tumor has been completely removed. (3) Deep infiltrative lesions can be completely excised, and cartilage and bone can be removed if they have been invaded. (4) Lesions that occur in dense scar tissue or in other poorly vascularized tissues cannot be treated by curettage and desiccation, radiation therapy, or chemosurgery, since healing is poor. Excision and flap coverage may be the only method for treatment in these conditions. (5) Recurrent lesions in tissues that have been exposed to maximum safe amounts of radiation can be excised and covered.

Small to moderate-sized lesions can be excised in one stage under local anesthesia. The visible and palpable margins of the tumor are marked on the skin with marking ink. The width of excision is then marked 3-5 mm beyond these margins. If the margins of the basal cell carcinoma are vague, the width of excision will have to be wider to ensure complete removal of the lesion. The lines of incision are drawn around the lesion as a circle. This tissue is excised, taking care to leave a margin of normal-appearing subcutaneous tissue around the deep margins of the tumor. Frozen sections may be obtained at the time of excision to aid in determining whether tumor-free margins have been obtained. This is minimized with experience. It is better to err on the side of removing more normal tissue than necessary rather than to risk including tumor at the margins. Closure of the wound is accomplished in the direction of minimal skin tension, usually along the skin lines. The dog-ears are removed appropriately.

Wounds resulting from the excision of some moderate-sized tumors and nearly all large tumors may require reconstruction of function and appearance with the use of local, regional, and free flaps. This can nearly always be performed in one stage with good frozen section control.

The disadvantages of surgical excision are as follows: (1) Certain large excisions and reconstruction require specialized training and experience to master the surgical techniques. (2) Whereas curettage and desiccation may be performed in the office, surgical excision often requires specialized facilities. (3) In lesions with vague clinical margins, an excessive amount of normal tissue may have to be excised to ensure complete removal even with the use of frozen section verification. (4) Reconstruction may need to wait until permanent pathologic diagnosis and margins are available in cases involving deep or specialized structures.

To overcome some of these objections, Mohs described in 1941 a new technique that allows for serial excisions and microscopic examination of chemically fixed tissue. Newer developments have obviated the cumbersome fixation techniques, but it may still take several hours to scan an area for suspected malignant cells. The procedure is nevertheless quite useful for recurrent lesions and in areas in which maximal preservation is desirable such as the face. Nonetheless, there are no prospective comparative studies to indicate that the microscopically controlled removal of tumor by the Mohs technique, which amounts to excision of the lesion with serial review by fresh frozen section, is superior to surgical excision. An additional problem is that there is no quality control because the excising physician is also the one who evaluates the pathology slides. Many of the more extensive lesions treated with the Mohs technique require complex reconstruction to rebuild noble structures that have needed resection.

Radiation therapy is as effective as any other in the treatment of basal cell carcinoma. Its advantages are as follows: (1) Structures that are difficult to reconstruct, such as the eyelids, tear ducts, and nasal tip, can be preserved when they are invaded by but not destroyed by tumor. (2) A wide margin of tissue can be treated around lesions with poorly defined margins to ensure destruction of nondiscernible extensions of tumor. (3) It may be less traumatic than surgical excision to elderly patients with advanced lesions. (4) Hospitalization is not necessary.

The disadvantages are as follows: (1) Only well-trained, experienced physicians can obtain good results. (2) Expensive facilities are necessary. (3) Improperly administered radiation therapy may produce severe sequelae, including scarring, radiation dermatitis, ulceration, and malignant degeneration. (4) In hair-bearing areas, epilation will result. (5) It may be difficult to treat areas of irregular contour (eg, the ear and the auditory canal). (6) Repeated treatments over a period of 4-6 weeks may be necessary.

Radiation therapy should not be used in patients under age 40 except in unusual circumstances, and it should not be repeated in patients who have failed to respond to radiation therapy in the past.

3. Squamous Cell Carcinoma

Squamous cell carcinoma is the second most common cancer of the skin in light-skinned racial groups and the most common skin cancer in darkly pigmented racial groups. As with basal cell carcinoma, sunlight is the most common causative factor in whites. The most common sites of occurrence are the ears, cheeks, lower lip, and backs of the hands. Other causative factors are chemical and thermal burns, scars, chronic ulcers, chronic granulomas (tuberculosis of the skin, syphilis), draining sinuses, contact with tars and hydrocarbons, and exposure to ionizing radiation. When a squamous cell carcinoma occurs in a burn scar, it is called a Marjolin ulcer. This lesion may appear many years after the original burn. It tends to be aggressive, and the prognosis is poor.

Because exposure to the sun is the greatest stimulus for the production of squamous cell carcinoma, most of these lesions are preceded by actinic keratosis on areas of the skin showing chronic solar damage. They may also arise from other premalignant skin lesions and from normal-appearing skin.

The natural history of squamous cell carcinoma may be quite variable. It may present as a slowly growing, locally invasive lesion without metastases or as a rapidly growing, widely invasive tumor with early metastatic spread. In general, squamous cell carcinomas that develop from actinic keratoses are more common and are of the slowly growing type, whereas those that develop from Bowen disease, erythroplasia of Queyrat, chronic radiation dermatitis, scars, and chronic ulcers tend to be more aggressive. Lesions that arise from normal-appearing skin and from the lips, genitalia, and anal regions also tend to be aggressive.

Early squamous cell carcinoma usually appears as a small, firm erythematous plaque or nodule with indistinct margins. The surface may be flat and smooth or may be verrucous. As the tumor grows, it becomes raised and, because of

progressive invasion, becomes fixed to surrounding tissues. Ulceration may occur early or late but tends to appear earlier in the more rapidly growing lesions.

Histologically, malignant epithelial cells are seen extending down into the dermis as broad, rounded masses or slender strands. In squamous cell carcinomas of low-grade malignancy, the individual cells may be quite well differentiated, resembling uniform mature squamous cells having intercellular bridges. Keratinization may be present, and layers of keratinizing squamous cells may produce typical round "horn pearls." In highly malignant lesions, the epithelial cells may be extremely atypical; abnormal mitotic figures are common; intercellular bridges are not present; and keratinization does not occur.

► Treatment

As with basal cell carcinomas, the method of treatment that will eradicate squamous cell carcinomas and produce the best aesthetic and functional results varies with the characteristics of the individual lesion. Factors that determine the optimal method of treatment include the size, shape, and location of the tumor as well as the histologic pattern that determines its aggressiveness.

The mainstay of treatment is surgery. Radiation has also been used in some circumstances. Because basal cell carcinomas are relatively nonaggressive lesions that rarely metastasize, failure to eradicate the lesion may result only in local recurrence. Although this may result in extensive local tissue destruction, there is rarely a threat to life. Aggressive squamous cell carcinomas, on the other hand, may metastasize to any part of the body, and failure of treatment may have fatal consequences. For this reason, total eradication of each lesion is the imperative goal of treatment.

The use of sentinel lymph node biopsy (SLNB) is usually reserved for patients with a high-risk squamous cell cancer or when the lesion is larger than 2 cm. This procedure maps the first node basin that any disease would travel to if metastatic. Palpable nodes of any type are a contraindication for SLNB.

Netscher DT, Leong M, Orengo I, et al: Cutaneous malignancies: melanoma and nonmelanoma types. *Plast Reconstr Surg.* 2011;127(3):37e-56e.

▼ IV. RECONSTRUCTIVE SURGERY

HEAD & NECK RECONSTRUCTION

Many head and neck tumors require surgical excision as a primary form of therapy. This often involves removal of large areas of composite tissue, such as the floor of the mouth, the maxilla, part of the mandible, or the lymph-bearing tissue of the neck. Reconstruction after such resections can be very challenging and may require special skill.

A salient advance in the complete treatment of the patient with a head or neck tumor is reconstruction, usually done in the same setting as oncologic resection. Free flaps with microvascular techniques are the most appropriate methods even though they require a high level of skill and are time consuming. The free flaps most commonly used following ablative procedures in the head and neck include the ALT flap or the radial forearm flap for resurfacing the floor of the mouth and the composite fibular flap, which includes fibula as well as skin, to reconstruct the mandible and the floor of the mouth. For larger defects, judicious use of the rectus abdominis muscle, latissimus dorsi, or other musculocutaneous flaps has also been helpful. For pharyngoesophageal reconstruction, either the tubed radial forearm flap or the free jejunum is most successful.

Because no two surgical resections for tumor in the head and neck are identical, the key to effective treatment is preoperative planning. Probable extent of resection, areas that will require preoperative or postoperative radiation therapy, incision and flaps created by neck dissections, and available donor areas must all be carefully assessed. New preoperative techniques are being used that are based off of preoperative CT scanning. From these scans, templates are created that show exactly where excisions should be made, and for mandibular reconstruction, the size, and bending of the plate can all be done preoperatively.

Useful musculocutaneous flaps in the head and neck are the sternocleidomastoid, platysma, trapezius, pectoralis major, and latissimus dorsi muscles. Useful axial skin flaps can be obtained from the forehead, deltopectoral, and cervicohumeral areas. When these flaps are insufficient or unavailable for the reconstructive needs of the patient, free tissue transfer must be used. Although many flaps have been developed for bone and soft tissue reconstructions, the ALT flap (cutaneous or myocutaneous), the radial forearm flap, and the osteoseptocutaneous fibula flap are the most useful free flaps for head and neck reconstruction. Healing is quick, so radiation, if necessary, may be started as early as 1 month after surgery.

BREAST RECONSTRUCTION

Reconstruction of the female breast after mastectomy is available to all patients in the United States, and new techniques continue to be developed providing women with more options. The insurance carriers now reimburse for this procedure as part of the treatment for breast cancer, and this includes symmetry surgery of the contralateral breast. Even women with significant defects in the anterior chest wall as a result of radical mastectomy and radiation therapy can undergo reconstructive surgery if they are otherwise appropriate candidates. Breast reconstruction can be performed immediately at the time of the mastectomy or in a delayed fashion after completion of the mastectomy and any adjuvant oncologic treatments. High-risk patients may be advised to delay their breast reconstruction to minimize complication risks and avoid any potential disruption of oncologic therapy. The methods of breast reconstruction include implant-based versus autologous reconstruction.

Heightened awareness of breast cancer and well-established screening guidelines have affected surgical treatment of the cancer and, subsequently, approaches to reconstruction of the breast. A skin-sparing, modified radical mastectomy, for example, may allow for an immediate reconstruction with autologous tissue that results in an aesthetically pleasing breast mound. Nipple-sparing mastectomy can allow for aesthetically pleasing reconstructions with maximal breast skin preservation in patients who are candidates. Lumpectomy followed by irradiation (breast-conservation therapy), initially indicated for relatively small tumors, has now expanded to larger tumors and may thus result in considerable distortion and concavity in the treated breast. In the appropriate patient, concomitant oncoplastic surgery, such as tailored bilateral reduction mammoplasty or local tissue rearrangement, may allow for a large lumpectomy while maintaining symmetry and contour.

▶ Implant-Based Reconstruction

Implant-based reconstruction includes single-stage direct-to-implant reconstruction and two-stage reconstruction with tissue expander placement, which is later replaced by implants during exchange procedure. The type of implants can be silicone or saline, smooth or textured, or round or anatomic shaped ("teardrop"). Tissue expanders and implants have traditionally been placed in subpectoral position under the pectoralis major muscle. Acellular dermal matrix (ADM) has been popularized as an adjunct to tissue expander or implant-based breast reconstruction for inferior pole support and coverage. Use of ADM can allow more intraoperative fill volume, expedite the expansion process, and improve cosmetic result with better definition of the inframammary fold. In two-stage breast reconstruction, a tissue expander is placed first and then expanded with percutaneous saline injections over a series of outpatient clinic visits that can take 6 weeks to several months. Once the expansion is completed, a second-stage exchange procedure is performed to replace the tissue expander with an implant of choice (Figure 43–10). When there is sufficient native breast skin available, a single-stage direct-to-implant reconstruction can be performed by placing the desired implant immediately after mastectomy.

Most recently, prepectoral implant-based breast reconstruction has been used by placing the tissue expander or implant above the pectoralis major muscle usually in conjunction with complete anterior coverage with ADM. While prepectoral implant-based breast reconstruction has the advantage of avoiding animation deformity of the pectoralis

A

B

▲ **Figure 43–10.** Implant-based breast reconstruction. **A:** Preoperatively. **B:** Postoperative following bilateral nipple-sparing mastectomy and implant-based reconstruction.

major muscle, it can only be safely accomplished when the mastectomy flap quality is thick. Prepectoral implant-based reconstruction lacks long-term results at this time and may require secondary fat grafting procedures to improve contour.

Breast implant-associated anaplastic large-cell lymphoma (BIA-ALCL) is a very rare treatable T-cell lymphoma that can develop around breast implants. The most common clinical presentation is late-onset swelling of the breast with seroma and more rarely with a mass. More recent data suggest association of BIA-ALCL with textured implants (both cosmetic and reconstructive). Workup includes ultrasound imaging and cytology evaluation of the peri-implant fluid for CD30. Treatment ranges from removal of implants and complete capsulectomy to adjuvant therapy such as chemotherapy.

Autologous Reconstruction

Autologous reconstruction can be performed by a variety of different methods, including latissimus flap with or without implant; abdominal tissue–based flaps, including pedicled TRAM, free TRAM flap, DIEP flap, or SIEA flap; or other non–abdominal-based free flaps, including superior gluteal artery perforator, profunda artery perforator (PAP) flap, and transvers upper gracilis flaps.

The latissimus dorsi myocutaneous flap is often used with an implant for reconstruction of the breast given the limited soft tissue volume on the back. The latissimus musculocutaneous unit is freed up completely except for its insertion at the humerus, thus preserving the neurovascular pedicle. It is transposed as a pendulum through the anterior chest wall. The superior portion of the latissimus dorsi is sutured to the pectoralis major muscle, and the lower edge is secured to the lower skin flap as far down as it will reach. The implant is then inserted, having been covered by the latissimus dorsi inferiorly and by two layers of muscle superiorly, including the latissimus dorsi and the pectoralis major. The skin island is used in its entirety, if necessary, or is deepithelialized appropriately, maintaining only the skin portion that is needed. This method is most suitable for patients who do not have a large amount of abdominal skin, are relatively thin, and do not object to the use of implants. However, smaller breast reconstruction may be achieved with latissimus dorsi flap alone without an implant if there is sufficient skin paddle volume.

Abdominal tissue–based autologous breast reconstruction produces the most natural breast mound reconstruction in appearance and feel, but it requires longer operating time, hospitalization, and recovery compared to tissue expander or implant-based breast reconstruction. The TRAM flap based on the superior epigastric vessels remains the standard for breast reconstruction (Figure 43–11). The incision at the donor site is similar to that of an abdominoplasty operation along the lower abdomen.

If the superior epigastric system has been violated, such as from surgery or trauma, or if there are other factors that would question the reliability of these vessels to adequately supply the volume and region of tissue required for the reconstruction, the surgeon may favor using the inferior epigastric system and transferring the TRAM as a free flap. Typical recipient vessels are the internal mammary or the thoracodorsal vessels. Again, past surgical history, previous or planned radiation, and anatomic variance may dictate reconstructive strategy regarding recipient vessels and whether to use the ipsilateral or contralateral inferior epigastric system.

Many surgeons have sought to further refine autologous reconstruction by decreasing donor site morbidity. TRAM flap reconstruction takes the rectus abdominis muscle, which can lead to increased postoperative pain and abdominal

A

B

▲ **Figure 43–11.** Breast reconstruction autologous.
A: Preoperatively. **B:** Postoperatively following left mastectomy and immediate transverse rectus abdominis myocutaneous flap reconstruction.

wall bulge or hernia. Modifications of the free TRAM flap have been made so that the rectus abdominis muscle is mostly spared, such as a muscle-sparing TRAM, or spared in its entirety, known as a deep inferior epigastric perforator (DIEP) flap. The same skin territory as the TRAM flap is used; however, the musculocutaneous branches that supply the skin are dissected away from the rectus abdominis muscle. In this manner, the muscle itself is spared and left in situ in an effort to preserve muscular function and reduce abdominal wall weakness. The deep inferior epigastric vessels are then divided, the flap is inset into the thoracic defect, and the flap vessels are anastomosed to recipient vessels along the chest wall. An extension of the DIEP has been the SIEA (superficial inferior epigastric artery) free flap. Although feasible in only a minority of patients, this artery allows for free flap reconstruction that completely avoids any disruption of the rectus muscle. This means minimal abdominal wall complications for the patient.

Secondary Procedures

In addition to reconstruction of the affected breast, many patients undergo secondary procedures that alter the contralateral breast to achieve symmetry or to create the nipple-areola complex. Such symmetry procedures are considered stages in postoncologic breast reconstruction.

The creation of the nipple-areola complex can be performed in cases of skin-sparing mastectomy. Current techniques for nipple reconstruction use adjacent flaps from the area where the nipple is to be positioned, taking skin and variable amounts of underlying fat from the skin paddle if an autologous flap has been used or elevating skin and lesser amounts of subcutaneous tissue in an implant-based reconstruction. The areola may be reconstructed with a full-thickness skin graft or be tattooed. Recently, three-dimensional nipple-areola complex tattoos have been used to create a visually realistic nipple and areola.

Fat grafting can be performed to improve the reconstructed breast contour or add more volume in both autologous and implant-based breast reconstruction. Typically, this is done at either the time of tissue expander to implant exchange, nipple creation, or other secondary procedures. However, one may require multiple fat grafting sessions to achieve desired volume enhancement, and complications such as oil cysts and fat necrosis can occur.

Effects of Postmastectomy Radiotherapy

The use of radiation therapy has continued to become more common for the treatment of breast cancer to reduce local recurrence risk. Unfortunately, the chronic soft tissue fibrosis and vascular compromise resulting from radiotherapy lead to long-term negative impact on the breast reconstruction outcome. Implant-based reconstruction has been shown to have significantly higher complication rates when radiation therapy is involved, such as capsular contracture, infection, extrusion, and failure. Autologous flap reconstruction generally tolerates radiotherapy better; however, the negative impact still applies with flap shrinkage, fibrosis, and cosmetic compromise. Some reconstructive surgeons have advocated using this option as a delayed reconstruction about 6 months to 1 year after completion of postmastectomy radiotherapy.

Colwell AS, Christensen JM: Nipple-sparing mastectomy and direct-to-implant breast reconstruction. *Plast Reconstr Surg.* 2017;140(5S):44S-50S.

Ganske I, Verma K, Rosen H, et al: Minimizing complications with the use of acellular dermal matrix for immediate implant-based breast reconstruction. *Ann Plast Surg.* 2013;71(5):464-470.

Sbitany H, Piper M, Lentz R: Prepectoral breast reconstruction: a safe alternative to submuscular prosthetic reconstruction following nipple-sparing mastectomy. *Plast Reconstr Surg.* 2017;140(3):432-443.

Spear SL, Seruya M, Rao SS, et al: Two-stage prosthetic breast reconstruction using AlloDerm including outcomes of different timings of radiotherapy. *Plast Reconstr Surg.* 2012;130(1):1-9.

Tan BK, Joethy J, Ong YS, et al: Preferred use of the ipsilateral pedicled TRAM flap for immediate breast reconstruction: an illustrated approach. *Aesthetic Plast Surg.* 2012;36(1):128-133.

CHEST WALL RECONSTRUCTION

When evaluating a chest wall defect, the etiology, location, size, layers of chest wall involved, and patient comorbidities must be considered when developing a reconstructive plan. The etiology of the wound may be oncologic, infectious, or congenital. If necrotic, nonviable, or infectious tissue is present, it must be debrided to a clean wound bed. Typically, the thoracic skeleton is reconstructed for stability if more than four consecutive ribs are removed or if the defect is greater than 5 cm. Respiratory function may be affected and vital structures placed at risk if the skeletal structure is not reconstructed in these cases. Patients with chronic obstructive pulmonary disease may be particularly affected if their skeletal structure is not reconstructed in these cases. Conversely, if the defect is posterior, the patient may be less affected by respiratory mechanics given the more rigid construct of the remaining adjacent posterior chest. Soft tissue coverage must be provided and any dead space must be obliterated, which may require local, regional, or free tissue transfer.

Sternal wounds are commonly reconstructed by plastic surgeons after sternal nonunion, drainage, or infection from open chest surgery. Depending on the etiology of the sternal wound and defect present, a number of different reconstructive options are available. If the patient has adequate soft tissue coverage but has sternal nonunion with painful clicking on exam from rubbing of the two sternal halves from osteotomy, the patient may require sternal fixation with plating, rewiring, or zip-tie closure. If a sternal wound is present with inadequate soft tissue coverage, local flaps can be used for reconstruction including a pectoralis major turnover flap based on the internal mammary perforators, pectoralis advancement flaps based on the thoracoacromial vessels, vertical rectus abdominus myocutaneous (VRAM) flap, or omental flap. A thorough history of prior chest surgical procedures must be taken into account given that many cardiac cases use the left and/or right internal mammary arteries, and this will limit the ability to use local flaps. For example, pectoralis turnover flaps would not be feasible following internal mammary harvest since the flap is based on the internal mammary artery. However, pectoralis advancement flap based on the thoracoacromial system would be safe to use in this setting. If an infected sternal wound is present, then the wound needs to be adequately debrided in conjunction with cardiac surgery to ensure source control prior to definitive reconstruction of the wound.

ABDOMINAL WALL RECONSTRUCTION

As with any other reconstruction, patient comorbidities, nutritional status, smoking status, presence of wound infection, wound size, and layers of abdominal wall involved must be considered in abdominal wall reconstruction. Prior to reconstruction, patient comorbidities should be optimized and risk stratified for evaluation of safety of elective surgical reconstruction. Nutrition should be optimized with protein and caloric support. Blood sugar levels should be less than 110 mg/dL. Smoking and nicotine use should be stopped at least 4 weeks preoperatively.

When considering reconstruction of the fascia for abdominal wall support, materials may include prosthetic, such as polypropylene mesh, or biologic, such as ADM or acellular porcine dermis, or a composite material combining both nonabsorbable and absorbable materials. Biologic mesh is often used if there is concern for contamination, history of infection, or placement of mesh onto bowel. Disadvantages of biologic mesh are increased rates of hernia recurrence and abdominal wall laxity. Prosthetic mesh has the advantage of durable strength but the disadvantage of adhesions to bowel, increased risk of enterocutaneous fistula formation, and persistent foreign body that can become stiff, colonized, or extrude. Mesh may be placed as an underlay, overlay, or interpositional support. Underlay, where the mesh is placed deep to the edges of the fascia, provides the most reliable abdominal wall mesh repair. Overlay is where the mesh is placed superficial to the fascia. Interpositional provides the least reliable abdominal wall mesh repair, where mesh is placed between the edges of the fascia.

Component separation allows for mobilization of the abdominal wall to provide advancement of the lateral abdominal wall medially. The procedure involves the incision of aponeuroses of the abdominal wall musculature to advance the rectus muscle medially: the external oblique aponeurosis is divided, external oblique dissected from the internal oblique, and posterior sheath dissected from the posterior aspect of the rectus muscle, which allows for advancement of the rectus/internal oblique/transversus abdominis muscles medially as a unit.

If component separation does not provide adequate abdominal wall coverage, additional options such as tissue expansion, regional flaps, and free flaps can be considered. Tissue expansion is often performed with insertion of an expander under the external oblique muscles bilaterally. If a large defect is present without ability to be treated with local options, a free ALT is often considered given the large flap size that may be harvested for coverage.

Boukovalas S, Sisk G, Selber JC: Abdominal wall reconstruction: an integrated approach. *Semin Plast Surg.* 2018;32(3):107-119.

PERINEAL RECONSTRUCTION

Perineal coverage, as with other types of reconstructive planning, requires consideration of patient comorbidities, wound size, location and layers of defect, and presence of infection. Many perineal wounds are from oncologic resection and often involve radiated wounds that require movement of nonradiated, well-vascularized tissue into the wound. Given the location of the wound, colonization with bacteria and yeast is common and risk for infection and wound breakdown is high. Wounds must be adequately debrided and source control must be obtained prior to reconstruction. Local pedicled flaps are often used to bring healthy, well-vascularized tissue into the area. Depending on the exact size and location of the wound, pedicled flaps, including the gracilis muscle flap with or without a skin paddle, pedicled ALT flap, pedicled VRAM flap with or without a skin paddle, and pudendal artery perforator flaps, can be used. Temporary urinary or fecal diversion may be necessary to prevent infection and/or breakdown of the reconstructed wound.

Weichman KE, Matros E, Disa JJ: Reconstruction of peripelvic oncologic defects. *Plast Reconstr Surg.* 2017;140(4):601e-612e.

LOWER EXTREMITY RECONSTRUCTION & SALVAGE

Probably one of the most difficult areas for which to provide wound coverage and closure is the lower extremity, particularly the distal leg and foot areas. Tenuous and unstable skin grafts or poorly vascularized local or cross-leg skin flaps were once the only tissues available for resurfacing of these parts of the body. When large segments of bone were exposed or missing or when infection had become established, these grafts or flaps often were inadequate and amputation was the only recourse. Use of musculocutaneous flaps, and particularly free flaps, has greatly improved coverage in the lower extremities.

Generally, wound problems in the lower leg, ankle, and foot involve orthopedic injuries, such as compound tibial or ankle fractures. Multiple classification systems are used, but the most popular are the Gustilo and Byrd systems. These take into account the degree of fracture as well as tissue loss and nerve and arterial involvement.

▶ Treatment

Treatment depends on the extent of tissue loss and the depth of the wound. Fairly extensive wounds around the knee and upper third of the leg can be reconstructed with a gastrocnemius muscle flap (usually the medial head) and a split-thickness skin graft. Soft tissue defects of the middle third of the leg can be reconstructed in a similar manner by the soleus muscle in many cases. Large middle third and distal third soft tissue defects are more difficult to reconstruct.

When they are complicated by extensive bone and soft tissue loss, free tissue transfer may be necessary. Although there are small muscles that end in tendons in the foot, such as the peroneus brevis, flexor hallucis longus, and extensor digitorum muscles, they can provide only limited coverage. If there is a suitable recipient artery remaining in the leg, better coverage is generally provided by a free muscle flap such as the gracilis muscle for small and medium-sized defects or the latissimus dorsi or rectus abdominis muscle for larger defects.

Large areas of the heel or the sole of the foot are difficult to replace because skin in these regions is specially adapted to bear the weight of the body without shearing or breaking down. Free muscle flaps surfaced with skin grafts have proven to be adequate, but protective sensation is missing. The use of free neurovascular axial skin flaps, such as the inferior gluteal thigh flap and the deltoid flap, may help provide coverage with some gross sensation. Neurosensory flaps—and specifically the sural flap, distally based on one of the lower septocutaneous perforators from the lateral aspect of the leg and supplied by the sural artery, which accompanies the sural nerve—have been used to resurface defects around the ankle and heel. The procedure provides good skin and fascia for a weight-bearing area such as the heel, but it usually does not provide protective sensibility.

Segmental defects of the tibia may be reconstructed with bone grafts or, if the gap is large, free bone flaps such as the contralateral fibula or iliac crest. It is also possible to reconstruct the soft tissue defect and then reconstruct the bony gap with a distraction osteogenesis technique (Ilizarov bone transport). This bone transport method consists of performing a cortical osteotomy proximal to the site of injury and then applying a distraction apparatus, which in effect lengthens the bone 1 mm per day by appropriate adjustment screws. Such lower extremity reconstruction requires a well-coordinated, cooperative effort between the plastic and orthopedic surgeons. Amputation may be recommended in cases with a constellation of extensive vascular injury, greater than 6 hours of warm ischemia time with irreversible damage to soft tissue, or a medically unstable patient. Prior indications for amputation, including loss of tibial sensation, are no longer absolute contraindications to replantation. The LEAP Study, or Lower Extremity Assessment Project, found that the greatest indicator of poor limb salvage outcomes was a poor social support network.

Osteomyelitis of the tibia or bones in the foot may be devastating and often uncontrollable. Probably because of poor vascularity in the area, even long-term antibiotic treatment has often failed to control bone infections in the leg. Recently, effective surgical treatment for bone infections has been developed. The bone is surgically debrided and covered with a microvascular free muscle flap such as the gracilis or rectus abdominis muscle. Apparently, the muscle tissue with its excellent blood supply not only covers the exposed bone but also assists natural defenses in controlling infection.

Antibiotics are also used, but the well-vascularized muscle flap appears to be the deciding factor in control of infection. Reconstruction of bony defects may be accomplished at a later date.

Higgins TF, Klatt JB, Beals TC: Lower Extremity Assessment Project (LEAP): the best available evidence on limb-threatening lower extremity trauma. *Orthop Clin North Am.* 2010;41(2):233-239.

NEUROMA PREVENTION & TREATMENT

Neuromas are disorganized bulbous nerve endings resulting from traumatic nerve injury and attempted growth of the nerve end to achieve repair. If a distal target is not present or available, the nerve ending has disorganized axonal sprouting. Often painful on presentation, neuromas can cause significant discomfort and disability to a patient. Traditionally, treatment of neuroma or attempted prevention of neuroma in amputation procedures has involved nerve end avulsion, crushing, cautery, or insertion into muscle. These methods unfortunately have high rates of neuroma development.

Newer methods of neuroma prevention include targeted muscle reinnervation and regenerative peripheral nerve interfaces. Targeted muscle reinnervation (TMR) involves selected growth of the cut nerve end into a motor nerve with ending in muscle. The motor nerve provides a pathway such that axonal sprouting is directed and prevents the disorganized growth of a neuroma. TMR can be performed preferably at the time of amputation to prevent neuroma growth or after neuroma has formed as a neuroma treatment. Regenerative peripheral nerve interfaces (RPNI) involve treatment or prevention of a neuroma with sharp excision and wrapping with a free muscle graft around a nerve end, providing a target for axonal growth. Amputees have experienced an approximate 70% reduction in neuroma symptoms after RPNI. Additionally, RPNI has been used for amplification of nerve signals for use of smart prosthetics. Both TMR and RPNI are in early stages of data collection but offer promising treatment modalities based on early results.

Woo SL, Kung TA, Brown DL, et al: Regenerative peripheral nerve interfaces for the treatment of postamputation neuroma pain: a pilot study. *Plast Reconstr Surg Glob Open.* 2016;4(12):e1038.

TRANSGENDER RECONSTRUCTION

Reconstruction of transgender patients is becoming increasingly more prevalent. Collaboration between medical teams is essential to ensure success with transgender surgery. Primary care, endocrinology, psychiatry, urology, gynecology, and plastic surgery are often involved in the multidisciplinary care of transgender patients. Different sets of guidelines have been developed to establish standard of care for transgender surgery, which often include living in society as a transgender person for at least 2 years, diagnosis of gender dysmorphia by at least two psychiatrists, and negative workup for a medical cause such as chromosomal, physical, or psychological abnormalities. Appropriate patient selection must be considered with a multidisciplinary approach to ensure patients have the appropriate support both at home and within the hospital.

Patients may elect to undergo no medical or surgical treatment; only hormonal/medical treatment; surgical treatment of one of multiple aspects of the body including facial surgery, "top surgery," or chest surgery; or genital/reproductive organ surgery.

Transgender female-to-male patients may take testosterone, which leads to significant changes in hormonal cycles as well as facial and body hirsutism. "Top surgery" includes performing bilateral mastectomies, either through a double incision with free nipple grafts or periareolar mastectomies. The goal of this procedure is to create a more muscular-appearing chest with removal of breast tissue, chest soft tissue contouring, and reduction and lateralization of the nipple-areola complex. Procedures to alter genitals and/or reproductive organs may include hysterectomy, vaginectomy, and creation of a neophallus. When a neophallus is created, urethral lengthening must be performed to allow connection of the native urethra to the urethroplasty within the neophallus. Different options can be used for phallus creation, which most commonly include a neurotized free radial forearm flap or pedicled ALT flap. At a later date, once the neophallus flap has healed, a prosthetic can be placed to allow for erection. Urology, gynecology, and plastic surgery must all be involved in these procedures given each expertise is required for successful reconstruction.

Transgender male-to-female patients may take estrogen or other hormonal therapy for feminization. Facial feminization includes facial contour procedures such as cheek and chin implants, reduction of prominent brow, reduction of thyroid cartilage, and rhinoplasty. Breast augmentation in one or two stages with tissue expander reconstruction allows for feminization of the chest. The difficulty with feminization of the male chest is that most cis-males have a broad chest compared to cis-females. Although less common than facial feminization or breast surgery, genital surgery can be performed where the penis can be inverted or bowel used to create a vaginal wall.

Schechter LS, Safa B: Introduction to phalloplasty. *Clin Plast Surg.* 2018;45(3):387-389.

▼ V. CRANIOFACIAL SURGERY

Craniofacial surgery includes procedures performed on patients of all ages, from pediatric to adult, and for many indications, from congenital defects to trauma and oncologic reconstruction.

TRAUMA

Because of the aesthetic and functional importance of the face, fractures of the facial bones, although rarely life threatening, are best treated by surgeons who have extensive experience with facial injuries and reconstruction. Soft tissue injury should be treated immediately with washout and repair; facial fractures should be treated within the first 7-10 days. If facial bone fracture fixation is not needed emergently, then allowing for facial edema to improve can be beneficial for exposure of the repair.

Facial bone fractures are usually caused by trauma from a blunt instrument, such as a fist or club, or by violent contact with the steering wheel, dashboard, or windshield during an automobile accident. Particularly in the latter case, the patient should be assessed for associated injuries. For example, cervical spine injuries are present in up to 12% of automobile accident patients and should be treated or stabilized before facial bone injuries are attended to. Injuries to the brain, eyes, chest, abdomen, and extremities must also be assessed and may require earlier treatment.

The diagnosis of facial fractures is made primarily on clinical examination. Ideally, the examination should be done immediately so that swelling will not obscure the findings. The mechanism and the line of direction of injury are important. If conscious, the patient should be asked about previous facial injuries, areas of pain and numbness, whether the jaw opens properly and the teeth come together normally, and whether vision in all quadrants is normal.

Most facial fractures can be palpated, or at least the abnormal position of bones can be noted. Beginning along the mandibular rims, one can feel for irregularities of the facial bones. The dental occlusion is noted. With bimanual palpation, placing the thumbs inside the mouth, one can elicit bony crepitus if there is an associated fracture. The maxilla and mid face can be rocked forward and backward between the thumb and the index finger in the presence of a midfacial fracture. Nasal fractures may be detected by palpation. Irregularities and step-offs along the infraorbital border, lateral orbital rim, or zygomatic arch regions indicate a depressed zygomatic fracture.

Radiologic studies are additional aids to the proper diagnosis of facial fractures. Rarely is a significant fracture seen on x-ray that is not also clinically evident. Helpful views include the Waters and submentovertex projections and oblique views of the mandible. The panorex view of the mandible is very useful to look at the condyles. CT scans of facial bones, with appropriate biplanar and three-dimensional reconstructions so that bones can be viewed through several planes, have essentially supplanted regular radiographs in the workup of the facially injured patient. They are helpful in assessing the extent of fractures, in particular in more posterior areas such as the ethmoid area, medial and inferior orbit, pterygoid plates, and base of the skull.

The bones of the nose are the most commonly fractured facial bones. Next in frequency are the mandible, the zygomatic-malar bones, and the maxilla.

▶ Frontal Bone Fractures

Frontal bone fractures require high-energy trauma, with a force of 800-1600 pounds. The frontal bone is composed of anterior and posterior tables that form the frontal sinus. The frontal sinus drains through the nasofrontal duct into the middle meatus of the nose. Treatment of frontal bone fractures is dependent on whether the fracture includes the anterior table and/or posterior table, the degree of fracture displacement, and involvement of the nasofrontal duct. If the anterior table is nondisplaced, then no operative intervention is necessary. If the anterior table is displaced with no posterior table involvement, then the anterior table can undergo reduction and stabilization. If the frontal duct is involved, the frontal sinus must undergo removal of mucosal lining and obliteration of the sinus to prevent mucocele. If the posterior table is displaced more than one width of the posterior table, then dural tear is more likely, which may be associated with cerebrospinal fluid (CSF) leak. Neurosurgery should be consulted if there is a concern for CSF leak, which may be indicated with rhinorrhea and posterior table displacement. If CSF leak does not resolve with more conservative measures or a lumboperitoneal shunt, cranialization may need to be performed in which the posterior table is removed, ducts are obliterated, and nasal and cranial cavities are separated with a pericranial flap.

▶ Nasal Fractures

Fractures may affect the nasal bones, cartilage, and septum. Fractures occur in two patterns, caused by lateral or head-on trauma. With lateral trauma, the nasal bone on the side of the injury is fractured and displaced toward the septum, the septum is deviated and fractured, and the nasal bone on the side away from the injury is fractured and displaced away from the septum, so that the upper part of the nose, as a whole, is deviated. Depending on the degree of violence, one or more of these displacements will be present, and the degree of comminution is variable. Head-on trauma gives rise to telescoping and saddling of the nose and broadening of its upper half as a result of the depression and splaying of the fractured nasal bones. This of course produces severe damage to the septum, which usually buckles or actually suffers a fracture.

Nasal fractures requiring reduction should be treated with a minimal delay because they tend to become fixed in the displaced position in a few days. The surgical approach depends on whether the fracture has resulted in deviation or collapse of the nasal bones. Local anesthesia is preferred; either topical tetracaine or cocaine intranasally or lidocaine for infiltration of the skin can be used. The nasal bones may be disimpacted with intranasal forceps or a periosteal elevator and aligned by external molding or pressure. Collapsed nasal fractures can be repositioned with Walsham nasal forceps, introduced into each nostril and placed on each side of the septum, which is then elevated to its proper position. A septal hematoma should be recognized and drained to prevent infection and subsequent necrosis of the cartilaginous septum with associated collapse of the entire nose. Compound fractures of the nose require prompt repair of the skin wound and, if possible, early reduction of the displaced nasal bones.

External splinting, which is essentially a protective dressing, and intranasal packing using nonadhering gauze are appropriate after reduction. The intranasal packing provides support for the septum in its reduced position and helps prevent development of a hematoma. It also provides counter-pressure for the external splint immobilizing the nasal bones and prevents them from collapsing. The packing is usually removed within 48 hours.

In severe comminuted nasal fractures, the medial canthal ligaments, which are easily felt by applying lateral traction to the upper eyelid, may have dislodged. If they have been avulsed, they should be reattached in position to prevent late deformities. For these severe fractures involving the entire naso-orbital ethmoid complex, the coronal approach, which offers wide exposure, allows for proper anatomic reduction of all small nasal fragments as well as repositioning of the canthal ligaments and correction and elevation of the tele-scoped bone fragments at the root of the nose and glabella. The lacrimal apparatus is commonly disrupted in these injuries and should be repaired and stented appropriately.

Mandibular Fractures

Mandibular fractures are most commonly bilateral, generally occurring in the region of the mid body at the mental foramen, the angle of the ramus, or the neck of the condyle. A frequent combination is a fracture at the mental region of the body with a condylar fracture on the opposite side. Displacement of the fragments results from the force of the external blow as well as the pull of the muscles of the floor of the mouth and the muscles of mastication. The diagnosis is suggested by derangement of dental occlusion associated with local pain, swelling, and often crepitation upon palpation. Appropriate x-rays confirm the diagnosis. Special views of the condyle, including tomograms, may be required. Sublingual hematoma and acute malocclusion are usually diagnostic of a mandibular fracture.

Restoration of functional dental occlusion is the most important consideration in treating mandibular fractures. In patients with an adequate complement of teeth, arch bars or interdental wires can be placed. Local nerve block anesthesia is preferable for this procedure, though certain patients may require general anesthesia. Intermaxillary elastic traction will usually correct minor degrees of displacement and bring the

teeth into normal occlusion by overcoming the muscle pull. When the fracture involves the base of a tooth socket with suspected devitalization of the tooth, extraction of the tooth should be considered. Particularly in the incisor region, such devitalized teeth may be a source of infection, leading to the development of osteomyelitis and nonunion of the fracture.

Patients with more severe mandibular injuries require anatomic reduction and fixation of the fracture by the open, direct technique. These include compound, comminuted, and unfavorable fractures. An unfavorable fracture is one that is inherently unstable because muscle pull distracts the fracture segments. In this situation, intermaxillary fixation alone is insufficient. Edentulous patients also benefit from the open technique, although proper dentures or dental splints are useful to maintain normal occlusion.

Metal wire fixation of fractured segments and intermaxillary fixation for 6 weeks was a proven and popular method of fracture treatment. The more recent resurgence in popularity of the screw-plate system is due to a number of advantages over wiring. The screw plate usually achieves rigid fixation in three dimensions, providing adequate stability; it eliminates the need for intermaxillary fixation in most cases; it is useful in complex, comminuted fractures; and it is quite easy to use after familiarity with the technique has been acquired.

With bilateral parasymphyseal fractures, anterior stabilization of the tongue may be lost, so that it may fall back and obstruct the airway. Anterior stabilization and splinting must be accomplished early in these cases.

Open reduction is rarely advised in condylar fractures; simple intermaxillary fixation for 4-6 weeks is sufficient. Indications for open reduction are severely displaced fractures, which may prevent motion of the mandible because of impingement of the coronoid process on the zygomatic arch. The endoscopic approach has increasingly been used for repair of condylar fractures. In children, the fracture may destroy the growth center of the condyle, resulting in maldevelopment of the mandible and gross distortion.

Zygomatic and Orbital Floor Fractures

Fractures of the zygomatic bones may involve just the arch of the zygomatic bone or the entire body of the zygoma, which forms the malar eminence, and the lateral wall and floor of the orbit. The "tripod fracture" characteristically occurs at the frontozygomatic and zygomaticomaxillary sutures as well as at the arch. However, it should be referred to as a tetrapod fracture because the anterior or posterior buttress of the maxilla is also involved in the fracture. Displacement of the body of the zygoma results in flattening of the cheek and depression of the orbital rim and floor.

Important diagnostic signs are subconjunctival hemorrhage; disturbances of extraocular muscle function, which may be accompanied by diplopia; and loss of sensation in the upper lip and alveoli on the involved side as a result of injury to the infraorbital nerve. Reduction of a displaced zygomatic fracture is seldom an emergency procedure and may be delayed until the patient's general condition is satisfactory for anesthesia. Local anesthesia will suffice only for reduction of fractures of the zygomatic arch. More extensively displaced fractures usually require general anesthesia. At least two-point fixation with direct interosseous wiring is necessary for these fractures. Here, again, delicate miniplates have been used with success, providing anatomic reduction and rigid fixation.

Simple depressed fractures of the zygomatic arch can best be elevated using the Gillies technique. Through a temporal incision above the hairline, an instrument is passed beneath the superficial layer of the deep temporalis fascia and under the arch and the body of the zygoma. The fracture can also be elevated percutaneously with a hook or screw in conjunction with overlying palpation to achieve accurate reduction. If the fracture is complex or comminuted, as is often the case with high-velocity injuries, repair through a coronal scalp approach may be necessary to obtain an anatomic and stable result.

Extensive disruption should be suspected in conjunction with the zygomatic fracture when significant diplopia and enophthalmos and posterior displacement of the globe are present. Orbital fat and extraocular muscles may herniate through the defect and become entrapped, giving rise to the signs and symptoms. A "blowout" fracture is similar disruption of the orbital floor due to blunt trauma to the globe but not associated with a fracture of the zygoma or orbital rim. Treatment in both cases demands exploration, reduction of herniated contents, and repair of the floor. The most direct approach is through a lower lid subciliary incision, which provides excellent visualization. A buccal transantral approach can be used, and blind antral packing for support has been described. This is quite hazardous, because bony spicules may be pushed into the ocular globe and perhaps cause injury or blindness. In cases of extensive communication or loss of bony fragments of the floor, use of local autogenous bone or cartilage as a scaffold may be performed. At times, in cases of extensive injuries to the floor, alloplastic material in the form of titanium mesh may be necessary.

Even with careful anatomic reduction and repair of the orbital floor, ocular problems such as enophthalmos may persist, possibly due to an undiagnosed fracture, such as a medial ethmoidal blowout fracture. These can be properly evaluated with CT scanning. Treatment requires reduction and repair of the defect. The injury can at times cause ischemia of herniated soft tissue and subsequent atrophy and scarring. This may result in enophthalmos, which is almost impossible to resolve completely.

Maxillary Fractures

Maxillary fractures range in complexity from partial fractures through the alveolar process to extensive displacement of the midfacial structures in conjunction with fractures of the frontonasal bones and orbital maxillary region and total craniofacial separation. Hemorrhage and airway obstruction require emergency care, and in severe cases, tracheostomy is indicated. Mobility of the maxilla can be elicited by palpation in extensive fractures. "Dish-face" deformity of the retrodisplaced maxilla may be disguised by edema, and CT may be necessary to determine the extent and complexity of the midfacial fracture. Treatment may have to be delayed because of other severe injuries. A delay of as long as 10-14 days may be safe before reduction and fixation, but the earliest possible restoration of maxillary position and dental occlusion is desirable to prevent late complications.

In the case of unilateral fractures or bilateral fractures with little or no displacement, splinting by intermaxillary fixation for 4 weeks may suffice. Fractures are usually displaced inferiorly or posteriorly and require direct surgical disimpaction and reduction and proper fixation with appropriate plates and screws. Early reduction may help control bleeding, as torn, stretched vessels are allowed to reestablish their normal tension. In certain severe cases, external traction may be necessary. Manipulation is directed toward restoring normal occlusion and maintaining the reduction with intermaxillary fixation to the mandible in association with direct plate fixation. Complicated fractures may require external fixation using a head cap and intraoral splints in conjunction with multiple surgical incisions for direct plate fixation. Coexisting mandibular fractures usually necessitate open reduction and fixation at the same time.

LeFort Fractures

LeFort fractures are midface fractures classified based on the fracture patterns: I, II, and III. The LeFort I fracture is a transverse fracture separating the inferior portion of the maxilla from the midface extending from the piriform aperture through the pterygoid plates. The LeFort II fracture is a pyramidal fracture that separates the maxilla and nasal complex from the cranium, traveling along the zygomatic orbital rim and through the pterygoid plates. The LeFort III fracture, also known as total craniofacial separation, is a fracture that separates the midface from the cranium, through the naso-orbital ethmoid complex, and extending through the orbits, zygomaticofrontal suture, and pterygoid plates. All LeFort fractures include fracture through the pterygoid plates.

Kim HS, Jeong EC: Orbital floor fracture. *Arch Craniofac Surg.* 2016;17(3):111-118.

Kyzas PA, Saeed A, Tabbenor O: The treatment of mandibular condyle fractures: a meta-analysis. *J Craniomaxillofacial Surg.* 2012;40(8):e438-452.

CONGENITAL

▶ Cleft Lip & Cleft Palate

Cleft lip, cleft palate, and combinations of the two are the most common congenital anomalies of the head and neck. The incidence of facial clefts has been reported to be 1 in every 650-750 live births, making this deformity second only to clubfoot in frequency as a reported birth defect.

The cleft may involve the floor of the nostril and lip on one or both sides and may extend through the alveolus, the hard palate, and the entire soft palate. A useful classification based on embryologic and anatomic aspects divides the structures into the primary and secondary palate. The dividing point between the primary palate anteriorly and the secondary palate posteriorly is the incisive foramen. Clefts can thus be classified as partial or complete clefts of the primary or secondary palate in various combinations. The most common clefts are left unilateral complete clefts of the primary and secondary palate and partial midline clefts of the secondary palate, involving the soft palate and part of the hard palate.

Most infants with cleft palate present some feeding difficulties, and breastfeeding may be impossible. As a rule, enlarging the openings in an artificial nipple or using a syringe with a soft rubber feeding tube will solve difficulties in sucking. Feeding in the upright position helps prevent oronasal reflux or aspiration. Severe feeding and breathing problems and recurrent aspiration are seen in Pierre Robin sequence, in which the palatal cleft is associated with a receding lower jaw and posterior and cephalic displacement of the tongue, obstructing the naso-oropharyngeal airway. This is a medical emergency and is a cause of sudden infant death syndrome. Nonsurgical treatment includes pulling the tongue forward with an instrument and laying the baby prone with a towel under the chest to let the mandible and tongue drop forward. Insertion of a small (No. 8) nasogastric tube into the pharynx may temporarily prevent respiratory distress and may be used to supplement the baby's feedings. Placement of an acrylic obturator or appliance has proved quite successful in alleviating the breathing difficulties by bringing the tongue down and permitting a better nasal airway. Several surgical procedures that bring the tongue and mandible forward have been described but should be employed only when conservative measures have been tried without success. Recently, the use of distraction of the mandible has shown some beneficial effects. However, it should be done with great caution in the neonate.

A. Treatment

Surgical repair of cleft lip is not considered an emergency. The optimal time for operation can be described as the widely accepted "rule of 10." This includes body weight of 10 lb (4.5 kg) or more and a hemoglobin of 10 g/dL or more. This is usually at some time after the 10th week of life. In most cases, closure of the lip will mold distortions of the cleft alveolus into a satisfactory contour. In occasional cases in which there is marked distortion of the alveolus, such as in severe bilateral clefts with marked protrusion of the premaxilla, preliminary maxillary orthodontic treatment may be indicated. This may involve the use of carefully crafted appliances or simple constant pressure by use of an elastic band.

General endotracheal anesthesia via an orally placed endotracheal tube is the anesthetic technique of choice. A variety of techniques for repair of unilateral clefts have evolved over many years. Earlier procedures ignored anatomic landmarks and resulted in a characteristic "repaired harelip" look. The Millard rotation advancement operation that is now commonly used for repair employs an incision in the medial side of the cleft to allow the Cupid's bow of the lip to be rotated down to a normal position. The resulting gap in the medial side of the cleft is filled by advancing a flap from the lateral side. This principle can be varied in placement of the incisions and results in most cases in a symmetric lip with normally placed landmarks. Bilateral clefts, because of greater deficiency of tissue, present more challenging technical problems. Maximum preservation of available tissue is the underlying principle, and most surgeons prefer approximation of the central and lateral lip elements in a straight-line closure, rolling up the vermilion border of the lip (Manchester repair).

Secondary revisions are frequently necessary in the older child with a repaired cleft lip. A constant associated deformity in patients with cleft lip is distortion of the soft tissue and cartilage structures of the ala and dome of the nose. These patients often present with deficiency of growth of the structures of the mid face. This has been attributed to intrinsic growth disturbances and to external pressures from the lip and palate repairs. Some correction of these deformities, especially of the nose, can be done at the initial lip operation. More definitive correction is done after the cartilage and bone growth is more complete. These may include scar revisions and rearrangement of the cartilage structure of the nose. Recent approaches involve degloving of the nasal skin envelope with complete exposure of the abnormal cartilage framework. These are then rearranged in proper position with or without additional grafts. Maxillary osteotomies, with LeFort I with advancement, will substantially correct the midfacial depression. A tight upper lip due to severe tissue deficiency can be corrected by a two-stage transfer of a lower lip flap known as an Abbe flap.

In utero repair of cleft lip deformities has recently become a topic of discussion. In utero repair affords the potential to provide a scarless repair and correct the primary deformity. Furthermore, scarless fetal lip and palate repairs may prevent the ripple effect of postnatal scarring with its resultant secondary dentoalveolar and midface growth deformities. While these suggestions make in utero repair attractive, the risk of fetal loss remains high. Preterm labor is a major complication and one that is directly related to the large hysterotomy required for fetal exposure. Due to the great risks associated with it, intrauterine fetal surgery is still largely reserved for severe malformations that cannot be helped significantly by postnatal intervention.

Palatal clefts may involve the alveolus, the bony hard palate, or the soft palate, singly or in any combination. Clefts of the hard palate and alveolus may be either unilateral or bilateral, whereas the soft palate cleft is always midline, extending back through the uvula. The width of the cleft varies greatly, making the amount of tissue available for repair also variable. The bony palate, with its mucoperiosteal lining, forms the roof of the anterior mouth and the floor of the nose. The posteriorly attached soft palate is composed of five paired muscles of speech and swallowing.

Surgical closure of the cleft to allow for normal speech is the treatment of choice. The timetable for closure depends on the size of the cleft and any other associated problems. However, the defect should be closed before the child undertakes serious speech, usually before age 2. Closure at 6 months usually is performed without difficulty and also aids in the child's feeding. If the soft palate seems to be long enough, simple approximation of the freshened edges of the cleft after freeing of the tissues through lateral relaxing incisions may suffice. If the soft palate is too short, a pushback type of operation is required. In this procedure, the short soft palate is retrodisplaced closer to the posterior pharyngeal wall utilizing the mucoperiosteal flaps based on the posterior palatine artery.

Satisfactory speech following surgical repair of cleft palate is achieved in 70%-90% of cases. Significant speech defects usually require secondary operations when the child is older. The most widely used technique is the pharyngeal flap operation, in which the palatopharyngeal space is reduced by attaching a flap of posterior pharyngeal muscle and mucosa to the soft palate. This permits voluntary closure of the velopharyngeal complex and thus avoids hypernasal speech. Various other kinds of pharyngoplasties have been useful in selected cases.

Fisher DM, Sommerlad BC: Cleft lip, cleft palate, and velopharyngeal insufficiency. *Plast Reconstr Surg.* 2011;128(4):342e-360e.

Mulliken JB: Repair of bilateral cleft lip and its variants. *Indian J Plast Surg.* 2009;42(suppl):S79-S90.

▶ Craniofacial Anomalies

These are congenital deformities of the hard and soft tissues of the head. Particular problems of the brain, eye, and internal ear are treated by the appropriate specialist. The craniofacial surgeon often needs the collaboration of these specialists when operating on such patients.

Serious craniofacial anomalies are relatively rare, although mild forms often go undiagnosed or are accepted as normal variants. A classification is therefore difficult, although many have been proposed. Tessier has offered a numerical

classification based on clinical presentation (Figure 43–12). He considers a cleft to be the basis of the malformation, which involves both hard and soft tissues. Other classifications are based on embryologic and etiologic features. With greater understanding and continued investigation, classification efforts will no doubt be more satisfactory.

There are well-known chromosomal and genetic aberrations as well as environmental causes that can lead to craniofacial deformity. The cause in most cases, however, is unknown. Arrest in the migration and proliferation of neural crest cells and defects in differentiation characterize most of these deformities. We describe some of the more common ones in brief terms.

Crouzon syndrome (craniofacial dysostosis) and Apert syndrome (acrocephalosyndactyly) are closely related, differing in the extremity deformities present in Apert syndrome. Both are caused by autosomal dominant mutations of *FGFR2* with variable expression. Both present with skull deformities due to premature closure of the cranial sutures. The cranial sutures most affected will determine the type of skull deformity. Exophthalmos, midfacial hypoplasia, and hypertelorism are also features of these two syndromes. Apert syndrome patients have syndactyly of both upper and lower extremities that requires syndactyly release with small local tissue flaps and skin grafts.

The facial organs and tissues proceed in great measure from the first and second branchial arches and the first branchial cleft. Disorders in their development lead to a spectrum of anomalies of variable severity. Treacher Collins syndrome (mandibulofacial dysostosis) is a severe disorder characterized by hypoplasia of the malar bones and lower eyelids, colobomas, and antimongoloid slant of the palpebrae. The mandible and ears are often quite underdeveloped. The presentation is bilateral and is an autosomal dominant trait. A unilateral deformity known as hemifacial microsomia presents with progressive skeletal and soft tissue underdevelopment. Hemifacial microsomia can be associated with upper bulbar dermoids, notching of the upper eyelids, and vertebral anomalies.

Some of these patients show mental delay, but in most cases, intelligence is not affected. The psychosocial problems are serious and most often related to how the patients look. Within the past two decades, craniofacial surgery has progressed so that previously untreatable deformities can now be corrected. With the anatomic work of LeFort as a basis, and guided by the incomplete attempts of Gillies and others, Paul Tessier, in the late 1960s, proposed a set of surgical techniques to correct major craniofacial deformities. Two basic concepts soon emerged from his work: (1) large segments of the craniofacial skeleton can be completely denuded of their blood supply, repositioned, and yet survive and heal; and (2) the eyes can be translocated horizontally or vertically over a considerable distance with no adverse effect on vision. The tendency today is to operate at approximately

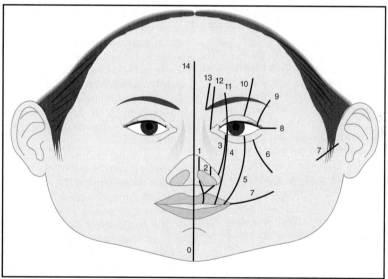

▲ **Figure 43–12.** Tessier classification of craniofacial clefts.

6-9 months of age for cranial vault remodeling and fronto-orbital advancement.

A coronal scalp incision is used to expose the skull and facial bones with an intracranial or extracranial approach. The cut bones are then reshaped, repositioned, and fixed with a combination of wires or miniplates and screws. The latter have the advantage of rigid fixation and less need to maintain large movements with bone grafts. Autogenous

inlay and onlay bone grafts can be used to improve contour. The entire operation is usually completed in one stage, and complications are surprisingly few. Miniplates have been used extensively in the past few years. In infants, fixation with absorbable suture material or the newer absorbable plates and screws has provided effective and stable fixation. They commonly resorb at 6-9 months. They do not interfere with imaging techniques such as CT or MRI, and they seem to have less impairment of craniofacial growth and development.

Craniofacial surgery has improved the treatment not only of major congenital deformities, but also of major complex facial fractures, chronic sequelae of trauma, isolated exophthalmos, fibrous dysplasia, and aesthetic facial sculpturing.

▶ Microtia

Microtia is absence or hypoplasia of the pinna of the ear, with a blind or absent external auditory meatus. The incidence of significant auricular deformity is about 1 in 8000 births and is usually spontaneous. Ten percent of these defects are bilateral, and boys are afflicted twice or three times as commonly as girls. Because the ear arises from the first and second branchial arches, the middle ear is always involved, and many patients have other disorders of the first and second arches. The inner ear structures are usually spared. Generally, correction of conductive hearing by an otologist has not been long lasting or helpful, and surgery for this problem is reserved for bilateral cases.

Different techniques have been described that vary in terms of required surgeries as well as technical complexity. The Brent and Nagata techniques are the most commonly used today, with the Brent technique requiring four stages and the Nagata only two. In any case, reconstruction of the external ear usually involves a multistage procedure beginning at preschool age. Autogenous rib cartilage or cartilage from the opposite ear is used to construct a framework to replace the absent ear. The cartilage is imbedded under the skin in the appropriate area, and after adjustments are made in local tissue to reposition or recreate the earlobe and conchal cavity, the framework is elevated posteriorly and the resulting sulcus grafted to obtain projection. In cases in which local tissue is poor or unavailable, the neighboring superficial temporalis fascia is dissected and placed over the cartilage framework. This is then skin grafted with adequate tissue.

The contralateral normal ear is occasionally altered to provide better symmetry. Excellent results have been achieved. Silastic frameworks for ear cartilage have also been used, and although their use eliminates donor site problems, rates of infection and extrusion have been unacceptable. More recently, a porous polyethylene construct has been used with better long-term results. A temporalis fascia flap is rotated to cover the allograft, and then a full-thickness skin graft is placed. They are quite useful in bilateral cases or when sufficient cartilage is not available.

Lesser deformities, such as overly large, prominent, or bent ears, are corrected by appropriate resection of skin and cartilage, "scoring" of the cartilage to alter its curve, and placement sutures to aid in contouring.

Cho BC, Kim JY, Byun JS: Two-stage reconstruction of the auricle in congenital microtia using autogenous costal cartilage. *J Plast Reconstr Aesthet Surg.* 2007;60(9):998-1006.

▼ VI. HAND SURGERY

Surgeons from both plastic surgery and orthopedic surgery specialize in hand surgery. Procedures in the field vary widely and can include treatment of trauma, nerve compression and injury, arthritis, tumor, and vascular, transplant, and congenital disorders. Knowledge of anatomy is essential in understanding hand surgery.

HAND EXAM

The hand exam can be broken into five main categories: (1) vascular perfusion, (2) nerve, (3) tendon, (4) soft tissue, and (5) bone.

Vascular perfusion is best evaluated through (1) color and capillary refill; (2) pulse oximetry, during which all digits should be evaluated to look for discrepancies; (3) palpable radial and ulnar pulse; (4) handheld Doppler examination of radial, ulnar, palmar arch, and ulnar and radial digital vascular bundles; and (5) the Allen test, which determines perfusion through the radial and ulnar arteries and can be performed with or without the Doppler.

Nerves should be evaluated for both sensory and motor function. Sensation in the radial (radial dorsal aspect of the hand and dorsal thumb, index, middle, and radial half of dorsal ring finger), median (volar thumb, index, middle, and radial side of volar ring finger), and ulnar (ulnar half of ring finger and all of small finger) nerve distributions should be tested in addition to radial and ulnar aspects of each digit. Sensation can be tested with light touch, sharp touch, and two-point static or dynamic discrimination. Motor function should be tested in radial, median, and ulnar nerve distributions.

Tendon function should be isolated when tested. For example, if there is suspected injury to the extensor pollicis longus, place the hand flat on the table and ask the patient to lift his or her thumb off the table. Tendon exam will be dependent on the concerned area of trauma or pathology.

The soft tissue of the hand should be evaluated as it can provide important information on injury to structures, pathology, and required treatment. Laceration over a particular anatomic area will point to possible injured vascular, neural, tendinous, or bony structures. If structures such as vessels, nerve, tendon, or bone are exposed with injury, then reconstructive planning of soft tissue coverage will need to be considered.

Examination of boney structures are best performed with x-ray and CT scan; however, exam can reveal suspicions for open or closed fracture and dislocation in the event of trauma or osteomyelitis in the event of chronic infection.

Almost all consultations of the hand require hand x-rays, which provide important information on bone structure, fractures, joint integrity, and foreign bodies. If soft tissue needs to be examined through imaging, additional imaging modalities, such as ultrasound, CT scan, or MRI must be obtained.

TRAUMA

▶ Traumatic Amputation

Traumatic amputation at the level of the digits, palm, wrist, or more proximal forearm or arm frequently presents to trauma centers. The first step on arrival to the emergency department must include primary and secondary surveys to ensure stability of a critically injured patient and any additional injuries. Amputations are distracting injuries that may result in missed identification of other critical injuries. Tourniquet, if present from placement in the field, should be removed for identification of any bleeding vasculature, and importantly to prevent further ischemia to distal musculature, which can be severely damaged with reperfusion injury. If a tourniquet has been in place for a significant amount of time with concern for reperfusion injury, fasciotomies should strongly be considered during replantation procedure. The tourniquet should not be replaced if pinpoint manual pressure can prevent hemorrhage, as this will preserve long-term muscle viability of the forearm.

Once primary and secondary surveys are performed, full hand exam must be completed to determine which structures are injured. Mechanism of injury, obtained by both the history and exam, should be noted. Replantation and revascularization after sharp injury has a greater chance of survival versus after a crush or avulsion injury, which often leads to irreversible damage to many critical structures including vascular intima, soft tissue, nerve, and bone.

X-rays are required for all amputations to evaluate for level of amputation of the bone, additional fractures or dislocations, and any foreign bodies. X-ray with the amputated part in the same frame is very helpful for use in planning and display in the operating room.

Amputations may be partial, with the piece not fully detached, or complete. Exam and imaging are critical to determine the involved structures of the amputation. A range of structures can be injured in partial amputations. If a digit is fully amputated, decision must be made for replantation versus revision amputation to provide adequate soft tissue coverage to the exposed critical structures. If a partial amputation involves damage to vascular structures, causing the distal part to be dysvascular, revascularization must be strongly considered.

Order of repair during replantations and revascularizations typically is (1) bone, (2) tendon, (3) nerve, (4) vessel (artery and vein), and (5) soft tissue. All patients should be consented for possible vein, nerve, and tendon grafts in case of damage to one of these structures. All patients must be aware of possible need for amputation in case of failed replantation or revascularization attempt.

Zhu H, Bao B, Zheng X: A comparison of functional outcomes and therapeutic costs: single-digit replantation versus revision amputation. *Plast Reconstr Surg.* 2018;141(2):244e-249e.

▶ Soft Tissue Loss

Soft tissue coverage of upper extremity trauma is dependent on the location, size, depth, and involved structures of the wound. Vessels, nerves, tendon, and bone require soft tissue coverage to prevent damage. The reconstructive ladder should be considered when developing a treatment plan in general; however, many functional and aesthetic results will be improved with more complex reconstructive options given the critical function of the hand and numerous critical structures. The volar surfaces of the finger tips, ulnar aspect of the thumb, and radial aspect of the index, middle, ring, and little fingers are particularly important to attempt to provide sensation, durable glabrous skin, and enough soft tissue to maintain length of the digit. Local or regional neurotized flaps are options to help achieve these goals.

▶ Fracture

All upper extremity injuries that have suspected bony injury must undergo plain films. Plain films provide information on fracture pattern, dislocation, baseline hand physiology including osteopenia or arthritis, and radiopaque foreign bodies. Fractures should be identified, including laterality, digit involved (thumb, index, middle, ring, or little), bone type (eg, metacarpal, proximal phalanx, middle phalanx, distal phalanx), open or closed, intra- or extra-articular, and degree of comminution.

If open, treatment will involve thorough washout; repair of injured structures and skin, reduction of bone by closed technique with or without pins or open technique (open reduction internal fixation [ORIF]) with pins, plate, or screws; and splinting or cast. If closed, the treatment will involve closed reduction and splinting initially. If the fracture pattern is unstable, the patient will require operative fixation with closed technique (closed reduction percutaneous pinning) or open technique (ORIF).

CONGENITAL

Congenital hand deformities can be classified into seven types as follows: type I, failure of formation (radial/ulnar clubhand); type II, failure of differentiation (syndactyly, camptodactyly, clinodactyly, and symbrachydactyly); type III, duplication (polydactyly); type IV, overgrowth (macrodactyly and hemihypertrophy); type V, undergrowth (brachysyndactyly or brachydactyly); type VI, constriction ring syndrome (constriction ring syndrome, in utero amputation at any level); and type VII, generalized skeletal deformities (Apert syndrome, Holt-Oram syndrome, thrombocytopenia-absent radius syndrome).

The most common hand anomaly is syndactyly, or webbing of the digits. This may be simple, involving only soft tissue, or complex, involving fusion of bone and soft tissue. The fusion may be partial or complete. Surgical correction involves separation and repair with local flaps and skin grafts. Correction should be done before growth disturbance of the webbed digits takes place. Other anomalies, such as polydactyly, or extra digits, and adactyly, or absence of digits, and ectrodactyly, or cleft hand, also exist.

Thumb hypoplasia can range from minor hypoplasia to aplasia or complete absence of a thumb. Reconstruction will depend on the severity of deformity, from no treatment in minor hypoplasia, to tendon transfer for opponensplasty when thenar musculature is hypoplastic, to great toe–to–thumb transfer when skeletal deficiency exists in the setting of a stable carpometacarpal joint, to index finger pollicization in the situation of a "pouce flottant," or floating thumb, or in complete aplasia.

Congenital ring constriction can range from mild induration of skin to lymphedema, vascular compromise to the extremity, and even amputation in utero. The ring constrictions are best treated by excision and Z-plasty either in stages or in a single-stage procedure if deemed safe from a vascular prospective.

Poland syndrome consists of a variable degree of unilateral chest deformity, including absence or abnormality of the pectoralis major muscle and symbrachydactyly. The hand deformity is treated according to the severity. The latissimus dorsi muscles can be transposed to replace the absent pectoralis major, simulating the sites of origin and insertion. In more severe cases and in women requiring breast/chest wall reconstruction, the transverse rectus abdominis island flap can be used to replace the deficit. An alternative treatment to autologous reconstruction is tissue expansion with implant-based reconstruction.

Greene WB: One-stage release of congenital circumferential constriction bands. *J Bone Joint Surg Am.* 1993;75(5):650-655.
Rayan GM, Upton J III: *Congenital Hand Anomalies and Associated Syndromes.* Berlin, Germany: Springer-Verlag; 2014.

VII. AESTHETIC SURGERY

Aesthetic surgery is an integral part of plastic surgery. In fact, the two terms have become almost synonymous even though aesthetic surgery is only one component of the field of plastic surgery. Increased interest and curiosity about the specialty results in part from increased demands for its services by an aging population but also from the development of more predictable, lasting, and safer techniques. A number of specialists other than plastic surgeons have also performed and contributed to cosmetic surgery. A skilled surgeon can perform such cosmetic operations safely and with maximum benefit to the patient.

Patient selection is probably as important for success as any other factor. Not all patients are good candidates for aesthetic procedures, and such operations are contraindicated in others. Age or poor general health of the patient may be a contraindication and a reason for delay or avoidance of purely elective procedures. Anatomic feasibility of the procedure and psychological makeup of the patient are important considerations, including patient understanding and expectations. Cosmetic changes in appearance will not save a failing marriage, help to procure a new job, or substantially improve a person's station in life, and thus, patients with such unrealistic expectations should not undergo aesthetic surgery. Surgery should be postponed for persons experiencing severe stress, such as divorce, death of a loved one, or other periods of emotional instability. The ideal candidate for cosmetic surgery is a person who has a realistic idea of what is to be accomplished, is not under pressure from others to have the operation done, and does not expect major changes in interpersonal relations or career potential following surgery. Personal satisfaction is a valid reason for seeking aesthetic refinements.

RHYTIDECTOMY

The combined effects of gravity, sun exposure, and loss of elasticity due to aging result in varying degrees of wrinkles and sagging of skin along the cheeks, jawline, neck, and elsewhere in the facial area. These natural signs of aging can be removed to a great extent by a rhytidectomy, or facelift procedure. Not all wrinkles can be removed, however; those in the forehead, around the eyes, in the nasolabial area, and around the lips are not significantly corrected without additional procedures.

Rhytidectomy is a major procedure requiring extensive incisions hidden in the scalp and in front of and behind the ears and occasionally in the submental region. The first such operations consisted of freeing up the skin and then stretching it and resuturing as it was drawn cephalad and laterally. This gave a masklike and unnatural appearance. Over the past few years, there has been a significant change in the concept of the facelift procedure, so that now it consists of elevation of the soft tissues, particularly the jowls and malar fat pads, to where they were at a younger age, giving more prominence to the cheek bones and better delineating the jawline. Undermining of the skin is done only to approach the soft tissues to be elevated, and the excess skin is then removed and reapproximated without tension. This approach to the mid face has given more natural and lasting results and also provides a three-dimensional type of restoration of the soft tissues, leading to a more youthful appearance.

For the double neck, extensive freeing up of the skin over the neck from the jawline down to the hyoid is performed, and the fat overlying the platysmal muscle is removed either by suctioning or directly with scissors. The platysma itself is tightened laterally as well as centrally to provide an effect similar to a hammock that will give a more defined neck and jaw angle.

Drains are used particularly in the neck, as well as a padded circumferential dressing to protect the face and provide light pressure during healing. The introduction of liposuction has been adapted to the neck but is not recommended for the face. In appropriate patients, liposuction in the neck does give fine definition to the chin and jawline and may substantially correct the double chin appearance or obtuse mental angle.

Either local or general anesthesia may be used for this procedure. Local vasoconstrictors are routinely used. Complications include hematoma, skin slough, injuries to branches of the facial nerve or greater auricular nerve, scars, and asymmetry.

BLEPHAROPLASTY

Blepharoplasty involves removal of redundant skin of the upper and lower eyelids and removal of periorbital fat protruding through sagging orbital septa. It is done alone or as part of a facelift procedure.

Incisions are made in the upper lids surrounding previously marked redundant skin, which is then removed. A subciliary incision is generally used in the lower lids. The orbicularis oculi muscle may be altered if necessary. The periorbital fat compartments are opened, and protruding fat is removed. The extent of redundant skin in the lower lid is gauged, and the skin is resected. External sutures are used. Minimal or no dressing is required. Local anesthesia in the form of lidocaine with epinephrine is usually adequate. Swelling and ecchymosis subside in 7-10 days, and sutures are removed in 3-4 days. In recent years, there have been significant changes in the concept of the blepharoplasty procedure. For the upper lids, the change consists of the recognition of senile ptosis due to either disruption or stretching of the levator mechanism. This can be corrected by imbrication of the levator mechanism with sutures. Complications include bleeding, hematoma formation, epidermal inclusion cysts, ectropion, and asymmetry. Patients are usually satisfied with the results. Recurrence is much less of a problem than with facelift procedures.

The lower eyelid operation has undergone even more changes. Less removal of fat but rather redistribution has gained wider acceptance. The subconjunctival removal of fat has been advocated and is particularly applicable to young patients with congenital fat hernias. The subconjunctival approach is also used in conjunction with the laser, which

has the effect of tightening the skin of the lower lid and ameliorating the periorbital wrinkles. Another important concept is the recognition of the proper position of the lower lid, especially the lateral canthal area. A youthful appearance is restored by elevating this to a more normal level.

RHINOPLASTY

Surgical alterations of nasal structures are done for relief of airway obstruction, usually secondary to trauma, and to reshape the nose because of undesirable characteristics, such as a prominent dorsal hump, bulbous or drooping tip, or overly large size. There is often a combination of problems.

Procedures are generally performed through intranasal incisions. The nasal skin is usually temporarily freed from its underlying bony and cartilaginous framework, so that the framework can be altered by removal, rearrangement, or augmentation of bone or cartilage. The skin is then redraped over the new foundation. The nasal septum and lower turbinate can also be altered to reestablish an open airway. A better understanding of nasal physiology has enabled surgeons to correct internal valve dysfunction by inserting spreader grafts, often following modification of the bony radix of the nose. Spreader grafts are small pieces of cartilage placed next to the septum and under the upper lateral cartilages, which serve to open up the internal valve for improved airflow.

Surgery can be done under local or general anesthesia; in either case, topical and injectable vasoconstrictors and anesthetic agents are commonly used. Hospitalization may or may not be indicated. Nasal packing is often used for hemostasis and support of the nasal mucosa during initial healing, as incisions are usually only minimally sutured with absorbable sutures. External nasal splints are placed to control swelling and provide some protection, particularly if osteotomy of the nasal bones is performed. Convalescence requires 10-14 days before most swelling and periorbital ecchymosis subside; however, several months are often required before completely normal sensation returns and all swelling resolves.

Nasal procedures are commonly performed, generally quite safe, and usually effective. Complications include bleeding, internal scarring, recurrence of airways obstruction, and irregularities of contour. Infections are rare except with the use of alloplastic nasal implants.

AUGMENTATION MAMMAPLASTY

In procedures for augmentation of the breasts, a silicone bag filled with saline solution or silicone is placed beneath the breast tissue in the submammary or subpectoral plane. Incisions are concealed in the periareolar margin, inframammary fold area, or axilla. Dissection is then carried out above or below the pectoralis major muscle, and the implant is placed in the pocket created. Drains are not generally used, and a padded dressing providing light pressure is applied. The subpectoral plane is generally preferred by most surgeons for augmentation mammaplasty because it does not interfere with mammography and the capsular contracture rate is lower.

After a prolonged investigation by the U.S. Food and Drug Administration, silicone gel–filled implants are available in the United States for cosmetic purposes. During the investigation, silicone gel–filled implants were found to be safe; however, definitive long-term data concerning these implants (eg, capsular contracture, deflation, and rupture rates) remain unknown. Nevertheless, patients and surgeons now have the opportunity to review the data and choose the type of implant used during breast augmentation.

Breast augmentation can be performed on an outpatient basis with local anesthesia, although this may not be satisfactory when subpectoral implants are used. General anesthesia is often used for augmentation procedures.

Although patient satisfaction is excellent in most cases, a significant rate of capsular contracture remains a problem (~10%). Scar tissue around the implant may contract in variable degrees even in the same patient. Control of this process is difficult even though the best possible environment for healing is provided (ie, appropriate implants are used, infection is controlled, bleeding is not present, debris is removed, and movement is restricted). Implants placed in the subpectoral position appear to be associated with a lesser degree of capsular contracture and less severe deformity if contracture occurs. Deflation of saline implants occurs at a rate of 1% per year.

Other complications include hematoma, infection, exposure of the implant, deflation or rupture of the implant, asymmetry of the breasts, and external scars. Breast function and sensation are usually not altered.

As discussed with breast reconstruction, data have emerged on the risk of anaplastic large-cell lymphoma (ALCL), which is a very rare lymphoma associated with textured implants. The lymphoma presents as a delayed seroma, which should be sent for cytology to test for CD30, a marker of ALCL. Treatment ranges from removal of implants with capsulectomy to adjuvant therapy such as chemotherapy.

REDUCTION MAMMOPLASTY

Reduction of hypertrophied breasts is most often completed for functional reasons because large breasts can cause poor posture, back and shoulder pain, and discomfort due to grooves from bra straps. Reduction mammoplasty, or breast reduction, is similar to mastopexy, since nearly all hypertrophic breasts are ptotic and must be lifted during correction. Enlargement can occur during puberty or later in life. Massive breasts can become a significant disability to the patient.

Although various techniques have been developed for breast reduction, nearly all require a pedicle to carry the nipple areola to its new position based on a pedicle. Breast

▲ **Figure 43–13.** Breast reduction inferior pedicle.

reductions can be classified based on the type of incision and the type of pedicle. Common incisions are vertical or wise-pattern/inverted T-shaped. Pedicle types include inferior (Figure 43–13), central mound, superior, medial, and McKissock or bipedicle. Vertical reduction mammoplasty, such as with the Hall-Findlay (medial pedicle) technique, has aroused considerable recent interest because of the decrease in amount of scarring. The incision runs circumferentially around the areola and vertically to or just past the inframammary fold. Liposuction may be performed for breast shaping along the inferior aspect. The Boston Modified Robertson breast reduction is an alternative technique where an inferior pedicle is used with only incisions along the inframammary fold and around the nipple-areola complex, eliminating the vertical scar. In extreme cases of gigantomastia and ptosis, a wide-based inferior pedicle is recommended to maximize perfusion to the nipple. However, free nipple-areola graft may still need to be considered if perfusion is inadequate.

General anesthesia is nearly always required because dissection is considerable, but blood loss can be minimized by the use of epinephrine as a vasoconstriction agent. Transfusions are rarely indicated, and postoperative drains are often not used. The procedure can be done on an outpatient basis. Although problems with nipple-areola loss, bleeding, infection, asymmetry, and scarring may occur, breast reduction patients are often among the most satisfied and appreciative of patients.

Hall-Findlay EJ: Vertical breast reduction with a medially-based pedicle. *Aesthet Surg J.* 2002;22(2):185-194.

Movassaghi K, Liao EC, Ting V, et al: Eliminating the vertical scar in breast reduction-Boston modification of the Robertson technique. *Aesthet Surg J.* 2006;26(6):687-696.

MASTOPEXY

Mastopexy is another common procedure used for correction of sagging or ptotic breasts. Although some breasts develop in a ptotic manner, most cases are caused by normal relaxation of aging tissues, gravity, and atrophy after pregnancy and lactation. It is not clear whether use of a brassiere alters this process in any significant manner. The degree of deformity is defined by the relationship of the areola to the inframammary fold and the direction of the nipple. A ptotic breast will have a nipple that is below the inframammary line and pointing down toward the toes.

Correction may be done with simultaneous reduction of the skin or augmentation. An incision must be made around the areola, and the breast tissue itself is imbricated, or better still, an inferiorly based flap of breast tissue is designed and placed underneath the remnant superior part of the breast and over the pectoralis major muscle, serving as an autoaugmentation as one brings the lateral breast columns together. This procedure gives a more lasting effect than merely decreasing the skin envelope. Attempts at making more lasting corrections of ptosis of the breasts through the periareolar incision, which decreases the scarring, have included wrapping the breast with prosthetic material such as polyglycolic meshes or, more recently, by wrapping it around with segments of pectoralis major muscle. Nonetheless, significant scarring may occur, particularly around the more visible periareolar incision.

General anesthesia is usually necessary, and recovery from mastopexy may take 7-10 days. Complications include bleeding, infection, tissue loss, altered sensation or loss of function of the nipple and areolar areas, scars, and asymmetry of the breasts.

Patient satisfaction with the results is often not as great as with other breast procedures. Satisfaction often depends on preoperative counseling and how well the patient is prepared to accept the resulting external scars.

GYNECOMASTIA

Gynecomastia is excess breast glandular tissue in men, which can be caused by a variety of etiologies including idiopathic, increased circulating estrogen, decreased circulating testosterone, chronic diseases, tumors, and drug side effects. Idiopathic etiology is the most common cause of gynecomastia. Increased circulating estrogen can occur from endogenous production from Leydig or Sertoli tumors; higher aromatization from obesity, aging, Klinefelter syndrome, testicular tumors, and hyperthyroidism; exogenous estrogen from topical or oral sources; and decreased estrogen metabolism from cirrhosis. Decreased circulating testosterone can occur from gonadal failure, Klinefelter syndrome, and defective androgen receptors. Chronic illness, cirrhosis, chronic renal failure, and HIV also can lead to gynecomastia. Common drugs associated with gynecomastia include hormones, anabolic steroids, protease inhibitors for HIV treatment, spironolactone, ketoconazole, isoniazid, digoxin, antipsychotics, antidepressants, marijuana, amphetamines, and heroin. Physical exam, including testicular exam, and lab workup, including thyroid-stimulating hormone, luteinizing hormone, human chorionic gonadotropin, and testosterone, in addition to standard preoperative labs, should be obtained.

Pseudogynecomastia is excess adipose tissue and may present similar to gynecomastia. Physical exam can help differentiate between the two conditions. Treatment of both conditions includes observation, weight loss if patient is obese, and surgery. Medical therapy, including tamoxifen, is less common. The surgical treatment is dependent on the stage of the gynecomastia. Rohrich and colleagues developed a staging system of four grades: grade I, minimal hypertrophy (< 250 g) with no ptosis; grade II, moderate hypertrophy (250-500 g) with no ptosis; grade III, severe hypertrophy (> 500 g) with minimal ptosis; and grade IV, severe hypertrophy with more severe ptosis. Liposuction is typically used alone for more mild cases and in conjunction with glandular excision in more severe cases. If a patient is extremely ptotic, skin may also require removal through a double incision procedure with free nipple graft.

Rohrich RJ, Ha RY, Kenkel JM, et al: Classification and management of gynecomastia: defining the role of ultrasound-assisted liposuction. *Plast Reconstr Surg.* 2003;111(2):909-923; discussion 24-25.

SUCTION-ASSISTED LIPECTOMY

Suction-assisted lipectomy, or liposuction, has now become the most common cosmetic surgical procedure performed in the United States. The use of a suction-assisted lipectomy with appropriate cannulas to remove localized excess fat deposits has become widespread. It is clear, however, that patient selection and judicious use of liposuction are necessary to avoid complications, including hypovolemia due to blood loss, hematoma formation, skin sloughs, and excess laxity of the skin and soft tissues. Used with discretion, liposuction can offer definition to areas of the abdomen, flanks, thighs, and buttocks. Results are generally quite dramatic with excellent patient satisfaction in properly selected cases.

As presently practiced, lipectomy consists of infiltration of a "wetting" or "tumescent" solution to provide vasoconstriction and anesthesia to the operative sites. A common mixture consists of a solution of lactated Ringer's with the addition of 1 mg of epinephrine per 1000 mL of Ringer's and 250 mg of plain lidocaine—the former to provide vasoconstriction and the lidocaine to provide a certain amount of anesthesia and thus reduce the depth of general anesthesia. Some surgeons perform the entire operation under local anesthesia, necessitating the use of larger amounts of lidocaine. Once the solution has been infiltrated sufficiently to produce the proposed effects, a small cannula is introduced through a small incision and suction is applied either with a syringe or with a suction machine. The fat layer that has been enlarged by the injection of tumescent solution dislodges easily and disrupts much faster than the blood vessels and the nerves.

Suction-assisted lipectomy is effective in removing abnormal bulges of localized fat throughout the body, particularly in the trochanters or the abdomen and flanks, but it is not considered a weight reduction technique. The procedure is safe when done by well-trained surgeons respecting sterility and technique and in adequately equipped operating rooms. Safety in the use of up to 35 mg of lidocaine per kilogram has been established by clinical studies. Fatalities are rare but have been reported with suction-assisted lipectomy due to pulmonary embolization, perforation of the intestines, or severe infections of the abdominal wall. Since the American Society of Plastic and Reconstructive Surgeons established safety guidelines, fatalities have decreased. High-volume liposuction (ie, > 5000 mL of aspirate) should be done in a hospital or accredited ambulatory facility and that performed with combined procedures should be carefully monitored. More common complications of suction-assisted lipectomy include irregularities of contour, dimpling, and, rarely, local infection at the entrance points.

Ultrasonic liposuction, external and internal, has also been advocated. External ultrasonic liposuction has the effect of a massage to disperse the infiltrated tumescent solution. Internal ultrasonic liposuction, on the other hand, emulsifies the fat with ultrasonic energy, which produces heat, so that this emulsified fat needs to be suctioned with standard suctioning equipment. The problems with ultrasonic liposuction include seroma formation, the need for larger portals of entrance, the possibility of burns of the skin or perforations of the skin, or end hits, if the cannula is misdirected.

ABDOMINOPLASTY

Abdominoplasty usually involves removal of a large ellipse of skin and fat down to the wall of the lower abdomen. Dissection is carried out in the same plane up to the costal margin. The naval is circumscribed and left in place. After the upper abdominal flap is stretched to the suprapubic incision, excess skin and fat are excised. The fascia of the abdominal wall midline can be tightened by plication. The umbilicus is brought up through an incision in the flap, and the wound is closed over drains. When the extent of excess abdominal tissue is severe and extends throughout the trunk, better results can be obtained with what is called a circumferential abdominoplasty, or lower body lift.

BODY CONTOURING AFTER MASSIVE-WEIGHT LOSS

In addition to abdominoplasty, other procedures usually classified as aesthetic surgery are various body contouring procedures that serve to remove excess tissue from the lower trunk, thighs, and upper arms. Patients with sagging tissue due to aging, pregnancies, multiple abdominal operations, or significant or massive weight loss are usually good candidates for body contouring procedures.

With the increased popularity of bariatric surgery, more people are seeking surgery to remove and correct large amounts of excess and redundant skin and soft tissue of the trunk and extremities. These types of procedures are not indicated as a treatment for obesity. This involves a complete regimen of diet, exercise, and lifestyle modifications.

Lower body lift, or when abdominoplasty incisions are carried posteriorly for complete circumferential excision of soft tissue, allows for excision of excess tissue of the abdomen, flanks, and back after massive weight loss. This requires changing the position of the patient at least on one occasion, with typically prone to supine position change. Proper markings preoperatively are essential in order to obtain a satisfactory and symmetric result.

Additional body contouring procedures include brachioplasty to remove excess skin from the upper arms, buttock lift, and thigh lift. Although these procedures can significantly improve the overall contour, the extensive incisions under tension are predisposed to wound dehiscence complications as well as significant external scarring. Careful preoperative planning and counseling of the patient is imperative in order to obtain a satisfactory result.

MULTIPLE CHOICE QUESTIONS

1. Normal skin has a ratio of type I to type III collagen of

    A. 2:1
    B. 4:1
    C. 1:2
    D. 1:4

2. The rectus abdominis flap is a Mathes and Nahai type ____ flap with ____ vascular pedicle source(s).

    A. II, a dominant and minor
    B. II, two dominant
    C. III, a dominant and minor
    D. III, two dominant
    E. IV, a segmental

3. Infantile hemangiomas are associated with which gene?

   A. *PIK3CA*
   B. *GLUT1*
   C. *RASA1*
   D. *PTEN*

4. When a patient with an upper extremity amputation presents to the emergency department, the first step is to

   A. Obtain x-ray
   B. Remove tourniquet
   C. Perform primary and secondary trauma surveys
   D. Proceed directly to the operating room

5. Anaplastic large-cell lymphoma (ALCL) is associated with which cytologic marker?

   A. CD10
   B. CD15
   C. CD20
   D. CD30

Hand Surgery

David M. Young, MD

Scott L. Hansen, MD

Gerard M. Doherty, MD

In industry and in the home, the hand is the most commonly injured part of the body. Disorders of the hand rarely jeopardize life but can significantly affect the ability to function.

INTRODUCTION

The prime functions of the hand are feeling (sensibility) and grasping. Sensibility is most important on the radial sides of the index, middle, and ring fingers and on the opposing ulnar side of the thumb, where one must feel and be able to pinch, pick up, and hold objects. The skin on the ulnar side of the small finger and its metacarpal, upon which the hand usually rests, must register the sensations of contact and pain to avoid burns and other trauma.

Mobility is critical for grasping. The upper extremity is a cantilevered system extending from the shoulder to the fingertips. It must be adaptable to varying rates and kinds of movements. Stability of proximal joints is essential for good skeletal control distally.

The specialization of the thumb has allowed humans to have superior aptitudes for defense, work, and dexterity. The thumb has exquisite sensibility and is a highly mobile structure with well-developed adductor and thenar (pronating) musculature. It is the most important digit of the hand, and every effort must be made to preserve its function.

The **position of function** of the upper extremity favors reaching the mouth and perineum and achieves a comfortable, forceful, and unfatiguing grip and pinch. The elbow is held at or near a right angle, the forearm neutral between pronation and supination, and the wrist extended 30 degrees with the fingers flexed to almost meet the opposed (pronated) tip of the thumb (Figure 44–1A). This is the desired position of the extremity if stiffness is likely to occur, and it should be maintained when joints are immobilized by splinting, arthrodesis, or tenodesis.

Opposite to the position of function is the **position of rest**, in which the flexed wrist extends the digits, making

grip and pinch awkward, uncomfortable, weak, and fatiguing (Figure 44–1B). The forearm is usually pronated, and the elbow may be extended. This habitus is assumed, without intention, after injury, paralysis, or the onset of a painful stimulus. For that reason, it is also called the **position of the injury**. Immobility in this position jeopardizes function.

ANATOMY

All references to the forearm and hand should be made to the radial and ulnar sides (not lateral and medial) and to the volar (or palmar) and dorsal surfaces. The digits are identified as the thumb, index finger, middle finger, ring finger, and small finger.

The skin is an elastic outer sleeve and glove of the arm and hand. Sacrifice of its surface area or elasticity by debridement and fibrosis can severely diminish the range of motion and constrict circulation. In the adult hand, the dorsal skin stretches about 4 cm in the longitudinal and in the transverse planes when the palm is flattened and spread. The long finger can have as much as 48 cm^2 of skin cover, and the whole hand (exclusive of digits) has 210 cm^2.

Fascia anchors the palmar skin to bone to make pinch and grip stable; the midlateral fibers of the Cleland and Grayson ligaments keep the skin sleeve from twisting around the digit (Figure 44–2). In the form of sheaths and pulleys, fascia holds tendons in the concavity of arched joints to convey mechanical efficiency and power. The fascial sleeve of the forearm, hand, and digits must sometimes be released along with skin to prevent or relieve congestion (eg, compartment syndrome). Any fascial compartment of the hand provides a space for infection or an avenue for its dissemination.

Each finger has three joints, the distal interphalangeal joint (DIP), the proximal interphalangeal joint (PIP), and the metacarpophalangeal joint (MCP). The thumb contains the interphalangeal, the MCP, and the carpometacarpal (CMC) joints. The wrist is the "key joint" of the hand, governing

▲ Figure 44–1. Positions of function **(A)** and rest (injury) **(B)**.

▲ **Figure 44–3.** Longitudinal *(top)* and transverse *(bottom)* arches.

motion of the digits, and may need to be included in the immobilization required for a major finger or hand problem. The position of the wrist governs the efficiency of extrinsic muscle contraction. The wrist is composed of a proximal and distal row of carpal bones. The proximal row contains the scaphoid, lunate, triquetrum, and pisiform, while the distal row contains the trapezium, trapezoid, capitate, and hamate. The stability of the digital joints and their planes of motion are governed by the length of the ligaments and the anatomy of their articulating surfaces. The longitudinal and transverse arches of the hand (Figure 44–3) are architectural

prerequisites to gripping, pinching, and cupping and are maintained by the active contraction and passive tone of intact muscles. The arches create the position of function. When the arches are collapsed, the hand assumes the position of injury. Loss of these arches is most often initiated by edema. They may be preserved by splinting in the position of function, elevation without constriction, and early restoration of active joint motion.

Each MCP and PIP joint has a distally anchored volar plate (Figure 44–4) in addition to collateral ligaments

▲ **Figure 44–4.** Volar plate.

▲ **Figure 44–2. A:** Cleland ligament. **B:** Transverse retinacular ligament.

Flexion

— MP joint

— IP joints

Extension

▲ **Figure 44–5.** Collateral ligaments.

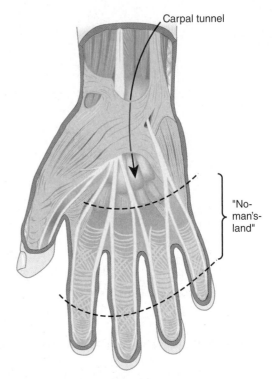

Carpal tunnel

"No-man's-land"

▲ **Figure 44–6.** Carpal tunnel and no man's land.

stabilizing the joint on either side (Figure 44–5). The thickened lateral portions of the volar plate form the checkrein ligaments, which prevent interphalangeal hyperextension.

The extrinsic flexor tendons are contained in fibrous **sheaths** to prevent bowstringing and preserve mechanical efficiency as the digits flex into the palm. Pulleys (hypertrophied sections of the sheath) resist the points of greatest tendency to bowstring. The retinacular pulley system contains five annular bands and three cruciform bands. Sheaths are inelastic and relatively avascular. Therefore, they crowd and congest any swollen, inflamed, or injured tendons and curtail glide by friction, constriction, and the generation of inelastic adhesions. The A-2 and A-4 pulleys must be maintained to prevent tendon bowstringing. These are located over the proximal and middle phalanges, respectively. The A-1, A-3, and A-5 pulleys are located over the MCP, PIP, and DIP joints, respectively. Five flexor tendon zones have been described. Zone II, or "**no man's land**," is the zone from the middle of the palm to just beyond the PIP joint, wherein the superficialis and profundus tendons lay ensheathed together and where recovery of glide is difficult after wounding (Figure 44–6).

Across the wrist, the dense volar transverse carpal ligament closes the bony carpal canal (**carpal tunnel**) through which passes all eight finger flexors as well as the flexor pollicis longus and median nerve (Figure 44–6). The **ulnar bursa** is the continuation of the synovium around the long flexors of the small finger through the carpal tunnel, encompassing the other finger flexors, which interrupted their separated bursa at the midpalm level. The **radial bursa** is the synovium around the flexor pollicis longus contained through the

carpal tunnel. These two bursas may intercommunicate. **Parona space** is the tissue plane over the pronator quadratus in the distal forearm deep to the radial and ulnar bursas.

The extensor tendons are ensheathed in six individual compartments at the wrist beneath the extensor retinaculum (Figures 44–7 and 44–8), which predisposes to adhesions. Its role as a pulley is not as vital.

The nerves of greatest importance to hand function are the musculocutaneous, radial, ulnar, and median nerves. The importance of the musculocutaneous and radial nerves combined is forearm supination and of the radial nerve alone is innervation of the extensor muscles. The ulnar nerve innervates 15 of the 20 intrinsic muscles. The median nerve provides sensation to the thumb, index finger, middle finger, and the radial aspect of the ring finger; through its motor innervation, it maintains most of the long flexors, the pronators of the forearm, and the thenar muscles. Figure 44–9 shows the sensory distribution of the ulnar, radial, and median nerves.

CLINICAL EVALUATION OF HAND DISORDERS

The presenting complaint must be assessed in complete detail with regard to its mechanisms of onset, evolution, aggravating factors, and relieving factors. Age, sex, hand dominance, occupation, preexisting hand problems, and relevant matters pertaining to the patient's general health must also be noted.

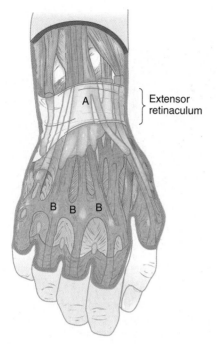

▲ **Figure 44–7.** **A:** Extensor retinaculum over six tendon compartments. **B:** Juncturae tendinum (conexus intertendineus).

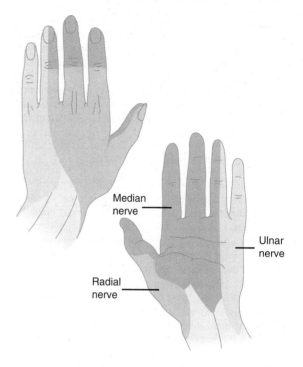

▲ **Figure 44–9.** Sensory distribution in the hand. Light-shaded area, ulnar nerve; diagonal area, radial nerve; darker area, median nerve.

A: Middle extensor tendon
B: Intrinsics
C: Lateral extensor tendon
D: Terminal extensor tendon

Dorsal   **Lateral**

▲ **Figure 44–8.** Extensor hood mechanism.

The examination should follow an orderly routine. Observe the neck, shoulders, both upper extremities, and the action and strength of all muscle groups, and be certain that all parts can pass painlessly and coordinately through a normal range of motion, starting with the head and neck and working down to the fingertips. Compare both upper extremities and keep detailed notes, diagrams, and measurements. Having the patient reach for the ceiling and simultaneously open and close both fists and then spread and adduct the fingers and, finally, oppose the thumbs sequentially to each fingertip will immediately demonstrate any abnormalities.

Observe habitus, wasting, hypertrophy, deformities, skin changes, skin temperature, scars, and signs of pain (including when the patient attempts to bear weight on the palms). Feel the wrist pulses and the sweat of the finger pads, and test reflexes and the sensibility of the median, ulnar, and radial nerves.

Serial x-rays and laboratory studies may clarify a problem with an indolent evolution (eg, Kienböck avascular necrosis of the lunate, causing unexplained wrist pain). Contralateral and multiple-view x-rays in different planes are often helpful. In addition, computed tomography (CT) scans, magnetic resonance imaging (MRI), bone scans, or all of these may aid in diagnosis. This is especially true in patients who have persistent bone and joint pain or limited motion or in patients who have not attained adult growth. In the case of wrist problems, arthrograms and arthroscopy may be of diagnostic value. MRI can be quite helpful in the diagnosis of subtle carpal bone problems.

The diagnosis is often made by noting the response to therapy. This is particularly true in the case of local corticosteroids injected at the site of noninfectious inflammatory conditions (eg, carpal tunnel syndrome, trigger finger).

GENERAL OPERATIVE PRINCIPLES

A bloodless field (eg, by tourniquet ischemia) is essential for accurate evaluation, dissection, and management of tissues of the hand. This is achieved by elevating or exsanguinating the extremity and then inflating a padded blood pressure cuff around the arm to 100 mm Hg above systolic pressure. This is readily tolerated by the unanesthetized arm for 30 minutes and by the anesthetized arm for 2 hours.

Incisions (Figure 44–10) must be either zigzagged across lines of tension (eg, must never cross perpendicularly to a flexion crease), termed Brunner incisions, or run longitudinally in "neutral" zones (eg, connecting the lateral limits of the flexion and extension creases of the digits), and whenever possible, must be designed so that a healthy skin-fat flap is raised over the zone of repair of a tendon, nerve, or artery.

Proper evaluation and treatment of an acute injury often requires extension of the wound. Normal structures can then be identified and traced into the zone of injury, where blood and devitalized tissue can make their identification difficult or impossible.

Constriction and tension by dressings must be avoided. The dressing should be applied evenly to the skin without wrinkles. The wound should be covered with a single layer of

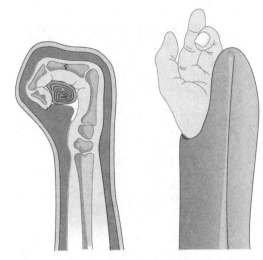

▲ **Figure 44–11.** Casting.

fine-mesh gauze followed by a moist spongy medium (fluffs, Rest-On, Kling, or Kerlix). Moisture facilitates the drainage of blood into the dressing, which should be applied with gentle pressure to restrict dead space.

Splinting and immediate elevation are paramount in controlling swelling and pain postoperatively. In general, plaster (fast-setting) or fiberglass is preferred because of its adaptability to specific requirements. More often than not, the wrist requires immobilization along with any other part of the hand (Figures 44–11 and 44–12).

It must be appreciated that effective immobilization of a finger most often requires concomitant immobilization of one or more adjacent fingers, usually in the position of

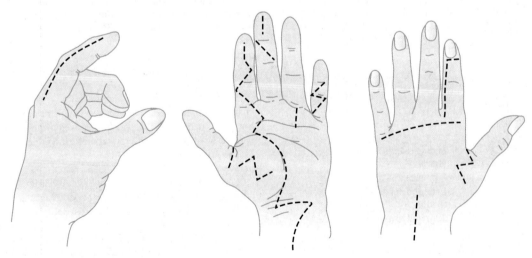

▲ **Figure 44–10.** Proper placement of skin incisions.

Cross section

▲ **Figure 44–12.** Casting.

function. Straight splints such as tongue blades involve a hazard of digital stiffness and distortion and should not be used across the MCP joint.

Persistence of pain signifies inadequate immobilization and, if throbbing is present, congestion. Congestion must be promptly relieved by elevation and sectioning of the cast and dressing and, if necessary, the skin and fascia.

CONGENITAL ANOMALIES OF THE HAND

Major congenital hand anomalies are not rare, with approximately 1 in 700 live births affected. When minor deformities are included, approximately 3% of all births are affected. Camptodactyly (bent finger), polydactyly (more than five fingers), and syndactyly (two or more fingers are joined together) are the most common malformations. Newborns with hand anomalies should be carefully examined for other malformations because multisystem syndromes can be present in 5% of patients (eg, vertebral, anal atresia, cardiac, trachea, esophageal, renal, and limb [VACTERL] syndrome with radial head dysphasia).

Anomalies may be inherited, caused by environmental factors (drugs, viral infections, irradiation, alcohol), or idiopathic. Major genetic or major environmental causes are infrequently found, suggesting that the cause of most defects is multifactorial.

In order to simplify an extremely complex clinical problem, the American Society for Surgery of the Hand (ASSH) and all major international hand societies have adopted a single classification system that divides anomalies into six main categories: failures of formation (absent digits, phocomelia [seal limb]), failures of differentiation (syndactyly),

duplication (polydactyly), undergrowth (brachydactyly), overgrowth (macrodactyly), and constriction ring syndrome (focal necrosis, intrauterine amputation). There is considerable overlap in the categories, as might be expected.

Ideally, surgery is performed early in the first 2 years of life, but timing is individually tailored to the problem.

Bates SJ, Hansen SL, Jones NF: Reconstruction of congenital differences of the hand. *Plast Reconstr Surg.* 2009;124:128e.
Chung MS: Congenital differences of the upper extremity: classification and treatment principles. *Clin Orthop Surg.* 2011;3:172.

TENDON DISORDERS OF THE HAND

Movement of the muscles of the hand and arm is transmitted into finger and wrist motion by the tendons. The tendons are strong, compact units that glide within their individual compartments. Disruption of the tendon by trauma or loss of tendon gliding by inflammation hinders tendon excursion and therefore limits active motion of the joints. Passive motion of the joint is still possible with an isolated tendon problem and distinguishes tendon disorders from joint disorders when both active and passive motions are limited.

Tendon disruption can result from any penetrating injury and can be diagnosed by physical examination. A tendon injury should be suspected when the patient is unable to actively move a joint. Certain tendon lacerations, such as an isolated flexor digitorum superficialis disruption, may be masked because the profunda tendon can still move the entire finger. Blocking of profunda function by blocking flexion in the neighboring fingers (the profunda tendons are joined in the palm) reveals the injury to the superficialis when the injured PIP joint cannot be flexed.

The state of the wound and the complexity of the injury are the principal issues the hand surgeon must weigh in choosing between a primary and secondary tenorrhaphy. Clean wounds generally favor primary tenorrhaphy. Primary tenorrhaphy is defined as one that is done within 24-72 hours after injury. When wounds are unstable, contaminated, or complicated by fracture or ischemia, formal tenorrhaphy may have to be delayed for weeks or months until the tendon bed is more favorable to healing and glide. However, interim tacking of the tendons—together, to tendon sheaths, or to bone—to maintain the fiber length of a muscle may be done as a preliminary procedure.

Preoperative treatment of fresh lacerations consists of wound closure, immobilization, and prophylactic antibiotics. Such cases can be deferred for definitive primary repair for 24 hours or more. The timing of delayed secondary procedures depends on the resolution of wound edema and fibrous callus (ie, how soft and pliable it is). After 6-8 weeks, tendons that retract over 2.5 cm may defy full excursion because muscle elasticity has been lost or because the tendon is recoiled and congealed in scar.

▲ **Figure 44–13.** Flexor tenorrhaphy by advancement or graft. Pulleys are saved.

▲ **Figure 44–14.** Mallet finger with swan-neck deformity.

Tenorrhaphy must be done without surface trauma along the tendon or its bed. The repair is made end to end or by weaving one tendon with the other, using a 3-0 or 4-0 braided synthetic polyester material, Prolene, or nylon sutures. A flexor tendon graft is anchored distally to bone (Figure 44–13). Tenodesis will occur if the surface of the tendon and the surface where adherence is desired are roughened. The position of immobilization should relieve tension on the tendon juncture. The duration of immobilization after tenorrhaphy is generally no more than 3-4 weeks. Controlled early, passive or active mobilization after tenorrhaphy may be initiated as early as 1 week to minimize excessive tendon scarring. This requires a very cooperative patient and close supervision by the hand therapist to avoid rupture of the repaired tendon.

Adhesions invariably form wherever tendons are even slightly inflamed or injured and can severely limit tendon function. Even so, adhesions are necessary for a tendon to reestablish continuity. With continuous active and passive movement over months, tendon glide can be increased with maturation and molding of the collagen in the adhesions. If the adhesions remain thick and tendon excursion is limited, surgical release of the tendon adhesions (tenolysis) needs to be performed. Successful surgery requires the release of all adhesions limiting tendon glide without rupturing the tendon repair. Movement of the tendon as soon as possible after surgery (within 24-48 hours) under the guidance of the hand therapist is critical to avoid recurrence of adhesions.

The access to tenolysis should be through an incision offering effective exposure and placed where the immediate active and passive joint motion that must follow will not jeopardize healing of the wound by undue stretching or direct pressure. Performing a concomitant procedure requiring immobilization such as a neurorrhaphy should be avoided. The patient must understand that joint mobilization after tendon surgery is a time-consuming process, often taking many weeks or months to achieve maximum recovery.

Mallet finger ("baseball" or "drop" finger) (Figure 44–14) is due to disruption of the extensor tendon to the distal phalanx. A distal joint that can be passively but not actively extended is diagnostic. The injury most commonly results from sudden forceful flexion of the digit when it is held in rigid extension. Either the extensor is partially or completely ruptured or the dorsal lip of the bone is avulsed. Less frequently, the injury is due to direct trauma such as a laceration. An x-ray should be taken to determine the presence and extent of any fracture.

Treatment requires 6-8 weeks of continuous splinting in full distal joint extension (not hyperextension) with or without 40 degrees of PIP joint flexion. Patient education and compliance are essential for good results. Joint fixation internally with a percutaneous Kirschner wire or externally with padded aluminum, plastic, or plaster splints is equally effective. A lacerated tendon should be repaired. When a significantly displaced fracture fragment represents one-third or more of the surface of the joint, it should be reduced by wiring or pinning. If there is sufficient articular surface disruption, one may consider joint fusion.

Swan-neck deformity (Figure 44–14) is a frequent complication of mallet finger, but it may also be the result of disparity of pull between the extrinsic flexors and extensor hood with or without attenuation of the DIP joint extensor. It is seen in congenitally hypermobile joints, spastic and rheumatoid states, and following resection of the superficialis tendon. The dorsal hood acts to extend the distal joint but is held back by its insertion at the base of the middle phalanx, which it therefore hyperextends. This in turn increases the tension on the profundus, which hyperflexes the DIP joint. If the mallet deformity is 25 degrees or less and there is some active distal joint extension, it may be treated by undermining and elevating the extensor hood at the PIP joint and severing its insertion on the base of the middle phalanx. Otherwise, the deformity may be corrected by tethering PIP joint extension with one slip of the flexor digitorum superficialis threaded through the flexor pulley of the proximal phalanx with the PIP joint flexed 20 degrees.

The **boutonnière,** or **"buttonhole," deformity** (Figure 44–15) appears as the opposite of the swan-neck deformity:

▲ **Figure 44–15.** Buttonhole deformity.

hyperextension of the DIP joint and flexion of the PIP joint. There is attenuation or separation of the dorsal hood, so that the middle extensor tendon becomes ineffective and the lateral extensor tendons shift volar to the PIP joint axis and the joint buckles dorsally. The entire extrinsic-intrinsic force on the hood passes onto the lateral extensor tendons, which flex the PIP joint and hyperextend the DIP joint. This deformity may develop suddenly or, more often, insidiously after closed blunt or open trauma over the dorsum of the PIP joint.

To avoid this complication, sutured extensor tendon lacerations and severe contusions over the PIP joint should always have the PIP joint alone splinted in extension for 3-4 weeks. Established deformities can be treated by such immobilization but more often require operative correction.

STENOSING TENOSYNOVITIS

In stenosing tenosynovitis, there is a disproportion between the clearance inside a tendon pulley or tunnel and the diameter of the tendon or tendons that must glide through it. Any pulley or tunnel may be implicated. The more common sites are as follows:

1. The proximal digital (A1) pulleys in the distal palm, causing **trigger finger** or thumb. There is local tenderness of the pulley; pain, which may be referred to the PIP joint; and (usually but not always) locking of the digit in flexion with a painful "pop" as it goes into extension (ie, as the bulge in the tendon or tendons passes through the tight pulley).

2. The pulley over the radial styloid housing the abductor pollicis longus and extensor pollicis brevis (first extensor compartment), causing **de Quervain's tenosynovitis**. Local tenderness and pain occur if these tendons are actively stretched (eg, Finkelstein test). The Finkelstein test is performed by having the patient bend the thumb into the palm and grasp with the fingers. The wrist is then bent ulnarly, and the first extensor compartment palpated. Pain in this area suggests de Quervain's tenosynovitis.

Relief of the symptoms can be achieved by local injections of triamcinolone mixed with lidocaine. Immediate surgery is justified if the constriction is so tight that the tendon is locked. Surgical section of the constricting tendon sheath is also indicated if symptoms persist or recur. When releasing the flexor tendon, care is taken not to resect more than the section of sheath restricting the tendon or else the tendon will pull away from the finger like a bowstring and weaken the grip.

Chesney A, Chauhan A, Kattan A, et al: Systematic review of flexor tendon rehabilitation protocols in zone II of the hand. *Plast Reconstr Surg.* 2011;127:1583.

Lee SK: Modern tendon repair techniques. *Hand Clin.* 2012;28:565.

McAuliffe JA: Tendon disorders of the hand and wrist. *J Hand Surg Am.* 2010;35:846.

▼ SKELETAL INJURIES OF THE HAND

Injuries to the bones and joints of the hand are the most common skeletal injuries treated by physicians. Recognition of the injury, appropriate diagnostic tests, and timely treatment are essential for minimizing the complications of these injuries. Some patients may neglect obvious fractures and dislocations in hope of spontaneous recovery. More subtle injuries to the wrist are more often neglected by the patient and sometimes even missed by physicians until further damage is done. The use of the fluoroscope, found in many offices, greatly enhances the surgeon's ability to diagnose fractures. The machine allows real-time assessment of the bones as part of the physical examination. A common late sequela of skeletal injury at the articular surfaces is osteoarthritis, which is difficult to treat. Patients with symptoms related to the hand or wrist but without a discernible cause should be referred early to a hand specialist.

METACARPALS & PHALANGES

▶ Fractures

Fractures of the metacarpal and phalangeal bones such as distal phalanx tuft of the fingers caught in closing doors and metacarpal shaft fractures of the ulnar side of the hand (boxer's fractures) create an obvious deformity and are easy to diagnose. Adequate x-rays of the specific site of the fracture with anteroposterior, lateral, and oblique views are essential for developing a treatment plan.

Fractures of the shaft can usually be treated with closed reduction and a cast or splint holding the hand in the position of function (Figure 44–1) for 3-4 weeks. Residual angulation of a metacarpal shaft fracture of up to 30 degrees in the fifth finger and 20 degrees in the fourth finger is functionally well tolerated, although a dorsal bump may be aesthetically unpleasant. However, even a small rotational misalignment of the fracture at the metacarpal bone results in scissoring of the fingers in flexion and causes severe dysfunction.

When fractures do not remain reduced, fixation with Kirschner pins placed through the skin is required. Placement of more than one pin is usually needed to keep the fracture reduced. The pins are removed after the fracture is healed. Displaced and comminuted fractures may require opening of the fracture site and reduction under direct visualization. Pins, lag screws, and small, low-profile metal plates and screws are used to maintain reduction. Metal plates provide strong support to the fracture site and allow earlier mobilization of the hand. However, plates are more invasive and occasionally interfere with tendon function due to excessive scar formation postoperatively.

Fractures through an articular surface need to be carefully evaluated. Nondisplaced fractures can be treated by casting. Displaced fractures require open reduction and accurate pin or lag screw fixation because discrepancies of the articular surface will eventually result in degenerative arthritis.

Fractures of the distal phalanx from crush injuries require attention to the disrupted nail bed. The nail is removed to decompress the painful subungual hematoma and provide irrigation of the open fracture and careful reapproximation of the nail matrix. Large disruptions in the nail matrix may result in deformity of the regenerating nail. The nail is replaced under the nail fold (eponychium) as a splint. A protective splint is placed over the finger to hold the distal fragment in extension.

An intra-articular fracture of the base of the thumb metacarpal bone with subluxation (displacement) of the metacarpal leaving a volar pyramidal shaped fragment attached to the trapezium is called a **Bennett fracture**. The anterior oblique ligament, responsible for stability of the thumb base, is left attached to the pyramidal fragment. The remainder of the thumb metacarpal is unstable and limits use of the thumb. The fracture must be reduced and stabilized with Kirschner pins, plate, or lag screws. Accurate reduction of the articular surface is crucial in reducing complications. However, despite adequate treatment, most patients eventually develop arthritis.

Dislocations

Dislocations are most common in the PIP joint. Injuries are classified according to the position of the distal digit as hyperextension, dorsal displacement, or volar displacement. The type of dislocation determines which structures, such as the volar plate, collateral ligaments, and extensor tendon, are likely to be disrupted.

The MCP and CMC joints are better protected by surrounding soft tissue but can still be dislocated. The MCP joint of the thumb is most frequently injured by forced abduction. The ulnar collateral ligament is torn, as occurs with forced use of a ski pole or as historically described in gamekeepers when twisting the neck of birds ("gamekeeper's thumb"). Of the CMC joints, the fifth is most commonly injured. A fracture analogous to a Bennett fracture (reverse Bennett fracture) can occur. Examination to determine injury to the deep motor branch of the ulnar nerve in this area should be done.

Radiographs are occasionally useful for diagnosis, but the physical examination is most important. Since pain often limits the extent of the examination, regional anesthesia with a wrist or finger block allows a more detailed examination. Partial tears of ligaments without dislocation or instability are treated by splints. Dislocations can usually be reduced, and the need for surgical therapy is determined by the stability of the joint after reduction. Stable reductions are treated with early mobilization to decrease stiffness.

Fracture dislocations usually require surgical repair. Instability after reduction can be treated by repair of the torn collateral ligament or volar plate. Severe dislocations of the PIP and MCP joints can result in interposition of disrupted soft tissue in the joint, making closed reduction impossible. The joint must be opened and the trapped soft tissue removed and repaired to correct the dislocation. A complete disruption of the ulnar collateral ligament in a gamekeeper's thumb injury can result in interposition of the adductor aponeurosis between the torn ends of the ulnar collateral ligament. The ends of the ligament must be reduced and repaired under direct vision.

WRIST & FOREARM INJURIES

Fractures

Fractures in the wrist and forearm usually result from falls on the outstretched hand. The distal radius is most commonly fractured. Many classification systems and eponyms have been used based on the extent and displacement of the fracture and involvement of the articular surface. The hyperextended wrist also exposes the scaphoid bone to injury in a fall. Since the scaphoid is crucial to wrist motion, displacement of the fracture is poorly tolerated. In addition, the blood supply enters the distal part of the bone and makes ischemic necrosis of the proximal fragment a problem.

Diagnosis of distal radius fractures is not difficult, but scaphoid fractures can easily be missed. Special radiographic views of the wrist or CT or MRI scans may be needed in difficult cases. If the clinical picture is suspicious but the radiographs are inconclusive, the wrist should be immobilized. Repeat radiographs in 7-10 days may demonstrate the fracture. Untreated scaphoid fractures lead to debilitating arthritis and collapse of the wrist.

Distal radius fractures are treated by reduction and immobilization. As with other fractures, articular irregularities and unstable fractures need to be treated by open reduction and internal fixation. Use of bone grafting and external fixation devices to initially treat the fracture has been advocated. Scaphoid fractures require careful and prolonged immobilization. Displaced fractures or nonhealing fractures require operative treatment with screw compression, bone grafts, and/or scaphoid replacement.

Dislocations & Sprains

Dislocations and ligamentous injuries of the wrist are the most difficult hand injuries to diagnose and treat. Wrist injuries often present as a painful wrist after minor trauma. Routine radiographs are often normal, and physical findings can be unimpressive. Still, these injuries can lead to chronic problems. Special stress radiographs, fluoroscopy, and physical maneuvers (scaphoid shift test) help delineate the injury.

The scaphoid lunate ligament is most often injured. Instability of the joint is best treated by repair or reconstruction of the ligament. Injury of the ligaments of the radiocarpal-radioulnar joint is likewise difficult to determine. Surgical treatment involves repair of the disrupted ligament.

Buijze GA, Ochtman L, Ring D: Management of scaphoid non-union. *J Hand Surg Am.* 2012;37(5):1095-1100.

Friedrich JB, Vedder NB: An evidence-based approach to meta-carpal fractures. *Plast Reconstr Surg.* 2010;126:2205.

Gaston RG, Chadderdon C: Phalangeal fractures: displaced/nondisplaced. *Hand Clin.* 2012;28:395.

Jones NF, Jupiter JB, Lalonde DH: Common fractures and dislocations of the hand. *Plast Reconstr Surg.* 2012;130:722e.

Khalid M, Jummani ZR, Kanagaraj K, et al: Role of MRI in the diagnosis of clinically suspected scaphoid fracture: analysis of 611 consecutive cases and literature review. *Emerg Med J.* 2010;27:266.

Neuhaus V, Jupiter JB: Current concepts review: carpal injuries - fractures, ligaments, dislocations. *Acta Chir Orthop Trauma-tol Cech.* 2011;78(5):395-403.

Sendher R, Ladd AL: The scaphoid. *Orthop Clin North Am.* 2013;44:107.

NERVE DISORDERS

Nerve disorders of the hands are conveniently organized into compression neuropathies, injuries of peripheral nerves, and various problems located more proximal to the upper extremities (spinal cord or central nervous system). For nerve dysfunction due to strokes, cerebral palsy, and spinal cord injury, readers are referred to more specific textbooks on hand surgery.

▶ Compression Neuropathies

Compression of the nerves of the upper extremities due to an increase in surrounding tissue pressure occurs in specific locations and causes predictable signs and symptoms. Tissue edema from a variety of causes such as crushing injuries, vascular disorders, and prolonged repetitive hand motions can compress nerves traveling within tight compartments of the arm and produce nerve ischemia. Prolonged ischemia results in axonal destruction and sensory and motor dysfunction.

The median nerve can be compressed by local structures at the elbow (pronator syndrome), the anterior interosseous branch, and the wrist (carpal tunnel syndrome). Compression of the median nerve at the elbow causes forearm pain and sensory changes in the radial four fingers. The anterior interosseous branch of the median nerve is purely a motor nerve, and lesions produce only weakness of thumb and index finger flexion and no pain. Carpal tunnel syndrome presents with weakness in the hand, sensory abnormalities of the fingers sparing the small finger and ulnar aspect of the ring finger, and exacerbation of symptoms on forced flexion of the wrist (Phalen sign) or tapping the nerve at the wrist (Tinel sign). Shoulder, elbow, and forearm pain is also common. Atrophy of thenar muscles occurs in long-standing cases.

The ulnar nerve can be compressed at the elbow (cubital tunnel syndrome) or the wrist (Guyon canal). Sensory abnormalities in the small finger and weakness of intrinsic hand muscles occur with compression in either area. Segmental nerve conduction velocity tests help to localize the abnormality to one site or the other. Compression of the radial nerve occurs most frequently from fractures of the humerus. Compression of the nerve along the proximal radius (radial tunnel syndrome) causes diffuse pain around the elbow but occurs rarely.

Abnormal findings on nerve conduction studies and clinical manifestations of nerve compression are adequate for diagnosis. Electromyography (EMG) demonstrating denervation patterns in the corresponding muscles or slowing of nerve conduction velocities indicates injury to the nerve. Although helpful, these tests only complement the physical examination, since electrodiagnostic tests can occasionally be inaccurate.

Early or mild cases of compression are treated by controlling tissue swelling. Resting the extremity with splints and using nonsteroidal anti-inflammatory medications as well as local injection of steroids often resolves the problem. If repetitive motions, such as typing, are thought to be the cause, changing the motion or hand position should help. If clinical manifestations are severe or if nonsurgical therapy fails, surgical decompression of the nerve is advocated.

Carpal tunnel syndrome is the most common type of compression neuropathy and one of the most common hand disorders. Surgical therapy of median nerve entrapment in the carpal tunnel or any of the compression neuropathies requires detailed knowledge of the anatomy. Division of the constricting structures results in partial or complete reversal of the symptoms. In the carpal tunnel, the median nerve is surrounded on three sides by carpal bones. Incision of the transverse carpal ligament, which forms the roof of the tunnel, decompresses the nerve. Occasionally, internal fibrosis of the nerve occurs and internal neurolysis with an operating microscope is required to allow the nerve to recover. Endoscopic release of the carpal tunnel through a smaller skin incision has been advocated.

▶ Nerve Injuries

Injury to individual peripheral nerves of the arm results in predictable and defined deficits. Proximal injuries involving the brachial plexus have more variable manifestations. Nerve conduction can be disrupted in the absence of structural changes due to compression, blunt injury, or ischemia (neuropraxia). More severe injury results in disruption of the axon with preservation of the epineurial covering of the nerve (axonotmesis). Both types of injury are followed by spontaneous recovery of function of good quality. Complete disruption of the nerve (neurotmesis), as with a laceration, requires surgical repair. Wallerian degeneration of the distal nerve occurs in both neurotmesis and axonotmesis, and recovery depends on the growth of the cut axon to the end organ. However, with neurotmesis, orientation of the proximal and distal axons is lost and recovery may be incomplete, especially in mixed motor and sensory nerves. Methods to differentiate sensory from motor fascicles have been used during repairs with some benefit.

A patient with loss of the radial nerve is unable to extend the fingers, wrist, and thumb. In addition, the patient will have sensory loss to the dorsum of the hand. Median nerve dysfunction causes problems with opposition of the thumb and grip of the fingers. Sensory loss is to the radial four digits and can significantly impair use of the hand. An ulnar neuropathy causes dysfunction of the intrinsic muscles of the hand, clawing of the ulnar two digits, and weakness in gripping smaller objects. Sensation is lost along the ulnar side of the hand.

Diagnosis of nerve injury is mainly by the physical examination. Understanding the functional anatomy of the peripheral nerves allows adequate evaluation of nerve loss. Electrodiagnostic studies are used to distinguish between partial and complete lesions and to follow functional recovery.

Obvious and complete disruption of the nerve is treated best by early surgical exploration and repair. An incomplete lesion or questionable disruption of nerve integrity is best treated with close observation, splinting to prevent contractures, and surgical exploration if no recovery occurs. Segmental loss of nerves requires nerve grafts, usually taken from a minor sensory nerve, such as the sural nerve, to bridge the gap. Results of primary repair are better than the results of grafts, and repairs done soon after injury are better than delayed repairs. Recovery of protective sensation of the hand is crucial for good functional recovery.

Motor dysfunction due to nerve damage can be treated by arthrodesis (stabilization of flail joints) and tendon transfers. Tendon transfers should utilize a muscle unit that is unaffected by the nerve injury, have direction of force and excursion similar to those of the damaged muscle, and produce no further deficits due to loss of the donor muscle. For radial nerve palsy, the pronator teres to extensor carpi radialis transfer provides wrist extension, the flexor carpi radialis to extensor digitorum communis transfer gives finger extension, and the palmaris longus or flexor digitorum superficialis of the fourth finger transfer to the extensor pollicis longus extends the thumb. Restoration of thumb opposition is most important with median nerve palsies, and the use of several donor muscles to achieve this result has been described including the extensor indices proprius and flexor digitorum superficialis from the middle or ring fingers. Tendon transfers to control claw deformity and strengthen key pinch are used for ulnar nerve palsies.

Gottschalk HP, Bindra RR: Late reconstruction of ulnar nerve palsy. *Orthop Clin North Am.* 2012;43:495.

Jones NF, Machado GR: Tendon transfers for radial, median, and ulnar nerve injuries: current surgical techniques. *Clin Plast Surg.* 2011;38:621.

Kang JR, Zamorano DP, Gupta R: Limb salvage with major nerve injury: current management and future directions. *J Am Acad Orthop Surg.* 2011;19:S28.

Ko JW, Mirarchi AJ: Late reconstruction of median nerve palsy. *Orthop Clin North Am.* 2012;43:449.

Lee SK, Wolfe SW: Nerve transfers for the upper extremity: new horizons in nerve reconstruction. *J Am Acad Orthop Surg.* 2012;20:506.

Mintalucci DJ, Leinberry CF: Open versus endoscopic carpal tunnel release. *Orthop Clin North Am.* 2012;43:431.

Watson JC: The electrodiagnostic approach to carpal tunnel syndrome. *Neurol Clin.* 2012;30:457.

HAND INFECTIONS

Small breaks in the skin or nails of the hand can lead to widespread infection and abscess. The original injury often cannot be identified. Poor venous and lymphatic drainage of the upper extremity, especially when held in a dependent position, aggravate the situation. Immunocompromised patients (diabetics, HIV-positive patients) are prone to develop extensive infections very quickly and should be treated more carefully.

The hallmark of infection (pain, swelling, and erythema) may be widespread in the hand and make localizing the infection difficult. Swelling of the dorsum of the hand is common even with palmar infections, and knowledge of the tissue planes of the hand is crucial to understanding how infections spread. Lymphatic streaks (lymphangitis) extending up the arm indicate rapid extension of the infection and must be treated urgently.

Oral antibiotics effective against *Staphylococcus* and common anaerobic organisms (ie, first-generation cephalosporins and penicillin) are adequate to treat most infections. Infections from animal bites (*Pasteurella multocida*) and human bites (oral flora) also respond to penicillin. The intravenous route is reserved for severe infections or for those not responsive to oral antibiotics. Once the situation improves, oral antibiotics are given for 7-10 days. Equally as important, the infected hand needs to be immobilized and elevated. Pillows and trapezes help to elevate the arm, but elbow slings aggravate the dependent position of the arm and should not be used. The best results are obtained when the patient is convinced that elevation of the extremity is beneficial.

Once treatment of a hand infection has begun, improvement within 24 hours is expected. If prompt improvement does not occur, an occult abscess may be present. Obvious abscesses should be drained at the point of maximum tenderness or the point of maximum fluctuance, where the overlying tissues are thinnest. The drainage wound should run parallel to and not across the paths of nerves, arteries, and veins. Wounds should be made long enough and should be zigzagged, when necessary, to avoid secondary contractures. Ultrasonography may be useful when a definite abscess cannot be located.

Pyogenic Granuloma

Pyogenic granuloma is a mound of granulation-like tissue 3-20 mm (or more) in diameter. It usually develops under a chronically moist dressing and may form around a suture. A small granuloma (6-7 mm in diameter) exposed to the air will soon dry up and epithelialize, whereas larger ones should be scraped flush with the skin under local anesthesia and covered with a thin split-thickness skin graft. If the granuloma is adjacent to the nail and the nail is acting as a foreign body aggravating the reaction, the nail must be removed.

Nail Infections

The nail fold is often traumatized and becomes secondarily inflamed, leading to a **paronychia** on the radial or ulnar side. The lesion is termed an **eponychia** if it involves the base of the nail, although the entire fold can be involved; and it is called a **subungual abscess** if pus develops and extends under the nail plate. Because of the early and unrelenting tissue tension that develops, these entities are quite painful. Early treatment before abscess formation consists of soaking, elevation, immobilization, and antibiotics. Most abscesses can be drained painlessly with a scalpel; the insensate necrotic skin cap should be cut through where it points (Figure 44–16). Sagittal incisions, which form a "trapdoor" of the eponychium, should be reserved for the long-standing case in which a dense fibrous callus of the nail fold must be excised. Occasionally, the nail must be basally excised or totally avulsed, after which the eponychial fold should be separated from the nail matrix by a thin, loose pack. Chronically wet nails of dishwashers may develop tissue changes and nail deformities, which are best treated by removing the nail plate. Fungal infections should be diagnosed and treated, and the fingers should be protected from water or excessive sweating.

Deep Space Abscess

A **felon** is an abscess in the pulp of the fingertip and is often deep and very painful. Untreated or inadequately drained abscesses may lead to osteomyelitis of the distal phalanx. Incision and drainage with disruption of the many vertical fibrous septa of the pulp space are required to adequately

▲ Figure 44–17. Cross-section of distal phalanx.

drain the abscess (Figure 44–17). The traditional fishmouth incision is no longer recommended for drainage since it may expose the underlying bone and because it often heals in a tender scar. Instead, lateral through-and-through incisions or direct incisions on the pulp, where the abscess points, have better results (Figure 44–18).

The **web spaces** are the path of least resistance for pus from infected distal palm calluses, puncture wounds, and infections of the lumbrical canals. Infection and abscess formation in the dorsum of the thumb web may be the result of extension from the volar thenar space (collar button). A dorsal incision is usually made between the fingers to drain both spaces. A dorsal incision in the web of the thumb may be zigzagged to prevent contracture (Figure 44–10).

The **midpalmar space** becomes infected by direct puncture or by extension of infections from the flexor sheaths of the index, middle, or ring fingers (Figure 44–6). Only the skin should be incised over the point of fluctuance. The rest of the dissection should be carried out by gentle spreading with a blunt clamp to avoid injury to arteries, nerves, and tendons. Infection spreads easily from this space along the lumbrical canals and to the thenar space.

A hypothenar space abscess is usually a product of a penetrating wound and should be drained at the point of greatest fluctuance. The same is true for a thenar space abscess, which may point in the palm rather than the thumb web.

Infection within the synovium of the flexor tendon is difficult to diagnose. **Pyogenic tenosynovitis** spreads easily down the tendon sheath to affect the other fingers. Untreated, the infection causes adhesions of the tendon to the surrounding soft tissues and permanently limits movement of the fingers.

▲ Figure 44–16. Incision and drainage of paronychia.

▲ Figure 44–18. Incision of felon (distal fat pad infection).

▲ **Figure 44–19.** Drainage and irrigation for septic tenosynovitis. The antibiotic solution drips in through the distal catheter and drains out through the proximal one.

The signs of flexor tendon infection described by Kanavel include fusiform swelling of the digit, severe pain on passive finger extension, a fixed flexed position of the finger, and most importantly, tenderness over the extent of the tendon sheath into the palm. Ultrasonography of the distal palm can also be helpful when the diagnosis is unclear. The probe is held across the palm and reveals swelling of the involved tendon and fluid around the tendon at the proximal flexor sheath.

Only unresponsive, tensely swollen, and toxic cases need immediate incision and drainage. With rest, elevation, and antibiotics, it is safe to observe most cases for several hours. The most common method of incision and drainage (Figure 44–19) is to make a short sagittal midline distal wound immediately over the tendon and introduce a small plastic catheter into the synovial bursa for irrigating with an antibiotic solution. The catheter should pass through the sheath and exit by a counterincision in the palm to allow for drainage of the fluid. Not all surgeons advocate placement of an irrigation catheter, however. When a catheter is placed, it should remain for only 24-48 hours. These incisions do not cross flexion creases. The hand should then be elevated and immobilized in the position of function and covered by a dressing. Phlegmonous tenosynovitis usually requires opening of the entire synovial sheath (often through a lateral midaxial digital incision or longitudinally across the wrist for extensor sheath infections) and, frequently, excision of necrotic tendon and sometimes amputation of a digit.

▶ **Other Infections**

Necrotizing soft tissue infections of the upper extremity are rare but devastating when they occur. The condition has been called many different names such as necrotizing fasciitis, Meleney ulcer, and streptococcal gangrene. The organisms responsible include *Clostridium* species, *Streptococcus pyogenes,* and mixed infections. The hallmarks are the rapid spread of infection and the extensive necrosis of soft tissue. Treatment includes wide debridement of the necrotic tissue and intravenous antibiotics.

Human bite wounds of the hand occur most often during altercations when the fist strikes an opponent's tooth. The MCP joint can be entered. The injury is often ignored by the patient until infection of the joint has begun. The joint must be explored and cleaned and the patient treated with antibiotics to cover oral flora (penicillin). Once the infection reaches the joint, destruction of the cartilage often occurs despite all therapy.

An inordinate amount of pain, with little or no swelling or induration, predating and accompanying the appearance of multiple tiny vesicles, suggests **herpes simplex (herpetic whitlow).** The vesicles may appear cyclically. They contain clear fluid and not pus and should be distinguished from paronychia. Antibiotics are not indicated in this self-limited viral infection. Acyclovir 5% ointment applied topically for 7 days decreases the severity and duration of symptoms but is of no value in prophylaxis.

Tuberculous infection of the hand is usually chronic and may be relatively painless. Some cultures take months to become positive. Tuberculosis commonly involves only one hand, which may be the only focus of infection in the body. Bones and joints may be infected, but the process more commonly involves the tendon synovium, which becomes matted to the tendons. Treatment is by synovectomy and antituberculous drug therapy for 6-12 months.

Leprosy causes neuritis of the median and ulnar nerves, resulting in sensory and motor loss to the hand. Crippling claw deformities develop as a result of intrinsic muscle palsy. Open sores appear on the hands as a result of trauma to anesthetic digits. Reconstructive surgery and occupational training are required.

Fungal infections involve primarily the nails. Tinea unguium (onychomycosis) may be caused by many organisms, including *Epidermophyton floccosum,* trichophyton, and *Candida albicans.* Prolonged treatment with antifungal drugs—griseofulvin systemically or nystatin topically—may be necessary, along with daily applications of fungicidal agents such as tolnaftate. Removal of the nail is advocated for chronic intractable cases.

McDonald LS, Bavaro MF, Hofmeister, et al: Hand infections. *J Hand Surg Am.* 2011;36:1403.

Nikkhah D, Rodrigues J, Osman, et al: Pyogenic flexor tenosynovitis: one year's experience at a UK hand unit and a review of the current literature. *Hand Surg.* 2012;17:199.

Ritting AW, O'Malley MP, Rodner CM: Acute paronychia. *J Hand Surg Am.* 2012;37:1068.

Shoji K, Cavanaugh Z, Rodner CM: Acute fight bite. *J Hand Surg.* 2013;38:1612.

INFLAMMATORY DISORDERS OF THE HAND

DUPUYTREN CONTRACTURE

▶ Palmar Fasciitis

The cause of Dupuytren contracture, which is common particularly among white populations of Celtic origin, is not known. It occurs in one of three types (acute, subacute, and chronic), predominately in males over 50 who have been in sedentary occupations, and is bilateral in about half of cases. There is a hereditary influence, and the incidence is higher among idiopathic epileptics, diabetics, alcoholics, and patients with chronic illnesses. The contracture may develop in people who do not work and (in laborers) in the hand that does the least work, so that it is not considered work related. It is frequently found in the plantar fascia of the instep and occasionally in the penis (Peyronie disease).

Dupuytren contracture manifests itself most commonly in the palm by thickening, which may be nodular, and therefore mistaken for a callosity, or may be cord-like, and therefore mistaken for a tendon abnormality because it passes into the digits and restricts their extension. This process typically involves the longitudinal and vertical components of the fascia but at times seems to exist apart from anatomically distinct fascia. The skin may fuse with the underlying fascia and become raised and hard, or it may be greatly shrunken and sometimes drawn into a deeply puckered crevasse. The disorder invades the palm at the expense of fat but is never adherent to vessels, nerves, or musculotendinous structures (though it may be adherent to flexor tendon sheaths). It has an unpredictable rate of progression, but the earlier it starts in life, the more destructive and recurrent it is apt to be.

Dupuytren fasciitis may involve any digit or web space, but it affects predominantly the ring and small fingers. In long-standing cases, the fingers may be drawn tightly into the palm, resulting in secondary contracture of joint capsule and ligaments, flexor sheaths, and atrophic muscles.

The most recent addition for the treatment of Dupuytren contracture is enzyme (collagenase) injection. Based on early studies, it appears that this treatment works best on MCP contractures rather than PIP contractures in patients with a well-defined cord. This treatment does require two office visits, one for the injection and a follow-up visit to manipulate and rupture the cord.

Surgery is indicated when the disorder has progressed sufficiently, especially when it causes more than 30 degrees of flexion at the MCP joint or any flexion contracture of the PIP joint. The patient must be warned about the increasing technical difficulty with progressive flexion and adduction contractures and the potential for recurrence after surgery. Fasciectomy is the surgical procedure that gives the best long-term results. In selected cases where only the longitudinal pretendinous fascial band is involved and the skin

moves freely over it, subcutaneous fasciotomy done through a small longitudinal incision may release a contracture quite well with only a few days of postoperative disability. In the occasional case with acute and rapid onset of a tender nodule, local triamcinolone may be used for subjective and even objective relief.

Depending on the amount of cutaneous shrinkage, skin grafts may be required for wound closure after fasciectomy. The overlying dermis has been implicated as an inductive mechanism in this process. Thus, skin grafting may diminish the recurrence rate in severe cases. The hopelessly contracted little finger must sometimes be amputated.

Motion should be started within 3-5 days after surgery. Dynamic splints and postoperative injection of corticosteroids into joints and the zone of surgery may help the well-motivated patient.

The potential complications of surgery are wound breakdown (loss of skin flaps), hematoma, fibrosis and stiffness, digital nerve injury, recurrence of contractures, and digital ischemia secondary to digital artery injury. Reflex sympathetic dystrophy, a painful, debilitating neurologic disorder of the hand, can occur after surgery and must be treated aggressively. In general, the functional reward for the patient is great at any age.

Brandt KE: An evidence-based approach to Dupuytren's contracture. *Plast Reconstr Surg.* 2010;126:2210.
Desai SS, Hentz: The treatment of Dupuytren disease. *J Hand Surg.* 2011;36:936.
Hentz VR, Watt AJ, Desai SS, et al: Advances in the management of Dupuytren disease: collagenase. *Hand Clin.* 2012;28:551.

DEGENERATIVE & RHEUMATOID ARTHRITIS

Arthritis of the hand is divided into two categories. **Degenerative changes** are usually due to some trauma resulting in damage to the bone or cartilage or to the supporting ligamentous structures. The increased wear to the joint results in inflammation and damage to the cartilage or underlying bone followed by reactive new bone formation (spurs). The wrists, hips, and knees are most commonly affected. **Rheumatoid arthritis** is a systemic disease characterized by synovial inflammation. The diseased synovium destroys adjacent tendons and joints in a specific way, leading to characteristic deformities in the hand.

Patients with degenerative arthritis complain of pain, aching, and stiffness in the area of the affected joint. Progression of the problem leads to immobility of the joint that affects the entire hand. Radiographic studies demonstrate joint narrowing and periosteal thickening early in the problem, progressing to bone spurs, loss of the articular surface, and bone destruction later. Patients with rheumatoid arthritis often present with very severe deformities without pain. Nodules around the olecranon and dorsum of the hand are often found. Both flexor and extensor tendons at the wrist can be inflamed, limiting tendon movement and resulting in rupture of the tendon. Involvement of the tendons and ligaments at the digits and MCP joints results in ulnar deviation of the digits, MCP joint destruction and dislocation, and swan-neck and boutonnière deformities. Destruction of the wrist joint is also common.

Arthritis is common among older patients and usually treated by primary care physicians and rheumatologists with anti-inflammatory medications and modification of the patient's activities. In most cases, it is only when symptoms greatly hinder the patient's lifestyle that they are referred to a hand surgeon. Physical therapy, splints, and medications are often no longer effective for these patients.

Surgical treatment of painful joints includes replacement with a prosthetic joint and partial or full fusion. Prosthetic joints of metal or Silastic permit near-normal movement but can become unstable and dislocate or degenerate over time. For a durable solution to the problem, fusion of the joint is recommended. Motion is severely limited, but pain relief is complete. There are more therapeutic options for the wrist, such as replacement, local fusion of only the affected carpal bone, or complete excision of the proximal row of carpal bones, leaving motion and stability to the distal carpal bones and ligaments.

Therapy for synovial inflammation in rheumatoid disease includes excision of the synovium to increase tendon excursion and prevent rupture, repair of ruptured tendons, and excision of painful nodules. Tendon-balancing procedures can help ulnar deviation of the MCP joints and improve joint movement. The most important concept of treating patients with rheumatoid hand disease is that often the patients have adapted well to their functional deficits. Correcting a physical deformity in a well-compensated patient may actually result in more problems for that patient.

Adams J, Ryall C, Pandyan A, et al: Proximal interphalangeal joint replacement in patients with arthritis of the hand: a meta-analysis. *J Bone Joint Surg Br.* 2012;94:1305.

Ono S, Entezami P, Chung KC: Reconstruction of the rheumatoid hand. *Clin Plast Surg.* 2011;38:713.

Schindele SF, Herren DB, Simmen BR: Tendon reconstruction of the rheumatoid hand. *Hand Clin.* 2011;27:105.

SCLERODERMA & LUPUS ERYTHEMATOSUS

These systemic diseases of unknown cause have distinctive—though not necessarily pathognomonic—manifestations in the hands.

Scleroderma initially produces joint stiffness, hyperhidrosis, and Raynaud phenomenon. Unchecked, it leads to marked tautness of skin and rigidity of joints with associated osteoporosis (even atrophy and ultimate resorption of the distal phalanges) and soft tissue calcifications.

Lupus erythematosus, which may be initiated or aggravated by certain drugs, foreign proteins, or psychic states, often causes polyarthritis indistinguishable from that of rheumatoid arthritis. It does not usually lead to similar joint destruction. Vasospasm in both lupus and scleroderma can cause severe ischemia of the hand and digits and may require therapy to prevent gangrene.

GOUT

Gout is a metabolic disorder of uric acid metabolism that affects about 1% of the population; approximately 50% of patients with gout have **cheiragra** (gouty hands).

The diagnosis is suggested by a rapid onset of severe pain and inflammatory signs about the joints and musculotendinous structure, simulating a phlegmonous infectious cellulitis with marked induration (most dramatically seen about the elbow). The usual duration of an attack is 5-10 days. The serum uric acid is elevated in 75% of cases. Gout may coexist with rheumatoid disease. The diagnosis is confirmed by identification of uric acid crystals in joint fluid or tissue biopsy.

In time, typical tophi form, consisting of toothpaste-like infiltrates of urate crystals, arising in multilobulated form about soft tissue structures that have been invaded. X-rays show characteristic punched-out lesions at the margins of articular cartilage.

Prophylactic treatment of gouty arthritis consists of diet, colchicine, allopurinol (a urate-blocking agent) or probenecid (a uricosuric agent), and avoidance of stress. Colchicine, 0.6 mg/h with a glass of water for 6-8 doses or to the point of gastrointestinal distress, is the time-honored means of interrupting an attack, but phenylbutazone, topical corticotropin gel, and systemic corticosteroids are also of value.

Surgical measures consist of drainage of abscessed tophi (seldom needed) and tophectomy. The latter procedure is more often of cosmetic rather than functional value. Tophectomy consists of removal of as much tophaceous material as can be fairly easily recovered. The surgeon should be careful not to destroy ligaments, tenoretinacular structures, nerves, and vessels in the process.

Porter SB, Murray PM: Raynaud phenomenon. *J Hand Surg Am.* 2013;38:375.

Tripoli M, Falcone AR, Mossuto C, et al: Different surgical approaches to treat chronic tophaceous gout in the hand: our experience. *Tech Hand Up Extrem Surg.* 2010;14:187.

Wasserman A, Brahn E: Systemic sclerosis: bilateral improvement of Raynaud's phenomenon with unilateral digital sympathectomy. *Semin Arthritis Rheum.* 2010;40:137.

BURNS & FROSTBITE OF THE HAND

▶ Thermal Burns

The hands are a common site of thermal (including frictional), electrical, chemical, and radiation burns. Function is imperiled in all instances by swelling and scar formation.

Prompt measures to preserve existing function are often urgently required. Burns over other areas of the body may be more life threatening and require more urgent attention, but burns of the hand should never be neglected. Delay in therapy leads to irreversible impairment and deformity that are impossible to correct later.

As in other areas of the body, thermal burns are grouped into three degrees. Superficial (first-degree) burns are red and painful; partial-thickness (second-degree) burns develop blisters; and full-thickness (third-degree) burns are insensate and appear like leather or charred tissue. The prognosis and therapy depend on the location, depth, and extent of the burn.

All burns to the hand cause swelling of the tissues, and the need for elevation of the arm to relieve pain and prevent stiffness cannot be overemphasized. Tetanus immunization should be given. Cold compresses may help alleviate the pain in first-degree burns. Second-degree burns must be watched more carefully. Large blisters restricting motion are broken. Otherwise, since they are sterile, they should be left intact. Treatment with thrice-daily washing and silver sulfadiazine is usually adequate. Patients with third-degree burns or superficial burns that fail to heal and patients unable to care for their burns at home should be admitted to the hospital.

Deeper burns require close observation and more extensive treatment. In the first few hours after injury, circumferential or near-circumferential burns may cause ischemia in the extremity. Because evaluation of sensory function and capillary refill is nearly impossible in these limbs, escharotomies should be performed if compartment syndrome is suspected. If done correctly, escharotomies have few complications, since these burns usually require surgical debridement anyway. Incisions are placed to avoid exposure of neurovascular structures.

Partial-thickness burns heal spontaneously. Deeper burns on the dorsum of the hand are best treated with early excision of the eschar and placement of skin grafts to prevent contractures. Palmar burns are best left to heal spontaneously because skin grafts function very poorly in this area. Some hand surgeons believe that excision and grafting of superficial burns should be performed to prevent contractures. This is true if adequate therapy has not been available. In burn units with good rehabilitation services, surgeons are treating superficial second-degree burns without surgery and obtaining results as good as with skin grafting. Pigskin, cadaver homografts, or a number of commercially available biologic dressings can be used to cover the wounds temporarily, decreasing pain and keeping the wound moist until autologous skin grafts are placed.

Neglected burns of the hands result in contracture deformities that often require extensive surgery to restore function. Delayed healing and wound contractures often result in a claw hand with MCP hyperextension and fusion of the digits with loss of the web space (syndactyly). Burns on the volar surface leave flexion contractures. Some contractures can be treated with release and skin grafting of the tissue gap. Web space contractures and released contractures with exposed tendons or nerves must be covered with skin or muscle flaps. Web space release is done with skin flaps from the dorsum folded down to create the space. Large flaps can be obtained by attaching the hand to the groin, allowing the tissue to adhere and vascularize before cutting the flap away from the groin. Recently, free tissue transfer from other parts of the body using microsurgical techniques has allowed more extensive reconstruction of severely burned hands.

Electrical Burns

Electrical burns of the upper extremity may not appear extensive on initial inspection. The skin may be burned only in a very small area of the entry point of the current or by ignited clothing. The current tends to spare the skin but damage underlying muscles, vessels, and nerves. Often, the extent of dead tissue is not evident for several days.

Initial treatment is the same as for thermal burns. Since muscle damage may be extensive, it is important to prevent renal failure from myoglobinuria by maintaining a high output of alkaline urine. Arteriography, fluorescein injections, and radionuclide studies may help delineate the extent of necrosis. Examination of the patient in the operating room is still the most accurate method of assessing the extent of tissue damage. All obviously dead tissue should be removed during the initial evaluation. Two or three days later, the patient is reexamined in the operating room and any additional debris is removed. The wounds are closed when only clearly viable tissue remains.

Frostbite

Frostbite occurs most often in people under the influence of alcohol or with psychiatric illness. The lower extremity is affected more often than the upper. Freezing tissue causes cellular death and vascular thrombosis. Hypothermia of the entire body must first be treated. The frozen part should be quickly rewarmed by immersion in warm water (40°C). Elevation of the extremity minimizes edema. Skin wounds are treated like burns with silver sulfadiazine cream. The extent of necrosis may not be obvious for several weeks, and debridement or amputation should be delayed until demarcation of the injury occurs. Sympathectomy may help ameliorate the sequelae of frostbite, such as cold sensitivity and pain. Children with frostbite may develop premature closure of phalangeal epiphyses, which creates growth disturbances of the bone.

Arnoldo BD, Purdue GF: The diagnosis and management of electrical injuries. *Hand Clin.* 2009;25:469.
Kreymerman PA, Andres LA, Lucas, et al: Reconstruction of the burned hand. *Plast Reconstr Surg.* 2011;127:752.

Mohr WJ, Jenabzadeh K, Ahrenholz DH: Cold injury. *Hand Clin.* 2009;25:481.

Moore ML, Dewey WS, Richard RL: Rehabilitation of the burned hand. *Hand Clin.* 2009;25:529.

MASSES OF THE HAND

Only 2% of all masses in the hand are malignant lesions; the majority are benign neoplasms, cysts, or a myriad of other masses. Although the clinician must be ever vigilant to identify malignancy, a mass of the hand is highly likely to be benign—excisional biopsies are thus reserved for subcutaneous lesions that are rapidly growing or for skin lesions that may be carcinomas. Otherwise, masses can be observed over a period of time to determine that they are not growing. They may be removed for functional or cosmetic reasons.

Ganglions are formed by herniation of the synovial lining of joints or tendons into the surrounding soft tissue. These cysts are filled with a viscous fluid thought to be modified joint fluid. Trauma to the wrist or hand may cause extrusion of the synovium, but it is more likely that the ganglion was already present and that trauma to that area merely brought the lesion to the surgeon's attention.

Ganglions can arise from any joint of the hand but most commonly appear on the dorsal wrist over the scapholunate ligament and the volar wrist near the radial artery. Tendon ganglions are most common on the flexor sheath at the metacarpal head (A1 pulley). Pain and tenderness are due to compression of adjacent nerves by the mass.

Ganglions have a typical appearance, and diagnosis is simple. If any doubt exists, aspiration with a large-bore needle of the viscous fluid confirms the diagnosis and occasionally cures the lesions. Injection of the empty sac with steroids and lidocaine may help to keep the mass from reappearing, but the majority recurs. Ganglions need not be treated unless they cause pain or interfere with hand function. Often, it is enough just to reassure the patient that the mass is benign.

Operative removal of ganglions should be done using loupe magnification and a tourniquet. The entire ganglion should be removed, including all attachments to the joint capsule and the underlying ligament, without injuring the surrounding structures. Prolonged splinting after removal of ganglions does not decrease recurrence rates but does cause hand stiffness. Unfortunately, despite careful surgical removal of the lesion, recurrence of ganglions is relatively common.

Epidermal cysts are rests of epidermis located in the subcutaneous tissue. Many are thought to be due to traumatic disruption of epidermal cells into the soft tissue (inclusion cyst). The cells proliferate just as skin does and form a cyst filled with creamy keratin, the remains of dead epidermal cells that usually desquamate from the skin. Infected cysts become inflamed and form abscesses. Removal of the entire cyst wall is required to prevent abscess formation.

Pyogenic granuloma may form in any chronic wound. Histologically, it consists of vascular tissue identical to granulation tissue. Just as for hypertrophic granulation tissue elsewhere on the body, excision or cautery of the material flush to skin level allows epidermis to migrate over the wound.

Giant cell tumors are benign, multilobulated, solid masses found on the lateral aspects of the finger. They are often attached to the tendon sheath. The mass may be quite complex and extend throughout the adjacent nerves, vessels, tendons, and ligaments. The entire lesion should be removed, but recurrence is relatively common.

The most common bone tumors are **enchondromas.** Multiple enchondromas (Ollier disease) are associated with other skeletal deformities. The lesion appears on x-ray as thinned cortical bone with speckled calcifications. Fractures through the tumors usually do not heal spontaneously. The tumor should be removed with a curette. Bone graft taken from the distal radius is used to fill the gap if needed.

A **carpal boss** is due to abnormal bone formation at the base of the second or third metacarpal bones and presents as a hard mass on the dorsum of the hand. The excess growth of bone can be removed if symptomatic.

Glomus tumors are composed of blood vessels and unmyelinated nerves of a heat-regulating arteriovenous malformation. They are usually found in the fingertip or under the fingernail and can be extremely painful. Local excision of the tumor is curative. Occasionally, when the tumor is large and disrupts the nail matrix, a split-thickness nail graft from another digit is needed to reconstruct the defect.

The most common malignant tumor of the hand is **squamous cell carcinoma**, though **basal cell carcinomas** and **melanomas** also occur. Subungual melanomas are often difficult to diagnose because they are difficult to examine. These tumors should be treated just the same as elsewhere on the body. Particular care should be taken to examine for spread of tumor in the lymphatic drainage at the supratrochlear and axillary nodes.

Other tumors include lipomas, fibromas, hemangiomas, arteriovenous malformations, neurofibromas, sarcomas, and various skin lesions. These tumors act no differently in the hand than elsewhere in the body. However, because of the close proximity of the nervous and vascular structures within the small spaces of the hand, these tumors cause compressive signs and symptoms sooner. CT scans or MRI help delineate the extent of soft tissue tumors and may help in preoperative planning.

Abzug JM, Cappel MA: Benign acquired superficial skin lesions of the hand. *J Hand Surg Am.* 2012;37:378.

English C, Hammert WC: Cutaneous malignancies of the upper extremity. *J Hand Surg Am.* 2012;37:367.

Gant J, Ruff M, Janz BA: Wrist ganglions. *J Hand Surg Am.* 2011;36:510.

Sookur PA, Saifuddin A: Indeterminate soft-tissue tumors of the hand and wrist: a review based on a clinical series of 39 cases. *Skeletal Radiol.* 2011;40:977.

COMPLEX HAND INJURIES

▶ Crush Injuries & Amputations

Advances in microvascular surgery have greatly increased our ability to treat complex hand injuries. Mangled and amputated digits, hands, as well as entire upper extremities have been replanted or repaired. Complex nerve repairs, microvascular free tissue transfers of muscle flaps, and toe-to-hand reconstructions have made it possible to restore more function to severely injured hands. The end result must be a sensate, painless, and useful extremity. Patients who undergo multiple surgical procedures and prolonged rehabilitation with only marginal results would have benefited from early amputation. A surgeon with extensive experience can best assess the patient's injuries, occupational requirements, and psychosocial needs to determine if salvage is worthwhile.

Complex hand injuries often result from improper use or malfunction of machinery. Heavy machinery in the workplace or motorized cutting tools at home, such as rotary saws, are often cited as the mechanism of injury. Sharply amputated or partially devascularized parts are most likely to be saved. Severe crushing or avulsion of the part produces wider nerve and vessel injury. The extent of this type of damage is difficult to determine and often impossible to repair.

The decision to try to salvage a damaged part must be individualized to each situation, but some general principles apply. The thumb is crucial to hand function, and all efforts are made to save the entire digit or as much length as possible. When multiple digits or half of the hand is damaged or amputated, a greater effort is made to repair the part. Children can recover function in badly damaged extremities far better than adults can, and any amputated parts in children should be replanted. Replantation of the entire arm at the elbow and above is controversial. The usefulness of these replanted limbs is limited by the slow nerve regeneration, and some hand surgeons believe that amputations in these cases result in better function.

Patients with complex hand injuries should be immediately referred to a regional center with the staff and facilities to manage the problems. Occasionally, in the rush to transfer patients with these very obvious injuries, intra-abdominal, neurologic, and other less obvious injuries have been overlooked. The entire patient must be evaluated and stabilized prior to transfer. A clean, moist dressing should be placed on the wound and the extremity elevated. The amputated part is wrapped in a plastic bag and placed in ice water. The amputated part should never be frozen.

The accepting hand surgeon evaluates the patient's overall condition, potential for rehabilitation, and personal wishes before coming to a decision. To revascularize or replant a part, the patient must be taken urgently to the operating room. Ischemia over 6 hours is often associated with failure of revascularization, but—depending on the metabolic needs of the constituent tissues—extremities that have undergone periods of ischemia longer than this can be successfully replanted.

Bone must first be stabilized with Kirschner wires or metal plates before vascular repairs are performed. Arterial and venous repairs are done with microscopic magnification, and the ischemic tissue is reperfused. Failure of a replanted part is more often due to venous outflow problems than arterial inflow. Systemic and local anticoagulants help to maintain perfusion but are not always needed. Leeches placed on the part release a potent local anticoagulant and can decrease venous congestion. Nerve and tendon repairs must also be performed. When there is inadequate local soft tissue to cover the repaired structures, muscle or skin flaps from a distant site must be transferred using microsurgical methods to the area. Although these operations are not life threatening, blood loss can be extensive and transfusions are sometimes required.

Secondary procedures to free tendon adhesions, reduce bulky flaps, and transfer tendons in motor nerve injuries may need to be done. Reconstruction of unsuccessful replantations is being done more often. The original method using toes to reconstruct thumbs has also been used to make fingers. These reconstructions give patients the ability to grasp objects. Because these digits are sensate, they can even perform fine movement tasks not possible with prosthetic devices. Patients with loss only of the thumb are better treated with transfer of the index finger to the thumb position (pollicization).

Partial or total loss of a single digit is less critical. Hand function is better without a stiff or painful digit. When a decision is made to amputate a digit, care must be taken to leave a painless stump with good sensate soft tissue coverage. The flexor tendon must not be sutured to the extensor tendon for soft tissue coverage, since this will cause the tendons to pull each other rather than move the joint. Local flaps to cover the stump are preferred to skin grafts or cross-finger flaps, since they usually provide better sensation. A short amputation stump on the long or ring finger is often bothersome because small objects such as coins tend to fall out of the palm, and a ray amputation eliminates the problem. For cosmetic purposes, ray amputations are far less noticeable than partial amputations. The loss of hand breadth with a ray amputation can decrease grip strength, however.

The loss of part of all of the hand can be compensated both functionally and cosmetically by a variety of prostheses. Their use involves careful adaptation to the requirements of the patient, who must receive appropriate training to ensure success.

INJECTION INJURIES OF THE HAND

High-pressure devices used in industry to apply material such as air, grease, paint, and oil cause a unique hand injury. The typical case is injection of the material into the index finger of the nondominant hand of a factory worker. A pinpoint injection site may be the only external evidence of injury, and the hand appears discolored or pale, or swollen due to the injected material.

The examination should include a careful hand evaluation and an x-ray to demonstrate the distribution of material or gas in the hand. All such cases require continued, unrelenting scrutiny, even if the part seems completely normal. If there is any evidence of retained foreign material, swelling, or ischemia, early surgical exploration is advocated to release the tourniquet effect of the skin and fascia and to remove as much of the material as possible without injuring healthy tissue. Prophylactic antisludging agents (dextran 40), corticosteroids, and antibiotics may help.

Often, the pressure forces the material to spread along the tendon sheaths throughout the hand and even into the forearm. Expansion of the foreign material in a closed space and the chemical irritation cause congestion, inflammation, vascular thrombosis, and gangrene. The injected material is difficult to remove completely, and a foreign-body response leads to fibrosis so extensive that it often destroys the function of the hand.

Davis Sears E, Chung KC: Replantation of finger avulsion injuries: a systematic review of survival and functional outcomes. *J Hand Surg Am.* 2011;36:686.

Friedrich JB, Vedder NB: Thumb reconstruction. *Clin Plast Surg.* 2011;38:697.

Hegge T, Neumeister MW: Mutilated hand injuries. *Clin Plast Surg.* 2011;38:543.

Leversedge FJ, More TJ, Peterson BC, et al: Compartment syndrome of the upper extremity. *J Hand Surg.* 2011;36:544.

Ninkovic M, Voigt S, Dornseifer U, et al: Microsurgical advances in extremity salvage. *Clin Plast Surg.* 2012;39:491.

▼ MINIMALLY INVASIVE HAND SURGERY

The goal of reconstructive hand surgery is return of normal function, including pain-free movement, normal active and passive range of motion, premorbid strength, and intact sensation. Yet the process of incising, dissecting, and sewing is associated with significant scarring and pain. Scarring is especially troublesome in the hand, since it leads to stiffness, ligamental tightening, and arthritis. As a result, any procedure in the hand that minimizes postoperative scarring or pain will contribute to an improved result.

Surgical care in the past decade has been revolutionized by the introduction and incorporation of minimally invasive surgical techniques. Laparoscopies and thoracoscopies have permitted the resection of hollow and solid organs through 1 cm incisions, reducing the need for laparotomies and thoracotomies. Likewise, urologists have employed cystoscopy for evaluation and treatment of bladder and kidney disorders, while orthopedic surgeons have used arthroscopy to similar effective ends in the knee, ankle, elbow, and shoulder.

Two areas of hand surgery incorporate minimally invasive techniques: Wrist arthroscopy has expanded the options for evaluating the chronically painful wrist, and endoscopic carpal tunnel release (ECTR) provides a less invasive method than open release for decompressing the median nerve. Although ECTR theoretically allows for a faster recovery, it may in fact offer only limited advantages.

WRIST ARTHROSCOPY

Diagnostic wrist arthroscopy was first successfully used in 1970. Over the past three decades, it has taken its place among traditional imaging techniques as a low-morbidity method for evaluating chronic wrist pain. As the hardware for examining the wrist has become more sophisticated and as hand surgeons have become more familiar with the arthroscopic view of the wrist, increasingly aggressive attempts have been made to use the arthroscope to treat as well as to diagnose wrist problems.

▶ Indications & Contraindications

Diagnostic wrist arthroscopy is a useful technique to evaluate patients with wrist pain, whether chronic or acute. In patients with chronic pain, this technique can be used to augment information offered by plain radiographs, CT, MRI, or wrist arthrography. It can confirm an uncertain diagnosis or be used to reevaluate a patient who has failed other treatments. In contrast, patients with acute symptoms—such as those suffering from mechanical wrist pain—may complain of pain localized over the joint, catching and popping sensations, and relief with rest. Here, the wrist can be manipulated during arthroscopy to localize the source of the symptoms. In general, the technique is useful for evaluating articular cartilage, ligaments, the triangular fibrocartilage complex (TFCC), and the synovium. Interestingly, diagnostic wrist arthroscopy may provide too comprehensive an examination. Only some of the lesions that are visualized during an examination may be responsible for a patient's symptoms. The hand surgeon must critically correlate arthroscopic findings with the patient's examination to arrive at the appropriate diagnosis.

Therapeutic wrist arthroscopy is useful for the treatment of ligament tears, TFCC lesions, articular cartilage lesions, subtle distal radius and carpus fractures, dorsal wrist ganglions, removal of isolated carpal bones up to and including the proximal carpal row, and disorders of the distal radioulnar joint. It is useful also in the management of lesions arising from rheumatoid arthritis. It has been successfully used in completing synovectomies, proximal row carpectomies in the case of scaphoid nonunion or scapholunate collapse, radial styloidectomy, and isolated symptomatic chondral defects.

Procedure

Equipment for diagnostic wrist arthroscopy includes an apparatus for elevating and distracting the wrist, an arthroscopic telescope, a video camera, a fluid infusion system, and both manual and powered instruments.

Either general or regional anesthesia may be used. A tourniquet is placed at the mid-arm to provide a blood-free field during the operation. The distal forearm, wrist, and hand are prepared into the operative field. Traction is applied to the hand, usually via sterile finger traps, and a distraction force is applied across the wrist.

Individual skin incisions are then made at standard portal sites determined by the goal of the operation. Portal sites are described according to their relationship with the radius and ulna, the carpal bones, and the extensor tendons. The relationship to the extensor tendons is indicated by listing the extensor compartments on either side of the incision. Typical portals include the 3-4 radiocarpal, through which the scaphoid and lunate facets can be visualized; the 4-5 radiocarpal, through which the TFCC and the ulnocarpal ligaments can be seen; and the 6R radiocarpal, through which the extensor carpi ulnaris tendon and ulnar wrist are approached. The midcarpal joint is approached through any of three portals, including the midcarpal ulnar, the midcarpal radial, and the scaphotrapezial-trapezoid.

Once abnormalities are identified, therapeutic wrist arthroscopy can be used to effect repairs. Partial ligament tears and tears of the TFCC can be debrided arthroscopically using knife blades and motorized shavers. Carpal bone resections can be completed with miniature osteotomes and powered saw blades.

Outcomes

Operations employing diagnostic and therapeutic wrist arthroscopy typically result in less swelling, less postoperative pain, and less stiffness than comparable open wrist procedures. There is a concomitant earlier return to function and work. Therapeutic wrist arthroscopy even of dorsal wrist ganglia, the most superficial of wrist abnormalities, is followed by fewer—or no more—recurrences than the open technique.

Complications

The rate of complications associated with diagnostic and therapeutic wrist arthroscopy is estimated to be 2% and is due to a variety of causes. The continuous traction necessary to properly distract the wrist can cause problems, including ligamental strain at the MCP joints with concomitant joint edema and stiffness and stretching of peripheral nerves. Establishment of the operative portals can damage articular cartilage, ligaments, tendons, cutaneous nerves, the radial artery, and cutaneous and deep veins. Such injuries include abrasions, contusions, lacerations, and transections. A high proportion of complications of therapeutic wrist arthroscopy are associated with inadequate relief of symptoms or a diminished return of function. A now less common complication of therapeutic wrist arthroscopy results from the fluid infusion. Forearm compartment syndromes have resulted from extravasation of infusion fluid during endoscopic repair of distal radius fractures; this problem is now avoided by circumferential compression of the forearm during the procedure.

ENDOSCOPIC CARPAL TUNNEL RELEASE

Endoscopic release of the transverse carpal ligament is an increasingly popular method of treating carpal tunnel syndrome. Advocates of the procedure claim that it is associated with decreased postoperative morbidity and earlier return to work. Others caution that there is little if any short-term difference between endoscopic and open carpal tunnel release, no long-term difference, and that endoscopic carpal tunnel release is associated with an increased likelihood of significant nerve injury.

Indications & Contraindications

Endoscopic carpal tunnel release is easier to perform in patients with larger wrists. Ease of access to the carpal tunnel correlates with the wrist circumference and the height and age of patients. Surgeons should be aware that the procedure is likely to be more difficult in small patients with small wrists and are advised to maintain a lower threshold for conversion to the open technique to avoid neurologic complications.

Absolute contraindications to endoscopic carpal tunnel release include masses in the carpal canal and other space-occupying lesions, abnormalities in canal anatomy, and wrist stiffness that precludes proper positioning.

Procedure

In the United States, most surgeons use one of two techniques—either Chow or Agee. The two differ primarily in the number of incisions, or portals, needed to gain access. The Chow technique, first described in 1989, employs two portals, while the Agee technique requires only one.

Either operation can be performed under local anesthesia with a brachial tourniquet. An initial transverse incision is made proximal to the wrist flexion crease between the palmaris longus and flexor carpi ulnaris tendons. The space between the transverse carpal ligament and the flexor tendons is defined with a dissector. In the Agee procedure, the endoscope is advanced under the transverse carpal ligament, radial to the hook of the hamate along the axis of the ring finger. The ligament is incised along its entire length, with care taken to avoid the Guyon canal and the superficial palmar arch. In the Chow operation, a second transverse incision is made just distal to the transverse carpal ligament along the axis of the ring finger. The wrist is dorsiflexed, and a slotted cannula is advanced into the proximal incision, deep to the transverse carpal ligament, and out the distal incision. The endoscope is then used to visualize the ligament while the knife divides it. The wounds are closed, and the patient's wrist placed in dorsiflexion.

▶ Outcomes

Several studies have compared open versus endoscopic carpal tunnel release, focusing on the incidence of recovery from symptoms, the time span until the patient returns to work, and the incidence of recurrence of symptoms. Overall, both techniques have equivalent outcomes.

Many of the most convincing studies are prospective randomized trials. One such study, comparing open and endoscopic carpal tunnel release among 32 hands in 29 patients, found no difference in postoperative recovery time or surgical result. The only significant difference noted by the authors was transient numbness on the radial side of the ring finger in three endoscopic carpal tunnel release patients.

In another study, the authors compared in a prospective randomized manner the early outcome of carpal tunnel release using either a conventional open carpal tunnel release procedure in 40 patients or a two-portal endoscopic release in 56 patients. They found no statistically significant difference between the groups in postoperative pain, recovery from paresthesias, or time taken to return to work. However, the endoscopic group demonstrated better grip strength recovery at 1 and 3 months. No surgical complications were observed in either group.

Nonrandomized studies have supported this trend. An analysis of 191 consecutive patients undergoing carpal tunnel release with an average 2-year follow-up showed that none of the patients undergoing open release had a recurrence, while 7% of patients undergoing endoscopic release had recurrences. Another study observed a higher incidence of incomplete release of the carpal tunnel with endoscopic techniques than with standard open releases.

The factors identified with poor outcomes in endoscopic carpal tunnel release are similar to those seen in open release. Less satisfactory results were present in workers' compensation cases; patients with normal motor latencies on nerve conduction studies; patients with preoperative hand weakness, widened two-point discrimination, myofascial pain syndrome, or fibromyalgia; and patients involved in litigation, those with multiple compressive neuropathies, and those with abnormal psychologic factors.

▶ Complications

Only a limited number of studies include a sufficient number of patients to compare complication rates and type between endoscopic and open carpal tunnel release. Overall, the types

and rates of complications between the two forms of release are similar. Nonetheless, isolated but severe complications from endoscopic release over the past decade tend to dramatize its risk.

The study by Boeckstyns and Sorensen is perhaps the most comprehensive to date. These authors analyzed 54 published series of endoscopic and open releases comprising 9516 and 1203 patients, respectively. Irreversible nerve damage from the procedure occurred in 0.3% of endoscopic and 0.2% of open releases, including such injuries as transection of the median nerve. While reversible nerve injuries were more common with endoscopic release than with open release (4.4% vs 0.9%, respectively, among prospective controlled and randomized studies), tendon lesions, reflex sympathetic dystrophy, hematoma, and wound problems were equally common with either technique.

A less compelling analysis—a retrospective survey of hand surgeons who had performed either open or endoscopic carpal tunnel release over the preceding 5 years—found major complications with both approaches, including median nerve lacerations, ulnar nerve lacerations, digital nerve lacerations, vessel lacerations, and tendon lacerations. Although the authors could not reach a conclusion about the rate of complications for one procedure versus the other, their results demonstrate the potentially devastating sequelae of carpal tunnel release even in experienced hands.

Carpal tunnel symptoms may persist or recur following either open or endoscopic release. In patients who have persistent symptoms following endoscopic release, many authors recommend open carpal tunnel release as definitive therapy.

Ahsan ZS, Yao J: Complications of wrist arthroscopy. *Arthroscopy.* 2012;28:855.

Herzberg G: Intra-articular fracture of the distal radius: arthroscopic-assisted reduction. *J Hand Surg.* 2010;35:1517.

Mintalucci DJ, Leinberry CF: Open versus endoscopic carpal tunnel release. *Orthop Clin North Am.* 2012;43:431.

Wolf JM, Dukas A, Pensak M: Advances in wrist arthroscopy. *J Am Acad Orthop Surg.* 2012;20:725.

MULTIPLE CHOICE QUESTIONS

1. All of the following are true about applying a cast to the hand, except

    A. The wrist should be extended 30 degrees.
    B. The fingers should be flexed.
    C. The thumb should be in the opposed (pronated) position.
    D. The hand should be in the position of rest.
    E. Fiberglass casting materials are preferred for their flexibility.

2. Incisions on the hand should be

   A. Never made on the palm
   B. Across lines of tension
   C. Only made along the medial and lateral surfaces of the fingers
   D. Zigzagged across lines of tension
   E. Carried perpendicularly across the wrist crease

3. Major congenital hand anomalies

   A. Occur in about 1 in 10,000 live births
   B. Can include camptodactyly
   C. Are rarely accompanied by other anomalies (< 1%)
   D. Are not known to be associated with environmental factors
   E. Are usually treated by surgery delayed until after age 15 years

4. Stenosing tenosynovitis

   A. Can be treated by local injections of corticosteroid
   B. Is usually best treated by early surgery
   C. Is always associated with a locked tendon that is trapped and frozen in the tendon sheath
   D. Can be confused with trigger finger or thumb, and must be differentiated
   E. Can be improved with immobilization

5. Management of carpal tunnel syndrome

   A. Typically requires emergent operation
   B. Cannot be done by endoscopic approaches
   C. Should usually include incision of the transverse carpal ligament, which forms the roof of the tunnel
   D. Is uncommon among hand disorders
   E. Should include surgery, not delayed by attempts at nonoperative treatment

Pediatric Surgery

Jonathan L. Hills-Dunlap, MD, MPH

Shawn J. Rangel, MD, MSCE

Considerations surrounding care of the pediatric surgical patient can differ markedly from that of their adult counterparts. This is not only due to differences in the pathophysiology of surgical diseases that affect neonates, infants, and children, but also differences in the physiologic demands of illness across different stages of development. Management of pediatric surgical diseases therefore requires an intimate understanding of not only the embryology and pathophysiology of pediatric surgical diseases, but also the unique physiologic requirement requirements of the pediatric population in response to stress and injury.

NEWBORN CARE

Neonatal Intensive Care

Care of surgical neonates, particularly premature and small for gestational age infants, continues to improve over time with advances in technology and medical therapy in neonatal intensive care units. Neonates with surgical disease often have comorbid conditions that threaten survival and necessitate multidisciplinary care.

Temperature is controlled by servoregulation, whereas pulse and blood pressure are continuously recorded. Ventilation is monitored by transcutaneous oxygen (O_2) and carbon dioxide (CO_2) electrodes or by indwelling arterial catheters. The metabolic consequences of prematurity and intrauterine growth retardation are monitored by frequent measurement of glucose, calcium, electrolytes, and bilirubin in microliter quantities of blood. Nutritional requirements for growth and development can be provided by enteral or parenteral routes. This kind of specialized care of critically ill newborns requires trained personnel and specialized equipment. The care of such babies is best accomplished in designated regional centers capable of providing pediatric surgical and neonatal intensive care.

Classification

Neonates are classified according to their gestational age and weight. A *premature infant* has a gestational age of less than 37 weeks, a *term infant* has a gestational age of 37-42 weeks, and a *postmature infant* has a gestational age of greater than 42 weeks. The gestational age of the infant is calculated from the date of the last normal menstrual period; however, clinical assessment of gestational age by morphologic and neurologic examination may be more accurate. For a term infant, normal birth weight is greater than 2500 g, whereas *low birth weight*, *very low birth weight*, and *extremely low birth weight* are defined by weights of 1500-2500 g, 1000-1500 g, and less than 1000 g, respectively.

Several clinical exam findings may be useful in assessing gestational age. Infants less than 37 weeks' gestational age may have (1) fine fuzzy hair with thin, semitransparent skin; (2) ears that lack cartilaginous support; (3) a breast nodule less than 3 mm in diameter; and (4) few transverse creases on the balls of the feet anteriorly. In males, the testicles may be undescended and reside in the inguinal canal, and the scrotum is small with few rugae. In females, the labia minora are relatively enlarged and the labia majora are small.

Premature infants may have several physiologic abnormalities depending on their gestational age at birth. Apneic and bradycardic episodes are common and may represent an immature central nervous system or, conversely, may represent signs of physiologic instability, most notably with sepsis. The lungs and retinas of preterm infants are very susceptible to oxygen toxicity. Retinopathy of prematurity from high oxygen levels may lead to blindness. Relatively brief exposures to high oxygen concentrations, often coupled with barotrauma from mechanical ventilation, may damage the lungs and result in bronchopulmonary dysplasia. Shunting across a patent ductus arteriosus is common and may lead to pulmonary hemorrhage and congestive heart failure. The premature infant also has a friable choroids plexus and is susceptible to intraventricular hemorrhage when stressed in the first week of life. The premature infant may be unable to tolerate oral feeding due to a weak suck reflex. Tube feeds or total parenteral nutrition may be required. Preterm infants have increased requirements for glucose, calcium, and sodium as well as a propensity for hypothermia, impaired bilirubin metabolism, polycythemia, and metabolic acidosis. These problems are accentuated in very low birth weight and especially extremely low birth weight infants.

A *small for gestational age* (SGA) infant is less than the tenth percentile for weight for the infant's gestational age. An SGA infant may be the product of a pregnancy complicated by placental, maternal, or fetal abnormalities. Although body weight is low, the body length and head circumference are age appropriate. Compared with the premature infant of equivalent weight, the SGA infant is developmentally more mature and faces different physiologic problems. Intrauterine malnutrition results in reduced body fat and decreased glycogen stores. Their relatively large surface area and high metabolic rate predisposes SGA infants to hypothermia and hypoglycemia. SGA infants also have an increased risk of meconium aspiration syndrome. Polycythemia (which may lead to complications of hyperviscosity syndrome) is common and necessitates close monitoring of hemoglobin and hematocrit. Due to their relatively mature organ development (compared to premature infants), retinopathy, intraventricular hemorrhage, and hyaline membrane disease are uncommon.

▶ Temperature Regulation

Neonates and infants are more susceptible to heat loss due to their relatively greater body surface area, decreased fat insulation, thinner skin, and immature thermoregulation mechanism compared to older children and adults. The rate of heat loss through conduction, convection, evaporation, and radiation can be four times greater in the infant compared to the adult and is exacerbated in the premature infant. Infants are homeotherms and will expend metabolic energy to maintain a constant body temperature at the expense of other bodily functions. Heat is generated by nonshivering thermogenesis, which increases the metabolic rate through the metabolism of brown adipose tissue. This mechanism can be impaired by medications (vasopressors and anesthetic agents) and by poor nutrition with depletion of brown adipose stores. Premature infants also have less brown adipose tissue. Exposure to cold environments increases metabolic work and caloric consumption. Due to limited energy reserves and thin skin, prolonged cold exposure may rapidly cause hypothermia. Catecholamine secretion in result to cold stimulus increases the metabolic rate (particularly in the myocardium), producing vasoconstriction with impaired tissue perfusion and increased lactic acid production.

With the considerations above, it is important to maintain the neonate in a thermally neutral environment, avoiding hypothermia and hyperthermia. This is best achieved by placing the infant in an enclosed incubator and regulating ambient temperature and humidity. An open radiant warmer can be used for infants requiring frequent care access. Either the ambient temperature of the incubator can be monitored and maintained at thermoneutrality or a servo system can be used. The latter regulates the incubator temperature according to the infant's skin temperature.

In the operating room, the temperature of the infant must be continuously recorded by placing a thermistor in the rectum or esophagus. Body heat may be conserved by use of a heating pad, circulated warm air around the child (bear-hugger), infrared lamp, and warm irrigation fluids. The operating room should be prewarmed and the temperature kept at 20-27°C. Wet sponges and drapes can exaggerate evaporative heat losses and should be avoided if possible. Warming and humidification of the inhalational anesthetic gases play an important role in maintaining thermoregulation in the operating room.

▶ Ventilation

At birth, inadequate respiratory effort should be assisted with positive pressure via mask and escalated to an endotracheal tube as necessary. Assisted ventilation is often necessary in the setting of underlying disease (eg, persistent fetal circulation and pulmonary hypertension), medications that suppress respiratory function (eg, opioids and sedatives), and physiologic changes associated with increased respiratory effort following a surgical procedure (eg, omphalocele closure).

Mechanical ventilation in the neonate is indicated when noninvasive means fail to support adequate respiratory function or when the airway must be protected. An uncuffed endotracheal tube should be used to minimize risk for subglottic stenosis. The tube diameter should approximate that of the fifth digit or the nares, usually between 2.5 and 4 mm. The term newborn usually requires a 3.5-mm tube. An orotracheal tube is preferred to a nasotracheal tube to minimize trauma and subsequent infection in the nasal passages. The trachea (from the glottis to the carina) is relatively short in the newborn, and placement of the tube into the right or left bronchus must be avoided. For infants, depth of tube placement can be estimated using an equation adding 6 to the patient's body weight in kilograms (eg, 7 cm from the lips in a 1-kg infant, 9 cm in a 3-kg infant). The presence of a small air leak indicates a small space between the endotracheal tube and airway and is ideally present to minimize laryngeal and tracheal trauma.

Most infant ventilators are time-cycled flow generators capable of delivering multiple modes, including continuous positive airway pressure (CPAP) and intermittent mandatory ventilation (IMV). IMV is a synthesis of simple mechanical ventilation and CPAP breathing that allows the baby to breathe independently between mandatory breaths provided by the ventilator while a continuous positive pressure is maintained in the airway. CPAP breathing helps keep the terminal airways open and is particularly useful when alveolar collapse develops, such as in hyaline membrane disease or with persistent atelectasis.

In general, O_2 saturation should be maintained above 92% and arterial Po_2 between 60 and 80 torr. The gas should be humidified by using a heated nebulizer because nonhumidified circuits can lead to insensible loses. In severe respiratory compromise, more complex ventilatory strategies are needed to maintain oxygenation and clearance of CO_2. High-frequency ventilation (jet and oscillatory modes) uses extremely high rates (up to 600 breaths/min) of low tidal volume ventilation to minimize the effects of high airway pressures. Inhaled nitric oxide (iNO) can be administered via the ventilatory circuit and may help relax the small airways and pulmonary vasculature. Allowing higher Pco_2 levels (permissive hypercapnia) is a frequently used strategy to reduce the risk of barotrauma from high airway pressures. If these ventilation strategies are inadequate, oxygenation and gas exchange can be accomplished using extracorporeal membrane oxygenation (ECMO). ECMO works by circulating blood through a bypass circuit where the blood is oxygenated and cleared of CO_2. The clinical need for ECMO has diminished with the increased widespread use of iNO, surfactant, and high-frequency ventilation and the adoption of permissive hypercapnia as a ventilatory strategy.

Arca MJ, et al: Current concepts in acute respiratory support for neonates and children. *Semin Pediatr Surg.* 2015;24:2.

▶ Fluids & Electrolytes

Careful fluid and electrolyte management is critical in the neonate to optimize cellular metabolism and tissue perfusion. This includes calculating fluid and electrolyte requirements necessary for supporting metabolic function, replacement of ongoing losses (eg, evaporative, third spacing, and external loss), and addressing any preexisting fluid deficits or excess. The patient's response to ongoing management is carefully monitored and adjusted accordingly.

Fluid status and acid-base balance can be assessed by noninvasive or invasive means. Physical exam findings consistent with dehydration include dry mucous membranes, absence of tears, delayed capillary refill, sunken eyes or a depressed fontanel, and loss of skin turgor. Clinical signs such as tachycardia, low urine output, hypotension, and a mottled skin appearance may indicate ongoing or evolving fluid deficits. Commonly used noninvasive modalities include pulse oximetry, transcutaneous CO_2 monitoring, and sphygmomanometry. For critically ill infants, invasive modalities may be necessary to assess adequacy of fluid status through central venous or arterial catheterization.

Indwelling arterial catheters can be placed in the radial, femoral, or temporal arteries, either percutaneously or by a cut-down incision. Central venous access may assist in cases where prolonged venous access is needed, parenteral nutrition is necessary, or when blood is frequently sampled. Such catheters may be placed via the umbilical vein or percutaneously via the saphenous, cephalic, median basilic, or temporal veins. Tunneled central venous access may be placed in the femoral, internal jugular, facial, or subclavian veins.

A. Calculating Maintenance Needs

In the newborn infant, the basic maintenance fluid requirement is the volume required for growth and replacement of ongoing losses from the skin, lungs, and stool. In the neonatal period, fluid losses primary occur through the skin and lungs, which is exacerbated in premature and very low birth weight infants. Requirements during the first 24 hours of life are unique because of the expanded extracellular fluid volume in the newborn, which decreases after 24 hours. Up to 10% of a newborn's birth weight is lost in the first 3-7 days, with the majority attributable to water loss, with minor contributions from meconium and urine. During the first 24 hours of life, initial fluid requirements are 60-80 mL/kg/d for normal weight infants, 80-100 mL/kg/d for low and very low birth weight infants, and 100-120 mL/kg/d or more for extremely low birth weight neonates. This requirement gradually increases to a minimum of 90-110 mL/kg/d by 4 days of life in normal infants. For children and adolescents, a commonly used method of calculating 24-hour fluid requirements is based on body weight, known as the Holliday-Segar method (Table 45–1). The "4-2-1 rule" is a simplified weight-based calculation, where children are provided an hourly fluid rate of 4 mL/kg up to 10 kg with an additional 2 mL/kg for every kilogram between 10 and 20 kg, and an additional 1 mL/kg for every additional kilogram above 20 kg. However, due to the many factors affecting maintenance requirements, modification of these guidelines may be necessary to optimize fluid and electrolyte needs in the individual patient.

Table 45–1. Calculation of maintenance fluid requirements.[1]

Body Weight	Fluid Volume per 24 h
1-10 kg	100 mL/kg
11-20 kg	1000 mL + 50 mL for each kg over 10 kg
> 20 kg	1500 mL + 20 mL for each kg over 20 kg

[1]Reproduced with permission from Norton, JA: *Surgery.* New York, NY: Springer; 2000.

B. Perioperative Fluid Management

Fluid, electrolyte, and acid-base abnormalities should be corrected in the neonate prior to operation if possible. In infants greater than 2 months of age, lactated Ringer's or normal saline is recommended for fluid resuscitation to reduce the risk of hyponatremia. Hypotonic fluids should generally be avoided outside of the neonatal period. Intraoperatively, fluid replacement consists of estimated maintenance requirement plus replacement of preexisting deficits (if uncorrected) and replacement of intraoperative losses.

Gastrointestinal losses from intestinal drainage and fistulas are directly measured and replaced with an appropriate electrolyte solution (Table 45–2). Protein-rich losses (eg, chest tube drainage of a chylothorax) can be replaced with colloid such as an albumin solution or fresh frozen plasma. Internal losses into body cavities or tissues (ie, third space losses) cannot be measured; replacement of these losses should be guided by careful monitoring of the patient's vital signs and urine output. Following an operation such as a laparotomy or thoracotomy, the fluid requirement may exceed 150 mL/kg/d for several days postoperatively. Isotonic fluids are typically recommended in the immediate postoperative period in patients over 2 months of age to replace third space losses.

C. Electrolyte Considerations

Electrolyte requirements for neonates, infants, and children vary by age. Normal electrolyte and energy requirements typically include sodium, potassium, magnesium, calcium, and phosphorus. Additional electrolytes such as bicarbonate may be necessary to correct acid-base abnormalities. Neonates may develop electrolyte abnormalities involving sodium, potassium, calcium, magnesium, and glucose, among others. Hyponatremia may result from excess administration of hypotonic fluids. Hypernatremia is commonly due to a free water deficit. Both hyponatremia and hypernatremia should be corrected cautiously in a monitored setting to avoid neurological complications. If there is no response to correction of a documented calcium deficiency, hypomagnesemia should be suspected and a serum magnesium level obtained. Generally, intravenous fluids should contain a minimum of 10% dextrose to prevent hypoglycemia. The treatment of hypoglycemia consists of giving 1-2 mL/kg of 50% glucose intravenously, followed by a continuous infusion of 10%-15% glucose solution at a rate set at maintenance fluid requirements.

Dell KR: Fluid, electrolytes, and acid-base homeostasis, in Martin RJ, Fanaroff AA, Walsh MC (eds): *Neonatal-Perinatal Medicine: Diseases of the Fetus and Infant*, 9th ed, Vol 1. St. Louis, MO: Elsevier Mosby; 2011, p. 669.

Padua AP, et al: Isotonic versus hypotonic saline solution for maintenance intravenous fluid therapy in children: a systematic review. *Pediatr Nephrol*. 2015;30:1163.

▶ Nutrition

Newborns require a relatively large caloric intake due to their high basal metabolic rate, caloric needs for normal growth and development, energy needs to maintain body temperature, and limited energy reserves. An infant requires 100-130 kcal/kg/d and 2-4 g/kg/d of protein to achieve a target daily weight gain of 10-15 g (Table 45–3). Thirty to forty percent of the total nonprotein calories should be provided as fat. These requirements decline with age but increase during periods of physiologic stress, during surgery, and in the presence of sepsis.

The best route of providing calories and protein is through the gastrointestinal tract. During the first year of life, human breast milk is the ideal nutritional source for

Table 45–2. Replacement of abnormal losses of fluids and electrolytes.

Type of Fluid	Electrolyte Content				Replacement
	Na⁺ (mEq/L)	K⁺ (mEq/L)	Cl⁻ (mEq/L)	HCO₃⁻ (mEq/L)	
Gastric (vomiting)	50 (20-90)	10 (4-15)	90 (50-150)	...	5% dextrose in half-normal (0.45%) saline plus KCl 20-40 mEq/L
Small bowel (ileostomy)	110 (70-140)	5 (3-10)	100 (70-130)	20 (10-40)	Lactated Ringer's
Diarrhea	80 (10-140)	25 (10-60)	90 (20-120)	40 (30-50)	Lactated Ringer's with or without HCO₃⁻
Bile	145 (130-160)	5 (4-7)	100 (80-120)	40 (30-50)	Lactated Ringer's with or without HCO₃⁻
Pancreatic	140 (130-150)	5 (4-7)	80 (60-100)	80 (60-110)	Lactated Ringer's with or without HCO₃⁻
Sweat Normal	20 (10-30)	4 (3-10)	20 (10-40)	...	...
Cystic fibrosis	90 (50-130)	15 (5-25)	90 (60-120)	...	...

Table 45–3. Caloric requirements of various age groups per 24 hours.[1]

Age	kcal/kg per 24 hours
Newborn term (0-4 days)	110-120
Low birth weight	120-130
3-4 months	100-106
5-12 months	100
1-7 years	75-90
7-12 years	60-75
12-18 years	30-60

[1]Reproduced with permission from Norton, JA: *Surgery.* New York, NY: Springer; 2000.

neonates and infants. If the gastrointestinal tract is functional, breast milk, standard infant formulas, blenderized meals, or prepared elemental diets can be given by mouth, through nasogastric or nasojejunal feeding tubes, or through surgically placed gastrostomy or jejunostomy tubes. Gastric feeding is typically preferred because it allows for normal digestive processes and hormonal responses, a greater tolerance for larger osmotic loads, a lower incidence of dumping, and fewer delays to initiation of feeds. The use of nasoduodenal or nasojejunal tubes is reserved for infants who cannot tolerate intragastric feeding (eg, delayed gastric emptying, gastroesophageal reflux, depressed gag reflex). Neonates who are critically ill or immediately postsurgery have less nutritional reserves than older children or adults. They require early enteral nutrition initiation, typically within 24-48 hours of fasting, to reduce the risk of hypoglycemia, pneumonia, and sepsis.

The multitude of nutritionally complete, low-viscosity liquid diets allows for multiple feeding options for neonates. Formulas exist for premature babies as well as children with lactose intolerance, galactosemia, protein intolerance, cystic fibrosis, renal failure, and short bowel syndrome, among others. Elemental diets are also made by mixing crystalline amino acids, oligosaccharides, and fats that can be completely absorbed in the small intestine with little residue.

B. Parenteral Nutrition

Parenteral nutrition is an essential and lifesaving intervention for many children who are unable to tolerate enteral feeding. There are several indications for parenteral nutrition in children, including prolonged ileus, high-output enterocutaneous fistulae, supplementation of oral feedings, short bowel syndrome, malabsorption syndromes, catabolic wasting states such as infections or tumors when gastric feedings are inadequate or not tolerated, inflammatory bowel disease, severe acute alimentary disorders (pancreatitis, necrotizing enterocolitis), chylothorax, and radiation enteritis, among others. When enteral nutrition is not adequate or feasible, initiation of parenteral nutrition is essential to promote growth, development, and recovery in children.

Parenteral nutrition can be delivered temporarily via peripheral veins, but concentrated glucose solutions (12.5% glucose or higher) may lead to thrombosis of peripheral vessels. For long-term alimentation, a central venous catheter (peripherally inserted central catheter or Broviac) is placed. The higher blood flow in these vessels ensures immediate dilution of the concentrated solution and allows for safe administration of more concentrated glucose solutions (15%-30%). Catheters may be placed percutaneously through the subclavian or internal jugular vein or inserted by cutdown into the external jugular, anterior facial, internal jugular, cephalic, brachial, or saphenous veins. For long-term use, Broviac (single-lumen) or Hickman (double-lumen) catheters, with Dacron cuffs positioned near the exit site of the skin, are preferred to minimize infection and to prevent dislodgment.

Parenteral nutrition solutions typically contain glucose (10%-40% solutions), amino acids (2%-5% crystalline amino acids or protein hydrolysate), electrolytes, vitamins, and trace minerals. The electrolyte composition of the protein solution should be known so that the desired composition of the final solution can be adjusted by appropriate additives according to the individual patient's requirements. A standard solution suitable for infants and young children must contain calcium, magnesium, and phosphate to allow for growth. Trace minerals are also added to the basic solution (Table 45–4). These solutions should be infused at a constant rate to reduce the risk of significant fluctuations of blood glucose and amino acid concentrations. If it is necessary to restrict the total fluid volume, more concentrated glucose solutions can be used in order to meet caloric needs.

There are numerous complications associated with prolonged parenteral nutrition administration. The most frequent problem is catheter-associated bloodstream infection. Although catheter removal will control the source of the infection, an initial trial of broad-spectrum antibiotics against gram-positive and gram-negative pathogens may be indicated. Catheter removal is required in the presence of worsening sepsis, recurrent positive blood cultures despite ongoing antibiotic treatment, and fungal infections. Catheter thrombosis is another common complication. Hyperglycemia or hypoglycemia can be minimized during parenteral nutrition administration with a constant infusion rate. Close monitoring of serum electrolytes (including calcium and phosphate) may be necessary several times a week initially, but the interval is decreased to once a week when the patient is stable. Patients must be observed for hyperammonemia and for vitamin or trace mineral deficiency.

Table 45–4. Total parenteral nutrition requirements.[1]

Component	Neonate	6 mo to 10 y	>10 y
Calories (kcal/kg/d)	90-120	60-105	40-75
Fluid (mL/kg/d)	120-180	120-150	50-75
Dextrose (mg/kg/min)	4-6	7-8	7-8
Protein (g/kg/d)	2-3	1.5-2.5	0.8-2.0
Fat (g/kg/d)	0.5-3.0	1.0-4.0	1.0-4.0
Sodium (mEq/kg/d)	3-4	3-4	3-4
Potassium (mEq/kg/d)	2-3	2-3	1-2
Calcium (mg/kg/d)	80-120	40-80	40-60
Phosphate (mg/kg/d)	25-40	25-40	25-40
Magnesium (mEq/kg/d)	0.25-1.0	0.5	0.5
Zinc (µg/kg/d)	300	100	3 mg/d
Copper (µg/kg/d)	20	20	1.2 mg/d
Chromium (µg/kg/d)	0.2	0.2	12 mg/d
Manganese (µg/kg/d)	6	6	0.3 mg/d
Selenium (mg/kg/d)	2	2	10-20 mg/d

[1]Reproduced with permission from Norton, JA: *Surgery*. New York, NY: Springer; 2000.

Progressive hepatomegaly and jaundice leading to liver dysfunction can occur after prolonged parenteral alimentation. Protective strategies to reduce the risk of liver dysfunction include "cycling" (giving full 24-hour volume of parenteral nutrition over shorter time periods) and augmenting with enteral feeding. Recently, an omega-3 fatty acid–based emulsion (Omegaven) was approved by the U.S. Food and Drug Administration for use in children with parenteral nutrition–associated liver disease.

Cowan E, et al: Fish oil-based lipid emulsion in the treatment of parenteral nutrition-associated liver disease. *Curr Opin Pediatr.* 2013;25:193.

Wessner S, et al: Review of nutritional assessment and clinical outcomes in pediatric surgical patients: Does preoperative nutritional assessment impact clinical outcomes? *J Pediatr Surg.* 2014;49:823.

▶ Blood Volume & Resuscitation

Circulating blood, plasma, and red blood cell (RBC) volumes are relatively high during the first few postnatal hours of life. Several hours after birth, plasma begins to shift out of the

Table 45–5. Blood volume based on age.

Preterm infants	85-100 mL/kg
Term infants	85 mL/kg
Age > 1 month	75 mL/kg
Age 3 months to adult	70 mL/kg

circulation, and total blood and plasma volumes decrease. The high RBC volume persists, slowly decreasing over approximately 7 weeks to reach normal adult levels. Age-related blood volume estimates are summarized in Table 45–5. Providers must be aware that routine lab draws can quickly result in symptomatic anemia in children as compared to adults.

Fetal hemoglobin, which persists for up to 6 months postpartum, is the main oxygen transport protein in newborn infants. The fetal liver is the major site of RBC production after 6-8 weeks' gestation, but the bone marrow becomes the primary site of hematopoiesis following birth. In neonates, the prothrombin time and the partial thromboplastin time may be slightly prolonged due to relative deficiencies of clotting factors. Coagulopathies may occur as a result of vitamin K deficiency, thrombocytopenia, inherited disorders, and temporary hepatic insufficiency due to immaturity, asphyxia, or infection. Although these coagulopathies are generally subclinical, it is standard to administer vitamin K intramuscularly to all neonates.

Blood lost during surgery varies greatly according to the complexity of the operative procedure, underlying disease, and effectiveness of hemostasis. Mild blood loss, amounting to less than 10% of the blood volume, usually does not require transfusion. It is imperative to develop methods for closely monitoring the amount of blood lost during operations since significant blood loss is often underestimated in the newborn, especially in the premature infant.

If a major surgical procedure is anticipated, the patient's blood should be typed and cross-matched in case transfusion is required. In infants with hematocrits greater than 50%, blood loss may be replaced by infusing lactated Ringer's solution or fresh frozen plasma (FFP) to compensate for losses of up to 25% of total blood volume. There are no national consensus transfusion guidelines, but blood losses greater than 25% are typically replaced with packed RBCs. Transfusion of 10 mL/kg of RBCs should raise the hematocrit 3%-4% on average. Transfused blood products should be prewarmed to body temperature to reduce the risk of hypothermia. With extensive blood loss and replacement, clotting factors and platelets can be rapidly depleted. A massive transfusion or "balanced" transfusion protocol should be initiated, which consists of replacing blood volume in a 1:1:1 ratio of RBCs to FFP to platelets. Cryoprecipitate may also be administered to replace low levels of fibrinogen.

Kasat K, et al: Neonatal red blood cell transfusions: searching for better guidelines. *Blood Transfus.* 2011;9:86.

Parker RI: Transfusion in critically ill children: indications, risks, and challenges. *Crit Care Med.* 2014;42:675.

► Perioperative Considerations

A. Gastrointestinal Decompression

The importance of gastric decompression in the surgical newborn cannot be overemphasized. The distended stomach carries the risk of aspiration and pneumonia. It may also impair diaphragmatic excursion, resulting in respiratory distress. Oxygenation and ventilation in a neonate with congenital diaphragmatic hernia may become progressively impaired as the herniated intestine becomes distended with air and fluid. The ability to reduce the prolapsed intestine into the abdominal cavity with gastroschisis, omphalocele, and diaphragmatic hernia may be impaired by intestinal distention. It is critical to avoid bag-mask ventilation in these patients, which can distend the stomach. A double-lumen (sump) tube is the preferred modality for gastric decompression. If a single-lumen tube is used, intermittent aspiration by syringe or machine is required. The correct position of the tube in the stomach is confirmed by carefully measuring the tube prior to insertion and by plain radiographs.

B. Preoperative Blood Sampling

Blood analyses should be restricted to laboratory studies that are essential for diagnosis and management. The volume of blood drawn for laboratory tests should be documented as these small volumes cumulatively represent significant blood loss in children, especially newborn infants. Generally, the only "routine" preoperative blood analyses for a neonate consist of a complete blood count and a blood specimen for type and crossmatch (in the case of major surgery). Electrolytes in the first 12 hours of life simply reflect the mother's electrolytes. Coagulation studies (eg, prothrombin time, partial thromboplastin time, activated clotting time) are rarely indicated.

C. Preoperative NPO Guidelines

The following are general guidelines as institutional practices vary considerably. Standard guiding principles weigh the risk of hypoglycemia associated with NPO (nothing by mouth) status and the tolerance of an NPO child with the surgical team's desire to reduce the risk of aspiration upon induction of general anesthesia. In the newborn period (and in early infancy), no solids or formula should be given within 4 hours prior to the procedure. Infants may have clear liquids (water, oral electrolyte mixtures, glucose water, or apple juice) and breast milk until 2 hours prior to the procedure.

▼ LESIONS OF THE HEAD & NECK

DERMOID CYSTS

Dermoid cysts are congenital subcutaneous lesions of skin and skin appendages commonly found on the scalp and eyebrows, or in the midline of the nose, neck, and upper chest. They present as painless, nonpulsatile, noncompressible nodules that are usually solitary and may be mobile or fixed to the skin and deeper structures. Dermoid cysts of the eyebrows and scalp may produce a depression in the underlying bone that appears as a smooth, punched-out defect on radiographs of the outer table of the skull. They rarely extend intracranially, although dermoid cysts located in the midline of the face and scalp may extend through the inner table of the skull. It is therefore imperative to obtain an ultrasound or cross-sectional imaging (magnetic resonance imaging [MRI] or computed tomography [CT]) to rule out a deep extension prior to operative intervention. Dermoid cysts of the midline neck may also resemble thyroglossal duct cysts. However, unlike thyroglossal duct cysts, dermoids do not move with swallowing or protrusion of the tongue. Many dermoids contain a thick, white ("cheesy") fluid that is a result of desquamation of the epithelial lining of the cyst well. Excision is generally recommended due to the propensity of the cysts to become infected or continue to grow with time. Incomplete removal leaving cyst wall behind has been associated with recurrence. Lesions arising near the eyebrows should be excised through an incision adjacent to the hairline. The eyebrows should not be shaved, nor should the incision go through any eyebrow follicles because a permanent glabrous area will develop. Tunneled endoscopic approaches originating from behind the hair line have also been reported to avoid facial scarring.

BRANCHIAL ANOMALIES

Branchial anomalies are remnants of the fetal branchial apparatus that can manifest as cysts, sinuses, fistulas, or cartilaginous remnants. These anomalies result from incomplete regression of branchial structures during embryogenesis. During the first month of fetal life, the primitive neck develops four external clefts and four pharyngeal pouches that are separated by a membrane. The dorsal portion of the first cleft becomes the external auditory canal; the other clefts are obliterated. The pharyngeal pouches persist as adult organs. The first pouch becomes the auditory tube, the middle ear cavity, and the mastoid air cells. The second pouch incompletely regresses and becomes the palatine tonsil and the supratonsillar fossa. The third pouch forms the inferior parathyroid glands and thymus, while the fourth forms the superior parathyroid glands.

A tract of branchial origin may form a complete fistula. Alternatively, one end may be obliterated to form an external

▲ **Figure 45–1.** Branchiogenic fistula from second branchial cleft origin. The fistula extends along the anterior border of the sternocleidomastoid muscle and courses between the internal and external carotid arteries and cephalad to the hypoglossal nerve to enter the tonsillar fossa.

or internal sinus, or both ends may resorb, leaving an aggregate of cells forming an internal cyst (Figure 45–1). Fistulas that arise above the hyoid bone and communicate with the external auditory canal represent persistence of the first branchial cleft. These tracts are always lined by squamous epithelium. Cysts and sinuses of second or third branchial origin are lined by squamous, cuboidal, or ciliated columnar epithelium. Fistulas that communicate between the anterior border of the sternocleidomastoid muscle and the tonsillar fossa are of second branchial origin, and those that extend into the piriform sinus are derived from the third branchial pouch. Cysts developing from branchial structures usually appear later in childhood as opposed to sinuses and fistulas. Branchial anomalies occur with equal frequency on each side of the neck, and 15% present as bilateral. Branchial cleft cysts account for approximately 20% of pediatric neck masses. Second branchial cleft abnormalities are most common, occurring six times more frequently than first cleft anomalies.

Clinical Findings

A sinus or fistulous opening along the anterior border of the sternocleidomastoid muscle may be noted at birth, and mucoid discharge may be present. A firm, cordlike tract may also be palpable under the skin. The patient may complain of a foul-tasting discharge in the mouth upon massaging the tract, but the internal orifice is rarely recognized. Some may present with an acute infection. Cysts typically present later

in childhood when a previously undiagnosed cyst becomes infected. They are characteristically found anterior and deep to the upper third of the sternocleidomastoid muscle, or they may be located within the parotid gland or pharyngeal wall, over the manubrium, or in the mediastinum. Sinuses and cysts are prone to become repeatedly infected, with associated cellulitis and abscess formation. Incomplete branchial sinuses appear as a dimple that contain cartilage and do not drain or communicate with the deep structures of the neck.

Differential Diagnosis

Granulomatous lymphadenitis from mycobacterial infections may produce draining sinuses, but these are usually distinguishable from branchial cleft anomalies by a chronic inflammatory reaction that precedes the onset of discharge. Suppurative lymphadenitis, most commonly due to *Staphylococcus aureus,* may also resemble an infected branchial remnant. However, treatment and complete healing of the lymphadenitis are curative, whereas a branchial remnant will persist after the infection resolves. Lymphatic malformations may transilluminate, while branchial cysts do not. Thyroglossal duct cysts, dermoid cysts, and parotid cysts (first branchial lesions) may also be mistaken for branchial anomalies.

Treatment

Nearly all branchial abnormalities should be excised early in life as recurrent infection is common. Neck swelling, airway compromise leading to respiratory symptoms, and the potential for malignancy are other considerations for excision. Asymptomatic, small cartilaginous remnants may be observed but should be removed if they become infected. Infected sinuses and cysts require antibiotic treatment and initial incision and drainage prior to definitive surgical excision. Every effort should be made to excise the entire cyst wall and fistula tract (including the skin punctum, if present) since recurrence and infection are the norm with incomplete removal. Excision should be undertaken cautiously, as the tracts may lie adjacent to the facial, hypoglossal, and glossopharyngeal nerves, as well as the carotid artery and internal jugular vein.

Erikci V, et al: Management of congenital neck lesions in children. *J Plast Reconstr Aesthet Surg.* 2014;67:e217.
Rosser JD, et al: Branchial cleft anomalies and thymic cysts. *Otolaryngol Clin North Am.* 2015;48:1.

PREAURICULAR LESIONS

Preauricular lesions arise from anomalous development of the auricle and include sinuses, cysts, pits, fissures, and cartilaginous rests. They are unrelated to branchial anomalies. The sinuses are typically short and end blindly. Excision is generally recommended due to the propensity of these anomalies to become infected. Superficial skin tags and cartilaginous rests are easily excised with minimal risk. Preauricular sinus tracts may be intimately associated with branches of the facial nerve, however, and so dissection should proceed with great caution. Infants with preauricular pits should undergo formal audiologic evaluation as these anomalies are associated with hearing loss.

LYMPHATIC MALFORMATIONS

Lymphatic malformations (LM) are benign, multilobular and multinodular cystic masses lined by lymph channel endothelial cells. They result from anomalous development or obstruction of embryonic lymphatics. They are not proliferative lesions and should be distinguished from hemangiomas. LMs can be categorized into three morphologic types depending on their histologic characteristics: macrocystic, microcystic, or mixed macrocystic and microcystic. They typically present as soft compressible masses with normal overlying skin. There may be a faint blue hue present underneath the skin. Fifty to sixty five percent appear at birth, and 90% are apparent by the second year of life. They are located most commonly in the posterior triangle of the neck (75%) (Figure 45–2) and axilla (20%), with the remainder located in the mediastinum, retroperitoneum, and groin. Cystic hygroma and lymphangioma are misnomers and should not be used to describe LM.

▶ Clinical Findings

Cervical LMs may extend beneath the clavicle into the axilla or mediastinum. These lesions grow along fascial planes and around neurovascular structures. They are infiltrative but not invasive. The majority of LMs are asymptomatic; however, occult LMs may present following an upper aerodigestive tract infection as a result of increased or infected lymph flow or following hemorrhage into the LM. Occasionally, very large lesions involving the floor of the mouth can cause hydrops in utero or asphyxiation at birth due to acute airway compromise. Large lesions may be recognized prenatally using ultrasound or MRI examination.

▶ Treatment

Treatment is generally tailored based on size, location, and extent of the LM and may include observation, pharmacotherapy, sclerotherapy, or surgery. LM can be treated medically or surgically, but surgical resection is considered to be the only potentially curative management. The preferred treatment depends on acuity, patient/parent preference, and provider experience. Image-guided, percutaneous intralesional injection of a sclerosing agent has become the preferred management for most macrocystic lesions. Commonly used sclerosing agents include ethanol, sodium tetradecyl sulfate, and doxycycline. Indwelling catheters can be placed for repeated drainage or sclerotherapy injections of large macrocystic lesions. Surgical resection is safe and has the highest likelihood for cure for lesions that are well-localized. Excision is typically carried out with bipolar cautery to ensure hemostatic dissection and to decrease the risk of a postoperative lymph leak and nerve injury. The recurrence rate following surgery can be as high as 50% since incomplete excision is the rule. Laser and radiofrequency ablative techniques have also been used to treat LM.

THYROGLOSSAL DUCT CYST

Thyroglossal duct cysts are the most common neck masses in children. During the fourth week of gestation, the thyroid gland develops from an evagination in the floor of the primitive pharynx located between the first pair of pharyngeal pouches. If the anlage of the thyroid does not descend normally, the gland may form at the base of the tongue or remain as a mass anywhere in the midline of the neck along its path of descent. If the thyroglossal duct persists, the epithelial tract can form a cyst, which usually communicates with the foramen cecum of the tongue. Because the thyroglossal duct descends through the second branchial arch anlage, which becomes the hyoid bone, the tract of a persistent thyroglossal duct often extends directly through the hyoid bone (Figures 45–3 and 45–4).

▶ Clinical Findings

The most common physical finding is a round, rubbery cystic mass in the midline of the neck just below the hyoid bone. The fluid in the cyst may be under pressure and resemble a solid tumor. Cysts and aberrant midline thyroid glands often

▲ **Figure 45–2.** Neonate with a complex lymphatic malformation involving the left neck and anterior thorax. (Used with permission from Steven J. Fishman, MD.)

▲ **Figure 45–3.** Thyroglossal cyst and duct course through the hyoid bone to the foramen cecum of the tongue.

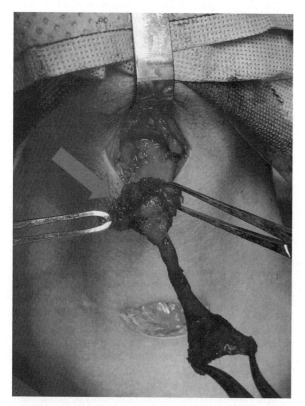

▲ **Figure 45–4.** Operative excision of a thyroglossal duct cyst. The course of the tract can be seen extending from the skin through the center of the hyoid bone (arrow). (Used with permission from Craig W. Lillehei, MD.)

move up and down with swallowing and with protrusion of the tongue. Infection may be the initial presentation of a thyroglossal cyst, with patients complaining of a bad taste secondary to pus draining into their mouths. Spontaneous drainage or incision and drainage of an abscess will often result in a chronically draining fistula.

▶ Differential Diagnosis

Lymphadenopathy, dermoid cysts, and branchial anomalies may all resemble thyroglossal duct cysts. Dermoid cysts do not move with swallowing. Lingual thyroids may be confused with a hypertrophied lingual tonsil or with a ranula, fibroma, angioma, sarcoma, or carcinoma of the tongue. Thyroglossal cysts may be distinguished from aberrantly located thyroid glands by ultrasound, needle aspiration, or radioiodine scintiscan.

▶ Treatment

Complete excision is generally recommended due to the risk of infection and malignant degeneration. Infection should be treated with antibiotics, and abscesses should be incised and drained before an attempt at definitive excision. The mid portion of the hyoid bone should be removed en bloc with the thyroglossal tract extending to the base of the tongue (Sistrunk procedure). Recurrences occur in approximately 10% of cases, with risk factors including previous infection and inadequate resection of the hyoid bone. In rare instances, the thyroglossal duct tract may contain all of a patient's normal functioning thyroid tissue. All patients undergoing excision of a thyroglossal duct cyst should therefor undergo ultrasound to document the presence of normal thyroid gland.

TORTICOLLIS

Torticollis is an abnormal contracture of the neck with resulting tilting of the head. The most common etiology is congenital muscular torticollis (CMT), which is characterized by the presence of a hard, nontender, fibrotic mass within the sternocleidomastoid muscle. It may be present at birth but is usually not apparent until the second to sixth weeks of life. CMT is often unilateral and affects both sexes equally. A history of breech delivery is present in 20%-30% of patients. Other etiologies of torticollis include familial (idiopathic), traumatic, infectious, and medication related.

▶ Clinical Findings

The clinical manifestations of torticollis occur when the sternocleidomastoid muscle is shortened and the mastoid process on the involved side is pulled down toward the clavicle and manubrium. As a result, the head is abducted to the ipsilateral side and rotated toward the contralateral shoulder.

The shoulder on the affected side is raised, and there may be cervical and thoracic scoliosis. Passive rotation of the head to the side of the involved muscle will be resisted and limited to varying degrees, and the muscle appears as a protuberant band. Due to persistent pressure when the patient is recumbent, the ipsilateral face and contralateral occiput may be flattened. Facial hemihypoplasia and plagiocephaly (flattening of the ipsilateral posterior skull) occur in untreated cases.

▶ Treatment

Torticollis is treated with physical therapy (active range-of-motion exercises), and surgery is rarely needed. The child's shoulders are held flat to a table and the head is tilted and rotated in a full range of motion. This exercise should be performed at least four times a day, usually for 2-3 months. In severe cases associated with facial or occipital skull deformities, both heads of the sternocleidomastoid muscle can be divided through a small transverse incision just above the clavicle. This procedure will not reverse the bony changes that have already developed but will prevent further deformity progression.

▼ CERVICAL LYMPHADENOPATHY

SUPPURATIVE LYMPHADENITIS

Infections of the upper respiratory passages, scalp, ear, or neck can produce secondary lymphadenitis. Acute bilateral lymphadenitis is typically viral in etiology, and most cases of acute unilateral lymphadenitis are caused by streptococcal and staphylococcal species. The clinical course of suppurative lymphadenitis may greatly overshadow a seemingly insignificant or (or even inapparent) primary infection. Scalp or ear infections can lead to suppurative lymphadenitis involving pre- or postauricular and suboccipital lymph nodes, whereas submental, oral, tonsillar, and pharyngeal infections can extend to the submandibular and deep jugular nodes.

▶ Clinical Findings

Symptoms typically include enlargement of regional lymph with associated pain and tenderness. Cervical involvement is most common, followed by occipital and submandibular nodes. Fevers are common, often intermittent, and may persist for days or weeks. Involved nodes may remain enlarged and firm for prolonged periods, or they may suppurate and produce surrounding cellulitis and edema. Subsequently, the nodes may involute or a fluctuant abscess may form, resulting in redness and thinning of the overlying skin. Infected, matted nodes may become so hard as to be indistinguishable (on palpation) from a solid mass.

▶ Differential Diagnosis

Suppurative lymphadenitis that neither resolves nor becomes suppurative can resemble granulomatous lymphadenitis, lymphoma, or metastatic tumor. Excisional biopsy may be required to differentiate these lesions. There will usually be a reduction in the size and firmness of suppurative adenitis, especially 1-2 weeks after antibiotic treatment has been started. Methicillin-resistant *S aureus* (MRSA) has become a common organism associated with suppurative lymphadenitis in the ambulatory setting. A high suspicion of an MRSA infection should be entertained in all children presenting with recurrent suppurative lymphadenitis.

▶ Treatment

All patients with suspected suppurative lymphadenitis should be treated with oral or intravenous antistaphylococcal and antistreptococcal antibiotics. In the subacute or chronic phase, the presence of pus in the node may be confirmed by needle aspiration. Abscesses should be incised and drained. In cases of documented MRSA infection, a prolonged course of either vancomycin or linezolid may be required for complete eradication even after drainage.

GRANULOMATOUS LYMPHADENITIS

Atypical mycobacteria account for the majority of confirmed causes of granulomatous lymphadenitis in the United States. *Mycobacterium avium-intracellulare* is the most commonly isolated organism, and patients often present with a non-suppurative area of matted nodes in the cervical, axillary, or inguinal regions. Tenderness and a draining sinus may also be present. Cat-scratch disease may cause a caseating lymphadenitis in regional lymph nodes (eg, epitrochlear and axillary nodes enlarge after an upper extremity cat scratch).

▶ Clinical Findings

The initial manifestation typically begins with a painless, progressive enlargement of regional lymph nodes. The duration of lymphadenopathy is usually 1-3 months or longer. The nodes may be large and mobile or, with progressive disease, may become matted, fixed, and finally caseate to form an abscess. Incision or skin breakdown over the involved nodes may result in a chronically draining sinus. In cases of tuberculosis, both sides of the neck or multiple groups of nodes are often involved, and a chest radiograph may indicate pulmonary involvement. In cases involving atypical mycobacterial lymphadenitis, pulmonary disease is rare and the cervical adenitis is nearly always unilateral. The tuberculin skin test is weakly positive in the majority of patients with atypical mycobacterial infection. Skin test antigens from the various strains of atypical mycobacteria are available. A positive skin test helps differentiate granulomatous adenitis from malignant lymphadenopathy.

Cat-scratch disease is usually acquired by a bite or scratch from a cat and is characterized by fever, malaise, musculoskeletal manifestations, and, occasionally, a pustular lesion at the site of the scratch. It is caused by a pleomorphic gramnegative bacillus (*Bartonella henselae*). Tender lymph node enlargement usually develops, with submandibular nodes being the most common site (92%). Regional lymphadenitis persists, producing painful, fixed suppurative nodes that may develop into a chronically draining sinus after 2-4 weeks.

▶ Treatment

Atypical tuberculous lymphadenitis typically requires surgical excision and/or antimycobacterial therapy. Azithromycin or trimethoprim-sulfamethoxazole may shorten the course of cat-scratch disease and prevent suppuration. When antibiotics are ineffective, excision of involved nodes should be performed before caseation occurs. Once the nodes become fluctuant or a draining sinus forms, a wedge of involved skin should be excised and the underlying necrotic nodes should be curetted out. The wound edges and skin should be closed primarily if possible. Excision and primary closure usually result in excellent healing with good cosmetic results.

▼ CONGENITAL CHEST WALL DEFORMITIES

PECTUS EXCAVATUM

Pectus excavatum is the most common congenital chest wall abnormality, representing approximately 90% of all chest wall deformities. The incidence is 1 in 350 live births, with a strong male predominance. The overwhelming majority of cases are sporadic, and approximately 10% are associated with genetic musculoskeletal disorders (Marfan, Ehlers-Danlos, and Noonan syndromes and idiopathic scoliosis). Sixteen percent of cases are associated with mitral value prolapse. Approximately 40% of patients have an affected relative, but no gene defect has been identified.

The cause of pectus excavatum remains unknown. Common theories include an unbalanced posterior growth of costal cartilages and abnormal costal cartilage structure. The result is a prominent posterior curvature of the inferior sternal body (Figure 45–5). The third, fourth, and fifth costal cartilages are most frequently affected. The severity of the defect varies from a barely discernable depression to an extreme defect where the xiphoid bone lies adjacent to the spine. The anomaly may also be associated with varying degrees of sternal rotation.

▶ Clinical Findings

Patients with pectus excavatum are typically round-shouldered with a stooped posture and have a relative abdominal

▲ **Figure 45–5.** Adolescent with a pectus excavatum deformity. Note that the most pronounced sternal curvature is in the lower half.

prominence and flared costal margins. The deformity is usually more pronounced during the pubertal growth spurt. Most children are asymptomatic, although occasionally patients may complain of dyspnea, chest wall discomfort, and easy fatigability. Although the defects can appear impressive on exam, they are rarely associated with measurable deficiencies in pulmonary and cardiac reserve. The primary complaint expressed by most patients is one of cosmetic concern, and many patients may refuse to participate in sports or other activities that may expose their deformity to peers.

▶ Treatment & Prognosis

There is no consensus around the optimal age for repair, with surgical management largely dependent on anatomic features and motivation on behalf of the patient. Younger children with increased chest wall flexibility make an operation technically easier. Drawbacks of an early opera- tion, however, include a higher risk of recurrence during the adolescent growth spurt and the inability of a young child to comprehend and assent to a predominantly cosmetic opera- tion. Measures of defect severity, including the Haller and correction indices, can be calculated from cross-sectional imaging to help guide decision making for surgery.

Historically, an open repair (Ravitch technique) was performed in which the abnormal cartilages are resected and the sternum is fractured and fixed in a corrected posi- tion. The Ravitch technique has been largely replaced by the minimally invasive Nuss procedure, where a curved sternal strut is passed under the chest wall muscles into each hemi- thorax. The strut is advanced across the mediastinum under the sternum via two small incisions in the midaxillary line. The strut is then passed upside down and then "flipped" into position, lifting the sternum and chest wall into a corrected position. The bar is left in place for 2-4 years, and then typi- cally removed as an ambulatory procedure. A good to excel- lent cosmetic outcome has been reported in more than 95% of patients following a Nuss repair. There is only weak evi- dence to suggest significant cardiopulmonary benefit after chest wall repair, except in rare instances when the deformity is excessive. The psychosocial benefits of repair are consid- erable, however, with many children reporting significant improvement in self-image and confidence.

PECTUS CARINATUM

Pectus carinatum is a chest wall defect associated with ster- nal protrusion and is approximately five times less common than pectus excavatum. As with pectus excavatum, there is a strong male predominance. The etiology is unknown, although the condition is thought to result from structural or connective tissue abnormalities, leading to overgrowth of costal cartilages and forward buckling of the sternum (Figure 45–6). Asymmetric forms with variable sternal rota- tion are common. The deformity has been noted to run in families, although no causative gene has been identified. It is associated with Marfan disease, neurofibromatosis, Poland syndrome, and vertebral anomalies. The deformity is typi- cally mild or nearly imperceptible in early childhood. Similar to pectus excavatum, the deformity often becomes increas- ingly pronounced during the pubertal growth spurt.

Bostanci K et al: Quality of life of patients who have undergone the minimally invasive repair of pectus carinatum. *Eur J Cardiotho- rac Surg.* 2013;43:122.

Lee RT, et al: Bracing is an effective therapy for pectus carinatum: interim results. *J Pediatr Surg.* 2013;48:184.

Nuss D, et al: Nuss bar procedure: past, present and future. *Ann Cardiothorac Surg.* 2016;5:422.

▲ **Figure 45–6.** Severe pectus carinatum deformity. (Reproduced with permission from O'Neill JA, Rowe MI, Grosted JL: *Pediatric Surgery,* 5th ed. Philadelphia, PA: Mosby/ Elsevier;1998.)

▶ Treatment & Prognosis

Historically, surgical repair was performed in moderate to severe cases to improve cosmetic appearance. Surgery has since been replaced by external bracing as the first-line treatment. Mild deformities can be observed over time for progression, particularly in early adolescence. Moderate to severe defects in adolescents should be treated, particularly when the patient indicates a desire for repair. Braces are typi- cally worn for 12-18 hours a day with maximum correction expected within 12-18 months.

STERNAL CLEFT

A sternal cleft anomaly occurs due to incomplete fusion of the two sternal bodies during embryonic development. The defect accounts for less than 1% of chest wall abnormalities. In its most severe form, the defect can be associated with protrusion of the pericardium and heart (ectopia cordis) and congenital heart lesions. Defects may be associated with extra- cardiac anomalies, including cleft lip, cleft palate, hydro- cephalus, central nervous system disorders, and pentalogy of Cantrell. Operative correction is typically performed in the neonatal period since the chest wall is so pliable.

Repair techniques include either suture approximation of the two sternal bodies or creation of a posterior sternal wall using chondral grafts.

SURGICAL RESPIRATORY CONDITIONS IN THE NEWBORN

The newborn is an obligate nasal breather, with ability to breathe through the mouth taking weeks or months to develop. Inspiration is accomplished chiefly by diaphragmatic excursion as intercostal and accessory muscles contribute relatively little. Impaired inspiration results in retraction of the sternum, costal margin, and neck fossae; the resulting paradoxical motion may contribute to respiratory insufficiency. The neonatal airway is relatively narrow and flaccid, is readily occluded by mucus or edema, and collapses easily under external pressure. Dyspneic infants tend to swallow large volumes of air, which may further impair diaphragmatic excursion due to distention of the stomach and small bowel.

Classification

A. Upper Airway Disorders

1. Micrognathia—Pierre Robin syndrome
2. Macroglossia—Muscular hypertrophy, hypothyroidism, lymphatic malformation, Beckwith-Wiedemann syndrome
3. Anomalous nasopharyngeal passage—Choanal atresia, Treacher Collins syndrome, Apert syndrome, and Crouzon syndrome
4. Tumors, cysts, or enlarged thyroid remnants in the pharynx or neck
5. Laryngeal or tracheal stenosis, webs, cysts, tumors, or vocal cord paralysis
6. Epiglottitis
7. Tracheomalacia
8. Tracheal stenosis with or without complete tracheal rings

B. Intrathoracic Airway Disorders

1. Atelectasis
2. Pneumothorax and pneumomediastinum
3. Pleural effusion or chylothorax
4. Pulmonary cysts, sequestration, and tumors
5. Congenital lobar emphysema
6. Diaphragmatic hernia or eventration
7. Esophageal atresia with or without tracheoesophageal fistula
8. Anomalies of the great vessels (eg, double aortic arch, aberrant left subclavian artery, anomalous origin of left pulmonary artery)
9. Mediastinal tumors and cysts (foregut duplications, thymomas, substernal goiter, lymphoma)

PIERRE ROBIN SYNDROME

Pierre Robin syndrome, also known as Pierre Robin sequence, is a congenital defect characterized by micrognathia, glossoptosis, and cleft palate. The etiology is unknown, but respiratory compromise arises indirectly as a result of mandibular hypoplasia mandible. The small lower jaw allows the tongue to be sucked back into the laryngeal airway where it could become occlusive. In severe cases, the occlusion can result in life-threatening asphyxiation.

Infants with mild occlusion should be kept in the prone position during care and feeding. Infants eventually learn how to keep the tongue from occluding the airway. Noninvasive respiratory support or nasopharyngeal airways can be effective in preventing occlusion of the larynx. A nasogastric or gastrostomy tube may be necessary for feeding. The majority of airway symptoms resolve by a year of age as a result of mandibular growth. If these conservative measures fail, surgical management should be considered. Surgical treatment includes mandibular distraction, glossopexy, and even tracheostomy in severe cases.

CHOANAL ATRESIA

Choanal atresia is a congenital blockage or obliteration of the posterior nasal aperture. The etiology remains unknown, but most cases involve bony or membranous obstruction. The majority of cases are associated with other congenital anomalies. Approximately two-thirds of cases are unilateral, and these cases are often asymptomatic. In contrast, neonates with bilateral involvement may present with severe respiratory distress, characterized by inspiratory stridor, chest wall retractions, and cyanosis that becomes worse with feeding. Symptoms tend to improve paradoxically with normal crying. The diagnosis is confirmed by the inability to pass a tube through the nares to the pharynx. With the baby in a supine position, contrast may be instilled into the nares, and lateral x-rays or CT scan of the head will demonstrate narrowing at the level of the pterygoid plate.

Cardiology and ophthalmology consultation are warranted if the diagnosis is confirmed.

Emergency treatment includes placement of an oral airway (placement of a nipple in the mouth with the tip cut off) and initiation of gavage feedings. Definitive treatment involves transnasal endoscopic resection of the posterior nasal septum with or without stenting. Endoscopic resection has largely replaced simple transnasal puncture as the latter technique has been associated with high recurrence rate.

TRACHEOMALACIA AND CONGENITAL TRACHEAL STENOSIS

Tracheomalacia is a functional obstruction that results from dynamic collapse of the trachea during respiration. Depending on the location, airway obstruction can occur during inspiration or expiration. It can be congenital or secondary to external compression by vascular anomalies, tumors, or a chronically dilated upper esophageal pouch in patients with esophageal atresia. There are three major types of congenital tracheal stenosis: segmental stenosis occurring anywhere in the tracheobronchial tree (50%); generalized hypoplasia (30%); and funnel-like narrowing (20%), usually tapering to a tight stenosis just above the carina.

▷ Diagnosis

The diagnostic approach to an infant with respiratory distress and possible distal tracheal obstruction must be carefully integrated with plans for management of the airway, since the compromised infant airway is easily occluded by edema or secretions. The diagnostic value of every procedure must be weighed against the threat of precipitating an acute airway obstruction from the procedure itself. Dynamic lesions such as tracheomalacia are best evaluated by endoscopy using a ventilating bronchoscope. Definitive diagnosis is made by bronchoscopy during spontaneous breathing. Fluoroscopy or cineradiography with barium in the esophagus has largely been abandoned. CT angiography may be necessary, and flow-volume curves can help define the level of obstruction (intrathoracic vs extrathoracic) and the type of obstruction (tracheomalacia vs stenosis). Tracheal stenosis lesions can sometimes be visualized using chest radiographs or fluoroscopy, but bronchoscopy is usually required to confirm the diagnosis. Dynamic airway CT protocols have also been used to characterize the location and severity of involved segments as well as the presence of vascular rings.

▷ Treatment

Noncritical tracheomalacia and stenotic lesions in infants and children should be managed conservatively if possible, preferably without intubation. Many infants improve over time when cartilage development leads to increased airway caliber. In children with symptomatic disease or airway obstruction, surgical management should be considered, especially in patients with a history of apparent life-threatening events attributable to airway compromise. Open and thoracoscopic tracheopexy have both been used to externally "stent open" the involved segments by suturing the trachea to the aorta, bronchus, or sternum. Posterior tracheopexy is a recently developed technique where the posterior wall of the trachea is sutured to the prevertebral fascia.

Mitchell ME, et al: Anterior tracheal suspension for tracheobronchomalacia in infants and children. *Ann Thorac Surg.* 2014;98:1246.

CONGENITAL DIAPHRAGMATIC HERNIA

Congenital diaphragmatic hernia (CDH) results from a defect in embryologic fusion, which allows herniation of abdominal viscera into the chest. The condition affects 2 in 10,000 live births and is associated with a significant burden of morbidity and mortality within the spectrum of pediatric general surgery (Figure 45–7). Anatomically, there are two types of CDHs. If diaphragmatic formation is incomplete, the pleuroperitoneal hiatus (foramen of Bochdalek) persists. Posterolateral (Bochdalek) hernias account for more than 95% of all cases, whereas anteromedial (Morgagni) hernias account for the remainder. Intestinal malrotation is a commonly associated condition. Disease severity and prognosis are closely related to the degree of pulmonary hypoplasia and associated pulmonary hypertension. ECMO may be required in severe cases to support cardiopulmonary function.

▲ **Figure 45–7.** Congenital posterolateral (Bochdalek) diaphragmatic hernia. Bowel, spleen, and liver sometimes herniate into the chest. Compromised lung development in utero negatively affects ventilation after birth.

Clinical Findings

A. Symptoms and Signs

Infants with large diaphragmatic defects are typically symptomatic immediately following delivery. Signs of respiratory distress, including tachypnea, grunting, severe retractions, and cyanosis, are common. Respiratory symptoms associated with smaller defects may not become apparent until the infant is several days or even months old. With moderate to large defects, herniation of abdominal viscera into the chest may result in a scaphoid abdomen, and breath sounds may be absent on the side of the hernia. Over 80% of CDHs occur on the left side (~80%-85%), and approximately 2% are bilateral. Other congenital anomalies are present with CDH in up to 50% of cases, including chromosomal abnormalities, neural tube defects, and congenital heart disease, among others.

B. Imaging Studies

The majority of CDH cases are diagnosed by prenatal ultrasound, although a small percentage are not diagnosed until birth. Following birth, a plain film may demonstrate several findings suggestive of the diagnosis, including a paucity of gas within the abdomen, a radiopaque hemithorax, loss of normal ipsilateral diaphragmatic contour, bowel in the thorax, mediastinal shift away from the side of the hernia, and a coiled nasogastric tube in the hemithorax. Right-sided hernias can be difficult to distinguish from diaphragmatic eventration. MRI or CT scan may be helpful in distinguishing between CDH and a cystic lung disease (eg, congenital cystic adenomatoid malformation).

Treatment

Initial optimization of medical management prior to surgical repair is critical to optimize survival. Immediate goals of care following delivery in a child with a known CDH include intubation, placement of a nasogastric tube on suction to prevent distention of the herniated bowel (which could further impair respiratory function), and initiation of adequate sedation and analgesia to prevent stress-induced exacerbation of pulmonary hypertension. Cardiovascular support with fluids and inotropic agents, ventilatory support (high-frequency ventilation may be required), and ECMO are supportive medical interventions. Surgery is performed once the infant has been stabilized medically, which may be several days or even weeks following birth. Surgical repair can be performed via laparotomy or thoracoscopically through small chest incisions. Successful use of minimally invasive techniques has been increasingly reported over the past decade; however, recurrence rates appear to be higher compared to historical data for open repair.

Open surgical repair is typically performed through a subcostal abdominal incision, although a thoracic incision may also be used. Herniated abdominal viscera are carefully reduced from the pleural space. Following reduction, the next step of the repair is to close the defect in its entirety while at the same time minimizing tension. Primary repair should be performed using nonabsorbable sutures. Larger defects may require a synthetic patch. The abdominal cavity may be too small and underdeveloped to accommodate the reduced viscera and permit closure of the abdominal wall. In such cases, abdominal wall skin flaps can be mobilized and closed over the protruding bowel. Other alternatives include use of synthetic or biological mesh to close the abdomen, or temporary silo placement to allow for gradual reduction of the viscera with staged closure of the abdominal wall.

Respiratory support and treatment of hypoxemia, hypercapnia, and acidosis are often required before and often after surgical repair of the defect. Persistent pulmonary hypertension may result in right-to-left shunt and produce severe hypoxemia. Nitric oxide is often used as a medical treatment to reduce the deleterious effects of severe pulmonary hypertension. Effects of nitrous oxide include pulmonary vasodilation, improved pulmonary perfusion, and decreased right-to-left shunting. Permissive hypercapnia ventilatory strategies have become a cornerstone of CDH management (high-frequency ventilation), with ECMO reserved for severe cases where adequate ventilation cannot be achieved by conventional methods. Hypoxemic myocardiopathy may require infusion of ionotropic agents to support cardiac output.

Prognosis

Postnatal survival rates have improved at tertiary care centers, with rates between 70% and 90% reported. Factors associated with decreased survival include prematurity (birth weight < 1500 g), severity of pulmonary hypoplasia and associated pulmonary hypertension, defect size, and associated cardiac and chromosomal anomalies. When diagnosed in utero, prognosis depends on the presence or absence of liver herniation, gestational age at diagnosis, and estimation of predicted lung volume (eg, the lung-to-head ratio). Long-term sequelae include restrictive or obstructive lung disease, and some children may require prolonged oxygen therapy. Gastroesophageal reflux is common due to deficiencies in periesophageal muscular tissue and an abnormal orientation of the gastroesophageal junction. Most patients respond to medical therapy, but refractory cases may require antireflux surgery or feeding via a gastrojejunostomy. Recurrent diaphragmatic hernia occurs in 10%-20% of infants and should be considered in any child with a history of CDH who presents with new gastrointestinal or pulmonary symptoms. Recurrence is most common when a prosthetic patch is used for the repair, especially when the patch is placed thoracoscopically.

With ongoing advancements in both prenatal diagnosis and postnatal care, more CDH newborns are being born at and receiving optimal care at tertiary facilities that are better equipped to care for these high-risk infants. Excluding infants with severe associated anomalies, the overall survival rate has been gradually increasing over the past 20 years.

FORAMEN OF MORGAGNI HERNIA

The foramen of Morgagni occurs at the junction of the septum transversum and the anterior thoracic wall. This defect of the central diaphragm is relatively rare, composing only 2% of all CDH cases. It may be parasternal, retrosternal, or bilateral in location. Unlike Bochdalek hernias, children with Morgagni hernia are often asymptomatic, and the defect is typically discovered later in life on a chest radiograph obtained for reasons unrelated to the hernia. A lateral chest radiograph demonstrating an air-filled mass extending into the anterior mediastinum is highly suggestive of the diagnosis. Repair is indicated even in the asymptomatic patient due to the risk of bowel obstruction. Operative principles include reduction of abdominal viscera, excision of the hernia sac, and closure of the defect by suturing the posterior rim of diaphragm to the posterior rectus sheath (there is no anterior diaphragm). A prosthetic patch closure may be required to achieve a tension-free repair. Open and laparoscopic approaches have been described. Unlike Bochdalek CDH, there is no associated pulmonary hypoplasia or pulmonary hypertension. However, Morgagni defects can be associated with the pentalogy of Cantrell, a disorder with considerable morbidity and mortality that is characterized by distal sternal cleft, epigastric omphalocele, apical pericardial defect, and congenital heart disease (usually a septal defect). Excluding patients with the pentalogy of Cantrell, survival is nearly 100%.

EVENTRATION OF THE DIAPHRAGM

Diaphragmatic eventration is a condition associated with an abnormally elevated, albeit intact, diaphragm. It may be congenital (idiopathic or associated with congenital myopathies or intrauterine infections) or acquired as a result of phrenic nerve injury during birth trauma or thoracic surgery. In the congenital form, there is variable thinning of diaphragmatic muscle, and distinction from CDH may be difficult on diagnostic evaluation. The elevated hemidiaphragm may produce abnormalities of chest wall mechanics with impaired pulmonary function. Respiratory symptoms may range from asymptomatic to significant distress, and recurrent infections are common. Gastrointestinal symptoms associated with obstruction may also be present, and gastric volvulus has also been reported.

Diagnosis is often made by plain chest radiograph. It is confirmed by dynamic fluoroscopy or sonographic evaluation, which demonstrates paradoxical movement of the diaphragm during spontaneous respiration. Asymptomatic eventrations may be observed. Eventration associated with respiratory symptoms requiring respiratory support should be repaired by plicating the diaphragm using interrupted nonabsorbable sutures.

Pierro M, et al: Understanding and treating pulmonary hypertension in congenital diaphragmatic hernia. *Semin Fetal Neonatal Med.* 2014;19:357.

Wynn J, et al: Outcomes of congenital diaphragmatic hernia in the modern era of management. *J Pediatr.* 2013;163:114.

Zani A, et al: Advances in the surgical approach to congenital diaphragmatic hernia. *Semin Fetal Neonatal Med.* 2014;19:364.

▼ GREAT VESSEL ANOMALIES

Tracheobronchial and esophageal compression may occur as a result of aortic arch anomalies or from pulmonary and subclavian arteries that are abnormally located or enlarged. The most common anomaly is an aberrant right subclavian artery, but the most clinically relevant anomaly is the double aortic arch, which can result in significant respiratory distress in young children (Figure 45–8). Affected children have a characteristic inspiratory and expiratory wheeze, stridor, or croup-like cough. Echocardiography or cross-sectional imaging (CT and MRI) is frequently used to establish the diagnosis, and esophagoscopy and bronchoscopy may be helpful in assessing the degree and level of compression. Surgical correction can be approached through the left or right chest. Following removal of the thymus to provide exposure, the aortic arch and its branches are skeletonized and the anatomy is established. In cases of a double aortic arch, the smallest arterial component is divided. Anomalous right subclavian arteries are managed by dividing them at their origin and restoring flow through anastomosis to the aortic arch or carotid artery. The accompanying fibrous bands and sheaths constricting the trachea and esophagus must also be divided.

▲ **Figure 45–8.** Anterior (left) and posterior (right) views of double aortic arch constricting the trachea and esophagus.

MEDIASTINAL MASSES

Mediastinal masses are relatively rare in children, but up to 40% are malignant. They can be classified according to the compartment of the mediastinum from which they arise (anterior, middle, or posterior compartments). The anterior mediastinum consists of the area between the sternum and the anterior aspect of the trachea and pericardium. The middle compartment contains the pericardium, trachea, major bronchi, and paratracheal spaces. The posterior segment extends from the posterior aspect of the trachea to the spine.

Forty to fifty percent of mediastinal masses are located within the posterior compartment and are most commonly neurogenic in origin. These include neuroblastoma, ganglioneuroblastoma, ganglioneuroma, neurofibroma, and neurofibrosarcoma. Posterior compartment masses also include foregut duplication and neurenteric cysts. Anterior masses make up one-third of cases and are most commonly teratomas and lymphomas. Teratomas may be cystic or solid, and approximately 20% are malignant. Other anterior compartment masses include thymomas and thyroid goiters. Middle compartment masses make up 10%-20% of mediastinal masses and include bronchogenic cysts, lymphoma, vascular tumors, cardiac tumors, and metastatic disease.

Symptoms associated with mediastinal masses include respiratory distress (via tracheal or lung compression), recurrent pulmonary infections (pneumonia), Horner syndrome, and pain.

LUNG MALFORMATIONS

There are four main categories of lung malformations: (1) congenital pulmonary airway malformation (CPAM); (2) bronchopulmonary sequestration (BPS); (3) congenital lobar emphysema (CLE); and (4) bronchogenic cyst. CPAM is the most common, and hybrid malformations with mixed histology can also be seen. Lung malformations arise when embryonic tissues that are destined to form bronchi and lung become isolated structures within or outside of the lung. These lesions can produce symptoms from their size and position, resulting in compression of bronchi or lung parenchyma, or from infection and abscess formation within the cyst and the adjacent normal lung. A growing number of congenital lung lesions are being diagnosed due to improvements in prenatal imaging. Lung malformations diagnosed prenatally warrant a postnatal CT angiogram to establish anatomy and identify the presence of systemic feeding vessels.

CONGENITAL PULMONARY AIRWAY MALFORMATION

CPAM was previously referred to as congenital cystic adenomatoid malformation. It is a hamartomatous lesion composed of multiple cystic and adenomatous elements resulting from proliferation of terminal bronchiolar structures that are in communication with the native airways. It is typically lined by a polypoid proliferation of bronchial epithelium surrounded by striated muscle and elastic tissue, but there is an absence of mucous glands and cartilage. Lesions are equally distributed among both lungs, but 75% of cases occur in the lower lobes. The arterial supply and venous drainage typically arise from the pulmonary circulation. Associated renal and nervous system anomalies may be present.

CPAMs are further categorized into five types based on size of the cysts and cellular characteristics: type 0 lesions originate from tracheal or bronchial tissue, with small cysts (< 0.5 cm); type 1 lesions are the most common (60%-70% of all CPAMS), originate from distal bronchi or proximal bronchioles, and are characterized by large cysts (> 2 cm); type 2 lesions (15%-20%) resemble dilated terminal bronchioles with multiple smaller cysts (0.5-2 cm); type 3 lesions (5%-10%) are often very large and can involve an entire or several lobes, with numerous small cysts (< 0.5 cm); and type 4 lesions (5%-10%) consist of alveolar lining cells with larger cysts (< 7 cm). Type 4 lesions have been associated with malignant degeneration (pleuropulmonary blastoma).

Clinical Findings

The majority of patients (75%) with CPAMS are asymptomatic at birth, and one-third of cases are diagnosed following the neonatal period. Recurrent pneumonia and spontaneous pneumothorax are common presentations. Large lesions can compress adjacent structures, resulting in pulmonary hypoplasia and esophageal obstruction with polyhydramnios. Compression of venous return to the heart may lead to fetal congestive heart failure, hydrops fetalis, and fetal death. Large lesions that do not result in hydrops can remain stable or involute during fetal life, producing surprisingly minimal or no respiratory symptoms at birth. Diagnosis can often made by chest radiograph, with CT and MRI used to further delineate anatomic characteristics and vascular supply.

Treatment

Prenatal intervention may be considered if the disorder is identified in utero in association with hydrops. Prenatal steroids, drainage procedures, in utero surgery, and early delivery are potential options, but generally the presence of hydrops is associated a poor prognosis. Asymptomatic children may be observed, but this remains controversial due to the risk of future infectious complications and malignant degeneration. It should be noted that the frequency of future infection and malignancy are not well established; however, surgical resection (pulmonary lobectomy or nonanatomic segmental resection) is generally recommended by the first year of life based on these considerations.

▲ **Figure 45–9.** Pulmonary sequestration involving the left lower lobe in an 8-month-old child. Note the large arterial blood supply arising from the aorta inferior to the diaphragm (arrow).

BRONCHOPULMONARY SEQUESTRATION

BPS is an anomaly of normal airway development where a segment or cluster of normally developed bronchioles and alveoli does not communicate with the airway. They are supplied by systemic rather than pulmonary arteries, which is pathognomonic for BPS (Figure 45–9). Sequestrations occur predominantly in the lower lobes of the lung, most commonly on the left side. Rarely, they may occur in the upper or middle lobes and even below the diaphragm. Arterial blood supply is typically from the lower thoracic or upper abdominal aorta. Sequestrations may be intralobar (75%) or extralobar (25%). Intralobar lesions drain through the pulmonary veins and are prone to recurrent infections because of their close proximity to (and compression of) normally aerated lung. Extralobar lesions typically drain into the azygous vein and are usually asymptomatic and have a separate pleural covering. BPS may be found in association with CDH. Histologic evidence suggests that these lesions have embryologic origin similar to that of bronchogenic cysts and CPAMs. However, unlike the latter, sequestrations rarely grow large enough to produce hydrops and in utero demise. Treatment is by resection of the extralobar sequestration or lobectomy in cases of intralobar sequestration.

CONGENITAL LOBAR EMPHYSEMA

CLE, also known as congenital alveolar overdistension, results from hyperinflation of one or more lobes. The left upper (40%-50%) and right middle (25%-30%) lobes are most frequently involved, and CLE is categorized into three forms: hypoplastic emphysema, polyalveolar lobe, and bronchial obstruction.

Hypoplastic emphysema is distinguished by a segment, lobe, or whole lung that has a reduced number of bronchial branches with a diminished number and smaller size of blood vessels. The number of alveoli is decreased, and air spaces are excessively large, with overall markedly reduced surface area for gas exchange. Polyalveolar lobe is characterized by a normal size and number of bronchial branches, but there is an abnormal number of alveoli from each respiratory unit. These alveoli are prone to expand excessively, producing emphysema, which encroaches on the surrounding normal lung.

Bronchial obstruction may occur from deficient bronchial cartilage support, redundant mucosa, bronchial stenosis, mucus plug, or bronchial compression by anomalous vessels or other mediastinal lesions. With inspiration, the bronchus opens to allow air into the lung, but on expiration, the bronchus collapses, trapping the air, and with each respiratory cycle, there is progressive expansion of the lobe.

▶ Clinical Findings

Approximately one-third of patients with CLE present with symptoms at birth and 50% by 4 weeks of age. It is rare for symptoms to develop after 6 months of age. Males are more commonly affected, and the incidence of CLE is approximately 1 in 25,000 births. Common symptoms include dyspnea, wheezing, grunting, coughing, cyanosis, and poor feeding. Increased anteroposterior dimension of the chest and retractions may be seen. The chest is hyperresonant, and decreased breath sounds may be noted over the affected lobe. A chest radiograph may demonstrate radiolucency and expansion of the affected lobe. Compressive atelectasis of adjacent lung, mediastinal shift, depression of the diaphragm, and anterior bowing of the sternum can be seen.

▶ Treatment & Prognosis

Symptomatic lesions require surgical resection. For patients undergoing resection, the need for an emergent thoracotomy or needle decompression should be anticipated with initiation of positive-pressure ventilation (may acutely result in overexpansion of the emphysematous lobe). Treatment of asymptomatic and mildly symptomatic cases is often unnecessary. Prognosis following surgical resection of CLE in most patients is excellent.

BRONCHOGENIC CYST

Bronchogenic cysts are characterized by a ciliated columnar epithelium lining and cartilaginous elements and are often filled with mucoid material. Bronchogenic cysts arise in the right lung three times more often than in the left and are more commonly found in the lower lobes. About 50% of cysts arise in the mediastinum (paratracheal and subcarinal locations) and do not communicate with the bronchi. They appear as radiopaque masses on chest radiographs. When located within the lung parenchyma, the cysts can communicate with the airways and consequently are prone to abscess formation. Partial compression of bronchi may produce hyperinflation of the involved lung, while complete obstruction produces atelectasis. Rarely, rupture of a cyst that communicates with bronchi may present as a tension pneumothorax. Squamous epithelial metaplasia has been reported. Treatment of a non-infected cyst is by excision. Infected cysts should be initially managed with antibiotic therapy and drainage (usually per-cutaneous) followed by resection.

Davenport M, et al: Long term respiratory outcomes of congenital thoracic malformations. *Semin Fetal Neonatal Med.* 2012;17:99.
Kunisaki SM, et al: Thoracoscopic vs open lobectomy in infants and young children with congenital lung malformations. *J Am Coll Surg.* 2014;218:261.
Puligandla PS, et al: Congenital lung lesions. *Clin Perinatol.* 2012; 39(2):331-347.

CONGENITAL GASTROINTESTINAL LESIONS

ESOPHAGEAL ANOMALIES AND TRACHEOESOPHAGEAL FISTULA

The trachea and esophagus are derived from the primitive foregut. Initially, they appear as a common ventral diverticulum at about the 19th day of gestation. Elongation and separation of the diverticulum into the airway and esophagus then occur in a caudal to cephalad direction. Incomplete separation

during this process results in esophageal atresia, tracheo-esophageal fistula, and associated anomalies (Figure 45–10).

Esophageal atresia (EA) with or without tracheoesophageal fistula (TEF) occurs in approximately 1 in 3500 live births. Approximately 30%-40% of newborns with such anomalies are born prematurely, likely secondary to the inability to swallow amniotic fluid (resulting in polyhydramnios).

▶ Classification

A. Esophageal Atresia With Tracheoesophageal Fistula

EA is categorized into several types depending on the associated presence and anatomic relationship of a TEF. Four types of EA are characterized with an associated TEF. Type C atresias are by far the most common (85%) and are associated with a blind proximal pouch and a fistula between the distal end of the esophagus and the distal one-third of the trachea. The remaining types are relatively rare, with type E atresias (4% of cases) characterized by an "H"-type TEF between the proximal esophagus and trachea (often present in the low cervical region), type B atresias (1%) characterized by a fistula between the proximal esophagus and the trachea and a blind distal esophagus without fistula, and type D atresias (1%) characterized by fistulas between both proximal and distal esophageal segments and the trachea.

B. Esophageal Atresia Without Tracheoesophageal Fistula and Other Anomalies

EA without TEF is the second most common type of EA (8% of cases) and is characterized by a blind proximal esophageal pouch and a blind (and often quite attenuated) distal esophagus. This type of EA is usually associated with a wide

▲ **Figure 45–10.** **A:** Pure (long-gap) esophageal atresia. **B:** Esophageal atresia with proximal tracheoesophageal fistula. **C:** Esophageal atresia with distal tracheoesophageal fistula. **D:** Esophageal atresia with proximal and distal fistulas. **E:** Tracheoesophageal fistula without esophageal atresia. (Reproduced with permission from Sabiston DC: *Textbook of Surgery.* Philadelphia, PA: Saunders/Elsevier; 1991.)

gap between the proximal and distal esophageal segments, which can make surgical correction challenging ("long gap" atresia). Less common anomalies include cartilaginous obstructive membranes present in the distal esophagus and laryngotracheoesophageal clefts of varying lengths.

Clinical Findings

Symptoms associated with EA include excessive oral secretions, coughing, choking, and cyanosis. Attempts at feeding will immediately result in choking, gagging, and regurgitation. Infants with an associated TEF may also have reflux of gastric secretions into the tracheobronchial tree, putting them at risk for aspiration pneumonia and even laryngospasm. Diagnosis may be delayed (several months to years) in the case of a small H-type TEF where infants are able to feed but develop recurrent upper respiratory infections due to aspiration.

The diagnosis of EA can be made by attempting to pass an orogastric tube into the stomach by way of the nose or mouth. If EA is present, the tube will coil in the upper esophageal pouch, which can be confirmed with a plain radiograph. If an associated TEF is present, air will be present in the stomach and bowel on plain films. Absence of air below the diaphragm usually means a type A atresia is present without a TEF. In cases where the diagnosis is uncertain, a small amount of water-soluble contrast material can be placed in the esophageal pouch via the orogastric tube and visualized under fluoroscopy.

Isolated TEFs are best diagnosed by esophageal endoscopy and bronchoscopy as contrast studies have been associated with lower sensitivity (Figure 45–11). Abdominal distention may be a prominent exam finding due to diversion of air through a fistula into the stomach and bowel. The position of the fistula is usually determined by bronchoscopy. Laryngotracheoesophageal cleft produces symptoms similar to those of TEF but of greater severity, particularly in cases where the cleft extends well below the larynx. Laryngoscopy may show the cleft between the arytenoids extending down the larynx. Bronchoscopy is the best means of outlining the cleft.

There is a 50% incidence of associated anomalies with EA, including cardiac (patent ductus arteriosus, septal defects), gastrointestinal (imperforate anus, duodenal atresia), genitourinary, and skeletal. The VACTERL association (*v*ertebral, *a*norectal, *c*ardiac, *t*racheoesophageal, *r*enal, and *l*imb anomalies) is present in 25% of cases. Isolated EA has been associated with trisomy 18 and 21. Evaluation of all children with EA should therefore include echocardiogram, ultrasound of the urogenital tract, skeletal films, careful anorectal exam, spine ultrasound (to rule out a tethered cord), and genetic testing.

Treatment

Once the diagnosis is suspected, a sump should be placed in the upper esophageal pouch and placed to continuous suction and the head of the bed elevated. An echocardiogram is

▲ **Figure 45–11.** Rigid bronchoscopy performed in a newborn with a tracheoesophageal fistula. The opening to the fistula can be seen in the posterior trachea just proximal to the carina (arrow). (Used with permission from Craig W. Lillehei, MD.)

obtained not only to identify associated cardiac anomalies, but also to establish the position of the aortic arch. A right-sided arch is present in 5% of infants and may change the operative approach from the standard right thoracotomy or thoracoscopic repair.

The goals of operative repair are to divide and ligate the TEF and repair the EA in a single stage, if possible. This is usually performed using a right posterolateral thoracotomy with an extrapleural dissection. A transpleural thoracoscopic approach can also be used in stable, near-term infants. H-type TEFs are usually approached through a left transverse cervical incision (the fistula is located above the thoracic inlet in two-thirds of cases). A feeding gastrostomy tube is placed in cases of long gap atresia where a single-stage repair cannot be performed. Gastrostomy may also be considered in premature infants and in the presence of other comorbidities that may impact feeding ability or tolerance (eg, severe congenital heart disease). A transanastomotic feeding tube may be placed by some surgeons to stent open the anastomosis, although this practice is not universally accepted. Enteral feeding is usually initiated following demonstration of a leak-free anastomosis by esophagram obtained on postoperative day 7.

Staged operations may be needed for infants who are extremely premature and those with severe aspiration pneumonitis, cardiac anomalies associated with hemodynamic instability, and long-gap EA where primary anastomosis is not possible. Long-gap atresia can pose a challenge to establishing esophageal continuity. The traditional approach is to place a feeding gastrostomy tube and delay repair for several months to allow growth of the esophageal ends. Strategies for repair of extremely long-gap EA include gastric pull-up procedures, colonic and jejunal interposition, and even permanent cervical esophagostomy. Recently, an innovative staged esophageal lengthening protocol has been successful in treating long-gap EA through sustained external traction on the esophageal ends.

Esophageal narrowing or webs in the distal esophageal segment can be treated with esophageal dilation, although several dilations may be necessary and not all lesions respond. Esophagoscopy and endoscopic excision of residual scar tissue may be required in addition to dilation. Lower esophageal strictures containing cartilage and those recalcitrant to endoscopic treatment often require resection and anastomosis.

▶ Prognosis

The survival rate for a full-term infant without associated anomalies is excellent. However, mortality rates are not insignificant, and death can occur as a result of pulmonary complications, associated anomalies, prematurity, and sepsis. Anastomotic leaks may occur due to anastomotic tension or poor blood supply. The extrapleural surgical approach helps prevent the development of empyema if an anastomotic leak occurs and confines a leak to a small localized area.

Swallowing is a reflex that must be reinforced early in infancy through the normal feeding mechanism. If establishment of esophageal continuity is delayed for more than 4-6 weeks, it may take many months to overcome oral aversion and learn to swallow. Babies with cervical esophagostomies should be encouraged to suck, eat, and swallow during gastrostomy feedings.

Dysphagia following EA repair is multifactorial and may occur for months or years. Anastomotic strictures are not uncommon and may require one or more dilations under anesthesia. Solid food may become lodged or impacted at the anastomotic site and require endoscopic removal. Peristalsis may also be impacted and lead to dysphagia, especially involving the distal esophageal segment in long-gap cases.

Many infants may develop respiratory symptoms associated with tracheomalacia. Tracheomalacia frequently improves with age and is rare after 5 years of age. In severe cases, however, the flaccid airway may lead to severe respiratory compromise and even cardiopulmonary arrest. Gastroesophageal reflux is common after successful repair and may result in recurrent aspiration pneumonitis, dysphagia, failure to thrive, and recurrent anastomotic stricture. Medical therapy with an H_2-blocker or proton pump inhibitor should be instituted in all patients after repair, and a surgical antireflux procedure may be necessary if medical therapy fails.

Bairdain S, et al: Foker process for the correction of long gap esophageal atresia: primary treatment versus secondary treatment after prior esophageal surgery. *J Pediatr Surg.* 2015;50:933.

Dellenmark-Blom M, et al: Health-related quality of life among children, young people and adults with esophageal atresia: a review of the literature and recommendations for future research. *Qual Life Res.* 2015;24:2433.

Kunisaki SM, et al: Surgical advances in the fetus and neonate: esophageal atresia. *Clin Perinatol* 2012;39:349.

Sulkowski JP, et al: Morbidity and mortality in patients with esophageal atresia. *Surgery.* 2014;156:483.

INTESTINAL OBSTRUCTION IN THE NEWBORN

Intestinal obstruction may be noted on prenatal ultrasound by the presence of polyhydramnios (increased amniotic fluid). The presence of polyhydramnios correlates with the level of the obstruction; it is most common with proximal gastrointestinal tract obstruction (eg, esophageal and duodenal atresia) and is rarely noted with obstructive lesions of the distal ileum (eg, atresia) and beyond.

Following birth, emesis is the principal symptom of intestinal obstruction and may be bile stained if the obstruction is distal to the ampulla of Vater. Bilious emesis in the newborn is a surgical emergency until proved otherwise. On physical examination, the presence and degree of abdominal distention are dependent on the level of the obstruction. There is typically little distention associated with duodenal lesions, whereas distal small bowel and colorectal obstruction can lead to marked abdominal distention. A careful perineal examination should be performed to determine whether the anus is present, patent, and in the normal location. Meconium, the first newborn stool, passes in the first 24 hours of life in 94% of normal full-term infants and by 48 hours in 98%. Failure to pass meconium may be indicative of a distal gastrointestinal tract obstruction. However, 30%-50% of newborn infants with intestinal obstruction will pass meconium, so this finding has relatively poor negative predictive value.

Depending on the underlying pathology, plain abdominal films may demonstrate dilated bowel loops, air-fluid levels, or a gasless abdomen. Unlike adult patients, one often cannot differentiate between small and large bowel by their usual markings in neonates and infants. If a distal gastrointestinal tract obstruction is suspected, a water-soluble contrast enema is the most useful study since it can be both diagnostic and therapeutic. An upper gastrointestinal series should be obtained with a small bowel follow-through if malrotation is suspected. There is seldom a role for additional imaging outside of plain films for complete obstructions of the duodenum and small bowel. These children should generally be explored without further imaging once they are hemodynamically stable and other life-threatening conditions (eg, cardiac anomalies) have been ruled out. Cross-sectional imaging modalities such as CT and MRI are usually not indicated in the workup of newborn intestinal obstruction.

▲ **Figure 45–12.** Hypertrophic pyloric stenosis. Note that the distal end of the hypertrophic muscle protrudes into the duodenum (arrow), accounting for the ease of perforation into the duodenum during pyloromyotomy.

Ultrasound is also seldom useful in the evaluation of intestinal obstruction outside of hypertrophic pyloric stenosis.

HYPERTROPHIC PYLORIC STENOSIS

Pyloric stenosis is the most common cause of gastric outlet obstruction in infants and the pediatric population in general. It results from hypertrophy of the circular muscle of the pylorus and the distal antrum of the stomach with progressive narrowing of the pyloric channel (Figure 45–12). The etiology remains largely unknown. Pyloric stenosis affects approximately 1 in 300 live births, is much more common in males (80%), and occurs more commonly in Caucasians and first-born infants. There also appears to be a strong genetic component. If one monozygotic twin is affected, the other will have the disorder in two-thirds of cases. Pyloric stenosis occurs four times more often in the offspring of mothers who had the disease as infants than in those whose fathers had the disease.

▶ Clinical Findings

A. Symptoms and Signs

The typical presentation is an infant who was previously feeding well and then developed progressive feeding intolerance and nonbilious, forceful ("projectile") postprandial emesis. Shortly after vomiting, the infant will attempt to feed again, often voraciously. With progressive poor feeding and dehydration, physical exam findings may include a sunken fontanel, dry mucous membranes, poor skin turgor, and weight loss. A mass in the mid to upper abdomen ("olive") representative of the enlarged pylorus may be palpable in infants who are relaxed. The severity of dehydration and electrolyte abnormalities (classically a hypochloremic hypokalemic metabolic alkalosis) can be quite variable among infants and is primarily dependent on duration of symptoms and treatment delay.

B. Imaging Studies

Abdominal ultrasound is the most sensitive and specific imaging test to confirm the diagnosis. Pyloric muscle thickness measuring 3 mm or more and a pyloric channel length at least 15 mm are strongly suggestive of the diagnosis. Lack of gastric emptying on dynamic ultrasound imaging provides further evidence to support the diagnosis. An upper gastrointestinal study (previous gold standard) is indicated if ultrasound is not available or if the exam is equivocal.

▶ Differential Diagnosis

Recurrent nonbilious vomiting in early infancy is most often due to overfeeding and gastroesophageal reflux. Other "surgical" causes are far less common and may include intracranial lesions, antral webs, pyloric duplications, duodenal stenosis, and malrotation with volvulus.

▶ Complications

Protracted vomiting with inadequate rehydration results in a hypokalemic hypochloremic metabolic alkalosis, progressive dehydration, and ultimately starvation if the disorder is not corrected. Gastritis and reflux esophagitis occur frequently. Aspiration of vomitus may produce pneumonia.

▶ Treatment & Prognosis

Definitive management is surgical, although surgery is not emergent and should be postponed until after dehydration, electrolyte derangement, and metabolic alkalosis have been corrected. Operative treatment includes an open or laparoscopic pyloromyotomy, in which the pylorus is incised along its entire length and spread widely exposing but not breaching the underlying mucosa (Figure 45–13).

There are three general operative approaches to pyloromyotomy: a right upper quadrant transverse skin incision, a circumumbilical or intraumbilical skin incision, or a laparoscopic approach. In the last technique, a laparoscope is placed through the umbilicus, and two working ports are placed directly through the abdominal wall in the right and left upper quadrants. If the mucosa is inadvertently entered (usually on the duodenal side) during the pyloromyotomy, the mucosal breach is closed with fine absorbable sutures, and an omental patch is placed to buttress the repair. Larger perforations are managed by closing the pyloromyotomy, rotating the pylorus 90 degrees, and repeating the myotomy on the opposite side.

Feeding can be resumed in most infants as soon as the infant recovers from anesthesia and is awake enough to feed. Nearly all patients with pyloric stenosis have moderate regurgitation after surgery, presumably due to gastric ileus, gastritis, gastroesophageal reflux, or all of the above. Parents should be informed of this, but the reinitiation of feeds

▲ **Figure 45–13.** Appearance of the pylorus following laparoscopic pyloromyotomy. The mucosa can be seen bulging out from within the split pyloric muscle fibers (**arrow**). (Used with permission from Craig W. Lillehei, MD.)

should not be delayed. An incomplete pyloromyotomy (usually on the antral side) may be suspected when vomiting persists beyond 1-2 weeks postoperatively. The possibility of an incomplete myotomy should be evaluated by upper gastrointestinal series because ultrasound will often demonstrate persistent hypertrophy.

Pyloric stenosis does not recur if the myotomy is adequate, and there is a uniformly excellent outcome.

Ein SH, et al: The ins and outs of pyloromyotomy: what we have learned in 35 years. *Pediatr Surg Int.* 2014;30:467.

Sullivan KJ, et al: Feeding post-pyloromyotomy: a meta-analysis. *Pediatrics.* 2016;137:1.

Svenningsson A, et al: Maternal and pregnancy characteristics and risk of infantile hypertrophic pyloric stenosis. *J Pediatr Surg.* 2014;49:1226.

CONGENITAL DUODENAL OBSTRUCTION

The duodenum is the second most common site of congenital intestinal obstruction behind only the stomach (pyloric stenosis). The etiology of duodenal obstruction can be categorized into intrinsic and extrinsic lesions. Intrinsic lesions include atresia, stenosis, and mucosal webs (complete or partial). Extrinsic obstruction can be due to an annular pancreas, preduodenal portal vein, choledochoceles, and peritoneal bands (Ladd bands) from malfixation. Duodenal atresia is due to failure of recanalization of the duodenum early in gestation rather than mesenteric vascular accidents (which are more commonly associated with small bowel atresias).

Atresia of the duodenum accounts for 50% of all small intestinal atresias. Multiple congenital anomalies are present in approximately half of all patients, with the most common being Down syndrome (30%) and congenital heart disease (20%). Annular pancreas is a developmental anomaly characterized by circumferential persistence of the gland around the duodenum at the site of the embryonic ventral anlage, leading to duodenal obstruction and an accessory pancreatic duct.

▶ Clinical Findings

In 80% of cases, duodenal obstruction occurs distal to the ampulla of Vater, resulting in bilious emesis shortly following birth. The upper abdomen is rarely distended, and passage of meconium is common.

Plain abdominal radiographs demonstrate an air-distended stomach and duodenum (double bubble sign). Gas in the small and large intestine indicates incomplete obstruction. An upper gastrointestinal series may be necessary to rule out malrotation with a midgut volvulus in neonates in whom the diagnosis remains in question.

▶ Treatment

Surgery is performed using an open or laparoscopic approach, with the former using a right upper transverse abdominal incision. A Kocher maneuver is initially performed, with complete mobilization of the third and fourth portions of the duodenum. A diamond-shaped duodenoduodenostomy is performed for duodenal atresia and annular pancreas. A mucosal web can be excised through a duodenotomy if technically feasible, taking care to avoid injury to the adjacent ampulla. The duodenum may be markedly dilated proximal to the obstruction, which may result in impaired dysmotility and feeding intolerance. This problem can be prevented (or managed) by a tapering duodenoplasty, which involves plication or resection of a portion of the antimesenteric wall to reduce luminal diameter. The remaining distal duodenal segment should be irrigated and assessed for additional obstructive lesions prior to reanastomosis. Mortality is related to prematurity and associated anomalies.

Kilbride H, et al: Congenital duodenal obstruction: timing of diagnosis during the newborn period. *J Perinatol.* 2010;30:197.

Li B, et al: Laparoscopic methods in the treatment of congenital duodenal obstruction for neonates. *J Laparoendosc Adv Surg Tech A.* 2013;23:881.

ATRESIA & STENOSIS OF THE JEJUNUM, ILEUM, & COLON

Atresia and intestinal stenosis of the jejunum, ileum, and colon are caused by a mesenteric vascular accident in utero, which may result from hernia, volvulus, or intussusception.

The accident results in aseptic necrosis and resorption of the involved bowel. The diagnosis is made on prenatal ultrasound in 50% of cases. Although atresia may occur in any portion of the intestine, most cases involve the distal ileum or proximal jejunum. Colonic atresia is rare, accounting for less than 1% of all intestinal atresias. Overall, atresias occur in 1 in 5000 live births.

Several types of atresias are recognized based on anatomic characteristics. Type I atresias are characterized by a short area of stenosis or a membranous web occluding the lumen (Figure 45–14). A more extensive infarct may leave a fibrous cord between the two bowel loops (type II), whereas type IIIa lesions are characterized by a V-shaped mesenteric defect with complete separation of the proximal and distal bowel ends. Type 4 lesions are characterized by multiple atresias. A type III variant (type IIIb) is commonly called apple peel or Christmas tree atresia, in which there is a blind-ending proximal jejunum, absence of a long length of mid small bowel, and a terminal ileum coiled around its tenuous

blood supply from an ileocolic vessel. Type IIIb lesions can be particularly challenging to manage secondary to their tenuous blood supply.

▶ Clinical Findings

Bilious emesis within the first 24-48 hours of life is the classic presentation of patients with intestinal atresias. Depending on the level of the obstruction, patients may develop abdominal distention in the case of distal obstructions or have a relatively normal exam with more proximal obstructions. Meconium may or may not be passed following birth depending on the timing and level of the intrauterine vascular accident. A contrast enema may be indicated to detect the level of obstruction, particularly in cases where multiple dilated loops of bowel seen on imaging are suggestive of a distal lesion.

▶ Treatment

There are three main goals of surgery: (1) to restore the continuity of the bowel; (2) to preserve as much intestinal length as possible; and (3) to retain the ileocecal valve if possible. A transverse upper abdominal incision is the standard approach to small bowel atresias, although periumbilical and laparoscopic techniques have also been described. The segment of proximal bowel leading up to the atresia may be markedly dilated and often has impaired peristaltic activity. It may become a source of functional obstruction if not excised or tapered to a more normal caliber of bowel. Resection with reanastomosis is the preferred approach as long as there is an adequate length of bowel remaining to support enteral nutrition. Tapering should be considered for dilated proximal bowel near the ligament of Treitz or in cases where maximal intestinal length should be preserved. The discrepancy between the caliber of the proximal and distal segments can be considerable and can often make the anastomosis technically challenging (Figure 45–15).

In contrast to duodenal atresia, associated anomalies are uncommon with small bowel and colonic atresias. Return of gastrointestinal function can be quite delayed following atresia repair, particularly in cases of duodenal atresia. Parenteral nutrition is therefore a common and necessary nutritional adjunct in these infants.

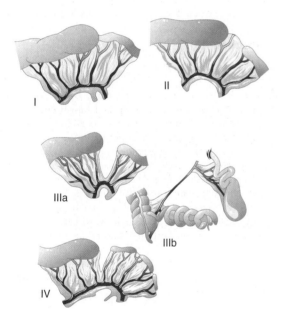

▲ **Figure 45–14.** The anatomic spectrum of intestinal atresia. Type I is a stenosis or mucosal web. Type II, a fibrous cord between two bowel ends. Type IIIa, blind-ending proximal and distal bowel loops with a V-shaped mesenteric defect. Type IIIb (apple peel deformity, Christmas tree deformity) consists of a blind-ending proximal jejunum, absence of a large portion of the midgut, and a terminal ileum that is coiled around its ileocolic blood supply. Type IV, multiple atresias of any kind. (Reproduced with permission from Sabiston DC: *Textbook of Surgery.* Philadelphia, PA: Saunders/Elsevier; 1991.)

Burjonrappa S, et al: Comparative outcomes in intestinal atresia: a clinical outcome and pathophysiology analysis. *Pediatr Surg Int.* 2011;27:437.

Haxhija EQ, et al: Management of isolated and associated colonic atresia. *Pediatr Surg Int.* 2011;27:411.

INTESTINAL ROTATION ABNORMALITIES

Abnormalities of intestinal fixation are congenital conditions that predispose the gut to twisting, with possible obstructive and ischemic sequelae. The fetal intestine

▲ **Figure 45–15.** Surgical repair of a type II jejunal atresia. Note the size mismatch that is typically present between the distal, smaller end (arrow) and the more dilated proximal end. (Used with permission from Craig W. Lillehei, MD.)

herniates out into the extraembryonic coelom at about 4-6 weeks of gestational age. At 10-12 weeks, the bowel returns to the abdominal cavity and becomes fixed to the retroperitoneum along a long diagonal axis. The duodeno-jejunal portion of the gut rotates posteriorly (counterclock-wise) 270 degrees relative to the superior mesenteric vessels and becomes fixed at the ligament of Treitz. The cecocolic portion of the gut also rotates 270 degrees, but in a clock-wise manner (anteriorly) to the superior mesenteric artery. The cecum then becomes fixed in the right lower quadrant of the abdomen.

Intestinal anomalies of rotation and fixation occur in approximately 1 in 200 live births and are twice as common in males. The normal process of intestinal rotation and fixa-tion creates a broad anchoring mesentery that prevents the occurrence of a midgut volvulus, which occurs in approxi-mately 1 in 6000 children.

▶ Classification

Abnormalities of intestinal fixation are classified as (1) non-rotation, (2) incomplete rotation, (3) reversed rotation, and (4) anomalous fixation of the mesentery.

A. Nonrotation

With nonrotation, no midgut rotation occurs. As a result, the small intestine is located predominantly on the right side of the abdomen and the colon in the left abdomen. The mesen-tery of the intestine is narrow due to a complete lack of fixa-tion, predisposing to a clockwise twisting of the bowel about the superior mesenteric vessels (midgut volvulus). Nonrota-tion is typically found in patients with anomalies of the ante-rior abdominal wall and diaphragm, including omphalocele, gastroschisis, and CDH.

B. Incomplete Rotation

Incomplete rotation (commonly referred to as *malrotation*) may affect the duodenojejunal segment, the cecocolic seg-ment, or both. In the most common form, the cecocolic limb lies in the left epigastrium and the duodenojejunal limb lies in the right epigastrium. Dense peritoneal bands (Ladd bands) extend from the right upper quadrant across the cecum and duodenum and may partially or completely obstruct the sec-ond or third portion of the duodenum. The intestinal mesen-tery is fixed posteriorly but is relatively narrow, and patients are at risk for midgut volvulus (Figure 45–16).

C. Reversed Rotation

In reversed rotation, the bowel rotates varying degrees in an abnormal clockwise direction about the superior mesenteric axis. The duodenojejunal limb is located anterior to the supe-rior mesenteric artery, and the cecocolic limb may be prear-terial or may be rotated clockwise or counterclockwise in a retroarterial position. The cecum may be right sided or left sided. The most frequent anomaly is retroarterial clockwise

▲ **Figure 45–16.** Malrotation of the midgut with volvulus. Note cecum at the origin of the superior mesenteric vessels. Fibrous bands cross and obstruct the duodenum as they adhere to the cecum. Midgut volvulus is untwisted in a counterclockwise direction.

rotation, which may be associated with partial obstruction of the proximal or mid portion of the colon.

D. Anomalous Fixation of Mesentery

Anomalies of mesenteric fixation are associated with "internal" hernias (mesenteric or paraduodenal in location), an excessively mobile cecum (cecal bascule), and obstructing adhesive bands in the absence of abnormal intestinal rotation. Excessive rotation of the duodenojejunal junction may result in superior mesenteric artery compression of the third portion of the duodenum.

▶ Clinical Findings

A. Symptoms and Signs

Depending on the location and extent of fixation, anomalies of intestinal rotation may cause symptoms associated with obstruction, peptic ulceration, or malabsorption. Seventy percent of patients who develop symptoms of intestinal obstruction are infants, and 70% of infants present in their first month of life. Bilious emesis can result from obstruction in the duodenum or jejunum as a result of Ladd bands or a midgut volvulus. Other symptoms may include vague or severe abdominal pain, lethargy, and failure to thrive. Older patients may have nonspecific symptoms due to intermittent or partial obstruction, usually due to partial fixation where complete obstruction cannot occur. These children may present thin and underweight because of chronic postprandial discomfort or malabsorption. Malabsorption with steatorrhea may result from partial venous and lymphatic obstruction, which is associated with coarse rugal folds in the small bowel. Depending on the level and extent of obstruction, abdominal distention may or may not be prominent. Bloody stools and signs of peritonitis may be present and are manifestations of intestinal ischemia. Peptic ulcer occurs in 20% of children, presumably as a result of antral and duodenal stasis.

B. Imaging Studies

Emergent radiographic valuation is required in cases of suspected midgut volvulus and should include upper gastrointestinal series with small bowel follow-through. Ultrasound with Doppler evaluation of mesenteric vessel position and cross-sectional imaging (CT and MRI) can also be used to establish the diagnosis but are associated with false-negative results and treatment delay. These tests should not be used in lieu of an upper gastrointestinal series in symptomatic children.

Upper gastrointestinal series is the gold standard for establishing the diagnosis of both malrotation and midgut volvulus. An upper gastrointestinal series may demonstrate distention of the duodenum, abnormal positioning of the duodenojejunal segment (usually to the right of the midline), failure of retroperitoneal duodenal position, and narrowing ("bird beak") at the point of obstruction. The proximal small bowel may be primarily located on the right side of the abdomen and the colon on the left. The identification of inverted superior mesenteric artery and superior mesenteric vein position on ultrasound or cross-sectional imaging is highly suggestive of malrotation.

▶ Treatment & Prognosis

Patients with suspected malrotation with midgut volvulus should undergo urgent laparotomy through a transverse right upper quadrant abdominal incision. The entire bowel should be eviscerated from the abdominal cavity to assess viability and intestinal fixation (Figure 45–17). Volvulized bowel should be untwisted in a counterclockwise direction. Division of any adhesive bands (Ladd bands) between the proximal colon, duodenum, and the right abdominal wall should be undertaken. Intermesenteric adhesions are often present to variable degrees, and these are incised to broaden the mesentery. An appendectomy is performed as a standard part of the Ladd procedure. Finally, the cecum is placed in the left lower quadrant, and the small bowel is oriented along the right side of the abdomen. In essence, one is creating nonrotated intestinal anatomy much like the anatomic situation in early fetal life. The Ladd procedure may be performed laparoscopically for cases of malrotation without suspected volvulus.

The morality rate for infants treated for intestinal rotation abnormalities is less than 5%; however, midgut volvulus is responsible for approximately 20% of all children with intestinal failure requiring chronic parenteral nutrition. The most common complication following a Ladd procedure is adhesive bowel obstruction (~5% of cases), whereas a recurrent volvulus is relatively rare (< 1% of cases).

▲ **Figure 45–17.** Operative findings in a newborn with malrotation and midgut volvulus. Note the 540-degree clockwise twist of the small bowel (arrow). (Used with permission from Craig W. Lillehei, MD.)

Graziano K, et al: Asymptomatic malrotation: diagnosis and surgical management: an American Pediatric Surgical Association outcomes and evidence based practice committee systematic review. *J Pediatr Surg*. 2015;50:1783.

Lodwick DL, et al: Current surgical management of intestinal rotational abnormalities. *Curr Opin Pediatr*. 2015;27:383.

MECONIUM ILEUS

Meconium ileus is an obstruction of the terminal ileum (and may also involve the colon) due to inspissated meconium. It is present in 10%-20% of infants born with cystic fibrosis and is the only clinically relevant manifestation of cystic fibrosis at birth. Although there is no clear correlation between pancreatic insufficiency and the development of inspissated meconium, meconium ileus also occurs in patients with pancreatic duct obstruction and pancreatic aplasia. Meconium obstruction with no apparent cause (idiopathic) has also been described in newborn infants.

Meconium ileus is categorized into simple and complex types. In simple meconium ileus, there are no associated gastrointestinal abnormalities. In complex types, associated gastrointestinal abnormalities may include intestinal atresias, volvulus, perforation, or the presence of a pseudocyst. Intestinal perforation in utero secondary to meconium ileus can lead to meconium peritonitis following birth.

▶ Clinical Findings

A. Symptoms and Signs

Infants born with meconium ileus may present with a very distended or benign-appearing abdomen. Typically, no meconium is passed, and bilious emesis may develop in the first few days of life.

B. Imaging Studies

Plain abdominal radiographs may demonstrate distended loops of bowel, and inspissated meconium may have a ground-glass appearance. Air mixed with the meconium produces the classic "soap bubble" sign, which is usually located in the right lower quadrant. A contrast enema will typically demonstrate a microcolon with meconium flecks. Reflux of contrast medium through the ileocecal valve (which is often not possible with the first enema) demonstrates a small terminal ileum containing "pellets" of inspissated mucus; more proximally, the bowel is progressively distended with packed meconium. Prenatal perforation (meconium peritonitis) may be evidenced by the presence of abdominal calcifications due to saponification of meconium in the peritoneal cavity.

▶ Complications

Meconium ileus may be complicated by a segmental volvulus due to the heavy, distended loops of distal ileum. If this occurs early in fetal life, the volvulus may progress to loss of the affected bowel segment. This can heal completely prior to birth, with abdominal calcifications on plain radiographs as the only evidence that it occurred. However, such in utero perforations often result in an intestinal atresia and complete bowel obstruction. Perforation later in gestation may lead to meconium peritonitis or a large meconium pseudocyst at birth.

Other complications of meconium ileus are related to the presence of cystic fibrosis when present. These infants are susceptible to pulmonary infections with chronic bronchopneumonia, bronchiectasis, atelectasis, and lung abscesses. Malabsorption due to pancreatic insufficiency may require pancreatic enzyme replacement. Rectal prolapse and intussusception may result from chronic constipation due to inspissated stools. Nasal polyps and chronic sinusitis are frequent. Biliary cirrhosis and bleeding varices from portal hypertension are late manifestations of bile duct obstruction by mucus.

▶ Treatment & Prognosis

Nonoperative treatment for simple meconium ileus is successful in 60%-80% of cases. Once the diagnosis is being considered, a nasogastric tube should be inserted and placed to continuous wall suction. A contrast enema can be both diagnostic and therapeutic. It should be performed with hypertonic water-soluble contrast agent (rather than barium) and monitored by fluoroscopic imaging. The infant must be well hydrated, and intravenous fluids must be continued during and after the procedure in order to prevent hypovolemia from the hypertonic contrast solution (which works by drawing water from the gut into the lumen of the bowel). Several contrast enemas may be required to evacuate all of the obstructive meconium. If this fails to relieve the obstruction after two or three attempts or if the infant develops signs of peritonitis or sepsis, surgery is indicated.

Operative management is pursued in cases of complex meconium ileus or failed attempts to relieve the obstruction by enema reduction (Figure 45–18). Traditionally, an ileotomy is made and the lumen of the bowel is irrigated with normal saline or a solution of gastrograffin or *N*-acetylcysteine. An alternative approach is to use the appendix as the conduit for administering the hypertonic fluid, followed by an appendectomy when the obstruction is cleared. All of the obstructing meconium should be removed or flushed distally to prevent a recurrent obstruction postoperatively. Compromised intestine is resected, and appendectomy is performed because of the high rate of appendicitis in patients with cystic fibrosis. Depending on the stability of the patient and condition of the bowel, the enterotomy can be primarily closed or the ileum can be brought out as a double-barrel stoma.

▲ **Figure 45–18.** Operative findings in a newborn with a high-grade small bowel obstruction due to meconium ileus. Note the dilated loops of small bowel, which appear dilated and dark due to the collection of inspissated meconium. (Used with permission from Craig W. Lillehei, MD.)

All patients should be evaluated for cystic fibrosis. Pancreatic enzyme replacement may be required. A formula low in long-chain fatty acids and high in medium-chain triglycerides may give better absorption and growth than standard formulas. The patient must be placed in an environment with high humidity to keep tracheobronchial secretions fluid. Up to 50% of patients with cystic fibrosis may develop a meconium ileus-like syndrome known as distal ileal obstruction syndrome. This is ileal obstruction due to inspissated stool. It can occur when patients are not compliant with their medications or become dehydrated. It is often successfully treated with hypertonic contrast enemas, although an operation may be required for the same indications as in meconium ileus.

Carlyle BE, et al: A review of pathophysiology and management of fetuses and neonates with meconium ileus for the pediatric surgeon. *J Pediatr Surg.* 2012;47(4):772-781.

HIRSCHSPRUNG DISEASE

Hirschsprung disease (HD) is a disorder caused by failure in the migration of intestinal ganglion progenitor cells into the distal bowel. As these cells migrate craniocaudally during development of the gastrointestinal tract, the absence of ganglion cells extends proximally from the anus for a variable distance depending on the extent of migration. The aganglionic bowel produces functional obstruction due to its inability to relax in response to distention. Aganglionosis most commonly extends to the sigmoid colon (75% of cases), but may also involve the terminal rectum only (10%). More proximal involvement is seen in approximately 15% of patients, with 5% of all patients found to have aganglionosis of the entire colon with variable involvement of the small bowel (total colonic aganglionosis). In rare cases, extensive involvement of the small bowel is found.

Males are affected four times more commonly than females, although females tend to have longer aganglionic segments. A familial association has been documented in up to 10% of cases, and the extent of aganglionosis tends to be consistent in familial cases. Approximately 10% of patients with HD have Down syndrome.

▶ Clinical Findings

A. Symptoms and Signs

The symptoms of HD vary widely in severity and are primarily due to the extent of aganglionosis. More than 90% of infants with HD will fail to pass meconium within 24 hours. Progressive abdominal distention, bilious emesis, and feeding intolerance usually follow. A rectal examination in the infant may be followed by expulsion of stool and flatus. In older children, chronic constipation and abdominal distention are characteristic, as well as diarrhea secondary to pseudo-incontinence and poor growth. Passage of flatus and stool requires great effort, and the stools are small in caliber. Children with constipation from HD often do not exhibit soiling of their diapers or undergarments, distinguishing this form of constipation from idiopathic constipation (encopresis).

B. Imaging Studies

Plain abdominal radiographs may demonstrate distal intestinal obstruction with dilated loops of bowel, but it is often difficult to distinguish small from large bowel in infants. A water-soluble contrast enema may be diagnostic and should be performed in all infants where the diagnosis is suspected. There should be no attempt to clean out the stool before the fluoroscopic examination because this can dilate the rectum and obscure the change in caliber between aganglionic and ganglionic bowel. The contrast enema often demonstrates a "transition zone," which is a contracted (aganglionic) segment that appears relatively narrow compared with the more dilated proximal bowel. However, the proximal aganglionic intestine can be dilated by impacted stool or enema, giving a false impression of the level of the normal colon. Irregular contractions in a saw-toothed pattern may also be seen in the aganglionic portion of the bowel, especially in the distal rectum.

During the contrast enema, lateral projection images should be obtained to examine the caliber of the rectum and proximal bowel that may otherwise be obscured by a redundant sigmoid colon on anteroposterior views. In neonates without HD, the rectum is typically wider than the rest of the colon (including the cecum). When the rectum is narrower than the more proximal colon (eg, sigmoid), then HD should be suspected. Radiographs of the abdomen should be repeated after 24-48 hours to asses progression of contrast.

In children with HD, the contrast agent will be retained for prolonged periods and may demonstrate little progression. It should be noted that these classic radiologic findings may be absent in long-segment or total-colon HD.

C. Additional Workup

Definitive diagnosis of HD is made by rectal biopsy. Mucosal and submucosal biopsies may be taken from the posterior rectal wall with a suction biopsy device at the bedside. Serial sections may demonstrate the characteristic lack of ganglion cells and proliferation of nerve trunks in Meissner's plexus. If the findings are equivocal from the suction rectal biopsy specimen, a full-thickness biopsy from the posterior rectum proximal to the dentate line can be performed under general anesthesia. Manometric studies may show a failure of relaxation of the internal sphincter following rectal distention by a balloon, although this test is generally only used in older children in whom the diagnosis is in question.

► Differential Diagnosis

Lower gastrointestinal obstruction in the newborn infant may be due to meconium plug syndrome, meconium ileus, anorectal malformations, or a variety of functional causes including hypermagnesemia, hypocalcemia, hypokalemia, and hypothyroidism. HD may also resemble functional constipation, especially with very-short-segment HD where only the very distal rectum is involved. However, stool is typically palpable in the lower rectum in patients with functional constipation, and a contrast enema shows uniformly dilated bowel to the level of the anus. However, short-segment HD may be difficult to differentiate from functional constipation on contrast enema, and rectal biopsy may be necessary.

► Treatment

Historically, surgical management of HD involved a staged approach with an initial diverting ("leveling") colostomy followed several months later by resection of the aganglionic segment and restoration of intestinal continuity. In many cases, it is now routine to perform a single-stage procedure without a protective colostomy in the newborn period (Figure 45–19). Exceptions include infants presenting with severe enterocolitis that cannot be managed with antibiotics and irrigations. At the time of surgery, frozen section analysis of colonic biopsies is performed to establish the level of aganglionosis in preparation for resection or diverting colostomy, depending on whether the operation will be a single- or multiple-staged procedure. There are three major types of pull-through procedures for HD, including the Swenson operation, the Duhamel operation, and the Soave operation. The main operative principles for all of these procedures are removal of most or all of the aganglionic bowel and anastomosing ganglionic bowel to the rectum just above the dentate line. In contrast to

▲ **Figure 45–19.** Operative findings in a newborn with Hirschsprung disease extending to the sigmoid colon. Note the transition in bowel caliber between the normal (dilated) and aganglionic colon (arrow). (Used with permission from Craig W. Lillehei, MD.)

the Swenson and Soave procedures, the Duhamel operation leaves a segment of full-thickness aganglionic rectum along which the ganglionic bowel is stapled, creating a mini-reservoir. The Swenson procedure includes a full-thickness dissection of the distal rectum, leaving no aganglionic bowel behind, whereas the Soave involves a partial-thickness distal dissection that leaves a muscular cuff behind that must be divided. Laparoscopy is typically used to mobilize the intra-abdominal portion of colon, and biopsies are obtained to identify the level of aganglionosis.

► Prognosis

Hirschsprung-associated enterocolitis (HAEC) occurs in 20%-60% of cases and is the primary cause of morbidity and mortality in neonates with HD. The cause is not known but seems to be related to the high-grade partial obstruction, poor motility in the residual ganglionic bowel, and hypertonic rectal sphincters. This tends to occur more frequently in infants but may appear at any age and even after complete resection of aganglionic bowel. There is no clear association between the length of aganglionosis and the occurrence of enterocolitis. Management includes broad-spectrum antibiotics, aggressive rehydration and correction of electrolyte abnormalities, and rectal irrigations.

Anastomotic leak with a pelvic abscess is rare but is a serious complication following pull-through procedures. Necrosis of the colonic pull-through segment and anastomotic stricture can occur if the bowel has not been mobilized sufficiently to prevent tension on the mesenteric blood supply.

Long-term patients who are properly treated for HD do well. Episodic constipation and abdominal distention may occur since the aganglionic internal anal sphincter is intact. Botox injections of the sphincter have been effective in managing this complication. Enterocolitis may occur even after definitive treatment, and patients diagnosed with HAEC should be treated with intravenous antibiotics, rectal irrigations, and bowel rest. Postoperative enterocolitis is more common in children with Down syndrome.

Demehri FR, et al: Hirschsprung-associated enterocolitis: pathogenesis, treatment and prevention. *Pediatr Surg Int.* 2013;29:873.

Rintala RJ, et al: Long-term outcomes of Hirschsprung's disease. *Semin Pediatr Surg.* 2012;21:336.

NEONATAL SMALL LEFT COLON SYNDROME (MECONIUM PLUG SYNDROME)

Small left colon syndrome is a distal intestinal obstruction associated with a narrow caliber left colon and a dilated transverse and right colon. Two-thirds of patients are male. Infants are typically otherwise healthy, although approximately 30%-50% are born to diabetic mothers and are large for gestational age.

▶ Clinical Findings

Rectal examination is typically normal. Similar to HD, little or no meconium is passed during the first 24-48 hours, and progressive abdominal distention is followed by emesis. Contrast enema shows a very small left colon, usually to the level of the splenic flexure. The colon and small bowel proximal to this point may be markedly distended. In about 30% of cases, a meconium plug is present at the junction of the narrow and dilated portion of the bowel. Contrast enema using water-soluble contrast is often both diagnostic and therapeutic.

▶ Differential Diagnosis

Small left colon syndrome may present similarly to HD and meconium ileus. These conditions rarely cause obstruction at the level of the splenic flexure, and when the colon readily decompresses without further obstruction, HD is unlikely. A plain abdominal radiograph will reveal multiple dilated loops of bowel. Water-soluble contrast enema is essential to differentiate the various causes of lower intestinal obstruction. When the left colon is narrow and contrast material refluxes into the dilated proximal colon, the diagnosis is more suggestive of small left colon syndrome.

▶ Treatment

A nasogastric tube should be inserted in the presence of emesis or marked distention. The diagnostic contrast enema is usually therapeutic as well, resulting in evacuation of copious meconium and decompression of the bowel. Incomplete evacuation of the meconium or persistent symptoms after the enema mandate a suction rectal biopsy to rule out HD.

INTUSSUSCEPTION

Telescoping of a segment of bowel (intussusceptum) into the adjacent segment (intussuscipiens) is the most common cause of intestinal obstruction in children between 6 months and 2 years of age (Figure 45–20). Intussusception may result in ischemia, necrosis, or perforation of the intussusceptum if mesenteric vascular flow is compromised. The most common involved segment of bowel is the terminal ileum, which intussuscepts into the right colon (ileocolic intussusception). The condition is more common in males, and 80% of patients present before 2 years of age. The cause is idiopathic in 90% of infants and children, whereas a pathologic lead point is identified in 10% of cases. Meckel diverticulum, polyps, hemangioma, enteric duplication, intramural hematoma (Henoch-Schönlein purpura), and intestinal lymphoma are common sources of pathologic lead points and are more common in patients older than 5 years of age. Postoperative intussusception can occur at any age and is usually ileoileal or jejunojejunal in nature.

▶ Clinical Findings

Patients are typically previously healthy and present with a history of intermittent crying and severe, crampy abdominal pain. The pain is episodic and may alternate with intervals of apparent well-being. Bilious emesis is a late finding and signifies the presence of a high-grade bowel obstruction. The child may become lethargic or somnolent. The combination of stool, blood from ischemic bowel, and mucosal sloughing can produce the so-called "currant jelly" stool.

▲ **Figure 45–20.** Intussusception.

A "sausage-like" mass may be palpable in the right upper quadrant of the abdomen in cases of ileocolic intussusception. Prolonged intussusception produces edema and hemorrhagic or ischemic infarction of the intussusceptum.

Imaging Studies

Abdominal ultrasound is the most sensitive test to confirm the diagnosis of intussusception. Identification of a "target" or "donut" sign is diagnostic. Plain abdominal films are less sensitive but may demonstrate findings suggestive of intestinal obstruction or a soft tissue mass on the right side of the abdomen.

Treatment & Prognosis

Enemas using air, saline, or water-soluble contrast are both diagnostic and therapeutic in up to 90% of cases (Figure 45–21). An enema should not be attempted until the patient has been resuscitated to allow an operative procedure to be performed safely. It is contraindicated if peritonitis is present. Air is pumped into the colon at a pressure of 60-120 mm Hg (never > 120 mm Hg). The reduction is usually performed under fluoroscopic guidance. A successful study reduces the intussusceptum and demonstrates reflux of air into the terminal ileum. Multiple attempts should be made to reduce the intussusception before committing to operative exploration.

▲ **Figure 45–22.** Operative findings in a 3-year-old child with a complete bowel obstruction due to ileocolic intussusception. The proximal portion of the intussuscepted segment (intussusceptum) is denoted by the blue arrow, and the leading edge of distal portion can be seen through the wall of the right colon (black arrow). (Used with permission from Craig W. Lillehei, MD.)

Operative management is required if the child has signs of bowel perforation or peritonitis or if enema reduction is unsuccessful. The operation may be performed either by laparotomy or laparoscopy. In the absence of gangrene, reduction is best accomplished by gentle retrograde compression of the intussuscipiens, not by putting traction on the proximal bowel (Figure 45–22). Resection of the intussusception is indicated if the bowel cannot be reduced or if the intestine is gangrenous. Intussusception recurs after 5%-15% of enema reductions and 1% of operative reductions.

Banapour P, et al: Surgical approach to intussusception in older children: influence of lead points. *J Pediatr Surg.* 2015;50:647.
Mandeville K, et al: Intussusception: clinical presentations and imaging characteristics. *Pediatr Emerg Care.* 2012;28:842.
Wei CH, et al: Laparoscopy versus open surgery for idiopathic intussusception in children. *Surg Endosc.* 2015;29:668.

ANORECTAL MALFORMATIONS (IMPERFORATE ANUS)

Anorectal malformations (ARMs) are congenital anomalies where the rectum and anus are malpositioned anteriorly and may or may not be associated with a fistula tract. ARMs have historically been referred to as "imperforate anus," although this is not an accurate description because, in many cases, there is a fistulous connection to the perineum or structures arising from the urogenital

▲ **Figure 45–21.** Contrast enema demonstrating obstruction to retrograde flow of barium by a filling defect (intussusceptum) in the mid-transverse colon. (Reproduced with permission from Norton, JA: *Surgery.* New York, NY: Springer; 2000.)

sinus. As a result, the rectum may empty anteriorly onto the perineum, into the vagina (in females) or urinary system (in males), or may end in a blind end without any connection. The normal continence mechanism for bowel control consists of an internal sphincter composed of smooth muscle and the striated muscle complex from the levator ani and external sphincter. The striated muscles assume a funnel shape, originating from the pubis, pelvic rim, and sacrum. These muscles converge at the perineum while interdigitating with the internal and external sphincters. Most of the striated muscle complex consists of horizontal muscles that contract against the wall of the rectum and anus, whereas longitudinal muscle fibers run in a cephalocaudal direction and elevate the anus.

▶ Classification & Clinical Findings

Physical examination of the perineum and, in some cases, imaging studies are used to categorize the level and nature of the ARM. When an orifice is visible at the perineum or vaginal introitus, the anomaly is referred to as a low ARM. In males, the absence of an obvious orifice at the perineal level suggests a high ARM (Figures 45–23 to 45–26) with a communication (fistula) between the anomalously located rectum and urethra or bladder neck. In females, a high ARM is represented by the persistence of a cloaca, which includes a common channel of variable length made up of the rectum and urogenital sinus. ARMs most commonly involve a fistula to the urethra in males and to the posterior vestibule of the vagina in girls.

Associated anomalies occur in 60%-70% of patients with ARMs. Imperforate anus is included in the VACTERL association (see Esophageal Anomalies). The possible constellation of anomalies includes EA, anomalies of the gastrointestinal tract, hemivertebrae or agenesis of one or more

A   B

▲ **Figure 45–24. A:** High female anatomic anomaly. Low vaginal fistula. **B:** High female anomaly. High vaginal fistula. (Reproduced with permission from Pena A: *Atlas of Surgical Management of Anorectal Malformations*. New York, NY: Springer-Verlag; 1990.)

A   B

▲ **Figure 45–25. A:** Low male anomaly. Perineal fistula. **B:** Low male anomaly. Rectobulbar urethra fistula. (Reproduced with permission from Pena A: *Atlas of Surgical Management of Anorectal Malformations*. New York, NY: Springer-Verlag; 1990.)

A   B

▲ **Figure 45–23. A:** Low female anomaly. Perineal fistula. **B:** Low female anomaly. Fourchette/vestibule fistula. (Reproduced with permission from Pena A: *Atlas of Surgical Management of Anorectal Malformations*. New York, NY: Springer-Verlag; 1990.)

A   B

▲ **Figure 45–26. A:** High male anomaly. Rectoprostatic urethra fistula. **B:** High male anomaly. Rectovesical neck fistula. (Reproduced with permission from Pena A: *Atlas of Surgical Management of Anorectal Malformations*. New York, NY: Springer-Verlag; 1990.)

sacral vertebrae (agenesis of S1, S2, or S3 is associated with corresponding neurologic deficits, resulting in neuropathic bladder and greatly impaired continence), genitourinary anomalies (up to 50% incidence with high imperforate anus), and anomalies of the heart and upper limbs or digits.

A. Low Anorectal Malformations

In low ARMs, the anus may be ectopically located anterior to its normal position, or it may be in the normal position with a narrow outlet due to stenosis or presence of a skin bridge over the anal opening ("bucket handle" deformity). A small fistula may extend from the anus anteriorly to open in the raphe of the perineum, scrotum, or penis in the male or the vulva in the female. These babies often have well-developed perineal and gluteal musculature and rarely have sacral vertebral anomalies.

B. High Anorectal Malformations

In high ARM anomalies, the rectum may end blindly (10%), but more commonly, there is a fistula to the urethra or bladder in the male or the persistent urogenital sinus in the female (cloaca). Patients with high ARMs often have deficient pelvic and gluteal innervation and musculature, a high incidence of sacral anomalies (caudal regression), and a poor prognosis for continence after surgical repair. The most severe of the high deformities in girls is a cloacal anomaly in which there is a common channel between the poorly developed pelvic structures (urogenital sinus and rectum) with a single perineal opening.

B. Imaging Studies

Imaging studies are generally used to characterize internal anatomy for high ARMs and to rule out associated anomalies. Radiographs are sometimes useful when the clinical impression is unclear. A lateral prone film of the pelvis with the baby inverted (invertogram), once commonly used, is an imperfect method of establishing the lower extent of the rectum because swallowed air may not have completely displaced the meconium from the rectum. Gas in the bladder is suggestive of a rectourinary fistula. Lower abdominal and perineal ultrasound, x-ray, CT, and MRI may be useful to define the pelvic anatomy and for surgical planning, particularly in cases of cloacal malformations where associated urogenital anomalies are common. Anomalies of the vertebrae and the urinary tract occur in two-thirds of all patients with high anomalies and in one-third of male patients with low anomalies. Vertebral abnormalities in females invariably indicate a high imperforate anus. Anomalies of the sacrum warrant an ultrasound or MRI of the lumbosacral area to identify spinal cord anomalies such as a tethered filum terminale.

Complications

Delay in diagnosis of imperforate anus may result in progressive bowel distention and perforation or severe, chronic constipation with encopresis in less severe cases. The presence of a rectourinary fistula allows reflux of urine into the rectum and colon, and absorption of ammonium chloride may cause acidosis. Colon contents can then reflux into the urethra, bladder, and upper tracts, potentially resulting in pyelonephritis.

Treatment

Definitive repair of ARMs can be done in the newborn period or delayed until 3-4 months of life, depending on the ability of the baby to remain decompressed through an existing fistula. Most patients should undergo operative repair within the first 2-3 months of life. The three main goals of operative management include relocation of the rectal opening to lie within the center of the muscle complex (including sphincter mechanism) and repair of any fistulous connections between the rectum and urogenital structures. The presence of associated life-threatening anomalies (cardiac anomalies) may warrant a diverting colostomy and delayed definitive repair.

A. Repair of Low Anorectal Malformations

Low ARMs can be repaired through a perineal approach using a muscle stimulator to determine the location of the muscle complex. A posterior sagittal incision is made in the midline just anterior to the fistula opening and extends through the muscle complex posteriorly. The rectal pouch is then mobilized posteriorly and anastomosed to create a new anal canal within the muscle complex (posterior sagittal anorectoplasty). Postoperative dilations are necessary to prevent postoperative stricturing and are usually initiated after 2-3 postoperative weeks and performed daily for 3-5 months to prevent stricture formation and to allow for growth.

B. High Anomalies

Historically, high ARMs were managed by a two- or three-stage repair, consisting of initial diverting colostomy and mucous fistula, followed by a posterior sagittal anorectoplasty 2-3 months later with or without closure of the colostomy (delaying colostomy closure would require a third operation). Single-stage repairs of high ARMs have become more common by combining posterior sagittal approaches with laparoscopic mobilization. High ARMs can be quite technically challenging to repair, especially in girls with complex cloaca malformations. The decision to proceed with a single-stage operation versus a staged repair with a protective colostomy must be carefully considered in each case.

Prognosis

Complications associated with ARM repair include damage to the pelvic nerves, urethra, and vaginal wall during perineal dissection and rectal mobilization. Complications associated with repair of urethra fistulas include a urethral diverticulum (produces a blind pouch prone to recurrent infection and stone formation) and urethral strictures. These result from division of the fistula tract too far away from and too close to the urethra, respectively.

Patients with imperforate anus tend to have varying degrees of constipation postoperatively, even following a technically perfect repair. This is believed to be due to poor colonic motility and usually responds well to careful dietary changes and laxative medications. Patients with low anomalies usually have good sphincter function and bowel control. Children with high anomalies have a much more variable prognosis as it pertains to fecal continence and need for bowel management. In the most severe cases, the muscle complex and associated sphincters are poorly developed. This may be further exacerbated by maldeveloped sacral nerve roots and absent or incomplete innervation. The children may need an antegrade continent enema procedure (eg, appendicostomy or cecostomy) to facilitate daily bowel emptying. Recently, sacral nerve stimulation has demonstrated promising results in the management of fecal and urinary incontinence in this cohort of children.

Bischoff A, et al: Update on the management of anorectal malformations. *Pediatr Surg Int.* 2013;29:899.

Bischoff A, et al: Laparoscopic-assisted PSARP: the advantages of combining both techniques for the treatment of anorectal malformations with recto-bladderneck or high prostatic fistulas. *J Pediatr Surg.* 2013;48:367.

Sulkowski JP, et al: Sacral nerve stimulation: a promising therapy for fecal and urinary incontinence and constipation in children. *J Pediatr Surg.* 2015;50:1644.

▼ GASTROINTESTINAL TRACT ABNORMALITIES

GASTROESOPHAGEAL REFLUX

The high-pressure zone in the distal esophagus is absent in newborns and young infants. The normal adult pattern of peristalsis and lower esophageal sphincter function begins to develop after several months of age. Therefore, many infants experience varying degrees of regurgitation after feeding, which is commonly referred to as gastroesophageal reflux (GER). Rarely, severe reflux may produce peptic esophagitis and interfere with the development of a normally competent sphincter. Unlike adults, children with symptomatic GER rarely have an associated hiatal hernia as a cause of their symptoms.

▶ Clinical Findings

A. Symptoms and Signs

Children with symptomatic GER typically have effortless regurgitation of feedings, particularly when the baby is placed in a recumbent position. With severe GER, persistent regurgitation may result in poor weight gain (failure to thrive), peptic esophagitis with blood-tinged emesis, and occult bleeding leading to anemia. Severe GER has also been associated with so-called *acute life-threatening events*, which are thought to be related to severe bronchospasm from aspirated gastric contents. Chronic intermitted reflux may also be associated with occult aspiration, leading to asthma and recurrent lower respiratory tract infections. Stricture formation of the lower esophagus and metaplasia of the esophageal mucosa, leading to Barrett esophagus, are late complications of severe, untreated GER. Almost half of infants and children with chronic, severe GER have neurologic disorders related to perinatal asphyxia or congenital nervous system anomalies. Abnormal motility of the esophagus, gastric dysmotility, and impaired gastric emptying are frequently present.

B. Diagnostic Studies

Establishing the diagnosis in neonates is challenging due to the lack of consensus around what constitutes pathologic reflux. In general, esophageal 24-hour pH monitoring is the most commonly used diagnostic modality as upper gastrointestinal evaluation is associated with a high rate of false-positive and false-negative exams. An upper gastrointestinal series is less sensitive but can be useful to rule out other anatomic abnormalities (eg, intestinal malrotation) and assess for esophageal strictures in cases of chronic GER. There is currently no role for esophageal manometry in neonates and young children except for cases where achalasia is suspected.

▶ Treatment

Nonoperative therapy with dietary and behavioral changes is successful in most cases. Feedings can be thickened with rice cereal, and symptoms of GER can be mitigated by maintaining an upright position in an infant seat or a prone position after feeding. Persistent symptoms or evidence of esophagitis can be treated with acid-suppressing medications (eg, H_2-blocker or proton pump inhibitor) with or without a prokinetic agent (eg, metoclopramide). If a prolonged trial of nonoperative therapy fails or if complications of reflux can be documented (ie, poor weight gain, esophagitis, stricture, asthma, recurrent aspiration pneumonia), operative management with antireflux surgery should be considered. The Nissen fundoplication is the standard surgical treatment, although many variations on fundoplication exist. To date, there remain few high-quality comparative effectiveness data to establish the relative benefit of medication versus surgical therapy or when operative therapy should be considered. The procedure can be performed using both open and laparoscopic techniques with equivalent functional results, although there is a cosmetic benefit associated with the minimally invasive approach.

McAteer J, et al: Antireflux procedures for gastroesophageal reflux disease in children: influence of patient age on surgical management. *JAMA Surg.* 2014;149:56.

Rothenberg SS: Two decades of experience with laparoscopic Nissen fundoplication in infants and children: a critical evaluation of indications, technique, and results. *J Laparoendosc Adv Surg Tech A.* 2013;23:791.

Vernon-Roberts A, et al: Fundoplication versus postoperative medication for gastro-oesophageal reflux in children with neurological impairment undergoing gastrostomy. *Cochrane Database Syst Rev.* 2013;8:CD006151.

ACUTE APPENDICITIS

Acute appendicitis is the most common abdominal surgical emergency in childhood and is responsible for the greatest relative burden of resource utilization among all pediatric surgical procedures. The diagnosis must be considered in all age groups presenting with abdominal pain, but the highest incidence is in patients 10-12 years of age. Complicated appendicitis composes nearly 30% of cases and is associated with prolonged hospital stay, increased complication rates, and significantly higher hospital cost.

Clinical Findings

The classic presentation includes the gradual onset of vague epigastric or periumbilical pain followed by anorexia, nausea, vomiting, and migration to the right lower quadrant. In children, the risk of perforation is higher than in adults (~30%), and this is more common in younger children who cannot verbalize their abdominal pain. Diarrhea and fever are more common in complicated appendicitis. On physical exam, right lower quadrant tenderness (McBurney point tenderness) is the most sensitive finding, although it is not specific for appendicitis. Right lower quadrant pain during palpation of the left lower quadrant (Rovsing sign), rebound tenderness, involuntary guarding due to spasm of the right hemirectus muscle, and pain with jumping are other common findings, although they are associated with relatively poor sensitivity and specificity.

A white blood cell (WBC) count with differential should be obtained in all patients with suspected appendicitis. The WBC count is greater than 10,000/µL (often with a left shift) in more than 80% of patients with appendicitis. Findings on flat and upright abdominal radiographs are often nonspecific, although infrequently they may demonstrate the presence of a fecalith. Ultrasound should be the initial diagnostic imaging study, and CT or MRI should be used as secondary studies in cases of an equivocal ultrasound or where classic history and physical examination findings are unclear. Combining WBC data with ultrasound findings may further improve the predictive value of these tests. Admission for serial abdominal examinations without cross-sectional imaging is another acceptable option.

Differential Diagnosis

Gastroenteritis is most commonly confused with appendicitis. Vomiting typically follows periumbilical pain in appendicitis but often precedes abdominal pain in gastroenteritis. In addition, the patient with gastroenteritis commonly has diffuse abdominal pain and frequent copious watery diarrhea. Intussusception, intestinal obstruction and volvulus, mesenteric adenitis, Meckel diverticulitis, Henoch-Schönlein purpura, ruptured ovarian cyst, and Crohn disease must also be considered in the differential diagnosis for children. In adolescent girls, information regarding the menstrual cycle and previous episodes of pelvic inflammatory disease and an accurate sexual history are important to exclude gynecologic causes of an acute abdomen. Ultrasound can be valuable for ruling out other right lower quadrant causes of pain, including ovarian torsion and ruptured ovarian cysts.

Treatment

Once the diagnosis is made, fluid resuscitation is initiated and intravenous antibiotics should be administered. Appendectomy is the definitive treatment, which should be performed via a laparoscopic or open operation within 24 hours of diagnosis to prevent risk of perforation. In cases of perforation diagnosed preoperatively, treatment options include an operation or percutaneous drainage with a delayed, interval appendectomy. For complicated appendicitis, the duration of antibiotics is highly variable among institutions, but the typical duration is 5-10 days or until the WBC count has normalized. Recently, nonoperative management strategies have been described in certain adult populations; studies to evaluate safety and efficacy of nonoperative management strategies in children are ongoing.

Anandalwar SP, et al: Influence of intraoperative findings on outcomes and resource utilization in children with complicated appendicitis. *JAMA Surg.* 2018 Jul 25. doi: 10.1097/SLA.0000000000003059. [Epub ahead of print]

Glass C, et al: Diagnostic evaluation of children with suspected appendicitis: wading through the evidence. *Semin Pediatr Surg.* 2016;25(4):198-203.

Serres SK, et al: Time to appendectomy and risk of complicated appendicitis and adverse outcomes in children. *JAMA Pediatr.* 2017;171(8):740-746.

DUPLICATIONS OF THE GASTROINTESTINAL TRACT

Duplications are rare malformations of the gastrointestinal tract that occur in approximately 1 per 100,000 live birth. Duplications most commonly involve the ileum (50%), followed by the esophagus (20%), colon, rectum, stomach, and duodenum. Intrathoracic (esophageal) and small bowel duplications are usually spherical, whereas colonic duplications are more often long and tubular (Figure 45–27). Duplications are typically on the mesenteric side of the intestine and may or may not share a common wall with the intestine.

Duplications can be characterized by location, with lesions in the foregut being most common (~35%), followed by midgut (~50%) and hindgut (~15%) lesions. Foregut duplications may involve the respiratory tract and proximal gastrointestinal tract extending form the pharynx to the second portion of the duodenum. Midgut duplications are found between this point in the duodenum to the mid-transverse colon, and hindgut lesion include duplications

▲ **Figure 45–27.** Duplications of the gastrointestinal tract. Duplications may be saccular or tubular. They usually arise within the mesentery, having a common wall with the intestine. Thoracoabdominal duplications arise from the duodenum or jejunum and extend through the diaphragm into the mediastinum.

of the distal transverse colon extending to the anus. Thoracoabdominal duplications can be found when the saccular component of a thoracic duplication extends through the esophageal hiatus or a separate diaphragmatic opening to empty into the duodenum or jejunum. A neurenteric cyst is a thoracic duplication associated with a cervical or thoracic vertebral anomaly in which the duplication communicates with the subarachnoid space. Associated anomalies are found in approximately one-third of cases and may include cardiovascular, neurologic, skeletal, urologic, and gastrointestinal anomalies. Malignant degeneration has been reported in intestinal duplications diagnosed later in life.

▶ Clinical Findings

A. Symptoms and Signs

Two-thirds of patients with enteric duplications are symptomatic in the first year of life, and approximately 80% will present with symptoms by 2 years of life. Duplications of the neck and mediastinum can produce respiratory symptoms by compression of the airway. Thoracic duplications may lead to pneumonia or hemoptysis by compressing or eroding into adjacent lung parenchyma. Intra-abdominal duplications may produce abdominal pain due to distention of the duplication cyst, peptic ulceration from ectopic gastric mucosa present in the duplication, or mechanical obstruction. Obstruction may result due to intussusception, segmental volvulus, or luminal compression. Less commonly, an asymptomatic duplication may be found during imaging for other indications (eg, appendicitis).

B. Imaging Studies

Several diagnostic studies have been used to diagnose duplication cysts, including plain films, CT, MRI, ultrasound, and fluoroscopic imaging. If intraspinal extension of a duplication is suspected, MRI is indicated to evaluate the extent of central nervous system involvement and aid in operative planning. Ultrasonography may show a cystic or tubular mass within the mediastinum or abdomen. A Meckel scan may visualize duplications associated with ectopic gastric mucosa, although these are relatively rare and often negative.

▶ Treatment

Duplication cysts should be removed given their propensity to become symptomatic over time. Isolated spherical duplications may be removed with or without resection of the adjacent bowel, depending on the extent of a common wall between the cyst and the involved intestine. Long tubular duplications of the colon and rectum can be managed by establishing an anastomosis between the proximal and distal ends of the cyst and adjacent bowel. Duplications that contain gastric mucosa and cannot be removed completely should be opened and the mucosal lining excised. Extension of a mediastinal duplication into the spinal canal requires assistance from a neurosurgeon for safe excision.

Erginel B, et al: Enteric duplication cysts in children: a single-institution series with forty patients in twenty-six years. *World J Surg.* 2017;41:620.

Laje P, et al: Prenatal diagnosis and postnatal resection of intraabdominal enteric duplications. *J Pediatr Surg.* 2010; 45(7):1554-1558.

OMPHALOMESENTERIC DUCT ANOMALIES

Omphalomesenteric duct anomalies arise from incomplete obliteration of the omphalomesenteric (vitelline) duct, which itself is a remnant of the embryonic yolk sac. When the entire duct remains intact, it is recognized postnatally as an omphalomesenteric fistula connecting the umbilicus to the distal small intestine. An umbilical sinus arises when the duct is obliterated at the intestinal end but communicates with the umbilicus at the distal end. When the mid portion of the duct persists but both ends are occluded, an umbilical cyst or intra-abdominal enterocystoma may develop. A fibrous band may also persist between the ileum and the umbilicus and potentially serve as a lead point for a segmental volvulus (Figures 45–28 and 45–29).

The most common omphalomesenteric duct remnant is a Meckel diverticulum, which is present in 1%-3% of the population. Meckel diverticula occur with equal frequency in both sexes and are usually asymptomatic. Most lesions are discovered as an incidental finding during unrelated intra-abdominal procedures or by abdominal imaging. A Meckel diverticulum may be lined wholly or in part by gastric, small intestinal, or colonic mucosa and may also contain pancreatic tissue. Heterotopic tissue is found in 5% of asymptomatic and 75% of symptomatic cases. In contrast to enteric duplications, Meckel diverticula are located on the antimesenteric border of the ileum, usually within 100 cm of the ileocecal valve. The lifelong risk of complications associated with a Meckel diverticulum is estimated to be 4%-6%, and 40% of cases leading to a complication present in children before 10 years of age.

Clinical Findings

The most common symptoms associated with omphalomesenteric remnants include rectal bleeding (40%), intussusception (20%), diverticulitis or peptic ulceration (15%), umbilical drainage due to a persistent sinus or fistula (15%), and intestinal obstruction (7%). Rectal bleeding is usually due to peptic ulceration of the adjacent ileum caused by ectopic gastric mucosa and usually does not involve the diverticulum itself. The majority of patients are under 2 years of age at the time of their initial bleeding episode. A history of previous rectal bleeding may be present in close to half

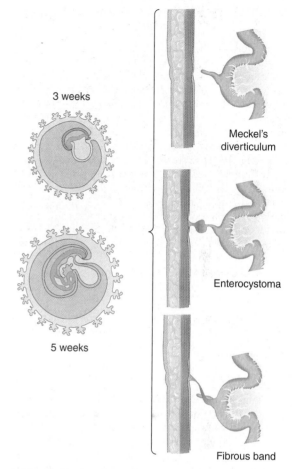

▲ **Figure 45–28.** Omphalomesenteric duct anomalies arise from the primitive yolk sac. Remnants include Meckel diverticulum, enterocystoma, and a fibrous band or fistulous tract between the ileum and the umbilicus.

of cases. Bleeding is often quite brisk, and younger children are at risk for hemorrhagic shock if the bleeding is not controlled. Diverticulitis or free perforation may present with abdominal pain and focal or generalized peritonitis similar to acute appendicitis.

Intestinal obstruction may develop as a result of a segmental volvulus around a persistent band between the umbilicus and ileum, as a result of internal herniation of bowel between the mesentery and a persistent vitelline or mesodiverticular vessel, or due to intussusception of the diverticulum. An infected umbilical sinus or omphalomesenteric fistula may present with purulent drainage, cellulitis, or an abdominal wall abscess.

Fluoroscopic studies using contrast are neither sensitive nor specific enough to identify a Meckel diverticulum. A technetium Tc-99m pertechnetate scintiscan (Meckel scan) may

▲ **Figure 45–29.** Meckel diverticulum. (Used with permission from Craig W. Lillehei, MD.)

localize a Meckel diverticulum if it is lined with gastric mucosa. Cimetidine is often used before initiating a Meckel scan to increase uptake of the tracer by heterotopic gastric mucosa.

▶ Treatment

Resection of Meckel diverticulum should be performed in symptomatic patients and can usually be accomplished by laparoscopy. An omphalomesenteric remnant with a narrow base may be treated by amputation and closure of the bowel defect (usually with a surgical stapler). Intestinal resection may be required with primary anastomosis in cases where the diverticulum has a wide base, when the diverticulum is associated with ectopic tissue extending to the adjacent small intestine, or when an inflammatory or ischemic process involves the adjacent ileum. There is no general consensus as to whether an incidental diverticulectomy performed during other abdominal operations is justified.

Sinha CK, et al: Meckel's scan in children: a review of 183 cases referred to two paediatric surgery specialist centres over 18 years. *Pediatr Surg Int.* 2013;29:511.

NECROTIZING ENTEROCOLITIS

Necrotizing enterocolitis (NEC) is the most common gastrointestinal surgical disorder associated with prematurity and is the leading cause of operative mortality in this population. The overall incidence of NEC is approximately 1 in 1000 live births, and median onset is 10 days following birth. The incidence of NEC has increased over time as therapeutic advances in neonatal intensive care have allowed ever more premature infants to survive. The pathophysiology of NEC has not been completely elucidated and is the focus of much ongoing basic and translational research. In general, NEC is thought to be the result of mucosal compromise and bacterial translocation after the introduction of enteral feedings. The process occurs nearly exclusively in premature infants and leads to bowel injury and inflammation. Necrosis and ulceration of intestinal mucosa ensue and, in severe cases, may progresses to full-thickness necrosis and perforation. Gas-producing bacteria present in the intestinal wall may lead to pneumatosis, a finding that may be noted on plain abdominal radiographs and on gross examination during laparotomy. The terminal ileum and right colon are most commonly affected, followed by the transverse and descending colon, proximal small bowel, and stomach. In the most extreme case, *NEC totalis* is found, where nearly the entirety of the small and large bowel is gangrenous and nonviable. Nearly 80% of NEC cases occur in premature infants weighing less than 2500 g at birth, and 50% are in neonates under 1500 g. Variable associations between NEC and perinatal events have been reported in epidemiologic studies, including premature rupture of membranes with amnionitis, breech delivery, intrauterine bradycardia, umbilical vessel catheterization with or without exchange transfusions, respiratory distress syndrome, sepsis, omphalitis, and congenital heart disease. The clustering of cases in nurseries suggests that an infectious agent may be responsible.

▶ Clinical Findings

Clinical findings associated with NEC include increased gastric residuals, bilious emesis, abdominal distention, bloody stools, and poor skin perfusion. Signs associated with NEC include apnea, bradycardia, hypoglycemia, and temperature instability. On examination, abdominal distention is the most frequent finding of early NEC, and the presence of abdominal wall erythema, edema, and a fixed abdominal mass may be a sign of bowel necrosis. The WBC count may be elevated or suppressed, and thrombocytopenia and progressive acidosis are suggestive of perforation and evolving sepsis.

Abdominal radiographs show small bowel distention early on, followed by pneumatosis intestinalis and even portal venous gas with more advanced disease. Serial plain films may show a fixed loop or loops of intestine. Perforation with pneumoperitoneum will develop in approximately 20% of cases. Infants who develop ascites without pneumoperitoneum should have paracentesis and examination of the fluid for bacteria.

▶ Treatment

Nonoperative treatment is the mainstay of early NEC without evidence of perforation. This includes bowel rest, nasogastric decompression, broad-spectrum antibiotics, parenteral nutrition, and correction of hypovolemia and electrolyte abnormalities. Indications for operative intervention include pneumoperitoneum, paracentesis with evidence of succus or stool, and progressive clinical deterioration in the setting of maximal medical therapy. The latter may include progressive (and uncorrectable) metabolic acidosis and the inability to ventilate due to abdominal distention. At laparotomy, all visibly necrotic bowel is resected and a stoma is created at a level of the proximal resection site. Severe disease may require extensive bowel resection, leading to short bowel syndrome and lifelong need for parenteral nutrition (Figure 45-30). Bedside drainage of the peritoneal cavity is an alternative treatment option in extremely low birth weight infants (< 1000 g) who are too unstable to transport to the operating room. Peritoneal drainage involves a small incision made in the right lower quadrant using local anesthesia and placement of a Penrose drain. Studies comparing laparotomy to drain placement for very low birth weight infants have demonstrated equivalent outcomes in mortality.

The overall survival rate for NEC is 70%-75% and primarily depends on birth weight, gestational age, and the need for operative management. Development of intestinal strictures occur in approximately 15% of cases as a late complication following operative therapy. For this reason, a contrast enema is used to evaluate the defunctionalized distal bowel before stoma closure. Short bowel syndrome and neurodevelopmental abnormalities have been characterized as long-term sequalae in severe cases of NEC.

Downard CD, et al: Treatment of necrotizing enterocolitis: an American Pediatric Surgical Association Outcomes and Clinical Trials Committee systematic review. *J Pediatr Surg.* 2012;47:2111.
Frost BL, et al: New medical and surgical insights into neonatal necrotizing enterocolitis: a review. *JAMA Pediatr.* 2017;171(1):83-88.

GASTROINTESTINAL BLEEDING

Severe gastrointestinal bleeding in children is rare but can be quite alarming and anxiety provoking for parents and caregivers. The diagnostic approach used in the evaluation of these children is similar to that used in adults, but the causes vary depending on the age of the child. The etiology is invariably benign (malignancy is exceedingly rare), and common symptoms can include hematemesis, hematochezia, or melena. Depending on the amount and chronicity of bleeding, the child may have sunken fontanelles, dry mucous membranes, and cool skin. Tachycardia, oliguria, and hypotension may be present. Laboratory tests will typically include hematocrit measurements and coagulation studies.

Upper Gastrointestinal Bleeding

The presence of melena and the presence of blood on passage of a nasogastric tube can help differentiate between upper and lower gastrointestinal bleeding. Upper gastrointestinal bleeding originates above the ligament of Treitz. Upper gastrointestinal bleeding in infants and young children is most often associated with gastric ulcers, but in older children, it may also be caused by duodenal ulcer, esophagitis, and esophageal varices (particularly in children with underlying liver disease). Evaluation following stabilization of the child begins with flexible esophagoduodenoscopy. Once the diagnosis is made, treatment is usually amenable to antacids (H_2-blockers, proton pump inhibitors). Variceal hemorrhage may require more aggressive intervention, including the use of octreotide, endoscopic varix sclerosis or band ligation, and, in extreme cases, transjugular intrahepatic portocaval shunt, mesocaval shunt, or liver transplantation.

Lower Gastrointestinal Hemorrhage

The causes of lower gastrointestinal bleeding in infants and children can be categorized in diagnostic age groups where the age of the patient, the amount of hemorrhage, and the color of the blood may provide insight into the source of bleeding.

Hemorrhage in the neonate may be caused by swallowed maternal blood during delivery, anorectal fissures, upper gastrointestinal bleeding secondary to gastritis or ulceration,

▲ **Figure 45–30.** Premature infant with necrotizing enterocolitis (NEC) with diffuse involvement of the entire small bowel and colon (NEC totalis). (Used with permission from Craig W. Lillehei, MD.)

NEC, and volvulus, among others. The Apt test for maternal blood, physical examination of the rectum and inguinal canal, and evaluation of the upper gastrointestinal tract can quickly rule out most of these causes. Bleeding from NEC is rarely life-threatening, and the diagnosis is commonly made based on the premature delivery of the infant and radiologic evaluation. If bleeding from malrotation with midgut volvulus is suspected, prompt laparotomy is indicated.

Anal fissures are the most common cause of rectal bleeding in infants and neonates. Other causes include intestinal volvulus, intussusception, intestinal duplication, Meckel diverticulum, milk or formula protein allergy, and infectious diarrhea. Contrast studies and appropriate stool cultures guide treatment. The differential in older children includes rectal prolapse and a variety of polyps of the colon (juvenile, Peutz-Jeghers, polypoid lymphoid hyperplasia, and, rarely, adenomatosis), in addition to causes similar to that of infants. Diagnostic modalities include traditional endoscopy and capsule endoscopy. Juvenile polyps are the single most common cause of lower gastrointestinal bleeding in children (20%-30%). Most juvenile polyps are solitary (80%) and often pass spontaneously without treatment. However, if bleeding continues to recur, endoscopic excision of polyps can be performed. Adolescents may manifest signs and symptoms of inflammatory bowel disease (ulcerative colitis, Crohn disease), familial adenomatous polyposis, and small vascular lesions such as telangiectasias. Diagnosis is made by colonoscopy, and treatment is disease specific.

Owensby S, et al: Diagnosis and management of upper gastrointestinal bleeding in children. *J Am Board Fam Med.* 2015; 28:134.

Pant C, et al: Emergency department visits for gastrointestinal bleeding in children: results from the Nationwide Emergency Department Sample 2006-2011. *Curr Med Res Opin.* 2015;31:347.

GASTROINTESTINAL FOREIGN BODIES

Aspiration of foreign bodies is the leading cause of accidental death in infants, and children less than 2 years old are at particular risk due to their tendency to place objects in their mouths. The type of foreign body and the location in the airway or gastrointestinal tract dictate the need, urgency, and approach to management.

▶ Esophageal Foreign Bodies

Typical foreign bodies found in the esophagus include coins, food, and small toys. The most common site of obstruction is at the level of the cricopharyngeus muscle, followed by the aortic arch and the gastroesophageal junction. Previous areas of repair/anastomosis (eg, EA) predispose to obstruction due to intrinsic narrowing. Common symptoms include drooling, feeding intolerance, dysphagia, emesis, and retrosternal pain. Respiratory symptoms may also occur. Perforation is rare but is more common with sharp objects and button batteries that are lodged in the esophagus. Magnets ("bucky balls") can conglomerize together within different loops of small bowel following ingestion and cause fistulas from prolonged pressure necrosis. The diagnosis of esophageal foreign bodies can be made by anteroposterior chest or lateral neck radiography if the ingested object is radiopaque. Otherwise, fluoroscopy, CT imaging, or esophagoscopy is indicated.

Due to the risk of erosion, aspiration, perforation, and stricture, impacted objects should be removed. Extraction can be performed using balloon catheter retrieval under fluoroscopic control or under direct visualization using esophagoscopy with general anesthesia. The latter technique is generally preferred if the nature of the object is unknown, if the object is sharp, or the ingestion occurred more than 24-48 hours ago. A Hopkins rod lens endoscopy system allows visualization of the object and retrieval with specially designed forceps for grasping small objects.

Ninety-five percent of foreign bodies that pass beyond the gastroesophageal junction proceed uneventfully through the gastrointestinal tract. Operative retrieval should be strongly considered for button batteries, multiple magnets or sharp objects, or objects longer than 5 cm, and for cases where ingested objects cause complete obstruction (eg, bezoars).

▶ Airway Foreign Bodies

The most commonly aspirated objects include peanuts and popcorn, and obstruction tends to occur at the level of the right main stem bronchus.

Symptoms commonly include ongoing or a history of coughing, choking, wheezing, dyspnea, tachypnea, drooling, and fatigue. Air trapping may result when the foreign body forms a ball-valve obstruction, leading to hyperinflation of the affected pulmonary lobe and mediastinal shift away from the affected side. On the other hand, complete obstruction may lead to loss of air volume with atelectasis and mediastinal shift to the ipsilateral side. Plain films of the chest in infants may demonstrate air trapping, although the foreign body is rarely visualized on radiographs.

Any child with symptoms, history, or imaging concerning for foreign body aspiration should undergo bronchoscopic evaluation under general anesthesia. Optical grasping forceps outfitted with fiberoptic lighting are used to retrieve foreign bodies in the proximal to mid-distal airways. Rarely, an unrecognized aspirated foreign body presents as chronic lung infection and may require removal of the affected pulmonary lobe.

Jayachandra S, et al: A systematic review of paediatric foreign body ingestion: presentation, complications, and management. *Int J Pediatr Otorhinolaryngol.* 2013;77:311.

Kramer RE, et al: Management of ingested foreign bodies in children: a clinical report of the NASPGHAN Endoscopy Committee. *J Pediatr Gastroenterol Nutr.* 2015;60:562.

LIVER & BILIARY TRACT DISORDERS

Jaundice in the first 2 weeks of infancy is usually due to indirect (unconjugated) hyperbilirubinemia, and common causes include "physiologic jaundice" (associated with breast-feeding), hemolysis due to Rh and ABO incompatibility, and infections. Jaundice that persists beyond the first 2 weeks in which both indirect and direct bilirubin levels are elevated should prompt a more thorough workup. The most common cause of prolonged jaundice in infancy is biliary atresia (approximately two-thirds of all cases), followed by various forms of hepatitis (30%) and choledochal cysts (5%). Intestinal obstruction can intensify jaundice by increasing the enterohepatic circulation of bilirubin. Finally, jaundice can be an early sign of sepsis in the newborn.

BILIARY ATRESIA

Biliary atresia is a condition characterized by absence of normal bile ducts draining the liver (sclerosing cholangiopathy). The atretic ducts consist of solid fibrous cords that may contain occasional islands of biliary epithelium. Biliary atresia is the most common cause of end-stage liver disease and the most common indication for liver transplantation in the pediatric age group. The etiology of biliary atresia remains unknown, but there is evidence that biliary atresia may develop after birth. This is supported by the observation that jaundice is not usually evident in the newborn period after 2 weeks of life. Furthermore, conjugated bilirubin is not cleared by the placenta as unconjugated bilirubin is, and jaundice due to conjugated hyperbilirubinemia with biliary obstruction has not been recognized in newborn infants.

The extent of duct involvement varies from case to case. There are three anatomic patterns of obstruction, including distal obstruction at the common bile duct (type I), proximal obstruction at the common hepatic duct (type II), and more proximal obstruction at the porta hepatis (type III; most common). Liver biopsy demonstrates proliferation of the bile canaliculi containing inspissated bile. Over time, the failure to excrete bile out of the liver results in progressive periportal fibrosis and obstruction of the intrahepatic portal veins, resulting in biliary cirrhosis and ultimately liver failure if untreated.

Clinical Findings

A. Symptoms and Signs

The typical presentation of a neonate with biliary atresia is a full-term infant with an uneventful neonatal course until jaundice is noted at 2-3 weeks of age. Stools may be normal or clay colored, and the urine may be dark. The stools contain an increased quantity of fat but are of normal consistency and not frothy. The liver may be of normal size early, but it becomes enlarged over time. Splenomegaly may develop due to portal hypertension in late disease. Ascites and portal hypertension do not manifest for several months and are signs of advanced cirrhosis.

B. Laboratory Findings

The workup of biliary atresia consists of fractionated bilirubin, liver and coagulation profiles, complete blood count, and metabolic and serologic screening. The bilirubin levels may vary considerably from day to day, but direct bilirubin levels greater than 3 mg/dL are common. Alkaline phosphatase levels are often elevated to 500-1000 units/L, and γ-glutamyltranspeptidase levels are greater than 300 units/L.

C. Imaging Studies

Ultrasonography may demonstrate absence or inability to visualize a contracted gallbladder. Hepatobiliary scintigraphy (eg, HIDA scan) can be used to examine the intensity of uptake within the liver and evidence of tracer secretion into the bowel (which rules out biliary atresia). However, scintigraphy is not routinely used because the test requires a 3- to 5-day delay following phenobarbital administration to optimize tracer uptake into the liver. Core needle biopsy has poor sensitivity and specificity for diagnosing biliary atresia. Therefore, all children suspected of having biliary atresia should undergo operative cholangiography with the intention of proceeding to exploration of the porta hepatis and portoenterostomy as necessary.

Other Causes

Other causes of obstructive jaundice include choledochal cyst, inspissated bile syndrome, and neonatal hepatitis. Choledochal cysts can be identified by the presence of a palpable mass in the right upper quadrant and ultrasonographic confirmation. Inspissated bile syndrome typically follows an episode of hemolysis in which a large bilirubin load is excreted into the bile ducts. The syndrome can be recognized by abdominal ultrasound. Hepatitis is most commonly of unknown cause. It may be due to a variety of infections, often of maternal origin, such as toxoplasmosis, cytomegalovirus, rubella syndrome, herpes simplex, coxsackievirus, or varicella. Serum should be tested for elevated antibody titers to these agents. Neonatal physiologic jaundice is self-limited and also responds to phototherapy.

Genetic metabolic diseases associated with jaundice include α_1-antitrypsin deficiency, galactosemia, and cystic fibrosis. Other rare causes include sepsis, parenteral alimentation cholestasis, Gilbert disease, and Alagille syndrome.

Treatment

When biliary atresia is the suspected cause of neonatal jaundice, surgical exploration is indicated as early as possible. Delayed treatment will result in progressive cirrhosis, and earlier operations (within the first 2-3 months of life) are associated with a greater likelihood of operative success. The procedure begins with an intraoperative cholangiogram to establish the diagnosis. This involves cannulating the gallbladder through a transverse abdominal incision or via laparoscopy and injecting water-soluble contrast into the biliary tree. If the image shows no excretion of contrast into the duodenum, the diagnosis is confirmed. A liver biopsy should be performed in all cases.

Confirmed biliary atresia is treated by a hepatic portoenterostomy (Kasai procedure). This involves a cholecystectomy and excision of the scarred bile ducts at the portal plate. A Roux-en-Y limb of jejunum is sutured to an area of the hilum to provide biliary drainage into the intestine. Empiric antibiotics may be used postoperatively to reduce the risk of cholangitis, which can result in scarring and need for revision or transplantation. Steroids have also been used both pre- and postoperatively in an effort to prevent ongoing hepatic fibrosis.

▶ Prognosis

Favorable long-term outcomes are associated with younger age at operation (< 2 months), absence of cirrhosis at the time of operation, and establishment of adequate bile flow. In general, one-third of infants undergoing the Kasai procedure will have excellent bile flow and will not develop liver failure, one-third will never have bile flow and will require early liver transplantation, and one-third have an initially good response (eg, bile flow) but then develop progressive biliary cirrhosis requiring liver transplantation. The average life span for infants with uncorrected biliary atresia without transplantation is 19 months. For those with established bile flow postoperatively, the most common complication is cholangitis, and this may be recurrent.

Chung PH, et al: Predictors for failure after Kasai operation. *J Pediatr Surg.* 2015;50:293.

Wang KS, et al: Newborn screening for biliary atresia. *Pediatrics.* 2015;136:e1663.

CHOLEDOCHAL CYST

A choledochal cyst arises from cystic dilation or a diverticulum of the biliary system. The incidence is geography dependent, ranging from 1:100,000 in Western countries to 1:13,000 in East Asia. There is a strong female predominance. The etiology is unknown, but many theories have been proposed, including infectious etiology, genetic factors, and biliary autonomic dysfunction.

Choledochal cysts are classified into one of five subtypes based on anatomy and distribution within the biliary tree. These include fusiform dilation of the extrahepatic bile duct (type I, 80% of all cases), saccular outpouching of the common bile duct (type II, < 2%), dilation of the common bile duct at its confluence with the duodenum (type III,

choledochocele < 4%), cystic dilation of both the intra- and extrahepatic bile ducts (type IV, ~20%), and lakes of multiple intrahepatic cysts with no extrahepatic component (type V, 10%). Type V cysts associated with hepatic fibrosis are termed Caroli disease.

If left untreated, choledochal cysts may eventually cause biliary obstruction, cholangitis, and cholangiocarcinoma. The risk of cholangiocarcinoma increases to 10%-15% after 10 years of follow-up and may increase even further throughout life.

▶ Clinical Findings

The typical presentation of a child with a choledochal cyst is right upper quadrant pain and jaundice. A right upper quadrant mass may be palpable on exam. Eighty percent of cases are diagnosed in the first decade of life. The cyst may become painful or infected over time, and rarely a child may develop bile peritonitis secondary to cyst perforation. Gallstones and cholangitis may develop due to biliary stasis.

The diagnosis is most often suggested by ultrasonography, although cross-sectional imaging including CT and MRI is frequently obtained to confirm the diagnosis and better characterize anatomy.

▶ Treatment

Treatment of choledochal cysts is complete excision with Roux-en-Y hepaticojejunostomy to restore biliary drainage. Cholecystectomy is always performed. Biliary cirrhosis and portal hypertension secondary to prolonged ductal obstruction may be assessed with liver biopsy. The results of choledochal cyst excision with hepaticojejunostomy reconstruction are excellent, but these children do require lifelong monitoring due to the risk of anastomotic stricture and intrahepatic stone formation.

Soares KC, et al: Pediatric choledochal cysts: diagnosis and current management. *Pediatr Surg Int.* 2017;33:637-650.

▼ INGUINAL & SCROTAL DISORDERS

INGUINAL HERNIA & HYDROCELE

Inguinal hernias are common in infancy and childhood, occurring in 1%-3% of all children. Unlike hernias in adulthood, these nearly always result from a patent processus vaginalis (indirect hernia) and not from a weakness in the floor of the inguinal canal (direct hernia). The processus vaginalis follows the descent of the testis into the inguinal canal. Failure of obliteration of the processus may lead to a variety of anomalies, including hernia, communicating hydrocele, noncommunicating hydrocele, hydrocele of the spermatic cord, and hydrocele of the tunica vaginalis (Figure 45–31).

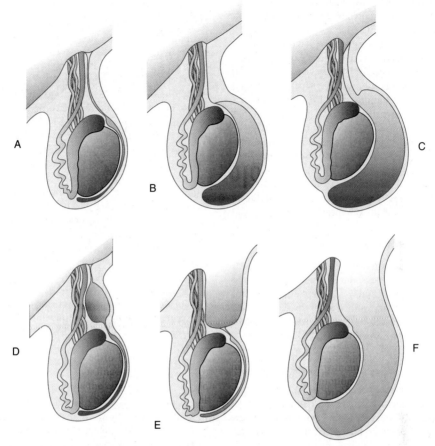

▲ **Figure 45–31.** Spectrum of inguinoscrotal disorders. **A:** Normal anatomy. The processus vaginalis is obliterated, and there is a small remnant, the tunica vaginalis, adjacent to the posterior surface of the testis. **B:** Scrotal hydrocele. **C:** Communicating hydrocele. Note the proximal patency of the processus vaginalis. **D:** Hydrocele of the spermatic cord. **E:** Inguinal hernia. **F:** Inguinoscrotal hernia. (Reproduced with permission from Rowe MI et al: *Essentials of Pediatric Surgery.* St. Louis, MO: Mosby/Elsevier; 1995.)

The processus vaginalis remains patent in over 80% of newborn infants. The incidence of a processus vaginalis decreases to 40%-50% by 2 years of age, and in adults, 25% are persistently patent. Visible herniation of bowel into a patent processus vaginalis develops in 1%-4% of children, with 25% apparent within the first year of life. Indirect inguinal hernias occur five times more commonly in males. Direct and femoral hernias also occur in children but are relatively rare.

Inguinal hernias are found involving the right groin in 60% of children, the left side in 30%, and bilaterally in 10%. Conditions associated with increased risk for inguinal hernias include prematurity, history of an abdominal wall defect (eg, gastroschisis), cryptorchidism, intersex anomalies, connective tissue disorders, and ascites.

► Clinical Findings

The diagnosis of hernia in infants and children is strongly suggested by the demonstration of an inguinal bulge originating from the internal ring. The bulge can be elicited during Valsalva (crying, coughing, straining). Having an assistant hold the infant's arms over his or her head and legs straight will often elicit crying and straining that will aid in the physical examination. Indirect signs, such as a wide external ring and the "silk glove" sign (palpable thickening of the spermatic cord), are not specific. One must always locate the position of the testis during examination for a hernia since an inguinal bulge due to an undescended or retractile testis may be mistaken for a hernia.

A hydrocele is fluid within the remnant processus vaginalis. It is characteristically an oblong, nontender soft mass. Hydroceles may involve the testicle only (testicular hydrocele), extend from the testicle into the inguinal region (inguinoscrotal hydrocele), be contained within a segment of the processus adjacent to the spermatic cord (hydrocele of the cord), or communicate with the peritoneal cavity (communicating hydrocele). With a noncommunicating hydrocele (the first three hydroceles described earlier), the processus vaginalis has closed proximally. The normal spermatic cord can usually be palpated above the level of the hydrocele. Transillumination may not be reliable in the newborn since intestine and fluid transilluminate equally well. A communicating hydrocele is suspected by a history of size variation throughout the day (smallest in the morning after lying recumbent, largest during the day after the upright posture or repeated straining).

Differential Diagnosis

A hydrocele under tension may be confused with an incarcerated inguinal hernia. The sudden appearance of fluid confined to the testicular area may represent a noncommunicating hydrocele secondary to torsion of the testis or testicular appendage, epididymo-orchitis, panserositis from a recent viral syndrome, or idiopathic scrotal edema.

Complications

The principle complication of an untreated inguinal hernia is incarceration (viscus stuck in sac) and strangulation of incarcerated contents (Figure 45–32). Compression of the spermatic vessels by an incarcerated hernia may produce hemorrhagic infarction of the ipsilateral testicle.

▲ **Figure 45–32.** Two-month-old infant boy with an incarcerated right inguinal hernia. Note the swelling and erythema involving the right scrotum. (Used with permission from Craig W. Lillehei, MD.)

Treatment

In general, hydroceles that do not communicate with the peritoneal cavity are physiologic, and the vast majority resolve by 12-18 months of age. Those that persist after 1 year or those that demonstrate changes in size (communicating hydroceles) should be repaired.

Inguinal hernias diagnosed in infancy and childhood should be repaired. In hospitalized premature infants, hernia repair may be deferred until the baby is ready to be discharged. High ligation of the hernia sac by obliteration of the internal ring (leaving enough space for the spermatic cord) is all that is required. Historically, it was recommended that premature infants undergo operative exploration of the contralateral inguinal canal in search of a clinically silent patent processus vaginalis. This approach has been replaced by laparoscopic exploration through the ipsilateral hernia sac. If a patent processus vaginalis is demonstrated, a second inguinal incision is made and the procedure is repeated as described earlier. A completely laparoscopic repair has been described, which has the advantage of simultaneous exploration of the contralateral side and virtually no manipulation of the spermatic cord. The incidence of complications from uncomplicated inguinal hernia repair (recurrence, wound infection, and damage to the spermatic cord) should be 2% or less.

An incarcerated hernia in an infant can usually be reduced initially before operation. This is accomplished by sedation and by elevation of the foot of the bed to keep intra-abdominal pressure from being exerted against the inguinal area. When the infant is well sedated, the hernia may be reduced by gentle constant pressure over the internal ring in a manner that milks the bowel into the abdominal cavity. This is a two-handed maneuver in which one hand "squeezes" the incarcerated mass while the other directs it posteriorly into the internal ring. If the bowel cannot be reduced, an urgent operation is required. If the hernia is reduced, operative repair can be performed immediately or be delayed for 24-48 hours to allow edema in the tissues to subside. An incarcerated ovary may not be able to be reduced but is usually asymptomatic, and repair can be performed on a semi-urgent basis. Bloody stools, edema, and red discoloration of the skin around the groin suggest a strangulated hernia, and reduction of the bowel should not be attempted. Emergency repair of incarcerated inguinal hernia can be technically difficult due to edematous and friable tissues. When gangrenous intestine is encountered, the bowel should be resected and an end-to-end intestinal anastomosis performed.

Bruzoni M, et al: Long-term follow-up of laparoscopic transcutaneous inguinal herniorraphy with high transfixation suture ligature of the hernia sac. *J Pediatr Surg.* 2015;50(10):1767-1771.

Lao OB, et al: Pediatric inguinal hernias, hydroceles, and undescended testicles. *Surg Clin North Am.* 2012;92:487.

UNDESCENDED TESTIS (CRYPTORCHIDISM)

In the seventh month of gestation, the testicles normally descend into the scrotum. Cryptorchidism is commonly used to refer to undescended, retractile, ectopic, or absent testes. Undescended testis occurs when there is arrested descent and fixation of testis retroperitoneally, in the inguinal canal, or just beyond the external ring in the upper scrotum. The incidence of undescended testis is 1%-2% in full-term neonates and up to 30% in premature infants. The right testis is affected most commonly. The majority are able to be located with palpation in the upper scrotum or inguinal canal, and less than 10% are intra-abdominal in location. A patent processus vaginalis is present in 60%-90% of patients with cryptorchidism, and approximately 25% have or will develop an associated inguinal hernia. Continued descent of the testes may progress after birth, but further descent is rare after 2 years of age.

Operative correction may be required as normal spermatogenesis requires cooler temperatures provided by the scrotal environment. When testes remain undescended, prolonged exposure to normal body temperature can result in degenerative changes in the seminiferous tubules. Such degenerative changes have been documented as early as 2 years of age. Unless the disorder is corrected, patients with bilateral cryptorchidism will become sterile as adults. There is also evidence of malignant transformation in adults with unrepaired cryptorchidism. The incidence of testicular cancer in a cryptorchid testis is higher than in the normal population and is not decreased by repair. Finally, cryptorchid testes are more susceptible to trauma and torsion, often have an associated inguinal hernia, and may cause adverse psychosocial effects.

Anomalies associated with cryptorchidism occur in about 15% of cases and may include a wide variety of syndromes such as Klinefelter, hypogonadotropic hypogonadism, and prune belly syndrome. Isolated anomalies of the collecting system may also be present, including horseshoe kidney, renal agenesis or hypoplasia, bladder exstrophy, ureteral reflux, and cloacal exstrophy.

▶ Clinical Findings

Physical examination often demonstrates a flat, "empty" hemiscrotum with absent rugae. Cryptorchidism must be differentiated from retractile testes. Due to active cremaster muscles of children under 3 years of age and the relatively small size of the testis, the gonad can retract into the external inguinal ring or inguinal canal. This is a retractile testis and is a normal variant. Retractile testes can usually be manually manipulated into the mid to lower scrotum and do not require operative intervention unless they remain in the area of the external ring. Ultrasound may demonstrate the presence of an intra-abdominal testis, although the study is generally unnecessary to establish the diagnosis of cryptorchidism.

▶ Treatment

Recommended timing of operative management remains controversial. In general, most would consider repair between 9 and 18 months of age if spontaneous descent has not occurred. An orchidopexy is performed to mobilize the testis from its ectopic location into the scrotum. This is usually possible with testis that can be palpated in the inguinal canal. Several techniques have been described to lengthen the spermatic cord structures, including complete skeletonization of the cremasteric muscles and division of the epigastric vessels to create a more direct path. If the testis is not palpable when the child is anesthetized, laparoscopy should be performed before making an inguinal incision. This allows for identification of an abdominal testis or the diagnosis of an absent or "vanishing" testis (usually due to in utero torsion). Intra-abdominal testes with a short blood supply can be brought into the scrotum by a two-stage repair, initially dividing the spermatic artery and vein (which limits mobility of the testicle) without mobilizing the testicle itself. This is followed 3-6 months later by a combined laparoscopic and groin procedure where the testicle is mobilized and positioned in the scrotum. The success of the staged procedure is based on dual blood supply between the spermatic vessels and the collateral blood supply via the vas deferens and the gubernaculum. The prognosis for fertility following orchidopexy in unilateral maldescent is between 80% and 90%, whereas fertility after bilateral orchidopexy is between 50% and 70%.

Ikraman J, et al: The undescended testis: clinical management and scientific advances. *Semin Pediatr Surg.* 2016;25:241.

TESTICULAR TORSION

Testicular torsion is a surgical emergency that occurs most commonly in early adolescence (age 13-14 years) but also is common during the neonatal period. There are two categories of testicular torsion depending on where the spermatic cord is torsed with respect to the tunica vaginalis. These include intravaginal torsion (bell-clapper deformity), which is the most common form, and extravaginal torsion, which occurs principally in neonates and in children with an undescended testis. Rarely, the testis may twist on a long epididymal mesentery. In children and adolescents, testicular torsion may be either idiopathic or posttraumatic in etiology.

▶ Clinical Findings

The typical presentation is acute onset of scrotal or testicular pain that may radiate to the lower abdomen. Progressive swelling, edema, and erythema of the hemiscrotum occur. The testis is often exquisitely tender to palpation. The spermatic cord may be foreshortened (resulting in an elevated testicle), the epididymis may lie anteriorly, and the cremasteric reflex may be absent.

The diagnosis of testicular torsion is based mainly on clinical examination, and ultrasound can be confirmatory in cases where the diagnosis is in question.

▶ Differential Diagnosis

Torsion of the testicular appendices (vestigial Müllerian duct structures) and epididymitis may mimic testicular torsion. With epididymitis, there is often pyuria, voiding symptoms, and fever. Torsion of the testicular appendices often has a gradual onset, and careful palpation may reveal point tenderness rather than diffuse tenderness. There may be a visible necrotic lesion on scrotal transillumination (blue dot sign). Incarcerated inguinal hernias can also mimic testicular torsion.

▶ Treatment

If the diagnosis is strongly suspected, the best "test" is operative scrotal exploration. Timing is essential, as reduction of the torsion is related to the likelihood of testicular ischemia and salvage. The testicular salvage rate if detorsion is performed within 6 hours after onset of symptoms is up to 90%-100%, versus less than 50% if delayed more than 12 hours, and less than 10% if delayed more than 24 hours. At exploration, an orchiopexy is performed in which the torsion is corrected and the gonad, if viable, is fixed to the hemiscrotum using a dartos pouch. A prophylactic contralateral orchiopexy is performed to prevent future torsion of the uninvolved testicle. Torsion of the testicular appendices tends to be self-limiting since necrosis and autoamputation usually occur. Treatment is conservative and includes warm baths, limited activity, and anti-inflammatory medications. If significant pain persists after 2-3 days and the appendix has not autoamputated, excision is indicated. Testicular salvage after neonatal testicular torsion is very rare.

DaJusta DG, et al: Contemporary review of testicular torsion: new concepts, emerging technologies and potential therapeutics. *J Pediatr Urol.* 2013;9:723.

▼ ABDOMINAL WALL DEFECTS

UMBILICAL HERNIA

A fascial defect at the umbilicus is frequently present in the newborn, particularly in premature infants. The incidence is highest in African American children. In most children (> 85%), the umbilical ring progressively diminishes in size and will close spontaneously by 5 years of age. Unlike inguinal hernias, protrusion of bowel through the umbilical defect rarely results in incarceration during childhood. Surgical repair is indicated if a child exhibits symptoms or signs of

incarceration at any age. In children with asymptomatic hernias, repair is indicated after 4-5 years of age. Both open and laparoscopic approaches are associated with excellent results.

OMPHALOCELE

Omphalocele is a defect of the midline abdominal wall and affects 1-4:10,000 live births. The abdominal viscera (commonly liver and bowel) are contained within a sac composed of peritoneum and amnion from which the umbilical cord arises (Figure 45–33). When there is no facial defect but rather an open umbilical ring with herniated abdominal contents, the condition is termed *hernia of the umbilical cord.* *Giant omphalocele* refers to a large facial defect with some portion of the liver outside of the body. Associated abnormalities are common, occurring in approximately 50% of infants. These include chromosomal abnormalities (trisomy 13, 18, 21), congenital heart disease (tetralogy of Fallot, atrial septal defect), Beckwith-Wiedemann syndrome, pentalogy of Cantrell, and prune belly syndrome.

▶ Treatment

The primary goal of surgery is to return the viscera to the abdominal cavity and close the abdominal wall defect. With an intact sac, emergency operation is not necessary, and a thorough physical examination and workup for associated anomalies can be performed. An orogastric tube should be placed on suction to minimize intestinal distention.

The success of primary closure depends on the size of the defect, abdominal and thoracic capacity, and the presence of associated comorbidities (eg, pulmonary insufficiency). Supplemental coverage with plastic wrap or a bowel bag can be used to prevent heat loss. If the viscera reduce but abdominal wall closure is not possible, there are three options: staged

▲ **Figure 45–33.** Neonate with omphalocele. The herniated liver and bowel can be seen within a sac composed of amnion and chorion. (Used with permission from Craig W. Lillehei, MD.)

repair, prosthetic patch repair, or delayed operative management with initial epithelialization. A staged repair aims to create a protective extra-abdominal extension of the peritoneal cavity, allowing gradual reduction of the viscera and gradual abdominal wall expansion using two parallel sheets of reinforced Silastic sheeting (or a spring-loaded silo bag) sutured to the fascial edges. The silo is progressively compressed to invert the amniotic sac and its contents into the abdomen and to bring the edges of the linea alba together by stretching the abdominal wall muscles. When abdominal relaxation is sufficient to allow the rectus muscles to come together, the silo is removed, the amnion is left inverted into the abdominal cavity, and the defect is closed.

Delayed operative management is appropriate for infants with severe associated anomalies or a giant omphalocele. The amnion is allowed to dry and form an eschar, and this process is facilitated by daily application of any number of agents including Silvadene or Betadine. The membrane becomes vascularized beneath the eschar, and contraction of the wound with skin growth covers the defect. This can be further facilitated by creation of a compression orthotic that allows for the gradual return of abdominal contents and re-creation of abdominal domain. A ventral hernia results, which is repaired electively when the patient is stable. The survival rate for infants with small omphaloceles is excellent. Complications may include abdominal compartment syndrome, infection, wound complications, respiratory failure, or pulmonary hypertension. Deaths associated with larger omphaloceles are principally from wound dehiscence with subsequent and ensuing infection or from associated anomalies.

GASTROSCHISIS

Gastroschisis is a defect in the abdominal wall characterized by variable evisceration of viscera without an associated sac (Figure 45–34). The incidence of gastroschisis is increasing, and currently, the condition affects between 4 and 5 per 100,000 live births in the United States. Gastroschisis is twice as common as omphalocele, and the fascial defect is usually smaller. The remnants of the amnion are usually reabsorbed. The skin may continue to grow over the remnants of the amnion, and there may be a bridge of skin between the defect and the cord. Unlike in omphalocele, the liver is virtually never present in the defect. The eviscerated bowel is often inflamed and edematous and may have a thick, matted membrane ("peel") covering. This is thought to be due to prolonged exposure to amniotic fluid and compression of the mesenteric blood supply at the abdominal defect.

▶ Complications

Over 70% of infants with this disorder are premature, and associated anomalies are far less common than with

▲ **Figure 45–34.** Neonate with gastroschisis. The defect is to the right of the umbilical cord, and there is no investing sac around the herniated bowel and stomach. (Used with permission from Craig W. Lillehei, MD.)

omphalocele (< 10% of cases). In approximately 10% of cases, associated intestinal atresias may be found and are thought to arise from infarcted segments of intestine that have herniated through the defect in utero. Closed or "vanishing" gastroschisis refers to the severe in utero complication where a substantial length of intestine is lost to in utero infarction. Many of these children will require lifelong parenteral nutrition or a multivisceral transplant.

▶ Treatment & Prognosis

Due to the exposed abdominal viscera, urgent abdominal wall closure is necessary. Smaller defects may be closed primarily; however, a staged approach is often required for moderate to large defects where a significant loss of abdominal domain is present. This can be performed using a silo reduction technique as described previously for gastroschisis. As bowel wall edema subsides, the bowel can be slowly reduced into the abdominal cavity over a period of several days. When the bowel has been completely reduced (usually 5-7 days), the silo is removed and the abdominal wall can then be closed. Alternatively, the umbilical remnant can be used as a "patch" dressing to allow primary closure without the need for formal operative intervention (sutureless closure).

The overall mortality rate for infants with gastroschisis is less than 5%. Prolonged postoperative ileus (> 2 weeks) is the rule, and total parenteral nutrition is necessary to support the infant's nutritional and fluid needs during that time. Primary repair of an associated intestinal atresia is not advisable during initial management of the gastroschisis. In many cases, the atretic ends are reduced and repaired 6 weeks later when the intra-abdominal inflammation has subsided.

Akinkuotu AC, et al: Giant omphaloceles: surgical management and perinatal outcomes. *J Surg Res.* 2015;198:388.

Gamba P, et al: Abdominal wall defects: prenatal diagnosis, newborn management, and long-term outcomes. *Semin Pediatr Surg.* 2014;23(5):283-290.

Lusk LA, et al: Multi-institutional practice patterns and outcomes in uncomplicated gastroschisis: a report from the University of California Fetal Consortium (UCfC). *J Pediatr Surg.* 2014;49:1782.

▼ VASCULAR ANOMALIES

Vascular anomalies are categorized into vascular tumors and vascular malformations. They can be congenital or acquired and can be distinguished by blood flow (high vs low) and histologic characteristics. Tumors exhibit endothelial hyperplasia, whereas vascular malformations exhibit normal endothelial turnover. Vascular anomalies are present in 2%-4% of children.

VASCULAR TUMORS (HEMANGIOMAS)

The most common vascular tumors in infants and children are benign infantile hemangiomas (Figure 45–35). Other less common vascular tumors include angiosarcomas,

▲ **Figure 45–35.** Newborn with a large infantile hemangioma involving the left chest wall. (Used with permission from Steven J. Fishman, MD.)

Kaposiform hemangioendotheliomas (which are locally aggressive), and pyogenic granulomas. Hemangiomas are much more common than vascular malformations. In the neonatal period, hemangiomas can be subclassified according to their growth phase. A rapid proliferating phase is usually seen during the first few years of life followed by an involuting phase that may last several years.

▶ Clinical Findings

Superficial dermal lesions (capillary hemangiomas, strawberry hemangiomas) are raised and profoundly erythematous, with an irregular texture. Deeper lesions (cavernous hemangiomas) are smooth and slightly raised, with a bluish hue or a faint telangiectatic pattern on the overlying skin. Mixed lesions are often noted. Twenty percent of patients have mixed lesions (eg, capillary-cavernous hemangiomas). Complications from hemangiomas consist of ulceration (during the proliferative phase), bleeding, scaring, infection, thrombocytopenia (Kasabach-Merritt syndrome), consumptive coagulopathy, and high-output heart failure.

▶ Treatment

Up to 50% of hemangiomas will spontaneously involute without treatment by 5 years of age, and the remainder will slowly involute by age 10-12 years. Topical β-blockers and intralesional steroid injections have both been used in the treatment of superficial hemangiomas. Medical therapy should be considered for infantile hemangiomas that are symptomatic (bleeding or ulcerated), compromise vital function, or may be associated with permanent disfigurement if left untreated. Oral propranolol has replaced oral corticosteroids as first-line treatment for infantile hemangiomas necessitating pharmacotherapy.

VASCULAR MALFORMATIONS

Vascular malformations, in contrast to vascular tumors, have normal endothelial cell turnover and tend to grow proportionally with the child. They are usually visible at birth but may take years or even decades to become clinically evident. Vascular malformations are categorized into low-flow and high-flow variants and further classified according to the type of vascular channel abnormality: capillary, lymphatic, venous, arterial, or combined malformations.

▶ Capillary Malformations

Capillary malformations present as sporadic, flat, pink singular cutaneous patches at birth. Examples include nevus flammeus (port wine stain), nevus flammeus neonatorum (angel's kiss), nevus flammeus nuchae (stork bite, salmon patch), angiokeratomas, and telangiectasias. They are prone to infection, and when such complications occur, they are treated aggressively with intravenous antibiotics. A compression garment should be used if anatomically feasible. Some lesions can be treated with excision or injection with sclerosing agents.

Lymphatic Malformations

LMs can present at birth as soft compressible benign masses with normal overlying skin but can also appear in older children or adults. Presentation may be quite variable and include cystic lesions in areas of major lymphatic channels, angiokeratoma, chylous leakage, osseous lesions of Gotham-Stout, lymphedema, and generalized lymphatic anomalies. Cystic hygroma and lymphangioma are misleading descriptions that should not be used to describe LMs. Diagnosis can be made prenatally via ultrasound or in the neonatal period with transillumination or CT imaging. Treatment depends on size, location, and presence of associated symptoms and complications and may include observation, drainage procedures, and surgical excision.

Venous Malformations

Venous malformations present along a wide spectrum of anatomic involvement, ranging from simple varicosities (soft, bluish, easily compressible) to complex lesions that involve different types of structures, including bone, muscle, and salivary glands, among others. Ninety percent are sporadic, and they are usually recognized at birth. Pain may result from thrombosis within a lesion. Cross-sectional imaging (CT or MRI) may be obtained for extensive lesions to characterize relation to adjacent strictures, particularly if surgical excision if being considered. Photocoagulation or Nd:YAG laser may be effective for superficial lesions. Resection is the definitive treatment since it can reduce bulk, improve contour and function, and control pain. Excision of larger lesions may be limited by anatomic boundaries, and multiple staged procedures may be required for complete excision. Blue rubber bleb nevus syndrome is a rare disorder consisting of multifocal venous malformations in the skin and gastrointestinal tract.

Arterial Malformations

Arterial and arteriovenous malformations are characterized by multiple small fistulas surrounded by abnormal tissue. They are most common in the head and neck region. Symptoms may include pain due to necrosis of adjacent skin and osseous structures. Selective embolization is used either as palliation or prior to surgery to limit hemorrhage. Excision, when possible, is the treatment of choice.

Combined Malformations

Combined vascular malformations and hypertrophy syndromes consist of Klippel-Trenaunay-Weber syndrome (combined capillary-lymphatic venous malformation associated with lower limb hypertrophy), Parkes-Weber syndrome (upper limb arteriovenous shunting), Maffucci syndrome (low-flow vascular malformations and multiple extremity enchondromas with hypoplastic long bones), and Sturge-Weber syndrome (upper facial port wine stain and vascular anomalies of the choroid plexus and leptomeninges).

Elluru RG, et al: Lymphatic malformations: diagnosis and management. *Semin Pediatr Surg.* 2014;23:178.

Wassef M, et al: Vascular anomalies classification: recommendations from the International Society for the Study of Vascular Anomalies. *Pediatrics.* 2015;136:e203.

TUMORS IN CHILDHOOD

NEUROBLASTOMA

Neuroblastoma is the most common extracranial solid tumor in the pediatric population, accounting for 6%-7% of all childhood cancers and 15% of the childhood cancer mortality burden. Neuroblastoma is exceeded in incidence only by leukemia and brain tumors, but the incidence is increasing. Neuroblastoma is a tumor of early childhood with approximately 60% of cases occurring within the first 2 years of life. Neuroblastoma is of neural crest origin and may originate anywhere along the distribution of the sympathetic chain. The most common sites for primary disease are the adrenal gland (40%) and the abdomen (25%), followed by the thorax (15%), neck (5%), pelvis, and occasionally the head. Neuroblastomas originate in the retroperitoneum in 75% of cases. They may reach massive size, causing obstruction, or violate tissue planes such that they envelop major blood vessels, their branches, and other structures (eg, ureters), which can render attempts at primary resection hazardous. The biologic behavior varies with the age of the patient, the site of primary origin, and the extent of the disease at diagnosis.

Clinical Findings

A. Symptoms and Signs

Symptoms are site specific. The most common symptoms are fever, malaise, and pain (from primary or metastatic disease). Nonspecific symptoms include growth retardation, weight loss, anorexia, nausea, and emesis. Children frequently appear ill at the time of diagnosis. Constipation and urinary retention are signs of pelvic disease. Orbital metastases commonly present with periorbital ecchymoses and proptosis ("raccoon eyes"). Spinal canal involvement may present with acute paralysis due to compression. Opsomyoclonus syndrome is an acute cerebellar encephalopathy characterized by ataxia, opsoclonus ("dancing eyes"), myoclonus, and dementia. It occurs in association with approximately

3% of all neuroblastomas and is usually associated with a good prognosis, although the neurologic abnormalities tend to persist after successful treatment of the primary tumor. Infants with stage IV-S disease (see later in text) may display cutaneous metastases ("blueberry muffin" lesions) or respiratory compromise secondary to massive hepatomegaly from tumor infiltration. Palpable lesions are often hard and fixed.

In infants, metastases confined to the liver or subcutaneous fat are frequent, but cortical bone metastases are unusual. Overall, 50% of children present with metastatic disease at diagnosis. In older children, metastases to lymph nodes and bone are found in over 70% of cases at diagnosis. Pain in areas of bony involvement and in joints with associated myalgia and fever mimics rheumatic fever. Eighty-five to 90% secrete high levels of the catecholamine metabolites (vanillylmandelic acid and homovanillic acid). Hypertension and diarrhea may occur as a result of catecholamine and vasoactive intestinal peptide secretion.

B. Imaging Studies and Staging

The goals of imaging are to define the extent of disease and determine the presence of metastases to distant sites (most commonly lymph nodes, bone, lung, and liver). CT imaging can identify the relationship between the tumor and surrounding structures to help establish resectability (Figure 45–36). Calcifications are present in up to 50% of abdominal neuroblastomas prior to chemotherapy. MRI is useful in assessing tumor within the spinal canal and spinal cord compression and has the added advantage of

▲ **Figure 45–36.** Five-month-old infant with neuroblastoma. Note the infiltrative nature of the tumor, which has grown to encase the major vessels of the celiac plexus. (Used with permission from Robert C. Shamberger, MD.)

Table 45–6. International Neuroblastoma Risk Group (INRG) staging system used for neuroblastoma.

Stage	Definition
L1	Localized tumor contained within one body compartment without IDRF; these include intraspinal tumors not meeting IDRF definition
L2	Locoregional tumor with one or more IDRFs; ipsilateral contiguous body compartments
M	Distant metastases excluding stage MS disease; contralateral contiguous body compartments
MS	L1 or L2 primary tumor in a patient < 18 months of age with metastases confined to skin, liver, and/or bone marrow and negative MIBG for bone/bone marrow

IDRF = image-defined risk factor; MIBG = metaiodobenzylguanidine.

being superior to CT in assessing vessel encasement, vessel patency, and spinal cord compression. Metaiodobenzylguanidine (MIBG) scintigraphy is very sensitive in detecting tumors that concentrate catecholamines and has been useful in the diagnosis of primary, residual, and metastatic disease in patients with neuroblastoma. For retroperitoneal tumors, an CT urogram may show displacement or compression of the adjacent kidney without distortion of the renal calices. Bone scans may be useful in detecting osseous metastases.

Neuroblastoma is staged using a pretreatment risk stratification based on image-defined risk factors (IDRFs) by anatomic region (Table 45–6). The International Neuroblastoma Risk Group (INRG) staging system uses imaging alone to categorize tumors as stage L1 (locoregional tumor without IDRFs), stage L2 (locoregional tumor with one or more IDRFs), stage M (distant metastatic disease with the exception of MS), and stage MS (INRG stage L1 or L2 tumor with metastatic disease confined to any combination of skin, liver, or bone marrow sites).

▶ Prognostic Factors

The INRG has established an international consensus stratification system for treatment guidelines based on seven clinical and biologic factors. These factors categorize patients into very low–, low–, intermediate–, and high-risk groups based on prognosis, therapeutic tumor response, and risk of tumor recurrence. Diagnosis before age 18 months is a favorable prognostic factor, whereas an adrenal primary lesion is a poor prognostic factor. Several molecular and cellular tumor characteristics are prognostically important, and *MYCN* amplification is associated with poor prognosis. Histologically, well-differentiated, stroma-rich tumors have a favorable prognosis.

Diagnosis & Treatment

Diagnosis is confirmed by tissue biopsy or bone marrow aspirate that demonstrates immature neuroblastic tissue. Biopsy specimens are sent for tumor markers, cytologic studies, and special stains. These data are then used for staging and prognostication, as well as for planning treatment.

The spectrum of treatment for neuroblastoma is complex and can include many combinations of surgery, chemotherapy, and radiation therapy depending on stage of disease. Stage L1 tumors typically undergo surgical resection prior to any other treatment. Stages L2 and M tumors may undergo induction chemotherapy prior to surgery. Induction chemotherapy may include a number of agents and combinations, including cyclophosphamide, vincristine, topotecan, cisplatin, doxorubicin, and etoposide. Supportive therapy is indicated for patients with stage MS tumors. For low-risk patients, surgery may be curative and chemotherapy may be avoided. Intermediate-risk patients typically receive both surgery and chemotherapy. Although surgical resection of all disease is the goal, it is not always possible. Radiotherapy may be used as an adjunct therapy for high-risk patients following incomplete surgical resection, for progressive tumors unresponsive to chemotherapy, and for life-threatening complications. The majority of deaths associated with neuroblastoma occur in patients with high-risk disease. Advancements in multimodal treatment have improved significantly over the past few decades; however, rates of 5-year survival remain modest at around 40%.

Davidoff AM: Neuroblastoma. *Semin Pediatr Surg.* 2012;21(1):2-14.
Nuchtern JG, et al: A prospective study of expectant observation as primary therapy for neuroblastoma in young infants: a Children's Oncology Group study. *Ann Surg.* 2012;256:573.

WILMS TUMOR (NEPHROBLASTOMA)

Wilms tumor (nephroblastoma) is the most common primary renal malignancy in childhood and the second most common abdominal tumor after neuroblastoma. Renal malignancies account for about 5% of all childhood cancers, and Wilms tumors accounts for 95% of renal malignancies. The tumor consists of heterogeneous embryonic tissues, including tubules and glomeruli, smooth and skeletal muscle fibers, spindle cells, cartilage, and bone. Two-thirds of children with nephroblastoma are diagnosed before 5 years of age, and the peak incidence is between 2 and 3 years of age.

The left kidney is affected slightly more often than the right, and in 5%-7% of cases, the tumors are bilateral. Wilms tumor is primarily a sporadic disease, although in 10% of cases, the disease occurs in association with a known syndrome, including multiple malformation syndromes, such as WAGR (*W*ilms tumor, *a*niridia, *g*enitourinary anomalies, and *m*ental retardation), Beckwith-Wiedemann, and Denys-Drash syndromes.

Clinical Findings

A. Symptoms and Signs

Most children present with an asymptomatic abdominal mass and are otherwise healthy. Other symptoms and signs may include abdominal pain (30%-40% of patients), hematuria, malaise, weakness, anorexia, weight loss, and fever. Hypertension is present in more than half of patients, and an abdominal mass can often be palpated on physical exam. Palpable in almost all cases, the mass is usually very large, firm, and smooth, and it does not ordinarily extend across the midline.

B. Diagnostic Studies

Imaging is required to determine the extent of the mass, involvement of the inferior vena cava, and presence of bilateral and metastatic disease and to confirm the presence of a contralateral kidney. Abdominal ultrasound is the initial study of choice, which can also assess for venous (inferior vena cava, renal vein) invasion. This information is further evaluated by a CT scan of the abdomen and chest, with the latter performed to rule out lung metastasis (Figure 45–37). MRI can also be used for additional imaging in certain cases. Laboratory testing includes a comprehensive metabolic panel to assess renal and liver function, complete blood count, coagulation studies, and urinalysis.

▲ **Figure 45–37.** Computed tomography scan of a 3-year-old child with a large Wilms' tumor involving the right kidney. Unlike neuroblastoma, Wilms' tumors tend to respect anatomic planes and typically do not cross the midline. (Used with permission from Robert C. Shamberger, MD.)

Differential Diagnosis

Abdominal masses may also be caused by hydronephrotic, multicystic, or duplicated kidneys and by neuroblastoma, teratoma, hepatoma, and rhabdomyosarcoma. Ultrasonography and CT scanning can usually distinguish nephroblastoma from these other tumors. Calcification occurs in 10% of cases of nephroblastoma and tends to be more crescent-shaped, discrete, and peripherally situated than the calcifications typical of neuroblastoma, which are finely stippled. Other renal cell tumors are rare. Wilms tumors usually do not cross the midline on cross-sectional imaging, which is particularly helpful to differentiate them from neuroblastoma when large tumors are present.

Treatment & Prognosis

Surgical excision is often accomplished without the need for preoperative treatment unless significant invasion into the inferior vena cava (and associated thrombus) is present. The aim of surgery is to completely resect the tumor (nephroureterectomy) without intraoperative spillage, and to accurately establish tumor stage. The major staging system used in the United States and Canada is the National Wilms Tumor Study (NWTS)/Children's Oncology Group (COG) system (Table 45–7). The staging system is based on surgical evaluation prior to the initiation of chemotherapy and without consideration for biologic, histologic, or genetic markers. Stage I is tumor confined to a kidney that has been completely excised; stage II is tumor extending beyond the kidney (perirenal tissues, renal vein or vena cava, biopsy, or local spill in the flank) and completely excised; stage III is residual, nonhematogenous tumor confined to the abdomen (lymph node metastases, preoperative or intraoperative diffuse peritoneal deposits, residual tumor at the surgical margins, or unresectable tumor); stage IV is hematogenous metastases (lung, liver, bone, and brain); and stage V is bilateral renal involvement.

Table 45–7. The National Wilms Tumor Study (NWTS)/Children's Oncology Group (COG) staging system (before chemotherapy).

Stage I: Tumor limited to kidney and completely excised. The surface of the renal capsule is intact and the tumor was not ruptured prior to removal. There is no residual tumor.
Stage II: Tumor extends through the perirenal capsule but is completely excised. There may be local spillage of tumor confined to the flank, or the tumor may have been biopsied. Extrarenal vessels may contain tumor thrombus or be infiltrated by tumor.
Stage III: Residual nonhematogenous tumor confined to the abdomen: lymph node involvement, diffuse peritoneal spillage, peritoneal implants, tumor beyond surgical margin either grossly or microscopically, or tumor not completely removed.
Stage IV: Hematogenous metastases to lung, liver, bone, brain, etc.
Stage V: Bilateral renal involvement at diagnosis; each kidney should be staged separately.

Chemotherapy is typically administered following surgery, with the choice of agents and duration based on tumor stage and histology. Radiation to the tumor bed is indicated if the tumor has extended beyond the capsule of the kidney to involve adjacent organs or lymph nodes or if intraoperative tumor spillage occurred. Very large tumors may be treated with neoadjuvant radiation and chemotherapy upfront prior to attempted surgical excision to reduce their size. A significant reduction in size usually occurs in 7-10 days, after which nephrectomy can be performed. Nephrectomy is accomplished through a long transverse or thoracoabdominal incision.

During operative exploration, palpation of the renal veins and inferior vena cava is critical to detect tumor thrombus. Treatment of bilateral disease is individualized with the goal of eradicating tumor while preserving the maximal amount of functional renal tissue. Suspicious lesions in the opposite kidney are biopsied. If the tumor is too large for safe resection, it is biopsied along with regional lymph nodes. Neoadjuvant chemotherapy with or without radiation therapy will usually result in a significant reduction in tumor size and allow subsequent resection. Metastatic foci in the lung or liver may be resected or treated with radiation therapy. Any residual tumor following radiation therapy, including multiple lesions, should be resected.

Overall 5-year survival for Wilms patients is greater than 85%, and survival strongly correlates with disease stage and tumor histology. The 4-year survival with respect to stage and histology is shown in Table 45–8. Tumor rupture with gross spillage portends a six-fold increase in risk of local recurrence.

Table 45–8. Event-free survival and late effects for children treated for Wilms tumor.

Survival	Risk of Late Effects*	
	Low	Moderate to High
Excellent (> 85%)	Stage I/II FHWT, LOH–	Stage I/II CCSK Stage III FHWT, LOH–
Good (75%-84%)		Stage IV FHWT, LOH– Stage II AHWT Stage III CCSK
Poor (< 75%)	Stage I/II FHWT, LOH+ Stage I AHWT Stage I-IV RCC	Stage III/IV FHWT, LOH+ Stage III/IV AHWT Stage V WT Stage IV CCSK Stage I-IV MRT Relapsed FHWT

AHWT = anaplastic histology Wilms tumor; CCSK = clear cell sarcoma of the kidney; FHWT = familial histology Wilms tumor; LOH = loss of heterozygosity; MRT = malignant rhabdoid tumor; WT = Wilms tumor.
[1]Late effects include disease relapse, development of a chronic health condition, secondary malignancies, congestive heart failure, and end-stage renal disease.

Fernandez CV, et al: Clinical outcome and biological predictors of relapse after nephrectomy only for very low-risk wilms tumor: a report from Children's Oncology Group AREN0532. *Ann Surg.* 2017;265(4):835-840.

Hamilton TE, et al: Wilms tumor: recent advances in clinical care and biology. *Semin Pediatr Surg.* 2012;21(1):15-20.

RHABDOMYOSARCOMA

Rhabdomyosarcoma (RMS) is the most common malignant soft tissue tumor in the pediatric population and is the third most common solid malignancy in children overall. RMS arises from embryonic mesenchyme, which has the potential to differentiate into muscle, fat, or fibrous tissue.

The age distribution typical of RMS diagnosis is bimodal, with the first peak occurring between 2 and 5 years of age and the second between 15 and 19 years. Two-thirds of all cases present before 6 years of age, and most cases appear to be sporadic. There is an increased incidence of RMS in patients with neurofibromatosis type I, Beckwith-Wiedemann syndrome, and Li-Fraumeni syndrome.

RMS is categorized into major four histologic subtypes: (1) embryonal RMS (intermediate prognosis, 59%); (2) botryoides and spindle cell (leiomyomatous) variants (favorable prognosis, 5%-9%); (3) alveolar (relatively poorer prognosis, 21%); and (4) sclerosing and spindle cell variants (relatively poor prognosis). Less common variants include undifferentiated RMS (8%), pleomorphic/anaplastic (1%), and RMS not otherwise specified (11%). Younger children are more likely to have embryonal histology, whereas older children more likely to have alveolar histology. Botryoid tumors present more commonly in young children from within visceral cavities (eg, vagina), whereas spindle cell types have a predilection for paratesticular sites. Alveolar tumors arise from the extremities, trunk, and perineum. Undifferentiated tumors arise from the extremity and head and neck sites.

▶ Clinical Findings

Clinical presentation varies with the site of origin of the primary tumor, the patient's age, and the presence or absence of metastatic disease. The most common presentation is an asymptomatic mass discovered by the patient or their parents. Symptoms are typically secondary to the effects of the tumor compressing adjacent structures. The most common site is the head and neck region (35%), and these are further subdivided into orbital (10%), parameningeal (15%), and non-parameningeal (10%) sites. Head and neck tumors are usually embryonal. Genitourinary RMSs (26%) are categorized into bladder and prostate types (10%) and nonbladder and nonprostate types, including paratesticular sites, perineum, vulva, vagina, and uterus (16%). The most common histologic type is embryonal, although botryoid tumors and spindle cell

Table 45–9. Intergroup Rhabdomyosarcoma Study Clinical Group staging system.[1]

Group I: Localized disease, completely removed
  a. Confined to muscle or organ of origin
  b. Infiltration outside organ or muscle of origin; regional nodes not involved.
Group II: Total gross resection with evidence of regional spread
  a. Grossly resected tumor with microscopic residual
  b. Regional disease with involved nodes, completely resected with no microscopic residual
  c. Regional disease with involved nodes, grossly resected, but with evidence of microscopic residual and/or histologic involvement of the most distal regional node in the dissection
Group III: Incomplete resection, or biopsy with presence of gross disease
Group IV: Distant metastases

[1]Adapted with permission from Neville HL et al: Preoperative staging, prognostic factors, and outcome for extremity rhabdomyosarcoma: a preliminary report from the Intergroup Rhabdomyosarcoma Study IV (1991–1997), *J Pediatr Surg* 2000 Feb;35(2):317-321.

tumors are seen more frequently here than in any other site. These tumors may be quite large when diagnosed, and there is a propensity for early lymphatic spread in genitourinary primary tumors. Bladder and prostate tumors frequently present with urinary retention or hematuria, whereas vaginal and uterine tumors present with vaginal bleeding or discharge and can present with a mass in the vaginal introitus. Extremity RMSs (1%) are more common in the lower extremities and are usually of the alveolar variety. There is a high incidence of regional nodal involvement and distal metastases.

Staging and clinical grouping of RMS are combined to determine a risk group for guiding treatment. Staging is determined by the TNM (tumor-node-metastasis) classification, whereas clinical grouping is established after tumor excision and determination of nodal status (Table 45–9). The clinical grouping system was developed by the Intergroup Rhabdomyosarcoma Study Group (IRSG) to stratify different extents of disease in order to compare treatment and outcome results. CT or MRI imaging is essential to evaluate the primary tumor and its relationship to surrounding structures for operative planning. Ultrasound, bone scan, bone marrow biopsy, and lumbar puncture are all commonly used diagnostic adjuncts.

▶ Treatment & Prognosis

Surgical management is site specific and includes complete wide excision of the primary tumor with negative margins (0.5 cm). Incomplete excision or tumor debulking is not beneficial, and severely mutilating or debilitating procedures should be avoided unless complete excision can be performed. Tumors not amenable to primary excision should be biopsied and then managed with neoadjuvant agents.

Secondary excision is then performed and is associated with better outcomes than partial or incomplete excision. Clinically suspicious lymph nodes are biopsied for staging purposes. Delayed primary excision should be performed following neoadjuvant treatment if posttreatment imaging suggests residual tumor.

All patients with RMS receive chemotherapy as part of their treatment regimen, and radiation treatment may also be used as an adjuvant therapy to improve local control. Five-year survival is 90% for stage I tumors; 77% for stage II, clinical group I or II tumors; 65% for stage II, clinical group III tumors; and 55% for stage III lesions (group I, II, or III). Stage IV tumors arising from favorable sites of origin are often curable, whereas those from unfavorable sites have a very poor prognosis. The prognosis for recurrent disease is poor.

Weiss AR, et al: Histologic and clinical characteristics can guide staging evaluations for children and adolescents with rhabdomyosarcoma: a report from the Children's Oncology Group Soft Tissue Sarcoma Committee. *J Clin Oncol.* 2013;31:3226.

TERATOMA

Teratomas are embryonal neoplasms derived from pluripotent cells containing tissue from at least two of three germ layers (ectoderm, endoderm, mesoderm). Approximately 80% are found in females, and approximately one in five teratomas are malignant. They are typically found in the midline, with the most common locations being sacrococcygeal (57%), gonadal (29%), mediastinal (7%), retroperitoneal (4%), cervical (3%), and intracranial (3%). Nongonadal teratomas typically present in infancy, whereas gonadal ones are often diagnosed during adolescence.

Serum α-fetoprotein (AFP) level may be elevated in tumors containing malignant endodermal sinus (yolk sac) elements, and elevated β-human chorionic gonadotropin (β-hCG) may be present with teratomas containing malignant choriocarcinoma tissue. Elevated AFP and β-hCG levels in histologically benign tumors indicate an increased risk of recurrence and malignant transformation, particularly with "immature" benign teratomas. Serial AFP levels can be followed after resection as a marker for recurrence.

▶ Sacrococcygeal Teratoma

Sacrococcygeal teratomas are rare tumors with an incidence of 1 in 40,000 live births. The tumors are far more common in females, although the rate of malignancy is higher in males. Sacrococcygeal teratomas typically present in the newborn period but can also be diagnosed by prenatal ultrasound (Figure 45–38). Complications during pregnancy may include high-output cardiac failure in the fetus due to arteriovenous shunting within the tumor. In severe cases, shunting may lead to hydrops fetalis and fetal

▲ **Figure 45–38.** Intraoperative positioning (prone) in preparation for a large sacrococcygeal teratoma resection in a newborn with a large sacrococcygeal teratoma. (Used with permission from Farokh Demehri, MD.)

demise. Sacrococcygeal teratomas are classified according to location (Altman classification): type I, predominantly external (47%); type II, external mass and presacral component (34%); type III, visible externally, but predominantly presacral (9%); and type IV, entirely presacral (10%).

Treatment involves complete excision of the tumor and coccyx. Type I and II lesions can be resected through a perineal approach, and type III and IV lesions are approached through a combined intra-abdominal and perineal resection. The majority of newborn sacrococcygeal teratomas are benign and do not require adjuvant therapy. Follow-up should include serial AFP measurement to ensure normalization (and to monitor recurrence). Greater than 90% of sacrococcygeal teratomas are benign, although the risk for malignancy increases sharply with older age at diagnosis. More than half of sacrococcygeal teratomas diagnosed after 2 months of age are found to be malignant. Malignant tumors are often treated with surgery and chemotherapy. The 5-year survival for malignant germ cell tumors arising from a sacrococcygeal teratoma is approximately 50%.

▶ Mediastinal Teratoma

Mediastinal teratomas account for approximately 20% of all pediatric mediastinal tumors. They usually arise in the anterior mediastinum, although intrapericardial and cardiac lesions have been reported. Symptoms include respiratory distress, chronic cough, chest pain, and wheezing. Males with β-hCG–producing tumors may display precocious puberty. Cardiac failure may develop from compression or pericardial effusion. Plain films of the chest may demonstrate a calcified anterior mediastinal mass. Ultrasonography delineates cystic and solid components. General anesthesia should not be induced until a CT evaluation of the airway has been obtained since the supine position coupled with a loss of airway tone from anesthetic agents may allow the anterior mass to obstruct the distal trachea, making rapid establishment of an airway nearly impossible. If significant airway compression is present, an awake needle biopsy under local anesthesia followed by radiation therapy or chemotherapy is indicated. Complete resection is definitive treatment.

Cervical Teratoma

Cervical teratomas are neonatal neck masses that may cause respiratory distress given their frequently large size. The rapid establishment of an endotracheal airway may be necessary, and tracheostomy can be hazardous due to distortion of landmarks. Calcifications may be evident on plain films, and a mixed cystic and solid appearance is characteristic on ultrasound. Cervical teratomas are most commonly benign, although malignant types have been reported, with the most common being a yolk sac tumor (endodermal sinus tumor). Treatment is complete excision, with malignant tumors also receiving radiation and chemotherapy in many cases.

Amies Oelschlager AM, et al: Teratomas and ovarian lesions in children. *Surg Clin North Am.* 2012;92(3):599-613.
Shalaby MS, et al: The long-term outcome of patients diagnosed with sacrococcygeal teratoma in childhood. A study of a national cohort. *Arch Dis Child.* 2014;99:1009.

LIVER NEOPLASMS

Tumors of the liver are uncommon in childhood and comprise only 1% of all childhood cancers. However, more than 70% of liver tumors in children are malignant. Most hepatic malignancies are of epithelial origin, whereas most benign lesions are vascular in nature.

1. Hepatoblastoma

Hepatoblastoma is the most common pediatric primary hepatic malignancy, accounting for nearly 50% of all liver masses in children and approximately two-thirds of all malignant liver tumors. The majority are seen in children under 4 years of age, and two-thirds are diagnosed prior to 2 years of age. Several congenital anomalies and syndromes have been associated with hepatoblastoma, including Beckwith-Wiedemann syndrome and familial adenomatous polyposis.

Clinical Findings

A. Symptoms and Signs

The most common clinical presentation is an abdominal mass in an otherwise healthy-appearing child. Less commonly, there may be obstructive gastrointestinal symptoms secondary to compression of the stomach or duodenum or acute pain secondary to hemorrhage into the tumor. Physical examination reveals a nontender, firm mass in the right upper quadrant or midline that moves with respiration. Advanced disease with larger tumors may be associated with weight loss, ascites, and failure to thrive. Approximately 10% of males present with isosexual precocity secondary to tumor secretion of β-hCG.

B. Laboratory Findings

Laboratory studies reveal nonspecifically elevated liver function tests and a mild anemia. Thrombocytosis is occasionally seen, and AFP levels are significantly elevated in up to 90% of cases. This tumor marker is also associated with other malignant tumors such as germ cell tumors. Serial serum AFP measurements are used to monitor patients for tumor recurrence following resection and adjuvant therapy. Levels of AFP should fall to normal after curative resection.

C. Imaging Studies

Abdominal ultrasound typically demonstrates a solid lesion involving a single lobe of the liver, with the right side being more common. Abdominal CT and MRI scans may be used to further characterize the mass for diagnosis and treatment planning. The typical CT appearance is a solitary hypoattenuating mass, and CT scans should be obtained using both arterial and portal venous phases to optimize diagnostic sensitivity. MRI may be useful in characterizing the relationship of the tumor to adjacent vascular structures. Chest CT should be obtained to rule out pulmonary metastasis.

Differential Diagnosis

It can be challenging to differentiate benign hepatic adenomas from hepatocellular carcinoma. Focal nodular hyperplasia is a well-circumscribed, nonencapsulated nodular liver mass that may appear similar to an adenoma or malignancy on ultrasonography and CT. A biopsy is often required to differentiate these diagnoses. Mesenchymal hamartomas are uncommon benign lesions presenting in the first year of life as asymptomatic large solitary masses (usually involving the right lobe). CT demonstrates a well-defined tumor margin and minimal to no contrast enhancement.

Treatment

The definitive diagnosis of hepatoblastoma requires tissue biopsy. Although this can be performed percutaneously, it is preferable to perform an open biopsy with assessment of resectability. If complete resection cannot be achieved, vascular access is obtained during the same anesthetic for neoadjuvant chemotherapy. Table 45–10 outlines the COG's postoperative staging system for pediatric hepatic

Table 45–10. Children's Oncology Group staging for hepatoblastoma.

Stage	Definition
I	Complete gross resection with negative margins
II	Complete gross resection with microscopic residual disease at resection margins
III	Biopsy or incomplete resection only (gross disease remains) or gross total resection with lymph node involvement or preoperative tumor rupture
IV	Distant metastatic disease

malignancies. However, hepatoblastoma staging is evolving toward the international consensus classification system using preoperative extent of disease (PRETEXT) groupings and annotations based on imaging studies, not surgical findings. Currently, the PRETEXT classification (developed by the European Liver Tumor Strategy Group) provides the best framework for planning these resections, which vary from segmentectomy to orthotopic liver transplantation.

Complete surgical resection is the major objective of therapy and represents the only chance for cure. Strategies to achieve this goal include: (1) initial primary resection; (2) delayed resection after neoadjuvant chemotherapy; or (3) total hepatectomy with liver transplantation. The timing of chemotherapy in relation to initial surgical resection is controversial among the major pediatric liver study groups. COG recommends initial primary resection at diagnosis for PRETEXT I or II tumors with preoperative radiographically clear venous margins. Lobectomy or extended lobectomy (trisegmentectomy) is typical, but segmental (nonanatomic) resection of small isolated tumors may be possible. Resections are usually performed through an extended subcostal or bilateral subcostal incision, although bulky lesions may require extension into the right hemithorax to gain adequate vascular control during dissection. Ascitic fluid is obtained for cytologic examination. If the lesion is deemed unresectable, the tumor is biopsied. If the lesion is deemed resectable following chemotherapy, lobectomy or trisegmentectomy is performed. Intraoperative cholangiography may be a useful intraoperative adjunct to characterize the anatomy of the biliary tree during resection.

Postoperative complications include hemorrhage, biliary fistula, subphrenic abscess, and injury to the biliary tree during dissection. Hepatic regeneration occurs quickly, and hepatic insufficiency is rare if more than 25% of the liver parenchyma remains following tumor resection. Hepatic transplantation is indicated for unresectable disease without evidence of metastatic disease.

The overall survival for all children with hepatoblastoma is approximately 50%, although it is quite variable across different stages. The best survival (90%) is seen in patients with stage I tumors who receive adjunctive chemotherapy after complete excision.

Aronson DC, et al: Malignant tumors of the liver in children. *Semin Pediatr Surg.* 2016;25(5):265-275.

Kremer N, et al: Management of hepatoblastoma: an update. *Curr Opin Pediatr.* 2014;26(3):362-369.

2. Hepatocellular Carcinoma

Hepatocellular carcinoma (HCC) is less common than hepatoblastoma and typically presents in older children. It is most commonly associated with preexisting conditions causing chronic liver inflammation, including hepatitis B–associated cirrhosis and other noninfectious causes of cirrhosis (tyrosinemia, biliary cirrhosis, α_1-antitrypsin deficiency, type 1 glycogen storage disease). Signs and symptoms on presentation can include a palpable abdominal mass or diffuse swelling, abdominal pain, weight loss, anorexia, and jaundice. The serum AFP level is elevated in 50%-60% of patients, although the absolute levels are typically lower than seen with hepatoblastoma. The approach to diagnostic staging and treatment are similar to those for hepatoblastoma. Unlike hepatoblastoma, only a minority of HCC cases are amenable to initial curative resection due to multicentricity, bilobar involvement, portal vein invasion, and lymphatic metastases. The fibrolamellar variant of HCC is associated with a relatively high rate of initial resectability and a better prognosis overall. The overall long-term survival for all cases is poor however (15%), and HCC is relatively chemoresistant.

3. Liver Hemangioma

Infantile hepatic hemangiomas are the most common benign liver tumors in childhood. They are typically diagnosed in the first 3-6 months of life. These tumors can be solitary (cavernous hemangioma), multiple (infantile hemangioendothelioma), or diffusely infiltrative involving the bulk of the liver. Infantile hemangioendotheliomas are commonly associated with hemangiomas in other parts of the body. Patients with a solitary hemangioma are frequently asymptomatic, but may present with a palpable mass or abdominal pain from intratumor hemorrhage or rupture. Infants with hemangioendothelioma typically present with massive hepatomegaly and high-output cardiac failure from arteriovenous shunting. The condition is associated with Kasabach-Merritt syndrome (thrombocytopenic coagulopathy due to platelet sequestration within the tumor). Diagnosis can often be established by ultrasound, although CT and MRI are typically used for surgical planning.

Treatment is not necessary in an asymptomatic child as most hemangiomas will spontaneously involute over time. Symptomatic, diffuse, or multifocal hemangiomas are treated with propranolol as a first-line agent. Patients without a response to propranolol may benefit from hepatic artery embolization. External-beam radiation has been shown to reduce the size of hemangiomas and improve symptoms. Considerations for surgery include ruptured hemangiomas with hemorrhage, masses with uncertain diagnoses, and symptomatic lesions refractory to conservative measures; however, the large size and diffuse involvement of many hemangiomas often preclude resection. Liver transplantation may also be considered in severe cases. Hemangioendotheliomas may undergo malignant degeneration into angiosarcoma.

Langham MR, et al: Current management of neonatal liver tumors. *Curr Pediatr Rev.* 2015;11:195.

Meyers RL, et al: Hepatoblastoma state of the art: pre-treatment extent of disease, surgical resection guidelines and the role of liver transplantation. *Curr Opin Pediatr.* 2014;26:29.

▼ PEDIATRIC TRAUMA

Accidental trauma is the leading cause of death among children age 18 years and younger. The initial trauma assessment is similar to adults, but a child's anatomy, physiology, and social behaviors are markedly different. Such differences must be accounted for during initial trauma survey. Patterns of injury vary by age, but head injury remains the primary cause of pediatric mortality in the United States.

Mortality due to trauma has decreased over the past few decades due to a combination of factors, including prevention and improved prehospital care. Pediatric trauma has a trimodal distribution of mortality. Early mortality is from severe injury to the central nervous system at the time of injury and can only be reduced by injury prevention. Mortality occurring within hours of injury is frequently due to evolving hemorrhagic injury to the brain (or associated edema and herniation), solid organ injury with associated hemorrhage, and intrathoracic trauma. Late mortality seen days to weeks after injury is due to sepsis and multiorgan failure.

NONACCIDENTAL TRAUMA

Maltreatment is a term that refers to either nonaccidental trauma (acts of commission) or neglect (acts of omission) that result in actual or potential harm to a child. *Nonaccidental trauma* (NAT) refers to any nonaccidental injury inflicted by a parent, guardian, or other caretaker. It is most readily recognized in the active form, characterized as "battered, bruised, beaten, broken, and burned." It is estimated that 1 million children annually in the United States suffer mistreatment that qualifies for reporting to the National Center on Child Abuse and Neglect. Up to 50% of children may experience recurrent NAT after the initial presentation, resulting in death in 5% and permanent disability in 35% when abuse is not initially recognized. More than 40% of deaths from child abuse occur before 12 months of age, and 70% of all deaths occur in children less than 3 years of age. Up to 10% of all traumatic injuries in children requiring inpatient hospitalization are associated with NAT.

Risk factors for caregiver-associated NAT include young age, single marital status, low income, lower education level, history of abuse while a child themselves, substance abuse, and psychiatric illness. Several patient characteristics have been associated with an increased risk for NAT, including congenital anomalies, developmental delay, and intellectual disability. The abuser is often someone who knows the child well, such as a parent, guardian, babysitter, or even a neighborhood child. Physical abuse cases of NAT are most commonly perpetrated by a patient's father, but neglect with failure to thrive from nutritional or emotional deprivation is usually attributable to the mother.

▷ Clinical Findings

Most cases of NAT occur in children less than 3 years of age. There may often be a discrepancy between the history furnished by caregivers and the magnitude of the injury. Several elements of the presentation should raise suspicion for NAT, including contradictory histories, delay in presentation following the apparent timing of injury, and a history of visits to different emergency departments for similar or recurrent injuries. History of a previous injury in the child or sibling and any injury in an infant less than 1 year of age should trigger high concern for NAT. Parents associated with NAT cases may be evasive or hostile. They may have open feelings of guilt or may be capable of complete concealment. The innocent spouse is usually more protective of the abusive caregiver than of the child.

The child may be withdrawn, apathetic, whimpering, and fearful and shows signs of neglect or failure to thrive. Multiple forms of injury may be noted at varying stages of healing. The child should be carefully examined from head to toe for signs of additional trauma. This includes evidence of bites, burns, and injuries to the skull and scalp (subgaleal hematoma from hair pulling). Retinal hemorrhage or detachment may follow blows to the head or shaking. Abdominal trauma may produce laceration to the liver, spleen, or pancreas or bowel perforation. Sexual abuse should be ruled out by determining whether the vaginal introitus or anus is bruised, lacerated, or enlarged and whether aspirated fluid contains sperm or prostatic acid phosphatase.

In cases where NAT is suspected, clinicians should have a low threshold to perform a formal radiographic skeletal survey. The bone most commonly fractured is the femur, followed by the humerus in the region of the diaphysis. Rib fractures and periosteal reactions in various stages of healing may be seen and are highly suggestive of NAT. Skull fractures are the most common fracture documented in infants less than 1 year old. Suture separation of the skull may indicate subdural hematoma. Neurologic injury may require evaluation with CT or MRI imaging.

▶ Treatment

Suspected victims of NAT should be admitted to hospital for treatment of injuries and protection until the case and home environment can be evaluated by child protective services (CPS). Consultation with several specialists may be required to complete a formal and comprehensive NAT assessment, including ophthalmology, neurology, neurosurgery, and orthopedic surgery. Bleeding disorders should be evaluated by a complete blood count and coagulation studies to ensure that multiple bruises are not due to coagulopathy. Serologic testing for syphilis or cultures (including pharyngeal) for gonorrhea should be performed for all cases of suspected sexual abuse. All injuries should be carefully documented radiographically and with photographs in the medical record.

It is required by law in every state for both the hospital and physicians caring for a child with suspected or documented NAT to report these cases to CPS. This process is usually facilitated through the hospital's social work department or dedicated team of child abuse specialists. The physician is responsible for overseeing the care of the child, but is also responsible to be a consultant to the parents; the physician should not assume the role of prosecutor or judge because many cases of suspected NAT are the result of accidental injury. A difficult task is to notify the parents regarding mandatory reporting without accusation or blame that NAT or neglect is suspected. The physician must tell the parents that the law requires reporting injuries that are unexplained or inadequately explained in view of the nature of the injury. A written referral should then be made to other professionals, such as child welfare personnel, hospital social workers, or psychiatrists. The referral should formally document the history of past injuries and the nature of current injuries, results of physical examination and laboratory and imaging studies, and a statement about why NAT is suspected. Child welfare personnel and social workers may have to assess the home environment and develop a plan to prevent future events. It may be necessary to place the child in a foster home (temporarily or permanently) while the investigation is proceeding and permanent plans for placement are established.

▶ Prognosis

Recognition of NAT is essential to prevent future morbidity and mortality. As many as 20% of NAT cases may go unrecognized during their initial medical evaluation. The overall mortality rate from NAT ranges from 2%-8%.

Approximately 40% of patients will have at least one documented recurrent NAT event, and over 10% have multiple events. Patients who experience NAT are at increased risk for physical and emotional behavioral problems, including substance abuse disorders, obesity, and psychiatric illness. Approximately 90% of children are eventually reunited with their parents and families.

Deans KJ, et al: Mortality increases with recurrent episodes of nonaccidental trauma in children. *J Trauma Acute Care Surg.* 2013;75:161.

Escobar MA, et al: Development of a systematic protocol to identify victims of non-accidental trauma. *Pediatr Surg Int.* 2016;32:377.

Finkelhor D, et al: Violence, crime, and abuse exposure in a national sample of children and youth: an update. *JAMA Pediatr.* 2013;167:614.

MULTIPLE CHOICE QUESTIONS

1. What would be the most common electrolyte and acid-base abnormality seen in a 5-week-old infant with ongoing emesis from pyloric stenosis?

   A. Hyperchloremic metabolic acidosis
   B. Hypernatremic metabolic acidosis
   C. Hyponatremic metabolic acidosis
   D. Hypochloremic metabolic alkalosis
   E. Hyponatremic metabolic alkalosis

2. What is the most appropriate diagnostic test for an otherwise healthy 2-month-old infant with new-onset bilious emesis?

   A. Ultrasound
   B. Upper gastrointestinal series
   C. Computed tomography (CT) scan of abdomen and pelvis
   D. Contrast enema
   E. Esophagram

3. Which of the following is the most appropriate management strategy for an otherwise healthy 2-year-old boy seen in the surgery clinic with an asymptomatic umbilical hernia?

   A. Repair the hernia electively within the next few weeks due to risk of incarceration.
   B. Inform the parents that repair is not indicated unless the hernia becomes symptomatic or enlarges over time.
   C. CT scan should be attained to determine the size of the hernia defect.
   D. Reassure the parents that repair is not needed until 4-5 years of age to allow for spontaneous resolution.
   E. Admit the child to the hospital for urgent repair.

4. The most common types of anorectal malformation (ARM) seen in boys and girls are:

    A. Rectoperineal fistula and rectovestibular fistula, respectively
    B. Rectovesical fistula and rectovestibular fistula, respectively
    C. Rectoperineal fistula and cloacal malformation, respectively
    D. Rectourethral fistula and rectovestibular fistula, respectively
    E. ARM without a fistula (blind-ending rectum) and rectourethral fistula and cloacal malformation, respectively

5. Which of the following is the most common extracranial solid tumor in the pediatric population?

    A. Wilms tumor (nephroblastoma)
    B. Hepatoblastoma
    C. Neuroblastoma
    D. Sacrococcygeal teratoma
    E. Rhabdomyosarcoma

Surgical Weight Management

James N. Luo, MD

Ali Tavakkoli, MD

THE OBESITY EPIDEMIC AND ETIOLOGY

Obesity has been a part of human society from time immemorial. One of the earliest documented references to human obesity can be seen in a limestone female figurine from the late Paleolithic period (c. 25,000 BC) found in Willendorf, Australia, in 1908, commonly referred to as the Venus of Willendorf. She is believed to be the matriarch of fertility. As human evolution progressed from thrift to abundance, the apparent selection advantage of excess body fat (eg, insulation, protection, efficient energy storage) was replaced by the health burdens of obesity. This shift has accelerated dramatically over the past half-century, and today, obesity and its attendant metabolic consequences have become a major health crisis worldwide.

Broadly defined, obesity is the excess accumulation of body fat and is commonly accepted as a body mass index (BMI; weight/height^2 [kg/m^2]) of > 30. BMI was adopted by the medical community after its earlier adoption by the insurance industry for actuarial use. Although its use has many imperfections (eg, a short muscular man may be classified as overweight or obese but not be burdened by the health risks of excess body fat), its relative simplicity renders it an attractive common measurement of body weight. It is estimated that from 1970 to 2005, the prevalence of obesity in the United States more than doubled, and it has continued to rise. The Centers for Disease Control and Prevention (CDC) estimates that, as of 2016, 39.8% of American adults and 18.5% of American youth (age 2-19 years) are obese. American adults between the age of 40 and 59 years have the highest overall obesity rate at 42.8%, whereas American adolescents (age 12-19 years) have the highest youth obesity rate at 20.6%. The burden of obesity is also not distributed equally, with certain ethnic groups bearing the brunt of it. Hispanic and non-Hispanic black Americans have the highest obesity rates at 47% and 46.8%, respectively. Non-Hispanic whites have an obesity rate of 37.9%, and non-Hispanic Asians have

the lowest obesity rate at 12.7%. Furthermore, the obesity rate also differs by gender, with women having higher obesity rates across all ethnic groups. Geographically, every state and territory of the United States had an obesity rate of 20% or greater in 2017, with states in the southeast bearing the heaviest burden. Although any BMI > 30 is considered obese, this is often further stratified into classes of severity. Table 46–1 summarizes the breakdown of obesity classification by BMI.

Although these classifications allowed us to more precisely study the health burdens of obesity, they do not take into account the regional distribution of body fat, which has been shown to be more important than the mere volume of body fat. When compared with peripheral fat, intra-abdominal and visceral obesity are both associated with greater risks of insulin resistance, hypertension, dyslipidemia, and cardiovascular diseases. This difference in the metabolic impact of obesity is likely to account for the elevated risks of metabolic disease development at lower BMIs in certain races, such as Asians, and is a frontier of active investigation.

The continued rise in obesity is having a direct and significant impact on the quantity and quality of human life. In aggregate, having a BMI > 35 is associated with a 94% increase in all-cause mortality. Individuals with a BMI > 40 can experience, on average, an 8-year reduction in life expectancy. This relationship between obesity and many of its preventable comorbidities also bears a heavy financial burden. The estimated obesity-related healthcare spending in the United States in 2008 was $147 billion, and the average individual medical spending of a person with obesity was nearly $1500 more than that of a normal-weight counterpart.

This dramatic impact can be attributed to the elevated risks that obesity bestows on the development of many chronic and morbid conditions such as hypertension, dyslipidemia, cardiovascular diseases, cerebrovascular diseases, and even cancer. The recognition that central obesity is associated with the development of these disorders has led to the concept of a "metabolic syndrome." There are differing

Table 46–1. Obesity classification.

BMI	Obesity Class
30.0-34.9	Class I
35.0-39.9	Class II
≥ 40.0	Class III (morbid obesity)

definitions for metabolic syndrome; nonetheless, broadly defined, it is the presence of abdominal or central obesity, insulin resistance, elevated lipids, and hypertension. The American Heart Association notes that metabolic syndrome entails a greater risk for future cardiovascular disease than any of its constituent disorders alone.

The exact cause behind the quick and dramatic rise of obesity remains somewhat uncertain and is likely to be multifactorial, involving genetic, environmental, and epigenetic elements. The rise in the abundance of relatively cheap and calorie-rich foods disrupted the balance between energy intake and expenditure. This imbalance led to the formation and accumulation of excess body fat. Further, the gradual decline in our daily physical activity, coupled with the adoption of a more sedentary lifestyle, also contributed to our present epidemic. Recurring evidence points to the strong and inverse relationship between obesity and physical activity, where even small increases in moderately vigorous physical activity can significantly diminish one's risk for obesity and its attendant metabolic consequences.

In addition to caloric excess and physical inactivity, a growing body of literature has demonstrated the previously underappreciated role that genetics plays in the development of obesity and metabolic disorders. It is postulated that many of these obesogenic genetic variations were selected and preserved by an environment that, for most of its harsh and food-scarce history, has favored the "thrift phenotype." These variants encumber patients with a genetic predisposition which then interacts with an obesity-promoting environment resulting in the disease process of obesity. This growing recognition of the complexity of obesity is beginning to shed light on the difficulties patients experience in losing weight and combating this disease.

Lavie C, et al: Healthy weight and obesity prevention: JACC Health Promotion Series. *J Am Coll Cardiol.* 2018;72(13):1506-1531.

NONSURGICAL TREATMENT OPTIONS FOR OBESITY: BEHAVIORAL AND MEDICAL

Our present armamentarium for combating obesity and its associated metabolic disorders can be broadly divided into three categories: behavioral, medical, and surgical. Each has its own advantages, challenges, and efficacies.

Behavioral Modifications

Behavioral modification for the treatment of obesity mainly consists of three approaches: dietary modification, physical exercise, and psychological therapy. Dietary modification is the mainstay of behavioral modification. The overarching goal of dietary modification is caloric reduction. There are a multitude of diet programs with differing macronutrient compositions (eg, low carbohydrate, low fat). There are also many commercially available diet programs. There is no evidence to demonstrate the superiority of one diet regimen over another. Specifically, it has been shown that it is the total calorie restriction of a diet regimen, rather than the relative macronutrient composition, that determines weight loss. Although this is true for weight loss, the impact of macronutrient composition on the reduction of specific metabolic disorders remains less clear, with some studies suggesting that among individuals with high cardiovascular risk, a Mediterranean diet supplemented with nuts or olive oil helps reduce cardiovascular mortality.

What has become evident is that weight loss with dieting alone is modest at best and difficult to sustain. With intense support and close follow-up, diet alone can achieve an average absolute weight loss of approximately 4-5 kg, and these losses are often not sustained once the intense support and follow-up are withdrawn. Dietary modification likely has the greatest impact on maintaining a healthy weight when it is employed as part of a multimodal regimen.

Physical exercise is another essential component of behavioral modification, with the overarching goal of increasing caloric expenditure. The typical recommendation sets a daily goal of > 10,000 steps and > 150 minutes of aerobic physical exercise per week. The weight loss outcome for exercise alone is similarly poor. Nonetheless, when employed in conjunction with dietary modification, the two potentiate each other to improve weight loss. Furthermore, regular physical exercise has been shown to improve cardiovascular health, independent of its effect on weight loss. Available evidence suggests that high-intensity exercise may be more effective in achieving weight loss; however, many obese patients are unable to participate in these higher intensity exercises due to existing cardiovascular and/or musculoskeletal comorbidities.

Psychological treatment of obesity is the least familiar component of behavioral modification. There exists a wide variety of psychosocial interventions used to combat obesity, ranging from individual approaches to group approaches. Among them, cognitive-behavioral therapy (CBT) is the most common. Similar to diet and exercise, increased frequency of psychosocial interventions is associated with improved weight loss. However, when used alone, CBT or group therapy only yields modest results.

Pharmacologic Intervention

The journey to identify the perfect weight loss medication dates back to at least the 19th century. There is currently no effective medical monotherapy for treating obesity. Rather, similar to behavioral modification, pharmacologic intervention can be used as an adjunct to a multimodal weight loss regimen. There are several U.S. Food and Drug Administration (FDA)-approved weight loss medications available today, with new agents under development. Because most of these medications have systemic effects that are either a part of or separate from their weight loss mechanism, prescribing them requires detailed understanding of their mechanism, efficacy, and potential side effects. It also requires expertise in the patient's overall weight loss management in order to judiciously and effectively use these agents to maximum effect.

Pharmacotherapy can be prescribed for patients with a BMI > 30 or BMI > 27 with related comorbidities. They are also increasingly being used for patients who experience inadequate initial weight loss or weight regain after bariatric surgery. Typically, one agent is tried for up to 3 months, and if no significant weight loss is seen, it is discontinued, and an alternative agent is considered. When used appropriately, pharmacologic adjuncts can help to increase compliance with dietary modification by suppressing appetite and/or increasing satiety.

Phentermine was introduced in 1959 and, together with fenfluramine (an amphetamine derivative), formed the combination agent "fen-phen." Fen-phen was quickly withdrawn from the market due to heart valve disease caused by the fenfluramine. Phentermine itself is a sympathomimetic amine that stimulates the release of norepinephrine and dopamine in order to increase basal metabolic rate and reduce appetite. It is approved for short-term (up to 3 months) use, with an average total-body weight loss (TBWL) of 5%-6%, most of which is seen in the first several weeks.

Orlistat (Xenical or Alli) was approved by the FDA in 1999. It inhibits pancreatic and gastric lipase, thereby causing fat malabsorption. It results in an average TBWL of 5%-10%. However, its use has been limited by its gastrointestinal intolerability (eg, diarrhea, fecal incontinence, flatulence) in many patients.

Phentermine/topiramate (Qsymia) is a newer combination drug that takes advantage of the mechanism of phentermine. Topiramate is a central nervous system agent that acts as a γ-aminobutyric acid (GABA) receptor agonist. Initially conceived as an antiepileptic agent, it is commonly used for migraines. Phentermine/topiramate was approved by the FDA in 2012, with an average TBWL of 7%-10%. Common side effects include headache, paresthesia, and dry mouth.

Bupropion sustained release (SR)/naltrexone SR (Contrave) is another combination medication that was approved by the FDA for weight loss in 2014, although each of the individual ingredients has been on the market for many years. Bupropion has been used widely for depression, and naltrexone has been used for opiate and alcohol withdrawal. Together, these two agents work synergistically to stimulate the hypothalamic release of α-melanocyte–stimulating hormone, which

functions as a potent anorectic neuropeptide. Average weight loss is modest (5%-6% of TBWL), and common side effects include headache, insomnia, constipation, and tremors.

Lorcaserin (Belviq) is another central nervous system modulator that was approved by the FDA for weight loss in 2012. It functions as a serotonin receptor (5-HT2C) agonist, which suppresses appetite via activation of the proopiomelanocortin (POMC) pathway, a hypothalamic anorexigenic pathway. Average TBWL is 5%-7%. Common side effects include headache, hallucination, and possible cardiovascular risks. The CAMELLIA-TIMI 61 (Cardiovascular and Metabolic Effects of Lorcaserin in Overweight and Obese Patients–Thrombolysis in Myocardial Infarction 61) trial published in *The New England Journal of Medicine* in 2018 randomized 12,000 overweight or obese patients with atherosclerotic cardiovascular diseases or risk factors to either lorcaserin (10 mg twice daily) or placebo. At 1 year, the patients who received lorcaserin experienced sustained weight loss of > 5% without a higher rate of major cardiovascular events when compared with the placebo group.

Whereas the earlier weight loss agents primarily targeted monoamine signaling cascades, more recent research has brought to light the diverse functions of gut peptides in regulating hunger and satiety. Glucagon-like peptide 1 (GLP-1) is a peptide secreted by the ileal L cells in response to food. It induces satiety, suppress appetite, and increases peripheral insulin sensitivity. **Liraglutide** (Saxenda) is a GLP-1 agonist that was initially approved by the FDA for type 2 diabetes. Its use for weight loss was approved in 2014. TBWL averages 7%-9%, with common side effects including diarrhea, nausea, and, rarely, pancreatitis.

Bohula EA, et al: Cardiovascular safety of lorcaserin in overweight or obese patients. *N Engl J Med.* 2018;379:1107-1117.

SURGICAL OPTIONS

▶ Overview

The modern practice of bariatric surgery is the product of more than a half-century of surgical evolution and innovation. Unlike the often lackluster efficacies of behavioral and pharmacologic interventions, surgical interventions have been repeatedly shown to deliver the most significant and sustained weight loss. Started as serendipitous observations and crude animal experiments, bariatric surgery has become a highly specialized subspecialty of general surgery, with specific surgical and medical expertise that must be mastered in order to deliver the most effective patient care.

Bariatric surgeries were traditionally divided into two categories: restrictive and malabsorptive, with some procedures employing both principals. Purely restrictive procedures, such as the gastric band, are intended to create a surgical bottleneck effect in the proximal gastrointestinal tract, thereby decreasing the volume of food that can be consumed at any one time. The theory is simple: by limiting the number of calories that can be physically consumed, weight loss should be the result of net caloric decrease. Malabsorptive procedures such as the jejunoileal bypass typically involved a rearrangement of the alimentary tract in order to decrease the absorptive surface area with which nutrients come into contract. Weight loss is achieved by a decrease in the number of calories extracted from food.

It has become increasingly clear that this simplified view of bariatric surgery is incorrect and that the procedures work through complex neurohormonal pathways that lead to durable weight loss and changes in appetite. The precise mechanism of weight loss in bariatric surgery continues to be an area of significant scientific interest and research, exploring novel hypotheses, such as surgery-induced changes in the microbiome and portal vein milieu, to name a few.

▶ Specific Operations

A. Jejunoileal Bypass

The first bariatric operation to be widely used was the jejunoileal bypass. Variations of this operation entered the literature in the early 1960s and gained popularity over the subsequent decade. In the classic version of this malabsorptive procedure, as described by J. Howeard Payne and colleagues, the jejunum is divided 14 inches (~35.5 cm) distal to the ligament of Treitz, and an end-to-side jejunoileostomy is constructed approximately 4 inches (~10 cm) proximal to the ileocecal valve (other variations used an end-to-end anastomosis) (Figure 46–1). This rearrangement bypasses 90%-95% of the small intestine. The jejunoileal bypass was extremely successful in achieving surgical weight loss. However, as postoperative data accumulated, it became clear that this procedure entailed a prohibitive degree of malnutrition, leading to severe side effects such as intractable diarrhea, macro- and micronutrient deficiencies, dehydration, and even liver and neurologic pathologies. This unacceptable morbidity profile led to the abandonment of this procedure in the 1970s.

B. Vertical Banded Gastroplasty

The early disappointment with the jejunoileal bypass turned efforts toward more restrictive approaches. Early gastric portioning was done via a double-row stapling technique across the proximal stomach, creating a narrow passageway for food to pass into the gastric body. Through a series of subsequent failures and improvements, the vertical banded gastroplasty (VBG) was introduced. In the VBG, four parallel rows of staples are laid vertically across the upper stomach, creating a narrow passageway for food to enter into the stomach body, similar to the gastric portioning (Figure 46–2). However,

▲ **Figure 46–1.** Jejunoileal bypass. The jejunum is divided distal to the ligament of Treitz, and an end-to-side jejunoileostomy is constructed.

the configuration of the portioning was altered to allow for the placement of a prosthetic band to further constrict food passage. The VBG gained much prominence in the 1980s. However, it soon became apparent that not only did it fail to achieve significant weight loss or maintain weight loss, it was also plagued by complications such as severe reflux, persistent nausea, stricture formation, and band erosion, leading to its abandonment.

C. Laparoscopic Adjustable Gastric Banding

Although the VBG did not live up to its initial promise, the efforts to develop a minimally invasive purely restrictive bariatric procedure continued. In the laparoscopic adjustable gastric banding (LAGB) procedure, an adjustable prosthetic band is placed around the upper stomach, creating an approximately 30-mL proximal gastric pouch (Figure 46–3). The degree of constriction is regulated with a saline-filled balloon within the band, the volume of which is adjusted via a subcutaneously placed port. The procedure was initially

▲ **Figure 46–3.** Laparoscopic adjustable gastric banding. An adjustable prosthetic band is placed around the supper stomach, creating an approximately 30-mL pouch. The degree of constriction is regulated with a saline-filled balloon within the band, and the volume of the balloon is adjusted via a subcutaneous port.

▲ **Figure 46–2.** Vertical banded gastroplasty. Staples are laid vertically across the upper stomach, creating a narrow passageway for enteric content. A prosthetic band is then placed to further constrict food passage.

developed as an open operation in Europe before being refined into a laparoscopic approach. LAGB gained considerable popularity in the early 2000s, in part from its lack of gastrointestinal rearrangement and the attendant complications. There are currently two FDA-approved LAGB devices in the United States. The LAP-BAND (ReShape Lifesciences) was approved in 2001 and has remained the most popular brand on the US market. The REALIZE Adjustable Gastric Band (Ethicon Endo-Surgery) was later approved in 2007.

Unlike other surgical bariatric procedures, the LAGB requires no complex gastrointestinal anatomic manipulation. It was marketed as a less invasive and safer alternative to the Roux-en-Y gastric bypass. Data from the Longitudinal Assessment of Bariatric Surgery (LABS) Consortium showed relatively low rates of 30-day postoperative adverse outcomes. In 1198 patients who underwent the LAGB, there were zero 30-day postoperative deaths, three venous thromboembolic events (0.3%), nine patients who required postoperative abdominal operations (0.8%), and one patient who required postoperative endoscopy (0.1%). These short-term encouragements notwithstanding, long-term weight loss with the LAGB proved disappointing. In a study of 301 patients undergoing LAGB, Carandina and colleagues reported excessive weight loss rates at 5, 10, and 15 years of 41.4%, 38.7%, and 35.1%, respectively. Furthermore, the long-term tolerance of

the LAGB was problematic. Vinzens and colleagues reported data on 343 patients with a mean follow-up of 13 years following LAGB, of whom 63% of patients had undergone subsequent revisional bariatric surgery. Reasons for revision included poor band tolerance, inadequate weight loss, and excessive weight regain. Overall, 41% of these patients reported poor band tolerances, 18.4% had band slippage, and 14.3% had gastric pouch dilation. Because of these and similar results, the popularity of the LAGB has diminished significantly in recent years, and today, it remains a viable albeit uncommon weight loss procedure, accounting for less than 5% of the over 200,000 weight loss procedures performed in the United States.

D. Roux-en-Y Gastric Bypass

Dr. Edward Mason is often credited as the "father of bariatric surgery," an accolade that he gained in large part from his early work in developing the gastric bypass. Since its introduction in the 1970s, it has undergone several iterations and revisions to arrive at its present status as the gold standard weight loss operation. The procedure starts with a small 20- to 30-mL pouch gastroplasty. Initially, gastrointestinal continuity was established using a loop of jejunum to create a gastrojejunostomy. However, the high incidence of postoperative bile reflux led to the adoption of a Roux-en-Y configuration. Today, the small gastric pouch is connected to a Roux limb of approximately 100-150 cm to form the alimentary limb. Digestive enzymes are reintroduced via a jejunojejunostomy. Although the Roux-en-Y gastric bypass (RYGB) was initially introduced as an open operation, today, it is most often performed laparoscopically. Several terms are important in understanding the anatomic basis of this operation (Figure 46–4):

- **Alimentary limb:** The Roux limb extending from the gastrojejunostomy to the jejunojejunostomy of the biliopancreatic limb, typically approximately 100-150 cm in length. Food transit occurs through this segment without interacting with the pancreaticobiliary enzymes necessary for proper digestion and absorption. The length of the

▲ **Figure 46–4.** Roux-en-Y gastric bypass. A small proximal gastric pouch is created and connected to the Roux limb forming the alimentary limb (A). The digestive enzymes transit through the biliopancreatic limb (BP) before mixing with the enteric content in the common channel (CC).

Roux limb has been the topic of significant clinical interest. Because it is a malabsorptive segment, many hypothesized that increasing its length would augment weight loss. However, clinical evidence supporting this hypothesis remains scant. Several studies comparing the long Roux limb (150 cm) have failed to demonstrate its weight loss superiority. In a retrospective analysis of 730 patients undergoing RYGB where 360 of them had a Roux limb of 150 cm, Dogan and colleagues reported no significant difference in post-RYGB weight loss between patients receiving a long Roux limb and those receiving the standard 100-cm Roux limb. Other studies suggest that a long Roux limb might offer more effective weight loss in the superobese (BMI > 50). For example, Ciovica and colleagues showed that, at 12 months, a 150-cm roux limb is associated a total weight loss of 68.5 kg, versus 55.3 kg for a 100-cm roux limb. Most studies also show that there is no significant difference in long-term vitamin and mineral absorption between long and short Roux limbs.

- **Biliopancreatic limb:** The limb of jejunum from the ligament of Treitz to the jejunojejunostomy, typically 30-60 cm in length. Through this limb, pancreaticobiliary secretion is introduced to the digesting food. Emerging research investigating the effect of the length of the biliopancreatic limb on weight loss suggests that a long biliopancreatic limb may induce greater weight loss. For example, in the ELEGANCE RE-DO trial, 146 patients who failed the gastric band were randomized to alimentary/biliopancreatic limbs of either 150 cm/75 cm or 75 cm/150 cm. At 48 months, the authors reported that those who had alimentary/biliopancreatic limbs of 75/150 cm (long biliopancreatic limb) experienced significantly more total weight loss. Further studies are needed to evaluate ideal biliopancreatic limb length for primary and revisional surgeries.

- **Common channel:** The remaining small intestine beginning from the biliopancreatic jejunojejunostomy.

E. Biliopancreatic Diversion with Duodenal Switch

Compared to RYGB, biliopancreatic diversion with duodenal switch (BPD/DS) involves a higher degree of malabsorption. It began as a renewed effort to further the malabsorptive approaches to bariatric surgery following the failure of the jejunoileal bypass. The initial BPD/DS involved an antrectomy followed by a gastrojejunostomy and a Roux-en-Y-jejunoileostomy. Because of its significantly shorter common channel, the malabsorptive capacity of the BPD/DS is much greater than the RYGB. Through several iterations, the current BPD/DS involves a vertical sleeve gastrectomy and transection of the duodenum distal to the pylorus, followed by a duodenojejunostomy incorporating the pylorus and a distal Roux-en-Y jejunoileostomy (Figure 46–5). In this procedure, the alimentary limb is typically 100-150 cm, similar to

(SADI) is an attempt to harness the weight loss and metabolic benefits of the BPD/DS while simplifying the surgical procedure. It begins with a sleeve gastrectomy and pylorus-preserving division of the duodenum, but instead of the more complex reconstruction, a single-anastomosis, end-to-side duodenoileostomy is performed (Figure 46–6). This leaves a common channel of typically approximately 250 cm, much longer than the typical length for a BPD/DS. Even longer common channels have been described in the effort to further decrease the magnitude of malnutrition. Early results are promising, but conclusive long-term studies remain absent. At present, it is being performed as an investigational

▲ **Figure 46–5.** Biliopancreatic diversion with duodenal switch. The procedure involves a vertical sleeve gastrectomy and transection of the duodenum distal to the pylorus. Gastrointestinal continuity is achieved by the creation of a gastrojejunostomy and a distal Roux-en-Y jejunoileostomy.

the RYGB. However, unlike the RYGB, the common channel typically does not exceed 100 cm in length. This creates a significantly more malabsorptive anatomy. The need for duodenal rearrangement makes this a more technically demanding operation.

Although the BPD/DS is effective, its technical complicity and long-term malnutrition have significantly limited its use. Consequently, a simpler alternative has been gaining ground in recent years. The single-anastomosis duodenoileal bypass

▲ **Figure 46–6.** Single-anastomosis duodenoileal bypass. The procedure involves a sleeve gastrectomy and pylorus-preserving division of the duodenum. This is followed by a single end-to-side duodenoileostomy.

procedure and as a revisional procedure for patients who have previously undergone sleeve gastrectomies.

F. Laparoscopic Sleeve Gastrectomy

Originally begun as the first stage of the BPD/DS operation, laparoscopic sleeve gastrectomy (LSG) became a standalone operation in the early 2000s and has since gained rapid popularity. The earliest sleeve gastrectomies were performed as the first stage of a staged BPD/DS in the super morbidly obese patients. Given the high perioperative risks in these patients, it was felt that the safest approach would be to perform the sleeve gastrectomy first and return subsequently to complete the BPD/DS. As early data emerged, it became apparent that the sleeve gastrectomy, in and of itself, produced significant weight loss, thus transforming it into an independent operation. It is technically much simpler than either the RYGB or the BPD/DS. In this procedure, a lateral gastrectomy is performed, leaving a lesser curve–based narrow tube ("sleeve") of stomach (Figure 46–7). Because it does not involve any intestinal rearrangement, the LSG is technically easier and is likely to be spared of the long-term malabsorptive complications of intestinal bypasses. Although on its surface, the LSG appears to be a restrictive procedure, the surgery works through multiple mechanisms, including neurohormonal ones, to exert its weight loss and other metabolic benefits.

▲ **Figure 46–7.** Laparoscopic sleeve gastrectomy. The procedure began as the first step of the biliopancreatic diversion with duodenal switch. A lateral gastrectomy is performed to create a lesser curve–based narrow tube ("sleeve").

The precise mechanism of these results remains an area of active investigation. Regardless of the mechanism, the LSG has been shown to deliver sustained long-term weight loss and improvement in diabetes as well as other metabolic disorder. Due to its efficacy coupled with its relative technical simplicity, the LSG is rapidly becoming the predominant bariatric procedure. At the time of this writing, the LSG is the most commonly performed bariatric operation in the United States.

► Efficacy

Unlike behavioral modification or pharmacotherapy, the efficacy of surgery in achieving sustained long-term weight loss has been well established. The efficacy of bariatric surgery is typically measured as the percentage of excess weight loss (EWL), although people are increasingly moving away from this metric and using TBWL or changes in BMI (as a percentage or absolute number) as a metric. For most patients undergoing bariatric surgery, a period of rapid weight loss is followed by some weight regain, after which, they will enter their maintenance weight. Pathologic weight regain is defined as > 20% of the maximal weight loss, and this can be seen in 15%-20% of patients. In patients undergoing the RYGB, the initial expected weight loss can be as high as 60%-80% EWL, with success defined as a minimal weight loss of > 50% EWL. As described earlier, BPD/DS produces the most dramatic surgical weight loss. Topart and Ritz reported in their series of 83 BPD/DS and 97 RYGB procedures that, at 3 years of follow-up, the mean EWL was 63.7% for RYGB and 84% for BPD/DS.

Adams and colleagues reported a large (n = 1156) prospective observational study comparing patients undergoing RYGB with nonsurgical controls. Two nonsurgical control groups were used: group 1 sought but did not receive surgery, and group 2 did not seek surgery. At 12 years, mean body weight change was 26.9% for the surgical patients and –2% and –0.9% for control groups 1 and 2, respectively. Furthermore, the odds ratios for the incidence of type 2 diabetes were also significantly lower for the surgical patients (0.08 vs control group 1 and 0.09 vs control group 2).

Unlike the more invasive surgical approaches, the LAGB produces a relatively more modest weight loss result. Early weight loss is typically around 40% EWL.

The LSG is the newest operation to gain popularity, but nonetheless, sufficient evidence has accumulated to suggest that it induces weight loss that is slightly less than that of RYGB, around 40%-50% EWL at 3- to 5-year follow-ups.

In a retrospective observational cohort study of 65,093 patients, Arterburn and colleagues reported that, at 5 years, the percent total weight loss for RYGB is greater than that for either LSG or LAGB. Table 46–2 summarizes the average expected weight loss for the most commonly performed bariatric surgical procedures. All of these procedures tend to

Table 46–2. Average weight loss for common bariatric procedures.

	Maximum Weight Loss (%TBWL)	5-Year Weight Loss (%TBWL)
LAGB[1]	13.7	11.7
LSG[1]	25.2	18.8
RYGB[1]	31.2	25.5
BPD/DS	44.8[2]	40.3[3]

BPD/DS, biliopancreatic diversion with duodenal switch; LAGB, laparoscopic adjustable gastric banding; LSG, laparoscopic sleeve gastrectomy; RYGB, Roux-en-Y gastric bypass; TBWL, total-body weight loss.
[1]Data from Arterburn D, Wellman R, Emiliano A, Smith SR, Odegaard AO, Murali S, Williams N, Coleman KJ, Courcoulas A, Coley RY, Anau J, Pardee R, Toh S, Janning C, Cook A, Sturtevant J, Horgan C, McTigue KM; PCORnet Bariatric Study Collaborative. Comparative Effectiveness and Safety of Bariatric Procedures for Weight Loss: A PCORnet Cohort Study. *Ann Intern Med.* 2018;169(11):741-750.
[2]Data from Søvik TT, Aasheim ET, Taha O, Engström M, Fagerland MW, Björkman S, Kristinsson J, Birkeland KI, Mala T, Olbers T. Weight loss, cardiovascular risk factors, and quality of life after gastric bypass and duodenal switch: a randomized trial. *Ann Intern Med.* 2011;155(5):281-91.
[3]Data from Risstad H, Søvik TT, Engström M, Aasheim ET, Fagerland MW, Olsén MF, Kristinsson JA, le Roux CW, Bøhmer T, Birkeland KI, Mala T, Olbers T. Five-year outcomes after laparoscopic gastric bypass and laparoscopic duodenal switch in patients with body mass index of 50 to 60: a randomized clinical trial. *JAMA Surg.* 2015;150(4):352-61.

reach a nadir weight around 12-18 months, followed by some degrees of weight regain by 5 years.

▶ Complications

Overall, bariatric surgery is a safe treatment modality for the right patient suffering from refractory obesity. Death following bariatric surgery is uncommon, especially in the era of laparoscopy. The LABS study reported a 30-day postbariatric surgery (RYGB and LAGB) mortality of 0.3%, with the most common cause of death being sepsis (33%), followed by cardiac causes (28%) and pulmonary embolism (17%). Kumar and colleagues compared the 30-day postoperative morbidity and mortality of LSG (n = 93,062) and RYGB (n = 41,080) using the 2015 Metabolic and Bariatric Surgery Accreditation and Quality Improvement Data Registry (MBSAQIP). They found mortality rates of 0.1% for LSG and 0.2% for RYGB (*P* < .001). Overall morbidity rates were 5.8% for LSG and 11.7% for RYGB (*P* < .001)

Common postbariatric complications can be categorized into early versus late complications. Early complications include those seen with other forms of gastrointestinal surgery: bleeding, infection, anastomotic leak, and delayed

return of bowel function. The most dreaded complication following bariatric surgery is leakage at the anastomosis or staple line. In theory, any gastrointestinal anastomosis or staple line has the potential for leak. However, this is a particularly challenging situation in bariatric patients because their body habitus renders their physical exam relatively unreliable, and a leak may not be immediately recognized. For the RYGB, the most common site of leak is the gastrojejunostomy. Although the LSG eliminated the need for intestinal rearrangement, its relatively long staple line along the greater curvature is also susceptible to leak. Management of leaks in bariatric surgery patients follows a similar set of principles as those used in nonbariatric gastrointestinal surgery. Early detection is paramount. In early postoperative patients with unexplained tachycardia, leukocytosis, or delayed gastric emptying, one must harbor a high index of suspicion for anastomotic leak. When identified, prompt source control is mandatory, whether it be interventional, endoscopic, or surgical. Delayed recognition of these proximal gastrointestinal leaks can lead to devastating consequence such peritonitis, sepsis, and even death. Early leaks (< 5 days after surgery) can often be managed by returning to the operating room for exploration, most often laparoscopically. This allows one to wash out the peritoneum, inspect the anastomosis and staple line, and repair or resect potential defects. Management of late leaks is often less straight forward. Management will often depend on the patient's clinical stability. A small leak in a patient who is otherwise stable may be managed with percutaneous drainage rather than reoperation. Some patients will also benefit from establishing enteral feeding access for enteral nutrition. Although historically anastomotic leaks are attributed to technical insufficiency, emerging experimental evidence suggests that it may be a much more complex biologic process, with the gut microbiome playing a significant role.

Late complications vary based on the type of bariatric procedure. The most serious long-term complication following the LAGB is band slippage or erosion. With the number of LAGB procedures worldwide continuing to decrease, this may represent a much rarer clinical entity in the future. Another potential complication of LAGB is long-term band tolerance. In a study examining 19,221 LAGB patients from New York State, Altieri and colleagues reported a total removal or revision rate that was as high as 34% over a 7-year period. Late complications associated with RYGB include gastrogastric fistula, stricture formation, marginal ulceration, and internal hernias. Anastomotic strictures can be difficult to diagnose on imaging, and definitive diagnosis often requires endoscopic interrogation. In general, anastomosis < 1 cm may cause symptoms and requires endoscopic dilation, with some patient requiring serial dilations. Dilations must be carried out with utmost caution given the risk of perforation. The rate of marginal ulcer formation after bariatric surgery varies dramatically in the literature, ranging from 1% to as high as 15%. Exact etiology remains elusive, with *Helicobacter pylori*, smoking, and use of nonsteroidal anti-inflammatory medications all believed to play a role. The first-line treatment is pharmacologic acid suppression, which leads to resolution in most cases. Refractory marginal ulcers are challenging and can lead to clinically significant bleeding, sometimes necessitating resection and reconstruction of the anastomosis.

Internal hernias are a serious complication following RYGB, which at times can be difficult to diagnose. The operation creates two new potential sites of herniation. One defect is at the site of the jejunojejunostomy where the space between the mesentery of the biliopancreatic limb and the mesentery of the jejunum creates a potential herniation site. A second defect is the space between the mesentery of the Roux limb and the transverse mesocolon, known as the Petersen defect. Many experts advocate the routine closure of these defects during the index operation in order to mitigate subsequent complications. A recent randomized controlled trial published by Sternberg and colleagues found a significantly lower incidence of reoperation for small bowel obstruction in the defect closure group (both jejunojejunostomy and Petersen defect) and supports the routine closure of these defects in RYGB. Management of internal hernias hinges on early recognition and prompt intervention. Because these patients can sometimes present with vague symptoms, a high index of suspicion is required on the part of the surgeon. Computed tomography (CT) remains the most effective diagnostic modality. In patients suspected of internal herniation, a CT of the abdomen and pelvis should be promptly obtained. In patients without other medical contraindications, oral and intravenous contrast should be used. Demonstration of a swirling of the mesenteric vessels is the most reliable indicator for the diagnosis of internal hernia (Figure 46–8).

▲ **Figure 46–8.** Axial computed tomography image of abdomen with intravenous and oral contrast. Swirl of mesenteric vessel with associated mesenteric edema (*arrow*).

Nutritional Consequence of Surgery

Long-term malnutrition was a complication that plagued early malabsorptive surgical attempts. Although modern procedures carry a much lower risk than their earlier counterparts, postbariatric surgical malnutrition remains a major source of morbidity and thus deserves special attention. Two aspects of bariatric surgery contribute to its malnutrition risks: first, the decrease in enteral nutritional intake can directly decrease the supply of many essential nutrients, and second, procedures that involve intestinal bypass and rearrangement can affect the absorptive capacity of certain vitamins and micronutrients.

A. Iron

An important building block of hemoglobin, iron absorption occurs mainly in the duodenum and proximal jejunum. Several mechanisms in bariatric surgery account for decreased iron absorption. First, gastric resection decreases the stomach's acid-producing capacity. Elevated gastric pH decreases the solubility and uptake of iron, which substantially reduces iron absorption. Second, procedures bypassing the proximal foregut will divert nutrients away from the iron-absorbing enterocytes. Third, patients tend to have diminished iron consumption due to their overall decrease of caloric intake, in particular, meat and dairy products. More than 30% of patients will experience iron deficiency 5 years following bariatric surgery. Therefore, current guidelines recommend prophylactic iron supplementation for all bariatric surgical patients.

B. Vitamin B_{12}/Folate

Hypovitaminosis B is most commonly seen following RYGB and BPD/DS. 20 to 35% of these patients will experience some degree of vitamin B_{12} deficiency at 5 years after surgery. Several mechanisms account for this, including decreased intrinsic factor production and increased gastric pH. In addition, although eventual enteric uptake of vitamin B_{12} occurs mostly in the ileum, the duodenum and proximal jejunum play an important role in this process. Vitamin B_{12} binding to intrinsic factors occurs in the proximal foregut. Thus, procedures that bypass the proximal foregut will substantially decrease vitamin B_{12} absorption. Unlike vitamin B_{12}, folate deficiency in bariatric surgical patients results largely from diminished dietary intake rather than malabsorption. Both hypovitaminosis B and folate deficiency will lead to macrocytic anemia. Because of the body's large store of vitamin B_{12}, its deficiency tends to manifest much later than folate deficiency. Both vitamin B_{12} and folate can be supplemented orally, although severe vitamin B_{12} deficiency may require intramuscular supplementation.

C. Fat-Soluble Vitamins

Vitamins A, D, E, and K are all at risk for deficiency following bariatric surgery, especially in procedures with greater malabsorptive potential such as BPD/DS. In these procedures, the malabsorption of dietary fat leads to decreased serum levels of fat-soluble vitamins. The prevalence of vitamins A and K deficiencies following BPD/DS can be as high as 65% and 60%, respectively. However, a significantly small proportion of these deficiencies result in clinical symptoms.

Vitamin D and Bone Metabolism

Decreased bone mineral density (BMD) is seen in 8%-13% of postbariatric surgical patients. Deficiencies in vitamin D and calcium are the two main culprits of this decrease in BMD. Calcium absorption occurs mainly in the duodenum and proximal jejunum; thus, bypassing these segments will result in a substantial decrease in calcium absorption. Up to 10% of postbariatric surgical patients will experience calcium deficiency. Similar to other fat-soluble vitamins, hypovitaminosis D is a consequence of decreased fat absorption following bariatric surgery. As many as 70% of bariatric surgical patients will experience vitamin D deficiency. Deficiencies in vitamin D and calcium result in higher bone turnover, which in turn leads to lower BMD. There is a more than twofold increase in the relative risk of fractures in bariatric surgical patients compared with the general population. Thus, careful attention to calcium and vitamin D supplementation and regular follow-up of calcium, vitamin D, and parathyroid hormone levels remain an important part of postsurgical surveillance.

▶ Expanding Surgical Indications and Patient Selection

As in all surgical procedures, proper patient selection in bariatric surgery is paramount. The most widely accepted criteria for bariatric surgery today are those from the 1991 National Institutes of Health (NIH) Consensus Development Conference on Gastrointestinal Surgery for Severe Obesity. Under this guideline, patients can qualify for bariatric operations if their BMI exceeds 40 or if their BMI is 35-40 and they have obesity-related comorbidities (eg, severe sleep apnea, Pickwickian syndrome, cardiovascular diseases, severe diabetes) or significant lifestyle hindrance due to obesity. The NIH consensus guidelines also underscore that patients choosing to undergo bariatric surgery must also have a clear and realistic understanding of what their postoperative life entails.

Many experts have criticized these criteria because they are likely outdated and may not reflect the risk and benefit calculations using today's techniques and technology. Because most insurance companies still rely on the 1991 NIH consensus guidelines, many patients who may benefit from earlier bariatric intervention are denied treatment. This prompted the American Society for Metabolic and Bariatric Surgery to release its own consensus statement in 2012 advocating that bariatric surgery should be made available for patients with class I obesity (BMI 30-35) who are suffering from metabolic or lifestyle comorbidities and have failed

nonsurgical interventions. The Second Diabetes Surgery Summit (DSS-II) was an international consensus conference aimed at developing guidelines for the use of bariatric and metabolic surgery for the treatment of type 2 diabetes. It concluded that metabolic surgery should be recommended for all class III obese patient with type 2 diabetes and for class II obese patients with poor glycemic control with medical and lifestyle interventions. In addition, it also concluded that metabolic surgery should be *considered* for class I obese patients with type 2 diabetes if glycemic control remains inadequate on optimal oral or injectable antiglycemic agents. Furthermore, it recommended that these BMI guidelines should be lowered by 2.7 kg/m² for patients of Asian ancestry because of the relatively higher proportion of visceral fat in Asian patients compared with their white counterparts.

Rubino F, et al: Metabolic surgery in the treatment algorithm for type 2 diabetes: a joint statement by International Diabetes Organizations. *Diabetes Care.* 2016;39(6):861-877.

METABOLIC EFFECTS OF SURGICAL WEIGHT LOSS

The complete review of the metabolic changes following bariatric surgery is beyond the scope of this chapter. Nonetheless, several important areas of metabolic alterations are worth highlighting. The metabolic consequences of obesity have been well established, and it appears that even modest weight loss can herald significant improvements in many obesity-related metabolic disorders. Although any type of meaningful weight loss can decrease the risk of developing these disorders, nonsurgical weight loss is frequently unsuccessful due to the high likelihood of weight regain. As such, we are gaining a greater appreciation for the metabolic improvements following bariatric surgery. In fact, in many cases, surgery is evolving into the standard of care for medically refractory obesity-related disorders.

Cardiovascular disease is the leading cause of death in the United States and remains a major source of the human and financial costs of obesity. Hypertension is observed in up to 50% of patients undergoing bariatric surgery. As many as 60%-70% of these patients will experience postoperative improvement or remission. Weight loss surgery has been shown to reduce the 10-year risk of a cardiac event by up to 40%.

Likely related to its effect on weight loss, bariatric surgery has been shown to bring about significant improvement in lipid profile. Approximately half of patients undergoing bariatric surgery have some degree of baseline dyslipidemia. Following surgery, more than 70% of patients experience either improvement or resolution of their dyslipidemia within 2 years. There is emerging evidence that many of the metabolic benefits of bariatric surgery are long lasting. The 7-year follow-up data from the LABS study showed improvement in obesity-related metabolic disorders following both

RYGB and LAGB. The prevalence of dyslipidemia was lower at 7 years following both procedures.

Although its cardiovascular and lipid-lowering effects are significant, the most dramatic metabolic improvement following bariatric surgery is arguably glycemic control. Intense research efforts are ongoing to improve the pharmacologic treatment of diabetes, but pharmacologic treatment has only had limited success thus far. Glycemic improvement is expected following weight loss regardless of the method used to achieve it. However, emerging data have confirmed that bariatric operations can improve glycemic control in a weight-independent manner. As many as 11 randomized trials have compared various bariatric operations to maximal medical therapy, and they have all confirmed the superiority of bariatric surgery over medial management of diabetes. Bariatric surgery can achieve type 2 diabetes remission in as many as 80% of patients. For these reasons, the DSS-II meeting recommended that not only should bariatric surgery be recommended in obese diabetic patients who fall under the current NIH consensus guidelines, it should also be considered for patients with class I obesity who have had inadequate glycemic control on optimal oral or injectable medications.

Several active lines of inquiry are devoted to elucidating the mechanisms behind the antidiabetic effects of bariatric surgery. A rapid improvement in hepatic insulin sensitivity is an important step after bariatric surgery and can occur before significant weight loss. Mechanisms behind this and other possible pathways driving these antidiabetic effects have shown several important changes after surgery, including an increase in postprandial GLP-1 secretion following RYGB, likely from an earlier ileal exposure to nutrients. However, emerging experimental data suggest that this is less likely than originally thought. The exclusion of the duodenum and proximal small intestine from nutrient flow is also believed to play a critical role. More recent animal studies have suggested that, after surgery, intestinal metabolism changes lead to alterations in the portal vein milieu, which can in turn modulate hepatic insulin sensitivity. Another theory espouses that the postoperative improvement in glycemic control is related to the elevated circulating bile acid levels found following RYGB. Definitive human evidence is still lacking, but understanding the precise mechanism(s) behind the antidiabetic effects of bariatric surgery is rapidly becoming the next frontier in metabolic research.

Dimitri Miras A, et al: Obesity surgery makes patients healthier and more functional: real world results from the United Kingdom National Bariatric Surgery Registry. *Surg Obes Relat Dis.* 2018;14(7):1033-1040.

WEIGHT LOSS DEVICES: AN EMERGING MARKET

Despite the success that bariatric surgery has had in weight loss and metabolic improvement, many patients remain hesitant to undergo an invasive surgical procedure. Moreover, many other patients suffering from obesity and metabolic disorders may not meet the stringent criteria to qualify for bariatric surgery, as described earlier. This has prompted the proliferation of many endoluminal weight loss devices hoping to achieve the weight loss and metabolic benefits of gastrointestinal manipulation without the need for surgery. Currently, there are three categories of devices on the market approved by the FDA for the treatment of obesity, and these are discussed in the following sections (not including the gastric band, which was discussed earlier).

Vagal Electrical Stimulation Systems

This device involves electrodes that are placed around the vagus nerve laparoscopically in order to modulate neural signaling between the brain and stomach. The device works by having a rechargeable internal (implanted subcutaneously) component that generates intermittent electrical pulses to block the signaling of the vagus nerve. Although the precise mechanism underlying this type of vagal-blocking therapy remains unclear, it is believed that vagal signaling disruption can modulate the feedback loop governing hunger and satiety. The ReCharge Trial randomized patients with BMI > 40 or > 35 with comorbidities to either vagal block or sham intervention. The 24-month outcomes were published in 2017. Among the 123 vagal-blocked patients who remained for the 2 years of follow-up, the mean EWL was 21%. The device has the same selection criteria as surgical bariatric procedures. Specific contraindications include patients with liver cirrhosis, portal hypertension, esophageal varices, and clinically significant hiatal hernia.

Implantable Gastric Balloon Systems

These devices are implanted inside the stomach in order to occupy space, thus producing a restrictive effect. They are approved for patients with a BMI of 30-40 and usually for a period of 6 months, after which they have to be removed. Several devices of this category have been approved by the FDA. The Orbera (Apollo Endosurgery) is a single balloon device that is placed endoscopically and inflated with saline. The device then sits in the gastric body and produces a space-occupying effect in order to restrict caloric intake. The balloon is endoscopically removed after 6 months. The ReShape system (ReShape Lifesciences), approved by the FDA in 2015, is also placed and removed endoscopically but has a different design that employs two independently inflated, noncommunicating balloons connected via a central silicone shaft. The dual-balloon design is proposed to decrease the risk of downstream balloon migration in the event that one of the balloons experiences a defect and deflates.

The Obalon system (Kensaq) is a relatively new system that compromises three smaller balloons that can be swallowed. Each balloon comes in the form of a small capsule when deflated. The patient swallows the capsule, and once the capsule reaches the stomach, it is inflated with air. Each fully inflated balloon occupies a volume of 250 mL. Up to three balloons may be placed in the first 3 months. The gas-filled balloons occupy space in the stomach and thus diminish its ability to accommodate food, creating early satiety. The balloons are removed endoscopically after 6 months, similar to other systems. The Obalon system is marketed for adult patients with a BMI between 30 and 40 who have failed adequate weight loss via diet and exercise.

In general, the balloon devices are intended for short-term placement with modest weight loss goals (10%-15% TBWL). Unlike the standard bariatric surgical procedures, the balloon devices have a lower BMI threshold for patient selection. Contraindications include prior gastrointestinal surgery, inflammatory diseases of the alimentary tract, large or symptomatic hiatal hernia, and patients taking daily medications that may damage the device (eg, aspirin, anti-inflammatory agents, anticoagulants). Although the effects of the balloon devices are not as significant or as durable as standard bariatric surgery, they can offer a unique solution to patients who have failed more conservative means of weight loss but do not qualify for surgery under the current guidelines.

▶ Gastric Emptying Systems

The only FDA-approved device of this category is the AspireAssist system (Aspire Bariatrics), which consists of an endoscopically placed gastrostomy tube that is attached to a port valve secured to the abdominal wall skin. Following a meal, the valve is opened and the consumed food is drained out via an external tubing. In approving the device, the FDA reviewed a clinical trial of 111 patients that showed patients lost, on average, 12.1% TBWL compared to the control group. The device is aimed at patients age 22 years or older with a BMI between 35 and 55 who have failed other conservative means of weight loss. It is contraindicated in patients with uncontrolled hypertension, bulimia, binge eating disorder, inflammatory bowel disease, gastric ulcer disease, pregnancy or lactation, and certain types of prior abdominal operations.

Vyas D, et al: Advances in endoscopic balloon therapy for weight loss and its limitations. *World J Gastroenterol.* 2017;23(14): 7813-7817.

WEIGHT MANAGEMENT IN ADOLESCENTS

Obesity and its related disorders in the adolescent population are a major and growing public health concern. The prevalence of obesity in children increased by more than 47% in the decades between 1980 and 2013. Nearly one-third of American children between 2 and 19 years of age are overweight or obese, and > 18% are obese (BMI ≥ 95th percentile for age). Several aspects are unique in the consideration of adolescent obesity. First, BMI is a rather poor measure of childhood obesity because, unlike adults, children have differing proportions of body fat. Second, youth are at risk for even more significant metabolic consequences given their still maturing bodily development. Finally, children with obesity experience a unique set of psychosocial challenges and require a specialized approach in addressing them.

There are also similarities between adolescent and adult obesity. Like adult obesity, behavioral or medical management alone has proven to be ineffective or short lived. In addition, surgery has been shown to be the only effective and durable treatment modality for many adolescents suffering from intractable obesity and its related metabolic disorders. However, because of the unique anatomic, physiologic, and psychological challenges of childhood obesity, bariatric surgery in this population requires several special considerations.

Patient selection in adolescent bariatric surgery can be difficult. There is currently no conclusive evidence-based guideline for selecting adolescent patients for weight loss surgery. Most centers rely on the adult guidelines and extrapolate the evidence to the younger population. There is also no agreed upon age recommendation for childhood weight loss surgery. Most experts agree that surgery should be reserved for patients in their mid to late teens, after they have reached 95% of adult stature. There are currently no data to allow us to make any meaningful assertions on surgery for patients younger than that age group. Furthermore, proper patient selection and follow-up must consider the unique psychosocial challenges of adolescent obesity. Because of these challenges, adolescent bariatric surgery should be approached in a multidisciplinary fashion with teams that include a specialized surgeon, pediatrician, psychologist or counselor, social worker, dietician, and exercise coaches.

Available data thus far suggest that bariatric surgery in adolescents has a similar effectiveness as in adults. An average of 50%-60% EWL can be expected in the first 2 years following surgery. Among postoperative teens, up to 70% experience type 2 diabetes resolution. Several studies have also shown that adolescents undergoing bariatric surgery experience an improvement in mental health following surgery, although some data suggest that this improvement is not necessarily maintained at 2 years. A recent prospective study of 242 adolescents was reported by Inge and colleagues in the *New England Journal of Medicine*, in which 161 patients underwent RYGB and 67 underwent LSG. The average age of the participants was 17 ± 1.6 years. They showed that, at 3 years, mean body weight decreased by 27% in all patients (28% in those who underwent RYGB and 26% in those who underwent LSG). Moreover, at 3 years, the remission rate was 95% for diabetes, 74% for elevated blood pressure, and 66% for dyslipidemia. They study also found that 57% of these patients developed elements of hypoferritinemia at 3 years.

Active investigations are underway to better elucidate the long-term risks and benefits of bariatric surgery in adolescent patients, and their data will help to better guide physicians in managing this growing disease.

Durkin N, et al: What is the evidence for paediatric/adolescent bariatric surgery? *Curr Obes Rep.* 2017;6(3):278-285.
Inge T, et al: Weight loss health status 3 years after bariatric
surgery in adolescents. *N Engl J Med.* 2016;374(20):113-123.

MULTIPLE CHOICE QUESTIONS

1. Which of the following patients would qualify for bariatric surgery under the 1991 National Institutes of Health
Consensus Guideline?

    A. A 55-year-old otherwise healthy male with a body
    mass index (BMI) of 37

    B. A 35-year-old female with BMI of 32 and hyperten-
    sion, diabetes, and obstructive sleep apnea

    C. A 50-year-old female with a BMI of 38 and a family
    history of type 2 diabetes, hypertension, and coronary
    artery disease

    D. A 38-year-old male with BMI of 36 and obstructive
    sleep apnea, type 2 diabetes, and dyslipidemia

    E. A 48-year-old female with a BMI of 34 and chronic
    low back pain

2. Which of the follow statements regarding the medical
and surgical treatments of obesity is correct?

    A. Surgery and intense medical therapy achieve compa-
    rable weight loss results when compared at 5 years.

    B. Surgery achieves greater weight loss and medical ther-
    apy achieves better glycemic control in obese diabetic
    patients.

    C. Surgery is the only treatment modality that has been
    shown to achieve sustained remission in hypertension
    and type 2 diabetes in obese patients.

    D. Bariatric surgery should only be offered to patients
    over the age of 18.

    E. There is never a role for surgery in the management
    of type 2 diabetes.

3. A 60-year-old man with a BMI of 38 and hypertension,
type 2 diabetes, and obstructive sleep apnea is interested
in undergoing bariatric surgery. After completing the
required preoperative evaluation, he wants to know what
he can expect following surgery. Which of the following
statements is correct in addressing his concerns?

    A. He can expect comparable weight loss results
    with Roux-en-Y gastric bypass (RYGB), sleeve
    gastrectomy, or gastric banding.

    B. With RYGB, the average patient experiences > 50%
    excess weight loss (EWL) at 2 years.

    C. The RYGB has a higher risk of long-term nutritional
    deficiency than the biliopancreatic diversion with
    duodenal switch.

    D. All patients undergoing laparoscopic sleeve
    gastrectomy experience up to 60% EWL.

    E. This patient does not meet criteria for bariatric
    surgery.

4. Which of the following statements regarding RYGB
procedure is *incorrect*?

    A. It is considered by most to be the gold standard for
    bariatric surgery.

    B. Most RYGB procedures today are performed
    laparoscopically.

    C. It is currently the most commonly performed
    bariatric surgery in the United States.

    D. Many patients undergoing RYGB experience an
    average of > 60% EWL.

    E. Internal hernias are serious complication following
    RYGB.

5. Which of the following statements regarding the use of
bariatric devices for weight loss is correct?

    A. There are currently no U.S. Food and Drug
    Administration–approved weight loss devices on the
    market in the United States.

    B. Implantable gastric balloons usually produce
    comparable weight loss outcomes to the laparoscopic
    sleeve gastrectomy.

    C. Implantable gastric balloons can be used for
    long-term weight loss if the patient is compliant with
    regular follow-up.

    D. The electric stimulation devices are contraindicated in
    patients with significant liver pathology or significant
    hiatal hernia.

    E. Unlike surgery, these devices present no significant
    risks to the patient.

Oncology

Michael S. Sabel, MD

More than 1.75 million individuals in the United States are expected to be diagnosed with invasive cancer in 2019, with more than 6,000,000 estimated cancer deaths. Currently, 21.7% of all deaths in the United States are due to cancer, ranking second only to heart disease as the leading cause of mortality in this country. Over the past 10 years, however, cancer death rates have decreased. This decline translates into more than 2.3 million fewer cancer deaths from 1991 to 2015, progress that has been driven by rapid declines in death rates for the four most common cancer types (lung, colorectal, breast, and prostate).

The surgeon is intimately involved in the care of cancer patients, since the majority will require surgical therapy at some time. Surgeons are often the first specialists to see newly diagnosed cancer patients or are often called upon to make the diagnosis in patients suspected of having cancer. As such, they will be responsible for orchestrating the patient's care, including coordination with medical oncologists and radiation oncologists. It is imperative that they have an in-depth knowledge of the different types of cancer and the different modalities available for treatment.

TUMOR NOMENCLATURE

Neoplasms are defined as benign or malignant according to the clinical behavior of the tumor. Benign tumors have lost normal growth regulation but tend to be surrounded by a capsule and do not invade surrounding tissues or metastasize.

Benign tumors are generally designated by adding the suffix -oma to the name of the cell of origin. Examples include lipoma and adenoma. The term *cancer* normally refers to malignant tumors, which can invade surrounding tissues or metastasize to distant sites in the host. The nomenclature of malignant tumors is typically based on the cell's embryonal tissue origins. Malignant tumors derived from cells of mesenchymal origin are called *sarcomas*. These include cancers that derive from muscle, bone, tendon, fat,

cartilage, lymphoid tissues, vessels, and connective tissue. Neoplasms of epithelial origin are called *carcinomas*. These may be further categorized according to the histologic appearance of the cells. Tumor cells that have glandular growth patterns are called adenocarcinomas, and those that resemble squamous epithelial cells are called squamous cell carcinomas. Cancers composed of undifferentiated cells that bear no resemblance to any tissues are designated as "poorly differentiated" or "undifferentiated" carcinomas.

▶ Tumor Grade

Beyond the type of cancer, it is important to classify tumors by their behavior and prognosis in order to determine appropriate therapy as well as evaluate different treatment modalities. Grading of a tumor is a histologic determination and refers to the degree of cellular differentiation. Separate pathologic grading systems exist for each histologic type of cancer. Depending on the type of tumor, these systems are based on nuclear pleomorphism, cellularity, necrosis, cellular invasion, and the number of mitoses. Increasing grades generally denote increasing degrees of dedifferentiation. While the grade of the tumor typically has less prognostic value than its stage, tumor grade has great clinical significance in soft tissue sarcoma, astrocytoma, transitional cell cancers of the genitourinary tract, and Hodgkin and non-Hodgkin lymphoma.

▶ Tumor Stage

Tumor staging establishes the extent of disease and has important prognostic and therapeutic implications in most types of cancer. Clinical staging is based on the results of a noninvasive evaluation, including physical examination and various imaging studies. Pathologic staging is based on findings in surgical tumor specimens and biopsies and allows for the evaluation of microscopic disease undetectable by imaging techniques. Pathologic staging may reveal more extensive tumor spread than the clinical evaluation and is the more reliable information. Clinicians must be careful when attempting to compare clinically and pathologically staged patients, as the two groups may have dramatically different outcomes.

As with grading, the staging systems vary with different tumor types. Two major staging systems are currently in use, one developed by the Union Internationale Contre le Cancer (UICC) and the other by the American Joint Committee on Cancer (AJCC). The UICC system is based on the TNM classification. *T* refers to the primary tumor and is based on the size of the tumor and invasion of surrounding structures. Tumors are characterized as T1 to T4 cancers, with the higher T stages for larger and more invasive tumors. *N* refers to regional lymph nodes, and classifications of N0 to N3 denote increasing degrees of lymph node involvement. Finally, *M* refers to distant metastatic disease, with M0 signifying no distant metastases and M1 and M2 indicating the presence of blood-borne metastatic disease.

The AJCC system divides cancers into stages 0 to IV, with higher stages representing more widespread disease and a poorer prognosis. The AJCC staging system is primarily based on the anatomic TNM system. Although TNM staging provides a good prediction of outcome when applied to groups, we are increasingly recognizing the importance of biologic subtypes when looking at individual patients. For this reason, biomarkers are now increasingly being incorporated into the AJCC staging system. In breast cancer, for example, the eighth edition of the AJCC staging manual now incorporates tumor grade, hormone receptor status, and human epidermal growth factor receptor 2 (HER2) status into parallel prognostic stage groups that recognize intrinsic tumor biology. The results of multigene panel testing (Oncotype DX), when available, may also be incorporated. As more level I evidence regarding biomarkers and multigene assays emerges, the AJCC staging system will likely continue to evolve.

▶ Cancer Epidemiology

Cancer epidemiology is the study of the distribution of cancer and its determinants among defined populations and is used to examine cancer etiology as well as the efficacy of prevention, detection, and treatment strategies. The most basic types of epidemiologic terms describe cancer rates or cancer deaths for specific populations over a certain period of time.

While absolute numbers of cancer cases may be useful for health care planning, they do not take into account the size or nature of the underlying population at risk. For this reason, the most commonly used population-based measures of cancer are incidence and mortality. **Cancer incidence rates** are defined as the number of new cancer cases diagnosed during a fixed time period divided by the total population at risk. **Cancer mortality rates** are defined similarly, with cancer deaths replacing new cancer cases. These rates are typically expressed as the number of events per 100,000 individuals per year.

Incidence and mortality rates are compared across populations or over time to identify causes as well as the effect of screening or treatment. However, other factors among populations may contribute to observed differences, and these must be taken into account. For most cancers, age is the strongest risk factor, and so comparison of cancer incidence between two populations must consider the age distributions of the two groups. Adjustment (or standardization) is the most common method used to account for such differences. Comparing age-adjusted cancer incidence rates ensures that any observed differences are not the results of differences in age distributions between the two populations. Incidence and mortality rates are often also adjusted for gender, race, or socioeconomic status.

Cancer incidence examines only those diagnosed with the disease during that time period; it does not include patients diagnosed earlier who are living with cancer. **Cancer prevalence** describes the number of people with the disease either at a single point in time (**point prevalence**) or within a defined period of time (**period prevalence**). Prevalence is more relevant to the public health burden of cancer because all prevalent cases involve accessing health care. The relationship among incidence, prevalence, and mortality is influenced by the fatality of the disease. If the disease is highly fatal and the interval between presentation and death is short, mortality rates will be similar to incidence rates. The number of deaths from cancer divided by the total number of people diagnosed with the cancer is known as the **cancer fatality rate,** although this is somewhat of a misnomer because they are not technically rates (they do not include time as a parameter).

Examining the fatality of cancer is obviously important when comparing treatments meant to improve outcome. **Overall survival** is the most global end point and is defined as the proportion of people alive at a specified period after being diagnosed with the disease. A period of 5 years is conventionally used as the time period (ie, 5-year survival). However, overall survival may not always reflect the success of treatment. Over that period of time, some patients may die of disease, but others may die of other causes. For this reason, epidemiologists often report on the **relative survival**. This is defined as the proportion of people with cancer who are alive for a designated time (eg, 5 years) divided by the proportion of people of similar age, race, and so on expected to be alive in the absence of cancer based on normal life expectancy. In addition, some patients may have a local or regional recurrence that is successfully treated, whereas others may experience recurrence with distant metastases but not succumb to them. For this reason, survival rates in cancer are often qualified by the patient's disease status.

Disease-free survival refers to the proportion of patients alive and without disease over a specific period of time. A patient who developed metastases but is still alive would be included in the overall survival rate but not the disease-free survival rate. Disease-free survival and overall survival may provide different pictures of the success of treatment. A therapy that improves disease-free survival but not overall survival may still be important if quality of life is improved. In some cancers, local or regional recurrences can be readily treated with minimal impact on overall survival. In these cases, disease-free survival may present an overly pessimistic picture of outcome. Therefore, it may be more relevant to compare **distant disease-free survival,** which refers to the proportion of people alive and without distant metastases, regardless of local recurrence. In some cases, it is difficult to assess the efficacy of a treatment by looking at overall survival or disease-free survival if there are deaths from competing causes. It may be more helpful to compare **disease-specific survival,** which is the percentage of people who have survived a disease since diagnosis or treatment and does not count patients who died from other causes.

It is important for the surgeon to understand the different methods for describing cancer survival as well as the differences between the definitions, because the appropriateness of the comparison will vary with the biology of the disease and the clinical question being asked.

Emin MD, Edge S, Greene F, et al. *AJCC Cancer Staging Manual,* 8th ed. New York, NY: Springer; 2017.

Giuliano AE, Connolly JL, Edge SB, et al: Breast cancer: major changes in the American Joint Committee on Cancer Eighth Edition Cancer Staging Manual. *CA Cancer J Clin.* 2017;67:290-303.

Siegel RL, Miller KD, Jemal A: Cancer statistics, 2018. *CA Cancer J Clin.* 2018;68:7-30.

ROLE OF THE SURGICAL ONCOLOGIST

The surgeon is often the first specialist to see a patient with suspected or newly diagnosed cancer and in many cases assumes responsibility for orchestrating the overall management of the cancer patient's care. The role of the surgeon involves not only the curative resection of the tumor but also obtaining tissue for diagnosis and staging, providing palliation for incurable patients, and preventing cancer by the prophylactic removal of organs. With improving imaging technologies, expanded use of neoadjuvant therapies, molecular staging, and increasing knowledge of the genetic predisposition to cancer, the role of the surgical oncologist is continuously evolving. It is therefore imperative for surgical oncologists to remain current on the newest approaches to cancer therapy and be prepared to adapt to the changing role of surgery.

▶ Diagnosis & Staging

A tissue diagnosis is critical to the care of all cancer patients. Depending on the type of tumor and its location, the method of biopsy will vary. Common diagnostic techniques include needle aspiration biopsy, core needle biopsy, incisional biopsy, and excisional biopsy.

Fine-needle aspiration biopsy (FNAB) is a rapid and minimally invasive technique for the biopsy of palpable superficial tumors. Deeper, nonpalpable lesions may also be sampled by this technique when FNAB is combined with various imaging modalities, such as ultrasonography or computed tomography (CT). FNAB involves aspiration of cells from a suspicious mass, followed by cytologic examination of the stained smear. FNAB is particularly useful in the diagnosis of enlarged lymph nodes, breast lumps, thyroid masses, and lung nodules.

Advantages to FNAB include the simplicity of the procedure and the low rate of complications. However, there are limitations. FNAB cytology requires an experienced cytopathologist for accurate interpretation. Because cytology does not demonstrate architecture, it does not allow the cytopathologist to accurately grade tumors or to differentiate between in situ and invasive disease. If this information is necessary, FNAB may be inadequate. Sampling errors can lead to false-negative results, so a negative FNAB should be interpreted cautiously. In addition, although rare, false-positive results can occur, so confirmation may be needed before definitive surgical intervention. For example, a mastectomy should never be performed on the basis of an FNAB of a breast lump without confirming the diagnosis by either preoperative core biopsy or frozen section analysis at the time of surgery.

Core needle biopsy uses a needle that removes a sliver of tissue for analysis. This technique provides more histologic information than FNAB because it allows the pathologist to see the histologic architecture of the sample rather than just the cellular characteristics. False-positive results are extremely rare. Although less so than with FNAB, sampling errors may occur, and a negative result must be weighed against clinical judgment. Core biopsies are also advantageous in that they easily allow for immunohistochemical staining for relevant biomarkers. This is highly important as neoadjuvant chemotherapy is increasingly used. Ultrasound and radiographic imaging may enable the clinician to sample deep-seated or nonpalpable masses. The technique may also be used during surgery to biopsy suspicious masses encountered at operation. Core needle biopsy is also increasingly being used to obtain tissue for genomic sequencing in patients with advanced disease.

When a larger tumor sample is necessary for accurate grading or staging or a needle biopsy provided inadequate information, an incisional or excisional biopsy is required. **Excisional biopsy** is the surgical removal of an entire gross lesion, whereas **incisional biopsy** involves sampling a representative portion of a suspicious lesion. In general, excisional biopsy is recommended whenever it is possible to excise the entire lesion without damage to surrounding structures. Incisional biopsy should be considered whenever a core biopsy fails to make the diagnosis but removing the tumor might compromise the subsequent operation (eg, a large [> 5 cm], deep soft tissue mass for which sarcoma is a possibility) or preclude delivery of neoadjuvant therapy.

Although biopsy techniques are usually simple, the surgeon must adhere to some specific principles when performing a biopsy for a suspected malignancy. The positioning of the needle tract or scar should be such that if further surgery is required, the biopsy site will be easily included in the excised specimen. Excisional biopsies of the breast should consider the cosmetic implications of a lumpectomy (and radiation) or the possibility of a subsequent mastectomy. The excision of skin or subcutaneous lesions on the extremities should be oriented in a way that allows for the following wide excision and lymphatic mapping if malignancy is discovered. Meticulous hemostasis is imperative, as the formation of a wound hematoma may make subsequent operation more difficult. The surgeon should carefully orient the pathologic specimen to allow the pathologist to evaluate margins in the context of the preresection anatomy, which may prove important in curative surgical procedures.

Once a diagnosis is made, the next step is typically to determine the extent of the cancer, or **staging.** This step begins with a complete history and physical examination, looking for signs or symptoms of advanced or metastatic disease. Laboratory or imaging studies may follow to determine not only the extent of the primary tumor but also the presence of regional or distant metastases. Patients with signs or symptoms of metastatic disease should undergo appropriate workup of their symptoms. For some tumor types, routine staging examinations are indicated. However, for many asymptomatic patients newly diagnosed with cancer, a full battery of staging studies is not necessary and not only will increase the cost of treatment but may also lead to false-positive findings, unnecessary biopsies, and inappropriate changes in therapy.

Surgeons are sometimes called upon to perform operations that provide staging information for various types of cancer. Such procedures are necessary when the clinical extent of the disease has a direct bearing on the choice of treatment modalities. Examples include laparoscopy for gastric or pancreatic cancer, a staging laparotomy for ovarian cancer, or mediastinoscopy for lung and esophageal cancer. Staging procedures can often help to avert highly morbid procedures in cases where there is little chance for cure.

▶ Curative Surgery

Surgical resections with curative intent can be divided into three categories: resection of a primary lesion, resection of isolated metastases, and resection of metastatic deposits. In each case, the clinician must strive to reach a balance between the chance for cure and the morbidity of the procedure. Each situation must be evaluated individually, and the patient's wishes must be paramount.

The guiding principle of cancer surgery is to remove the entire tumor with adequate margins so as to prevent local recurrence and potentially distant recurrence. What constitutes an adequate margin varies among tumor types. Various tumors require different disease-free margins in order to achieve optimal chances for a cure. For a tumor that appears adherent or fixed to adjacent structures, **en bloc resection** is mandatory, and any attachment should be considered malignant in nature. Appropriate preoperative imaging of the tumor is often necessary to be prepared in the operating room for the possible resection of small or large bowel, bladder, or other adjacent organs.

It is important that the surgeon have knowledge of other modalities that may be integrated into the management plan to allow for a less extensive surgical procedure. Radiation and chemotherapy are commonly used in combination with surgery and are referred to as adjuvant therapies if used after complete resection with no demonstrable local or systemic disease. While their use has in some cases diminished the extent of resection necessary for local control (breast, sarcoma, head and neck), it is important to note that these modalities do not compensate for inadequate margins in controlling local disease. Every attempt should be made to achieve widely negative margins surgically, even if it requires a second operation, rather than assuming radiation will "clean up" residual disease.

If these modalities are used in the preoperative setting, they are called neoadjuvant therapies. In many cases, neoadjuvant therapy has dramatically improved outcomes, as with pediatric rhabdomyosarcoma or locally advanced or inflammatory breast cancer. In some cases, neoadjuvant therapy can convert an unresectable tumor to resectable, whereas in other cases, it can decrease the extent of surgery necessary to obtain control or decrease the likelihood of positive margins. Neoadjuvant therapy is commonly used in the treatment of esophageal cancer, rectal cancer, pancreatic cancer, breast cancer, and sarcoma. It is important the surgeon consider the possibility of neoadjuvant therapy when performing a biopsy, staging the patient, or planning surgery.

The regional lymph nodes represent the most prevalent site of metastases for solid tumors, and in most cases, involvement of the regional nodes represents the most important prognostic factor. Removal of the regional lymph nodes not only provides important prognostic information that may help guide adjuvant therapy, but also provides regional control, preventing regional recurrence and the associated complications. For this reason, the removal of the regional lymph nodes is often performed at the time of resection of the primary cancer. More controversial is whether the removal of regional lymph nodes can improve survival. These controversies concern both the extent and the timing of the procedure. For example, the extent of lymphadenectomy at the time of gastrectomy for stomach cancer has been hypothesized to have an impact on improving overall survival. This has not, however, been borne out in prospective randomized trials. It may be that extended lymphadenectomy results in more accurate staging of patients at a cost of increased morbidity and minimal effect, if any, on overall survival. The relative benefit of nodal dissection may also vary with the efficacy of adjuvant therapies, such as chemotherapy or radiation therapy. How extensive a lymph node dissection to perform at the time of definitive resection varies with tumor type and, in many cases, remains controversial.

For many nonvisceral solid tumors, such as melanoma or breast cancer, elective node dissections were performed in clinically node-negative patients at the time of their primary tumor resection. Unfortunately, this exposed many node-negative patients to the morbidity of a node dissection, and a clear survival benefit could not be demonstrated in prospective randomized studies. This practice has been replaced with lymphatic mapping and sentinel lymph node biopsy. Mapping agents (a radioactive tracer or a blue dye) are injected around the site of the tumor prior to surgery. These travel to the lymph nodes that first receive drainage from the site of the primary and thus are the most likely to harbor cancer. Only the sentinel nodes (those nodes that are blue or radioactive) are removed and carefully examined for micrometastases. This has dramatically improved our ability to stage the regional lymph nodes, helping to guide adjuvant therapies, while minimizing morbidity. Classically, node-negative patients could safely avoid further surgery, whereas node-positive patients underwent a completion lymph node dissection. This approach has also changed recently. In breast cancer, the American College of Surgeons Oncology Group (ACoSOG) Z0011 trial demonstrated that a subset of breast cancer patients with positive sentinel lymph nodes did not benefit from completion lymph node dissection. In melanoma, the Multicenter Selective Lymphadenectomy Trial II (MSLT-II), demonstrated that sentinel lymph node–positive patients could safely be observed with serial ultrasounds of the involved basin as an alternative to completion node dissection.

The surgeon plays a much more limited role when the patient has metastatic disease; nonetheless, the resection of "isolated" metastases in patients with solid malignancies is sometimes a consideration when technically feasible. The selection of candidate patients for surgical resection requires a thorough evaluation of the extent of known disease, likelihood of additional metastatic disease, length of time between the primary and the distant recurrence (disease-free interval), medical status of the patient, and feasibility of resecting the metastatic site with a negative margin. Ultimately, this process identifies a small subset of patients who would be surgical candidates. Although there are no prospective randomized trials documenting the survival benefit of surgical resection of metastatic disease, there is considerable retrospective evidence indicating that this approach can result in long-term benefit. The resection of lung metastases in patients with osteogenic or soft tissue sarcomas has been associated with an approximately 20%-25% overall survival rate at greater than 5 years. There is also a large body of retrospective evidence documenting the benefit of resecting colorectal metastases to the liver, resulting in a 25%-40% overall 5-year survival rate, depending on the extent of liver involvement. A similar benefit has been demonstrated in an aggressive surgical approach to metastatic melanoma. Another question in stage IV disease is when to resect the primary tumor. Typically, resection of the primary cancer when the patient already has metastatic disease was only done for palliation or to prevent future complications. This approach is changing, however. For some cancers, such as colon cancer, resection of the primary tumor in the face of metastatic disease to prevent obstruction or bleeding is less necessary due to the improved efficacy of systemic agents. Conversely, in some cancers, such as renal cell carcinoma and possibly breast cancer, there is evidence that resection of the primary tumor may improve outcome in stage IV patients. One of the roles of the surgical oncologist is to know when it is appropriate to offer this option.

▶ Palliation

Surgical intervention is sometimes required in the patient with unresectable advanced cancer for palliative indications such as pain, bleeding, obstruction, malnutrition, or infection. The decision to operate must balance several factors, including the likelihood of adding significantly to the quality of life of the patient, the expected survival of the individual, the potential morbidity of the procedure, and whether there are alternative methods of palliation.

Malnutrition is a common problem in the cancer patient, especially one with advanced, unresectable disease. Commonly, the surgeon is involved in placement of vascular access for hyperalimentation, or if the gastrointestinal tract is functional, the placement of gastrostomy or jejunostomy tubes for enteral nutrition. Occasionally, the surgeon is involved in palliating pain due to a metastatic lesion compressing upon an organ or adjacent nerves. Examples include cutaneous or subcutaneous melanoma metastases, a large ulcerating breast cancer, or a recurrent intra-abdominal sarcoma mass. The surgeon must assess the relative risk-to-benefit ratio in resecting a symptomatic mass, knowing that it will not impact the overall survival of the patient. If the quality of life of the individual can be improved at an acceptable operative risk, then the surgical intervention is warranted.

Finally, the surgeon may be called upon to manage oncologic emergencies. Acute hemorrhage and obstruction of a hollow viscus represent the most common potential oncologic emergencies. In these cases, surgeons may have to emergently intervene in the care of a cancer patient or, in some instances, use nonsurgical approaches (eg, stents or angiography).

▶ Prophylaxis

With our improved understanding of inherited genetic mutations and the identification of patients who are predisposed to cancer, surgical therapy has expanded beyond the therapy of established tumors and into the prevention of cancer. Prophylaxis is not a new concept in surgical oncology. Patients with chronic inflammatory diseases are known to be at high risk of subsequent malignant transformation. This typically prompts close surveillance and surgical resection at the first identification of premalignant changes. One of the earliest examples of this is the recommendation for total proctocolectomy for subsets of patients with chronic ulcerative colitis.

The ability to perform genetic screening for relevant mutations has allowed for prophylactic surgery to be implemented prior to the onset of symptoms or histologic changes. Familial adenomatous polyposis (FAP) syndrome, defined by the diffuse involvement of the colon and rectum with adenomatous polyps, almost always predisposes to colorectal cancer if the large intestine is left in place. With the identification of the gene responsible for FAP, the adenomatous polyposis coli (APC) gene, members of families in which an APC mutation has been identified can have genetic testing prior to polyps becoming evident and be considered for prophylactic proctocolectomy. Medullary thyroid cancer (MTC) is a well-established component of multiple endocrine neoplasia syndrome type 2A (MEN 2A) or type 2B (MEN 2B). Mutations in the RET protooncogene are present in almost all cases of MEN 2A and MEN 2B. Family members of MEN patients can be screened for the presence of a RET mutation, and those with the mutation should undergo total thyroidectomy at a young age (6 years for MEN 2A, infancy for MEN 2B). The role of prophylactic mastectomies has been greatly expanded with the identification of BRCA1 and BRCA2, which can be associated with a lifetime probability of breast cancer of between 40% and 85%. Other prophylactic operations are listed in Table 47–1. However, potential benefits of prophylactic surgeries must be weighed against quality-of-life issues and the morbidity of the surgery. A detailed discussion must be held with each patient considering prophylactic surgery regarding the risks and benefits, so today's surgical oncologist needs a clear understanding of genetics and inherited risk.

CYTOTOXIC CHEMOTHERAPY

The goal of chemotherapeutic regimens is to deliver pharmacologic agents systemically to eradicate all tumor cells. The ideal tumor drug would kill cancer cells without harming normal tissues. No such agent exists, and most drugs affect normal cells to some extent. The success of chemotherapy

Table 47–1. Examples of prophylactic operations in surgical oncology.

Prophylactic Surgery	Potential Indications
Bilateral mastectomy	BRCA1 or BRCA2 mutation Atypical hyperplasia or lobular carcinoma in situ Familial breast cancer Radiation therapy to the chest before age 30
Bilateral oophorectomy	BRCA1 or BRCA2 mutation Familial ovarian cancer
Thyroidectomy	RET proto-oncogene mutation Multiple endocrine neoplasia type 2A (MEN 2A) Multiple endocrine neoplasia type 2B (MEN 2B) Familial non-MEN medullary thyroid carcinoma (FMTC)
Hysterectomy with or without salpingo-oophorectomy	Lynch syndrome
Total proctocolectomy	Familial adenomatous polyposis or antigen-presenting cell mutation Ulcerative colitis Hereditary nonpolyposis colorectal cancer germline mutation
Gastrectomy	CDH1

relies on the normal cell's greater capacity for repair and survival relative to tumor cells.

Even a single cancer cell can potentially reproduce to form a lethal tumor. For this reason, the goal of curative chemotherapy must be the complete eradication of all tumor cells. Tumor burden is important in chemotherapy. A large cancer may harbor more than 10^9 tumor cells. If a tolerable dose of an effective drug killed 99.99% of these cells, the tumor burden would still be 10^5 cells. The remaining cells, while clinically undetectable, are likely to continue to grow and lead to a clinical recurrence of cancer. For this reason, most chemotherapy protocols rely on repeated administrations of drugs in order to achieve maximal cell killing. Tumor cells may avoid the cell-killing effects of a particular drug because of their stage in the cell cycle, residence in an area protected from the drug (central nervous system), or an inherent resistance to the drug.

Drug resistance plays a large role in chemotherapy failures. Several mechanisms of tumor resistance are known. The multidrug resistance (MDR) gene encodes a protein that actively pumps drugs out of tumor cells. This gene confers resistance on a variety of antitumor drugs, including antibiotics and plant-derived compounds. Other tumor mechanisms of resistance include the alteration of target enzymes, increased production of a target enzyme to overwhelm the drug, and an increased capability for DNA repair. Tumor resistance to a given chemotherapeutic agent can often be overcome by the administration of multiple drugs.

▶ Principles of Chemotherapy Use

A. Curative Chemotherapy

Hematologic malignancies are typically treated by chemotherapy, radiation, or both, with surgery used primarily for diagnosis and staging. However, surgery is the primary treatment for nonhematologic malignancies, although there are some exceptions. Anal cancer is cured in approximately 80% of patients with the Nigro protocol—fluorouracil (FU)/mitomycin C and radiation therapy—as first-line treatment. Testicular cancer, even when metastatic, is curable with bleomycin/etoposide/cisplatin in approximately 85% of patients.

B. Adjuvant Treatment

Although all visible tumor may be removed at the time of surgery, microscopic tumor deposits may still be present locally or may have spread to distant locations. Chemotherapy is most effective against very small tumors and microscopic tumor deposits. Therefore, adjuvant chemotherapy is often given to improve the likelihood of cure after surgical resection.

The benefit gained from adjuvant chemotherapy can be thought of in terms of absolute benefit or relative benefit (Figure 47–1). For example, after colectomy for stage III colon cancer, the chance of cure is approximately 50%. This can be increased to approximately 70% by adjuvant FU/leucovorin. This represents a 40% relative benefit (40% more patients are cured with chemotherapy than without chemotherapy) but a 20% absolute benefit (20% of the patients who take the chemotherapy will have altered their outcome). Another way to look at this is that with a 20% absolute benefit, 80% of patients experience the inconvenience and side effects of chemotherapy without gaining any improvement themselves. The decision to receive adjuvant chemotherapy is a balance between the expected benefit of treatment, the patient's comorbid conditions and general health, and the patient's wishes.

C. Neoadjuvant Treatment

Neoadjuvant chemotherapy is usually given to facilitate surgical resection by shrinking the primary tumor, or it may convert an unresectable tumor into a resectable tumor. In some cases, this treatment has been shown to prolong survival. Another advantage to neoadjuvant chemotherapy is that it allows the oncologist to observe the primary tumor to determine if it is sensitive to a particular chemotherapeutic regimen. During the course of cancer treatment, it is important to define the progress and outcomes resulting from therapy. The terms complete and partial response are often used as end points to evaluate the efficacy of a particular therapeutic regimen. A **complete response** is defined as the absence of demonstrable cancer. A **partial response** refers to a reduction of tumor mass by greater than 50%. The patient's response to neoadjuvant chemotherapy can be an important predictor of outcome.

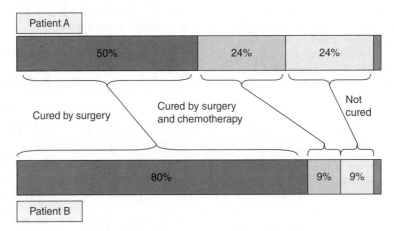

▲ **Figure 47–1.** Benefits of adjuvant chemotherapy. For 100 patients treated with adjuvant chemotherapy, some will be cured by surgery alone (dark red bar), some will die of other causes (gray bar), and some will die of their cancer (light red bar). Adjuvant therapy will prevent a cancer death in a portion of those patients (medium red bar). Adjuvant chemotherapy will result in a relative benefit of 50% for both patient A and patient B, meaning treatment will reduce the likelihood of dying of cancer by 50%. However, the absolute benefit is different for both patients. For patient A, who has a high likelihood of dying of disease, the absolute benefit is 24%. For patient B, who has a good prognosis, the absolute benefit is only 9%.

D. Chemotherapy for Metastatic Disease

The majority of patients who are receiving chemotherapy have metastatic disease that is not curable. For these patients, treatment with chemotherapy is intended to prolong survival, improve quality of life, or both. Response rates range from 20% to 75% depending on the tumor type and chemotherapy regimen. However, even a complete remission is rarely durable. Most partial or complete remissions last only months.

As with all therapies, the decision to use chemotherapy must balance the potential benefits with the risks, toxicities, and the patient's general health and condition. There is little to be gained by treating an asymptomatic patient if no prolongation of survival is expected. A detailed discussion must be held with each individual patient; some patients are more willing than others to tolerate the side effects of chemotherapy. Since the disease is not curable, treatment with single agents, which are less toxic than combination chemotherapy, is often considered, with more willingness to reduce doses for toxicity.

▶ Classes of Chemotherapeutic Agents

With all forms of curative chemotherapy, the goal is elimination of all tumor stem cells. Cells that are incapable of further division cannot cause progression of a tumor, and the sterilization of a tumor cell is as good as a kill. Chemotherapeutic drugs are generally classified as cell cycle–specific drugs, which are toxic to actively proliferating cells, or cell cycle–nonspecific drugs, which are capable of killing cells that are not dividing during drug exposure. These two classifications are not absolute, and many drugs may overlap between the two categories.

In order to achieve maximal cell killing, most therapeutic protocols use combination chemotherapy. Agents with differing mechanisms of action and different toxic side effects are used, allowing for relatively high doses of multiple agents. This method of combining agents helps to combat tumor cell resistance and increase the tumor cell killing while avoiding the compounding of toxic effects.

A. Alkylating Agents

These agents exert their effects by the transfer of alkyl groups to various cellular components, most importantly by the alkylation of DNA. Alkylators can cause DNA strand breaks, cross-linking of DNA strands, or miscoding of DNA during replication. The alkylating agents are considered cell cycle–nonspecific agents but tend to have their greatest effect on proliferating cells. Normal cells are able to avoid many of the lethal effects of alkylating agents because of their ability to repair DNA. The alkylating agents are effective in treatment of the hematologic malignancies and in a variety of solid tumors such as breast, melanoma, lung, and endometrial cancers. Included in this class are the nitrosoureas (eg, carmustine, semustine, lomustine), cyclophosphamide, chlorambucil, mechlorethamine, dacarbazine, and procarbazine.

B. Platinum Analogs

The platinum analogs are similar to the alkylating agents. They bind DNA to form interstrand and intrastrand cross-links, leading to inhibition of DNA synthesis and transcription. The mechanisms of cancer cell resistance are also similar to those of alkylating agents: decreased cellular uptake of the drugs, increased activity of DNA repair enzymes, and increased thiol-containing proteins. In addition, resistance to both cisplatin and carboplatin has been associated with a deficiency of mismatch repair (MMR) genes. It is not known why this mechanism of resistance appears to be specific to cisplatin and carboplatin, but the efficacy of the newest platinum analog, oxaliplatin, is not affected by MMR gene deficiency.

C. Antimetabolites

Rapidly dividing cells require increased synthesis of nucleic acid precursors. This increased synthesis can be exploited pharmacologically by the antimetabolites. These drugs are analogs of nucleic acids or nucleic acid precursors. The antimetabolites may be incorporated into the nucleic acids of a cell and serve as a false messenger. Antimetabolites can shut down the cellular synthetic machinery by binding to and inhibiting enzymes important in the production of nucleic acids. Since this class of drugs affects all rapidly proliferating cells, they are relatively toxic to normal tissues that have a high rate of cell turnover. Antimetabolites are most effective in the hematologic malignancies but are also used in the treatment of solid tumors such as breast and gastrointestinal cancers. They include methotrexate, mercaptopurine, thioguanine, fluorouracil, and cytarabine.

D. Antimicrotubule Agents

A variety of antitumor drugs are derived from natural plants (and are also known as plant alkaloids). Vincristine, vinblastine, docetaxel, and paclitaxel work by binding tubulin and poisoning the assembly of microtubules in the mitotic spindle. This leads to mitotic arrest in metaphase, and these compounds are effective only on rapidly dividing cell populations. The plant alkaloids are most useful for hematologic malignancies and breast, renal, testicular, and head and neck cancers.

E. Topoisomerase Inhibitors

These plant derivatives exert their antitumor effects by binding to and inhibiting various forms of the enzyme topoisomerase. Topoisomerases are responsible for the maintenance of DNA structure and are also important in the cleavage and religation of DNA strands. Inhibition of these enzymes leads to DNA strand breakage and structural damage. The topoisomerase inhibitors are also cell cycle–specific agents and have their greatest activity against rapidly proliferating cells. Examples include etoposide, teniposide, and topotecan. These drugs are used in the treatment of hematologic malignancies and lung, bladder, prostate, and testicular cancers.

F. Antibiotics

Most of the drugs in this class are derived from the soil fungus *Streptomyces*. All the antibiotics exert their antitumor effects by interference with the synthesis of nucleic acids. Most of the drugs in this class intercalate in DNA, blocking DNA synthesis and inducing strand breakages. The antibiotics are considered cell cycle–nonspecific, and they have antitumor activity against a wide variety of solid tumors. Included in this class of drugs are doxorubicin, dactinomycin, plicamycin, mitomycin, and bleomycin.

▶ Side Effects of Chemotherapy

Most side effects from chemotherapeutic regimens are the result of toxicities to rapidly dividing normal cell populations, particularly bone marrow and epithelial cells. Bone marrow suppression is an adverse effect of many of these drugs, resulting in neutropenia, thrombocytopenia, and even anemia. Mucosal ulcerations and alopecia also occur in patients treated with cell cycle–specific agents. Intractable nausea and vomiting is another common side effect that can severely affect quality of life. Testicular or ovarian failure can result from chemotherapy, leading to sterility. Many of these drugs also are powerful teratogens and should be avoided in pregnant patients. Finally, many of the alkylating agents have been implicated in the development of secondary cancers, especially hematologic malignancies.

REGIONAL THERAPY

Systemic chemotherapy is limited by toxicity to the host. Regional delivery of chemotherapeutic agents via arterial cannulation allows for high levels of drugs in the region of the primary tumor while decreasing systemic toxicity.

Isolated limb perfusion is a technique for the delivery of chemotherapeutic agents to an extremity with locally advanced cancer and is of benefit primarily in the treatment of extremity melanoma and sarcoma. In this approach, a tourniquet is applied to the extremity to occlude venous outflow. The major artery perfusing the limb is then isolated, cannulated, and perfused with hyperthermic chemotherapeutic agents using a pump oxygenator as for cardiopulmonary bypass. The perfusion is done in the operating room and lasts for approximately 1 hour. The cannula is then removed. Most protocols involve only a single treatment. Melphalan, an alkylating agent, is the most common agent used today in the treatment of both sarcomas and melanomas. In patients with extensive in-transit melanoma confined to an extremity, isolated limb perfusion can provide regional control and palliation. In patients with unresectable extremity sarcomas, preoperative limb perfusion may

shrink the tumor and allow for a limb-sparing resection. While improving regional control, this therapy has yet to show a definitive survival benefit. An alternate approach is isolated limb infusion, which involves using minimally invasive techniques to access the vessels along with a tourniquet to minimize systemic uptake.

Another approach is isolated hepatic artery infusion for the treatment of colorectal cancer metastatic to the liver. Metastatic tumors derive nearly all of their blood supply from the hepatic artery, while the normal liver parenchyma derives more than two-thirds of its blood supply from the portal system. This permits the delivery of higher doses of chemotherapeutic agents to the tumor relative to the normal hepatocytes. The drug most commonly used in this protocol is floxuridine, which is almost completely extracted on its first pass through the liver, resulting in relatively low systemic toxicity. Hepatic artery infusion requires the surgical placement of a catheter into the hepatic artery, which is connected to an implanted or external infusion pump for continuous treatment. Hepatic artery infusion has been used for unresectable colorectal metastases as well as an adjuvant to hepatic resection. Although there are clearly improved tumor responses in comparison to systemic therapy, the data are less clear on overall survival benefits. Some studies, however, have suggested an improved survival and have stimulated further investigation.

TARGETED THERAPIES

An expanding knowledge of molecular biology is revolutionizing the field of oncology, truly personalizing care for each individual patient with cancer. Molecular diagnostics is increasingly allowing us to customize the selection and dosing of traditional agents to maximize benefit and minimize toxicity. Molecular oncology is changing the way we approach drug discovery and development, leading to the development of targeted therapies. A targeted therapy is a drug with a focused mechanism that specifically acts on a well-defined target or biologic pathway. Inactivation of this target/pathway results in regression or destruction of the malignant cell. Targeted therapies are broadly classified as either monoclonal antibodies or small molecules. The name of a targeted therapy lets you know the type of agent; names that end with *–mab* are monoclonal antibodies, whereas small molecules end with *–ib*.

The ideal target is one that is expressed (and can be measured) on cancer cells but not significantly expressed in vital organs and tissues. It is preferably crucial to the malignant phenotype, and its inhibition results in a clinical response in patients whose tumor expresses the target. Several different types of targeted therapies have been approved for use, including signal transduction inhibitors, gene expression modulators, apoptosis inducers, and angiogenesis inhibitors. Table 47–2 lists many of the targeted therapies that have been approved for cancer therapy.

Table 47–2. Targeted therapeutic agents for cancer.

Drug Name	Brand Name	Target	Used in the Treatment of
Afatinib	Gilotrif	EGFR, HER2	NSCLC
Alectinib	Alencensa	ALK	NSCLC
Alemtuzumab	Campath	CD52	B-cell CLL
Axitinib	Inlyta	KIT, PDGFRβ, VEGFR	Renal cell carcinoma
Belinostat	Beleodaq	HDAC	Peripheral T-cell lymphoma
Bevacizumab	Avastin	VEGF	Glioblastoma, NSCLC, colorectal cancer, renal cell carcinoma
Bexarotene	Targretin	Retinoid X receptors	CTCL
Blinatumomab	Blincyto	CD19/CD3	ALL
Bortezomib	Velcade	Proteasome	Multiple myeloma, mantle cell lymphoma
Bosutinib	Bosulif	ABL	CML
Brentuximab	Adcetris	CD30	HL, anaplastic large-cell lymphoma
Brigatinib	Alunbrig	ALK	NSCLC
Cabozantinib	Cabometyx or Cometriq	FLT3, KIT, MET, RET, VEGFR2	Medullary thyroid cancer, renal cell carcinoma
Carfilzomib	Kyprolis	Proteasome	Multiple myeloma
Ceritinib	Zykadia	ALK	NSCLC
Cetuximab	Erbitux	EGFR	SCCa of the head and neck, colorectal cancer
Cobimetinib	Cotellic	MEK	Melanoma
Crizotinib	Xalkori	EML4-ALK	NSCLC
Dabrafenib	Tafinlar	BRAF	Melanoma, NSCLC
Daratumumab	Darzalex	CD38	Multiple myeloma
Dasatinib	Sprycel	SRC-family protein kinases	CML, ALL
Denosumab	Xgeva	RANKL	Giant cell tumor of the bone
Dinutuximab	Unituxin	B4GALNT1 (GD2)	Pediatric neuroblastoma
Erlotinib	Tarceva	EGFR	NSCLC, pancreatic cancer
Everolimus	Afinitor	Immunophilin FK binding protein-12	Renal cell carcinoma, astrocytoma, breast cancer, pancreatic neuroendocrine tumors
Gefitinib	Iressa	EGFR	NSCLC
Ibrutinib	Imbruvica	BTK	Mantle cell lymphoma, CLL
Idelalisib	Zydelig	PI3K	CLL, follicular B-cell NHL, small lymphocytic lymphoma
Imatinib mesylate	Gleevec	Bcr-abl, c-kit, PDGFR	GIST, DFSP, ALL, CML
Ixazomib	Ninlaro	Proteasome	Multiple myeloma
Lapatinib	Tykerb	EGFR, ErbB2, Erk-1 and Erk-2 AKT kinases	Breast cancer
Lenvatinib	Lenvima	VEGFR2	Renal cell carcinoma, thyroid cancer
Midostaurin	Rydapt	FLT3	Acute myeloid leukemia
Necitumumab	Portrazza	EGFR	Squamous NSCLC
Neratinib	Nerlynx	HER2	Breast cancer

(Continued)

Table 47–2. Targeted therapeutic agents for cancer. (*Continued*)

Drug Name	Brand Name	Target	Used in the Treatment of
Nilotinib	Tasigna	Bcr-abl, c-kit, PDGFR	CML
Niraparib	Zejula	PARP	Ovarian cancer, fallopian tube cancer, peritoneal cancer
Obinutuzumab	Gazyva	CD20	CLL
Ofatumumab	Arzerra	CD20	B-cell CLL
Olaparib	Lynparza	PARP	Ovarian cancer
Olaratumab	Lartruvo	PDGFRα	Soft tissue sarcoma
Osimertinib	Tagrisso	EGFR	NSCLC
Palbociclib	Ibrance	CDK4, CDK6	Breast cancer
Panitumumab	Vectibix	EGFR	Colorectal cancer
Panitumumab	Vectibix	EGFR	Colorectal cancer
Panobinostat	Farydak	HDAC	Multiple myeloma
Paxopanib	Votrient	VEGF, c-kit, PDGFR	Renal cell carcinoma, soft tissue sarcoma
Pertuzumab	Perjeta	HER2/neu	Breast cancer
Ponatinib	Iclusig	ABL, FGFR1-3, FLT3, VEGFR2	CML, ALL
Ramucirumab	Cyramza	VEGFR2	Colorectal cancer, gastric cancer, NSCLC
Regorafenib	Stivarga	KIT, PDGFRβ, RAF, RET, VEGFR	Colorectal cancer, GIST, hepatocellular carcinoma
Ribociclib	Kisqali	CDK4, CDK6	Breast cancer
Rituximab	Rituxan	CD20	B-cell NHL, CLL
Romidepsin	Istodax	HDACs	CTCL
Rucaparib	Rubraca	PARP	Ovarian cancer
Sorafenib	Nexavar	VEGFR, PDGFR, KIT, RAF	Renal cell carcinoma, hepatocellular carcinoma
Sunitinib	Sutent	PDGFR, VEGFR	Renal cell carcinoma, GIST, pancreatic neuroendocrine tumors
Temsirolimus	Torisel	mTOR	Renal cell carcinoma
Tositumomab	Bexxar	CD20	NHL
Trametinib	Mekinist	MEK	Melanoma, NSCLC
Traztuzumab	Herceptin	HER2/neu	Breast cancer, gastric adenocarcinoma
Tretinoin	Vesanoid	Retinoic acid receptors	Acute promyelocytic leukemia
Vandetanib	Caprelsa	EGFR, VEGFR2	Medullary thyroid
Vemurafenib	Zelboraf	*BRAF* V600E	Melanoma (*BRAF* V600E mutation)
Venetoclax	Venclexta	BCL2	CLL
Vismodegib	Erivedge	PTCH	Basal cell carcinoma
Vorinostat	Zolinza	HDACs	CTCL
Ziv-aflibercept	Zaltrap	PlGF, VEGF-A/B	Colorectal cancer

ALL, acute lymphoblastic leukemia; CLL, chronic lymphocytic leukemia; CML, chronic myelogenous leukemia; CTCL, cutaneous T-cell lymphoma; DFSP, dermatofibrosarcoma protuberans; EGFR, epidermal growth factor receptor; GIST, gastrointestinal stromal tumor; HDAC, histone deacetylase; HER2, human epidermal growth factor receptor 2; HL, Hodgkin lymphoma; NHL, non-Hodgkin lymphoma; NSCLC, non–small-cell lung cancer; PDGFR, platelet-derived growth factor receptor; SCCa, squamous cell carcinoma; VEGFR, vascular endothelial growth factor receptor.

Trastuzumab is an immunoglobulin (Ig) G antibody that binds to the juxtamembrane portion of the extracellular domain of the HER2/neu receptor and has become an important option for patients with HER2/neu–positive breast cancer. HER2/neu is an epidermal growth factor receptor that has a functional intracellular tyrosine kinase and, when overexpressed, can lead to increased proliferation, increased metastatic potential, and resistance to therapeutic agents. Although the binding of trastuzumab to the HER2/neu protein may lead to antibody-dependent cell-mediated cytotoxicity, the more important function appears to be the disruption of the downstream signaling through the intracellular tyrosine kinase. Another monoclonal antibody that targets HER2 is **pertuzumab.** Because pertuzumab targets a different subdomain on the HER2 receptor, the combination provides a dual blockade and can improve outcomes compared to single-agent therapy.

Another way to target cancer cells is through the use of small molecules. The development of **imatinib mesylate** is the classic example of a small-molecule targeted therapy. Imatinib is an adenosine triphosphate–binding selective inhibitor of *bcr-abl*, and its use has been associated with durable, complete responses in the treatment of Philadelphia chromosome–positive chronic myelogenous leukemia as well as the treatment of gastrointestinal stromal tumors. The latter characteristically express an activating mutation in the c-kit receptor tyrosine kinase (*RTK*) gene.

Perhaps the most noteworthy example of the impact of targeted therapies is in the treatment of melanoma. It was discovered that 40%-60% of melanoma patients harbor a specific mutation in the *BRAF* gene, and 90% of these mutations involve a substitution of glutamic acid for valine at amino acid 600 (the V600E mutation). This gene codes for the protein kinase BRAF, a component of the mitogen-activated protein (MAP) kinase pathway. Two U.S. Food and Drug Administration (FDA)–approved agents, **vemurafenib** and **dabrafenib**, selectively inhibit the kinase activity of this mutated *BRAF*. Dramatic results have been seen in patients with advanced melanoma who harbor the *BRAF* V600E mutation. Another targeted therapy used in combination with dabrafenib is **trametinib**, which blocks MEK, an alternate protein downstream of BRAF in the MAP kinase pathway. The combination not only improves outcomes, but also decreases the toxicity of treatment compared with single-agent therapy.

Finally, a new trend in oncology is the use of next-generation sequencing and what is being referred to as **precision medicine** or **personalized medicine**. Traditionally, treatment choices have been centered around the type of tumor. However, over the past decade, the feasibility and cost of next-generation sequencing has improved to the point where it is possible to obtain rapid and accurate sequencing of many genes at one time. This genomic data can then be used to design treatments based on disease-driving molecular alterations of an individual's specific tumor. Some studies have suggested as many as 30% of cases where genomic data identified a mutation that could be targeted by an existing targeted therapy, often a therapy not classically used for that tumor type. This represents a shift from treating tumors based on histology to treating tumors based on molecular alterations, regardless of histology. Ongoing studies are examining whether sequencing and personalized oncology improve outcomes.

HORMONAL THERAPY

Hormones are normally involved in the differentiation, stimulation, and control of certain tissues, including but not limited to lymphoid tissue, the uterus, the prostate, and the mammary glands. Tumors arising from these tissues may also be stimulated or inhibited by hormones, and so manipulation of the hormonal balance can be beneficial in the systemic therapy of these cancers. In some cases, hormones themselves are used as cancer therapies. For example, the administration of estrogen to a man ultimately suppresses the production of testosterone, which is a useful effect in the treatment of prostate cancer. Corticosteroids, particularly the glucocorticoids, have a powerful suppressive effect on lymphoid cells, making them useful in the treatment of acute leukemias, lymphomas, myeloma, and other myeloproliferative disorders. In most cases, however, hormonal therapy involves blocking the effects of hormones that stimulate proliferation.

▶ Estrogen & Androgen Inhibitors

One approach to hormonal therapy is to block the hormone receptor on the cell. Selective estrogen receptor modulators (SERMs) are medications that mimic the structure of estrogen. Because the estrogen receptor complex varies among tissue types, SERMs can have different effects on different tissues, sometimes inhibiting the actions of estrogen and sometimes behaving like estrogen. The most well-known SERM is tamoxifen (Nolvadex), which is used not only to treat estrogen-sensitive breast cancer, but also to prevent breast cancer in high-risk individuals. Because it also has some proestrogen properties, side effects of tamoxifen can include an increased risk of uterine cancer and deep vein thrombosis. Raloxifene (Evista) is a newer SERM that has been approved for prevention and treatment of postmenopausal osteoporosis and is used in the chemoprevention of breast cancer for postmenopausal women.

Flutamide (Eulexin) is a testosterone antagonist used in the treatment of prostate cancer. It works by blocking translocation of the androgen receptor to the nucleus. Although hormonal therapy for prostate cancer is palliative, it can be quite effective in slowing the progression of disease. Hormonal therapy can add several years to the life expectancy of patients with unresectable or metastatic disease. Flutamide is most effective when used in combination with surgical or pharmacologic castration.

Gonadotropin-Releasing Hormone Analogs

The most definitive way to block the production of testosterone and estrogen is by surgical castration. The pharmacologic equivalent of castration can be accomplished with gonadotropin-releasing hormone (GnRH) analogs. Normally, GnRH leads to the production of luteinizing hormone (LH) and follicle-stimulating hormone (FSH), the physiologic stimulators of sex hormone production. Analogs of GnRH lead to constant stimulation, which inhibits LH and FSH release and leads to decreased synthesis of the sex steroids. Leuprolide (Lupron) is commonly used to decrease testosterone levels in the treatment of unresectable prostate cancer. Goserelin (Zoladex) is often used in premenopausal women with hormone receptor–positive breast cancer.

Aromatase Inhibitors

Postmenopausal women have functionally inactive ovaries; however, estrogens are still produced to a lesser extent in extragonadal tissues, primarily the conversion of adrenal steroids in fat cells by the enzyme aromatase. Aromatase inhibitors, such as anastrozole (Arimidex), exemestane (Aromasin), and letrozole (Femara), eliminate functional estrogen in this population of women and are an effective hormonal treatment of breast cancer. A number of studies have demonstrated the benefit of aromatase inhibitors in postmenopausal women with hormone receptor–positive breast cancer, either as first-line therapy or after the use of tamoxifen.

RADIATION THERAPY

Radiation therapy may be used alone or in combination with surgery and chemotherapy and may be given with curative or palliative intent. Some tumors, such as head and neck cancers, prostate cancer, and Hodgkin disease, can often be cured by irradiation alone, eliminating the need for surgical resection or chemotherapy. More commonly, locoregional control of tumors involves surgical resection combined with localized radiation. The theoretical advantage of combining these two therapies is based on the mechanisms by which they fail to achieve their purpose. Surgical failures occur at the margins of tumors, whereas radiation therapy fails in the center of tumors, where the malignant cells are numerous and hypoxic conditions exist. Radiation failures are rare at the periphery of tumors, where cell numbers are low and oxygenation is high. Depending on tumor histology and location, radiation therapy can be used as a surgical adjunct either preoperatively or postoperatively. Preoperative radiation can shrink tumors and increase the chances for complete surgical resection in cancers such as sarcomas, rectal cancers, and superior sulcus lung cancers.

Principles of Radiation Therapy

Ionizing radiation is defined as energy with sufficient strength to cause the ejection of an orbital electron from an atom when the radiation is absorbed. Ionizing radiation can take either an electromagnetic form, as high-energy photons, or particulate forms, such as electrons, protons, neutrons, alpha particles, or other particles. Most radiation therapies use either photons or electrons. Electrons interact directly with tissue, causing ionization, in contrast to photons, which affect tissues by the electrons that they eject. Electron beams deliver a high skin dose and exhibit a rapid fall-off after only a few centimeters and are therefore commonly used to treat superficial targets such as skin cancers or lymph nodes within a few centimeters of the surface of the body. More commonly, electromagnetic radiation (high-energy photons) is used to treat cancer. This consists of either gamma rays (photons created from the decay of radioactive nuclei) or x-rays (photons created by interaction of accelerated electrons with electrons and nuclei of atoms in an x-ray tube target).

To quantify the interaction of radiation on tissues, one must first measure the ionization produced in air by the beam of radiation. This quantity is known as **exposure** and is measured in roentgens (R). One can then correct for the presence of soft tissue and calculate the **absorbed dose**: the amount of energy absorbed per unit mass. This quantity was previously measured in rads but today is typically measured as joules per kilogram, or gray (Gy) units: 100 rad = 100 cGy = 1 Gy. As photons enter tissue, the dose increases at first and then begins to fall off because radiation falls off with the square of the distance from the source (a law of physics known as the inverse-square law).

The effect on biological tissues when they encounter ionizing radiation comes from ejected electrons interacting either directly with target molecules within the cell or indirectly with water to produce free radicals (eg, hydroxyl radicals) that subsequently interact with target molecules. During their brief life span, electrons and free radicals interact with molecules in a random fashion. If they interact with molecules that are not crucial to cell survival, the effect of the radiation will be harmless. If they react with biologically important molecules, the effect will be detrimental. Molecular oxygen prolongs the life of reactive radicals, increasing the likelihood that it will have a detrimental effect. This is why tumor hypoxia tends to increase resistance to radiation.

Although ionizing radiation may damage many molecules with the cell, the most critical injury with respect to cell death appears to be DNA damage in the form of single-strand or double-strand breaks. Cells have relatively efficient repair mechanisms for single-strand breaks in DNA, but double-strand breaks in DNA are much more difficult for cells to repair, although not impossible. Therefore, the ability of ionizing radiation to kill cells is dependent not only on the generation of enough DNA double-strand breaks to overwhelm repair pathways, but also on the time the cell has to repair those breaks prior to the next mitotic cell division.

This phenomenon is known as **sublethal damage repair** in which increased cell survival is observed if a dose of radiation is divided into two fractions separated by a time interval. As the time interval between the fractions increases, the surviving fraction of the cells also increases as the cells are able to repair double-strand DNA breaks. Of course, in clinical radiation therapy, the goal is to kill the cancer cells but spare the normal cells. Delivering a single large dose of radiation will have a high rate of tumor cell killing, but the concordant killing of the normal tissue cells may limit the clinical utility due to normal tissue toxicity. This has led to the development of multifraction regimens commonly used today, typically delivering daily fractions of 1.8-2.5 Gy. *Fractionation* of radiation dose spares normal tissues because of their greater ability to repair sublethal damage between dose fractions and repopulate with cells if the overall time is sufficiently long.

▶ Modes of Delivery

A. Teletherapy

Radiation is administered by two methods: an external machine (teletherapy) or the implantation of radioactive sources in or around the tumor (brachytherapy). In the past, teletherapy radiation was delivered using cobalt-60, a radioisotope produced in nuclear reactors. Although cobalt machines were very reliable, their usefulness is restricted by limited penetration to deep tumors without significant skin toxicity and difficulty in confining the dose to normal tissues. Today, external radiation is most often administered using a linear accelerator capable of producing higher energy photons without the geometric disadvantages associated with cobalt-60 units.

No matter the source, the beam of radiation needs to be modified to get optimal delivery of the desired dose to the tumor while minimizing dose to the normal tissues. Typically, the beam of radiation is rectangular. Collimators are thick shielding devices made from materials with a high atomic number. Primary collimators at the head of the machine create a rectangular beam, and additional devices such as wedges, compensators, blocks, or multileaf collimators are used to further modify the beam to desired specifications. Wedges or compensators can optimize the dose distribution if the treatment surface is curved or irregular in shape. The beam can also be shaped using individually fashioned blocks custom-made for each patient's anatomy and tumor size and shape. In modern linear accelerators, multileaf collimators have replaced handmade blocks and allow automated and precise field shaping without the use of cumbersome handmade blocks.

B. Brachytherapy

Brachytherapy involves the placement of radioactive sources into or next to the target tissue. It takes advantage of the inverse-square law, which states that the intensity of electromagnetic radiation dissipates as the inverse square of the distance from the source. Thus, if radioactive sources can be placed so that the tumor is within a centimeter of the sources, the dose received by normal tissues just 2 cm distant from the source and 1 cm distant from the tumor would be one-fourth of the dose received by the tumor. This can allow delivery of a high dose to the tumor with only a modest dose to normal tissue.

There are many implantation techniques for brachytherapy. The surgical approach to the target volume may be interstitial (eg, prostate seed implantation), intracavitary (eg, gynecologic applicators), transluminal (eg, endoscopic applications), or surface mold techniques (eg, eye plaques for ocular melanoma). The implants may be permanent or temporary, and the dose may be delivered using low, medium, or high dose rates. Many modern applications use afterloading techniques that place treatment applicators and load radioactive sources afterward to reduce radiation exposure for therapy personnel.

▶ Complications of Radiation Therapy

A. Acute Radiation Effects

Acute radiation effects are those toxicities that occur within a few weeks to months of radiation therapy. They occur mainly in self-renewing tissues that are characterized by actively proliferating stem cells producing progeny that divide and differentiate into mature functioning cells. This includes bone marrow, skin and its appendages, and mucosal surfaces of the oropharynx, esophagus, stomach, intestines, rectum, bladder, and vagina. Once the normal life span of the mature cells expires, the normal turnover and replacement with new cells do not occur because of radiation killing of the dividing stem cells. Acute toxicity is influenced by both fraction size and the time interval between fractions. The more rapidly a given dose is delivered during the overall treatment period, the more severe the acute effects will be. A decrease in fraction size or prolongation of the interval between fractions allows the cell populations to repair and repopulate, decreasing the severity of acute toxicity.

Head and neck irradiation is one of the most toxic in the acute period due to significant mucositis of the oral cavity, oropharynx, larynx, and cervical esophagus. Skin and the salivary glands are also affected. Mucositis, yeast super-infection, desquamation, pain, xerostomia, odynophagia, dysphagia, dehydration, and malnutrition are all common clinical scenarios that radiation oncologists manage when delivering head and neck radiotherapy. Other common acute effects observed during radiation therapy directed at other anatomic sites include dysphagia and cough from thoracic radiation; nausea, vomiting, and diarrhea from abdominal radiation; and dysuria, proctitis, and perineal desquamation and pain from pelvic radiation.

B. Late Radiation Effects

Late effects are those toxicities that occur months to years after radiotherapy and are more commonly permanent. Mitotically inactive tissues without the capacity for self-renewal are commonly involved. The mechanism causing late effects may include direct damage to the parenchymal cells within an organ or indirect effects due to microvascular damage. Each organ is characterized by a **tolerance dose**, a radiation dose above which the risk of organ complications increases rapidly. These normal tissue tolerances are the true dose-limiting factors in clinical radiation therapy, because late complications can be permanent and in some cases life threatening.

The types of late complications induced by radiation can vary. For the brain, late toxicity may mean necrosis of the brain tissue, while in the kidney it may mean nephrotic syndrome and organ failure. The tolerance doses for different organs vary over a large range, from a few grays for sterility from testicular irradiation to over 100 Gy for necrosis or perforation of the uterus. Late complications may include fibrosis, necrosis, ulceration and bleeding, chronic edema, telangiectasias and pigmentation changes, cataract formation, nerve damage, lung pneumonitis and fibrosis, pericarditis, myocardial damage, bone fracture, liver or kidney failure, sterility, intestinal obstruction, and fistula and stricture formation.

IMMUNOTHERAPY

▶ Principles of Antitumor Immune Responses

Immunotherapy refers to treatments designed to kill tumor cells through immune mechanisms. There are two broad types of antitumor immune responses, one involving the humoral arm of the immune system and the other involving the cellular arm. Humoral immunity involves antibody production by mature B lymphocytes. Cell-mediated immunity involves stimulation of cytotoxic (CD8+) T cells through a major histocompatibility complex (MHC) class I–restricted process and stimulation of helper (CD4+) T cells through an MHC class II–restricted process. The humoral and cell-mediated immune responses overlap in that the activation of a B-cell response usually requires the presence of helper T cells.

Essential to the generation of an immune response through either arm of the immune system is the ability of antigen-presenting cells (APCs), most commonly dendritic cells (DCs) but also monocytes and macrophages, to process and present tumor-associated peptide antigens. Proteins are phagocytosed by APCs and partially digested into smaller polypeptides. These small-peptide antigens are then bound to MHC molecules on the cell surface. These unique antigen–MHC complexes can then be recognized by naïve T lymphocytes through the T-cell receptor (TCR). Activation of a naïve T-cell requires two signals. The first comes from the recognition of the antigen–MHC molecule by the TCR. The second signal comes from the binding of co-stimulatory molecules on the T cell to their ligands on the APC. Most commonly, this involves the binding of CD28 on the T cells to B7.1 and B7.2 on the APC. These two signals then result in activation, proliferation, and differentiation of the T cell. There are different types of T cells. There are two types of helper (CD4+) T cells. The Th1 helper T cells produce cytokines that help promote a cellular response (interleukin [IL]-2, interferon [IFN]-γ, tumor necrosis factor α, and granulocyte-macrophage colony-stimulating factor). These help with the activation of cytotoxic (CD8+) T cells, which again need recognition of antigen being presented on MHC class I molecules as well as co-stimulatory molecules. Once activated, cytolytic T cells destroy tumor cells via TCR recognition of tumor-specific antigen presented on MHC class I molecules at the tumor cell surface. Antigen-specific T cells bind to the MHC I receptor–tumor antigen complex and destroy the tumor cell via the release of granules containing granzyme B and perforin and via induction of the Fas/Fas ligand apoptosis. Cytotoxic T cells can only recognize antigen expressed on the tumor surface in the context of the MHC class I molecule.

The second type of helper T cell (Th2) secretes B-cell stimulatory cytokines (IL-4, IL-5, and IL-10), which results in the proliferation and differentiation of plasma cells. As opposed to a cellular response, for an antibody response, the antigens do not have to be presented on class I MHC receptors. Tumor cells can then be killed by a variety of methods. Antibody-dependent cell-mediated cytotoxicity involves the attachment of tumor-specific antibodies to tumor cells and the subsequent destruction of the tumor cell by the natural killer (NK) cell. Complement-dependent cell-mediated cytotoxicity involves the recognition and attachment of complement-fixing antibodies to tumor-specific surface antigens followed by complement activation. A third mechanism of tumor destruction, opsonization, results when tumor-specific antibodies attach to their target antigens on tumor cell surfaces, thus marking them for engulfment by macrophages.

In addition to the mechanisms to generate and propagate an immune response, the immune system also has several mechanisms to limit that response. One mechanism includes negative costimulatory molecules like cytotoxic T lymphocyte-associated antigen 4 (CTLA-4) and PD-1 that serve to attenuate T-cell activation. CTLA-4 is immediately upregulated on activated T cells and dampens TCR signaling by competing with the co-stimulatory molecule CD28 for the B7 ligands. PD-1 is also expressed upon activation. When it binds to its ligand, PD-L1, it leads to a negative feedback loop to attenuate local T-cell responses.

Other cells of the immune system serve to suppress an immune response, including myeloid-derived suppressor cells, regulatory T cells, and subsets of DCs that possess a regulatory function. Several immunosuppressive cytokines within the tumor microenvironment (IL-6, IL-10, and transforming growth factor-β) also function to suppress an immune response. These regulatory functions are necessary to prevent lymphoproliferative disorders, excess tissue damage, and autoimmune diseases. However, neoplasms may also take advantage of this, creating an immunosuppressive network within the tumor microenvironment that protects the tumor from immune attack.

The generation of an effective anticancer immune response therefore requires a series of stepwise events to be initiated. These seven steps are often referred to as the *cancer-immunity cycle*. This includes (1) the release of cancer-specific antigens from cancer cells, (2) presentation of these antigens by APCs, (3) activation of T cells, (4) trafficking of T cells to tumors, (5) infiltration of T cells into the tumor microenvironment, (6) recognition of cancer cells by the T cell, and (7) the killing of cancer cells.

Immunotherapy generally takes two forms: passive and active. Passive immunotherapy involves therapeutic agents that directly or indirectly mediate tumor killing. Examples include the use of monoclonal antibodies or adoptive (cellular) immunotherapy.

Active immunotherapy, on the other hand, is the delivery of materials designed to augment and propagate the cancer-immunity cycle. This can further be broken down to specific and nonspecific active immunotherapies. Specific immunotherapies seek to initiate an immune response to cancer-specific antigens, whereas nonspecific immunotherapy seeks to stimulate the immune cycle in general to augment a preexisting immune recognition.

▶ Passive Immunotherapy (Monoclonal Antibodies)

The development of monoclonal antibodies with unique specificity to tumor antigens has allowed for multiple attempts to use them as cancer therapy. In addition to their relative selectivity and minimal toxicity, they are easily mass produced for widespread application. In some cases, monoclonal antibodies work primarily through the immune system (antibody-dependent cell-mediated cytotoxicity), whereas in other cases, they behave more as targeted therapies (see earlier section on targeted therapies). Examples of monoclonal antibodies that are primarily immunotherapies include rituximab and alemtuzumab. Rituximab (Rituxan) is an anti-CD20 monoclonal antibody that is approved for the treatment of relapsed or refractory low-grade or follicular non-Hodgkin lymphoma. Alemtuzumab (Campath) targets CD52, which is present on both B and T cells and is used in the treatment of B-cell chronic lymphocytic leukemia.

▶ Adoptive Immunotherapy

Adoptive cellular immunotherapy is the passive administration of cells with antitumor activity to the tumor-bearing host. Tumor-infiltrating lymphocytes (TILs) are lymphocytes that infiltrate growing tumors and recognize tumor-associated antigens. These can be isolated from tumor specimens or the blood and expanded ex vivo by growing them in the presence of IL-2. TILs have been isolated from virtually all types of tumors; however, there are significant challenges in isolating and expanding TILs.

Rather than finding naturally occurring T cells that recognize tumor, a newer approach is to modify T cells from the patient to recognize tumor antigens and then delivering these back to the patient. One method is to transduce lymphocytes with a retrovirus that encodes for TCRs that already recognize cancer antigens. This is referred to as modified TCR therapy and has been shown to be clinically effective in melanoma and sarcoma, although with limited benefit.

A second approach is to generate chimeric antigen receptor T cells, or CAR-T cells. Chimeric antigen receptors are not TCRs; instead, they consist of fusion molecules composed of an antibody specific for a tumor antigen and signaling molecules that trigger T-cell effector functions. CAR-T cells target antigens on the cell surface, whereas genetically modified TCR cells target antigens that are part of the intracellular proteome. The ideal target for CAR-T therapy is a cell surface marker that is ubiquitously expressed on the tumor cells, is essential for tumor survival (so there can be no tumor escape), and has minimal off-target expression on essential cells. As an example, CAR-T cells that recognize CD19, which is expressed on most of the B-lineage cells, have been highly successful in treating certain B-cell malignancies. To date, CAR-T therapy for solid tumors has proven more challenging.

▶ Active Immunotherapy

As opposed to passive immunotherapy, active immunotherapy aims to stimulate the patient's immune system against the cancer. Instead of administering antibodies or effector cells, an agent is given to the patient to initiate or augment an antitumor immune response.

▶ Cytokines

Cytokines are naturally occurring soluble proteins produced by mononuclear cells of the immune system that can affect the growth and function of cells through interaction with specific cell-surface receptors. There have been over 50 cytokines isolated to date, and several have subsequently been approved by the FDA for clinical use, including interferon-α and IL-2.

The interferons (IFN-α, IFN-β, and IFN-γ) were originally described as proteins produced by virally infected cells that serve to protect against further viral infection through a variety of effects. These include the increased antigen presentation via increased expression of MHC and antigens, enhancement of NK cell function, and the enhancement of antibody-dependent cell-mediated cytotoxicity. In addition, the interferons exert direct antiangiogenic, cytotoxic, and cytostatic effects. Although the anticancer effects of IFN-β and IFN-γ have been disappointing, several hematologic and solid tumors have proved responsive to IFN-α, including chronic myelogenous leukemia, cutaneous T-cell lymphoma, hairy cell leukemia, and Kaposi sarcoma.

IL-2 was originally described as the "T-cell growth factor" because it is required for the differentiation and proliferation of activated T cells. As such, it seems like an ideal choice for immunotherapy. The major drawback of IL-2 is the significant dose-related toxicity. IL-2 leads to significant interstitial edema and vascular depletion and lymphoid infiltration into vital organs, possibly resulting in severe hypotension and ischemic damage to the heart, liver, kidneys, and bowel, which limits the use of IL-2 to patients with excellent performance status, normal pulmonary and cardiac function, and no active infections. Despite these limitations, IL-2 has proved to be an effective therapy in patients with metastatic melanoma and metastatic renal cell carcinoma.

▶ Specific Active Immunotherapy (Vaccines)

The goal of cancer vaccines is to generate a host immune response to known or unknown tumor-associated antigens. Many different vaccine strategies have been under investigation, each with advantages and disadvantages in regard to clinical feasibility, cost, the number of antigens available, and the mechanism of response (cellular, humoral, or both). Some vaccine strategies use specific peptide antigens. These are highly purified and therefore are easy to standardize, distribute, and administer. Unfortunately, immunizing a patient against a single antigen has several drawbacks that limit the potential clinical benefit. If a peptide vaccine does stimulate a response, it may not be the "right" peptide for many patients. Even commonly expressed tumor antigens are not present on all patients' tumors, or they may be present in varying degrees. In addition, the T cell's recognition of an antigen depends on the presentation of that antigen on a specific MHC molecule. Only certain human leukocyte antigen (HLA) phenotypes can present any given peptide to induce an immune response, so they will function only on a limited subset of patients. A classic example is that of the MART-1/Melan-A antigen in melanoma. The antigen is expressed by 80% of melanomas, but the peptide only binds to HLA-A2. Because only about 45% of Caucasians have HLA-A2, only

36% (80% of 45%) of melanoma patients given a MART-1/Melen-A vaccine would see a benefit. Finally, a cancer can escape immune recognition rather simply if a population of cells stops expressing that antigen or the MHC molecule.

For many cancers, only a few tumor-associated antigens have been defined; these may not be present in a large percentage of patients. Using the patient's cancer as the vaccine precludes the need to identify specific antigens. Autologous tumor cell vaccines are created from cancer cells harvested from the patient, altered to be more immunogenic, and irradiated, before being returned to the patient to stimulate a tumor-specific immune response. This approach is limited to individuals with sufficient tumor to prepare a vaccine. Trials are restricted to patients with bulky nodal or accessible distant metastatic disease who have a poor overall prognosis to begin with. Furthermore, the technical complexities inherent in procuring tumor and preparing a vaccine have made it difficult to conduct multi-institutional trials to test the efficacy of these vaccines.

Because many tumor-associated antigens are shared among a large number of patients, it is possible that one could create a vaccine from cultured cell lines that would stimulate an antitumor immune response in any patient who shared some of those antigens. This is the principle behind allogeneic tumor cell vaccines. This approach offers several advantages over autologous vaccines: Allogeneic vaccines are readily available, even for patients who lack sufficient tumor to produce an autologous tumor cell vaccine, and can be standardized, preserved, and distributed in a manner akin to any other therapeutic agent.

▶ Checkpoint Inhibition

As described earlier, the immune system has natural checks and balances to prevent an immune response from getting out of hand, which could lead to attacks on normal cells (autoimmune disorders) or lymphoproliferative disorders. Cancer may take advantage of these suppressive mechanisms to avoid immune surveillance. The newest form of immunotherapy, and to date the most effective, has been checkpoint inhibition. This involves the use of drugs meant to interrupt the negative feedback loop and augment an immune response. These drugs have resulted in remarkable outcomes in a variety of cancers, including some that have not classically been thought of as immunogenic.

Activated T lymphocytes express the molecule CTLA-4, which exerts a suppressive effect on the induction of immune response through its interactions with the B7 ligands (B7-1 or CD80, B7-2 or CD86) on APCs. Blocking the binding of CTLA-4 through the use of monoclonal antibodies can therefore enhance antitumor T-cell responses. Ipilimumab (Yervoy), a monoclonal antibody to CTLA-4, has been shown to cause tumor regression and improve survival in patients with metastatic melanoma and renal cell carcinoma.

It is also approved in the adjuvant setting in the treatment of high-risk melanoma.

PD-1 is a receptor expressed on the surface of activated mature T cells and NK cells as well as B cells, monocytes, and normal tissues. It acts via interactions with its ligand, PD-L1 (B7-H1), primarily in T-cell modulation in peripheral tissues and plays a crucial role in the maintenance of peripheral tolerance. The binding of PD-1 on T cells to PD-L1 can prevent T-cell function and lead to anergy. Although this helps prevent autoimmune disorders, it can also serve as one mechanism by which cancer cells evade immune attack. This can be interrupted by either the use of an anti–PD-1 monoclonal antibody or an anti–PD-L1 monoclonal antibody. Multiple trials have demonstrated antitumor activity in a number of cancers, including melanoma, renal cell carcinoma, non-small-cell lung cancer, breast cancer, Merkel cell carcinoma, squamous cell carcinoma of the head and neck, and others. Several checkpoint inhibitors in use today are listed in Table 47–3.

Checkpoint inhibitors may be used in combination, either with other checkpoint inhibitors or other active immunotherapy agents. For example, the combination of CTLA-4 blockade with PD-1 blockade improves both the objective response rate and overall survival of patients with advanced melanoma. Checkpoint inhibitors can also be combined with other immune-stimulating agents, chemotherapy, or targeted therapies, and multiple ongoing clinical trials are exploring the efficacy of these combinations. However, the checkpoint inhibitors do have significant toxicity, particularly those related to immune-related adverse events. These adverse events include pulmonary pneumonitis, colitis, hepatitis, endocrinopathies (hypophysitis or hypothyroidism), and dermatologic complications. These can sometimes be life threatening and require cessation of therapy and treatment with immunosuppressants.

SPECIFIC TYPES OF MALIGNANT NEOPLASMS

SOFT TISSUE SARCOMA

Soft tissue sarcomas account for approximately 1% of all new cancer diagnoses. Almost half of all patients diagnosed with the disease eventually die as a result of the cancer. Soft tissue sarcomas can occur anywhere in the body, but most originate in an extremity (41%), the trunk (10%), the retroperitoneum (16%), visceral sites (21%), or the head and neck (12%). Soft tissue sarcomas originate from a wide variety of mesenchymal cell types and include malignant fibrous histiocytoma, liposarcoma, rhabdomyosarcoma, leiomyosarcoma, and desmoid tumors. Although the histopathology of these tumors is highly variable, with some exceptions, they tend to behave in a fashion dictated by tumor grade rather than the cell of origin.

Most soft tissue sarcomas arise de novo, and rarely do they result from malignant degeneration of a benign lesion. There are several familial syndromes in which patients are genetically predisposed to the formation of soft tissue sarcomas, including Li-Fraumeni syndrome, Recklinghausen disease, and Gardner syndrome. Other proven risk factors exist that may increase the chances of sarcoma formation. External radiation therapy can increase the incidence of sarcomas by 8- to 50-fold. Chronic extremity lymphedema also increases the risk for lymphangiosarcoma. A classic example is the development of upper extremity lymphangiosarcomas in the lymphedematous arm of women treated for breast cancer (Stewart-Treves syndrome). Other less clear associations link chronic tissue trauma and occupational chemical exposures with an increased risk for sarcoma formation.

Grade is a significant prognostic factor in sarcoma and one of the few malignancies where grade is factored into

Table 47–3. Checkpoint inhibitors used for cancer immunotherapy.

Drug Name	Brand Name	Target	Used in the Treatment of
Ipilimumab	Yervoy	CTLA-4	Melanoma, RCC
Nivolumab	Opdivo	PD-1	Melanoma, colorectal cancer, SCCa of the head and neck, hepatocellular carcinoma, HL, NSCLC, RCC, urothelial carcinoma
Pembrolizumab	Keytruda	PD-1	Melanoma, cHL, colorectal cancer, gastric cancer, NSCLC, SCCa of the head and neck, urothelial cancer
Atezolizumab	Tecentriq	PD-L1	Urothelial carcinoma, NSCLC
Avelumab	Bavencio	PD-L1	Merkel cell carcinoma, urothelial cancer
Durvalumab	Imfinzi	PD-L1	Urothelial cancer, NSCLC

cHL, classical Hodgkin lymphoma; HL, Hodgkin lymphoma; NSCLC, non–small-cell lung cancer; RCC, renal cell carcinoma; SCCa, squamous cell carcinoma.

the staging system. Grade is determined by the French Federation Nationale des Cetres de Lutte Contre le Cancer (FNCLCC) system and incorporates the differentiation (which is highly dependent on the histologic subtype), the mitotic count, and the degree of tumor necrosis (Table 47–4). Because grading is based on the cellular architecture and invasive nature of the tumor, FNAB is not a typically useful biopsy technique for the initial diagnosis of a sarcoma. If a tumor is small (< 3 cm) and superficial, excisional biopsy should be performed. All extremity biopsy incisions should be oriented longitudinally, as the biopsy incision scar should be excised in a subsequent definitive

resection of the tumor. Core needle biopsies may be performed for large, palpable, superficial tumors. For large, deep tumors or those adjacent to vital structures, where core needle biopsy is not advised or failed, incisional biopsy should be considered. The incision should be centered over the mass, tissue flaps should not be raised, and meticulous hemostasis should be ensured, all to prevent the dissemination of tumor cells into adjacent tissue planes.

There are different staging systems for soft tissue sarcoma depending on where the cancer is in the body, as location can impact prognosis (eg, retroperitoneal sarcomas have a worse prognosis than extremity or trunk sarcomas). The major features of the staging system for soft tissue sarcomas include the grade of the tumor, its size, and the presence of nodal or metastatic disease. The staging for trunk/extremity sarcoma and retroperitoneal sarcomas is shown in Table 47–5. Sarcomas generally metastasize by the hematogenous route. Lymph node involvement is rare with most soft tissue sarcomas, although it may occur with epithelioid sarcoma, clear cell sarcoma, angiosarcoma, rhabdomyosarcoma, or synovial sarcoma. The vast majority of metastases from extremity sarcomas are to the lung, whereas the majority of retroperitoneal tumors metastasize to the liver.

Table 47–4. FNCLCC grading for soft tissue sarcoma.

Tumor Differentiation[1]	
Differentiation Score	**Definition**
1	Resembles normal adult mesenchymal tissue, may be confused with a benign lesion, such as well-differentiated liposarcoma
2	Histologic typing is certain, such as myxoid liposarcoma
3	Synovial sarcoma, osteosarcoma, Ewing sarcoma/PNET, sarcomas of doubtful tumor type, embryonal and undifferentiated sarcomas
Mitotic Count	
Mitotic Count Score	
1	0-9 mitoses per 10 HPF
2	10-19 mitoses per 10 HPF
3	≥ 20 mitoses per 10 HPF
Tumor Necrosis	
Necrosis Score	
0	No necrosis
1	< 50% tumor necrosis
2	≥ 50% tumor necrosis
Grade (based on sum of differentiation, mitotic count, and necrosis scores)	
GX	Grade cannot be assessed
G1	Total score of 2 or 3
G2	Total score of 4 or 5
G3	Total score of 6, 7, or 8

FNCLCC, French Federation Nationale des Cetres de Lutte Contre le Cancer; HPF, high-power field; PNET, primitive neuroectodermal tumor.
[1]Tumor differentiation is histology specific.

▶ Treatment of Extremity Sarcomas

Magnetic resonance imaging (MRI) is the imaging modality of choice for any suspected extremity sarcoma because it is most accurate in defining the extent of the tumor and invasion of surrounding structures. MRI is also used for follow-up imaging to assess response in patients undergoing therapy, as well as for local and regional recurrence. A chest x-ray or chest CT should be obtained in order to evaluate for pulmonary metastases in patients with high-grade tumors.

Surgery remains the primary therapy for localized extremity sarcomas, but multimodality therapy is recommended to minimize the likelihood of recurrence or the need for amputation. Historically, amputation was the only form of curative surgical therapy for large extremity sarcomas, but multimodality therapy has allowed for a high rate of limb preservation. Today, fewer than 5% of patients with extremity soft tissue sarcoma require amputation, which is generally reserved for patients whose tumors do not respond to preoperative therapy and cannot be resected adequately, have no evidence of metastatic disease, and have a good prognosis for rehabilitation.

A pseudocapsule composed of tumor cells surrounds sarcomas, and local invasion along fascial planes and neurovascular structures is common. It is important not to dissect along the pseudocapsule, which is associated with high local recurrence rates, but rather obtain a wide (2-cm) margin of normal tissue. This may need to be compromised in the immediate vicinity of functionally important neurovascular structures. If the tumor involves these structures, nerve grafts and arterial reconstruction with autologous or

Table 47–5. AJCC eighth edition staging system for soft tissue sarcoma.

DEFINITIONS OF AJCC TNM

Definition of Primary Tumor (T)

T Category	T Criteria
TX	Primary tumor cannot be assessed
T0	No evidence of primary tumor
T1	Tumor 5 cm or less in greatest dimension
T2	Tumor more than 5 cm and less than or equal to 10 cm in greatest dimension
T3	Tumor more than 10 cm and less than or equal to 15 cm in greatest dimension
T4	Tumor more than 15 cm in greatest dimension

Definition of Regional Lymph Node (N)

N Category	N Criteria
N0	No regional lymph node metastasis or unknown lymph node status
N1	Regional lymph node metastasis

Definition of Distant Metastasis (M)

M Category	M Criteria
M0	No distant metastasis
M1	Distant metastasis

Staging Group for Trunck or Extremity Sarcoma

When T is...	And N is...	And M is...	And grade is...	Then the stage group is...
T1	N0	M0	G1, GX	IA
T2, T3, T4	N0	M0	G1, GX	IB
T1	N0	M0	G2, G3	II
T2	N0	M0	G2, G3	IIIA
T3, T4	N0	M0	G2, G3	IIIB
Any T	N1	M0	Any G	IV
Any T	Any N	M1	Any G	IV

Staging Group for Retroperitoneal Sarcoma

When T is...	And N is...	And M is...	And grade is...	Then the stage group is...
T1	N0	M0	G1, GX	IA
T2, T3, T4	N0	M0	G1, GX	IB
T1	N0	M0	G2, G3	II
T2	N0	M0	G2, G3	IIIA
T3, T4	N0	M0	G2, G3	IIIB
Any T	N1	M0	Any G	IIIB
Any T	Any N	M1	Any G	IV

Used with the permission of the American College of Surgeons. Amin MB, Edge SB, Greene FL, et al. (Eds.) *AJCC Cancer Staging Manual,* 8th Ed. Springer New York, 2017.

prosthetic conduits may be required. Large soft tissue defects often require the construction of myocutaneous flaps to improve function and cosmesis. Soft tissue sarcomas rarely invade bone or skin, and wide resections of these structures are infrequently necessary.

Following wide local excision, metal clips should be placed at all margins of the resection in order to guide subsequent radiotherapy. For patients with T1 tumors located superficially in an area where it is not difficult to obtain widely negative margins, postoperative radiation therapy may not be necessary. For most other lesions, postoperative radiation is almost always recommended, with either external beam radiation or brachytherapy. Radiation should be started 4-8 weeks after surgery, as delay can result in a lower local control rate. Preoperative radiotherapy may have some advantages in patients with large tumors. Lower doses can be delivered to an undisturbed tumor bed, which may also have better oxygenation, and larger tumors may decrease in size, allowing for limb-sparing procedures. Preoperative radiation is associated with an increase in short-term wound complications but a decrease in long-term tissue fibrosis and edema. The optimal mode and sequence for treatment have yet to be defined and often require a multidisciplinary approach.

Adjuvant chemotherapy remains controversial. Chemotherapy can be given either preoperatively or postoperatively. Preoperative chemotherapy is sometimes recommended because in addition to the early treatment of micrometastatic disease, it allows for assessment of tumor response, which helps avoid prolonged therapy in patients not responding. However, although disease-free survival may be improved, there are conflicting data on overall survival. A recent meta-analysis of randomized trials suggested there may be a small survival benefit for extremity sarcomas, and so its use has increased.

The vast majority of localized recurrences in soft tissue sarcomas occur in the first 2 years after resection, necessitating close follow-up during that period. A local recurrence is not indicative of systemic disease and, in the absence of evidence of metastases, should be treated aggressively in the same manner as a primary tumor. The resection of pulmonary metastases should be considered in patients who have fewer than four radiographically detectable lesions and who have achieved apparent local control following resection of the primary tumor. In such circumstances, disease-free survival can approach 25%-35%.

▶ Treatment of Retroperitoneal Sarcomas

Retroperitoneal sarcomas compose approximately 15% of all soft tissue sarcomas, with liposarcoma, malignant fibrous histiocytoma, and leiomyosarcoma being the three most common types. They usually present as a large abdominal mass. Nearly half are over 20 cm in size at diagnosis. Once they compress or invade contiguous structures, they can cause symptoms such as abdominal pain or nausea and vomiting. Workup should include CT of the abdomen and pelvis to evaluate the mass as well as CT of the lung and liver to look for metastases. CT-guided core biopsy is the sampling technique of choice, with open or laparoscopic incisional biopsy reserved for inconclusive core biopsies.

As with extremity sarcomas, surgery represents the primary treatment, with the goal being en bloc resection with a rim of normal tissue. Although retroperitoneal tumors are generally large at presentation and often invade vital structures, the majority of these tumors are resectable. Retroperitoneal sarcomas rarely invade surrounding organs, but an intense desmoplastic reaction makes it difficult to assess the extent of tumor, so often these organs need to be resected rather than risk positive margins. The kidney, colon, pancreas, and spleen are the most commonly resected organs.

Although adjuvant radiation therapy is standard in extremity sarcoma, evidence supporting its use in retroperitoneal sarcoma is less convincing. Because of the low tolerance to radiation of the abdominal and retroperitoneal organs, delivery of adequate radiotherapy is often difficult. There is encouraging evidence for intraoperative radiation therapy to the tumor bed, but this technique is still considered investigational and can be performed only in select centers. Although complex, preoperative radiation may be beneficial because it uses lower radiation doses, is less injurious to the small bowel, and can increase respectability by shrinking the tumor and creating a thickened capsular structure around the lesion.

Brennan MF, Antonescu CR, Alektiar KM, et al: *Management of Soft Tissue Sarcoma*. New York, NY: Springer; 2016.
Wong SL: Sarcomas of soft tissues and bone. In Mulholland MW, et al (eds): *Scientific Principles and Practice*, 6th ed. Philadelphia, PA: Lippincott Williams & Wilkins; 2017.

MELANOMA

The incidence of melanoma is unfortunately rising. The reasons for this rise are not clear but are most likely related to an increased exposure to ultraviolet radiation from sunlight. Individuals whose first sunburn occurred at an early age or have had three or more sunburns before age 21 have an increased incidence of melanoma, as do individuals who use tanning beds. Other risk factors include freckles, a fair complexion, reddish or blond hair, blue eyes, a first-degree relative with melanoma, and the presence of multiple or dysplastic nevi.

The best approach to melanoma is to prevent it from occurring, through sun avoidance and sun protection with sunscreens with a sun protection factor (SPF) of 30 or higher. Second to prevention, the most significant impact on melanoma comes from early recognition and diagnosis. The prognosis of melanoma is inversely and dramatically related to the depth of invasion at diagnosis (Breslow thickness), emphasizing the importance of early diagnosis of this disease. Lesions that are suspicious for melanoma can be identified by their clinical characteristics, often referred to as the ABCDs of melanoma, and include asymmetry (A), irregular borders (B), color variation (C), and a difference (D) or change in the lesion. Diagnosed early, well over 90% of primary melanomas can be cured with surgical excision alone. Patients presenting with thicker lesions or regional nodal metastases have a significantly poorer prognosis. The AJCC staging system is presented in Table 47–6.

There are several distinct categories of melanoma; the four most common are superficial spreading, nodular, lentigo maligna, and acral lentiginous melanoma.

Superficial spreading melanoma is the most common presentation, accounting for nearly 70% of all melanomas. These usually occur in sun-exposed areas of the body or in individuals with multiple dysplastic nevi. They generally arise in preexisting nevi and can occur at any age after puberty. The superficial spreading subtype tends to grow in a radial pattern during the earlier stages and converts to a vertical growth pattern during the later stages of development.

Nodular melanomas account for between 15% and 25% of all melanomas. These tend to occur in older individuals and are more common in men. Nodular melanomas generally develop de novo, not in a preexisting nevus. They usually are dome shaped with distinct borders and often resemble a blood blister. Nodular melanomas occur most commonly on the head, neck, and trunk. They lack a significant horizontal growth phase and tend to be deep at the time of diagnosis.

Lentigo maligna melanoma has less propensity to metastasize and thus has a more favorable prognosis relative to the other subtypes. However, it can be locally aggressive, with high recurrence rates after excision. These lesions account for 4%-10% of melanomas and occur in an older population. Lentigo maligna lesions almost always develop in sun-exposed areas. They have a long horizontal growth phase and often have very convoluted borders.

Acral lentiginous melanomas account for between 2% and 8% of melanomas in Caucasians but for 30%-60% of melanomas in blacks, Asians, and Hispanics. These lesions do not occur in sun-exposed areas; instead, they occur on the sole of the foot, the palm, beneath the nail beds, and in the perineal region. Acral lentiginous melanomas are often large, with an average diameter of 3 cm at the time of diagnosis. They develop relatively rapidly over the course of months to several years and tend to behave very aggressively. The clinical characteristics of these melanomas are often unmistakable, with variegations in color and convoluted borders. Ulceration of these lesions is common.

► Treatment of Primary Melanoma

Any suspected melanoma should be removed by punch or excisional biopsy. Given the importance of Breslow thickness, shave or curette biopsies are contraindicated. If the biopsy specimen reveals melanoma, a formal excision with adequate margins is required. Because microscopic tumor cells frequently surround primary melanomas, excision with narrow margins is associated with an unacceptably high rate of local recurrence. The current standard for lesions less

Table 47–6. AJCC eighth edition staging system for melanoma.

DEFINITIONS OF TNM

Definition of Primary Tumor (T)

T Category	Thickness	Ulceration status
TX: primary tumor thickness cannot be assessed (e.g., diagnosis by curettage)	Not applicable	Not applicable
T0: no evidence of primary tumor (e.g., unknown primary or completely regressed melanoma)	Not applicable	Not applicable
Tis (melanoma *in situ*)	Not applicable	Not applicable
T1	≤ 1.0 mm	Unknown or unspecified
T1a	< 0.8 mm	Without ulceration
T1b	< 0.8 mm 0.8–1.0 mm	With ulceration With or without ulceration
T2	> 1.0–2.0 mm	Unknown or unspecified
T2a	> 1.0–2.0 mm	Without ulceration
T2b	> 1.0–2.0 mm	With ulceration
T3	> 2.0–4.0 mm	Unknown or unspecified
T3a	> 2.0–4.0 mm	Without ulceration
T3b	> 2.0–4.0 mm	With ulceration
T4	> 4.0 mm	Unknown or unspecified
T4a	> 4.0 mm	Without ulceration
T4b	> 4.0 mm	With ulceration

Definition of Regional Lymph Node (N)

	Extent of regional lymph node and/or lymphatic metastasis	
N Category	Number or tumor-involved regional lymph node	Presence of in-transit, satellite, and/or microsatellite metastases
NX	Regional nodes not assessed (e.g., SLN biopsy not performed, regional nodes previously removed for another reason) **Exception:** pathological N category is not required for T1 melanomas, use cN.	No
N0	No regional metastases detected	No
N1	One tumor-involved node or in-transit, satellite, and/or microsatellite metastases with no tumor-involved nodes	
N1a	One clinically occult (i.e., detected by SLN biopsy)	No
N1b	One clinically detected	No
N1c	No regional lymph node disease	yes
N2	Two or three tumor-involved nodes or in-transit, satellite, and/or microsatellite metastases with one tumor-involved node	
N2a	Two or three clinically occult (i.e., detected by SLN biopsy)	No
N2b	Two or three, at least one of which was clinically detected	No
N2c	One clinically occult or clinically detected	Yes

(Continued)

Table 47–6. AJCC eighth edition staging system for melanoma. (*Continued*)

N3	Four or more tumor-involved nodes or in-transit, satellite, and/or microsatellite metastases with two or more tumor-involved nodes, or any number of matted nodes without or with in-transit, satellite, and/or microsatellite metastases	
N3a	Four or more clinically occult (i.e., detected by SLN biopsy)	No
N3b	Four or more, at least one of which was clinically detected, or presence of any number of matted nodes	No
N3c	Two or more clinically occult or clinically detected and/or presence of any number of matted nodes	Yes

Definition of Distant Metastasis (M)

	M Criteria	
M Category	**Antomic site**	**LDH level**
M0	No evidence of distant metastasis	Not applicable
M1	Evidence of distant metastasis	See below
M1a	Distant metastasis to skin, soft tissue including muscle, and/or nonregional lymph node	Not recorded or unspecified
M1a(0)		Not elevated
M1a(1)		Elevated
M1b	Distant metastasis to lung with or without M1a sites of disease	Not recorded or unspecified
M1b(0)		Not elevated
M1b(1)		Elevated
M1c	Distant metastasis to non-CNS visceral sites with or without M1a or M1b sites of disease	Not recorded or unspecified
M1c(0)		Not elevated
M1c(1)		Elevated
M1d	Distant metastasis to CNS with or without M1a, M1b, or M1c sites of disease	Not recorded or unspecified
M1d(0)		Normal
M1d(1)		Elevated

Suffixes for M category: (0) LDH not elevated, (1) LDH elevated. No suffix is used if LDH is not recorded or is unspecified.

Pathological (pTNM)

When T is...	And N is...	And M is...	Then the pathological stage group is...
Tis	N0	M0	0
T1a	N0	M0	IA
T1b	N0	M0	IA
T2a	N0	M0	IB
T2b	N0	M0	IIA
T3a	N0	M0	IIA
T3b	N0	M0	IIB
T4a	N0	M0	IIB
T4b	N0	M0	IIC
T0	N1b, N1c	M0	IIIB
T0	N2b/c, N3b/c	M0	IIIC
T1a/b, T2a	N1a, N2a	M0	IIIA
T1a/b, T2a	N1b/c N2b	M0	IIIB
T2b, T3a	N1a/b/c, N2a/b	M0	IIIB
T1a/b, T2a/b, T3a	N2c, N3a/b/c	M0	IIIC
T3b, T4a	Any N ≥ N1	M0	IIIC
T4b	N1a/b/c, N2a/b/c	M0	IIIC
T4b	N3a/b/c	M0	IIID
Any T, Tis	Any N	M1	IV

Pathological Stage 0 (melanoma *in situ*) and T1 do not require pathological evaluation of lymph nodes to complete pathological staging; use cN information to assign their pathological stage.

than 1 mm in depth is excision with 1-cm margins. Melanomas between 1 and 2 mm in thickness should be excised with 2-cm margins, but a smaller margin (10-15 mm) may be acceptable in areas where it is difficult to get 2 cm without the need for a skin graft or exceptionally tight closure. Melanomas deeper than 2 mm should be excised with a 2-cm margin. The resection should be carried down to the underlying fascia, although the fascia need not be excised.

Melanomas generally metastasize by the lymphatic route in a predictable and orderly fashion. Any palpable nodes must be considered suspicious for metastatic involvement, easily verified with an FNAB. About 5%-10% of patients have clinical evidence of nodal metastases upon initial presentation and should undergo a therapeutic lymph node dissection at the time of their wide excision. Some patients may benefit from neoadjuvant therapy, either with immunotherapy or targeted therapy, prior to surgery.

Many patients will have microscopic disease in the lymph nodes that will not be apparent on physical examination. In the past, substantial controversy surrounded elective lymph node dissection of the draining nodal basin for melanoma. The practice gained dramatic acceptance, however, with the advent of the sentinel lymph node biopsy, which is based on the anatomic concept that lymphatic fluid from defined regions of skin drains specifically to an initial node or nodes ("sentinel nodes") prior to disseminating to other nodes in the same or nearby basins. Sentinel lymph node biopsy allows for a more detailed histologic examination of the sentinel lymph nodes and helps avoid the morbidity of lymph node dissection in patients who are pathologically node negative. Patients with a positive sentinel node are over six times more likely to die of their disease than those with a negative sentinel lymph node, making the predictive impact of sentinel node status much greater than any other prognostic factor. Evidence also suggests that early removal of micrometastatic disease from the lymph nodes, as compared with waiting for regional recurrence to perform a lymph node dissection, may improve survival.

For patients who are clinically node negative, sentinel lymph node biopsy has become the standard of care in the staging and treatment of melanoma and should be performed at the time of the wide excision for primary melanomas thicker than 1.0 mm. It should be selectively applied for tumors between 0.8 and 1.0 mm when other worrisome features are present, such as ulceration, angiolymphatic invasion, or a mitotic rate greater than 1. Melanomas less than 0.8 mm are very unlikely to have regional metastases and do not typically require sentinel lymph node biopsy unless they have very worrisome features or if the deep margin is involved by tumor. The dominant drainage basins can be identified by lymphoscintigraphy, which involves intradermal injection of technetium-99m (^{99m}Tc) sulfur colloid in the area around the tumor and a gamma camera to image the sites of lymph node drainage. In the operating room, blue dye (isosulfan or methylene) is injected in a similar fashion. Any lymph nodes that have evidence of ^{99m}Tc uptake on a handheld gamma probe, have evidence of blue dye, or are clinically suspicious should be excised. After removal of the nodes, they are analyzed by serial thin-sectioning, routine hematoxylin and eosin staining, and immunohistochemical staining. Using these methods of analysis, the pathologist is able to detect even minute numbers of metastatic melanoma cells in the sentinel node. Until recently, patients with a positive sentinel lymph node biopsy have been recommended to undergo a completion lymph node dissection of the entire basin. However, the recent prospective randomized MSLT-II trial demonstrated that although completion lymph node dissection may improve regional control, it does not improve overall survival compared to close observation. Today, patients with a positive sentinel lymph node may opt to avoid completion lymph node dissection and undergo serial monitoring of the basin with ultrasound. Patients who develop an abnormal node should have FNAB confirmation of recurrence and, if distant staging is negative, then return to the operating room for completion lymph node dissection.

Traditional chemotherapy regimens have proved largely ineffective in the treatment of melanoma. For decades, the only available adjuvant therapy for melanoma was the cytokine IFN alfa-2b (Intron A), although this was controversial because the duration of therapy is long (12 months), the toxicities are substantial, and some of the data regarding the overall survival benefit are conflicting. Today, however, several systemic therapies that have proven highly effective in the management of stage IV disease have demonstrated benefit in the adjuvant setting in prospective, randomized trials.

For patients with node-positive disease, adjuvant immunotherapy with a checkpoint inhibitor has been shown to be effective. This includes monoclonal antibodies against CTLA-4 (ipilimumab) or PD-1 (nivolumab or pembrolizumab). Nivolumab is the most commonly used adjuvant immunotherapy and has been shown to prolong relapse-free survival and decrease toxicity compared with ipilimumab. Another option is targeted therapy. All patients with high-risk melanoma should undergo testing for the *BRAF* V600 driver mutation. When present, these patients are candidates for adjuvant therapy with the combination of dabrafenib plus trametinib, which was shown in a randomized trial to improve both relapse-free and overall survival.

Although melanoma is relatively radioresistant, there may be some benefit to regional control after node dissection with radiation in patients with gross extracapsular extension or multiple involved lymph nodes.

▶ Local Recurrence & In-Transit Metastasis

Although rare with appropriate surgery, an isolated local recurrence can be treated with a repeat wide excision with

2-cm margins. Approximately 2%-3% of melanoma patients will develop in-transit metastasis, which is the appearance of metastasis along the path from the primary tumor to its regional nodal basin, that is lymphatic in nature. The management of in-transit metastasis is dictated by the number and the size of the lesions. If few in number, surgical excision with a margin of surrounding normal cutaneous and subcutaneous tissue is appropriate; however, this becomes unlikely with multiple lesions.

For most patients with in-transit recurrence, the risk of distant recurrence is high, and so systemic therapy, either immunotherapy or targeted therapy, is often the first line of therapy. For patients who are poor candidates for these therapies or have resistant disease isolated to the extremity, regional therapy is an option. Hyperthermic isolated limb perfusion is a way of isolating the blood circuit to the extremity and administering chemotherapeutic agents regionally at a concentration 15-25 times higher without resulting in systemic side effects. Melphalan has been used as a standard drug for hyperthermic isolated limb perfusion secondary to its efficacy and low regional toxicity. Although this has not been shown to improve survival, the use of hyperthermic isolated limb perfusion provides a significant palliation of locoregional symptoms when other options are not available. Less complicated, but also effective, is isolated limb infusion. This involves using minimally invasive techniques to access the vessels along with a tourniquet to minimize systemic uptake. Another option for the management of local or in-transit recurrence is intralesional therapy. Talimogene laherparepvec is an oncolytic virus containing the gene for granulocyte-macrophage colony-stimulating factor that can be directly injected into a tumor. In addition to a direct oncolytic effect, it can induce an immune response that eradicates additional lesions that have not been injected.

Regional and systemic recurrence of melanoma can be latent, and recurrence 10 years after the original diagnosis is not uncommon. This fact necessitates close lifelong followup of these patients. Patients with a past history of melanoma have a dramatically increased risk of developing a second primary lesion and require diligent screening for other lesions.

Faries MB, Thompson JF, Cochran AJ, et al: Completion dissection or observation for sentinel-node metastasis in melanoma. *N Engl J Med.* 2017;376(23):2211-2222.

Long GV, Hauschild A, Sanitnami M, et al: Adjuvant dabrafenib plus trametinib in stage III BRAF-mutated melanoma. *N Engl J Med.* 2017;377(19):1813-1823.

Morton DL, Thompson JF, Cochran AJ, et al: Final trial report of sentinel node biopsy versus nodal observation in melanoma. *N Engl J Med.* 2014;370:5995-5609.

Sabel MS, Johnson TM, Bichakjian CK: Cutaneous neoplasms. In Mulholland MW, et al (eds): *Scientific Principles and Practice*, 6th ed. Philadelphia, PA: Lippincott Williams & Wilkins; 2017.

Weber, J, Mandala M, Del Vecchio M, et al: Adjuvant nivolumab versus ipilimumab in resected stage III or IV melanoma. *N Engl J Med.* 2017;377(19):1824-1835.

LYMPHOMA

Lymphomas are malignant neoplasms that originate from the lymphoid tissues. Two distinct categories of lymphoma exist: Hodgkin and non-Hodgkin. Hodgkin lymphoma (HL) accounts for approximately 10%, whereas non-Hodgkin lymphoma (NHL) accounts for the remainder. The two types not only have different morphologic characteristics but also differ in their clinical behavior and their response to various therapeutic regimens. It is not possible to differentiate HL and NHL on clinical grounds; surgical biopsy is necessary. In the diagnosis of a suspected lymphoma, excisional biopsy of the entire lymph node or nodes is imperative, as the architecture has a bearing on the diagnosis and the subsequent treatment of the tumor.

1. Hodgkin Lymphoma

HL may occur at any age but is generally a disease of young adults. Although it can be seen across the age spectrum, the median age is 39, and it is most frequently seen in the group 20-34 years of age. Incidence rate have stayed flat for several decades, but fortunately, mortality rates have steadily declined, from 1.3 cases per 100,000 in 1975 to 0.3 cases per 100,000 in 2014. Over this period, the 5-year survival has improved from 70% to 85%.

In HL, the cancer cells form only a small fraction of the tumor, surrounded by a reactive inflammatory background consisting of lymphocytes, eosinophils, neutrophils, histiocytes, and plasma cells. The malignant cells are multinucleate giant cells or large mononuclear cells and are referred to as Hodgkin and Reed-Sternberg (HRS) cells. It is the pattern of the lymphocytic infiltrate that determines the classic subtypes of HL. HL is subdivided into classical and nodular lymphocyte-predominant HL, with the latter having a more indolent biology. Classical HL is further subdivided into four histologic subtypes based on morphology, the abundance of HRS cells, and the background infiltrate (Table 47–7).

The cause of HL is not well understood; however, epidemiologic studies have revealed certain patterns of disease clustering. The incidence appears to be higher with a lower number of siblings, early birth order, siblings with HL, a decreased number of playmates, certain HLAs, single-family dwellings, and patients who have undergone tonsillectomy. The incidence is increased also in persons with immunodeficiencies and autoimmune disorders. This pattern suggests that an oncogenic virus may cause HL. Epstein-Barr virus (EBV) is detected in HRS cells in a majority of HL specimens from the developing world; however, this is less frequent in North America and Western Europe.

Most patients present with enlarging but painless lymph nodes, often in the lower neck or supraclavicular region. Mediastinal involvement is common; however, these nodes can grow quite large before a diagnosis is made, either secondary to symptoms (cough or dyspnea) or routine chest

Table 47–7. Classic subtypes of Hodgkin lymphoma.

Subtype	Characteristics
Nodular sclerosis	Most common form (70% of Hodgkin lymphoma) Characterized by lacunar-type HRS in an inflammatory background of band-forming sclerosis Mediastinal adenopathy in 80% of cases Better prognosis than other types
Mixed cellularity	Common (20%-25% of Hodgkin lymphoma) HRS cells scattered in a diffuse, mixed, inflammatory background without sclerosing fibrosis Often presents with disseminated disease
Lymphocyte rich	Uncommon (5% of Hodgkin lymphomas) Scattered HRS cells within a background of small lymphocytes Peripheral adenopathy without bulky mediastinal involvement Caught early with excellent outcomes
Lymphocyte depleted	Rare (< 1% of Hodgkin lymphoma) Diffuse infiltration of HRS cells without significant inflammatory infiltrate More aggressive disease course. Often seen in association with HIV

HRS, Hodgkin and Reed-Sternberg cells.

Table 47–8. Lugano classification for Hodgkin and non-Hodgkin lymphoma.

Stage	Stage Description
Limited Stage	
I	Involvement of a single lymphatic site (ie, nodal region, Waldeyer ring, thymus, or spleen)
IE	Single extralymphatic site in the absence of nodal involvement
II	Involvement of 2 or more lymphatic sites on the same side of the diaphragm
IIE	Contiguous extralymphatic extension from a nodal site with or without involvement of other nodal regions on the same side of the diaphragm
II bulky[1]	Stage II with disease "bulk"
Advanced Stage	
III	Involvement of lymph node regions on both sides of the diaphragm; nodes above the diaphragm with spleen involvement
IV	Diffuse or disseminated involvement of 1 or more extralymphatic organs, with or without associated lymph node involvement Noncontiguous extralymphatic organ involvement in conjunction with nodal stage II disease or any extralymphatic organ involvement in nodal stage III disease Any involvement of the cerebrospinal fluid, bone marrow, liver, or multiple lung lesions (other than by direct extension)

[1]Stage II bulky may be early or advanced depending on histology and prognostic factors. "Bulk" varies according to the lymphoma histology and anatomy.

Note: For Hodgkin lymphoma, there is an A or B designation with stage group. A/B is not used for non-Hodgkin lymphoma. A indicates asymptomatic; B indicates any B symptoms (fevers, night sweats, unexplained weight loss).

x-ray. About 25% of patients will have systemic symptoms, called B symptoms, including weight loss, fever, and drenching night sweats. Both bulky mediastinal disease (> 10 cm) and B symptoms are associated with a poorer prognosis. Some patients will present with pruritis without obvious skin pathology and resistant to topical agents. This can sometimes be a clue to clinically occult HL.

Staging

For many years, the Ann Arbor staging system had been used to stage HL; however, this was based on interventions such as bone marrow biopsy or staging laparotomy (splenectomy, wedge liver biopsy, and dissection of the para-aortic, iliac, splenic hilar, and hepatic portal lymph nodes) that were commonly used. Today, with the advent of fluorodeoxyglucose (FDG) positron emission tomography (PET)- CT, the staging system has changed accordingly. The **Deauville scale** established a consensus on simple, reproducible criteria for PET interpretation. The most modern staging system for both HL and NHL today is the Lugano classification (Table 47–8). This classifies patients as having limited or advanced disease based on histology and other prognostic factors.

Treatment

HL has changed from a uniformly fatal disease to one that is curable in the majority of patients with the advent of combination chemotherapy and radiation. Today, the 5-year relative survival for patients under 19 years of age is 96.4%, and for patients between 20 and 64 years, it is 89.9%.

Treatment is guided by both the stage of disease as well as stratification into favorable and unfavorable prognostic factors. Because many patients were more likely to die from long-term complications of the treatment than the lymphoma itself, the focus has been to minimize the risks of therapy while maintaining the excellent outcomes. For early-stage classical HL, chemotherapy consists of ABVD (doxorubicin, bleomycin, vinblastine, and dacarbazine) and involved-field radiation. Increasingly, select patients with an excellent response on PET after chemotherapy may be spared the radiation. Patients with early classical HL with unfavorable prognostic features may require additional cycles of ABVD in combination with either involved-field radiotherapy or extended-field radiotherapy.

Although ABVD remains the standard regimen for advanced classical HL, an intensified seven-drug combination of escalated BEACOPP (bleomycin, etoposide, doxorubicin, cyclophosphamide, vincristine, procarbazine, and prednisone) is also an option. A multivariate analysis comparing escalated BEACOPP versus ABVD showed a significant benefit to progression-free survival and a small but significant overall survival benefit with BEACOPP, but with greatly increased toxicity. The response rates, toxicity, and patient comorbidities must be weighed when deciding on a regimen, and ABVD remains the most commonly used regimen in the United States.

Although most patients with classical HL are cured with first-line therapy, significant percentages of patients either fail to respond (refractory disease) or relapse. In this case, salvage therapy typically involves an alternate chemotherapy regimen. High-dose chemotherapy and autologous hematopoietic cell transplantation (HCT) should be considered for patients with early relapse (within 12 months), second relapse, or a generalized systemic relapse, even after 12 months. For patients who fail this approach or are not candidates for high-dose chemotherapy with HCT, there are unfortunately few good treatment options. These patients should consider clinical trials of newer approaches, such as antibody-drug conjugates or immunotherapy.

2. Non-Hodgkin Lymphoma

NHL encompasses a wide spectrum of lymphoid-derived tumors. NHL may originate from B cells, T cells, NK cells, histiocytes, or DCs. Clinicians, geneticists, and pathologists have made several attempts to develop a universal, clinically relevant classification system for the subtypes of NHL. The most widely accepted classification system is the World Health Organization classification (Table 47–9).

As opposed to HL, the prevalence of NHL rises with age. The incidence of NHL had been increasing in Europe and North America but has stabilized. This, however, may vary among specific subtypes. Several risk factors have been identified that predispose patients to the development of disease, including immune disorders, infections, lifestyle, genetics, race, family history, and occupational factors. Patients with congenital disorders such as ataxia-telangiectasia, Wiskott-Aldrich syndrome, and celiac disease have an increased incidence of lymphoma. Certain acquired conditions also predispose patients to lymphoma, including prior chemotherapy or radiotherapy, immunosuppressive therapy, viral infection (EBV, HIV, human T-cell lymphoma virus), *Helicobacter pylori* gastritis, Hashimoto thyroiditis, and Sjögren syndrome. Obesity has been found to be a risk factor for diffuse large B-cell lymphoma.

Classically, NHL presents as nontender enlargement of lymph nodes. NHL sometimes behaves indolently, with waxing and waning lymphadenopathy for years. Others behave aggressively. These tend to present with a rapidly growing mass and systemic B symptoms. However, nearly one-third of

all cases originate outside the lymph nodes. These extranodal malignancies develop in organs that normally have nests of lymphoid tissue (mucosal surfaces, bone marrow, and skin). In these cases, the presentation may reflect the location. Patients with gastrointestinal lymphoma, for example, may present with anorexia, weight loss, nausea, bowel changes, or early satiety. They may even present emergently with obstruction, perforation, or gastrointestinal hemorrhage.

▶ Diagnosis & Staging

A biopsy is necessary for the diagnosis and classification of NHL. This requires a tissue biopsy, possibly from a core needle biopsy or preferably excision of an intact lymph node. This allows histologic, immunologic, molecular, and possibly genetic assessment to classify the lymphoma. Surgeons are often called upon to perform a lymph node biopsy for diagnosis, often urgently in cases where treatment needs to be initiated promptly. For patients with peripheral adenopathy, surgical biopsy is preferred because peripheral lymph nodes are easily accessed and because surgical biopsy has a high diagnostic yield with low morbidity. When a superficial surgical biopsy is not possible, CT-guided core needle biopsies or laparoscopic biopsies usually obtain enough material to make a diagnosis. In certain subtypes of NHL, which lack adenopathy, other specimens or tissues, such as cerebrospinal fluid, pleural or pericardial fluid, or ascites, can be obtained. Although splenectomy is rarely indicated for diagnosis, some subtypes, such as splenic marginal zone lymphoma, are more likely to involve the spleen and less likely to be present in the lymph nodes. In these rare cases, splenectomy may be indicated.

After pathologic diagnosis, the staging evaluation for NHL consists of a detailed history and physical examination, routine laboratory tests, a bone marrow biopsy, and full body imaging. The preferred imaging modality for staging a patient with NHL depends on the FDG avidity of the subtype. PET/CT is preferred for FDG-avid lymphomas, whereas CT alone is preferred for those considered to be nonavid (eg, chronic lymphocytic leukemia/small lymphocytic lymphoma). The current staging system for both HL and NHL is the Lugano classification (see Table 47–8), with some differences. For example, the presence of B symptoms is included in the staging of HL but not NHL, because it is not an independent prognostic factor. Staging of NHL is less useful than HL because fewer patients present with localized disease.

▶ Treatment

In general, the treatment of NHL is highly dependent on the subtype. Treatment modalities include chemotherapy, radiation therapy, immunotherapy (monoclonal antibodies, immune checkpoint inhibitors, and CAR-T cells), and

Table 47–9. World Health Organization classification of lymphoid neoplasms.

Mature B-cell neoplasms	Mature T- and NK-cell neoplasms
Chronic lymphocytic leukemia/small lymphocytic lymphoma	T-cell prolymphocytic leukemia
Monoclonal B-cell lymphocytosis	T-cell large granular lymphocytic leukemia
B-cell prolymphocytic leukemia	Aggressive NK-cell leukemia
Splenic marginal zone lymphoma	Systemic EBV1 T-cell lymphoma of childhood
Hairy cell leukemia	Hydroa vacciniforme–like lymphoproliferative disorder
Lymphoplasmacytic lymphoma	Adult T-cell leukemia/lymphoma
Waldenström macroglobulinemia	Extranodal NK-/T-cell lymphoma, nasal type
Monoclonal gammopathy of undetermined significance (MGUS), IgM	Enteropathy-associated T-cell lymphoma
μ, γ, and α heavy-chain disease	Monomorphic epitheliotropic intestinal T-cell lymphoma
MGUS, IgG/A	Hepatosplenic T-cell lymphoma
Plasma cell myeloma	Subcutaneous panniculitis-like T-cell lymphoma
Solitary plasmacytoma of bone	Mycosis fungoides, Sézary syndrome
Extraosseous plasmacytoma	Primary cutaneous CD301 T-cell lymphoproliferative disorders
Monoclonal immunoglobulin deposition diseases	Lymphomatoid papulosis
Extranodal marginal zone lymphoma of mucosa-associated lymphoid	Primary cutaneous anaplastic large-cell lymphoma
tissue lymphoma	Peripheral T-cell lymphoma, NOS
Nodal marginal zone lymphoma	Nodal peripheral T-cell lymphoma with TFH phenotype
Follicular lymphoma	Anaplastic large-cell lymphoma, ALK positive
In situ follicular neoplasia	Anaplastic large-cell lymphoma, ALK negative
Duodenal-type follicular lymphoma	Breast implant–associated anaplastic large-cell lymphoma
Pediatric-type follicular lymphoma	**Hodgkin lymphoma**
Primary cutaneous follicle center lymphoma	Nodular lymphocyte-predominant Hodgkin lymphoma
Mantle cell lymphoma	Classical Hodgkin lymphoma
In situ mantle cell neoplasia	Nodular sclerosis classical Hodgkin lymphoma
Diffuse large B-cell lymphoma (DLBCL), not otherwise specified (NOS)	Lymphocyte-rich classical Hodgkin lymphoma
Germinal center B-cell type	Mixed cellularity classical Hodgkin lymphoma
Activated B-cell type	Lymphocyte-depleted classical Hodgkin lymphoma
T-cell/histiocyte-rich large B-cell lymphoma	**Posttransplant lymphoproliferative disorders (PTLD)**
Primary DLBCL of the central nervous system (CNS)	Plasmacytic hyperplasia PTLD
Primary cutaneous DLBCL, leg type	Infectious mononucleosis PTLD
EBV1 DLBCL, NOS	Florid follicular hyperplasia PTLD
DLBCL associated with chronic inflammation	Polymorphic PTLD
Lymphomatoid granulomatosis	Monomorphic PTLD (B- and T-/NK-cell types)
Primary mediastinal (thymic) large B-cell lymphoma	Classical Hodgkin lymphoma PTLD
Intravascular large B-cell lymphoma	**Histiocytic and dendritic cell neoplasms**
ALK-positive large B-cell lymphoma	Histiocytic sarcoma
Plasmablastic lymphoma	Langerhans cell histiocytosis
Primary effusion lymphoma	Langerhans cell sarcoma
Burkitt lymphoma	Indeterminate dendritic cell tumor
High-grade B-cell lymphoma, with MYC and BCL2 and/or BCL6	Interdigitating dendritic cell sarcoma
rearrangements	Follicular dendritic cell sarcoma
High-grade B-cell lymphoma, NOS	Fibroblastic reticular cell tumor
B-cell lymphoma, unclassifiable	Disseminated juvenile xanthogranuloma
	Erdheim-Chester disease

NK, natural killer; TFH, T-follicular helper.

targeted therapies. NHL can be functionally divided into two groups: indolent (low-grade) and aggressive (high-grade) lymphomas. Smaller, differentiated cells characterize the indolent lymphomas, and this class tends to have a follicular architecture. Although the course of these lymphomas is not very aggressive and they have a long median survival, they are not usually curable in advanced clinical stages. Patients with localized disease, although the minority, can be treated with radiation therapy only with curative intent. Most patients have disseminated disease, which tends to be chronic relapsing and remitting. The current therapies for systemic indolent lymphomas are rarely curative, and the goal of treatment is generally directed at palliation of symptoms. At present, a "watch and wait" approach to treatment is recommended for asymptomatic patients. After diagnosis, asymptomatic patients are followed up clinically until they progress to more aggressive disease, major symptoms, or organ dysfunction. Withholding chemotherapy does not reduce survival in patients with NHL, and it probably improves quality of life.

The aggressive lymphomas behave differently and demand a different therapeutic approach. Histologically, the aggressive lymphomas spread more diffusely throughout the lymph nodes and consist of larger, less differentiated cell types. This class of lymphomas demonstrates a very rapid growth rate and an increased rate of early mortality. Despite their aggressive nature, these lymphomas have a better chance for cure than their more indolent counterparts. The treatment is typically guided by the prognostic factors (International Prognostic Index score). The most common form of chemotherapy for the initial treatment of aggressive NHL is the CHOP regimen (cyclophosphamide, doxorubicin, prednisone, and vincristine). The CD20 monoclonal antibody rituximab is often added for patients with B-cell lymphoma. There are other monoclonal antibodies to CD20 that may also be used, and these are listed in Table 47–2. Radiotherapy may be used after chemotherapy for areas of bulky disease. Patients with high-risk lymphoma benefit from more intensive regimens of chemotherapy and targeted therapy and potentially high-dose therapy with HCT. This approach should also be considered for patients who relapse or fail to enter remission after induction chemotherapy.

Outside of the initial diagnosis, surgery is rarely a component of therapy for NHL. The treatment of gastric lymphomas has been controversial. Mucosa-associated lymphoid tissue (MALT)–type gastric lymphomas typically have an indolent behavior, and the most widely accepted initial therapy is the eradication of *H pylori* using regimens combining antibiotics and proton pump inhibitors. For patients with MALT-type gastric lymphoma who are *H pylori* negative or do not respond to antibiotic/proton pump inhibitor therapy, radiation therapy to the stomach and perigastric lymph nodes obtains high complete response rates and excellent long-term survival. Although surgery had previously been used in the treatment of gastric lymphomas, there are now sufficient data to suggest that nonoperative management permits a better quality of life with no impact on overall survival. When the disease has spread, the use of chemotherapy is similar to that used for other indolent, advanced lymphomas.

High-grade gastric lymphoma is treated with aggressive polychemotherapy, usually combined with rituximab. Again, surgery used to play a more prominent role but has greatly diminished. It was assumed that the increased risk of perforation and bleeding with chemotherapy could be prevented by pretreatment gastric resection, but modern series have failed to demonstrate that benefit and actually show a high degree of postsurgical complications that may delay the start of chemotherapy. Surgery is limited to patients who have complications or who cannot be managed by standard regimens.

Splenectomy in patients with lymphomatous splenic involvement has not demonstrated therapeutic benefit and should be reserved for patients with symptomatic splenomegaly, pain from recurrent splenic infarctions, and hematologic depression from hypersplenism.

Armitage JO, Gascoyne RD, Lunning MA, et al: Non-Hodgkin lymphoma. *Lancet.* 2017;390:298-310.

Shanbhag, S, Ambinder RF: Hodgkin lymphoma: a review and update on recent progress. *CA Cancer J Clin.* 2018;68:116-132.

Swerdlow SH, Campo E, Pileri SA: The 2016 revision of the WHO classification of lymphoid neoplasms. *Blood.* 2016;127(20):2375-2390.

MULTIPLE CHOICE QUESTIONS

1. The proportion of people with cancer who are alive, divided by the proportion of people of a similar age expected to be alive in the absence of cancer, is known as the

   A. Overall survival
   B. Disease-free survival
   C. Disease-specific survival
   D. Relative survival

2. The ideal target for a targeted therapy would include all of the following characteristics except

   A. Can be measured on cancer cells
   B. Crucial to the malignant phenotype
   C. Inhibition leads to regression or death
   D. Expressed on vital organs and tissues

3. Which of the following is true regarding immunotherapy with checkpoint inhibitors?

   A. CTLA-4 is upregulated on activated T cells and serves to dampen the T-cell response.
   B. When PD-1 on tumor cells binds to PD-L1 on T cells, it leads to T-cell anergy.
   C. The checkpoint inhibitors have only proven effective in melanoma and renal cell carcinoma.
   D. Checkpoint inhibitors have minimal toxicity but can cause significant immunosuppression that may require cessation of therapy.

4. Regarding soft tissue sarcoma, which of the following is correct?

   A. The presence of nodal metastases is considered stage IV disease for sarcoma of the trunk, extremities, or retroperitoneum.
   B. For a patient presenting with a new mass, when sarcoma is suspected, excisional biopsy is always the preferred method of diagnosis.

C. Twenty percent of patients with extremity sarcoma may require amputation for surgical therapy.

D. The most common site for soft tissue sarcoma is on the extremity.

5. Which of the following statements regarding the surgical treatment of melanoma is true?

A. Sentinel lymph node biopsy is recommended for any invasive melanoma but not for melanoma in situ.

B. When a sentinel lymph node is positive for melanoma, close observation with ultrasounds of the basin is an acceptable alternative to completion node dissection.

C. Excision of the primary lesion with negative histologic margins is associated with a very low local recurrence rate.

D. In-transit recurrences, even multiple, require surgical excision because there are few alternative options for management.

48

Abdominal Organ Transplantation

Joshua S. Jolissaint, MD

Stefan G. Tullius, MD, PhD

Solid organ transplantation is the standard of care for patients with end-stage organ disease. The field of transplantation is exceedingly complex and requires multidisciplinary collaboration to navigate the intricacies of patient selection, perioperative care, and operative technique. Relevant aspects include careful evaluation of patients prior to transplantation, determining the potential benefits of the procedure, and assessing any inherent risks. Prolonged waiting times due to discrepancies between organ supply and demand mandate careful consideration of all available organs, and novel preservation methods may allow for the use of previously unavailable or marginal organs. High morbidity and mortality rates for patients awaiting transplantation are currently one of the most challenging areas in the field of transplantation. This chapter will focus on these topics as they relate to liver, kidney, and pancreas transplantation.

ORGAN DONORS AND SELECTION CRITERIA

In 2017 alone, 34,770 solid organ transplantations were performed in the United States, which included more than 28,000 transplants from deceased donation: almost 20,000 kidney, more than 8000 liver, and just over 1000 pancreas transplants (either as simultaneous kidney/pancreas, pancreas after kidney, or isolated pancreas transplants; Organ Procurement and Transplantation Network [OPTN] data from https://optn.transplant.hrsa.gov/data/view-data-reports/national-data/). The demand for organs exceeds the available supply by far, and there are currently more than 125,000 patients awaiting transplantation. Moreover, the number of waitlisted patients has doubled over the past two decades, and more than 6000 patients die each year while awaiting transplantation. Among abdominal organs transplanted, there has been a decline in patients listed for pancreas and liver transplants; in contrast, patients listed for renal transplants have steadily increased by approximately 3% per year.

Deceased Donor Transplantation

The overwhelming majority of abdominal transplants are from deceased donors, a practice that has allowed solid organ transplantation to become an established therapy for end-stage organ failure. Within this category, 80%-90% of deceased donor transplants are from patients with brain death (BD), defined as cessation of brainstem reflexes, and the remainder are from patients after a declaration of death has been made by circulatory criteria (so-called donor after cardiac death [DCD]). Rates for donation after cardiac death have increased over the past decade. Circulatory death ultimately leads to prolonged warm ischemia times as compared to BD, an inevitability that must be considered during perioperative planning and when analyzing outcomes. Specific time intervals between discontinuation of life support and cardiac arrest have therefore been proposed to prevent detrimental consequences to organ quality. For kidney transplant recipients from DCDs, there is a higher rate of delayed graft function, but rates of patient and graft survival are comparable and without a risk of increased complications. However, among liver transplants, DCDs have a fivefold higher potential for nonanastomotic biliary stricture, either due to the ischemic insult itself or due to impaired biliary epithelial regeneration, in addition to higher rates of graft loss and overall mortality. Although specific criteria such as donor age, time from extubation to circulatory arrest, and hemodynamics impact outcomes, DCD organs have allowed for an increase in the availability of transplants with outcomes mostly comparable to those of donor after BD (DBD) organs. Given the risks associated with prolonged warm ischemia time, novel preservation methods may be particularly advantageous for DCD organs.

Living Donor Transplantation

Patients in need of a kidney transplant and, to a lesser extent, a liver transplant may also receive an organ from a living donor. Donations may be in the form of a **directed** donation, as from a biological relative, an unrelated relative, or a friend. Donations may also be **nondirected** or **altruistic**, in which the donor may not specify the recipient of the donor organ, or **paired**, in which two ABO-incompatible donor–recipient pairs "trade" their organs to assure compatibility. These paired kidney exchanges have increased vastly during recent years and have made extensive desensitization therapies almost obsolete. Both survival and graft function after living donor kidney transplantation exceed that of deceased donor transplantation, and the elective nature of the operation makes it an ideal scenario for patients. It is also important to note that long-term donor mortality and rates of development of end-stage renal disease (ESRD) are comparable to those of nondonors. The incidence of ESRD among living kidney donors has actually been reported to be lower than that of the general population, attributed to careful screening and the good health of these patients preoperatively. As in the general population, risk factors for a lower glomerular filtration rate are older age and higher body mass index. In the rare situation of patients requiring dialysis after donation, priority listing for a kidney transplant is provided to avoid prolonged waiting times. Notably, more recent studies following donors after nephrectomy have suggested an increased risk of hypertension and resulting microalbuminuria.

Approximately 370 living donor liver transplants (LDLTs) were performed in 2017 in the United States (based on OPTN data from https://optn.transplant.hrsa.gov/data/view-data-reports/national-data/). LDLTs are more frequently performed in some Asian countries due to a less well-developed deceased donor transplant system. Numerous studies have been performed to determine which patients would benefit from LDLT. LDLT provides a survival benefit for patients with hepatocellular carcinoma and a Model for End-Stage Liver Disease (MELD) score greater than 15; however, there is no benefit for patients with a MELD score less than 15 or for patients with hepatitis C virus. Overall, outcomes after LDLT may be marginally better than after deceased donor liver transplants at experienced centers. In contrast to living donor renal transplant, LDLT has significantly higher reported rates of morbidity and mortality, with the Adult-to-Adult Living Donor Liver Transplant study quoting a 40% rate of complications and 0.04% rate of perioperative mortality. Notably, biliary complications are significantly higher with LDLTs, possibly due to disruption of blood supply to the donor and recipient bile ducts with hilar dissection. Among donors alone, the risk of any complication at 6 years has been reported to be between 40% and 51%, with infections and bile leaks being the most common 90-day complications and hernias being the most common long-term problem. The rate of serious complications leading to lasting disability is approximately 1%. This higher rate of perioperative adverse events has been well publicized, leading to some reticence on behalf of both institutions and donors themselves to pursue this option.

Abecassis MM, Fisher RA, Olthoff KM, et al: Complications of living donor hepatic lobectomy–a comprehensive report. Am J Transplant. 2012;12(5):1208-1217.

Callaghan CJ, Charman SC, Muiesan P, et al: Outcomes of transplantation of livers from donation after circulatory death donors in the UK: a cohort study. BMJ Open. 2013;3(9):e003287.

Chen C-L, Kabiling CS, Concejero AM: Why does living donor liver transplantation flourish in Asia? Nat Rev Gastroenterol Hepatol. 2013;10(12):746-751.

Dhital KK, Iyer A, Connellan M, et al: Adult heart transplantation with distant procurement and ex-vivo preservation of donor hearts after circulatory death: a case series. Lancet. 2015; 385(9987):2585-2591.

Gill J, Rose C, Lesage J, et al: Use and outcomes of kidneys from donation after circulatory death donors in the United States. J Am Soc Nephrol. 2017;28(12):3647-3657.

Girlanda R: Deceased organ donation for transplantation: challenges and opportunities. World J Transplant. 2016;6(3):451-459.

Hart A, Smith JM, Skeans MA, et al: OPTN/SRTR 2016 annual data report. Am J Transplant. 2018;18:1-96.

Ibrahim HN, Foley R, Tan L, et al: Long-term consequences of kidney donation. N Engl J Med. 2009;360(5):459-469.

Kim PTW, Testa G: Living donor liver transplantation in the USA. Hepatobiliary Surg Nutr. 2016;5(2):133-140.

Muzaale AD, Massie AB, Kucirka LM, et al: Outcomes of live kidney donors who develop end-stage renal disease. Transplantation. 2016;100(6):1306-1312.

Steinbrook R: Organ donation after cardiac death. N Engl J Med. 2007;357(3):209-213.

Thiel GT, Nolte C, Tsinalis D, et al: Investigating kidney donation as a risk factor for hypertension and microalbuminuria: findings from the Swiss prospective follow-up of living kidney donors. BMJ Open. 2016;6(3):e010869.

Tullius SG, Rabb H: Improving the supply and quality of deceased-donor organs for transplantation. N Engl J Med. 2018; 378:1920-1929.

Wadei HM, Heckman MG, Rawal B, et al: Comparison of kidney function between donation after cardiac death and donation after brain death kidney transplantation. Transplant J. 2013; 96(3):274-281.

TRANSPLANT IMMUNOLOGY

The core tenet of transplant immunology and immunosuppressive therapy is the alloimmune response from the recipient once exposed to the graft, resulting in T-cell–mediated, or in the presence of preformed antibodies, humoral (B-cell) mediated allograft rejection. The major histocompatibility complex (MHC) is the strongest and by far most relevant of the antigens involved. There are at least seven loci that code for genes involved in the MHC, with each locus being highly polymorphic and allowing for as many as 50 or more discrete antigens. The human leukocyte antigen (HLA) categorization is further subdivided into **class I** (HLA-A, -B, and -C) and **class II** (HLA-DP, -DQ, -DR). Class I molecules are present on all nucleated cells; they have a 44-kDa heavy chain (α chain) and a 12-kDa light chain (β2-microglobulin) and present to CD8 coreceptors, facilitating the activation of cytotoxic T cells. Class II molecules are composed of heterodimers of α1 and α2 and β1 and β2 proteins, constitutively expressed on antigen-presenting cells (APCs). Class II molecules interact with CD4 coreceptors, thereby activating helper T cells. The HLA mismatch between donor and recipient is relevant in assessing the rigor of alloimmunity.

▶ Types of Rejection

Hyperacute rejection manifests within minutes to hours based on preformed antibodies directed against tissue antigens or in response to ABO blood group incompatibility. ABO antigens are present on vascular endothelial cells, among others, and preformed antibodies can target these antigens, resulting in hemagglutination and vessel thrombosis. In clinical practice, hyperacute rejection is largely excluded by pretransplant in vitro tests such as mixed lymphocyte reactions. **Acute rejections** are predominantly T-cell mediated and can occur within 1 week up to several years after transplantation. If left untreated, acute rejection will invariably lead to graft loss. **Antibody-mediated rejection (AMR)** are a distinct pathologic entity defined by the formation of donor-specific anti-HLA antibodies, vasculitis, and complement deposition. Antibodies can be present at the time of transplantation or develop de novo at any time; they are attributed to cross-reactivity to another antigen, insufficient immunosuppression, or nonadherence to a prescribed immunosuppressive regimen. **Chronic rejection** is the most common reason for progressive allograft failure after transplantation. The process remains ill-defined, with both alloantigen-specific and nonspecific causes. There are multiple theories attempting to explain the pathways leading to chronic rejection, including consequences of ischemia-reperfusion injury, brain death, insufficiently treated rejection episodes, and endothelial disruption leading to local hypoxia, all of which lead to mononuclear cell infiltration with structural changes, including fibrosis and obliterative vasculopathy, as a result of an endothelial-to-mesenchymal transition. Despite major advances in immunosuppression, the pathogenesis of and, consequently, the ability to prevent chronic allograft rejection continue to elude researchers.

▶ Alloimmune Responses

Lymphocyte activation can occur through (1) the direct recognition of intact HLA antigens expressed on donor tissue and presented by donor APCs (**direct allorecognition**), (2) presentation of peptides derived from HLA antigens by recipient APCs (**indirect allorecognition**), and (3) presentation of intact MHC complexes acquired from other dendritic or endothelial cells by recipient APCs (**semi-direct allorecognition**).

Direct recognition dominates in the early posttransplant period, with recipient APCs recognizing foreign antigens on the allograft, resulting in acute cellular rejection if left untreated. The indirect pathway of rejection is more prevalent at later stages as recipient APCs are able to acquire previously phagocytosed peptides that are being released from foreign cells either through necrosis or apoptosis.

T-cell immunity requires three signals for activation. In the first signal, an APC presents an antigenic peptide to the T-cell receptor (TCR)–CD3 complex. The second signal has some heterogeneity, with a critical interaction between CD28 and CD154, which are expressed on T cells, and their ligands, CD80/86 (or B7) and CD40, expressed on APCs. The costimulatory binding leads to downstream activation of the calcium–calcineurin–nuclear factor of activated T cells (NFAT) pathway, the protein kinase C–nuclear factor-κB (NF-κB) pathway, and Ras–MAP kinase–AP-1 pathway, all of which results in the production of cytokines and interleukins that support the clonal expansion of T cells in addition to the production of antibodies by B cells. The third signal is the result of inflammatory cytokines such as interleukin (IL)-12 or interferon-α/β, which direct differentiation into phenotypes such as Th1, Th2, and Th17 CD4+ cells.

As part of the humoral immune response, B cells can recognize donor antigens, and with the assistance of CD4+ T-helper cells, they turn into antibody-producing plasma cells. These antibodies can directly cause graft damage via activation of the complement cascade, natural killer (NK) cells, or eosinophils or indirectly cause damage by serving as APCs and presenting donor antigens for T-cell activation.

Curtsinger JM, Mescher MF: Inflammatory cytokines as a third signal for T cell activation. *Curr Opin Immunol.* 2010; 22(3):333-340.

Kumbala D, Zhang R: Essential concept of transplant immunology for clinical practice. *World J Transplant.* 2013;3(4):113-118.

Loupy A, Lefaucheur C: Antibody-mediated rejection of solid-organ allografts. *N Engl J Med.* 2018;379(12):1150-1160.

Tullius SG, Hancock WW, Heemann U, et al: Reversibility of chronic renal allograft rejection. Critical effect of time after transplantation suggests both host immune dependent and independent phases of progressive injury. *Transplantation.* 1994;58(1):93-99.

Wedel J, Bruneau S, Kochupurakkal N, et al: Chronic allograft rejection: a fresh look. *Curr Opin Organ Transplant.* 2015;20(1):13-20.

IMMUNOSUPPRESSION

In the absence of available alloantigen-specific treatments, chemical immunosuppression targets multiple biochemical pathways to effectively prevent organ rejection while minimizing the toxicities associated with each

▲ **Figure 48–1.** Targets of immunosuppression. ATG, antithymocyte globulin; AZA, azathioprine; BSX, basiliximab; CaN, calcineurin; FKBP, FK-binding protein; MMF, myocofenolate mofetil; mTOR, mammalian target of rapamycin; NFAT, nuclear factor of activated T cells; RAPA, rapamycin. (Used with permission from Michelle Long, Harvard University.)

drug (Figure 48–1). Many patients are treated with dual maintenance therapy, consisting of a calcineurin inhibitor (predominantly tacrolimus, but also cyclosporine A for some indications) and either an antimetabolite (eg, mycophenolate mofetil [MMF], azathioprine) or a mammalian target of rapamycin (mTOR) inhibitor (eg, sirolimus). Triple maintenance immunosuppression adds corticosteroids (eg, prednisone). Steroid withdrawal and avoidance approaches have been tested successful in patients who are either of low immunologic risk or who have low risk for recurrent disease. Many patients receive an induction treatment with a polyclonal T-cell antibody or a monoclonal antibody targeting the IL-2 receptor (IL-2R) or CD52. Induction treatments (1) blunt the immune response during the initial encounter with the antigen, (2) facilitate the aforementioned steroid withdrawal or avoidance protocols, and (3) allow for a delay in the introduction of a calcineurin inhibitor and consequent early exposure to nephrotoxicity.

Induction Treatment

A. Polyclonal Antithymoblast or Antilymphocyte Globulin and Antithymocyte Globulin

Antilymphoblast globulin and **antithymocyte globulin (ATG)** are polyclonal antibody preparations derived by immunizing animals against human lymphocytes and collecting and purifying the resulting antibodies. ATG depletes circulating lymphocytes with effects against T cells, but also against circulating B cells and NK cells. The effect of ATG is a profound immunosuppression that lasts for weeks to months and is used for both induction treatments and steroid-resistant acute rejections. Interestingly, a full and detailed mechanism of ATG remains limited and hypothetical.

Side effects include fevers and chills, neutropenia, and thrombocytopenia. Fever, chills, and malaise occur due to mediator release by T cells and circulating mononuclear cells, specifically tumor necrosis factor-α, IL-1, and IL-6. Clinical symptoms are frequently similar to those associated with an acute viral infection (the common cold); these effects are often transient and occur primarily following the first or second dose of the treatment and can be attenuated by pretreatment with corticosteroids, acetaminophen, and diphenhydramine. Neutropenia and thrombocytopenia result from direct antibody binding to these cell types, causing depletion. This effect is also transient and tends to resolve in 24-48 hours; however, it may be necessary to monitor neutrophil and platelet counts during therapy and withhold or reduce doses of the treatment if counts drop to low levels. Although rare, patients may experience serum sickness with hemodynamic instability involving prolonged hypotension and vasopressor support, which ultimately may lead to allograft loss.

B. Monoclonal Antibody Therapy

Monoclonal antibodies have the ability to selectively inhibit the expansion of T-cell clones that are activated at the time of transplantation, without affecting existing T-cell immunity to other antigens (eg, common viruses). **Basiliximab** binds to CD25, the high-affinity subunit of the TCR for IL-2. **Alemtuzumab**, a recombinant DNA-derived humanized IgG antibody, binds to CD52, a protein present on the surface of mature lymphocytes, resulting in a profound lymphocyte-depleting effect. Clinical trials in kidney transplant recipients on established maintenance immunosuppression with tacrolimus and MMF have shown that alemtuzumab reduces the rate of biopsy-proven rejection over 1 year compared with either ATG or basiliximab in both low- and high-risk patients, as stratified by repeated transplants, panel reactive antibodies greater than 20%, and African American race. At 3 years, the rate of acute rejections was lower only for patients who received alemtuzumab in the low-risk group, but not the high-risk group. Follow-up studies showed promising potential to use alemtuzumab as a method of reducing the use of calcineurin inhibitor (CNI, see below). Initial investigations using alemtuzumab as induction, followed by either sirolimus alone or sirolimus and MMF as maintenance immunosuppression, demonstrated an unacceptably high rate of rejection. Studies are ongoing, but preliminary data do suggest the possibility of CNI and prednisone-free maintenance regimens. Alemtuzumab remains of interest as an induction treatment; however, there is concern for humoral autoimmunity and potent and long-lasting T-cell depletion, which has been correlated with higher rates of autoimmune thyroid disorders in patients treated with alemtuzumab for multiple sclerosis.

Currently, ATG is used as the most common induction therapy in the United States, whereas IL-2R antagonists are more common in Europe. Guidelines from Kidney Disease: Improving Global Outcomes (KDIGO) and the Transplantation Society recommend induction therapy with a combination of immunosuppressants (grade 1A) and that patients should be started on IL-2R antagonists (eg, basiliximab) preferentially over lymphocyte-depleting antibodies (eg, ATG). For recipients with high immunologic risk 18 years of age or older, the guidelines recommend induction therapy with a lymphocyte-depleting agent such as ATG.

C. Calcineurin Inhibitors

Cyclosporine A is a cyclic undecapeptide that binds to cytosolic cyclophilin in lymphocytes; this complex, in turn, inhibits calcineurin, a protein that activates NFAT and subsequently decreases the transcription of IL-2. **Tacrolimus**, or **FK506**, is a macrolide drug with a comparable mode of action. Both drugs also interfere with the release of IL-1 by macrophages as well as the proliferation of B lymphocytes. Blood levels must be carefully monitored because both agents have broad side effect profiles including nephrotoxicity and neurotoxicity at supratherapeutic levels. Cyclosporine has been pivotal for organ transplantation since introduced clinically in the 1970s. Over the past several decades, tacrolimus has become the CNI of choice, with clinical studies showing more potent immunosuppressive capacities and slightly less toxic side effects.

D. Antimetabolites

Established antimetabolic immunosuppressants include azathioprine and MMF. These drugs inhibit nucleic acid synthesis by pathways that limit the ability of activated lymphocytes to expand clonally. In general, these drugs are used as maintenance immunosuppressants but are not effective at reversing active acute rejection.

Azathioprine, a purine analog, frequently causes neutropenia and thrombocytopenia in a dose-dependent fashion. **Mycophenolic acid,** with the most common form being **MMF**, is an inhibitor of inosine monophosphate dehydrogenase, a critical enzyme in the de novo synthesis pathway of purines. Lymphocytes depend on this metabolic pathway, whereas other cells are able to use a salvage pathway for synthesis. MMF is therefore more specific for lymphocytes and has largely replaced azathioprine for use in combination with CNIs and corticosteroids for triple therapy immunosuppression. The main side effect of MMF is gastrointestinal distress, which may manifest as nausea, vomiting, diarrhea, constipation, and/or abdominal pain. To prevent these effects, mycophenolic acid also comes in an enteric-coated form, known as **Myfortic**.

E. Inhibitors of Mammalian Target of Rapamycin

Sirolimus (or rapamycin) is a macrocyclic triene antibiotic produced by a species of *Streptomyces*. The drug was originally developed as an antifungal and antitumor agent but was found to have significant immunosuppressive properties. Rapamycin binds to the cytosolic protein FK-binding protein 12 (FKBP12). This complex subsequently inhibits mTOR and has an antiproliferative effect on lymphocytes. Gastrointestinal side effects are frequent, in addition to wound-healing problems associated with its inhibition of smooth muscle proliferation. Hyperlipidemia and, rarely, oral ulceration are additional side effects. Based on their antitumor effects, mTOR inhibitors are considered in recipients with a cancer history. Another potential benefit may be the T-regulatory sparing effect of mTOR inhibitors, supporting their addition to tolerance protocols.

F. Costimulation Blockade

Cytotoxic T-lymphocyte–associated antigen-4 (CTLA-4) is homologous to CD28 and binds with higher affinity to B7, inhibiting T cells. This has led to the development of **belatacept**, a fusion protein of CTLA-4 and the Fc fragment of IgG, which binds to B7 and inhibits T-cell activation. Phase II and III clinical trials have demonstrated that belatacept results in superior renal function with similar patient and graft survival and a decrease in the side effect profile for transplanted patients. During the phase III Belatacept Evaluation of Nephroprotection and Efficacy as First-Line Immunosuppression (BENEFIT) trial, patients who were Epstein-Barr virus (EBV) seronegative were found to have an increased risk of posttransplant lymphoproliferative disorder, and thus, maintenance therapy with belatacept has been restricted to EBV-seropositive recipients. In 2016, 7-year follow-up data from the same BENEFIT patient population were analyzed based on an intent-to-treat basis, and patients treated with belatacept were found to have a significantly lower rate of death and graft loss compared to patients treated with a cyclosporine regimen. Interestingly, rates of acute rejections by 84 months were significantly higher in patients treated with belatacept; reported results indicated rates of 24.4%, 18.3%, and 11.4% with more intensive belatacept, less intensive belatacept, and cyclosporine treatment, respectively.

G. Corticosteroids

Corticosteroids, particularly glucocorticoids such as prednisone, Solu-Medrol, and methylprednisolone, bind to a cytosolic glucocorticoid receptor that translocates to the cell nucleus, binding to response elements that then modulate gene expression. This mechanism inhibits the transcription factor NF-κB, genes coding for IL-2, and other cytokines and reduces both T-cell proliferation and the clonal expansion of B cells. Side effects of corticosteroids include weight gain, cushingoid features (eg, moon facies, lipodystrophy with a prominent back hump, abdominal obesity), hypertension, hyperlipidemia, hyperglycemia, and acne.

Typically, high doses of intravenous corticosteroids (eg, methylprednisolone) are given at the time of engraftment, with the dose tapered to a maintenance dosage of 0.1-0.2 mg/kg of oral prednisone. Recently, there has been interest in early withdrawal and steroid-free protocols given their multitude of side effects. This treatment may be appropriate and effective for selected low-risk renal transplant recipients. Corticosteroid-free protocols for higher risk candidates, including those with known sensitization to HLA and patients undergoing second renal transplants, are more controversial.

▶ Treatment of Acute Rejection

The incidence of acute rejections in the first year after kidney transplant is approximately 8%-9% for all allograft recipients, with a higher risk of acute rejections for recipients of deceased donor renal transplants. Recent data suggest there may be variability in the frequency of rejection depending on induction strategy, with patients receiving no induction being at significantly higher risk of acute rejection. Rates of acute rejection for liver transplant vary by age, with patients between the ages of 18 and 34 having a greater than 20% probability within the first year, which tapers to approximately 8%-10% after age 50. The incidence after pancreas transplant varies based on the type of transplant performed, with the incidence after simultaneous pancreas and kidney transplant being 12.3%, after pancreas transplant alone being 16.5%, and after pancreas transplant after kidney transplant being 18.3%.

Corticosteroids are the first-line therapy for acute rejections, typically consisting of three or more daily doses between 200 and 500 mg of intravenous methylprednisolone (steroid pulses). Depending on the severity of the rejection, steroid pulses will resolve 50%-80% of allograft rejection episodes. For acute rejection episodes that do not respond to corticosteroids, second-line therapy involves treatment with an antilymphocyte agent such as ATG. For T-cell–mediated rejections, current options include treatment with ATG, alemtuzumab, plasma exchange, or intravenous immunoglobulin (IVIG).

▶ Antibody-Mediated Rejection

AMR has evolved as one of the main barriers to improving long-term outcomes. Willicombe and colleagues reported a 10.2% incidence of AMR after alemtuzumab induction and a far inferior allograft survival for patients who developed AMR. This phenotype has more severe microvascular inflammation with increased C4d deposition within graft capillaries. Further research has demonstrated an association between donor-specific antibodies (DSAs) and C4d deposition, showing that anti-HLA antibodies that bind complement lead to a greater than fourfold risk of graft loss after transplantation. Belatacept may ultimately serve as a treatment for this process given its inhibition of T-cell activation and, thus, T-cell–dependent antibody responses via CD28. A recent study by Bray and colleagues demonstrated lower rates of DSA development among belatacept-treated patients compared to those treated with cyclosporine. Based on this post hoc analysis, additional studies are currently underway. Additional therapies include plasmapheresis, IVIG, and rituximab, an antibody-targeting CD20; more recently, the proteasome inhibitor bortezomib and the complement inhibitor eculizumab have shown favorable results in the treatment of refractory AMR.

▶ Limitations of Immunosuppression

Although the vast majority of patients enjoy an overwhelmingly improved quality of life for many years after transplantation, side effects of immunosuppression remain an unsolved issue. Moreover, long-term graft survival remains unsatisfactory, with particular relevance for heart and lung transplantation, which remain stagnant at 50%-60% graft survival at 5 years. One significant limitation to long-term survival involves the current options for immunosuppression, particularly medications with significant collateral toxicities. Unfortunately, there are also significant barriers to drug development, including regulatory barriers of the U.S. Food and Drug Administration, lack of biopharmaceutical experience, risk aversion to developing new therapeutics, and a lack of research infrastructure. Going forward, it will be important to develop clinical trial consortia and more focused attention on drug development to better improve transplant outcomes.

▶ Tolerance

Recently, a growing body of research has focused on using the immunomodulatory effects of hematopoietic stem cells of donor origin to induce tolerance in recipients after organ transplantation. Initial clinical reports on 10 patients who received granulocyte colony-stimulating factor–induced hematopoietic stem cell transplants from haploidentical donors demonstrated achievement of tolerance in six patients. This was followed by a subsequent report on 16 patients who received total lymphoid irradiation followed by CD34+ donor bone marrow cells, with 12 of 16 patients ultimately completely weaned from immunosuppression. Unfortunately, these models are currently limited to haploidentical living donors. Most recently, enriched hematopoietic stem cells and tolerogenic CD8+/TCR– graft cells have been used to establish chimerism and induce tolerance. Of the initial 15 patients reported, 11 patients maintained durable chimerism and were fully withdrawn from immunosuppression within 1 year. Although there has been substantial progress in tolerance induction, broader clinical applications are on the horizon. Further research is expected to focus on combining approaches of achieving chimerism with the application of regulatory T cells. Additional future goals will also need to find ways to apply tolerance protocols in recipients of organs from deceased doors.

Bray RA, Gebel HM, Townsend R, et al: De novo donor-specific antibodies in belatacept-treated vs cyclosporine-treated kidney-transplant recipients: post hoc analyses of the randomized phase III BENEFIT and BENEFIT-EXT studies. *Am J Transplant.* 2018;18(7):1783-1789.

Cohen JA, Coles AJ, Arnold DL, et al: Alemtuzumab versus interferon beta 1a as first-line treatment for patients with relapsing-remitting multiple sclerosis: a randomised controlled phase 3 trial. *Lancet.* 2012;380(9856):1819-1828.

Coles AJ, Twyman CL, Arnold DL, et al: Alemtuzumab for patients with relapsing multiple sclerosis after disease-modifying therapy: a randomised controlled phase 3 trial. *Lancet.* 2012; 380(9856):1829-1839.

Costelloe L, Jones J, Coles A: Secondary autoimmune diseases following alemtuzumab therapy for multiple sclerosis. *Expert Rev Neurother.* 2012;12(3):335-341.

Djamali A, Kaufman DB, Ellis TM, et al: Diagnosis and management of antibody-mediated rejection: current status and novel approaches. *Am J Transplant.* 2014;14(2):255-271.

Friend PJ: Alemtuzumab induction therapy in solid organ transplantation. *Transplant Res.* 2013;2(Suppl 1):S5.

Garces JC, Giusti S, Staffeld-Coit C, et al: Antibody-mediated rejection: a review. *Ochsner J.* 2017;17(1):46-55.

Geissler EK, Schnitzbauer AA, Zülke C, et al: Sirolimus use in liver transplant recipients with hepatocellular carcinoma: a randomized, multicenter, open-label phase 3 trial. *Transplantation.* 2016;100(1):116-125.

Halloran PF: Immunosuppressive drugs for kidney transplantation. *N Engl J Med.* 2004;351(26):2715-2729.

Hanaway MJ, Woodle ES, Mulgaonkar S, et al: Alemtuzumab induction in renal transplantation. *N Engl J Med.* 2011;364(20):1909-1919.

Kandaswamy R, Stock PG, Gustafson SK, et al: OPTN/SRTR 2016 annual data report: pancreas. *Am J Transplant.* 2018;18:114-171.

Kawai T, Cosimi AB, Spitzer TR, et al: HLA-mismatched renal transplantation without maintenance immunosuppression. *N Engl J Med.* 2008;358(4):353-361.

Kidney Disease: Improving Global Outcomes (KDIGO) Living Kidney Donor Work Group: KDIGO clinical practice guideline on the evaluation of living kidney donors. *Transplantation.* 2017;Suppl 8S:S1-S109.

Kim WR, Lake JR, Smith JM, et al: OPTN/SRTR 2016 annual data report: liver. *Am J Transplant.* 2018;18:172-253.

Leung DYM, Bloom JW, Bloom JW: Update on glucocorticoid action and resistance. *J Allergy Clin Immunol.* 2003;111(1):3-22; quiz 23.

Leventhal J, Abecassis M, Miller J, et al: Chimerism and tolerance without GVHD or engraftment syndrome in HLA-mismatched combined kidney and hematopoietic stem cell transplantation. *Sci Transl Med.* 2012;4(124):124ra28.

Mohty M: Mechanisms of action of antithymocyte globulin: T-cell depletion and beyond. *Leukemia.* 2007;21(7):1387-1394.

Scandling JD, Busque S, Dejbakhsh-Jones S, et al: Tolerance and withdrawal of immunosuppressive drugs in patients given kidney and hematopoietic cell transplants. *Am J Transplant.* 2012;12(5):1133-1145.

Stegall MD, Morris RE, Alloway RR, et al: Developing new immunosuppression for the next generation of transplant recipients: the path forward. *Am J Transplant.* 2016;16(4):1094-1101.

Tanriover B, Jaikaransingh V, MacConmara MP, et al: Acute rejection rates and graft outcomes according to induction regimen among recipients of kidneys from deceased donors treated with tacrolimus and mycophenolate. *Clin J Am Soc Nephrol.* 2016;11(9):1650-1661.

Vincenti F, Rostaing L, Grinyo J, et al: Belatacept and long-term outcomes in kidney transplantation. *N Engl J Med.* 2016; 374(4):333-343.

Willicombe M, Roufosse C, Brookes P, et al: Antibody-mediated rejection after alemtuzumab induction: incidence, risk factors, and predictors of poor outcome. *Transplantation.* 2011;92(2):176-182.

Zeiser R, Leveson-Gower DB, Zambricki EA, et al: Differential impact of mammalian target of rapamycin inhibition on CD4 CD25 Foxp3 regulatory T cells compared with conventional CD4 T cells. *Blood.* 2008;111(1):453-462.

KIDNEY TRANSPLANTATION

The first successful kidney transplant was performed at the Peter Bent Brigham Hospital in Boston by Dr. Joseph Murray (1954) between identical twins and demonstrated the surgical feasibility of organ transplantation. The same group went on to successfully transplant kidneys from genetically disparate donors and later effectively applied chemical immunosuppression.

In the United States, patients may be listed for kidney transplantation with advanced chronic kidney disease (CKD) documented by a glomerular filtration rate or creatinine clearance ≤ 20 mL/min or once dialysis has been initiated. Absolute contraindications to transplantation include active infections, active malignancies, active substance abuse, medication nonadherence, and active untreated psychiatric disorders. There are many potential relative contraindications that require a targeted patient assessment; these may include untreated ischemic cardiac disease and life expectancy. Age cutoffs vary by institution; however, historically, clinical trials in organ transplantation have not included patients over the age 65. Despite this, approximately 20% of renal transplant recipients are greater than 65 years old. Clinical studies have shown a decreased frequency of acute allograft rejection in the elderly. Research regarding immunosenescence and the outcomes of renal transplant in traditionally older patients is ongoing, with a growing amount of elderly transplant recipients.

The prominent discrepancy between demand and supply in renal transplantation has resulted in prolonged waiting times and rising morbidity and mortality rates for patients awaiting transplantation. Since 2010, there has been a 277% increase in deceased donor renal transplantation through patients who died of an opioid overdose. There is hope that current initiatives will successfully combat the opioid epidemic in the United States. A new Kidney Allocation System (KAS) was implemented in December of 2014 and emphasizes additional opportunities to transplant highly sensitized patients while linking organ placement with estimated posttransplant survival (EPTS).

The new KAS is predicated upon a continuous donor quality metric known as the Kidney Donor Profile Index (KDPI). The KDPI ranges from 0% to 100% and incorporates 10 donor factors that estimate the potential for graft longevity (with a lower percentage corresponding to a lower risk of graft failure). This metric is paired with the EPTS score, which is based on age, time on dialysis, diabetic status, and prior organ transplant. Together, donors with a KDPI of less than 20% are paired with patients with the top 20% of EPTS scores, who receive priority transplantation before other candidates. Within this system, older recipients, patients who have been on the waitlist for a prolonged period, and patients with diabetes may benefit from what were previously considered to be expanded criteria donor (ECD) allografts (Figure 48–2).

ECDs include donors with factors such as older age, hypertension, diabetes, high-risk behaviors, and cardiac death (as opposed to brain death). These ECD allografts, by definition, have inferior outcomes compared to standard deceased donation; however, they can still have good results, with 3-month and 1-rear graft survival rates of 90% and 82%, respectively, compared to standard criteria deceased donation survival rates of 94% and 89%, respectively. However, the success of ECD transplants is directly related to both donor quality, as measured by the Kidney Donor Risk Index and cold ischemia time, and also recipient characteristics, such as race, diabetes, age, and circulating DSAs at the time of transplantation. Nevertheless, older patients or those whose health deteriorates faster on dialysis will benefit from the transplantation of less than optimal allografts.

When comparing DCD versus DBD allografts, DCD kidneys have a significantly higher risk of delayed graft function and primary nonfunction primarily due to prolonged

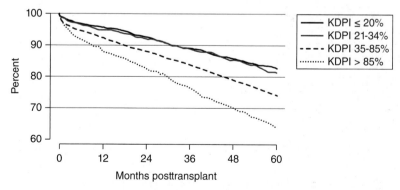

▲ **Figure 48–2.** Graft survival among adult deceased donor kidney transplant recipients, 2011, by kidney donor profile index (KDPI). Graft survival estimated using unadjusted Kaplan-Meier methods. (Reproduced with permission from Hart A, Smith JM, Skeans MA, et al: OPTN/SRTR 2016 Annual Data Report: Kidney, *Am J Transplant.* 2018 Jan;18 Suppl 1:18-113.)

warm ischemia time; however, for functioning kidneys, the long-term graft function is comparable. Based on Scientific Registry of Transplant Recipients data on all kidney transplants through 2014, the 1- and 5-year unadjusted allograft survival rates from all deceased donors were 93.4% and 72.4%, respectively, and this is similar for both DCD and DBD allografts. For living donor recipients, allograft survival is significantly higher, at 97.2% and 84.6% at 1 and 5 years, respectively.

Concerted efforts have been made to increase the use of kidneys from older donors, donors after cardiac death, and donors at increased risk for infection, such as those with a history of intravenous drug use, hepatitis B virus, and/or hepatitis C virus.

► Operative Technique

During kidney transplantation, grafts are positioned heterotopically (transplantation into a location other than the normal anatomic position), and the native kidney is, in general, not removed. In adults, the allograft is preferably transplanted into the right or left iliac fossa with vascular anastomoses to the external iliac vessels (Figure 48–3). The ureter is anastomosed to the bladder.

1. A modified Gibson incision is made that involves a curvilinear skin incision, beginning at the pubic symphysis and extending superolaterally. An incision is then made at the border between the fascia of the external oblique and the lateral edge of the rectus abdominus, which when pulled aside, allows access to the posterior rectus sheath.

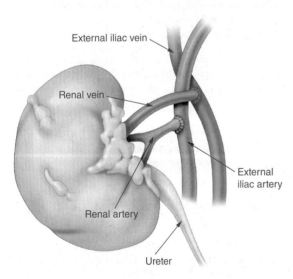

External iliac vein

Renal vein

Renal artery

External iliac artery

Ureter

▲ **Figure 48–3.** Renal transplant after arterial and venous anastomoses. The ureter will be anastomosed to the recipient's bladder, thereby preventing urinary reflux with the Lich-Gregoire or Leadbetter-Politano techniques (not shown).

Dividing the posterior rectus sheath or going below the arcuate line (where the posterior sheath is missing) provides access to the retroperitoneal space.

2. The peritoneum is then mobilized medially. The inferior epigastric artery and vein, along with the round ligament (in females), will be encountered, ligated, and divided during this step. The spermatic cord in males is identified, isolated with a vessel loop, and preserved.

3. The external or common iliac artery and vein are dissected free; the allograft renal artery and vein are anastomosed to the recipient iliac artery and vein, respectively, usually as an end-to-side vascular anastomosis with nonabsorbable suture. An end-to-end anastomosis of the renal artery to the internal iliac artery is an alternative; however, this is complicated by higher rates of arterial thrombosis linked to torsion or kinking of the internal iliac/renal artery.

4. After establishing perfusion, the ureter is transplanted into the bladder. Generally, a cystotomy is created, and the donor ureter is spatulated and anastomosed using absorbable suture (usually PDS, or polydioxanone suture). This may be performed either via an inferolateral submucosal tunnel (Leadbetter-Politano technique) or with an anterolateral mucosal dissection (Lich-Gregoir technique).

5. Ureteral stents may be placed, but this is at the discretion of the surgeon and based on a balance of infectious complications and confidence with the anastomotic quality.

6. The anastomoses are inspected, and the incision is closed.

In small children or patients with previous transplants or surgeries in the groin challenging the surgical exposure, kidneys may also be placed intra-abdominally and anastomosed to the common or external iliac artery and vein.

► Complications

Complications after renal transplantation can include events typical to all operations, such as postoperative bleeding and surgical site infections. Operation-specific complications can be vascular or urologic in nature. Vascular complications have variable incidence, depending on how they are classified, but can include renal artery stenosis, arteriovenous fistula formation, pseudoaneurysm formation, or renal artery/vein thrombosis. The most feared complication is renal artery/vein thrombosis, which occurs in less than 1% of patients, but generally occurs in the immediate posttransplant period and is often heralded by an immediate drop in urine output in addition to a sharp rise in blood urea nitrogen (BUN) or serum creatinine levels. Other indicators, although less frequent, include pain over the graft site or hematuria; risk factors include a history of hypercoagulopathy or technical errors in anastomosis creation (eg, creation of an intimal flap or arterial kinking). Diagnosis is made with an immediate duplex ultrasonography, which will demonstrate a cessation of vascular flow into the allograft. Complete ABO incompatibility, hyperacute rejection, and subsequent hemagglutination will invariably lead to graft thrombosis; however, in the era of meticulous preoperative testing, this outcome is rarely, if ever, observed.

Urologic complications can be seen in up to 5% of patients and include urinary leak or urinary obstruction. Urinary leak is often due to distal ureter ischemia, increased urinary pressure from obstruction, or technical errors in anastomosis creation but may also be seen from the renal pelvis related to the back-table preparation of the kidney or surgical errors during procurement. Signs and symptoms of urine leak include a decrease in urine output, fever, or fullness and tenderness around the graft site. Ultrasonography or a computed tomography (CT) can support the diagnosis by demonstrating a perigraft anechoic fluid collection (urinoma). However, those findings may be nonspecific. Elevated creatinine or BUN in the fluid collection or an extravasate detected on CT urogram confirms a leak. Small leaks and urinomas may be treated with percutaneous nephrostomy, ureteral stent placement, and percutaneous urinoma drainage. If this strategy is unsuccessful in allowing the ureteral anastomosis or the leakage to heal, surgical reexploration and repair may be necessary. Urinary obstruction in the early postoperative period may be secondary to hematoma formation, postoperative edema, or technical errors such as ureteral kinking or narrowing of the anastomosis. Long-term urinary obstruction after transplantation may be linked to distal ischemia of the ureter and consequent stricture or stenosis. Duplex ultrasonography will demonstrate hydronephrosis, and initial treatment is similar to urinary leak with percutaneous nephrostomy and ureteral stenting. Failed conservative management may necessitate operative intervention and anastomotic revision.

Akbar SA, Jafri SZH, Amendola MA, et al: Complications of renal transplantation. *RadioGraphics*. 2005;25(5):1335-1356.

Akoh JA: Kidney donation after cardiac death. *World J Nephrol*. 2012;1(3):79-91.

Aubert O, Kamar N, Vernerey D, et al: Long term outcomes of transplantation using kidneys from expanded criteria donors: prospective, population based cohort study. *BMJ*. 2015;351:h3557.

Batabyal P, Chapman JR, Wong G, et al: Clinical practice guidelines on wait-listing for kidney transplantation. *Transplant J*. 2012;94(7):703-713.

Chute DF, Sise ME: Effect of the opioid crisis on the donor pool for kidney transplantation: an analysis of national kidney deceased donor trends from 2010–2016. *Am J Nephrol*. 2018;47(2):84-93.

Colvin MM, Smith CA, Tullius SG, et al: Aging and the immune response to organ transplantation. *J Clin Invest*. 2017;127(7):2523-2529.

Gruessner AC, Jie T, Papas K, et al: *Schwartz's Principles of Surgery*. 10th ed. New York, NY: McGraw-Hill Education; 2014.

Heaphy ELG, Goldfarb DA, Poggio ED, et al: The impact of deceased donor kidney risk significantly varies by recipient characteristics. *Am J Transplant*. 2013;13(4):1001-1011.

Huang E, Segev DL, Rabb H: Kidney transplantation in the elderly. *Semin Nephrol*. 2009;29(6):621-635.

Kasiske BL, Cangro CB, Hariharan S, et al: The evaluation of renal transplantation candidates: clinical practice guidelines. *Am J Transplant*. 2001;1(Suppl 2):3-95.

Kidney Allocation System. https://optn.transplant.hrsa.gov/learn/professional-education/kidney-allocation-system/.

Merrill JP, Murray JE, Harrison JH, et al: Successful homotransplantation of the human kidney between identical twins. *J Am Med Assoc*. 1956;160(4):277-282.

Metzger RA, Delmonico FL, Feng S, et al: Expanded criteria donors for kidney transplantation. *Am J Transplant*. 2003;3(s4):114-125.

Nieto T, Inston N, Cockwell P: Renal transplantation in adults. *BMJ*. 2016;355:i6158.

Reyna-Sepúlveda F, Ponce-Escobedo A, Guevara-Charles A, et al: Outcomes and surgical complications in kidney transplantation. *Int J Organ Transplant Med*. 2017;8(2):78-84.

Wang JH, Skeans MA, Israni AK: Current status of kidney transplant outcomes: dying to survive. *Adv Chronic Kidney Dis*. 2016;23:281-286.

Wolfe RA, Ashby VB, Milford EL, et al: Comparison of mortality in all patients on dialysis, patients on dialysis awaiting transplantation, and recipients of a first cadaveric transplant. *N Engl J Med*. 1999;341(23):1725-1730.

LIVER TRANSPLANTATION

Indications for liver transplantation include acute hepatic failure; complications from cirrhosis or chronic liver disease that may include ascites, variceal bleeding, and hepatopulmonary syndrome; metabolic conditions such as hemochromatosis; and glycogen storage diseases. Between 2004 and 2015, hepatocellular carcinoma was the most common indication for liver transplantation, composing 18.5% of waitlist registrants and totaling over 109,000 patients. The **MELD score**, although initially created to evaluate 3-month prognosis for patients undergoing transjugular intrahepatic portosystemic shunting, incorporates serum creatine, bilirubin, and international normalized ratio (INR) and has been shown to predict survival. This model was subsequently adopted by the transplant community as a method to objectify the organ allocation process, prioritizing sicker patients for transplantation. One absolute contraindication for transplantation is a MELD score of less than 15 because risks of transplantation may not outweigh any benefit. Other contraindications include debilitating cardiovascular disease, metastatic cancer or extrahepatic malignancies, noncompliance, and lack of social support.

There has been substantial controversy surrounding current allocation models, notably between predicted and actual waitlist deaths. To realign donor allocation, the National Liver Review Board was tasked with assigning "exception points" to patients' MELD scores; however, this

Table 48–1. The Child-Pugh Scoring system.

Clinical and Laboratory Criteria	Points		
	1	2	3
Encephalopathy	None	Mild to moderate	Severe
Ascites	None	Mild to moderate	Severe
Bilirubin (mg/dL)	< 2	2-3	> 3
Albumin (g/dL)	> 3.5	2.8-3.5	< 2.8
Prothrombin time prolongation (s)	< 4	4-6	> 6
International normalized ratio (INR)	< 1.7	1.7-2.3	> 2.3
Child-Pugh class A: 5-6 points, 10% operative mortality			
Child-Pugh class B: 7-9 points, 30%-31% operative mortality			
Child-Pugh class C: 10-15 points, 76%-82% operative mortality			

Note. Mortality rates are for major abdominal surgery.
Data from Garrison RN, Cryer HM, Howard DA, et al: Clarification of risk factors for abdominal operations in patients with hepatic cirrhosis, *Ann Surg.* 1984 Jun;199(6):648-55.

did not solve the problem of donor shortage. The OPTN has undertaken the creation of a new model with eight mathematically optimized districts and the assignment of 3 MELD points for patients within a 150-mile radius of the donor hospital. However, there is still concern among the transplant community that this model may not fairly distribute organs, with some arguing that more organs would be allocated to wealthy, urban, high socioeconomic status areas. Despite frequently lower MELD scores, low socioeconomic areas have substantially higher waitlist mortality than more densely populated areas with more accessible tertiary care facilities. However, patients are encouraged to travel outside their respective donor service areas, a luxury that is limited almost exclusively to high socioeconomic status patients. Waitlist outcomes may be purely due to transplant center availability and density; thus, reorganizing the current 58 donor service area boundaries and establishing allocation models based on acuity or changing the geographic distribution may help equalize organ distribution. Liver allocation is currently still in flux, and new proposals that will align geographic disparities and patients' needs continue to be discussed. Those discussions will likely also impact the allocation of other organs.

The **Child-Pugh score** was originally designed to predict operative outcomes of cirrhotic patients undergoing portosystemic shunt therapy for bleeding esophageal varices and has since been used to assess the operative risk for any cirrhotic patients undergoing surgery. The scoring system uses bilirubin, albumin, INR, presence of ascites, and encephalopathy to grade patients as Child class A, B,

or C; immediate perioperative mortality increases with each class, with mortality exceeding 76%-82% for Child class C patients (Table 48–1). The utility of using the MELD versus Child-Pugh score has been debated, with the main drawback of the Child-Pugh score being the subjectivity of the ascites and encephalopathy assessments; regardless, both scores appear equally valid in the appropriate scenario.

▶ **Operative Technique**

Unlike in renal transplantation, the recipient's native organ is, in general, removed prior to **orthotopic transplantation** (transplantation into the normal anatomic position), with the exception of auxiliary liver transplants in cases of acute liver failure. The phases of the operation can thus be divided into the initial hepatectomy, followed by the liver transplantation.

A. Recipient Hepatectomy

1. A bilateral subcostal incision is made approximately two fingerbreadths below the costal margin (also known as a "chevron" incision).

2. The falciform ligament is ligated between ties and divided to better expose the porta hepatis.

3. The cystic duct and artery are ligated and divided.

4. The right and left hepatic arteries are ligated and divided high within the porta hepatis to maximize the length available for anastomosis.

5. The common bile duct and the portal vein are dissected circumferentially, but division is saved until just prior to the hepatectomy.

6. The left triangular ligament is divided, allowing the left lobe to be retracted to the right.

7. The remainder of the gastrohepatic ligament is divided exposing the lesser sac and the caudate lobe.

8. The peritoneal attachments between the caudate lobe and the inferior vena cava (IVC) are divided.

9. The retroperitoneum is divided to the left of the IVC to allow for a retroperitoneal mobilization.

10. The right hepatic lobe is dissected from the diaphragm and right abdominal side wall to expose the bare area of the liver; this allows exposure of the right adrenal vein for ligation and division.

11. The retroperitoneal plane previously dissected is continued from right to left, also creating a retrocaval plane.

12. Once the liver is fully mobilized, the portal vein is divided and the supra- and infrahepatic IVC are controlled with clamps prior to division.

B. Venovenous Bypass

1. Venovenous bypass is rarely required in modern transplantation; however, it may be required for patients with portal bleeding, which limits the ability to perform the recipient hepatectomy.

2. The objective is to maintain systemic pressure during caval occlusion with a bypass from the portal and left femoral veins to the left axillary vein.

C. Liver Transplantation

1. The allograft is transplanted with a segment of the supra- and infrahepatic IVC, which allows for a "bicaval" anastomosis between the donor and recipient segments (Figure 48–4).

2. Alternatively, during the "piggyback technique," the recipient vena cava is not divided. The donor suprahepatic vena cava is anastomosed to the recipient hepatic veins. The intrahepatic cava is then ligated.

3. After the caval anastomosis, the portal venous anastomosis is performed, and the liver is perfused.

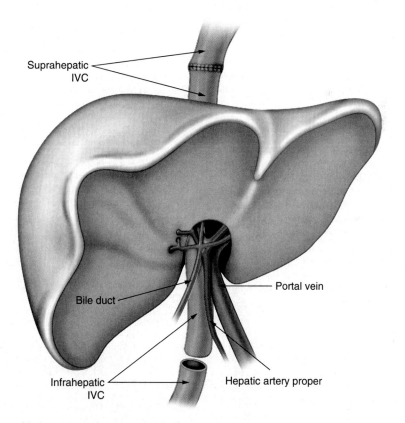

Suprahepatic IVC

Portal vein

Bile duct

Infrahepatic IVC

Hepatic artery proper

▲ **Figure 48–4.** Bicaval hepatic transplantation. IVC, inferior vena cava.

4. This anastomosis is then followed by the arterial anastomosis; donor and recipient arteries can arise from the bifurcation of the right and left hepatic arteries, the bifurcation of the gastroduodenal artery and the hepatic artery proper, or the bifurcation of the common hepatic and splenic arteries.

5. Finally, the biliary anastomosis is performed, preferably in an end-to-end or side-to-side fashion between the donor and recipient common bile ducts; however, a Roux-en-Y hepaticojejunostomy can also be performed.

    a. An anastomosis between the donor and recipient common bile ducts is referred to as a choledochocholedochostomy and is the preferred and most common biliary anastomosis performed due to sphincter of Oddi preservation, which, at least in theory, decreases the risk of ascending cholangitis. This also allows for endoscopic evaluation of the common duct via endoscopic retrograde cholangiopancreatography (ERCP).

    b. Alternatively, a choledochojejunostomy may be performed in patients with biliary disease such as primary sclerosing cholangitis, primary biliary surgery, prior biliary surgery, or a size mismatch between donor and recipient bile ducts. This anastomosis adds additional time and challenges an endoscopic bile duct evaluation.

6. The anastomoses are inspected, and the abdomen is closed.

▶ Complications

The incidence of complications after liver transplantation exceeds that of renal transplantation, and vigilance must be kept in monitoring these patients in the perioperative period, most of whom had some degree of coagulopathy and volume disturbance before transplant. These complications can be grouped into graft-related complications, such as postoperative bleeding, vascular thrombosis, and biliary complications, and medical complications, such as pulmonary, renal, and infectious complications.

As in all intra-abdominal operations, bleeding is a possibility after transplantation, with an elevated risk in liver transplant recipients linked to coagulopathy secondary to hepatic dysfunction. Rates of hemorrhage requiring reoperation have been reported in up to 20% of patients and are linked to the amount of transfused blood products intraoperatively, hepatitis B virus–related liver disease, MELD score, and preoperative partial thromboplastin time. Vascular complications may occur in up to 15% of patients and include hepatic artery thrombosis (HAT), anastomotic stenosis, and pseudoaneurysm formation. Notably, vascular complications are higher in living compared to deceased donor liver transplants (13% vs 7%, respectively). HAT alone has been reported to occur in 8%-12% of orthotopic liver transplants, and risk factors include the duration of the hepatectomy, arterial anomalies, arterial reconstructions, and size of the arteries. HAT is a significant concern postoperatively because it can lead to graft loss and mortality. Should patients experience these complications postoperatively, therapeutic considerations may include attempting endovascular thrombolysis or angioplasty and stenting; performing an immediate open surgical revascularization; and lastly, retransplantation. This approach is dictated by the time interval between HAT and transplantation; early HAT is often treated with reintervention; unsuccessful surgical or endoscopic revision will be followed by retransplantation.

Biliary complications include primarily bile leaks (early) and biliary obstructions (late), which are attributed to ischemic-type biliary lesions. Sphincter of Oddi dysfunction or recurrence of primary disease may occur in up to 32% of patients after transplantation. These complications are specific to the type of anastomosis performed and whether T-tubes are used during creation of the anastomosis. T-tube use during choledochocholedochostomy, while allowing for direct evaluation of the biliary tree, is associated with higher rates of overall complications, including postoperative cholangitis. Additional complications unrelated to the use of T-tubes include anastomotic leaks and strictures. Patients undergoing choledochojejunostomy have the additional risk of intestinal perforation, bleeding, and ascending cholangitis, while retaining the risk of anastomotic leaking and stricture.

Patients with bile leaks are often managed endoscopically (ERCP with sphincterotomy and bile duct stenting) with treatment success in the clear majority. For patients unable to have an ERCP performed, including those with a choledochojejunostomy, a percutaneous transhepatic catheter may be placed to allow for biliary diversion and healing of the anastomosis. If these radiologic and endoscopic interventions fail, surgical correction may be necessary. As with bile leaks, biliary strictures may be managed endoscopically with stent and balloon dilation if necessary.

Adler JT, Yeh H: Social determinants in liver transplantation. *Clin Liver Dis.* 2016;7(1):15-17.

Angermayr B, Cejna M, Karnel F, et al: Child-Pugh versus MELD score in predicting survival in patients undergoing transjugular intrahepatic portosystemic shunt. *Gut.* 2003;52(6):879-885.

Flavin CM: *Redesigning Liver Distribution: OPTN/UNOS Liver and Intestinal Organ Transplantation Committee.* 2016. https://optn.transplant.hrsa.gov/governance/public-comment/redesigning-liver-distribution/

Friedman LS: Surgery in the patient with liver disease. *Trans Am Clin Climatol Assoc.* 2010;121:192-204; discussion 205.

Garrison RN, Cryer HM, Howard DA, et al: Clarification of risk factors for abdominal operations in patients with hepatic cirrhosis. *Ann Surg.* 1984;199(6):648-655.

Gerber DA, Baliga P, Karp SJ: Allocation of donor livers for transplantation. *JAMA Surg.* 2018;153(9):787.

Kochhar G, Parungao JM, Hanouneh IA, et al: Biliary complications following liver transplantation. *World J Gastroenterol.* 2013;19(19):2841-2846.

Martin P, DiMartini A, Feng S, et al: Evaluation for liver transplantation in adults: 2013 practice guideline by the American Association for the Study of Liver Diseases and the American Society of Transplantation. *Hepatology.* 2014;59(3):1144-1165.

Neeff H, Mariaskin D, Spangenberg H-C, et al: Perioperative mortality after non-hepatic general surgery in patients with liver cirrhosis: an analysis of 138 operations in the 2000s using Child and MELD scores. *J Gastrointest Surg.* 2011;15(1):1-11.

Nemes B, Gaman G, Gelley F, et al: Technical risk factors for hepatic artery thrombosis after orthotopic liver transplantation: the Hungarian experience. *Transplant Proc.* 2013;45(10):3691-3694.

Peng Y, Qi X, Guo X: Child-Pugh versus MELD score for the assessment of prognosis in liver cirrhosis: a systematic review and meta-analysis of observational studies. *Medicine (Baltimore).* 2016;95(8):e2877.

Piardi T, Lhuaire M, Bruno O, et al: Vascular complications following liver transplantation: A literature review of advances in 2015. *World J Hepatol.* 2016;8(1):36-57.

Puliti Reigada CH, de Ataide EC, de Almeida Prado Mattosinho T, et al: Hepatic artery thrombosis after liver transplantation: five-year experience at the State University of Campinas. *Transplant Proc.* 2017;49(4):867-870.

Schrem H, Klußmann A, Focken M, et al: Post-operative hemorrhage after liver transplantation: risk factors and long-term outcome. *Ann Transplant.* 2016;21:46-55.

Yang JD, Larson JJ, Watt KD, et al: Hepatocellular carcinoma is the most common indication for liver transplantation and placement on the waitlist in the United States. *Clin Gastroenterol Hepatol.* 2017;15(5):767-775.e3.

PANCREAS TRANSPLANTATION

Diabetes is currently the leading cause of renal failure, blindness, and nontraumatic amputations (from diabetic foot sepsis) with an immense burden on the American healthcare system. Although injectable insulin has drastically improved both the quality of life and life expectancy for diabetics, the ability of the pancreas to physiologically regulate and treat variations in serum glucose levels is unmatched by current pharmaceuticals or technology. It is worthwhile to note significant innovations and advancements in insulin delivery, including a fully automated, bihormonal, "bionic" pancreas, which, at least in small studies, has shown improved mean glucose levels and fewer hypoglycemic episodes compared to injectable insulin. A functioning pancreas transplant, however, allows for both improved quality of life through cessation of insulin injections and achievement of a euglycemic insulin-independent state.

The main disadvantage to pancreas transplantation, aside from surgical complications, is immunosuppression, such that the American Diabetes Association recommends pancreas transplantation, either as a simultaneous pancreas-kidney transplant or after a kidney transplant (pancreas after kidney), for patients with type 1 diabetes mellitus (DM) and concomitant ESRD. Given the side effects associated with immunosuppression, pancreas transplantation is considered for patients with frequent and severe metabolic complications of diabetes (labile serum glucose with ketoacidosis or hypoglycemia or diabetic retinopathy and neuropathy), difficulties with insulin administration, and/or failure of insulin administration. Patients with type 1 DM and no evidence of CKD may be considered for pancreas transplantation alone (PTA) with evidence of impaired hypoglycemic awareness (eg, fear, seizures, accidents, job loss) and multiple life-threatening hypoglycemic events despite a trial of continuous glucose monitoring or insulin pump therapy. Finally, pancreatic islet transplantation, during which a donor pancreas is enzymatically digested and the islets infused percutaneously into the portal venous circulation, is currently under clinical and experimental investigation as another option for patients with type 1 DM. The main difference compared to a PTA is the avoidance of a major operation with its potential complications. Success, measured in insulin independence, is highly variable, and ranges between 23% and greater than 90%, depending on the institution. Although traditionally considered a contraindication, certain patients with type 2 DM have been transplanted with favorable outcomes by some. Selection criteria require refinement but include hypoglycemic unawareness and low C-peptide levels, among others.

Allo-islet cell transplantation is an attractive alternative to whole pancreas transplantation because the procedure avoids, in general, surgical complications. While great progress has been achieved, unresolved aspects will need to be addressed in the future to establish the procedure as a clinical routine. Most relevant are an optimization of the islet isolation process, the progressive loss of islets over time, and the necessity of frequent retransfusions requiring multiple islet cell donors

Pancreatic auto-islet transplantation is an evolving field but used for patients with refractory pancreatitis who ultimately proceed with total pancreatectomy as a method to preserve some measure of insulin independence.

▶ Operative Technique

Pancreas transplants are placed into a **heterotopic** location, and the recipient pancreas is not explanted.

A. Deceased Donor Pancreatectomy

1. The lesser sac is entered by dividing the gastrocolic ligament and retracting the stomach superiorly.

2. The gastroduodenal and right and left gastric arteries are ligated and divided; the common bile duct is divided.

3. A Kocher maneuver is performed, and attention is then turned to freeing the splenic attachments, which allows for lateral-to-medial dissection of the remainder of the pancreas.

4. The pancreas is removed en bloc with the spleen and duodenum, given the shared blood supply; care is taken to preserve the splenic artery, superior mesenteric artery (SMA), and portal vein with sufficient length; ideally, a patch of aorta is removed with the SMA to facilitate anastomotic creation, but this may not always be possible.

5. Prior to transplantation, the splenic artery and SMA are connected using a reversed segment of donor iliac artery to create a Y-graft, which allows for a single inflow anastomosis.

B. Pancreas Transplantation

1. The abdomen is entered via a low midline laparotomy with dissection turned toward the right lower quadrant, between the cecum and the retroperitoneum.

2. The right iliac fossa is preferred due to more superficial vessels and a better position of the pancreas, avoiding a position lateral to the mobilized sigmoid colon on the left.

3. The vascular anastomosis is performed between the Y-graft and the recipient's distal aorta, common iliac artery, or external iliac artery; the donor portal vein is anastomosed to the distal IVC, the recipient common iliac vein, or the external iliac vein.

4. Next, the pancreatic exocrine secretions are drained by anastomosing the donor duodenum to the recipient small intestine, either in continuity or via a Roux-en-Y enteric limb or the bladder.
   a. For bladder drainage, the anterior and lateral attachments of the bladder are dissected free, and the duodenum is anastomosed to the dome of the bladder.
   b. For enteric drainage, a loop of mid-jejunum, approximately 70-100 cm past the ligament of Treitz, is mobilized, and a side-to-side anastomosis between the duodenum and jejunum is performed (Figure 48–5).

5. The anastomoses are inspected, and the abdomen is closed.

► Complications

As with both kidney and liver transplantation, pancreas allografts are susceptible to vascular graft thrombosis. At a rate of about 6%, thrombosis can ultimately lead to graft failure. Salvage attempts at therapy can include both percutaneous/endovascular and surgical thrombectomy; however, frequently, retransplantation may be necessary. The approach will again depend on the time interval between surgery and the vascular complication. For this reason,

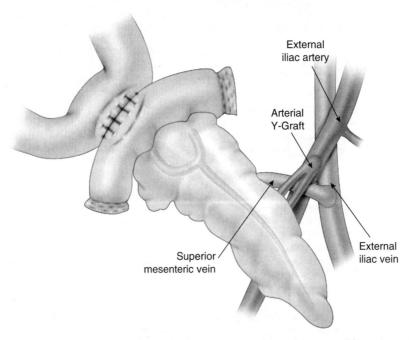

▲ **Figure 48–5.** Pancreatic transplantation with enteric drainage. Arterial Y-graft is created from donor iliac artery and connects the donor superior mesenteric and splenic arteries. The superior mesenteric vein and the arterial Y-graft can be anastomosed to the distal inferior vena cava/aorta; the common iliac artery or common iliac vein; or, as on this illustration, the external iliac artery or external iliac vein.

anticoagulation is often recommended in the form of aspirin postoperatively.

Bladder drainage can be associated with significant dehydration and metabolic acidosis from a loss of bicarbonate in the urine, in addition to urinary tract infections, hematuria, and nephrolithiasis. Bladder calculi may develop due to the exposed suture material and may require cystoscopy with suture or staple removal. For this reason, absorbable sutures are used to create the anastomosis, thus mitigating this risk. Patients may develop urinomas/urinary leaks from the enteric-bladder anastomosis. These can often be managed conservatively with bladder catheters. Up to 10%-20% of patients with bladder drainage are converted to enteric drainage.

Leakage of the enteric exocrine drainage my cause peritonitis and pancreatitis. This complication may require interventional or surgical drainage with washout, enteric diversion, or removal of the transplanted pancreas. Pancreatitis may also occur based on quality or graft injury and represents a severe complication, with symptoms of an acute abdomen and acute hemorrhage. Donor selection is thus critically contributory to the success of pancreas transplantation.

Ahearn AJ, Parekh JR, Posselt AM: Islet transplantation for type 1 diabetes: where are we now? *Expert Rev Clin Immunol.* 2015;11(1):59-68.

Ciancio G, Burke GW: Type 2 diabetes: is pancreas transplantation an option? *Curr Diab Rep.* 2014;14(11):542.

Farney AC, Rogers J, Stratta RJ: Pancreas graft thrombosis. *Curr Opin Organ Transplant.* 2012;17(1):87-92.

Jolissaint JS, Langman LW, DeBolt CL, et al: The impact of bacterial colonization on graft success after total pancreatectomy with autologous islet transplantation: considerations for early definitive surgical intervention. *Clin Transplant.* 2016;30:11.

Robertson RP, Davis C, Larsen J, et al :Pancreas and islet transplantation in type 1 diabetes. *Diabetes Care.* 2006;29(4):935.

Russell SJ, El-Khatib FH, Sinha M, et al: Outpatient glycemic control with a bionic pancreas in type 1 diabetes. *N Engl J Med.* 2014; 371(4):313-325.

CONCLUSION

Transplantation is the gold standard for several end-stage conditions. When successful, these operations can be curative and improve both life expectancy and quality of life. Each transplant carries both immediate and long-term risks, in addition to the currently inevitable risks of long-term immunosuppression. Risks and benefits of each operation benefit from a case-by-case multidisciplinary discussion, with considerations given to the patient's overall health, treatment adherence, and social support. Once transplanted, each organ has the power to drastically improve a patient's life.

MULTIPLE CHOICE QUESTIONS

1. Compared to other types of kidney transplants, transplants from donors after cardiac death have

   A. Comparable rates of delayed graft function and graft survival
   B. Higher rates of delayed graft function with comparable rates of graft survival
   C. Higher mortality rates
   D. Higher rates of acute rejection in the immediate postoperative period

2. Compared to other types of liver transplants, transplants from donors after cardiac death have

   A. Higher rates of acute rejection in the immediate postoperative period
   B. Higher rates of nonanastomotic biliary stricture and graft loss
   C. Higher rates of biliary anastomotic stenosis with comparable rates of graft loss
   D. Lower rates of mortality

3. Since 2010, there has been a 277% increase in deceased donor renal transplantation due to

   A. Increased efforts to promote organ donation in the public
   B. Outreach at the hospital level after trauma
   C. Opioid overdoses
   D. Paired organ donation

4. Venovenous bypass during liver transplantation requires a bypass between which of the following vessels

   A. Superior mesenteric vein, common iliac vein, left axillary vein
   B. Superior mesenteric vein, splenic vein, left axillary vein
   C. Portal vein, inferior vena cava, left brachial vein
   D. Portal vein, femoral vein, and left axillary vein

5. Alemtuzumab has not been widely accepted as an induction agent for immunosuppression due to

   A. Higher rate of posttransplant lymphoproliferative disorder in Epstein-Barr virus–seronegative patients
   B. Inconclusive long-term ability to prevent acute rejection
   C. Higher rates of short-term acute rejection
   D. Higher rates of chronic allograft rejection

Appendix: Answers to Multiple Choice Questions

CHAPTER 2

1A. Beneficence and nonmaleficence are synonyms

2E. Both A and C are true

3C. Technical skills

4D. Are separate organizations that credential surgeons, and educate surgeons, respectively, as primary parts of their missions

5E. A, B, and C

CHAPTER 3

1A. Is an approach to categorizing patients preoperatively to assess their risk for an operative procedure

2D. Should include a pain assessment to aid in the management of postoperative pain

3C. Can be modified by risk-based interventions

4E. Both A and C are true

5C. Can have frailty measured by a variety of means that predict the risk of complications

CHAPTER 4

1E. Hypocalcemia

2D. Discharge the patient with a prescription for pain medication and a plan for follow-up in 2 weeks

3C. Cancel the operation with the plan for improved preoperative preparation

4E. All of the above except for D

5D. Evaluation of the patient, intubation for protection of airway, transfer to a higher level of care, transfusion with 2 units of FFP and 2 units of matched packed RBCs, antibiotic administration, and computed tomography of the abdomen

CHAPTER 5

1C. Surgical technique does not play a role in leading to infection

2E. Both A and D

3A. Inadequate fluid resuscitation

4D. Bladder pressure measurement to assess for increased abdominal pressures

5C. Urinary tract infection

CHAPTER 6

1B. Inflammation. An acute wound is defined by its ability to normally progress, in a predictable and timely manner, through all of the phases of wound healing; coagulation, inflammation, fibroplasia, angiogenesis, and remodeling. A protracted inflammatory phase is the usual mechanism for the formation of a chronic wound. All clinical efforts should be made to reduce chronic wound inflammation in an effort to support healing.

2C. Macrophage. The macrophage is the most important source of growth factor signals for wound healing. Experimental studies show that wound healing is most impaired in the absence of macrophages. Although fibroblasts are the main source of collagen synthesis and endothelial cells are required for revascularization, they are dependent on macrophage signaling to stimulate and direct tissue repair. A platelet is not a cell.

3E. Tco_2 < 30 mm Hg. Wounds will not heal when the tissue concentration of oxygen falls below 30 mm Hg. It is the most powerful predictive measure of delayed or impaired wound healing. Vitamin C deficiency may result in impaired collagen cross linking (scurvy) and weak scars. Low serum albumin predicts increased wound complications, like wound infection. The microangiopathy of radiated tissue indirectly reduces perfusion and therefore, Tco_2 levels. Finally, smoking impairs wound healing through the vasoconstrictive effects of chronic nicotine and relative hypoxia as well.

4C. A moist wound environment. A moist or even wet wound environment is critical to normal wound healing. The cellular and molecular biological activity within a wound requires hydration to proceed. Clinical use of dry dressings to support wound debridement, for example, should be limited. Similarly, poor dressing resulting in repeated trauma and mechanical instability to the wound is often overlooked as a source for wound healing failure. Wound infection is the most clinically important, and expensive, impediment to surgical wound healing. Foreign bodies in the wound, such as synthetic surgical meshes, also delay normal wound healing. Finally, experimental and clinical data support that obesity contributes to abnormal wound healing, primarily through a metabolic pathway, and secondarily by increasing the risk of wound infection.

5D. Early fascial dehiscence and wound failure. Pollock and Evans showed in a classic clinical study that 94% of incisional hernias were the result of 1.2 cm fascial dehiscence before POD 30. The majority of the time, these were clinically occult wound closure failures, progressing to incisional hernias over the subsequent 3 years. It is no longer believed that many incisional hernias are the result of abnormal scar formation or suture breaking, stretching or even pulling through the fascia. Poor technique certainly will contribute to incisional hernia formation, but the fundamental mechanism is early fascial dehiscence.

CHAPTER 7

1B. In bipolar electrosurgery, the current flows from the handpiece to the return electrode

2C. The length of the path between the two poles in the circuit

3B. Fire depends upon the presence of an oxygen source, an ignition source and fuel

4C. Muscle and nerve stimulation ceases at 100 kHz

5C. Destroys tumor tissue by generating heat with the application of electromagnetic waves

CHAPTER 8

1B. Narrowing the spectrum of antibiotic coverage based on cultures

2C. Requires the use of alcohol-containing skin preparation solutions

3E. A and C

4A. NSSSIs are generally self-limited and non-threatening

CHAPTER 9

1C. Anion gap metabolic acidosis with appropriate respiratory compensation. As above, values from an arterial blood gas are typically reported in this order: pH, pCO_2, paO_2, and HCO_3^-.

This patient's pH is normal, but near-acidotic. HCO_3^- and pCO_2 are both low. Decreased HCO_3^- will cause acidosis, while decreased pCO_2 will cause alkalosis, thus the patient's primary disorder is metabolic. His calculated anion gap is 22. The pCO_2 is within the 36-40 mm Hg range of appropriate compensation predicted by Winter's formula, thus no concurrent respiratory disorder exists. Therefore, this patient has an anion gap metabolic acidosis with appropriate respiratory compensation. Respiratory compensation for metabolic disorders is rapid (note his hyperventilation), hence the normal pH.

If respiratory compensation were inappropriate, one would need to consider another, simultaneous process, in addition to alkalosis, for example, the respiratory acidosis that occurs in the later stages of salicylate poisoning, when central respiratory drive has been suppressed.

Note the patient's $\Delta\Delta$ = 2.5. Considering this finding in isolation, one would conclude that the patient has a mixed anion-gap metabolic acidosis and metabolic alkalosis. This underscores the need to take into account all of the patient's data when making determinations of acid-base status. There is no additional evidence of a metabolic alkalosis, thus this additional disturbance is unlikely.

2A. Hypophosphatemia. Refeeding syndrome occurs when a malnourished patient (eg, an elderly or alcohol-dependent patient, or a patient who has experienced recent weight loss) begins to consume calories or begins to receive intravenous glucose administration. Insulin levels rise, causing electrolytes which have shifted to the extracellular space during a period of starvation to shift back to the intracellular space for use in the construction of new proteins and cells. Refeeding also leads to increased intracellular requirements for PO_4^{3-} and Mg^{2+} due to increased ATP production and glucose metabolism, decreasing serum levels of these electrolytes even further. This all leads to hypokalemia, hypomagnesemia, and hypophosphatemia, any one of which may be fatal. For these reasons, electrolytes must be closely monitored and aggressively repleted in patients at risk for refeeding syndrome.

3C. FENa < 1%. In oliguric patients, FENa < 1% is indicative of prerenal azotemia and intravascular volume depletion.

BUN:Cr ratio > 20 is indicative of hypovolemia. FENa > 1% is indicative of intrinsic renal causes of oliguria, and should prompt workup including microscopic urine analysis and renal ultrasonography. Post-renal obstruction should be investigated if clinically suspected (eg, caused by benign prostatic hypertrophy in this 70-year-old male). See Table 9-5.

FENa is unreliable in patients taking diuretics. In such cases, FEUN should be calculated:

$$FEUN = 100 \times \frac{(UN_U \times Cr_P)}{(Cr_U \times BUN)}$$

where U: urine, P: plasma, UN: urea nitrogen, BUN: blood urea nitrogen, Cr: creatinine.

Table 9–5. Common laboratory values distinguishing between oliguric prerenal and intrinsic renal failure.

Test	Prerenal Value	Intrinsic Venal Value	Postrenal Value
FENa	< 1%	≥ 1%	
FEUN	< 35%	≥ 35%	
BUN:Cr ratio	> 20	< 10	10–20

4D. All of the above. Stored blood products are anticoagulated with trisodium citrate, which chelates Ca^{2+} from stored blood, disrupting the clotting cascade. In the setting of massive transfusion, such as this patient has undergone, normal hepatic metabolism of trisodium citrate may be overwhelmed, and Ca^{2+} (along with Mg^{2+}) may be chelated from the blood, leading to hypocoagulability, hypocalcemia, and hypomagnesemia. Furthermore, stored pRBCs contain high levels of K^+, the result of lysis of red blood cells. This is especially true of the older pRBCs often utilized in massive transfusion situations. For these reasons, serum electrolytes must be closely monitored and controlled in the setting of massive transfusion.

5B. Mixed metabolic alkalosis and AG metabolic acidosis. The patient is acidotic, with a normal pCO_2, low-normal HCO_3^-, and high anion gap. Therefore, this patient has an anion-gap metabolic acidosis. Given the clinical circumstances, the most likely etiology of her metabolic acidosis is lactic acidosis caused by septic shock.

Note that the patient's pH is significantly below the lower limit of normal, despite the normal pCO_2 and low-normal HCO_3^-. This should prompt concern for a mixed acid-base disorder. Her $\Delta\Delta = 2$, indicating a coexistent metabolic alkalosis. The several days of gastric suctioning provides a ready explanation for this component of her mixed acid-base disorder.

CHAPTER 10

1C. Albumin. Albumin is a poor indicator of nutrition status, as it is a negative acute-phase protein and may be low because of an underlying inflammatory process. Albumin is also sensitive to volume status and may be inaccurate because of dehydration or volume overload. The 2012 Academy of Nutrition and Dietetics/ASPEN clinical characteristics to identify malnutrition in adults specifically do not use circulating proteins because of these issues. Unintentional weight loss, prolonged inadequate energy intake, and fat wasting (as well as muscle wasting, presence of edema, and reduced functional status) are all more reliable markers of malnutrition.

2D. Burns. Energy requirements above basal needs are approximately 10% for elective operations, 10% to 30% for trauma, 50% to 80% for sepsis, and 100% to 200% for burns. Burns covering more than 40% total body surface area (TBSA) are typically followed by a period of severe stress, characterized by an exaggerated catabolic state. Increases in catecholamine, glucocorticoid, glucagon, and dopamine secretion are thought to initiate the cascade of events leading to the acute hypermetabolic response with its ensuing catabolic state. Appropriate nutrient delivery can be accomplished by feeding 1.2 to 1.4 times the measured resting energy expenditures (REEs).

3C. When gastric residuals are checked, tube feeds should only be held if the residual volume is greater than 500 mL. A major change in monitoring tolerance to EN is the approach to monitoring gastric residual volumes (GRVs). Traditionally, GRV have been used to monitor gastric emptying to determine risk of aspiration pneumonia. However, two large randomized trials in critically ill patients determined that not checking residuals and holding for a gastric residual greater than 500 mL was not associated with increased risk of aspiration. Based on these and other data, ASPEN recommends no longer checking GRVs, but if a clinical scenario prompts GRV monitoring, EN should only be held for GRV greater than 500 mL. Technical complications occur in about 5% of enterally fed patients and include clogging of the tube; esophageal, tracheal, bronchial, or duodenal perforation; and tracheobronchial intubation with tube feeding aspiration.

4C. PICC. Tunneled catheters and ports may remain in place for years if there are no complications. Percutaneously placed central catheters generally are designed to stay in for 10 to 14 days. PICCs are appropriate for short-term therapies, up to 12 weeks.

5B. Multiple chest tubes with air leaks. Indirect calorimetry is the best way to determine energy requirements in severely burned patients and in patients with altered body composition, including those who are amputees, morbidly obese, or underweight. However, indirect calorimetry requires accurate measurement of CO_2 production. Patients with multiple chest tubes with air leaks are not candidates for indirect calorimetry because the loss of expired air through the air leaks will lead to inaccurate measurement of CO_2 production and inaccurate measurement of energy expenditure.

CHAPTER 11

1D. Stop all over-the-counter herbal remedies. Although the use of herbal medications has been around for many years, none have been approved by the FDA. Many times the pharmacology of these remedies is unknown and the remedies may not contain the correct amounts of active ingredients stated on the label. It is estimated that up to 12% of patients are using these herbal drugs.

2B. The initial assessment should be done at a minimum the day before surgery for patients undergoing procedures of high surgical invasiveness. The timing of the preoperative evaluation by an anesthesiologist depends primarily on the planned degree of the surgery. Even healthy patients undergoing a surgical procedure that involves a high degree of surgical invasiveness that may include the risks of a high volume of blood loss, prolonged surgical time, special positioning requirements, etc, should be seen at least a day before the planned procedure. Patients with significant comorbidities should be seen in a PAC at least the day before surgery no matter the degree of surgical invasiveness as it is necessary to ascertain the degree of control of the comorbidities.

3D. Surgery should be delayed for up to 1 year. The risk of stent thrombosis makes it necessary to place patients who have had a drug-eluting stent placed on antiplatelet agents such as clopidogrel and aspirin. Stopping these drugs prematurely to allow for the performance of an elective surgical procedure requires careful consideration of the risk of bleeding as well as the risk of stent thrombosis if the antiplatelet agents are both stopped. At a minimum aspirin should be continued. Emergent procedures that involve a high risk of bleeding require that the clopidogrel be stopped, but continuing the low-dose aspirin is recommended.

4D. None of the above. There is no way to be 100% of preventing intraoperative awareness. Anesthesiologists performing strict equipment check before beginning an anesthetic to ensure that vaporizers have sufficient agent levels, that there is an agent concentration monitor as part of the anesthesia monitoring system, and frequent observation that IV lines are patent and intact when intravenous medications are used is one way to eliminate the preventable components. Stable vital signs throughout a case are not always a reliable sign that a patient may not suffer from intraoperative awareness. Finally the processed EEG BIS monitor has been shown to be no more effective in preventing awareness than careful monitoring of end-tidal agent concentration.

5C. Obesity. The RCRI factors of (1) ischemic heart disease, (2) heart failure, (3) high-risk surgery, (4) diabetes mellitus, (5) renal insufficiency, and (6) cerebral vascular diseases are a validated set of independent predictors of cardiac risk for patients. There RCRIs were derived from a single-center prospective group of patients undergoing elective major noncardiac surgery. The anesthesiologist in a pre-op clinic will screen for these factors and recommend further studies based on the presence or absence of RCRIs. Patients with no RCRIs had a very low (0.4%) cardiac risk while patients with three or more risk factors have a 5.4% risk of an adverse cardiac event and warrant further testing or optimization of the factor(s).

CHAPTER 12

1E. A, B, and C

2B. Can contribute to coagulopathy

3E. A, B, and C

4B. Hypotension and warm skin

5D. All of the above

CHAPTER 13

1A. Can be related to products of coagulation and inflammation that are washed out from the damaged tissues

2B. PSV includes a set inspiratory time

3B. Positive sputum cultures

4D. GCS < 14

5B. Prophylactic antibiotics

CHAPTER 14

1C. Should have an initial assessment including airway, breathing and circulation

2D. Should bypass the trauma room and go directly to the operating room

3E. A, B, and C are all correct

4E. From gunshot wounds below the nipple line typically require laparotomy for evaluation and management

5E. All are correct

CHAPTER 15

1E. All of the above

2C. Can cause an increase in glycolsysis and insulin production

3E. All of the above

4A. Benefits from early consideration with functional position splinting and active motion

5B. Inhalational injury

CHAPTER 16

1B. Take her to the operating room immediately for an emergent biopsy. Invasive fungal sinusitis is usually seen in immunocompromised patients, such as the patient described here. It is caused by uncontrolled infiltrative growth of usually nonpathogenic fungal organisms such as *Rhizopus* or *Aspergillus* species. Even with prompt diagnosis, aggressive surgical therapy, and modern antifungal agents, the disease still carries a significant mortality rate (up to 30%). The index of suspicion for invasive fungal sinusitis must be high for any immunocompromised patient, as the symptoms can be subtle and the disease rapidly progressive. If invasive fungal sinusitis is suspected, biopsies should be taken of the suspicious areas and sent for immediate pathologic examination. Note that this can often involve calling a pathologist in from home in the middle of the night or on a weekend, if they are not in-house. In the case presented here, the likelihood of the child cooperating with an examination and biopsy is low, thus an emergent posting to the operating room is the most prudent action.

2E. All of the above. Acute angioedema is characterized by localized swelling of subcutaneous and submucosal tissue of the head and neck. The swelling usually begins with mild facial involvement but may progress to involve the oral cavity, tongue, pharynx, and larynx. The underlying pathophysiology of angioedema involves vasoactive mediators such as bradykinin and histamine, causing interstitial edema through endothelial-mediated vasodilation of arterioles with subsequent capillary and venule leakage. Drug-induced angioedema has classically been associated with the use of angiotensin-converting enzyme inhibitors (ACE inhibitors), although many other medications can also cause this phenomenon. Other drugs known to be associated with angioedema include rituximab, alteplase, fluoxetine, laronidase, lepirudin, angiotensin II receptor blockers (ARBs), and tacrolimus.

3A. Immediately superior to the cricoid cartilage. The patient described has Ludwig angina, an uncommon life-threatening condition characterized by cellulitis involving the submental, sublingual, and submandibular spaces. The source of the infection is odontogenic and spreads rapidly. The infection is usually polymicrobial with aerobic and anaerobic gram-positive cocci and gram-negative rods. Airway compromise in these patients is common, and should be of primary concern. A cricothyroidotomy is performed through the cricothyroid membrane which spans the midline area between the cricoid cartilage inferiorly and the thyroid cartilage superiorly. It can be easily palpated just inferior to the thyroid cartilage, and has no major blood vessels or structures. In patients with significant anterior neck adipose tissue, after a long vertical incision, the inferior aspect of the thyroid cartilage can be palpated in the wound. While an emergency tracheotomy can be performed through the second or third intertracheal ring space, this often involves either going through or dissecting part of the thyroid gland off the tracheal wall. As the thyroid's blood supply is quite robust, the bleeding encountered can be significant. Therefore, in an emergency situation the cricothyroid space is preferred.

4C. Both adductor and abductor synkinesis. Innervation to the larynx is provided by the vagus nerve (cranial nerve X). The recurrent laryngeal nerves branch from the vagus nerve and provide motor innervation to all of the intrinsic muscles of the larynx except the cricothyroid muscle. All of the intrinsic muscles of the larynx serve to tense the vocal folds or adduct the vocal folds except one—the paired posterior cricoarytenoid muscles. Current understanding of peripheral nerve injury and regeneration presents the following scenario when the nerve supply to the larynx is injured. After nerve injury, when a new nerve supply is introduced (ansa cervicalis) neuronal axon regrowth results in reinnervation of the target muscles but in a random pattern. Since only one of the muscles abducts the vocal folds, reinnervation is more likely to result in a tonically adducted vocal fold. Therefore, over several months, the vocal fold usually assumes a more midline position, leading to improved speech and swallowing.

5D. Plan for a definitive resection of the primary site with ipsilateral neck dissection and possible adjuvant radiotherapy after depending on pathological results. This patient is a very high risk for local recurrent disease without further therapy. Oral cavity cancer is treated with primary definitive up-front surgery (with 1 cm clinical margins) and for any lesions with a depth of invasion of 4 mm or more, there is a considerable (>20%) risk of nodal metastasis and an ipsilateral neck dissection is indicated. An oral cavity squamous cell carcinoma with a depth of invasion of 10 mm is staged T3 and should be considered for adjuvant radiotherapy. Should the patient have 2 or more involved lymph nodes on analysis of the neck dissection specimen, this would be a definite indication for adjuvant radiotherapy.

CHAPTER 17

1D. TSH

2D. Both A and C

3B. Is less likely to spread to lymph nodes than is papillary thyroid cancer

4A. Vitamin A toxicity

5D. Osteoporosis with a T-score of 2.8

CHAPTER 18

1C. Caused at least in part by estrogen stimulation of breast tissue

2D. A personal history of breast cancer

3B. Identifies cancer without node involvement in about 80% of detected cases

4A. A painless mass identified by the patient

5D. Can be reliably detected by sentinel lymph node biopsy in women with clinically uninvolved axillary lymph nodes

CHAPTER 19

1C. Mostly arise from bone or cartilage

2D. Iodine deficiency

3B. Ureteral obstruction with transdiaphragmatic urine leak

4A. Spontaneous bacterial mediastinitis of sarcoidosis

5D. Effectively cured by double lung transplantation with a 10-year graft survival exceeding 85%

CHAPTER 20

1C. Atherosclerosis tends to occur diffusely in small coronary vessels. Myocardial tissue extracts 70%-80% of arterial blood oxygen at rest, unlike other organs which can extract additional oxygen during periods of increased demand. The myocardium recruits additional blood flow by vasodilation and recruitment of an extensive capillary bed via a feedback mechanism from adenosine diphosphate and other byproducts of metabolism, increasing oxygen delivery to match consumption. Atherosclerosis, or the formation of intra-arterial cholesterol plaques, tends to occur in the more proximal and larger epicardial vessels, leaving the distal vasculature relatively unobstructed. This allows revascularization by either percutaneous or surgical techniques.

2D. Typical symptoms are exertional dyspnea, angina or syncope. Senile calcific aortic stenosis occurs in the eighth decade of life in patients with tricuspid (normal) aortic valves. While dilation of the ascending aorta is a normal part of the aging process, aneurysms of the ascending aorta are associated with bicuspid aortic valves, related to abnormalities in elastin fiber formation. Rheumatic heart disease affects the mitral valve most commonly. It is unusual for a patient with rheumatic heart disease to present with isolated aortic stenosis but not mitral valve disease, whereas the opposite is fairly common. Indications for surgery in aortic stenosis are the presence of symptoms, which are exercise intolerance, angina, syncope, and dyspnea.

3C. Asymptomatic with a prolapsed anterior mitral leaflet. Indications for surgery in patients with mitral regurgitation include heart failure symptoms, left ventricular dilation and reduced left ventricular systolic function. In asymptomatic patients without symptoms and normal ventricular function and size, surgery could be recommended if the likelihood of durable repair is high. Repair of posterior leaflet prolapse is much more common than in prolapse of the anterior leaflet. Mitral replacement would entail either a bioprosthetic with limited durability, or a mechanical valve and a lifelong requirement for anticoagulation. Moderate mitral regurgitation is typically addressed incidentally at the time of other cardiac surgery, including coronary bypass grafting or aortic valve replacement.

4D. Malperfusion of the abdominal viscera can occur with either Stanford type A or type B aortic dissections. Due to gradual and progressive breakdown of elastin fibers, the ascending aorta dilates as part of the natural aging process. Indications for replacement of the ascending aorta include size of 5-5.5 cm in asymptomatic patients, 4.5 cm in patients with know Marfan syndrome, interval growth of 1 cm in 1 year, or 4.5 cm when incidental to other cardiac surgery including aortic valve replacement or coronary bypass grafting. Stanford type A dissections involve the ascending aorta, which can cause sudden death from intrapericardial rupture and tamponade, aortic valve insufficiency from prolapse, or coronary malperfusion and myocardial infarction. Stanford type B dissections are distal to the ascending aorta and thus not within the pericardial space and not directly adjacent to the aortic valve or coronary ostia. Malperfusion from an aortic dissection occurs when the intimal flap occludes any branch of the aorta causing ischemia. Both Stanford type A and B can cause malperfusion of the abdominal viscera, depending on the extent and geometry of the dissection.

5A. Beta-blockers improve survival in patients with advanced heart failure from a variety of proposed mechanisms, including up-regulation of beta-receptors in the myocardium. Heart failure incidence is increasing related to aging population and the rising incidence of diabetes as well as obesity. Deaths from coronary artery disease and myocardial infarctions are decreasing from improved medical care. Temporary mechanical circulatory support increases a heart transplant candidate to status 1A, while implantable mechanical circulatory support results in status 1B. Patients with chronic heart failure on oral medical treatment are status 2. Following heart transplantation, right ventricular dysfunction is the most frequent complication, as the donor's untrained right ventricle is required to maintain circulation in a recipient with pulmonary hypertension, which is often present from long standing heart failure.

CHAPTER 21

1B. Left-to-right shunting through a VSD causes a volume load on the right ventricle. Ventricular septal defects are classified by their location in the ventricular septum. The most common type is perimembranous. Left-to-right shunting through a VSD causes a volume load on the left ventricle as blood returns from the lungs. The right ventricle does not experience a volume load, but is pressure loaded. Certainly, as PVR decreases after birth, congestive heart failure may develop in a previously asymptomatic patient with a large VSD as left-to-right shunting increases. Knowledge of the expected location of the conduction system is paramount in the surgical repair of a VSD. The AV node is an atrial structure that lies at the apex of an anatomic triangle (known as the triangle of Koch) formed by the coronary sinus, the tendon of Todaro, and the septal attachment of the tricuspid valve. The node then gives rise to the bundle of His, which penetrates the AV junction beneath the membranous septum. The bundle of His then bifurcates into right and left bundle branches, which pass along either side of the muscular ventricular septum. In the presence of a perimembranous VSD, the bundle of His passes along the posterior and inferior rim of the defect, generally on the left ventricular side. The bundle of His tends to run along the posterior and inferior margin of inlet VSDs as well. The conduction tissue is usually remote from outlet and trabecular VSDs.

2A. Neonate with prenatal diagnosis of aortic coarctation who develops acidosis, oliguria, and diminished pedal pulses 8 hours after birth. In scenario A, the neonate described has inadequate systemic perfusion as demonstrated by oliguria and acidosis. With a prenatal diagnosis of aortic coarctation, one must be suspicious at 8 hours after birth that ductal closure has caused a critical narrowing of the aortic isthmus as it involutes. This patient will benefit by reopening the ductus arteriosus with PGE1. The patient described in option B is likely experiencing pulmonary overcirculation with congestive heart failure. Initiating PGE1 would be expected to exacerbate this problem. In option C, a 6-week-old child's ductus would not be expected to reopen with prostaglandins. Also, the etiology of the heart failure symptoms described is due to myocardial ischemia and surgical correction of the coronary anomaly is required. PGE is not appropriate. In option D, the vascular ring described is likely causing a mechanical airway obstruction. Again, surgical intervention is required. PGE therapy has no role in this situation.

3C. Balloon atrial septostomy. d-transposition of the great arteries typically requires two or more levels of mixing in order to maintain adequate saturations. This may involve mixing at the atrial level (via an ASD), ventricular level (via a VSD), or at the level of the great arteries (via a PDA). In the situation described, the infant requires an additional level of mixing. This may be due to the absence of additional (intracardiac) shunts, or they may be too small if present. Emergent balloon atrial septostomy in the catheterization laboratory is indicated. The other options are not appropriate at this time.

4C. Coronary AV fistula. Coronary AV fistula is the most common major coronary anomaly. The second most common is ALCAPA.

5B. Isolated pulmonary stenosis in a neonate. Isolated aortic coarctation in a neonate is well managed with a primary extended end-to-end anastomosis and is almost always primarily approached surgically. Isolated pulmonary stenosis is typically primarily treated with balloon pulmonary valvuloplasty. This approach has been highly successful. The patient in option C is best managed with a trial of Indocin, followed by bedside surgical ligation if the ductus fails to close with medical management. Larger patients with PDAs requiring closure are frequently treated with catheter-based closure with excellent results. Perimembranous VSDs are best closed surgically. Device closure of VSDs in this location is associated with prohibitively high rates of complete heart block along with the risk of impairing the function of the aortic and/or tricuspid valve.

CHAPTER 22

1A. Absence of esophageal peristalsis. Esophageal manometry is the gold standard for establishing the diagnosis of esophageal achalasia. The classic manometric findings are (1) absence of esophageal peristalsis and (2) partial or absent relaxation of the LES in response to swallowing. Dysphagia for both solid and liquid food is the most common symptom, experienced by virtually every patients. Heartburn is present in about 50% of patients. The low intraluminal pH in achalasia patients it is not due to GERD, but rather to stasis and fermentation of undigested food in the distal esophagus.

2D. The surgical treatment consists of LES myotomy, resection of the diverticulum or its suspension. Although rare, Zenker diverticulum is more common than the epiphrenic diverticulum. It is a protrusion of pharyngeal mucosa through a weak zone in the Killian's triangle, secondary to abnormalities of the UES sphincter. Dysphagia occurs very frequently. As the pouch enlarges, its contents can be inhaled into the respiratory tree causing chronic cough and pneumonia. Finally, the established treatment consists of eliminating the functional obstruction performing a UES myotomy, associated with resection or suspension of the diverticulum.

3D. Upper endoscopy, esophageal manometry, and 24-hour pH monitoring. Upper endoscopy visualizes the mucosal surface of the esophagus, determines the presence and degree of esophagitis, and allows biopsies. Esophageal manometry is mandatory to evaluate the function of both the esophageal body and LES, and is essential for proper placement of the pH probe for ambulatory pH monitoring. The 24-hour pH monitoring is the gold standard for the diagnosis of GERD, as measures reflux of acid from the stomach into the esophagus and correlates it to the symptoms.

4B. Is defined as metaplastic columnar epithelium with intestinal metaplasia.

Barrett esophagus (BE) is defined as the presence of at least 1 cm of metaplastic columnar epithelium that replaces the stratified squamous epithelium normally lining the distal esophagus. Currently, the presence of intestinal metaplasia—columnar epithelium with *goblet cells*—is also needed for the diagnosis of BE. About 10%-15% of patients with GERD will develop BE. Patient usually become asymptomatic over time due to the decreased sensitivity of the metaplastic epithelium.

5D. All of the above. In patients with early esophageal cancer (pT1a), an esophagectomy can be avoided, because of the very low risk of lymph nodes metastasis (0%-3%), and EMR and RFA are very effective. In case of locally advanced esophageal cancer (T3-4 N0-3, T2 N1-3), chemoradiation followed by surgery is the best treatment. In patients with distant metastases, survival is very poor and treatment modalities focus on the palliation of symptoms. Endoscopic stenting is one of the most successful options in the treatment of dysphagia.

CHAPTER 23

1D. Abdominal ultrasound. Ultrasound is the best test for detecting most gallbladder disease, including acute cholecystitis. Classic findings for cholecystitis include presence of gallstones, gallbladder wall thickening, and pericholecystic fluid. Ultrasound also allows for assessment for choledocholithiasis and the common bile duct can be visualized and the diameter measured. A dilated common bile duct (CBD) along with a direct hyperbilirubinemia is highly concerning for choledocholithiasis. Normal CBD diameter is up to 4 mm in patients through their 40s. Thereafter, every decade, normal CBD diameter increases by 1 mm maximum. Thus, a patient in their 50s may have a normal CBD up to 5 mm in diameter, and a patient in their 70s may have a normal CBD up to 7 mm in diameter.

2D. NG tube decompression and continued observation. The most common cause of a small bowel obstruction is due to adhesive disease, and the majority of these cases can be treated with nonoperative therapy. This includes NG tube decompression, bowel rest, electrolyte replacement, and ambulation. After 48 hours, there should be signs of a resolving obstruction. If this fails, surgery may be required to find the point of obstruction and release it. Early postoperative patients are managed differently in that the observational period is extended to 2 to 3 weeks before consideration of surgery, providing there are no signs of perforation or ischemia. This period of time is extended due to the increased difficulty of operating on early postoperative patients secondary to advanced inflammation, where there is increased risk of enterotomies and other complications. These patients should be provided with parental nutrition and observed as long as their condition is stable.

3C. In a complete closed-loop obstruction, serum lactate can be normal. Mechanical SBO is the most frequently encountered surgical disorder of the small intestine and, in the United States, is most commonly due to intra-abdominal adhesions from a previous surgery. However, worldwide, the most common cause is a hernia. The risk of readmission for SBO is greatest for patients undergoing lower abdominal surgery (~ 9% long term). Diagnosis can be made with CT scan or small bowel series, and the majority of patients can be successfully treated nonoperatively (~ 80%) with resolution of symptoms in ~ 48 hours. Symptoms of strangulation constitute an indication for surgical interventions, including abdominal pain out of proportion to exam findings (typically a late finding). Serum lactate levels are 90% sensitive and 87% specific for the presence of bowel ischemia. However, it is possible for patients with a closed-loop obstruction to have normal lactate. This is because obstruction of venous drainage prevents the lactic acid produced by the affected enterocytes from reaching systemic circulation.

4E. Cholinesterase inhibitor. This patient has the stigma of a colonic pseudo-obstruction, also known as Ogilvie syndrome. The patient is to be admitted to the hospital, and his plan of care should include intravenous fluids, eventually nasogastric decompression, and bowel rest. Pharmacologic treatment is recommended as the first line of treatment unless the patient presents with evidence of toxic megacolon, perforation, and/or obstruction. It is contraindicated after 72 hours of observation without improvement and/or in case of worsening clinical picture. The anticholinesterase inhibitor neostigmine, at a dose of 1 to 2 mg, has been shown to significantly reduce the colonic distention within 30 minutes from its administration. In about 40% of patients, a second dose may be required. The most important adverse reaction of neostigmine is bradycardia. Therefore, its administration requires cardiac monitoring. Overall, the success rate of nonoperative management is about 80%. If no improvement is seen within 6 days, operative intervention should be considered. In patients at high risk, a cecostomy may be considered; otherwise, an exploratory laparotomy with possible colonic resection should be done promptly. In case of hemodynamic instability, worsening clinical picture, or soilage of the abdominal cavity, extensive resection with end ileostomy or a colostomy may need to be performed.

5C. Admission to hospital, bowel rest, IV fluids, colonoscopy. This patient has the clinical and radiologic signs of a sigmoid volvulus. A volvulus is the result of a torsion of the colon around its mesenteric base. About 50% of patients with a sigmoid volvulus have 360 degrees of torsion, usually 15 to 25 cm, from the anal verge. The patients are usually elderly with psychiatric or neurologic disease or institutionalized. The clinical presentation is consistent, with nausea, vomiting, abdominal distention and pain, obstipation, and constipation. The diagnosis of a sigmoid volvulus can be made with a plain abdominal radiograph that shows dilation of the sigmoid with a coffee bean appearance. Although no longer in use, barium enema was showing the shape of a bird's beak or an ace of spades at the point of obstruction. A CT scan of oral and IV contrast may be also helpful. The treatment of sigmoid volvulus depends on the patient's clinical presentation. Unstable patients with peritoneal signs, increased WBC, acidosis, and radiologic signs of perforation and/or strangulation are recommended for an emergent laparotomy with sigmoid resection with or without colostomy depending on the clinical presentation and soilage of the abdominal cavity. Stable patients without evidence of systemic compromise and strangulation/perforation are recommended for a decompressive colonoscopy/flexible sigmoidoscopy with the additional goal of resolving the torsion. Once the obstruction point is passed, a rectal tube is left in place for 8 to 72 hours. Decompression alone relieves the obstruction. Surgery should be followed electively within the same admission. Colonic resection is the procedure of choice.

CHAPTER 24

1B. Fever over 37.8°C (100.0°F)

2A. Intraperitoneal

3C. Reversal of low-flow state

4B. 4 days

5B. CT scan of the abdomen with intravenous contrast

CHAPTER 25

1D. May include a posterior gastric artery that is typically a branch of the splenic artery

2B. Associated mortality rate is as high as 56%

3B. Requires resection of uninvolved margins of stomach, duodenum, and regional lymph nodes

4A. Can impair the appropriate relaxation of the pylorus

5C. Consists of multimodal medical treatment including triple and quadruple therapy

CHAPTER 26

1B. The common hepatic artery typically arises from the superior mesenteric artery, ascends in the hepatoduodenal ligament, and gives rise to the right gastric, gastroduodenal, and proper hepatic arteries.

2D. Serum creatinine

3B. Laceration greater than 3 cm deep into the parenchyma

4D. Budd-Chiari syndrome

5B. End-to-side portocaval shunt

CHAPTER 27

1D. Oral cholecystography

2D. Intestin

3B. Are nearly always present in people with chronic cholecystitis

4A. Diverticulitis

5C. Should usually include draining the biliary tree

CHAPTER 28

1D. The uncinate process lies anterior to the superior mesenteric artery

2D. Parotid gland

3B. Can be complicated by pancreatic necrosis

4A. Is unresectable at the time of diagnosis in most people

5C. May be treated by enucleation of the pancreatic lesion

CHAPTER 29

1D. The gastrosplenic ligament carries the short gastric vessels.

2D. Both A and C

3B. Is at greatest risk in young children

CHAPTER 30

1D. The appendix is fixed retrocecally in 65% of adults

2D. A, B, and C

3B. Are most commonly neuroendocrine (carcinoid) tumors

CHAPTER 31

1A. Intra-abdominal adhesions. Sixty percent to 75% of cases of mechanical SBO are secondary to adhesions, related to prior abdominal surgery. Lower abdominal and pelvic surgery appears to be associated with a higher incidence of adhesions than the upper abdominal surgery. Congenital bands are rarely seen in children.

2D. All of the above. A nasogastric tube should be inserted early in order to relieve symptoms, avoid aspiration, and monitor the fluid and electrolyte losses. Depending on the level and duration of obstruction, fluid and electrolyte deficit vary. The exact volume of fluid and electrolytes must be calculated individually for each patient. In some cases, in which there is preoperative evidence of free space in the abdomen for the trocar placement, laparoscopy finds a good indication. Laparoscopic adhesiolysis reduces the risk of further adhesions thanks to the reduced peritoneal trauma.

3C. Deep venous thrombosis can be a cause. Acute mesenteric ischemia is characterized by severe and diffuse abdominal pain that is often unresponsive to narcotics. Mesenteric arterial embolism accounts for about 50% of cases. The main cause is atrial fibrillation. Venous thrombosis can be a consequence of venous stasis (as in portal hypertension) or hypercoagulability (congenital disorders, oral contraceptives). Deep venous thrombosis may cause pulmonary embolism but not mesenteric thrombosis.

4D. Carcinoid syndrome develops in the presence of liver metastases. *Adenomas* are the most common benign tumors of the small intestine. The duodenum is the most common site of involvement, and the lesion most commonly noted is the villous adenoma. These lesions tend to involve the region of the ampulla of Vater. Malignant tumors tend to increase in frequency from proximal to distal, with the exception of adenocarcinomas which are most frequent in the duodenum. Adenocarcinoma is the most common histologic type (45%), followed by carcinoids (30%), lymphomas (15%), sarcomas, and GISTs (10%). Peutz–Jeghers syndrome is characterized by diffuse gastrointestinal hamartomas and mucocutaneous pigmentation. The malignant potential of this polyposis is very small.

Carcinoid tumors produce symptoms secondary to hormone production, including hot flashes, bronchospasms and arrhythmias. This constellation of symptoms, called carcinoid syndrome, occurs when the liver is not able to metabolize the active substances produced by the carcinoid tumor.

5A. Ileosigmoid fistula is a common complication of perforating CD of the terminal ileum. Typically, the inflamed terminal ileum adheres to the sigmoid colon that is otherwise healthy. Ileovesical fistulae occur in approximately 5% of CD patients. Although hematuria and fecaluria are virtually diagnostic of ileovesical fistula, these symptoms are absent in almost 30% of cases. Enterovaginal and ECF are rare fistulas caused by perforating small bowel disease draining through the vaginal stump in a female who has previously undergone a hysterectomy or through the abdominal wall, usually at the site of a previous scar.

CHAPTER 32

1D. Inferior hypogastric plexus near Denonvillier fascia

2C. Bowel rest, intravenous fluids, broad spectrum antibiotics, and percutaneous drainage

3D. Exploratory laparotomy

4D. Right hemicolectomy

5C. Dehydration

CHAPTER 33

1D. Infralevator

2D. Anal fissure

3A. Can be distinguished from prolapsed hemorrhoids based on exam showing concentric folds of the mucosa

4A. Are typically treated with a regimen of chemotherapy and radiation therapy after diagnosis

5C. Can be managed by palliation of macroscopic lesions of operation

CHAPTER 34

1D. Lotheissen-McVay repair. The Lotheissen-McVay repair, which brings the conjoined tendon posteriorly and inferiorly to the Cooper ligament, is the only one of the repairs listed that obliterates the opening through which a femoral hernia travels. Because this repair by its very nature has a greater degree of tension than the other four, it should always be accompanied by a relaxing incision in the anterior rectus sheath.

2E. A defect in collagen synthesis. During the first year after repair, a recurrence is most commonly the result of a technical error. The first four options are the most common reasons why early failures occur. Although a defect in collagen may play a role in predisposing someone to develop a hernia in the first place, the mechanical factors listed are overwhelmingly the most common reasons for hernia recurrence early after repair.

3C. Lichtenstein repair. The Lichtenstein repair was developed specifically as a repair that would be associated with less tension on the repair, since tension is one of the major causes of failure of a repair. It is the only one repair listed that employs mesh in the repair. Although the Shouldice repair is reported to have a very low recurrence rate in the hands of those surgeons who employ it, it is far less commonly used than the Lichtenstein repair, which is also both easier and faster to perform.

4E. Lower Cost. Laparoscopic hernia repair is most commonly employed in younger, healthier individuals who desire to resume full physical activity sooner postoperatively to return to work or athletics. This group of patients can also best tolerate general anesthesia and a longer operative time. Pain is also reported to be less with the minimally invasive surgery (MIS) approach than open technique. The increased cost of the MIS approach relates to the slightly longer operative time and material expense, such as trocars, to access the abdomen and balloons to expand the preperitoneal space if that is the surgical approach used.

5A. Femoral hernia. A femoral hernia has the most rigid, distinct, and unyielding borders, which include the ileopubic tract, inguinal ligament, lacunar ligament, and femoral vein. It is also generally of smaller orificial diameter and is unable to expand. The remainder of the groin hernias have a larger opening that is able to enlarge further with time. However, all groin hernias can become incarcerated and strangulated.

6C. Develop a wound infection. Several comorbidities have been demonstrated to increase the risk of incisional hernia formation after an abdominal operation: poor surgical technique, advanced age, obesity, pulmonary disease, smoking, diabetes, previous radiation, blood loss greater than 1000 mL, poor nutrition, steroid use, and immunocompromise. The greatest risk of incisional hernia, as high as 80%, is found in patients who develop a wound infection.

CHAPTER 35

1D. Plasma free metanephrines. Plasma free metanephrines or 24-hour urinary fractionated metanephrines are the most sensitive and specific test for diagnosis of pheochromocytoma/paraganglioma.

2C. Fine-needle biopsy of the adrenal tumor. Fine-needle biopsy of an adrenal tumor is almost never necessary, is associated with significant false positive and false negative results, can be dangerous (for pheochromocytoma) and risks seeding of tumor (adrenocortical cancer).

3B. A feminizing tumor. Feminizing adrenal tumors are rare, large, and almost always adrenal cortical cancer. Laparoscopic resection would be both difficult and risk local recurrence and seeding of the cancer. In contrast, metastatic cancer to the adrenal gland can usually be resected safely by laparoscopy.

4E. 5-HIAA. Adrenal tumors do not secret 5-HIAA as do some carcinoid tumors.

5D. Stress dose steroids and subsequent steroid taper are needed in all patients postoperatively. Stress dose steroids and steroid taper are not routinely needed when unilateral adrenalectomy is performed for pheochromocytoma given cortisol production will be maintained by the contralateral gland perioperatively.

CHAPTER 36

1D. Typically occurs with at least a 50% reduction in arterial diameter, which correlates with a 75% narrowing of cross-sectional area

2D. Pain occuring at rest

3B. Can be caused by a major arterial dissection

4A. Should not be performed when the carotid artery is completely occluded

5C. Is defined as a localized dilation of an artery to at least 1.5 times its normal diameter

CHAPTER 37

1C. Thermal ablation is an effective approach to the treatment of saphenous veins. The 2011 consensus opinion recommends thermal ablation to surgical or chemical ablation for GSVs. Selective treatment of incompetent perforating veins is not recommended in patients with simple varicose veins, though is an option for pathologic perforating veins. Vein absorption occurs over the course of months.

2D. A and B. Three months of anticoagulation are similarly recommended in patients with PE or proximal DVT of the leg provoked by a nonsurgical transient risk factor and in patients with PE or an isolated distal DVT of the leg provoked by surgery or by a nonsurgical transient risk factor. This is recommended over a longer or shorter duration of anticoagulation. Patients with unprovoked DVT should be considered for an extended duration therapy.

3D. Upper extremity venous duplex ultrasound. Upper extremity venous duplex ultrasound is both sensitive and reliable in the diagnosis of axillary-subclavian vein thrombosis. A chest x-ray is obtained to exclude the presence of cervical ribs which can contribute to the compression of the subclavian vein, but cannot be used solely in diagnosis. A CT venogram is not an appropriate initial evaluation modality. A CT angiogram will not properly image the subclavian vein.

4B. Up to 40% of presentations have associated acute DVT. Up to 40% of patients with superficial thrombophlebitis have been reported to have associated acute DVT. Generalized edema is present only if the deep veins are involved. Ambulation is encouraged along with NSAIDs, local heat, elevation, and support stockings. Most episodes of septic thrombophlebitis respond to conservative management and do not require operative treatment.

5C. Venous duplex scans aid in ruling out venous insufficiency and venous obstruction. The distribution of edema from lymphedema is centered around the ankle and is most pronounced on the dorsum of the foot. It often involves the toes, a characteristic not seen in venous stasis disease. Venous duplex scans are helpful in ruling out venous causes of edema, especially in patients with unilateral edema. Due to its minimal risk and ability to provide information on lymph transport and reflux, lymphoscintigraphy is the gold standard for evaluation of lymphatic function. Diuretics are not effective in the long-term treatment of lymphedema, though may be useful for acute exacerbations.

CHAPTER 38

1D. Is normally maintained at a stable level by displacement of cerebrospinal fluid (CSF)

2D. Trendelenburg position

3B. Is accompanied by initial hyporeflexia

4A. Occurs with axonal regeneration after wallerian degeneration at a rate of 1 mm/d

5C. Can cause symptoms related to the compression of the pituitary stalk causing increased prolactin levels

CHAPTER 39

1C. Medically manage the patient's pain and nausea and arrange an urgent ophthalmology consult. Sudden onset of severe unilateral eye pain with decreased visual acuity, a dilated, unreactive pupil, hazy cornea, and elevated intraocular pressure is the classic presentation of acute angle-closure glaucoma. This is a vision threatening condition that must be managed urgently. It is necessary to treat the patient's pain and nausea and lower the patient's intraocular pressure with topical, oral, and IV medications; however, definitive treatment consists of performing a peripheral iridotomy.

2C. Obtain a maxillofacial CT scan and start on intravenous (IV) antibiotics. Acute onset of eyelid swelling with the additional signs of eyelid warmth and redness is highly suggestive of an infectious process. Double vision and limitation of extraocular movement on the affected side indicates that there is orbital involvement. Imaging is indicated to rule out abscess formation and IV antibiotics should be initiated. Oral antibiotics would be appropriate for a preseptal cellulitis; however, there are signs of orbital involvement in this case. Thyroid ophthalmopathy is a common cause of chronic, progressive unilateral proptosis and herpes zoster ophthalmicus can present with eyelid swelling and a vesicular rash.

3D. HSV keratitis classically presents with a dendritic corneal lesion. Ocular HSV infection is most commonly caused by HSV-1 and presents with eye irritation, reduced vision, and a dendritic corneal lesion on fluorescein staining. Herpes zoster virus (HZV) infection typically presents differently from HSV, often with vesicular skin lesions around the eye. If a vesicular lesion is found on the tip of the nose (Hutchinson sign) this is suggestive of intraocular involvement with HZV. Postherpetic neuralgia can be a painful sequela of HZV, not HSV.

4C. Nonexudative "dry" macular degeneration. VEGF targeting agents are used to treat a variety of ophthalmic conditions including diabetic macular edema, exudative macular degeneration, and other diseases in which neovascularization occurs such as neovascular glaucoma. VEGF-targeting agents are not used in nonexudative or "dry" macular degeneration.

5C. Instill tetracaine 0.5% and irrigate with approximately 2 L of saline (or any other immediately available fluid) immediately. Ocular burns with the alkali ammonia are serious because of rapid penetration of ocular tissue and the significant tissue damage caused. Immediate steps should be taken to make the patient comfortable and irrigate the eye with large volumes of saline. Ophthalmology can be consulted while the patient is being irrigated and eventually, after the pH has normalized, topical dilating drops and antibiotic ointments may be instilled.

CHAPTER 40

1A. Prenephros

2A. Just outside the external ring

3D. Have a history of urinary tract infections

4A. Hyperoxaluria

5C. Transurethral prostatectomy

CHAPTER 41

1D. Luteal cyst

2D. Carcinoma occurs most frequently in women between the ages of 20 and 30 years

3B. Consists of radiation therapy and chemotherapy for advanced disease

4A. Are present in 20%-30% of women of reproductive age

5D. A, B, and C

CHAPTER 42

1C. An open fracture is defined as an osseous disruption with a break in the overlying skin and soft tissues resulting in communication between the fracture and the external environment. Open fractures can be classified using the Gustillo and Anderson classification: Grade 1, clean skin opening less than 1.0 cm, Grade 2, traumatic wound greater than 1.0 cm but less than 10 cm in size, and Grade 3, extensive soft tissue injury requiring flap and/or vascular repair. Antibiotic treatment, tetanus prophylaxis and urgert irrigation and debridement in the operation is necessary. Fractures should be stabilized with internal or external fixation and/or splinting to minimize additional soft tissue injury.

2D. Pelvic fractures are among the most serious orthopaedic injuries, resulting in life-threatening hemorrhage, neurologic and genitourinary injury. Hemodynamically unstable patients have a mortality of 40%-50%. Immediate care of the patient with a pelvic fracture must address the retroperitoneal hemorrhage, pelvic ring stability and injuries to the GU system. General resuscitation principles are applied and active bleeding from the pelvic can be controlled by wrapping a pelvic binder or sheet circumferentially around the pelvis to close down the pelvic volume.

3A. Traumatic knee dislocations can be limb-threatening because of disruption to the popliteal vasculature. If the knee remains dislocated at presentation, immediate reduction should be performed. Postreduction neurologic and vascular exam is critical. If there is any indication of abnormal arterial inflow (ABI < 0.9, diminished or absent pulses, delayed capillary refill) then arteriography is indication. If the limb is frankly ischemic, emergent vascular exploration is indicated.

4C. Supracondylar humerus fractures are among the most common injuries in children ages 4-8 years. The typical mechanism is a hyperextension injury after a fall onto an outstretched arm. If displaced, supracondylar fractures require urgent reduction and stabilization in the operating room. The anterior interosseous nerve is the most commonly injured with extension type fractures. Most nerve injuries represent neuropraxias that resolve with observation over the subsequent 3-6 months.

CHAPTER 43

1B. 4:1. The ratio of type I to type III collagen in normal skin is 4:1. During the proliferative phase of healing, skin has increased presence of type III collagen. During the maturation and remodeling phase, type III collagen is replaced by type I, thus approaching the normal 4:1 type I to type III collagen ratio.

2D. III, two dominant. The rectus abdominis muscle has two dominant pedicle vascular sources, including the deep superior epigastric vessels and deep inferior epigastric vessels, with classification as a Mathes and Nahai type III flap.

3B. *GLUT1*. Infantile hemangiomas are associated with the *GLUT1* gene. *PIK3CA* is associated with overgrowth syndromes, such as CLOVES syndrome (congenital lipomatous overgrowth, vascular malformations, epidermal nevi,

spinal/skeletal/scoliosis syndrome). *RASA1* gene is associated with capillary malformations. *PTEN* is a tumor suppressor gene that is associated with many tumors. In terms of vascular anomaly syndromes, the *PTEN* mutation is associated with Bannayan-Riley-Ruvalcaba syndrome, which is an autosomal dominant syndrome that includes macrocephaly, genital lentiginosis, gastrointestinal polyps, and arteriovenous fistulas.

4C. Perform primary and secondary trauma surveys. Initial management of an upper extremity amputation should be to perform a primary and secondary trauma survey. The patient's airway, breathing, and hemodynamic status are paramount. A secondary survey to identify additional injuries is important because an amputation can be a distracting injury for both the patient, given significant pain and emotional trauma, as well as to the medical team. More critical injuries should not be missed prior to management of the amputation. Once the primary and secondary survey have been performed, the tourniquet should be removed to allow for evaluation of bleeding vessels as well as to allow perfusion to distal musculature. If there is concern for significant length of time of tourniquet use, fasciotomies should be performed to prevent reperfusion ischemia and subsequent Volkmann contracture.

5D. CD30. Anaplastic large-cell lymphoma (ALCL) is a rare lymphoma associated with the use of textured implants in breast reconstruction. Presentation is typically delayed seroma, which should be sent for both Gram stain/culture and cytology to test for ALCL. The cytologic marker positive in ALCL is CD30.

CHAPTER 44

1D. The hand should be in the position of rest

2D. Zigzagged across lines of tension

3B. Can include camptodactyly

4A. Can be treated by local injections of corticosteroid

5C. Should usually incision of the transverse carpal ligament, which forms the roof of the tunnel

CHAPTER 45

1D. Hypochloremic metabolic alkalosis

2B. Upper gastrointestinal series

3D. Reassure the parents that repair is not needed until 4-5 years of age to allow for spontaneous resolution

4D. Rectourethral fistula and rectovestibular fistula, respectively

5C. Neuroblastoma

CHAPTER 46

1D. A 38-year-old male with BMI of 36 and obstructive sleep apnea, type 2 diabetes, and dyslipidemia

2C. Surgery is the only treatment modality that has been shown to achieve sustained remission in hypertension and type 2 diabetes in obese patients

3B. With RYGB, the average patient experiences > 50% excess weight loss (EWL) at 2 years

4C. It is currently the most commonly performed bariatric surgery in the United States

5D. The electric stimulation devices are contraindicated in patients with significant liver pathology or significant hiatal hernia

CHAPTER 47

1D. Relative Survival

2D. Expressed on vital organs and tissues

3A. CTLA-4 is upregulated on activated T cells and serves to dampen the T-cell response

4D. The most common site for soft tissue sarcoma is on the extremity

5B. When a sentinel lymph node is positive for melanoma, close observation with ultrasounds of the basin is an acceptable alternative to completion node dissection

CHAPTER 48

1B. Higher rates of delayed graft function with comparable rates of graft survival

2B. Higher rates of nonanastomotic biliary stricture and graft loss

3C. Opioid overdoses

4D. Portal vein, femoral vein, and left axillary vein

5B. Inconclusive long-term ability to prevent acute rejection

Index

Page numbers followed by *t* and *i* indicate tables and illustrations, respectively. Drugs are listed under their generic names; when a trade name is listed, the entry is cross-referenced to the generic name.

H_2 blocking agents